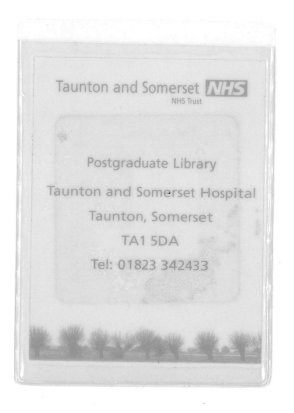

The Treatment of Epilepsy

The Treatment of Epilepsy

Edited by

Simon D. Shorvon

MA MB BChir MD FRCP

Professor in Clinical Neurology, Institute of Neurology
University College London
Consultant Neurologist, National Hospital for
Neurology and Neurosurgery
Queen Square
London WC1N 3BG, UK
Past Vice President, International League
against Epilepsy

David R. Fish

MA MB BS MD FRCP

Professor in Clinical Neurophysiology and Epilepsy
Institute of Neurology, University College London
Queen Square, London WC1N 3BG, UK

Foreword by Giuliano Avanzini

MD

Professor of Medicine and Director of the Department of
Clinical Neurosciences
Istituto Nazionale Neurologico "C Besta"
Via Celoria 11. 20133, Milano, Italy
President of the International League Against Epilepsy

Emilio Perucca

MD PhD FRCP(Edin)

Professor of Medical Pharmacology
Department of Internal Medicine and Therapeutics
University of Pavia
Piazza Botta 10
27100 Pavia, Italy
and
Consultant Clinical Pharmacologist
Institute of Neurology
C. Mondino Foundation
27100 Pavia, Italy

W. Edwin Dodson

MD, FAAP, FAAN

Professor of Neurology and Pediatrics
Associate Vice Chancellor and Associate Dean
Washington University School of Medicine
St Louis Children's Hospital
660 South Euclid Avenue
Campus Box 8077
St Louis, MO 63110-1093, USA
Past President of the Epilepsy Foundation in America

Second edition

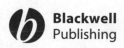
Blackwell
Publishing

© 1996, 2004 by Blackwell Science Ltd
a Blackwell Publishing company
Blackwell Science, Inc., 350 Main Street, Malden, Massachusetts 02148-5020, USA
Blackwell Publishing Ltd, 9600 Garsington Road, Oxford OX4 2DQ, UK
Blackwell Science Asia Pty Ltd, 550 Swanston Street, Carlton, Victoria 3053, Australia

First published 1996
Second edition 2004
Reprinted 2005

Library of Congress Cataloging-in-Publication Data

The treatment of epilepsy/edited by Simon D. Shorvon . . . [et al.].—2nd ed.
     p.   ;   cm.
Includes bibliographical references and index.
    ISBN 0-632-06046-8
  1. Epilepsy—Treatment.
    [DNLM: 1. Epilepsy—drug therapy. 2. Epilepsy—surgery. 3. Anticonvulsants—thera-
peutic use.   WL 385 T7831 2003]   I. Shorvon, S.D. (Simon D.)
  RC372.T67 2003
  616.8'5306—dc21   2003013250

ISBN 0-632-06046-8

A catalogue record for this title is available from the British Library

Set in Sabon by SNP Best-set Typesetter Ltd, Hong Kong
Printed and bound by Replika Press Pvt. Ltd, India

Commissioning Editor: Stuart Taylor
Managing Editor: Rupal Malde
Production Editor: Rebecca Huxley
Production Controller: Kate Charman

For further information on Blackwell Publishing, visit our website:
http://www.blackwellpublishing.com

Contents

Contributors   vii

Foreword by Giuliano Avanzini   xi

Preface to the Second Edition   xii

Preface to the First Edition   xiv

The Drug Treatment of Epilepsy Between 1938 and 1955, with Special Reference to *Epilepsia*, the Journal of International League Against Epilepsy   xvi

SECTION 1: Introduction   1

1 Definitions and Classification of Epilepsy   3
W.E. Dodson

2 Epidemiology and Prognosis of Epilepsy and its Treatment   21
L. Forsgren

3 Sudden Death in Epilepsy   43
L. Nashef and Y. Langan

4 Aetiology of Epilepsy   50
E. Beghi

5 Differential Diagnosis of Epilepsy   64
M. Cook

6 Mechanisms of Epileptogenesis   74
G. Avanzini and S. Franceschetti

7 Mechanisms of Drug Resistance in Epilepsy   84
S.M. Sisodiya

8 Antiepileptic Drug Discovery   89
S.H. White

9 Mechanisms of Antiepileptic Drug Action   96
M.C. Walker and A. Fisher

10 Drug Interactions in Epilepsy   120
E. Spina and M.G. Scordo

SECTION 2: Principles of Medical Treatment   137

11 General Principles of Medical Treatment   139
E. Perucca

12 Management of Newly Diagnosed Epilepsy   161
Y.M. Hart

13 Management of Epilepsy in Remission   174
D. Chadwick

14 Management of Epilepsy in Infants   180
C. Chiron

15 Management of Epilepsy in Children   190
W.-L. Lee and H.-T. Ong

16 Management of Epilepsy in the Elderly Person   201
R.C. Tallis

17 Management of Epilepsy in People with Learning Disability   215
E. Brodtkorb

18 Emergency Treatment of Seizures and Status Epilepticus   227
M.C. Walker and S.D. Shorvon

19 Treatment of Epilepsy in General Medical Conditions   244
J.M. Parent and M.J. Aminoff

20 Treatment of Psychiatric Disorders in Epilepsy   255
E.S. Krishnamoorthy

21 The Ketogenic Diet   262
E.H. Kossoff and E.P.G. Vining

22 Complementary and Alternative Treatments in Epilepsy   269
T.E. Whitmarsh

23 Reproductive Aspects of Epilepsy Treatment   277
T. Tomson

24 Genetic Counselling in Epilepsy   290
F. Zara

25 Diagnosis and Treatment of Non-Epileptic Seizures   307
J.R. Gates

SECTION 3: Drugs Used in the Treatment of Epilepsy   315

26 The Choice of Drugs and Approach to Drug Treatments in Partial Epilepsy   317
S.D. Shorvon

27 Acetazolamide   334
M.Y. Neufeld

28 Carbamazepine   345
M. Sillanpää

29 Clobazam   358
M.A. Dalby

30 Clonazepam   365
S. Sato and E.A. Boudreau

31 Short-Acting and Other Benzodiazepines   374
L.J. Greenfield Jr and H.C. Rosenberg

32 Ethosuximide   391
T.A. Glauser

33 Felbamate   403
I.E. Leppik

34 Fosphenytoin   410
R.E. Ramsay and F. Pryor

35 Gabapentin   418
T.R. Browne

36 Lamotrigine   425
F. Matsuo

37 Levetiracetam   443
A. Sadek and J.A. French

38 Oxcarbazepine   451
E. Faught and N. Limdi

39 Phenobarbital, Primidone and Other Barbiturates   461
R. Michelucci and C.A. Tassinari

40 Phenytoin   475
M.J. Eadie

41 Piracetam   489
S.D. Shorvon

42 Pregabalin   496
E. Ben-Menachem and A.R. Kugler

43 Rufinamide   500
V. Biton

44 Tiagabine   507
R. Kälviäinen

45 Topiramate   515
J.H. Cross

46 Valproate   528
S. Arroyo

47 Vigabatrin   540
G. Krämer

48 Zonisamide   548
M. Seino and B. Fujitani

49 Other Drugs More Rarely Used in the Treatment of Epilepsy   560
H. Meierkord

50 Antiepileptic Drugs in Clinical Trials   568
P.N. Patsalos and J.W.A.S. Sander

SECTION 4: Presurgical Evaluation of Epilepsy and Epilepsy Surgery   **577**

51 Introduction to Epilepsy Surgery and its Presurgical Assessment   579
S.D. Shorvon

52 The Scalp EEG in Presurgical Evaluation of Epilepsy   599
D.R. Fish

53 Invasive EEG in Presurgical Evaluation of Epilepsy   609
D.K. Nguyen and S.S. Spencer

54 MEG in Presurgical Evaluation of Epilepsy   635
H. Stefan, C. Hummel and R. Hopfengärtner

55 MRI in Presurgical Evaluation of Epilepsy   640
C.E. Elger and J. von Oertzen

56 PET and SPECT in Presurgical Evaluation of Epilepsy   652
B. Sadzot and W. van Paesschen

57 New Physiological and Radiological Investigations in the Presurgical Evaluation of Epilepsy   665
A. Salek-Haddadi, I. Merlet, F. Mauguière, H. Meierkord, K. Buchheim, D.R. Fish, M.J. Koepp and E.L. So

58 Psychological Testing in Presurgical Evaluation of Epilepsy   699
J. Djordjevic and M. Jones-Gotman

59 The Role of Psychiatric Assessment in Presurgical Evaluation   716
E.S. Krishnamoorthy

60 Surgery of Hippocampal Sclerosis   723
J.G. Ojemann and T.S. Park

61 Resective Surgery of Neoplastic Lesions for Epilepsy   728
N.M. Wetjen, K. Radhakrishnan, A.A. Cohen-Gadol and G. Cascino

62 Resective Surgery of Vascular and Infective Lesions for Epilepsy   742
N.D. Kitchen, A. Belli and J.A. Sen

63 Surgery of Cortical Dysgenesis for Epilepsy   763
S.M. Sisodiya

64 Surgery of Post-Traumatic Epilepsy   775
K.S. Firlik and D.D. Spencer

65 Paediatric Epilepsy Surgery   779
J.A. Lawson and M.S. Duchowny

66 Hemispherectomy for Epilepsy   790
J.-G. Villemure and V. Bartanusz

67 Corpus Callosum Section for Epilepsy   798
J.R. Gates and L. De Paola

68 Multiple Subpial Transection for Epilepsy   812
R. Selway and R. Dardis

69 Awake Surgery for Epilepsy   824
A.N. Miles and G.A. Ojemann

70 Stereotactic Surgery for Epilepsy   833
A.W. McEvoy, B.M. Trivedi and N.D. Kitchen

71 Complications of Epilepsy Surgery   849
C.E. Polkey

72 Anaesthesia for Epilepsy Surgery   861
M. Smith

73 Vagus Nerve Stimulation   873
S.C. Schachter

74 Future Surgical Approaches to Epilepsy   884
K.E. Nilsen and H.R. Cock

Index   893

Colour plates are found between pp. 670–671

Contributors

Michael J. Aminoff
Professor of Neurology, School of Medicine, Room 794-M, University of California, San Francisco, CA 94143-0114, USA

Santiago Arroyo
Associate Professor of Neurology, Medical College of Wisconsin and Director, Comprehensive Epilepsy Program and EEG Laboratory, Froedtert Hospital, 9200 West Wisconsin Avenue, Milwaukee, WI 53226, USA

Giuliano Avanzini
President of the International League Against Epilepsy, Professor of Medicine and Director of the Department of Clinical Neurosciences. Istituto Nazionale Neurologico "C Besta", Via Celoria 11.20133, Milano, Italy

Viktor Bartanusz
Chief Resident, Neurosurgery Service, Centre Hospitalier Universitaire Vaudois, 1011 Lausanne, Switzerland

Ettore Beghi
Chief, Neurophysiology Unit and Epilepsy Center, University of Milano-Bicocca, Monza, Italy

Antonio Belli
Honorary Research Fellow, The National Hospital for Neurology and Neurosurgery, Queen Square, London WC1N 3BG, UK

Elinor Ben-Menachem
Associate Professor, Neurologkliniken, Sahlgrenska Sjukhuset, 41345 Goteburg, Sweden

Victor Biton
Director, Arkansas Epilepsy Program, 2 Lile Court, Suite 100, Little Rock, AR 72205, USA

Eilis A. Boudreau
Portland VA Medical Center P3H5RD, 3710 SW US Veteran Hospital Road, Portland, OR 97239, USA

Eylert Brodtkorb
Professor of Neurology, Senior Consultant, Department of Neurology, Trondheim University Hospital, 7006 Trondheim, Norway

Thomas R. Browne
Professor of Neurology, Department of Neurology, Boston University School of Medicine, 36 Riddle Hill Road, Falmouth, MA 02540, USA

Katharina Buchheim
Neurologische Klinik und Poliklinik, Universitätsklinikum Charité, Humboldt-Universität zu Berlin, Schumannstrasse 20/21, 10117 Berlin, Germany

Gregory Cascino
Professor of Neurology, Department of Neurology, Mayo Clinic, 200 First Street SW, Rochester, Minnnesota 55905, USA

David Chadwick
Professor of Neurology, Department of Neurology, Walton Centre for Neurology and Neurosurgery, Fazakerley Road, Lower Lane, Liverpool L9 7LJ, UK

Catherine Chiron
Child Epileptologist, Neuropediatric Department, Hôpital Saint Vincent de Paul, 82 Avenue Deufert-Rochereau, 75674 Paris, Cedex 14, France

Hannah R. Cock
Senior Lecturer and Honorary Consultant Neurologist, Clinical Neurosciences, St Georges Hospital Medical School, Cranmer Terrace, London SW17 0RE, UK

Aaron A. Cohen-Gadol
Department of Neurosurgery, 1-229 Joseph, Saint Mary's Hospital, 1218 2nd Street SW, Mayo Clinic, Rochester, MN 55906, USA

Mark Cook
Professor of Neurology and Director, Department of Neurology, St Vincent's Hospital and University of Melbourne, Melbourne, Victoria 3065, Australia

J. Helen Cross
Senior Lecturer and Honorary Consultant in Paediatric Neurology, Neurosciences Unit, Institute of Child Health, The Wolfson Centre, Mecklenburgh Square, London WC1N 2AP, UK

Mogens A. Dalby
Consultant Neurologist, Neurological Department, Aarhus University Hospital, Norregade 44, 8000 Aarhus C, Denmark

Ronan Dardis
Senior Registrar in Neurosurgery, Department of Neurosurgery, King's College Hospital, Denmark Hill, London SE5 9RS, UK

Luciano De Paola
Universiadade Federal do Parana, Servico de EEG, Curitiba PR-CEP, CEP 80.060-900, Brazil

Jelena Djordjevic
Montreal Neurological Institute, 3801 University Street, Montreal, QC H3A 2B4, Canada

W. Edwin Dodson
Professor of Neurology and Pediatrics, Associate Vice Chancellor and Associate Dean, Washington University School of Medicine, St Louis Children's Hospital, 660 South Euclid Avenue, Campus Box 8077, Saint Louis, MO 63110-1093, USA

Michael S. Duchowny
Director of the Comprehensive Epilepsy Program, Miami Children's Hospital, Neuroscience Center, 3200 SW 62nd Avenue, Miami, FL 33155-3009, USA

CONTRIBUTORS

Mervyn J. Eadie
Emeritus Professor, University of Queensland, University of Brisbane Hospital, Brisbane, 4068, Australia

Christian E. Elger
Professor of Neurology and Director, Klinik fuer Epileptologie, Universitaet Bonn, Sigmund-Freud Strasse 25, 53127 Bonn, Germany

Edward Faught
Professor and Vice Chairman, Department of Neurology, University of Alabama, Epilepsy Center, 1719 6th Avenue South, CIRC 312, Birmingham, Alabama 352-0021, USA

Katrina S. Firlik
Clinical Assistant Professor, Yale University School of Medicine, Greenwich Neurosurgery, 75 Holly Hill Lane, Greenwich, CT 06830, USA

David R. Fish
Professor in Clinical Neurology, Institute of Neurology, University College London, Queen Square, London WC1N 3BG, UK

Andrew Fisher
Postdoctoral Research Fellow, Institute of Neurology, National Hospital, Queen Square, London WC1N 3BG, UK

Lars Forsgren
Head, Department of Pharmacology and Clinical Neuroscience, Department of Neurology, Umeå University Hospital, S-901 85 Umeå, Sweden

Silvana Franceschetti
Istituto Nazionale Neurologico, via Celoria 11, 20133 Milan, Italy

Jacqueline A. French
Professor of Neurology, Neurological Institute, Hospital of the University of Pennsylvania, 3400 Spruce Street, Philadelphia, PA 19104, USA

Buichi Fujitani
International Affairs, Dainippon Pharmaceutical Co. Ltd, 6–8 Doshomachi, 2-Chome, Chuo-ku, Osaka, 541-0045, Japan

John R. Gates
President, Minnesota Epilepsy Group, 310 Smith Avenue North, Suite 300, St Paul, MN 55102, USA

Tracey A. Glauser
Department of Neurology, C-5, Children's Hospital Medical Center, 3333 Burnet Avenue, Cincinnati, Ohio 45229-3039, USA

L. John Greenfield Jr
Assistant Professor of Neurology and Pharmacology, Department of Neurology, Medical College of Ohio, Toledo, Ohio 43614, USA

Yvonne M. Hart
Consultant Neurologist, Department of Neurology, Radcliffe Infirmary, Woodstock Road, Oxford OX2 6HE, UK

Ruediger Hopfengärtner
Department of Neurology, Epilepsy Center (ZEE), University Erlangen-Nuernberg, Schwabachanlage 6, 91054 Erlangen, Germany

Cornelia Hummel
Department of Neurology, Epilepsy Center (ZEE), University Erlangen-Nuernberg, Schwabachanlage 6, 91054 Erlangen, Germany

Marilyn Jones-Gotman
Professor, Montreal Neurological Hospital and Institute, 3801 University Street, Montreal H3A 2B4, Canada

Reetta Kälviäinen
Head of Outpatient Clinic, Leader of the Clinical Epilepsy Research Project, Department of Neurology, Kuopio University Hospital, PO Box 1777, 70211 Kuopio, Finland

Neil David Kitchen
Consultant Neurosurgeon, National Hospital for Neurology and Neurosurgery, Queen Square, London WC1N 3BG, UK

Mathias J. Koepp
Senior Lecturer in Neurology, Institute of Neurology, National Hospital for Neurology and Neurosurgery, Queen Square, London WC1N 3BG, UK and National Society for Epilepsy, Chesham Lane, Chalfont St Peter, Buckinghamshire SL9 0RJ, UK

Eric H. Kossoff
Assistant Professor of Pediatrics and Neurology, Pediatric Epilepsy Centre, Johns Hopkins Hospital, Baltimore, MD 21287, USA

Gunter Krämer
Medical Director, Swiss Epilepsy Centre, Bleulerstrasse 60-8008, Zurich, Switzerland

Ennapadam S. Krishnamoorthy
Vice Chairman, T.S. Srinivasan Institute of Neurological Sciences and Research, Public Health Centre, Chennai, India and K. Gopalakrishna Department of Neurology, VHS Medical Centre, Chennai, India

Alan R. Kugler
Pfizer Global Research and Development, Ann Arbor Laboratories, 2800 Plymouth Road, Ann Arbor, MI 48105-2430, USA

Yvonne Langan
Specialist Registrar in Neurology, Royal Victoria Infirmary, Newcastle-Upon-Tyne, UK

John A. Lawson
Consultant, Child Neurologist, Sydney Children's Hospital, Randwick, 2031, Australia

Wei-Ling Lee
Senior Consultant, Department of Neurology, National Neuroscience Institute, 11 Jalan Tan Tock Seng, Singapore, 308433

Ilo E. Leppik
Director of Research, MINCEP Epilepsy Care, 5775 Wayzata Blvd, Suite 255, Minneapolis, 55416-1221, USA

Nita Limdi
Assistant Professor of Neurology, Department of Neurology, University of Alabama, Epilepsy Center, 1719 6th Avenue South, CIRC 312, Birmingham, Alabama 352-0021, USA

Fumisuke Matsuo
Professor of Neurology, University of Utah, Medical Centre, EEG Laboratory, 50N Medical Drive, Salt Lake City 84132, USA

François Mauguière
Professor of Neurology, Epilepsy and Functional Neurology Department, Hôpital Neurologique, 59 Boulevard Pinel, 69003 Lyon, France

Andrew W. McEvoy
Research Fellow in Neurosurgery, Institute of Neurology and Department of Surgical Neurology, the National Hospital for Neurology and Neurosurgery, Queen Square, London WC1N 3BG, UK

Hartmut Meierkord
Neurologische Klinik und Poliklinik, Universitätsklinikum Charité, Humboldt-Universität zu Berlin, Schumannstrasse 20/21, 10117 Berlin, Germany

Isabelle Merlet
Full Researcher, Functional Neurology and Epilepsy Department, Hopital Neurologique, 59 Boulevard Pinal, 69003 Lyon, France

Roberto Michelucci
Deputy Head, Department of Neurosciences, Division of Neurology, Bellaria Hospital, Via Altura 3, 40139 Bologna, Italy

Andrew N. Miles
Consultant Neurosurgeon, Western Australia Comprehensive Epilepsy Service and Department of Neurosurgery, Royal Perth Hospital, Perth, 6001, Australia

Lina Nashef
Consultant Neurologist, King's College Hospital and Kent and Canterbury Hospital, Denmark Hill, London SE5 9RS, UK

Miri Y. Neufeld
Clinical Associate Professor of Neurology, Tel-Aviv University and Director, EEG and Epilepsy Unit, Department of Neurology, Tel-Aviv Sourasky Medical Center, 6 Weizmann Street, Tel-Aviv 64239, Israel

Dang K. Nguyen
Associate Professor of Neurology, Notre-Dame Hospital, 1560 Sherbrooke East, Montreal H2L 3M1, Canada

Karen E. Nilsen
Research Fellow, Clinical Neurosciences, St Georges Hospital Medical School, Cranmer Terrace, London SW17 0RE, UK

George A. Ojemann
Professor of Neurological Surgery, Department of Neurological Surgery, University of Washington, Department of Neurological Surgery, Box 356470-RR-744, 1959 NE Pacific Street, Seattle, WA 98195, USA

Jeffrey G. Ojemann
Associate Professor of Pediatric Neurosurgery, Washington University School of Medicine, St Louis Children's Hospital, 1 Children's Place, St Louis, MO 63110, USA

Hian-Tat Ong
Consultant, Department of Paediatrics, National University Hospital, 5 Lower Kent Ridge Road, Singapore 119074

Jack M. Parent
Department of Neurology, University of Michigan Medical Center, 4412 Kresge III Building, 200 Zina Pitcher Place, Ann Arbor, MI 48109-0585, USA

Tae Sung Park
Professor of Neurosurgery, Washington University School of Medicine, St Louis Children's Hospital, 1 Children's Place, St Louis, MO 63110, USA

Philip N. Patsalos
Professor of Clinical Pharmacology, Pharmacology and Therapeutics Unit, Department of Clinical and Experimental Epilepsy, Institute of Neurology, University College London, Queen Square, London WC1N 3BG, UK

Emilio Perucca
Professor of Medical Pharmacology, Department of Internal Medicine and Therapeutics, University of Pavia, Piazza Botta 10, 27100 Pavia, Italy and Consultant Clinical Pharmacologist, Institute of Neurology, C. Mondino Foundation, 27100 Pavia, Italy

Charles E. Polkey
Professor of Functional Neurosurgery, Department of Neurosurgery, Kings Healthcare NHS Trust, Denmark Hill, London SE5 9RS, UK

Flavia Pryor
Project Director, Neurology Service—127, Miami VA Medical Center, 1201 NW 16th Street, Miami, FL 33125, USA

Kurupath Radhakrishnan
Professor and Head, Department of Neurology, Sree Chitra Tirunal Institute for Medical Sciences and Technology, Trivandrum—695 011, Kerala, India

R. Eugene Ramsay
Director, International Centre for Epilepsy, Professional Arts Centre, Suite 410, 1150 NW 14th Street, Miami, FL 33136, USA

Howard C. Rosenberg
Professor and Chair, Department of Pharmacology and Therapeutics, Medical College of Ohio, Toledo, OH 43699-0008, USA

Ahmed Sadek
Neurological Institute, Hospital of the University of Pennsylvania, 3400 Spruce Street, Philadelphia, PA 19104, USA

Bernard Sadzot
Professor of Neurology, Department of Neurology, CHU B35, 4000, Liege, Belgium

Afraim Salek-Haddadi
Clinical Research Fellow, Department of Clinical and Experimental Epilepsy, Institute of Neurology, University College London, Queen Square, London WC1N 3BG, UK

Josemir Sander
Professor and Consultant Neurologist, Department of Clinical and Experimental Epilepsy, Institute of Neurology, Queen Square, London WC1N 3BG, UK

Sasumo Sato
Chief, EEG Section, National Institute of Neurological Disorders and Stroke, National Institutes of Health, Building 10, Room 5C101, MSC-1404 NIH, 9000 Rockville Pike, Bethesda, MD 20892, USA

Steven C. Schachter
Associate Professor of Neurology, Harvard Medical School, Medical Director, Office of Clinical Trials and Research, Beth Israel Deaconess Medical Center, 330 Brookline Avenue, KS478, Boston, MA 02215, USA

Maria Gabriella Scordo
Research Fellow, Department of Clinical and Experimental Medicine and Pharmacology, Section of Pharmacology, University of Messina, Policlinico Universitario, Via Consolare Valeria, 89125 Messina, Italy

Masakazu Seino
National Shizuoka Medical Institute of Neurology, Epilepsy Center, 886 Urushiyama, Shizuoka 420-8688, Japan

Richard Selway
Consultant in Functional Neurosurgery, Department of Neurosurgery, King's College Hospital, Denmark Hill, London SE5 9RS, UK

Jon A. Sen
Senior House Officer in Neurosurgery, 5 Swan Road, Starcross, Exeter, Devon EX6 8QW, UK

Simon D. Shorvon
Professor of Clinical Neurology, Institute of Neurology, University College London, Queen Square, London WC1N 3BG, UK

Matti Sillanpää
Professor of Child Neurology, Departments of Child Neurology and Public Health, Turku University Hospital, 20520 Turku, Finland

Sanjay M. Sisodiya
Clinical Senior Lecturer and Honorary Consultant Neurologist, Institute of Neurology, University College London, Queen Square, London WC1N 3BG, UK

Martin Smith
Consultant in Neuroanaesthesia and Neurocritical Care, National Hospital for Neurology and Neurosurgery, Queen Square, London WC1N 3BG, UK

Elson Lee So
Professor of Neurology, Director of EEG Section, Mayo Clinic and Mayo Medical School, 2001st Street SW, Rochester, MN 55905, USA

Dennis D. Spencer
Professor, Chairman, Yale University School of Medicine, Section of Neurology, 333 Cedar Street, PO Box 208082, New Haven CT 06520-8082, USA

Susan S. Spencer
Professor of Neurology, Yale University School of Medicine, Laboratory of Clinical Investigation and Neurology, PO Box 208018, New Haven, CT—6520-8018, USA

Edoardo Spina
Associate Professor of Pharmacology, Department of Clinical and Experimental Medicine and Pharmacology, Section of Pharmacology, University of Messina, Policlinico Universitario, Via Consolare Valeria, 98125 Messina, Italy

Herman Stefan
Professor of Neurology, Department of Neurology, Epilepsy Center (ZEE), University Erlangen-Nuernberg, Schwabachanlage 6, 91054 Erlangen, Germany

Raymond C. Tallis
Professor of Geriatric Medicine, Department of Geriatric Medicine, Clinical Sciences Building, Hope Hospital, Manchester M6 8HD, UK

Carlo Alberto Tassinari
Professor of Neurology, Department of Neurosciences, Division of Neurology, Bellaria Hospital, Via Altura 3, 40139 Bologna, Italy

Torbjörn Tomson
Professor of Neurology, Department of Neurology, Karolinska Hospital, S-17176, Stockholm, Sweden

Bijal M. Trivedi
Research Fellow, Institute of Neurology, University College London, Queen Square, London WC1N 3BG, UK

Wim van Paesschen
Professor in Neurology, UZ Gasthuisberg, Neurology, Herestraat 49, 3000 Leuven, Belgium

Jean-Guy Villemure
Head of Neurosurgery, Neurosurgery Service, Centre Hospitalier Universitaire Vaudois, CH-1011, Lausanne, Switzerland

Eileen P.G. Vining
Professor of Pediatrics and Neurology, Director, Pediatric Epilepsy Center, Johns Hopkins Hospital, Baltimore, MD 21287, USA

Joachim von Oertzen
Senior Neurologist, Klinik fuer Epileptologie, Universitaet Bonn, Sigmund-Freud Strasse 25, 53127 Bonn, Germany

Matthew C. Walker
Senior Lecturer and Honorary Consultant Neurologist, Institute of Neurology, University College London National Hospital, Queen Square, London WC1N 3BG, UK

Nicholas M. Wetjen
Neurosurgery Resident, Department of Neurosurgery, 1–229 Joseph, St Mary's Hospital, 1218 2nd Street SW, Mayo Clinic, Rochester, MN 55905, USA

Steve H. White
Professor of Pharmacology and Therapeutics, University of Utah, Anticonvulsant Development Plan, Department of Pharmacology and Toxicology, Salt Lake City, Utah 84112, USA

Thomas E. Whitmarsh
Consultant Physician, Glasgow Homeopathic Hospital, 1053 Great Western Road, Glasgow G12 0XQ, UK

Federico Zara
Laboratory of Neurogenetics, Istituto G. Gaslini, Largo Gaslini 5, 16147 Genova, Italy

Foreword

I tell the people whose pathways will lead them to theoretical or pure science never to lose sight of the main purpose of medicine, which is to preserve health and cure diseases. I tell the people whose careers will lead them to practice medicine never to forget that, just as theory is destined to enlighten practice, practice must in its turn be of profit to science.

These words were written by Claude Bernard more than one century ago, but can be equally applied to the subsequent development of epileptology. The value of integrating the observations of basic and clinical scientists in improving our understanding of epilepsy and its treatment is convincingly demonstrated by this textbook, whose comprehensive approach has been particularly appreciated by the epileptological community ever since it first came out in 1996. The first edition rapidly became a substantial resource for everybody working in the field as it contained all of the information useful for devising epilepsy treatments on the basis of a sound scientific rationale. Given the major advances that have taken place over the last 8 years, we are grateful to the editors for having completed the demanding task of updating the book in such an outstanding manner.

Since the first demonstration of the involvement of nicotinic receptors in a rare form of genetic epilepsy in 1995, further evidence has been provided concerning the pathophysiological role of ionic channel structural and functional alterations. This has led to the productive concept of epileptogenic channelopathies and highlighted the power of combining neurophysiological and biomolecular techniques. The subsequent wave of investigations stimulated by these results have analysed the effects of antiepileptic drugs on ion channels and receptors, and identified new molecules that can counteract epileptic discharges by modulating transmembrane ionic currents. The number of novel antiepileptic drugs described in this second edition has been substantially increased, and their strengths and limitations in clinical practice are exhaustively reviewed.

When appropriately chosen—based on the specific type of epilepsy—the rational use of currently available antiepileptic drugs allows satisfactory seizure control in about two-thirds of patients. However, this still leaves a considerable number whose seizures are not satisfactorily alleviated by established drugs, which can not only cause various side-effects but, most importantly, merely treat the symptom rather than the underlying epileptogenic disorder. Exciting new prospects are offered by advances in molecular studies that could lead to the development of more selective and even individually tailored pharmacological agents. Unfortunately, we are much less optimistic about future progress in preventing the epileptogenic process, which is currently the main challenge facing epilepsy research. Attempts to use the available *antiepileptic* drugs as *antiepileptogenic* agents have so far been largely disappointing because their anti-ictogenic effectiveness in counteracting seizures is not paralleled by an ability to modify the underlying disorder. Comparisons of human and animal studies have shown that brief seizure episodes can set in motion a cascade of events leading to sprouting and neo-synaptogenesis that may account for the tendency of epilepsy to evolve towards a condition of medical intractability. The biological factors responsible for the epileptogenic process will need to be further characterized before therapeutic strategies capable of preventing disease progression can be developed.

A considerable proportion of drug-refractory patients can benefit from surgical treatment, the indications for which have been greatly clarified by the rigorous protocols and guidelines developed by a number of qualified centres throughout the world. The readers of this book will therefore greatly appreciate the updated information it contains concerning presurgical investigations and indication criteria.

The optimal management of epilepsy not only depends on the availability of effective therapeutic agents, but also on their rational use, the prerequisites of which include a precise diagnosis, a suitable means of evaluating the results (in terms of seizure control and side-effects), and a trustful interaction between patients and physicians. During its almost centennial history, the International League Against Epilepsy (ILAE) has made a substantial contribution to this end as a result of its mission of promoting the prevention, diagnosis and treatment of the epilepsies, and the advocacy and care of everybody affected by them all over the world. ILAE Commissions are currently producing guidelines, position papers and educational material that are being made widely available by means of an ever-growing number of educational and training courses held in many parts of the world, their publication in the ILAE journal *Epilepsia*, the most authoritative scientific publication in the field, and the synergistic work of the ILAE with the International Bureau for Epilepsy and the World Health Organization that has led to the launching of a joint Global Campaign Against Epilepsy. The outstanding scientific quality and comprehensiveness of this textbook perfectly reflect the ILAE mission by significantly contributing to the dissemination of updated information on which to base optimal epilepsy treatments. I am therefore particularly pleased at having been given the privilege of presenting its second edition to the international epileptologic community, and proud of recognizing in it the mark of the ILAE to whose life the editors and authors have made, and continue to make, an invaluable contribution.

Giuliano Avanzini
2004

Preface to the Second Edition

The first edition of this book was published in 1996. In the 8 years that have since passed much has happened in the science of epilepsy and its treatment. Advances in therapy fall into four main themes, and these four themes run through this second edition. The first, and perhaps of greatest importance, has been the rise of molecular genetics—a tidal wave that has swept across all of medicine and which has left few areas of clinical therapeutics dry, and certainly not that of epilepsy. The impact on clinical practice is only just beginning to be realized, and when the third edition of this book is (hopefully) published, no doubt change will be even greater. Molecular genetics has lead to—and will surely lead to more—designer drugs, treatment predicated on new molecular targets, and therapies designed to interfere with specific molecular processes. Similarly, the understanding of the genetic and molecular basis of drug responsiveness may result in matching patient genetic profiles to specific therapies with greater predictive accuracy. This is what makes the science of contemporary epilepsy exciting, and it has thus been our intention to cover these nascent developments in this volume. On a more pragmatic level, the second major change in epilepsy therapeutics since the publication of the first edition has been the consolidation into clinical practice of a range of novel antiepileptic drugs, and the gathering of more substantial and well-evidenced information about the established medicaments. This development too is covered in this second edition, where for instance eight more chapters have been added, devoted to new individual drugs. The scientific quality of drug evaluation has also greatly improved in the past decade, and we hope that this improvement is reflected in the chapters of this book, designed to provide accurate and relevant information in a concise but comprehensive manner. The use of clinical protocols for therapy, with a strong emphasis on hard evidence rather than the more traditional clinical anecdote, is a welcome change, and one covered in the text. The third major change in epilepsy management through this period has been a contextual change, with more attention being paid to patient-centred issues, to individuality, to patient preference and to the individual clinical circumstances in which epilepsy manifests. This dual focus on evidence-based protocols and on patient-centred therapy is a powerful combination. The final thematic change in this edition is the attempt to integrate more closely the investigatory advances in epilepsy—which have had their greatest impact on surgical rather than medical therapy—with the specific modes of surgical therapy. Although the advances in investigatory technique have been less dramatic than in previous decades, and many techniques are still research-focused, the utility of individual techniques needs to be clearly defined and backed up with an evidence base. The text concentrates on this theme.

The editorship of this volume has also changed. Professor Fritz Dreifuss, who was a founding editor in the first edition, died on 18 October 1997. Fritz was a top-notch epileptologist, whose encyclopaedic knowledge and understanding of epilepsy was unmatched. He was an outstanding individual, who combined the application of science with incredible energy and compassion, and also a marvellous teacher—a defining period of my own career was spent as a visiting fellow in his unit in Virginia. He was a member of the ILAE Executive Committee for 12 years, serving as both President and Secretary General, and in these posts was a formidable advocate for epilepsy. It is our wish to dedicate this edition to the memory of Professor Dreifuss.

Professor David Thomas also has stepped down as editor. David is the chief of neurosurgery at University College London, a heavyweight intellectually and professionally who was the progenitor and guiding light of the epilepsy surgery programme at the National Hospital for Neurology and Neurosurgery at Queen Square, my home base. The second edition, though, has indeed been fortunate to replace giants by giants. Professors Emilio Perucca and Ed Dodson have both kindly joined the editorship and their influence on the book has been substantial and enlightening. Both are, of course, renowned international figures in epilepsy, and bring a new perspective from different continents and from different specialisms, and both have enriched the volume greatly. With the new editors come new contributors, and over half of the 108 contributors to this edition are also new and 28 new chapters have been added, reflecting the changing patterns of therapy.

The underpinning principles of the book, though, remain unscathed by the passage of time. The primary objective is unchanged—namely to provide a systematic review of the whole field of contemporary therapy in epilepsy. The emphasis is, as before, on a text that provides practical information, useful for the clinician but which is comprehensive, accurate and concisely given. We have asked the contributors to examine the evidential basis of both conventional and experimental therapies, and have attempted to cover all therapeutic options. As in the first edition, the editors have worked fiercely to avoid overlap or repetition, and summary tables have been used to present information, especially in relation to drug therapy in an easily digested form. It remains the basic purpose of the book to guide clinical practice and rational therapy, and to be a source of reference for clinicians at every level.

The spirit of internationalism which was strongly emphasized in the first edition is also the central plank of the second. The international focus of clinical epilepsy is, of course, the International League Against Epilepsy (ILAE), and the spirit of the ILAE remains central to this book. The league has expanded since the first edition was published. There were then chapters in 48 countries and now there are 93. The individual membership of the ILAE has also grown by 50%. A remarkable feature of modern medicine is the rapid speed at which information is disseminated throughout the world. In epilepsy, this has been in no small part due to the international scientific meetings of the ILAE and to *Epilepsia*, its house journal. The upward levelling of epilepsy practice in all countries owes much to both these ILAE activities. It is our hope that this book will, by providing an authoritative overview, contribute to this process. We are fortunate to have a foreword to this volume by the current President of the ILAE, Professor Giuliano Avanzini, himself a highly distinguished epileptologist and clinician scientist, and a longstanding friend and colleague. Contributors to the book are from 19 countries in five continents, and many too have been deeply involved in ILAE work. The historical preface of this edition concerns treatment in the years 1938–1955 (in the first edition, the preface covered the years 1850–1937) and in this edition this history is taken from the perspective of *Epilepsia*, a reflection of the burgeoning importance of the journal and of the ILAE.

The book has inevitably expanded in size. It now approaches 1000 pages, which is a distinctly mixed blessing. Heavy may be the book to handle, but heavy most assuredly was the task of production, and of maintaining momentum and coherence of style and content. The editors have reason to be greatly thankful for the efforts of the publishers, led—as in the first edition—by Dr Stuart Taylor, in managing the processes of production and publication. Stuart has been a friend and advisor for many years, and now must know more about publishing in epilepsy than any other. Without his persistence and advice, the first edition might well have proved to be the last. In this task he has been very ably assisted by a number of editorial colleagues including Rebecca Huxley, Rupal Malde and Geraldine Jeffers and it has been a joy to work with each—their expertise and professionalism is exceptional, and my heartfelt thanks goes out to them and to all the production team. At Queen Square, Ms Juliet Solomon has also greatly helped the organisation and conception of the book and has been a stalwart friend. Also, Dr Matthew Walker provided enormous assistance and expert help with the editing of the surgical sections. His expertise in this latter task has moulded the whole section to the great benefit of the book, and without his help the book would have been seriously diminished. This book evolved partly during my Directorship at the National Neuroscience Institute in Singapore, and there Ms Michelle Lian was magnificent in her efforts to assist in the development of the book. Her assistance made the book viable and life bearable there. Thanks too need to be given to the chapter authors for writing to such a high standard and for giving freely of their knowledge and their time. In this age of publication overload (and impact factors), writing chapters can be a thankless task and yet most have worked with humour and with grace. Finally, I must thank my own patients in London, and those of the other contributors. It is the experience gleaned from our clinical practice—most definitely a two-way process—that distinguishes this book, and in turn it is our greatest hope that the book will also assist in the application of advanced knowledge for the benefit of this practice.

Simon Shorvon, for the editors
London 2004

Preface to the First Edition

Epilepsy is one of the oldest recorded diseases. Throughout its history strange and varied methods of therapy have been employed. Medicaments, potions, ointments, amulets, enemas, exorcism, magic, spiritualism, magnetism, galvanism, dietary regimens, surgical and physical and moral and behavioural therapies have all been popular; reputations have been made (less often broken) and are still being made by therapeutic manoeuvres, yet none has provided the cure. Within this compass have been some effective therapies but others which are ill-directed, useless, misleading, and at times frankly fraudulent. Epilepsy is, of course, a difficult taskmaster for the inquisitive. Its fluctuating nature, its ready influence by environmental factors, its easy confusion with hysterical disorders, its multifactorial causation and its tendency to spontaneous remission, all render judgements of treatment difficult. Such confounding factors allowed ineffective and fashionable therapies to flourish in the past, and today marketing and commercial pressures add to the difficulties of evaluation.

This book is an attempt to catalogue the contemporary treatment of epilepsy in the late 1990s, both medical and surgical, in a comprehensive, concise, balanced and practical manner. Each chapter has been commissioned from an acknowledged authority, known personally to the editors as knowledgeable, intellectually honest and capable of clear communication. We have covered all matters of importance to those treating patients with epilepsy, and provide clear clinical advice on these issues. We have avoided unsupported speculation and highly biased opinion, but have asked our contributors to be as up-to-date as is compatible with our evidence-based exigencies. These are difficult and challenging requirements, which, I hope, have been largely realized.

What are the boundaries of the volume? When bromide was introduced in 1857, a new era can be said to have been entered, with a treatment that was indubitably effective. Ironically, one can note that similar claims had been made many times before in earlier and less competitive times, and the single most important lesson of history is surely scepticism. In our historical chapter, we have surveyed treatment from the time of the introduction of bromides to the outbreak of World War II, a fascinating period which provides the context for today's therapeutic approaches. From about 1940 onwards, more scientific methods were adopted to devise and assess therapy, and more rigid standards were set for proof of effectiveness. Various new therapies were introduced, but most have not stood the test of time. Even as recently as 1970, the orthodox practitioner in most countries could still offer only phenytoin and phenobarbitone as effective options for most epileptic patients.

There has been, however, in the past decade or so, a sea change, almost a revolution in the field, and a wide range of highly effective new therapeutic possibilities has become available. Not only has a series of new medicaments been introduced, but new approaches to drug therapy have become possible, and also with improvements in the investigation of epilepsy, much more effective and ambitious surgical treatment. This expansion in the options for effective treatment, both medical and surgical, is enormously welcome, but brings its own problems. The physician now has to make much more difficult decisions about treatment because of the greater range of therapeutic choices and also because the evidence on which to base rational therapy is more complex, at times contradictory, and not all readily accessible. In this book we have addressed these issues.

Our principal objective is to provide a systematic review of the whole field of contemporary therapy. We have included individual chapters on all licensed medications, on drugs in an advanced stage of clinical trial, on all specific surgical therapies of value in epilepsy, and also chapters on treatment in specific clinical situations. The contributors were asked to examine the evidential basis of both conventional and experimental therapies, and to provide a clear assessment of this. We have attempted, therefore, to encompass all therapeutic options, and their relative values in the varied clinical circumstances of the person with epilepsy. In this sense, the book should be a useful platform for all doctors treating epilepsy. Although the book is primarily about the treatment of epilepsy, we have also included an initial section of six chapters, the purpose of which is to place therapy in context. In these chapters we have also highlighted those areas in which rapid advances are being made, for herein will the context of treatment also change (the chapters on pathophysiology, the developmental basis of epilepsy, diagnosis and prognosis, and on economic cost, for example).

The information contained within the pages of this book is sufficiently comprehensive to act as a reference for specialists, and concise enough for more general clinical usage. It is very much a hands-on text, and, we hope, a constant companion. The aim of the book is to guide clinical practice and rational therapy and to be a source of reference. It has been designed for doctors in adult and paediatric medicine, both generalists and also specialists in the fields of neurology, neurosurgery, psychiatry, paediatrics, alienist medicine and in learning difficulty. It will also appeal to practitioners of the paramedical specialties who are involved in the management of epilepsy.

One remarkable fact about modern epileptology is its internationalism. In countries all around the world, the same issues about the treatment of epilepsy arise, the same therapeutic questions are debated, and there is a large and surprising measure of agreement on specific points. The international nature of epilepsy is in no small part due to the endeavours of the International League Against Epilepsy (ILAE) which has chapters now in 48 countries and nearly

10 000 members, and whose meetings are a forum for the dissemination of information about epilepsy and its treatment. The influence of the league has left no area of epilepsy untouched. We are therefore greatly honoured, in this book, to Dr E.H. Reynolds, the current president of the ILAE, for contributing a foreword. A distinguished and accomplished physician, Dr Reynolds is also a mentor and a friend, and a person whose influence on modern British and international epileptology has been benevolent and all-embracing. Our contributors are from four continents and provide a truly international perspective. Almost all are active in the ILAE, and the text reflects to a great extent the current interest and research of ILAE members. Matching this internationalism, nearly half of the chapters are by contributors (from various countries and continents) whose training was partly at the National Hospital for Neurology and Neurosurgery at Queen Square in London. Our preliminary historical chapter looks at the history of epilepsy therapy (from 1857 to 1939) using the National Hospital as an historical mirror, and as epilepsy is still an important area of contemporary neurology at Queen Square, subsequent chapters also reflect current practice at the National Hospital. This is another thread which runs through the book and gives to the volume, at least in part, a specific flavour which I hope provides the text with an interesting perspective.

A book of 63 chapters will always pose a challenge for its editors and its publisher. In this volume, we have heavily edited some individual contributions, and worked assiduously in conjunction with the authors to avoid repetition or overlap. Where overlap has been permitted between chapters, this is because individual authors have taken differing (and occasionally conflicting) approaches which are, in the editors' view, sufficiently instructive to allow inclusion.

We have also added editorial tables in places to ease comprehension and in particular to make the information contained in the text easy to follow and readily accessible to the reader, often a busy clinician. Also, we have tried to provide a uniform style, and a high quality of writing. To assemble chapters on such a disparate subject from authorities around the world, to edit and to produce a pleasing and useful book has been a major task. In this, the editors have been expertly helped by Dr Stuart Taylor from Blackwell Science, the publishers, whose skill and expertise were the essential ingredients of the successful completion of our work. We are enormously grateful to Dr Taylor, not least for his humour and forbearance in executing (a seemingly, at times, well-chosen word) the task, also to Lorna Dickson, our production editor who has worked absolutely tirelessly on this project, and other members of the design and production team at Blackwells; they have all been pre-eminent in their work. Finally, we would like to thank the chapter authors for their outstanding contributions, their patients for providing the experience on which our current therapeutics is based, and epileptologists around the world, ILAE members and others, who have stimulated our thoughts and actions in the field of epilepsy treatment.

Every effort has been made in the preparation and editing of this book to ensure that the details given (for instance of drug dosages and pharmacokinetic values) are correct, but it is possible that errors have been overlooked. The reader is advised to refer to published information from the pharmaceutical companies and other reference works to check accuracy.

S.D. Shorvon, for the editors
London, 1996

The Drug Treatment of Epilepsy Between 1938 and 1955, with Special Reference to *Epilepsia*, the Journal of the International League Against Epilepsy

S.D. Shorvon

In the first edition of this textbook, I wrote a historical introduction which attempted in its own small way to describe the history of the treatment of epilepsy between 1857 and 1939. This was written largely from the perspective of the National Hospital, Queen Square. This perspective was chosen for a number of reasons; the well-documented archives of the hospital, its cutting edge position in epilepsy during this period, the presence of world renowned academic physicians and surgeons who provided leadership in epilepsy matters and not least because of my own institutional allegiance. The history was largely well received—an exception was the reviewer in the *BMJ* who objected to the perspective, suspecting neocolonial sympathies I presume, an impression I hope that is entirely unjustified. This has encouraged me to attempt a survey of the next phase of the history of treatment in epilepsy—the years 1938–55. 1857 was chosen as the start of the first edition history because it was, of course, the year of the first appearance of bromide on the epilepsy stage. Locock's observations were made on 15 patients, and so effective was the therapy that within a few years bromide was used worldwide for the control of epilepsy. Bromide, one can hazard to say, was the first very effective pharmaceutical, and it ushered in a new era for epilepsy patients. 1939 was chosen as the end of this chapter for several obvious reasons. The world was to descend in that fateful year into the century's darkest period, as the destruction of war spread across the planet. Research in epilepsy ceased as attention turned to more pressing matters. In parallel and partly because of the war, the era of research leadership by the National Hospital at Queen Square also largely came to an end. Research at the hospital turned mainly to other topics, many related to the urgent needs of combatants. 1939, therefore, seemed a fitting time to pause.

All history has a perspective, and that is why—partly—no histories concur. If language is responsible for the artificiality of truth, so history, the fossilization of language, can never be objective. It is therefore important to be transparent and the perspective should be clear. In this preface, I will move from the perspective of the archive of one London hospital to that of the published word—and in particular to that of the journal, *Epilepsia*. This is justified because the journal became, during the period under review, a force in scientific communication in epilepsy, and also the mouthpiece for the bureaucracy of the international epilepsy movement which also developed greatly during this period. I have therefore, in preparing this chapter, plundered the *Epilepsia* archives heavily and relied upon the version of truth proclaimed therein. *Epilepsia*

in this period was very clearly fashioned by the world view of its second editor, William Lennox (actually *de facto* editor from 1939 to 1952), and his influence keenly felt. I apologize in advance for this undoubtedly flagrant bias (and kneel before future *BMJ* reviewers for forbearance and understanding)—but nevertheless feel that history with a clear perspective is probably better than one with none. Other scientific journals have also been helpful (for instance the *British Medical Journal*, *The Lancet*, the *New England Journal of Medicine*, *Archives of Neurology and Psychiatry*, the *Journal of Pediatrics*, *Diseases of the Nervous System*, the *Journal of the American Medical Association* and so on) whose pages in those days not infrequently turned to the problems of epilepsy. This story is therefore an amalgam, but one solidly embedded in the pages of the journal of the International League, and the distinctive bias of its editor.

1938 was the year in which the first clinical reports of the anticonvulsant effects of phenytoin were published, indeed 'a year of jubilee for epileptics' as Lennox wrote [1], and the second series of *Epilepsia* had been launched in the previous year. 1938 seems therefore an appropriate starting point for this history. I have chosen to end this history in 1955, as this was when the third series of *Epilepsia* came to a close. This period of 1938–55 was tumultuous in obvious ways, a new world order was created and the hegemony of the USA in science as well as in other fields was established, reflected for instance by the 45% of Nobel prizes for physiology or medicine which were awarded to American scientists (Great Britain was a distant second with 14%) and the 60% of all new drug discoveries which originated in the USA between 1941 and 1963. This was a period in medicine of great advance. The pharmaceutical industry developed dramatically to become a major economic force. Antibiotics were introduced into medicine (tetracycline, chloramphenicol, streptomycin, penicillin produced by deep fermentation) and infectious disease was thought to have been defeated. The first antipsychotics, adrenergic drugs, B vitamins, steroids and vaccines for polio were introduced. Knowledge of the biochemistry and neurophysiology of the brain had advanced enormously, with the discovery of electroencephalography, the citric acid cycle, the metabolism of carbohydrates, hormone action, vitamins and nutrition. In this period, the advances in epilepsy seem rather overshadowed by these discoveries, but were nevertheless of importance. In the theatre of epilepsy history, the introduction of phenytoin played the starring role but other developments were important supporting actors (Table 1), and here I will briefly review the therapeutic progress of

Table 1 New anticonvulsant drugs marketed in the USA between 1938 and 1955

Year of introduction (US)	Trade name	Scientific name	Manufacturing company
1938	Dilantin	Phenytoin	Parke, Davis
1946	Tridione	Trimethadione	Abbott
1947	Mesantoin	Mephenytoin	Sandoz
1949	Paradione	Paramethadione	Abbott
1950	Thiantoin	Phenthenylate	Lilly
1951	Phenurone	Phenacemide	Abbott
1952	Gemonil	Metharbital	Abbott
1952	Hibicon	Benzchlorpropamide	Lederle
1953	Milontin	Phensuximide	Parke, Davis
1954	Mysoline	Primidone	ICI

Table 2 Officers of the ILAE and members of the Executive Committee between 1935 and 1955

President	Lennox WG (1935–49); McDonald Critchley (1949–53); Walker EA (1953–57)
Vice President	Muskens LJJ (1935–37); Stauder KH (1937–46); Ledeboer BCh (1946–49); Stubbe-Teglbjaerg HP (1949–53); Gibbs FA (1949–53); Williams D (1953–57); Niemeyer P (1953–57)
Secretary	Schou HI (1935–49)
Secretary-general	Ledeboer BCh (1949–57)
Treasurer	Tyler Fox J (1935–46); Williams D (1946–53); Stubbe-Taglbjaerg HP (1953–57)
Editor of *Epilepsia*	Schou HI (1935–46); Lennox WG (1946–52); Merlis J (1952–57)
President-elect	Gastaut H (1953–57)
Hon. President	Lennox WG (1949–53)

Table 3 Member chapters of the ILAE from its resuscitation in 1935–55

1935	3 chapters: America, Britain, Scandinavia
1936	5 chapters: America, Britain, Czechoslavakia, Holland, Scandinavia
1946	5 chapters: America, Argentina, Britain, Holland, Scandinavia
1949	6 chapters: America, Argentina, Britain, France, Holland, Scandinavia
1950–2[a]	11 chapters: America, Argentina, Belgium, Brazil, Britain, Canada, France, Holland, Israel, Japan, Scandinavia
1953	10 chapters: Argentina, Brazil, Chile, France, Great Britain, Holland, Japan, Peru, Scandinavia, United States and Canada
1954[b]	11 chapters: Argentina, Brazil, Canada, Chile, France, Great Britain, Holland, Japan, Peru, Scandinavia, United States

[a] The membership of these years seems rather confused. *Epilepsia* in 1952 mentions the 11 chapters listed above, whereas the report of the Secretary General in *Epilepsia* in 1953 fails to mention Belgium or Israel (in the Secretary General's report of 1954, Belgium is still said to be ineligible and Israel is said to be about to form a chapter).

[b] A report of the Uruguayan chapter is also published in *Epilepsia* 1954, without any evidence that the chapter was officially admitted to the ILAE.

these years. History is after all prologue, and what was learnt in those days will surely be of future utility.

Epilepsia: 1909–45

The International League Against Epilepsy (ILAE) had been created on 2 September 1909, at a meeting in Budapest. It was an ambitious exercise with great plans and hopes, as Marie put it in his description of the programme for League action (*Epilepsia* series 1, volume 1, 1910, pp. 229–31):

> . . . le programme est vaste et grandiose, bien susceptible de passionner les philanthropes et les savants de tous pays.

These sentiments still resonate today and then, as now, the publication of a journal, *Epilepsia*, and the organization of international congresses were the enduring outward signs of the ILAE's work. In these early years, the ILAE began to take shape. By the general assembly in Zurich in 1911, there were chapters in 16 countries with a total of 96 members. Congresses were held every year, and *Epilepsia* (see below) was becoming a major scientific journal. The onset of war in 1914 resulted in the complete collapse of all this endeavour and the ILAE and *Epilepsia* went into hibernation for over 20 years. However, other international medical societies were more tenacious, and in the interwar years international medical meetings be-

came commonplace. In 1931, at the International Neurological Congress in Bern, a futile attempt to resuscitate the ILAE was made with six countries meeting to discuss its resuscitation. It was not until July 1935, however, during the next meeting of the International Neurological Congress held in London to mark the centenary of the birth of Hughlings Jackson, that a second attempt was made, this time with more success. Thirty-two doctors representing 14 countries met at the Lingfield Colony, and the decision was made to reconstitute the ILAE. At an adjourned meeting on 2 August 1935, William Lennox was appointed president and a committee formed. At this first meeting, a decision was made to restart the publication of *Epilepsia* under the editorship of H.I. Schou. Membership was set at 15 shillings for a 4-year period and included a subscription to *Epilepsia*. By 1937 there were 247 members (84 in the US branch, 102 in the British branch, 31 in the Scandinavian branch and 30 members from countries outside the three branches). Over the next 20 years, the executive structure developed (Table 2), the number of chapters grew (Table 3), the regular congresses were held (Table 4) and *Epilepsia* published.

The publication of *Epilepsia* is now, and has always been, the cardinal effectuation of the ILAE. In spite of this, however, the journal has had a decidedly chequered history. Its publication has ceased on three occasions (twice due to world wars, and the third time in a crisis of confidence) and its editorial policy and format changed several

Table 4 International congresses of the International League Against Epilepsy before 1955

1909	Budapest
1910	Berlin
1912	Zurich
1913	London
1914	Bern (cancelled because of the outbreak of war)
1939	Copenhagen[a]
1946	New York[b]
1949	Paris[a]
1953	Lisbon[a]

[a] Held jointly with the International Neurological Congress.
[b] A joint meeting of the American Branch of the ILAE with the Association for Research in Nervous and Mental Disease.

Table 5 The four series of *Epilepsia*: how complex can a numbering system get?

Series I	Volume 1	1 issue: 1909–10
	Volume 2e	4 issues: 1910–11
	Volume 3e	4 issues and a Supplement: 1911–12
	Volume 4e	4 issues: 1912–13
	Volume 5e	6 issues: 1914–15
Series II	Volume I–III	4 issues: 1937, 1938, 1939, 1940
	Volume II	4 issues: 1941, 1942, 1943, 1944
	Volume III	4 issues: 1945, 1946, 1947, 1948
	Volume IV	2 issues: 1949, 1950
Series III	Volume 1	1952
	Volume 2	1953
	Volume 3	1954
	Volume 4	1955
Series IV	Volume 1	5 issues: 1959–60
	Volume 2–18	4 issues a year: 1961–77
	Volume 19–35	6 issues a year: 1978–94
	Volume 36–	12 issues a year: 1995–present

Note: *Epilepsia* has had a confusing system of numbering its issues caused by the interruption of publication on three occasions (creating 4 'series') and changes in editorial policy. The original conception was of a single volume annually, each comprising four quarterly issues. Actually in 7 years of its existence, only five volumes were produced. When series II was initiated in 1937, it was planned to have one volume covering a 4-year period, with one issue a year. This scheme was followed between 1937 and 1948, but the last volume (IV) comprised only two issues before publication again ceased. When *Epilepsia* was resuscitated again in 1952, it was intended to publish one volume in a single issue each year. This plan was followed for 4 years and again publication ceased. Series IV was launched in 1959, with one volume a year comprising varying numbers of issues. The first volume actually occupied 2 years. The term 'series IV' was dropped in 1974, although the volume numbering (i.e. 1974 = volume 15) was continued.

times. It was published in four series with a highly confusing set of volume and issue numbers (Table 5). Over the period in question, however, it emerged as an important force in the promotion of scientific knowledge in epilepsy, and not least its treatment.

The first 'series', published between 1909 and 1915, was a highly successful exercise. Five volumes were produced with over 2014 published pages. The aim of the journal was clearly scientific, and the journal contained important and original papers and reviews, in English, French and German, by many leading medical scientists. A bibliography of epilepsy publications was also published annually. The destructiveness of war is its tragedy, and the premature termination of this phase of the development of *Epilepsia* was a calamity for science and epilepsy.

The second series of *Epilepsia* was inaugurated in 1937. It was decided that it should have a rather different role and form, reflecting the changing emphasis of the ILAE. As the editor H.I. Schou wrote in the first issue:

> The first aim of the reorganised League must be the social care of epileptics and not so much scientific research into epilepsy. The new edition of *Epilepsia* must follow these lines. It must be the organ for our League. . . . The editors desire to express the hope that it will become a useful connecting link between the different countries of the world, which especially in our time need connection. Thereby it should become a stimulus to the care of epileptics in the countries not so well provided for in this respect.
> (*Epilepsia* second series, 1937, 1: 12)

Perhaps as a result, the second series was a low key production by comparison with the first. The 14 annual issues (in four volumes) comprised compilations of statements of ILAE intentions and desires, the constitution of the branches, reports from the branches, programmes of the branches' annual meetings (usually rather lame affairs) and summaries from different countries of epilepsy statistics (though usually hardly justifying this term). In the second issue (1938), Lennox and colleagues provided the first literature summary—of 171 articles published in English in the medical journals of 1936—using the quarterly *Cumulative Index Medicus*. This was intended to be published annually, but 1939 and 1940 were missed. In 1941, the literature review reappeared and increasingly became the central feature of all the remaining issues.

By 1939, the ILAE was making some progress. It had 337 members and four chapters, and the publication of *Epilepsia* was according to Lennox, 'the first and foremost enterprise' of the League. The next international meeting was held on 26 August 1939 in Copenhagen (in association with the International Neurological Congress) and was eagerly awaited. However, progress was brought to an abrupt end, again by the coming of war. The German forces began their blitzkrieg whilst the Copenhagen congress was in session. Poland was invaded on 1 September, and as Lennox records:

> The banquet was a tragic affair. There were brave speeches for freedom but silence on the part of German colleagues. Delegates who were neighbours of Germany began leaving for whatever fate might meet them. The League was again broken. . . . [Little international European activity was possible and] the responsibility for the yearly issue of *Epilepsia* was left on our [the American] doorstep, where it remained for 10 years, supported by the American Branch (but then the trunk) of the League.

Epilepsia continued to be published annually, but as the official editor (H.I. Schou) in Denmark was unable to carry out the work due to the deprecations of war, Lennox stood in as acting editor.

The treatment of epilepsy between 1938 and 1945

Lennox's literature reviews and the summaries of epilepsy practice in the different countries (notably in the USA in these years) in *Epilepsia* provide an excellent vantage point to view the progress of epilepsy therapy in the years 1938–45. The first literature review was published in 1938 (actually a review of the year 1936). Thirteen articles on treatment were reviewed, and these were concerned with bromides, phenobarbital, prominal, antirabies vaccine, ergotamine tartrate, subarachnoid air injections, non-dehydrating doses of Epsom Salt, X-irradiation, atropine, fluid restriction and the keto-genic diet. In 1939, Lennox published his annual review of epilepsy in America [2]. He again described treatment. Barbiturate, bromide and borotartrate were still the mainstay of treatment, but he also reported the experimental results of other therapies. Of these, the most interest was in the effects of ketosis and the ketogenic diet (this had been of recurring interest throughout the 1930s), vital dyes and of phenytoin. The list of therapies mentioned by Lennox in *Epilepsia* in 1938/9 and also in a standard neurology textbook of the time by Kinnear Wilson (published in 1940 [3], although Kinnear Wilson had died in 1937, just before the first report of phenytoin) are shown in Table 6. These give an impression of the cast of medicines for epilepsy at the point that phenytoin appeared on the epilepsy stage.

The potential for brilliant red dyes were reported by Cobb, Cohen and Ney (1938 [4]), following a paper presented at the Boston Society for Psychiatry and Neurology in 1936. The use of the dye has an interesting history, Cobb and colleagues were trying to stain, *in vivo*, cerebral tissue subjected to anoxia. The dye would not take and so an attempt was made to increase the uptake of the dye by chemically induced convulsions. They observed that the dyes inhibited convulsions, and they were then evaluated in camphor-induced seizures in rabbits and mice. Subsequently six children were treated with daily intravenous injections of a 1% solution of brilliant vital red, until their skin was bright pink. Five had a reduction in the number of seizures while in the pink condition and one remained seizure free. Lennox [5] reported that Osgood and Robinson treated 13 institutionalized boys with improvements in eight, and Kajdi and Taylor used 2–20 cc of 1% methyl blue IV in 22 cases of status with excellent results. Aird [6] reported positive results in six further cases, and postulated that the dye worked by rendering the blood–brain barrier impermeable to 'convulsive toxins' in the systemic circulation. Further experimentation continued for some years later, in spite of the obvious unpleasantness of this treatment, a colourful but futile interlude in the history of epilepsy therapy.

In his review, Lennox introduced a much more enduring topic:

Not content with the generally complacent attitude towards anti-convulsant drugs, Putnam of Harvard determined to go broadside through many untried ones. To that end he devised a standardised method of producing convulsions in a cat by means of a measured electric current. Putnam and Merritt found three

Table 6 The drugs used in the treatment of epilepsy in the mid-1930s in America and Great Britain

Lennox (USA)	Kinnear Wilson (Great Britain)
	Drugs of definite benefit
Bromides (various preparations and combinations including gold and sodium tetrabromide)	Bromide—ammonium, potassium, sodium, lithium, calcium, calcium bromine galactogluconate
Phenytoin (first mentioned in 1937)	Bromide combinations—bromocarpine, bromopin, brominol, bromalin, Gelieau's dragees, sedobrol, ozerine, trench's remedy
Phenobarbitone	Phenobarbitone (Luminal)
Prominal	Prominal
	Borax, sodium biborate
Borotartrate	Double tartrate of borax and potassium
Ergotamine, ephedrine, prostigmine	Belladonna (usually with bromide, Luminal or caffeine)
Brilliant vital red, methyl blue	Nitroglycerine (usually combined with strychnine and a small dose of sodium bromide)
Ketogenic diet, fluid restriction	Ketogenic diet
Antirabies vaccine	
	Drugs thought to be of doubtful benefit
	Zinc, iron, digitalis, strophanthus, calcium, opiates, hypnotics, dialacetin
	Drugs for status epilepticus
	Bromide and opiates (orally or rectally), IV luminal, chloral (rectally), chloroform, drainage of the CSF, bromide (orally, rectally, intrathecally)

Note: Lennox's list is derived from his annual review of epilepsy in America in 1937 and 1938 (see text), and reflects US practice in those years. The list of Kinnear Wilson is derived from his standard textbook [3]. Kinnear Wilson died in 1937, leaving the book in a near finished state, and his list reflects British practice in the mid-1930s, before the introduction of phenytoin.

drugs, diphenyl hydantoin, acetophenone and benzophenone, which were more effective than either bromide or phenobarbital in protecting animals from electrically induced convulsions. (Looking ahead a year, the authors have proved the value of the drug sodium diphenyl hydantoinate clinically. It is more effective than phenobarbital in stopping the various types of seizures, and is without the depressive effect on the mentality, but has a more marked toxic action on the skin. This finding promises to be a therapeutic advance of real importance.) [2]

By the 1940 issue of *Epilepsia*, phenytoin had become centre stage in Lennox's annual review of epilepsy in America [5]. Other drugs mentioned, but with far less interest or enthusiasm, were phenobarbitone, bromides, gold, luminal, brilliant vital red, methyl blue (for status), epival sodium, chloral hydrate, luminal, ephedrine sulphate and the ketogenic diet. However, on the subject of phenytoin, Lennox waxed lyrical:

The big news of the year is the discovery and clinical use of sodium diphenyl hydantoinate (Dilantin Sodium). Merritt and Putnam, working at the Neurological Unit of the Boston City Hospital, report the results of treating 200 non-institutionalised cases of epilepsy. Of 118 patients who received treatment from 2 to 11 months, grand mal attacks had been absent in 58%, and in an additional 27% there were greatly reduced . . . results were relatively poor for petit mal. . . . Benefit. . . . was most dramatic in patients having psychomotor attacks. Besides being more effective than phenobarbital or bromides in controlling grand mal and psychomotor seizures, dilantin has the great advantage of having only a weak hypnotic effect. [5]

Herewith was phenytoin announced to the world community, and I will return to this drug below. In the subsequent issues of *Epilepsia*, Lennox's reviews mention various other treatment approaches. The older drugs such as bromide and barbiturate therapy, and the ketogenic diet, continued to occupy much space and were clearly widely recommended, as were phenytoin and (in the later years) tridione. Other treatments were also written up. Amongst the most interesting were the effects of X-irradiation and of metrazol-induced or electrically induced convulsions — both therapies were of recurring interest throughout these years and were enthusiastically endorsed by many authors, although not Lennox himself. Benzedrine and caffeine were also widely recommended to counteract the sedative effects of the barbiturate, bromide and hydantoin drugs, and both were included in many proprietary combination tablets [7]. Vasodilator therapy was also written up, using a variety of substances including acetylcholine, amyl nitrite, doryl and the 'fourth substance of the arteriolenstaff', reflecting the interest in alterations in cerebral blood flow in the pathogenesis of epilepsy. The insufflation of the cerebrospinal fluid spaces with air was also, curiously, repeatedly reported in the continental literature. Other medical therapies, reviewed by Lennox, which have not survived the ravages of time included: the use of thyroid extract, pancreatic extract, vitamin B, strychnine, boric acid, pyridine, ammonium chloride, ethyl phenyl sulphone and glutamic acid.

The ketogenic diet

Of all the ancillary therapies being championed in the 1930s, the ketogenic diet requires special mention, as it remains of marginal interest right up to the present time (see Chapter 21). Lennox [1] records his version of how the ketogenic diet was introduced. In the 1920s, a New York corporate lawyer consulted an osteopathic physician concerning his son who had severe epilepsy. A water diet was recommended, which consisted of starvation of 3 or 4 weeks. Dramatically, the seizures were relieved. This observation was relayed to Dr H. Rawle Geyelin of the New York Presbyterian Hospital who treated a further 26 patients by starvation. Twenty patients improved. The lawyer then asked Stanley Cobb to investigate this further, and in 1922 Cobb recruited William Lennox, then a young missionary; and this was the start of Lennox's illustrious career in epilepsy. In 1921, Wilder at the Mayo clinic had suggested that a ketogenic diet would be as effective as fasting and could be maintained for a much longer period, and Lennox and Cobb and others then pursued this therapy with great vigour. In 1922 Wilder and Winter showed that ketosis occurred when the ratio of fatty acids to glucose was greater than 2 : 1 and they recommended that to maintain ketosis over a prolonged period, a diet of ketotic to antiketotic ratio of at least 3 : 1 was needed. This became standard therapy.

Over the next 10 years, Lennox and Cobb and others experimented with various modifications and attempted to understand the specific mechanisms (e.g. hyperpnoea, fluid deprivation, the role of glucose, ketone bodies, pH changes, etc.). In the 1930s, the diet was popular. Peterman [8], an enthusiast, reported the results in 500 children, and that the ketogenic diet plus dehydration, and if necessary phenobarbital, did control seizures in half the children and brought improvement in an added 20%. It was realized by then that the diet was much more effective in children than in adults. As late as 1947 Peterman [9] wrote 'the new drugs [i.e. phenytoin *et al.*] . . . are no more effective than the ketogenic diet' and that 'the epileptic should not be given false hopes by articles in the popular literature to the effect that he may now be cured with a few pills or capsules'. In his review of the year's progress, Lennox [2] also reported that Helmhotz and Goldstein had updated their results at the Mayo clinic and treated 501 children over 15 years. Of the 409 idiopathic cases, 267 children had given the diet an adequate trial and of these 84 (31%) had been rendered free of attacks for a year or more, and 73 of the 84 were reported currently to be on a normal diet. In 1977, Livingstone and his colleagues [10] reported their 40 years' experience with the diet in myoclonic seizures in children and stated that it completely controlled seizures in 54% of patients and caused marked improvement in 26%. In 1947, Keith [11] reviewed therapy in 300 consecutive children and concluded that the use of the ketogenic diet with drugs was the most satisfactory method of treatment — and better than phenobarbital or phenytoin or both together. His observation of 190 patients treated over a 9-year period and followed for a further 15 years showed 35% to 'have remained well for between 4 and 22 years' [11].

Diphenylhydantoin (phenytoin)

The introduction of phenytoin was of course a major step in the history of epilepsy, neurology and clinical pharmacology. It transformed the treatment of epilepsy, it changed the conceptual basis of epilepsy practice, the approach to drug discovery, the role of the pharmaceutical company in epilepsy, the organization of epilepsy care and indeed the whole international epilepsy movement. I doubt whether any other single treatment, with the possible exception of phenobarbital, has had such an enduring and worldwide impact on the medical or social aspects of the disease.

As Friedlander points out in his excellent review (from which this account is heavily drawn [12]), the discovery of phenytoin—as innovative as indeed it was—should be considered within the context of the times. There had of course been an enormous growth in organic chemistry in the previous 30 years. The chemical structure of drugs was well understood, as was the concept of manufacturing families of drugs which might have similar functions (e.g. the hydantoins and barbiturates—Fig. 1). Phenytoin was not the first hydantoin to be synthesized which had known antiepileptic effects. Phenylethylhydantoin (Nirvanol) was an important precursor. It has a hydantoin ring and the same attached radicals as phenobarbital. It was in general use as a hypnotic in the 1920s and 1930s and although there was little doubt that it was clinically effective in epilepsy, it was not widely used because of toxicity. By the early 1930s, it had also been recognized that Nirvanol was a racemic mixture and that the drug toxicity could be reduced by removing the laevo derivative without altering beneficial effects [12,13], but the drug was not tested in any large clinical trial. Mesantoin was the second antiepileptic drug (AED) (after phenytoin) to be introduced into wide practice, and became very popular. It is in fact metabolized *in vivo* into phenylethylhydantoin (Nirvanol), and had Nirvanol been properly assessed clinically in the 1930s, it is quite possible that it would have pre-empted phenytoin. Nevertheless, the knowledge that the hydantoin drugs were antiepileptic must surely have contributed to the submission of phenytoin to Merritt and Putnam for testing.

The concept of screening drugs in an experimental model of epilepsy was not new when Merritt and Putnam initiated their work on phenytoin. It had long been recognized that certain chemicals were convulsant in animals, and experiments with these compounds had been widely undertaken since the late 19th century. Camphor for instance was introduced as a chemical convulsant in animals in 1877, and even Metrazol (pentylenetetrazol), which was subsequently to become a standard for chemical-convulsant screening, was recognized to be a convulsant in 1926, and metrozol-induced convulsions were used therapeutically in the 1930s and 1940s. Nor was the use of chemical convulsants to assess potential AEDs new. Thujone, camphor and metrazol were studied by Lennox in the 1920s [14], and Keith reported the protectant effects of ketone bodies and related acids and alcohols on thujone-induced seizures in rabbits ([15–17] acetone, ethylacetoacetate, diacetone alcohol). However, as Putnam noted [18], they were difficult to use, and it was probably the inconsistency of chemically induced convulsion which dissuaded Merritt and Putnam from pursuing chemical models in their subsequent work [14,19]. The fact that convulsions could be induced by the application of electrical current directly to the brain had been demonstrated in the latter half of the 18th century according to Brazier [20], and this model too had been used to assess treatment. Albertoni [21] for instance had shown that bromide reduced these convulsions. Viale [22], Krasnogorsky [23] and Spiegel *et al.* [24–26] all developed experimental models with convulsions induced by electrical stimulation through the intact skull. Putnam noted that his own method was based on a modification (by Frederick Gibbs) of these methods [18], and also recorded that Fulton and Keller used cortical excitability to electrical stimulation to investigate the effects of anaesthetics. It seems likely that these experiments were the precursors of his own.

The intellectual milieu in which Putnam and Merritt made their contributions is worth briefly recording. Boston had in the 1920s and 1930s become a major centre of epilepsy research (and had certainly by then overtaken London, the focus of the earlier work described in the first edition of this book). In 1922, Stanley Cobb had

	Barbiturates			Hydantoins		
	R1	R2	R3		R1	R2	R3
Veronal (barbital)	Et	Et	H	(Too toxic)	Et	Et	H
Phenobarbital	Ph	Et	H	Nirvanol	Ph	Et	H
Mebaral. prominal	Ph	Et	Me	Mesantoin	Ph	Et	Me
(Not synthesized)	Ph	Ph	H	Phenytoin	Ph	Ph	H

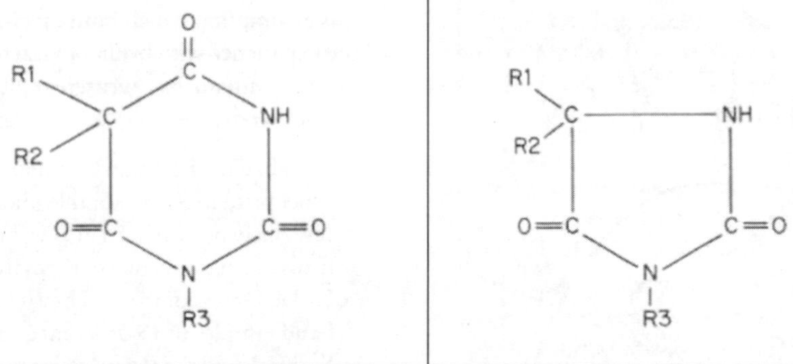

Fig. 1 Comparison of the structure of early barbiturate and hydantoin drugs—showing their similarity. The barbiturates, hydantoins, oxalolidine diones, succinimides and phenacemide are all based on the ureide moiety with different side-chains (R1,R2-C-CO-NH-CO-R3) This was well recognized by medicinal chemists at the time who deliberately synthesized ureide derivatives in the hope of finding improved clinical action.

formed a laboratory for experimental physiology at Harvard, with Lennox as an assistant. In 1930–31, the neurological unit at the Boston City Hospital opened and Cobb was appointed director. Epilepsy became the main focus of research. When Cobb moved to Harvard in 1934, Tracey Jackson Putnam was appointed as his successor. Putnam was the son of Jackson Putnam, Professor of Diseases of the Nervous System at Harvard. He appointed H. Houston Merritt as 'my faithful Chef de Clinique, in charge of my Outpatient Department'. At the Boston City Hospital at that time were also Frederick and Erna Gibbs. The intellectual power assembled at that time in Boston applied to epilepsy research was indeed formidable. These brilliant people (Cobb, Lennox, Gibbs, Putnam and Merritt) worked in a setting that, as Friedlander [12] suggested, mixed the 'essential ingredients of a liberal setting and an environment which placed high priority on intellectual enquiry'.

The idea that a systemic survey of potential drugs should be undertaken seems to have originated in 1935 according to Cobb *et al.* [4]. Merritt and Putnam over the next few years developed an experimental model using electroshock which was based on that of Spiegel who in turn derived his method from Krasnogorsky in Moscow. Spiegel recognized that his technique could be used to 'Study . . . the effect of drugs or other therapeutic measures upon convulsive reactivity' [25] and did himself present a comparative study of the protection against electroshock convulsions afforded by the various salts of bromide [26]. Putnam and Merritt [18] mention that their researches 'continued the work of Spiegel', but in a very systematic and comprehensive fashion.

Merritt and Putnam's apparatus (Fig. 2) was similar to Spiegel's. Their work began in 1936–37. The method involved the administration of an electric current to cats via scalp and mouth electrodes. The stimulator consisted of a 45-volt battery, discharging through a commutator operated by a motor and through a potentiometer of

50 ohms. The amount of current that produced a tonic-clonic seizure was recorded as a control (the convulsive threshold), and then some hours after the administration of a test drug. Each drug was rated:

0 = no change in convulsive threshold;
1+ = elevation of the convulsive threshold by 5–15 mA;
2+ = elevation of the convulsive threshold by 20–30 mA;
3+ = elevation of the convulsive threshold by 30–50 mA;
4+ = elevation of the convulsive threshold by greater than 50 mA.

The discovery of phenytoin itself has an interesting history, which was well rehearsed in the subsequent 50 years. In its retelling, facts may have been jumbled and Friedlander's paper on the subject is a model of historical detective work [12].

Putnam wrote in 1937 [18] that he was interested in studying conjugated phenols following the work of Harrison, Mason and Resnik, who had shown that the phenols were responsible for the motor depression of uraemia.

Accordingly, a large number of phenol-compounds were studied. These included phenyl, cresyl and tolyl sulfonates, benzoates, ketones and esters of such radicals as carbamic, malic, barbituric acids and hydantoin. The compounds which appear to have the greatest anticonvulsant activity combined with the least relative hypnotic effect of those tested so far are diphenylhydantoin, acetophenone and benzophenone. [18]

Diphenylhydantoin had been originally synthesized in 1908 by Blitz [27], and again in 1923 by Dox and Thomas, organic chemists searching for hypnotic drugs in the Parke, Davis laboratories [28]. They noted that hydantoins had a similar ring structure to barbituric acid and that like barbiturates, aliphatic substitutions on the 5 position conferred hypnotic properties but not aromatic substitutions. They prepared and tested diphenylhydantoin but found it had no hypnotic action and thus ignored it. It was widely accepted that, because most effective antiepileptic substances in use at the time were also sedatives (e.g. bromide, phenobarbitone, methylethylphenylbarbituric acid, phenylmethylbarbituric acid), the antiepileptic effect must be related to the sedative effect. It was this assumption which Putnam challenged, perhaps on the basis of the experience with brilliant vital red (which has no sedative action at all). Putnam has written that, having designed his screening methodology,

I combed the Eastman Chemical Company's catalogue, and other price lists, for suitable phenyl compounds that were not obviously poisonous. I also wrote to the major pharmaceutical firms . . . the only one of them that showed any interest was Parke, Davis company. They wrote back to me that they had on hand samples of 19 different compounds analogous to phenobarbital, and that I was welcome to them. [29]

The 19 compounds were those which Dox had prepared. Dox sent Putnam seven compounds in 1936 and phenytoin was the first on the list (Table 7).

Putnam started to use the drug experimentally in 1936 and reported his findings in the 28 May issue of *Science* in 1937 [18]. The first eight patients treated were reported to the Parke, Davis Company in August 1937, and the first clinical trials were reported in June 1938 at the annual meeting of the American Medical Association. Clinical observations in the first 200 patients were published in

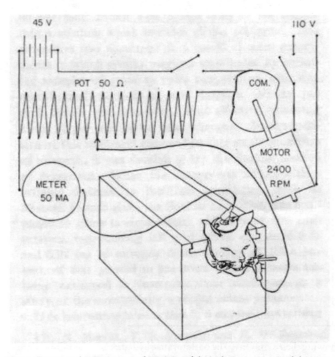

Fig. 2 Diagram by Putnam and Merritt of their drug testing model (as published in their first report of this model in [18]).

Table 7 Seven compounds sent to Dr T.J. Putnam from the Parke, Davies laboratories on 24 April 1936

5,5,-diphenylhydantoin
N-phenylbarbital
N-phenyl-ethylpropylbarbituric acid
N-p-methoxyphenylbarbital
N-p-ethoxyphenylbarbital
N-benzylbarbital
N-p-tolylbarbital

From the Parke, Davis and Co research files—cited in [83].

September 1938, and were not all that encouraging. Of the 200 patients, minor toxic symptoms were reported in 15% and more serious reactions in 5%. Merritt and Putnam recorded then that phenytoin was:

> without doubt . . . considerably more toxic than bromides and the barbituric compounds . . . [and thus] . . . it is worth trying with proper precautions in patients who have not responded to less toxic modes of therapy, such as bromides, the barbituric acid compounds or the ketogenic diet. [30]

In 1938, others were also trialling the drug. Kimball gave it to children and was the first to report gum hypertrophy [31]. A year later, a presentation made to the American Psychiatric Association and published 4 months later [32] was more upbeat. Two hundred and sixty-seven patients were reported, who had been treated for between 2 and 22 months. Of 227 patients with grand mal, 74% had seizures controlled or greatly improved compared with 59% of 104 patients with petit mal and 85% of 39 patients with psychomotor seizures. Dilantin sodium was added to the catalogue price list of Parke, Davis in June 1938. In 1939, the AMA council added Dilantin into *New and Nonofficial Remedies* as indicated in 'epileptic patients who are not benefitted by phenobarbital or bromides and in those in whom these drugs induced disagreeable side reactions'. The drug was included on the basis of 13 different clinical trials, which included a total of 595 treated patients; Merritt and Putnam's patients comprised therefore only one-third [30,33–35].

Within a few years, though, the drug had become extremely popular, and its importance realized. Cohen *et al.* [36] for instance summed up contemporary opinion in 1940 in a paper submitted to the American Psychopathological Association [12] in which they concluded that the history of drug treatment in epilepsy could be divided into three epochs, the first of bromide, the second of phenobarbital and 'the third era is very recent in origin and is characterized by the introduction in 1938 of Dilantin Sodium'.

Over the next decade, Putnam and Merritt continued to test a large number of test drugs, using their screening programme. In 1945, they published in *Epilepsia* that they had tested over 700 compounds and they listed in their paper the results on 618 [37]. Seventy-six compounds were given a 4+ rating. They could be grouped into seven categories on the basis of their structure: barbiturates, benzoxazoles, hydantoins, ketones and phenyl ketones, oxazolidinediones, phenyl compounds with sulfur, and phenyl glycol. Of these drugs, phenytoin and four others were selected for clinical

trial. None of the other four (5-phenyl-5-isopropoxymethylhydantoin, ethyl-phenylsulfone, 5-methyl-5-phenylhydantoin, 5,5-diphenylenehydantoin) showed clinical benefits greater than phenytoin and so were not pursued after the initial trials. What distinguishes Merritt and Putnam's work from their predecessors is the systematic approach which they adopted to screening compounds. This was an enduring legacy and mass animal screening became part of the developmental programme of all the major pharmaceutical companies and drug development programmes in epilepsy. Ironically, it is now recognized that Merritt and Putnam's method does not reliably measure seizure threshold, and furthermore phenytoin does not actually usually increase threshold; one can muse on how many of the drugs rejected by Merritt and Putnam on the basis of this test might have in fact proved useful in epilepsy.

The process of mass screening was developed by Goodman and colleagues, who undertook extensive studies of 'the physiology and therapy of experimental convulsive disorders' and developed a battery of tests using electrically and chemically induced seizures [38–40]. By the mid-1960s, maximal electroshock (MES) and pentylenetetrazol (metrazol)-induced convulsions were considered the only models necessary for AED evaluation, because their effects correlated with all aspects of clinical epilepsy, and thousands of compounds were screened using these experimental models. The National Institutes of Health (NIH) AED screening programme is the apogee of this approach. Between 1975 and 1995, the NIH programme screened 16 000 chemicals using MES and also the pentylenetetrazol tests. Of these 16 000 compounds, 2700 were shown to have AED action, 130 were evaluated in advanced studies, 11 entered clinical trials, six had been filed for approval and one had reached the market (felbamate). One can estimate that over 5 million animal experiments were carried out. The limitations of such an approach are many and include: (a) existing drugs have been produced by similar models and so this method may miss drugs with alternative mechanisms of action; (b) the MES test is an acute seizure model and as such will miss drugs which have a delayed action or disease-modifying properties; and (c) the epileptic brain differs from the normal brain so a model of seizure activity may not be wholly appropriate. The small number of drugs marketed in the NIH programme may reflect these limitations, but the huge impact that Merritt and Putnam's method had is quite clear.

1945–54: *Epilepsia* and epilepsy treatment in the postwar decade

In 1945, the war was over and the world began recovering. It was a changed place. Political and economic ascendancy had shifted finally across the Atlantic, and the rubble of Britain and Europe were hardly fertile grounds for scientific work. The first business meeting of the ILAE since 1939 was held on 13 December 1946, and the next congress was held in Paris in 1949.

The 1946 issue of *Epilepsia* contained Lennox's literature review of 1945, in which 222 publications were considered. Twenty-seven articles on drug treatment were abstracted. Nine were primarily concerned with phenytoin and two with its methylated variant, two bromide and phenobarbital, two the 'fourth substance of the Arteriolenstaff' injected intravenously in the prodromal period, four tridione, one chorionic gonadotropin therapy in hypopituitarism after head injury, one sulfoxides and sulfones, one acetylcholine, one glutamic acid and four electroshock therapy. Thus, apart from the introduction of phenytoin, epilepsy treatment had not made dramatic progress during the war years. The fate of the 'fourth substance' is unclear—it was a material isolated from the cells of the small blood vessels (in the placenta, spleen, lungs) and was a vasodilator. It could be given only by intravenous means, and nitrites and nitroglycerine were considered more practical for clinical use [41]. This approach reflects the interest at the time in the potential role of cerebral blood flow changes in epilepsy, a preoccupation which was to resurface periodically in subsequent years.

In the subsequent annual reviews (1947–50), the literature came to be dominated by reviews of hydantoins (phenytoin and its derivatives such as mesantoin and thyphenytoin), the newer barbiturates and oxazolidine diones (tridione and dimethylethyloxazolidine dione). Phenurone made its debut in the 1950 review [42,43], and was to become widely used in the next decade. Also interesting was the observation of Loewe and Goodman [44] of the high potency of marijuana in protection against MES, a potency comparable with phenytoin, another line of treatment more recently revived. Amongst other drugs reported to show promise between 1945 and 1949, but which were not widely taken up, were: nicotine, vitamins A and D, glutamic acid, potassium mono- and diphosphate, creatinine, thyroid therapy, papaverine hydrochloride and the antihistamines. Here too was the first report in *Epilepsia* of paraldehyde in status, although this had been mentioned by Wilson in his textbook of 1940 [3]. Several reviews from France were also cited, providing not very complimentary snapshots of therapeutic progress there. Guiot [45] wrote that barbiturate was considered superior to phenytoin and also recommended belladonna, caffeine, picrotoxin (actually a convulsant) and cerebrospinal fluid drainage. Gobbi [46] described 'Wander', a new antiepileptic combination tablet comprising atropine, caffeine, phenobarbital, phenytoin and calcium bromide, about which Lennox commented 'shotgun preparations are hardly new'. Others wrote up the beneficial effects of the removal of molar teeth and the induction of a turpentine abscess.

The 1950 issue of *Epilepsia* was the last of the second series, and there was another hiatus. No journal appeared in 1951, and the third series of *Epilepsia* was inaugurated in 1952. The second series of *Epilepsia* had all too obviously run out of steam, and the hiatus allowed a re-evaluation of the role of the journal. The new editor (J. Merlis) was evidently unhappy with the internalized nature of the journal of little enduring interest, comprising as it did simply society reports and a literature review, and strove to alter this. There was thought to be a divergence of opinion within the ILAE executive. Ledeboer (the then secretary-general) wrote in his 1953 secretary-general's report:

> Personally I would prefer that inserting of original articles be not the main thing. These articles could also be published in all other periodicals appearing all over the world and they would have more readers then. It would be very advisable if the unique position of the journal *Epilepsia* for all epileptologists could return . . . *Epilepsia* should indeed be more evidently the journal of the International League and its branches. Therefore it should contain more reports from these branches. (*Epilepsia* 1953, third series, 2: 104)

Regardless of this view, the third series took a very different stance from that of its predecessor, as the editors wrote with striking modernity in their introduction to volume 1 in 1952:

> With this issue, *Epilepsia* inaugurates a new editorial policy. Any publication must have a *raison d'être*; as an annual abstract journal, *Epilepsia* has lost much of its significance. Abstracts of the literature pertinent to epilepsy are now available from many sources, and although coverage may be incomplete in any one publication, the usefulness of *Epilepsia* becomes more and more limited. Similarly annual review and report of progress in the field appear regularly elsewhere. . . . *Epilepsia* would like to offer its pages to people who wish to express their considered thoughts. . . . In this issue you will find critical reviews, a symposium, a report on research in epilepsy, abstracts of original contributions, an annual bibliography. . . . The things you read in this issue are in the nature of trial balloons. You may wish to puncture some, and release new ones. The future of *Epilepsia* now lies in the hands (and minds) of its contributors. (*Epilepsia* 1952, third series, 1: preface)

The journal had therefore largely returned to the purpose and format of its first series. It was now again a journal of primarily scientific intent; and the internal business of the ILAE and its chapters were relegated to briefer mention. The result was undoubtedly a great improvement, but the process of modernization had to wait until the fourth series (in 1959) to be finally completed. In the 1952 edition, there were interesting articles on the classification of epilepsy (F. MacNaughton), consciousness and cerebral localization (S. Cobb), the role of alcohol in convulsive seizures (R. Berry), the mechanism of action and metabolism of anticonvulsants (J. Toman and J. Taylor), a symposium on seizure mechanisms and reviews on research.

By 1952, a higher profile was being given to research into epilepsy, as the postwar economic climate improved. In the USA, the Veterans Association set up a centre for epilepsy and initiated a landmark follow-up project on head-injured veterans of World War II. The new National Institute of Neurology and Blindness was set up by the NIH. The American branch of the ILAE established a research committee in 1951 and their first report was published in *Epilepsia* in 1952. This document was divided into three sections, reflecting the interests of the time: electroencephalography, experimental epilepsy, anticonvulsant and convulsant agents. The latter section provided an up to date summary of contemporary treatment in the USA, by Harold Himwich from Galesburg, Illinois [47]. It is worth dwelling on this document here as Himwich provides a useful summary of contemporary practice (at least in the USA). He admitted that: 'to a large degree, even today the choice and dosage of drugs remains largely a matter of trial and error. Thus among our urgent problems of current interest is a better understanding of drug actions'. He lists drugs in general use with comments, and also drugs in the experimental phase of development (Table 8).

A major emphasis was placed on understanding the mechanisms of action of the drugs—the first evidence of a concern which grew steadily in the following 50 years. Acetylcholinergic mechanisms were the focus of most interest, with work also on steroid and adrenergic actions. The use of an animal model of epilepsy to investigate the antiepileptic potential of compounds, pioneered by

Table 8 Contemporary drug treatment in 1952 in the USA (listed in a Report by the Committee on Research of the American League Against Epilepsy)

Drug	Comments by the committee chairman
Bromide	Still frequently employed against grand mal seizures, but not helpful in other kinds of epilepsy
Phenobarbital	The mainstay of treatment for many years and today in general use for grand mal and to a lesser extent petit mal
Methylbarbital (Mebaral)	The only other barbiturate which can duplicate the anti-epileptic effect of phenobarbital. . . . some recent work . . . suggests that Mebaral [anyway] forms phenobarbital within the body
Diphenylhydantoin (Dilantin)	Superior to bromides and phenobarbital in many instances in the treatment of grand mal seizures
Trimethadione (Tridione)	[A drug which has] unique properties in the control of the petit mal triad
Paradione	A homolog of trimethadione . . . somewhat less potent but also less toxic
Benzedrine and dexedrine	Stimulants employed in overcoming the sedative effects of such anti-epileptics as trimethadione and phenobarbital. In addition they have been useful in the treatment of some patients with petit mal
Mesantoin	A drug of recent origin which 'is of value in psychomotor seizures' which acts via an intermediary compound which turns out to be 'the old drug Nirvanol'
Phenacetlyurea (Phenurone)	The best drug now available for all the three major types of epilepsy
Drugs in an experimental phase of development	Antihistamines, spirobarbiturates, aureomycin, desoxycorticosterone acetate, succinimide compounds, new barbiturates and anticholinesterases (parathione, tetraethyl pyrophosphate, octamethyl pyrophosphoramide)

From [48].
Compare with Table 6 for an impression of how therapy had evolved over two decades.

Merritt and Putnam, had also been highly influential. Himworth considered that such models would be useful for determining relative efficacy, dosage and the value of certain combinations—a prediction that has been realized at least in part. On the clinical side, the arbitrariness of therapy was recognized. Himwich also noted that:

> experience teaches in many instances a combination of anti-epileptic drugs works better than any single one. At present we do not possess a rational basis either for the mixtures used or the dosages employed . . . *plus ça change.*

Mention was also made of the dangers of sudden withdrawal of barbiturate, clearly recognized at the time, especially in barbiturate addiction.

Mesantoin

Mesantoin (methyl hydantoin, methphenytoin) was introduced into practice in 1945 (Fig. 3) and was the first of the phenytoin analogues to achieve wide usage. Mesantoin is N-methylated at position 3 in the hydantoin ring and has an ethyl group substitution in place of the phenyl group at position 5. This provides a broader spectrum of activity in animal models but also a lower therapeutic index. By 1949, observations from various series were being reported, often of patients who were treatment failures with dilantin. Excellent results were claimed, few side-effects and indeed stimulatory properties to counteract drug-induced somnolence. However, the first reports too of aplastic anaemia, pancytopenia and fatal skin reactions were also being made—a fact which did not stop the manufacturers Sandoz widely advertising its use (in the pages of *Epilepsia*) for routine cases of epilepsy as late as 1955. There were many reports of its value in the epilepsy literature reviews from 1945 onwards. The largest series of patients was of Kozol [48] and

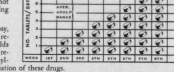

Fig. 3 Contemporary advertisement from *Epilepsia* for mesantoin.

Loscalzo [49]. In the first, 200 patients were treated for periods ranging between 2 months and 4 years. Seventy per cent had grand mal seizures and about half were taking mesantoin alone. Of the patients, 132 (66%) experienced a great reduction in seizures, and 43 (22%) had some benefit. Only 12% were reported to have no change in seizures. Loscalzo [49] reported similar findings in a series of 224 patients treated for 1–7 years. Complete control in grand mal seizures was obtained in 305 and partial control in another 52%. Psychomotor seizures did nearly as well, but mesantoin was noted in this series, as in others, to be ineffective in petit mal. General toxicity was thought to be less with mesantoin than with phenytoin. Loscalzo [49] reported sedation in 16%, skin rash with fever and lymphadenopathy in 9% and gum hyperplasia in 3%. Hirsutism and skin pigmentation were rare. However, Abbot and Schwab [50] found a fall in the leucocyte count below 2500 in 23% of 79 treated patients and in view of this and the relatively high number of fatalities linked to mesantoin therapy due to exfoliative dermatitis, aplastic anaemia, pancytopenia and hepatic failure, recommended that the drug should be considered contraindicated in therapy in all but exceptional cases.

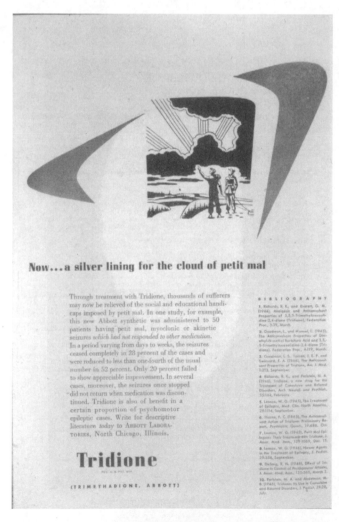

Fig. 4 Contemporary advertisement from *Epilepsia* for Tridione. A fantasy of new horizons and care-free life. There is no mention of the risks of idiosyncratic reaction.

Trimethadione (Tridione)

Trimethadione was synthesized in 1944 by Spielman [51] in his search for drugs with analgesic properties. Its anticonvulsant effects in animals were reported in the same year [52], and in human subjects by 1946 [53–57]. It was licensed for therapy in 1946 (Fig. 4). It was recognized immediately that the drug was particularly effective in petit mal. Again, it was frequently the subject of the *Epilepsia* reviews. Perlstein and Andelman [56] for instance reported that 11 out of 14 patients with petit mal were greatly improved, and three out of seven with grand mal. Lennox [55] reported dramatic results in 166 patients with the petit mal triad, of whom > 80% improvement was noted in 63% in petit mal, 64% of astatic attacks and 70% of myoclonic jerks. Worldwide acceptance of Tridione was very rapid and faster than with phenytoin—perhaps because there was no alternative therapy—and as Lennox wrote in 1960 'Workers had a repetition of the thrill experienced with Dilantin only 7 years before' [1]. Lennox estimated that amongst his 131 patients with petit mal, the annual mean rate of attacks fell from 3500 per year to about 1500 on Tridione—which assuming 100 000 patients in the USA, was a reduction of over 200 million attacks a year. Tridione given IV controlled status in 16 out of 17 cases in one series [58]. Trimethadione is metabolized to dimethadione in the liver and in chronic therapy the ratio of trimethadione to dimethadione is 1:20 and it is likely that the effects of the drug are due largely to the active metabolite. The major side-effect of Tridione is hemeralopia —a visual disturbance which is manifest by a glare when going into a brightly lit environment. Objects look indistinct and colours faded. When severe, the effect is that of a blinding snowstorm. The symptoms were recognized to appear within a few days of initiating therapy and wear off within 8–10 weeks of stopping therapy. The mechanism is obscure, although thought at the time to be retinal in origin [59]. This curious effect is rare in younger children. Rash also occurs in 14% of patients, and other more minor gastric and neurological side-effects are common. Interestingly, seizures were also reported in the earliest literature to be markedly exacerbated in some patients. The rosy picture of medical progress was clouded however by reports of nephrotic syndrome [60], renal failure, fatal dermatitis and fatal blood dyscrasia [61]. The nephrotic syndrome was usually reversible, although two fatalities had been recorded by 1957 [62]. In 1947, within a year of the introduction of the drug, two deaths from aplastic anaemia were reported—and by 1957, a further 11 had been recorded [62]. Davis and Lennox [63] found neutropenia (white count less than 2500/cm^3) in 6.3% of 222 patients. In Davidoff's series, six out of the 75 patients experienced severe blood reactions [64]. Indeed, the jury in a coroner's court in London in 1948 were of the opinion that the drug should be scheduled as a poison. Some side-effects were not recognized in this period, including the unique precipitation of a myasthenic syndrome. By far the most serious omission though was surely the failure to recognize the very strong teratogenic effects of the oxalolidine diones (trimethadione and paradione). Trimethadione results in significant congenital deformity, growth retardation, and/or mental retardation in 30–50% of exposed fetuses—and yet this fact was completely overlooked until 1970. One shudders to contemplate the numbers of adolescent and young adult girls that must have been treated for petit mal over these years, and the tragic unrecognized consequences. To paraphrase Lennox, was this drug worth that risk?

Primidone (5-ethyl-5-phenyl-hexahydropyrimidine-4, 6-dione; Mysoline)

Over 2500 barbiturate compounds have been synthesized since barbituric acid was first produced in 1864. Of these only a small fraction have been shown to have anticonvulsant action—and none has been demonstrated to be so significantly superior to phenobarbital that it has replaced the parent drug in practice. Primidone, though, is perhaps the closest competitor. It was introduced into clinical practice in Britain in 1952 and in the US in 1954 (see Chapter 39 for a fuller description of primidone). As primidone is metabolized largely to phenobarbital *in vivo*, many now consider the drug to have no advantages over phenobarbital, but it was recognized in the early 1950s that primidone suppressed generalized seizures in mice before there was time for significant production of phenobarbital [65]—and it seems likely on the basis of this evidence, that the parent drug does indeed have independent antiepileptic activity. Primidone was also the first non-American drug licensed during this period. The first clinical report, of 40 patients, was by Handley and Stewart [66]. Timberlake *et al.* [67] published what must be one of the first meta-analyses, the results in 742 patients in 12 studies including 96 of their own cases. Good or complete control was found in 60% of grand mal cases 56% of patients with psychomotor seizures and 33% in those with petit mal. The side-effects of primidone were recognized early to be similar to that of phenobarbital—with the usual anecdotal claim that it was less sedative—and with the early recognition that the first few doses could produce a severe reaction (see Chapter 39). In the 1953 edition of *Epilepsia*, Mysoline was being activity advertised. 'Calm after storm' as the advertisements put it, with reassuring pictures of a sailor mending his boat (Fig. 5). Its notable features, according to the advertisements, were its low toxicity, its notable absence of hypnotic effects, its well-tolerated nature and its beneficial effect on general behaviour, performance and sociability.

Other drugs licensed in between 1945 and 1955

Paramethadione (Paradione)

This is a close structural analogue of trimethadione, with a methyl group substituted for one of the two methyl groups at position 5. It performs somewhat better than trimethadione in animal experiments and was pursued for this reason. Davis and Lennox [68] wrote up 85 patients, 73 of whom had taken paramethadione and trimethadione successively. Paramethadione controlled petit mal rather better and grand mal rather worse in this highly uncontrolled study. There was also less depression of the white count and less hemeralopia with paramethadione compared to trimethadione, although drowsiness was somewhat more common. Fatal side-effects, although they did occur, seem also to be less reported. On the basis of all this evidence, the drug should have replaced Tridione in the therapy of petit mal, but in practice this did not occur. It is not clear why this was, but as both drugs were marketed by Abbott, perhaps internal competition made no commercial sense (Fig. 6); the drug was withdrawn from the US market in 1994. Other oxalolidine diones were also investigated in the 1940s and 1960s but were not licensed, including malidone [69].

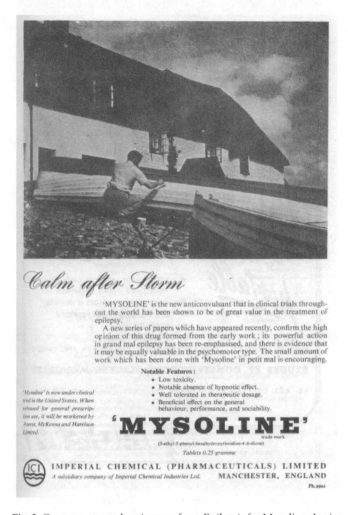

Fig. 5 Contemporary advertisement from *Epilepsia* for Mysoline. Again, a fantasy of peace and naturalness. The emphasis on better tolerability, lack of sedation and positive effect on behaviour and performance seem spurious now.

Phensuximide (Milontin)

This is another analogue of trimethadione, with ethyl groups replacing both methyl groups on position 5. It is noticeable that animal toxicology in dogs and mice was reported with this drug [70], an indication that safety was becoming a greater issue. Large clinical studies were also carried out and suggested that phensuximide had similar efficacy to tridione [70,71], although subsequent work did not confirm this. Phensuximide and its demethylated metabolites have short half-lives which may account for its modest effect. Millichap [72] carried out what was an early placebo-controlled trial where, in 20 patients, he alternated phensuximide and placebo therapy and showed that phensuximide reduced petit mal attacks by 54–56% (depending on the order in which the compounds were administered). Over time, phensuximide was also shown to have a toxic profile similar to that of trimethadione, with possibly a higher incidence of idiosyncratic reactions. It can cause serious renal, hepatic and haematological reactions and also an unusual encephalopathy at high doses. Because of this its use has diminished, although it spawned over the next few years a family of related compounds of which ethosuccimide is still widely prescribed today.

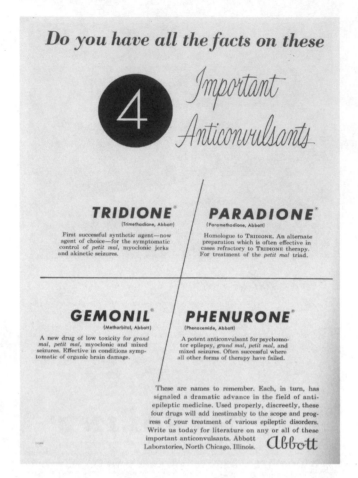

Fig. 6 Contemporary advertisement from *Epilepsia* for the Abbott stable of epilepsy drugs. Three have severe toxicity which was not mentioned in this advertisement, although the advice was to use the drugs discreetly! Later advertisements for phenurone (headed: Why Abbott advertises Phenurone) do emphasize toxicity, and in these advertisements, Abbott make a virtue of the fact that they take a responsible attitude to advertising.

Metharbital (Gemonil)

This was licensed in the US in 1952, and is a diethyl methyl derivative of barbituric acid. It is one of the few barbiturate products which has anticonvulsant activity similar to that of phenobarbital but was claimed to be less sedative although on anecdotal evidence and in the complete absence of comparative trials. It is demethylated *in vivo* to barbital. It never seems to have attracted much of a market, and this is perhaps because of the lack of any obvious clinical advantage over phenobarbital. It is interesting to note that the barbiturates (phenobarbital, primidone or metharbital) are much safer in terms of severe or fatal idiosyncratic reactions than the hydantoins, suximides or oxalolidine diones—a fact seldom commented upon at the time.

Phenacemide (phenylacetlyurea; Phenurone)

This is a straight chain (open ring) analogue of phenytoin which has a broad spectrum of action in experimental animals. It was intro-

duced with some enthusiasm in 1951, and was thought by Himwich [47] to be the best drug for all three types of epilepsy (petit mal, grand mal and psychomotor attacks). Davidson and Lennox [73] reported the effects in 178 patients resistant to other forms of therapy, of whom 25% experienced a reduction in seizures of 50% or more. It is metabolized by *para*-hydroxylation and then glucuronidation, but the hydantoin ring structure is not closed. Effective as an antiepileptic phenacemide certainly is, but it also proved very quickly to be highly toxic. The warning signs were there even in the first reports, and one of the patients reported by Davidson and Lennox died of hepatic failure. Tyler and King [74], writing from the laboratories of Abbott the manufacturers, analysed the results of 1562 patients who were submitted by doctors who were supplied with the drug by the company. Great improvement was noted in 38% of patients with petit mal, 39% with grand mal and 36% with psychomotor seizures. However, 36 patients developed blood dyscrasia and six patients died of hepatitis (four patients) or blood dyscrasia (two patients [75])—a 0.4% risk of death. In addition to the hepatic and haematological effects, phenacemide can also severely affect behaviour, causing aggression, destructiveness, irritability and depression-related effects noted initially by Tyler and King [74] and reiterated by every observer since. Surprisingly, the drug has remained on the formulary despite its impressive toxicity.

Phethenylate (sodium phenylthienyl hydantoin; Thiantoin)

This made a brief appearance in the formulary, licensed in 1950 and withdrawn in 1952. It was withdrawn without much in the way of published assessment, a short foray into the sulfurated hydantoin group.

Benzchlorpropamide (Hibicon)

This was another short-lived drug [76], licensed in the US in 1952 and withdrawn in 1955, despite early claims about its safety (Fig. 7).

Acetazolamide (Diamox)

This was first reported by Merlis in the abstracts of the American League Against Epilepsy meeting in 1954 ([77] Fig. 8). Forty-seven chronic epileptics were reported to have been given the drug with 80–100% relief in 29, 40–80% in six and no effect in 12 patients. It was recognized even then that the main action of Diamox was the inhibition of carbonic anhydrase, and the idea that it might have anticonvulsant action may have derived from the earlier work on the antiepileptic potential of ketosis, fasting and acidosis, or the fact that hyperventilation (and the lowering of carbon dioxide levels in the blood) had long been recognized to exacerbate petit mal. Diamox also induces a pink colour in the plasma, and this was reminiscent of the effect of brilliant vital red. Whatever the reasons, Bergstrom *et al.* [78] initiated a study which was reported in 1956 [79]. Seizures were reduced by 50% or more in 54% of 126 patients and in 27% by 90% or more. The beneficial effects were noted in all seizure types. Other reports followed [80] and the drug still has a useful place in adjunctive therapy today. The toxicity of Diamox was not recorded at the time, but noted later.

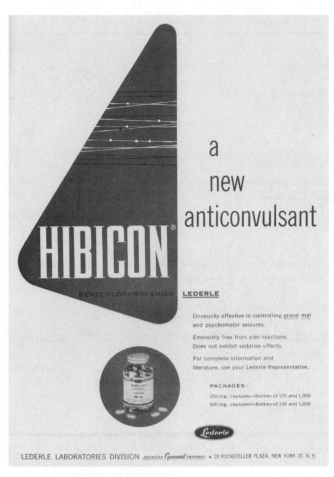

Fig. 7 Contemporary advertisement from *Epilepsia* for Hibicon, emphasizing its safety. The drug was withdrawn from practice a year or so later.

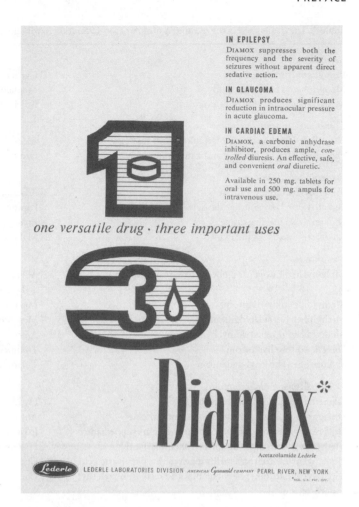

Fig. 8 Contemporary advertisement from *Epilepsia* for Diamox.

Epilepsy therapy in 1955

By 1955, the new format of *Epilepsia* was fully established. The journal now contained a number of full scientific original articles as well as reviews. The annual reports of the chapters were now relegated to a small part of the journal. In November 1955, a review of the available pharmaceutical preparations in the treatment of epilepsy, by Saunie and Vaille [81], was published in which the structural similarities of the barbiturates, hydantoins, oxazolidine diones, pyrimidine diones, succinimide and benzylamide were emphasized. This is interesting, for by now all drugs were being tested using the MES method of Merritt and Putnam, and this method undoubtedly was leading to the self selection of compounds related to each other. With this article was also published, for the first time, an international list of AEDs (Table 9). A comparison with Kinnear Wilson's list (Table 6), published 25 years earlier, shows how far treatment had evolved in this period, which was a phase of great expansion in the pharmaceutical industry. Cost was also a factor in those days, and Lennox's list of drug costs compares costs in 1960 (Table 10).

Postscript

What can we learn from this story of drug discovery and develop-

ment in those tempestuous postwar years? Of the 10 drugs licensed between 1938 and 1954 (Table 1), only two—phenytoin and primidone—remain in widespread use, and the others have fallen, not so much because of lack of effect but rather because of their toxicity and their lack of advantage over other standard therapy. This is not a particularly ringing endorsement of the methods of drug evaluation.

At the preclinical level, the 'big news' as Lennox put it was the systematic evaluation of drugs using the feline electroshock model. As outlined above, the idea of assessing drugs using animal models was not new, and nor indeed was a method using electroshock, but the achievement was the vigour in which this method was applied systematically. The obvious drawbacks of this approach have been mentioned, but it is worth emphasizing again the fact that a single method tends to select drugs with similar modes of action. Thus, almost all of the 10 drugs are closely chemically related (Fig. 1), and have similar profiles of action. How many drugs with different actions or with distinctive structures were overlooked by the overreliance on Putnam and Merritt's method will never be known, but one cannot help regretting what must have been lost opportunities. The concept that the method measures how much drugs elevate the 'epilepsy threshold' was also wrong and, as so often, much of the testing edifice was built on a spurious theoretical foundation. Despite these flaws, Putnam and Merritt's approach was a very real

Table 9 The drugs used in the treatment of epilepsy in 1955 (taken from the international list of antiepilepsy drugs published in *Epilepsia* 1955)

Barbiturates
Phenylethyl barbituric acid — Gardenal, luminal, phenobarbital, phenobarbitone
Methylphenyl barbituric acid — Mephebarbital, rutonal
Methylphenylethyl barbituric acid — Isonal, meberal, prominal

Combinations with barbiturate
Phenylethyl barbituric acid, belladonna and caffeine — Alepsal
Phenylethyl barbituric acid and amphetamine — Ortenal

Oxazolidine diones
Trimethyl oxazolidine dione — Absentaol, epidione, mino-alleviatin, petilep, trimethadione, tridione
Dimethylethyl oxazolidine dione — Paramethadione, Paradione
Diphenyl oxazolidine dione — Epidon
Allylmethyl oxazolidine dione — Malidone

Hydantoins
Diphenyl hydantoin (or diphenyl hydantoin sodium) — Alleviatin, alepsin, antipil. Antisacer, comitiona, convulsin, dihydan, dilantin, diphentoin, ditoinate, epamin, epaneutin, petoin, phnytoine, solantyl
Methyldiphenyl hydantoin — Melantoine
Methylphenylethyl hydantoin — Mesantoin, phenantoin, sedantoinal
Methyldibromophenylethyl hydantoin — Anirrit
Dimethyldithio hydantoin — Thiomedan
Sodium phenylthienyl hydantoin — Thiantoin, phethenylate

Combinations with hydantoins
Diphenyl hydantoin and phenobarbital — Hydantoinal, comitoina compound
Diphenyl hydantoin, phenobarbital and caffeine — Antisacer compound, apilep
Diphenyl hydantoin, Phenobarbital and desoxyephedrine — Isosolantyl, phelantin
Methylphenylethylhydantoin and phenobarbital — Hydantal
Diphenyl hydantoin and methylphenylethyl barbituric acid — Comital, mebaroin
Diphenyl hydantoin, phenobarbital and methylphenylethyl barbituric acid — Comital L

Other types
Phenylacetylurea — Epiclase, fenilep, phenacemide, phenurone
Phenylethylhexahydropyrimidine dione — Mysoline, primidone
Benzchlorpropamide — Hibicon, posedrine
Methylaphaphenyl succinimide — Lifene, milontin
Acetazolamide — Diamox
Alkaline borotartrates — Several preparations
Glutamic acid (or glutamic acid-HCl) — Acidulin, Glutan-HCl, Glutamicol
Bromides — Large numbers of preparations (in three categories: alkaline bromides and alkaline earths: polybromide; organicbromides; bromide in combination with other agents; alkaline borotartrates)

achievement, and dominated the experimental assessment of drugs for generations to come.

The clinical evaluation of drugs in this period is also worth reflecting upon. To the complacent modern reader, the uncontrolled nature of the clinical studies may seem primitive or even shocking. The literature reviews of *Epilepsia* are littered with case series where the new potential therapy was tried in small numbers of patients, for varying lengths of times at varying dosages and with results expressed in varying ways (often unquantified). There seems to have been no attempt to standardize clinical assessment, which is paradoxical considering the converse way that experimental assessment had been (over)standardized. Licensing too was possible on the basis of experience in only a few patients; thus I doubt whether any of the newly licensed drugs in this period had been given to more

than a few hundred patients prior to launch, and probably even less experimental animals. Clinical testing was thus a much shorter process than today, and drugs were introduced and licensed with remarkable speed. Phenytoin for instance was licensed within 1–2 years of the first discovery of its antiepileptic effect, and tridione even earlier. This apparent insouciance may have reflected the lack of regulatory requirement in this period to show clear efficacy—this requirement had to wait until the Kefauver–Harris amendments to the Food, Drug and Cosmetic Act in 1962. I encountered one study only where any sort of control was in place (the comparison of tridione and paradione tried sequentially in the same group of patients, mentioned above). Nevertheless, all of the drugs which were licensed during these years had undoubted antiepileptic activity. Thus, an uncomfortable question inevitably arises—to what extent

Table 10 Annual cost of anticonvulsant drugs in available between 1938 and 1955

Drug	Dose (mg)	Cost (US$)	Manufacturer
Bromide	4000	20	–
Dexedrine (dextro-amphetamine sulfate)	10	44	SKF
Diamox (acetozolamide)	1000	175	Lederle
Dilantin (phenytoin)	400	29	Parke, Davis
Gemonil (metharbital)	400	29	Abbott
Mebaral (mephobarbital)	500	49	Winthrop-Stearns
Mesantoin (mephenytoin)	600	71	Sandoz
Milontin (phensuximide)	2000	92	Parke, Davis
Mysoline (primidone)	1500	142	Ayerst
Paradione (paramethadione)	900	66	Abbott
Phenobarbital	200	11	–
Phenurone (phenacemide)	1500	57	Abbott
Tridione (trimethadione)	900	57	Abbott

Note: The cost is expressed in 1960 prices (derived from [1]).

are controlled studies superior to the open observations of experienced physicians? The answer is not known, but I suspect the pendulum has swung too far today, and a more mixed approach to drug evaluation (with open as well as blinded and controlled trials) might result in a faster and more intelligent assessment.

Although it may be true that a small number of patients only is needed to demonstrate efficacy in the case of a strong anticonvulsant, it is also true that many more patients are needed before one can be sure that a drug has no severe idiosyncratic side-effects. The speed of introduction and the small number of exposed patients seem to have reflected a general lack of interest in this issue. Certainly, the attitude to risk-taking in this period seems to differ from that today. Lennox could for instance write about phenurone (a 1:250 chance of death)—is the risk too great? Today, felbamate was withdrawn from the formulary rapidly, and with great alarm, with a risk of death of about 1:5000. Lennox again: 'physicians to epileptics are mariners who sail in a sea of cross currents (individual susceptibility) between Scylla (no results) and Charybdis (toxic reactions)'—one senses his opinion that trade winds could blow the ship closer to danger than would today be allowed. The regulatory environment of the times was however changing. In 1938, in the USA, the Federal Drug and Cosmetic Act of 1938 required a demonstration of drug safety before a drug could be licensed, and there was no such requirement before 1938. However, this regulation seems to have had little meaning in a period when rapid licensing was obtained for drugs such as mesantoin, trimethadione, paradione, dimethadione, phenthenylate, phenacemide, benzchlorpropamide and phensuximide all of which resulted in non-infrequent serious sometime fatal side-effects. Similarly, toxicology or mutagenicity were also seldom reported, and even when frequent and severe, the teratogenic potential of drugs was completely overlooked (e.g. of the oxazolidine diones). A number of other drugs also proved highly toxic during this period, and were withdrawn from use, e.g. thiantoin (phenthenylate), 3-methyl-5-phenyl hydantoin (Nuvarone), sodium 5,5-phenyl thienyl hydantoin (Phelantin), atrolactamide (Themisone)—but often only having been given without much initial concern.

The evolution of the pharmaceutical industry, particularly in the last years of this period is also worthy of comment. In the 1930s, the European pharmaceutical industry had the edge over that in the US, and led in many areas. The war effort changed all this. There was a running down of research and a virtual standstill in innovation as war interrupted academic and industrial work, and the physical destruction of the postwar years in Europe further hampered economic recovery. The initiative (and many scientists) had passed to the USA. Several of the companies innovative in the epilepsy field had also developed large research and development departments in the early years (for instance Abbott and Parke Davis; although interestingly their lack of research and development investment in the late 1940s and 1950s led to their massive decline in the 1960s and 1970s). The companies also developed large and specialized marketing departments, as the advertisements in the medical press attest. It was in this period too that the financial viability of the journals became dependent on the revenue from advertisement, and the rapid increase in advertising space and influence is readily apparent in the pages of *Epilepsia*. The antiepileptic market itself was never going to be large enough to encourage the industry to prioritize drug discovery in this area, but, from an early stage, it was recognized that AEDs often had other actions (e.g. as hypnotics or analgesics). It was probably this fact which helped maintain interest in what in global terms was a relatively minor indication. The massive expansion of the pharmaceutical industry was to follow in subsequent decades, but the seeds of their future growth were planted in these postwar years. The extraordinary scientific development of organic chemistry was undoubtedly the stimulus for much of this activity, and the advance in chemical knowledge during these years was surely one of the greatest achievements of the 20th century. The methods for analysing and synthesizing chemicals with defined structure greatly stimulated the development of AEDs. It was recognized that the existing AEDs all shared a ureide moiety, and a range of derivatives were produced with a ureide base. Phenobarbital, phenytoin and the other hydantoins, the oxalolidine diones, the succinimide and phenacemide all share the same ureide core—and these classes vary by a (simple) substitution in one position only. The expansion of each family is by the addition of side-chains—often simply phenyl, ethyl, methyl or allyl elements. The fact that the ureides monopolized the AED field during this period was a deliberate consequence of the then dominant approach to medicinal chemistry. The focus moved on only several decades later, when interest shifted to the benzodiazepines, valproate and the tricyclic drugs [82].

Finally, what of the role of *Epilepsia*? The only enduring contribution of the second series was the provision of literature reviews, and this must have been useful and instructive to many readers, in the pre-computer, pre-Medline age. Other bibliographies did exist, but the unique contribution of *Epilepsia* was the printing of abstracts. This contributed to what was a remarkably rapid dissemination of information about drug action in the period under review. Thus, for instance, within a few year of the introduction of phenytoin in the USA, papers on the drug were appearing from Britain, Scandinavia, Italy, Germany, Spain, Portugal, eastern Europe, South America and even China. The globalization of medicine and medicines was clearly apparent even in these early years. How much of this was due to the role of the medical journals (including *Epilepsia*) or to the activities of the pharmaceutical industries is not clear, although I suspect the former were very influential. The position of *Epilepsia* as an organ in which original science is published was lost during the second series (especially sad in view of the impressive start made by the first series) and it was not until the third, and particularly recently in the fourth series, that this position has been regained.

This period of 17 years was a time of great activity in epilepsy, and despite—or possibly because of—the carnage of the world wars, there was at the end of our period great optimism. As Lennox wrote 'the mid-twentieth century for the epileptic, as for so many persons who are sick, [was] a time of thankfulness and expectation' [1]. Others will judge how justified this expectation is, but the therapeutic advances of the period seem less definitive now than they did then. Nevertheless, this period opened by the 'year of jubilee' and the discovery of phenytoin, was an interesting and important one which shaped the progress of epilepsy therapy for many years.

Acknowledgements

I am very grateful to Ms Michelle Lian for help with the references and organization of this chapter.

References

1 Lennox WG. *Epilepsy and Related Disorders*. Boston: Little, Brown, 1960.
2 Lennox W. Progress in the study of epilepsy in America in 1937. *Epilepsia* 1939; 196–208.
3 Kinnear Wilson SA. *Neurology*. London: Edward Arnold, 1940.
4 Cobb S, Cohen ME, Ney J. Brilliant Vital Red as an anticonvulsant. *Arch Neurol Psychiatr* 1938; 37: 463–5.
5 Lennox W. Study of epilepsy in America in 1938. *Epilepsia* 1940; 279–90.
6 Aird RB. Mode of action of brilliant vital red in epilepsy. *Arch Neurol Psychiatr* 1939; 42: 700–23.
7 Cohen B, Myerson A. Effective use of phenobarbital and benzedrine sulphate (amphetamine sulphate) in treatment of epilepsy. *Am J Psychiatr* 1938; 95: 371 (Sept).
8 Peterman MG. Therapy of epilepsy in children. *Am J Psychiat* 1936; 92: 1433–8.
9 Peterman MG. Idiopathic epilepsy in childhood. *Nerv Child* 1947; 6: 49–51.
10 Livingstone S, Pauli LL, Pruce I. Ketogenic diet in the treatment of childhood epilepsy. *Dev Med Child Neurol* 1977; 19: 833–4.
11 Keith HM. Results of treatment of recurring convulsions, epilepsy. *Proc Mayo Clinic* 1947; 22: 14–16.
12 Friedlander WJ. Putnam, Merritt and the discovery of Dilantin. *Epilepsia* 1986; 27 (Suppl. 3): S1–21.
13 Sobotka H, Holzman MF, Kahn J. Optically active 5,5′-disubstituted hydantoins. *J Am Chem Soc* 1932; 54: 687–702.
14 Lennox WG, Nelson R, Beetham WP. Studies in epilepsy: VI. Factors affecting convulsions induced in rabbits. *Arch Neurol Psychiatr* 1929; 21: 625–36.
15 Keith HM. Influence of various factors on experimental convulsions. *Proc Staff Meet Mayo Clin* 1930; 5: 204–5.
16 Keith HM. The effect of various factors on experimentally produced convulsions. *Am J Dis Child* 1931; 41: 532–43.
17 Keith HM. Further studies of the control of experimentally produced convulsions. *J Pharmacol Exp Ther* 1932; 46: 449–55.
18 Putnam TJ, Merritt HH. Experimental determination of the anticonvulsant properties of some phenyl derivatives. *Science* 1937; 85: 525–6.
19 Pollock LJ, Finkelman I, Tigay E. The action of pyridine, some of its derivatives and phenyl cinchoninic acid in preventing convulsions produced by Metrazol. *Trans Am Neurol Assoc* 1941; 67: 6–10.
20 Brazier MAB. The history of electrical activity of the brain as a method for localizing sensory function. *Med Hist* 1963; 7: 199–211.
21 Albertoni P. Untersuchunger uber die wirkung einiger arzneimittel auf de effegbarkeit des grosshirns nebst beiträgen zur therapie der epilepsie. *Arch Exp Pathol Pharmakol* 1882; 15: 248–88.
22 Viale G. Acces epileptiforme chez le chien par application peripherique du courant alternatif. *Compt Rend Soc Biol* 1929; 102: 464–5.
23 Krasnogorsky NI. Convulsions called forth in the dog by conditioned reflex stimulation, and the resulting psychoneurotic state of the animal. XV International Physiological Congress, Leningrad and Moscow, August 1935. *Summaries of communications* 9:7. Moscow–Leningrad: State Publishing House for Biological and Medical Literature, 1935: 213–14.
24 Spiegel EA, Spiegel-Adolf M, Wohl MG. New biophysical methods. *JAMA* 1936: 106: 1301.
25 Spiegel EA. Quantitative determination of reactivity by electric stimulation of the brain with the skull intact. *J Lab Clin Med* 1937; 22: 1274–6.
26 Spiegel EA. Therapeutic procedures in experimental convulsions and catalepsy. I. Quantitative determination of the convulsive reactivity by electric stimulation of the brain with the skull intact (with special reference to the effects of the bromids). *Trans Am Ther Soc* 1937; 37: 37–44.
27 Biltz H. Constitution of the products of the interaction of substituted carbamides of Benzil. *Berl Dtsch Chem Gesamte* 1908; 41: 1379–93 (Abstracted in *Chem Abstr* 1908; 2: 2252).
28 Dox AW, Thomas A. 5,5-arylbarbituric acids. *J Am Chem Soc* 1923; 45: 1811–16.
29 Putnam TJ. The demonstration of the specific anti convulsant action of diphenylhydantoin and related compounds. In: Ayd FJ, Blackwell B, eds. *Discoveries in Biological Psychiatry*. Philadelphia: JB Lippincott, 1970: 85–90.
30 Merritt HH, Putnam TJ. Sodium diphenyl hydantoinate in the treatment of convulsive disorders. *JAMA* 1938; 111: 1068–73.
31 Kimball OP. The treatment of epilepsy with sodium diphenyl hydantoinate. *JAMA* 1939; 112: 1244–5.
32 Merritt HH, Putnam TJ. Further experiences with the use of sodium diphenyl hydantoinate in the treatment of convulsive disorders. *Am J Psychiatr* 1940; 96: 1023–7.
33 Merritt HH, Putnam TJ. Sodium diphenyl hydantoinate in the treatment of convulsive seizures. Toxic symptoms and their prevention. *Arch Neurol Psychiatr* 1939; 42: 1053–8.
34 Merritt HH, Putnam TJ. Sodium diphenyl hydantoinate in the treatment of convulsive seizures. Toxic symptoms and their prevention. *Trans Am Neurol Assoc* 1939; 65: 158–62.
35 Council of pharmacy and chemistry. Dilantin sodium. *J Am Med Assoc* 1939; 113: 1734–5.
36 Cohen B, Showstack N, Myerson A. The synergism of phenobarbital, dilantin sodium and other drugs in the treatment of institutional epilepsy. *JAMA* 1940; 114: 480–4.
37 Merritt HH, Putnam TJ. Experimental determination of anticonvulsive activity of chemical compounds. *Epilepsia* 1945; 5 (Series 11): 51–75.

38 Goodman LS, Toman JEP, Swinyard EA. Anticonvulsant drugs; mechanisms of action and methods of assay. *Arch Int Pharmacodyn Ther* 1949; 78: 144–62.

39 Swinyard EA. Laboratory assay of clinically effective antiepileptic drugs. *J Am Pharm Assoc* 1949; 38: 201–4.

40 Swinyard EA, Brown WC, Goodman LS. Comparative assays of antiepileptic drugs in mice and rats. *J Pharmacol Exp Ther* 1952; 106: 319–30.

41 Stauder KH. Zur behandlung des epileptischen anfalls. *Med Wschr* 1944; 91: 289–90.

42 Gibbs FA, Everett GM, Richards RK. Phenurone in epilepsy. *Dis Nerv Syst* 1949; 10 (2): 47–9 (Feb).

43 Zeifert M. Phenurone in epilepsy. *Dis Nerv Syst* 1949; 10: 245–8.

44 Loewe S, Goodman LS. Anticonvulsant action of marihuana-active substances. *Fed Proc* 1947; 6: 352.

45 Guiot G. Traintment de l'epilepsie essentielle. *Prog Med* 1946; 21: 496.

46 Gobbi E. Un nouvel antiepileptique: L'amtosacer compositum "Wander" Praxis 1946; 51/52: 875–7.

47 Himwich HE. Report of committee on research 111. Anticonvulsant and convulsant agents. *Epilepsia* 1992; third series (1): 145–52.

48 Kozol HL. Mesantoin in treatment of epilepsy. *Arch Neurol Psychiatr* 1950; 63: 235–48.

49 Loscalzo AE. Mesantoin in the control of epilepsy. *Neurology (Minneap.)* 1952; 2: 403–11.

50 Abbott JA, Schwab RS. Mesantoin in the treatment of epilepsy; a study of its effects on the leukocyte count in seventy-nine cases. *N Engl J Med* 1954; 250: 197–9.

51 Spielman MA. Some analgesic agents derived from oxazolidine-2,4-dione. *J Am Chem Soc* 1944; 66: 1244–5.

52 Everett GM, and Richards R. Comparative anticonvulsive action of 3,5,5 trimethyloxazolidine 2-4 dione (Tridione), Dilantin and phenobarbital. *J Pharmacol Exp Ther* 1944; 81: 402–7.

53 Goodman LS, Toman JEP, Swinyard EA. The anticonvulsant properties of Tridione. Laboratory and clinical investigations. *Am J Med* 1946; 1: 213–28.

54 Lennox WG. The petit mal epilepsies. Their treatment with Tridione®. *JAMA* 1945; 129: 1069–75.

55 Lennox WG. Tridione® in the treatment of epilepsy. *JAMA* 1947; 134: 138–43.

56 Perlstein MA, Andelman MB. Tridione®. Its use in convulsive and related disorders. *J Pediatr* 1946; 29: 20–40.

57 Perlstein, MA. Tridione therapy. *Am J Psychiat* 1947; 104: 247–53 (Oct).

58 Thorne FC. The anticonvulsant action of tridione: preliminary report. *Psychiatr Quart* 1945; 19: 686–91.

59 Sloan LL, Gilger AP. Visual effects of Tridione. *Am J Ophthalmol* 1947; 30: 1387–405.

60 Barnett HL, Simons DJ, Wells RE Jr. Nephrotic syndrome occurring during Tridione therapy. *Am J Med* 1948; 4: 760–4.

61 Denhoff E, Laufer MW. Clinical studies of the effects of 3,5,5-trimethyloxazolidine-2-4-dione (Tridione) on the hematopoietic system, liver and kidney. *Pediatrics* 1950; 5: 695–707.

62 Wells CE. Trimethadione: Its dosage and toxicity. *Arch Neurol Psychiatr* 1957; 77: 140–5.

63 Davis JP, Lennox WG. Effect of trimethyloxazolidine dione and of dimethyloxazolidine dione on seizures and on blood. *Res Publ Assoc Res Nerv Ment Dis* 1947; 26: 423–36.

64 Davidoff E. Clinical and electroencephalographic observations concerning the effect of Tridione in epileptic patients. *Am J Psychiatr* 1948; 104: 10: 600–7 (Apr).

65 Goodman LS, Swinyard EA, Brown WC, Schiffman DO, Grewal MS, Bliss EL. Anticonvulsant properties of 5-phenyl-5-ethyl-hexahydropyrimidine-4,6 dione (Mysoline®), a new anti-epileptic. *J Pharmacol Exp Ther* 1953; 108: 428–36.

66 Handley R, Stewart ASR. Mysoline®: A new drug in the treatment of epilepsy. *Lancet* 1952; 1: 742–4.

67 Timberlake WH, Abbott JA, Schwab RS. Mysoline®: Effective anticonvulsant with initial problems of adjustment. *N Engl J Med* 1955; 252: 304.

68 Davis JP, Lennox WG. A comparison of Paradione and Tridione in the treatment of epilepsy. *J Pediatr* 1949; 34: 273–8.

69 Butter AJM. Tridione compared with malidone in the treatment of petit mal. *J Neurol (Lond)* 1952; 15: 37.

70 Zimmerman FT. Use of methylphenylsuccinimide in treatment of petit mal epilepsy. *AMA Arch Neurol Psychiatr* 1951; 66: 156–62.

71 Davidson DT, Lombroso C, Markham CH. Methylphenylsuccinimide (Milontin) in epilepsy. *N Engl J Med* 1955; 253: 173–5.

72 Millichap J. Milontin: a new drug in the treatment of petit-mal. *Lancet* 1952; 2: 907–10.

73 Davidson DT, Lennox WG. Phenacetylurea phenurone in epilepsy. *Dis Nerv Syst* 1950; 129: 261.

74 Tyler MW, King EQ. Phenacimide in the treatment of epilepsy *JAMA* 1951; 147: 17–21.

75 Livingston S, Pauli LL. Phenacemide in the treatment of epilepsy: Results of treatment of 411 patients and review of literature. *N Engl J Med* 1957; 256: 588–91.

76 Kaplan LA, Maslanka S. Hibicon: a new anticonvulsant. *Dis Nerv Syst* 1952; 15: 88.

77 Merlis S. Diamox: a carbonic anhydrase inhibitor: its use in epilepsy. *Epilepsia* 1954; third series, 4: 117.

78 Bergstrom WH, Garzolli RF, Lombroso CT, Davidson DT, Wallce WM. Observations on the metabolic and clinical effects of carbonic anhydrase inhibitors. *Am J Dis Child* 1952; 84: 771.

79 Lombroso CT, Davidson DT, Grossi-Bianchi MI. Further evaluation of acetazolamide (Diamox) in the treatment of epilepsy. *JAMA* 1956; 160: 268.

80 Golla FI, Jodge RS. The control of petit mal by acetazolamide. *J Ment Sci* 1957; 103.

81 Saunie R, Vaille C. Pharmaceutical preparations in the treatment of epilepsy. *Epilepsia* 1955; third series 4: 116–23.

82 Camerman A, Camerman N. Diphenylhydantoin and diazepam: Molecular structure similarities and steric basis of anticonvulsant activity. *Science* 1970; 168: 1457–8.

83 Glazko AJ. Discovery of phenytoin. *Ther Drug Monit* 1986; 8: 490–7.

Section 1
Introduction

1

Definitions and Classification of Epilepsy

W.E. Dodson

More than a century and a half ago, Hughlings Jackson defined epileptic seizures as the result of an occasional, sudden and excessive discharge of grey matter [1], a definition that has stood the test of time. Over the years, the motor, sensory and autonomic phenomena that are produced by epileptic brain discharges have been identified and classified. Today, as in Jackson's time, seizures remain important signals to the possibility of underlying brain disorders that need to be identified and treated. Seizures are symptoms of abnormal brain function.

Epilepsy, like a seizure, is a symptom of abnormal brain function. Epilepsy is present when seizures are recurrent and are not due to easily reversed, transient metabolic or toxic disorders. Seizures are fundamental elements of epilepsy. Although a causative brain disease can be identified in some cases, in a majority of cases no cause can be found and the best diagnosis possible is only descriptive. Of course the goal in all cases is to identify the aetiology and pathoanatomical basis for the symptoms, but this is achieved in fewer than half of all cases. To summarize: there are two levels of descriptive diagnosis. The most elementary is according to the type of epileptic seizure. The more comprehensive system of descriptive diagnosis categorizes types of epilepsy or epileptic syndromes. The descriptive classifications of seizures and epilepsy are the subjects of this chapter.

Classification of seizure types

The currently used classification of seizures was published in 1981 [2] (Table 1.1). It evolved from a seminal version that was undertaken in 1968 and reported in 1969 [3] and 1970 [4]. The 1981 product was the result of combined videotaping and EEG recordings of seizures which were reviewed and categorized in workshops convened between 1975 and 1979. Unlike previous schemes, the 1981 classification did not consider evidence of brain pathology, age and aetiology, but instead restricted the basis for classification to clinical seizure types plus EEG data.

The primary dichotomy in classifying seizure types depends on whether the seizure arises in a restricted part of the brain in one hemisphere or appears to involve both hemispheres from the onset [2]. These lead to the root distinction of partial vs. generalized seizure types. A third category, known as unclassified, is provided for cases that lack sufficient information for categorization.

Partial seizures

Partial seizures are subdivided into three groups—simple partial, complex partial or partial secondarily generalized according to whether consciousness is impaired or the seizure evolves into a generalized convulsion as the epileptic brain discharge extends to involve both hemispheres. Partial seizures are classified as simple if consciousness is unimpaired during the episode. The label complex partial is applied if consciousness is impaired at any point during the ictus. Note that consciousness need only be impaired, not fully lost, to qualify the seizure as complex partial. Secondary generalization of the partial seizure is typically dramatic and in many cases overshadows the preceding partial seizure. For this reason many secondarily generalized seizures with partial onset often go unappreciated by inexperienced observers only to be reclassified accurately after more details are elicited [5]. For this reason, it is always important to ask the patient and witness(es) to describe in detail, step by step, the sequence of events that led up to a convulsion.

Simple partial seizures

The components of epileptic seizures can include any brain-modulated bodily function. Hence, seizures include any movement, sensation, perception or emotion of which humans are capable. However, the behavioural elements of seizures typically are situationally inappropriate, fragmentary manifestations of brain activity and thereby stand apart from smoothly integrated, situationally appropriate behaviours generated by normal brain functioning.

Movements or motor signs in partial seizures depend on the region of brain in which the epileptic discharge takes place. If the seizure is confined to a discrete area, isolated twitching or jerking occurs. If the discharge spreads to contiguous cortical areas, the movement often extends step-wise to involve adjacent functional groups. The progressive extension of an epileptic discharge through the motor strip results in an anatomically contiguous spread of the epileptic jerking called a jacksonian march or jacksonian seizure. (This type of seizure is named after Hughlings Jackson who first drew attention to this pattern of seizure progression. On the basis of these observations he deduced the somatotopographic representation of the motor cortex.) Partial seizures that affect speech centres may lead to speech arrest. The phenomenon of ictal repetition of syllables or phrases is called epileptic pallilalia. Non-stop partial seizures often lasting days or longer are called epilepsia partialis continua.

Transient localized paralysis lasting minutes to hours following a partial or secondary generalized motor seizure, is called a Todd's paralysis. In some cases, focal postictal paralysis may be the only clue indicating that a generalized seizure had a partial onset.

Sensory symptoms that are produced by seizures also reflect the normal function of the brain region where the discharge is occurring. Frequently felt sensations include pins-and-needles and numb-

Table 1.1 The international classification of epileptic seizures

I. Partial (focal, local) seizures

Clinical seizure type	EEG seizure type	EEG interictal expression
A. *Simple partial seizures* (consciousness not impaired)	Local contralateral discharge starting over the corresponding area of cortical representation (not always recorded on the scalp)	Local contralateral discharge
1. With motor signs (a) Focal motor without march (b) Focal motor with march (jacksonian) (c) Versive (d) Postural (e) Phonatory (vocalization or arrest of speech)		
2. With somatosensory or special-sensory symptoms (simple hallucinations, e.g. tingling, light flashes, buzzing) (a) Somatosensory (b) Visual (c) Auditory (d) Olfactory (e) Gustatory (f) Vertiginous		
3. With autonomic symptoms or signs (including epigastric sensation, pallor, sweating, flushing, piloerection and pupillary dilatation)		
4. With psychic symptoms (disturbance of higher cerebral function). These symptoms rarely occur without impairment of consciousness and are much more commonly experienced as complex partial seizures (a) Dysphasic (b) Dysmnesic (e.g. *déjà vu*) (c) Cognitive (e.g. dreamy states, distortions of time sense) (d) Affective (fear, anger, etc.) (e) Illusions (e.g. macropsia) (f) Structured hallucinations (e.g. music, scenes)		
B. *Complex partial seizures* (with impairment of consciousness; may sometimes begin with simple symptomatology)	Unilateral or frequently bilateral discharge, diffuse or focal in temporal or frontotemporal regions	Unilateral or bilateral generally asynchronous focus; usually in the temporal or frontal regions
1. Simple partial onset followed by impairment of consciousness (a) With simple partial features (A.1.–A.4.) followed by impaired consciousness (b) With automatisms		
2. With impairment of consciousness at onset (a) With impairment of consciousness only (b) With automatisms		
C. *Partial seizures evolving to secondarily generalized seizures* (this may be generalized tonic-clonic, tonic, or clonic)	Above discharges become secondarily and rapidly generalized	
1. Simple partial seizures (a) Cvolving to generalized seizures		
2. Complex partial seizures (b) Cvolving to generalized seizures		
3. Simple partial seizures evolving to complex partial seizures evolving to generalized seizures		

Table 1.1 *Continued*

II. Generalized seizures (convulsive or non-convulsive)

Clinical seizure type	EEG seizure type	EEG interictal expression
A.		
1. *Absence seizures* (a) Impairment of consciousness only (b) With mild clonic components (c) With atonic components (d) With tonic components (e) With automatisms (f) With autonomic components (b–f may be used alone or in combination)	Usually regular and symmetrical 3 Hz but may be 2–4 Hz spike-and-slow-wave complexes and may have multiple spike-and-slow-wave complexes. Abnormalities are bilateral	Background activity usually normal although paroxysmal activity (such as spikes or spike-and-slow-wave complexes) may occur. This activity is usually regular and symmetrical
2. *Atypical absence* May have: (a) Changes in tone that are more pronounced than in A1 (b) Onset and/or cessation that is not abrupt	EEG more heterogeneous; may include irregular spike-and-slow-wave complexes, fast activity or other paroxysmal activity. Abnormalities are bilateral but often irregular and asymmetrical	Background usually abnormal; paroxysmal activity (such as spikes or spike-and-slow-wave complexes) frequently irregular and asymmetrical
B. *Myoclonic seizures* Myoclonic jerks (single or multiple)	Polyspike and wave, or sometimes spike and wave or sharp and slow waves	Same as ictal
C. *Clonic seizures*	Fast activity (10 c/s or more) and slow waves; occasional spike-and-wave patterns	Spike-and-wave or polyspike-and-wave discharges
D. *Tonic seizures*	Low voltage, fast activity or a fast rhythm of 9–10 c/s or more decreasing in frequency and increasing in amplitude	More or less rhythmic discharges of sharp and slow waves, sometimes asymmetrical. Background is often abnormal for age
E. *Tonic-clonic seizures*	Rhythm at 10 or more c/s decreasing in frequency and increasing in amplitude during tonic phase, interrupted by slow waves during clonic phase	Polyspike and waves or spike-and-wave, or, sometimes, sharp-and-slow-wave discharges
F. *Atonic seizures* (Astatic) (combinations of the above may occur, e.g. B and F, B and D)	Polyspikes and wave or flattening or low-voltage fast activity	Polyspikes and slow wave

III. Unclassified epileptic seizures

Includes all seizures that cannot be classified because of inadequate or incomplete data and some that defy classification in hitherto described categories. This includes some neonatal seizures, e.g. rhythmic eye movements, chewing and swimming movements

Reproduced with permission from [2].

ness. Sensory seizures that originate in visual cortex or auditory cortex produce visual and auditory hallucinations, respectively. As emphasized in the 1981 classification [2], epileptic hallucinations vary in sophistication from ill-formed patterns of light and sound to well-structured images and recognizable sounds such as music [2]. Ictal olfactory hallucinations tend to be vague but are generally disagreeable. Hallucinated tastes are frequently metallic. Vertiginous symptoms, such as hallucinated rotation or spinning, are relatively common. Unlike vertigo of vestibular origin, epileptic vertigo usually is not associated with nausea or severe anxiety and is rarely incapacitating.

When simple partial sensory seizures precede complex partial or secondarily generalized seizures, the premonitory experience is called an aura. Attributed to Galen, the term aura was derived from the Greek word αερ or air meaning breeze as it was used by a 13-year-old boy who described a sensation that began on his lower leg and 'climbed upwards in a straight line' [6]. Subsequently, the term aura has been applied generally to include any premonitory ictal sensation.

Psychic symptoms

Psychic symptoms are among the most intriguing consequences of partial seizures. These result from discharges that interrupt higher cortical processes and are often associated with impaired consciousness and thereby become components of complex partial seizures.

The most common psychic symptoms are affective, especially the feeling of fear, or in the extreme, terror. These experiences frequently are accompanied by autonomic manifestations including mydriasis, change in skin colour, piloerection and other signs. When epileptic fear or anxiety occurs, the affected person may run to escape or to find a caretaker, seeking assistance. Children who experience ictal fear go to a parent and display fearful facial expressions.

Other affective symptoms include anger, rage, extreme pleasure, sexual sensations and, rarely, ecstasy. These experiences are typically brief and paroxysmal, beginning without warning or provocation, and ceasing abruptly as if an electrical switch were turned on and off. The result is a time course of emotion that is substantially shorter than normal. Furthermore, seizure-generated affect is usually inappropriate to the social context of the moment. Seizure-induced laughter characteristically sounds automatic, mirthless, hollow or vacuous and is not socially infectious like normal mirthful laughter. Seizures that are manifest by laughter are called gelastic from the Greek word for laughter.

Ecstatic seizures, also known as Dostoevsky seizures, are so rare that it is debated whether they truly occur [7]. Named after the great author Fyodor Dostoevsky (*The Brothers Karamazov*), they have attracted widespread attention and generally are felt to represent aura [8,9]. Described as brief moments of feeling 'a contentedness which is unthinkable under normal conditions, and unimaginable for those who have not experienced it', Dostoevsky went on to say, 'At such times I am in perfect harmony with myself and with the entire universe. Perception is so clear and so agreeable that one would give 10 years of his life, and perhaps all of it for a few seconds of such bliss' [7].

Memory distortions are also reported frequently by people who experience complex partial seizures. Representing heightened perceptions of familiarity, *déjà vu* and *déjà entendu* refer to the intuition that an experience was previously seen or heard, respectively. *Jamais vu* and *jamais entendu* indicate the opposite: the experience is unfamiliar and was never before seen or heard. Panoramic vision is a rapid remembrance of previous life experiences.

Dysphasic psychic epileptic symptoms involve speech. Speech disturbances can occur as either an active part of the seizure (as when words or phrases are repeated) or postictally as transient neurological deficits due to cortical neuronal exhaustion. The latter produce receptive and expressive aphasias of the types seen in cortical deficits of other causes.

Cognitive psychic symptoms include dreamy states, distorted perception of time and reality as well as detachment or depersonalization in which the person feels as if he is outside his body.

Illusions are distorted perceptions. The visual illusions of an object's being too large or too small are called macropsia and micropsia, respectively. Analogous distortions affect hearing, resulting in macro- and microacusia. Illusions can affect any simple or complex sensory modality. Examples include monocular diplopia and altered appreciation of limb size and weight.

Complex partial seizures

The *sine qua non* of complex partial seizures is impairment of consciousness. Premonitory sensory or psychic aura (simple partial seizures) frequently forewarn and lead into the complex partial episode. The nature of the sensory experience provides important clues about the origin of the seizure. However, many complex partial seizures begin with sudden impairment of consciousness.

Automatisms—repetitive, patterned, semipurposeful spontaneous movements—are another common feature of complex partial seizures. Gastaut described automatisms as 'more or less coordinated adapted (eupractic or dyspractic) involuntary motor activity occurring during the state of clouding of consciousness either in the course of or after an epileptic seizure, and usually followed by amnesia for the event' [4]. Pathophysiologically, automatisms appear when bilateral cortical dysfunction lasts long enough to release the expression of patterned movements that are represented at lower brain levels but which are normally held in check by cortical inhibition [10,11]. Whereas automatisms result from bilateral cortical dysfunction, consciousness is impaired when they occur.

Automatisms are either perseverated continuation of a previous movement or represent a novel behaviour. The most common ones include chewing or swallowing movements categorized as 'eating'; expressions of emotion (usually fear) categorized as 'mimicry'; picking at or fumbling with garments (gestural automatisms); walking, often in circles (cursive seizures), categorized as 'ambulatory'; and finally verbal or repeated items of speech (also called epileptic pallilalia) [4].

Generalized seizures

Generalized seizures are produced by epileptic discharges that affect both hemispheres simultaneously. When this occurs consciousness usually is lost or impaired.

Absence seizures

In absence seizures, consciousness is lost and regained in an abrupt off–on pattern. Behaviour or movement that is occurring at the onset may be perseverated but usually ceases instantly as the person begins to stare. During the staring, the eyes may gaze straight ahead or deviate upward while the eyelids twitch faintly and rhythmically. Rarely lasting more than 30 s, absence seizures are usually quite brief, often less than 5 s. As one cause of episodic staring behaviour, absence seizures need be differentiated from normal daydreaming or complex partial seizures. The latter typically have a longer duration and last more than 60 s in untreated cases. In daydreaming, consciousness is intact, although responses to questions or commands may be delayed or slow. In absence and complex partial seizures, consciousness is impaired.

A good way to assess clinically whether consciousness is impaired is to present the person with several words and then ask him to repeat what was just said. For example, say to the person, 'Ball, yellow, girl' followed by 'What did I say?' Even young children usually respond correctly to this type of elementary request if consciousness is unimpaired. Repeatedly asking 'Are you alright?' usually does not help to determine whether consciousness was altered during brief staring episodes because if the questioning is repeated enough times, eventually the episode ends and the person answers appropriately. When staring due to daydreaming cannot be differentiated from epileptic staring on clinical grounds, video EEG recordings of the episodes usually solve the problem [12,13].

Atypical absence seizures

Like typical absence, atypical absence seizures begin and end abruptly. Although no single feature differentiates typical from atypical absence, atypical absence seizures are more likely to be associated with the following features: longer duration, decreased postural tone and tonic activity. Atypical absence seizures are more likely to occur in patients with interictal abnormalities on EEG, multiple seizure types and mental retardation. Although the 1981 classification noted that the onset and cessation of atypical absence was not as abrupt as typical absence, subsequent investigation found that both types begin and end suddenly. However, postural changes and other features of atypical episodes tend to evolve gradually [2,13,14].

Myoclonic seizures

Myoclonus is a sudden brief involuntary movement that can originate from many regions and levels of the central nervous system [15]. When used in the context of epilepsy, myoclonus epilepsy refers to several progressive disorders in which either epileptic or non-epileptic myoclonus is a prominent feature. Myoclonic seizures are myoclonic jerks that result from epileptic discharges in the brain. In the 1981 classification, myoclonic jerks were defined as 'sudden, brief, shock-like contractions'. As pointed out by Dreifuss [16], myoclonic seizures occur in many different epileptic syndromes such as benign and severe myoclonic seizures of infancy, symptomatic epilepsies due to systemic storage diseases or defects in energy metabolism. On the other hand, non-epileptic myoclonus occurs in spinal disease, cerebellar degeneration, uremic encephalopathy, subcortical (brainstem) myoclonus and other syndromes. Occurring singly or repeated serially, myoclonic seizures may be generalized or limited to part of the body or a single muscle. Generalized myoclonic seizures that affect the body have been called massive epileptic myoclonus, a term that was put into use after the 1981 classification was published.

In practice, the terms myoclonic jerks, myoclonus, myoclonic epilepsy and myoclonus epilepsy are confusing because various authorities apply the terms for different purposes. The term myoclonic epilepsy is used by some authors to describe a particular type of epilepsy and by others to define a group of several epilepsies in which patients have myoclonic seizures plus other features. This ambiguous terminology led Jeavons to comment in 1977 [17] that application of the term 'myoclonic' had become so confusing that he recommended defining the term whenever it was applied to seizures or epilepsy.

In some cases the epileptic origin of the muscular jerking cannot be discerned on routine EEG but requires event-locked (also called jerk-locked) averaging of cortical potentials for the epileptic discharge to be visualized [18,19].

Clonic seizures

Clonic seizures are represented by repetitive, rhythmic jerking which is exemplified in common tonic-clonic seizures. In isolation, a single clonic movement is characterized by a rapid phase of contraction followed by a slower relaxation. In clonic seizures this results in an alternating pattern of jerk-relax, jerk-relax, and so on. Note, however, that the progression of some generalized seizures evolve with the sequence of clonic-tonic-clonic phases.

Tonic seizures

These are defined as rigid violent muscular contractions of axial and limb musculature which typically last 30s or less with mydriasis plus eye deviation upwards or to the side. Tonic seizures end abruptly with variable to no postictal symptoms. During the seizure, the face is often distorted by the contraction and respiration is disrupted, often leading to cyanosis. Other variable features include slowly progressive alterations of tone, and versive movements with rotation, twisting or turning. As pointed out by Dreifuss, these need to be differentiated from non-epileptic dystonia [16]. Isolated tonic seizures seem to be most common during sleep and may go unrecognized.

Tonic-clonic seizures

The tonic-clonic seizure is the formal name for a generalized convulsion, historically called a grand mal seizure. Readily recognized by lay persons as a seizure or fit, it is characterized by a sudden fall and dramatic, violent, involuntary shaking or muscular spasms of the limbs and body (Table 1.2). The episode begins suddenly with the simultaneous loss of consciousness and contraction of body musculature—the tonic phase during which the person becomes rigid and falls *en bloc*, often traumatizing the head or extensor surfaces of the body. The tonic contraction first involves flexion and then extension of the axial muscles [20]. Contractions of axial muscles can be sufficiently forceful as to cause compression fractures of the vertebrae [21]. Contraction of respiratory musculature leads to forced exhalation and vocalization in the form of a cry or moan. The eyes deviate upwards and pupils dilate. Incontinence can occur during the tonic phase or later when postictal exhaustion leads to

Table 1.2 Behavioural stages of generalized convulsive seizures

Prodrome
Aura
Tonic phase
Clonic phase
Postictal unconsciousness and hypotonia
Postictal neurological deficit (Todd's paralysis)
Sleepiness
Return to normal functioning

relaxation of sphincters. During the tonic phase the individual may bite himself and respiration is disrupted, leading to cyanosis. During the tonic phase the EEG most often is characterized by high-frequency spike activity.

During the maximal tonic contraction of body and limb muscles, the initial rigidity gradually evolves into irregular tremulous shaking similar to what is seen in supramaximal muscular exertion. This in turn evolves into generalized jerking—the clonic phase. In the clonic phase, generalized flexor spasms alternate with relaxation causing irregular respiration, sometimes with grunting. Salivation is profuse and when combined with lack of swallowing and an irregular respiratory pattern leads to frothing at the mouth.

The oscillatory contractions during the clonic phase gradually slow and stop marking the end of the convulsion and the beginning of the postictal period. Although convulsions are frightening and seem to last a long time, few last longer than 60 s. Those seizures that do last longer than 60 s tend to be prolonged [22,23].

The postictal phase is characterized by diffuse hypotonia, slow deep respirations and unresponsiveness. Over time, consciousness slowly returns but is clouded at first as awareness emerges from unconsciousness into partial comprehension with confusion. If the person is restrained or handled forcefully, he may resist combatively. The subsequent recovery over minutes to hours are marked by sleepiness, variable headache and complaints of musculoskeletal soreness upon awakening. Persistent back pain may indicate that a vertebral compression fracture occurred during the seizure.

Atonic seizures

Atonic seizures produce sudden reduction or loss of postural tone affecting posture to varying degrees. When extensive, postural control is lost and the person drops or slumps to the ground, producing so-called drop attacks or astatic seizures. The latter term, astatic seizures, was not part of the 1981 classification but has become widely used since. In part this has occurred because most drop attacks are not due to atonic seizures *per se*, but rather represent massive myoclonic seizures or combinations of atonic and myoclonic seizures that forcefully thrust down the person. Drop attacks or astatic seizures often result in loss of teeth plus lacerations and contusions of the head and face. Some atonic seizures alter tone in a restricted part of the body causing head nods, head drops or lapses of limb posture. If consciousness is lost in atonic or in astatic seizures, the lapse is quite brief. The difference between partial or brief atonic seizures and so-called epileptic negative myoclonus is unclear [15,24]. As emphasized in the 1981 classification [2], other non-epileptic disorders can cause drops or lapse of posture. Other causes include cataplexy and brainstem ischaemic attacks.

Seizures not classified by the 1981 classification

Epileptic prodrome is the term applied to disturbances in mood and affect that precede seizures by hours to days. More often noted by companions or family members than by the person who has epilepsy, the behavioural characteristics such as irritability and meanness cause the observers to look forward to the seizure after which the person's affect and mood normalize [25].

Classification of epilepsies and epileptic syndromes

The epilepsies, also called epileptic syndromes or types of epilepsy, are characterized by other features in addition to seizure type (Table 1.3). From the Greek *syn* plus *dramein*, to run with, the word syndrome indicates a group of signs and symptoms that occur together. Thus, epileptic syndromes are constellations of epileptic seizures plus concurrent or serially linked symptoms and signs. Seizures are the seminal elements that comprise an epilepsy, but other features largely differentiate the overall disorder or type of epilepsy. As Professor Fritz E. Dreifuss was fond of saying, 'Seizures are to epilepsy as a cough is to pneumonia'.

The current classification of epilepsies is empirical. It is the work product of expert epileptologists who spent countless hours viewing video recordings of seizures, discussing their observations and deliberating about whether clinically similar groups of patients represent discrete clinical entities. At the time the syndromes were being codified, knowledge regarding the genetic neurobiological basis of epilepsy was rudimentary.

Individual metabolic and genetic causes of seizures can produce many different patterns of epilepsy. For example, the epileptogenicity of pyridoxine deficiency was recognized in the 1950s, but it took many years to fully appreciate the heterogeneity of epilepsy syndromes that result from pyridoxine dependency states [26,27]. As a prototype for other epileptogenic diseases, pyridoxine dependency illustrates the principle that discordance between current syndromic classifications of epilepsy and the neurobiology of epilepsy is more often the rule than the exception. Numerous examples illustrate the principle that for a particular genetic or congenital aetiology of epilepsy, the age of onset, not a specific epileptic syndrome, is the characteristic feature.

Initially pyridoxine dependency was felt to cause only neonatal seizures and drug-resistant neonatal status epilepticus. However, over time the spectrum of epileptic disorders attributable to pyridoxine dependency expanded to include epilepsies with onsets ranging from *in utero* to early childhood. Many types of seizures and epileptic syndromes were the result. Seizure types included partial, multifocal, hemiclonic, infantile spasms, myoclonic and generalized convulsive seizures in infants and young toddlers [28]. The syndromes include uncategorized encephalopathic disorders with partial and generalized seizures along with West syndrome and Lennox–Gastaut syndrome (LGS) [29–31]. Furthermore, some cases of infantile and early childhood onset epilepsy caused by pyridoxine dependency respond temporarily to antiepileptic drugs [32,33]. Inadequately treated, pyridoxine dependency has been linked to progressive brain atrophy and catastrophic neurological outcomes [34,35].

Contemporary genetic discoveries further substantiate the variability of clinical pictures that can result from individual genetic mutations: clinical heterogeneity of epileptic phenotypes caused by a single gene mutation has turned out to be the rule. For example, a single gene mutation that causes the syndrome of generalized epilepsy with febrile seizures plus (GEFS+) produces different epileptic syndromes, some benign and some severe, in different family members [36]. Thus, the relationships between epileptic genotypes and phenotypes has turned out to be highly variable and to a large extent unpredictable. Moreover, variability in the

Table 1.3 International classification of epilepsies and epileptic syndromes

1 Localization-related (focal, local, partial epilepsies and syndromes)
  1.1 Idiopathic (with age-related onset)
- Benign childhood epilepsy with centrotemporal spike
- Childhood epilepsy with occipital paroxysms
- Primary reading epilepsy

  1.2 Symptomatic epilepsy
- Chronic epilepsia partialis continua of childhood (Kojewnikow's syndrome)
- Syndromes characterized by seizures with specific modes of precipitation

  1.3 Cryptogenic

2 Generalized epilepsies and syndromes
  2.1 Idiopathic (with age-related onset—listed in order of age)
- Benign neonatal familial convulsions
- Benign neonatal convulsions
- Benign myoclonic epilepsy in infancy
- Childhood absence epilepsy (pyknolepsy)
- Juvenile myoclonic epilepsy (impulsive petit mal)
- Epilepsy with grand mal (GTCS) seizures on awakening
- Other generalized idiopathic epilepsies not defined above
- Epilepsies with seizures precipitated by specific modes of activation

  2.2 Cryptogenic or symptomatic (in order of age)
- West syndrome (infantile spasms, Blitz–Nick–Salaam–Krämpfe)
- Lennox–Gastaut syndrome
- Epilepsy with myoclonic-astatic seizures
- Epilepsy with myoclonic absences

  2.3 Symptomatic
    2.3.1 Non-specific aetiology
- Early myoclonic encephalopathy
- Early infantile epileptic encephalopathy with suppression-burst
- Other symptomatic generalized epilepsies not defined above

    2.3.2 Specific syndromes
- Epileptic seizure may complicate many disease states Under this heading are diseases in which seizures are a presenting or predominant feature

3 Epilepsies and syndromes undetermined whether focal or generalized
  3.1 With both generalized and focal seizures
- Neonatal seizures
- Severe myoclonic epilepsy in infancy
- Epilepsy with continuous spike-waves during slow-wave sleep
- Acquired epileptic aphasia (Landau–Kleffner)
- Other undetermined epilepsies not defined above

  3.2 Without unequivocal generalized or focal features. All cases with generalized tonic-clonic seizures in which clinical and EEG findings do not permit classification as clearly generalized or localization-related such as in many cases of sleep-grand mal (GTCS) are considered not to have unequivocal generalized or focal features

4 Special syndromes
  4.1 Situation-related seizures (Gelegenheitsanfälle)
- Febrile convulsions
- Isolated seizures or isolated status epilepticus
- Seizures occurring only when there is an acute metabolic or toxic event due to factors such as alcohol, drugs, eclampsia, non-ketotic hyperglycaemia

Reproduced with permission from [49].

genotype–phenotype relationships operates in both directions. A single epileptic genetic mutation does not breed true because the same mutation produces different types of epilepsy. Conversely, a single type of epilepsy or epileptic syndrome has many causes, not just one. As a result, the diagnosis and treatment of epilepsy is intrinsically fraught with a high degree of uncertainty and unpredictability.

The lessons illustrated by pyridoxine dependency, chromosomal disorders and single gene disorders that cause 'pure' epilepsy indicate that syndromic classifications need to be taken with a grain of salt. As pointed out by several authorities, syndromes lack clear limits and the boundaries are continuing subjects of debate [37]. In many cases syndromes serve better as descriptive after-the-fact categories of outcomes than as diagnostic entities on which to base prognosis.

Despite the tribulation of limited neurobiological validity, syndromic diagnosis is clinically useful. The value of classifying syndromes, as with classifying seizure types, is that a standard lexicon facilitates communication among professionals as well as lay persons. In some cases syndromic classification provides a basis for fashioning symptomatic treatments. Whereas looking at a seizure and trying to comprehend what is wrong with the brain may be akin to seeing someone smile and trying to guess what is funny, standardized naming of epileptic outcomes for clinically similar groups underpins effective dialogue about the clinical epiphenomenon that are being observed. However, the highly variable relationships between aetiologies and epileptic phenotypes predicates the futility of highly detailed, intricate classification.

To summarize, both seizures and syndromes are symptoms of underlying brain disorders. Both are empirical and descriptive, not aetiological. As a general rule, individual syndromes have many different aetiologies.

There are several impediments to diagnosing epileptic syndromes that result in some patients' disorders being unclassified. When seizures first appear the clinical picture is often incomplete [38,39]. Consequently, some syndromes become discernible only over time after the disorders evolve a sufficient number of features to become distinctive and diagnosable. Like an unprocessed photographic print dipped into developing solution, over time the clinical picture becomes visible as additional features appear.

Nowhere is the importance of time for sufficient development of distinctive clinical features more apparent than with encephalopathic childhood epilepsies such as infantile spasms and LGS. These disorders materialize from a wide variety of premorbid conditions, arising in normal as well as compromised children. Similarly, many epilepsies that evolve into severe epileptic syndromes begin innocently as febrile seizures or occasional idiopathic generalized tonic-clonic convulsions in early childhood.

Other factors that appear to affect the evolution of epileptic syndromes include treatment(s), the timing of treatment and the response to treatment. Each can contribute to the eventual clinical syndrome individually and in concert with other factors. Of course, when information about the current clinical picture is incomplete or erroneous, the diagnosis is likely to be missed. Nonetheless, once syndromic diagnoses are established, 80% hold up over time [39].

The major groupings in the current classification of epilepsies have been validated consensually. In various studies, between a third and close to all cases of new onset epilepsy have been categorized according to the 1989 international classification [39–47]. In one study where patients were reclassified 2 years later, classifications changed in 14%; 4% of changes resulted from evolution of the syndrome; 10% of relabelling resulted from acquisition of new information [16,20,45,48].

The associated clinical features which have been used to define the epilepsies are listed in Table 1.4. Among these, intellectual capacity, motor function and natural history merit special emphasis. Certain syndromes include mental retardation in a high proportion of affected people. When mental subnormality is a key component of a syndrome, the intellectual deficit can either antedate the appearance of epilepsy or develop only after chronic epilepsy with numerous seizures. Conversely, in some syndromes, normal intellect is an expected feature.

In classifying the epilepsies, the major division depends on whether the principal seizure type is partial and has localized onset or is generalized. The second axis of categorization is aetiological. Is the disorder symptomatic, idiopathic or cryptogenic? Symptomatic epilepsies, also called secondary epilepsies, are those caused by known brain disorders. Cryptogenic epilepsies are those in which a cause is presumed but not identified.

Idiopathic epilepsies have no apparent cause, but are believed to be due to 'hereditary predisposition' [49]. In other words, they are thought to be genetic. Defining characteristics of idiopathic epilepsies include age of onset, clinical features, plus characteristic EEG patterns from both interictal and ictal recordings.

In addition to the extensive classification of syndromes presented in the 1989 classification, the authors also described four anatomically defined localization-related epilepsies: temporal lobe, frontal lobe, parietal lobe and occipital lobe. These anatomical groups are considered next, with the major features of each group briefly listed.

Table 1.4 Factors used to characterize the epilepsies or epileptic syndromes

Seizure type
EEG patterns — both ictal and interictal
Age of onset and remission
Natural history
Associated clinical features
Familial predisposition
Response to or aggravation by specific medications

Temporal lobe epilepsies

• Simple partial seizures with autonomic, psychic or certain sensory manifestations include epigastric rising, olfactory and auditory sensations or illusions.
• Complex partial seizures usually lasting more than 1 min, beginning with initial motor arrest followed by oroalimentary and other automatisms. Other features are amnesia for the episode, postictal confusion and gradual recovery to normal.
• Seizures occur in clusters or in isolation.
• Interictal EEG features range from normal to abnormal with various irregularities including spikes, sharp waves, or slowing localized to, but not restricted to, the temporal lobe region.
• Ictal EEG abnormalities include appropriately localized alteration of background rhythms, low amplitude fast activity, spikes or rhythmic slow activity.

The temporal lobe syndromes were further subdivided into two groups: medial basal (amygdalo-hippocampal) and lateral temporal (neocortical). Symptoms pointing to the former location include rising epigastric discomfort, autonomic signs like pallor, flushing, mydriasis, irregular respiration or respiratory arrest, abdominal borborygmi, eructation, plus fearful, olfactory and gustatory auras. Symptoms of lateral temporal seizures included auditory and/or visual sensory experiences, psychic dreamy states and dysphasias if the speech areas in the dominant temporal lobe were involved.

Frontal lobe epilepsies

Frontal lobe epilepsies are prone to misdiagnosis as psychogenic episodes. They are manifest as simple partial, complex partial and partial secondarily generalized seizure types. As defined in the 1989 classification the notable features of frontal lobe seizures are summarized in Table 1.5.

When seizures originate in specific areas of the frontal lobes they produce symptoms that reflect the normal functions that are mediated by that region. Thus clinical features of seizures provide clues as to which area(s) of cortex are involved. Many seizures that originate in the frontal lobes are complex partial.

Supplementary motor seizures result in fencing postures, focal tonic movement, speech arrest, vocalization.

Cingulate seizures are complex partial and include affective and autonomic changes plus gestural automatisms.

Anterior frontopolar seizures include psychic features, adversive head and eye movements and tend to cause abrupt loss of consciousness.

Orbitofrontal seizures begin with motor or gestural automatisms, olfactory symptoms and autonomic signs.

Table 1.5 Features of frontal lobe seizures [49]

Brief duration
Complex partial with little or no postictal confusion
Rapid secondary generalization
Prominent tonic or postural movements
Frequent complex gestural automatisms at onset
Frequent falling when discharges are bilateral

Dorsolateral frontal seizures are tonic or clonic with eye and head deviation and speech arrest.

Opercular frontal lobe seizures involve taste, speech and oral-buccal movements. Auras attributed to this area include fear plus gustatory, laryngeal and epigastric sensations. Motor features include chewing, swallowing, speech arrest or clonic facial twitching. Salivation and other autonomic features are produced by seizures from this region.

Motor cortex seizures tend to be simple partial and reflect the physiological role of the cortex that is producing the seizure. If after the seizure a postictal, so-called Todd's paralysis occurs, it is an important clue that the seizure originated in the motor area.

Parietal lobe epilepsies

Seizures that originate in the parietal lobe are often sensory at the onset with variable secondary generalization and infrequent evolution to complex partial [49]. Thus the sensory components may be discretely localized or spread to contiguous areas. Sensations that have been described are mostly tactile and include tingling, electricity, crawling, stiffness, cold, or pain or unpleasant dysaesthesias. Visual hallucinations of parietal origin are usually structured. Partial seizures originating in the parietal lobes have variable tendencies to secondarily generalize. Postictally transient neurological deficits that follow parietal lobe seizures are typical of the signs and symptoms that result from permanent parietal damage of other causes. These include asomatognosia, cortical sensory deficits, spatial disorientation and dyscalculia [49].

Occipital lobe epilepsies

Like parietal lobe seizures, when seizures originate in the occipital lobes, they reflect the usual function of that brain region and often involve eye movements, head turning and/or visual hallucinations [49]. Hallucinations that are generated posteriorly tend to be unstructured lights, colours and flashes whereas anterior occipital and temporal-occipital regions generate more structured images or visual distortions such as macropsia or micropsia. Depending on the areas of cortical involvement, visual abnormalities may be restricted to discrete portions of the visual fields.

Localization-related (focal, local, partial) epilepsies and syndromes

Localization-related syndromes account for approximately 60% or more of the epilepsies [19,44–46]. In children, 23% are idiopathic and 77% are symptomatic or cryptogenic.

Idiopathic localization-related epilepsies

Benign partial epilepsy of childhood

The syndrome of benign partial epilepsy of childhood (BPEC) is also called benign rolandic epilepsy (BRE) and benign epilepsy of childhood with centrotemporal spikes (BECTS). The natural history is favourable for normal neurological and cognitive function plus eventual remission of epilepsy in more than 97% [50]. It is characterized by the onset of usually infrequent partial seizures between

ages 3 and 13 years. The temporal distribution of seizure favours nocturnal occurrence but seizures occur any time of day [51]. An autosomal dominant variant has been described [52]. The medical history is positive for prior febrile seizures in 10% or less, and family history is positive for seizures of various types in 40%. According to some physicians half of these cases do not warrant treatment [53].

Although patients with BPEC are typically lesion-free, findings that have been reported in patients who manifest the phenotype include hippocampal atrophy [54], cortical dysplasia [55], lesions of corpus callosum, porencephalic cysts and toxoplasmosis [56]. Of course once a lesion is found, the diagnosis of BPEC usually needs to be changed.

The distinctive seizure type is simple partial often with onset in the face and orobuccal area variably followed by secondary generalization. The ictus may be sensory or motor or a combination of the two. Ictal phenomena include clonic jerking, speech arrest, drooling and unilateral tonic or clonic convulsions or merely episodic dysarthria and drooling [57,58]. In most cases consciousness is preserved until the seizures secondarily generalize [59]. Typically, examination is normal whereas the EEG is demonstrably abnormal due to focal spikes which originate most often in the centrotemporal regions, although on repeated EEG recordings, the spikes often wander [60]. When centrotemporal spikes are discovered incidentally in EEGs of children who have not had seizures, most of the children do not go on to have seizures subsequently [61]. In approximately 25% of cases, the EEG occasionally reveals generalized spike-waves [62].

Although the natural history of typical BPEC is for remission of epilepsy and normal development [63,64], numerous reports describe children whose courses deviate from a benign pattern in terms of seizure frequency, seizure severity and occurrence of neuropsychological problems [65–68]. Fejerman et al. described 26 children who had atypical evolutions of their epilepsies after presenting with typical clinical pictures of BPEC [69]. Twelve developed atypical benign partial epilepsy; three developed acquired epileptic aphasia (Landau–Kleffner syndrome); seven had bouts of status epilepticus; and five evolved mixed pictures of these atypical patterns.

The overlap of BPEC with other epileptic syndromes of childhood illustrates how the boundaries between syndromic entities are blurred and often indistinct. Some cases that present as BPEC evolve into more complicated clinical problems blending into phenotypes overlapping with LGS, Landau–Kleffner and electrical status epilepticus in slow-wave sleep (ESES) [70–72]. There are cases that have been labelled atypical benign partial epilepsy (ABPE) or pseudo-Lennox syndrome. Atypical features include bouts of status epilepticus, atypical absence seizures, atonic seizures [69,73] and cognitive and behavioural impairment combined with an EEG pattern of slow spike-wave—all of this along with the core feature of partial seizures. Some investigators have correlated the occurrence of cognitive impairment in BPEC to the abundance of paroxysmal EEG activity [74].

Benign partial epilepsy in infancy

Benign partial epilepsy in infancy as first described by Watanabe et al. in 1987 consists of complex partial seizures appearing in infancy with normal interictal EEG patterns awake and asleep [75]. Subsequently infants were identified who had both complex partial seizures and secondarily generalized seizures in various combinations [5,76] and later still cases were found with vertex spike-wave patterns during sleep [77]. Among those who had developed normally through the age 2 years, 90% continued to develop normally when evaluated at age 5 years [78].

Childhood epilepsy with occipital paroxysms

Described by Gastaut in 1950, this disorder has prominent occipital epileptiform spike-wave activity that appears after eye closure and is suppressed by eye opening [79,80]. Clinical features include visual symptoms such as hemianopsias and amaurosis, abstract and complex structured visual hallucinations along with seizures (simple and complex partial, and/or generalized convulsions) and prominent postictal symptoms with migraine headaches accompanied by nausea and vomiting. Subsequent reports indicated that the original cases described by Gastaut were rare and differed from the norm. The picture that emerged as more typical had variable features that included cases of severe epilepsy, epilepsy confounded by cognitive difficulties and lesional/symptomatic aetiologies which in some cases such as mitochondrial encephalopathy with lactic acidaemia and stroke (Melas) were progressive [81] These exceptions notwithstanding, authoritative opinions regarding this condition emphasized an excellent prognosis. Key features include onset around age 5 years of episodic vomiting, eye deviation and impaired consciousness with variable secondary generalized convulsions. Most seizures are nocturnal. Most affected children have occipital spikes on EEG, but 20% may have spikes elsewhere or not at all [82].

Reading epilepsy

This rare, benign, non-progressive syndrome is characterized by reading-provoked sensorimotor symptoms affecting the oral-buccal-lingual-facial muscles that are involved in reading aloud [83]. However, reading aloud usually is not required to trigger the seizures. As a result, some authorities have recommended renaming the condition language-induced epilepsy [84]. The condition is accompanied by a positive family history of a similar disorder in as many as one fourth of cases. Described by observers as myoclonic, jerking or tonic movements of the jaw, patients report sensations such as stiffness, numbness or tightness during the seizures. A pubertal or postpubertal disorder, the average age of onset is 17 years with symptoms starting as young as 10 years of age in some people [85]. Cases have been described that overlap clinically with BPEC, with juvenile myoclonic epilepsy (JME) and with absence epilepsy [86–88].

Symptomatic localization-related epilepsy

There are many causes of symptomatic epilepsy and most lead to localization related forms of epilepsy. These are considered in Chapter 4 where the many causes of epilepsy are addressed. However, one condition, epilepsia partialis continua, is considered here next because of its distinctive clinical presentation.

Chronic epilepsia partialis continua of childhood (Kojewnikow's syndrome)

This eponym is linked to two variants of epilepsia partialis continua (continuous partial seizures) and received special mention among various motor seizures in the 1989 classification [49,89,90]. The first type is characterized by a stable neurological picture that is punctuated by infrequent bouts of epilepsia partialis continua that are not linked to progressive brain disease. The second type is linked to progressive diseases caused by various progressive aetiologies. The clinical picture is one of progressive loss of motor and eventually mental function that follows prolonged periods of epilepsia partialis continua. In these cases the localization of the partial seizures migrates, leaving in its wake paralysis of the affected areas [91]. Rasmussen's encephalitis is one type of the progressive form. A wide variety of aetiologies have been linked to Kojewnikow's syndrome including neoplasia, inborn errors of metabolism (cytochrome C oxidase-induced Leigh disease), [92] immunoallergic paraneoplastic syndromes [93] and infections [94–96].

Generalized epilepsies and syndromes

Idiopathic generalized epilepsies (with age-related onset)

Benign neonatal familial convulsions

Although most seizures in the neonatal period are symptomatic of perinatal problems, especially hypoxia and ischaemia, idiopathic benign seizures rarely occur in otherwise normal, full-term newborns. Cases occur on both a familial and sporadic basis [97,98].

Inherited in an autosomal dominant pattern, benign familial neonatal seizures typically appear in the first 2 weeks of life [99,100]. The most common semiology is a generalized tonic phase followed by variable patterns of clonic and autonomic activity [101,102]. Approximately 10% have subsequent epilepsy [103].

In the 1990s the disorder was linked to mutations in two genes (*KCNQ2* and *KCNQ3*) which determine the structure and function of potassium channels and hence influence brain excitability [104]. Other genetic causes are likely to be found.

Benign neonatal convulsions

Also called fifth-day fits, benign neonatal convulsions appear in previously normal newborns [99,104]. Seizure types include apnoeic, partial or generalized clonic, but not tonic. EEG interictal patterns include normal, focal or multifocal spikes and bursts of theta activity in the central regions, so-called theta pointu alternant. Ictal patterns are mainly rhythmic spikes or rhythmic slow waves [104]. The typical picture is clusters of seizures of 1–3 min duration that occur for 24–48 h and then cease. During the cluster of convulsive activity, the seizures are said to be resistant to antiepileptic drugs. For the majority of affected newborns the natural history includes normal development and permanent remission of seizures. However, approximately 10% have ongoing problems. A few are delayed developmentally, have febrile seizures and/or have persistently epileptiform EEGs. North *et al.* [105] noted that in Australia the syndrome of fifth-day fits was 'epidemic' during the 1970s but disappeared thereafter.

Benign myoclonic epilepsy in infancy

This rare condition appears in infancy in normal children although symptomatic cases have been reported. Features include generalized axial, massive myoclonic seizures, interictal EEG pattern of generalized spike-waves and a mixed picture developmentally. Persistent uncontrolled seizures are associated with developmental stagnation and psychomotor retardation. It is unclear whether this is a phenotypic variant of severe myoclonic epilepsy of infancy (see below) [106,107].

Childhood absence epilepsy (pyknolepsy)

Appearing in the early and middle years of childhood with the onset of absence seizures, this disorder is characterized by female predominance, usually normal intellect and at least a 40% chance of remission. In this disorder, the absence seizures are quite brief, so brief that in some cases they go unrecognized as seizures for long periods. The seizures also tend to occur in clusters. Although absence seizures are the predominant seizure type, other types of seizures occur infrequently. The classical EEG pattern is monotonous, generalized 3 Hz spike-wave. As defined clinically this condition overlaps with several others, especially JME [108]. In a series of 194 patients with typical clinical features and EEG, approximately one-third also had generalized tonic-clonic seizures (GTCS) at some point and absence status occurred in 15%. When followed up after age 18 years, approximately 20% were still having seizures [109].

In population-based studies, absence epilepsies account for fewer than 3% of newly diagnosed seizure disorders. Whereas in paediatric populations, they account for 15–20% [40,41,43,110]. Although children with absence epilepsies as a group have above-average IQ in some studies [111], some investigators have found an overrepresentation of academic and behavioural problems associated with childhood absence epilepsy [112]. Based on the work of Metrakos and Metrakos [113], childhood absence epilepsy is generally felt to be inherited as an autosomal dominant with variable penetrance.

Boundaries in generalized epilepsies that appear in adolescence are indistinct, suggesting underlying neurobiological relationships [114]. Olsson and Hagberg [115] identified two groups of children with absence epilepsy. One group who had the onset of seizures before age 12 years responded to therapy quickly, had a low chance of GTCS and a high remission rate. On the other hand, juvenile onset after age 12 years was associated with a high risk of GTCS and a high relapse rate after discontinuation of antiepileptic therapy. Both groups responded well to antiepileptic drug therapy. In up to one-third of patients with JME, their epilepsy begins with absence seizures in early to mid childhood—well before the peripubertal onset of myoclonic jerks that are diagnostic for JME [116]. When JME presents in this fashion with absence seizures and an EEG pattern of 3 Hz spike-wave, it is impossible to differentiate from childhood absence epilepsy.

Certain cases of childhood absence epilepsy that were preceded by febrile seizures have been linked to mutations in the γ-aminobutyric acid A (GABA-A) receptor [117].

Juvenile myoclonic epilepsy (JME)

JME, also known as impulsive petit mal or Janz syndrome, includes the following: myoclonic jerks, general tonic-clonic seizures and absence seizures [118,119]. Initially thought to originate in the peripubertal period when the myoclonias usually appear, subsequent studies revealed that in approximately 15–30% of people with the disorder experience the onset of absence seizures in childhood in which case absence seizures always predate the appearance of myoclonic seizures [117,120–122]. Seizure precipitants that have been mentioned include sleep deprivation, stress, alcohol intake and menses, but the main precipitant is sleep deprivation [123]. Interictal EEG patterns vary from 3 Hz spike-wave to faster patterns of poly spike-wave at 4–6 Hz, but EEG patterns may be asymmetrical and misleading [121,124]. Photosensitivity is present in approximately one-third [124].

The genetics of JME have been the subject of controversy [125–127]. Initial reports of linkage to chromosome 6 were not substantiated consistently. Recently, a mutation in a gene for the GABA-A receptor has been reported in a family with autosomal dominant inheritance of JME [128].

JME often goes unrecognized or misdiagnosed. The most common source of these errors is the failure to identify the myoclonic jerks (myoclonias) that are required for the diagnosis or to misinterpret them as partial seizures [129]. Epileptic in origin, the myoclonias are accompanied by polyspikes and spike-wave EEG discharges. Although the jerks can be disruptive and numerous, occurring repeatedly over minutes to hours, consciousness remains intact.

A notable feature of the jerks is that most patients do not report them voluntarily and may attribute them to early morning clumsiness, nervousness or restlessness when in fact the jerks are surprisingly forceful and dramatic. For this reason, the possibility of myoclonias, especially after awakening, should be the subject of direct inquiry if JME is suspected or in anyone who presents with generalized convulsions [130].

The typical natural history includes responsiveness to therapy with valproic acid and vulnerability to the exacerbation of absence seizures when treated with traditional antiepileptic drugs that modulate use-dependent sodium conductance such as phenytoin and carbamazepine [131]. Whereas seizures may be completely prevented with medication, they usually recur if medication is discontinued [132].

Epilepsy with grand mal seizures (GTCS) on awakening

This condition overlaps considerably with other generalized epilepsies especially with JME in which most affected people also have GTCS on awakening. The EEG pattern is generalized spike-wave [121]. Whether this syndrome represents a discrete entity or simply the leftovers from other disorders has been debated for years [133]. At best, the syndrome is indistinct because as noted in the 1989 classification 'If other seizures occur, they are mostly absence or myoclonic . . .' [49].

Cryptogenic or symptomatic generalized epilepsies (in order of age)

West syndrome (infantile spasms, Blitz–Nick–Salaam–Krämpfe)

The term infantile spasms is used to describe a seizure type as well as an epileptic syndrome, an ambiguity that is avoided by the appellation West syndrome. Synonyms for infantile spasms include Blitz–Nick–Salaam–Krämpfe, massive myoclonic spasms, lightning spasms, flexion spasms, jackknife convulsions and infantile myoclonic epilepsy. West syndrome includes three features: infantile spasms, developmental arrest and an EEG pattern of hypsarrhythmia.

The EEG is almost always abnormal in these patients [134]. Approximately two-thirds of patients have a pattern of hypsarrhythmia. One-third have focal abnormalities. Fewer than 2% of patients with infantile spasms have normal EEGs and if the EEG is normal the diagnosis should be questioned. Young infants who have spasms without EEG paroxysms have an innocent condition called benign infantile myoclonus that does not require treatment [135]. Hypsarrhthymia is a severe epileptic EEG abnormality. There are 'mountainous' high amplitude, asynchronous delta slow waves intermixed with multifocal spikes or polyspikes and wave complexes.

The onset of infantile spasms occurs before age 12 months in 85% of cases, and spasms usually cease by age 5 years only to be replaced by other types of seizures [135–138]. In approximately 30% of cases other types of seizures, mostly partial, precede the spasms; in 40% of cases other seizure types appear after the spasms begin [137]. The ictal movements include mixtures of flexion and extension, purely flexor movements, or pure extension which accounts for 22% of spasms studied by video-EEG monitoring. In full form, flexor spasms cause flexion of the neck and trunk with adduction of the shoulders and outstretched arms and variable flexion of the lower extremities, so-called salaam fits. Males account for the majority of patients. Aggressive, effective treatment is believed to reduce the chance of developmental stagnation and subsequent retardation [139,140]. Currently, the optimal therapy of infantile spasms appears to be adrenocorticotrophic hormone (ACTH) that is initiated within 1 month of the onset of the spasms or aggressive therapy with antiepileptic drugs [139–147].

Spasms vary from subtle to dramatic in intensity. Often when they first appear they are subtle, but as the child grows older, they tend to become more intense and occur in clusters during which the infant cries. The clusters are most common on awakening.

The aetiology of West syndrome is diverse. In approximately two-thirds of cases the condition is symptomatic of identifiable brain disorders; in approximately one-third, the aetiology is idiopathic or cryptogenic. The most common aetiologies are perinatal asphyxia and tuberous sclerosis. However, any aetiology that results in brain malformation or brain tissue destruction can produce this epileptic picture. Idiopathic cases have the best prognosis [140].

Brain imaging is abnormal in 80% of children with West's syndrome [147,148]. The most common abnormalities are atrophic lesions (50%), followed by malformations, atrophy plus calcification, calcifications and porencephaly, respectively. Occurring almost exclusively in females, Aicardi's syndrome includes agenesis of the corpus callosum, chorioretinitis, vertebral anomalies, cortical heterotopias and severe mental handicap [149–151].

The prognosis in West's syndrome is related to the underlying brain disorder and to the therapy [140,144,152]. Patients with idiopathic, cryptogenic infantile spasms who receive optimal therapy have the best prognosis. Those with severe encephaloclastic disorders have the worst. Among all patients with West's syndrome, 20% die before age 5 years and between 75% and 93% have been reported to be mentally retarded; at least 50% have persistent epilepsy and half of these individuals develop LGS.

Lennox–Gastant syndrome (LGS)

LGS is an age-dependent syndrome that includes early childhood onset epilepsy with either mental retardation before seizures start or developmental stagnation leading to retardation that accumulates while epilepsy remains uncontrolled [153,154]. The syndrome overlaps clinically with other severe myoclonic epileptic syndromes [155,156]. Approximately 25% of cases of LGS evolve from infantile spasms or West's syndrome [138,157].

In LGS, tonic and atypical absence seizures are the most common types, occurring in 71% and 49% of patients, respectively. GTCS and astatic seizures (drop attacks) occur in approximately one-third of patients whereas partial seizures occur in about one-fourth [158]. The distinctive interictal EEG pattern is slow spike-wave with frequencies of ≤2.5 Hz. During sleep, bursts of 10 Hz activity occur.

Whereas LGS is classified among symptomatic-cryptogenic disorders, the condition shares many features with myoclonic astatic epilepsy, also called Doose's syndrome [159]. Multiple seizure types typify both syndromes and the evolutions of the disorders resulting in mental retardation when seizures are uncontrolled are similar. Not surprisingly, there has been debate and confusion about the boundaries of LGS and other myoclonic epilepsies with encephalopathy [156,160].

Epilepsy with myoclonic astatic seizures

This disorder is also called myoclonic astatic epilepsy of early childhood. It usually appears in children who were previously normal. Even though it is listed here among cryptogenic or symptomatic conditions, it is an idiopathic disorder with a strong genetic component and a positive family history of epilepsy reported in more than one-third [160]. The epilepsy usually starts with GTCS occurring with or without fever. Over time other seizure types appear. These include myoclonic seizures, astatic seizures (usually atonic), atypical absence seizures and GTCS but not daytime tonic seizures. However, in Doose's 1992 report, 30% of 109 cases had tonic seizures, most of which were nocturnal [161]. Minor motor status occurred in 36%. The EEG is abnormal due to generalized patterns of spike and wave, 4–7/s rhythms and photosensitivity but not multifocal patterns [107,162,163]. The prognosis for normal development is related to the extent of seizure control. The risk of mental deterioration is increased by onset of epilepsy before the age of 2 years, bouts of minor motor status, tonic seizures, failure to respond to anticonvulsant therapy and the failure to develop a normal alpha rhythm on the EEG. Children with persistent frequent seizures experience developmental stagnation that results in eventual mental handicap.

Epilepsy with myoclonic absences

This uncommon disorder is characterized by absence seizures that are accompanied by dramatic bilateral myoclonic jerks that occur in synchrony with an EEG pattern of 3 Hz spike-wave. The onset is in middle childhood, and a male predominance has been described [109,164]. Approximately half of the affected children have intellectual handicap and karyotypic abnormalities are common [165]. However, in the absence of structural brain abnormalities, development may be normal [166].

Symptomatic generalized epilepsies and syndromes: non-specific aetiology (age-related onset)

The next four conditions overlap considerably phenotypically and share many aetiologies, including a wide range of inborn errors of metabolism and structural brain abnormalities such as hemimegalencephaly and other disorders of neuronal migration. All are associated with a high risk of severe developmental impairment, persistent epilepsy and are generally resistant to treatment. As a group they support the general concept that the earlier the onset of symptomatic epilepsy, the more extensive the neuropathology is likely to be and the more grave the prognosis [167–169]. Taken collectively, these syndromes which include early myoclonic encephalopathy, early infantile epileptic encephalopathy with suppression burst, West's syndrome and LGS comprise a spectrum of age-dependent epileptic encephalopathies through which the severely epileptic child graduates from one syndrome to the next as brain maturation leads to evolving epileptic phenotypes [170].

Early myoclonic encephalopathy

With onset in the first 3 months of life, this syndrome results from various metabolic, malformative and encephaloclastic diseases that affect the brains of newborns. More than half of patients who manifest this severe epileptic phenotype do not live 12 months [171]. If they do survive infancy, the clinical picture often evolves into infantile spasms or West's syndrome. All affected infants are profoundly handicapped developmentally. The EEG pattern is burst-suppression [49]. As described by Aicardi [172] the seizures present as variable and erratic multifocal myoclonic jerks, but as the infants' brains mature, tonic spasms typical of West's syndrome become predominant, only to be superseded by LGS as the child ages.

Early infantile epileptic encephalopathy with suppression-burst

Beginning before the age of 6 months, this disorder is characterized by tonic axial spasms and burst-suppression EEG patterns. It is also know as Ohtahara syndrome [170]. The same continuum of aetiologies produce this syndrome as produce early myoclonic encephalopathy, but tonic spasms rather than myoclonic seizures predominate in Ohtahara syndrome [173]. For this reason, some regard this syndrome as an early onset variant of West's syndrome [174]. Often evolving into West's syndrome, the seizures are therapy resistant and psychomotor retardation is the rule.

Epilepsies and syndromes undetermined whether focal or generalized

Neonatal seizures

Classification schemes for neonatal seizures and epilepsies do not conform to the same patterns as seizures and epilepsy in older patients. These are considered separately in Chapter 14.

Severe myoclonic epilepsy in infancy

First described by Dravet in 1978 [175], the disorder has its onset before the age of 1 year when it presents with febrile convulsions, either generalized clonic or hemiclonic, that are often prolonged. Like fever, hot baths can also precipitate seizures in affected infants [176]. Prior to the onset of the epilepsy, development is normal but encephalopathy eventually develops [177]. After a variable number of febrile seizures, afebrile seizures of various types appear. These include myoclonic seizures either focal or generalized with concomitant EEG patterns of generalized spike-wave or poly spike-wave, atypical absence seizures, GTCS and partial seizures in about half of affected children. Initially the interictal EEG is normal but over time it becomes progressively epileptic with generalized fast spike-wave, focal and multifocal abnormalities. When severe, the myoclonic seizures cause the children to fall down and thus qualify for the descriptor astatic seizures. As seizure frequency increases, development stagnates, resulting in mental subnormality. Ataxia appears in half of these children [164]. The seizures continue despite aggressive therapy with antiepileptic medications and are associated with shortened life expectancy. Recently, severe myoclonic epilepsy in infancy has been linked to mutations in the sodium channel gene *SCN1A* [178].

Several disorders have been described that are linked to severe myoclonic epilepsy of infancy because they evolve from febrile seizures and have mutations in the sodium channel gene. Collectively the epilepsies have been named GEFS+ [179,180]. Other disorders such as high voltage slow-wave grand mal syndrome (HVSW-GM) overlap clinically but whether the molecular pathogenetic mechanisms overlap remains to be determined [181]. Other clinically overlapping syndromes include early infantile epilepsy with GTCS, cases of myoclonic astatic epilepsy and childhood absence epilepsy with GTCS [182].

Epilepsy with continuous spike-waves during slow-wave sleep

This condition is defined by an EEG pattern of continuous spike-wave during 85% or more of slow-wave sleep [183]. Synonyms and abbreviations include ESES and continuous spikes and waves during slow-wave sleep (CSWS). The central features are cognitive and behavioural deterioration that follow the appearance of various types of epileptic seizures [184,185]. The types of seizures that have been described include partial, absence, astatic and generalized tonic-clonic.

Several syndromic phenotypes have been described with ESES including typical Landau–Kleffner syndrome of acquired epileptic aphasia (see below) and frontal opercular syndrome, variants of BPEC plus less discrete clinical pictures [186,187]. Some investigators feel that Landau–Kleffner syndrome and ESES represent the same condition [188]. Frontal opercular syndrome consists of episodic dysarthria, dysphagia, drooling and variable degrees of hand apraxia and hemi- or monomelic paralysis [189,190]. ESES occurs on both an idiopathic/cryptogenic and symptomatic basis with several reports noting cases caused by polymicrogyria and by shunted hydrocephalus [191,192].

Acquired epileptic aphasia (Landau–Kleffner syndrome)

Appearing in early childhood, usually before age 5 years, in previously normal children, the syndrome of acquired epileptic aphasia [193] presents abruptly or subacutely, with mutism, apparent deafness, behavioural abnormalities, an epileptiform EEG pattern and seizures in approximately two-thirds [49,194,195]. However, hearing is normal when evaluated by evoked response audiometry pointing to verbal auditory agnosia as the proper diagnosis instead of deafness [196]. Multiple types of seizures occur including partial, generalized tonic-clonic and absence. Typically, the EEG is abnormal due to generalized or multifocal spike and spike-wave patterns although clinical investigations with positron emission tomography, magnetoencephalography and occasional EEG studies point to temporal lobe dysfunction [197–199]. In sleep, continuous spikes and waves during slow-wave sleep are common. For this reason, some investigators have concluded that ESES and acquired epileptic aphasia represent the same condition [189]. The seizures tend to be resistant to drug therapy but abate with advancing age. Between 25% and 50% of patients experience much improved normal language function when followed up in adolescence or later, but an EEG pattern of ESES lasting longer than 36 months [200,201] or persistently abnormal EEG patterns have been linked to continual language impairment [202,203].

Special syndromes: situation-related seizures (Gelegenheitsanfälle)

Febrile convulsions

Febrile seizures are the most common epileptic syndrome, occurring in more than 3% of children. Fever from any cause can provoke seizures in susceptible infants and toddlers. The seizures may be partial or generalized, brief or lengthy, single or repeated. Interictal EEGs are either normal or have non-specific irregularities. Following febrile seizures, the risk of subsequent afebrile seizures (epilepsy) is increased from two- to seven-fold in various studies [204–207]. Although heightened risk of later epilepsy has been linked to many historical and demographic factors in affected children, since 1995 genetic discoveries about the links between febrile seizures and later epilepsy have provided insight into the neurobiology of epilepsy. Various family members who are affected by the same, single point mutation, develop a heterogeneous array of epileptic syndromes [180,208].

Genetic studies in febrile seizures have identified several mutations that lead to febrile seizures and later generalized epilepsy, a group of disorders that has become known as GEFS+ [209]. Recently discovered causes of GEFS+ include mutations involving two genes for voltage-gated sodium channels (*SCN1A* and *SCN1B*) [210,211] along with mutations of the genes that encode GABA-A receptor [212,213]. In addition, digenic inheritance has been described [214]. However, among familial GEFS+ cases, mutations affecting *SCN1A* and *SCN1B* accounted for only 17% of cases indicating that many more genetic mechanisms await discovery [215].

To date most of the discoveries regarding inherited forms of epilepsy have resulted from investigations of families where epilepsy occurs as the result of mutated genes that are inherited according to simple mendelian genetics. Berkovic and Scheffer have estimated that 95% of genetic epilepsies are inherited in complex patterns due to the combined effects of single or multiple genes that interact with environmental and experiential variables [216]. These conditions are in addition to the many chromosomal abnormalities that increase susceptibility to epilepsy [217].

References

1 Jackson JH. On the anatomical, physiological and pathological investigation of epilepsies. *West Riding Lunatic Asylum Med Reports* 1873; 3: 315–39.
2 Commission on Classification and Terminology of the International League Against Epilepsy. Proposal for revised clinical and electroencephalographic classification of epileptic seizures. *Epilepsia* 1981; 22: 489–501.
3 Gastaut H. Clinical and electroencephalographical classification of epileptic seizures. *Epilepsia* 1969; 10 (Suppl.): 2–13.
4 Gastaut H. Clinical and electroencephalographic classification of epileptic seizures. *Epilepsia* 1970; 11: 102–13.
5 Watanabe K, Negoro T, Aso K. Benign partial epilepsy with secondarily generalized seizures in infancy. *Epilepsia* 1993; 34: 635–8.
6 Temkin O. *The Falling Sickness. A History of Epilepsy from the Greeks to the Beginnings of Modern Neurology.* Baltimore: Johns Hopkins Press, 1943: 36.
7 Gastaut H. Fyodor Mikhailovitch Dostoevsky's involuntary contribution to the symptomatology and prognosis of epilepsy. *Epilepsia* 1978; 19: 186–201.
8 Cirignotta F, Todesco CV, Lugaresi E. Temporal lobe epilepsy with ecstatic seizures (so-called Dostoevsky epilepsy). *Epilepsia* 1980; 21: 705–10.
9 Kiloh LG. The epilepsy of Dostoevsky. *Psychiatr Dev* 1986; 4: 31–44.
10 Penry JK, Porter RJ, Dreifuss RE. Simultaneous recording of absence seizures with video tape and electroencephalography. A study of 374 seizures in 48 patients. *Brain* 1975; 98 (3): 427–40.
11 Mizrahi EM. Neonatal seizures: problems in diagnosis and classification. *Epilepsia* 1987; 28 (Suppl. 1): S46–55.
12 Carmant L, Kramer U, Holmes GL, Mikati MA, Riviello JJ, Helmers SL. Differential diagnosis of staring spells in children: a video-EEG study. *Pediatr Neurol* 1996; 14: 199–202.
13 Holmes GL, McKeever M, Adamson M. Absence seizures in children. clinical and electroencephalographic features. *Ann Neurol* 1987; 21: 268–73.
14 Yaqub BA. Electroclinical seizures in Lennox–Gastaut syndrome. *Epilepsia* 1993; 34: 120–7.
15 Dulac O, Plouin P, Shewmon A. Myoclonus and epilepsy in childhood: 1996 Royaumont meeting. *Epilepsy Res* 1998; 30: 91–106.
16 Dreifuss FE. Classification of epileptic seizures. In: Engel J Jr, Pedley TA, eds. *Epilepsy: a Comprehensive Textbook.* Philadelphia: Lippincott-Raven, 1997: 517–32.
17 Jeavons PM. Nosological problems of myoclonic epilepsies in childhood and adolescence. *Dev Med Child Neurol* 1977: 193–8.
18 Shibasaki H. Somatosensory evoked potentials, jerk-locked EEG averaging and movement-related potentials in myoclonus. *Electroencephalogr Clin Neurophysiol* 1987; 39 (Suppl.): 281–90.
19 Barrett G. Jerk-locked averaging. technique and application. *J Clin Neurophysiol* 1992; 9: 495–508.
20 Fisch BJ. Generalized tonic-clonic seizures. In: Wyllie E, ed. *The Treatment of Epilepsy: Principles and Practice.* Philadelphia/London: Lea & Febiger 1993: 425–42.

21 Vasconcelos D. Compression fractures of the vertebrae during major epileptic seizures. *Epilepsia* 1973; 14: 323–8.

22 Porter RJ. Clinical phenomenology of seizure spread. *Epilepsia* 1990; 31: 617.

23 Bromfield ED, Porter RJ, Kelly K, Sato S *et al*. Progression to generalized tonic-clonic seizures. *Epilepsia* 1989; 30: 724–5.

24 Nanba Y, Maegaki Y. Epileptic negative myoclonus induced by carbamazepine in a child with BECTS. Benign childhood epilepsy with centrotemporal spikes. *Pediatr Neurol* 1999; 21: 664–7.

25 Gowers WR. *Epilepsy and Other Chronic Convulsive Diseases: Their Causes Symptoms and Treatment*, 2nd edn. London: J & A Churchill, 1901.

26 Gospe SM. Pyridoxine-dependent seizures: findings from recent studies pose new questions. *Pediatr Neurol* 2002; 26: 181–5.

27 Baxter P. Pyridoxine-dependent and pyridoxine-responsive seizures. *Dev Med Child Neurol* 2001; 43: 416–20.

28 Nabbout R, Soufflet C, Plouin P, Dulac O. Pyridoxine dependent epilepsy: a suggestive electroclinical pattern. *Arch Dis Child Fetal Neonatal Med* 1999; 81: F125–9.

29 Miyasaki K, Matsumoto J, Muras S *et al*. Infantile convulsion suspected of pyridoxine responsive seizures. *Acta Path Jap* 1978; 28: 741–9.

30 Bankier A, Turner M, Hopkins IA. Pyridoxine dependent seizures—a wider clinical spectrum. *Arch Dis Child* 1983; 58: 415–18.

31 Stephenson JBP, Byren KE. Pyridoxine responsive epilepsy: expanded pyridoxine dependency? *Arch Dis Child* 1983; 58: 1034–6.

32 Goutieres F, Aicardi J. Atypical presentations of pyridoxine-dependent seizures: a treatable cause of intractable epilepsy in infants. *Ann Neurol* 1985; 17: 117–20.

33 Mikati MA, Trevathan E, Krishnamoorthy KS, Lombroso CT. Pyridoxine-dependent epilepsy. EEG investigations and long-term follow-up. *Electroencephalogr Clin Neurophysiol* 1991; 78: 215–21.

34 Gospe SMJ, Hecht ST. Longitudinal MRI findings in pyridoxine-dependent seizures. *Neurology* 1998; 51: 74–8.

35 Chou ML, Wang HS, Hung PC, Sun PC, Huang SC. Late-onset pyridoxine-dependent seizures: report of two cases. *Chung-Hua Min Kuo Hsiao Erh Ko I Hsueh Hui Tsa Chih* 1995; 36: 434–7.

36 Scheffer IE, Berkovic SF. Generalized epilepsy with febrile seizures plus. A genetic disorder with heterogeneous clinical phenotypes. *Brain* 1997; 120: 479–90.

37 Aicardi J. Epileptic encephalopathies of early childhood. *Curr Opin Neurol Neurosurg* 1992; 5: 344–8.

38 Watanabe K. The localization-related epilepsies: some problems with subclassification. *Jpn J Psychiatry Neurol* 1989; 43: 471–5.

39 Berg AT, Shinnar S, Levy SR, Testa FM. Newly diagnosed epilepsy in children: presentation at diagnosis. *Epilepsia* 1999; 40: 445–52.

40 Manford M, Hart YM, Sander JW, Shorvon SD. The National General Practice Study of Epilepsy. The syndromic classification of the International League Against Epilepsy applied to epilepsy in a general population. *Arch Neurol* 1992; 49: 801–8.

41 Viani F, Beghi E, Atza MG, Gulotta MP. Classifications of epileptic syndromes: advantages and limitations for evaluation of childhood epileptic syndromes in clinical practice. *Epilepsia* 1988; 29: 440–5.

42 Jallon P, Loiseau P, Loiseau J. Newly diagnosed unprovoked epileptic seizures: presentation at diagnosis in CAROLE study. Coordination Active du Reseau Observatoire Longitudinal de l'Epilepsie. *Epilepsia* 2001; 42: 464–75.

43 Waaler PE, Blom BH, Skeidsvoll H, Mykletun A. Prevalence, classification, and severity of epilepsy in children in western Norway. *Epilepsia* 2000; 41: 802–10.

44 Kwong KL, Chak WK, Wong SN, So KT. Epidemiology of childhood epilepsy in a cohort of 309 Chinese children. *Pediatr Neurol* 2002; 24: 276–82.

45 Shinnar S, O'Dell C, Berg AT. Distribution of epilepsy syndromes in a cohort of children prospectively monitored from the time of their first unprovoked seizure. *Epilepsia* 1999; 40: 1378–83.

46 Murthy JM, Yangala R, Srinivas M. The syndromic classification of the International League Against Epilepsy: a hospital-based study from South India. *Epilepsia* 1998; 39: 48–54.

47 Sillanpaa M, Jalava M, Shinnar S. Epilepsy syndromes in patients with childhood-onset seizures in Finland. *Pediatr Neurol* 1999; 21: 533–7.

48 Berg AT, Shinnar S, Levy SR, Testa FM, Smith-Rapaport S, Beckerman B. How well can epilepsy syndromes be identified at diagnosis? A reassessment 2 years after initial diagnosis. *Epilepsia* 2000; 41: 1269–75.

49 Commission on Classification and Terminology of the International League against Epilepsy. Proposal for revised classification of epilepsies and epileptic syndromes. *Epilepsia* 1989; 30: 389–99.

50 Bouma PA, Bovenkerk AC, Westendorp RG, Brouwer OF. The course of benign partial epilepsy of childhood with centrotemporal spikes: a meta-analysis. *Neurology* 1997; 48: 430–7.

51 Stephani U. Typical semiology of benign childhood epilepsy with centrotemporal spikes (BCECTS). *Epileptic Disord* 2000; 2 (Suppl. 1): S3–4.

52 Scheffer IE. Autosomal dominant rolandic epilepsy with speech dyspraxia. *Epileptic Disord* 2000; 2 (Suppl. 1): S19–22.

53 Peters JM, Camfield CS, Camfield PR. Population study of benign rolandic epilepsy: is treatment needed? *Neurology* 2002; 57: 537–9.

54 Gelisse P, Genton P, Raybaud C, Thiry A, Pincemaille O. Benign childhood epilepsy with centrotemporal spikes and hippocampal atrophy. *Epilepsia* 1999; 40 (9): 1312–15.

55 Sheth RD, Gutierrez AR, Riggs JE. Rolandic epilepsy and cortical dysplasia: MRI correlation of epileptiform discharges. *Pediatr Neurol* 1997; 17: 177–9.

56 Santanelli P, Bureau M, Magaudda A, Gobbi G, Roger J. Benign partial epilepsy with centrotemporal (or rolandic) spikes and brain lesion. *Epilepsia* 1989; 30: 182–8.

57 Deonna TW, Roulet E, Fontan D, Marcoz JP. Speech and oromotor deficits of epileptic origin in benign partial epilepsy of childhood with rolandic spikes (BPERS). Relationship to the acquired aphasia–epilepsy syndrome. *Neuropediatrics* 1993; 24: 83–7.

58 Kramer U, Ben-Zeev B, Harel S, Kivity S. Transient oromotor deficits in children with benign childhood epilepsy with central temporal spikes. *Epilepsia* 2001; 42: 616–20.

59 Lerman P. Benign partial epilepsy with centro-temporal spikes. In: Roger J, Bureau M, Dravet C, Dreifuss F, Perret A, Wolf P, eds. *Epileptic Syndromes in Infancy, Childhood and Adolescence*, 2nd edn. London: John Libbey & Company 1992: 189–200.

60 Camfield P, Gordon K, Camfield C, Tibbles J, Dooley J, Smith B. EEG results are rarely the same if repeated within six months in childhood epilepsy. *Can J Neurol Sci* 1995; 2: 297–300.

61 Verrotti A, Greco R, Altobelli E *et al*. Centro-temporal spikes in non-epileptic children: a long-term follow up. *J Paediatr Child Health* 1999; 35: 60–2.

62 Gelisse P, Genton P, Bureau M *et al*. Are there generalised spike waves and typical absences in benign rolandic epilepsy? *Brain Dev* 1999; 21: 390–6.

63 Beaussart M, Faou R. Evolution of epilepsy with rolandic paroxysmal foci: a study of 324 cases. *Epilepsia* 1978; 19: 337–42.

64 Loiseau P, Duche B, Cohadon S. The prognosis of benign localized epilepsy in early childhood. *Epilepsy Res Suppl* 1992; 6: 75–81.

65 Gunduz E, Demirbilek V, Korkmaz B. Benign rolandic epilepsy: neuropsychological findings. *Seizure* 1999; 8 (4): 246–9.

66 Ong HT, Wyllie E. Benign childhood epilepsy with centrotemporal spikes: is it always benign? *Neurology* 2000; 54: 1182–5.

67 Massa R, de Saint-Martin A, Carcangiu R *et al*. EEG criteria predictive of complicated evolution in idiopathic rolandic epilepsy. *Neurology* 2001; 57: 1071–9.

68 Aicardi J. Atypical semiology of rolandic epilepsy in some related syndromes. *Epileptic Disord* 2000; 2 (Suppl. 1): S5–9.

69 Fejerman N, Caraballo R, Tenembaum SN. Atypical evolutions of benign localization-related epilepsies in children: are they predictable? *Epilepsia* 2000; 41: 380–90.

70 Aicardi J, Chevrie JJ. Atypical benign partial epilepsy of childhood. *Dev Med Child Neurol* 1982; 24: 281–92.

71 Doose H, Hahn A, Neubauer BA, Pistohl J, Stephani U. Atypical 'benign' partial epilepsy of childhood or pseudo-Lennox syndrome. Part II: family study. *Neuropediatrics* 2001; 32: 9–13.

72 Deonna T, Ziegler AL, Despland PA. Combined myoclonic-astatic and 'benign' focal epilepsy of childhood ('atypical benign partial epilepsy of childhood'). A separate syndrome? *Neuropediatrics* 1986; 17: 144–51.

73 Hahn A, Pistohl J, Neubauer BA, Stephani U. Atypical 'benign' partial

epilepsy or pseudo-Lennox syndrome. Part I. Symptomatology and long-term prognosis. *Neuropediatrics* 2001; 32: 1–8.

74 Deonna T, Zesiger P, Davidoff V, Maeder M, Mayor C, Roulet E. Benign partial epilepsy of childhood: a longitudinal neuropsychological and EEG study of cognitive function. *Dev Med Child Neurol* 2000; 42: 595–603.

75 Watanabe K, Yamamoto N, Negoro T *et al.* Benign complex partial epilepsies in infancy. *Pediatr Neurol* 1987; 3: 208–11.

76 Okumura A, Hayakawa F, Kuno K, Watanabe K. Benign partial epilepsy in infancy. *Arch Dis Child* 1996; 74: 19–21.

77 Capovilla G, Beccaria F. Benign partial epilepsy in infancy and early childhood with vertex spikes and waves during sleep: a new epileptic form. *Brain Dev* 2000; 22: 93–8.

78 Okumura A, Hayakawa F, Kato T, Kuno K, Negoro T, Watanabe K. Early recognition of benign partial epilepsy in infancy. *Epilepsia* 2000; 41: 714–17.

79 Gastaut H. Benign epilepsy of childhood with occipital paroxysms. In: Roger J, Bureau M, Dravet C, Dreifuss F, Perret A, Wolf P, eds. *Epileptic Syndromes in Infancy, Childhood and Adolescence*, 2nd edn. London: John Libbey & Company, 1992: 201–17.

80 Lugaresi E, Cirignotta F, Montagna P. Occipital lobe epilepsy with scotosensitive seizures. the role of central vision. *Epilepsia* 1984; 25: 115–20.

81 Roger J, Bureau M. Up-date. In: Roger J, Bureau M, Dravet C, Dreifuss F, Perret A, Wolf P, eds. *Epileptic Syndromes in Infancy, Childhood and Adolescence*, 2nd edn. London: John Libbey & Company, 1992: 205–15.

82 Panayiotopoulos CP. Benign childhood epileptic syndromes with occipital spikes: new classification proposed by the International League Against Epilepsy. *J Child Neurol* 2000; 15: 548–52.

83 Wolf P. Reading epilepsy. In: Roger J, Bureau M, Dravet C, Dreifuss F, Perret A, Wolf P, eds. *Epileptic Syndromes in Infancy, Childhood and Adolescence*, 2nd edn. London: John Libbey & Company, 1992: 281–98.

84 Koutroumanidis M, Koepp MJ, Richardson MP *et al.* The variants of reading epilepsy. A clinical and video-EEG study of 17 patients with reading-induced seizures. *Brain* 1998; 121: 1409–27.

85 Radhakrishnan K, Silbert PL, Klass DW. Reading epilepsy. An appraisal of 20 patients diagnosed at the Mayo Clinic, Rochester, Minnesota, between 1949 and 1989, and delineation of the epileptic syndrome. *Brain* 1995; 118: 75–89.

86 Valenti MP, Tinuper P, Cerullo A, Carcangiu R, Marini C. Reading epilepsy in a patient with previous idiopathic focal epilepsy with centrotemporal spikes. *Epileptic Disord* 1999; 1: 167–71.

87 Wolf P, Mayer T, Reker M. Reading epilepsy. Report of five new cases and further considerations on the pathophysiology. *Seizure* 1998; 7: 271–9.

88 Singh B, Anderson L, al Gashlan M, al-Shahwan SA, Riela AR. Reading-induced absence seizures. *Neurology* 1995; 45: 1623–4.

89 Wallace SJ. Management issues in severe childhood epilepsies. *Seizure* 1995; 4: 215–20.

90 Bancaud J, Bonis A, Trottier S, Talairach J, Dulac O. Continuous partial epilepsy: syndrome and disease. *Rev Neurol (Paris)* 1982; 138: 803–14.

91 Coppola G, Plouin P, Chiron C, Robain O, Dulac O. Migrating partial seizures in infancy: a malignant disorder with developmental arrest. *Epilepsia* 1995; 36: 1017–24.

92 Elia M, Musumeci SA, Ferri R *et al.* Leigh syndrome and partial deficit of cytochrome c oxidase associated with epilepsia partialis continua. *Brain Dev* 1996; 18: 207–11.

93 Shavit YB, Graus F, Probst A, Rene R, Steck AJ. Epilepsia partialis continua. A new manifestation of anti-Hu-associated paraneoplastic encephalomyelitis. *Ann Neurol* 1999; 45: 255–8.

94 De Sciscio G, Mennonna P, Ammannati F, Bindi A, Zappoli F, Rossi L. Continuous partial epilepsy in a case of cerebral abscess of long duration. *Riv Patol Nerv Ment* 1982; 103: 277–84.

95 Antunes NL, Boulad F, Prasad V, Rosenblum M, Lis E, Souweidane M. Rolandic encephalopathy and epilepsia partialis continua following bone marrow transplant. *Bone Marrow Transplant* 2000; 26: 917–19.

96 Bartolomei F, Gavaret M, Dhiver C *et al.* Isolated, chronic, epilepsia partialis continua in an HIV-infected patient. *Arch Neurol* 1999; 56: 111–14.

97 Arpino C, Domizio S, Carrieri MP, Brescianini DS, Sabatino MG, Curatolo P. Prenatal and perinatal determinants of neonatal seizures occurring in the first week of life. *J Child Neurol* 2001; 16: 651–6.

98 Mizrahi EM, Clancy RR. Neonatal seizures. Early-onset seizure syndromes and their consequences for development. *Ment Retard Dev Disabil Res Rev* 2000; 6: 229–41.

99 Quattlebaum TG. Benign familial convulsions in the neonatal period and early infancy. *J Pediatr* 1979; 95: 257–9.

100 Pettit RE, Fenichel GM. Benign familial neonatal seizures. *Arch Neurol* 1980; 37: 47–8.

101 Hirsch E, Velez A, Sellal F *et al.* Electroclinical signs of benign neonatal familial convulsions. *Ann Neurol* 1993; 34: 835–41.

102 Ronen GM, Rosales TO, Connolly MED, Anderson VE, Leppert M. Seizure characteristics in chromosome 20 benign familial neonatal convulsions. *Neurology* 1993; 43: 1355–60.

103 Poulin P. Benign idiopathic neonatal convulsions (familial and nonfamilial). In: Roger J, Bureau M, Dravet C, Dreifuss F, Perret A, Wolf P, eds. *Epileptic Syndromes in Infancy, Childhood and Adolescence*, 2nd edn. London: John Libbey & Company, 1992: 3–11.

104 Lerche H, Biervert C, Alekov AK *et al.* A reduced K+ current due to a novel mutation in KCNQ2 causes neonatal convulsions. *Ann Neurol* 1999; 46: 305–12.

105 North KN, Storey GN, Henderson-Smart DJ. Fifth day fits in the newborn. *Aust Paediatr J* 1989; 25: 284–7.

106 Dravet C, Bureau M, Roger J. Benign myoclonic epilepsy in infants. In: Roger J, Bureau M, Dravet C, Dreifuss F, Perret A, Wolf P, eds. *Epileptic Syndromes in Infancy, Childhood and Adolescence*, 2nd edn. London: John Libbey & Company, 1992: 64–74.

107 Aicardi J, Gomes AL. The myoclonic epilepsies of childhood. *Clev Clin J Med* 1989; 56 (Suppl. 1): S34–S39.

108 Porter RJ. The absence epilepsies. *Epilepsia* 1993; 34 (Suppl. 3): S42–8.

109 Dieterich E, Baier WK, Doose H, Tuxhorn I, Fichsel H. Longterm follow-up of childhood epilepsy with absences. I. Epilepsy with absences at onset. *Neuropediatrics* 1985; 16: 149–54.

110 Freitag CM, May TW, Pfafflin M, Konig S, Rating D. Incidence of epilepsies and epileptic syndromes in children and adolescents: a population-based prospective study in Germany. *Epilepsia* 2001; 42: 979–85.

111 Farwell JR, Dodrill CB, Batzel LW. Neuropsychological abilities of children with epilepsy. *Epilepsia* 1985; 26: 395–400.

112 Wirrell EC, Camfield CS, Camfield PR, Dooley JM, Gordon KE, Smith B. Long-term psychosocial outcome in typical absence epilepsy. Sometimes a wolf in sheep's clothing. *Arch Pediatr Adolesc Med* 1997; 151: 152–8.

113 Metrakos JD, Metrakos K. Genetic factors in the epilepsies. In: Alter R, Hauser WA, eds. *The Epidemiology of Epilepsy: a Workshop*. NINDS monograph no. 14. Washington DC. US Government Printing Office, 1972: 97–102.

114 Reutens DC, Berkovic SF. Idiopathic generalized epilepsy of adolescence: are the syndromes clinically distinct? *Neurology* 1995; 45: 1469–76.

115 Olsson I, Hagberg G. Epidemiology of absence epilepsy. III. Clinical aspects. *Acta Paediatr Scand* 1991; 80: 1066–72.

116 Asconape J, Penry JK. Some clinical and EEG aspects of benign juvenile myoclonic epilepsy. *Epilepsia* 1984; 25: 108–14.

117 Wallace RH, Marini C, Petrou S *et al.* Mutant GABA (A) receptor gamma-2-subunit in childhood absence epilepsy and febrile seizures. *Nat Genet* 2001; 28: 49–52.

118 Janz D. Juvenile myoclonic epilepsy. Epilepsy with impulsive petit mal. *Cleve Clin J Med* 1989; 56 (Suppl.) (Part 1): S23–33.

119 Janz D. Epilepsy with impulsive petit mal (juvenile myoclonic epilepsy). *Acta Neurol Scand* 1985; 72: 449–59.

120 Panayiotopoulos CP, Obeid T, Tahan AR. Juvenile myoclonic epilepsy: a 5-year prospective study. *Epilepsia* 1994; 35: 285–96.

121 Wirrell EC, Camfield CS, Camfield PR, Gordon KE, Dooley JM. Long-term prognosis of typical childhood absence epilepsy: remission or progression to juvenile myoclonic epilepsy. *Neurology* 1996; 47: 912–18.

122 Murthy JM, Rao CM, Meena AK. Clinical observations of juvenile myoclonic epilepsy in 131 patients: a study in South India. *Seizure* 1998; 7: 43–7.

123 Frucht MM, Quigg M, Schwaner C, Fountain NB. Distribution of seizure precipitants among epilepsy syndromes. *Epilepsia* 2000; 41: 1534–9.

124 Appleton R, Beirne M, Acomb B. Photosensitivity in juvenile myoclonic epilepsy. *Seizure* 2000; 9: 108–11.

125 Greenberg DA, Durner M, Keddache M *et al*. Reproducibility and complications in gene searches: linkage on chromosome 6, heterogeneity, association, and maternal inheritance in juvenile myoclonic epilepsy. *Am J Hum Genet* 2000; 66: 508–16.

126 Serratosa JM, Delgado-Escueta AV, Medina MT, Zhang Q, Iranmanesh R, Sparkes RS. Clinical and genetic analysis of a large pedigree with juvenile myoclonic epilepsy. *Ann Neurol* 1996; 39: 187–95.

127 Sander T, Hildmann T, Janz D *et al*. The phenotypic spectrum related to the human epilepsy susceptibility gene 'EJM1'. *Ann Neurol* 1995; 38: 210–17.

128 Cossette P, Liu L, Brisebois K *et al*. Mutation of GABRA1 in an autosomal dominant form of juvenile myoclonic epilepsy. *Nat Genet* 2002; 31: 184–9.

129 Panayiotopoulos CP, Tahan R, Obeid T. Juvenile myoclonic epilepsy. Factors of error involved in the diagnosis and treatment. *Epilepsia* 1991; 32: 672–6.

130 Montalenti E, Imperiale D, Rovera A, Bergamasco B, Benna P. Clinical features, EEG findings and diagnostic pitfalls in juvenile myoclonic epilepsy: a series of 63 patients. *J Neurol Sci* 2001; 184: 65–70.

131 Genton P. When antiepileptic drugs aggravate epilepsy. *Brain Dev* 2000; 22: 75–80.

132 Delgado-Escueta AV, Enrile-Bacsal F. Juvenile myoclonic epilepsy of Janz. *Neurology* 1984; 34: 285–94.

133 Janz D, Wolf P. Epilepsy with grand mal on awakening. In: Engel J Jr, Pedley TA, eds, *Epilepsy: a Comprehensive Textbook*. Philadelphia: Lippincott-Raven, 1997: 2347–54.

134 Kellaway P, Frost JD, Hrachovy RA. Infantile spasms. In: Paolo L, Morselli CE, Pippenger J, Kiffin P, eds. *Antiepileptic Drug Therapy in Pediatrics*. New York: Raven Press, 1983: 115–36.

135 Lombroso CT, Fejerman N. Benign myoclonus of early infancy. *Ann Neurol* 1977; 1: 138–43.

136 Jeavons PM, Harper JR, Bower BD. Long-term prognosis in infantile spasms. A follow-up report on 112 cases. *Dev Med Child Neurol* 1970; 12: 413–21.

137 Kurokowa T, Goya N, Fukuyama Y, Suzuki M, Seki T, Ohtahara S. West syndrome and Lennox–Gastaut syndrome: a survey of natural history. *Pediatrics* 1980; 65: 81–8.

138 Matsumoto A, Wantanabe K, Negoro T *et al*. Long-term prognosis after infantile spasms: a statistical study of prognostic factors in 200 cases. *Dev Med Child Neurol* 1981; 23: 51–65.

139 Lombroso CT. Differentiation of seizures in newborns and early infancy. In: Paolo L, Morselli PL, Pippenger CE, Penry JK, eds. *Antiepileptic Drug Therapy in Pediatrics*. New York: Raven Press, 1983, 85–102.

140 Singer WD, Rabe EF, Haller JS. The effect of ACTH therapy upon infantile spasms. *J Pediatr* 1980; 96: 485–9.

141 Snead OC III, Benton JW Jr, Hosey LC *et al*. Treatment of infantile spasms with high-dose ACTH. Efficacy and plasma levels of ACTH and cortisol. *Neurology* 1989; 39: 1027–31.

142 Baram TZ, Mitchell WG, Tournay A, Snead OC, Hanson RA, Horton EJ. High-dose corticotropin (ACTH) versus prednisone for infantile spasms: a prospective, randomized, blinded study. *Pediatrics* 1996; 97: 375–9.

143 Riikonen R. ACTH therapy of West syndrome: Finnish views. (Review, 37 refs.) *Brain Dev* 2001; 23: 642–6.

144 Chiron C, Dulac O, Luna D *et al*. Vigabatrin in infantile spasms. *Lancet* 1990; 335: 363–4.

145 Chiron C, Dumas C, Jambaque I, Mumford J, Dulac O. Randomized trial comparing vigabatrin and hydrocortisone in infantile spasms due to tuberous sclerosis. *Epilepsy Res* 1997; 26: 389–95.

146 Mikati MA, Lepejian GA, Holmes GL. Medical treatment of patients with infantile spasms. *Clin Neuropharmacol* 2002; 25: 61–70.

147 Lagenstein I, Willig RP, Kuhne D. Cranial computed tomography (CCT) findings in children treated with ACTH and dexamethasone: first report. *Neuropadiatrie* 1979; 10: 370–84.

148 Singer WD, Haller JS, Sullivan LR *et al*. The value of neuroradiology in infantile spasms. *J Pediatr* 1982; 100: 47–50.

149 Bertoni JM, von Loh S, Allen RJ. The Aicardi syndrome: report of 4 cases and review of the literature. *Ann Neurol* 1979; 5: 475–82.

150 Curatolo P, Libutti G, Dallapiccola B. Aicardi syndrome in a male infant. *J Pediatr* 1980; 96: 286–7.

151 Willis J, Rosman NP. The Aicardi syndrome versus congenital infection: diagnostic considerations. *J Pediatr* 1980; 96: 235–9.

152 Huttenlocher PR. Dendritic development in neocortex of children with mental defect and infantile spasms. *Neurology* 1974: 203–10.

153 Gastaut H, Roger J, Soulayrol R, Tassinari CA, Regis H, Dravet C. Childhood epileptic encephalopathy with diffuse slow spike-waves (otherwise known as 'petit mal variant') or Lennox syndrome. *Epilepsia* 1966; 7: 139–79.

154 Aicardi J, Chevrie JJ. Myoclonic epilepsies of childhood. *Neuropediatrie* 1971; 3: 177–90.

155 Aicardi J. The problem of the Lennox syndrome. *Dev Med Child Neurol* 1973; 15: 77–81.

156 Ohtahara S. Lennox–Gastaut syndrome. Considerations in its concept and categorization. *Jpn J Psychiatry Neurol* 1988; 42: 535–42.

157 Riikonen R. A long-term follow-up study of 214 children with the syndrome of infantile spasms. *Neuropediatrics* 1982; 13: 14–23.

158 Aicardi J. The Lennox–Gastaut syndrome. *Int Pediatr* 1988; 3: 1552–7.

159 Doose H. Myoclonic astatic epilepsy of early childhood. In: Roger J, Dravet C, Bureau M, Dreifuss FE, Wolf P, eds. *Epileptic Syndromes in Infancy, Childhood and Adolescence*. London: John Libbey Eurotext Ltd, 1985: 78–88.

160 Henriksen O. Discussion of myoclonic epilepsies and Lennox–Gastaut syndrome. In: Roger J, Dravet C, Bureau M, Dreifuss FE, Wolf P, eds. *Epileptic Syndromes in Infancy, Childhood and Adolescence*. London: John Libbey Eurotext Ltd, 1985: 100–4.

161 Doose H. Myoclonic astatic epilepsy of early childhood. In: Roger J, Bureau M, Dravet C, Dreifuss F, Perret A, Wolf P, eds. *Epileptic Syndromes in Infancy, Childhood and Adolescence*, 2nd edn. London: John Libbey & Company, 1992: 103–14.

162 Doose H. Myoclonic-astatic epilepsy. *Epilepsy Res Suppl* 1992; 6: 163–8.

163 Dravet C, Bureau B, Guerrini R, Giraud N, Roger J. Severe myoclonic epilepsy in infants. In: Roger J, Bureau M, Dravet C, Dreifuss F, Perret A, Wolf P, eds. *Epileptic Syndromes in Infancy, Childhood and Adolescence*, 2nd edn. London: John Libbey & Company, 1992: 75–88.

164 Tassanari CA, Bureau M, Thomas P. Epilepsy with myoclonic absences. In: Roger J, Bureau M, Dravet C, Dreifuss F, Perret A, Wolf P, eds. *Epileptic Syndromes in Infancy, Childhood and Adolescence*, 2nd edn. London: John Libbey & Company, 1992: 151–60.

165 Elia M, Guerrini R, Musumeci SA, Bonanni P, Gambardella A, Aguglia U. Myoclonic absence-like seizures and chromosome abnormality syndromes. *Epilepsia* 1998; 39: 660–3.

166 Verrotti A, Greco R, Chiarelli F, Domizio S, Sabatino G, Morgese G. Epilepsy with myoclonic absences with early onset: a follow-up study. *J Child Neurol* 1999; 14: 746–9.

167 Itoh M, Hanaoka S, Sasaki M, Ohama E, Takashima S. Neuropathology of carly-infantile epileptic encephalopathy with suppression-bursts; comparison with those of early myoclonic encephalopathy and West syndrome. *Brain Dev* 2001; 23: 721–6.

168 Ohtahara S, Ohtsuka Y, Oka E. Epileptic encephalopathies in early infancy. *Indian J Pediatr* 1997; 64: 603–12.

169 Yamatogi Y, Ohtahara S. Early-infantile epileptic encephalopathy with suppression-bursts, Ohtahara syndrome; its overview referring to our 16 cases. *Brain Dev* 2002; 24: 13–23.

170 Aicardi J. Syndromic classification in the management of childhood epilepsy. *J Child Neurol* 1994; 9 (Suppl. 2): 14–18.

171 Ohtsuka Y, Kobayashi K, Ogino T, Oka E. Spasms in clusters in epilepsies other than typical West syndrome. *Brain Dev* 2001; 23: 473–81.

172 Aicardi J. Early myoclonic encephalopathy (neonatal myoclonic encephalopathy). In: Roger J, Bureau M, Dravet C, Dreifuss F, Perret A, Wolf P, eds. *Epileptic Syndromes in Infancy, Childhood and Adolescence*, 2nd edn. London: John Libbey & Company, 1992: 13–23.

173 Murakami N, Ohtsuka Y, Ohtahara S. Early infantile epileptic syndromes with suppression-bursts: early myoclonic encephalopathy vs. Ohtahara syndrome. *Jpn J Psychiatry Neurol* 1993; 47: 197–200.

174 Lombroso CT. Early myoclonic encephalopathy, early infantile epileptic encephalopathy, and benign and severe infantile myoclonic epilepsies: a critical review and personal contributions. *J Clin Neurophysiol* 1990; 7: 380–408.

175 Dravet C. Les épilepsies graves de l'enfant. *Vie Med* 1978; 8: 543–8.

176 Oguni H, Hayashi K, Awaya Y, Fukuyama Y, Osawa M. Severe

myoclonic epilepsy in infants—a review based on the Tokyo Women's Medical University series of 84 cases. *Brain Dev* 2001; 23: 736–48.

177 Yakoub M, Dulac O, Jambaque I, Chiron C, Plouin P. Early diagnosis of severe myoclonic epilepsy in infancy. *Brain Dev* 1992; 14: 299–303.

178 Claes L, Del-Favero J, Ceulemans B *et al.* De novo mutations in the sodium-channel gene SCN1A cause severe myoclonic epilepsy of infancy. *Am J Hum Genet* 2001; 68: 1327–32.

179 Scheffer IE, Wallace R, Mulley JC, Berkovic SF. Clinical and molecular genetics of myoclonic-astatic epilepsy and severe myoclonic epilepsy in infancy (Dravet syndrome). *Brain Dev* 2001; 23: 732–5.

180 Sugawara T, Mazaki-Miyazaki E, Fukushima K *et al.* Frequent mutations of SCN1A in severe myoclonic epilepsy in infancy. *Neurology* 2002; 58: 1122–4.

181 Kanazawa O. Refractory grand mal seizures with onset during infancy including severe myoclonic epilepsy in infancy. *Brain Dev* 2001; 23: 749–56.

182 Doose H, Lunau H, Castiglione E, Waltz S. Severe idiopathic generalized epilepsy of infancy with generalized tonic-clonic seizures. *Neuropediatrics* 1998; 29: 229–38.

183 Dalla Bernardina B, Tassinari CA, Dravet C, Bureau M, Beghini G, Roger J. Benign focal epilepsy and 'electrical status epilepticus' during sleep. *Rev Electroencephalogr Neurophysiol Clin* 1978; 8: 350–3.

184 Tassinari CA, Rubboli G, Volpi L *et al.* Encephalopathy with electrical status epilepticus during slow sleep or ESES syndrome including the acquired aphasia. *Clin Neurophysiol* 2000; 111 (Suppl. 2): S94–S102.

185 Guilhoto LM, Machado-Haertel LR, Manreza ML, Diament AJ. Continuous spike-wave activity during sleep. Electroencephalographic and clinical features. *Arq Neuropsiquiatr* 1997; 55: 762–70.

186 Veggiotti P, Beccaria F, Guerrini R, Capovilla G, Lanzi G. Continuous spike-and-wave activity during slow-wave sleep: syndrome or EEG pattern? *Epilepsia* 1999; 40: 1593–601.

187 Kobayashi K, Murakami N, Yoshinaga H, Enoki H, Ohtsuka Y, Ohtahara S. Nonconvulsive status epilepticus with continuous diffuse spike-and-wave discharges during sleep in childhood. *Jpn J Psychiatry Neurol* 1988; 42: 509–14.

188 Hirsch E, Marescaux C, Maquet P *et al.* Landau–Kleffner syndrome. A clinical and EEG study of five cases. *Epilepsia* 1990; 31: 756–67.

189 Shafrir Y, Prensky AL. Acquired epileptiform opercular syndrome. A second case report, review of the literature, and comparison to the Landau–Kleffner syndrome. *Epilepsia* 1995; 36: 1050–7.

190 Tachikawa E, Oguni H, Shirakawa S, Funatsuka M, Hayashi K, Osawa M. Acquired epileptiform opercular syndrome. A case report and results of single photon emission computed tomography and computer-assisted electroencephalographic analysis. *Brain Dev* 2001; 23: 246–50.

191 Guerrini R, Genton P, Bureau M *et al.* Multilobar polymicrogyria, intractable drop attack seizures, and sleep-related electrical status epilepticus. *Neurology* 1998; 51: 504–12.

192 Veggiotti P, Beccaria F, Papalia G, Termine C, Piazza F, Lanzi G. Continuous spikes and waves during sleep in children with shunted hydrocephalus. *Childs Nerv Syst* 1998; 14: 188–94.

193 Landau WM, Kleffner FR. Syndrome of acquired aphasia with convulsive disorder in children. *Neurology* 1957; 7: 523–30.

194 Kale U, el-Naggar M, Hawthorne M. Verbal auditory agnosia with focal EEG abnormality: an unusual case of a child presenting to an ENT surgeon with 'deafness'. *J Laryngol Otol* 1995; 109: 431–2.

195 Deonna TW. Acquired epileptiform aphasia in children (Landau–Kleffner syndrome). *J Clin Neurophysiol* 1991; 8: 288–98.

196 Tharpe AM, Olson BJ. Landau–Kleffner syndrome: acquired epileptic aphasia in children. *J Am Acad Audiol* 1994; 5: 146–50.

197 da Silva EA, Chugani DC, Muzik O, Chugani HT. Landau–Kleffner syndrome: metabolic abnormalities in temporal lobe are a common feature. *J Child Neurol* 1997; 12: 489–95.

198 Cole AJ, Andermann F, Taylor L *et al.* The Landau–Kleffner syndrome of acquired epileptic aphasia: unusual clinical outcome, surgical experience, and absence of encephalitis. *Neurology* 1988; 38: 31–8.

199 Wioland N, Rudolf G, Metz-Lutz MN. Electrophysiological evidence of persisting unilateral auditory cortex dysfunction in the late outcome of Landau and Kleffner syndrome. *Clin Neurophysiol* 2001; 112: 319–23.

200 Robinson RO, Baird G, Robinson G, Simonoff E. Landau–Kleffner syndrome: course and correlates with outcome. *Dev Med Child Neurol* 2001; 43: 243–7.

201 Rossi PG, Parmeggiani A, Posar A, Scaduto MC, Chiodo S, Vatti G. Landau–Kleffner syndrome (LKS). Long-term follow-up and links with electrical status epilepticus during sleep (ESES). *Brain Dev* 1999; 21: 90–8.

202 Soprano AM, Garcia EF, Caraballo R, Fejerman N. Acquired epileptic aphasia. Neuropsychologic follow-up of 12 patients. *Pediatr Neurol* 1994; 11: 230–5.

203 Mantovani JF, Landau WM. Acquired aphasia with convulsive disorder. Course and prognosis. *Neurology* 1980; 30: 524–9.

204 Nelson KB, Ellenberg JH. Predictors of epilepsy in children who have experienced febrile seizures. *New Eng J Med* 1976; 295: 1029–33.

205 Nelson KB, Ellenberg JH. Prognosis in children with febrile seizures. *Pediatrics* 1978; 61: 720–7.

206 Annegers JF, Hauser WA, Elveback LR, Kurland LT. The risk of epilepsy following febrile convulsions. *Neurology* 1979; 29: 297–303.

207 Annegers JF, Hauser WA, Shirts SB, Kurland LT. Factors prognostic of unprovoked seizures after febrile convulsions. *N Engl J Med* 1987; 316: 493–8.

208 Lerche H, Weber YG, Baier H *et al.* Generalized epilepsy with febrile seizures plus: further heterogeneity in a large family. *Neurology* 2001; 57: 1191–8.

209 Meisler MH, Kearney J, Ottman R, Escayg A. Identification of epilepsy genes in human and mouse. *Annu Rev Genet* 2001; 35: 567–88.

210 Alekov AK, Rahman MM, Mitrovic N, Lehmann-Horn F, Lerche H. Enhanced inactivation and acceleration of activation of the sodium channel associated with epilepsy in man. *Eur J Neurosci* 2001; 13: 2171–6.

211 Wallace RH, Scheffer IE, Parasivam G *et al.* Generalized epilepsy with febrile seizures plus. Mutation of the sodium channel subunit SCN1B. *Neurology* 2002; 58: 1426–9.

212 Baulac S, Huberfeld G, Gourfinkel-An I *et al.* First genetic evidence of GABA (A) receptor dysfunction in epilepsy: a mutation in the gamma-2-subunit gene. *Nat Genet* 2001; 28: 46–8.

213 Harkin LA, Bowser DN, Dibbens LM *et al.* Truncation of the GABA (A)-receptor gamma2 subunit in a family with generalized epilepsy with febrile seizures plus. *Am J Hum Genet* 2002; 70: 530–6.

214 Baulac S, Picard F, Herman A *et al.* Evidence for digenic inheritance in a family with both febrile convulsions and temporal lobe epilepsy implicating chromosomes 18qter and 1q25-q31. *Ann Neurol* 2001; 49: 786–92.

215 Wallace RH, Scheffer IE, Barnett S *et al.* Neuronal sodium-channel alpha1-subunit mutations in generalized epilepsy with febrile seizures plus. *Am J Hum Genet* 2001; 68: 859–65.

216 Berkovic SF, Scheffer IE. Genetics of the epilepsies. *Epilepsia* 2001; 42 (Suppl. 5): 16–23.

217 Singh R, Gardner RJ, Crossland KM, Scheffer IE, Berkovic SF. Chromosomal abnormalities and epilepsy: a review for clinicians and gene hunters. *Epilepsia* 2002; 43: 127–40.

Epidemiology and Prognosis of Epilepsy and its Treatment

L. Forsgren

Epidemiological studies of epilepsy provide fundamental information on magnitude of the disorder, its causes and its consequences. They can also quantify the impact of important variables such as the risk for further seizures, the chance of becoming seizure free, and the risk of dying from seizures. Furthermore, they can identify factors that are associated with a low or high risk for intractability.

Prevalence studies of well-characterized epilepsy populations provide valuable information for planning purposes. How many have epilepsy? How many have mild or severe epilepsy? How frequent is epilepsy in different ages? How many have concomitant disorders, and of what type? This and related information make it possible to estimate the number affected, the levels of care needed and the resources that will be required.

Incidence studies are also of value for planning, especially for estimating the investigational resources needed. Another great value of incidence studies is to identify aetiological factors, to generate hypotheses and to evaluate how risk can be reduced. Incidence studies can provide important information on prognostic factors, but compared to prevalence studies, they are more complex, expensive and therefore relatively uncommon.

The epilepsy population studied should be representative of the general population with epilepsy. From a global perspective, however, it is difficult for a study from a single country to be representative since around the world epilepsy differs in many aspects such as aetiology, distribution of risk factors and age composition. Epidemiological studies on certain aspects of epilepsy are lacking from some parts of the world. For example, studies on mortality in epilepsy have only been reported from a few of the developed countries. While the effect of a factor such as age can be adjusted for in the analysis to allow comparability between studies, for many other factors adjustment is impossible. Nonetheless, combining information from many population-based studies on all continents is needed to give a global picture of common and unique aspects of epilepsy.

There are many sources for identifying epilepsy populations; these include diagnostic registries at hospitals and EEG laboratories as well as registries of groups with conditions that increase the risk for epilepsy such as mental retardation. When registries which partly overlap have identified the vast majority of persons with epilepsy in the study area, the study is considered to be population-based (or community-based) and thus representative of the general epilepsy population in the study area. The use of hospitals as the sole source for identification can bias the sample resulting in an underestimation of the number affected and an overestimation of severe cases.

Categorizing countries as developed and developing is sensitive and sometimes misleading because all countries change and are in

that sense developing. Other indicators for developed countries are industrialization and market economies. In this chapter countries in Europe, North America and Australia are classified as developed and the countries of Central and South America, Africa and Asia as less developed. Of course this is an oversimplification since some countries in the less developed parts of the world are socio-economically more advanced than some of the more developed countries.

General epidemiology

The size of the epilepsy population, prevalence

In order to compare the prevalence of epilepsy in different groups, the definition of epilepsy should be the same across studies. The definition of epilepsy recommended by international guidelines for epidemiological studies of epilepsy states that seizures should be recurrent (i.e. at least two seizures should have occurred) and unprovoked by any immediate identified cause [1]. To be able to generalize results, ascertainment of cases within the study area should be complete, a goal that is achieved more or less, but never fully. Estimates of the size of the epilepsy population exist for all continents, based on studies that applied established definitions of epilepsy and ascertained a reasonable number of cases. Epidemiological studies of epilepsy are mainly interested in people with active epilepsy. Active epilepsy refers to cases who fulfil the criteria for epilepsy and who have had at least one seizure during the last 5 years. Some studies also include people whose last seizures occurred more than 5 years previously if they are still being treated with antiepileptic drugs (AED).

More developed countries

Population-based European studies including all ages have been performed in Poland, Italy, Faeroes (Denmark) and on Iceland, the latter two studies being large. These studies report the prevalence of active epilepsy to be 4.8–7.8 per 1000 inhabitants. In Scandinavia and the Baltic countries prevalence rates are 3.6–5.3 in children and 5.5 and 6.3 in adults (Table 2.1). In North America extensive epidemiological studies on epilepsy have been performed on the population of Rochester in Minnesota, where the 1980 prevalence rate was 6.8, the same as that reported from the southern states. Studies on children and adolescents found prevalence rates of 4.7 and 5.7. A small study from Australia found a prevalence of 7.5. Thus overall prevalence rates of epilepsy are similar in Europe, North America and Australia, around 7/1000; rates in children are slightly lower [2–20] (Table 2.1).

Table 2.1 Prevalence of active epilepsy in more developed countries

Country, year (study)	Prevalence per 1000 people			Number of cases
	Not age-adjusted	Age-adjusted[a]	Age	
Poland, 1974 (2)	7.8	8.0	All ages	33
Italy, 1983 (3)	6.2	6.7	All ages	278
Italy, 1991 (4)	5.1		All ages	51
Faeroes (Denmark), 1986 (5)	7.6	7.8	All ages	333
Iceland, 1999 (6)	4.8	4.8	All ages	428
United States[b], 1986 (7)	6.8	7.0	All ages	160
United States, 1991 (8)		6.8	All ages	383
Australia, 1985 (9)	7.5		All ages	35
Finland, 1989 (10)	6.3		Adults	1233
Sweden, 1992 (11)	5.5	5.7	Adults	713
Sweden, 1996 (12)	4.2		Children 0–16 years	155
Norway, 2000 (13)	5.3		Children 6–12 years	205
Finland, 1997 (14)	3.9		Children 0–15 years	329
Lithuania, 1997 (15)	4.3		Children 0–15 years	378
Estonia, 1999 (16)	3.6		Children 0–19 years	560
Italy, 1987 (17)	4.5		Children 5–14 years	178
Spain, 1991 (18)	3.7		Children 6–14 years	124
United States, 1978 (19)	5.7		Children 6–16 years	23
United States, 1983 (20)	4.7		Children 0–19 years	1159

[a] Age-adjusted to the US population.
[b] Includes 22% with 'possible epilepsy'.

Less developed countries

Studies from countries in South and Central America, Africa and Asia report larger differences in prevalence rates of active epilepsy than found in more developed countries [21–33]. Several studies from South and Central America find prevalence rates much higher than in other parts of the world. Many of these studies are small but large studies also report high rates although in the largest study [21] the rate was similar to that of more developed countries (Table 2.2).

Several African studies report high prevalence rates. Many of these studies are small or include cases with provoked and/or inactive epilepsy. Larger population-based studies find prevalence rates comparable to what is found in more developed countries (Table 2.2). The country in Asia with the largest number of studies is India. A meta-analysis of 20 studies [29] in India found an overall prevalence of 5.3 with a 95% CI of 4.3–6.4. A similar rate has been found in other studies in India while slightly higher rates have been reported from other Asian countries (Table 2.2).

It is often claimed that epilepsy is more common in the less developed parts of the world. From the literature this appears likely for South and Central America, possibly so for sub-Saharan Africa and less likely for Asia. From the age-specific prevalence rates it can be estimated that globally more than 10 million children, 28–29 million adults and close to 3 million elderly have active epilepsy. This means that children constitute one-quarter, adults two-thirds and the elderly 6–7% of the global epilepsy population. In total, at the beginning of this millennium, approximately 42 million people have active epilepsy. Of these 82% live in less developed countries. Since the largest population increase occurs in the elderly, both in more and less developed countries, it is expected that the elderly will constitute a growing part of the epilepsy population.

Gender

Is epilepsy more frequent in males or females? Most studies have found epilepsy to be more common in males [2–7,10,11]. However, there are exceptions. In a study from the USA covering a 50-year period, prevalence was higher for males between 1940 and 1970 but more common in females in 1980 [8]. The increase in prevalence of active epilepsy during the 50-year period was largely due to an increasing prevalence in females. Studies in children often report higher prevalence in males [13–17] but higher rates have also been found in females [12]. Interestingly, the larger prevalence studies from South America report higher rates in females [21,23] or no difference [22]. In Asia most [29–31] but not all [32] studies report slightly higher rates in males. In Africa the situation is the same with most [24,25,27], but not all [26], studies finding slightly higher rates in males. The difference in prevalence found between genders is rarely statistically significant [3,10] and in individual studies one almost invariably finds that the dominance by females and males shifts between age groups. Thus, from available studies it can be concluded that epilepsy probably is slightly more common in males but several studies find the opposite and therefore uncertainty remains as to whether there is a true gender difference of active epilepsy.

Table 2.2 Prevalence of active epilepsy in less developed countries

Country, year (study)	Prevalence per 1000 people	Age	Number of cases
Ecuador, 1992 (21[a])	6.7–8.0	All ages	575
Chile, 1992 (22)	17.7	All ages	314
Bolivia, 1999 (23)	11.2	All ages	112
Nigeria, 1987 (24)	5.0	All ages	101
Ethiopia, 1990 (25)	5.2	All ages	316
Tanzania, 1992 (26)	10.2	All ages	185
Tunisia, 1993 (27)	4.0	All ages	141
South-Africa, 2000 (28)	6.7	Children 2–9 years	45
India, 1999 (29)	5.3	All ages	3207
India, 1998 (30)	4.6	All ages	301
India, 2000 (31)	4.9	All ages	1175
Pakistan, 1994 (32)	10.0	All ages	241
Turkey, 1997 (33)	7.0	All ages	81

[a] Single seizures and afebrile provoked seizures included.

Ethnicity

Almost all studies come from racially homogeneous populations. A study of childhood epilepsy in the USA found higher rates in the black than in the white population [20]. The difference was found for all childhood ages but especially in children below age 10 years. In a population with all ages included, rates were higher in the black population, both for males and females, except for children aged 5 years or younger [7]. In an area in England with a large South Asian population, the prevalence was 4.5 per 1000. A lower rate was found in the population with South Asian origin, 3.6 per 1000, compared with 7.8 in the rest of the population [34]. The low rate found in the Asian population may be due to selective migration and/or stigma and denial. The effect of ethnicity on the frequency of epilepsy is difficult to assess due to confounding of socioeconomic factors.

Socioeconomic factors

Using an index for material deprivation with the key variables unemployment, no car in the household, overcrowded households and households not owner occupied, a strong correlation was found between the prevalence of epilepsy and social deprivation in a study from Wales [35]. The correlation remained when patients with co-existing psychiatric illness or learning disability were excluded from the analysis. Social deprivation can be both a cause and a consequence of epilepsy. The authors interpreted the correlation found to go in the direction of epilepsy being a consequence of social deprivation since a high correlation with prevalence was found already in those under age 20 years, at a time when the drift down the social scale due to epilepsy should be minor.

In Ecuador, Pakistan and Turkey prevalence was higher in rural than in urban areas [21,32,33]. A meta-analysis of 20 studies from India found the opposite, a higher prevalence in urban than in rural areas [29]. It is unknown how differences in prevalence between rural and urban areas are related to socioeconomic factors since poverty exists both in the countryside and in urban and suburban slums.

Seizure types

Modern epidemiological studies on seizure types have used the International Classification of Epileptic Seizures [36]. In more developed countries patients with partial seizures (PS) or localization-related epilepsies account for 33–65% of the epilepsy population; those with generalized seizures account for 17–60%; and in 2–8% seizures are unclassifiable [3–6,8]. Many generalized convulsive seizures have a focal onset and rapidly generalize precluding observation of focal onset. When EEG is added to the analysis of seizure type a proportion of generalized seizures can be reclassified as partial, secondarily generalized. In a study from Iceland 35% of patients had PS on clinical grounds but data from the EEG increased the proportion to 50% [6].

Studies in adults find that 55–60% have PS or localization-related epilepsies, 26–32% have primarily generalized seizures and 8–17% have seizures that are unclassifiable [10,11]. In studies of childhood epilepsy 36–66% have focal seizures/epilepsies, 30–62% have primarily generalized seizures and 2–4% have unclassifiable seizures [12–17,20]. Another study found localization-related epilepsies account for 50% of the epilepsies in people up into their 30s and account for 75% of epilepsy among people aged 75 years and older [8].

Summarizing studies from developed countries, PS are more common than generalized seizures in both children and adults although the preponderance of PS is more pronounced in adults. However, in clinical practice generalized seizures are most often encountered since hospital contact is more likely to occur when seizures are generalized. However, it should be remembered that most of these seizures are secondarily generalized, following a focal onset.

The distribution of seizure types in less developed countries is as follows: focal seizures in 11–55%, generalized seizures in 26–86%, and unclassifiable in 0–19% of patients [21–26,29,31]. Combining EEG results with clinical diagnosis increases the proportion of seizures classified as partial from 20 to 26% in Ethiopia and from 34 to 53% in Bolivia [23,25].

Prevalence of epileptic syndromes

In the last 10 years several population-based epidemiological studies have identified the occurrence of epileptic syndromes based on the International Classification of Epilepsies and Epileptic Syndromes [37]. This classification is based on seizure/epilepsy type (partial/focal/localization-related or generalized) and aetiology (idiopathic, cryptogenic or symptomatic). Two studies have investigated childhood epilepsy in the Baltic countries. In Estonia idiopathic epileptic syndromes had the highest prevalence rate, 1.2 per 1000 [16]. The most frequent idiopathic syndromes were generalized tonic-clonic seizures (GTCS) on awakening (0.6 per 1000) and benign childhood epilepsy with centrotemporal spikes (BECT) and absence epilepsy (each 0.3 per 1000). The prevalence rate for cryptogenic epilepsies was 1.0 per 1000 with localization-related epilepsies as the most common cryptogenic syndrome (0.9 per 1000), followed by Lennox–Gastaut syndrome (LGS) (0.1 per 1000) and West's syndrome (0.05 per 1000). The prevalence rate for symptomatic epileptic syndromes was 0.5 per 1000 [16]. In Lithuania cryptogenic epilepsies were most frequent (1.8 per 1000) [15]. Localization-related epilepsies were most frequent in Lithuania (2.1 per 1000) followed by generalized epilepsies (1.3 per 1000). In many it was not possible to determine whether seizures were partial or generalized (0.7 per 1000) [15]. The rate for West's syndrome was the same as in Estonia and the rate for LGS slightly higher.

Three Scandinavian studies in children reported on the distribution of epileptic syndromes [12–14]. Localization-related syndromes were found in 41–54%, and were the most frequent syndromes of children in Sweden and Norway [12,13]. Generalized syndromes were found in 37–48%, being the most frequent syndromes in Finland [14]. A specific syndrome could not be identified in 5–10% of patients in these studies. BECT was common in Sweden and Norway, found in 17% in both countries, and in 5% in Finland. Absence epilepsies were found in 6–8%, juvenile myoclonic epilepsy (JME) in 1–5%, West's syndrome in 0.5–8% and LGS in 2–6% [12–14]. A study on Iceland including all ages found BECT to be the most frequent syndrome (4%), followed by JME (3%), absence epilepsies (2%) and LGS (2%) [6].

New cases with epilepsy, incidence

Incidence studies measure how many new patients develop epilepsy. Incidence is expressed as the number of new cases observed annually in 100 000 people (or person-years). Incidence studies should be prospective in order to identify aetiological factors where possible. Studies often have to go on for years in order to collect a sufficient number of cases. As seen, the number of cases included in incidence studies (Table 2.3) is often smaller than in prevalence studies (Tables 2.1 and 2.2). Due to logistic and economical reasons incidence studies are relatively rare.

There is often a delay of months to years between the initial seizure(s) and contact with the health authorities and diagnosis. Thus, annual incidence rates in most studies provide information on the proportion of newly diagnosed cases regardless of whether the initial seizure(s) occurred prior or during the investigation period. A synonymous term for incidence rate used in this way is the first

Table 2.3 Annual incidence of epilepsy

Country, year (study)	Incidence per 100 000 person-years	Age	Number of cases	Comments
Faeroes, 1986 (5)	43	All ages	118	
France, 1990 (38)	44	All ages	494	SS[a] included
Iceland, 1996 (39)	47	All ages	42	
Sweden, 1996 (40)	56	Adults > 16 year	160	SS[a] included
Switzerland, 1997 (41)	46	All ages	176	SS[a] included
United Kingdom[c], 2000 (42)	46	All ages	31	
United States[d], 1993 (43)	48	All ages	275	
United States, 1999 (44)	52	All ages	157	
Ecuador, 1992 (21)	122–190	All ages	137	SS[a] & APS[b] included
Chile, 1992 (22)	113	All ages	102	
Martinique, 1999 (45)	64	All ages	246	SS[a] included
Tanzania, 1992 (26)	73	All ages	122	
Ethiopia, 1997 (46)	64	All ages	139	
China, 1985 (47)	25	All ages	16	
India, 1998 (30)	49	All ages	32	

[a] Single seizures included.
[b] Afebrile provoked seizures.
[c] Incidence 57 with SS[a] included.
[d] Data for the period 1975–84.

attendance rate. The index seizure is 'the diagnostic seizure', the seizure leading to the diagnostic contact. Some studies on the incidence of epilepsy include single unprovoked seizures. In studies on seizure prognosis it is important to be aware whether the starting point is the time of the first seizure or the time of diagnosis.

More developed countries

In the USA, France, Iceland, Faeroes and Sweden annual incidence rates are around 50/100 000 (Table 2.3). Higher rates, 60–80/100 000, were found in studies from the UK, with acute provoked seizures included [48,49].

Less developed countries

Studies from Chile and Ecuador have reported the highest incidence rates worldwide (Table 2.3). The two existing studies on incidence of epilepsy from Africa report slightly higher incidence rates than found in more developed countries (Table 2.3). However, when incidence is adjusted for age using the USA population, the incidence in Africa is similar to that found in more developed countries, around 50/100 000. The two incidence studies from Asia show rates to be similar to more developed countries (India) or lower (China) (Table 2.3). A surprisingly low adjusted incidence—25/100 000, or 35/100 000 if adjusted—was reported from China. However, the study was small with an upper 95% CI above 50/100 000.

Age-specific incidence

The highest incidence is found in young children and the elderly. Based on data from the USA, Iceland, Faeroes and Sweden [5,39,40,43,50] the curve for the age-specific incidence is U-shaped with the lowest incidence in people in their 30s and the highest incidence in the elderly (Fig. 2.1). Only a few studies have addressed age-specific incidence in less developed countries, but they show the incidence to be higher in children and (with a single exception)

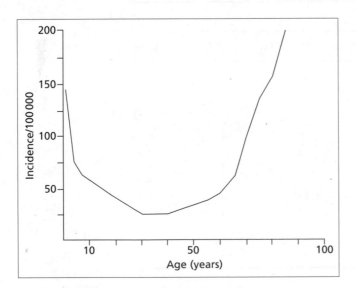

Fig. 2.1 Age-specific incidence of epilepsy based on studies from the USA, Iceland, Faeroes and Sweden (single unprovoked seizures included in the Swedish studies) ([5,39,40,43,50]).

lower in the elderly compared with more developed countries [21,22,26,46]. Based on the global demography and available population-based studies with information on the age-specific incidence it can be estimated that globally 3.5 million people develop epilepsy annually. About 40% of these are children under the age of 15 years, another 40% are adolescents and adults 15–64 years old, and close to 20% are elderly. Thus, the majority of people who develop epilepsy do so after childhood.

Cumulative incidence

The cumulative incidence is the summation of age-specific incidence and gives the proportion of a population that develops a disease during a specified period. In Iceland the cumulative incidence was 1% up to age 15, 1.9% by age 55 and 3.6% by age 75 years [39]. In the USA the cumulative incidence was 1.2% up to age 24, 3% up to age 74 and 4.4% up to age 85 years [43]. When single unprovoked seizures were included, the cumulative incidence increased to 4.1% up to age 74 years. In Sweden the cumulative incidence, single unprovoked seizures included, up to age 74 years was identical, 4.1%, and 5.8% up to age 84 years [40]. Thus, approximately every 30th person is expected to have epilepsy during some part of his or her life, and every 25th will have at least one unprovoked seizure.

Gender

In prevalence studies and most incidence studies epilepsy is more common in males than females [5,39,46,47], although the difference is rarely statistically significant [5]. Other studies find minor or no difference between gender [30,40,43,51] and a few find a higher frequency in females [21,26].

Ethnicity and socioeconomic factors

In an incidence study in an urban area in the USA, new onset epilepsy was more common in black than white children [52]. Febrile and other provoked seizures, and neonatal seizures were included in the epilepsies. This study also reported an excess of epilepsy in both black and white children living in lower socioeconomic areas.

Seizure types in incidence populations

Partial seizures are most common, found in 51–68% of incidence populations [5,22,38,43,51]. In studies where lower frequencies are found, the most likely explanation is that a proportion of PS with secondary generalization were misclassified as generalized [39,46]. Seizures were generalized in 16–69% and unclassifiable in 0–17% [5,22,38,39,44,46,51].

Incidence of epileptic syndromes

In France localization-related syndromes had the highest incidence, 15 per 100 000 (13.6 symptomatic and 1.7 idiopathic), which corresponds to 60% of incident cases with epilepsy [38]. Among childhood onset syndromes BECT was most frequent (6%) followed by absence syndromes (5%), West's syndrome (3%) and JME (2%). In a study from the USA on the incidence of epileptic syndromes the annual incidence was 52 per 100 000, higher than in France and elsewhere thus indicating a high degree of case ascertainment [44]. This study also found localization-related syndromes to be most frequent, found in 69% and an incidence of 35 per 100 000. Generalized syndromes were found in 12%. Specific childhood syndromes were rare. Absence epilepsies were found in 2%, BECT in 1% and JME in less than 1%.

Many cases were classified in unspecific categories. In 18% it could not be determined whether the syndromes were focal or generalized. Another 43% had generalized symptomatic or cryptogenic localization-related syndromes. The limitations of the syndromic classification were discussed in relation to its application in a population-based study in the UK [53]. A large proportion, 37% of 508 patients with repeated unprovoked seizures, had syndromes that lacked clear-cut focal and generalized features. An additional 29% belonged to the unspecific category of cryptogenic localization-related syndromes. Localization-related syndromes were found in 50% and generalized syndromes in 13%. Absence syndromes were found in 3%, JME in 2% and BECT in 1% [53]. In Iceland JME was found in 7%, BECT in 5% and West's syndrome in 2% [39]. An incidence study limited to adults found 72% to have localization-related syndromes, 16% generalized syndromes and 12% syndromes undetermined as to whether they were focal or generalized [40]. Some studies have focused on specific syndromes. The annual incidence of absence epilepsy for children 0–15 years is 7 per 100 000 [54]. The annual incidence of West's syndrome is between 0.3 and 0.5 per 1000 live births [50,55–57].

The finding of localization-related syndromes as the most common form of epilepsy is congruent with incidence studies showing the majority of patients having PS [5,22,38,43,51].

Causes of epilepsy

The aetiologies of epilepsy are best explored in population-based studies of newly diagnosed patients. Prevalence studies are less well suited for aetiological analysis because the most severe causes of epilepsy with increased mortality will be underrepresented as will those with the most benign epilepsies that rapidly enter remission. Given the different habits and life conditions for people living in various countries, it is expected that risk factors and their relative importance differ within and between countries and continents.

The cause of epilepsy is unknown in the majority of patients. Population-based studies from Europe and the USA do not identify an aetiology in 54–69% of patients (Table 2.4) according to studies of newly diagnosed patients many decades ago before modern neuroradiological techniques were available. For this reason one would anticipate that recent studies, where the majority of patients are extensively investigated with modern imaging, would yield higher proportions with identified aetiologies. However, results from the most recent population-based studies have been inconsistent. Studies from Iceland [39] and Sweden [40,50] report the lowest and highest proportions, respectively, of identified aetiologies (Table 2.4).

The most commonly identified aetiology in all population-based studies from more developed countries is stroke, accounting for approximately every sixth patient who develops epilepsy. Other common causes are neoplasm and congenital disorders. Congenital disorders mainly include patients who in addition to epilepsy have a central nervous system (CNS) disorder presumed present at birth, also causing mental retardation, cerebral palsy and/or a developmental malformation of the brain. Other fairly common causes of epilepsy are trauma and degenerative disorders. The most common neurodegenerative disorder causing epilepsy is Alzheimer's disease which causes GTCS in 10–16% of patients [58,59]. These often occur during the late stage of the disease [59,60], a stage where many also develop myoclonic seizures [58]. Partial seizures have also been reported in Alzheimer's disease [60]. A population-based

Table 2.4 Population-based studies estimating the proportion (in per cent) of identified presumed causes of epilepsy

| Aetiology | Study | | | | |
	Iceland (39)	Sweden[ab] (40,50)	U.K.[bc] (51)	U.S.A (43)	Range
Vascular	14	21	15	11	11–21
Ischemia		18			
Haemorrhage		3			
Trauma	0	2	3	6	0–6
Neoplasm	7	7	6	4	4–7
Infection	2	0	2	3	0–3
Degenerative	2	5		4	2–5
Congenital	5	7		8	5–7
Other	0	4	13[d]	0	0–13
Remote or progressive symptomatic	31	46	39	35	31–46
Idiopathic	69	54	61	65	54–69

[a] Frequencies based on combining studies on children and adults.
[b] Includes single seizures.
[c] Includes 15% with acute provoked afebrile seizures.
[d] Includes 6% with alcohol-related seizures.

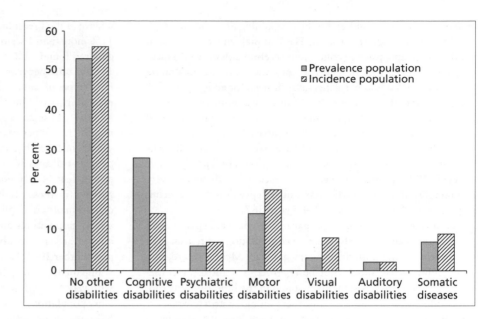

Fig. 2.2 Major disabilities associated with epilepsy in adults 17 years and older ([11,40]).

case–control study with incident cases of a first unprovoked seizure found that diagnosis of either Alzheimer's disease or a diagnosis of other dementia was associated with at least a six-fold increased risk for unprovoked seizures [61]. The risk was the same for generalized seizures as for PS.

In less developed countries the proportion with unknown causes is large, over 70%, in population-based incidence studies [26,45,46]. Whereas the same aetiologies for epilepsy are found in all countries, some of these aetiologies, e.g. head trauma, infections, pre- and perinatal causes, may be more common in less developed countries; however, there are additional causes. For example, neurocysticercosis is an infection of the CNS contracted by eating pork or fruits and vegetables contaminated by the pork tapeworm *Taenia solium*, which is endemic in South America, parts of Africa, India and China. In a recent study from Ecuador on newly diagnosed patients with epilepsy, the proportion with identified causes was comparable to more developed countries [62], but neurocysticercosis was found in 8%. Thus, neurocysticercosis accounts for a small fraction of the epilepsies and should be regarded as one of several factors responsible for the high incidence of epilepsy in South America.

Associated disabilities (comorbidities)

A few epidemiological studies provide information on other impairments/disabilities in epilepsy populations. Most people with epilepsy do not have other disabilities, but conditions that cause epilepsy often also produce other disabilities. For some, the other disabilities have a minor impact compared to epilepsy, for others they may be the major disability.

The frequency of associated disabilities differs in newly diagnosed populations compared with populations where a majority have had epilepsy for many years. In a prevalence study of epilepsy 47% had no other disabilities, compared with 44% in an incidence population [11,40]. The most common disabilities associated with epilepsy in patients with established epilepsy is cognitive disabilities followed by motor disabilities. In newly diagnosed patients motor

disabilities are most common, followed by cognitive disabilities (Fig. 2.2).

Learning disabilities

Learning disability is the most common associated disability in epilepsy, both in children and adults. The term most often used for learning disability/cognitive disturbance in epidemiological studies of epilepsy is mental retardation. Mental retardation is found in 38–49% of children [12,13,63,64] and in 23% of adults [11] with active epilepsy. The picture is the same in less developed countries. In a population-based study in India 23% of those with epilepsy were mentally retarded [65] and in Ethiopia 8% were severely mentally retarded [25].

The degree of mental retardation is clearly related to the risk for epilepsy. Among children with mild mental retardation (IQ 50–70) epilepsy is found in 7–18% [63,66,67] and in 35–44% of children with severe mental retardation (IQ < 50) [63,67,68]. In a population with mental retardation including all ages, active epilepsy was found in 20% corresponding to a prevalence rate of 1.2/1000 people [69]. This study also shows a clear relationship between the degree of mental retardation and frequency of epilepsy with epilepsy occurring in 11% of the mildly mentally retarded and increasing in moderate, severe and profoundly retarded to 12%, 23% and 59%, respectively [69]. In another study frequency of epilepsy increased from 9% in mild mental retardation to 43% in profound mental retardation [70].

Cognitive disability is also found in people with epilepsy due to stroke, or due to dementia. In adults with newly diagnosed unprovoked seizures, 18% were demented [40]. With a growing ageing population the coming decades will see the group with epilepsy and concomitant dementia increase substantially.

Motor disabilities

Motor disabilities are also common in epilepsy populations. Cerebral palsy is the most common motor disability in patients with epilepsy, not just in children but also in adults, affecting 16–21% and 9%, respectively [11–13,63]. The vast majority, 89–100%, of children with epilepsy and concurrent cerebral palsy are also mentally retarded [12,13,63]. Likewise, the combination of mental retardation and cerebral palsy increases the risk for epilepsy to 48% compared with 11% when either of these disabilities occur alone [71]. Epilepsy is more frequent in the most severe form of cerebral palsy, tetraplegia, occurring in 94% compared to 23% in patients with hemiplegia [72,73]. A hospital-based study including all forms of cerebral palsy found 42% of patients with cerebral palsy to have epilepsy [74]. Spastic tetraplegia is associated with more severe mental retardation and earlier onset of epilepsy than spastic hemiplegia, 1 month to 2.5 years vs. 3–4.5 years [67].

The comorbid neurological impairments when epilepsy, mental retardation or cerebral palsy occur in combination is a reflection of the severity of the underlying brain damage. Mental retardation and cerebral palsy should not be regarded as causes (or consequences) of epilepsy as sometimes stated in the literature. Instead, any combination of these three disorders should, with a few rare exceptions, be considered as different manifestations of a prior brain insult, usually one that occurred early in life.

Around 6% of adults with epilepsy have motor disabilities other than those connected with cerebral palsy, mostly in the form of hemiplegia caused by stroke [11].

Other associated disabilities

In adults with epilepsy other major disabilities were severe psychiatric disorders in 6%, severe visual impairment in 3% and severe hearing impairment in 2%. Other major somatic diseases (cardiovascular, pulmonary, renal, systemic) were found in 7% [11]. A Finnish study compared concurrent illnesses in adults with childhood onset epilepsy followed up for 35 years, with controls. The case–control comparison included patients with only epilepsy and no other neurological impairment. At the time of the investigation two-thirds of the epilepsy patients no longer had active epilepsy (5-year seizure remission without medication). Psychiatric disorders, but not somatic disorders, were more frequent in patients than in controls, 23% vs. 7% [64]. However, the frequency of somatic disorders was substantially higher in those who had died, than in controls.

Seizure frequency

The severity of epilepsy depends on several factors, e.g. seizure frequency, seizure type and duration of individual seizures. Seizure frequency is among the most important determinants of severity. In unselected epilepsy populations the severity varies from patients who after having two seizures are started on AED treatment and become seizure free (or even have no further seizures without AED treatment) to the other extreme with patients who from an early age have multiple daily seizures throughout life. Thus, epilepsy populations are extremly heterogeneous in seizure frequency.

In a population-based study of children 0–16 years with active epilepsy, almost half (48%) had no seizure in the preceding year, 23% had 1–11 seizures per year, 8% had 12–51 seizures per year, 12% had 52–364 seizures per year and 8% had daily seizures (>364 per year) [12]. In a study of children 0–15 years of age 53% had no

seizure in the preceding year, 30% up to 1 seizure per month and 17% more than 1 seizure per month [14]. A study of 6–12-year-old children found 31% seizure free in the preceding year, 29% with 1–12 seizures per year and 40% with more than 12 seizures per year [13]. In people more than 16 years old 44% had no seizure in the preceding year. One-third (32%) had less than one seizure per month (1–11 seizures per year), 13% had one to several seizures per month (12–50 per year), 11% had weekly seizures (more than 50 years) and 2.7% had more than 300 seizures per year [11]. Among people of all ages 36% of patients were seizure free during the preceding year [6]. The differences in the proportion of seizure-free patients in these studies are partly explained by differences in definition of active epilepsy. Summarizing the studies, in unselected seizure populations an estimated 40–50% have been seizure free during the last year, about 30% have up to one seizure per month and another 20–30% more than monthly seizures.

In patients with epilepsy and mental retardation the proportion with very frequent seizures is much larger than in the general epilepsy population. About 10% have daily seizures and another 15% have one seizure or more per week, which means that one-quarter have at least weekly seizures [69].

Studies from less developed countries find a larger proportion of people with epilepsy having frequent seizures. In Ethiopia where the seizure frequency was known for 91%, 10% had daily seizures, 27% weekly seizures, 47% monthly seizures and 16% yearly seizures but less than one per month [25]. In Bolivia 21% of patients with active epilepsy had weekly seizures, 53% monthly seizures, 21% yearly seizures, but less than one per month, and 6% less than one seizure per year [23]. The large proportion with high seizure frequency is probably due to the lack of antiepileptic treatment because in Ethiopia less than 2% received treatment and in Bolivia only 11% [23,25]. Part of the explanation for the large proportion with high seizure frequency in less developed countries may also be underascertainment of patients with low-seizure frequency.

Epidemiological time trends

The incidence of epilepsy was relatively stable in the population of Rochester in Minnesota, USA, for a 50-year period from 1935 to 1984 [43,75]. However, a major change occurred in the age-specific incidence. The incidence in children younger than age 10 years decreased successively by 40–50% between 1935 and 1984 with a slight increase during the last decade studied, 1975–1984 [43,75]. The reason for this decrease is unknown but improved ante- and perinatal care may be partly responsible. A decreasing incidence in children was also found in the UK where the cumulative incidence by age 5 years declined from 4 per 1000 in children born 1946 [76] to 2.9 per 1000 in children born 1958 [77]. In Sweden the incidence (neonatal seizures excluded) in children 0–15 years was 124 per 100 000 in 1973 and 73 per 100 000 in 1986, a more than 40% decrease in incidence [50,55]. Part of this decrease may be due to inclusion of non-epileptic events in the earlier study. However, a statistically significant decrease in incidence in children 0–20 years old was also reported from the UK in a study including single seizures and afebrile provoked and unprovoked seizures [48]. Incidence decreased by more than half, falling from 152 per 100 000 in 1974–83 to 61 per 100 000 in 1984–93.

The study from Rochester also found an increase in incidence in those over the age of 60 years that almost doubled during the 50-year study period [43]. In incidence studies of adults in Sweden, an increase from 34 per 100000 in 1986 to 56 in 1994 was noted [40,78]. The incidence in people younger than 60 years was the same in the two studies while a considerable increase was found in older age groups. Part of this increase can be due to a true increase in incidence but more complete case ascertainment in the latter study is also a likely explanation. The secular trend with an increased incidence in the elderly may be due to better survivorship from stroke, a group with increased risk for epilepsy, and due to more accurate case ascertainment. No information on trends exists from less developed countries.

Prognosis of seizures

The hope of patients, relatives and treating physicians is that future seizures can be prevented with a treatment that does not harm, and seizure freedom is maintained when treatment is stopped. Unfortunately, this is but one of many possible outcomes of epilepsy. Epidemiological population-based studies provide data that help formulate realistic expectations and prognosis for patients with specific characteristics. However, it has to be remembered that in the individual person the prognosis may deviate substantially from what studies tell us to expect.

Many studies have been published on the prognosis of seizures in epilepsy. Almost all that were published before 1970 were cross-sectional studies in hospital populations. These were biased by an overrepresentation of patients with severe epilepsy and the seizure prognosis observed was considerably worse than for general epilepsy populations. The prognostic data presented will therefore mainly include results from population-based studies on cohorts with incident or newly diagnosed patients. Hospital-based studies on newly diagnosed patients using multiple sources for identification are likely to have included most cases with epilepsy and are also included. For specific rare forms of epilepsy only hospital-based data exist.

The Guidelines for Epidemiologic Studies on Epilepsy defines epilepsy in remission as a prevalent case of epilepsy with no seizures for 5 or more years [1]. Depending on whether the patient is receiving AED treatment or not at the time of ascertainment, remission is further specified as occurring with or without treatment. Follow-up is short in many studies and remission is often given for shorter periods than 5 years. Terminal remission refers to patients still in remission at the end of a follow-up period. Temporary remission refers to patients where remission has occurred for a defined period earlier during the follow-up period, followed by a relapse. Permanent remission is not well defined but could be used for patients in terminal remission for a long period, e.g. 20 years, and judged to be very unlikely to relapse. The term could also be used for patients with specific syndromes with good prognosis once a certain age is reached, e.g. in patients with BECT after age 18 years. Cumulative remission refers to the proportion that has been in remission at any time during the follow-up period, i.e. both patients in temporal and terminal remission. Some studies have used the term temporary remission for cumulative remission. Studies on remission should be analysed by life-table techniques.

Early prognosis

The risk for a second seizure following a first unprovoked seizure has been investigated by several studies and these studies are discussed in detail in Chapter 12. When two unprovoked seizures have occurred the person per definition has epilepsy and the national laws regulating different aspects in relation to epilepsy are applicable, e.g. driving regulations. While a minority will have a second seizure following a first seizure, the proportion with a third or fourth unprovoked seizure following a second is considerably higher, 73% and 76%, respectively [79]. Seizure recurrence following a first, second or third seizure mainly occurs within 1 year [79].

Late prognosis, overall remission

What is the chance of achieving long-term remission? In population-based studies from more developed countries on incident or newly diagnosed cohorts with epilepsy the vast majority of patients are treated with AED. Thus, these studies give the prognosis of treated epilepsy and not the natural prognosis of epilepsy. Results from studies are very similar despite some variation in methods (Table 2.5). At 10 years follow-up 5-year cumulative remission was 58–65% in studies from the USA and the UK including all ages [80–82] and from Sweden including adults [86]. Terminal 5-year remission at 10 years follow-up was 61% [80]. Higher remission rates are found in children where 74–78% achieve 3–5 years remission at 12–30 years follow-up [84,85]. In a prospective study with patients mainly collected by paediatric neurologists, 10% of children developed intractable epilepsy with more than monthly seizures during 18 of the first 24 months following diagnosis [87]. The only study including all ages with a follow-up exceeding or of similar length as the childhood studies found a terminal 5-year remission rate of 70% at 20 years [80]. Fifty per cent were seizure free without antiepileptic treatment and 20% with treatment. Another study from the same area and partly including the same study population found a cumulative 5-year remission at 10 and 20 years follow-up of 58 and 75%, respectively, and a terminal 5-year remission at 10 years of 54% [88]. Based on these studies it can be concluded that at least two of three patients will eventually receive long-term remission, and about three of four in the childhood onset population.

Large hospital-based studies on cohorts with newly diagnosed patients provide data on remission periods of 1–2 years. Based on three studies 1-year remission at 3 years follow-up was 84–91%, and 64–97% at 5 years. The corresponding rates for 2-year remission was 57–71% and 79–90% [89–91]. A 2-year remission of 61% at 4 years follow-up was found in a population-based study from the UK [48].

Time to enter remission

All studies on incident or newly diagnosed patients find that most patients enter seizure remission early. The longer patients continue to have seizures the lower the probability for subsequent remission. Curves from studies depicting the relationship between remission and years after diagnosis have the same form with minor deviations (Fig. 2.3).

Table 2.5 Population-based studies on epilepsy prognosis

Country, year (reference)	In remission (%)[a]	Years of remission	Follow-up (year)	Number followed	Ages (years)	Comments
USA, 1979 (80)	65, 61	5	10	458	All	Incidence cohort, pop[b]
	76, 70	5	20			
UK, 1995,97 (81,82)	86, 68	3	7	564	All	Incidence cohort, pop[b]
	68, 54	5	7			
	82	3	7	397		SS' & APS[d] excluded
	62	5	7			SS' & APS[d] excluded
UK, 1983,95 (83,48)	74	4	10	184	All[e]	SS' & APS[d] included
Sweden, 1987 (84)	78	3	12	68	Child	Incidence cohort, pop[b]
Finland, 1993 (85)	76	3	30	178	Child	Inc & prev cohort, pop[b]
	74	5	30			
Sweden, 2001 (86)	64	3	10	107	Adults	SS[c] included
	58	5	10			

[a] Left and right column refers to temporary and terminal remission, respectively.
[b] Population-based.
[c] Single seizures.
[d] Acute provoked afebrile seizures.
[e] Incident and prevalent cases in a population-based study.

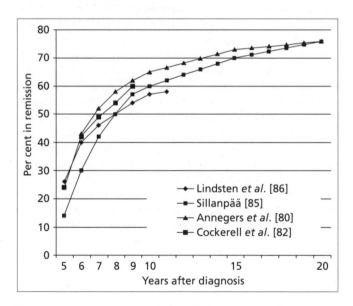

Fig. 2.3 Cumulative 5-year remission of epilepsy by years after diagnosis. Population-based studies.

Initial seizure frequency

The seizure frequency during the first 6 months greatly affects the chance to achieve long-term remission. In the National General Practice Study of Epilepsy (NGPSE) study a 1-year remission by 6 years follow-up was found in 95% of patients with up to two seizures during the first 6 months following diagnosis, and lower, 75% for patients with 10 or more seizures during the same period [42]. The corresponding rates for 5-year remission by 6 years were

47% and 24%. Studies of childhood onset epilepsy found similar results [84,85]. In children high initial seizure frequency also predicts the development of intractable epilepsy, defined as more than one seizure per month for at least 18 months, despite trial with at least three different AED during the first 2 years following diagnosis [87]. Only 12% of children achieved 1-year remission during a mean follow-up period of 38 months.

Studies focusing on the number of seizures before diagnosis or the start of AED treatment have inconsistent findings. In the NGPSE study, having had more than 10 seizures before the diagnostic seizure was associated with an increased chance of remission [42]. However, a hospital-based study found having more than 20 seizures before the start of antiepileptic treatment resulted in a lower proportion with remission than in those with less than 20 seizures [91]. Another hospital-based study found a high frequency of GTCS before treatment (two or more/month) to predict a lower chance to achieve remission [89]. A third hospital-based study, a study with single seizures included, found a higher chance to achieve long-term remission for those with only one seizure before treatment than those with two or more seizures [90]. This is what can be expected because of differences in the proportion at risk for further seizures between these groups, as reported from studies of recurrence following a first, second or third seizure (see above).

Predictors of seizure remission

Gender

There are syndromes with sex-linked inheritance where epilepsy is common and prognosis well defined, e.g. Rett syndrome and fragile X syndrome. These disorders are rare and have little impact on the influence of gender for seizure prognosis for the general epilepsy population. All studies in large epilepsy populations have found that gender has no influence on seizure prognosis [42,48,80,83,88,90,91].

Age at onset

The age at onset of epilepsy is not a significant predictor of remission. In Rochester, Minnesota, the proportion that achieved 10-year remission decreased with increasing age at onset [80]. Another study on partly the same population found age at first seizure not to be a predictor in the univariate analysis but the multivariate analysis showed diagnosis of epilepsy before age 16 years to be a significant predictor for achieving 5-year remission without antiepileptic treatment [88]. Other studies found small or no effect [48,83] [82]. In a Swedish adult population the age at diagnostic seizure (<50 vs. 50 years and older) was not a significant predictor of remission [86]. Large hospital-based studies in Italy and the UK did not find age on onset of seizures to predict achieving 1–3 years remission [89–91]. One study of childhood onset epilepsy found that age at onset was not a significant prognostic factor [84] for remission while another study reported a reduced risk for development of intractability in children with onset of epilepsy between ages 5 and 9 years [87].

Aetiology

Overall, idiopathic epilepsy has a better prognosis than symptomatic epilepsy. Studies on aetiology as a potential predictor for seizure prognosis have used the term idiopathic for cases with epilepsy of unknown cause and not as has been proposed for specific epileptic syndromes [37]. A study from Rochester, Minnesota, reported higher 5-year remission rates without medication for idiopathic epilepsy (36% and 42% after 10 and 15 years, respectively) than in the remote symptomatic group (remission rates 19% and 30%) [80]. However, after 20 years 5-year remission was slightly more frequent in the remote symptomatic group (54%) than in the idiopathic group (47%), a change the authors interpreted to be due to increased mortality in the remote symptomatic group leaving a subgroup with better prognosis. The difference was even larger at 20 years when all cases in remission (with and without medication) were included; 74% of the idiopathic cases and 90% of the remote symptomatic cases were in remission for 5 or more years. Another study that included part of the same population also found idiopathic aetiology to be a significant predictor for 5-year remission [88].

In a Finnish study of childhood onset epilepsy, remote symptomatic aetiology was a predictor for seizure intractability [85]. On the contrary, two studies from the UK on partly overlapping study populations reported no difference in 2- and 4-year remission between idiopathic and symptomatic cases [48,83]. However, the majority of symptomatic cases in these studies had acute provoked seizures. The British NGPSE study and a Swedish study did not find aetiology to be a significant predictor for remission, with more than 60% of both the idiopathic and remote symptomatic groups achieving cumulative 5-year remission at 9 or 10 years follow-up [42,81,82,86].

Some hospital-based studies found idiopathic epilepsy to have significantly better prognosis than remote symptomatic epilepsy with 74% and 60% in the respective groups achieving cumulative 1-year remission at 5 years follow-up [91]. Another study found no effect [90].

Comorbidities

Patients with other neurological dysfunctions besides epilepsy, believed to have been present from birth, have been analysed separately in some studies. Mental retardation and cerebral palsy make up the vast majority of cases in this group, often called the neurodeficit group or the group with early brain damage. This group has the worst prognosis for seizure remission. In Rochester, Minnesota, 5-year remission at 20 years was found in less than half, 46%, and this was achieved without medication in only 15%, and 30% at 10 and 20 years follow-up, respectively [80]. Conversely, the absence of early brain damage was a significant predictor for achieving cumulative 5-year remission [88]. Studies on childhood onset epilepsy have also found the neurodeficit group to have less chance of achieving long-term seizure remission [84,85]. By 12 years, 3-year seizure remission occurred in 79% of children without neurodeficit and in 39% of children with neurodeficit [84].

To summarize studies on incident/newly diagnosed epilepsy cohorts, we find that when epilepsy is due to early brain damage severe enough to cause other neurological impairments, i.e. mental retardation and/or cerebral palsy, aetiology is clearly a predictor for long-term seizure prognosis. Almost all studies find long-term seizure remission to be more common in those with epilepsy of unknown aetiology (idiopathic) than patients with symptomatic/cryptogenic aetiology.

Specific aetiological factors

Stroke

Following stroke, early seizures (ES) occur in 1.8% during the first 24 h [92] and in 4.1% to 6% within the first week [93,94] and in 4.4% to 5.2% during the first 2 weeks [95,96]. Early seizures should be classified as acute provoked seizures if they occur during the first week following stroke and thus all seizures in three of the five studies belong to this category [1]. Most ES, defined as acute provoked seizures that occur during the first week after the stroke, occur largely during the first 24 h in 78–87% of population-based studies [92,93]. A hospital-based study found 98% to have their ES during the first 48 h [95].

By 5 years after a stroke, approximately 12% of patients will have seizures, either early, late or both [92,93]. Early seizures increase the risk for late unprovoked seizures by eight times [92,93]. However, most patients with ES do not go on to have late unprovoked seizures or epilepsy. At 5-year follow-up 36% with ES went on to have seizures. Without ES only 7% developed epilepsy [92]. Overall, 21% of patients with ES who survived 1 week after cerebral epilepsy, developed epilepsy [94]. Epilepsy is more common following a late seizure, found in almost 55–60% after ischaemic stroke [94,96]. Early seizures do not predict 30-day mortality [92,93,95] when stroke severity has been accounted for. Status epilepticus occurs in one-quarter of stroke patients who have ES [93].

The characteristics of the stroke affect the occurrence and prognosis of seizures. Haemorrhagic stroke more often results in seizures than ischaemic stroke. Population-based studies report ES in 2–3% with ischaemic stroke, in 3–7% with haemorrhagic stroke and in 6–8% with subarachnoidal haemorrhage (SAH) [92,93]. The occurrence of ES also depends on location of the lesion being more common in lobar/cortical lesions (7%) than deep lesions (1%) [93]. When subtype and location of lesion are combined ES occurs in 14% with lobar/cortical haemorrhage, in 8% with SAH, in 6% with lobar/cortical ischaemia, in 4% with deep haemorrhage, and in <1% with deep ischaemia [93]. When ischaemic stroke patients are followed for 5 years the cumulative risk for seizures increased during the whole 5-year period and reached 10% [92]. After primary intracerebral haemorrhage and subarachnoid haemorrhage all seizures occurred by the third year, with a cumulative risk of 26% and 34%, respectively. Following ischaemic stroke, a hospital-based study reported seizures occurring within the first 2 weeks in 5% and after 2 weeks in 4% [96]. The corresponding rates for haemorrhagic stroke was 8% and 3%. Epilepsy occurred in 55% with ischaemic stroke and seizures after 2 weeks, and in all with haemorrhagic stroke and seizures after 2 weeks.

Early seizures due to stroke are mostly focal, but generalized seizures without obvious focal onset occur in 25–50% [92,93].

Trauma

Seizures following head trauma occur in 4–5% [97,98]. Early seizures occur in 2–3% and are more common in children than adults [97,98]. Late unprovoked seizures (late is defined as occurring more than 1 week after the insult) occur in 2% [98] and three-quarters of these will be recurrent, i.e. epilepsy [98]. Late seizures follow ES in 10–15%, mostly in adults with moderate to severe head injury [97]. In multivariate analysis ES do not predict late seizures [98]. The risk for seizures varies according to the severity of head trauma and time since head trauma. For all degrees of head trauma the elevated risk decreases with time. Mild head trauma (loss of consciousness or amnesia <30 min) results in a very minor increase for late seizures, which are only seen during the first 5 years following trauma [98]. Moderate head trauma (loss of consciousness or amnesia 30 min to 24 h, or skull fracture) causes a three-fold increase in seizures compared to the general population during the first 10 years following trauma but not thereafter. Severe head trauma (loss of consciousness or amnesia >24 h, brain contusion or intracranial haematoma) increases risk 17-fold, and the increased risk persists beyond 10 years.

CNS infections

CNS infections predispose to subsequent epilepsy that may appear many years later. In the USA CNS infections account for 15% of all acute provoked seizures (febrile convulsions excluded), corresponding to a yearly incidence of 5 per 100 000 [99]. A population-based study of people followed up an average of more than 10 years found ES in 19% [100] and by 20 years 7% had late unprovoked seizures. The majority, 58%, of late seizures occurred in patients with previous ES. However, most patients, 87%, with ES did not have later unprovoked seizures. In 98% (all but one patient) late seizures were recurrent. Thus, prophylactic antiepileptic treatment is unwarranted in CNS infections and ES, but should probably be started after a late unprovoked seizure.

Viral encephalitis with ES carries the highest risk for later epi-

lepsy, found in 10% by 5 years and 22% by 20 years follow-up [100]. Without ES, the cumulative risk of epilepsy after viral encephalitis is 10% by 20 years. The corresponding rates for bacterial meningitis is 13% with ES and 2% without ES, and 2% for aseptic meningitis at 20 years follow-up. The low cumulative incidence epilepsy following bacterial meningitis without ES and following aseptic meningitis is no greater than expected in the general population [100].

Seizures in patients with human immunodeficiency virus (HIV) infections have been reported in 3–5% in a prospective study, and in 11–17% in retrospective studies [101–104]. Most first seizures appear in advanced stages of acquired immune deficiency syndrome (AIDS). An aetiology can be identified in the majority and include cerebral toxoplasmosis, tuberculoma, cryptococcosis, progressive multifocal leukoencephalopathy and toxic-metabolic factors. Thus, most of these seizures are classified as acute provoked seizures. In the majority of patients seizures are recurrent [101]. A considerable portion of seizures is expected to be HIV related in countries where HIV infections are abundant, i.e. in many less developed countries.

Neurological examination

Since early brain damage causing neurodeficits is a strong predictor for long-term seizure prognosis it is not surprising that studies have found neurological abnormalities to be associated with increased risk for persistent epilepsy. This has been substantiated in childhood onset epilepsy [84,85] and in a hospital-based study of newly diagnosed cases [89,90].

Seizure type

By 20 years follow-up, 5-year remission was found in 85% of cases with idiopathic GTCS (50% off medication) and in 80% with absences, in Rochester, Minnesota [80]. Remission was lower, 65%, in patients with complex partial seizures (CPS) (35% off medication) although the CPS figures may be low due to under-ascertainment of mild cases. At 20 years follow-up, the highest remission rates, 77%, occurred in patients with generalized seizures and seizure onset before age 20 years. The lowest remission rate, 59%, was found in patients with PS and onset after age 20 years. In other studies seizure type was an inconsistent predictor for remission [42,48,82,83,86,87]. However, hospital-based studies on newly diagnosed cases have reported that multiple seizure types [90] and partial seizures [89] worsen long-term seizure prognosis.

Status epilepticus

In childhood onset epilepsy followed for 30 years, status epilepticus is a predictor for not achieving remission [85]. Prior acute symptomatic or neonatal status epilepticus, but not unprovoked or febrile status epilepticus, predispose to the development of intractable epilepsy [87].

EEG

In data from Rochester, Minnesota, multivariate analysis found that the absence of generalized epileptiform activity on the first EEG was a significant predictor for cumulative 5-year remission [88]. Whereas focal epileptiform activity and generalized non-epileptiform activity were not of prognostic value in children with epilepsy, focal slowing on the EEG was a predictor for development of intractable epilepsy [87].

Prognosis for specific epilepsies and syndromes

In children early development of intractable epilepsy occurred in 35% with cryptogenic/symptomatic generalized epilepsy, followed by 13% with localization-related symptomatic epilepsy and in 3% with idiopathic syndromes [87]. The more common specific epilepsies and syndromes where prognosis is known have their onset during childhood.

West's syndrome

Between 30 and 50% of children with this condition will become seizure free during long-term follow-up. Other seizure types besides spasms arise in 50–70% and 20–50% evolve into LGS [105]. Among people with West's syndrome followed for 20–35 years or until death, 33% of surviving patients have a terminal 2-year seizure remission. However, 31% died, mainly before age 10 years [106]. Intelligence was normal in 17% and only slightly impaired in another 7%. The aetiology of infantile spasms is a strong predictor for cognitive outcome with mental retardation occurring in 30–50% with cryptogenic aetiology and in 80–95% with symptomatic aetiology [105].

Lennox–Gastaut syndrome (LGS)

In 20–29% LGS develops without a preceding seizure disorder; in 13–40% it is preceded by infantile spasms; and in 40–50% by other seizure types [107,108]. After more than 10 years follow-up 5–13% are seizure free and 8% are not mentally retarded. In one study a better cognitive prognosis was found for patients with cryptogenic LGS [108] but no difference between aetiological groups was found by another study [107].

Absence epilepsy

The prognosis in absence epilepsies differs widely depending on the inclusion criteria and length of follow-up. In absence epilepsy with onset before age 10 years 90% achieved remission for 2 years or more when followed up for at least 20 years [109]. GTCS occurred in 16% of patients with onset before 9 years. In children with onset of absence epilepsy between 9 and 16 years (mean and median 12 years) only 37% achieved long-term remission and GTCS occurred in 79%. Another study where children were 1–14 years old at seizure onset and followed up for an average of 20 years, 65% achieved terminal 1-year remission off AED, 72% if cases still treated are included [110]. Among this same group 15% evolved a clinical picture of JME, or 44% of those without remission. Predictors for development of JME were slow response to treatment, absence status, family history of generalized seizures and background slowing on EEG.

Juvenile myoclonic epilepsy (JME)

Myoclonic jerks are the first seizure type in about 80%, GTCS in 15% and absences in the remainder [111]. Between 44 and 63% of people with JME become seizure free on antiepileptic treatment, mostly on valproic acid [112,113]. Recurrence of seizures is common when AED are discontinued, often necessitating treatment for several decades or lifelong [114].

Benign epilepsy of childhood with centrotemporal spikes (BECT)

The seizure prognosis in BECT is excellent with seizure freedom in 95% 5 years after onset and terminal remission without antiepileptic treatment in 100% by late teenage years [115]. A few case reports have been published with recurrence of seizures in adults following a childhood history of BECT. These rare patients may have developed a separate epileptic disorder as adults, not related to BECT.

Relapse after achieving remission

Relapse can occur despite achieving long-term remission and a mean annual relapse incidence of 1.6% has been reported [80]. Relapse occurred in 8% during the first 5 years following 5-year remission and in 15% at 10 years after remission. By 20 years following remission almost one-quarter (24%) had relapsed. Relapse by 20 years was most frequent in patients with CPS (32%) and became more common with increasing age. In patients aged 9 years or younger at diagnosis 13% had relapses following 5-year remission. and 22% when diagnosed at age 10–19 years, and to 32% and 45% when diagnosed at 20–59 years and 60 and above, respectively.

Mortality

To witness a seizure for the first time, especially a generalized convulsive seizure, is a frightening experience where many think the seizing person is dying. Despite this, patients, their relatives and physicians often are reluctant to discuss the risk of death in epilepsy. The physician may be unaware of an increased mortality in epilepsy, or, even when knowledgeable, the physician may feel that it is inappropriate to disclose this information for fear of creating unnecessary worry.

If, when, and how to inform about mortality in epilepsy are delicate matters that must be based on facts. During the last 10 years several studies on mortality in epilepsy have been published. These studies provide important information on an aspect of epilepsy that has largely not been addressed during the 1970s to the early 1990s. During these years population-based studies showed the prognosis of epilepsy to be much better than previous studies from tertiary referral centres and epilepsy hospitals with an overrepresentation of patients with severe epilepsy. This resulted in an optimistic picture of epilepsy that has been very important in providing a positive and hopeful view on epilepsy to patients, relatives and the general public. However, large subgroups of patients with severe epilepsy and increased mortality exist (see Chapter 3).

Methods used in epidemiological studies of mortality in epilepsy

Studies of mortality should strive for inclusion of all cases that develop epilepsy. This is best achieved in incidence studies where all new cases during a specified period are identified. Prospective identification of cases increases the chances for nearly complete ascertainment since the identification net in prospective studies is not entirely built on conventional registers. In addition to conventional registries, cases can in prospective studies be identified through key persons working where diagnostic registries are incomplete such as in wards for old and demented persons. Thus, epidemiological investigations of mortality in epilepsy should be population-based incidence studies. The results presented below mainly come from such studies. Studies requiring large numbers of patients are difficult to obtain in population-based studies, but higher numbers may be identified by including hospital populations, although the study population is not fully representative of the general epilepsy population.

Measures of mortality

Mortality rate (death rate) is the number of deaths during a specified period divided by the number of persons at risk of dying during the period. Studies on mortality rates in epilepsy often use death certificates to identify deaths related to epilepsy. One has to be cautious in interpreting results from studies based on death certificates since these are unreliable due to both false positives and false negatives [116]. For this reason mortality rates of epilepsy reported in this chapter are often supported by information from other sources such as medical records in addition to death certificates.

Mortality in epilepsy is often expressed as the ratio between the observed and expected numbers of death—the standardized mortality ratio (SMR). Expected deaths are calculated by measuring the death rates of a reference population with an age distribution that is similar to the study population. When there is no difference in mortality between the study and reference population the SMR is 1. The 95% CI provides an estimate of the significance of the calculated SMR. The SMR cannot be compared between studies when age distributions and age- and sex-specific death rates differ.

Proportionate mortality ratio gives the percentage of deaths in persons with epilepsy that are due to any one cause. Studies on proportionate mortality provide information on the distribution of various causes of death. However, in studies on proportionate mortality the frequency of deaths is not provided for a reference population. This makes it difficult to know if certain causes of death are under- or overrepresented in the epilepsy population.

Overall mortality in population-based studies

There are six population-based studies of mortality, five encompassing entire epilepsy populations [117–123] and one limited to adults [124]. In all studies mortality was presented as SMR (Table 2.6). All but one study [117] was based on incident/newly diagnosed patients. Most studies included persons who had only had a single unprovoked seizure at the time of the formation of the study cohort [120–124]. In one study 15% of the patients had acute symptomatic non-febrile seizures [120,121]. The SMR in this subgroup was 2.9 and similar to the whole group. SMRs in population-based studies vary from 1.6 to 4.1 (Table 2.6), which means that in unselected epilepsy populations the excess mortality is 60% to 310% of that in the control population without epilepsy.

The mortality rate for patients with known epilepsy in Poland was 7.8 per 100 000 person-years, and lower, 2.3 per 100 000 person-years, if information was based only on death certificates that reported epilepsy [117]. The mortality rate in Rochester, Minnesota, based on death certificates, was 0.68 per 100 000 person-years when epilepsy was listed as the underlying cause of death, and 2.4 if based on any mention of epilepsy on the death certificate [125].

Two studies have reported on mortality after childhood onset epilepsy. A population-based cohort of children with active epilepsy (245 cases, 61% incident, 39% prevalent) was identified in Finland between 1961 and 1964. When followed up 35 years later 90% (220 cases) of the cohort could be traced and 44 were dead, corresponding to a mortality rate of 6.2 per 1000 patient-years (95% CI 5.7–6.7) [126]. Several deaths occurred during adult age. The mortality rate in incident cases was 4.8 (95% CI 4.4–5.3) and in prevalent cases 8.4 (95% CI 7.8–9.0). The difference in mortality between incident and prevalent cases was significant with a relative

Table 2.6 Standardized mortality ratios (with 95% confidence intervals) in population-based studies of epilepsy, by aetiology

Country, year (reference)	Aetiology			
	All	Idiopathic	Remote symptomatic	Neurodeficit
Poland, 1974 (117)	1.8			
United States, 1980 (118)	2.3 (1.9–2.6)	1.8 (1.4–2.3)	2.2 (1.8–2.7)	11.0 (6.9–16.4)
United States, 1984 (119)	2.1 (1.9–2.5)	1.6 (1.3–1.9)	2.8 (2.4–3.4)	7.0 (4.6–10.2)
United Kingdom, 1994 (120)	3.0 (2.5–3.7)	1.6 (1.0–2.4)	4.3 (3.3–5.5)	50.0 (10–146)
United Kingdom, 2001 (121)	2.6 (2.1–3.0)	1.3 (0.9–1.9)	3.7 (2.9–4.6)	25.0 (5.1–73)
Iceland, 1997 (122)	1.6 (1.2–2.2)	1.3 (0.8–1.9)	2.3 (1.4–3.5)	
France, 1999 (123)	4.1 (2.5–6.2)	1.5 (0.4–3.9)[a]	6.5 (3.8–10.5)	
Sweden, 2000 (124)	2.5 (1.6–3.8)	1.1 (0.5–2.4)	3.3 (2.4–4.5)	
Range (SMR)	1.6–4.1	1.1–1.8	2.2–6.5	

[a] Includes all cases with seizures of unknown aetiology: idiopathic and cryptogenic.

risk of death among incident cases of 0.53 (95% CI 0.31–0.90, $P = 0.03$) [89].

A study from Australia reported on mortality in children with epilepsy where deaths occurred during childhood [127]. All children aged 1–14 years, who died and had a diagnosis of epilepsy or seizures, or another neurological diagnosis known to be associated with epilepsy, or died accidentally or unexpectedly, were identified from a database, and their diagnosis of epilepsy was confirmed or refuted based on a review of their medical records. A history of epilepsy, either active or inactive, was found in 93 of 1095 children who died. Based on an assumed prevalence of childhood epilepsy of 7/1000 the authors estimated the mortality rate to 3.1/1000 patient-years (95% CI 2.0–4.8) in children with epilepsy. The mortality rate in children without epilepsy was 0.23/1000 (95% CI 0.22–0.25), which results in a relative risk of 13.2 (95% CI 8.5–21).

The explanation for how childhood onset epilepsy mortality rates differ 100-fold between studies from Poland and the USA [117,125] and studies in Finland and Australia [126,127] is an effect of whether the total population [80,88] or the epilepsy population [126,127] was used in the denominator. When the epilepsy population constitutes the denominator the rate produced is also called the case-fatality rate.

Overall mortality in selected epilepsy populations

Mortality has also been studied in selected epilepsy populations. The selection bias in these studies differs widely, ranging from very selected populations to populations that approach the general epilepsy population. SMRs from nine studies in selected epilepsy populations varied from 1.9 to 15.9 [128–136]. The SMRs in these selected populations are generally higher than in population-based studies with ratios of 3 or more in six of nine studies [128–136], compared to ratios of 2–2.5 in most population-based studies. Selected epilepsy populations contain more people with severe epilepsy than unselected general epilepsy populations. Thus, the higher SMRs found in the selected populations indicate that mortality is related to seizure frequency and severity. This is supported in a study where SMR was higher in persons with moderate to severe epilepsy than in persons with few or no seizures [129].

Mortality by aetiology

The classification used by most studies investigating the effects of aetiology of epilepsy on mortality categorizes patients either as belonging to the group with unknown aetiology (idiopathic), or to the group with seizures due to conditions resulting in static encephalopathy (remote symptomatic). Patients with seizures and a CNS lesion presumed present at birth, e.g. cerebral palsy or mental retardation, have either been included in the remote symptomatic group [122,124] or classified as a separate entity—neurodeficits [118] or congenital deficits [120,121]. The term postnatal acquired secondary epilepsy is synonymous with remote symptomatic aetiology with the neurodeficit group excluded [118,119]. Progressive CNS disorders, e.g. brain tumours and neurodegenerative disorders, have often been included in the remote symptomatic group [118,120,122,124]. In a recent study [123] and according to guidelines [1] these cases were classified as a separate entity. This

study was also the only study to use cryptogenic epilepsies in the classification [123].

In population-based studies the mortality is lower in the idiopathic group than in the remote symptomatic group (Table 2.6). Most studies report little or no increase in mortality in the idiopathic group [120–124]. In the remote symptomatic group mortality was two to six times greater than in general population. The group with neurodeficits carries the highest mortality with SMRs between 7 and 50 [118–121]. An increased mortality in children with neurodeficits was reported in a Swedish cohort with a mixture of incident and prevalent children with epilepsy, and followed up for 12 years [84]. Eleven per cent of children with neurodeficit died compared with 2.5% in children without neurodeficit [84].

Mortality by age and gender

The majority of studies [117,118,122,124] report higher mortality in males than females with epilepsy. Age is another factor affecting the relative mortality. The relative mortality of epilepsy populations compared with reference populations is higher at all ages. Most studies have found an inverse relation between SMR and age. The highest SMRs are found in children, and decreasing SMRs are found with increasing age [117,118,120,129]. The high SMR in children and young adults with epilepsy is partly a reflection of two factors, the low mortality in the reference population and the high mortality in children with epilepsy and neurodeficits [84,116].

Although the highest SMRs are found in children the highest excess mortality is found in the elderly. In the Rochester, Minnesota, study [118] the lowest excess mortality due to epilepsy, 6/1000, was found in children, where the SMR is highest [116]. The highest excess mortality, 47/1000, or eight times higher than in children, was found in the oldest age group, 75 years and older [116]. In Iceland 81% of the study population had idiopathic epilepsy. When mortality was analysed by age at onset of epilepsy, no increase in mortality was found in any age group with idiopathic epilepsy [122].

Mortality by duration of epilepsy

The increase in mortality is most marked during the initial years following diagnosis. In the Rochester, Minnesota, study, when all types of epilepsy were included, the SMR was significantly increased during the first 10 years after diagnosis and after 25 years [118]. In the NGPSE in the UK [120,121] SMR significantly increased during the first 4 years following diagnosis, and especially so during the first year (SMR 6.6, 95% CI 4.8–8.7). This first year rate is comparable to a French study, with an SMR of 4.1 (95% CI 2.5–6.2) [123]. In a study from Iceland [122] the mortality was significantly increased during the first 14 years, but only marginally beyond the first 4 years. A significantly increased mortality was found during the first 2 years in a Swedish study [124], with the increase most marked during the first year (SMR 7.3, 95% CI 4.4–12.1). A late increase after 9–11 years was also found. In two study populations (Rochester, Minnesota and NGPSE) the overall mortality decreased with longer follow-up [118–121].

In studies of cases with an established epilepsy of several years duration there is an underrepresentation of patients with life-threatening causes of epilepsy causing increased mortality during the first year(s) following onset of seizures. Despite these early deaths, increased mortality has been reported from the majority of studies of selected populations with longstanding epilepsy [128–136] as compared with population-based incident populations [118–124]. The increased mortality in longstanding epilepsy due to less life-threatening aetiologies supports the assumption that other determinants besides aetiology contribute to mortality. Seizure frequency and seizure severity could be some of these factors (see Chapter 3).

Relative survivorship (RS)

The two- to three-fold increase of overall mortality in the epilepsy population can produce an impression of death being a more common outcome in epilepsy than it actually is. Another view is provided by the RS which is the proportion of observed to expected number of survivors. The decline in RS is highest during the first years after diagnosis, i.e. during the period with highest mortality. The decline becomes successively less pronounced. The RS at 5, 10 and 15 years following diagnosis was 91, 85 and 83% in one study [137]. Another study found the RS 20–30 years following diagnosis to be 66% in patients with remote symptomatic epilepsy, and over 95% in idiopathic epilepsies [122,137]. The importance of aetiology for the prognosis is illustrated by a study of childhood onset epilepsy where the RS to the age of 40 years was 73% (95% CI 65–81%) in those with remote symptomatic epilepsy and 87% in those with idiopathic epilepsy (95% CI 77–96%) [126].

Mortality by seizure type

Generalized tonic-clonic seizures (GTCS)

In studies assessing the effect of seizure type on mortality GTCS refers to seizures with no signs/symptoms indicating a focal seizure onset [118,122,124]. Idiopathic GTCS refers to patients without a known predisposing cause and are likely to have primary GTCS, although patients with secondary GTCS may be included inadvertently. A significantly increased mortality was reported from the USA for idiopathic GTCS with SMRs of 3.5 and 2.4 through 5 and 30 years following diagnosis, respectively [118]. In Iceland mortality was not increased in patients with idiopathic GTCS without generalized spike-wave activity on the EEG (SMR 1.0) [122]. The use of EEG criteria in the Icelandic study excluded a large portion of the primary GTCS from the idiopathic GTCS group. In Swedish males with GTCS following either idiopathic or remote symptomatic 'epilepsy there was a statistically significant risk for death' (SMR 3.9, 95% CI 2.3–6.8) [124]. Rates for GTCS in the cited studies are not fully comparable due to differences in inclusion [118,122,124].

Partial seizure (PS) with or without secondary generalization

Data regarding the relationship between PS and mortality rates have been inconsistent. In some studies mortality was not significantly increased in patients with complex PS with or without generalization or in idiopathic cases with PS (all types combined) [118,122]. However, one study reported increased mortality in PS in both males and females (SMR 2.1, 95% CI 1.2–3.6) [124].

Other seizure types

A significantly increased mortality was reported for myoclonic seizures (SMR 4.1) while no deaths were observed in patients with absence seizures with or without GTCS [118].

Cause-specific mortality

Population-based studies with control population

Population-based studies have found that persons with epilepsy have a significantly increased mortality due to cerebrovascular disease, SMR 2.6–4.2, and neoplastic disorders, SMR 2.9–4.8 [118,120,121,124], and pneumonia, SMR 3.5–10.3 [118,120,121]. The increased risk for death in neoplasm remained after exclusion of brain tumours [118,120,121]. An increased mortality due to accidents and non-heart/cerebrovascular circulatory disorders has also been reported [118]. Suicide is very uncommon in population-based studies of epilepsies [118,120,121,124].

Studies on selected populations with control population

In a large hospital-based study where an estimated 80% of the patients on which calculations were based had true epilepsy, mortality was increased for most causes examined [135]. Suicide was significantly more common than expected (SMR 3.5, 95% CI 2.6–4.6). Except for heart disease mortality was also increased for all causes examined in a long-term residential care unit for patients with epilepsy [130]. A later study in the same institution found an increased mortality for neoplasm (SMR 2.0, 95% CI 1.3–2.9) where only one of the 29 tumours was a brain tumour [131]. Circulatory diseases, including ischaemic heart disease and cerebrovascular disease, did not increase mortality (SMR 0.8, 95% CI 0.5–1.1). No suicides occurred [131].

Studies of proportionate mortality

The distribution of causes of death in epilepsy has been reported in several papers. The study populations differ widely, ranging from population-based [117,118,121,123] to general hospital-based [135] to highly specialized institutions [130,131,138]. The results are therefore very difficult to compare between studies.

Cerebrovascular disease accounts for 12–17% of epilepsy mortality except in patients from a long-term residential centre for persons with epilepsy where cerebrovascular disease was a less common cause (5–6%) of death [130,131] (Table 2.7). A substantial difference exists in the proportion of different causes of death also when population-based studies are compared [117,118,121,123] (Table 2.7). These differences can partly be due to different lengths of follow-up. For example in one study deaths due to brain tumours accounted for 53% of the mortality after 1 year following the epilepsy diagnosis [123]. Other studies on incident cases with a longer follow-up have found much lower proportions of deaths due to brain tumours, 9–15% [117,118,121]. Lower proportions were also reported from other than incident populations, 0.6–4% [130,131,135].

Table 2.7 Causes of death in epilepsy (proportionate mortality ratios,%)

Cause of death	Study						
	Poland [117]	US [118–19]	UK [121]	France [123]a	Sweden [135]	UK [130]	UK [131]
Cerebrovascular	12	14	12	17	14	6	5
Heart disease	16	19	8		16	10	19
Neoplasm, all	24	20	26		16	12	26
Brain tumours	15	8	9	53	4	0.6	0.8
Pneumonia	8	8	14		5	12	25
Suicide	7	1.6	0.5		1.3	3.3	0
Accidents	4	6			3	7	3
Seizure related	10	6	3			31	12
SUDEPb	4		0.5				6
Other	15	25	16	30	41	18	5

a Unprovoked seizures + progressive symptomatic.
b Sudden unexpected death in epilepsy.

Epilepsy and seizure-related mortality

When a person with epilepsy dies, death may be unrelated to the epilepsy disorder, be related to the underlying cause of epilepsy, or be seizure related. Seizure-related deaths comprise death during status epilepticus, accidents and drowning caused by seizures and sudden unexpected death in epilepsy (SUDEP). Suicide in persons with epilepsy is sometimes considered to be epilepsy-related. The relation between suicide and the epilepsy must be evaluated individually since suicide is not uncommon among persons who do not have epilepsy.

The pathophysiological mechanisms in SUDEP are presently unknown but believed to be seizure related [139,140]. Many studies on SUDEP have been published during the last decade and these are covered elsewhere (Chapter 3). It is enough to say here that the rates of SUDEP vary between different epilepsy populations, from 0.35 per 1000 person-years in an unselected population-based study [141], to around 1 per 1000 person-years in fairly unselected epilepsy populations [142–144], 1.5–6 per 1000 person-years in more selected populations [135,145–148], and around 1 per 100 annually in patients referred to epilepsy surgery [149] or with continued seizures following surgery [150]. In the only population-based study of SUDEP 1.7% of all deaths in the epilepsy cohort and 8.6% of deaths in ages 15–44 years was due to SUDEP [141]. In the ages 20–40 years SUDEP exceeded the expected rate of sudden death in the general population by nearly 24 times.

Two studies from a long-term residential care unit for patients with epilepsy found 20–31% of deaths to be due to epilepsy [130,131]. The 20% mortality reported in one of these studies appears to have been seizure-related deaths [131]. In an epilepsy hospital 35% had a possibly seizure-related death with a large proportion of deaths due to drowning (hospital next to a lake). Nineteen per cent of seizure-related deaths remained when drowned cases were excluded [138]. Studies of childhood onset epilepsy in Finland and Australia report 22–45% of deaths to be seizure related [126,127]. In the incident subgroup of a Finnish population-based study seizure-related mortality was 45% [126], which is very high compared to other incidence cohorts where

0.9–5.5% of deaths were seizure related [119–121]. A study of mortality in patients with epilepsy and mental retardation (prevalence population) found only 7% of deaths to be seizure related despite higher mortality in patients with frequent and severe seizures [134]. This may indicate that seizure frequency/severity in patients with neurodeficits are variables that in most cases represent markers of the severity of the underlying aetiology that contribute to mortality, and less often are directly responsible for death.

Overall it is reasonable to conclude that epilepsy doubles or triples mortality in people with epilepsy mainly due to the underlying causes of epilepsy and less often as a direct result of seizures. Thus, the potential to reduce mortality in epilepsy through reduction or elimination of seizures may be limited in the general epilepsy population but substantial in adolescents and younger adults with intractable epilepsy where SUDEP most often occurs [141,150].

There is no ready explanation for the late rise in mortality found in the Rochester, Minnesota, study 25–29 years after onset of epilepsy [118]. It may be seizure related, due to underlying diseases, due to late effects of antiepileptic treatment, or due to a combination of these and other factors. The increased mortality observed during the first 5 years following remission of seizures also indicates the contribution of non-seizure-related factors to mortality in epilepsy [118].

Epilepsy mortality in less developed countries

No studies have specifically investigated mortality in epilepsy populations of less developed countries. However, important information concerning mortality can be found in publications on epilepsy in less developed countries. A study from Sri Lanka identified deaths related to convulsive disorders through death certificates. Part of the study population seems to have had acute provoked seizures. Among patients over the age of 5 years 47% of deaths were due to malnutrition. The authors interpreted this group to be 'patients with frequent seizures who are neglected and become malnourished'. Seizure-related deaths were common. Drowning was the cause of death in 12%, status epilepticus in 6% and burns in 2.6% [151].

In Tanzania 164 patients with epilepsy identified and started on antiepileptic treatment between 1959 and 1971 were followed up in 1990 [152]. No antiepileptic treatment was available between 1973 and 1990. The majority were dead at follow-up and the majority of deaths with known cause were seizure related, mostly status epilepticus (15%), drowning (13%) and burns (6%). Compared to mortality in the general population, the mortality in patients with epilepsy was much increased. A substantial part of this increase was caused by seizures, although the retrospective nature of the study makes evaluation of causes of death uncertain. Mortality among untreated patients was similar to that for the group who were treated. The authors commented, 'Other factors such as good nutrition, family care and medical care were less available for epilepsy patients as compared with non-epileptic individuals. This indicates that the long-term survival of the epilepsy patients remained poor regardless of AED therapy, suggesting general neglect of the epilepsy patients in their society' [152].

In Ethiopia 20 patients in a prevalence population with epilepsy died during an observation period of 2 years with 45% of the deaths being seizure related, mainly status epilepticus [25]. The crude annual death rate was doubled in the epilepsy population compared to the general population of the study area [46]. This difference becomes even larger when age is controlled for, resulting in an SMR of 2.9.

A study from Kenya reported 78% of deaths in patients with epilepsy to be seizure related (status epilepticus, burns and falls) with the highest mortality occurring in young adults [153]. This study and the studies from Sri Lanka, Tanzania and Ethiopia consist of large proportions of patients not on treatment with AED. In contrast, another 1-year long study from Kenya among patients treated with AED found six deaths, none of which was seizure related [154]. A similar 1-year long study of treated patients from Ecuador found that three died, none seizure related [155]. Although small, these studies indicate that AED treatment is likely to reduce seizure-related mortality.

Mortality trends over time

During the last century a major improvement in the standard of living and availability of medical care has taken place including the introduction of new AED and epilepsy surgery. Although one would anticipate that this has decreased mortality in epilepsy, it is difficult to know for certain because of the lack of reliable data on epilepsy mortality over time. Studies evaluating trends in epilepsy mortality are based on death certificates causing the methodological problems discussed above.

The annual mortality rates for epilepsy declined from the 1950s to the 1970s [156]. A study of epilepsy mortality in the UK and the USA for 1959–94 found similar secular trends for both countries and for both sexes [157]. Epilepsy mortality declined profoundly after 1950 among people younger than age 20. A less marked decline was found in adults while mortality in the elderly declined between 1959 and 1974 but then increased. A marked birth cohort effect was found, with a fall with each successive birth cohort indicating that aetiological risk factors varied by generation [157]. The birth cohort effect could be due to a decrease in incidence in epilepsy which, as mentioned earlier, has been found for childhood epilepsy. The increase in mortality during the last decades in the elderly with epilepsy could be an effect of the high incidence of epilepsy in the elderly, which almost doubled during a 50-year interval (see the section on trends earlier in this chapter).

Prognosis in largely untreated populations

The natural history of epilepsy can be derived from untreated or largely untreated epilepsy populations. In less developed countries the vast majority of patients with epilepsy do not receive pharmacological treatment [158] for their epilepsy and would thus be suitable for the study of natural prognosis. In practice, however, once a patient with epilepsy is identified in a study it would be unethical to withhold AED treatment. A prospective study of the natural history is no longer possible once long-term prophylactic treatment is initiated. An analysis of epilepsy prognosis based on retrospective information in societies with high illiteracy rate and lack of calendars may have limited accuracy.

If epilepsy was a truly chronic condition not associated with increased mortality, the prevalence rate of active epilepsy would be similar to the cumulative incidence rate, but in fact it is much lower. To what extent can this discrepancy be explained by increased mortality and by seizure remission? It is known that mortality is increased in epilepsy, both in more and less developed countries (see above). The relative mortality may be similar in developed and developing countries, increasing 2–3 times. However, the highest mortality of general populations is found in less developed countries and multiplying that mortality 2–3 times means that the mortality is much higher in epilepsy populations of less developed countries than in epilepsy populations elsewhere. Yet a large proportion, probably the majority of untreated people with epilepsy anywhere in the world, leave the epilepsy population not because of death but because they remit spontaneously.

Does treatment affect the natural history of epilepsy?

When to start treatment with AED has been discussed widely due to concern that delay may reduce the possibility of seizure remission. However, studies of largely untreated populations with longstanding epilepsy in developing countries indicate otherwise. In Kenya over half of the epilepsy population became seizure free and another quarter had their seizure frequency reduced by at least 50% once treatment was initiated [154]. Long duration of epilepsy or a large number of seizures did not affect outcome. Similar results have been reported from Malawi, Ecuador and India [159,160]. In the study from India a majority of untreated patients with a mean duration of epilepsy of 7 years became seizure free [161]. Thus these studies indicate that the duration of epilepsy before treatment does not affect the likelihood of remission. However, the conclusion is not clear-cut because a lifetime total of more than 30 GTCS significantly decreased the chance for remission [161].

References

1 Commission on Epidemiology and Prognosis, International League Against Epilepsy. Guidelines for epidemiologic studies on epilepsy. *Epilepsia* 1993; 34: 592–6.

2 Zielinski JJ. *Epidemiology and Medicosocial Problems of Epilepsy in Warsaw. Final Report on Research Program no. 19–P–58325–F–01.* Warsaw: Psychoneurological Institute, 1974.

3 Granieri E, Rosati G, Tola R *et al.* A descriptive study of epilepsy in the district of Copporo, Italy, 1964–1978. *Epilepsia* 1983; 24: 502–14.

4 Maremmani C, Rossi G, Bonuccelli U, Murri L. Descriptive epidemiologic study of epilepsy syndromes in a district of northwest Tuscany, Italy. *Epilepsia* 1991; 32: 294–8.

5 Joensen P. Prevalence, incidence, and classification of epilepsy in the Faroes. *Acta Neurol Scand* 1986; 74: 150–5.

6 Olafsson E, Hauser WA. Prevalence of epilepsy in rural Iceland: a population-based study. *Epilepsia* 1999; 40: 1529–34.

7 Haerer AF, Anderson DW, Schoenberg BS. Prevalence and clinical features of epilepsy in a biracial population. *Epilepsia* 1986; 27: 66–75.

8 Hauser WA, Annegers JF, Kurland LT. Prevalence of epilepsy in Rochester, Minnesota: 1940–1980. *Epilepsia* 1991; 32: 429–45.

9 Beran RG, Hall L, Michelazzi J. An accurate assessment of the prevalence ratio of epilepsy adequately adjusted by influencing factors. *Neuroepidemiology* 1985; 4: 71–81.

10 Keränen T, Riekkinen PJ, Sillanpää M. Incidence and prevalence of epilepsy in adults in eastern Finland. *Epilepsia* 1989; 30: 413–21.

11 Forsgren L. Prevalence of epilepsy in adults in northern Sweden. *Epilepsia* 1992; 33: 450–8.

12 Sidenvall R, Forsgren L, Heijbel J. Prevalence and characteristics of epilepsy in children in Northern Sweden. *Seizure* 1996; 5: 139–46.

13 Waaler PE, Blom BH, Skeidsvoll H, Mykletun A. Prevalence, classification, and severity of epilepsy in children in western Norway. *Epilepsia* 2000; 41: 802–10.

14 Eriksson KJ, Koivikko MJ. Prevalence, classification, and severity of epilepsy and epileptic syndromes in children. *Epilepsia* 1997; 38: 1275–82.

15 Endziniene M, Pauza V, Miseviciene I. Prevalence of childhood epilepsy in Kaunas, Lithuania. *Brain Dev* 1997; 19: 379–87.

16 Beilmann A, Napa A, Sööt A, Talvik I, Talvik T. Prevalence of childhood epilepsy in Estonia. *Epilepsia* 1999; 40: 1011–19.

17 Cavazzuti GB. Epidemiology of different types of epilepsy in school age children of Modena, Italy. *Epilepsia* 1980; 21: 57–62.

18 Sangrador CO, Luaces RP. Study of the prevalence of epilepsy among school children in Valladolid, Spain. *Epilepsia* 1991; 32: 791–7.

19 Baumann RJ, Marx MB, Leonidakis MG. Epilepsy in rural Kentucky: prevalence in a population of school age children. *Epilepsia* 1978; 19: 75–80.

20 Cowan LD, Bodensteiner JB, Leviton A, Doherty L. Prevalence of the epilepsies in children and adolescents. *Epilepsia* 1989; 30: 94–106.

21 Placencia M, Shorvon SD, Paredes V *et al.* Incidence and prevalence in an Andean region of Ecuador. *Brain* 1992; 115: 771–82.

22 Lavados J, Germain L, Morales A, Campero M, Lavados P. A descriptive study of epilepsy in the district of El Salvador, Chile, 1984–1988. *Acta Neurol Scand* 1992; 85: 249–56.

23 Nicoletti A, Reggio A, Bartoloni A *et al.* Prevalence of epilepsy in rural Bolivia. A door-to-door survey. *Neurology* 1999; 53: 2064–9.

24 Osuntokun BO, Adeuja AOG, Schoenberg BS *et al.* Prevalence of the epilepsies in Nigerian Africans: a community-based study. *Epilepsia* 1987; 28: 272–9.

25 Tekle-Haimanot R, Forsgren L, Abebe M *et al.* Clinical and electroencephalographic characteristics of epilepsy in rural Ethiopia: a community-based study. *Epilepsy Res* 1990; 7: 230–9.

26 Rwiza HT, Kilonzo GP, Haule J *et al.* Prevalence and incidence of epilepsy in Ulanga, a rural Tanzanian district: a community-based study. *Epilepsia* 1992; 33: 1051–6.

27 Attia-Romdhane N, Mrabet A, Ben Hamida M. Prevalence of epilepsy in Kelibia, Tunisia. *Epilepsia* 1993; 34: 1028–32.

28 Christianson AL, Zwane ME, Manga P, Rosen E, Venter A, Kromberg JGR. Epilepsy in rural South African children—prevalence, associated disability and management. *S Afr Med J* 2000; 90: 262–6.

29 Sridharan R, Murthy BN. Prevalence and pattern of epilepsy in India. *Epilepsia* 1999; 40: 631–6.

30 Mani KS, Rangan G, Srinivas HV, Kalyanasundaram S, Narendran S, Reddy AK. The Yelandur study: a community-based approach to epilepsy in rural India—epidemiological aspects. *Seizure* 1998; 7: 281–8.

31 Radhakrishnan K, Pandian JD, Santhoshkumar T *et al.* Prevalence, knowledge, attitude, and practice of epilepsy in Kerala, South India. *Epilepsia* 2000; 41: 1027–35.

32 Aziz H, Ali SM, Frances P, Khan MI, Hasan KZ. Epilepsy in Pakistan: a population-based epidemiologic study. *Epilepsia* 1994; 35: 950–8.

33 Aziz H, Guvener A, Akhtar SW, Hasan KZ. Comparative epidemiology of epilepsy in Pakistan and Turkey: population-based studies using identical protocols. *Epilepsia* 1997; 38: 716–22.

34 Wright J, Pickard N, Whitfield A, Hakin N. A population-based study of the prevalence, clinical characteristics and effect of ethnicity in epilepsy. *Seizure* 2000; 9: 309–13.

35 Morgan CLI, Ahmed Z, Kerr MP. Social deprivation and prevalence of epilepsy and associated health usage. *J Neurol Neurosurg Psychiatry* 2000; 69: 13–17.

36 Commission on Classification and Terminology of the International League Against Epilepsy. Proposal for revised clinical and electroencephalographic classification of epileptic seizures. *Epilepsia* 1981; 22: 489–501.

37 Commission on Classification and Terminology of the International League Against Epilepsy. A revised proposal for the classification of epilepsies and epileptic syndromes. *Epilepsia* 1989; 30: 389–99.

38 Loiseau J, Loiseau P, Guyot M, Duché B, Dartigues J-F, Aublet B. Survey of seizure disorders in French southwest. I. Incidence of epileptic syndromes. *Epilepsia* 1990; 31: 391–6.

39 Olafsson E, Hauser WA, Ludvigsson P, Gudmundsson G. Incidence of epilepsy in rural Iceland—a population-based study. *Epilepsia* 1996; 37: 951–5.

40 Forsgren L, Bucht G, Eriksson S, Bergmark L. Incidence and clinical characterization of unprovoked seizures in adults: a prospective population-based study. *Epilepsia* 1996; 37: 224–9.

41 Jallon P, Goumaz M, Haenggeli C, Morabia A. Incidence of first epileptic seizures in the canton of Geneva, Switzerland. *Epilepsia* 1997; 38: 547–52.

42 MacDonald BK, Cockerell OC, Sander JWAS, Shorvon SD. The incidence and lifetime prevalence of neurological disorders in a prospective community-based study in the UK. *Brain* 2000; 123: 665–76.

43 Hauser WA, Annegers JF, Kurland LT. Incidence of epilepsy and unprovoked seizures in Rochester, Minnesota: 1935–1984. *Epilepsia* 1993; 34: 453–68.

44 Zarrelli MM, Beghi E, Rocca WA, Hauser WA. Incidence of epileptic syndromes in Rochester, Minnesota: 1980–1984. *Epilepsia* 1999; 40: 1708–14.

45 Jallon P, Smadja D, Cabre P, Le Mab G, Bazin M, and EPIMART Group. EPIMART: Prospective incidence study of epileptic seizures in newly referred patients in a French Caribbean island (Martinique). *Epilepsia* 1999; 40: 1103–9.

46 Tekle-Haimanot R, Forsgren L, Ekstedt J. Incidence of epilepsy in rural central Ethiopia. *Epilepsia* 1997; 38: 541–6.

47 Li S, Schoenberg BS, Wang C, Cheng X, Zhou S, Bolis CL. Epidemiology of epilepsy in urban areas of the People's Republic of China. *Epilepsia* 1990; 31: 391–6.

48 Cockerell OC, Eckle I, Goodridge DMG, Sander JWA, Shorvon SD. Epilepsy in a population of 6000 re-examined: secular trends in first attendance rates, prevalence, and prognosis. *J Neurol Neurosurg Psychiatry* 1995; 58: 570–6.

49 Wallace H, Shorvon S, Tallis R. Age-specific incidence and prevalence rates of treated epilepsy in an unselected population of 2052 922 and age-specific fertility rates of women with epilepsy. *Lancet* 1998; 352: 1970–3.

50 Sidenvall R, Forsgren L, Blomquist HK, Heijbel J. A community-based prospective incidence study of epileptic seizures in children. *Acta Paediatr* 1993; 82: 62–5.

51 Sander JWAS, Hart YM, Johnson AL, Shorvon SD. National general practice study of epilepsy: newly diagnosed epileptic seizures in a general population. *Lancet* 1990; 336: 1267–71.

52 Shamansky SL, Glaser G. Socioeconomic characteristics of childhood seizure disorders in the New Haven area: an epidemiologic study. *Epilepsia* 1979; 20: 457–74.

53 Manford M, Hart YM, Sander JWAS, Shorvon SD. The National General Practice Study of Epilepsy. The syndromic classification of the Interna-

tional League Against Epilepsy applied to epilepsy in a general population. *Arch Neurol* 1992; 49: 801–8.

54 Olsson I. Epidemiology of absence epilepsy. *Acta Paediatr Scand* 1988; 77: 860–6.

55 Heijbel J, Blom S, Bergfors PG. Benign epilepsy of children with centrotemporal EEG foci. A study of incidence rate in outpatient care. *Epilepsia* 1975; 16: 657–64.

56 Sidenvall R, Eeg-Olofsson O. Epidemiology of infantile spasm in Sweden. *Epilepsia* 1995; 36: 572–4.

57 Riikonen R, Donner M. Incidence and aetiology of infantile spasms from 1960 to 1976: a population study in Finland. *Dev Med Child Neurol* 1979; 21: 333–43.

58 Hauser WA, Morris ML, Heston LL, Anderson VE. Seizures and myoclonus in patients with Alzheimer's disease. *Neurology* 1986; 36: 1226–30.

59 Romanelli MF, Morris JC, Ashkin K, Coben LA. Advanced Alzheimer's disease is a risk factor for late-onset seizures. *Arch Neurol* 1999; 47: 847–50.

60 Mendez MF, Catanzaro P, Doss RC, Arguello R, Frey II WH. Seizures in Alzheimer's disease: clinicopathologic study. *J Geriatr Psychiatry Neurol* 1994; 7: 230–3.

61 Hesdorffer DC, Hauser WA, Annegers JF, Kokmen E, Rocca WA. Dementia and adult-onset unprovoked seizures. *Neurology* 1996; 46: 727–30.

62 Carpio A, Hauser WA, Lisanti N, Roman M, Aguirre R, Pesantez J. Etiology of epilepsy in Ecuador. *Epilepsia* 2001; 42 (Suppl. 2): 122.

63 Steffenburg U, Hagberg G, Viggedal G, Kyllerman K. Active epilepsy in mentally retarded children. I. Prevalence and additional neuroimpairments. *Acta Paediatr* 1995; 84: 1147–52.

64 Jalava M, Sillanpää M. Concurrent illnesses in adults with childhood-onset epilepsy: a population-based 35-year follow-up study. *Epilepsia* 1996; 37: 1155–63.

65 Koul R, Razdan S, Motta A. Prevalence and pattern of epilepsy (Lath/Mirgi/Laran) in rural Kashmir, India. *Epilepsia* 1988; 29: 116–22.

66 Blomquist HK, Gustavsson K-H, Holmgren G. Mild mental retardation in children in a northern Swedish county. *J Ment Defic Res* 1981; 25: 169–86.

67 Airaksinen EM, Matilainen R, Mononen T, Mustonen K, Partanen J, Jokela V, Halonen P. A population-based study of epilepsy in mentally retarded children. *Epilepsia* 2000; 41: 1214–20.

68 Gustavson K-H, Holmgren G, Jonsell R, Blomquist HK. Severe mental retardation in children in a northern Swedish county. *J Ment Defic Res* 1977; 21: 161–80.

69 Forsgren L, Edvinsson S-O, Blomquist HK, Heijbel J, Sidenvall R. Epilepsy in a population of mentally retarded children and adults. *Epilepsy Res* 1990; 6: 234–48.

70 Jacobson JW, Janicki MP. Observed prevalence in multiple mental disabilities. *Ment Retard* 1983; 21: 87–94.

71 Hauser WA, Shinnar S, Cohen H, Inbar D, Benedetti MD. Clinical predictors of epilepsy among children with cerebral palsy and/or mental retardation. *Neurology* 1987; 37 (Suppl. 1): 150.

72 Edebol-Tysk K. Epidemiology of spastic tetraplegic cerebral palsy in Sweden. I. Impairment and disabilities. *Neuropediatrics* 1989; 20: 41–5.

73 Uvebrant P. Hemiplegic cerebral palsy. Aetiology and outcome. *Acta Paediatr Scand* 1988; 345 (Suppl.): 1–82.

74 Hadjipanayis A, Hadjichristodoulou C, Youroukos S. Epilepsy in patients with cerebral palsy. *Dev Med Child Neurol* 1997; 39: 659–63.

75 Annegers JF, Hauser WA, Lee JR, Rocca WA. Secular trends and birth cohort effects in unprovoked seizures in Rochester, Minnesota: 1935–1984. *Epilepsia* 1995; 36: 575–9.

76 Britten N, Wadsworth MEJ, Fenwick PBC. Stigma in patients with early epilepsy: a national longitudinal study. *J Epidemiol Community Health* 1984; 38: 291–5.

77 Kurtz Z, Tookey P, Ross E. Epilepsy in young people: 23 year follow up of the British national child development study. *BMJ* 1998; 316: 339–42.

78 Forsgren L. Prospective incidence study and clinical characterization of seizures in newly referred adults. *Epilepsia* 1990; 31; 292–301.

79 Hauser WA, Rich SS, Lee JRJ, Annegers JF, Anderson VE. Risk of recurrent seizures after two unprovoked seizures. *N Engl J Med* 1998; 338: 429–34.

80 Annegers JF, Hauser WA, Elveback LR. Remission of seizures and relapse in patients with epilepsy. *Epilepsia* 1979; 30: 729–37.

81 Cockerell OC, Johnson AJ, Goodridge DMG, Sander JWAS, Shorvon SD. Remission of epilepsy: results from the National General Practice Study of Epilepsy. *Lancet* 1995; 346: 140–4.

82 Cockerell OC, Johnson AJ, Goodridge DMG, Sander JWAS, Shorvon SD. Prognosis of epilepsy: a review and further analysis of the first nine years of the British National General Practice Study of Epilepsy, a prospective population-based study. *Epilepsia* 1997; 38: 31–46.

83 Goodridge DMG, Shorvon SD. Epileptic seizures in a population of 6000. II: Treatment and prognosis. *BMJ* 1983; 287: 641–7.

84 Brorson L-O, Wranne L. Long-term prognosis in childhood epilepsy: survival and seizure prognosis. *Epilepsia* 1987; 28: 324–30.

85 Sillanpää M. Remission of seizures and predictors of intractability in long-term follow-up. *Epilepsia* 1993; 34: 930–6.

86 Lindsten H, Stenlund H, Forsgren L. Remission of seizures in a population-based adult cohort with a newly diagnosed unprovoked epileptic seizure. *Epilepsia* 2001; 42: 1025–30.

87 Berg AT, Shinnar S, Levy SR, Testa FM, Smith-Rapaport S, Beckerman B. Early development of intractable epilepsy in children. *Neurology* 2001; 56: 1445–52.

88 Shafer SQ, Hauser WA, Annegers JF, Klass DW. EEG and other early predictors of epilepsy remission: a community study. *Epilepsia* 1988; 29: 590–600.

89 Elwes RDC, Johnson AL, Shorvon SD, Reynolds EH. The prognosis for seizure control in newly diagnosed epilepsy. *N Engl J Med* 1984; 311: 944–7.

90 Collaborative Group for the Study of Epilepsy. Prognosis of epilepsy in newly referred patients: a multicenter prospective study of the effects of monotherapy on the long-term course of epilepsy. *Epilepsia* 1992; 33: 45–51.

91 Kwan P, Brodie MJ. Early identification of refractory epilepsy. *N Engl J Med* 2000; 342: 314–19.

92 Burn J, Dennis M, Bamford J, Sandercock P, Wade D, Warlow C. Epileptic seizures after a first stroke: the Oxfordshire community stroke project. *BMJ* 1997; 315: 1582–7.

93 Labovitz DL, Hauser WA, Sacco RL. Prevalence and predictors of early seizure and status epilepticus after first stroke. *Neurology* 2001; 57: 200–6.

94 So EL, Annegers JF, Hauser WA, O'Brien PC, Whisnant JP. Population-based study of seizure disorders after cerebral infarction. *Neurology* 1996; 46: 350–5.

95 Kilpatrick CJ, Davis SM, Tress BM, Rossiter SC, Hopper JL, Vandendriesen ML. Epileptic seizures in acute stroke. *Arch Neurol* 1990; 47: 157–60.

96 Bladin CF, Alexandrov AV, Bellavance A *et al.* Seizures after stroke. A prospective multicenter study. *Arch Neurol* 2000; 57: 1617–22.

97 Annegers JF, Grabow JD, Groover RV, Laws Jr ER, Elveback LR, Kurland LT. Seizures after head trauma: a population study. *Neurology* 1980; 30: 683–9.

98 Annegers JF, Hauser WA, Coan SP, Rocca WA. A population-based study of seizures after traumatic brain injuries. *N Engl J Med* 1998; 338: 20–4.

99 Annegers JF, Hauser WA, Lee JR-J, Rocca WA. Incidence of acute symptomatic seizures in Rochester, Minnesota, 1935–1984. *Epilepsia* 1995; 36: 327–33.

100 Annegers JF, Hauser WA, Beghi E, Nicolosi A, Kurland LT. The risk of unprovoked seizures after encephalitis and meningitis. *Neurology* 1988; 38: 1407–10.

101 Pasqual-Sedano B, Iranzo A, Marti-Fabregas J *et al.* Prospective study of new-onset seizures in patients with human immunodeficiency virus infection. *Arch Neurol* 1999; 56: 609–12.

102 Chadha DS, Handa A, Sharma SK, Varadarajulu P, Singh AP. Seizures in patients with human immunodeficiency virus infections. *J Assoc Physicians India* 2000; 48: 573–6.

103 Wong MC, Suite NDA, Labar DR. Seizures in human immunodeficiency virus infection. *Arch Neurol* 1990; 47: 640–2.

104 Levy RM, Bredesen DE. Central nervous diseases in acquired immunodeficiency syndrome. *J Aquired Defic Syndr Hum Retrovirol* 1988; 1: 41–64.

105 Wong M, Trevathan E. Infantile spasms. *Pediatr Neurol* 2001; 24: 89–98.

106 Riikonen R. Long-term outcome of West syndrome: a study of adults with a history of infantile spasms. *Epilepsia* 1996; 37: 367–72.

107 Rantala H, Putkonen T. Occurrence, outcome, and prognostic factors of infantile spasms and Lennox–Gastaut syndrome. *Epilepsia* 1999; 40: 286–9.

108 Goldsmith IL, Zupanc ML, Buchhalter JR. Long-term seizure outcome in 74 patients with Lennox–Gastaut syndrome: effects of incorporating MRI head imaging in defining the cryptogenic subgroup. *Epilepsia* 2000; 41: 395–9.

109 Loiseau P, Duche B, Pedespan J-M. Absence epilepsies. *Epilepsia* 1995; 36: 1182–6.

110 Wirrell EC, Camfield CS, Camfield PR, Gordon KE, Dooley JM. Long-term prognosis of typical childhood absence epilepsy: remission or progression to juvenile myoclonic epilepsy. *Neurology* 1996; 47: 912–18.

111 Sundqvist A. Juvenile myoclonic epilepsy: events before diagnosis. *J Epilepsy* 1990; 3: 189–92.

112 Sharpe C, Buchanan N. Juvenile myoclonic epilepsy: diagnosis, management and outcome. *Med J Aust* 1995; 162: 133–4.

113 Kleveland G, Engelsen B. Juvenile myoclonic epilepsy: clinical characteristics, treatment and prognosis in a Norwegian population of patients. *Seizure* 1998; 7: 31–8.

114 Shinnar S, Berg AT, Moshe SL *et al.* Discontinuing antiepileptic drugs in children with epilepsy: a prospective study. *Ann Neurol* 1994; 35: 534–45.

115 Astradsson A, Olafsson E, Ludvigsson P, Bjorgvinsson H, Hauser WA. Rolandic epilepsy: an incidence study on Iceland. *Epilepsia* 1998; 39: 884–6.

116 Hauser WA, Hesdorffer D. *Epilepsy: Frequency, Causes and Consequences.* New York: Demos Publications, 1990.

117 Zielinski JJ. Epilepsy and mortality rate and cause of death. *Epilepsia* 1974; 15: 191–201.

118 Hauser WA, Annegers J, Elveback L. Mortality in patients with epilepsy. *Epilepsia* 1980; 21: 399–412.

119 Annegers JF, Hauser JF, Shirts SB. Heart disease mortality and morbidity in patients with epilepsy. *Epilepsia* 1984; 25: 699–704.

120 Cockerell O, Johnson A, Sander JWAS, Hart Y, Goodridge D, Shorvon S. Mortality from epilepsy: results from a prospective population based study. *Lancet* 1994; 344: 918–21.

121 Lhatoo SD, Johnson AL, Goodridge DM, MacDonald BK, Sander JWAS, Shorvon SD. Mortality in epilepsy in the first 11–14 years after diagnosis: multivariate analysis of a long-term, prospective, population-based cohort. *Ann Neurol* 2001; 49: 336–44.

122 Olafsson E, Hauser WA, Gudmundsson G. Long-term survival of people with unprovoked seizures. A population-based study. *Epilepsia* 1998; 39: 89–92.

123 Loiseau J, Picot M-C, Loiseau P. Short-term mortality after a first epileptic seizure: a population-based study. *Epilepsia* 1999; 40: 1388–93.

124 Lindsten H, Nyström L, Forsgren L. Mortality in an adult cohort with newly diagnosed unprovoked epileptic seizure. A population-based study. *Epilepsia* 2000; 41: 1469–73.

125 Hauser WA, Annegers JF, Rocca WA. Descriptive epidemiology of epilepsy: contributions of population-based studies from Rochester, Minnesota. *Mayo Clin Proc* 1996; 71: 576–86.

126 Sillanpää M, Jalava M, Kaleva O, Shinnar S. Long-term prognosis of seizures with onset in childhood. *N Engl J Med* 1998; 338: 1715–22.

127 Harvey AS, Nolan T, Carlin JB. Community-based study of mortality in children with epilepsy. *Epilepsia* 1993; 34: 597–603.

128 Alström CH. A study of epilepsy in its clinical, social and genetic aspects. *Acta Psychiatr Neurol Scand* 1950; Suppl. 63: 1–284.

129 Henriksen B, Juul-Jensen P, Lund M. The mortality of epilepsy. In: Brackenridge RDC, ed. *Proceedings of the 10th International Congress of Life Insurance Medicine.* London: Pitman, 1970: 139–48.

130 White SJ, McLean AEM, Howland C. Anticonvulsant drugs and cancer. A cohort study in patients with severe epilepsy. *Lancet* 1979; 2: 458–61.

131 Klenerman P, Sander JWAS, Shorvon SD. Mortality in patients with epilepsy: a study of patients in long term residential care. *J Neurol Neurosurg Psychiatry* 1993; 56: 149–52.

132 Nashef L, Fish DR, Sander JWAS, Shorvon SD. Incidence of sudden unexpected death in an adult outpatient cohort with epilepsy at a tertiary referral centre. *J Neurol Neurosurg Psychiatry* 1995; 58: 462–4.

133 Nashef L, Fish DR, Garner S, Sander JWAS, Shorvon SD. Sudden death in epilepsy: a study of incidence in a young cohort with epilepsy and learning difficulty. *Epilepsia* 1995; 36: 1187–94.

134 Forsgren L, Edvinsson S-O, Nyström L, Blomquist KH. Influence of epilepsy on mortality in mental retardation: an epidemiologic study. *Epilepsia* 1996; 37: 956–63.

135 Nilsson L, Tomson T, Farahmand B, Diwan V, Persson PG. Cause-specific mortality in epilepsy: a cohort study of more than 9000 patients once hospitalized for epilepsy. *Epilepsia* 1997; 38: 1062–8.

136 Shackleton DP, Westendorp RGJ, Kasteleijn-Nolst Trenité DGA, Vandenbroucke JP. Mortality in patients with epilepsy: 40 years of follow up in a Dutch cohort study. *J Neurol Neurosurg Psychiatry* 1999; 66: 636–40.

137 Hauser WA, Kurland LT. The epidemiology of epilepsy in Rochester, Minnesota, 1935 through 1967. *Epilepsia* 1975: 16: 1–66.

138 Iivanainen M, Lehtinen J. Causes of death in institutionalized epileptics. *Epilepsia* 1979; 20: 485–92.

139 Nashef L, Walker F, Allen P, Sander JWAS, Shorvon SD, Fish DR. Apnoe and bradycardia during epileptic seizures: relation to sudden death in epilepsy. *J Neurol Neurosurg Psychiatry* 1996; 60: 297–300.

140 Lathers CM, Schraeder PL, Boggs JG. Sudden unexplained death and autonomic dysfunction. In: Engel J Jr, Pedley TA, eds. *Epilepsy: A Comprehensive Textbook,* Philadelphia: Lippincott-Raven Publishers, 1997: 1943–55.

141 Ficker DM, So EL, Shen WK *et al.* Population-based study of the incidence of sudden unexplained death in epilepsy. *Neurology* 1998; 51: 1270–4.

142 Leestma JE, Walzak T, Hughes JR, Kalelkar MB, Teas SS. A prospective study of sudden unexpected death in epilepsy. *Ann Neurol* 1989; 26: 195–203.

143 Jick SS, Cole TB, Mesher RA, Tennis P, Jick H. Sudden unexpected death in young persons with primary epilepsy. *Pharmacoepidemiol Drug Saf* 1992; 1: 59–64.

144 Tennis P, Cole TB, Annegers JF, Leestma JE, McNutt M, Rajput A. Cohort study of incidence of sudden unexplained death in persons with seizure disorders treated with antiepileptic drugs in Saskatchewan, Canada. *Epilepsia* 1995; 36: 29–36.

145 Lip GYH, Brodie MJ. Sudden death in epilepsy: an avoidable outcome. *J R Soc Med* 1992; 85: 609–11.

146 Timmings PL. Sudden unexpected deaths in epilepsy: a local audit. *Seizure* 1993; 2: 287–90.

147 Leestma JE, Annegers JF, Brodie MJ, Brown S, Schraeder P, Siscovick D. Sudden unexplained death in epilepsy: observations from a large clinical development program. *Epilepsia* 1997; 38: 47–55.

148 Nilsson L, Farahmand B, Persson PG, Thiblin I, Tomson T. Risk factors for sudden, unexpected death in epilepsy — a case control study. *Lancet* 1999; 353: 888–93.

149 Dasheiff RM. Sudden unexpected death in epilepsy: a series from an epilepsy surgery program and speculation on the relationship to sudden cardiac death. *J Clin Neurophysiol* 1991; 8: 216–22.

150 Sperling MR, Feldman H, Kinman J, Liporace JD, O'Connor MJ. Seizure control and mortality in epilepsy. *Ann Neurol* 1999; 46: 45–50.

151 Senanyake N, Peiris H. Mortality related to convulsive disorders in a developing country in Asia: trends over 20 years. *Seizure* 1995; 4: 273–7.

152 Jilek-Aall L, Rwiza HT. Prognosis of epilepsy in a rural African community: a 30-year follow-up of 164 patients in an outpatient clinic in rural Tanzania. *Epilepsia* 1992; 33: 645–50.

153 Snow RW, Williams REM, Rogers JE, Mung'ala VO, Peshu N. The prevalence of epilepsy among a rural Kenyan population. *Trop Geogr Med* 1994; 46: 175–9.

154 Feksi AT, Kaamugisha J, Sander JWAS, Gatiti S, Shorvon SD. Comprehensive primary health care antiepileptic drug treatment programme in rural and semi-urban Kenya. *Lancet* 1991; 337: 406–9.

155 Placencia M, Sander JWAS, Shorvon SD *et al.* Antiepileptic drug treatment in a community health care setting in northern Ecuador: a prospective 12-month assessment. *Epilepsy Res* 1993; 14: 237–44.

156 Massey EW, Schoenberg BS. Mortality from epilepsy. *Neuroepidemiology* 1985; 4: 65–70.

157 O'Callaghan FJK, Osmond C, Martyn CN. Trends in epilepsy mortality in England and Wales and the United States, 1950–1994. *Am J Epidemiol* 2000; 151: 182–9.

158 Meinardi H, Scott RA, Reis R, Sander JWAS. The treatment gap in epilepsy: the current situation and the ways forward. *Epilepsia* 2001; 42: 136–49.

159 Watts AE. A model for managing epilepsy in a rural community in Africa. *BMJ* 1989; 298: 805–7.

160 Placencia M, Sander JWAS, Roman M *et al.* The characteristics of epilepsy in a largely untreated population in rural Ecuador. *J Neurol Neurosurg Psychiatry* 1994; 57: 320–5.

161 Mani KS, Rangan G, Srinivas HV, Srindharan VS, Subbakrishna DK. Epilepsy control with phenobarbital or phenytoin in rural south India: the Yelandur study. *Lancet* 2001; 357; 1316–20.

3 Sudden Death in Epilepsy

L. Nashef and Y. Langan

Overview and historical perspective

Mortality is increased in epilepsy. Overall standardized mortality ratios (SMRs)[1] in population-based cohorts are 2–3 times that of the general population [1–4]. Much of the excess mortality is due to associated or underlying disease, but there is also a small excess due to epilepsy itself. Causes of death in epilepsy are listed in Table 3.1; those that are epilepsy related are to some extent preventable.

Sudden unexpected death in epilepsy (SUDEP), where an otherwise well person with epilepsy dies unexpectedly with no cause found at autopsy, is the single most important category of epilepsy-related deaths [5–9]. Given that the cause of death is not immediately apparent it is also the most difficult for relatives and indeed physicians to comprehend. It is also referred to as sudden unexplained death in epilepsy. As discussed below, the evidence suggests that most, but probably not all, SUDEP deaths are related to epileptic convulsions.

The recognition that ictal deaths could be due to intrinsic mechanisms as well as accidents was well recognized in the 19th and early 20th century [10–15]. Spratling described epilepsy as 'a disease which destroys life suddenly and without warning through a single, brief attack, unaided by an accident to the patient at the moment, such as suffocation or fracture of the skull from falling, and does so in from 3 to 4% of all who suffer from it'. Munson, like Spratling, based his observations on his experience at the Craig Colony. In his series, some 40 deaths out of each hundred were epilepsy related, and status deaths were relatively common. Nocturnal deaths were considered accidental and amenable to intervention. Munson noted that there was 'a definite and fairly large group where neither accident of any kind nor suffocation can be assigned as the cause of death which seemed to be intrinsic rather than extrinsic'. He also highlighted the frequent presence of pulmonary oedema, 'a frequent dangerous condition following all forms of the epileptic attack, even single grand mal seizures'. He concluded that 'death is imminent at the time of seizures, unless help is at hand. The cause may be traumatic, suffocation may take place, or deaths may occur without any apparent cause . . . the moral [being that] the epileptic should be by himself as little as possible'. Sudden death in epilepsy only became the focus of attention again during the last decade. The success of the self-help group, Epilepsy Bereaved, and the efforts of

medical researchers in the field contributed to this change. The pharmaceutical industry has been particularly instrumental in furthering the 're-emergence' of SUDEP. Sudden unexpected deaths were inevitably observed during large drug trial programmes, leading to industry-sponsored research and education in this field. Such support helped emphasize that these deaths were essentially epilepsy and not drug related, while at the same time reinforcing the importance of seizure control.

SUDEP is now acknowledged as a real entity; but this is only the beginning. The challenge is to set out effective strategies for prevention and emulate the success in reducing cot deaths. This can be achieved with better understanding of pathophysiological mechanisms and risk factors.

Definitions

The usual definition of sudden death applies with the additional requirement that deaths are not classified as SUDEP cases if there is a clear structural or toxicological cause for death. Some have favoured excluding definite peri-ictal deaths. This is not practically possible. Most SUDEP cases are unwitnessed and it is not possible to distinguish with certainty between deaths occurring during or shortly after an epileptic seizure and those unrelated to any epileptic event. There is often physical and circumstantial evidence suggesting that an epileptic seizure has taken place [16], but such evidence may also be present with anoxic events. Epileptic seizures may also occur without the usual stigmata of tongue biting or incontinence. Similarly, where an event is witnessed, an epileptic basis is not excluded even if a convulsive seizure is not observed. *The definition we favour is sudden, unexpected, witnessed or unwitnessed, non-traumatic and non-drowning death in epilepsy, with or without evidence for a seizure and excluding documented status epilepticus, where postmortem examination does not reveal a cause for death* [78].

This is a workable definition which allows for these deaths to be conveniently grouped together but makes no assumption about the underlying mechanism or mechanisms. The definition, however, requires an autopsy. This is usually performed in the UK, and we believe this practice should continue. This is not the case in all countries including the USA. Because autopsies are not always performed, it has been suggested that, for the purpose of epidemiological studies of SUDEP, deaths in those with epilepsy should be classified into cases with a clear alternative cause of death and (a) definite; (b) probable (all criteria but no autopsy); or (c) possible SUDEP cases (Table 3.2).

This strict definition, however, has its limitations. As pointed out by Hauser [17], it precludes research and assessment of increased

---

[1] Standardized mortality ratio is the ratio of deaths observed in a group to the number of deaths that would be expected to have occurred during a follow-up period if the group in question had experienced the same age- and sex-specific death rates as in the control population.

Table 3.1 Causes of death in epilepsy

Unrelated to epilepsy
Death from underlying/associated disease
Epilepsy related
  Seizure related
    status epilepticus
    trauma, burns or drowning consequent to a seizure
    the majority of sudden unexpected deaths in epilepsy
    deaths in a seizure with severe aspiration/airway obstruction by
      food, etc.
    deaths provoked by habitual seizures due to coexisting
      cardiorespiratory disease
  Deaths due to medical or surgical treatment of epilepsy
  Suicides

Table 3.2 SUDEP with categories denoting level of certainty

Sudden unexpected death of someone suffering from epilepsy (defined as recurrent unprovoked epileptic seizures) occurring while the victim is in a reasonable state of health, during normal activities and in benign circumstances, with no other obvious medical cause of death found

Definite SUDEP
Meet above criteria with sufficient description of death circumstances and autopsy

Probable SUDEP
As above but no autopsy

Possible SUDEP
Either, case suggestive of SUDEP, but information incomplete or there is a competing plausible explanation for the death, e.g. bath deaths

Not SUDEP
Either other cause of death clearly established or circumstances make SUDEP highly improbable

Adapted from [51].

risk, suggested by descriptive mortality series, in those with other coexisting pathology [18]. Older individuals, for example, with ischaemic heart disease, may well be more at risk of dying during habitual seizures.

Pathophysiological mechanisms

Animal and stimulation studies support an important role for ictal apnoea/hypoventilation. In Simon's [19] first sheep model of ictal sudden death, animals that died were those with a greater rise in pulmonary vascular pressure and hypoventilation. In the second study of tracheostomized sheep, which excluded airway obstruction, central apnoea and hypoventilation were observed in all animals, causing or contributing to death in two. A third animal also developed heart failure with significant pathological cardiac ischaemic changes [20].

A detailed study of the circumstances of death, already referred to, in largely unwitnessed SUDEP cases, concluded that indirect evidence for an epileptic seizure was present in the majority [16]. In a separate case–control study of SUDEP cases [21], 12 of 15 witnessed cases occurred in the context of a convulsive seizure with respiratory compromise observed in all witnessed cases. Thus, most, but probably not all, SUDEP deaths are likely to have occurred as a consequence of cardiorespiratory compromise during or immediately after a convulsive epileptic seizure. Different possible mechanisms are not mutually exclusive and indeed may be contributory in a given case. There is strong evidence in favour of hypoventilation being a common occurrence in epileptic seizures and this is likely to be a significant mechanism in SUDEP. Peri-ictal apnoea, both central and obstructive, is well documented, so are pulmonary oedema, excessive bronchial/oral secretions and hypoxia. Pulmonary oedema is frequently found at postmortem in SUDEP cases as is, less frequently, oedema of other organs. Hypoxia has been clearly observed even in partial seizures [22,23]. Thus, respiratory compromise during or shortly after seizures is likely to be an important mechanism which can predispose to secondary cardiac tachyarrhythmia or transient bradycardia [22]. The latter may occur as part of a cardiorespiratory reflex in the presence of apnoea. Bradycardia can also occur secondary to the seizure discharge as has been observed in complex partial seizures of temporal lobe origin where an epileptic partial seizure evolves into cardiac syncope [24,25]. Although sinus tachycardia very frequently occurs during epileptic seizures, both partial and generalized, systematic studies have shown more serious ictal and interictal tachyarrhythmias to be rare [26]. Scott and Fish [27] reviewed 5-year ictal data on 589 consecutive patients being assessed for epilepsy surgery and found only two out of more than 1500 complex partial seizures showing a significant period of asystole (13 and 15 s). This compared to previous observation of 39% with central apnoea. In this context, Mameli *et al.*'s animal model recorded cardiac autonomic changes during activation of brainstem arrhythmogenic trigger zones and showed that cardiac changes were transient and not life-threatening unless accompanied by alteration in metabolic parameters [28,29].

We wish to stress that emphasizing respiratory compromise should not be understood to negate the importance of cardiac mechanisms whether primary or secondary. First it is important to recognize that cases of cardiac arryhthmias may be misdiagnosed as epilepsy and wrongly certified as epilepsy-related deaths. In Langan's case–control study [21,30,31] one sudden death among some 150 cases identified, though certified as epilepsy related, was due to familial long QT syndrome.

In SUDEP, pathological studies have reported cardiac changes of uncertain significance [32,33] (see below). Furthermore, of particular interest is the possibility that the same condition causing epilepsy may predispose to sudden cardiac death. Examples include cases with neurodeficit and other malformations in early life as well as the elderly where the epilepsy may be a symptom of widespread vascular disease. In Rett's syndrome, for example, a neurodevelopmental disorder caused by mutations in the X-linked methyl CpG binding protein 2 (*MeCP2*) gene, clinical manifestations include epilepsy and an increased risk of sudden death (26% of deaths in one study) [34]. Affected individuals have been found to have decreased heart rate variability and longer corrected QT intervals when compared with aged-matched controls [35].

That the same channelopathy may cause both familial long QT syndromes and epilepsy has already been postulated [9,36] and we are now at the stage of being able to test this hypothesis with a study underway. A channelopathy could predispose to both primary cardiac sudden death in patients with epilepsy as well as death during epileptic seizures. Support for this comes from anecdotal reports of familial SUDEP and the findings of Nilsson et al.'s case–control study [37] of a higher *relative risk* of SUDEP among patients with idiopathic epilepsy, despite absolute numbers being proportionately less (see below). Also of interest is Donner et al.'s [38] paediatric series of SUDEP cases with 30% classified as having idiopathic epilepsy. This may well be shown to be a significant mechanism in a minority of SUDEP cases.

Suffocation used to be considered a major cause of death in epilepsy but has been rejected in recent years as too simplistic an explanation. Petechial haemorrhages found at autopsy are not specific for asphyxia and are known to occur secondary to hypoxia with raised venous pressure. Nevertheless, position may still be an important contributory factor exacerbating hypoxia during postictal coma, particularly if normal respiratory drive, in response to hypercapnoea or hypoxia, is impaired. The study of ictal recordings in humans with techniques used in polysomnography [22,39] observed central apnoea more commonly than obstructive apnoea. Studies in EEG/video telemetry units are likely to underestimate intrinsic/positional and extrinsic obstructive apnoea because of intervention from attending staff. The interview study of the circumstances of death in SUDEP, already referred to, reported that the position of the head was such that respiratory obstruction could have contributed to death in 11/26 cases [16]. In another interesting study, among 42 cases of SUDEP, 71% were found prone, only 4% were supine and 25% were found in other positions [40].

To our knowledge there is only one reported case of SUDEP occurring during depth EEG/video telemetry. Death occurred during a secondary generalized seizure captured on video [41]. Respiratory parameters were not recorded, but the persistence of pulse artefact seen on one of the intracranial depth EEG electrode channels for 120 s after complete EEG flattening indicated adequate perfusion until the late stages of the terminal event. This would be consistent with apnoea occurring prior to any cardiac compromise. The EEG changes of bursts of activity followed by total flattening were not typical of hypoxia and are likely to have occurred prior to any respiratory compromise. We are not aware of systematic ictal studies which may give an indication of the frequency with which this recognized pattern of postictal EEG suppression occurs after generalized convulsive seizures. One can speculate that such a pattern may reflect secondary endogenous opioid or other transmitter release previously suggested by J.W.A.S. Sander as a potential contributory mechanism for SUDEP through postictal apnoea.

Near-miss SUDEP events have been observed. In the Langan case–control study there were six reports of near-miss events having occurred in the past among individuals who subsequently died. Reports of 'near-miss' events were obtained only when it was possible to carry out detailed interviews of bereaved relatives. Those interviewed reported previous events where there was concern about postictal cardiorespiratory function and where it was necessary to summon medical assistance, actively stimulate or resuscitate the individual. In the interview study of Nashef et al. [16] in one of 26 SUDEP cases, near-miss events requiring resuscitation had been reported. There is one report of a near-miss event during video-EEG monitoring. The patient developed persistent apnoea in the context of a convulsive seizure and subsequently had a cardiac arrest with successful resuscitation. This individual had had an arrest in the past [42]. We believe that such events are underreported and their recognition may help identify individuals at particular risk.

Studies of heart rate variability (HRV) in epilepsy are of interest given the predictive value of reduced HRV in relation to mortality in other conditions. HRV reflects the sympathetic (low frequency), parasympathetic (high frequency) autonomic systems and the relationship between them (low-frequency/high-frequency ratio). Seizure type and focus, underlying pathology, medication and laterality may all influence HRV [43–46].

General and neuropathological changes

Pulmonary oedema and congestion of other organs are frequently seen in SUDEP cases at postmortem. Pulmonary oedema is a pathological hallmark and is almost a *sine qua non* of SUDEP [47]. Pulmonary oedema was also observed in Simon's sheep model of sudden death [19,20]. Findings of cardiac perivascular and interstitial fibrosis [32], and of increased heart weights relative to height, have been observed, the increase being significant in males [48]. Opeskin et al. [33] performed detailed cardiac examination on 10 SUDEP victims and 10 controls and found no increase in morphological cardiac conduction system abnormalities in the SUDEP group and neither was there any difference in the level of coronary artery stenoses. They qualified their findings by stating that the subtle abnormalities of the conduction system identified in some of the epilepsy-related deaths could still have contributed to death. Neuropathological studies indicate a higher incidence of macroscopic abnormalities in SUDEP cases [48–50]. This was taken as an indication of a greater risk for symptomatic epilepsies, but this has not been supported by case–control studies, one of which as already mentioned shows an increased relative risk in idiopathic epilepsy. The frequent presence of a neuropathological substrate for the epilepsy in SUDEP cases may simply be a reflection of the increased risk inherent in the associated epilepsy which tends to be more severe. Ischaemic changes in the central nervous system are not frequently seen in SUDEP cases, and would not be expected where the terminal event is brief. Such changes, however, are occasionally observed in unwitnessed cases which would otherwise fulfil the definition above. This suggests that some of these deaths occur over a longer time course than a few minutes [50].

Incidence studies

The incidence of sudden death in the general population is some 5–10/100 000 among those under 45 years of age and 300/100 000 among the elderly [51]. Useful recent review articles on different aspects of sudden death are to be found in *Cardiac Electrophysiology Reviews* [52]. Ficker et al. [53] studied all deaths in persons with epilepsy in Rochester, USA, diagnosed between 1935 and 1994. The study, which included 1535 people and 25 939.7 person-years, reported a SUDEP incidence of 0.35 in 1000 person-years. The number of SUDEP cases was small compared to the total number of deaths (535) in the whole cohort. There were seven definite, two probable and one possible SUDEP cases and six unclassified deaths. Among the 15–44-year age group, seven of 81 deaths or 8.6% were classified as SUDEP. Annegers [51] using population-based data from a study from Allegheny County, PA, USA [54], and a prevalence figure for epilepsy of 0.7/1000, estimated the incidence of sud-

45

den death among people with epilepsy to be 188.6/100 000 compared with only 4.6/100 000 for the general population, a risk that was 40-fold higher for younger individuals with epilepsy than that of the general population. The increase is observed in younger age groups (adolescents and young adults), but a similar increase in older age groups would be lost within much higher death rates. More data is required on incidence in children and the elderly [55–57]. Children were not included in the Langan case–control study although SUDEP cases in this age group were certainly brought to the attention of the investigators and detailed information is available where interviews were carried out. Appleton [58], while emphasizing difficulties involved in retrospective and coroner-based studies to estimate the incidence of SUDEP in children, observed that conclusions from adult studies should not necessarily be applied to the paediatric population with epilepsy in whom SUDEP may be a somewhat different entity. This may well be true. Cases where the same pathology may predispose to epilepsy and to sudden cardiac death, for example, may be more common in children with epilepsy than in a young adult population (Table 3.3). Donner et al. [38] identified 27 SUDEP cases under the age of 18 over a 10-year period in Ontario, Canada. Fourteen children had symptomatic epilepsy (52%), five had cryptogenic epilepsy (18%) and eight had idiopathic epilepsy (30%).

O'Donoghue and Sander [59] reviewed incidence studies published before 1996. A more recent multicentre study reported an incidence of 1.21/1000 patient-years [60]. Overall, cohorts with more severe epilepsy seen at tertiary centres have rates of approximately 1/250 person-years or more. In controlled patients SUDEP rate are low at some 1/2500 person-years [61]. Higher rates in intractable cohorts do not mean that sudden deaths do not occur in patients with less 'severe' epilepsy (see case–controls studies below). In the detailed interview study already referred to, 8/26 SUDEP cases had experienced less than 10 GTCS in a lifetime. Hauser [17] estimated that 'only 30% occur[red] in intractable cases'.

It may be argued that successful epilepsy surgery would prevent SUDEP. Elevated long-term mortality after epilepsy surgery has long been reported. Half to two-thirds of deaths reported in older series were seizure related or suicides [62,63]. In a recent observational study of 248 people who underwent diagnostic evaluation for epilepsy surgery [64], those not operated on had a significantly higher mortality than the surgical group. Furthermore, a significantly higher proportion of those who died were noted to have ongoing seizures at last recorded follow-up compared to survivors. In a study of postoperative mortality among 393 patients following epilepsy surgery, 199 patients were fully controlled, with no deaths observed in 701 person-years of follow-up. On the other hand, 194 patients experienced postoperative seizures with 11 deaths, including six SUDEP, observed during 801 person-years of follow-up [65].

Table 3.3 Estimate of SUDEP annual incidence in young adults with epilepsy (see text)

Controlled cohorts	1:2500 [61]
General population with epilepsy	Minimum 0.35/1000 [53]
Multicentre cohort	1.21/1000 [60]
Intractable cohorts	1:250 [59]

Complete seizure control in this study, through surgery, appeared to abolish the risk of SUDEP. Another explanation is that some cases with failed surgery had different pathophysiology. Both explanations are likely to be valid and are not mutually exclusive. In another study with 2815 person-years of follow-up after temporal lobectomy for epilepsy, and excluding deaths from surgical complications, SMR was 3.7 (95% CI 2.5–5.3). The excess mortality was epilepsy related and included six SUDEP cases, two status epilepticus, two drowning, two aspiration and one accidental death. SUDEP incidence was 1/455 person-years, lower than would be expected for an intractable cohort. In this study, temporal lobectomy for epilepsy appeared to reduce but did not normalize mortality in epilepsy. Causes of death observed suggest that the residual excess mortality was related to ongoing seizures in a proportion of patients. In some partial seizures were significantly improved but infrequent generalized seizures occurred postoperatively [66]. Another group with severe epilepsy is that of patients undergoing vagal nerve stimulation who had an elevated sudden death rate of 4.5/1000 for definite/probable SUDEP (6/1000 if possible cases were included). This is comparable to that expected in an intractable cohort. Interestingly this rate seemed to decrease with longer follow-up [67,68].

Risk factors and case–control studies

Descriptive cohorts

Descriptive studies reported the following putative risk factors: youth, male sex, remote symptomatic epilepsy, structural findings on neuropathology, severe epilepsy, unwitnessed seizures, alcohol abuse, abnormal EEGs with epileptiform changes and greater variations, mental handicap, psychotropic medication, African-Americans, lack of compliance with treatment, abrupt medication changes and low antiepileptic drug (AED) levels [69,70]. These should only be considered variables for further study.

Case–control studies

A risk factor emerging from an early case–control study was that of convulsive seizures [71]. This has been confirmed by other studies including a US multicentre study, which enrolled 4578 patients and prospectively followed them for 16 463 patient-years, comparing potential risk factors in SUDEP cases and in controls. SUDEP, with 20 definite and probable cases observed, accounted for 18% of all deaths. Of note is that there were a further eight possible SUDEP cases and five cases with insufficient information. Tonic-clonic seizures, treatment with more than two anticonvulsant medications and full-scale IQ of less than 70 were independent risk factors for SUDEP [60].

The landmark case–control study from Stockholm looked at 57 SUDEP cases aged 15–70 years on treatment for at least 1 year [37]. A higher risk of SUDEP was observed with (a) more frequent seizures (odds ratio of 10.16 (95% CI 2.94–35.18)) for those with >50 seizures per year compared to 2; (b) polytherapy (odds ratio of 9.89 (95% CI 3.20–30.60)) for those on three AEDs compared to monotherapy; and (c) frequent changes in medication (odds ratio of 6.08 (95% CI 1.99–18.56)) for those with frequent medication changes (3–5 per year) compared to those where medication remained stable. (d) The risk was also greater in patients with longer disease duration and idiopathic epilepsy.

Langan's large UK-based case–control study included 154 SUDEP cases, of whom 23 were witnessed [21,30]. Risk of SUDEP was greater if a generalized tonic-clonic seizure occurred in the last 3 months (odds ratio 10.3 (5.6–19.2)), with increasing number of AEDs taken (odds ratio 4.3 (2.1–8.90 for four AEDs when compared with 1–2)). Those who had never had drug therapy were at increased risk when compared with those who had taken one to two drugs (odds ratio 11.6 (4.3–39.4)). Recent AED reduction or withdrawal, i.e. in the last 3 months, also increased the risk of SUDEP (odds ratio 2.7 (1.1–6.5)). Carbamazepine was associated with a slightly higher odds ratio of 2 (1.1–3.6) (see below). This study importantly also provides evidence for what has long been suspected, namely that supervision appeared to have a protective effect. There was a decreased risk of SUDEP if the bedroom was shared with someone capable of giving assistance (odds ratio 0.38 (0.2–0.8)) and if special precautions such as the use of listening devices were taken (odds ratio 0.3 (0.1–0.86)). These results are supported by an older study from a residential school for pupils with epilepsy and learning difficulty where, during the period under study, SUDEP cases occurred either during school holidays or after the pupils left the school. Awake night staff and listening monitors insured prompt response to seizures [72].

AED treatment and risk of SUDEP

A consistent factor in case–control studies is that uncontrolled seizures increase the risk of SUDEP. Although it is not possible on ethical grounds to test this prospectively in a double-blind study, it is logical to assume that, as with surgery, successful prevention of seizures with AEDs would reduce the risk of SUDEP. We believe this to be the case.

There are, however, specific issues in drug treatment that require further clarification in relation to drug levels, compliance and abrupt withdrawal, polytherapy and choice of AED. These are important since, unlike the pathological substrate for the epilepsy, they are amenable to manipulation during routine management.

Both anecdotally and on the basis of Langan's finding of an increased risk with recent AED reduction or withdrawal, we believe that abrupt medication changes whether prescribed or otherwise should be avoided whenever possible.

A study from Australia which compared AED levels in 44 cases of sudden unexpected deaths in epilepsy with levels in a control group of epilepsy patients dying of other causes did not observe a difference between the two groups [73]. So-called subtherapeutic levels if stable and if the epilepsy is fully controlled are unlikely to be important in themselves.

Whether polytherapy *per se* is a risk factor, or whether it is simply a surrogate for seizure severity remains uncertain. Medication, however, could theoretically alter the post-ictal phase and increase the risk of respiratory depression.

A question that frequently arises is whether one particular AED is associated with a higher risk. This did not emerge with older descriptive series, which simply reflected prescribing practices. Walczak *et al.*'s study [60] did not identify any specific association with any particular AED. Further analysis of Nilsson *et al.*'s case–control study [18,74] suggested an increased risk, not with

carbamazepine *per se*, but with levels greater than the common target range in patients with frequent dose changes and polytherapy. The number of cases with higher levels however was only six among 33 on carbamazepine and 57 SUDEP cases in total. Timmings [75] had previously reported, in a review of the Cardiff Epilepsy Unit Data, that carbamazepine was disproportionately represented in patients suffering SUDEP, and Langan's case–control study also showed a small excess risk associated with carbamazepine treatment just reaching significance. Rare cases of heart block secondary to carbamazepine are well documented in predisposed individuals; the significance of these findings, however, to the majority of cases with epilepsy is uncertain. Seizure severity, as opposed to frequency or seizure type, has not been corrected for as a variable. A plausible explanation is that during the time course of these studies, patients with more severe epilepsy/seizures have been more likely to be prescribed higher doses of carbamazepine, a mainstay of epilepsy treatment in the last two decades. A precautionary note, however, relates to AED treatment not always being appropriate to the epilepsy syndrome; certainly in the interview study some of the patients who died whilst on carbamazepine had been patients with uncontrolled primary generalized epilepsy where a broad-spectrum drug would have been more likely to be successful.

We would like to emphasize that treatment interventions, whether surgical or medical, have the potential to worsen seizure frequency and severity [66,76,77]. Seizure severity in particular is not usually assessed and indeed scales of seizure severity have addressed the risk of injury during seizures but not the extent of associated cardiorespiratory distress.

Clinical implications

Although based on incomplete evidence, the following strategies for the prevention of SUDEP cases would be reasonable:
• Seizure prevention, particularly generalized tonic-clonic seizures: this should be achieved through active medical and surgical treatment, avoiding seizure precipitants and through patient and physician education.
• Avoiding abrupt medication changes.
• Ensuring prompt response to seizures with advice on first aid and positioning/stimulating the patient if there is any respiratory compromise or postictal hypoventilation. This can only be achieved with adequate supervision which would undermine independence for patients with epilepsy. Supervision would need to be appropriate to the severity of the epilepsy and depend on informed patient choice.
• Reversing any treatment intervention that appears to worsen control of the epilepsy, whether seizure frequency or severity including the post-ictal phase.

Future research

Much has been achieved but much remains to be done. Below we outline some of the areas we feel are worthy of further study and hope that researchers will be able to take some of these ideas further.

Epidemiology

Although further unselected descriptive epilepsy cohorts are unlike-

Table 3.4 Strategies for preventing SUDEP (see text)

Prevention of convulsions
Avoiding abrupt medication changes/non-compliance
Ensuring prompt response to seizures
Reversing treatment interventions that worsen epilepsy
control

ly to be informative, studies aiming to better define risk in relation to specific epilepsy syndromes are needed.

Correct internationally agreed certification of epilepsy deaths is vital both for accurate data on SUDEP and other epilepsy-related deaths. We need to be able to monitor trends in this field to assess the effect of any interventions. Well-conducted autopsies should be encouraged.

Mechanisms

The possible role of channelopathies and potential overlap between paroxysmal cardiac and central nervous system disorders need to be investigated. Other aspects requiring further study include the postictal EEG suppression pattern, its frequency, predisposing factors, relation to apnoea and intrinsic mechanisms of seizure termination, peri-ictal P_{CO_2} and postictal respiratory drive. Scales of seizure severity which take into account cardiorespiratory parameters need further development. Studies of near-miss events are also lacking.

Therapeutics

Further studies of aspects of AED administration and withdrawal discussed above as well as other treatment modalities are still needed. This applies particularly to AEDs, the mainstay of current epilepsy management.

Seizure prediction, detection and supervision

Issues of prevention and supervision need further discussion between patients, carers and health workers. To minimize loss of independence, better methods of seizure prediction and detection need to be developed, coupled with advice on response to seizures (Table 3.4).

Treatment gap

Health service delivery issues and treatment gaps in many parts of the world need to be addressed. The results of the UK national sentinel audit of epilepsy-related deaths is of interest in this regard.

References

1 Hauser WA, Annegers JF, Elveback LR. Mortality in patients with epilepsy. *Epilepsia* 1980; 21: 399–412.
2 Hauser WA, Hesdorffer DC. Mortality. In: Hauser WA, Hesdorffer DC, eds. *Epilepsy: Frequency, Causes and Consequences.* Maryland: Epilepsy Foundation of USA, 1990: 297–326.
3 Cockerell OC, Johnson AL, Sander JWAS, Hart YM, Goodridge DM, Shorvon SD. Mortality from epilepsy: Results from a prospective population-based study. *Lancet* 1994; 344: 918–21.
4 Nashef L, Sander JWAS, Shorvon SD. Mortality in epilepsy. In: Pedley T, Meldrum BS, eds. *Recent Advances in Epilepsy 6.* Edinburgh: Churchill Livingstone, 1995, 271–87.
5 Jay GW, Leestma JE. Sudden death in epilepsy. A comprehensive review of the literature and proposed mechanisms. *Acta Neurol Scand* 1981; 63 (Suppl. 82): 5–66.
6 Lathers CM, Schraeder PL, eds. *Epilepsy and Sudden Death.* New York: Marcel Dekker, 1990.
7 Brown SW. Sudden death and epilepsy: clinical review. *Seizure* 1992; 1: 71–3.
8 Nashef L. Sudden unexpected death in epilepsy: incidence, circumstances and mechanisms. MD thesis, University of Bristol, 1995.
9 Nashef L, Brown S eds. *Epilepsy and Sudden Death.* Proceedings of the International Workshop on Sudden Death in Epilepsy, London, 28/10/96. *Epilepsia* 1997; 38 (Suppl. 11): 11.
10 Delasiauve LJF. Terminaisons. In: *Traite De L'Epilepsie.* Paris: Victor Masson, 1854; 165–73.
11 Bacon GM. On the modes of death in epilepsy. *Lancet* 1868; 1: 555–6.
12 Gowers WR. Prognosis. In: *Epilepsy and Other Chronic Convulsive Diseases: their causes, symptoms and treatment.* American Academy of Neurology Reprint Series. New York: Dover Publications, 1885: 199–200.
13 Geysen MH. De la mort inopinee ou rapide chez les epileptiques (These). Faculté de Medicine et de Pharmacie de Lyon 1895; Series 1 No. 1114.
14 Spratling WP. Prognosis. In: *Epilepsy and its Treatment.* Philadelphia: WB Saunders, 1904: 304.
15 Munson JF. Death in epilepsy. *Medical Record* 1910; January 8; 58–62.
16 Nashef L, Garner S, Sander JWAS, Fish DR, Shorvon SD. Circumstances of death in sudden death in epilepsy: interviews of bereaved relatives. *J Neurol Neurosurg Psychiatry* 1998; 64(3): 349–52.
17 Hauser AW. *Sudden Unexpected Death in Patients with Epilepsy: issues for further study.* Proceedings of the International Workshop on Sudden Death in Epilepsy, London, 28/10/96, Nashef L, Brown S, eds. *Epilepsia* 1997; 38 (Suppl. 11): S26–S29.
18 Nilsson L, Tomson T, Farahmand BY, Diwan V, Persson PG. Cause specific mortality in epilepsy: a cohort study of more than 9,000 patients once hospitalised for epilepsy. *Epilepsia* 1997; 38: 1062–8.
19 Simon RP. Epileptic sudden death: animal models. *Epilepsia* 1997; 38 (Suppl. 11); S35–S36.
20 Johnston SC, Siedenberg R, Min JK, Jerome EH, Laxer KD. Central apnea and acute cardiac ischemia in a sheep model of epileptic sudden death. *Ann Neurol* 1997; 42(4): S88.
21 Langan Y, Nashef L, Sander JWAS. Sudden unexpected death in epilepsy: a series of witnessed deaths. *J Neurol Neurosurg Psychiatry* 2000; 68: 211–13.
22 Nashef L, Walker F, Allen P, Sander JWAS, Shorvon SD, Fish DR. Apnoea and bradycardia during epileptic seizures: relation to sudden death in epilepsy. *J Neurol Neurosurg Psychiatry* 1996; 60: 297–300.
23 Blum AS, Ives JR, Goldberger AL *et al.* Oxygen desaturations triggered by partial seizures: implications for cardiopulmonary instability in epilepsy. *Epilepsia* 2000; 41(5): 536–41.
24 Jallon P. Epilepsy and the heart. *Rev Neurol* 1997; 153(3): 173–84.
25 Jallon P. Arrhythmogenic seizures. *Epilepsia* 1997; 38 (Suppl. 11); S43–S47.
26 Blumhardt LD, Smith PEM, Owen L. Electrographic accompaniments of temporal lobe epileptic seizures. *Lancet* 1986; 1: 1051–5.
27 Scott CA, Fish DR. Cardiac asystole in partial seizures. *Epileptic Disord* 2000; 2(2): 89–92.
28 Mameli O, Melis F, Giraudi D *et al.* The brainstem cardioarrhythmogenic triggers and their possible role in sudden epileptic death. *Epilepsy Res* 1993; 15: 171–8.
29 Mameli O. *Epilepsia* 1997; 38 (Suppl. 11): S58.
30 Langan Y, Nashef L, Sander JWAS. Case–control study of sudden death in epilepsy. American Academy of Neurology (AAN) Meeting, 2000. *Neurology* 2000; 54 (Suppl. 3), A146 (abstract).
31 Langan Y, Nashef L, Sander JWAS. Sleeping alone increases the risk of sudden unexpected death in epilepsy (SUDEP). American Epilepsy Society, December 2000. *Epilepsia* 2000; 41 (Suppl. 7): 90 (abstract).

32 Natelson BH, Suarez RV, Terrence CF, Turizo R. Patients with epilepsy who die suddenly have cardiac disease. *Arch Neurol* 1998; 55: 857–60.

33 Opeskin K, Thomas A, Berkovic SF. Does cardiac conduction pathology contribute to sudden unexpected death in epilepsy? *Epilepsy Res* 2000; 40(1): 17–24.

34 Kerr AM, Armstrong DD, Prescott RJ, Doyle D, Kearney DL. Rett syndrome—analysis of deaths in the British survey. *Eur Child Adolesc Psychiatry* 1997; 6 (Suppl. 1): 71–4.

35 Guideri F, Acampa M, Hayek G, Zapella M, Di Perri T. Reduced heart rate variability in patients affected with Rett syndrome. A possible explanation for sudden death. *Neuropediatrics* 1999; 30: 146–8.

36 Hartmann HA, Colom LV, Sutherland ML, Noebels JL. Selective localization of cardiac SCN5a Na$^+$ channels in limbic regions of rat brain. *Nature Neurosci* 1999; 2: 593–5.

37 Nilsson L, Farahmand BY, Persson PG, Thiblin I, Tomson T. Risk factors for sudden unexpected death in epilepsy: a case-control study. *Lancet* 1999; 353: 888–93.

38 Donner EJ, Smith CR, Snead OC III. Sudden unexplained death in children with epilepsy. *Neurology* 2001; 57(3): 430–4.

39 Walker F, Fish DR. Recording respiratory parameters in patients with epilepsy. *Epilepsia* 1997; 38 (Suppl. 11); S41–S42.

40 Kloster R, Engelskjon T. Sudden unexpected death in epilepsy: a clinical perspective and a search for risk factors. *J Neurol Neurosurg Psychiatry* 1999; 67: 439–44.

41 Bird JM, Dembny KAT, Sandeman D, Butler S. Sudden unexplained death in epilepsy: an intracranially monitored case. *Epilepsia* 1997; 38 (Suppl. 11); S52–S56.

42 So EL, Sam MC, Lagerlund TL. Post-ictal central apnoea as a cause of SUDEP: evidence from near-SUDEP incident. *Epilepsia* 2000; 41: 1494–7.

43 Massetani R, Strata G, Galli R *et al*. Alterations of cardiac function in patients with temporal lobe epilepsy: Different roles of EEG-ECG monitoring and spectral analysis of RR variability. *Epilepsia* 1997; 38 (Suppl. 11); S363–369.

44 Tomson T, Kenneback G. Arrhythmia, heart rate variability and antiepileptic drugs. *Epilepsia* 1997; 38 (Suppl. 11); S48–S51.

45 Ahern GL, Sollers JJ, Lane RD *et al*. Heart rate and heart rate variability changes in the intracarotid sodium amobarbital test. *Epilepsia* 2001; 42(7): 912–21.

46 Hennessy MJ, Tighe MG, Binnie CD, Nashef L. Sudden withdrawal of carbamazepine increases cardiac sympathetic activity in sleep. *Neurology* 2001; 57(9): 1650–4.

47 Terrence CF, Rao GR, Perper JA. Neurogenic Pulmonary edema in unexpected unexplained death of epileptic patients. *Ann Neurol* 1981; 9: 458–64.

48 Leestma JE. A pathological review. In: Lathers CM, Schraeder PL, eds. *Epilepsy and Sudden Death*. New York: Marcel Dekker, 1990: 61–88.

49 Freytag E, Lindenberg R. Medicolegal autopsies on epileptics. *Arch Pathol* 1964; 78: 274–86.

50 Thom M. Neuropathologic findings in postmortem studies of sudden death in epilepsy. *Epilepsia* 1997; 38 (Suppl. 11): S32–S34.

51 Annegers JF. United States perspective on definitions and classification epilepsy and sudden death. *Epilepsia* 1997; 38 (Suppl. 11); S9–S12.

52 Lazzara R (ed). Syncope and sudden death. *Cardiac Electrophysiol Rev* 2001; 5.

53 Ficker DM, So EL, Annegers JF, O'Brien PC, Cascino GD, Belau PG. Population-based study of the incidence of sudden unexplained death in epilepsy. *Neurology* 1998; 51: 1270–4.

54 Neuspiel DR, Kuller LH. Sudden and unexpected natural death in childhood and adolescence. *JAMA* 1985; 254: 1321–5.

55 Luhdorf K, Jensen LK, Plesner AM. Epilepsy in the elderly: life expectancy and causes of death. *Acta Neurol Scand* 1987; 76: 183–90.

56 Harvey AS, Hopkins IJ, Nolan TM, Carlin JB. Mortality in children with epilepsy: an epidemiological study. AES proceedings. *Epilepsia* 1991; 32 (Suppl. 3): 54.

57 Keeling JW, Knowles SAS. Sudden death in childhood and adolescence. *J Pathol* 1989; 159: 221–4.

58 Appleton RE. Sudden unexpected death in epilepsy in children. *Seizure* 1997; 6(3): 175–7.

59 O'Donoghue MF, Sander JWAS. The mortality associated with epilepsy, with particular reference to sudden unexpected death: a review. *Epilepsia* 1997; 38 (Suppl. 11); S15–S19.

60 Walczak TS, Leppik IE, D'Amelio M *et al*. Incidence and risk factors in sudden unexpected death in epilepsy: a prospective cohort study. *Neurology* 2001; 56(4): 519–25.

61 Medical Research Council (MRC) Antiepileptic Drug Withdrawal Study Group. Randomized study of antiepileptic drug withdrawal in patients in remission. *Lancet* 1991; 337: 1175–80.

62 Jensen I. Temporal lobe epilepsy. Late mortality in patients treated with unilateral temporal lobe resections. *Acta Neurol Scand* 1975; 52: 374–80.

63 Taylor DC, Marsh SM. Implications of long-term follow-up studies in epilepsy: with a note on the cause of death. In: Penry JK, ed. *Epilepsy, the Eighth International Symposium*. New York: Raven Press, 1977: 27–34.

64 Vickery BG. Mortality in a consecutive cohort of 248 adolescents and adults who underwent diagnostic evaluation for epilepsy surgery. *Epilepsia* 1997; 38 (Suppl. 11): S67.

65 Sperling MR, Feldman H, Kinman J, Liporace JD, O'Connor MJ. Seizure control and mortality in epilepsy. *Ann Neurol* 1999; 46(1): 45–50.

66 Hennessy MJ, Langan Y, Elwes RDC, Binnie CD, Polkey CE, Nashef L. A study of mortality after temporal lobe epilepsy surgery. *Neurology* 1999; 53: 1276.

67 Annegers JF, Coan SP, Hauser WA, Leestma J, Duffell W, Tavern B. Epilepsy, vagal nerve stimulation by the NCP System, mortality and sudden unexpected unexplained death. *Epilepsia* 1998; 39(2): 206–12.

68 Annegers JF, Coan SP, Hauser WA, Leestma J. Epilepsy, vagal nerve stimulation by the NCP system, all cause mortality and sudden unexplained death. *Epilepsia* 2000; 41(5): 549–53.

69 Bowerman DL, Levisky JA, Urich RW, Wittenberg PH. Premature deaths in persons with seizure disorders—subtherapeutic levels of anticonvulsant drugs in postmortem blood specimens. *J Forensic Sci* 1978; 23(3): 522–6.

70 Lund A, Gormsen H. The role of antiepileptics in sudden death in epilepsy. *Acta Neurol Scand* 1985; 72: 444–6.

71 Birnbach CD, Wilensky AJ, Dodrill CB. Predictors of early mortality and sudden death in epilepsy. A multidisciplinary approach. *J Epilepsy* 1991; 4: 11–17.

72 Nashef L, Fish DR, Garner S, Sander JWAS, Shorvon SD. Sudden death in epilepsy – a study of incidence in a young cohort with epilepsy and learning difficulty. *Epilepsia* 1995; 36(12): 1187–94.

73 Opeskin K, Burke MP, Cordner SM, Berkovic SF. Comparison of antiepileptic drug levels in sudden unexpected deaths in epilepsy with deaths from other causes. *Epilepsia* 1999; 40(12): 1795–8.

74 Nilsson L, Bergman U, Diwan V, Farahmand BY, Persson PG, Tomson T. Antiepileptic drug therapy and its management in sudden unexpected death in epilepsy: a case-control study. *Epilepsia* 2001; 42(5): 667–73.

75 Timmings PL. Sudden unexpected death in epilepsy: is carbamazepine implicated? *Seizure* 1998; 7(4): 289–91.

76 Genton P, McMenamin J. *Can Antiepileptic Drugs Aggravate Epilepsy?* Proceedings of a symposium held at the 22nd International Epilepsy Congress, June 29, 1997, Dublin Ireland. *Epilepsia* 1998; 39 (Suppl. 3).

77 Perucca E, Grant L, Avanzini G, Dulac O. Antiepileptic drugs as a cause of worsening seizures. *Epilepsia* 1998; 39: 5–17.

78 Nashef L. *Sudden Unexpected Death in Epilepsy: Terminology and Definitions. Epilepsy and Sudden Death*. Proceedings of the International Workshop on Sudden Death in Epilepsy, London 28/10/96. *Epilepsia*, eds Nashef L, Brown S. 1997: 38 (Suppl. 11); S6–S8.

4 Aetiology of Epilepsy

E. Beghi

The development of therapeutic strategies for the treatment and prevention of epilepsy requires information about the aetiology of the disease. Epilepsy is a heterogeneous symptom complex whose common feature is hyperexcitability in the central nervous system (CNS). This dynamic process is a reflection of complex functional changes occurring in the anatomy and physiology of the brain in the presence of environmental and genetic factors. Whereas genetic and external influences on the susceptibility to epilepsy coexist, the occurrence of seizures, the clinical phenomena caused by the epileptic process, reflect complex interactions between genetic and environmental factors in the individual. On the basis of the differing gene–environment interactions, several epileptic syndromes have been identified [1] and the international classification of the epilepsies must be considered a dynamic instrument susceptible to modifications with increasing knowledge of the genetic and external mechanisms underlying brain hyperexcitability.

Methodological issues in the assessment of the aetiology of epilepsy

A correct understanding of the process leading to the identification of aetiological factors in epilepsy is needed before deducing that the occurrence of epileptic seizures in the presence of a brain insult (e.g. head trauma) establishes that particular brain insult as the causative factor. First, the origin of the epileptic seizure(s) should be clearly identified, with reference to the presence of the most common seizure precipitants, in order to separate provoked from unprovoked seizures. Second, the frequency and characteristics of epilepsy and epileptogenic factors in the general population should be assessed to define the fraction of epilepsies possibly caused by a given risk factor and the risk of epilepsy attributable to that factor. Third, the extent of the diagnostic work-up and the validity of the diagnostic tests must be considered before classifying a patient's epilepsy as idiopathic, cryptogenic or symptomatic. Fourth, the possibility should be considered that even when seizures appear due to a well-established epileptogenic factor they may be caused by unknown or independent factors.

Definitions

Epilepsy is the occurrence of repeated unprovoked seizures [2]. An unprovoked seizure is a seizure occurring in the absence of precipitating factors. By contrast, a provoked (acute symptomatic) seizure is a seizure occurring in close temporal relationship with an acute systemic, toxic or metabolic insult, which is expected to be the underlying cause. Unprovoked seizures include events occurring in the absence of a recognized aetiological or risk factor (idiopathic and cryptogenic seizures) and events occurring in patients with antecedent stable (non-progressing) CNS insults (remote symptomatic seizures). The difference between provoked and unprovoked seizures is relevant to the extent of assessment for a causative epileptogenic factor.

Incidence and prevalence of idiopathic, cryptogenic and symptomatic epilepsy

The study of the incidence, prevalence and characteristics of epilepsy in well-defined populations has several advantages, including the calculation of the fraction of epilepsy attributable to known aetiological factors (remote symptomatic epilepsies), the frequency of well-established risk factors for unprovoked seizures (e.g. head trauma, CNS infection, degenerative disorders, stroke, febrile seizures, cerebral palsy and mental retardation) and the fraction of known aetiology attributable to each given factor (attributable risk). On this basis, the aetiology of epilepsy in populations with differing distribution of aetiological factors may be different in terms of the proportion of cases with remote symptomatic seizures and risk of epilepsy attributable to each factor. This is particularly important in developing countries where exposure to epileptogenic conditions differs from industrialized countries [3].

Extent, validity and reliability of the diagnostic assessment

The identification of the aetiology of seizures is based on the extent and quality of diagnostic assessment, including biochemical and neuroimaging tests. These factors are subject to professional interpretation and thus require proofs of validity and reliability.

Assessment of the cause–effect relationship

Finding a correlation between a risk factor or brain abnormality and epilepsy does not necessarily establish a causal association. In order for a given variable to be considered a risk factor for epilepsy, the association should fulfil the following conditions [4]:

1 Temporal sequence: the exposure must precede epilepsy in time.
2 Strength: a greater risk of epilepsy is present among those exposed compared to those non-exposed; and the larger the difference of the exposure the greater the strength of the association.
3 Consistency: the association should be reproducible in different populations and under different conditions.
4 Biological gradient: the evidence of a dose–response effect.
5 Biological plausibility: the association between epilepsy and exposure should be consistent with a recognized biological mechanism.

Genetic epidemiology studies

Epilepsy has multiple genetic and non-genetic environmental causes. Several models of gene–environment interaction have been identified which link susceptibility genes, environmental risk factors and the disease [5]. These include the following:

1 Genotype increases expression of risk factor.
2 Genotype exacerbates effect of risk factor.
3 Risk factor exacerbates effect of genotype.
4 Both genotype and risk factor are required to increase risk.
5 Genotype and risk factor influence risk independently.

Aetiology of epilepsy from well-defined populations

Prevalence and incidence of epilepsy and distribution of epilepsies with known aetiology

Prevalence of epilepsy ranges from less than 3 to more than 40 cases per 1000 population [6], depending on the nature and socioeconomic status of the populations, the extent of case ascertainment and the study design and methods. Limited data prevent strict comparisons of prevalence between developed and developing countries, but overall a documented aetiology is present in 21–56% of cases, with modest differences between developed and developing countries (Table 4.1). In developed countries, the incidence of epilepsy ranges from 24 to 53 cases per 100 000 people per year. The corresponding incidence in developing countries is two to three

times higher [6]. The percentage of incident cases with known epilepsy from developed and developing countries ranges from 14 to 52% (Table 4.2).

Among 1056 cases from a well-defined population the most common aetiologies were the following: cerebrovascular disorders 6%; head trauma 5%; developmental disorders 5%; infections 4%; tumours 2%; and degenerative disorders 1% [7]. In the same population, the proportion of cases with newly diagnosed epilepsy assigned to specific aetiological categories varied significantly with age (Fig. 4.1). In another population-based study of newly diagnosed epileptic seizures, remote symptomatic seizures were present in 21% of cases [8]. The proportion of cases with symptomatic epilepsy increased with age. In patients over 60 years vascular disease was the most common aetiological factor (15%), followed by cerebral tumours (11%).

In surgical series, mesial temporal sclerosis (MTS) has been found in up to 70% of cases with medically refractory epilepsy [9]. The increasing reports of MTS in more recent years reflect a more intensive diagnostic investigation including modern neuroimaging. A relationship between MTS and febrile seizures has been postulated, but not clearly established. A variety of early insults, such as trauma and infection, or the presence of hamartomas and heterotopias are of aetiological importance.

Acute symptomatic seizures

Seizures are commonly encountered in people who do not have epilepsy. Factors provoking seizures in non-epileptic individuals in-

Table 4.1 Prevalence of epilepsy in developed and developing countries, with known aetiology in per cent

Author (year)	Area	Prevalence[a] (per 1000)	Known aetiology (%)
Grudzinska (1974)	Zabrze, Poland	3.4	51.6
Beaussart (1980)	Pas-de-Calais, France	8.0	30.0
Goodridge (1983)	Tonbridge, UK	5.3 (17.5)	25.4
Granieri (1983)	Copparo, Italy	6.4	39.6
Li (1985)	Six cities, China	4.4	21.1
Haerer (1986)	Copian County, USA	6.8 (10.4)	30.0
Sridharan (1986)[b]	Benghazi, Libya	2.3	17.5
Osuntokun (1987)	Igba-Ora, Nigeria	5.0	49.5
Bharucha (1988)	Bombay, India	3.7 (4.8)	22.7
Hauser (1991)	Rochester, USA	2.7–6.8	25.0
Maremmani (1991)	Vecchiano, Italy	5.2	43.1
Lavados (1992)	El Salvador, Chile	18.5	29.6
Rwiza (1992)	Ulanga, Tanzania	12.1	25.3
Mendizabal (1996)	Guatemala (rural village)	5.8 (8.5)	56.2
Reggio (1996)	Riposto, Italy	2.7 (5.8)	48.0
Aziz (1997)	Rural and urban Pakistan	9.8	38.4
Aziz (1997)	Rural and urban Turkey	7.1	31.9
Karaagac (1999)	Silivri, Turkey	10.2	53.1
Olafsson (1999)	Iceland	4.8	38.0
Wright (2000)	Bradford, UK	4.5 (7.3)	29.5

[a] Active epilepsy (lifetime prevalence in parenthesis).
[b] Only subjects >15 years.

Table 4.2 Incidence of epilepsy in developed and developing countries, with known aetiology in per cent

Author (year)	Area	Incidence (per 100 000/year)	Known aetiology (%)
Grudzinska (1974)	Zabrze, Poland	21.5	51.6
Beaussart (1980)	Pas-de-Calais, France	40–45	30.0
Granieri (1983)	Copparo, Italy	38.3	39.1
Lavados (1992)	El Salvador, Chile	108.1	29.6
Rwiza (1992)	Ulanga, Tanzania	73.3	25.3
Hauser (1993)	Rochester, USA	44.0	35.0
Olafsson (1996)	Rural Iceland	47.0	14.0
Tekle-Haimanot (1997)	Rural Ethiopia	64.0	13.7

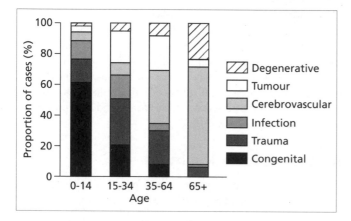

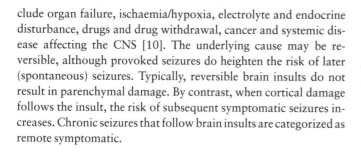

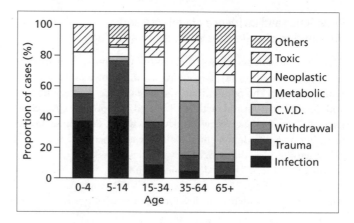

Fig. 4.1 Proportion of cases of newly diagnosed epilepsy to specific aetiological categories within age groups among those with assigned aetiologies. From [53] with permission.

Fig. 4.2 Acute symptomatic seizures: aetiology by age, Rochester, Minnesota, 1935–84. From [11] with permission.

clude organ failure, ischaemia/hypoxia, electrolyte and endocrine disturbance, drugs and drug withdrawal, cancer and systemic disease affecting the CNS [10]. The underlying cause may be reversible, although provoked seizures do heighten the risk of later (spontaneous) seizures. Typically, reversible brain insults do not result in parenchymal damage. By contrast, when cortical damage follows the insult, the risk of subsequent symptomatic seizures increases. Chronic seizures that follow brain insults are categorized as remote symptomatic.

Common causes of acute symptomatic seizures

In a study done in a well-defined population, the age-adjusted incidence rate of symptomatic seizures was about 40 per 100 000 person-years [11]. The rate was higher in men than in women (52 vs. 29 per 100 000/year). The rate was highest in the first year of life during which metabolic, infectious and encephalopathic factors were the predominant aetiologies. The rate decreased in childhood and early adulthood, with a nadir at 25–34 years. Then, the risk tended to increase with age producing a second peak at age 75 and older which is mostly accounted for by cerebrovascular disorders. The cumulative incidence of provoked seizures was almost 4% up to the age of 80. The most common precipitating causes were, in decreasing order, head trauma, cerebrovascular disease (16% each),

infection (15%), alcohol or drug withdrawal (14%) and metabolic disturbances (9%). The distribution of these causes varied with age (Fig. 4.2).

Acute symptomatic status epilepticus accounts for about one-half of cases with status epilepticus in the community with an overall incidence rate of 18 per 100 000 per year [12]. Acute symptomatic cases are associated primarily with anoxic encephalopathy, CNS infection and cerebrovascular disease.

Several acute and chronic metabolic and endocrine disorders may cause dysfunction of the CNS and induce acute symptomatic seizures. Electrolyte disorders that cause seizures include hyponatraemia and hypomagnesaemia. Epileptic seizures occur among the neurological manifestations of renal failure and its treatment, including uraemic encephalopathy, dialysis disequilibrium syndrome and dialysis encephalopathy. Pulmonary disease is also associated with seizures. Because the prevalence of asthma and epilepsy is relatively high, the two disorders may coexist in the same patient. In rare instances, epilepsy may result from chronic cerebral injury after recurrent severe hypoxic episodes during asthmatic attacks, and during acute asthma exacerbations seizures occur infrequently due to hypoxia or due to theophylline overdose. Endocrine disorders associated with epileptic seizures include pituitary neoplasms or hypoplasia, inappropriate secretion of antidiuretic hormone (ADH) syndrome, hyper/hypothyroidism, hyper/hypoparathyroidism and diabetes mellitus. Seizures are a common manifestation of non-ketotic hyperglycaemia; partial motor seizures or epilepsia partialis continua is often the first recognized feature of the disease. Seizures occurring in the context of symptomatic hypoglycaemia are also frequent and may result from several causes in patients with diabetes. Comatose survivors of cardiopulmonary arrest may present different types of seizures or status epilepticus, which result from global anoxic-ischaemic encephalopathy. Only myoclonic status epilepticus appears to correlate with a poor prognosis. Epilepsy and epileptic seizures may be manifestations of coeliac disease.

Seizures associated with lethargy, confusion and visual symptoms may be the first sign of hypertensive encephalopathy. This condition is secondary to cerebral oedema in the posterior parietal and occipital lobes with leucoencephalopathy [13]. Similar findings are reported with eclampsia and are generally reversible with blood pressure control.

Drugs and toxic agents

A wide range of substances, including drugs and illicit compounds, increase the risk of acute symptomatic seizures and epilepsy (Table 4.3). Seizures were recorded in less than 1% of 32 812 consecutive patients prospectively monitored for drug toxicity [14]. As many as 15% of drug-related seizures present as status epilepticus [15]. Drug overdose has been reported in 2% of children and 3% of adults with status epilepticus in a population-based survey [16].

Several factors are implicated in the pathophysiology of drug-induced seizures [17]. They include intrinsic epileptogenicity of the specific agent, factors influencing drug serum levels and CNS levels including lipid solubility, molecular weight, ionization, protein and binding. Patient-related factors should also be considered, including genetic susceptibility to the convulsant action of drugs,

Table 4.3 Substances reported to cause seizures[a]

Psychotropic	**Iodine contrast media******
Antidepressants	
Fluoxetine**	**Antibacterial agents**
Maprotiline****	Penicillins****
Bupropion****	Isoniazid***
Amitriptyline***	Mefloquine***
Imipramine***	Nalidixic acid**
Nortriptyline***	Norfloxacine**
Desipramine***	Cyprofloxacine**
Doxepin***	
Protriptyline***	**Antiviral agents**
MAOIs[b],**	Zidovudine***
	Aciclovir**
Antipsychotic	Ganciclovir**
Clozapine****	Foscarnet**
Phenothiazines***	
Haloperidol**	**Antineoplastic and immunosuppressant agents**
	Ciclosporin****
Hypnotic and tranquillizers	Iphosphamide***
Meprobamate (withdrawal)**	Chlorambucil***
	Busulphan***
Antiepileptic drugs	
Phenytoin*	**Respiratory agents**
Carbamazepine*	Theophylline****
Vigabatrin*	Phenylpropanolamine***
Ethosuximide*	
Gabapentin*	**Cardiovascular agents**
Benzodiazepines (withdrawal)****	β-blockers*
Barbiturates (withdrawal)****	Mexyletine*
Analgesics and anaesthetics	**Alcohol******
Meperidine****	
Propofol***	**Illicit drugs**
Lidocaine**	Cocaine****
Etomidate*	Amphetamines****
Enflurane*	Phencyclidine***
Naloxon*	Heroin**

[a] Modified from [17].
[b] Monoamine oxidase inhibitors.
Epileptogenic potential: high (****), intermediate (***), low (**), minimal (*).

antiepileptic drug interactions, impairment of the hepatic or renal drug metabolism, blood–brain barrier breakdown and intentional overdosage. However, the mechanisms of drug-induced seizures are poorly understood and the possibility exists of a chance occurrence of seizures, especially in patients with unsatisfactory seizure control receiving concurrent treatments.

A variety of agents are seizure-inducing including psychotropic drugs, non-psychotropic drugs and antiepileptic drugs [17–19]. Antipsychotic drugs lower seizure threshold and may precipitate seizures even in people without a history of seizure disorders. Factors implicated in the occurrence of seizures include high daily dose, rapid titration and concomitant brain pathology.

The risk of seizures differs according to the drug class. The aliphatic phenothiazines (e.g. chlorpromazine, promazine, trifluperazine) have the highest epileptogenic potential. The use of clozapine is associated with a 1–3% risk of seizures and with interictal epileptiform abnormalities in a relevant fraction of patients with seizures [20,21]. The piperazine phenothiazines (acetophenazine, fluphenazine, perphenazine, prochloperazine, trifluoperazine) have a less potent epileptogenic activity. Other antipsychotic agents, including haloperidol, pimozide, thioridazine and risperidone, exhibit the lowest epileptogenic effects. Patients with epilepsy are at higher risk of seizures induced by antipsychotic agents. In patients with epilepsy a drug interaction leading to an enhanced metabolism of the antiepileptic drugs may also be implicated. The risk of seizures with antidepressant drugs ranges between < 1 and 4% [22] and varies with the drug category. Agents accompanied by a high risk of seizures include clomipramine and second-generation antidepressants, amoxapine, maprotiline and bupropione [23]. The probability of seizures with tricyclic antidepressants other than clomipramine is lower and generally associated with an acute overdose. Selective serotonin reuptake inhibitors (fluoxetine, sertraline, paroxetine), monoamine oxidase inhibitors and trazodone are accompanied by a low risk of seizures.

The narcotic analgesic meperidine is metabolized in the liver to normaperidine, a potent proconvulsant, which tends to accumulate after prolonged administration and renal failure. Lidocaine-related neurotoxicity is common with intravenous use, especially with advanced age, congestive heart failure, shock, renal and hepatic failure. Seizures have been reported after administration of intravenous contrast media and may occur in as many as 15% of patients with brain metastases [24].

Neurotoxic reactions may occur frequently with β-lactam antibiotics (semisynthetic penicillins and cephalosporins) [25]. Penicillins and other β-lactam antibiotics probably increase CNS excitability by antagonizing γ-aminobutyric acid (GABA). There is considerable variability in the neurotoxic potential of the various agents. Benzylpenicillin, cefazolin and imipenem/cilastatin have the higher neurotoxic potential. Factors increasing the risk of seizure include excessive dose, decreased renal function, damage of the blood barrier, pre-existing CNS disorders and concurrent use of nephrotoxic agents or drugs lowering the seizure threshold. Isoniazide-induced seizures have been reported, mostly in patients with a history of epilepsy. Isoniazide probably provokes seizures by antagonizing pyridoxal phosphate (the active form of pyridoxine), which is involved in GABA biosynthesis. Seizures have also been reported in elderly patients receiving aminoglycosides, metronidazole, quinolones and amantadine. Quinolones (nalidixic acid, nor-floxacin, ciprofloxacin) probably enhance seizure activity by inhibiting GABA binding to membrane receptors.

Zidovudine and other antiviral agents have been followed by the occurrence of seizures in patients infected with human immunodeficiency virus (HIV). However, the risk of seizures attributable to these agents is ill-defined as HIV-infected patients have several concurrent risk factors for seizures.

The alkylating agents (especially chlorambucil and busulfan) tend to provoke seizures with high doses. The immunosuppressant agent ciclosporin exerts an epileptogenic action by producing a CNS structural lesion.

The epileptogenic potential of theophylline is well-known. Seizures and status epilepticus have been repeatedly reported with theophylline, often attributable to inadvertent or intentional overdosing. However, some patients may develop seizures with therapeutic drug concentrations. The exact mechanism of theophylline-induced seizures is unknown, although it may be related to antagonism of adenosine.

β-blockers and other antiarrhythmic agents have been reported to precipitate seizures, particularly in overdose.

Cimetidine has been occasionally found to induce seizures, especially in elderly individuals. Hypocalcaemia due to impaired parathyroid hormone levels has been implicated in cimetidine neurotoxicity. Levodopa, insulin, thiazide diuretics, lidocaine, salicylates, chemotherapeutic agents, L-asparaginase and baclofen have been reported to cause seizures on several occasions.

Seizures may be precipitated after sudden withdrawal of any antiepileptic drug, particularly benzodiazepines and barbiturates.

Excessive alcohol consumption and alcohol abstinence syndrome are risk factors for a generalized tonic-clonic seizure and epilepsy. The risk of a first generalized tonic-clonic seizure in chronic alcoholics is increased almost seven-fold when compared to non-alcoholics [26]. For a daily alcohol intake of less than 50 g/day the risk is non-significant. However, the risk of seizures increases directly as the daily alcohol intake rises. The odds ratio (OR) is 3.0 (95% CI 1.7–5.4) for a daily intake of 51–100 g/day, 7.9 (95% CI 2.9–21.9) for 101–200 g/day, and 16.6 (95% CI 1.9–373.4) when the intake is more than 200 g/day. Although alcohol withdrawal has been repeatedly implicated in the occurrence of seizures, the mechanism is unknown [27].

Illicit drugs such as cocaine, phencyclidine, amphetamines and heroin, can cause seizures. Past and present heroin use has been shown to be a risk factor for provoked and unprovoked seizures (OR 2.8; 95% CI 1.5–5.7) [28]. By contrast, marijuana use in men appeared to be a protective factor against seizures (OR 0.4; 95% CI 0.2–0.8) and against provoked seizures occurring within 90 days (OR 0.2; 95% CI 0.1–0.8). The amphetamine derivative 3,4-methylenedioxymethamphetamine (MDMA), colloquially called 'ecstasy', can cause seizures, rhabdomyolysis and liver dysfunction.

Carbon monoxide poisoning leading to carboxyhaemoglobin levels above 50% may be followed by seizures. Organic solvent exposure and poisoning with heavy metals may cause seizures in individuals with no history of epilepsy and they may exacerbate seizures in patients with epilepsy.

Table 4.4 Risk for epilepsy in genetic disorders

Category	No increase in risk	Slight increase in risk (5–20%)	High risk (>20%)
Chromosome disorders	Cri-du-chat syndrome Sex chromosome disorders	Trisomy 21 syndrome Other chromosome anomalies	Fragile X syndrome Trisomy 13 syndrome Trisomy 18 syndrome Wolf-Hirschhorn syndrome
Contiguous gene disorders		Prader–Willi syndrome	Angelman's syndrome Miller–Dieker syndrome
Metabolic disorders	Endocrine disorders Exocrine disorders Glycogen storage disease Mucopolysaccharidoses	Acute intermittent porphyria Leukodystrophies	Amino acid disorders Glycogen storage disorders Homocystinuria Krabbe's disease Leigh's syndrome Menkes disease Mitochondrial disorders Organic acidurias Peroxisomal disorders Pyridoxine-dependent seizures
Genetic syndromes			
Short stature	Bloom's syndrome Cockayne's syndrome Dubowitz's syndrome Hallermann–Streiff syndrome Noonan's syndrome	Brachmann–de Lange syndrome Robinow's syndrome Rubinstein–Taybi syndrome Smith–Lemli–Opitz syndrome Xeroderma pigmentosum (de Sanctis–Cacchione variant)	
Early overgrowth	Marshall–Smith syndrome Smith–Golabi–Behmel syndrome Sotos' syndrome Weaver's syndrome	Bannayan–Riley–Ruvalcaba syndrome Beckwith–Wiedemann syndrome Cohen's syndrome	Borjeson–Forssman–Lehmann syndrome
Skeletal dysplasias	Achondroplasia Apert's syndrome Metaphyseal dysplasias Osteochondrodysplasias Osteopetrosis Saethre–Chotzen syndrome	Albright's osteodystrophy Crouzon's syndrome Hypophosphatasia Pfeiffer's syndrome	Christian's syndrome
Facial defects	Moebius sequence Oculo-auriculo-vertebral syndromes Treacher–Collins syndrome Other branchial arch syndromes	FG syndrome Langer–Giedion syndrome Progressive hemifacial atrophy	Acrocallosal syndrome Cardiofaciocutaneous syndrome Coffin–Lowry syndrome
Connective tissue disorders	All except homocystinuria		
Neurocutaneous disorders	Neurofibromatosis-2	Neurofibromatosis-1	Encephalocraniocutaneous lipomatosis Epidermal naevus Hemimegalencephaly Incontinentia pigmenti Sturge–Weber syndrome Tuberous sclerosis
Ectodermal/mesodermal dysplasias	All disorders		
Disorders of brain development	Posterior fossa disorders		Agenesis of corpus callosum syndromes Holoprosencephaly Lissencephaly Other disorders of neuro proliferation, migration and connectivity

Continued.

Table 4.4 *Continued*

Category	No increase in risk	Slight increase in risk (5–20%)	High risk (>20%)
Neurodegenerative disorders	Ataxias Parkinson's disease and variants	Alzheimer's disease Hallervorden–Spatz disease Wilson's disease	Ceroid lipofuscinosis Dentatorubropallidoluysian atrophy (myoclonus epilepsy form) Juvenile onset Huntington's disease Neuroacanthocytosis Rett's syndrome

From [67] with permission.

Gene–environment relationship in epilepsy

Mechanisms of inheritance in epilepsy

Inheritance in epilepsy follows four different patterns which can be summarized as follows:

1 Epileptic seizures occurring in the context of multiorgan hereditary disorders.
2 Idiopathic epilepsies with simple mendelian inheritance.
3 Epilepsies with complex inheritance.
4 Idiopathic epilepsies associated with cytogenetic (chromosomal) abnormalities [29].

Patients with genetic or chromosomal syndromes associated with epilepsy account for 2–3% of all cases of epilepsy. Epilepsies with simple mendelian inheritance and epilepsies with cytogenetic abnormalities account for about 1% of total epilepsies. Epilepsies with complex inheritance include the majority of the epileptic syndromes and are the result of complex as yet unknown mechanisms reflecting a gene–environment interaction. Advances in molecular genetics are beginning to provide the means for understanding the genetic basis of these epilepsies. Genetic disorders associated with epilepsy are summarized in Table 4.4.

Epilepsy secondary to multiorgan hereditary disorders

Chromosome disorders include additions, deletions or rearrangement of chromosomal material. The most common chromosome disorder is Down's syndrome with an approximate incidence of 1:650 live births. Usually due to trisomy 21, triplication of 21q22.3 results in the typical phenotype. Epilepsy is present in up to 10% of cases and EEG abnormalities in more than 20%. Fragile X syndrome has an incidence of 1:1500 males while 1:1000 females are carriers. The X chromosome shows a fragile site at Xq27.3. Seizures are present in one-quarter of cases and EEG abnormalities in one-half. Wolf–Hirschhorn syndrome is a severe condition characterized by systemic malformations and epilepsy in 70–100% of cases. The genetic defect is a partial monosomy 4p. Other conditions with a high risk for epilepsy include trisomy 13 and 18 which produce gross brain malformations.

Three disorders characterized by deletions of contiguous genes have been identified. Angelman's syndrome is a condition characterized by multiple malformations, seizures, EEG abnormalities and 'puppet-like' movements due to truncal ataxia causing titubation. Seizures are present in 85–90% of cases. In most cases a deletion is present at chromosome 15q11–q13. In contrast to Angelman's syndrome, seizures are present in 15–20% of patients with Prader–Willi syndrome, another complex entity, which results from paternally inherited deletions of 15q11–q13 and in systemic malformations and mental retardation. A third contiguous gene disorder is Miller–Dieker syndrome with a microdeletion involving the 17p13.3 band and a specific facial phenotype.

Several inherited metabolic disorders cause epilepsy (Table 4.4). These can cause intermittent or persistent hypoglycaemia, hyperammonaemia, hypocalcaemia, hyperglycinaemia, metabolic acidosis, ketoacidosis, abnormal amino acid or oligosaccharide profile, mucopolysaccharides or lipid storage, and lead to secondary structural abnormalities. In these conditions, both metabolic derangement and structural abnormalities contribute to the occurrence of seizures. Intrinsic genetic mutations, usually transmitted as simple mendelian traits, represent the underlying causes. About one-quarter of cases have clinical manifestations at birth and almost all are expressed by the end of puberty. Dysmorphic features are at times present. Seizure types are diverse. In these cases, treatment must be primarily directed at bringing the metabolic defect under control.

Among the disorders of energy metabolism, seizures have been reported in mitochondrial encephalomyopathies, a heterogeneous group of multisystem disorders resulting from mitochondrial DNA point mutations. Seizures are a common feature of myoclonus epilepsy and ragged red fibres (MERRF) and mitocondrial encephalopathy with lactic acidosis and stroke-like episodes (MELAS). MERRF is due to a point mutation in the tRNA gene of maternally derived mitochondrial genome. MELAS is another maternally inherited disorder with both partial and generalized seizures, due to an mtDNA point mutation, an adenine-to-guanine transition in the tRNA gene at nt3243. As with other clinical features, the frequency and severity of seizures vary within the syndrome and among affected individuals within a family.

Among the lysosomal storage disorders (lipidoses), epilepsy is a prominent feature of Krabbe's disease and some forms of Gaucher's disease. Seizures are also common in peroxisomal disorders like Zellweger's syndrome and neonatal adrenoleukodystrophy.

Neurocutaneous disorders are important recognizable causes of epilepsy. Neurofibromatosis, the best-known clinical entity, is characterized by the presence of abnormal cortical architecture (heterotopias), systemic or peripheral nerve changes (neurofibromatosis type 1) or by neoplastic lesions of Schwann cells, meningeal cells and glia (neurofibromatosis type 2). In neurofibromatosis type 1 the incidence of epilepsy is about 5–11%. Tuberous sclerosis is an autosomal dominant multisystem disorder of cell migration resulting in hamartoma formation. More than 90% of patients with tuberous sclerosis from clinical series have seizures of various types, mental retardation and clinical deterioration during their lifetime. Sturge–Weber syndrome is a sporadic disorder of the vasculature of the face and head associated with leptomeningeal angiomas and calcifications. Seizures are reported in more than 20% of cases. The presence of seizures is correlated to mental retardation and lack of independence.

Genetic disorders of brain development encompass a wide range of conditions characterized by interruptions in the development of the human brain at various stages. While cortical developmental disorders usually cause epilepsy, it is unknown what proportion of epilepsy is attributable to disorders of brain development. In addition, except for some specific syndromes, there are no clinical features which distinguish these disorders. Generalized abnormalities of cortical development tend to present with generalized seizures while focal or multifocal malformations are most commonly associated with focal seizures. There are many classification schemes for cortical malformations.

According to the stage in embryological development, cortical malformations can be classified in three major groups: malformations due to abnormal neuronal and glial proliferations, malformations due to abnormal neuronal migration and malformations due to abnormal cortical organization (postmigrational) [30]. Within each group, generalized and localized malformations are identified. The most common and better identified conditions include focal cortical dysplasia (disruption of cortical lamination with poorly differentiated glial elements), hemi-megaloencephaly (predominantly unilateral cerebral hemisphere pathology associated with an enlarged hemisphere), focal transmantle dysplasia (abnormal brain tissue extending through the entire cerebral mantle from the pia to the ventricular surface), lissencephaly (absence of normal sulcation), heterotopia (abnormal location of normal brain cells), polymicrogyria (shallow and small gyri separated by shallow sulci or wide gyri) and schizencephaly (grey matter-lined clefts in the cerebral hemispheres extending from the pia to the ependymal lining). Brain developmental abnormalities are reported in up to 50% of children and 20% of adults referred to epilepsy centres for intractable epilepsy. A screening for lissencephaly reported a prevalence rate of 11.7 per million births [31].

Seizures and EEG abnormalities are commonly found in several neurodegenerative disorders.

One of these, Rett's syndrome, is characterized by autistic dementia, gait apraxia, stereotyped hand movements, and bizarre attacks involving hyperventilation, limb and truncal jerking and profuse sweating. Likewise, seizures are a frequent clinical feature in patients with Huntington's disease starting in childhood or adolescence or with Wilson's disease with juvenile onset.

Other neurodegenerative disorders cause progressive myoclonus epilepsies, a group of epilepsies of various aetiologies, characterized by myoclonic seizures, tonic-clonic seizures and progressive neurological deterioration with ataxia and dementia [32]. Progressive myoclonus epilepsies account for approximately 1% of cases in referral centres and are mostly due to inherited metabolic abnormalities [33]. Series from different countries reveal marked geographical and ethnic variability in the occurrence of the specific subgroups of progressive myoclonus epilepsies. There are no data on the incidence and prevalence of these conditions, except for

Unverricht–Lundborg disease, which has an estimated incidence in excess of 1:20 000 in Finland [34].

Mitochondrial encephalopathies and lipidoses are among the most common causes of progressive myoclonus epilepsy [32]. The most common forms of progressive myoclonus epilepsies include Unverricht–Lundborg disease, MERRF, MELAS, Lafora's disease, lysosomal storage diseases (lipidoses), neuronal ceroid lipofuscinoses and dentatopallidoluysian atrophy. Unverricht–Lundborg disease is an autosomal recessive condition linked to the long arm of chromosome 21 where the gene for the protein cystatin B has been identified. The disease has a high incidence in the Baltic region, southern Europe and North Africa.

Lafora's disease, an autosomal recessive condition mostly reported from southern Europe, is characterized by the presence of Lafora bodies, polyglucosan inclusions in neurones and a variety of other sites. Among the lipidoses, sialidosis type I is an autosomal recessive disorder characterized by the deficiency of α-neuraminidase. Neuronal ceroid lipofuscinoses are autosomal recessive conditions with infantile, juvenile and adult onset, which are genetically distinct and represented in geographical clusterings. The metabolic defect is unknown. Dentatopallidoluysian atrophy has distinct pathological features associated with a variety of phenotypes, mainly identified in Japan.

Idiopathic epilepsies with simple mendelian inheritance

Several epilepsy syndromes result from mendelian inheritance of single gene mutations (Table 4.5). Molecular geneticists have classified these epilepsies as ion channelopathies, with mutations identified in genes encoding the α_4 or the β_2 subunit of the neuronal nicotinic acetylcholine receptor (CHRNA4; CHRNB2), GABA receptors (GABARB3), voltage-gated potassium channels (KCNA1, KCNQ2, KCNQ3) and voltage-gated sodium channel auxiliary subunits (SCN1A, SCN1B). They include an ever increasing number of generalized and partial epilepsies that include the following [35].

• Generalized epilepsy with febrile seizures plus include a spectrum of different phenotypes having in common the presence of febrile seizures and mild to severe generalized epilepsies. In these patients different seizure patterns are present, including tonic-clonic seizures, absence, myoclonic or atonic seizures, and rarely partial seizures. Myoclonic-astatic epilepsy or severe myoclonic epilepsy of infancy are present in the more severe cases. The pattern of inheritance is autosomal dominant with about 60% penetrance.

Table 4.5 Idiopathic epilepsies with simple mendelian inheritance

Disease	Gene	Locus
Autosomal dominant nocturnal	CHRNA4	20q
frontal lobe epilepsy	CHRNB2	1q
Benign familial neonatal	KCNQ2	20q
convulsions	KCNQ3	8q
Generalized epilepsy with febrile	SCN1B	19q
seizures plus	SCN1A	2q

From [29] with permission.

• Familial adult myoclonic epilepsy has been described in families from Japan and is characterized by the adult onset of myoclonic jerks in the four limbs (increasing with age), finger tremors, photosensitivity and rare generalized tonic-clonic seizures.

• Familial autosomal recessive idiopathic myoclonic epilepsy of infancy has been described in an Italian family; the phenotype is characterized by the occurrence of myoclonus at different paediatric and adult ages, accompanied by febrile and afebrile generalized tonic-clonic seizures.

• X-linked infantile spasms occur in male infants aged 2–6 months and present with infantile spasms, developmental arrest and hypsarrythmia on EEG.

• Benign familial neonatal convulsions tend to occur between the second or third day and last until the ninth or tenth day of life in about 90% of cases. Seizures tend to recur in later years in the remainder.

• In benign familial infantile convulsions partial seizures begin between 4 and 8 months, tend to occur in clusters lasting 2–4 days and are characterized by psychomotor arrest, cyanosis, deviation of the head, tonic contraction and bilateral clonic jerks. The ictal EEG shows occipitoparietal fast activity, which becomes at times generalized.

• Autosomal dominant nocturnal frontal lobe epilepsy follows an autosomal dominant inheritance with 70% penetrance and is characterized by the occurrence of clusters of motor seizures preceded by an aura, which is perceived by the patient while arising from sleep. Awareness of the seizure may be retained.

• Familial temporal lobe epilepsy includes two separate varieties of variable severity, the lateral and the mesial temporal lobe epilepsy. The former is characterized by the occurrence of auditory and visual hallucinations and the latter by *déjà vu*, perceptual changes and autonomic phenomena.

• Autosomal dominant rolandic epilepsy with speech dyspraxia is a rare syndrome following a dominant inheritance with anticipation and is characterized by typical rolandic seizures associated with speech apraxia.

• Autosomal recessive rolandic epilepsy with paroxysmal exercise-induced dystonia and writer's cramp has been described in a consanguineous Italian family: this condition is characterized by rare orofaciobrachial seizures, with interictal EEG centrotemporal spikes. The phenotype is also defined by the occurrence of childhood exercise-induced dystonia and writer's cramp (the latter persisting into adolescence).

• Familial partial epilepsy with variable foci is a syndrome presenting with different partial seizures in different family members.

Idiopathic epilepsies with complex inheritance [36]
(Table 4.6)

Epilepsies with complex, non-mendelian, genetic transmission include idiopathic generalized and partial epilepsies. The term 'complex' indicates a hereditary pattern which does not follow a simple mode of inheritance but involves multiple contributing factors. These disorders may have more than one genetic aetiology and phenotypes can be caused by mutations at different genetic loci. In these cases, multiple interacting loci contribute to the pathogenesis of the disease, by altering interactions between proteins. In this context, the concept of epilepsy syndromes as discrete entities which are

Table 4.6 Idiopathic epilepsies with complex inheritance

Disease	Gene
Generalized	
Infantile absence epilepsy	?3p, ?8q24
Juvenile absence epilepsy	
Juvenile myoclonic epilepsy	6p, ?15q
Epilepsy with generalized tonic clonic seizures only	?6p
Benign myoclonic epilepsy of infancy	
Myoclonic-astatic epilepsy	
Partial	
Benign rolandic epilepsy	?15q14
Benign epilepsy of childhood with occipital spikes	

clinically homogeneous and biologically distinct can be hardly sustained. By contrast, the emerging idea is that of a neurobiological continuum, with idiopathic epilepsies that are largely genetic at one end, and symptomatic epilepsies that are predominantly acquired at the other [37]. Thus, the interaction between genes and environment affects the risk of disease in susceptible individuals and defines the phenotype.

The idiopathic generalized epilepsies due to genetic causes account for about 40–60% of all epilepsy and most have complex inheritance patterns. These include infantile absence epilepsy, juvenile absence epilepsy, juvenile myoclonic epilepsy and epilepsy with generalized tonic-clonic seizures only. The latter accounts for 25–31% of all epilepsies. The corresponding numbers for infantile absence epilepsy, juvenile absence epilepsy and juvenile myoclonic epilepsy are 4–11%, 8–9% and 3–7%, respectively. In families with multiple affected individuals the majority have idiopathic generalized epilepsies or febrile seizures, but the specific syndrome often differs from that of the proband. Within the same family, two individuals are more likely to have similar syndromes if they have a close genetic relationship. Studies in twins have shown that affected monozygotic pairs have the same syndrome, but dizygotic pairs, like ordinary siblings, tend to have different syndromes.

In childhood and juvenile absence epilepsy concordance rates for absence seizures are significantly higher among monozygous than dizygous twins. The typical EEG pattern (normal background with interspersed bursts of bilaterally synchronous 2.5–3.5 Hz spike-wave complexes) is inherited as an autosomal dominant trait with age-dependent penetrance. Although a clear pattern of inheritance is not present, absence seizures and EEG patterns can be explained by the interaction between genetic and environmental factors. The locus for typical childhood absence epilepsy has not yet been located although mapping to chromosome 1p and 8q was reported in single families with absence seizures associated to myoclonic or generalized tonic-clonic seizures.

Several diverse models of inheritance have been proposed for juvenile myoclonic epilepsy, including monogenic autosomal dominant and recessive, digenic and polygenic. In the families with juvenile myoclonic epilepsy other idiopathic generalized epilepsies can be found, including childhood and juvenile absence epilepsy, and epilepsy with generalized tonic-clonic seizures only, as well as typical EEG traits (4–6 polyspike-wave complexes) in otherwise asymptomatic individuals. Although initial evidence of a susceptibility gene for juvenile myoclonic epilepsy pointed to chromosome 6p, at present data are inconsistent about chromosome 6p and juvenile myoclonic epilepsy since linkage to chromosome 15q was also reported.

Epilepsy with generalized tonic-clonic seizures only

The risk of epilepsy is increased in the family members of patients with epilepsy with generalized tonic-clonic seizures only. Other forms of idiopathic generalized epilepsy can usually be found in the family members. A susceptibility gene can be present on chromosome 6p in patients with grand mal on awakening.

Benign partial epilepsy with centrotemporal spikes (rolandic epilepsy) is the most common syndrome in the group of idiopathic partial epilepsies with complex inheritance. Unilateral motor or sensory seizures appear at the age of 5 to 10 years, generally during

Table 4.7 Prenatal and perinatal risk factors for epilepsy. Measure is OR for case–control studies and RR for cohort studies

Parameter	Lilienfeld (1954, 1955) Pasamanick (1955)	Henderson (1964)	Chevrie (1977)	Rocca (1987)
Case ascertainment	Specialty clinics	Specialty clinics	Clinic	Medical records
Study design	Case–control	Case–control	Case–control	Case–control
Obstetric complications	$1.62^{a,c}/1.13^{b,c}$	$1.7^{b,c}$	1.27^{ns}	
Toxaemia, pre-eclampsia, eclampsia		$0.99^{b,c}$		
Prematurity	$2.3^{a,d}/1.38^{b,d}$			
Pre- or perinatal abnormality			1.84^{f}	
Low birth weight	$4.9^{a}/1.2^{b}$	$1.4^{b,c}$		
Neonatal seizures		$3.0^{b,c}$		∞/ns^{c}
Neonatal abnormalities (seizures, asphyxia)	$1.6^{a,c,d}/1.2^{b-d}$	$9.3^{b,c}$	2.21^{g}	
Small for gestational age				
Delivery problems		$1.1^{b,c}$	1.74^{g}	
Maternal haemorrhage	12.4^{a}	$3.6^{b,c}$		
Hypoxia				

From [38] with permission.
[a] White only.
[b] Black only.
[c] Without associated defects (cerebral palsy, mental retardation, central nervous system malformations).
[d] Without maternal complications.
[e] Perinatal risk factors.
[f] $P < 0.01$.
[g] $P < 0.05$.
ns, not significant.

Table 4.7 *Continued*

Parameter	Bergamasco (1984)	Rantakallio (1986)	van den Berg (1969)	NCPP (1982–87)
Case ascertainment	Delivery rooms mothers	Birth cohort	Birth cohort	Pregnant
Study design	Historical cohort	Cohort	Cohort	Cohort
Obstetric complications		20		ns
Toxaemia, pre-eclampsia, eclampsia				ns
Prematurity				ns
Pre- or perinatal abnormality				
Low birth weight			2.1	ns
Neonatal seizures				22.4
Neonatal abnormalities (seizures, asphyxia)		5.6		
Small for gestational age			2.8	1.7
Delivery problems		17.4^{a}		ns
Maternal haemorrhage				ns
Hypoxia	5.1			ns

[a] Perinatal risk factors.
NCPP, National Collaborative Perinatal Project; ns, not significant.

sleep. Unconfirmed reports suggested that in this syndrome the EEG trait is inherited in an autosomal dominant fashion. Genetic factors have also been implicated in benign occipital epilepsy, a benign syndrome occurring mostly at age 4–8 years and characterized by visual and adversive seizures eventually evolving into unilateral or generalized tonic-clonic seizures, hemiclonic or partial complex seizures, and migraine-like headaches.

Acquired causes of epilepsy

Prenatal and perinatal risk factors

Pre- and perinatal risk factors include toxaemia and eclampsia during pregnancy, low birth weight, asphyxia and other neonatal abnormalities, and other less defined conditions [38]. Although the role of these factors in the aetiology of epilepsy seems established, most of the earlier studies yielded relative risks (RRs) or ORs below 10, which indicate, at best, a moderate association between pre- and perinatal factors and subsequent epilepsy (Table 4.7). Even in a more recent population-based study on the risk factors for idiopathic generalized seizures the association with specific factors was not clinically relevant [39]. The only significant factors included multiparity (OR 3.2 and 7.1 for women with two and three antecedent pregnancies, respectively), maternal age >35 years (OR 2.8) and enduring manual labour (OR 2.5). These results may be explained by the use of differing definitions of pre- and perinatal factors, the study populations, the methods of ascertainment of the cause–effect relationship and the sample size.

Cerebral palsy and mental retardation

Mental retardation and cerebral palsy are comorbid markers of neurological impairment, which explains their significant association with epilepsy, but they are not causes of epilepsy. Epilepsy occurred in 34% of children with cerebral palsy and cerebral palsy was present in 19% of children developing epilepsy in the US National Collaborative Perinatal Project, a study which followed newborns up to age 7 years [40]. In the same cohort the risk of mental retardation was 5.5 times higher among children developing epilepsy following a febrile seizure than in children with a febrile seizure alone [41]. Furthermore, these studies revealed that when perinatal asphyxia caused epilepsy it also produced cerebral palsy [42]. Mental retardation (IQ ≤ 70) was present in 27% of children with epilepsy. Seizures are present in about 50% of children with mental retardation *and* cerebral palsy.

CNS infections

CNS infections are a major risk factor for epilepsy. Seizures may be the presenting or the only symptom, or may be one component of a diffuse brain involvement. Using the incidence of epilepsy expected in the general population for reference, the risk of epilepsy among individuals with encephalitis or meningitis is increased almost seven-fold [43]. This increased risk is highest during the first 5 years after infection and tends to decrease thereafter, but it remains elevated up to 15 years. The low proportion of postinfectious epilepsies can be explained by the low incidence of encephalitis which is the most common cause of postinfectious epilepsy. The risk of

epilepsy varies according to the infection type, being highest with encephalitis (16.2), intermediate with bacterial meningitis (4.2) and lowest (non-significant) with aseptic meningitis (2.3). The presence of early seizures (i.e. during the acute phase of the infection) greatly influences the risk of subsequent unprovoked seizures. As encephalitis and bacterial meningitis are more prevalent in infants, children and young adults, most of the postinfectious epilepsies tend to occur in younger individuals. Infection-related seizures tend to be partial onset. Although brain abscesses are highly epileptogenic (up to 37% of supratentorial lesions) [44], the attributable risk is negligible because of the rarity of this condition which has an annual incidence: 0.3–1.2 cases per 100 000 population.

Infectious agents causing diseases in which seizures are a presenting or principal symptom include herpes simplex virus, cytomegalovirus, Epstein–Barr virus, HIV and arboviruses [45]. Toxoplasma can produce non-specific symptoms and signs of intracranial mass lesions and seizures in patients with acquired immune deficiency syndrome (AIDS).

Although immunizations have been repeatedly proposed as causes of epilepsy, epidemiological studies failed to link epilepsy and any other serious neurological condition to vaccine exposure [46]. In one report, an increase in febrile seizures has been observed during the second week after measles–mumps–rubella immunization [47].

In developing countries infectious causes of epilepsy have higher prevalence rates of epilepsy in rural compared to urban areas. In these countries, infectious diseases are common. Neurocysticercosis is a major cause of symptomatic epilepsy in developing countries [48]. Cerebral malaria, tuberculosis and toxoplasmosis are also common.

Dementia

Dementing disorders are common in the elderly with an overall prevalence in persons 65 years and older of 6% [49] and increase exponentially as a function of age in the 65–85-year age range [50]. Alzheimer's disease is the most common cause of dementia in the Western hemisphere, followed by multi-infarct dementia. Compared to non-demented individuals matched for age and sex, patients with Alzheimer's disease have a six-fold heightened risk of unprovoked seizures [51] and people with other types of dementia have an eight-fold increased risk. Seizures may occur as early as 3 months after the diagnosis of Alzheimer's disease or up to 9 years afterwards. The range is even wider in other dementias (<1 month to 22 years) suggesting a lack of correlation with the duration of the disease. This finding is in contrast with clinical series showing that seizures tend to occur in the late stages of the disease. Partial onset seizures are the prevailing type in Alzheimer's disease and generalized onset seizures tend to predominate in other dementing disorders. Myoclonus is another common finding in patients with Alzheimer's disease occurring in about 10% of autopsy-verified cases and is a late manifestation [52].

Based on the increased life expectancy of the general population, the number of individuals affected by Alzheimer's disease and other dementias is going to increase and so will the proportion of epilepsy attributed to dementing disorders.

Cerebrovascular disease

Stroke is the most commonly identified cause of epilepsy in the elderly [53]. Silent stroke may also explain the occurrence of some cryptogenic epilepsies in aged individuals.

A wide range of percentages of persons developing seizures after stroke has been reported and is mostly due to different study populations and methodology. In a population-based study of seizure disorders after cerebral infarction, early seizures occurred in 6% of patients [54]. In patients with early seizures cerebral infarcts were more likely located in the anterior hemisphere (OR 4.0; 95% CI 1.2–13.7). The standardized morbidity ratio (SMR)[1] for epilepsy was 5.9 (95% CI 3.5–9.4). The SMR for an initial late seizure was 6.4 (95% CI 4.2–9.3). About two-thirds of patients with initial late seizures developed epilepsy within 5 years. The SMR of developing initial late seizures or epilepsy was highest during the first year and tended to decrease during the ensuing 3 years. There was an inverse correlation between age and risk of seizures with a peak in patients aged less than 55 years. The corresponding risks were higher after recurrent stroke. Early seizures and recurrent strokes were the only factors shown by multivariate analysis to predict initial late seizures and epilepsy.

A history of stroke has been found to be associated with an increased lifetime occurrence of epilepsy (OR 3.3; 95% CI 1.3–8.5) [55]. Among the other vascular determinants, only a history of hypertension was associated with the occurrence of unprovoked seizures (OR 1.6; 95% CI 1.0–2.4). The risk of unprovoked seizures rises to 4.1 (95% CI 1.5–11.0) in subjects having a history of both stroke and hypertension [56]. Compared to ischaemic stroke, haemorrhagic stroke (subarachnoid haemorrhage and, to a lesser extent, primary intracerebral haemorrhage) is followed by a higher risk of seizures [57]. Another risk factor for seizures after ischaemic stroke is a lesion including the total anterior circulation. The cumulative probability of developing seizures after a first stroke is about 6% after 1 year and rises to 11% at 5 years, with significant differences across stroke subtypes (cerebral infarction 4 and 10%; primary cerebral haemorrhage 20 and 26%; subarachnoid haemorrhage 22 and 34%). The risk of epilepsy among survivors of subarachnoid haemorrhage caused by ruptured cerebral aneurysm is highest in patients with acute symptomatic seizures (RR 7.0; 95% CI 2.3; 21.6) and those with severe neurological sequelae (RR 2.5; 95% CI 0.9–6.3) [58].

Vascular malformations

Arteriovenous malformations cause epilepsy in 17–40% of cases. Factors associated with the development of epilepsy include the size and depth of the malformation, age at diagnosis, presentation with haemorrhage and surgical intervention [59]. Large and/or superficial malformations are more epileptogenic.

Other vascular disorders

Seizures also occur in several connective tissue disorders, most

frequently in systemic lupus erythematosus, and in patients with vasculitis involving the brain. In these conditions, often seizures are not due to the primary disease process, but rather are due to to secondary complications, like arterial hypertension, renal failure or atherosclerosis.

Demyelinating disorders

Several clinical series reported an association between epilepsy and multiple sclerosis. In a small population-based study, patients with multiple sclerosis had a three-fold increase (SMR 3.0; 95% CI 0.6–8.8) in the risk of epilepsy compared to the general population [60]. Although non-significant, the increased risk of epilepsy in patients with multiple sclerosis is consistent with clinical series. The cumulative risk of epilepsy after multiple sclerosis is 1.1% at 5 years, 1.8% by 10 years and 3.1% by 15 years. The mean interval until the onset of epilepsy is about 7 years after the onset of multiple sclerosis. Convulsive status epilepticus has been reported more frequently in patients with multiple sclerosis. Although in some patients epilepsy precedes multiple sclerosis by years or decades, there is no evidence of an increased risk of epilepsy prior to the onset of the symptoms due to multiple sclerosis.

Head trauma

Head trauma is an important cause of epilepsy. The occurrence of epilepsy after head injury depends on the severity of the trauma and the area of the brain that is affected. The kinetic energy imparted to the brain tissue produces pressure waves which disrupt tissue and lead to histopathological changes, including gliosis, axon retraction balls, wallerian degeneration, neurological scars and cystic white matter lesions. In addition, iron liberated from haemoglobin generates free radicals that disrupt cell membranes and have been implicated in post-traumatic epileptogenesis [61]. Iron and other compounds have also been found to provoke intracellular calcium oscillations.

In the civilian population, traumatic events provoking concussion as defined by either loss of consciousness or post-traumatic amnesia but no evidence of tissue disruption, usually are not followed by epilepsy [62]. The risk for seizures tends to increase according to the severity of traumatic brain injury (Table 4.8). Five years after concussion, the cumulative probability of post-traumatic epilepsy is 0.7% after mild injuries, 1.2% after moderate injuries and 10% after severe injuries. The excessive risk is highest during the first year and diminishes during the ensuing years. After 10 years, only severe injuries still exhibit an increased risk of seizures. The 30-year cumulative incidence of seizures is 2.1% for mild injuries, 4.2% for moderate injuries and 16.7% for severe injuries. Compared to mild injuries, the risk of seizures after severe injuries is 30 times higher during the first year and eight times higher by year 5. The highest risk of post-traumatic epilepsy occurs following missile wounds, brain volume loss being highly predictive. Additional risk factors for epilepsy after penetrating head injuries include focal neurological signs, haematoma, the presence of metal fragments and the location of the lesion [63]. The risk factors for seizure occurrence after traumatic civilian brain injury include, in decreasing order of importance, brain contusion and/or subdural haematoma, linear fracture and age older than 5 years, depressed fracture, loss of

[1] Defined here as the ratio between the incidence of epilepsy among patients with ischaemic stroke and the incidence of epilepsy in the general population.

61

Table 4.8 Standardized incidence ratios for seizures among 4541
patients with traumatic brain injury, according to the severity
of the injury

Severity of injury[a]	Number of cases		Standardized incidence ratio (95% CI)
	Observed	Expected	
Mild	28	18.4	1.5 (1.0–2.2)
Moderate	30	10.5	2.9 (1.9–4.1)
Severe	39	2.3	17.0 (12.3–23.6)
Total	97	31.2	3.1 (2.5–3.8)

[a] Patients with mild injuries had a loss of consciousness or post-traumatic
amnesia for less than 30 min, with no skull fracture; those with moderate
injuries had a loss of consciousness or post-traumatic amnesia for 30 min
to 24 h or a skull fracture; and those with severe injuries had a brain
contusion or intracranial haematoma or a loss of consciousness or post-
traumatic amnesia for more than 24 h.
From [62] with permission.

consciousness or post-traumatic amnesia for more than 24 h,
seizures occurring during the first week and age 65 years or older.

Brain tumours

Brain tumours are responsible for 1–6% of epilepsy according to
studies performed before modern imaging became available. Thus,
these studies probably underestimated the role of neoplasia in
epileptogenesis. The incidence of epilepsy associated with primary
brain tumours is related to tumour pathology, speed of growth and
location. Seizures are more often the presenting symptoms in low-
grade tumours than in rapidly invasive tumours. The mechanisms
of epileptogenesis in patients with brain tumours include impaired
vascularization of the surrounding cerebral cortex, morphological
neuronal alterations, changes in the excitatory and inhibitory
synaptic mechanisms and genetic susceptibility [64].

The epileptogenicity of tumours is related to their location. In
large neurosurgical series epilepsy was present in approximately
50% of patients with supratentorial tumours [65]. Individuals with
tumours in the centrotemporoparietal region have the highest incidence of epilepsy. Epilepsy is more frequent in patients with superficial and cortical tumours than those with deep and non-cortical
tumours. Age at seizure onset, seizure type, duration of epilepsy,
neurological finding and response to antiepileptic drugs are not useful in predicting the nature of the underlying lesion. Although it
is reported that most seizures caused by brain tumours are partial
and associated with abnormal clinical and electrophysiological
changes, there is no evidence that sensitivity and specificity of
seizure type, neurological examination and EEG are higher in brain
tumours than in other causes of epilepsy.

Neurosurgery

Surgery on the brain *per se* may be a risk factor for seizures. Based
on information derived from clinical series, in patients with no prior
seizures, a 17% cumulative incidence of postoperative seizures was
observed over 5 years [66]. The risk of late postoperative seizures is
greater in patients with younger age, early postoperative seizures
and severe neurological deficit. It also varies with the underlying
pathology and increases with the number of surgical interventions.

References

1 Commission on Classification and Terminology of the International League Against Epilepsy. Proposal for revised classification of epilepsies and epileptic syndromes. *Epilepsia* 1989; 30: 389–99.
2 Commission on Epidemiology and Prognosis, International League Against Epilepsy. Guidelines for epidemiologic studies on epilepsy. *Epilepsia* 1993; 34: 592–6.
3 Shorvon SD, Farmer PJ. Epilepsy in developing countries: a review of epidemiological, sociocultural and treatment aspects. *Epilepsia* 1988; 29 (Suppl. 1): S36–S54.
4 Schlesselman JJ, ed. *Case-control Studies. Design, Conduct, Analysis.* New York: Oxford University Press, 1982.
5 Ottman R. An epidemiologic approach to gene–environment interaction. *Genet Epidemiol* 1990; 7: 177–85.
6 Hauser WA. Incidence and prevalence. In: Engel J Jr, Pedley TA, eds. *Epilepsy: a Comprehensive Textbook.* Philadelphia: Lippincott-Raven Publishers, 1997: 47–57.
7 Hauser WA, Annegers JF, Kurland LT. Prevalence of epilepsy in Rochester, Minnesota: 1940–1980. *Epilepsia* 1991; 32: 429–45.
8 Sander JWAS, Hart YM, Johnson AL et al. National General Practice Study of epilepsy: newly diagnosed epileptic seizures in a general population. *Lancet* 1990; 336: 1267–71.
9 Babb TL, Brown WJ. Pathological findings in epilepsy. In: Engel J Jr, ed. *Surgical Treatment of the Epilepsies.* New York: Raven Press, 1997: 511–40.
10 Delanty N, Vaughan CJ, French JA. Medical causes of seizures. *Lancet* 1998; 352: 383–90.
11 Annegers JF, Hauser WA, Lee JR-J, Rocca WA. Incidence of acute symptomatic seizures in Rochester, Minnesota, 1935–1984. *Epilepsia* 1995; 36, 327–33.
12 Hesdorffer DC, Logroscino G, Cascino G, Annegers JF, Hauser WA. Incidence of status epilepticus in Rochester, Minnesota, 1965–1984. *Neurology* 1998; 50: 735–41.
13 Hinchey J, Chaves C, Appignani B et al. A reversible posterior leuko-encephalopathy syndrome. *N Engl J Med* 1996; 334: 494–500.
14 Porter J, Jick M. Drug-induced anaphylaxis, convulsions, deafness, and extrapyramidal symptoms. *Lancet* 1977; i: 1582–6.
15 Messing RO, Closson RG, Simon RP. Drug-induced seizures: a 10-year experience. *Neurology* 1984; 34: 1582–6.
16 De Lorenzo RJ, Hauser WA, Towne AR et al. A prospective, population-based epidemiologic study of status epilepticus in Richmond, Virginia. *Neurology* 1996; 46: 1029–35.
17 Garcia PA, Allredge BK. Drug-induced seizures. *Neurol Clin* 1994; 12: 85–99.
18 Franson HL, Hay DP, Neppe V et al. Drug-induced seizures in the elderly. Causative agents and optimal management. *Drugs Aging* 1995; 7: 38–48.
19 Perucca E, Gram L, Avanzini G, Dulac O. Antiepileptic drugs as a cause of worsening seizures. *Epilepsia* 1998; 39: 5–17.
20 Pacia SV, Devinsky O. Clozapine-related seizures: experience with 5,629 patients. *Neurology* 1994; 44: 2247–9.
21 Silvestri RC, Bromfield EB, Khoshbin S. Clozapine-induced seizures and EEG abnormalities in ambulatory patients. *Ann Pharmacother* 1998; 32: 1147–51.
22 Rosenstein DL, Nelson JC, Jacobs SC. Seizures associated with antidepressants: a review. *J Clin Psychiatry* 1993; 54: 289–99.
23 Skowron DM, Stimmel GL. Antidepressants and the risk of seizures. *Pharmacotherapy* 1992; 12: 18–22.
24 Nelson M, Bartlett RJW, Lamb JT. Seizures after intravenous contrast media for cranial computer tomography. *J Neurol Neurosurg Psychiatry* 1989; 52: 1170–5.
25 Schliamser SF, Cars O, Norrby SR. Neurotoxicity of beta-lactam antibiotics: predisposing factors and pathogenesis. *Antimicrob Chemother* 1991; 27: 405–25.

26 Leone M, Bottacchi E, Beghi E *et al*. Alcohol use is a risk factor for a first generalized tonic-clonic seizure. *Neurology* 1997; 48: 614–20.

27 Ng SK, Hauser WA, Brust JC, Susser M. Alcohol consumption and withdrawal in new-onset seizures. *N Engl J Med* 1988; 319: 666–73.

28 Ng SKC, Brust JCM, Hauser WA, Susser M. Illicit drug use and the risk of new-onset seizures. *Am J Epidemiol* 1990; 132: 47–57.

29 Johnson MR, Sander JWAS. The clinical impact of epilepsy genetics. *J Neurol Neurosurg Psychiatry* 2001; 70: 428–30.

30 Kuzniecky RI, Jackson GD. Developmental disorders. In: Engel J Jr, Pedley TA, eds. *Epilepsy: a Comprehensive Textbook*. Philadelphia: Lipincott-Raven Publishers, 1997: 2517–32.

31 de Rijk van Andel J, Arts W, Hofman A *et al*. Epidemiology of lissencephaly type I. *Neuroepidemiology* 1991; 10: 200–4.

32 Berkovic SF. Progressive myoclonic epilepsies. In: Engel Jr J, Pedley TA, eds. *Epilepsy: a Comprehensive Textbook*. Philadelphia: Lippincott-Raven Publishers, 1997: 2455–68.

33 Roger J. Progressive childhood epilepsy in childhood and adolescence. In: Roger J, Bureau M, Dravet C, Dreifuss FE, Perret A, Wolf P, eds. *Epileptic Syndromes in Infancy, Childhood and Adolescence*, 2nd edn. London: John Libbey, 1992: 381–400.

34 Norio R, Koskiniemi M. Progressive myoclonus epilepsy: genetic and nosological aspects with reference to 107 Finnish patients. *Clin Genet* 1979; 15: 382–98.

35 Scheffer IE, Berkovic SF. Genetics of the epilepsies. *Curr Opin Pediatr* 2000; 12: 536–42.

36 Serratosa JM. Idiopathic epilepsies with a complex mode of inheritance. *Epilepsia* 1999; 40 (Suppl. 3): 12–16.

37 Berkovic SF, Andermann F, Andermann E, Gloor P. Concepts of absence epilepsies: discrete syndromes or biological continuum? *Neurology* 1987; 37: 993–1000.

38 Hauser WA, Hesdorffer DC, eds. *Epilepsy: Frequency, Causes and Consequences*. New York: Demos Publications, 1990.

39 Monetti VC, Granieri E, Casetta I *et al*. Risk factors for idiopathic generalized seizures: a population-based case control study in Copparo, Italy. *Epilepsia* 1995; 36: 224–9.

40 Nelson KB, Ellenberg JH. Antecedents of seizure disorders in early childhood. *Am J Dis Child* 1986; 140: 1053–61.

41 Nelson KB, Ellenberg JH. Prognosis among children with febrile seizures. *Pediatrics* 1978; 61: 720–7.

42 Susser M, Hauser WA, Kiely JL, Pnaeth N, Stein Z. Quantitative estimates of prenatal and perinatal risk factors for perinatal mortality, cerebral palsy, mental retardation and epilepsy. In: Freeman J, ed. *Prenatal and Perinatal Factors Associated with Brain Disorders*. Washington, DC: NIH Publication No. 85-1149, 1985: 359–439.

43 Annegers JF, Hauser WA, Beghi E, Nicolosi A, Kurland LT. The risk of unprovoked seizures after encephalitis and meningitis. *Neurology* 1988; 38: 1407–10.

44 Koszewski W. Epilepsy following brain abscess. The evaluation of possible risk factors with emphasis on new concept of epileptic focus formation. *Acta Neurochir* 1991; 113: 110–17.

45 Labar Dr, Harden C. Infection and inflammatory diseases. In: Engel J Jr, Pedley TA, eds. *Epilepsy: a Comprehensive Textbook*. Philadelphia: Lippincott-Raven Publishers, 1997: 2587–96.

46 Gale JL, Thapa PB, Wassilak SG, Bobo JK, Mendelman PM, Foy HM. Risk of serious acute neurological illness after immunization with diphteria-tetanus-pertussis vaccine. A population-based case-control study. *JAMA* 1994; 271: 37–41.

47 Griffin MR, Ray WA, Mortimer EA, Fenichel GM, Schaffner W. Risk of seizures after measles-mumps-rubella immunization. *Pediatrics* 1991; 88: 881–5.

48 Carpio A, Escobar A, Hauser WA. Cysticercosis and epilepsy: a critical review. *Epilepsia* 1998; 39: 1025–40.

49 Lobo A, Launer LJ, Fratiglioni L *et al*. Prevalence of dementia and major subtypes in Europe: a collaborative study of population-based cohorts. *Neurology* 2000; 54 (Suppl. 5): S4–S9.

50 Fratiglioni L, Launer LJ, Andersen K *et al*. Incidence of dementia and major subtypes in Europe: a collaborative study of population-based cohorts. *Neurology* 2000; 54 (Suppl. 5): S10–S15.

51 Hesdorffer DC, Hauser WA, Annegers JF, Kokmen E, Rocca WA. Dementia and adult-onset unprovoked seizures. *Neurology* 1996; 46: 727–30.

52 Hauser WA, Morris ML, Heston LL, Anderson VE. Seizures and myoclonus in patients with Alzheimer's disease. *Neurology* 1986; 36: 1226–30.

53 Hauser WA, Annegers JF, Kurland LT. Incidence of epilepsy and unprovoked seizures in Rochester, Minnesota: 1935–1984. *Epilepsia* 1993; 34: 453–68.

54 So EL, Annegers JF, Hauser WA, O'Brien PC, Whisnant JP. Population-based study of seizure disorders after cerebral infarction. *Neurology* 1996; 46: 350–5.

55 Li X, Breteler MB, de Bruyne MC, Meinardi H, Hauser WA, Hofman A. Vascular determinants of epilepsy: the Rotterdam study. *Epilepsia* 1997; 38: 1216–20.

56 Ng SKC, Hauser WA, Brust JCM, Susser M. Hypertension and the risk of new-onset unprovoked seizures. *Neurology* 1993; 43: 425–8.

57 Burn J, Dennis M, Bamford J, Sandercock P, Wade D, Warlow C. Epileptic seizures after a first stroke: the Oxfordshire community stroke project. *Br Med J* 1997; 315: 1582–7.

58 Olafsson E, Gudmundsson G, Hauser WA. Risk of epilepsy in long-term survivors of surgery for aneurysmal subarachnoid hemorrhage: a population-based study in Iceland. *Epilepsia* 2000; 41: 1201–5.

59 Crawford PM, West CR, Shaw MDM, Chadwick DW. Cerebral arterovenous malformations and epilepsy: factors in the development of epilepsy. *Epilepsia* 1986; 27: 270–5.

60 Olafsson E, Benedikz J, Hauser WA. Risk of epilepsy in patients with multiple sclerosis: a population-based study in Iceland. *Epilepsia* 1999; 40: 745–7.

61 Willmore LJ. Post-traumatic epilepsy: cellular mechanisms and implications for treatment. *Epilepsia* 1990; 31 (Suppl. 5): S67–S73.

62 Annegers JF, Hauser WA, Coan SP, Rocca WA. A population-based study of seizures after traumatic brain injuries. *N Engl J Med* 1998; 338: 20–4.

63 Salazar AM, Jabbari B, Vance SC *et al*. Epilepsy after penetrating head injury: I. Clinical correlates: A report of the Vietnam Head Injury Study. *Neurology* 1985; 35: 1406–14.

64 Cascino GD. Epilepsy and brain tumors: implications for treatment. *Epilepsia* 1990; 31 (Suppl. 3): S37–S44.

65 Le Blanc F, Rasmussen T. Cerebral seizures and brain tumors. In: Vinken PJ, Bruyn GW, eds. *Handbook of Clinical Neurology*. Amsterdam: North-Holland, 1974: 295–301.

66 Foy PM, Copeland GP, Shaw MDM. The natural history of postoperative seizures. *Acta Neurochir* 1981; 57: 15–22.

67 Nance MA, Hauser WA, Anderson VE. Genetic diseases associated with epilepsy. In: Engel J Jr, Pedley TA, eds. *Epilepsy: a Comprehensive Textbook*. Philadelphia: Lippincott-Raven Publishers, 1997: 197–209.

5 Differential Diagnosis of Epilepsy

M. Cook

Episodic disorders of consciousness or behaviour are a common cause of visits to emergency departments, family physicians and neurologists. Whilst the diagnosis of an epileptic disorder may be straightforward, it is frequently difficult, especially if the event is unwitnessed, or if the history is incomplete. Among the wide variety of neurological and non-neurological conditions that may be mistaken for epilepsy the most frequent and challenging distinction is between epileptic events and syncope or presyncope.

In my experience, 20–30% of new patients attending a specialty epilepsy clinic have a diagnosis other than epilepsy. A number of studies have shown that syncope is commonly misdiagnosed as epilepsy, largely through ignorance of the complex prodrome that may occur, and the sometimes dramatic nature of a clinical event that shares many features with epileptic convulsions [1]. Syncope is the most common diagnosis, followed by migraine, pseudoseizures, hyperventilation and vertigo. Less common disorders that are confused with epilepsy include cerebral ischaemia, or paroxysmal symptoms of demyelinating disease, raised intracranial pressure, Tourette's syndrome and other movement disorders are confused with epileptic seizures. Patients presenting with behavioural symptoms most often have a primary psychiatric diagnosis, but are often suggested to be suffering a seizure disorder. The surprising abundance of misdiagnosed epilepsy has been confirmed in a number of studies, and is cause for much concern [2].

Epilepsy remains primarily a clinical diagnosis. Incorrect diagnosis is often catastrophic for the patient, resulting in significant restriction in social activity and employability, as well as perhaps administration of unnecessary medication, with all the problems that brings with it. Loss of driving privileges is often the most immediate and traumatic component for patients whose livelihood may depend on a valid driver's licence. From all perspectives, the diagnosis of epilepsy requires great clinical skill and judgement, and it is incumbent on the clinician to attach a definite diagnosis only if certain.

General approach to episodic disturbances

Since an enormous variety of conditions can cause episodes of transiently disturbed consciousness or function, the major component of clinical management consists of separating out the various causes. Determining the nature of events can be very challenging, particularly when the event has been unwitnessed or when the patient is an inadequate historian otherwise.

Obtaining a clear account of the nature of the attack is the most important single component of the assessment, ascertaining precisely the circumstances of the event, any warning that was suffered, the duration of the attack, exactly what occurred during the event,

nature and speed of recovery as well as whether there were any focal or lateralizing signs after the event. There is no substitute for a detailed history of the attack from both the patient and any eyewitnesses, as well as obtaining a detailed account of the circumstances of the event. For instance, what was the patient engaged in the day and evening prior to the event? Was there sleep deprivation or other medical problems? Was there unusual stress or anxiety [3]? Obtaining an eyewitness account is crucial and the telephone is an invaluable device in this regard, particularly now mobile telephones are so widely owned. Dramatic disparity is often noted between the eyewitness's and patient's stories. Whereas the patient may recall a simple fall or brief loss of consciousness, an eyewitness may provide a detailed account of generalized convulsion with postictal confusion, tongue biting and so on. Patients are often amnestic for the circumstances of the event. In other situations they may deliberately try to conceal it. Clinical examination may provide useful information, but is most often non-contributory. Supportive investigations including EEGs and structural imaging may provide additional evidence for the diagnosis, but interpreting all these factors requires the greatest clinical skill and judgement. EEG is most often normal interictally in the adult patient with epilepsy; conversely, around 20% of people have minor and irrelevant abnormalities on interictal traces which are frequently misinterpreted as confirming a diagnosis of epilepsy [4,5].

Events that occur under particular circumstances should always raise the suspicion of syncope. There are obvious causes, such as venesection, painful surgical procedures and watching unpleasant movies, but mechanical causes such as cough, urination or defaecation may also provoke syncope; the difference between syncope and epilepsy is detailed below. Episodes of loss of consciousness occurring with postural change are more likely to be syncopal. Shock, fright or extreme emotion may precipitate syncope also but are frequently recognized to be non-epileptic events. Other physical alterations such as change in head position, rolling in bed, looking up at a high shelf or bench precipitating an attack would suggest a vestibular basis. Relationship to eating might establish a hypoglycaemic basis.

Events that occur during sleep, even if only some of the time, are almost always epileptiform. Sleep disorders and other movement abnormalities might occasionally be confused but non-epileptic events never occur during sleep, though some patients maintain they were asleep when they occurred; this can be difficult to resolve without video-EEG monitoring [6]. Seizures are sometimes linked to particular phases of the menstrual cycle, and whilst once interpreted as a functional element, this is very common in women with organic episodes and should always be taken seriously.

Episodes that occur when under emotional stress, when the

patient is experiencing difficult circumstances, particularly in the cognitively impaired might relate to behavioural problems rather than seizure activity. However, the distinction is sometimes difficult particularly when it is suggested that the behavioural alterations are a feature of the postictal state.

The symptoms in the immediate moments prior to the event are diagnostically critical. Those who describe focal neurological symptoms, such as clonic jerks, olfactory or gustatory hallucinations, rising epigastric aura, intense *déjà vu* or similar phenomena are much more likely to be having seizures. However, some symptoms can be fairly non-specific such as light headedness and dizziness. True vertigo is rarely a feature of epileptic attacks, but it is not always easy to distinguish vertigo from brief seizures. A visual aura can be epileptiform but most often is migrainous. If a typical account of shimmering scotomatous deficit evolving over some minutes with or without a headache following and possibly associated with other neurological symptoms are described, then migraine becomes a strong possibility.

The duration of attacks is probably the best single guide when considering the nature of turns. Epileptic events are almost always seconds to minutes in duration. Migrainous neurological symptoms are usually 15–20 min in duration; the subsequent headache can last for hours but may occasionally be absent. With epileptic events there is often some warning and gradual build-up to maximal deficit whereas with ischaemic vascular episodes the onset is abrupt and deficit typically maximal at the outset with gradual resolution. Since consciousness is usually unimpaired in focal cerebrovascular events involving the hemispheres, altered consciousness during attacks of this type is also more suggestive of an epileptic aetiology. Generalized tonic-clonic seizures typically last 40–90 s but occasionally are longer. Reports of attacks lasting hours, whether considered to be complex partial events or generalized tonic-clonic attacks, should always raise the suspicion of non-epileptic episodes. Whilst status epilepticus both convulsive and non-convulsive are certainly possibilities, it is a relatively uncommon event amongst people with chronic seizures. After an event, rapid recovery, perhaps with sweatiness or nausea and vomiting, are more typical of syncope. Partial and generalized tonic-clonic seizures are usually followed by a period of confusion. Occasionally there is marked alteration in mood and behaviour postictally; less often a true psychosis occurs postictally which, though typically self-limiting, sometimes dominates the presentation.

Activity during the event often helps clarify the nature of the attack. If absences are typical with abrupt cessation of activity and prompt resumption of activity at the end of the few-second-long episode, then the diagnosis is usually clear. Classical complex partial seizures with a warning followed by loss of contact, oral and manual automatisms and postictal confusion, sometimes with lateralizing signs noted during or after the event, are obviously clear-cut. Generalized convulsive activity can be more difficult to distinguish from syncope. With generalized tonic-clonic seizures people may or may not have a warning, the event usually lasts less than a minute or two, tongue biting and incontinence are common and there is often marked confusion postictally. The total absence of confusion after a generalized convulsive event should immediately raise the suspicion that the event was not epileptic. After the event and confusion has settled patients may strenuously deny that anything occurred, certainly that consciousness was impaired. They

sometimes become convinced that others around them, most particularly their family, are conspiring to make a diagnosis of epilepsy in these circumstances. Particularly in the elderly, this denial sometimes takes on delusional proportions.

During a seizure well-organized motor activity is uncommon, though automatisms can sometimes be preservative and simple activities are continued, although in an incomplete and sometimes clumsy manner. The purposeless nature of motor activity during the events usually draws the attention of those around the patient. The description of normal performance of complex activity such as driving a car or riding a bicycle suggests the attacks are non-epileptic. More often these partial events are truly simply partial in nature, and patients are able to continue normal activity. Partial seizures of temporal lobe origin are usually associated with altered consciousness, at least to some degree, though this is often not perceived by the patient. There are rare accounts of patients suffering generalized tonic-clonic convulsions and being able to recall events around them after the episode. This rare phenomena is usually related to generalized motor convulsive activity resulting from lesions in the frontal or parietal cortex where consciousness can sometimes be preserved despite the bilateral symmetry of the motor activity [7].

Similarly, seizures of extratemporal origin, particularly those originating in the frontal lobes, sometimes have bizarre features that may be similar to non-epileptic events. Furthermore, video-EEG monitoring with scalp electrodes can be unremarkable during these events, obscuring the issue diagnostically. Helpful clues are the stereotypic nature of attacks that often cluster, and that may occur during sleep. If unusual events occur in association with a structural cerebral pathology the diagnosis is usually clear. Great caution must be exercised diagnosing non-epileptic events in patients with bizarre clinical events that have a structural pathology demonstrated on MRI, particularly if it is extratemporal in location.

Prolonged 'absences', typically occurring whilst driving, are a common reason for referral to the epilepsy clinic. The patient describes driving or walking some distance, and then finding themselves at their destination (or just missing it), and not able to recall how they got there. If they have made the trip without difficulty, arrived at their destination and there is no sign of damage to the vehicle, it is highly unlikely such activity occurred during a seizure. These patients—and the referring doctors—are typically very anxious about the event (in contrast to many patients who have had complex partial events whilst driving!). It can be difficult to provide satisfactory reassurance that this is a benign phenomenon experienced to some degree by very many people.

Neurological examination is rarely helpful in patients who present with episodic disorders. Stigmata of a phakomatosis, the finding of a significant hemi-atrophy, lateralized weakness or reflex change and, of course, transiently lateralizing signs immediately postictally can be very useful. Acutely after a seizure perhaps the most useful physical sign is the observation of petechiae over the upper trunk and face particularly sometimes a quite striking phenomenon but usually subtle. Tongue bites and evidence of incontinence might be present if the patient is seen early enough. Although most tongue bites are lateral after epileptic seizures, the tip of the tongue and occasionally even the lips or cheeks can be bitten. Injuries such as fractures and bruising are not so helpful, often occurring through loss of consciousness with syncope for example. Shoulder dislocation, particularly posterior dislocation, and crush-fractured vertebrae are highly suggestive that a seizure has occurred, and are never seen in syncope or non-epileptic events. Back pain or radicular pain postevent should always be investigated with X-rays of the region; these injuries are often not diagnosed correctly and can lead to significant problems in returning to normal activity. Tests for vestibular abnormalities might be performed and sometimes provoke attacks.

Cardiac examination might disclose features to suggest an alternative aetiology for episodic disorders. Cardiac bruits, valvular heart disease, cardiomegaly or postural hypotension, tics and other movement abnormalities might be detected during the physical examination.

Occasionally patients have seizures whilst being examined. Most often these episodes are non-epileptic. Hyperventilation might be induced deliberately having informed the patient of your purpose, but other floridly non-epileptic attacks are sometimes brought on by simple tests, such as deep tendon reflexes, fundoscopy or suggestion. One needs to exercise great caution interpreting such events but most often they provide strong primary evidence as to the true nature of the episodes. Vulnerable patients with epilepsy may be easily induced to have non-epileptic events in some circumstances, particularly if they believe the organic nature of events is being questioned. There is considerable pressure to 'perform' for some, whether during the examination and history or video-EEG monitoring. Thus, the use of suggestion and other provocative procedures should only be performed in special circumstances [8].

Laboratory tests, such as biochemistry and haematological screens, add little to the diagnosis of epilepsy. Occasionally a primary metabolic disturbance such as hyponatraemia is found, but this almost always occurs in a specific clinical setting and in the context of other recognized metabolic abnormalities. Elevation in creatine kinase (CK) and white blood cell count might transiently occur after a seizure [9]. Serum prolactin levels rise transiently after seizures, reaching a peak at about 15 min after the event and returning to normal after around an hour. Obtaining a blood prolactin level can be useful in the diagnosis of events of uncertain type, provided it is done close enough to the episode. Prolactin levels are elevated following generalized convulsions in about 90% of cases, following complex partial seizures in probably only about 50% and not elevated following simple partial episodes. There is some uncertainty as to how prolactin changes might be interpreted in other settings, such as syncope and migraine. Also, numerous medications and other pathological conditions can cause changes in prolactin levels, although generally these do not cause transient fluctuations like seizures do [10,11]. Although in principal serum prolactin ought to be a useful test, it is difficult to implement because of the time scale and the fact that most seizures do not occur in circumstances where obtaining an acute sample is possible. At times though, serum prolactin estimation provides useful supportive information. It is not appropriately used as the primary diagnostic modality [9].

Other tests that can be useful include structural imaging, CT scan or MRI. Visualization of a focal cerebral pathology involving the cortex may provide useful supportive evidence for a diagnosis of epilepsy, but finding a structural pathology does not prove attacks are epileptiform. Conversely, not finding a structural pathology does not exclude a diagnosis of epilepsy, even if the symptomatology is focal. The sensitivity of MRI scans particularly with quantitative measures is now so great that it is uncommon in focal seizures of long standing not to find a relevant abnormality. However, in some patients abnormalities are never demonstrated perhaps because they are too small or subtle, or do not exist. The aetiology of these seizure types is often unknown and many appear to have a relatively good prognosis.

Functional imaging tests such as SPECT and PET are more appropriately used in conjunction with video-EEG monitoring or as part of surgical work-up in specialty epilepsy units. They are rarely helpful in a diagnostic setting.

EEGs and video-EEG monitoring are extremely useful tests that need careful interpretation. Unfortunately EEGs show an enormous range of minor abnormalities, benign variants, artefactual change and other confusing features that are often misinterpreted as evidence that there is a cerebral disturbance of some sort [4,6,8,12]. Whilst EEG can provide confirmation of precisely the type of epilepsy, and occasionally the location of a structural pathology, more often it leads to erroneous diagnosis of epilepsy when minor changes are misinterpreted. The EEG should never be substituted for a good clinical history; EEG changes, even if epileptiform should be interpreted cautiously. There is a very strong case to be made for not doing studies like EEG if the primary diagnosis is non-epileptic, provided there are strong clinical grounds for an alternative diagnosis. Video-EEG monitoring is as close to a gold standard as is available. Actually capturing events, witnessing directly the physical accompaniment of the attacks and observing the EEG changes which occur with this, often allows a specific diagnosis or the exclusion of epilepsy. However, simple partial events, extratemporal episodes, particularly from the frontal lobes even if associated with altered consciousness, are sometimes not associated with changes on the EEG. On the other hand, generalized convulsions always, and most complex partial events usually, show diagnostic EEG change. Simple partial events, particularly those involving sensorimotor cortex, are very often normal, even if the seizure activity is continuous.

Repeated observations over time also help make the correct diagnosis. Clinicians often feel obliged to arrive at the correct diagnosis immediately and at first consultation in episodes where alteration in consciousness has occurred. Whilst there are good reasons for this, and obviously serious causes need to be excluded rapidly, when the diagnosis is unclear, it is much better to leave the diagnosis open, because an erroneous diagnosis of epilepsy has serious implications for the patient. The concern with unexplained episodes of altered consciousness generally relates to safety during driving and perhaps in the workplace, and these activities might need to be restricted if the nature of episodes is uncertain but this will depend on the specific circumstances of the patient, the frequency of attacks and their character. Even if these do need to be restricted to some degree, this is a much better precaution than the so-called 'therapeutic trial' of anticonvulsant that often gives rise to uncertain and confusing results, sometimes leading to the *de facto* diagnosis of epilepsy. Much more harm is done through the incorrect diagnosis of epilepsy than keeping an open mind and reviewing the situation when more information is to hand, after implementing appropriate safety precautions.

Syncope

Epidemiologically syncope has many features in common with epilepsy. It appears often in late childhood and teenagers, with a second peak in the elderly. The lifetime incidence of syncope is 3–5% [13–15], without sex preference. Neurocardiogenic (vasovagal) syncope is commonest in early life; cardiac causes become more common later on. Whereas syncope due to cardiac disease is potentially life threatening, syncope due to other causes is generally benign.

There are a variety of causes of syncope, but in over 25% no cause can be identified [16,17]. There has been considerable interest in the syndrome of ictal arrhythmias, with a syncopal event complicating a perhaps subclinical epileptic discharge. Well reported in a relatively small number of cases, this situation is probably a rare cause of syncope. In patients studied with video-EEG monitoring, it is rare to see symptomatic syncope complicating the frequently observed but usually minor disorders of cardiac rhythm that may occur during the ictus. When this does occur, it is more likely in patients with temporal lobe foci. It may be the presenting feature of the seizure syndrome, and is thought to require cardiac pacing as well as anticonvulsant therapy if symptomatic [18–21].

Any seizure that occurs in unusual circumstances should be regarded with suspicion. These are sometimes erroneously diagnosed as reflex seizures. An excellent example is the patient who arrives with a referral describing seizures that only occur during or immediately after venesection (often when having blood taken for anticonvulsant levels!). Episodes occurring during micturition, defaecation, coughing or with valsalva, whether during weightlifting or deliberate, should immediately raise suspicion [22]. Often the precipitant for a syncopal event is not obvious and the patient will reveal it only if specifically questioned. Male patients particularly may be embarrassed to disclose painful or emotional precipitants, especially if they perceive that the circumstances are relatively minor. Good examples of this include syncopal events occurring in cinemas during violent or bloody scenes, during venepuncture, or watching minor surgical procedures. Even visiting hospitals, discussing medical procedures, reading an unpleasant book or reminiscing on a painful or unpleasant experience can be sufficient stimuli. The latter particularly applies to children, and events that have occurred under these circumstances should be considered syncopal until proven otherwise [23]. It is of course more obvious if the patient is undergoing a surgical procedure, or has seizures in the setting of some acute medical illness, but it is surprising how often epilepsy is misdiagnosed under such circumstances, with unintended repercussions for the patient. Syncopal events related to primary cardiac disease less often have a well-defined aura than syncope due to neurocardiogenic episodes [24–26]. Cardiogenic syncope leads to sudden collapse and usually lacks situational precipitants.

In the lead up to syncope the patient is often unwell, has been sleep deprived or is 'run down'. It may be in the cooling down period after vigorous exercise, with a combination of vasodilatation and erect immobility, resulting in transient hypotension. At home, events are often in the kitchen, when prolonged standing is common, or in the bathroom again associated with standing immobile for long periods but also with micturition or defaecation. Standing in a hot shower, in supermarket queues and waiting for tickets, standing at church or at assembly are also common situations. Patients may be in a crowded warm environment such as a cinema or club. Alcohol has often been consumed, and this is frequently associated with a late night. The patient is often standing at the onset of the event, but syncope may occur whilst seated and rarely whilst recumbent. In the latter situation there is often some specific precipitant (i.e. pain). Familial predisposition to syncope is common, and migraine frequently coexists in these patients.

At the onset of the event frequent symptoms are nausea, often with a rising quality, light headedness and sweating. There is often the urge to get outside into cool air. Anxiety and claustrophobia may dominate the account. Patients often describe 'I knew I had to get out' or 'I had to get some air quickly'. Witnesses may observe pallor and sweating, and may report the subject to be confused or semi-responsive. The event may progress no further than this, so-called 'presyncope' or go on to a more typical event with collapse. Immediately prior to loss of consciousness symptoms such as an auditory disturbance with noises 'sounding distant' or 'as if from down a tunnel' are frequently reported, then flaccid collapse. More complex auditory and visual hallucinations are surprisingly common, seen in 36 and 60%, respectively, of Lempert's series [24]. Visual hallucinations are sometimes quite complex, and may involve figures and scenes, and be associated with familiarity or even *déjà vu* [26,27]. 'Out of body experience' has been described [28]. Auditory hallucinations are usually of ringing or roaring, sometimes voices are described, and as with partial seizures these often have a familiar but unidentifiable quality about them.

Generalized stiffening and then clonic limb movements are frequently described by witnesses. The limb movements are usually asynchronous but multifocal, and sometimes seen to involve one limb or side asymmetrically, rarely exclusively. Facial involvement with the myoclonic limb movement is common. Head turning is rarely seen. Estimates of the frequency of tonic and clonic components range from 40 to 90%, and depend on the quality of the witnessed account [24,29]. Medical or paramedical personnel are perhaps most prone to confuse the events with epileptic convulsions. Eyes are usually open during the event, and sometimes oral and perseverative manual automatisms can occur. Automatisms of this type may also be seen in the presyncopal phase [25].

Typically the duration of the convulsive activity is less than 15–20 s, but rarely prolonged convulsive activity may be provoked. This is more likely if the subject is held upright during the event, or if there is an underlying cause that persists. Urinary incontinence is not uncommon in syncope, but tongue biting is rare. Respiration is seen to cease briefly in some instances. On recovering the patient is usually quite lucid, though this may be complicated by head trauma, and in the elderly confusion postictally can be marked. Lateralized neurological signs should not be seen. Vomiting and marked diaphoresis are often reported in the postictal phase, the patient often appears grey and unwell. Cyanosis is rare, in contrast to epileptic events [22,30]. Whilst typically patients rapidly regain awareness and alertness postictally, they are often washed-out and prefer to sleep in this period. The marked confusion and drowsiness that follow epileptic convulsions are not usually confused with these features, but sometimes it is a difficult distinction, particularly if the patient sustained a significant blow to the head during the episodes. Syncopal episodes often occur in clusters, sometimes one after another, frequently as the patient is helped up from the first collapse. Where the sitting position is forced through restraint, such as with a car seatbelt, quite prolonged reflex anoxic seizures sometimes occur. A similar situation may be observed after cardiopulmonary arrest, when delayed seizures may be prolonged and recurrent [30].

Examination is typically unrewarding, patients usually have normal resting blood pressure and appropriate postural responses between episodes. Even if measured immediately after the event no abnormality is the rule, though contributing factors should be looked for including a primary arrhythmia, hypotension, inappropriate bradycardia and carotid sinus hypersensitivity. Fall-related injuries may be noted, usually in the form of facial trauma.

If the history is typical, extensive investigation should generally be avoided in patients with syncope. However, if there is diagnostic uncertainty, or if the events are frequent, cause anxiety, limiting activity or if a cardiac arrhythmia is suspected, then investigations are appropriate. If the event can be induced by reproducible stimulus (i.e. venepuncture or pain) then it may be practical to induce an event when under EEG/ECG monitoring in order to document the typical features of neurocardiogenic syncope with ictal bradycardia or asystole associated with profound slowing of EEG patterns. Routine ECG tracing, echocardiography and chest X-ray may be indicated. Because events are rarely frequent enough for spontaneous episodes to be recorded during inpatient monitoring, ambulatory studies with Holter monitoring, or more recently implantable loop recorders, may be more appropriate. Loop recording can be done for periods of up to 18 months, and is clearly the investigation of choice in many of these patients. A recent study demonstrated a surprisingly high rate of primary cardiac arrhythmias in patients misdiagnosed as suffering refractory epilepsy [31].

Tilt table testing has been available for some time, but its use remains controversial, particularly in relation to provocative drugs used to increase the sensitivity of the test, and interpretation of the results. Although this is a valuable adjunct to diagnosis in many patients, the wide range in results between centres should be recognized [32]. Carotid sinus massage may be helpful in the diagnosis, but this finding has low specificity in the elderly population where it is most often found. Cerebral imaging may be useful in some cases, and finding a cerebral cortical pathology suggesting an epileptic basis will be helpful in the management of a patient with refractory syncope.

Treatment of syncope depends on the cause. Where a clear cardiac cause is demonstrated, specific therapy is obviously indicated. However, most people have neurocardiogenic syncope, and their treatment consists primarily of reassurance and avoidance of precipitating circumstances. When typical premonitory symptoms are recognized, preventative measures should be promptly undertaken. Usually this consists of lying or sitting with the head between the knees, and rising cautiously and slowly after the episode seems to have abated. Attention to hydration is an important element in many, as may be avoiding alcohol. Other drugs, such as antihypertensives, may require adjustment. Therapeutic data from large randomized controlled trials relating to neurocardiogenic syncope are limited. Evidence for the use of lipophilic β-blockers remains controversial. Serotonin reuptake inhibitors [33], angiotensin-converting enzyme inhibitors [34] and midodrine [35] are the only agents that have been shown to be effective in randomized controlled trials. Elastic stockings, with or without fludrocortisone, are used widely, but like disopyramide, have not been shown to be effective. Cardiac pacing has been shown to be effective in two small, randomized controlled trials [36] for the treatment of refractory neurocardiogenic syncope, and is gaining increasing acceptance.

Non-epileptic seizures (NES)

NES has become the preferred term to describe the events referred to often as pseudoseizures, psychogenic seizures or hysterical seizures, as it lacks the pejorative implications of the other terms. Definition of these episodes is difficult; convulsive activity is witnessed but has no electrical correlate and is felt to reflect psychological stresses of some sort, though these are rarely specifically identified [37]. These episodes may be extremely difficult to distinguish from epileptic events, even by experienced observers. As a result one of the most useful applications of video-EEG monitoring has been to recognize and clarify these events. Although in some series up to 40% of patients with refractory seizures have NES, a more realistic proportion is 5–10% [8,12,37,38]. NES consume a disproportionate amount of resources at epilepsy centres—the patients present frequently and dramatically, often have inpatient stays and seek more consultations with neurologists. They typically consume more medications than those with organic seizures alone. Often they receive health benefits of some sort, are unemployed and require high levels of care at home [37].

There is no consensus on the mechanism of these events from a psychiatric point of view, and often no specific psychiatric diagnosis can be made; the disorder itself seems to be the sole clinical manifestation of the problem [39]. In Munchausen's syndrome by proxy, descriptions of seizures are given in a child which are fabricated by the caretaker and constitute a form of child abuse; this represents a difficult situation [40].

The clinical features of NES vary enormously. Whilst often precipitated by emotional stress or specific circumstance, this is not always the case. There is sometimes a family history of epilepsy, of epilepsy earlier in life or of personal encounters with epileptics, perhaps in a paramedical situation or as a carer. Events are usually very disruptive and dramatic, typically lead to multiple hospital admissions and have a propensity to occur in public where they may be readily observed. Though there are many reports of a high rate of coexistence of NES and epilepsy, this is in fact a very uncommon occurrence [38].

The events themselves may consist of loss of contact, flaccid collapse and immobility, or florid motor activity often with side-to-side head shaking, pelvic thrusting and back arching. Variability from event to event is common, making the lack of stereotypy a valuable clinical feature. The prolonged duration of many of the episodes is the most obvious clue to their non-organic nature. It is not uncommon for episodes to wax and wane for 30 min to hours in duration. Crying and screaming may be striking features of the episodes, and complex organized activity may be seen. Eyes are usually held closed during the episodes. Cyanosis is infrequent, but can be seen in some patients who may have what appears to be an adult version of breath-holding attacks. Tongue biting and urinary incontinence are sometimes reported, but rarely confirmed, symptoms that are frequently reported by patients with a long history of the disorder. Interestingly, almost exclusively this group of patients reports faecal incontinence. After the event recovery is usually rapid and often accompanied by emotional distress. Not all events resolve rapidly though, and prolonged unresponsiveness with normal vital signs may follow. The lack of tachycardia during this phase is a helpful feature diagnostically, but may be complicated by the sometimes frenetic motor activity of the episode.

Typically many anticonvulsant medications have been prescribed without benefit. Furthermore some patients have been treated urgently with parenteral benzodiazepines or even paralysis plus intubation in a critical care setting. In many centres NES is the commonest cause of uncontrolled seizures in the intensive care environment, and should always be considered as the diagnosis when a patient with chronic seizures presents in status without obvious cause.

Some non-epileptic events are embellished organic syndromes such as syncope or hyperventilation. The clinical scenario occurs in a hysterical or anxious person who experiences syncopal symptoms, hyperventilates and then evolves into a very complex and clearly non-organic behaviour which attracts attention while the prodrome becomes lost in the drama.

Confirming the diagnosis may be a challenge until VEEG monitoring makes the diagnosis. Patients who refuse monitoring, or those who have no events whilst monitored, present a very difficult diagnostic problem, but most will have typical events in hospital. Often they can be encouraged by suggestion to produce episodes. Some centres have used other provocative manoeuvres such as saline injection, but this may make interpretation of the events more difficult, because there is considerable pressure on the patient to 'perform', and typical attacks may not be evoked [41,42]. As part of the illness involves the drama and frequency of the seizures, usually outpatient VEEG monitoring will be sufficient to make the diagnosis [12,41].

Important traps in the diagnosis of NES are frontal lobe seizures and simple partial seizures. Seizures originating in the frontal lobe can be bizarre, frequent and associated with preserved awareness, and they are often refractory to medication. The stereotypic nature of the events, many of which may occur from sleep, and usually some response to acute parenteral therapy provide clues. VEEG may not demonstrate significant change during these episodes though, and movement artefact frequently obscures interpretation.

Simple partial seizures may also be difficult to prove when events are not accompanied by scalp EEG changes. In these situations the finding of a relevant structural abnormality on imaging studies supports the diagnosis of seizures, but negative imaging studies do not exclude it.

Management of NES is complex and difficult [37,39]. Engaging the patient in a therapeutic relationship is the most valuable component, followed by an explanation of the non-electrical basis of the events, and recognizing that the condition causes disability. Confirming this belief with the patient takes much of the tension out of the situation. Confronting patients with a diagnosis of functional illness does little for their long-term care, and often leads to presentation to multiple hospitals, with consequent polytherapy. A face-saving compromise is often required, with an agreement by the patient to reduce or withdraw anticonvulsant therapy, avoid hospitalization and where appropriate to seek help from a psychiatrist to address underlying issues, such as depression. Accepting the care of one neurologist, or at least of one centre, is a major component of the clinical management plan [43]. Although controversy exists as to whether these patients should be managed by neurologists at all, in my view psychiatrists have little to offer these patients, and the temptation to treat with anticonvulsants is too great in the primary care setting.

Panic disorder

Panic attacks can appear very similar to seizures. They are episodes of fear or discomfort that are often accompanied by somatic symptoms such as palpitations, dizziness, light headedness and epigastric sensation [44,45]. The attacks have an abrupt onset, typically reaching a peak within 10 min. Fearful patients want to escape and feel that the episodes indicate a life-threatening disorder. The attacks can be situational, but most often occur spontaneously without a clear precipitant. As with seizures, attacks can be nocturnal and cluster, occurring many times daily after long breaks between episodes.

Lifetime prevalence has been estimated at around 2%, with a higher risk for women. There is a significant familial incidence. Although the condition is usually diagnosed in young adults, it has been described in children and the elderly. Highly variable in severity, these episodes are often disruptive, and overlap considerably with other psychiatric syndromes, particularly agoraphobia and depression. At least 50% of patients with panic disorder develop a significant depressive illness during their life; the majority are depressed when they present for treatment [46,47].

Management consists of reassurance directed at specific unfounded concerns regarding underlying illnesses and psychiatric therapy of the phobic and depressive elements [48].

Migraine

Migraine is surprisingly often mistaken for epilepsy, particularly when the headache is mild or absent [47]. Migrainous aura may have visual, sensory or motor features that may be suggestive of seizure activity, and alertness is sometimes impaired. Postictal headache is also common in epilepsy, and this can make the distinction more complicated than anticipated.

Some unusual types of seizures, particularly those that originate in the occipital lobe, can be difficult to distinguish from migraines because features such as visual disturbance occur in both disorders [49,50]. Since there is no diagnostic test for migraine, the diagnosis is clinical. Migraines are more common amongst those who suffer syncope and there is often some overlap with the symptoms. Although visual disturbances are the most common neurological feature of migraine, sensory or motor change, speech disturbance, amnesia or confusion and even loss of consciousness may occur.

Migraine may have specific triggers such as foods, medication, emotional stress or visual stimuli. Sensory or visual symptoms generally build up slowly and typically spread over minutes, progressing stepwise from one affected cortical region to the next, with resolution of the symptoms as a new area is involved. Typical symptom duration is 15–30 min though occasionally episodes last longer and may not be followed by headache.

Whereas epilepsy and migraine are both common, one might anticipate encountering them occasionally in the same patient. This has been studied by a number of authors [51] with differing results. There seems to be no excess of epilepsy amongst patients with migraine overall [52]. None the less the distinction of migraines from seizures can be difficult. Some authors have postulated that migraines might be a seizure equivalent [53]. In some patients migraines trigger seizures [54], but this is rare.

Postictal migraine is well recognized and may have some lateralizing value [52,55]. Seen in focal and generalized syndromes, it more often occurs after a tonic-clonic convulsion. The increased cerebral blood flow that is induced by seizure activity is felt to be responsible for this headache. Often these types of headaches occur in patients who suffer migraines at other times. However, the patient who presents with new onset headache and seizure obviously requires the exclusion of an acute neurological problem such as intracranial haemorrhage or infection.

Seizures of occipital origin have many features of migraine, with visual hallucinations or amaurosis often complicated by headache. Benign partial epilepsy with occipital paroxysms is a syndrome of childhood to teenage years [56,57]. Hallucinations are typically simple in nature but can be complex and followed by complex partial or generalized convulsions [58] after which come the headache with nausea and vomiting. The diagnosis depends on observing the distinctive interictal EEG pattern. Occipital seizures resulting from structural pathologies, such as coeliac disease and mitochondrial encephalomyelopathies, may share these features [59].

Non-specific EEG changes occur with migraine, but specific epileptiform abnormalities are rare [56]. Finding interictal spikes in patients with migraine suggest an alternative diagnosis, such as benign occipital epilepsy in children or the possibility of a structural lesion in adults. As a rule, EEG is not useful in typical migraine. Minor abnormalities seen during episodes need to be interpreted with great caution.

The diagnosis of migraine is clinical and rests on recognizing the typical progression of symptoms, the duration of attack (tens of minutes rather than seconds), and gradual resolution. Response to anticonvulsant therapy is an unreliable basis for making the diagnosis.

Sleep disorders

A review of the many abnormalities that arise from sleep is outside the scope of this brief review. However, sleep disorders such as periodic limb movements of sleep, REM sleep disorders, narcolepsy and cataplexy can be confused with seizures [60]. On the other hand some epilepsies arise exclusively from sleep and there is a propensity for partial seizures to occur in sleep or shortly after waking [61]. Benign rolandic epilepsy is an example of a seizure syndrome that is associated with sleep.

The parasomnias, including sleep walking, night terrors, restless legs, nocturnal myoclonus, bruxism, paroxysmal nocturnal dystonia and REM sleep disorder, can be more difficult to differentiate from seizures [62,63] whereas disorders with hypersomnolence rarely present diagnostic problems. Sleep disorders are common, particularly in the elderly.

Although the classic tetrad of narcolepsy involves excessive daytime sleepiness, cataplexy, hypnogogic or hypnopompic hallucinations and sleep paralysis, not every component occurs in a given individual. The diagnosis is based on sleep latency studies in which REM sleep begins abnormally early. Cataplexy, sudden episodes of sleep and hallucinations are sometimes misidentified as seizures

[64]. Rarely, cataplexy precipitated by laughter is mistaken for a gelastic seizure.

Paroxysmal nocturnal dystonia presents as an often dramatic movement disorder from sleep with arousal and then vigorous motor activity, episodes typically lasting 30–60 s followed quickly by sleep [65]. They are usually amnestic for the episodes. Many patients originally diagnosed with this condition have since been recognized to have frontal lobe epilepsies. The diagnosis is made all the more difficult by movement artefact obscuring EEG traces made during the episodes.

Night terrors (pavor nocturnus) is a childhood parasomnia. Children wake from sleep screaming and crying inconsolably for many minutes, after which they go back to sleep and are amnestic for the episode. Rarely night terrors persist into adult life. If the diagnosis is in doubt, ictal EEG recordings can confirm that these do not have an epileptic basis [66].

Bruxism, or tooth grinding, can be a very striking nocturnal phenomenon. It is a benign disorder that requires no specific therapy.

Periodic movements of sleep are so distinctive that it is rare for them to be confused with seizures [67]. They are characterized by repetitive flexion and extension, sometimes quite vigorously, of hip, knee, ankle and toe for a period of 30 s or so. The episodes frequently recur throughout the night troubling the bed partner but not the patient.

The REM behaviour disorders are much more complicated. These episodes occur from REM sleep and consist of the individual acting out components of dreams. Sometimes dramatic and prolonged, the activity can be complex, violent or aggressive and accompanied by agitation and vocalizations. Typically recurrent the attacks present a serious risk of injury for the partner. Causes include structural brain injury, such as subarachnoid haemorrhage. In some situations REM behaviour disorder might be difficult to distinguish from postictal confusion [68].

Although most parasomnias can be distinguished from epileptic disorders by their distinctive clinical features, polysomnography allows definitive diagnosis in most instances [69].

Vertigo

Vertigo with brief episodes of dysequilibrium is often misinterpreted as seizure activity. This is because many patients describe the episode as involving loss of awareness, though this is not confirmed by witnesses. Whilst vertigo may rarely occur as a feature of focal seizures, especially those originating in frontal or parietal regions [70,71], other non-specific symptoms, such as light-headedness and dizziness, are more often reported as a feature of convulsive episodes.

In vertigo due to peripheral vestibular causes the episodes are often provoked by head movement, as in benign positional vertigo, and are associated with nausea and vomiting. Sometimes eye signs can be seen during the attacks. Although witnesses typically observe consciousness to be preserved during episodes of vertigo, it is not uncommon for patients to report the sensation of loss of awareness briefly during a severe brief vertiginous episode. In so far as attacks sometimes lead to falls, they imitate epilepsy. Careful history, provocative manoeuvres such as the Hallpike test and, sometimes, vestibular testing may be required to make the diagnosis. As true vertigo is such an uncommon feature of epileptic seizures, the description should immediately arouse suspicion.

Movement disorders

A number of movement disorders can imitate epilepsy. Paroxysmal choreoathetosis or dystonia, both kinesogenic and non-kinesogenic forms [72], are movement abnormalities with striking posturing or chorea that are precipitated by sudden movement, surprise or startle, stress or rapid movement. Some forms are aggravated by alcohol, caffeine and fatigue. Whereas these may be unilateral and consciousness is preserved during the attacks, the episodes may be mistaken for focal motor seizures. Thus the description of hemitonic seizures with preserved consciousness should raise the possibility of a paroxysmal dyskinesia and similar symptoms might be secondary to demyelinating disease, or other primary cerebral pathologies. So-called tonic seizures of multiple sclerosis may be unilateral or bilateral, and are sometimes precipitated by movement. Occasionally these entail what is interpreted as clonic movements, particularly as the attacks resolve [73]. Inability to speak during the episode may be interpreted by witnesses as altered awareness. The abrupt onset and extent of the attacks, as well as the lack of focal onset and typical rhythmic activity at the onset, are clues as to the true nature of the episodes. However, occasionally seizures, particularly those of frontal lobe origin, can cause abrupt tonic posturing. Startle seizures, with asymmetric posturing and collapse, occur in cognitively impaired patients [74]. Often a hemiparesis is present, and other seizure types have also been observed. The startle attacks might progress to more obvious convulsive seizure activity. Startle seizures can be mistaken for non-organic events and for paroxysmal dyskinesias.

Cerebral ischaemia

Vascular disturbances typically produce an abrupt onset of negative motor and/or sensory phenomena, speech disturbance or visual abnormality. When this occurs in an elderly person, at risk for cerebrovascular disease, the diagnosis is usually clear. Recurrent episodes of limb weakness, speech disturbance or paraesthesia in a limb have much in common with focal seizures. Ischaemic attacks tend to be maximal at the onset, last seconds to minutes, do not affect consciousness and do not progress to more typical seizure activity. Neuroimaging including echocardiography and carotid doppler or angiographic studies might allow a definitive diagnosis. Clonic jerking of the limb has been reported with transient ischaemic episodes and there may be some overlap here with seizure activity occasionally resulting from cortical ischaemia [75].

In general cerebral ischaemia presents no great challenges in differentiation from seizure activity. However, the most frequent seizures in the elderly are complex partial and thus can be missed by the unwary evaluator.

Endocrine and metabolic abnormalities

Disturbances of hormones, glucose, fluids and electrolytes can causes seizures, or seizure-like events [76,77]. When occult abnormalities such as insulinomas present with seizures, the diagnosis can be challenging.

The most common cause of transiently altered awareness due to endocrine abnormality is hypoglycaemia related to insulin therapy of diabetes. This can cause confusional episodes, generalized tonic-clonic convulsions and sometimes episodes imitating focal seizures. Although hypoglycaemia is common, it usually presents to the primary treating doctor rather than to a neurologist.

Hypoglycaemic episodes can be mistaken for vasovagal syncope or seizures. Besides insulin therapy, other causes of hypoglycaemia include alcohol, insulin-producing tumours, rare inborn metabolic abnormalities such as the congenital deficiencies of gluconeogenic enzymes and renal or hepatic disease [78,79]. Reactive hypoglycaemia may occur postprandially, or in association with other enzyme abnormalities such as hereditary fructose intolerance.

The symptoms of hypoglycaemia include altered vision, diaphoresis, confusion, coma and altered behaviour in addition to partial and generalized seizures. Behaviour during hypoglycaemia can be extremely bizarre and out of character. Irritability and aggression are common. Peri-oral and peripheral paraesthesia, dysarthria, ataxia, tremor and palpitations are common features. Occasionally true vertigo occurs. Some patients describe the symptoms as 'anxiety', or in otherwise non-specific terms. Hunger might be marked.

The relationship of symptoms to eating or fasting provides clues about the cause. The diagnosis is confirmed by measurement of serum glucose at the time of the event. Sometimes the rate of change of serum glucose levels is more important than the absolute glucose level.

Hyperglycaemia can also cause seizure-like activity and focal seizures are well described as features of hyperglycaemic states [80], sometimes in association with other neurological symptoms, such as movement disorders or lateralized weakness [81].

Hypocalcaemia can produce paraesthesia, carpopedal spasm, laryngeal stridor or convulsions [82]. Consciousness is preserved unless a generalized tonic-clonic seizure occurs. Hypocalcaemic sensory disturbances are sometimes misinterpreted as an aura.

Seizures rarely complicate a number of other endocrine abnormalities, including hypocalcaemia, hypo- and hyperthyroidism, generally only when the disorders are extreme. Pheochromocytoma and other catecholamine-producing tumours can produce paroxysmal symptoms that might be mistaken for presyncope, anxiety or seizures. Flushing and palpitations due to pheochromocytoma usually last longer than the autonomic features of seizures. Menopausal symptoms such as hot flushes and paroxysmal sweating are sometimes misinterpreted as seizure related. Seizures might be aggravated by hormonal change, such as in those who suffer seizures in relation to the menstrual cycle but again this is generally fairly clear [83].

Transient global amnesia

Transient global amnesia is an illness of uncertain aetiology. Some authorities feel it represents cerebrovascular disease, others attribute it to migraine and still others regard it as an epileptiform phenomenon [84]. Most would agree, however, that it is not an epileptic event. These stereotypic events are quite characteristic and easily recognized by the experienced clinician [85]. Amnesic episodes are recurrent in 8%.

The patient typically presents in a confused state, unsure of what they are doing or where they are going. Although they have little awareness of their current circumstances they typically retain personal information. The episodes can last up to hours, after which small islands of memory start to return of what went on during the amnestic period. However, some never recover any memory for the time that was involved. As a result these episodes typically cause great anxiety to those around them.

Although slightly perplexed or agitated during the attacks, no focal neurological abnormalities are found. EEGs and structural imaging are normal, and blood tests provide no clues. However, the description of events is so characteristic that the diagnosis is generally straightforward. Most patients have a history of migraine, and sometimes the episodes are followed by headache [86]. Rare causes include lacunar stroke seizures. If the seizure was not recognized then the most striking feature of a seizure might be a postictal confusional state afterwards but it is generally global and lacks the peculiar specificity of the true transient global amnestic attack [87].

Patients with transient global amnesia need no further investigation and no other specific therapy besides strong reassurance.

References

1 Smith D, Defalla BA, Chadwick DW. The misdiagnosis of epilepsy and the management of refractory epilepsy in a specialist clinic. *QJM* 1999; 92: 15–23.

2 Chadwick D, Smith D. The misdiagnosis of epilepsy. *BMJ* 2002; 324: 495–6.

3 Kanner AM, Balabanov A. Depression and epilepsy: how closely related are they? *Neurology* 2002; 58: S27–S39.

4 Hughes JR, Gruener G. The success of EEG in confirming epilepsy—revisited. *Clin Electroencephalogr* 1985; 16: 98–103.

5 Reuber M, Fernandez G, Bauer J, Singh DD, Elger CE. Interictal EEG abnormalities in patients with psychogenic nonepileptic seizures. *Epilepsia* 2002; 43: 1013–20.

6 Benbadis SR, Lancman ME, King LM, Swanson SJ. Preictal pseudosleep: a new finding in psychogenic seizures. *Neurology* 1996; 47: 63–7.

7 Bell WL, Walczak TS, Shin C, Radtke RA. Painful generalised clonic and tonic-clonic seizures with retained consciousness. *J Neurol Neurosurg Psychiatry* 1997; 63: 792–5.

8 Cragar DE, Berry DT, Fakhoury TA, Cibula JE, Schmitt FA. A review of diagnostic techniques in the differential diagnosis of epileptic and nonepileptic seizures. *Neuropsychol Rev* 2002; 12: 31–64.

9 Shah AK, Shein N, Fuerst D, Yangala R, Shah J, Watson C. Peripheral WBC count and serum prolactin level in various seizure types and nonepileptic events. *Epilepsia* 2001; 42: 1472–5.

10 Meierkord H, Shorvon S, Lightman SL. Plasma concentrations of prolactin, noradrenaline, vasopressin and oxytocin during and after a prolonged epileptic seizure. *Acta Neurol Scand* 1994; 90: 73–7.

11 Meierkord H, Shorvon S, Lightman S, Trimble M. Comparison of the effects of frontal and temporal lobe partial seizures on prolactin levels. *Arch Neurol* 1992; 49: 225–30.

12 Boon P, Michielsen G, Goossens L et al. Interictal and ictal video-EEG monitoring. *Acta Neurol Belg* 1999; 99: 247–55.

13 Youde J, Ruse C, Parker S, Fotherby M. A high diagnostic rate in older patients attending an integrated syncope clinic. *J Am Geriatr Soc* 2000; 48: 783–7.

14 Savage DD, Corwin L, McGee DL, Kannel WB, Wolf PA. Epidemiologic features of isolated syncope: the Framingham Study. *Stroke* 1985; 16: 626–9.

15 Wong KT, So LY. Syncope in children and adolescents of Hong Kong. *J Paediatr Child Health* 2002; 38: 196–8.

16 Mathias CJ, Kimber JR. Postural hypotension: causes, clinical features, investigation, and management. *Ann Rev Med* 1999; 50: 317–36.

17 Mathias CJ, Deguchi K, Schatz I. Observations on recurrent syncope and presyncope in 641 patients. *Lancet* 2001; 357: 348–53.

18 Reeves AL, Nollet KE, Klass DW, Sharbrough FW, So EL. The ictal bradycardia syndrome. *Epilepsia* 1996; 37: 983–7.

19 Liedholm LJ, Gudjonsson O. Cardiac arrest due to partial epileptic seizures. *Neurology* 1992; 42: 824–9.

20 Lim EC, Lim SH, Wilder-Smith E. Brain seizes, heart ceases: a case of ictal asystole. *J Neurol Neurosurg Psychiatry* 2000; 69: 557–9.

21 Tinuper P, Bisulli F, Cerullo A et al. Ictal bradycardia in partial epileptic seizures: Autonomic investigation in three cases and literature review. *Brain* 2001; 124: 2361–71.

22 Sheldon R, Rose S, Ritchie D et al. Historical criteria that distinguish syncope from seizures. *J Am Coll Cardiol* 2002; 40: 142–8.

23 Kapoor WN. Syncope. *N Engl J Med* 2000; 343: 1856–62.

24 Lempert T, Bauer M, Schmidt D. Syncope: a videometric analysis of 56 episodes of transient cerebral hypoxia. *Ann Neurol* 1994; 36: 233–7.

25 Lempert T. Recognizing syncope: pitfalls and surprises. *J R Soc Med* 1996; 89: 372–5.

26 Benke T, Hochleitner M, Bauer G. Aura phenomena during syncope. *Eur Neurol* 1997; 37: 28–32.

27 Whinnery JE, Whinnery AM. Acceleration-induced loss of consciousness. A review of 500 episodes. *Arch Neurol* 1990; 47: 764–76.

28 Lempert T, Bauer M, Schmidt D. Syncope and near-death experience. *Lancet* 1994; 344: 829–30.

29 Petch MC. Syncope. *BMJ* 1994; 308: 1251–2.

30 Krumholz A, Stern BJ, Weiss HD. Outcome from coma after cardiopulmonary resuscitation: relation to seizures and myoclonus. *Neurology* 1988; 38: 401–5.

31 Zaidi A, Clough P, Cooper P, Scheepers B, Fitzpatrick AP. Misdiagnosis of epilepsy: many seizure-like attacks have a cardiovascular cause. *J Am Coll Cardiol* 2000; 36: 181–4.

32 Fitzpatrick AP, Zaidi A. Tilt methodology in reflex syncope: emerging evidence. *J Am Coll Cardiol* 2000; 36: 179–80.

33 Di Girolamo E, Di Iorio C, Sabatini P, Leonzio L, Barbone C, Barsotti A. Effects of paroxetine hydrochloride, a selective serotonin reuptake inhibitor, on refractory vasovagal syncope: a randomized, double-blind, placebo-controlled study. *J Am Coll Cardiol* 1999; 33: 1227–30.

34 Zeng C, Zhu Z, Liu G et al. Randomized, double-blind, placebo-controlled trial of oral enalapril in patients with neurally mediated syncope. *Am Heart J* 1998; 136: 852–8.

35 Perez-Lugones A, Schweikert R, Pavia S et al. Usefulness of midodrine in patients with severely symptomatic neurocardiogenic syncope: a randomized control study. *J Cardiovasc Electrophysiol* 2001; 12: 935–8.

36 Sutton R. How and when to pace in vasovagal syncope. *J Cardiovasc Electrophysiol* 2002; 13: S14–S16.

37 Kuyk J, Leijten F, Meinardi H, Spinhoven, Van Dyck R. The diagnosis of psychogenic non-epileptic seizures: a review. *Seizure* 1997; 6: 243–53.

38 Benbadis SR, Agrawal V, Tatum WO. How many patients with psychogenic nonepileptic seizures also have epilepsy? *Neurology* 2001; 57: 915–17.

39 Brown RJ, Trimble MR. Dissociative psychopathology, non-epileptic seizures, and neurology. *J Neurol Neurosurg Psychiatry* 2000; 69: 285–9.

40 Barber MA, Davis PM. Fits, faints, or fatal fantasy? Fabricated seizures and child abuse. *Arch Dis Child* 2002; 86: 230–3.

41 McGonigal A, Oto M, Russell AJ, Greene J, Duncan R. Outpatient video EEG recording in the diagnosis of non-epileptic seizures: a randomised controlled trial of simple suggestion techniques. *J Neurol Neurosurg Psychiatry* 2002; 72: 549–51.

42 Zaidi A, Crampton S, Clough P, Fitzpatrick A, Scheepers B. Head-up tilting is a useful provocative test for psychogenic non-epileptic seizures. *Seizure* 1999; 8: 353–5.

43 Bowman ES. Nonepileptic seizures: psychiatric framework, treatment, and outcome. *Neurology* 1999; 53: S84–S88.

44 Hirschfeld RM. Panic disorder: diagnosis, epidemiology, and clinical course. *J Clin Psychiatry* 1996; 57 (Suppl. 10): 3–8.

45 Weissman MM. The hidden patient: unrecognized panic disorder. *J Clin Psychiatry* 1990; 51 (Suppl.): 5–8.

46 Marzol PC, Pollack MH. New developments in panic disorder. *Curr Psychiatry Rep* 2000; 2: 353–7.

47 Parker C. Complicated migraine syndromes and migraine variants. *Pediatr Ann* 1997; 26: 417–21.

48 Pollack MH, Marzol PC. Panic: course, complications and treatment of panic disorder. *J Psychopharmacol* 2000; 14: S25–S30.

49 Muranaka H, Fujita H, Goto A, Osari SI, Kimura Y. Visual symptoms in epilepsy and migraine: localization and patterns. *Epilepsia* 2001; 42: 62–6.

50 Panayiotopoulos CP. Visual phenomena and headache in occipital epilepsy: a review, a systematic study and differentiation from migraine. *Epileptic Disord* 1999; 1: 205–16.

51 Lance JW, Anthony M. Some clinical aspects of migraine. A prospective survey of 500 patients. *Arch Neurol* 1966; 15: 356–61.

52 Leniger T, Isbruch K, von den DS, Diener HC, Hufnagel A. Seizure-associated headache in epilepsy. *Epilepsia* 2001; 42: 1176–9.

53 Jonas AD. The distinction between paroxysmal and non-paroxysmal migraine. *Headache* 1967; 7: 79–84.

54 Niedermeyer E. Migraine-triggered epilepsy. *Clin Electroencephalogr* 1993; 24: 37–43.

55 Bernasconi A, Andermann F, Bernasconi N, Reutens DC, Dubeau F. Lateralizing value of peri-ictal headache: A study of 100 patients with partial epilepsy. *Neurology* 2001; 56: 130–2.

56 Brinciotti M, Di Sabato ML, Matricardi M, Guidetti V. Electroclinical features in children and adolescents with epilepsy and/or migraine, and occipital epileptiform EEG abnormalities. *Clin Electroencephalogr* 2000; 31: 76–82.

57 Andermann F, Zifkin B. The benign occipital epilepsies of childhood: an overview of the idiopathic syndromes and of the relationship to migraine. *Epilepsia* 1998; 39 (Suppl. 4): S9–S23.

58 Walker MC, Smith SJ, Sisodiya SM, Shorvon SD. Case of simple partial status epilepticus in occipital lobe epilepsy misdiagnosed as migraine: clinical, electrophysiological, and magnetic resonance imaging characteristics. *Epilepsia* 1995; 36: 1233–6.

59 Kuzniecky R. Symptomatic occipital lobe epilepsy. *Epilepsia* 1998; 39 (Suppl. 4): S24–S31.

60 Silber MH. Sleep disorders. *Neurol Clin* 2001; 19: 173–86.

61 Labar DR. Sleep disorders and epilepsy: differential diagnosis. *Semin Neurol* 1991; 11: 128–34.

62 Dement WC, Carskadon MA, Guilleminault C, Zarcone VP. Narcolepsy. Diagnosis and treatment. *Prim Care* 1976; 3: 609–23.

63 Culebras A. Update on disorders of sleep and the sleep-wake cycle. *Psychiatr Clin North Am* 1992; 15: 467–89.

64 Zeman A, Douglas N, Aylward R. Lesson of the week: Narcolepsy mistaken for epilepsy. *BMJ* 2001; 322: 216–18.

65 Sellal F, Hirsch E. Nocturnal paroxysmal dystonia. *Mov Disord* 1993; 8: 252–3.

66 Schenck CH, Mahowald MW. REM sleep parasomnias. *Neurol Clin* 1996; 14: 697–720.

67 Montagna P, Lugaresi E, Plazzi G. Motor disorders in sleep. *Eur Neurol* 1997; 38: 190–7.

68 Schenck CH, Mahowald MW. Parasomnias. Managing bizarre sleep-related behavior disorders. *Postgrad Med* 2000; 107: 145–56.

69 Ferini-Strambi L, Zucconi M. REM sleep behavior disorder. *Clin Neurophysiol* 2000; 111 (Suppl. 2): S136–S140.

70 Kluge M, Beyenburg S, Fernandez G, Elger CE. Epileptic vertigo: evidence for vestibular representation in human frontal cortex. *Neurology* 2000; 55: 1906–8.

71 Fried I, Spencer DD, Spencer SS. The anatomy of epileptic auras: focal pathology and surgical outcome. *J Neurosurg* 1995; 83: 60–6.

72 Vidailhet M. Paroxysmal dyskinesias as a paradigm of paroxysmal movement disorders. *Curr Opin Neurol* 2000; 13: 457–62.

73 Blakeley J, Jankovic J. Secondary causes of paroxysmal dyskinesia. *Adv Neurol* 2002; 89: 401–20.

74 Manford MR, Fish DR, Shorvon SD. Startle provoked epileptic seizures: features in 19 patients. *J Neurol Neurosurg Psychiatry* 1996; 61: 151–6.

75 Schulz UG, Rothwell PM. Transient ischaemic attacks mimicking focal motor seizures. *Postgrad Med J* 2002; 78: 246–7.

76 Messing RO, Simon RP. Seizures as a manifestation of systemic disease. *Neurol Clin* 1986; 4: 563–84.

77 Delanty N, Vaughan CJ, French JA. Medical causes of seizures. *Lancet* 1998; 352: 383–90.

78 Grant CS. Insulinoma. *Surg Oncol Clin N Am* 1998; 7: 819–44.

79 Pourmotabbed G, Kitabchi AE. Hypoglycemia. *Obstet Gynecol Clin North Am* 2001; 28: 383–400.

80 Roze E, Oubary P, Chedru F. Status-like recurrent pilomotor seizures: case report and review of the literature. *J Neurol Neurosurg Psychiatry* 2000; 68: 647–9.

81 Aquino A, Gabor AJ. Movement-induced seizures in nonketotic hyperglycemia. *Neurology* 1980; 30: 600–4.

82 Riggs JE. Neurologic manifestations of electrolyte disturbances. *Neurol Clin* 2002; 20: 227–39, vii.

83 Lambert MV. Seizures, hormones and sexuality. *Seizure* 2001; 10: 319–40.

84 Zeman AZ, Hodges JR. Transient global amnesia. *Br J Hosp Med* 1997; 58: 257–60.

85 Hodges JR, Warlow CP. Syndromes of transient amnesia: towards a classification. A study of 153 cases. *J Neurol Neurosurg Psychiatry* 1990; 53: 834–43.

86 Tosi L, Righetti CA. Transient global amnesia and migraine in young people. *Clin Neurol Neurosurg* 1997; 99: 63–5.

87 Hodges JR, Warlow CP. The aetiology of transient global amnesia. A case-control study of 114 cases with prospective follow-up. *Brain* 1990; 113 (Pt 3): 639–57.

6

Mechanisms of Epileptogenesis

G. Avanzini and S. Franceschetti

More than one and a half centuries ago, Hughlings Jackson defined epileptic seizures as the result of an occasional, sudden and excessive discharge of grey matter [1]. This statement can be viewed as the endpoint of a series of previous studies of animal electricity started by Luigi Galvani (1791) [2] and von Humbolt (1797) [3], which were subsequently pursued by means of cortical stimulation experiments by Fritsch and Hitzig (1870) [4] and the clinical observations of Todd (1849) [5]. However, the scientific soundness and anticipatory ideas of Jackson's work actually marks the beginnings of the modern era of epileptology. Since then, increasingly refined investigational techniques have provided a great deal of information about how epileptic discharges are generated and propagated within the central nervous system, and about the many different ways in which they manifest clinically.

As in the case of many other pathological conditions, experimental models made a major contribution to our understanding of epileptogenesis. The term 'experimental models' should be restricted to animals presenting spontaneous or experimentally induced epileptic seizures, whereas *in vitro* or computer models are more properly called models of epileptogenic mechanisms. This is not just a question of semantics because the relevance of experimental results to the advances made in our understanding of epilepsy depends on how suitably the experiment has been designed for its purpose. Operationally, it is enough to say that an experimental preparation should only be referred to as a model (of epilepsy, of seizures, of epileptogenic mechanisms) if it faithfully reproduces the clinical and EEG characteristics of human epilepsies or seizures, or the biological changes that are known to be associated with them. Over the last few years, animal experiments have been effectively supplemented by studies of human brain specimens surgically removed for the treatment of drug refractory epilepsies.

Experimental studies have shown that seizures can be induced by a number of different agents that affect excitatory or inhibitory neurotransmission, intrinsic cell excitation mechanisms or the ionic microenvironment.

A key to the investigation of cellular epileptogenic mechanisms came from the finding by Matsumoto and Ajmone Marsan [6] who were among the first to observe them in penicillin cortical foci. They found that neurones belonging to an epileptic neuronal aggregate consistently discharged in the form of protracted bursts (Fig. 6.1) that were named paroxysmal depolarization shifts (PDS). In normal brain, this phasic type of cell discharge can also be seen in some intrinsically bursting cell subpopulations of the neocortex and area 3 of Ammon's horn (CA3) in the hippocampus, which are involved in synchronizing cortical activity. In both experimental epileptogenic foci and epileptic human tissue, spontaneous or stimulus-evoked PDSs have been found to occur with a high probability in neurones that ordinarily are non-bursting. Therefore PDSs can be considered reliable hallmarks of an active epileptogenic process (see [7] for review).

Epileptogenic procedures, such as the blockade of γ-aminobutyric acid (GABA)-mediated inhibitory neurotransmission by bicuculline, picrotoxin and penicillin or the potentiation of excitatory amino acid (EAA)-mediated transmission by the kainate, ibothenate or N-methyl-D-aspartate (NMDA) receptors agonists, induce generalized phasic PDS-like activity in cortical cells (Fig. 6.1). Similar effects can also be obtained by means of epileptogenic agents acting on the intrinsic mechanisms responsible for membrane excitability such as Na^+ or Ca^{2+} depolarizing current activators (e.g. veratridine or Ca^{2+} chelators) or the inhibitors of hyperpolarizing K^+ currents (e.g. tetraethylammonium, intracellular Cs^{2+}, 4-aminopyridine).

In this chapter, particular attention will be given to the epileptogenic mechanisms that putatively account for naturally occurring animal and human epilepsies.

Membrane ion channels

The excitability of nerve cells depends on the movement of ions through specific voltage-dependent or receptor-activated membrane channels. The kinetics of transmembrane ion currents have been extensively investigated by means of various types of voltage clamp recordings. The effects of ion currents on cell membrane potential can be detected by means of current clamp recordings.

Ion channels are heterooligomeric membrane proteins typically consisting of 2–6 subunits, including transmembrane segments that are assembled in a variable number of domains (see Fig. 6.2 which shows the subunit structures forming ligand- and voltage-gated channels). Figure 6.2 also shows the disposition of N and C terminals from the extracellular side of the membrane in ligand-gated channels (receptors), and from the cytoplasmatic side in voltage-gated channels. The N terminal region is important in beginning the process of subunit association that leads to channel assembly, a process that is also influenced by accessory subunits and by a large number of different environmental influences. It leads to the formation of channels with different degrees of permeability to the various ions and different opening and closing kinetics, depending on the type of subunits assembled, their stoichiometric characteristics and the relative position of each subunit within the heterooligomeric complex.

The identification of the molecular structure of the various subunits and their corresponding coding genes has revealed a surprising multiplicity of distinct subunits whose assembly can lead to a considerable number of channel subtypes with different properties

[8]. One suitable experimental approach that has greatly contributed towards defining the structure–function relationships of the channels is to express them in cell lines that do not have endogenous channels by injecting messenger RNA isolated from tissue or synthesized using cloned complementary DNA. These procedures allow the precise measurement of ion currents by voltage or patch-clamp techniques developed by Neher and Sakmann [9], and make it possible to analyse the changes of the ion currents resulting from the mutated channels in isolation.

When investigating how ionic channels determine neuronal excitability it must be remembered that epileptic seizures result either from discharges generated in different parts of the neo- or paleocortices (partial seizures), or from discharges which seem to arise diffusely from both hemispheres with the possible involvement of thalamic structures (generalized seizures). The topographic expression pattern of putative epileptogenic processes should therefore be investigated at structural as well as cellular and subcellular levels.

Voltage-gated channels

These ion channels undergo voltage-dependent conformational changes leading to transitions from the closed to open state or vice versa.

Na+ channels

The molecular structure of the pore-forming α subunit of Na+ channels is shown in Fig. 6.2 in two dimensions. Each domain contains six transmembrane segments, the fourth one being the voltage sensor, and the loop between the fifth and sixth forming the ion-selective pore. The cytoplasmic loop between the third and fourth domain is the inactivation point. This structure correlates with the functional properties demonstrated by electrophysiological recordings which have been used to characterize the activation and inactivation kinetics of the main, transient component of Na+ current (I_{NaT}) and of the persistent component of Na+ current (I_{NaP}), produced by the fraction of Na+ channels that fail to inactivate. Experiments with toxins that block Na+ channel inactivation (thus

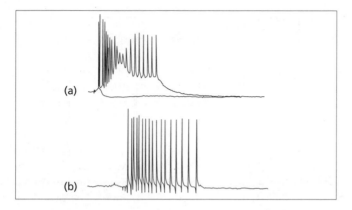

Fig. 6.1 Examples of paroxysmal discharges evoked in pyramidal neurones of the area CA1 (cornu Ammonis 1) in hippocampal slices. In (a), the paroxysmal response was synaptically evoked by stimulating the afferent fibbers during the perfusion with bicuculline, a drug suitable to block GABA$_A$-mediated neurotransmission. In (b), the paroxysmal discharge, occurring spontaneously during the perfusion with high extracellular K+ concentration, which reduces the driving force for this ion, exemplifies the 'epileptic' activities that can be induced by experimental manipulations of ionic currents.

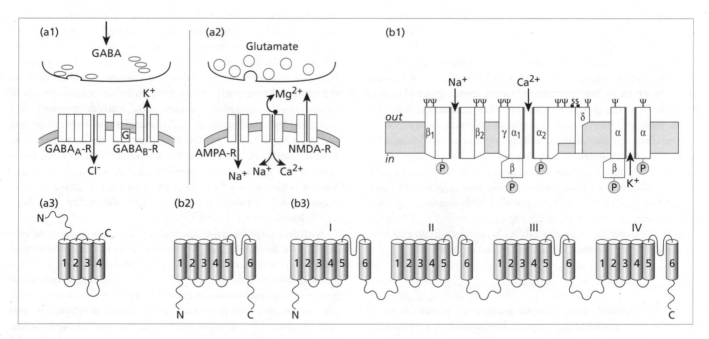

Fig. 6.2 Ligand-gated (a) and voltage-gated (b) channel involvement in paroxysmal depolarization shift (PDS) generation. First row schematic representation of GABAergic (a₁) and glutamatergic (a₂) synapses and of Na+, Ca2+ and K+ channels (b₁). Flat and round vesicles are respectively recognizable in GABA and glutamate containing presynaptic endings. Ionotropic receptors (R) are depicted on the postsynaptic membrane (GABA$_C$-R not shown). The inferior part of the figure shows a schematic representation of the molecular structure of pore-forming subunits of ligand-gated (a₃), and voltage-gated K+ (b₂) and Na+/Ca2+ (b₃) channels.

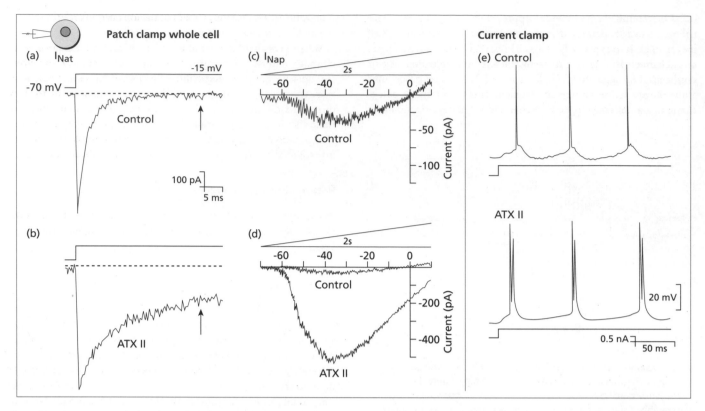

Fig. 6.3 Na+ currents studied with whole cell patch-clamp recording. Stepwise commands evoke transient Na+ current I_{Nat} (a); the slowly inactivating (persistent) component of the current (I_{Nap}) can be analysed in isolation using a slow ramp command (b). Note the slowing of fast inactivation (c) and the increase of the persistent component of the current (c, arrow and d) in presence of the sea anemone toxin ATX II that impairs Na+ channel inactivation. The ATX II-induced I_{Nap} enhancement is able to switch cell firing from individual spike to double spike bursting mode (current-clamp recording, inset e). Modified from [10].

considerably enhancing its persistent component) have demonstrated that this effect switches the firing of neocortical pyramidal neurones from regular spikes to bursts (Fig. 6.3, [10]).

The possibility that Na+ ions play a role in the pathophysiology of epilepsy was first suggested on the basis of indirect arguments, such as the blocking of Na+ currents by antiepileptic drugs [11] and particularly on the persistent fraction of Na+ current [12,13], and on the basis of observations of significant alterations in the ratio between different Na+ channel subtypes in human tissue surgically resected for the treatment of refractory temporal lobe epilepsy [14]. Subsequently, several groups found direct evidence of genetically determined changes in Na+ channel molecular structure in cases of familial generalized epilepsies with febrile seizures (GEFS+) [15–19] and in cases with severe myoclonic epilepsy of infancy (SMEI) [20]. Interestingly, the GEFS+ mutation significantly increases the time required for Na+ current inactivation.

K+ channels

Unlike Na+ and Ca2+ channels, which are large monomeric proteins including four homologous repeats, K+ channels are assembled from four proteins whose schematic structure with six transmembrane domains is shown in Fig. 6.2. The resulting structure is similar to that of Na+ and Ca2+ channels, but the number of possible subtypes is much higher because of the large number of potential combinations. Most K+ channel genes are conserved across verte-

brate families. As many as 40 genes coding for different K+ channels have been identified in simple organisms such as the nematode *Coenorabitis elegans*, whose nervous system consists of only 302 neurones [21]. Although it is assumed that there are subtle functional differences between the different subtypes, the currents flowing through K+ channels can be grouped into a limited number of physiological categories. Besides the 'delayed rectifier', first described by Hodgkin *et al.* [22], several other hyperpolarizing currents carried by K+ ions have been identified and classified on the basis of their activation and inactivation kinetics. Most K+ channels are voltage sensitive, so that membrane depolarization directly activates K+ currents. Ca2+ or Na+ entry into the cell activates other types of K+ channels, resulting in Ca2+-dependent and Na+-dependent K+ currents.

With the exception of the 'anomalous' rectifying currents, K+ currents move the membrane potential towards values that are more negative. This reduces the probability of cell discharge and/or limits the amplitude and duration of depolarizing events, whereas membrane depolarization after an excitatory event (i.e. an action potential) is prerequisite for further action potential generation. This was first recognized by Hodgkin *et al.* [22], who coined the term 'delayed rectifier' to indicate the characteristics of the depolarizing K+ current in the giant axon of the squid. The definition was intended to denote the fact that the increase in membrane conductance (rectification) due to the opening of the corresponding K+ channel is delayed in comparison with that of the Na+ channel relative to the beginning of the depolarizing pulse current used to evoke the action potential. In general, it is expected that the rich repertoire of K+ channels with which the neurone is endowed modulates membrane excitability and shapes excitatory events in a highly sophisticated manner.

Potassium currents limit the sustained depolarization underlying PDS and limit the high-frequency burst discharges of action potentials characterizing the neurones belonging to epileptic neurone aggregates. This is probably due to the combined influence of both voltage-dependent and Ca^2- or Na^+-activated K+ currents. On the other hand, epileptiform discharges can be easily obtained in *in vitro* preparations by perfusion with K+ blockers such as extracellular tetraethylammonium and intracellular Cs^+, or simply by increasing the K+ concentration in extracellular fluid. The latter reduces the strength of the outward K+ currents by decreasing the intra/extracellular K+ concentration gradient that provides the driving force for K+ outflow.

Among K+ currents, the M type of K+ current (I_M) is of particular interest in distancing the membrane potential from the threshold for the generation of the high-frequency discharges of action potentials because it is active at the resting potential. In benign neonatal familial convulsions (BNFC), Biervert *et al.* [23] and Wang *et al.* [24] have demonstrated the pathogenic role of a genetically determined I_M defect. These studies showed that two K+ channel subunits (KCNQ2 and KCNQ3) contribute to the native M current (Fig. 6.4). Mutations of either of the genes coding for these subunits (respectively located at the 20q13 and 8q24 chromosomal loci) impair the M current and cause the BNFC phenotype. As shown in Fig. 6.4, the M current depends on a slowly activating and inactivating K+ conductance whose range of activation (–60 to –20 mV) makes the I_M particularly suitable for controlling subthreshold membrane excitability and the responsiveness to synaptic inputs.

These types of studies have stimulated a new interest in K+ currents as possible targets for new antiepileptic drugs (see [25]).

Ca^{2+} channels

Like Na^+ channels, the Ca^{2+} α subunit is a large monomeric protein that includes four homologous domains (Fig. 6.2), and multiple channel types coexist in the same cell. Calcium currents differ in their sensitivity to depolarization and display different inactivation kinetics. Therefore, they differentially contribute to membrane excitability depending on the specific channel assembly and on which membrane potential they activate. A variety of 'high-voltage-activated' (HVA) Ca^{2+} currents, needing sustained membrane depolarization to activate, has been described in different neuronal subtypes, as well as in other excitable membranes. In addition, a low-threshold activated, namely the transient (I_T) Ca^{2+} current, which is inactive at resting membrane potential, and de-inactivated with membrane hyperpolarization, has been found to be particularly pronounced in some regions of the central nervous system such as the inferior olivary nucleus and the thalamic nuclei (see [26] for a review).

The different types of Ca^{2+} currents that can be activated at various membrane potentials are particularly effective in depolarizing the membrane. As a result a possible role of Ca^{2+} currents in sustaining the depolarization underlying PDS has been hypothesized repeatedly but has been difficult to prove experimentally. The main evidence for the involvement of Ca^{2+} channels in the pathogenesis of epilepsy comes from experimental studies of the generalized nonconvulsive epilepsies that occur in rats. These animal models include the genetic absence epilepsy rat from Strasbourg (GAERS) [27], WAG/Rij (Wistar albino Glaxo rat of Rijswijk) [28] and other mutant mice named tottering, lethargic, stargazer and ducky mice with absence epilepsy, cerebellar degeneration and ataxia (see [29] for a review).

Experiments carried out in our laboratory [30–33] indicate that overexpression of the low-threshold Ca^{2+} current in reticular thalamic nucleus (Rt) cells could be responsible for GAERS spike-wave discharges according to a mechanism further specified below. Although no genetic basis for this Ca^{2+} channel dysfunction has yet been demonstrated in GAERS, mutations have been found in the genes that code for the $α1_A$, β4, γ2 and α2δ subunits of the calcium channel in mutant tottering, lethargic, stargazer and ducky mice with spike-waves [29]. Furthermore, the role of the I_T current in the generation of spike-wave discharges has recently been confirmed by experiments in mice lacking one α subunit of T-type Ca^{2+} channel [34].

Investigations aimed at confirming the role of Ca^{2+} channel mutation in the most frequent types of human, non-convulsive generalized epilepsies (childhood and juvenile absence epilepsies) have been so far inconclusive. However, a mutation of the gene

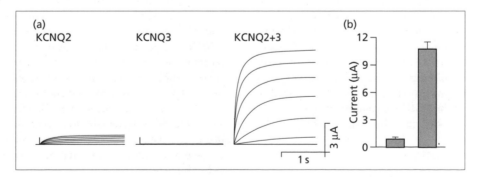

Fig. 6.4 Both KCNQ2 and KCNQ3 K+ channel subunits, whose gene mutations result in BNFC, contribute to the native I_M. (a) Currents recorded in *Xenopus* oocytes after individual injection of KCNQ2 mRNA, KCNQ3 mRNA; note the extremely small K+ current evoked in both cases (especially in the cell injected with KCNQ3 mRNA). After the injection of an equimolar ratio of KCNQ2 and KCNQ3 mRNAs the same protocol evokes a full developed K+ current that, evaluated by suitable protocols, shows the characteristics of the M-current (modified from [24]). (b) Histogrammatic representation of the average current response to a voltage step to 0 mV from –70 mV in the same conditions as in (a).

CACNA1A coding for particular Ca^{2+} channel (PQ-type) has been recently reported in a child with early onset absence epilepsy and cerebellar ataxia [35].

Ligand-gated channels

Ligand-gated channels or receptors are molecular complexes that include a pore region or ionophore, which becomes permeable to some ions when the relevant ligand binds to a specific site. Ligand-gated channels are categorized on the basis of the ligand (neurotransmitter or neuromodulator), with a number of functionally distinct subtypes being differentiated in each category on the basis of pharmacological (affinity for artificial ligands) or physiological criteria (selective ion permeability). Growing knowledge of the molecular structure of receptor subunits is providing more rational grounds for defining subtypes on the basis of their structure–function relationships.

Ion currents flowing through the receptor-associated ionophores can affect membrane potential and cell excitability. For this reason, ligand-gated channels have been implicated in epileptogenesis and have been considered as possible targets for drug therapy. Pharmacological agents acting on receptors could affect not only the primary epileptogenic process, but also its effect on the regions postsynaptic to the epileptogenic area.

EAA receptors

The amino acids glutamate and aspartate are the two main excitatory neurotransmitters in the cerebral cortex. They act through various receptor subtypes whose subunit composition determines the selective ionic permeability and kinetics of the respective ionic currents (see [36] for a review). Two main receptor types have been identified and named after the two ligands: α-amino-3-hydroxy-5-methyl-4-isoxazole-propionic acid (AMPA) and NMDA (Fig. 6.2). The ionophores associated with both receptor types are permeable to Na^+, but the NMDA receptor is also permeable to Ca^{2+} and is blocked by Mg^{2+} in a voltage-dependent manner. Consequently, the inward flux of Na^+ and Ca^{2+} can only be activated by ligand–receptor interaction when the membrane potential is depolarized enough to remove the Mg^{2+} block. In that case, the NMDA-dependent depolarization is so powerful that it significantly enhances and prolongs the excitatory postsynaptic potentials. The potential epileptogenic effect of EAA systems is demonstrated by the action of a number of EAA agonists (kainic and hybotenic acids, NMDA), which are currently used to induce epilepsy in experimental animals. In dysplastic human cortex, structural changes in EAA receptors lead to AMPA or NMDA epileptogenic hyperactivity [37]. Moreover in temporal lobe epilepsy circuits are rearranged leading to a selective facilitation of the NMDA-dependent excitatory postsynaptic potentials. This will be further discussed below.

GABA receptors

Two types of GABA ionotropic receptors (A and C) are coupled to Cl^- ionophores, whereas the metabotropic $GABA_B$ receptor is coupled to a K^+ channel, and can indirectly modulate membrane excitability. The inflow of Cl^- and outflow of K^+ promoted by GABA binding to ionotropic receptors both lead to a membrane hyperpolarization that results in inhibitory postsynaptic potentials (IPSPs). GABA-mediated IPSPs are very effective in preventing neuronal discharges because they are associated with a dramatic drop in membrane input resistance. Ubiquitously present in the cerebral cortex, local inhibitory circuits consisting of Golgi type 2 GABAergic neurones provide a mechanism for controlling the main population of pyramidal neurones. Although $GABA_A$ blockers such as bicuculline, penicillin and picrotoxin are epileptogenic in experimental studies, in human epilepsies, the evidence for decreased GABAergic neurones in brain tissue resected for treatment of refractory epilepsy [38,39] has been inconsistent. Moreover, the idea of the functional impairment of structurally intact GABAergic circuitry proposed by Sloviter [40], under the attractive name of the 'dormant basket cell hypothesis', was also not confirmed by recordings made of human hippocampi during presurgical evaluation of refractory temporal lobe epilepsy [41], because enhanced rather than impaired inhibition was found. Furthermore, hyperexcitable dentate gyri removed from patients with temporal lobe epilepsy retain bicuculline-sensitive synaptic inhibition [42]. A more recent analysis of tissue specimens from cortical dysplasias revealed significant derangement in GABAergic circuitry [43], the significance of which is still unclear. However, mutations of GABA receptors have been implicated in two genetic epilepsies. One variant of GEFS+ has recently been reported to be associated with a mutation of the *GABRG2* gene that codes for the γ2 subunit of the $GABA_A$ receptor [16,44]. A defect in the *GABRB3* gene that codes for the β3 $GABA_A$ receptor subunit is thought to account for epilepsy in Angelman's syndrome [45].

Acetylcholine (ACh) receptors

These are ubiquitously present in the central nervous system, but their role in controlling brain excitability is less well understood than that of the receptors in the peripheral nervous system, where ACh is the main excitatory neurotransmitter at neuromuscular junctions. As it could be obtained in very large quantities from the electric organ of the *Torpedo marina*, the ACh receptor was the first to be purified and characterized [46]. Its pore region has a pentameric structure consisting of various hetero- or homologous combinations of eight α and three β subunits.

Phillips *et al.* [47] identified a large Australian family including 27 members affected by autosomal dominant nocturnal frontal lobe epilepsy (ADNFLE) with a linkage at locus 20q 13.2 in 1995. Subsequently, Steinlein *et al.* [48] discovered the mutation of the *CHRNA4* gene that codes for the α4 subunit of the nicotinic ACh receptor, and thus provided the first demonstration of a human epilepsy due to a genetically determined channel alteration. Mutations of the *CHRNB2* gene that code for the β2 subunit of ACh receptors lead to similar phenotypes. The effect of these mutations on ACh receptor gating remains to be determined, as does their role in neuronal hyperexcitability. Since the α4 subunit is widely distributed in mammalian brain, it is puzzling how the mutation causes focal epilepsy.

Circuit involvement in epileptogenesis

Although an alteration in neuronal excitability is a primary prerequisite for epileptogenesis, epileptic discharges are not simply due to the abnormal activity of individual neurones. They also require the synchronous activation of large populations of hyperexcitable neurones. Furthermore, epileptic discharges propagate through normal and pathological fibre connections during the course of a seizure. The role of neuronal circuitry in the generation and spread of epileptic discharges therefore needs to be considered.

Intrinsically bursting-operated circuits

The special role of the physiologically intrinsically bursting neocortical and hippocampal neurones mentioned in the introduction not only depends on the power of their excitatory output, but also on their pattern of connectivity, which makes them particularly suitable for the synchronization of large populations.

Layer V intrinsically bursting pyramidal neurones of the neocortex

Chagnac-Amitai and Connors [49] have shown that one-third of the layer V pyramidal neurones of rat neocortex are endowed with intrinsically bursting properties. The axon collaterals of these neurones run tangentially to the cortical surface and establish synaptic connections with a large number of neighbouring pyramidal neurones. Pyramidal intrinsically bursting neurones consistently fire in association with highly synchronized electrocorticographic potentials, thus demonstrating synchronizing ability. It has been shown that the discharges of neocortical intrinsically bursting neurones are determined by the persistent fraction of the Na$^+$ current [50,51]. Consequently, it can be expected that inherited or acquired changes in Na$^+$ channels, especially those affecting Na$^+$ channel inactivation, may also enhance the intrinsically bursting-dependent synchronizing mechanism. Taken together, the available data suggest that the synchronizing circuitry of neocortical layer V intrinsically bursting pyramidal neurones plays an important role in recruiting the critical mass of neurones required to create an epileptogenic area.

Intrinsically bursting neurones of CA3

All CA3 neurones have an intrinsically determined bursting property which, unlike that of neocortical intrinsically bursting neurones, is Ca^{2+}-dependent. However, in functional terms, CA3 and neocortical intrinsically bursting neurones are similar insofar as their connectivity patterns enable them to synchronize the activity of synaptically connected neuronal populations. The anatomical basis is Shaeffer's collateral of CA3 neuronal axons, which connect extensively with the dendrites of the pyramidal neurones of Cornu Ammonis area 1 (CA1).

The effectiveness of this synaptic organization can be easily demonstrated in vitro in hippocampal slices by placing a stimulation electrode on the CA3 stratum radiatum, after which the synchronized CA1 output is conveyed to the hippocampal-entorhinal circuitry. There is no evidence of primary functional or anatomical CA3 neuronal alterations in human epilepsies, but it can be assumed that any change in Ca^{2+} channel function leading to a Ca^{2+} current enhancement increases the effectiveness of CA3-dependent synchronization of hippocampal activities. However, it is clear that CA3 and its efferent connections can be secondarily involved as a consequence of other circuit changes occurring in

human mesial temporal lobe epilepsy, as is discussed in the next paragraph.

Seizure-dependent circuit rearrangements

The mesial temporal structures are interconnected by fibre systems that create the reverberating loop involving entorhinal cortex–dentate gyrus–CA3–CA1 (subiculum)–entorhinal cortex. Dreier and Heinemann [52] have developed a technique for preparing in vitro slices including the full circuit and demonstrated that it is necessary and sufficient to sustain persistent epileptic activities.

The most striking evidence of epileptogenic hippocampal plasticity was provided in 1969 by Goddard [53], who demonstrated that repetition of electrical stimulation of the amygdala that initially did not evoke epileptic discharges gradually led to greater seizure susceptibility and then spontaneous seizures, a process named kindling. The discovery of kindling was the starting point for a number of experimental studies aimed at defining the biological basis of epileptogenic plasticity. Another important milestone was established by Sutula et al. [54], who first demonstrated that kindling results in sprouting of a mossy fibre pathway that reorganizes synaptic connections in the dentate gyrus. They observed a similar picture in surgically resected hippocampi from patients with epilepsy [55]. These findings have been confirmed by a number of other investigators, including Babb et al. [56] from whose work Fig. 6.5 has been taken. Mossy fibre sprouting had been previously observed after experimentally induced status epilepticus accompanied by extensive neural damage [57]. However, the kindling experiments demonstrated that repeated brief seizures can induce sprouting in the absence of extensive brain damage [58]. In human mesial temporal lobe epilepsy, mossy fibre sprouting is consistently associated with hippocampal sclerosis and cell loss. The degeneration of mossy cells in the hippocampal hilus significantly contributes to the circuitry rearrangement (schematically illustrated in Fig. 6.5 [56]).

Sprouted mossy fibres make ectopic synaptic contacts, and thereby create an excitatory feedback circuit [59–61]. The excitatory effect of the aberrant recurrent fibres is further enhanced by the facilitation of NMDA receptor-mediated conductance, which has been demonstrated in dentate granule cells from the surgically excised human epileptic temporal lobe tissue [62]. Recurrent axon collaterals also make synaptic contacts with inhibitory interneurones, leading to an enhanced inhibition [63] that, rather than preventing the generation of epileptic discharges, contributes to it by promoting synchrony [64]. Although the main dentate granule axon target is CA3, it is not known to what extent the sprouted collaterals of granule axons contribute to the enhanced excitability in postsynaptic neurones inside CA3, or contribute to hyperexcitability elsewhere in the hippocampal-entorhinal circuit, such as in CA1 [65].

The study of circuit reorganization in mesial temporal lobe epilepsy has provided important insights into its biological basis but a number of questions remain unanswered.

Comparisons of human and animal studies have shown that brief seizures can set in motion a cascade of events leading to sprouting and neosynaptogenesis, which may account for the tendency of mesial temporal lobe epilepsy to progress towards medical intractability. In both humans and experimental animal models of epilepsy kainic- and pilocarpine-induced epilepsy exhibits a bipha-

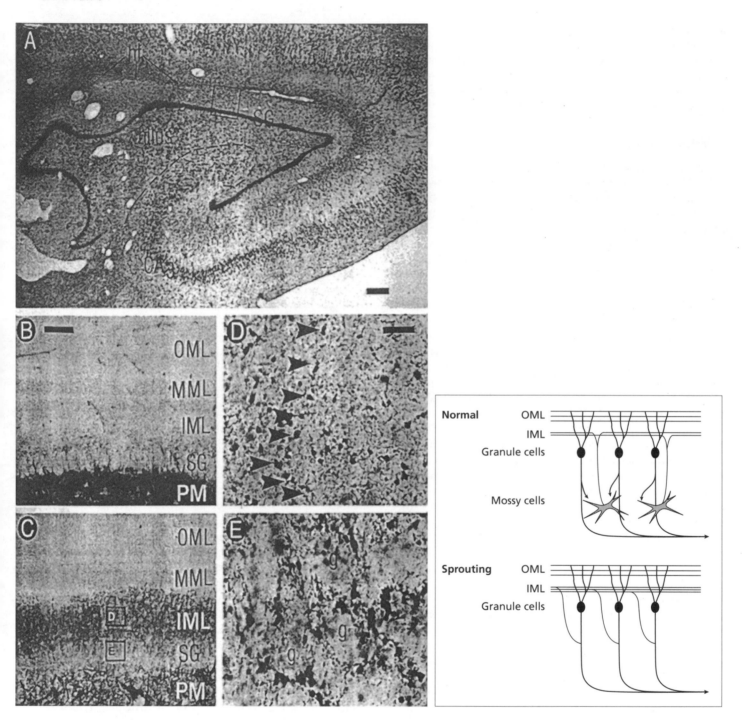

Fig. 6.5 Evidence for circuitry rearrangements in human hippocampus surgically removed from patients with mesial temporal lobe epilepsy and hippocampal sclerosis. Left (a) Coronal section of normal human hippocampus stained with cresyl violet. Dashed line segregates the CA4 pyramidal neurones from the hilus of the dentate gyrus (SG = stratum granulosum). (b) Adjacent section. Magnification of boxed area in (a) stained with the Timm method for heavy metals: the dense stain is strictly limited to the zinc-containing granule cells of polymorph layer (PM), whereas supragranular layer (SG), inner, mesial and outer molecular layers (IML, MML, OML) are completely devoid of staining. (c) The corresponding area from a surgically removed hippocampus of a patient with temporal epilepsy and hippocampal sclerosis shows a second band of zinc-containing axons in the IML. (d) Timm stain puncta in IML from boxed area in (c). (e) Timm stain puncta in SG from boxed area in (c). From [56]. Right: schematic representation of granule axon sprouting in hippocampal sclerosis. The newly formed axon collaterals occupy the inner molecular layer devoid of the mossy fibres due to the degeneration of the hilar mossy cells.

sic time course, with a prolonged latent interval between the initial event and the chronic epileptic phase during which the activation of Ca^{2+}-dependent proteases, protein kinase C, Ca^{2+}/calmodulinkinase systems and immediate early genes [66] promote circuit remodelling. The most frequent antecedent, the clinical history of mesial temporal lobe epilepsy, is a prolonged febrile seizure during the first 2 years of life that can be compared to the status epilepticus induced by kainic acid and pilocarpine in experimental animals. Once established, the aberrant hippocampal circuitry creates a condition of hyperexcitability that leads to chronic epilepsy that is often difficult to treat.

However, this theory is not supported by a number of other observations. First of all, experimental interventions that prevent sprouting do not prevent the acquisition of epileptic properties [67]. Second, although PDS-like discharges can be recorded easily from dentate granule cells in sclerotic hippocampal slices, recordings from the epileptogenic hippocampi of patients indicate that bursting neurones are only rarely encountered and that it is difficult to demonstrate synchrony [68,69]. Third, the role of the putatively seizure-dependent cell loss in determining the sprouting is still unclear, as is the role of excess of zinc caused by the sprouting of zinc-containing mossy fibres upon glutamatergic and GABAergic synaptic transmission [70]. Finally, the relevance of seizure-stimulated neurogenesis in the adult dentate gyrus to human mesial temporal lobe epilepsy [71] remains to be clarified.

Thalamocortical circuitry

It has long been known that thalamocortical circuits play a role in the generation of spikes and waves [72,73]. The results obtained in GAERS presenting with absences associated with 7 Hz spike-wave complexes have shed light on the rhythmogenic thalamic mechanisms responsible for the paroxysmal discharges [31–33,74].

A key role is played by the reticular thalamic nucleus, a laminar structure enfolding the anteroventral and lateral aspects of the dorsal thalamus that is entirely made up of GABAergic neurones. Reticular thalamic neurones have a low threshold Ca^{2+} current (I_T) that is particularly effective in generating sequences of 7–9 Hz Ca^2/K^+-dependent bursts [30,75]. The resulting rhythmic GABAergic output feeds into the thalamocortical relay neurones, which are thereby recruited to fire rhythmically with a reciprocal time relationship. A simplified sequence of the events occurring during a spike-wave discharge is schematically illustrated in Fig. 6.6.

The Ca^{2+}-dependent burst intrinsically generated in reticular thalamic neurones gives rise to a particularly strong $GABA_B$-mediated IPSP [76] in thalamocortical relay neurones: the resulting membrane hyperpolarization de-inactivate I_T, and a rebound burst is released during the depolarization phase of the IPSP. The thalamocortical relay excitatory output propagates to the cortex where both regularly spiking and intrinsically bursting pyramidal neurones are synchronously excited. Experiments in GAERS have shown that selective reticular thalamic lesions or local injections of the Cd^{2+}, an inorganic Ca^{2+} blocker, suppress or severely decrease ipsilateral spike-wave activity [31]. Patch-clamp recordings from GAERS reticular thalamic neurones have shown a genetically determined enhancement of I_T in comparison with control rats. This enhancement may lead to a strong GABA-mediated output towards

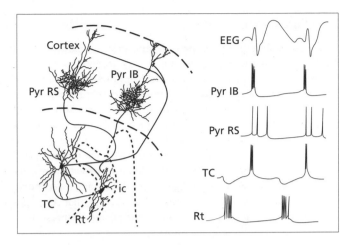

Fig. 6.6 Schematic representation of the reverberating thalamocorticothalamic circuit putatively responsible for spike-wave discharges in GAERS. An enhancement of low-threshold Ca^{2+} current in reticular neurones (Rt) gives rise to particularly pronounced burst-hyperpolarization sequences which induce rhythmic IPSPs in thalamocortical (TC) neurones. The resulting membrane hyperpolarization allows activation of low-threshold Ca^{2+} current in TC neurones that sustain rebound burst in reciprocal time relationship with Rt. The TC excitatory output propagates to the cortex where both regular spiking and intrinsically bursting pyramidal neurones (PyrRS, PyrIB) are excited simultaneously and send their rhythmic output back to thalamic Rt and TC neurones. The synchronous discharges of cortical neurones is 'seen' by the EEG scalp electrodes as rhythmic sharp-wave complexes. From [32].

thalamocortical relay neurones and thus play a central role in the pathogenesis of spike-waves in GAERS [33].

Other reported changes in glutamate and GABA-mediated transmission in GAERS also contribute to spike-wave generation [77,78]. The feedback excitation from the thalamocortical relay and cortex, which is transported along the thalamoreticular-thalamic and corticoreticular-thalamic fibres, reaches the reticular-thalamic neurones during the late part of after-hyperpolarization and promotes the reactivation of a low-threshold burst that starts the next cycle. The increased I_T in reticular thalamic cells appears during the course of postnatal GAERS development before the onset of absence and spike-wave expression. It could be at the root of the abnormally intense oscillatory activity that is initiated and sustained by reticular thalamic neurones that secondarily involve the interconnected structures. The resulting use-dependent changes involving glutamatergic and GABAergic neurotransmission in the neocortex may progressively enhance the oscillatory properties of the circuit towards the critical level reached during the first month of postnatal life, when the paroxysmal discharges become detectable.

Although a number of facts implicate Ca^{2+} channel dysfunction in the pathophysiology of GAERS absence epilepsy, it does not necessarily account for all types of experimental and human absence epilepsies. Any type of thalamic or cortical dysfunction that overactivates the involved thalamocortical circuit could theoretically lead to oscillatory activity that is capable of inducing spike-wave discharges. Recent evidence indicates that a non-inactivating Na^+ current component may act synergistically with the T-type Ca^{2+} current [79].

Other fibre systems

Corticocortical connections provide epileptic discharges with a number of propagation pathways that may account for the large variety of epileptic phenomena. Specific mention should be made of the role of frontal *callosal* projections in the interhemispheric synchronization of epileptic discharges. Marcus and Watson [80] reported that bilateral frontal homotropic epileptogenic foci in rhesus monkeys produced bilateral discharges resembling bilateral synchronous spike-wave complexes, but symmetrical foci located in other parts of the cortex were usually independent. They obtained different types of pseudo-generalized discharges depending on the location of the bilateral frontal loci, a finding that correlates well with the marked tendency towards the bilateral expression of seizures with a frontal origin in humans.

Conclusions

Many different types of experimental manipulations affecting the excitable properties of neurones can induce epileptic discharges in various *in vivo* and *in vitro* models of epilepsy.

Over the last few years, a number of abnormalities involving voltage-dependent and ligand-operated channels have been found to be relevant to human epilepsies. This has led to a greater understanding of how these elementary alterations can affect brain circuitry in some common types of human epilepsies. The data relating to seizure-related brain plasticity are particularly interesting because they shed further light on the biological basis for the tendency of mesial temporal lobe epilepsy to progress towards a medical intractability. We can expect further exciting progress in the not too distant future.

References

1 Jackson JH. On the anatomical, physiological and pathological investigation of epilepsies. *West Riding Lunatic Asylum Medical Reports* 1873; 3: 315–39.
2 Galvani L. De viribus electricitatis in motu muscularis commentarius. *De Bononiensi Scientiarum et Artium Instituto atque Academia* 1791: 363–418.
3 von Humboldt A. *Versuche über die Gereizte Muskel-under-Nervenfaser, oder Galvanismus, nebst Vermuthungen über den Chemischen Process des Lebens in der Thier und Pflanzenwelt.* Posen and Berlin: Decker and Rottman, 1797.
4 Fritsch GT, Hitzig JE Über die Elektrische Erregbarkeit des Grosshirns. *Arch Anat Physiol Wiss Med* 1870; 37: 300–32.
5 Todd RB. On the pathology and treatment of convulsive diseases. *London Medical Gazette* 1849; 8: 661–71; 724–9; 766–72; 815–22; 837–46.
6 Matsumoto H, Ajmone Marsan C. Cortical cellular phenomena in experimental epilepsy. Interictal manifestations. *Exp Neurol* 1964; 9: 286–304.
7 Prince DA. Neurophysiology of epilepsy. In: Cowan WM, Hall ZW, Kandel ER, eds. *Annual Review of Neuroscience.* Palo Alto California: Annual Reviews Inc., Vol. 1, 1978: 395–415.
8 Green W, Millar N. Ion channel assembly. *Trends Neurosci* 1995; 18: 280–7.
9 Neher E, Sakmann B. Single-channel current recorded from the membrane of denervated frog muscle fibres. *Nature* 1976; 260: 779–802.
10 Mantegazza M, Franceschetti S, Avanzini G. Anemone toxin (ATXII) induced increase in persistent sodium current: effects on the firing properties of rat neocortical pyramidal neurones. *J Physiol* 1998; 507: 105–16.
11 Löscher W. New vision in the pharmacology of anticonvulsion. *Eur J Pharmacol* 1998; 342: 1–13.
12 Chao TI, Alzheimer C. Effects of phenytoin on the persistent Na$^+$ current of mammalian CNS neurones. *NeuroReport* 1995; 6: 1778–80.
13 Taverna S, Sancini G, Mantegazza M, Franceschetti S, Avanzini G. Inhibition of transient and persistent Na$^+$ current fractions by the new anticonvulsant topiramate. *J Pharmacol Exp Ther* 1999; 288: 960–8.
14 Lombardo AJ, Kuzniecky R, Powers RE, Brown GB. Altered brain sodium channel transcript levels in human epilepsy. *Mol Brain Res* 1996; 35: 84–90.
15 Wallace RH, Wang DW, Singh R *et al.* Febrile seizures and generalized epilepsy associated with a mutation in the Na$^+$-channel β1 subunit gene SCN1B. *Nat Genet* 1998; 19: 366–70.
16 Wallace RH, Marini C, Petrou S *et al.* Mutant GABAA receptor gamma2-subunit in childhood absence epilepsy and febrile seizures. *Nat Genet* 2001; 28; 49–52.
17 Baulac S, Gourfinkel-An I, Picard F *et al.* A second locus for familial generalized epilepsy with febrile seizures plus maps to chromosome 2q21-q33. *Am J Hum Genet* 1999; 65: 1078–85.
18 Escayg A, MacDonald BT, Meisler MH *et al.* Mutations of SCN1A, encoding a neuronal sodium channel, in two families with GEFS+2. *Nat Genet* 2000; 24: 343–54.
19 Sugawara T, Tsurubuchi Y, Agarwala KL *et al.* A missense mutation of the Na$^+$ channel α_{II} subunit gene Na$_V$ 1.2 in a patient with febrile and afebrile seizures causes channel dysfunction. *PNAS* 2001; 98: 6384–9.
20 Claes L, Del-Favero J, Ceulemans B, Lagae L, Van Broeckhoven C, De Jonghe P. De novo mutations in the sodium-channel gene SCN1A cause severe myoclonic epilepsy of infancy. *Am J Hum Genet* 2001; 68: 1327–32.
21 Wei A, Jegla T, Salkoff L. Eight potassium channel families revealed by the *C. elegans* genome project. *Neuropharmacology* 1996; 35: 805–29.
22 Hodgkin AL, Huxley AF, Katz B. Ionic current underlying activity in the giant axon of the squid. *Arch Sci Physiol* 1949; 3: 129–50.
23 Biervert C, Schroeder BC, Kubisch C *et al.* A potassium channel mutation in neonatal human epilepsy. *Science* 1998; 279: 403–6.
24 Wang HS, Pan Z, Shi W *et al.* KCNQ2 and KCNQ3 potassium channel subunits: molecular correlates of the M-channel. *Science* 1998; 282: 1890–3.
25 Rogawski MA. KCNQ2/KCNQ3 K$^+$ channels and the molecular pathogenesis of epilepsy: implications for therapy. *TINS* 2000; 23: 393–8.
26 Zhang JF, Randall AD, Ellinor PT *et al.* Distinctive pharmacology and kinetics of cloned neuronal Ca^{2+} channels and their possible counterparts in mammalian CNS neurons. *Neuropharmacology* 1993; 32: 1075–88.
27 Vergnes M, Marescaux C, Micheletti G *et al.* Spontaneous paroxysmal electroclinical patterns in rat: a model of generalized nonconvulsive epilepsy. *Neurosci Lett* 1982; 33: 97–101.
28 Coenen AML, Drinkenburg WHIM, Inoue M, Van Luijtelaar ELJM. Genetic models of absence epilepsy, with emphasis on the WAG/Rij strain of rats. *Epilepsy Res* 1992; 12: 75–87.
29 Burgess DL, Noebels JL. Voltage-dependent calcium channel mutations in neurological disease. *Ann N Y Acad* 1999; 868: 199–212.
30 Avanzini G, de Curtis M, Panzica F, Spreafico R. Intrinsic properties of nucleus reticularis thalami neurones of the rat studies in vitro. *J Physiol* 1989; 416: 111–22.
31 Avanzini G, Vergnes M, Spreafico R, Marescaux C. Calcium-dependent regulation of genetically determined spike and waves by the reticular thalamic nucleus of rats. *Epilepsia* 1993; 34: 1–7.
32 Avanzini G, de Curtis M, Pape HC, Spreafico R. Intrinsic properties of reticular thalamic neurons relevant to genetically determined spike-wave generation. In: Delgado-Escueta AV, Wilson WA, Olsen RW, Porter RJ, eds. *Jasper's Basic Mechanisms of the Epilepsies*, 3rd edn. *Advances in Neurology*, Vol 79, Philadelphia: Lippincott Williams & Wilkins, 1999: 297–309.
33 Tsakiridou E, Bertollini L, de Curtis M, Avanzini G, Pape HC. Selective increase in T-type calcium conductance of reticular thalamic neurons in a rat model of absence epilepsy. *J Neurosci* 1995; 15: 3110–17.
34 Kim D, Song I, Keum S *et al.* Lack of the burst firing of thalamocortical relay neurons and resistance to absence seizures in mice lacking α (1G) T-type Ca^{2+} channels. *Neuron* 2001; 31: 3–4.
35 Jouvenceau A, Eunson LH, Spauschus A *et al.* Human epilepsy associated with dysfunction of the brain P/Q-type calcium channel. *Lancet* 2001; 358: 801–7.
36 Seeburg PH. The molecular biology of mammalian glutamate receptor channels. *TINS* 1993; 16: 359–65.

37 Najm IM, Ying Z, Babb T, Mohamed A *et al*. Epileptogenicity correlated with increased *N*-methil-D aspartate receptor subunit NR2A/B in human focal cortical dysplasia. *Epilepsia* 2000; 41: 971–6.

38 Lloyd KG, Munari C, Bossi L, Stoeffels C, Talairach J, Morselli PL. Biochemical evidence for the alterations of GABA-mediated synaptic transmission in pathological brain tissue (stereo EEG or morphological definition) from epileptic patients. In: Morselli PM, Lloyd KG, Loscher W *et al*., eds. *Neurotransmitters, Seizures and Epilepsy*. New-York: Raven Press, 1981; 325–38.

39 Sherwin AL, Van Gelder NM. Biochemical markers of metabolic abnormalities in human focal epilepsy. In: Delgado-Escueta AV, Ward AA, Woodbury D, eds. *Basic Mechanisms of the Epilepsies*. New York: Raven Press, 1985; 1011–32.

40 Sloviter RS. Permanently altered hippocampal structure, excitability, and inhibition after experimental status epilepticus in the rat: the 'dormant basket cell' hypothesis and its possible relevance to temporal lobe epilepsy. *Hippocampus* 1991; 1: 41–66.

41 Wilson CL, Engel JJ. Electrical stimulation of the human epileptic limbic cortex. *Adv. Neurol* 1993; 63: 103–12.

42 Isokawa M, Avanzini G, Finch DM, Babb TL, Levesque MF. Physiologic properties of human dentate granule cells in slices prepared from epileptic patients. *Epilepsy Res* 1991; 9: 242–50.

43 Spreafico R, Battaglia G, Arcelli P *et al*. Cortical dysplasia. An immunocytochemical study of three patients. *Neurology* 1998; 50: 27–36.

44 Baulac S, Huberfeld G, Gourfinkel-An I *et al*. First genetic evidence of GABAA receptor dysfunction in epilepsy: a mutation in the gamma2-subunit gene. *Nat Genet* 2001; 28: 46–8.

45 Minassian BA, DeLorey TM, Olsen RW *et al*. Angelman syndrome: correlations between epilepsy phenotypes and genotypes. *Ann Neurol* 1998; 43: 485–93.

46 Noda M, Takahaschi T, Tanabe T *et al*. Structural homology of torpedo californica acetylcholine receptors subunits. *Nature* 1983; 302: 528–32.

47 Phillips HA, Scheffer IE, Berkovic SF, Hollway GE, Sutherland GR, Mulley JC. Localization of a gene for autosomal dominant nocturnal frontal lobe epilepsy to chromosome 20q13.2. *Nat Genet* 1995; 10: 117–18.

48 Steinlein O, Schuster V, Fischer C, Haussler M. Benign familial neonatal convulsions: confirmation of genetic heterogeneity and further evidence for a second locus on chromosome 8q. *Human Genet* 1995; 95: 25–9.

49 Chagnac-Amitai Y, Connors BW. Synchronized excitation and inhibition driven by intrinsically bursting neurons in neocortex. *J Neurophysiol* 1989; 62: 1149–62.

50 Franceschetti S, Guatteo E, Panzica F, Sancini G, Wanke E, Avanzini G. Ionic mechanisms underlying burst firing in pyramidal neurons: intracellular study in rat sensorimotor cortex. *Brain Res* 1995; 69: 6127–39.

51 Mantegazza M, Franceschetti S, Avanzini G. Anemone toxin (ATXII) induced increase in persistent sodium current: effects on the firing properties of rat neocortical pyramidal neurones. *J Physiol* 1998; 507: 105–16.

52 Dreier JP, Heinemann U. Regional and time dependent variations of low Mg^{2+} induced epileptiform activity in rat temporal cortex slices. *Exp Brain Res* 1991; 87: 581–96.

53 Goddard GV. The development of epileptic seizures through brain stimulation at low intensity. *Nature* 1969; 214: 1020–1.

54 Sutula T, He XX, Cavazos J, Scott G. Synaptic reorganization in the hippocampus induced by abnormal functional activity. *Science* 1988; 239: 1147–50.

55 Sutula T, Cascino G, Cavazos J, Parada I, Ramirez L. Mossy fibers synaptic reorganization in the epileptic human temporal lobe. *Ann Neurol* 1989; 31: 322–30.

56 Babb TL, Kupfer WR, Pretorius JK, Crandall PH, Levesque MF. Synaptic reorganization by mossy fibers in human epileptic fascia dentata. *Neuroscience* 1991; 42: 351–63.

57 Tauck DL, Nadler JV. Evidence of functional mossy fiber sprouting in hippocampal formation of kainic acid-treated rats. *J Neurosci* 1985; 5: 1016–22.

58 Represa A, LaSalle LG, Ben-Ari Y. Hippocampal plasticity in the kindling model of epilepsy in rats. *Neurosci Lett* 1989; 99: 345–55.

59 Isokawa M, Levesque, M, Babb T, Engel J Jr. Single mossy fiber axonal systems of human dentate granule cells: studies in hippocampal slices from patients with temporal lobe epilepsy. *J Neurosci* 1993; 13: 1511–22.

60 Franck J, Pokorny J, Kunkel D, Schwartzkroin P. Physiologic and morphologic characteristics of granule cell circuitry in human epileptic hippocampus. *Epilepsia* 1995; 36: 543–58.

61 Okazaki M, Evanson D, Nadler J. Hippocampal mossy fiber sprouting and synapse formation after status epilepticus in rats: visualization after retrograde transport of biocytin. *J Comp Neurol* 1995; 352: 515–34.

62 Isokawa M, Levesque M, Fried I, Engel J Jr. Glutamate currents in morphology identified human dentate granule cells in temporal lobe epilepsy. *Am Physioll Soc* 1997; 3355–69.

63 Nusser Z, Hàjos N, Somogyi P, Mody I. Increased number of synaptic $GABA_A$ receptors underlies potentiation at hippocampal inhibitory synapses. *Nature* 1998; 395: 172–7.

64 Engel JJr, Williamson PD, Wieser HG. Mesial temporal lobe epilepsy. In: Engel J Jr, Pedley TA, eds. *Epilepsy: a comprehensive textbook*. Philadelphia: Lippincott-Raven Press, 1997: 2417–26.

65 Lehmann TN, Gabriel S, Kovacs R *et al*. Alterations of neuronal connectivity in area CA1 of hippocampal slices from temporal lobe epilepsy patients and from pilocarpine-treated epileptic rats. *Epilepsia* 2000; 41 (Suppl. 6): 190–4.

66 Ben-Ari Y, Represa A. Brief seizure episodes induce long-term potentiation and mossy fibers sprouting in the hippocampus. *TINS* 1990; 13: 312–18.

67 Longo BM, Mello LE. Blockade of pilocarpine- or kainate-induced mossy fiber sprouting by cycloheximide does not prevent subsequent epileptogenesis in rats. *Neurosci Lett* 1997; 226: 163–6.

68 Colder BW, Frysinger RC, Wilson CL, Harper RM, Engel J Jr. Decreased neuronal burst discharge near site of seizure onset in epileptic human temporal lobes. *Epilepsia* 1996; 37: 113–21.

69 Colder BW, Wilson CL, Frysinger RC, Chao LC, Harper RM, Engel J Jr. Neuronal synchrony in relation to burst discharge in epileptic human temporal lobes. *J Neurophysiol* 1996; 75: 2496–508.

70 Mody I. Ion channels in epilepsy. *Int Rev Neurobiol* 1998; 42: 199–225.

71 Parent J, Yu T, Leibowitz R, Geschwind D, Sloviter R, Lowenstein D. Dentate granule cell neurogenesis is increased by seizures and contributes to aberrant network reorganization in the adult rat hippocampus. *J Neurosci* 1997; 17: 3727–38.

72 Jasper H, Kershman J. Electroencephalographic classification of the epilepsies. *Arch Neurol Psychiatr* 1941; 45: 903–43.

73 Jasper H, Droogleever-Fortuyn J. Experimental studies of the functional anatomy of the petit mal epilepsy. *Assoc Res Nerv Ment Disord Proc* 1947; 26: 272–98.

74 de Curtis M, Avanzini G. Thalamic regulation of epileptic spike and wave discharges. *Funct Neurol* 1994; 9: 307–26.

75 Huguenard JR, Prince DA. A novel T-type current underlies prolonged Ca^{2+}-dependent burst firing in GABAergic neurons of rat thalamic reticular nucleus. *J Neurosci* 1992; 12: 3804–17.

76 Crunelli V, Lereshe N. A role for GABA-B receptors in excitation inhibition of thalamocortical cells. *Trends Neurosci* 1991; 14: 16–21.

77 Spreafico R, Mennini T, Danober L *et al*. GABA-A receptor impairment in the genetic absence epilepsy rats from Strasbourg (GAERS): an immunocytochemical and receptor binding autoradiographic study. *Epilepsy Res* 1993; 15: 229–38.

78 Avanzini G, de Curtis M, Franceschetti S, Sancini G, Spreafico R. Cortical versus thalamic mechanisms underlying spike and wave discharges in GAERS. *Epilepsy Res* 1996; 26: 37–44.

79 Parri HR, Crunelli V. Sodium current in rat and cat thalamocortical neurons: role of a non-inactivating component in tonic and burst firing. *J Neurosci* 1998; 18: 854–67.

80 Marcus EM, Watson CW. Symmetrical epileptogenic foci in monkey cerebral cortex: mechanisms of interaction and regional variations in capacity for synchronous. *Arch Neurol* 1968; 18: 99–116.

Mechanisms of Drug Resistance in Epilepsy

S.M. Sisodiya

Whilst for most patients with epilepsy, seizures come under control easily, in about one-third of adult and childhood cases, seizures continue to occur despite antiepileptic drug (AED) treatment. Comparatively little study has been undertaken to examine the causes of resistance to treatment. Cases are labelled medically refractory, are possibly considered for surgery or gravitate in specialist clinics, receiving successive novel or trial AEDs. More recently, increasing attention has been paid to the possible mechanisms of resistance to AED treatment, partly as a result of consideration of similar problems in cancer. Only a rational understanding of the underlying mechanisms can provide solutions to the problem of drug resistance. In this chapter, the problem and potential causes are considered.

The problem of resistance to drug treatment

For the majority of patients with epilepsy, seizures are well controlled, often with the first AED given. In about one-third of patients, epilepsy remains uncontrolled, despite a variety of AEDs being prescribed [1]. Such uncontrolled epilepsy carries significant risks for the affected individual. Mortality is increased, especially when generalized tonic-clonic seizures continue to occur [2], and physical and psychosocial morbidity are also increased. The burden to society is significant. In the UK alone, where 80 000 people have refractory epilepsy, the cost of epilepsy overall is at least £2000 million/year [3]. For a small proportion of patients with refractory epilepsy, surgical treatment is possible and offers a chance of remission of epilepsy and cure. However, surgery is not feasible for most patients with refractory epilepsy. There is an urgent need for other treatment options in this group of patients.

There are a number of simple causes of apparent drug resistance that must be excluded. These include misdiagnosis of another condition (syncopal, cardiac, neurological, metabolic or psychiatric) as epilepsy, particularly syncope [4] and non-epileptic attack disorder, which are most likely to be alternative diagnoses for apparently drug-resistant epilepsy. In addition, epilepsy may have been correctly diagnosed, but the most appropriate treatment not initiated: use of the wrong AED for a given syndrome may lead to poor control. Inadequate drug levels, usually from non-compliance, may also lead to poor control. If these causes are excluded, by careful history examination and appropriate investigation, the epilepsy may be refractory.

The term 'refractory epilepsy' lacks a precise definition, and can be debated. Most clinicians would consider as refractory epilepsy that had not been controlled by any of three first-line AEDs usually employed for a given epilepsy syndrome. Control ideally means cessation of seizures: the 50% reduction in seizure frequency benchmark used in trials is of little practical benefit to patients [5]; only seizure-freedom is associated with significant improvement in quality of life [6]. For children, however, even a reduction in seizure frequency may be of benefit in allowing cognitive and psychosocial development to occur [7].

Taking as an operative definition failure to respond to three first-line AEDs, overall about one-third of patients are resistant to AEDs. Whilst epilepsy of almost any type, including the primary generalized epilepsies, may be refractory [8], resistance to drug treatment is unevenly distributed amongst the many causes of epilepsy. MRI has uncovered many structural associations of resistant epilepsy: for example, epilepsy caused by hippocampal sclerosis, brain malformations and dysembryoplastic neuroepithelial tumours is very likely to be drug-resistant [9–11]. However, MRI studies have not explained why the epilepsy caused by or associated with these structural abnormalities is refractory to drug treatment.

There are many possible causes of refractory epilepsy. It is likely to be a multifactorial process. For example, seizure-related processes such as changes in brain connectivity, cerebral reorganization secondary to hypoxia and kindling have been suggested as possible mechanisms [12] but without extensive experimental evidence. Comparisons of responsive and refractory cohorts have identified some phenomena associated with resistance, such as remote symptomatic aetiology, early onset (before 1 year of age), multiple seizure types and high seizure frequency prior to initiation of treatment [8,13,14]. However, surprisingly little research has been undertaken into the basis of these phenomena or the molecular basis of drug resistance. More recently, disease-modified channel activity has been demonstrated [15] and may possibly contribute to altered cellular response to AEDs, and to resistance to AED treatment. There has been some recent interest in autoimmune diatheses in refractory epilepsy [16]. It is of interest that mutations in a ligand-gated ion channel thought to cause epilepsy actually render that channel more sensitive to an AED that may be effective in that epilepsy [17]. There is no proof yet of the truth of the converse, that disease-causing mutations (or polymorphisms) in other receptors or channels actually directly render the individuals harbouring those mutations more resistant to treatment. It is likely that there are a range of mechanisms that underlie resistance: some may generate certain aspects of resistance, whilst others may be specific to a given epilepsy type or syndrome. No mechanism is yet completely understood.

Drug-resistant epilepsy has a number of characteristics. Most individuals with refractory epilepsy are resistant to most, and often all, AEDs. The underlying type of epilepsy or its cause does not seem to influence the range of AEDs to which an individual is resistant. Notably, most AEDs share certain physical attributes: most are planar and lipophilic. Occasionally, the institution of novel therapy leads to temporary improvement, with the common observation that seizures eventually recrudesce. An AED that may once have been relatively effective can subsequently prove ineffective, for example when the original AED is reintroduced after a trial of another AED. These phenomena suggest the involvement of non-specific dynamic mechanisms of resistance to AEDs. One type of general mechanism will be considered in more detail in this chapter.

Drug resistance parallels in cancer: overexpression of drug resistance proteins

Drug resistance is not unique to epilepsy or indeed neurology. It may occur in other chronic conditions such as arthritis. Resistance has been studied most comprehensively in oncology. Laboratory studies show that resistance to anticancer drugs at a cellular level involves many mechanisms including reduced drug uptake, increased drug metabolism, alterations in intended drug targets, altered survival mechanisms, especially reduced induction of apoptosis and increased transport of anticancer drugs from the cell. Transport-based resistance mechanisms have been amongst the most intensively studied [18]. Many anticancer drugs are derived from natural product toxins. A number of innate host transporters have evolved to protect cells and organisms from such toxins by removing the toxins from cells or their environment. These transporters are widely distributed amongst living organisms and tend to share highly conserved amino acid and structural sequences. They possess the general ability to transport toxins across biomembranes, usually in an energy-dependent fashion, having as their substrates a wide range of molecules. Amongst the best studied of such transporters are members of the ABC (adenosine triphosphate binding cassette) superfamily, including P-glycoprotein or MDR1 (multidrug resistance protein 1). A transmembrane protein, MDR1 reduces organelle, intracytoplasmic or compartmental accumulation of a range of structurally unrelated compounds by active transport across vesicular or cellular membranes. The transported compounds are typically large and hydrophobic. Other members of the ABC transporter family have been identified and linked to drug resistance, including for example, multidrug resistance-associated protein, MRP1 [19], and subfamily members MRP2–6 [20]; sPgp, the bile salt export pump [21]; and *ABCG2* (mitoxantrone resistance gene [22]).

In cancer cells, MDR1 overexpression can be constitutive, present before exposure to anticancer drugs, and in this situation is related to the cell type of origin of the malignancy and may be associated with chromosomal rearrangements [23]. It may also be increased or induced by exposure to anticancer drugs which may select out resistant cells, a phenomenon commonly utilized *in vitro*. Constitutive MDR1 expression confers intrinsic resistance while induction or selection of MDR1 overexpression by exposure to chemotherapy confers acquired drug resistance.

The precise contribution of MDR1 expression to clinical drug resistance has not been elucidated. There are a limited number of examples of the clear relation of drug resistance to the documented overexpression of MDR1, and fewer proven examples of the benefit of inhibition of MDR1 in clinical oncological practice [24]. The clinical application of a molecular understanding of drug resistance protein overexpression is only beginning. The field has been hampered previously by an overestimation of the singular importance of MDR1 alone, by difficulties in the determination of its overexpression in biopsy samples and by a relative lack of sophistication in its inhibition and the selection of patients for consideration of such inhibition. In addition, most cancers are progressive, evolving conditions with a defined end (cure or death), whilst epilepsy is a chronic condition. Whilst the toxicity of drug resistance protein inhibitors given acutely in pulses may be acceptable in cancer, the same may not apply with chronic use in epilepsy. In cancer cells studied *in vitro*, the pattern of expression of various drug resistance proteins may change with time and with exposure to anticancer drugs. Parallels between cancer and epilepsy must therefore not be drawn too far. Nevertheless, the study of drug resistance in cancer provides clues to some mechanisms for resistance that might be explored in epilepsy.

Physiological expression of drug resistance proteins

The best studied drug resistance proteins are MDR1 and MRP1. MDR1 in particular generates xenobiotic barriers. MDR1 expression can be detected immunohistochemically in the intestine, limiting absorption of drugs and toxins, in the liver and kidney, promoting toxin export, in the testis, generating a privileged environment for sperm production, in the placenta, protecting the fetus, and in the blood–brain barrier, regulating the constitution of the cerebrospinal fluid [18,25]. The activity of MDR1 in these locations is affected by inherited functional polymorphisms. Thus absorption of digoxin, an MDR1 substrate, may be affected by polymorphisms in the *MDR1* gene [26]. Such analyses may be complicated where MDR1 substrates are also substrates for metabolizing enzyme systems such as the P450 cytochrome oxidases, functional polymorphisms which may also be important. One *MDR1* gene polymorphism (C3435T) is in a wobble position but has clear functional effects. More *MDR1* expression and activity is associated with CC homozygosity at this position, with reduced expression and functional restriction associated with TT homozygosity. Polymorphism frequency at this position demonstrates significant ethnic variation [27]. In caucasians, the genotype frequencies at this position are: TT, 25%; CT, 50%; and CC, 25% [28]. It is interesting to recall that epilepsy is refractory in about 30% of patients. The TT homozygous genotype is associated with an increased risk of renal cell carcinoma, probably because this type is associated with lower P-glycoprotein activity and consequent increased exposure to nephrotoxins.

The precise localization of MDR1 normally in the blood–brain barrier has been an area of some debate. The prevailing opinion is that expression is within the endothelial cells, MDR1 contributing to the blood–brain barrier [29]. An alternative school proposes that expression occurs on astrocytic end-feet [30]. Whilst the latter is unlikely to be the case in normal human brain, glia may affect MDR1 expression and activity [31]. The importance of MDR1 in the function of the blood–brain barrier has been demonstrated by the generation of knockout mice lacking the murine orthologues of MDR1. Such mice develop normally and are viable, but brain penetration of a number of drugs (e.g. domperidone, loperamide and ivermection) is increased, with possible neurotoxicity [32]. MDR1 is thus likely to have an important physiological function. It is likely that normal human cerebral parenchyma (glia, neurones) lacks MDR1 expression, at least as can be detected using immunohistochemistry with its inherent limitations. MDR1 is able to transport a wide variety of planar lipophilic molecules. It can transport both phenytoin and phenobarbital, albeit these molecules are relatively weak substrates [33,34].

MRP1 has been less well studied. Its expression in human brain has been shown [35,36]. It is expressed in the choroid plexus epithelium. The range of substrates of MRP1 is different from that of MDR1 [19]. It is believed to be able to transport organic anions, glutathione-conjugated molecules and leukotrienes that are active at drug permeability barriers. MRP1 is also known to transport drug glucuronides and epoxides, into which active conjugate carbamazepine is metabolized. MRP1 also protects the oropharyngeal mucosa and the testicular tubules.

Animal models of drug resistance in epilepsy

As for refractory epilepsy in humans, AED resistance in animal models has received little attention. Mice bred for their proneness to ethanol withdrawal convulsions are more resistant to various AEDs including phenytoin [37], whilst the genetically-susceptible E1 mouse has delayed phenytoin-induced upregulation of voltage-dependent sodium channels compared to normal mice [38]. These aspects have received little further attention. The model best studied is the amygdala-kindled phenytoin-resistant Wistar rat, studied by Löscher and his group. This is the only widely available model of pharmacoresistance. Drug responders and non-responders can be selected out on the basis of the effect of phenytoin on the afterdischarge threshold. In a series of detailed experiments, this group demonstrated that the non-responders were non-responsive to a range of AEDs, not just phenytoin even if they were selected on the basis of non-responsiveness to phenytoin [39]. They also showed that a wide range of environmental factors could not explain this phenomenon, and that there was probably a polygenic contribution to this resistance to the effects of phenytoin [40,41]. The precise molecular basis has not yet been determined. However, the model is versatile, and may reveal some molecular factors involved in drug resistance.

The use of knockout mouse models often provides useful information in the study of the function of given proteins. However, use of these models is limited in the study of drug resistance because of the redundancy of transport molecules—another transport protein may take over the function, albeit less effectively, of one that has been knocked out [32]. Thus failure of knockout to affect AED kinetics cannot be taken to prove that the protein knocked out does not transport AEDs.

Evidence for overexpression of drug resistance proteins in human epilepsy

A few studies have demonstrated increased expression of the drug transport proteins MDR1 and MRP1 in pathological human brain tissue. Tishler *et al.* first reported increased endothelial and glial MDR1 protein and mRNA expression in surgically-resected brain tissue from patients with refractory temporal lobe epilepsy [34]. Using engineered cell lines overexpressing MDR1 *in vitro*, they demonstrated that phenytoin was a transport substrate for MDR1, albeit with low affinity, making MDR1 overexpression a plausible candidate mediating drug resistance in human epilepsy. Lazarowski *et al.* [42] showed expression of MDR1 in resected tissue from a single case of tuberous sclerosis, but without any comparable control tissue. In these studies, the tissue examined had been exposed to the stress of seizures and AEDs, both of which may potentially increase expression of MDR1 [33,43].

Malformations of cortical development are an important cause of refractory epilepsy. Most cases of particular types of malformation will at some stage go on to cause epilepsy. Occasionally such malformations are found by chance in fetal postmortem brain tissue that has never been exposed to AEDs, giving the opportunity to study expression of drug resistance proteins before the onset of epilepsy in cases where epilepsy is likely to develop. In a proportion of such cases containing nodular heterotopia, polymicrogyria and lissencephaly, MDR1 expression was found not only in lesional capillary endothelium, as expected, but also in lesional glia [44]. Glia do not normally express MDR1. This suggests constitutive overexpression can occur in potentially epileptogenic pathologies, raising the possibility that *MDR1* overexpression may contribute to drug resistance in epilepsy, and also suggesting that drug resistance may be a constitutive feature of epilepsy due to such pathologies. The relationship between the malformations, their aetiology and the causation of *MDR1* overexpression has not been explored.

In three other pathologies commonly causing refractory epilepsy, hippocampal sclerosis, focal cortical dysplasia (FCD) and dysembryoplastic neuroepithelial tumours, we have shown the presence of known mediators of drug resistance, MDR1 and MRP1, in lesional glia and, for focal cortical dysplasia, in a proportion of lesional dysplastic neurones [45]. Normal human glia and neurones do not have detectable expression of either protein under normal conditions on immunohistochemistry [34,46]. Whether expression occurs below the threshold for detection with immunohistochemistry is not known: 'overexpression' rather than a novel cellular phenotype is a more conservative interpretation of these findings. In the case of dysplastic neurones in FCD, the MRP1-positive phenotype *may* be part of an overall cytological abnormality, as these dysplastic neurones are known to express a number of unusual phenotypes [47].

The distribution of immunostaining in these pathologies causing, or capable of causing, refractory epilepsy is intriguing. Immunoreaction appears most marked in glia and their processes around vessels and around dysplastic neurones. As described, MDR1 contributes to the blood–brain barrier, whilst MRP1 has a role in regulating cerebrospinal fluid constitution [36]. The normal endothelial blood–brain barrier may be disrupted in seizures [48], and glial overexpression may thus represent a 'second barrier'. There is strong cytoplasmic localization of immunostaining. This may obscure any underlying membranous labelling, such localization of MDR1 and MRP1 being most likely to be capable of drug export from interstitial cerebrospinal fluid, but intracellular activity of both proteins has also been demonstrated to be important [20,49–51].

The study of fixed material cannot determine whether the proteins detected are functionally active. Absence or inhibition of MDR1 and MRP1 can lead to excessive cerebrospinal fluid penetration of a range of molecules [32,36], and overexpression is associated with resistance to anticancer treatment in some neurological malignancies [52]. Given the known transport capacity of MDR1 in particular, it is possible that MDR1 and MRP1 overexpressed in the pattern observed might lower local interstitial AED concentration and thereby reduce their antiepileptic effects. Neuronal MRP1 expression might also modulate other effects of AEDs. A recent report suggests carbamazepine may not be a substrate for MDR1 [53]. However, the use of an MDR1 mouse knockout model, whole brain carbamazepine assays and rhodamine efflux assays do not conclusively exclude the possibility that carbamazepine may be a substrate for MDR1 (or other drug resistance proteins), particularly when MDR1 in epileptogenic brain tissue is locally overexpressed and may alter local interstitial carbamazepine concentration.

Conclusions

The study of drug resistance in epilepsy has just begun. There is evidence that drug transport proteins known to contribute to anticancer drug resistance are overexpressed in brain tissue from patients with refractory epilepsy. There is also evidence that some AEDs are substrates for MDR1-mediated transport. It is also unlikely that other AEDs are not substrates for one or other of the 50 or so transporters now recognized. Whilst the parallels between cancer and epilepsy are limited, the neuroscience community could benefit from the experience of cancer researchers, because drug resistance is likely to be a complex and adaptive phenomenon, as might be expected of a biological response crucial to the survival of an organism in a changing toxin-laden environment. Study of the basis of drug resistance in epilepsy may reveal new aspects of epileptogenesis, allow early prediction of poor response to AED treatment, enhance understanding of normal brain function and should offer new approaches to the rational treatment of epilepsy in general. Much more detailed analysis of drug resistance in epilepsy is now needed. In the final analysis, inhibition of drug resistance may not be possible in epilepsy, but studying its basis should reveal other means by which it might be overcome, for example by design of AEDs that are not substrates for brain-expressed resistance mechanisms.

References

1 Sander JW. Some aspects of prognosis in the epilepsies: a review. *Epilepsia* 1993; 34: 1007–16.

2 Nashef L, Shorvon SD. Mortality in epilepsy. *Epilepsia* 1997; 38: 1059–61.

3 Cockerell OC, Hart YM, Sander JW, Shorvon SD. The cost of epilepsy in the United Kingdom: an estimation based on the results of two population-based studies. *Epilepsy Res* 1994; 18: 249–60.

4 Zaidi A, Clough P, Scheepers B, Fitzpatrick A. Treatment resistant epilepsy or convulsive syncope? *BMJ* 1998; 317: 869–70.

5 Walker MC, Sander JW. Difficulties in extrapolating from clinical trial data to clinical practice: the case of antiepileptic drugs. *Neurology* 1997; 49: 333–7.

6 Sperling MR, Feldman H, Kinman J, Liporace JD, O'Connor MJ. Seizure control and mortality in epilepsy. *Ann Neurol* 1999; 46: 45–50.

7 Duchowny M, Jayakar P, Resnick T et al. Epilepsy surgery in the first three years of life. *Epilepsia* 1998; 39: 737–43.

8 Gelisse P, Genton P, Thomas P, Rey M, Samuelian JC, Dravet C. Clinical factors of drug resistance in juvenile myoclonic epilepsy. *J Neurol Neurosurg Psychiatry* 2001; 70: 240–3.

9 Guerrini R, Andermann F, Canapicchi R, Roger J, Zifkin BG, Pfanner P, eds. *Dysplasias of Cerebral Cortex and Epilepsy*. New York: Lippincott-Raven, 1996.

10 Semah F, Picot MC, Adam C et al. Is the underlying cause of epilepsy a major prognostic factor for recurrence? [see comments] *Neurology* 1998; 51: 1256–62.

11 Daumas-Duport C, Varlet P, Bacha S, Beuvon F, Cervera-Pierot P, Chodkiewicz JP. Dysembryoplastic neuroepithelial tumors: nonspecific histological forms—a study of 40 cases. *J Neurooncol* 1999; 41: 267–80.

12 Regesta G, Tanganelli P. Clinical aspects and biological bases of drug-resistant epilepsies. *Epilepsy Res* 1999; 34: 109–22.

13 Casetta I, Granieri E, Monetti VC et al. Early predictors of intractability in childhood epilepsy: a community-based case-control study in Copparo, Italy. *Acta Neurol Scand* 1999; 99: 329–33.

14 MacDonald BK, Johnson AL, Goodridge DM, Cockerell OC, Sander JW, Shorvon SD. Factors predicting prognosis of epilepsy after presentation with seizures. *Ann Neurol* 2000; 48: 833–41.

15 Chen K, Aradi I, Thon N, Eghbal-Ahmadi M, Baram TZ, Soltesz I. Persistently modified h-channels after complex febrile seizures convert the seizure-induced enhancement of inhibition to hyperexcitability. *Nat Med* 2001; 7: 331–7.

16 Peltola J, Kulmala P, Isojarvi J et al. Autoantibodies to glutamic acid decarboxylase in patients with therapy-resistant epilepsy. *Neurology* 2000; 55: 46–50.

17 Picard F, Bertrand S, Steinlein OK, Bertrand D. Mutated nicotinic receptors responsible for autosomal dominant nocturnal frontal lobe epilepsy are more sensitive to carbamazepine. *Epilepsia* 1999; 40: 1198–209.

18 Ling V. Multidrug resistance: molecular mechanisms and clinical relevance. *Cancer Chemother Pharmacol* 1997; 40 (Suppl.): S3–S8.

19 Hipfner DR, Deeley RG, Cole SP. Structural, mechanistic and clinical aspects of MRP1. *Biochim Biophys Acta* 1999; 1461: 359–76.

20 Tan B, Piwnica-Worms D, Ratner L. Multidrug resistance transporters and modulation. *Curr Opin Oncol* 2000; 12: 450–8.

21 Strautnieks SS, Bull LN, Knisely AS et al. A gene encoding a liver-specific ABC transporter is mutated in progressive familial intrahepatic cholestasis. *Nat Genet* 1998; 20: 233–8.

22 Bates SE, Robey R, Knutsen T et al. New ABC transporters in multidrug resistance. *Emerging Therapeutic Targets* 2000; 4: 561–80.

23 Knutsen T, Mickley LA, Ried T et al. Cytogenetic and molecular characterization of random chromosomal rearrangements activating the drug resistance gene, MDR1/P-glycoprotein, in drug-selected cell lines and patients with drug refractory ALL genes chromosomes. *Cancer* 1998; 23: 44–54.

24 Fishman MN, Sullivan DM. Application of resistance reversal agents in hematologic malignancies. *Curr Clin Pract Hematol* 2001; 5: 343–58.

25 Tanabe M, Ieiri I, Nagata N et al. Expression of P-glycoprotein in human placenta: relation to genetic polymorphism of the multidrug resistance (MDR)-1 gene. *J Pharmacol Exp Ther* 2001; 297: 1137–43.

26 Hoffmeyer S, Burk O, von Richter O et al. Functional polymorphisms of the human multidrug-resistance gene: multiple sequence variations and correlation of one allele with P-glycoprotein expression and activity in vivo. *Proc Natl Acad Sci USA* 2000; 97: 3473–8.

27 Ameyaw MM, Regateiro F, Li T et al. MDR1 pharmacogenetics: frequency of the C3435T mutation in exon 26 is significantly influenced by ethnicity. *Pharmacogenetics* 2001; 11: 217–21.

28 Cascorbi I, Gerloff T, Johne A et al. Frequency of single nucleotide polymorphisms in the P-glycoprotein drug transporter MDR1 gene in white subjects. *Clin Pharmacol Ther* 2001; 69: 169–74.

29 Beaulieu E, Demeule M, Ghitescu L, Beliveau R. P-glycoprotein is strongly expressed in the luminal membranes of the endothelium of blood vessels in the brain. *Biochem J* 1997; 326 (Pt 2): 539–44.

30 Golden PL, Pardridge WM. Brain microvascular P-glycoprotein and a revised model of multidrug resistance in brain. *Cell Mol Neurobiol* 2000; 20: 165–81.

31 Gaillard PJ, van der Sandt IC, Voorwinden LH et al. Astrocytes increase the functional expression of P-glycoprotein in an in vitro model of the blood–brain barrier. *Pharm Res* 2000; 17: 1198–205.

32 Schinkel AH. P-glycoprotein, a gatekeeper in the blood–brain barrier. *Adv Drug Deliv Rev* 1999; 36: 179–94.

33 Schuetz EG, Beck WT, Schuetz JD. Modulators and substrates of P-glycoprotein and cytochrome P4503A coordinately up-regulate these proteins in human colon carcinoma cells. *Mol Pharmacol* 1996; 49: 311–18.

34 Tishler DM, Weinberg KI, Hinton DR, Barbaro N, Annett GM, Raffel C.

MDR1 gene expression in brain of patients with medically intractable epilepsy. *Epilepsia* 1995; 36: 1–6.

35 Rao VV, Dahlheimer JL, Bardgett ME *et al*. Choroid plexus epithelial expression of MDR1 P glycoprotein and multidrug resistance-associated protein contribute to the blood-cerebrospinal-fluid drug–permeability barrier. *Proc Natl Acad Sci USA* 1999; 96: 3900–5.

36 Wijnholds J, deLange EC, Scheffer GL *et al*. Multidrug resistance protein 1 protects the choroid plexus epithelium and contributes to the blood–cerebrospinal fluid barrier. *J Clin Invest* 2000; 105: 279–85.

37 Crabbe JC, Kosobud A. Sensitivity and tolerance to ethanol in mice bred to be genetically prone or resistant to ethanol withdrawal seizures. *J Pharmacol Exp Ther* 1986; 239: 327–33.

38 Sashihara S, Yanagihara N, Izumi F, Murai Y, Mita T. Differential up-regulation of voltage-dependent Na+ channels induced by phenytoin in brains of genetically seizure-susceptible (E1) and control (ddY) mice. *Neuroscience* 1994; 62: 803–11.

39 Loscher W, Rundfeldt C, Honack D. Pharmacological characterization of phenytoin-resistant amygdala-kindled rats, a new model of drug-resistant partial epilepsy. *Epilepsy Res* 1993; 15: 207–19.

40 Ebert U, Loscher W. Characterization of phenytoin-resistant kindled rats, a new model of drug-resistant partial epilepsy: influence of genetic factors. *Epilepsy Res* 1999; 33: 217–26.

41 Ebert U, Rundfeldt C, Lehmann H, Loscher W. Characterization of phenytoin-resistant kindled rats, a new model of drug-resistant partial epilepsy: influence of experimental and environmental factors. *Epilepsy Res* 1999; 33: 199–215.

42 Lazarowski A, Sevlever G, Taratuto A, Massaro M, Rabinowicz A. Tuberous sclerosis associated with MDR1 gene expression and drug-resistant epilepsy. *Pediatr Neurol* 1999; 21: 731–4.

43 Vilaboa NE, Galan A, Troyano A, de Blas E, Aller P. Regulation of multidrug resistance 1 (MDR1)/P-glycoprotein gene expression and activity by heat-shock transcription factor 1 (HSF1). *J Biol Chem* 2000; 275: 24970–6.

44 Sisodiya SM, Heffernan J, Squier MV. Over-expression of P-glycoprotein in malformations of cortical development. *Neuroreport* 1999; 10: 3437–41.

45 Sisodiya SM, Lin WR, Squier MV, Thom M. Multidrug-resistance protein 1 in focal cortical dysplasia. *Lancet* 2001; 357: 42–3.

46 Seetharaman S, Barrand MA, Maskell L, Scheper RJ. Multidrug resistance-related transport proteins in isolated human brain microvessels and in cells cultured from these isolates. *J Neurochem* 1998; 70: 1151–9.

47 Garbelli R, Munari C, De Biasi S *et al*. Taylor's cortical dysplasia: a confocal and ultrastructural immunohistochemical study. *Brain Pathol* 1999; 9: 445–61.

48 Yaffe K, Ferriero D, Barkovich AJ, Rowley H. Reversible MRI abnormalities following seizures. *Neurology* 1995; 45: 104–8.

49 Van Luyn MJ, Muller M, Renes J *et al*. Transport of glutathione conjugates into secretory vesicles is mediated by the multidrug-resistance protein 1. *Int J Cancer* 1998; 76: 55–62.

50 Merlin JL, Bour-Dill C, Marchal S, Ramacci C, Poullain MG, Giroux B. Modulation of daunorubicin cellular resistance by combination of P-glycoprotein blockers acting on drug efflux and intracellular drug sequestration in Golgi vesicles. *Cytometry* 2000; 41: 62–72.

51 Meschini S, Calcabrini A, Monti E *et al*. Intracellular P-glycoprotein expression is associated with the intrinsic multidrug resistance phenotype in human colon adenocarcinoma cells. *Int J Cancer* 2000; 87: 615–28.

52 Abe T, Mori T, Wakabayashi Y *et al*. Expression of multidrug resistance protein gene in patients with glioma after chemotherapy. *J Neurooncol* 1998; 40: 11–18.

53 Owen A, Pirmohamed M, Tettey JN, Morgan P, Chadwick D, Park BK. Carbamazepine is not a substrate for P-glycoprotein. *Br J Clin Pharmacol* 2001; 51: 345–9.

8 Antiepileptic Drug Discovery

S.H. White

Epilepsy affects more than 50 million persons worldwide and consists of more than 40 clinical syndromes [1]. At the present time, treatment strategies are symptomatic in nature and aimed at the suppression of clinical seizures with one or more of the available antiepileptic drugs (AEDs). In the 1990s nine new AEDs were approved for the add-on treatment of partial seizures. This was an exciting era for the physician treating patients suffering from intractable seizure disorders. Likewise, for the patient with epilepsy these new drugs provided renewed hope for complete seizure control and lessening of their AED-associated side-effect profile. Never before had there been so many new and novel AEDs available for the management of epilepsy. As with any other class of drugs, the discovery and development of new AEDs relies heavily on the preclinical employment of animal models to establish efficacy and safety prior to their introduction in human volunteers. Obviously, the more predictive the animal model for any given seizure type or syndrome, the greater the likelihood that an investigational AED will demonstrate efficacy in human clinical trials. Herein lies one of the most often discussed issues in the current-day AED discovery process: what is the most appropriate animal model to employ when attempting to screen for efficacy against human epilepsy?

This chapter will review the different approaches employed in the AED discovery process and how each of these has led to the successful identification of clinically effective AEDs. In addition, it will address some of the issues surrounding the development of more appropriate models of pharmacoresistant seizures. An extensive discussion of these issues is beyond the scope of this chapter. Where possible, the reader will be referred to pertinent reviews for a more detailed discussion.

Characteristics of the ideal model system

In a perfect world, the 'ideal' screening model should reflect similar pathophysiology and phenomenology to human epilepsy. In addition, seizures should evolve spontaneously in a developmental time frame consistent with the human condition. Furthermore, since new drugs are needed to treat the 'therapy-resistant' population, the ideal model should display a pharmacological profile that is resistant to existing AEDs. Given the limitless potential of combinatorial chemistry to identify potential therapeutic leads, it would be preferable if a given animal model were amenable to high volume screening. Unfortunately, human epilepsy is a heterogeneous neurological disorder that encompasses many seizure phenotypes and syndromes. As such, it is highly unlikely that any one animal model will ever predict the full therapeutic potential of an investigational AED. This necessitates the evaluation of an investigational AED in several syndrome-specific model systems.

The current era of AED discovery

Since 1974, the National Institutes of Neurological Disorders and Stroke (NINDS) has played a pivotal role in stimulating the discovery and development of new chemical entities for the symptomatic treatment of human epilepsy. The efforts of NINDS have largely been heralded by the Anticonvulsant Drug Development Program, which since its inception has accessioned over 24 000 investigational AEDs from academic and pharmaceutical chemists worldwide. Typically, the majority of investigational AEDs have evolved from one of several different strategies. These include: (a) random drug screening and efficacy-based AED discovery; (b) structural modification of a clinically effective pharmacophore; and (c) mechanistic-based AED development. The initial characterization of their anticonvulsant and behavioural toxicity profile has been established through a contract with the University of Utah Anticonvulsant Screening Project using a battery of well-defined animal models [2–5]. The current era of AED discovery was ushered in by Merritt and Putnam in 1937 when they demonstrated the feasibility of using the maximal electroshock seizure (MES) model to identify the anticonvulsant potential of phenytoin [6]. Since then, a number of animal models has been employed in the search for more efficacious and more tolerable AEDs. Since 1993, these approaches have led to the successful development of nine clinically effective drugs including felbamate (1993), gabapentin (1993), lamotrigine (1994), fosphenytoin (1996), topiramate (1996), tiagabine (1997), levetiracetam (1999), zonisamide (2000) and oxcarbazepine (2000). Despite this apparent success, there continues to be a significant need for more efficacious and less toxic AEDs. This is particularly true for that population of patients whose seizure disorder falls in that category often referred to as 'therapy resistant'. Indeed, the percentage of patients with partial epilepsy that fall into this category has not changed significantly since the early 1970s and remains relatively stable between 25 and 40% [7]. This is not to say that the new drugs are without value. In fact, some of these second-generation AEDs have provided significant benefit to patients with partial epilepsy in the form of greater efficacy, better tolerability, more favourable pharmacokinetics and greater long-term safety. Some have subsequently been found to possess potential long-term safety concerns (e.g. felbamate and vigabatrin). For those patients that continue to experience uncontrolled seizures at the expense of intolerable adverse drug reactions, there is a clear and immediate need for more efficacious and better tolerated AEDs. It is within this realm that the AED discovery process confronts its greatest challenges and ignites significant debate. Unfortunately, as scientists and clinicians continue to debate the merits of one approach over another, the patient with 'therapy-resistant' seizures continues to suffer from both inadequate seizure control and unwarranted adverse drug effects. The remainder of this chapter will review the current systematic screening process employed by the Anticonvulsant Screening Project at the University of Utah and discuss some of its inherent advantages and limitations. Subsequent discussion will focus on some of the emerging models that may be more likely to identify the truly 'novel' AED for the treatment of pharmacoresistant partial epilepsy.

Identification of anticonvulsant activity

As shown in Fig. 8.1, the University of Utah Anticonvulsant Screening Project employs three primary screens in their initial identification studies. These include the MES, subcutaneous pentylenetetrazol (scPTZ), and 6 Hz psychomotor seizure tests. Each of these evoked seizure models provides valuable information regarding the potential anticonvulsant spectrum of an investigational AED.

The MES and scPTZ tests

The MES and scPTZ seizure models continue to represent the two most widely used animal seizure models employed in the search for new AEDs [5,8,9] and presently remain as the primary screens of the Anticonvulsant Screening Project (Fig. 8.1). As mentioned above, Merritt and Putnam successfully employed the MES test in a systematic screening programme to identify phenytoin [6]. This observation when coupled with the subsequent success of phenytoin in the clinical management of generalized tonic-clonic seizures provided the validation necessary to consider the MES test as a reasonable model of human generalized tonic-clonic seizures. In 1944, Everett and Richards [10] demonstrated that PTZ-induced seizures

could be blocked by trimethadione and phenobarbital but not by phenytoin. A year later, Lennox demonstrated that trimethadione was effective in decreasing or preventing petit mal attacks in 50 patients but was ineffective or worsened grand mal attacks in 10 patients [11]. Trimethadione's success in the clinic and its ability to block threshold seizures induced by PTZ provided the necessary correlation to establish the PTZ test as a model of petit mal or generalized absence seizures. With these observations, the current era of AED screening using the MES and scPTZ tests was launched.

The MES and scPTZ tests are routinely conducted with either mice or rats. For the MES test, individual animals receive an electrical stimulus that is delivered through either corneal or pinneal electrodes for 0.2 s duration. The stimulus is of sufficient intensity (e.g. 50 mA in mice and 150 mA in rats) to induce a tonic extension seizure characterized by hindlimb extension. This stimulus intensity is typically five to 10 times greater than the threshold current necessary to evoke a maximal seizure. An investigational drug is said to offer protection in the MES test if it displays an ability to block the hindlimb tonic extensor component of the seizure.

In the scPTZ test, PTZ is administered subcutaneously in a dose sufficient to produce a minimal clonic seizure of the vibrissae and/or forelimbs that persists for at least 5 s. A drug is said to be effective in the scPTZ test if it is able to block the minimal clonic seizure described above. It is important to note that higher doses of PTZ can produce myoclonic jerks, repeated clonic seizures of the vibrissae, forelimbs and hindlimbs without loss of righting reflex, clonic seizures of the limbs with loss of righting reflex and loss of righting reflex followed by tonic extension of the forelimbs and hindlimbs [12]. This is important to note because these different endpoints have been shown to be associated with markedly different pharmacological profiles [12,13]. For example, ethosuximide and pheny-

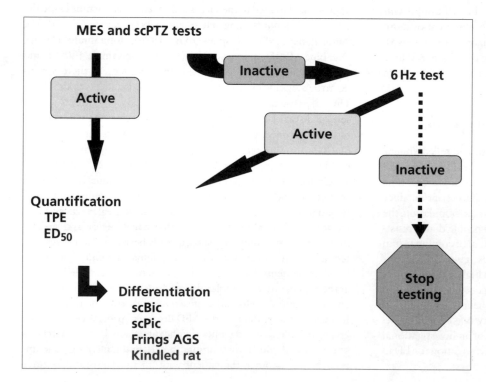

Fig. 8.1 Schematic diagram depicting the initial identification screen of the University of Utah Anticonvulsant Screening Project. Once accessioned, an investigational AED is screened for efficacy in both the MES and scPTZ tests. The activity of those compounds with demonstrated efficacy and minimal behavioural toxicity is quantitated at the time to peak anticonvulsant effect. Compounds found inactive in the MES and scPTZ tests are subsequently evaluated in the 6 Hz seizure test. The activity of those compounds with demonstrated efficacy in the 6 Hz test is then quantitated at their respective time to peak effect. All compounds found active in one or more of these three identification screens are then differentiated on the basis of their activity in the subcutaneous bicuculline (scBic) test, the subcutaneous picrotoxin (scPic) test, the Frings audiogenic seizure-susceptible (AGS) mouse, and the hippocampal kindled rat model of partial epilepsy.

toin (two AEDs with markedly different clinical profiles) will both block tonic extension seizures induced by scPTZ [13].

The anticonvulsant activity of those AEDs found to be active at non-toxic doses in the initial identification studies is then quantitated in a larger population of mice or rats. For these studies, the MES and scPTZ tests are routinely conducted at the predetermined time to peak effect of the investigational drug following oral or intraperitoneal administration to either mice or rats. Numerous technical, biological and pharmacokinetic factors have been identified which can 'qualitatively' affect the results obtained in a drug test [12,14,15]. It is important to note that these factors, albeit important, are not likely to contribute to missing an active drug in the MES and scPTZ tests. However, they may certainly contribute to false conclusions regarding potency and duration of action of an active drug and they should be kept in mind when designing an experimental protocol.

The MES and scPTZ tests are easily conducted with a minimal investment in equipment and technical expertise. They provide valuable data regarding the potential anticonvulsant activity of an investigational drug and with one exception (i.e. levetiracetam) all of the currently available AEDs have been found to be active in one or both of these tests (Table 8.1). Furthermore, both tests are amenable to high-volume screening with widely available relatively inexpensive normal rodents. This becomes an important issue for any AED discovery programme when attempting to screen hundreds to thousands of candidate substances in an attempt to identify the one or two novel therapeutic entities to carry forward into further development.

Although amenable to high-volume screening, the MES and scPTZ tests fail to meet any of the remaining criteria described above. For example, there are now several examples wherein the pharmacology can be affected by the disease state and since the MES and scPTZ tests are conducted in 'pathologically normal' rodents, there is no guarantee that they will be equally effective in 'pathologically abnormal' rodents. The best example to illustrate this point is levetiracetam. As mentioned above, the MES and scPTZ tests failed to identify levetiracetam's anticonvulsant activity. Subsequent investigations demonstrated that levetiracetam was active in 'pathologically abnormal' models of partial and primary generalized seizures [16–20]. In this regard, levetiracetam appears to represent the first 'truly' novel AED identified in recent years. The identification and subsequent development and launch of levetiracetam as an efficacious AED for the treatment of partial seizures underscores the need for flexibility when screening for efficacy and the need to incorporate levetiracetam-sensitive models into the early evaluation process.

As shown in Table 8.1, neither of these seizure models possesses a pharmacological profile consistent with therapy-resistant human epilepsy. For example, the MES test is sensitive to all of the first-generation AEDs with demonstrated clinical efficacy in the treatment of generalized tonic-clonic seizures (e.g. phenytoin, carbamazepine, valproate and phenobarbital). Likewise, the scPTZ test is sensitive to those first-line AEDs used in the management of generalized absence seizures (i.e. ethosuximide, valproate and the benzodiazepines). This is partly due to the fact that these two models were developed and initially validated using the older, established AEDs phenytoin, phenobarbital and trimethadione [4,8]. This particular validation process led to their selection on the basis that these two model systems displayed a pharmacological profile consistent with established medical practice at the time (see [4,8] for historical review and discussion). At that time, one must keep in mind, there was a limited armamentarium of AEDs available and

Table 8.1 Correlation between clinical utility and efficacy of the established and second-generation AEDs in experimental animal models[a]

Experimental model	Tonic and/or clonic generalized seizures Partial seizures	Clinical seizure type	
		Myoclonic/generalized absence seizures	Generalized absence seizures
MES (tonic extension)[b]	CBZ, PHT, VPA, PB [FBM, GBP, LTG, TPM, ZNS]		
scPTZ (clonic seizures)[b]		ESM, VPA, PB[c], BZD [FBM, GBP, TGB[c], VGB[c]]	
Spike-wave discharges[d]			ESM, VPA, BZD [LTG, TPM, LVT]
Electrical kindling (focal seizures)	CBZ, PHT, VPA, PB, BZD [FBM, GBP, LTG, TPM, TGB, ZNS, LVT, VGB]		
6 Hz (44 mA)[e]	VPA [LVT]		

[a] BZD, benzodiazepines; CBZ, carbamazepine; ESM, ethosuximide; FBM, felbamate; GBP, gabapentin; LTG, lamotrigine; LVT, levetiracetam; PB, phenobarbital; PHT, phenytoin; TGB, tiagabine; TPM, topiramate; VPA, valproic acid; ZNS, zonisamide; VGB, vigabatrin.
[b] Data summarized from [5].
[c] PB, TGB, and VGB block clonic seizures induced by scPTZ but are inactive against generalized absence seizures and may exacerbate spike-wave seizures.
[d] Data summarized from GBL, GAERS and *lh/lh* spike-wave models [33–36].
[e] Data summarized from [21].
[ ] Second-generation AEDs.

several of the drugs possessed significant liability in the form of teratogenesis and safety (e.g. trimethadione, bromide and phenobarbital). As such, there was a clear need for additional options for the physician and patient alike.

One might ask then what, if any, benefit these two tests might provide when screening for novel AEDs. First, both tests provide some insight into the central nervous system bioavailability of a particular investigational AED. Furthermore, both models are nonselective with respect to mechanism of action. As such, they are very well suited for the early evaluation of anticonvulsant activity because neither model assumes that a particular drug's pharmacodynamic activity is dependent on its molecular mechanism of action. Lastly, both model systems display clear and definable seizure endpoints and require minimal technical expertise. This coupled with lack of dependence on molecular mechanism make them ideally suited to screen large numbers of chemically diverse entities. Levetiracetam taught the community that lack of efficacy in either of these tests does not translate into lack of human efficacy. As such, there is no longer any reason to limit further screening on the basis of results obtained in the MES and scPTZ. In fact, there is no *a priori* reason to assume that a novel AED will be active in the MES, scPTZ or other acute seizure tests.

The 6 Hz seizure test

As discussed above, levetiracetam is unique among all of the clinically available AEDs in that it is inactive in either the MES or scPTZ tests. As such, levetiracetam clearly exemplifies why there is a continued need to identify and characterize new screening models so as to minimize the risk of missing other potentially novel AEDs. To this end, the Anticonvulsant Screening Project is currently utilizing the 6 Hz psychomotor seizure model in its early identification studies (Fig. 8.1 [5,21]).

While the high-frequency, short-duration stimulation employed in the MES test has become a standard for screening AEDs, it was only one of several electroshock paradigms initially developed in the 1940s and 1950s [22]. An alternative stimulation paradigm was the low-frequency (6 Hz) long-duration (3 s) corneal stimulation model which was stated to produce 'psychic' or 'psychomotor' seizures. Instead of the tonic extension seizure characteristic of the MES test, the 6 Hz seizure was reported to involve a minimal, clonic phase followed by stereotyped, automatistic behaviours reminiscent of human partial seizures [23–25]. At the time of its initial description, the authors were attempting to validate the 6 Hz model as a screening test for partial seizures; however, the pharmacological profile was not consistent with clinical practice [25]. For example, phenytoin was found to be inactive in the 6 Hz seizure test. This observation led the authors to suggest that it was no more predictive of clinical utility than the other models available at the time (i.e. the MES and scPTZ tests). Subsequent investigations in our laboratory confirmed the relative insensitivity of the 6 Hz test to phenytoin and extended the observation to include carbamazepine, lamotrigine and topiramate [21]. The relative resistance of some patients to phenytoin and other AEDs in today's clinical setting and the lack of sensitivity of the MES and scPTZ to levetiracetam prompted studies to re-evaluate the 6 Hz seizure test as a potential screen for therapy-resistant epilepsy [21]. Subsequent investigations demonstrated that levetiracetam was able to afford protection

Table 8.2 Effect of stimulus intensity on the anticonvulsant efficacy of phenytoin, lamotrigine, ethosuximide, levetiracetam and valproic acid in the 6 Hz seizure test

Antiepileptic drug	ED50 (mg/kg, ip)		
	22 mA	32 mA	44 mA
Phenytoin	9.4 (4.7–14.9)	>60	>60
Lamotrigine	4.4 (2.2–6.6)	>60	>60
Ethosuximide	86.9 (37.8–156)	167 (114–223)	>600
Levetiracetam	4.6 (1.1–8.7)	19.4 (9.9–36.0)	1089 (787–2650)
Valproic acid	41.5 (16.1–68.8)	126 94.5–152)	310 (258–335)

From [21] with permission.

against the 6 Hz seizure at a stimulus intensity where other AEDs display little to no efficacy (Table 8.2). This observation clearly demonstrates the potential utility of this model as a screen for novel AEDs that may be useful for the treatment of therapy-resistant partial seizures.

Differentiation of anticonvulsant activity

Once the efficacy of an investigational AED is established using either the MES, scPTZ or 6 Hz seizure test, a battery of tests are employed to characterize further the anticonvulsant potential of the test substance. These include assessing the ability of the investigational AED to block audiogenic seizures in the Frings audiogenic seizure-susceptible mouse, limbic seizures in the hippocampal kindled rat and acute clonic seizures induced by the γ-aminobutyric acid A (GABA$_A$) receptor antagonist bicuculline the Cl$^-$ channel blocker picrotoxin [3,5,8].

Of the tests mentioned thus far, the kindled rat is the only chronic model currently employed by the Anticonvulsant Screening Project. Kindling refers to the process whereby there is a progressive increase in electrographic and behavioural seizure activity in response to repeated stimulation of a limbic brain region such as the amygdala or hippocampus with an initially subconvulsive current [26]. The kindled rat is a useful chronic model for identifying those AEDs that are likely to be useful for the treatment of difficult-to-control seizure types such as complex partial seizures [27]. In addition to its utility in AED discovery, the kindled rat also provides a means of studying complex brain networks that may contribute to seizure spread and generalization from a focus [28]. The kindling process is associated with a progressive increase in seizure severity and duration, a decrease in the focal seizure threshold and neuronal degeneration in limbic brain regions that resemble human mesotemporal lobe epilepsy. The electrographic and behavioural components of the kindled seizure begins locally at the site of stimulation and quickly becomes secondarily generalized. In 1972, Racine proposed a behavioural scoring system that is still in use today [29]. The Racine scale provides a quantitative efficient mechanism through which to assess the effect of an investigational AED on the focal (stages 1 and 2) or secondarily generalized (stages 3–5) seizure. In addition to the behavioural seizure, one can assess whether the drug of interest also affects the electrographic seizure.

Of the various kindling paradigms described in the literature, the Anticonvulsant Screening Project employs the rapid hippocampal kindling model of Lothman *et al.* [28]. This particular model offers some distinct advantages for the screening and evaluation of new anticonvulsant substances. For example, this particular kindling model provides a framework for assessing, in a temporal fashion, drug efficacy in a focal seizure model. For most drug studies, the candidate substance is evaluated for its ability to block the evoked kindled motor seizure (seizure scores of 3–5) and limbic behavioural seizure (seizure score between 1 and 2) and to affect changes in the after-discharge duration. The kindled rat is also an important tool that can be used to identify drugs that prevent or attenuate the development of a seizure focus (i.e. antiepileptogenic vs. anticonvulsant drugs). Thus, in an acquisition paradigm, animals begin receiving the test substance prior to initiation of the kindling process. The relevance of a drug's ability to delay or prevent the development of kindling to human epileptogenesis remains unknown. Valproic acid, phenobarbital, levetiracetam, topiramate and several N-methyl-D-aspartate (NMDA) antagonists are among some of the drugs found to delay the acquisition of kindling. Of these, valproic acid has been examined for its ability to prevent the development of post-traumatic epilepsy following closed head injury [30,31]. In this study, valproic acid was quite effective in preventing the acute seizures but it failed to prevent the development of epilepsy. Although not conclusive, this finding would suggest that the kindling model is perhaps not a predictive model of trauma-induced epilepsy. Whether it is more predictive of other acquired epilepsies is not known at the present time.

Pharmacological profile and potential clinical utility

Although not predictive of therapy-resistant epilepsy, the pharmacological profile of the MES, scPTZ and kindled rat tests does provide some insight into the potential clinical utility of drugs that are found to be active in one or both of these tests. For example, the pharmacological profile of the MES test clearly supports its utility as a predictive model for human generalized tonic-clonic seizures. To date, all of the drugs that have demonstrated efficacy in the MES test and were subsequently evaluated in the clinic have been found to possess activity against generalized tonic-clonic seizures. In contrast, the lack of any demonstrable efficacy by tiagabine, vigabatrin and levetiracetam in the MES test argues against its utility as a predictive model of partial seizures. Consistent with this conclusion is the observation that NMDA antagonists are very effective against tonic extension seizures induced by MES; however, they were found to be without benefit in patients with partial seizures [32].

Historically, positive results obtained in the scPTZ seizure test were considered suggestive of potential clinical utility against generalized absence seizures. This interpretation was based largely on the finding that drugs active in the clinic against partial seizures (e.g. ethosuximide, trimethadione, valproic acid, the benzodiazepines) were able to block clonic seizures induced by scPTZ; whereas drugs such as phenytoin and carbamazepine which were ineffective against absence seizures were also inactive in the scPTZ test. Based

on this argument, phenobarbital, gabapentin and tiagabine should all be effective against spike-wave seizures and lamotrigine should be inactive against spike-wave seizures. However, clinical experience has demonstrated that this is an invalid prediction. For example, the barbiturates, gabapentin and tiagabine all aggravate spike-wave seizure discharge; whereas lamotrigine has been found to be effective against absence seizures. As such, the overall utility of the scPTZ test in predicting activity against human spike-wave seizures is limited. Thus, before any conclusion concerning potential clinical utility against spike-wave seizures is made, positive results in the scPTZ test should be corroborated by positive findings in other models of absence such as the γ-butyrolactone [33] seizure test, the genetic absence epileptic rat of Strasbourg [34] and the lethargic (*lh/lh*) mouse [35,36]. As summarized in Table 8.1, the pharmacological profile of these three models more reasonably predicts efficacy against spike-wave seizures than the scPTZ test. Another important advantage of all three of these models is that they accurately predict the potentiation of spike-wave seizures by drugs that elevated GABA concentrations (e.g. vigabatrin and tiagabine), drugs that directly activate the $GABA_B$ receptor and the barbiturates.

The 6 Hz seizure test appears to offer some advantage over the MES, scPTZ and kindled rat models. In particular, the pharmacological profile of the 6 Hz test clearly differentiates itself from the other models. For example, as the stimulus intensity is increased from the CC_{97} (convulsive current required to evoke a seizure in 97% of the mice tested) to twice the CC_{97}, the pharmacological profile shifted from being relatively non-discriminating to being very discriminating (Table 8.2). For example, at the CC_{97} (22 mA) all of the AEDs tested (phenytoin, lamotrigine, ethosuximide, levetiracetam and valproic acid) were active at doses devoid of behavioural toxicity. In contrast, at a current intensity twice the CC_{97} (44 mA), the 6 Hz seizure was resistant to ethosuximide, phenytoin and lamotrigine but sensitive to levetiracetam and valproic acid. As such, the 6 Hz test may represent a potential therapy-resistant model wherein seizures can be acutely evoked in normal mice. Such a model would provide a rather inexpensive alternative to the extremely labour-intensive and expensive chronic models such as kindling.

Of the four models discussed in some detail, the kindled rat model offers perhaps the best predictive value. For example, it is the only model that adequately predicted the clinical utility of the first- and second-generation AEDs including tiagabine and vigabatrin. Furthermore, the kindled rat is the only model that accurately predicted the lack of clinical efficacy of NMDA antagonists [37]. Given the predictive nature of the kindled rat, one might legitimately ask why this model or a similarly predictive chronic model is not utilized as a primary screen rather than a secondary screen for the early identification and evaluation of novel AEDs. The answer is primarily one of logistics. Any chronic model such as kindling is extremely labour-intensive and requires adequate facilities and resources to surgically implant the stimulating/recording electrode, to kindle and to house sufficient rats over a chronic period of time. Furthermore, unlike the acute seizure models, the time required to conduct a drug study with a chronic model far exceeds the time required to conduct a similar study with the MES, scPTZ or 6 Hz seizure test, thereby severely limiting the number of AEDs that can be screened in a timely manner.

Recommendations

Activity of a test substance in one or more of the electrical and chemical tests described above will provide some insight into the overall anticonvulsant potential of the compound. However, a concern voiced in recent years is that the continued use of the MES and scPTZ tests in the early evaluation of an investigational AED are likely to identify 'me too' drugs and are unlikely to discover those drugs with different mechanisms of action. It is anticipated that the inclusion of a kindling model into the initial identification screen will provide a mechanism to identify those novel compounds that are active in a chronic model that might be missed by the acute models currently employed in the initial identification screens. In this regard, it will be of further interest to assess whether the 6 Hz screen identifies molecules that will be inherently active in the kindled rat model.

A review of the data summarized in Table 8.1 clearly demonstrates the importance of employing multiple models in any screening protocol when attempting to identify and characterize the overall potential of a candidate AED substance. For example, levetiracetam is inactive in the traditional MES and scPTZ tests, yet it demonstrates excellent efficacy in the model of genetic absence epilepsy in rats from Strasbourg (GAERS) model of primary generalized seizures and in the kindled rat model [38]. Likewise, the efficacy of tiagabine and vigabatrin against human partial seizures was not predicted by the MES test, but by the kindled rat model [39,40]. Furthermore, as mentioned above, exacerbation of spike-wave seizures would not have been predicted by the scPTZ test but by the other models (i.e. 6 Hz, GAERS and the *lh/lh* mouse) wherein both drugs have been shown to increase spike-wave discharges [36]. These examples serve to illustrate the limitations of some of the animal models while emphasizing their overall utility in predicting both clinical efficacy and potential seizure exacerbation. What is clear is the need to evaluate each investigational AED in a variety of seizure and epilepsy models. Only then will it be possible to gain a full appreciation of the overall spectrum of activity for a given investigational drug.

What is the future of AED discovery and development?

Since its inception in 1975, the Anticonvulsant Screening Project, Utah, has screened over 24 000 investigational AEDs. In addition to the compounds that have been successfully developed, a number of additional compounds are in various stages of clinical development. Each of these drugs has brought about substantial benefit to the patient population in the form of increased seizure control, increased tolerability and better safety and pharmacokinetic profiles. Unfortunately for 25–40% of epilepsy patients, there still remains a need to identify therapies that will more effectively treat their therapy-resistant seizures. As such, there is a continued need to identify and incorporate more appropriate models of refractory epilepsy into the AED screening process. At the present time, there are several model systems that could be suggested including: the phenytoin-resistant kindled rat [41], the carbamazepine-resistant kindled rat [42], the 6 Hz psychomotor seizure model [21,25] and the *in vitro* low magnesium hippocampal slice preparation [43]. Unfortunately, it will take the successful clinical development of a drug with demonstrated clinical efficacy in the management of refractory epilepsy before any one of these (or other) model systems will be clinically validated. Nonetheless, this should not prevent the community at large from continuing the search for a more effective therapy using the models that we have available. In fact, until there is a validated model, it becomes even more important to characterize and incorporate several of the available models into the drug discovery process while at the same time continuing to identify new models of refractory epilepsy.

At the present time, there are no known therapies that are capable of modifying the course of acquired epilepsy. Attempts to prevent the development of epilepsy following febrile seizures, traumatic brain injury and craniotomy with the older established drugs have been disappointing (see [30,31] for review). At the same time, discoveries at the molecular level have provided greater insight into the pathophysiology of certain seizure disorders. As such, it may be possible in the not so distant future to identify a treatment strategy that will slow or halt the progressive nature of epilepsy and prevent the development of epilepsy in susceptible individuals. However, any successful human therapy will necessarily be identified and characterized in a model system that closely approximates human epileptogenesis. At the present time, there are several potential chronic animal models wherein spontaneous seizures develop secondary to a particular insult or genetic manipulation (for review and references, see [7,44]). If we are to be successful in identifying a novel, disease-modifying therapy in the near future, we must become intentional in our efforts to characterize and incorporate such models of epileptogenesis into our screening protocols.

Summary

This chapter has focused on the present-day process employed by the University of Utah Anticonvulsant Screening Project to evaluate the anticonvulsant efficacy of an investigational AED. An attempt has been made to identify and discuss the advantages and limitations of this approach and the various animal model systems employed. Lastly, the rationale and need to broaden the scope of AED screening protocols to include models of therapy resistance and epileptogenesis has also been discussed in context with the continuing need to identify more efficacious drugs for the 25–40% of patients that remain refractory to the currently available AEDs. The real future of epilepsy research lies in our ability to couple a greater understanding of the pathophysiology of epilepsy at the molecular level with the identification and development of a truly novel therapy that modifies the course of epilepsy or prevents the development of epilepsy in the susceptible individual.

References

1 Jacobs MP, Fischbach GD, Davis MR *et al.* Future directions for epilepsy research. *Neurology* 2001; 57(9): 1536–42.
2 White HS, Woodhead JH, Franklin MR *et al.* General principles: Experimental selection, quantification, and evaluation of antiepileptic drugs. In: Levy RH, Mattson RH, Meldrum BS, eds. *Antiepileptic Drugs*, 4th edn. New York: Raven Press, 1995: 99–110.
3 White HS, Wolf HH, Woodhead JH *et al.* The National Institutes of Health Anticonvulsant Drug Development Program: Screening for Efficacy. In: French J, Leppik I, Dichter MA, eds. *Antiepileptic Drug Development. Advances in Neurology*, Vol. 76. Philadelphia: Lippincott-Raven Publishers, 1998: 29–39.

4 Kupferberg H. Animal models used in the screening of antiepileptic drugs. *Epilepsia* 2001; 42 (Suppl. 4): 7–12.

5 White HS, Woodhead JH, Wilcox KS *et al.* Discovery and preclinical development of antiepileptic drugs. In: Levy RH, Mattson RH, Meldrum B, Perucca E, eds. *Antiepileptic Drugs*, 5th edn. Philadelphia: Lippincott, 2002: 36–48.

6 Putnam TJ, Merritt HH. Experimental determination of the anticonvulsant properties of some phenyl derivatives. *Science* 1937; 85: 525–6.

7 Loscher W. Current status and future directions in the pharmacotherapy of epilepsy. *TIPS* 2002; 23(3): 113–18.

8 White HS, Johnson M, Wolf HH *et al.* The early identification of anticonvulsant activity: role of the maximal electroshock and subcutaneous pentylenetetrazol seizure models. *Ital J Neurol Sci* 1995; 16: 73–7.

9 White HS, Wolf HH, Woodhead JH *et al.* The National Institutes of Health Anticonvulsant Drug Development Program: Screening for efficacy. In: French J, Leppik I, Dichter MA, eds. *Antiepileptic Drug Development. Advances in Neurology*. Philadelphia: Lippincott-Raven Publishers, 1997: 29–39.

10 Everett GM, Richards RK. Comparative anticonvulsive action of 3,5,5-trimethyloxazolidine-2,4-dione (Tridione), Dilantin and phenobarbital. *J Pharmacol Exp Ther* 1944; 81: 402–7.

11 Lennox WG. The petit mal epilepsies. Their treatment with Tridione. *JAMA* 1945; 129: 1069–74.

12 Loscher W, Honack D, Fassbender CP *et al.* The role of technical, biological and pharmacological factors in the laboratory evaluation of anticonvulsant drugs. 3. Pentylenetetrazole seizure models. *Epilepsy Res* 1991; 8(3): 171–89.

13 Piredda SG, Woodhead JH, Swinyard EA. Effect of stimulus intensity on the profile of anticonvulsant activity of phenytoin, ethosuximide and valproate. *J Pharmacol Exp Ther* 1985; 232(3): 741–5.

14 Swinyard EA, Woodhead JH, White HS *et al.* General principles: Experimental selection, quantification, and evaluation of anticonvulsants. In: Levy R, Mattson R, Meldrum B, Penry JK, Dreifuss FE, eds. *Antiepileptic Drugs*, 3rd edn. New York: Raven Press, 1989: 85–102.

15 Loscher W, Fassbender CP, Nolting B. The role of technical, biological and pharmacological factors in the laboratory evaluation of anticonvulsant drugs. II. Maximal electroshock seizure models. *Epilepsy Res* 1991; 8(2): 79–94.

16 Gower AJ, Noyer M, Verloes R *et al.* Ucb L059, a novel anti-convulsant drug: pharmacological profile in animals. *Eur J Pharmacol* 1992; 222(2–3): 193–203.

17 Loscher W, Honack D. Profile of ucb-L059, a novel anticonvulsant drug, in models of partial and generalized epilepsy in mice and rats. *Eur J Pharmacol* 1993; 232(2–3): 147–58.

18 Gower AJ, Hirsch E, Boehrer A *et al.* Effects of levetiracetam, a novel antiepileptic drug, on convulsant activity in two genetic rat models of epilepsy. *Epilepsy Res* 1995; 22(3): 207–13.

19 Klitgaard H, Matagne A, Gobert J *et al.* Levetiracetam (ucb LO59) prevents limbic seizures induced by pilocarpine and kainic acid in rats. *Epilepsia* 1996; 37 (Suppl. 5): 118.

20 Loscher W, Honack D, Rundfeldt C. Antiepileptogenic effects of the novel anticonvulsant levetiracetam (ucb L059) in the kindling model of temporal lobe epilepsy. *J Pharmacol Exp Ther* 1998; 284(2): 474–9.

21 Barton ME, Klein BD, Wolf HH *et al.* Pharmacological characterization of the 6 Hz psychomotor seizure model of partial epilepsy. *Epilepsy Res* 2001; 47(3): 217–27.

22 Swinyard EA. Electrically induced seizures. In: Purpura DP, Penry JK, Tower DB, Woodbury DM, Walter RD, eds. *Experimental Models of Epilepsy: A Manual for the Laboratory Worker*. New York: Raven Press, 1972: 433–58.

23 Toman JEP. Neuropharmacologic considerations in psychic seizures. *Neurology* 1951; 1: 444–60.

24 Toman JEP, Everett GM, Richards RK. The search for new drugs against epilepsy. *Tex Rep Biol Med* 1952; 10: 96–104.

25 Brown WC, Schiffman DO, Swinyard EA *et al.* Comparative assay of antiepileptic drugs by 'psychomotor' seizure test and minimal electroshock threshold test. *J Pharmacol Exp Ther* 1953; 107: 273–83.

26 Goddard GV, McIntyre DC, Leech CK. A permanent change in brain function resulting from daily electrical stimulation. *Exp Neurol* 1969; 25(3): 295–330.

27 Loscher W. Animal models of intractable epilepsy. *Prog Neurobiol* 1997; 53(2): 239–58.

28 Lothman EW, Salerno RA, Perlin JB *et al.* Screening and characterization of antiepileptic drugs with rapidly recurring hippocampal seizures in rats. *Epilepsy Res* 1988; 2: 366–79.

29 Racine RJ. Modification of seizure activity by electrical stimulation: II. Motor seizure. *Electroenceph Clin Neurophysiol* 1972; 32: 281–94.

30 Temkin NR, Jarell AD, Anderson GD. Antiepileptogenic agents: how close are we? *Drugs* 2001; 61(8): 1045–55.

31 Temkin NR. Antiepileptogenesis and seizure prevention trials with antiepileptic drugs: meta-analysis of controlled trials. *Epilepsia* 2001; 42(4): 515–24.

32 Meldrum BS. Excitatory amino acid receptors and their role in epilepsy and cerebral ischemia. *Ann N Y Acad Sci* 1995; 757: 492–505.

33 Snead OC. Pharmacological models of generalized absence seizures in rodents. *J Neural Transm* 1992; 35: 7–19.

34 Marescaux C, Vergnes M. Genetic absence epilepsy in rats from Strasbourg (GAERS). *Ital J Neurol Sci* 1995; 16: 113–18.

35 Hosford DA, Clark S, Cao Z *et al.* The role of $GABA_B$ receptor activation in absence seizures of lethargic (*lh/lh*) mice. *Science* 1992; 257: 398–401.

36 Hosford DA, Wang Y. Utility of the lethargic (*lh/lh*) mouse model of absence seizures in predicting the effects of lamotrigine, vigabatrin, tiagabine, gabapentin, and topiramate against human absence seizures. *Epilepsia* 1997; 38(4): 408–14.

37 Loscher W, Honack D. Responses to NMDA receptor antagonists altered by epileptogenesis. *Trends Pharmacol Sci* 1991; 12(2): 52.

38 Klitgaard H, Matagne A, Gobert J *et al.* Evidence for a unique profile of levetiracetam in rodent models of seizures and epilepsy. *Eur J Pharmacol* 1998; 353(2–3): 191–206.

39 Rogawski MA, Porter RJ. Antiepileptic drugs: pharmacological mechanisms and clinical efficacy with consideration of promising developmental stage compounds. *Pharmacol Rev* 1990; 42: 223–86.

40 Suzdak PD, Jansen JA. A review of the preclinical pharmacology of tiagabine: a potent and selective anticonvulsant GABA uptake inhibitor. *Epilepsia* 1995; 36(6): 612–26.

41 Loscher W, Reissmuller E, Ebert U. Anticonvulsant efficacy of gabapentin and levetiracetam in phenytoin-resistant kindled rats. *Epilepsy Res* 2000; 40(1): 63–77.

42 Nissinen J, Halonen T, Koivisto E *et al.* A new model of chronic temporal lobe epilepsy induced by electrical stimulation of the amygdala in rat. *Epilepsy Res* 2000; 38(2–3): 177–205.

43 Armand V, Rundfeldt C, Heinemann U. Effects of retigabine (D-23129) on different patterns of epileptiform activity induced by low magnesium in rat entorhinal cortex hippocampal slices. *Epilepsia* 2000; 41(1): 28–33.

44 Loscher W. Animal models of epilepsy for the development of antiepileptogenic and disease-modifying drugs. A comparison of the pharmacology of kindling and models with spontaneous recurrent seizures. *Epilepsy Res* 2002; (in press).

9 Mechanisms of Antiepileptic Drug Action

M.C. Walker and A. Fisher

Despite a burgeoning in epilepsy research, we are still a long way from understanding the mechanisms underlying seizure generation and epileptogenesis. Antiepileptic drugs have been developed either through serendipity, such as the fortuitous discovery of the antiepileptic effects of bromides and phenobarbital, or through screening in animal epilepsy models. Indeed, the recent growth in antiepileptic drug development has been due to extensive screening of over 22 500 compounds in animal epilepsy models. Designing antiepileptic drugs with specific mechanisms of action is a recent approach that has not been particularly fruitful; first, because the drugs then turn out to have separate mechanisms of actions (e.g. lamotrigine and gabapentin), and secondly, because most of these drugs have been ineffective or have had unacceptable side-effects (e.g. *N*-methyl-D-aspartate or NMDA antagonists). Because of this, the mode of action of antiepileptic drugs is multifarious, and often poorly defined. Most antiepileptic drugs have a number of putative targets, and it is often not possible to discern which are the most germane. There may be many complex effects, even when an antiepileptic drug ostensibly has one target (e.g. tiagabine inhibiting γ-aminobutyric acid or GABA uptake). Rather than describe the possible mechanisms underlying each antiepileptic drug in turn (this is covered in individual chapters), we have described the more important targets of antiepileptic drugs, and which drugs affect those targets. Those that are most relevant to our present armamentarium of antiepileptic drugs are sodium channels, calcium channels and the GABAergic system. Other putative and potential targets include potassium channels, the glutamatergic system and other amines. The efficacy of antiepileptic drugs has been mainly examined in animal models of seizures, later in this chapter we shall describe in more detail the more commonly used models that are used to determine antiepileptic efficacy.

Main targets

Sodium channels

Sodium channels provide the major target for a number of antiepileptic drugs (Table 9.1). Voltage-gated sodium channels are responsible for the rising phase of the action potential in excitable cells and membranes, and are thus critical for action potential generation and propagation [1]. The sodium channel exists in three principle conformational states: (a) at hyperpolarized potentials the channel is in the resting closed state; (b) with depolarization the channels convert to an open state that conducts sodium ions; and (c) the channel then enters a closed, non-conducting, inactivated state. This inactivation is removed by hyperpolarization (Fig. 9.1). In this manner, depolarization results in a transient inward sodium current

that rapidly inactivates. There is also a slow inactivated state which occurs with sustained depolarizations, and from which the channel recovers at hyperpolarized potentials over a matter of seconds [1].

The sodium channel consists of a 260-kDa α subunit that forms the sodium selective pore (Fig. 9.2). This α subunit consists of four homologous domains (I–IV) that each consist of six α-helical transmembrane segments (S1–6). The S4 segments are responsible for the voltage-dependent activation, as these are highly charged. Inactivation is mediated by a 'hinged lid' consisting of the intracellular loop connecting domains III and IV that can only close following voltage-dependent activation [1].

In the central nervous system, the α subunit is associated with two auxiliary β subunits ($β_1$ and $β_2$) that influence the kinetics and voltage dependence of the gating. There are at least 10 different sodium channel isoforms ($Na_v1.1$–1.9 and Na_x). Five of these isoforms are present in the central nervous system—$Na_v1.1$–1.3, $Na_v1.5$ (in the limbic system) and $Na_v1.6$; these isoforms have some functional differences that are of physiological importance (see below). In addition the sodium channel can be modulated by protein phosphorylation, which affects the peak sodium current, and the speed and voltage dependence of channel inactivation [1].

Many drugs including certain anaesthetics and antiarrhythmics exert their therapeutic effect by preferential binding to the inactivated state of the sodium channel [1]. This has two effects: first to shift the voltage dependence of inactivation towards the resting potential (i.e. the channels become inactive at less negative membrane potentials), and second to delay the return of the channel to the resting, closed conformation following hyperpolarization. Phenytoin, lamotrigine and carbamazepine have a similar mode of action [2,3]. All bind in the inner pore of the sodium channel, and their binding is mutually exclusive [2]. There may, however, be differences in the fashion in which drugs interact with adjacent amino acids that can partly explain drug-specific effects [4,5]. In addition the kinetics of antiepileptic drug interactions with the sodium channel differ, so that, for example, carbamazepine binds less potently, but faster than phenytoin [6]. How does this binding mediate their anticonvulsant effect? The conventional view has been that such binding prevents sustained repetitive firing [7]. The rate at which an axon can 'fire' is critically determined by the rate at which the sodium channels change from the inactivated state to the resting, closed state ready to be opened by a subsequent depolarization. If this time is delayed, then the 'refractory period' is prolonged. Thus phenytoin, carbamazepine and lamotrigine all prolong the 'refractory period' and so inhibit sustained repetitive firing. In addition, since these drugs bind to channels in their inactive state, then the greater the number of channels that have entered this state, the greater the drug binding. This results in a 'use-dependent' phenomenon in

Table 9.1 Drugs that act on voltage-gated sodium channels

Main action
Carbamazepine
Lamotrigine
Oxcarbazepine
Phenytoin

Importance unknown
Topiramate
Valproate
Zonisamide

**Only at high
concentrations**
Phenobarbitone
Benzodiazepines

which repetitive firing results in greater amounts of the drug bound and so greater inhibition. The slow onset of these drugs can be explained by the slow binding of these drugs to the sodium channel (i.e. the brevity of a single action potential does not permit substantial drug binding) [8]. Although an action on sustained repetitive firing may be one potential antiepileptic action, an action on persistent sodium currents is possibly of greater importance [9,10].

The persistent sodium current consists of rare late openings of sodium channels following a depolarization. Certain receptor subtypes, such as $Na_v1.6$ are more prone to these late openings. Epileptiform activity is reflected, at a cellular level, by persistent depolarizations (paroxysmal depolarizing shifts), and persistent sodium currents can be a significant component of these persistent depolarizations. Prolonged late openings would permit significant drug binding, and thus phenytoin, carbamazepine and lamotrigine should affect the persistent current to a much greater degree than

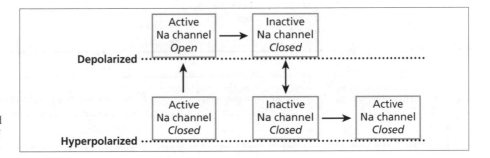

Fig. 9.1 Voltage dependence of sodium channel. In the activated state, the channel is opened by depolarization. The channel then inactivates, and hyperpolarization is necessary for reactivation of the channel.

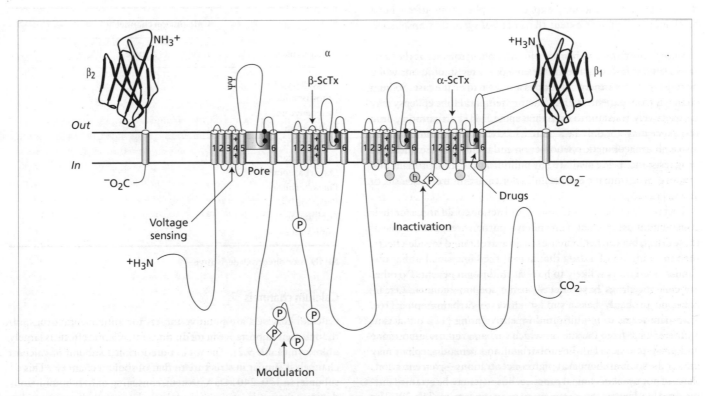

Fig. 9.2 The primary structure of the voltage-gated sodium channel consisting of four homologous six α-helical transmembrane segments (S1–6). P, sites of demonstrated protein phosphorylation by protein kinase A (PKA) (circles) and protein kinase C (PKC) (diamonds); between 5 and 6, pore-lining segments; +4+, S4 voltage sensors; h, inactivation particle in the inactivation gate loop; stippled circles, sites implicated in forming the inactivation gate receptor. Putative site of drug action is shown. From [1].

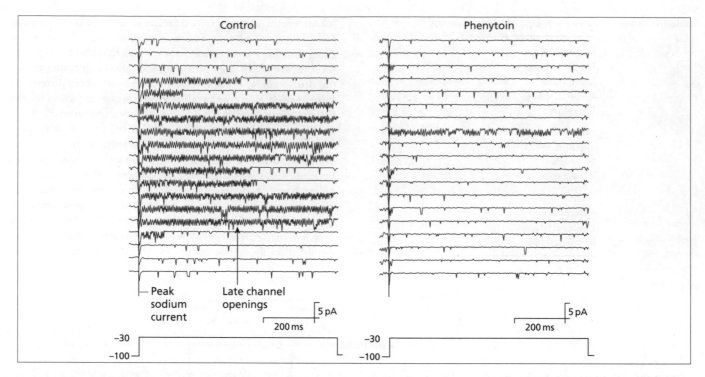

Fig. 9.3 Using outside-out patches from neuronal cultures; each record shows a consecutive trace. Sodium channels open with depolarization (peak current), followed by late channel openings. Phenytoin reduces the initial peak current, but more impressively reduces the late channel openings. From [10].

the peak sodium current during an action potential. This is indeed the case (Fig. 9.3), and may explain why phenytoin affects burst behaviour to a greater extent than normal synaptic transmission [10].

Since lamotrigine, carbamazepine and phenytoin act at the same site in similar fashions, then if the epilepsy is resistant to one will it be resistant to the others? This does not seem to be the case. Sodium channels from patients with refractory temporal lobe epilepsy may be selectively resistant to carbamazepine [11]. Furthermore, drug resistance may not only be a pharmacodynamic phenomenon, but also a pharmacokinetic phenomenon and there is some evidence of drug resistance being mediated by multidrug-resistant proteins that 'remove' drug from the extracellular fluid and thus from their site of action [12–15].

That the drugs have a similar mode of action could argue for their concomitant use. So that if an epilepsy partially responds to one of these drugs, but further increases in dose are limited by side-effects, then the addition of a drug that acts at the same site, but has dissimilar side-effects is likely to have an additional benefit. Do other antiepileptic drugs have effects on the sodium channel? Oxcarbazepine probably has a similar effect to carbamazepine [16]. Valproate seems to inhibit rapid repetitive firing [17], but acts at a different site from the site on which carbamazepine, lamotrigine and phenytoin act [18]. Phenobarbital and benzodiazepines may inhibit the sodium channel at high concentrations—concentrations that are not usual in clinical practice, but that may be attained during drug loading for the treatment of status epilepticus [19,20]. The new antiepileptic drugs, topiramate and zonisamide, also have actions on sodium channels, the exact nature and importance of which are unclear [21–23].

Table 9.2 Action of antiepileptic drugs on calcium channels

Anticonvulsant	Calcium ion channel			
	L-type	N-type	P/Q-type	T-type
Carbamazepine	*			
Ethosuximide				*
Fosphenytoin	*			*
Gabapentin	?		*	
Lamotrigine		*	?	
Levetiracetam		*		
Oxcarbazepine (MHD)		*	*	
Phenobarbitone	*	*		*
Phenytoin	*			*
Topiramate	*	*		
Zonisamide				*

MHD, monohydroxy derivative.

Calcium channels

Calcium channels are putative targets for antiepileptic drugs, although their importance in mediating antiepileptic effects is largely unknown (Table 9.2). The main pore-forming subunit of calcium channels is similar in structure to that of sodium channels. This α_1 subunit is a 170–240 kDaA protein, consisting of four homologous domains that each consist of six α-helical transmembrane segments [24]. The pore-forming segments and the mechanism of inactivation are similar to that of the sodium channels [24]. Cloning has uncovered 10 subtypes of the α_1 subunit; these have been named α_{1A-I}

and α_{1s} (this only exists in skeletal muscle), but have now been labelled $Ca_v1.1–1.4$ (L type), $Ca_v2.1–2.3$ (P/Q, N and R type) and $Ca_v3.1–3.3$ (T type). In addition there are associated subunits, $\alpha_2\delta$ and β, that promote channel expression, and affect channel kinetics. There is a third auxillary subunit, the γ subunit, that is expressed in skeletal muscle, but its expression and relevance in brain are controversial [24].

In brain, there are four main classes of voltage-gated calcium channel expressed, L-, P/Q-, N- and T-type channels [24]. L-, P/Q- and N-type channels are high voltage activated channels that require significant depolarization before activation, whilst the T-type channel is a low voltage activated channel and is activated at relatively hyperpolarized potentials.

The L-type channels are expressed mainly postsynaptically and are involved in postsynaptic calcium entry upon neuronal depolarization. L-type channels inactivate only slowly (long-lasting channels), thereby permitting sustained calcium entry [24]. L-type channels are typically blocked by dihydropyridines (e.g. nifedipine), and are regulated by protein phosphorylation and by calcium autoregulation [24]. Calcium entry through L-type channels is the major contributor of calcium to trigger the after-hyperpolarization (see below) in certain neuronal subtypes, particularly in the hippocampus [25]. The somatic expression of L-type receptors means that they are ideally placed to open during the depolarization that occurs with an action potential [26]. Calcium entering through L-type calcium channels may also have other effects including gene regulation and the expression of long-term synaptic potentiation with strong stimulation [27]. Blockade of L-type calcium channels has a variety of effects on epileptic discharges, and can have both anticonvulsant and proconvulsant effects, possibly by inhibiting synaptic potentiation, yet also inhibiting after-hyperpolarization [28,29]. L-type calcium antagonists are proconvulsant in absence epilepsy models [30]. L-type antagonists may, however, inhibit epileptogenesis by inhibiting the calcium entry that secondarily activates various genes necessary for the epileptogenic process [31,32]. Some antiepileptic drugs have been proposed to antagonize L-type calcium channels including phenytoin [25,30], carbamazepine [33], topiramate [34] and phenobarbital at high, anaesthetic doses [35]. The relevance of this to their antiepileptic effect is difficult to predict, but this antagonism may contribute to their side-effects including the proabsence effect of phenytoin and carbamazepine.

N- and P/Q-type channels are expressed at synaptic boutons where they mediate calcium entry necessary for neurotransmitter release [26]. These channels are rapidly inactivating, resulting in brief calcium transients. This calcium entry then triggers exocytosis of the presynaptic vesicles. N and P/Q channels are primarily regulated by G-proteins; they are thus modulated by G-protein-linked receptors such as $GABA_B$ receptors [24]. Inhibiting these calcium channels inhibits neurotransmitter release. Multiple types of these channels are present at excitatory synapses [36], but specific subtypes are present at inhibitory synapses [37]. N-type antagonists may, in the hippocampus, preferentially inhibit GABA release onto interneurones (D.M. Kullmann and D. Rusakov, personal communication), and thus could prevent the inhibition of inhibitory neurones (i.e. they could have antiepileptic potential). The following antiepileptic drugs have been proposed to inhibit N-type calcium channels: lamotrigine [38,39], levetiracetam [40], phenobarbital at

high doses [35] and topiramate [34]. Lamotrigine may also inhibit P-type channels [38]. Although oxcarbazepine only has some weak effect on L-type channels [41], the monohydroxy derivative (its main metabolite) inhibits high voltage activated calcium channels that are not L-type (presumably P/Q or N type) [42]. Gabapentin's effect on high voltage activated calcium channels is complex and novel. Gabapentin shows strong and specific binding for the $\alpha_2\delta$ auxillary subunit [43]. Via this mechanism, it inhibits P/Q-type calcium channels [44–46]. Gabapentin may also inhibit some peripheral L-type channels in a use dependent manner, but the significance of this for the central nervous system is, at present, unknown [44].

T-type channels are activated at relatively hyperpolarized potentials. They open with small depolarization (low voltage activated), and then rapidly inactivate. T-type channels undoubtedly contribute to the generation of spike-wave discharges associated with absence epilepsy [47]. Hyperpolarization of thalamocortical cells results in the activation of T-type channels that are then opened by the subsequent repolarization leading to calcium entry that further depolarizes, leading to action potential generation. Spike activity in the thalamocortical neurones results in the recruitment of neocortical neurones which, via reticular thalamic neurones, inhibit and so hyperpolarize thalamocortical neurones (Fig. 9.4). Ethosuximide, an effective antiabsence drug, has been proposed to inhibit specifically T-type calcium channels [48]. This hypothesis has recently been challenged in a study that found that ethosuximide has no effect on calcium currents, but instead modulates neuronal bursting by decreasing the persistent sodium current, and perhaps the calcium-dependent potassium current [49]. More recent studies using cloned channels have, however, demonstrated that ethosuximide does inhibit T-type calcium channels at therapeutically relevant concentrations [50]. A possible explanation for these opposing findings is that ethosuximide binds to inactivated T-type channels. Since T-type channels are inactivated at depolarized potentials, then ethosuximide's efficacy is dependent on voltage and will show use dependence [50]. Thus, the inefficacy of ethosuximide at T-type channels found in one study [49] could be explained by the relatively hyperpolarized potentials that were used (this would result

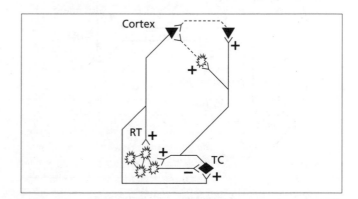

Fig. 9.4 The thalamocortical circuit proposed to underlie spike-wave discharges. RT, reticular thalamic neurones; TC, thalamocortical neurones. Filled, excitatory neurones; open, inhibitory neurones. RT hyperpolarize TC thus activating T-calcium currents that result, on depolarization, in burst firing and so excitation of cortical neurones. These in turn feedback onto RT and so the cycle continues.

in most T-type channels being in the active state, ethosuximide-insensitive state) [50]. Nevertheless, ethosuximide's mode of action is probably more complex than just inhibition of T-type channels [49]. Zonisamide, another drug with antiabsence effects, has been found to inhibit T-type calcium channels [51]. T-type channels can be subdivided into three types, and the expression of these vary between brain regions [24]. The pharmacological sensitivity of T-type calcium currents differs between peripheral neurones, central nervous system and neuroendocrine cells [52]. Phenytoin and the barbiturates inhibit T-type currents in dorsal root ganglion (valproate has a weak effect), but have minimal effect on thalamic T-type currents [52]. Furthermore, the low voltage activated calcium current is not necessarily confined to T-type channels [53]. Thus some of the effect of phenytoin on low voltage activated calcium currents in hippocampal neurones [54] could be due to an effect of phenytoin on other calcium channel subtypes [53]. Some T-type channels may play a part in the bursting of 'epileptic' neurones in the hippocampus, and thus drugs that reduce these T-type channels could be effective in partial epilepsy [54,55].

GABA and GABA receptors

GABA is the major inhibitory neurotransmitter in the brain. It is formed and degraded in the GABA shunt (Fig. 9.5). Glutamic acid decarboxylase (GAD) converts glutamate to GABA. Promotion of GABA synthesis has been proposed to contribute to the action of some antiepileptic drugs including valproate [56]. GABA is degraded by GABA transaminase to succinic semialdehyde; α-ketoglutarate accepts the amino group in this reaction to become glutamate (Fig. 9.5). GABA is transported into vesicles by the vesicular transporter, VGAT, which has been cloned [57]. Since this transporter is absent from some GABAergic synapses, then other

vesicular transporters probably also exist [58]. GABA acts at three specific receptor types: GABA$_A$, GABA$_B$ and GABA$_C$ receptors [59]. GABA$_C$ receptors are present almost exclusively within the retina where they are responsible for fast chloride currents [59].

GABA$_A$ receptors

GABA$_A$ receptors are expressed postsynaptically within the brain (presynaptic GABA$_A$ receptors have been described within the spinal cord). GABA$_A$ receptors are constructed from five of at least 16 mammalian subunits, grouped in seven classes: α, β, γ, δ, σ, ε and π [60]. This permits a vast number of putative receptor isoforms. The subunit composition determines the specific effects of allosteric modulators of GABA$_A$ receptors, such as neurosteroids, zinc and benzodiazepines [60]. The subunit composition also determines the kinetics of the receptors and can affect desensitization [61]. Importantly the subunit composition of GABA$_A$ receptors expressed in neurones can change during epileptogenesis, and these changes influence the pharmacodynamic response to drugs [62]. GABA$_A$ receptor activation results in the early rapid component of inhibitory transmission. Since GABA$_A$ receptors are permeable to chloride and, less so, bicarbonate, the effects of GABA$_A$ receptor activation on neuronal voltage are dependent on the chloride and bicarbonate concentration gradients across the membrane [63]. In neurones from adult animals, the extracellular chloride concentration is higher than the intracellular concentration resulting in the equilibrium potential of chloride being more negative than the resting potential. Thus GABA$_A$ receptor activation results in an influx of chloride and cellular hyperpolarization. This chloride gradient is maintained by a membrane potassium/chloride co-transporter, KCC2 [64]. Absence of this transporter in immature neurones results in a more positive reversal potential for chloride, and thus GABA$_A$ receptor activation in these neurones produces neuronal depolarization [64,65]. During excessive GABA$_A$ receptor activation intracellular chloride accumulation can result in depolarizing GABA$_A$ receptor-mediated responses. Repetitive stimulation can also have a further paradoxical effect in which the hyperpolarizing GABA$_A$ receptor-mediated potential is followed by a prolonged depolarizing potential. This depolarizing potential is partially mediated through an extracellular accumulation of potassium extruded by activation of KCC2 [66]. Thus under certain circumstances GABA$_A$ receptors can mediate excitation rather than inhibition. Drugs that inhibit carbonic anhydrase such as acetazolamide and topiramate will reduce the intracellular bicarbonate and thus can reduce these depolarizing GABA responses [67].

Benzodiazepines are specific modulators of GABA$_A$ receptors and act at GABA$_A$ receptors that contain a α_1, α_2, α_3 or α_5 subunit in combination with a γ subunit [60]. Drugs acting at the benzodiazepine site have different affinities for the different α subunit containing GABA$_A$ receptors, and this specificity can affect pharmacodynamic response [68]. This is due perhaps to the varied distribution of these receptors in the brain. Thus the α_1 subunit containing receptors seems to have mainly a sedative effect, and is perhaps responsible for this side-effect of benzodiazepines [68]. This also explains why zolpidem, a drug that has great affinity for GABA$_A$ receptors containing the α_1 subunit, has marked sedative effects and weak anticonvulsant efficacy [69]. More selective ligands could thus result in benzodiazepine agonists that have less

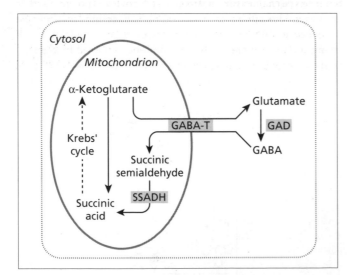

Fig. 9.5 GABA shunt. α-ketoglutarate and succinic acid are two intermediaries in the Krebs' cycle within the mitochondria. Outside the mitochondria, glutamate is converted to GABA by glutamic acid decarboxylase (GAD). GABA is converted by GABA-transaminase (a mitochondrial enzyme) into succinic semialdehyde and then by succinic semialdehyde dehydrogenase (SSADH) to succinic acid; α-ketoglutarate is converted in this reaction to glutamate.

sedative effect and greater anticonvulsant potential. The benzodiazepine's main effect is to increase the affinity of GABA$_A$ receptors for GABA, and to increase the probability of receptor opening [70,71]. There has also been the suggestion that benzodiazepines can increase the conductance of high-affinity GABA$_A$ receptors [72].

Barbiturates are less selective than benzodiazepines, and potentiate GABA$_A$ receptor-mediated currents. The potentiation is partly mediated by prolonging receptor opening times [70,73]. In addition, at high concentrations, they can directly activate the GABA$_A$ receptor [60]. This partly explains their anaesthetic effect at high concentrations. Other anaesthetic agents, such as propofol, have similar effects on GABA$_A$ receptors [60]. Topiramate can also potentiate GABA$_A$ receptors by an unknown mechanism of action [74].

GABA$_A$ receptors have other modulatory sites, and can be modulated by zinc [60]. Neurosteroids can also modulate GABA$_A$ receptors [60], and variations in neurosteroid levels may explain why seizures occasionally cluster around the time of menstruation [75]. Ganaxolone, a neurosteroid, was, however, dropped from clinical trials due to lack of efficacy [76].

On occasion GABA$_A$ receptor agonists can have paradoxical proepileptic effects perhaps due to: GABA being excitatory in some circumstances (see above), synchronization of neurones through the interneuronal network [77,78] or preferential potentiation of GABAergic inhibition of GABAergic interneurones leading to paradoxical disinhibition. GABA$_A$ receptor agonists can also exacerbate absence seizures [79]. Absence seizures are generated within a recurrent loop between the thalamus and neocortex, and their generation is dependent upon oscillatory behaviour mediated by GABA$_A$ receptors, GABA$_B$ receptors, T-type calcium channels and glutamate receptors [79–81]. One hypothesis is that hyperpolarization of the thalamocortical neurones in the thalamus mediated by GABAergic inhibition leads to activation of T-type calcium currents which open on neuronal depolarization, resulting in repetitive spiking. This activates neurones in the neocortex which in turn stimulate the thalamic reticular nucleus leading to GABAergic inhibition of the thalamocortical (relay) neurones (Fig. 9.4), and so the cycle continues [79,81]. Within this circuit, clonazepam preferentially inhibits the thalamic reticular neurones, perhaps due to the higher expression of α_3 containing GABA$_A$ receptors [82]. Non-specific GABA$_A$ receptor agonists, GABA$_B$ receptor agonists or agonists of specific GABA$_A$ receptors can all hyperpolarize thalamocortical neurones and so can have a proabsence effect [79]. This also occurs through the potentiation of GABAergic inhibition with ganaxalone [83].

GABA$_B$ receptors

GABA$_B$ receptors are expressed both pre- and postsynaptically [84,85]. They are G-protein-coupled receptors, and consist of dimers of either GABA$_{B1a}$ or GABA$_{B1b}$ and GABA$_{B2}$ subunits. Activation of GABA$_B$ receptors results in inhibition of adenylyl cyclase, inhibition of voltage-gated calcium channels and activation of G protein-linked inwardly rectifying potassium channels (GIRKs). The postsynaptic effect is a prolonged hyperpolarization leading to the late component of inhibitory neurotransmission. At many synapses postsynaptic GABA$_B$ receptors are located far from the re-

lease site, and are only activated by GABA spill-over during simultaneous release of GABA from multiple synapses [86]. Although the effects of this would be to decrease the excitability of the system, GABA$_B$ receptor activation may enhance the oscillatory nature of certain structures [86]. Indeed, activation of postsynaptic GABA$_B$ receptors in the thalamus has been proposed to underlie the generation of absence seizures [87]. The presynaptic effect of GABA$_B$ receptors is not only to inhibit GABA release at inhibitory synapses as a process of autoregulation, but also to inhibit glutamate release at excitatory synapses [85], and thus the effect on the network is complex and difficult to predict. Results with GABA$_B$ receptor agonists have been variable, but they seem to have a proabsence effect [79]; conversely, GABA$_B$ receptor antagonists have antiabsence effects but can be proconvulsant in other seizure models [88].

GABA uptake and breakdown

Other means of positively modulating GABAergic activity are to inhibit GABA uptake or inhibit GABA breakdown. GABA is mainly metabolized by GABA transaminase to succinic semialdehyde; glutamate is synthesized in this reaction (see above). Vigabatrin irreversibly inhibits GABA transaminase. This results in an increase in intracellular GABA that can produce an increase in vesicular GABA, and so inhibitory transmission [89]. In addition, vigabatrin results in an increase in extracellular GABA that can be partly explained by decreased GABA uptake [90]. GABA released into the extracellular space is transported into neurones and glial cells via Na$^+$/Cl$^-$-coupled GABA transporters (GAT) that can transport GABA against an osmotic gradient [91]. In human and rat, four GAT proteins have been identified and cloned: GAT-1, GAT-2, GAT-3 and BGT-1 [91]. GAT-1 is predominantly present on presynaptic GABAergic terminals and glia, and is the most prevalent GABA transporter in the rat forebrain. In contrast, GAT-3 is localized exclusively to astrocytes and glia, and GAT-2 has a more diffuse distribution. GABA uptake and GAT expression change during development, and are also regulated by protein kinase C (activated by a variety of G-protein receptors), a direct effect of GABA and tyrosine phosphatase [92–95].

Amongst the most potent of GABA transporter inhibitors is nipecotic acid. Nipecotic acid proved to be a useful tool *in vitro*, but had poor penetration across the blood–brain barrier [96,97]. Nipectoic acid was thus only effective in animal epilepsy models, if it was administered intracerebrally. In order to improve the blood–brain penetration of nipecotic acid and similar compounds, a lipophilic side chain was linked to them via an aliphatic chain [98]. This markedly increased the potency and the specificity of these compounds for the GAT-1 transporter as well as increasing brain penetration [99]. These compounds, in contrast to nipecotic acid, are not substrates for the transporter [100]. One such compound, tiagabine (R-[-]-1-[4,4-*bis*(3-methyl-2-thenyl)-3-butenyl]-3-piperidinecarboxylic acid), was selected because of its good preclinical profile [101]. Tiagabine is thus a GAT-1 specific, non-transportable, lipid-soluble GABA uptake inhibitor.

Microdialysis studies have demonstrated an increase in extracellular brain GABA concentrations in various brain regions following systemic or local administration of tiagabine [102–105]. There does, however, appear to be significant differences in the effect of tiagabine on extracellular GABA between brain areas, perhaps secondary to different levels and expression of the different GATs. Thus the thalamus seems to be less sensitive to the effects of tiagabine than the hippocampus [102]; indeed, the dose of tiagabine that results in an increase in thalamic GABA is much higher than that necessary to mediate an antiepileptic effect and is of the order that has a possible proconvulsive effect [104,105]. Tiagabine, in contrast to vigabatrin, has no effect on total brain GABA [106]. This and the failure of tiagabine to accumulate in the retina, again in contrast to vigabatrin, may mean that tiagabine will not cause the concentric visual field defects associated with vigabatrin [107].

Although many explanations of vigabatrin's and tiagabine's mode of action concentrate on raising the extracellular GABA concentration, these drugs have other important effects. The time-course of the GABA transit in the synaptic cleft is partly (and variably) determined by GABA uptake; tiagabine can thus prolong the synaptic GABA transient. In addition, by decreasing GABA uptake there is greater spill-over of GABA from the synaptic cleft onto extrasynaptic receptors. Each of these mechanisms can have an effect on inhibition, and there is no consensus as to the relative importance of each.

Increasing extracellular GABA can have two opposing effects. $GABA_A$ receptors containing the δ subunit have a high affinity and less propensity to desensitize [108], and receptors expressing this subunit are present extrasynaptically [109]. Extracellular GABA can thus cause a tonic current mediated by such receptors; this has been demonstrated in cerebellar granule cells in which the extrasynaptic $GABA_A$ receptors contain the α_6 and δ subunits [110,111]. Extracellular GABA in these neurones thus results in a somatic hyperpolarizing current—a form of tonic inhibition [110,111]. Such an effect can also be seen in dentate granule cells, although the subunit composition of the $GABA_A$ receptors mediating this effect is not known (Fig. 9.6 [112,113]). A second effect of increasing extracellular GABA is to desensitize synaptic $GABA_A$ receptors [112,114]. This can result in smaller amplitude $GABA_A$ receptor-mediated currents [112,114]. Thus vigabatrin increases tonic inhibition, but decreases synaptically mediated inhibition (Fig. 9.6 [112]).

The effects of inhibiting GABA uptake on the time-course of GABA in the synaptic cleft are dependent upon the extent to which the time-course is governed by uptake as opposed to just diffusion, and is thus dependent upon the affinity, on-rate and density of GABA transporters and the geometry of the cleft and the extracellular space. GABA uptake varies with age and location. Inhibiting GABA uptake has no effect on inhibitory postsynaptic current (IPSC) kinetics at early ages, whilst prolonging IPSCs at later age groups [115]. Even within the hippocampus GABA uptake shows marked regional variations [116]. The effect of changing the time-course of the GABA transient is not immediately predictable. Importantly at some synapses the decay of the $GABA_A$ receptor-mediated IPSC/P is determined mainly by the spatiotemporal profile of the GABA concentration rather than the kinetics of the $GABA_A$ receptors [117]. At these synapses, prolonging the time-course of the synaptic GABA transient prolongs the duration of the IPSC/P [117,118]. This results in an effect on the current that is similar to benzodiazepines or barbiturates, although mechanistically different. In contrast, studies at other synapses and in different neurones have found no change in the decay of miniature IPSP/Cs (or even small IPSP/Cs) with block of GABA uptake, but have found

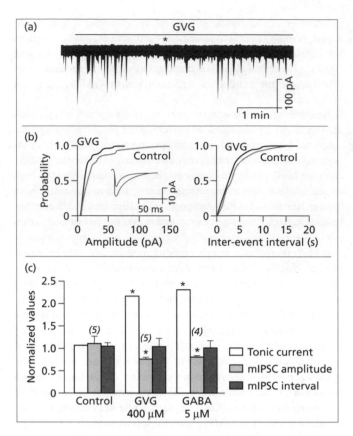

Fig. 9.6 Acute vigabatrin (GVG) or GABA reduce miniature inhibitory postsynaptic currents (pIPSC) amplitudes, but increase tonic inhibition. (a) GVG (400 µmol) applied to an untreated slice produced an increase in tonic current that was apparent after a couple of minutes (asterisk) and increased gradually throughout the experiment. (b) GVG reduced the mIPSC amplitude in all cases, without affecting the interevent interval. (c) The tonic current was increased by GVG or GABA, whilst the mIPSC amplitude reduced by GVG or GABA (experiments performed with $GABA_B$ receptors blocked). After [112].

a prolongation of large amplitude IPSCs [119,122,124]. Blockade of GABA uptake in large evoked IPSC/Ps affects the late, but not early decay [120,121]. The discrepancy between the effects on miniature IPSC/Ps compared with large amplitude IPSC/Ps can be explained by hypothesizing that the decay of small IPSC/Ps and the initial decay of the IPSC/P are determined by single channel kinetics and/or diffusion from the cleft [120–122]. Release of GABA from many sites, however, can result in spill-over to GABA receptors beyond the activated synapses, and this spill-over is enhanced by a decrease in GABA uptake [119,123]. Indeed, enhancing the amplitude of a slow GABA transient could convert it from desensitizing into a range that results in channel opening [124].

Spill-over of neurotransmitter can enhance not only $GABA_A$ receptor-mediated transmission, but also $GABA_B$ receptor-mediated effects. $GABA_B$ receptors are possibly remote to the synaptic cleft [119]. Thus, despite the presence of postsynaptic $GABA_B$ receptors, GABA released by a single interneurone usually activates postsynaptic $GABA_A$ receptors alone (Fig. 9.7 [86]); indeed, spontaneous IPSCs typically lack a $GABA_B$ receptor-mediated component [125]. Synchronous release of GABA from several interneurones, such as

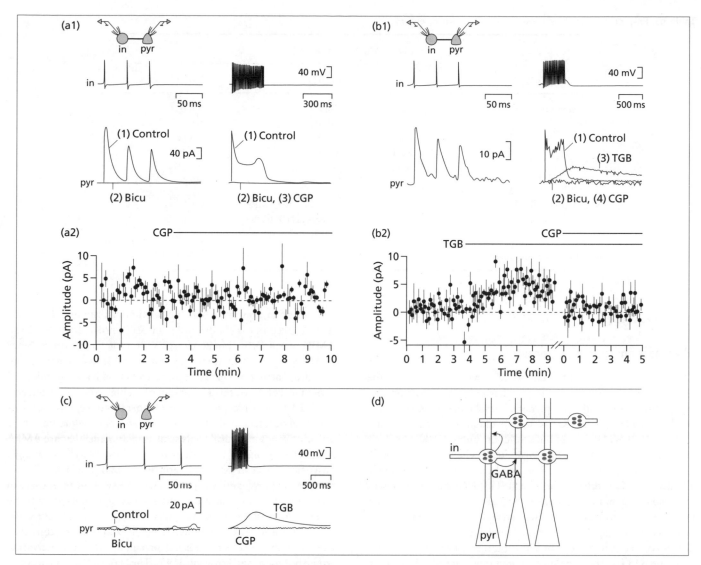

Fig. 9.7 Activation of GABA$_B$Rs by release of GABA from a single interneurone. (a1) Dual recording from a connected interneurone/pyramidal cell (in/pyr) pair. Three action potentials triggered in the interneurone elicit three inhibitory postsynaptic currents in the pyramidal cell. A train of action potentials (100 Hz) from the interneurone elicits an outward current in the pyramidal cell. Both types of responses are completely blocked by the GABA$_A$R antagonist bicuculline. Addition of the GABA$_B$R antagonist CGP62349 (2 µmol) has no further effect. (a2) Summary graph of the time course of the amplitude of the response, after application of bicuculline, for eight experiments. (b1) Similar experiment to the one illustrated in (a1), with the difference that the GABA uptake-blocker tiagabine (TGB; 10 µmol) was applied after perfusion of bicuculline. Under these conditions the AP train elicits a long-lasting outward current, which is abolished by CGP62349. (b2) Summary graph of the time course of the amplitude of the response, after application of bicuculline, for six experiments. (c) Dual recording from a non-connected in/pyr cell pair. After application of tiagabine, a train of APs in the interneurone elicits an outward current that can be blocked by CGP62349. (d) Schematic diagram illustrating extrasynaptic GABA$_B$R activation by diffusion of GABA on both postsynaptic and neighbouring pyramidal cells. After [86].

occurs with either strong stimulation or synchronous neuronal activity, can, however, activate postsynaptic GABA$_B$ receptors [86,119]. Blocking GABA uptake results in activation of GABA$_B$ receptors by GABA released by even a single interneurone (Fig. 9.7 [86]). Thus blocking GABA uptake can result in an enhancement of postsynaptic GABA$_B$ receptor-mediated inhibition. A defect in GABA uptake has been hypothesized to be the substrate for genetic absence epilepsy in one rat model [126,127]. It is thus not surprising that tiagabine and vigabatrin can worsen absence seizures, and can induce absence status epilepticus in humans [128–130]. Enhancement of GABA$_B$ receptor activation will not only have a postsynap-

tic effect, but also a presynaptic effect and will decrease the release of GABA from GABAergic terminals (decreasing inhibition), and glutamate from glutamatergic terminals (decreasing excitation). The overall effect on the network is thus difficult to predict.

Repetitive stimulation and bursts of neuronal activity such as occur during seizure activity can both cause GABA$_A$ receptor-mediated depolarizing responses (see above), and these could potentiate rather than inhibit epileptic activity. Tiagabine potentiates these depolarizing responses [131,132], and thus the concern is that through this mechanism tiagabine could in some circumstances enhance seizure activity.

Table 9.3 Properties of ion channel associated glutamate receptors

	Non-NMDA receptors		
	Kainate	*AMPA*	NMDA receptors
Subunits	GluR5	GluR1	NR1
	GluR6	GluR2	NR2A
	GluR7	GluR3	NR2B
	KA1	GluR4	NR2C
	KA2		NR2D
			NR3
Associated ion conductance		Na^+ (Ca^{2+} for AMPA receptors lacking the GluR2 subunit)	Ca^{2+}, Na^+
EC50 for glutamate		500 μmol	2–3 μmol

Other targets

Glutamate and glutamate receptors

Glutamate is a non-essential amino acid that does not cross the blood–brain barrier, but is readily synthesized by various biochemical pathways from different precursors including α-ketoglutarate (an intermediate of the Krebs' cycle), glutamine, ornithine and proline [133]. GABA transaminase contributes to the synthesis of glutamate (Fig. 9.5). Thus vigabatrin, which inhibits GABA transaminase, as well as inhibiting the breakdown of GABA may also decrease the synthesis of glutamate [134]. Glutamate is present in abundance in brain tissue, and is the major excitatory transmitter in the central nervous system. Glutamate is transported into vesicles by a specific vesicular transporter, and exhaustion of vesicular glutamate has been proposed to be a possible mechanism of seizure termination [135]. Abnormalities of glutamate uptake have been hypothesized to contribute to seizure generation, and thus drugs that modulate glutamate uptake may have an antiepileptic effect. Glutamate is present in the brain in large concentrations (10 mmol), but this is predominantly intracellular glutamate [133]. The extracellular glutamate is maintained at concentrations 5000 times lower than this (approximately 2 μmol) [136] by high affinity glutamate uptake into predominantly glia. Glutamate acts at three distinct receptor types: NMDA, non-NMDA (consisting of α-amino-3-hydroxy-5-methylisoxazole [AMPA] and kainic acid [KA] sensitive receptors) and metabotropic glutamate receptors. These receptor subtypes have very different properties (Table 9.3).

AMPA and kainate receptors

Non-NMDA receptors are mainly associated with channels that are permeable to sodium ions, and are responsible for fast excitatory neurotransmission. The receptors consist of four subunits; receptors comprising GluR1–4 subunits are the AMPA receptors and those comprising GluR5–7 and KA1–2 are the kainate receptors [137]. AMPA receptors lacking the GluR2 component are also permeable to calcium ions. Relatively large concentrations of glutamate result in channel opening and a rapid depolarization. The

concentration that gives half the maximum response (EC_{50}) for AMPA receptors is of the order of 500 μmol glutamate [138]. AMPA receptors are putative targets for antiepileptic drugs. Since AMPA receptors mediate most excitatory transmission in the brain, then drugs acting at these receptors are likely to have physiological consequences. Nevertheless, topiramate at high concentrations acts at AMPA/kainate receptors [139]; whether this is responsible for its antiepileptic effect or dose-related side-effects is unknown. There are other drugs in clinical trials such as talampanel that are AMPA receptor antagonists [140]. Kainate receptors, as well as having a postsynaptic role in exciting interneurones and principal cells, are also present presynaptically [141]. These presynaptic receptors can increase or decrease neurotransmitter release depending on subtype and target. In addition, axonal kainate receptors can affect axonal excitability leading to ectopic action potentials [142]. It is thus difficult to predict whether the effect of kainate receptor activation would be pro- or anti-ictogenic [143]. The agonist KA is, however, a powerful convulsant, thus kainate antagonists would perhaps be expected to have antiseizure effects [143]. Of interest is that interneurones may express a different kainate receptor subtype from that expressed on principal cells, raising the possibility that kainate receptor subtype-specific agonists and antagonists may provide a powerful approach to modulate the excitability of the system [143]. Indeed there has been a report of a GluR5-specific antagonist with antiepileptic effects in pilocarpine-induced seizures [144], yet there is a separate study demonstrating that GluR5 agonists can be antiepileptic [145]. This dichotomy demonstrates the difficulties in predicting the effects of kainate receptor antagonists and agonists.

NMDA receptors

NMDA receptors are associated with channels that are permeable to calcium and sodium ions. NMDA receptors are composed of multiple NR1 subunits in combination with at least one subtype of NR2 subunit (NR2A, B, C or D) and occasionally NR3 subunit [146]. The receptor has high affinity sites for both glycine and glutamate as well as sites for polyamines and zinc. Relatively low concentrations of glutamate are necessary to activate the receptor.

NMDA receptors typically have an EC_{50} for peak response of the order of 2–3 µmol glutamate (i.e. orders of magnitude lower than that of AMPA receptors [138]. NMDA receptors may thus be influenced by the ambient glutamate concentration and can thus be activated extrasynaptically by glutamate spill-over during excessive synaptic activity such as occurs during seizures. NMDA receptor responses decay slowly leading to a persistent depolarization that lasts for hundreds of milliseconds [147] that can thus contribute to burst firing. NMDA activation by glutamate does not necessarily result in any detectable current flow, because at negative potentials the ionic pore is tonically blocked by magnesium. This block is released by depolarization. During normal synaptic activity, the time-course of the non-NMDA excitatory postsynaptic potential (EPSP) is substantially shorter than the latency for NMDA receptor activation. Even if activation of non-NMDA receptors should result in a sufficient depolarization to release the magnesium block, by the time most NMDA receptors are activated by glutamate, most neurones will have repolarized to such an extent that the magnesium block will be in place and no current will flow through the NMDA receptors [147]. If, however, the NMDA receptor activation occurs coincident with neuronal depolarization, then the resultant depolarization will result in removal of the magnesium block and current flow. The NMDA receptor thus acts as a coincidence detector. The resultant influx of calcium through NMDA receptors has secondary consequences, affecting the phosphorylation of proteins that can produce long-term synaptic potentiation, modulation of other receptors and, if excessive, even cell death. NMDA receptors would seem an ideal target for antiepileptic drugs, both to prevent burst firing, proepileptogenic synaptic plasticity and neuronal death during prolonged epileptic activity (i.e. status epilepticus).

NMDA receptors, however, have numerous physiological roles in learning and motor control. This has meant that many of the NMDA receptor antagonists tried in epilepsy or for neuroprotection have had unacceptable side-effects. Interestingly, the adverse effects associated with NMDA receptor antagonists may be more prevalent in people with epilepsy, perhaps due to receptor modifications that occur with epileptogenesis. Nevertheless some presently available antiepileptic drugs may have modulatory effects on NMDA receptors. NMDA receptors have binding sites not only for glutamate, but also for zinc, glycine and polyamines. These sites modulate receptor function by affecting rates of desensitization, affinity for glutamate and channels opening. The glycine site has also been proposed to be essential for NMDA receptor activation. Thus felbamate, a drug that acts at the glycine site of the NMDA receptor, modulates NMDA receptor function [148]. Remacemide and its *des*-glycine metabolite may have a variety of effects on the NMDA receptor acting both as channel blockers and modulators [149]. NMDA receptors can also be modulated by other factors, such as pH, redox state and phosphorylation, that may provide additional drug targets. In addition, drugs that influence glutamate uptake can affect NMDA receptor activation, and so could possess antiepileptic activity [150].

Metabotropic glutamate receptors

Metabotropic glutamate receptors are G-protein-linked receptors that can be classified into three groups [151]. Group I receptors are mainly expressed postsynaptically where they enhance postsynap-

tic calcium entry, calcium release from internal stores and depolarization through inhibition of potassium currents. Group I receptors may thus play a part in neurodegeneration. Group I antagonists have neuroprotective and antiepileptic potential [152]. Presynaptic group I receptors can enhance neurotransmitter release. In contrast presynaptic group II and group III metabotropic glutamate receptors inhibit both GABA and glutamate release. The selectivity of some group II receptors for GABA synapses onto interneurones results in agonists inhibiting the inhibition of interneurones (i.e. decreasing the excitability of the system). Indeed group II and group III agonists have had antiepileptic effects in genetic epilepsy models and kindling [153–156], and may prove useful as antiepileptic drugs.

Potassium channels

Potassium channels form one of the most diverse groups of ion channels [157]. There are persistent potassium currents that determine the resting potential of neurones, but in addition there are a multitude of voltage-gated potassium channels. The voltage-gated potassium channels influence the resting potential and thus the excitability of neurones. They also repolarize neurones following action potentials, and so partly determine action potential width—a factor that can influence transmitter release. In addition, the rate of inactivation of potassium channels, which are activated during an action potential, influences the propensity for rapid repetitive firing. Voltage-gated potassium channels are thus critical for determining neuronal excitability.

Voltage-gated channels are assembled from four α subunits, and the diversity of possible α subunits leads to a multitude of combinations with different properties. The α subunits vary in size; the largest have six transmembrane segments (similar to a single domain of the sodium and calcium channels). Analogous to sodium channels, the voltage-sensing segment is S4 and the pore is composed of S5 and S6; in contrast to sodium channels, the mechanism of fast inactivation depends on an N-terminal structure that, like a ball and chain, occludes the pore. There is also a slower form of inactivation, which is poorly understood. There are smaller α subunits, which consist of two transmembrane segments, that make up the inward rectifying potassium channels. Auxillary β subunits can also combine with the α subunits and can influence channel kinetics and possibly receptor expression.

Conventionally, the voltage-gated potassium channels in the brain can be divided into: channels that rapidly activate and inactivate (A-type channels), and channels that open upon depolarization but do not significantly inactivate (delayed rectifier channels). There are also potassium channels that close upon depolarization but are open at the resting potential (inward rectifying channels); these channels do not inactivate in the same fashion as the other voltage-gated potassium channels, but the channels are rather blocked by internal ions at depolarized potentials. There are a variety of inward rectifying channels: some are G-protein linked and are opened by activation of G-protein-linked receptors (e.g. $GABA_B$ receptors), whilst some are opened by rises in intracellular adenosine triphosphate (ATP). There are other potassium channels that are similar in structure to the voltage-gated potassium channel, but are opened by intracellular calcium (calcium-activated potassium channels that mediate the after-hyperpolarization) or by cyclic nucleotides (mainly present in the retina where they mediate photoreceptor responses). There are also specific potassium channels that are inactivated by acetylcholine—termed M-type channels.

Although modulation of potassium channels would seem to be an ideal target for antiepileptic drugs, most drugs have no or poorly characterized effects on potassium channels. Phenytoin may selectively block delayed rectifier potassium channels [158], although how this contributes to its antiepileptic effect is unknown; indeed, such an effect may be proconvulsant. Drugs that potentiate potassium channels would be expected to have an antiepileptic effect by decreasing the excitability of neurones. Potentiation of specific potassium channels has indeed been proposed to contribute to the action of some presently available antiepileptic drugs. Thus gabapentin potentiates ATP activated inward rectifying potassium channels [159], and topiramate and acetazolamide induce a membrane hyperpolarization that is blocked by the potassium channel blocker, barium [67]. The after-hyperpolarization induced by calcium-dependent potassium channels also reduces neuronal excitability, and ethosuximide may mediate some of its effect by potentiating such channels [49].

Retigabine, a putative antiepileptic drug, has, as perhaps its main mode of action, potentiation of potassium channels. Retigabine induces a hyperpolarizing shift in the activation curves of KCNQ2/3 channels and probably other potassium channels from the same family that are responsible for the M current in neurones [160–163]. Interestingly mutations of KCNQ2/3 are responsible for benign neonatal seizures. The extent to which other antiepileptic drugs affect potassium channels remains unknown, but it is likely that modulation of potassium channels will be a future target for antiepileptic drug development.

Although separate from potassium channels, there is a specific cation conductance I_h that may play a critical role in epileptogenesis [164]. This channel is permeable to both potassium and sodium, and thus will tend to depolarize from the resting potential. I_h is activated at hyperpolarized potentials and inactivates at depolarized potentials. It may play a part in terminating thalamic oscillations and the generation of spike-wave discharges, as enhancement of I_h can depolarize thalamocortical neurones thus inactivating T-type calcium channels [165]. There is also a high density of I_h in dendrites where it shunts excitatory inputs, inhibiting transmission of excitation to the soma. Lamotrigine has recently been shown to cause a depolarizing shift in the inactivation curve of I_h, thus enhancing this current in dendrites [164]. This may have two potentially antiepileptic effects: (a) in the hippocampus it would inhibit excitatory transmission to the soma; and (b) in the thalamus, it would inhibit oscillations and thus may explain the efficacy of lamotrigine against absences.

Monoamines

It has been well established that monoamines play an integral role in epileptic phenomena. Experiments carried out in excised epileptic brain tissue have shown alterations in both catecholaminergic and indoleaminergic activity compared to non-epileptic tissue. In addition, monoamine content has been shown to differ in the cerebrospinal fluid of epileptic patients compared to non-epileptic patients [166]. Indeed, experimentally induced attenuation of

monoamine content has been directly implicated in the onset and propagation of many seizure disorders [167–170] whereas experimentally induced accretion of monoaminergic activity has been shown to retard the development of epileptiform activity [171–173]. The role of GABA in the epilepsies has been well characterized but little is known of the input that other monoamines have to play in, or following, seizure generation.

This section will examine the role that dopamine, noradrenaline (NA) and 5-hydroxytryptamine (5HT) play in the epileptic brain and how their concentrations are affected following anticonvulsant administration.

Dopamine

It is generally accepted that alterations in central dopamine levels are responsible, in part, for the onset and continuance of many seizure disorders (see [174] for a review). In the midbrain, inhibition of the substantia nigra (SN) has been shown to attenuate seizures in many animal models of seizure disorders. The SN projects dopaminergic neurones to the caudate putamen and, in turn, receives GABAergic afferents from the caudate putamen via one of two pathways. The first pathway, commonly known as the direct pathway, offers a direct monosynaptic GABAergic projection from the caudate putamen to the SN. The second pathway (indirect pathway) involves a GABAergic projection from the caudate putamen to the lateral globus pallidus. The globus pallidus then projects GABAergic efferents to the subthalamic nucleus that finally exerts glutamatergic tone onto the SN.

Both the SN and the caudate putamen have been thought to play major roles in the interruption and triggering of seizure generation, respectively. Seizure control appears to be partly regulated by the direct pathway and its ability to potentiate GABAergic activity within the SN. The antiepileptic profile of the indirect pathway is exemplified following the attenuation of seizure activity after local administration of NMDA antagonists either in the SN or the subthalamic nucleus. It would appear that both these pathways acting through the SN control seizure propagation, despite the fact that they exert opposite effects on SN neuronal activity.

As yet it remains undetermined just how these pathways interact to control seizures or whether or not anatomical subpopulations of striatal efferents have the propensity to control specific types of seizure.

The prefrontal cortex is also served by dopaminergic neurones that have their soma located in the ventral tegmental area (VTA). Innervation of the prefrontal cortex from the VTA has been thought to be responsible for the modulation of cognitive processes in humans [175] in addition to having a role to play in inhibiting spontaneous prefrontal neuronal firing [176]. In the primate cortex, dopamine terminals have been shown to colocalize with glutamate terminals on dendritic spines of pyramidal neurones. Furthermore, dopaminergic terminals have been found to exist in close proximity to the dendrites of inhibitory interneurones. Thus, it appears that dopamine has the potential to provide a regulatory control over the degree of excitatory input into the cortex [177]. Indeed, dopamine has been shown to attenuate the spontaneous firing of rodent prefrontal neurones [178] possibly via an enhancement of the frequency and amplitude of spontaneous IPSCs [179].

Noradrenaline

NA in the central nervous system is formed by the α-hydroxylation of dopamine and is considered to be primarily an inhibitory neurotransmitter. Attenuating synaptic NA levels have been shown to exert proconvulsant effects in models of seizure disorder [180] whereas increasing NA neurotransmission has been shown to reduce seizure activity [181]. Furthermore synaptic noradrenergic activity has been shown to retard the kindling process (i.e. epileptogenesis) [182]. It has been proposed that the anticonvulsant activity of sodium valproate and carbamazepine can be partly attributed to their ability to heighten noradrenergic activity [183–185].

5-Hydroxytrytamine

5HT mediates its actions in the mammalian central nervous system through seven classes of receptor ($5HT_{1-7}$). Within this classification there are at least four subtypes ($5HT_{1-4}$) which are thought to modify neuronal excitability and/or neurotransmitter release [186,187].

In the brain, the prominent 5HT cell bodies are located in the raphe nuclei which send ascending projections to the hippocampus [188]. 5HT has been shown to either inhibit or excite GABAergic interneurones in the CA1 region of the hippocampus following stimulation of $5HT_{1A}$ and/or $5HT_3$ receptors [189–191] and this has been proposed to modify excitatory responses within this region.

Serotonergic neurotransmission has been shown to influence the generation of certain types of seizure disorder in various experimental models including hippocampal kindling [192] and systemic administration of proconvulsants [193]. One report comparing monoamines and their metabolites in brain tissue from epileptic patients undergoing temporal lobe resections for seizure control found that the compensatory activation of serotonergic neurotransmission that exists in human epilepsy generated an increase in 5HT turnover as reflected in cerebrospinal fluid 5-hydroxyindoleacetic acid (5HIAA) levels. Despite the increase in 5HT turnover rate in this study it was reported to be insufficient for blocking seizure activity [166]. Furthermore, pharmacological agents which enhance and facilitate 5HT neurotransmission have been shown to provide anticonvulsant effects in a wide range of experimental models of seizure disorder, including the genetically epilepsy-prone rat model of generalized tonic-clonic epilepsy (GEPR) [194]. Drugs such as the selective serotonin reuptake inhibitor (SSRI) fluoxetine have been shown to augment the synaptic concentration of 5HT and may be effective against generalized tonic seizures [195]. Antiepileptic drugs such as carbamazepine [173], sodium valproate [196] and zonisamide [197] have all been shown to elevate extracellular hippocampal 5HT levels in rodents. Lamotrigine has also been shown to elevate synaptic 5HT levels by inhibiting its uptake in synaptosomal preparations from rodent cortex [198].

Effects of antiepileptic drugs

Carbamazepine, phenytoin, valproate and zonisamide are four of the most commonly cited antiepileptic drugs associated with alterations in monoaminergic neurotransmission. All of these antiepileptic drugs are thought to mediate their actions, at least in part, via a blockade of Na^+ channels [17,18,199–201]. It has been well established that blockade of Na^+ ion channels inhibits neuronal firing. However, at therapeutically relevant concentrations carbamazepine, phenytoin, valproate and zonisamide have been found to enhance monoamine neurotransmission [196,197,202,203]. Moreover, therapeutically relevant concentrations of carbamazepine and zonisamide have been shown to facilitate basal monoamine release without affecting basal glutamate release, and inhibited the depolarization-induced release of glutamate and monoamines [204]. This effect appears to be biphasic in that at supratherapeutic levels carbamazepine and zonisamide reduced brain monoamine concentrations [205,206]. The finding that carbamazepine produced a concentration-dependent increase in $3^{[H]}$ 5HT overspill without affecting Ca^{2+} [173] or K^+ evoked neurotransmission [207] suggests that carbamazepine-induced 5HT release is not dependent on depolarization or exocytosis.

It is interesting to note that coadministration of zonisamide with either phenytoin or valproate increased brain concentrations of dopamine and 5HT compared to treatment with zonisamide alone [208]. It has previously been shown that zonisamide does not affect the pharmacokinetic properties of valproate [209] and therefore it would be interesting to discover whether polypharmacy involving zonisamide as add-on therapy to existing valproate treatment would yield greater clinical benefit than that seen with valproate monotherapy.

Animal models

Animal testing is designed to tell us two things: whether a compound has antiepileptic activity, and secondly what is the nature of its antiepileptic action. It is in this last respect that animal models have given us some insight into mechanisms of action and differences between the antiepileptic drugs. Thus, animal models for epileptic disorders have played and continue to play a pivotal role in the discovery and development of antiepileptic drugs. Moreover, these models have provided researchers with a greater depth of understanding of the cognitive and physiological changes associated with the epileptic brain. However, the wealth of information uncovered has to be carefully interpreted in the light of the limitations of each of these models.

First, it is important to remember that human epilepsy is not a disease *per se*, but is instead more accurately defined as a collection of numerous, diverse syndromes which ultimately converge to elicit partial or generalized paroxysmal discharges in the brain. The occurrence of spontaneous, recurrent seizures may be considered a model of epilepsy; whilst acutely induced seizures must be considered as a separate entity. Unfortunately, many of the models cited in the literature as being representative of the neurophysiological abnormalities that occur in the human epileptic brain are, in fact, a more accurate portrayal of acute seizures. Furthermore, such is the desire to understand the underlying neurophysiology of the epilepsies that many experiments are carried out in animals with 'normal' brains. The validity of the mechanistic conclusions drawn from experiments performed on non-epileptic brains should be viewed with caution. Indeed, drugs such as glutamate antagonists have highlighted subtle neurophysiological differences that exist between experimental models of seizure disorder and human epilepsy.

Glutamate antagonists have been shown to be effective in seizure blockade in the laboratory [210,211] but are either ineffective or elicit serious side-effects when given clinically [212–214]. If these discrepancies exist in brains that are supposed to be representative of human epilepsy, then these differences are going to be more apparent in subjects with non-epileptogenic neurophysiology.

Any model of epileptic disorder has to be able to provide an accurate assessment of antiepileptic drugs both in terms of the drug's antiepileptic efficacy and with regard to any adverse effects evident at therapeutic doses. Unfortunately, there are many diverse epileptic disorders to characterize. This is borne out by the fact that no one model is currently believed to be truly representative of human epilepsy. With this in mind, it is generally agreed that preclinical evaluation and development of any putative antiepileptic drug must exhibit its effects in several animal models before being presented for clinical trials.

A number of criteria have been outlined which a potentially new model of epileptic disorder should fulfil. First, providing a greater susceptibility to generate acute ictal activity is, by itself, insufficient if the model is to be truly characteristic of a seizure disorder. The model must have the capacity to readily exhibit recurrent, spontaneously occurring seizures of high frequency but without endangering the animal so that both acute and chronic studies can be carried out. Secondly, there should be no distinguishable traits in clinical phenomenology or aetiology between the seizure type(s) observed in the laboratory and those seen in human epilepsies. Therefore, if there appears to be a genetic or age-specific disposition with regard to the manifestation of a specific seizure disorder then it must be incorporated in the animal model. In addition, seizure types characterized by the model should elicit paroxysmal EEG alterations that are correlates of the electrical abnormalities seen in human seizures. This allows a direct evaluation to be made of a drug's potential anticonvulsant profile. Thirdly, standard antiepileptic drugs should exhibit similar pharmacological properties between the seizure type being modelled and that seen in the human condition. One report has suggested that experimental use of the model in question should be designed in such a manner that animals are segregated into subgroups based on the differences in efficacy following standard antiepileptic treatment. This is believed to be a more accurate reflection of the situation seen in the clinic whereby patients who share the same type of seizure disorder differ in their response to standard drug therapy [215]. However, the same report also suggested that standard antiepileptic drugs should be either inactive or weakly active in blocking the seizures [215]. This apparent paradox is explained by the fact that seizures in models that are easily suppressed by standard antiepileptic treatment are unlikely to detect novel antiepileptic drugs that may find their clinical niche in the treatment of refractory epilepsy. A high proportion of currently available antiepileptic drugs were developed following the attenuation of seizures generated by the maximal electroshock (MES) or pentylenetetrazol (PTZ) tests. However, these tests alone do not always give an accurate assessment of the anticonvulsant profile of a drug. For example, vigabatrin and tiagabine are ineffective in blocking seizures in the MES model whereas novel antiepileptic drugs such as gabapentin, lamotrigine, topiramate and zonisamide have little or no effect in the PTZ test. These drugs are widely employed in the clinic in managing seizure disorders. Relying too heavily on these models may be at the expense of detecting novel

antiepileptic drugs. Leviteracetam provides us with a classic example of the dangers of placing too much emphasis on the MES and PTZ tests for antiepileptic drug screening. This drug was found to be completely ineffective in both the MES and PTZ tests [216], and in acute tests involving maximal dosing of chemoconvulsants such as bicuculline, picrotoxin and 3-mercaptopropionic acid [217]. Leviteracetam also differs from classical antiepileptic drugs in its lack of efficacy against clonic convulsions induced by administration of the glutamate agonists NMDA, AMPA and KA. Despite exhibiting a lack of effect in a wide range of tests traditionally used to screen drugs for their potential anticonvulsant properties, the drug was subsequently found to be efficacious in other models of epileptic disorders. Leviteracetam offers protection against seizure activity in audiogenic mice [218] and amygdala kindled rats [219]. In humans, the drug is found to be useful as an adjunct to traditional antiepileptic drugs for refractory partial epilepsy and appears to be well tolerated. It is probably not surprising that certain chronic epilepsies appear to remain refractory to drug treatment when the same seizure models (MES and PTZ tests) have been used as the criteria by which most of the currently clinically used antiepileptic drugs have been selected.

At present there appears to be no model that fulfils all of the criteria outlined above. Some recently discovered genetic models closely resemble the idiopathic human epilepsies but they too have their shortcomings. The remainder of this section will deal with some of the most commonly used animal models of epileptic disorders for drug testing and a discussion of their strengths and weaknesses.

Acute seizure models

The advantages of acute seizure model are reproducibility, and the ability to perform high throughput screening. The disadvantages are that the seizures do not mirror epilepsy (i.e. spontaneous seizure occurrence) and the seizures occur in 'normal', non-epileptic brains (see above). There have been a variety of acute seizure models developed either using electrical stimulation or convulsant drugs. The two that have been most widely used are the MES and PTZ models. Other convulsants include a variety of GABA$_A$ receptor antagonists, glutamate agonists and muscarinic agonists. Here we will describe the more commonly used models for drug screening.

MES test

One of the seminal discoveries of the last 150 years of epilepsy research was the discovery that electrical stimulation in animals subsequently generated seizures. The MES model is one of the most commonly used models of this type. The MES test involves either bilateral corneal or transauricular electrical stimulation and subsequently induces tonic hind limb extension and flexion followed by clonus. Traditionally, drugs that exhibit an affinity in blocking seizures generated by this model find their clinical niche in blocking primary and secondary generalized tonic-clonic epilepsies. In conjunction with the PTZ model, the MES test is responsible for the discovery of most of the currently employed antiepileptic drugs used to treat the human epilepsies. Indeed, phenytoin is one of the most effective drugs at blocking seizures induced by the MES model. In addition, some of the recently developed antiepileptic drugs such as topiramate and zonisamide also exhibit high potencies in blocking

MES-induced seizures. The affinity of these drugs in this model may be explained by studies that have attempted to correlate the preclinical anticonvulsant profile of standard and novel antiepileptic drugs with their mechanisms of action. Drugs that display high affinity in blocking voltage-sensitive sodium channels (e.g. carbamazepine, lamotrigine, phenytoin) appear to have greatest affinity at blocking MES-induced seizures. In addition, there is evidence that some drugs that enhance $GABA_A$ receptor-mediated inhibitory neurotransmission (e.g. benzodiazepines, phenobarbital) also elicit marked anticonvulsant efficacy in this test. Unfortunately, this model does not readily recognize the anticonvulsant properties of drugs such as ethosuximide or tiagabine. Moreover, vigabatrin administered to rats at doses as high as 2000 mg/kg failed to block seizures induced by this model [214].

PTZ test

PTZ reliably produced tonic-clonic convulsions in a wide range of animal species. Its popularity rose when it was considered a rapid and efficient method of screening new drugs for their potential anticonvulsant properties. Following high doses of the drug (>80 mg/kg) the drug induces myoclonic jerks that are sustained and propagate to form generalized tonic-clonic seizures. It has been widely accepted that drugs that are effective against PTZ-induced seizures have a potential therapeutic role to play in combating generalized absence and myoclonic seizures. However, phenobarbital, which was found to be active against seizures induced by PTZ, was subsequently found to be ineffective in human absence seizures [220]. This, once more, highlights the need for screening drugs in several models of epileptic disorders for complete evaluation. In this instance, it has been suggested that PTZ may be more beneficial in identifying drugs with activity against myoclonic seizures [220]. The PTZ model was responsible for the discovery of the anticonvulsant properties of the drug valproate. Subsequent clinical trials confirmed its anticonvulsant benefits in epileptic patients and now the drug is regularly prescribed to treat partial and generalized seizures. Moreover, it appears that drugs which act on $GABA_A$ receptors (e.g. phenobarbital), or block thalamic T-type calcium ion channels (e.g. ethosuximide), have the propensity to block PTZ-induced seizures.

Bicuculline

Bicuculline is an alkaloid convulsant that acts as a competitive antagonist at postsynaptic $GABA_A$ receptors. Systemic administration produces severe and continuous tonic-clonic seizures whereas partial seizure generation occurs following focal administration. In accordance with KA and pilocarpine (see below), one of the main disadvantages of this model is the age specificity required for the degree of seizure onset and propagation. Although seizure activity can be generated following administration of this drug throughout development, clonic seizures have been shown to only occur in rat pups >12 days of age [221]. Moreover, rat pups <8 days old have been shown to express behavioural seizures without having an EEG correlate [221,222].

Phenobarbital is the only classical antiepileptic drug that displays any effect, albeit moderate, against bicuculline-evoked seizures. The lack of affinity of the classical antiepileptic drugs in the cessation of seizures evoked by this model implies that bicuculline may be employed to represent refractory seizure disorders.

6 Hz seizure model

Low-frequency (6 Hz) corneal stimulation provides an alternative source of assessing the efficacy of antiepileptic drugs, and has been introduced for drug screening, because of the failure of the above screening models to detect the antiepileptic potential of levetiracetam. This model typically produces psychomotor seizures which differ from the high-frequency MES test in that the seizure intensity is reduced and the seizure propagation is not as widely pronounced. This culminates in the generation of seizures which appear to be brief and clonic in nature and is followed by the appearance of stereotypical behaviour [223]. Previous work has shown that while phenobarbital was effective, phenytoin displayed a lack of activity in the cessation of seizure episodes induced by this model [224]. As many patients appear to exhibit resistance to phenytoin treatment it was suggested that this model may be a useful test for screening drugs which have a role to play in treating refractory epilepsies. Indeed, in an examination of classical and novel antiepileptic drugs using this model carbamazepine, phenobarbital, trimethadione, ethosuximide, felbamate, lamotrigine and tiagabine exhibited partial efficacy whereas only levetiracetam and valproic acid were shown to display complete protection [223].

Chronic seizure models

Chronic models of seizures fall into three main types—the kindling models, post-status epilepticus models and the genetic models. The advantage of these models is that they can reproduce the epileptic state in which spontaneous seizures can take place. Furthermore, kindling and post-status epilepticus models reflect an epileptogenic process, and thus using these models it may be possible to determine the antiepileptogenic potential of antiepileptic drugs. Significant disadvantages include variability, expense and the necessity for long-term monitoring that makes a high throughput screening programme difficult.

Kindling

The kindling model is the phenomenon whereby repeated focal application of initially subconvulsive electrical stimulation or chemical stimuli subsequently generates intense partial or generalized convulsive seizures. Usually, kindling is initiated by electrical stimulation of the amygdala, but most regions of the forebrain can be kindled. Once the animal has recovered from the trauma of the surgery, it is exposed usually to daily electrical impulses usually in the form of 0.2–1.0 mA at 60 Hz for 2 s. Typically, these seizures pass through several behavioural stages of epileptiform activity and were originally documented by Racine: class 1, facial clonus; class 2, facial clonus and rhythmic head nodding; class 3, facial clonus, head nodding and contralateral forelimb clonus; class 4, facial clonus, head nodding, forelimb clonus and rearing; and class 5, facial clonus, head nodding, forelimb clonus, rearing and falling [225]. These seizures are concurrently associated with a gradual lengthening of the hyperexcitability and after-discharge with each stimulus train. One of the main advantages of the kindling model is that it allows researchers the benefits of assessing the anticonvulsant properties of drugs in combating seizures elicited via stimulation of the limbic system and neocortex. In contrast, the MES- or PTZ-induced seizures use different anatomical pathways. In addition, the possibility exists that the underlying mechanisms involved in evoking seizures in 'normal' brains, conventionally investigated using MES and PTZ models, may differ from those induced in an hyperexcitable brain. A further advantage in the kindling model is the ability to observe changes in the duration of the after-discharge as well as alterations in behavioural response following drug treatment, and to assess the potential of drugs to retard the epileptogenic process. However, inducing kindling in an animal is a time-consuming and laborious task compared with the more convenient chemical seizure models. Antiepileptic drugs seem to differ in their effects on different stages of kindling [226–234]. For example, valproate, phenobarbital and benzodiazepines inhibited acquisition of the kindled state [226]. Other drugs such as phenytoin and carbamazepine do not have such effects or at least only very weak effects on kindling development [226–228]. Carbamazepine, valproate and diazepam suppress kindled seizures once they have developed [227,234]. Phenytoin was not effective at suppressing kindled seizures, but did prevent spontaneous seizures in kindled animals [227,228]. Of the newer antiepileptic drugs, topiramate delayed seizure acquisition in kindling and inhibited kindled seizures in a dose-dependent fashion [229,231]. Although lamotrigine did not inhibit amygdala kindled seizure development at a low dose (5 mg/kg) in rats, a higher dose (15 mg/kg) enhanced kindling development, possibly exhibiting a 'proepileptogenic' effect [232]. In animals that were not treated with lamotrigine during kindling, kindled seizures were inhibited by lamotrigine. If, however, lamotrigine was administered during kindling development, it was ineffective in suppressing kindled seizures and even had proconvulsant effects. With acute treatment, levetiracetam inhibited kindling acquisition—an effect that persisted after acute treatment was discontinued—and suppressed seizures in fully kindled animals [233]. The persistent effect on kindling development associated with acute levetiracetam treatment may provide a different and as yet unclear parameter for potential antiepileptogenic effects of antiepileptic drugs.

These studies are often difficult to interpret as it is not always clear that inhibiting the kindling process is independent of the ability to suppress after-discharges following stimulation. Also opinions on the clinical relevance of kindling and how it relates to the human epileptic brain are still unresolved [235].

Post-status epilepticus

The muscarinic agonist pilocarpine is one of the most commonly used models of status epilepticus in the laboratory. Typically, an animal is administered the drug either intraperitoneally or subcutaneously and seizure activity occurs approximately 30 min later. The animals experience facial automatisms followed by head weaving and motor limbic seizures (rearing, forelimb clonus and salivation). The EEG pattern following pilocarpine administration displays a series of stages similar to that seen in human status epilepticus [236].

Neuropathologically, pilocarpine induces cell loss in the hippocampus, entorhinal cortex, amygdala and the hilus of the dentate gyrus [237]. Following status epilepticus there is a latent period of a few weeks followed by the development of spontaneous recurrent seizures. Phenobarbital, carbamazepine and phenytoin are found to be effective in the cessation of the spontaneous seizures whereas ethosuximide has been found to be completely ineffective, suggesting that this may be a useful model of partial epilepsy [238].

Kainic acid (KA) is another chemoconvulsant commonly used to induce status epilepticus. KA is a glutamate analogue that generates widespread neuronal damage via a mechanism that is thought to involve the activation of excitatory amino acid receptors. Local administration of the neurotoxin is rapidly followed by acute seizures that are typically displayed as facial myoclonus. This is followed by heightened seizure duration, complete with generalized motor clonus before a latent period similar to that seen with the pilocarpine model. After a latent period of 2–3 months, the seizures return with a behavioural profile similar to those observed in temporal lobe epilepsy.

Pathologically, KA generates lesions similar to those seen in humans with mesial temporal sclerosis. These lesions typically include loss of GABAergic interneurones in the dentate hilus and cell death of pyramidal neurones within the CA1 and CA3 regions of the hippocampus [239]. Furthermore, as reported in human epileptic hippocampus seizures, there is profound sprouting of mossy fibres in the dentate gyrus. The sustained epileptic profile and recurrence of persistent spontaneous seizures in animals exposed to KA can be more accurately described as being an example of a chronic, rather than an acute, model of epileptic disorder. Standard antiepileptic drugs exhibit variable activity against KA-induced seizures. Benzodiazepines appear to possess anticonvulsant activity when given acutely whereas there appears to be little, if any, effect of phenytoin, carbamazepine or valproate on acute seizures [240]. Prolonged electrical stimulation protocols can also induce status epilepticus. There are a number of these models that are distinguishable by the stimulation protocol used and the brain area stimulated.

The major weakness of the status epilepticus models is the age-dependent effects seen following administration with either drug. For example, systemic administration of either pilocarpine or KA to young rodents does not result in seizure-induced hippocampal damage, despite the presence of severe tonic-clonic seizures [241,242]. In addition, young rats do not display the full gamut of pathological or long-term behavioural effects that are observed in older rats [243].

Genetic models

Until recently, genetic models of epileptic disorders had to rely on animals with an inherent susceptibility to display seizure activity. However, recent advances have made it possible to study the effects of genetic modification and how these subtle changes lead to epileptogenesis at the cellular level. Moreover, a greater understanding of the anatomical and physiological adaptations that occur following the expression of the 'epileptic gene' may pave the way for improved pharmacotherapy of seizure disorders especially if distinct parallels can be drawn between genetic models and the human condition.

Genetic models of non-convulsive epilepsy

Spontaneous point mutations have resulted in the generation of mice that develop spike-wave discharges with accompanying behavioural abnormalities within the first few weeks after birth (tottering, stargazer and lethargic mutants). These mice have proved to be useful genetic models for childhood absence epilepsy [244].

Tottering mouse

The tottering mouse (tg/tg) was discovered as a spontaneous, recessive mutation in 1957 and has subsequently been shown to exhibit features of generalized epilepsy—namely absence-like seizures with accompanying paroxysmal 6–7 Hz spike-waves that can last between 0.3 and 10 s. The mutation develops in adolescent mice ($P > 17$ days) with full seizure activity manifested at approximately 4 weeks of age. The mutation involves a non-conservative proline to leucine amino acid substitution near the α_{1A} pore-forming subunit of the P/Q-type voltage-gated calcium ion channel [244]. This mutation presents itself phenotypically in the form of cerebellar ataxia and paroxysmal dyskinaesias involving the brainstem nuclei and cerebellum [245,246]. Despite no evidence of gross morphological defects in the brainstem nuclei or the cerebellum, tottering mice have been shown to have gene-linked heightening of noradrenergic tone originating from the locus coeruleus with a proliferation of terminal fields in the hippocampus and cerebellum [247]. Moreover, lesioning the noradrenergic nerve terminals by the selective neurotoxin 6-hydroxydopamine has been reported to provide partial protection against the expression of seizures and ataxia in these mice [248].

Electrophysiological studies have shown that a 60% reduction in current density occurs in mutant Purkinje cells with more modest effects on the kinetics of the P/Q current 249. Atypical P/Q channel functioning in the tottering mouse has been shown to contribute towards a reduction in excitatory synaptic transmission without a concomitant reduction in inhibitory neurotransmission in somatosensory thalamic neurones [250]. Voltage-gated calcium channels in the cerebellum are closely associated with excitatory vs. inhibitory synapses [251]. Aberrant P/Q channel functioning may lead to an imbalance within the thalamic circuitry if excitatory and inhibitory inputs are differentially affected by a reduction in current density.

There also exists the possibility that α_{1A} defects indirectly influence the function of other voltage-gated calcium ion channels as a slight increase in the expression of the α_{1C} subunit of L-type channels in Purkinje cells was reported in tottering mice [252]. The manifestation of movement disorders in these mice appears to involve the overexpression of α_{1C} subunits as the dyskinaesias were reportedly prevented by administration of specific antagonists for L-type calcium channels [252].

Two additional tottering mutants have been identified including leaner (tg^{la}) and rolling Nagoya (tg^{rol}). The leaner mutant phenotype is developed within 2 weeks following birth and is displayed as ataxia, rigidity and the manifestation of absence seizures [253] whereas the rolling Nagoya mutant experiences poor motor control leading to falling and rolling with stiffness of the tail and hindlimbs [254].

The leaner mutation is a single glycine to alanine substitution in the splice donor consensus sequence that causes abnormal splicing of this intron into either a smaller fragment by exon skipping or a larger product that contains the whole intron [244]. This aberrant splicing in the leaner mouse was thought to result in deletion of the C-terminal of the α_{1A} subunit. Leaner mice experience slow selective degeneration of cerebellar neurones that may be attributed to

the reduction of current density in tg^{la} Purkinje cells and concomitant changes in voltage dependency with regard to activation and inactivation [249].

Stargazer mouse

Stargazer mice have mutations in the γ_2 subunit of the voltage-gated calcium channel and have spike-wave discharges of 5–7 Hz. The γ_2 subunit is essential for synaptic targeting of the AMPA receptor, and its role in calcium channels is controversial [255]. The gene Cacng2, which is abnormally expressed in stargazers, encodes a 36-kDa protein with wide distribution in the central nervous system. The mutation itself involves a transposan insertion in the second intron that results in a marked reduction of normal transcription. The manifestation of ictal activity occurs after 2 weeks of age and is behaviourally expressed by ataxia and impaired vestibular functioning. Stargazer mice, like the tottering mutants, have their seizure activity immediately terminated by ethosuximide but differ from tottering mice in that there are no noradrenergic abnormalities associated with its spike-wave discharges. However, stargazer mice have been found to display far more pronounced mossy fibre sprouting in the molecular layer of the dentate gyrus compared to their tottering counterpart [256]. In addition, stargazers have reduced cerebellum expression of the neurotrophic factor brain-derived neurotrophic factor [257] and an undeveloped GABA$_A$ receptor profile [258] suggesting that cerebellum maturation in stargazers is impaired. It remains unclear how these events relate to the generation of spike-wave discharges in these mice.

Lethargic mouse

A mutation in the β_4 voltage-gated calcium channel subunit gives rise to the lethargic mouse mutant (gene Cacnb4^{lh}). This mutation destabilizes the mRNA, generates exon skipping and aberrant translation that culminates in the lack of β_4 protein in lethargic mice [259]. It is perhaps surprising that the Cacnb4^{lh} mutation does not have more widespread phenotypic consequences especially when it is considered that the β_4 subunit is not exclusively associated with any particular β_1 subunit. The lack of pathogenic changes in the brain may be attributed to compensation by other β subunits. Indeed, increased β_1 expression has been reported in lethargic mice [260]. Generalized spike-wave cortical discharges occur at 5–6 Hz with a duration of 0.6–5 s. Ataxia, focal myoclonus and loss of motor control are typically expressed 1 month postnatally. Increased absence seizures following administration of GABA$_B$ agonists could be reversed with the introduction of GABA$_B$ antagonists [261]. This discovery combined with reports of increased GABA$_B$ receptor density in neocortical plasma membranes of lethargic homozygotes [262] highlights the important epileptogenic role that GABA$_B$ transmission plays in the brains of these mice. The lethargic model has been proposed to be superior to the high-dose PTZ model in predicting efficacy of antiepileptic drugs against human absence seizures [129].

Genetic absence epilepsy rats from Strasbourg (GAERS)

GAERS display EEG paroxysms that are typical of human absence seizures including unresponsiveness to mild stimuli [79]. The occurrence of bilateral and synchronous spike-wave discharges occurs in approximately 30% of animals 30 days postnatally with the manifestation of seizure activity occurring in all animals at 4 months. Initially the seizure episodes are infrequent and transient but increase to one a minute by the age of 6 months [263]. Drugs that are effective in the treatment of human absence epilepsy are also efficacious in suppressing the spike-wave discharges in GAERS whereas drugs that are typical used in the treatment of convulsant or focal seizures in humans are ineffective in these rats [264]. The main differences between this model and the human phenotype are the higher frequency of spike-wave discharges (7–11 Hz) without the appearance of polyspikes and the behavioural and EEG components of these seizures persisting into adulthood [79]. The cortex and thalamus are thought to play major roles in the generation of seizure activity in GAERS as cortical lesions suppress thalamic spike-wave discharges and lesions of the thalamus encompassing the specific relay and reticular nuclei suppress ipsilateral epileptogenesis [265]. GABA neurotransmission appears to play an integral part in seizure manifestation in GAERS. $GABA_A$ and $GABA_B$ agonists have been reported to prolong and intensify episodes of seizure activity, respectively [264,266]. This suggests that abnormal GABAergic transmission contributes to the seizure profile seen in GAERS. Indeed autoradiography studies have shown that there are significantly fewer $GABA_A$ receptors in the CA2 region of the GAER hippocampus compared to control [267]. By contrast, the density of $GABA_B$ receptors was found to be comparable in GAERS and control, non-epileptic rats [268]. Recent evidence has uncovered a role of intrathalamic nuclei and their rhythmic recruitment during seizure activity via mechanisms that seem to rely on delayed glutamatergic excitation modulated by GABAergic influences [269].

Genetic models of convulsive seizures

DBA/2 J mice

The DBA/2 J mouse strain displays sound-induced seizures between the ages of 2 and 4 weeks. After this time the vulnerability to experience audiogenic seizures declines. At 7–8 weeks old these mice exhibit a low threshold for seizure activity in the MES test despite being completely free of audiogenic seizure activity. An audiogenic mouse in response to a loud stimulus will initially startle followed by running and leaping phases that unfortunately impede the collection of good EEG data. Another disadvantage of this model is the high fatality rate often seen following repetitive seizing in these mice [270]. Furthermore, the audiogenic mouse seizure model has no clinical correlate although it does provide a valuable insight into the genetic factors leading to seizure activity.

The epilepsy (EL) mouse

The EL mouse was developed in 1954 and is susceptible to convulsive seizures usually induced by vestibular stimulation (spinning) and is considered to portray accurately complex partial seizures with secondary generalizations [271,272]. Seizures originate in either the parietal cortex [273] or the hippocampus [274] and then generalize to other brain regions. EL mice are prone to seize in response to chemoconvulsants including PTZ [275]. The seizure susceptibility of the EL mouse is thought to involve disinhibition in the dentate gyrus via a decrease in GABA-mediated inhibition [276] and an age-dependent heightening of excitatory neurotransmission in the CA3 region of the hippocampus [277].

The spontaneous epileptic rat (SER)

The mating of the tremor rat (tm) with the zitter (zi) rat strain has resulted in the development of the SER. These rats are homozygous for both mutant genes and display spontaneous and frequent absence-like seizures, spongiform encephalography and tonic convulsions [278]. After 8 weeks of age, SER spontaneously show tonic convulsions and absence seizures characterized by low voltage fast activity and sudden ataxia with concomitant 5–7 Hz spike wave discharges in cortical and hippocampal EEG [279,280]. SER appear to have hyperexcitability in hippocampal CA3 neurones, displayed as a long-lasting depolarization shift induced by a single stimulation of mossy fibres [281]. Enhanced calcium influx in the CA3 region of the hippocampus possibly via an abnormality in the calcium ion channel is thought to contribute to epileptogenesis in these rats [282]. In vitro studies have shown that suppression of epileptiform bursting in hippocampal CA3 neurones of SER can be achieved by the application of vigabatrin [283] and topiramate [284]. The suppression of aberrant CA3 excitability by vigabatrin is mediated via GABA increase due to GABA transaminase inhibition, acting directly on $GABA_A$ receptors [283]. Topiramate exerts its anticonvulsant effects via several mechanisms, one of which involves inhibition of presynaptic excitatory neurotransmission and/or direct blockade of postsynaptic glutamate receptors in CA3 pyramidal neurones [284].

Genetically epilepsy-prone rat (GEPR)

The GEPR also displays audiogenic seizures, but also has seizures following various electrical and chemical stimuli. As with the DBA/2 J mice, the GEPR rat seizures are age dependent with increased susceptibility noted between 2 and 4 weeks postnatally. Whereas the totterer mouse strain, as previously mentioned, has heightened noradrenergic tone in the locus coeruleus, hippocampus and cerebellum, and a concomitant increase in receptor number in these regions compared to controls, GEPR have the opposite. Reduced noradrenergic drive and metabolism has been reported in the cerebellum and brainstem of GEPR. Other neurotransmitter abnormalities in the GEPR rat include a depression of brain 5HT activity [195] and an increase in cholinergic tone in the basal ganglia [285]. At present it is unclear whether these neurochemical abnormalities are directly responsible for the generation of seizure activity or merely as a consequence of the hyperactivity seen in the brain of these rats.

The genetic models allow investigators to selectively create cellular or molecular abnormalities in animals and to thereby directly assess the role that each has to play in refractory epileptic disorders. However, genetic models with reflex seizures are considered to have limited human correlates with only 5% or fewer of epileptic patients experiencing seizures in response to sensory stimulation.

In vitro models

Hippocampal brain slices offer investigators the potential to investigate and characterize the basic physiology of the neuronal circuitry involved in certain epileptic disorders. It also affords researchers the luxury of investigating the basic pharmacological properties of drugs without the hindrance of the blood–brain barrier or the confounding effects following administration of general anaesthetics. As a result, brain slice experiments have provided valuable insights into the ionic and electrophysiological mechanisms underlying the paroxysmal depolarizing shift and helped elucidate the physiological properties involved in the generation of longer epileptiform discharges, and its role in epileptogenesis. The major disadvantage of isolated brain slice or tissue culture experiments is that they cannot portray the behavioural and electronic complexities that are indicative *in vivo* of those seen in the human condition. Nevertheless epileptiform discharges induced in slice preparations can be insensitive to specific antiepileptic drugs, and have thus been proposed as a method of screening compounds that could possess anticonvulsant potential in cases of drug resistance [286].

Conclusions

Epilepsy research has advanced considerably through the study of animal models of epilepsy. This approach has led to the identification of the new generation of antiepileptic drugs. Unfortunately, the models can only go so far in providing a better understanding of the human epileptic brain.

If we are to enhance clinical management of epilepsy then we need to identify and develop novel antiepileptic drugs with more favourable pharmacological properties. Most drugs are effective in one or more models but it remains difficult to predict drug efficacy, tolerability and safety in humans by extrapolating data from animal models. In the last three decades many compounds have been found that displayed anticonvulsant properties in one or more models but subsequently failed in clinical trials. The widespread screening of compounds continues to be necessary, as we still have a poor understanding of the mechanisms underlying epilepsy and seizure generation. Indeed, the precise mechanisms underlying the efficacy of our presently available drugs remain uncertain.

Furthermore, there is little evidence that our present therapies are antiepileptogenic, independent of their ability to terminate seizures. Indeed our present drugs are developed to treat the symptom, seizures, rather than to modify the disease process [235].

References

1 Catterall WA. From ionic currents to molecular mechanisms: the structure and function of voltage-gated sodium channels. *Neuron* 2000; 26: 13–25.

2 Kuo CC. A common anticonvulsant binding site for phenytoin, carbamazepine, and lamotrigine in neuronal Na+ channels. *Mol Pharmacol* 1998; 54: 712–21.

3 Lang DG, Wang CM, Cooper BR. Lamotrigine, phenytoin and carbamazepine interactions on the sodium current present in N4TG1 mouse neuroblastoma cells. *J Pharmacol Exp Ther* 1993; 266: 829–35.

4 Ragsdale DS, McPhee JC, Scheuer T, Catterall WA. Common molecular determinants of local anesthetic, antiarrhythmic, and anticonvulsant block of voltage-gated Na+ channels. *Proc Natl Acad Sci USA* 1996; 93: 9270–5.

5 Yarov-Yarovoy V, Brown J, Sharp EM, Clare JJ, Scheuer T, Catterall WA. Molecular determinants of voltage-dependent gating and binding of pore-blocking drugs in transmembrane segment IIIS6 of the Na(+) channel alpha subunit. *J Biol Chem* 2001; 276: 20–7.

6 Kuo CC, Chen RS, Lu L, Chen RC. Carbamazepine inhibition of neuronal Na+ currents: quantitative distinction from phenytoin and possible therapeutic implications. *Mol Pharmacol* 1997; 51: 1077–83.

7 Macdonald RL, Kelly KM. Antiepileptic drug mechanisms of action. *Epilepsia 36 Suppl* 1995; 2: S2–12.

8 Kuo CC, Bean BP. Slow binding of phenytoin to inactivated sodium channels in rat hippocampal neurons. *Mol Pharmacol* 1994; 46: 716–25.

9 Lampl I, Schwindt P, Crill W. Reduction of cortical pyramidal neuron excitability by the action of phenytoin on persistent Na+ current. *J Pharmacol Exp Ther* 1998; 284: 228–37.

10 Segal MM, Douglas AF. Late sodium channel openings underlying epileptiform activity are preferentially diminished by the anticonvulsant phenytoin. *J Neurophysiol* 1997; 77: 3021–34.

11 Reckziegel G, Beck H, Schramm J, Urban BW, Elger CE. Carbamazepine effects on Na+ currents in human dentate granule cells from epileptogenic tissue. *Epilepsia* 1999; 40: 401–7.

12 Rizzi M, Caccia S, Guiso G et al. Limbic seizures induce P-glycoprotein in rodent brain: functional implications for pharmacoresistance. *J Neurosci* 2002; 22: 5833–9.

13 Loscher W, Potschka H. Role of multidrug transporters in pharmacoresistance to antiepileptic drugs. *J Pharmacol Exp Ther* 2002; 301: 7–14.

14 Sisodiya SM, Lin WR, Harding BN, Squier MV, Thom M. Drug resistance in epilepsy: expression of drug resistance proteins in common causes of refractory epilepsy. *Brain* 2002; 125: 22–31.

15 Tishler DM, Weinberg KI, Hinton DR, Barbaro N, Annett GM, Raffel C. MDR1 gene expression in brain of patients with medically intractable epilepsy. *Epilepsia* 1995; 36: 1–6.

16 McLean MJ, Schmutz M, Wamil AW, Olpe HR, Portet C, Feldmann KF. Oxcarbazepine: mechanisms of action. *Epilepsia 35 Suppl* 1994; 3: S5–S9.

17 McLean MJ, Macdonald RL. Sodium valproate, but not ethosuximide, produces use- and voltage-dependent limitation of high frequency repetitive firing of action potentials of mouse central neurons in cell culture. *J Pharmacol Exp Ther* 1986; 237: 1001–11.

18 Xie X, Dale TJ, John VH, Cater HL, Peakman TC, Clare JJ. Electrophysiological and pharmacological properties of the human brain type IIA Na+ channel expressed in a stable mammalian cell line. *Pflugers Arch* 2001; 441: 425–33.

19 Backus KH, Pflimlin P, Trube G. Action of diazepam on the voltage-dependent Na+ current. Comparison with the effects of phenytoin, carbamazepine, lidocaine and flumazenil. *Brain Res* 1991; 548: 41–9.

20 Kendig JJ. Barbiturates: active form and site of action at node of Ranvier sodium channels. *J Pharmacol Exp Ther* 1981; 218: 175–81.

21 DeLorenzo RJ, Sombati S, Coulter DA. Effects of topiramate on sustained repetitive firing and spontaneous recurrent seizure discharges in cultured hippocampal neurons. *Epilepsia* 2000; 41 Suppl 1: S40–S44.

22 McLean MJ, Bukhari AA, Wamil AW. Effects of topiramate on sodium-dependent action-potential firing by mouse spinal cord neurons in cell culture. *Epilepsia* 2000; 41 Suppl 1: S21–S24.

23 Schauf CL. Zonisamide enhances slow sodium inactivation in Myxicola. *Brain Res* 1987; 413: 185–8.

24 Catterall WA. Structure and regulation of voltage-gated Ca2+ channels. *Ann Rev Cell Dev Biol* 2000; 16: 521–55.

25 Tanabe M, Gahwiler BH, Gerber U. L-type Ca2+ channels mediate the slow Ca2+-dependent afterhyperpolarization current in rat CA3 pyramidal cells in vitro. *J Neurophysiol* 1998; 80: 2268–73.

26 Elliott EM, Malouf AT, Catterall WA. Role of calcium channel subtypes in calcium transients in hippocampal CA3 neurons. *J Neurosci* 1995; 15: 6433–44.

27 Raymond CR, Redman SJ. Different calcium sources are narrowly tuned to the induction of different forms of LTP. *J Neurophysiol* 2002; 88: 249–55.

28 Empson RM, Jefferys JGR. Ca2+ entry through type Ca2+ channels helps terminate epileptiform activity by activation of a Ca2+ dependent afterhyperpolarization in hippocampal CA3. *Neuroscience* 2001; 102: 297–306.

29 Straub H, Kohling R, Frieler A, Grigat M, Speckmann EJ. Contribution of L-type calcium channels to epileptiform activity in hippocampal and neocortical slices of guinea-pigs. *Neuroscience* 2000; 95: 63–72.

30 van Luijtelaar EL, Ates N, Coenen AM. Role of L-type calcium channel modulation in nonconvulsive epilepsy in rats. *Epilepsia* 1995; 36: 86–92.

31 Ikegaya Y, Nishiyama N, Matsuki N. L-type Ca²⁺ channel blocker inhibits mossy fiber sprouting and cognitive deficits following pilocarpine seizures in immature mice. *Neuroscience* 2000; 98: 647–59.

32 Hassan H, Grecksch G, Ruthrich H, Krug M. Effects of nicardipine, an antagonist of L-type voltage-dependent calcium channels, on kindling development, kindling-induced learning deficits and hippocampal potentiation phenomena. *Neuropharmacology* 1999; 38: 1841–50.

33 Ambrosio AF, Silva AP, Malva JO, Soares-da-Silva P, Carvalho AP, Carvalho CM. Carbamazepine inhibits L-type Ca²⁺ channels in cultured rat hippocampal neurons stimulated with glutamate receptor agonists. *Neuropharmacology* 1999; 38: 1349–59.

34 Zhang X, Velumian AA, Jones OT, Carlen PL. Modulation of high-voltage-activated calcium channels in dentate granule cells by topiramate. *Epilepsia* 2000; 41 Suppl 1: S52–S60.

35 Gross RA, Macdonald RL. Barbiturates and nifedipine have different and selective effects on calcium currents of mouse DRG neurons in culture: a possible basis for differing clinical actions. The 1987 S. Weir Mitchell award. *Neurology* 1988; 38: 443–51.

36 Wheeler DB, Randall A, Tsien RW. Roles of N-type and Q-type Ca²⁺ channels in supporting hippocampal synaptic transmission. *Science* 1994; 264: 107–11.

37 Poncer JC, McKinney RA, Gahwiler BH, Thompson SM. Either N- or P-type calcium channels mediate GABA release at distinct hippocampal inhibitory synapses. *Neuron* 1997; 18: 463–72.

38 Stefani A, Spadoni F, Siniscalchi A, Bernardi G. Lamotrigine inhibits Ca²⁺ currents in cortical neurons: functional implications. *Eur J Pharmacol* 1996; 307: 113–16.

39 Wang SJ, Huang CC, Hsu KS, Tsai JJ, Gean PW. Inhibition of N-type calcium currents by lamotrigine in rat amygdalar neurones. *Neuroreport* 1996; 7: 3037–40.

40 Lukyanetz EA, Shkryl VM, Kostyuk PG. Selective blockade of N-type calcium channels by levetiracetam. *Epilepsia* 2002; 43: 9–18.

41 Schmutz M, Brugger F, Gentsch C, McLean MJ, Olpe HR. Oxcarbazepine: preclinical anticonvulsant profile and putative mechanisms of action. *Epilepsia* 1994; 35 Suppl 5: S47–S50.

42 Stefani A, Pisani A, De Murtas M et al. Action of GP 47779: the active metabolite of oxcarbazepine, on the corticostriatal system. II. Modulation of high-voltage-activated calcium currents. *Epilepsia* 1995; 36: 997–1002.

43 Gee NS, Brown JP, Dissanayake VUK, Offord J, Thurlow R, Woodruff GN. The novel anticonvulsant drug, gabapentin (neurontin), binds to the alpha(2)[IMAGE] subunit of a calcium channel. *J Biol Chem* 1996; 271: 5768–76.

44 Alden KJ, Garcia J. Differential effect of gabapentin on neuronal and muscle calcium currents. *J Pharmacol Exp Ther* 2001; 297: 727–35.

45 Fink K, Meder W, Dooley DJ, Gothert M. Inhibition of neuronal Ca²⁺ influx by gabapentin and subsequent reduction of neurotransmitter release from rat neocortical slices. *Br J Pharmacol* 2000; 130: 900–6.

46 Fink K, Dooley DJ, Meder WP et al. Inhibition of neuronal Ca²⁺ influx by gabapentin and pregabalin in the human neocortex. *Neuropharmacology* 2002; 42: 229–36.

47 McCormick DA, Contreras D. On the cellular and network basis of epileptic seizures. *Ann Rev Physiol* 2001; 63: 815–46.

48 Coulter DA, Huguenard JR, Prince DA. Characterization of ethosuximide reduction of low-threshold calcium current in thalamic neurons. *Ann Neurol* 1989; 25: 582–93.

49 Leresche N, Parri HR, Erdemli G et al. On the action of the anti-absence drug ethosuximide in the rat and cat thalamus. *J Neurosci* 1998; 18: 4842–53.

50 Gomora JC, Daud AN, Weiergraber M, Perez-Reyes E. Block of cloned human t-type calcium channels by succinimide antiepileptic drugs. *Mol Pharmacol* 2001; 60: 1121–32.

51 Suzuki S, Kawakami K, Nishimura S et al. Zonisamide blocks T-type calcium channel in cultured neurons of rat cerebral cortex. *Epilepsy Res* 1992; 12: 21–7.

52 Todorovic SM, Lingle CJ. Pharmacological properties of T-type Ca²⁺ current in adult rat sensory neurons: effects of anticonvulsant and anesthetic agents. *J Neurophysiol* 1998; 79: 240–52.

53 Avery RB, Johnston D. Multiple channel types contribute to the low-voltage-activated calcium current in hippocampal CA3 pyramidal neurons. *J Neurosci* 1996; 16: 5567–82.

54 Yaari Y, Hamon B, Lux HD. Development of two types of calcium channels in cultured mammalian hippocampal neurons. *Science* 1987; 235: 680–2.

55 Su H, Sochivko D, Becker A et al. Upregulation of a T-type Ca²⁺ channel causes a long-lasting modification of neuronal firing mode after status epilepticus. *J Neurosci* 2002; 22: 3645–55.

56 Loscher W. Anticonvulsant and biochemical effects of inhibitors of GABA aminotransferase and valproic acid during subchronic treatment in mice. *Biochem Pharmacol* 1982; 31: 837–42.

57 McIntire SL, Reimer RJ, Schuske K, Edwards RH, Jorgensen EM. Identification and characterization of the vesicular GABA transporter. *Nature* 1997; 389: 870–6.

58 Chaudhry FA, Reimer RJ, Bellocchio EE et al. The vesicular GABA transporter, VGAT, localizes to synaptic vesicles in sets of glycinergic as well as GABAergic neurons. *J Neurosci* 1998; 18: 9733–50.

59 Bormann J. The 'ABC' of GABA receptors. *Trends Pharmacol Sci* 2000; 21: 16–19.

60 Mehta AK, Ticku MK. An update on GABAA receptors. *Brain Res Rev* 1999; 29: 196–217.

61 Bianchi MT, Haas KF, Macdonald RL. Structural determinants of fast desensitization and desensitization-deactivation coupling in GABAa receptors. *J Neurosci* 2001; 21: 1127–36.

62 Brooks KA, Shumate MD, Jin H, Rikhter TY, Coulter DA. Selective changes in single cell GABA(A) receptor subunit expression and function in temporal lobe epilepsy. *Nat Med* 1998; 4: 1166–72.

63 Macdonald RL, Olsen RW. GABA_A receptor channels. *Ann Rev Neurosci* 1994; 17: 569–602.

64 Rivera C, Voipio J, Payne JA et al. The K+/Cl– co-transporter KCC2 renders GABA hyperpolarizing during neuronal maturation. *Nature* 1999; 397: 251–5.

65 Ben-Ari Y, Tseeb V, Raggozzino D, Khazipov R, Gaiarsa JL. Gamma-aminobutyric acid (GABA): a fast excitatory transmitter which may regulate the development of hippocampal neurones in early postnatal life. *Prog Brain Res* 1994; 102: 261–73.

66 Smirnov S, Paalasmaa P, Uusisaari M, Voipio J, Kaila K. Pharmacological isolation of the synaptic and nonsynaptic components of the GABA-mediated biphasic response in rat CA1 hippocampal pyramidal cells. *J Neurosci* 1999; 19: 9252–60.

67 Herrero AI, Del Olmo N, Gonzalez-Escalada JR, Solis JM. Two new actions of topiramate: inhibition of depolarizing GABA(A)-mediated responses and activation of a potassium conductance. *Neuropharmacology* 2002; 42: 210–20.

68 McKernan RM, Rosahl TW, Reynolds DS et al. Sedative but not anxiolytic properties of benzodiazepines are mediated by the GABA(A) receptor alpha1 subtype. *Nat Neurosci* 2000; 3: 587–92.

69 Crestani F, Martin JR, Mohler H, Rudolph U. Mechanism of action of the hypnotic zolpidem in vivo. *Br J Pharmacol* 2000; 131: 1251–4.

70 Study RE, Barker JL. Diazepam and (–)-pentobarbital: fluctuation analysis reveals different mechanisms for potentiation of gamma-aminobutyric acid responses in cultured central neurons. *Proc Natl Acad Sci USA* 1981; 78: 7180–4.

71 Rogers CJ, Twyman RE, Macdonald RL. Benzodiazepine and beta-carboline regulation of single GABAA receptor channels of mouse spinal neurones in culture. *J Physiol* 1994; 475: 69–82.

72 Eghbali M, Curmi JP, Birnir B, Gage PW. Hippocampal GABA(A) channel conductance increased by diazepam. *Nature* 1997; 388: 71–5.

73 Twyman RE, Rogers CJ, Macdonald RL. Differential regulation of gamma-aminobutyric acid receptor channels by diazepam and phenobarbital. *Ann Neurol* 1989; 25: 213–20.

74 White HS, Brown SD, Woodhead JH, Skeen GA, Wolf HH. Topiramate modulates GABA-evoked currents in murine cortical neurons by a non-benzodiazepine mechanism. *Epilepsia* 2000; 41 Suppl 1: S17–S20.

75 Reddy DS, Rogawski MA. Enhanced anticonvulsant activity of neuroactive steroids in a rat model of catamenial epilepsy. *Epilepsia* 2001; 42: 337–44.

76 Monaghan EP, Navalta LA, Shum L, Ashbrook DW, Lee DA. Initial

human experience with ganaxolone, a neuroactive steroid with antiepileptic activity. *Epilepsia* 1997; 38: 1026–31.

77 Velazquez JL, Carlen PL. Synchronization of GABAergic interneuronal networks during seizure-like activity in the rat horizontal hippocampal slice. *Eur J Neurosci* 1999; 11: 4110–18.

78 Kohling R, Vreugdenhil M, Bracci E, Jefferys JG. Ictal epileptiform activity is facilitated by hippocampal GABAA receptor-mediated oscillations. *J Neurosci* 2000; 20: 6820–9.

79 Danober L, Deransart C, Depaulis A, Vergnes M, Marescaux C. Pathophysiological mechanisms of genetic absence epilepsy in the rat. *Prog Neurobiol* 1998; 55: 27–57.

80 Crunelli V, Leresche N. Childhood absence epilepsy: genes, channels, neurons and networks. *Nat Rev Neurosci* 2002; 3: 371–82.

81 Huguenard JR. Neuronal circuitry of thalamocortical epilepsy and mechanisms of antiabsence drug action. *Adv Neurol* 1999; 79: 991–9.

82 Browne SH, Kang J, Akk G *et al*. Kinetic and pharmacological properties of GABAA receptors in single thalamic neurons and GABAA subunit expression. *J Neurophysiol* 2001; 86: 2312–22.

83 Snead OCI. Ganaxolone, a selective high-affinity steroid modulator of the alpha-aminobutyric acid-A receptor, exacerbates seizures in animal models of absence. *Ann Neurol* 1998; 44: 688–91.

84 Couve A, Moss SJ, Pangalos MN. GABAB receptors: a new paradigm in G protein signaling. *Mol Cell Neurosci* 2000; 16: 296–312.

85 Mott DD, Lewis DV. The pharmacology and function of central GABAB receptors. *Int Rev Neurobiol* 1994; 36: 97–223.

86 Scanziani M. GABA spillover activates postsynaptic GABA(B) receptors to control rhythmic hippocampal activity. *Neuron* 2000; 25: 673–81.

87 von Krosigk M, Bal T, McCormick DA. Cellular mechanisms of a synchronized oscillation in the thalamus. *Science* 1993; 261: 361–4.

88 Vergnes M, Boehrer A, Simler S, Bernasconi R, Marescaux C. Opposite effects of GABAB receptor antagonists on absences and convulsive seizures. *Eur J Pharmacol* 1997; 332: 245–55.

90 Jolkkonen J, Mazurkiewicz M, Lahtinen H, Riekkinen P. Acute effects of gamma-vinyl GABA on the GABAergic system in rats as studied by microdialysis. *Eur J Pharmacol* 1992; 229: 269–72.

91 Borden LA. GABA transporter heterogeneity: pharmacology and cellular localization. *Neurochem Int* 1996; 29: 335–6.

92 Bernstein EM, Quick MW. Regulation of gamma-aminobutyric acid (GABA) transporters by extracellular GABA. *J Biol Chem* 1999; 274: 889–95.

93 Law RM, Stafford A, Quick MW. Functional regulation of gamma-aminobutyric acid transporters by direct tyrosine phosphorylation. *J Biol Chem* 2000; 275: 23986–91.

94 Beckman ML, Bernstein EM, Quick MW. Multiple G protein-coupled receptors initiate protein kinase C redistribution of GABA transporters in hippocampal neurons. *J Neurosci* 1999; 19: RC9.

95 Quick MW, Corey JL, Davidson N, Lester HA. Second messengers, trafficking-related proteins, and amino acid residues that contribute to the functional regulation of the rat brain GABA transporter GAT1. *J Neurosci* 1997; 17: 2967–79.

96 Horton RW, Collins JF, Anlezark GM, Meldrum BS. Convulsant and anticonvulsant actions in DBA/2 mice of compounds blocking the reuptake of GABA. *Eur J Pharmacol* 1979; 59: 75–83.

97 Croucher MJ, Meldrum BS, Krogsgaard-Larsen P. Anticonvulsant activity of GABA uptake inhibitors and their prodrugs following central or systemic administration. *Eur J Pharmacol* 1983; 89: 217–28.

98 Ali FE, Bondinell WE, Dandridge PA *et al*. Orally active and potent inhibitors of gamma-aminobutyric acid uptake. *J Med Chem* 1985; 28: 653–60.

99 Borden LA, Murali DT, Smith KE, Weinshank RL, Branchek TA, Gluchowski C. Tiagabine, SK & F 89976-A, CI-966: and NNC-711 are selective for the cloned GABA transporter GAT-1. *Eur J Pharmacol* 1994; 269: 219–24.

100 Braestrup C, Nielsen EB, Sonnewald U *et al*. R-N-[4,4-bis(3-methyl-2-thienyl)but-3-en-1-yl]nipecotic acid binds with high affinity to the brain gamma-aminobutyric acid uptake carrier. *J Neurochem* 1990; 54: 639–47.

101 Andersen KE, Braestrup C, Gronwald FC *et al*. The synthesis of novel GABA uptake inhibitors. 1. Elucidation of the structure-activity studies leading to the choice of R-1-[4,4-bis(3-methyl-2-thienyl)-3-butenyl]-3-

102 piperidinecarboxylic acid (tiagabine) as an anticonvulsant drug candidate. *J Med Chem* 1993; 36: 1716–25.

102 Dalby NO. GABA-level increasing and anticonvulsant effects of three different GABA uptake inhibitors. *Neuropharmacology* 2000; 39: 2399–407.

103 Fink-Jensen A, Suzdak PD, Swedberg MD, Judge ME, Hansen L, Nielsen PG. The gamma-aminobutyric acid (GABA) uptake inhibitor, tiagabine, increases extracellular brain levels of GABA in awake rats. *Eur J Pharmacol* 1992; 220: 197–201.

104 Ipponi A, Lamberti C, Medica A, Bartolini A, Malmberg-Aiello P. Tiagabine antinociception in rodents depends on GABA(B) receptor activation: parallel antinociception testing and medial thalamus GABA microdialysis. *Eur J Pharmacol* 1999; 368: 205–11.

105 Richards DA, Bowery NG. Comparative effects of the GABA uptake inhibitors, tiagabine and NNC-711: on extracellular GABA levels in the rat ventrolateral thalamus. *Neurochem Res* 1996; 21: 135–40.

106 Sills GJ, Butler E, Thompson GG, Brodie MJ. Vigabatrin and tiagabine are pharmacologically different drugs. A pre-clinical study. *Seizure* 1999; 8: 404–11.

107 Sills GJ, Patsalos PN, Butler E, Forrest G, Ratnaraj N, Brodie MJ. Visual field constriction: Accumulation of vigabatrin but not tiagabine in the retina. *Neurology* 2001; 57: 196–200.

108 Saxena NC, Macdonald RL. Assembly of GABAA receptor subunits: role of the delta subunit. *J Neurosci* 1994; 14: 7077–86.

109 Nusser Z, Sieghart W, Somogyi P. Segregation of different GABAA receptors to synaptic and extrasynaptic membranes of cerebellar granule cells. *J Neurosci* 1998; 18: 1693–703.

110 Brickley SG, Cull CS, Farrant M. Development of a tonic form of synaptic inhibition in rat cerebellar granule cells resulting from persistent activation of GABAA receptors. *J Physiol Lond* 1996; 497: 753–9.

111 Brickley SG, Revilla V, Cull-Candy SG, Wisden W, Farrant M. Adaptive regulation of neuronal excitability by a voltage-independent potassium conductance. *Nature* 2001; 409: 88–92.

112 Overstreet LS, Westbrook GL. Paradoxical reduction of synaptic inhibition by vigabatrin. *J Neurophysiol* 2001; 86: 596–603.

113 Nusser Z, Mody I. Selective modulation of tonic and phasic inhibitions in dentate gyrus granule cells. *J Neurophysiol* 2002; 87: 2624 8.

114 Bianchi MT, Haas KF, Macdonald RL. Structural determinants of fast desensitization and desensitization-deactivation coupling in GABAa receptors. *J Neurosci* 2001; 21: 1127–36.

115 Draguhn A, Heinemann U. Different mechanisms regulate IPSC kinetics in early postnatal and juvenile hippocampal granule cells. *J Neurophysiol* 1996; 76: 3983–93.

116 Engel D, Schmitz D, Gloveli T, Frahm C, Heinemann U, Draguhn A. Laminar difference in GABA uptake and GAT-1 expression in rat CA1. *J Physiol 512* (Pt 3), 1998; 643–9.

117 Nusser Z, Naylor D, Mody I. Synapse-specific contribution of the variation of transmitter concentration to the decay of inhibitory postsynaptic currents. *Biophys J* 2001; 80: 1251–61.

118 Williams SR, Buhl EH, Mody I. The dynamics of synchronized neurotransmitter release determined from compound spontaneous IPSCs in rat dentate granule neurones in vitro. *J Physiol* 1998; 510 (Pt 2): 477–97.

119 Isaacson JS, Solis JM, Nicoll RA. Local and diffuse synaptic actions of GABA in the hippocampus. *Neuron* 1993; 10: 165–75.

120 Dingledine R, Korn SJ. Gamma-aminobutyric acid uptake and the termination of inhibitory synaptic potentials in the rat hippocampal slice. *J Physiol* 1985; 366: 387–409.

121 Roepstorff A, Lambert JD. Factors contributing to the decay of the stimulus-evoked IPSC in rat hippocampal CA1 neurons. *J Neurophysiol* 1994; 72: 2911–26.

122 Thompson SM, Gahwiler BH. Effects of the GABA uptake inhibitor tiagabine on inhibitory synaptic potentials in rat hippocampal slice cultures. *J Neurophysiol* 1992; 67: 1698–701.

123 Rossi DJ, Hamann M. Spillover-mediated transmission at inhibitory synapses promoted by high affinity alpha6 subunit GABA(A) receptors and glomerular geometry. *Neuron* 1998; 20: 783–95.

124 Overstreet LS, Jones MV, Westbrook GL. Slow desensitization regulates the availability of synaptic GABA(A) receptors. *J Neurosci* 2000; 20: 7914–21.

125 Otis TS, Mody I. Differential activation of GABAA and GABAB receptors

by spontaneously released transmitter. *J Neurophysiol* 1992; 67: 227–35.

126 Richards DA, Lemos T, Whitton PS, Bowery NG. Extracellular GABA in the ventrolateral thalamus of rats exhibiting spontaneous absence epilepsy: a microdialysis study. *J Neurochem* 1995; 65: 1674–80.

127 Sutch RJ, Davies CC, Bowery NG. GABA release and uptake measured in crude synaptosomes from Genetic Absence Epilepsy Rats from Strasbourg (GAERS). *Neurochem Int* 1999; 34: 415–25.

128 Coenen AM, Blezer EH, van Luijtelaar EL. Effects of the GABA-uptake inhibitor tiagabine on electroencephalogram, spike-wave discharges and behaviour of rats. *Epilepsy Res* 1995; 21: 89–94.

129 Hosford DA, Wang Y. Utility of the lethargic (lh/lh) mouse model of absence seizures in predicting the effects of lamotrigine, vigabatrin, tiagabine, gabapentin, and topiramate against human absence seizures. *Epilepsia* 1997; 38: 408–14.

130 Kovacs I, Szarics E, Nyitrai G, Blandl T, Kardos J. Matching kinetics of synaptic vesicle recycling and enhanced neurotransmitter influx by Ca^{2+} in brain plasma membrane vesicles. *Neurochem Int* 1998; 33: 399–405.

131 Jackson MF, Esplin B, Capek R. Activity-dependent enhancement of hyperpolarizing and depolarizing gamma-aminobutyric acid (GABA) synaptic responses following inhibition of GABA uptake by tiagabine. *Epilepsy Res* 1999; 37: 25–36.

132 Jackson MF, Esplin B, Capek R. Inhibitory nature of tiagabine-augmented GABAA receptor-mediated depolarizing responses in hippocampal pyramidal cells. *J Neurophysiol* 1999; 81: 1192–8.

133 McGeer PL, Eccles JC, McGeer EG, eds. *Molecular Neurobiology of the Mammalian Brain*, 2nd edn. New York: Plenum Press, 1987: 175–96.

134 Hassel B, Johannessen CU, Sonnewald U, Fonnum F. Quantification of the GABA shunt and the importance of the GABA shunt versus the 2-oxoglutarate dehydrogenase pathway in GABAergic neurons. *J Neurochem* 1998; 71: 1511–18.

135 Staley KJ, Longacher M, Bains JS, Yee A. Presynaptic modulation of CA3 network activity. *Nat Neurosci* 1998; 1: 201–9.

136 Lerma J, Herranz AS, Herreras O, Abraira V, Martin del Rio R. In vitro determination of extracellular concentration of amino acids in the rat hippocampus. A method based on brain dialysis and computerizd analysis. *Brain Res* 1986; 384: 145–55.

137 Hollman M, Heinemann S. Cloned glutamate receptors. *Annu Rev Neurosci* 1994; 17: 31–108.

138 Patneau DK, Mayer ML. Structure–activity relationships for amino acid transmitter candidates acting at the N-methyl-D-aspartate and quisqualate receptors. *J Neurosci* 1990; 10: 2385–99.

139 Gibbs JW, III, Sombati S, DeLorenzo RJ, Coulter DA. Cellular actions of topiramate: blockade of kainate-evoked inward currents in cultured hippocampal neurons. *Epilepsia* 2000; 41 Suppl 1: S10–S16.

140 Chappell AS, Sander JW, Brodie MJ *et al*. A crossover, add-on trial of talampanel in patients with refractory partial seizures. *Neurology* 2002; 58: 1680–2.

141 Kullmann DM. Presynaptic kainate receptors in the hippocampus: slowly emerging from obscurity. *Neuron* 2001; 32: 561–4.

142 Semyanov A, Kullmann DM. Kainate receptor-dependent axonal depolarization and action potential initiation in interneurons. *Nat Neurosci* 2001; 4: 718–23.

143 Ben Ari Y, Cossart R. Kainate, a double agent that generates seizures: two decades of progress. *Trends Neurosci* 2000; 23: 580–7.

144 Smolders I, Bortolotto ZA, Clarke VR *et al*. Antagonists of GLU(K5)-containing kainate receptors prevent pilocarpine-induced limbic seizures. *Nat Neurosci* 2002; 5: 796–804.

145 Khalilov I, Hirsch J, Cossart R, Ben Ari Y. Paradoxical anti-epileptic effects of a GluR5 agonist of kainate receptors. *J Neurophysiol* 2002; 88: 523–7.

146 Cull-Candy S, Brickley S, Farrant M. NMDA receptor subunits: diversity, development and disease. *Curr Opin Neurobiol* 2001; 11: 327–35.

147 Edmonds B, Gibb AJ, Colquhoun D. Mechanisms of action of glutamate receptors and the time course of excitatory synaptic currents. *Annu Rev Physiol* 1995; 57: 495–519.

148 White HS, Harmsworth WL, Sofia RD, Wolf HH. Felbamate modulates the strychnine-insensitive glycine receptor. *Epilepsy Res* 1995; 20: 41–8.

149 Subramaniam S, Donevan SD, Rogawski MA. Block of the N-methyl-D-aspartate receptor by remacemide and its des-glycine metabolite. *J Pharmacol Exp Ther* 1996; 276: 161–8.

150 Rusakov DA, Kullmann DM. Extrasynaptic glutamate diffusion in the hippocampus: ultrastructural constraints, uptake, and receptor activation. *J Neurosci* 1998; 18: 3158–70.

151 De Blasi A, Conn PJ, Pin J, Nicoletti F. Molecular determinants of metabotropic glutamate receptor signaling. *Trends Pharmacol Sci* 2001; 22: 114–20.

152 Chapman AG, Nanan K, Williams M, Meldrum BS. Anticonvulsant activity of two metabotropic glutamate group I antagonists selective for the mGlu5 receptor: 2-methyl-6-(phenylethynyl)-pyridine (MPEP), and (E)-6-methyl-2-styryl-pyridine (SIB 1893). *Neuropharmacology* 2000; 39: 1567–74.

153 Abdul-Ghani AS, Attwell PJ, Singh KN, Bradford HF, Croucher MJ, Jane DE. Anti-epileptogenic and anticonvulsant activity of L-2-amino-4-phosphonobutyrate, a presynaptic glutamate receptor agonist. *Brain Res* 1997; 755: 202–12.

154 Attwell PJ, Singh KN, Jane DE, Croucher MJ, Bradford HF. Anticonvulsant and glutamate release-inhibiting properties of the highly potent metabotropic glutamate receptor agonist (2S, 2′R, 3′R)-2-(2′, 3′-dicarboxycyclopropyl)glycine (DCG-IV). *Brain Res* 1998; 805: 138–43.

155 Chapman AG, Talebi A, Yip PK, Meldrum BS. Anticonvulsant activity of a mGlu(4alpha) receptor selective agonist (1S, 3R, 4S)-1-aminocyclopentane-1:2:4-tricarboxylic acid. *Eur J Pharmacol* 2001; 424: 107–13.

156 Moldrich RX, Jeffrey M, Talebi A, Beart PM, Chapman AG, Meldrum BS. Anti-epileptic activity of group II metabotropic glutamate receptor agonists (−)-2-oxa-4-aminobicyclo[3.1.0]hexane-4,6-dicarboxylate (LY379268) and (−)-2-thia-4-aminobicyclo[3.1.0]hexane-4,6-dicarboxylate (LY389795). *Neuropharmacology* 2001; 41: 8–18.

157 Jan LY, Jan YN. Cloned potassium channels from eukaryotes and prokaryotes. *Ann Rev Neurosci* 1997; 20: 91–123.

158 Nobile M, Lagostena L. A discriminant block among K+ channel types by phenytoin in neuroblastoma cells. *Br J Pharmacol* 1998; 124: 1698–702.

159 Freiman TM, Kukolja J, Heinemeyer J *et al*. Modulation of K+-evoked [3H]-noradrenaline release from rat and human brain slices by gabapentin: involvement of KATP channels. *Naunyn Schmiedebergs Arch Pharmacol* 2001; 363: 537–42.

160 Main MJ, Cryan JE, Dupere JR, Cox B, Clare JJ, Burbidge SA. Modulation of KCNQ2/3 potassium channels by the novel anticonvulsant retigabine. *Mol Pharmacol* 2000; 58: 253–62.

161 Rundfeldt C. The new anticonvulsant retigabine (D-23129) acts as an opener of K+ channels in neuronal cells. *Eur J Pharmacol* 1997; 336: 243–9.

162 Rundfeldt C, Netzer R. The novel anticonvulsant retigabine activates M-currents in Chinese hamster ovary-cells transfected with human KCNQ2/3 subunits. *Neurosci Lett* 2000; 282: 73–6.

163 Tatulian L, Delmas P, Abogadie FC, Brown DA. Activation of expressed KCNQ potassium currents and native neuronal M-type potassium currents by the anti-convulsant drug retigabine. *J Neurosci* 2001; 21: 5535–45.

164 Poolos NP, Migliore M, Johnston D. Pharmacological upregulation of h-channels reduces the excitability of pyramidal neuron dendrites. *Nat Neurosci* 2002; 5: 767–74.

165 Luthi A, McCormick DA. Periodicity of thalamic synchronized oscillations: the role of Ca2+-mediated upregulation of Ih. *Neuron* 1998; 20: 553–63.

166 Naffah-Mazzacoratti MG, Amado D, Cukiert A *et al*. Monoamines and their metabolites in cerebrospinal fluid and temporal cortex of epileptic patients. *Epilepsy Res* 1996; 25(2): 133–7.

167 Racine RJ. Modification of seizure activity by electrical stimulation: II. Motor seizure. Electroenceph. *Clin Neurophysiol* 1972; 32: 281–94.

168 Corcoran ME. Characteristics of accelerated kindling after depletion of noradrenaline in adult rats. *Neuropharmacology* 1988; 27: 1081–4.

169 Bentue-Ferrer P, Bellisant E, Decombe R, Allain H. Temporal profile of aminergic neurotransmitter release in striatal dialysates in rats with post-ischaemic seizures. *Exp Brain Res* 1994; 437: 437–43.

170 Shouse MN, Langer J, Bier MJ *et al*. The alpha 2-adrenergic agonist clonidine suppresses seizures whereas the alpha 2-adrenergic antagonist ida-

zoxan promotes seizures in amygdala-kindled kittens: a comparison of amygdala and pontine microinfusion effects. *Epilepsia* 1996; 37: 709–17.

171 Bjorkland A, Lindvall O. Grafts of locus coeruleus in rat amygdala-piriform cortex suppress seizure development in hippocampal kindling. *Exp Neurol* 1989; 106: 125–32.

172 Yan QS, Jobe PC, Dailey JW. Further evidence of anticonvulsant role for 5-hydroxytryptamine in genetically epilepsy-prone rats. *Br J Pharmacol* 1995; 115: 1314–18.

173 Dailey JW, Reith ME, Yan QS, Li MY, Jobe PC. Carbamazepine increases extracellular serotonin: lack of antagonism by tetrodotoxin or zero Ca^{2+}. *Eur J Pharm* 1997; 328: 153–62.

174 Starr MS. The role of dopamine in epilepsy. *Synapse* 1996; 22: 159–94.

175 Okubo Y, Suhara T, Suzuki K *et al.* Decreased prefrontal dopamine D1 receptors in schizophrenia revealed by PET. *Nature* 1997; 385 6617: 634–6.

176 Ferron A, Thierry AM, LeDouarin C, Glowinski J. Inhibitory influence of the mesocortical dopamine system on spontaneous activity or excitatory response induced from the thalamic mediodorsal nucleus in the rat medial prefrontal cortex. *Brain Res* 1984; 302: 257–65.

177 Williams GV, Goldman-Rakic PS. Modulation of memory fields by dopamine D1 receptors in prefrontal cortex. *Nature* 1995; 376: 572–5.

178 Thierry AM, LeDouarin C, Penit J, Ferron A, Glowinski J. Variation in the ability of neuroleptics to block the inhibitory influence 1986.

179 Zhou F-M, Hablitz JJ. Dopamine modulation of membrane and synaptic properties of interneurons in rat cerebral cortex. *J Neurophysiol* 1999; 81: 967–76.

180 McIntyre DC, Edson N. Kindling-based status epilepticus: effect of norepinephrine depletion with 6-hydroxydopamine. *Exp Neurol* 1989; 77: 700–4.

181 Libet B, Gleason CA, Wright EW, Feinstein B. Suppression of an epileptiform type of electrocortical activity in the rat by stimulation in the vicinity of the locus coeruleus. *Epilepsia* 1977; 18: 451–62.

182 Kokaia M, Cenci MA, Elmer E, Nilsson OG, Kokai K, Bengzon J. Seizure development and noradrenergic release in kindling epilepsy after noradrenergic reinervation of the subcortically deafferented hippocampus by superior cervical ganglion or fetal locus coeruleus grafts. *Exp Neurol* 1994; 130: 351–61.

183 Olpe HR, Jones RS. The action of anticonvulsant drugs on the firing of locus coeruleus neurons: selective, activating effect of carbamazepine. *Eur J Pharmacol* 1983; 91: 107–10.

184 Baf MH, Subhash NM, Lakshmane KM, Roa BS. Alterations in monoamine levels in discrete regions of rat brain after chronic administration of carbamazepine. *Neurochem Res* 1994; 19: 1139–43.

185 Baf MH, Subhash NM, Lakshmane KM, Roa BS. Sodium valproate induced alterations in monoamine levels in different regions of the rat brain. *Neurochem Int* 1994; 24: 67–72.

186 Hoyer D, Clarke DE, Fozard JR *et al.* International Union of Pharmacology classification of receptors for 5-hydroxytryptamine (serotonin). *Pharmacol Rev* 1994; 46: 157–203.

187 Torres GE, Holt IL, Andrade R. Antagonists of 5HT4 receptor-mediated responses in adult hippocampal neurons. *J Pharm Exp Ther* 1994; 271: 255–61.

188 Moore RY, Halaris AE. Hippocampal innervation by serotonin neurons of the midbrain raphe in the rat. *J Comp Neurol* 1975; 164: 171–84.

189 Van den Hoof P, Galvin M. Electrophysiology of the 5HT1A ligand MDL 73005EF in the rat hippocampal slice. *Eur J Pharmacol* 1991; 196: 291–8.

190 Schmitz D, Empson RM, Heinemann U. Serotonin reduces inhibition via 5HT1A receptors in area CA1 of rat hippocampal slices in vitro. *J Neurosci* 1995; 15: 7217–25.

191 Ropert N, Guy N. Serotonin facilitates gabaergic transmission in the CA1 region of rat hippocampus in vitro. *J Physiol* 1991; 441: 121–36.

192 Wada Y, Nakamura M, Hasegawa H, Yamaguchi N. Role of serotonin receptor subtype in seizures kindled from the feline hippocampus. *Neurosci Lett* 1992; 141: 21–4.

193 Lazarova M, Bendotti C, Samanin R. Studies on the role of serotonin in different regions of the rat central nervous system on pentlyenetetrazole-induced seizures and the effect of di-n-propylacetate. *Naunyn-Schmiedebergs Arch Pharmacol* 1983; 322: 147–52.

194 Jobe PC, Picchioni AL, Chin L. Role of brain 5-hydroxytryptamine in audiogenic seizures in the rat. *Life Sci* 1973; 13: 1–13.

195 Dailey JW, Mishra PK, Ko KH, Penny JE, Jobe PC. Serotonergic abnormalities in the central nervous system of seizure-naive genetically epilepsy-prone rats. *Life Sci* 1992; 50(4): 319–26.

196 Biggs CS, Pearce BR, Fowler LJ, Whitton PS. Regional effects of sodium valproate on extracellular concentrations of 5-hydroxytryptamine, dopamine, and their metabolites in the rat brain: an in vivo microdialysis study. *J Neurochem* 1992; 59(5): 1702–8.

197 Okada M, Kaneko S, Hirano T *et al.* Effects of zonisamide on extracellular levels of monoamine and its metabolite, and on Ca^{2+} dependent dopamine release. *Epilepsy Res* 1992; 13(2): 113–19.

198 Southam E, Kirkby D, Higgins GA, Hagan RM. Lamotrigine inhibits monoamine uptake in vitro and modulates 5-hydroxytryptamine uptake in rats. *Eur J Pharm* 1998; 358: 19–24.

199 McLean M, MacDonald RL. Carbamazepine and 10,11 epoxycarbamazepine produces use- and voltage-dependent limitation of high frequency repetitive firing of action potentials of mouse central neurons in cell culture. *J Pharmacol Exp Ther* 1986; 238(2): 727–38.

200 Rock DM, MacDonald RL, Taylor CP. Blockade of sustained repetitive action potentials in cultured spinal cord neurons by zonisamide (AD 810: CI 912) a novel anticonvulsant. *Epilepsy Res* 1989; 3(2): 138–43.

201 Van den Berg RJ, Kok P, Voskuyl RA. Valproate and sodium currents in cultured hippocampal neurons. *Exp Brain Res* 1993; 93(2): 279–87.

202 Sudha S, Lakshmana MK, Pradhan N. Chronic phenytoin induced impairment of learning and memory with associated changes in brain acetylcholine esterase and monoamine levels. *Pharmacol Biochem Behav* 1995; 52(1): 119–24.

203 Okada M, Kawata Y, Kiryu K *et al.* Effects of non-toxic and toxic concentrations on phenytoin on monoamines levels in rat brain. *Epilepsy Res* 1997a; 28(2): 155–63.

204 Okada M, Kawata Y, Mizuno K *et al.* Interaction between Ca^{2+}, K^+, carbamazepine and zonisamide on hippocampal extracellular glutamate monitored with a microdialysis electrode. *Br J Pharmacol* 1998; 124(6): 1277–85.

205 Okada M, Kaneko S, Hirano T *et al.* Effects of zonisamide on dopaminergic system. *Epilepsy Res* 1995; 22(3): 193–205.

206 Okada M, Hirano T, Mizuno K *et al.* Biphasic effects of carbamazepine on the dopaminergic system in rat striatum and hippocampus. *Epilepsy Res* 1997; 28(2): 143–53.

207 Dailey JW, Reith ME, Steidley KR, Milbrandt JC, Jobe PC. Carbamazepine-induced release of serotonin from rat hippocampus in vitro. *Epilepsia* 1998; 39(10): 1054–63.

208 Nagamoto I, Akasaki Y, Uchida M *et al.* Effects of combined administration of zonisamide and valproic acid or phenytoin to nitric oxide production, monoamines and zonisamide concentrations in the brain of seizure-susceptible EL mice. *Brain Res Bull* 2000; 52(2): 211–18.

209 Kimura M, Tanaka N, Kimura Y, Miyake K, Kitaura T, Fukuchi H. Pharmacokinetic interaction of zonisamide in rats. Effect of zonisamide on other antiepileptics. *Biol Pharm Bull* 1993; 16(7): 722–5.

210 Manjarrez J, Alvarado R, Camacho-Arroyo I. Differential effects of NMDA antagonist micro-injections into the nucleus reticularis pontis caudalis on seizures induced by pentylene-tetrazol in the rat. *Epilepsy Res* 200; 46: 39–44.

211 Wasterlain CG, Liu H, Mazarati AM *et al.* Self-sustaining status epilepticus: a condition.

212 Loscher W. Pharmacology of glutamate receptor antagonists in the kindling model of epilepsy. *Prog Neurobiol* 1998; 54: 721–41.

213 Sveinbjornsdottir S, Sander JW, Upton D *et al.* The excitatory amino acid D-CPP-ene (SDZ EAA-494) in patients with epilepsy. *Epilepsy Res* 1993; 16: 165–74.

214 Löscher W, Schmidt D. Strategies in antiepileptic drug development: is rational drug design superior to random screening and structural variation? *Epilepsy Res* 1994; 17: 95–134.

215 Löscher W. Animal models of intractable epilepsy. *Prog Neurobiol* 1997; 53: 239–58.

216 Klitgaard H, Matagne A, Gobert J, Wulfert E. Evidence for a unique profile of levetiracetam in rodent models of seizures and epilepsy. *Eur J Pharmacol* 1998; 353(2–3): 191–206.

217 Klitgaard H. Levetiracetam: the preclinical profile of a new class of antiepileptic drugs? *Epilepsia* 2001; 42 Suppl 4: 13–18.

218 Gower AJ, Noyer M, Verloes R, Gobert J, Wulfert E. ucb L059, a novel anti-convulsant drug: pharmacological profile in animals. *Eur J Pharmacol* 1992; 222(2–3): 193–203.

219 Löscher W, Hönack D. Profile of ucb L059, a novel anticonvulsant drug, in models of partial and generalised epilepsy in mice and rats. *Eur J Pharmacol* 1993; 232(2–3): 147–58.

220 White HS. Clinical significance of animal seizure models and mechanisms of action studies of potential antiepileptic drugs. *Epilepsia* 1997; 38(suppl.1): s9–s17.

221 de Feo MR, Mecarelli O, Ricci GF. Bicuculline- and allylglycine-induced epilepsy in developing rats. *Exp Neurol* 1985; 90: 411–21.

222 Baram TZ, Snead OC, Bicuculline induced seizures in infant rats: ontogeny of behavioral and electrocortical phenomena. *Brain Res Dev Brain Res* 1990; 57: 291–5.

223 Barton ME, Klein BD, Wolf HH, White S. Pharmacological characterization of the 6 Hz psychomotor seizure model of partial epilepsy. *Epilepsy Res* 2001; 47: 217–27.

224 Brown WC, Schiffman DO, Swinyard EA, Goodman LS. Comparative assay of antiepileptic drugs by 'psychomotor' seizure test and minimal electroshock threshold test. *J Pharmacol Exp Ther* 1953; 107: 273–83.

225 Racine R, Coscina DV. Effects of midbrain raphe lesions or systemic p-chlorophenylalanine on the development of kindled seizures in rats. *Brain Res Bull* 1979; 4(1): 1–7.

226 Silver JM, Shin C, McNamara JO. Antiepileptogenic effects of conventional anticonvulsants in the kindling model of epilespy. *Ann Neurol* 1991; 29: 356–63.

227 Wada JA, Osawa T, Sato M, Wake A, Corcoran ME, Troupin AS. Acute anticonvulsant effects of diphenylhydantoin, phenobarbital, and carbamazepine: a combined electroclinical and serum level study in amygdaloid kindled cats and baboons. *Epilepsia* 1976; 17: 77–88.

228 Turner IM, Newman SM, Louis S, Kutt H. Pharmacological prophylaxis against the development of kindled amygdaloid seizures. *Ann Neurol* 1977; 2: 221–4.

229 Amano K, Hamada K, Yagi K, Seino M. Antiepileptic effects of topiramate on amygdaloid kindling in rats. *Epilepsy Res* 1998; 31: 123–8.

230 Wauquier A, Zhou S. Topiramate: a potent anticonvulsant in the amygdala-kindled rat. *Epilepsy Res* 1996; 24: 73–7.

231 Morimoto K, Sato H, Yamamoto Y, Watanabe T, Suwaki H. Antiepileptic effects of tiagabine, a selective GABA uptake inhibitor, in the rat kindling model of temporal lobe epilepsy. *Epilepsia* 1997; 38: 966–74.

232 Postma T, Krupp E, Li XL, Post RM, Weiss SR. Lamotrigine treatment during amygdala-kindled seizure development fails to inhibit seizures and diminishes subsequent anticonvulsant efficacy. *Epilepsia* 2000; 41: 1514–21.

233 Loscher W, Honack D, Rundfeldt C. Antiepileptogenic effects of the novel anticonvulsant levetiracetam (ucb L059) in the kindling model of temporal lobe epilepsy. *J Pharmacol Exp Ther* 1998; 284: 474–9.

234 Leviel V, Naquet R. A study of the action of valproic acid on the kindling effect. *Epilepsia* 1977; 18: 229–34.

235 Walker MC, White HS, Sander JW. Disease modification in partial epilepsy. *Brain.* 2002; 125: 1937–50.

236 Walton NY, Treiman DM. Response of status epilepticus induced by lithium and pilocarpine to treatment with diazepam. *Exp Neurol* 1988; 101(2): 267–75.

237 Turski WA, Cavalheiro EA, Schwartz M, Czuczwar SJ, Kleinrok Z, Turski L. Limbic seizures produced by pilocarpine in rats: behavioural, electroencephalographic and neuropathological study. *Behav Brain Res* 1983; 9(3): 315–35.

238 Leite JP, Cavalheiro EA. Effects of conventional antiepileptic drugs in a model of spontaneous recurrent seizures in rats. *Epilepsy Res* 1995; 20(2): 93–104.

239 Sloviter RS. Possible functional consequences of synaptic reorganization in the dentate gyrus of kainate-treated rats. *Neurosci Lett* 1992; 137(1): 91–6.

240 Sperk G. Kainic acid seizures in the rat. *Prog Neurobiol* 1994; 42(1): 1–32.

241 Priel MR, dos Santos NF, Cavalheiro EA. Developmental aspects of the pilocarpine model of epilepsy. *Epilepsy Res* 1996; 26: 115–21.

242 De Bruin VM, Marinho MM, De Sousa FC, Viana GS. Behavioural and neurochemical alterations after lithium-pilocarpine administration in young and adult rats: a comparative study. *Pharmacol Biochem Behav* 2000; 65(3): 547–51.

243 Wozniak DF, Stewart GR, Miller JP, Olney JW. Age-related sensitivity to kainate neurotoxicity. *Exp Neurol* 1991; 114(2): 250–3.

244 Fletcher CF, Lutz CM, O'Sullivan TN et al. Absence epilepsy in tottering mutant mice is associated with calcium channel defects. *Cell* 1996; 87: 607–17.

245 Noebels JL, Sidman RL. Inherited epilepsy: spike-wave and focal motor seizures in the mutant mouse tottering. *Science* 1979; 204: 1334–6.

246 Campbell DB, Hess EJ. Cerebellar circuitry is activated during convulsive episodes in the tottering (tg/tg) mutant mouse. *Neuroscience* 1998; 85: 773–83.

247 Levitt P, Noebels JL. Mutant mouse tottering: selective increase of locus ceruleus axons in a defined single-locus mutation. *Proc Natl Acad Sci USA* 1981; 78: 4630–4.

248 Noebels JL. A single gene error of noradrenergic axon growth synchronizes central neurones. *Nature* 1984; 310: 409–11.

249 Wakamori M, Yamazaki K, Matsunodaira H et al. Single tottering mutations responsible for the neuropathic phenotype of the P-type calcium channel. *J Biol Chem* 1998; 273(52): 34857–67.

250 Caddick SJ, Wang C, Fletcher CF, Jenkins NA, Copeland NG, Hosford DA. Excitatory but not inhibitory synaptic transmission is reduced in lethargic (Cacnb4^{lh}) and tottering (Cacna1a^{tg}) mouse thalami. *J Neurophysiol* 1999; 81: 2066–74.

251 Doroshenko PA, Woppmann A, Miljanich G, Augustine GJ. Pharmacologically distinct presynaptic calcium channels in cerebellar excitatory and inhibitory synapses. *Neuropharmacology* 1997; 36: 865–72.

252 Campbell DB, Hess EJ. L-type calcium channels contribute to the tottering mouse dystonic episodes. *Mol Pharmacol* 1999; 55: 23–31.

253 Heckroth JA, Abbott LC. Purkinje cell loss from alternating sagittal zones in the cerebellum of leaner mutant mice. *Brain Res* 1994; 658(1–2): 93–104.

254 Tamaki Y, Oda S, Kameyama Y. Postnatal locomotion development in a neurological mutant of rolling mouse Nagoya. *Dev Psychobiol* 1986; 19: 67–77.

255 Chen L, Chetkovich DM, Petralia RS et al. Stargazin regulates synaptic targeting of AMPA receptors by two distinct mechanisms. *Nature* 2000; 408 6815: 936–43.

256 Qiao X, Noebels JL. Developmental analysis of hippocampal mossy fiber outgrowth in a mutant mouse with inherited spike-wave seizures. *J Neurosci* 1993; 13(11): 4622–35.

257 Qiao X, Hefti F, Knusel B, Noebels JL. Selective failure of brain-derived neurotrophic factor mRNA expression in the cerebellum of stargazer, a mutant mouse with ataxia. *J Neurosci* 1996; 16(2): 640–8.

258 Thompson CL, Tehrani MHJ, Barnes EM Jr, Stephenson FA. Decreased expression of GABAA receptor α_6 and α_3 subunits in stargazer mutant mice: a possible role for brain-derived neurotrophic factor in the regulation of GABAA expression? *Brain Res Mol Brain Res* 1998; 60: 282–90.

259 McEnery MW, Copeland TD, Vance CL. Altered expression and assembly of N-type calcium ion channel a$_{1A}$ and a subunits in epileptic lethargic (lh/lh) mouse. *J Biol Chem* 1998; 273(34): 21435–8.

260 Vance CL, Begg CM, Lee WL, Haase H, Copeland TD, McEnery MW. Differential expression and association of calcium channel a$_{1A}$ and subunits in lethargic (lh/lh) mouse. *J Biol Chem* 1998; 273(23): 14495–502.

261 Hosford DA, Clark S, Cao Z et al. The role of GABA$_B$ receptor activation in absence seizures of lethargic (lh/lh) mice. *Science* 1992; 257(5068): 398–401.

262 Lin FH, Cao Z, Hosford DA. Increased number of GABA$_B$ receptors in the lethargic (lh/lh) mouse model of absence epilepsy. *Brain Res* 1993; 608: 101–6.

263 Vergnes M, Marescaux C, Depaulis A, Micheletti G, Warter JM. Ontogeny of spontaneous petit mal-like seizures in Wistar rats. *Dev Brain Res* 1986; 30: 85–7.

264 Marescaux C, Vergnes M, Paulus A. Genetic absence epilepsy in rats from Strasbourg—a review. *J Neural Transm Suppl* 1992; 35: 37–69.

265 Noebels JL, Fariello RG, Jobe PC, Lasley SM, Marescaux C. Genetic models of generalized epilepsy. In: Engell Jr J, Pedley TA, eds. *Epilepsy: A comprehensive textbook*, Vol. 1. Philadelphia: Lippincott-Raven 1997; 457–65.

266 Marescaux C, Vergnes M, Bernasconi R. GABA$_B$ receptor antagonists:

potential new anti-absence drugs. *J Neural Transm* Suppl 1992; 35: 179–88.

267 Snead OC, Depaulis A, Banerjee PK, Hechler V, Vergnes M. The GABAA receptor complex in experimental absence seizures in rat: an autoradiographic study. *Neurosci Lett* 1992; 140: 9–12.

268 Spreafico R, Mennini T, Danober L *et al.* GABA$_A$ receptor impairment in the genetic absence epilepsy rats from Strasborg (GAERS): an immunocytochemical and receptor binding autoradiographic study. *Epilepsy Res* 1993; 15(3): 229–38.

269 Seidenbecher T, Pape HC. Contribution of intralaminar thalamic nuclei to spike and wave discharges during spontaneous seizures in a genetic rat model of absence epilepsy. *Eur J Neurosci* 2001; 10(3): 1103–12.

270 Seyfried TN, Glaser GH. A review of mouse mutants as genetic models of epilepsy. *Epilepsia* 1985; 26(2): 143–50.

271 Suzuki J, Namamoto Y. Seizure patterns and electroencephalograms of E1 mouse. *Electroencephalogr Clin Neurophysiol* 1977; 43: 299–311.

272 Seyfried TN, Brigand JV, Flavin HJ, Frankel WN, Rise ML. Genetic and biochemical correlates of epilepsy in the EL mouse. *Neuroscience* 1992; 18: 9–20.

273 Ishida N, Kasamo K, Nakamoto Y, Suzuki J. Epileptic seizure of EL mouse initiates at the parietal cortex: Depth EEG observations in freely moving condition using buffer amplifier. *Brain Res* 1993; 608: 52–7.

274 Mutoh K, Ito M, Tsuda H *et al.* Depth EEG in mutant epileptic E1 mice: Demonstration of secondary generalization of the seizure from the hippocampus. *Electroencephalogr Clin Neurophysiol* 1993; 86: 205–12.

275 Sugaya E, Ishige A, Sekiguchi K *et al.* Pentylenetetrazole-induced convulsion and effect of anticonvulsants in mutant inbred El mice. *Epilepsia* 1986; 27(4): 354–8.

276 Ono T, Fueta Y, Janjua NA *et al.* Granule cell disinhibition in dentate gyrus of genetically seizure susceptible EL mice. *Brain Res* 1997; 745: 165–72.

277 Fueta Y, Kawano H, Ono T, Mita T, Fukata K, Ohno K. Regional differences in hippocampal excitability manifested by paired-pulse stimulation of genetically epileptic El mice. *Brain Res* 1998; 779: 324–8.

278 Kuramoto T, Mori M, Yamada J, Serikawa T. Tremor and zitter, causative mutant genes for epilepsy with spongiform encephalography in spontaneously epileptic rat (SER), are tightly linked to synaptobrevin-2 and prion protein genes, respectively. *Biochem Biophys Res Comm* 1994; 200(2): 1161–8.

279 Serikawa T, Yamada J. Epileptic seizures in rats homozygous for two mutations, zitter and tremor. *J Hered* 1986; 77: 441–4.

280 Sasa M, Ohno Y, Ujihara H *et al.* Effects of antiepileptic drugs on absence-like and tonic seizures in the spontaneously epileptic rat, a double mutant rat. *Epilepsia* 1988; 29: 505–13.

281 Ishihara K, Sasa M, Momiyama T *et al.* Abnormal excitability of hippocampal CA3 pyramidal neurons of spontaneously epileptic rats (SER), a double mutant. *Exp Neurol* 1993; 119: 287–90.

282 Amano T, Amano H, Matsubayashi H, Ishihara K, Serikawa T, Sasa M. Enhanced Ca^{2+} influx with mossy fiber stimulation in hippocampal CA3 neurons of spontaneously epileptic rats. *Brain Res* 2001; 910: 199–203.

283 Hanaya R. Sasa M, Kiura Y, Serikawa T, Kurisu K. Effects of vigabatrin on epileptiform abnormal discharges in hippocampal CA3 neurons of spontaneously epileptic rats (SER). *Epilepsy Res* 2002; 50: 223–31.

284 Hanaya R, Sasa M, Vjihara H *et al.* Suppression by topiramate of epileptiform burst discharges in hippocampal CA3 neurons of spontaneously epileptic rats in vitro. *Brain Res* 1998; 798: 274–82.

285 Laird HE, Hadjiconstantinou M, Neff NH. Abnormalities in the central cholinergic transmitter system of the genetically epilepsy-prone rat. *Life Sci* 1986; 39(9): 783–7.

286 Bruckner C, Stenkamp K, Meierkord H, Heinemann U. Epileptiform discharges induced by combined application of bicuculline and 4-aminopyridine are resistant to standard anticonvulsants in slices of rats. *Neurosci Lett* 1999; 268: 163–5.

10 Drug Interactions in Epilepsy

E. Spina and M.G. Scordo

The concomitant use of drugs in current medical practice has created the problem of drug interactions and sequelae of undesirable or even toxic reactions. A drug interaction occurs when the effectiveness or toxicity of a drug is altered by the concomitant administration of another drug. In a few cases drug interactions may prove beneficial, leading to increased efficacy or reduced risk of unwanted effects, and therefore certain drug combinations may be used advantageously in clinical practice. However, more often, drug interactions are of concern because the outcome of concurrent drug administration is diminished therapeutic efficacy or increased toxicity of one or more of the administered compounds.

Drug interactions represent a common clinical problem associated with the use of antiepileptic agents. These agents are usually given for prolonged periods and often in combination with other antiepileptics or medications used for the management of comorbid associated disorders [1,2]. The treatment of epilepsy with a single medication is a satisfactory therapeutic strategy in about 70% of patients. In most of the remaining patients better control can be achieved with long-term antiepileptic polytherapy. Antiepileptic drugs are also increasingly used to treat other non-epileptic conditions such as mood disorders, migraine and pain, thereby increasing the possibility of combined use with other compounds. The pharmacokinetic properties of antiepileptic drugs make these agents particularly susceptible to drug interactions. Many of the older antiepileptics have a low therapeutic index, and even a relatively small change in their plasma concentrations (due to inhibition or induction of their metabolism or protein binding displacement) may easily result in loss of efficacy or signs of intoxication. In addition, some exert a major influence on the activity of the hepatic drug metabolizing enzymes, stimulating or inhibiting their activity, thereby leading to a wide variety of interactions with other drugs that are also eliminated by biotransformation. On the other hand, most antiepileptics undergo extensive hepatic metabolism, and are vulnerable to the effect of other drugs with inducing or inhibiting properties. Compared with older agents, new antiepileptic drugs appear to have clear advantages in terms of a lower interaction potential [3].

The purpose of this chapter is to provide a concise overview on the principles and mechanisms of drug interactions involving antiepileptic drugs. Drug interactions are usually divided into two types: pharmacokinetic and pharmacodynamic. Pharmacokinetic interactions consist of changes in the absorption, distribution, metabolism or excretion of a drug and/or its metabolites, or in the quantity of active drug that reaches its site of action, after the addition of another chemical agent. Pharmacodynamic interactions occur when two drugs act at the same or interrelated receptor sites, resulting in additive, synergistic or antagonistic effects. While this classification is useful for didactic purposes, it should be pointed out that many interactions are multifactorial in nature and may involve a complex sequence of events both at pharmacokinetic and pharmacodynamic level. In general, pharmacokinetic interactions have been more extensively investigated, largely due to the fact that changes in drug concentrations are more easily quantifiable than changes in pharmacodynamic response.

Pharmacokinetic interactions

Mechanisms of pharmacokinetic drug interactions

Pharmacokinetic drug interactions may occur at the level of drug absorption, distribution, metabolism and excretion. However, pharmacokinetic interactions of antiepileptics arise most frequently as a consequence of drug-induced changes in hepatic metabolism, through enzyme inhibition or induction, and less frequently from changes in plasma protein binding. Very few relevant interactions involving other mechanisms seem to occur in clinical practice. For example, coadministration of antacids containing magnesium hydroxide or aluminium hydroxide has been reported to cause a moderate decrease in the absorption of phenytoin and gabapentin, resulting in diminished plasma concentrations and, possibly, reduced efficacy [4]. Moreover, as some of the new antiepileptics, notably gabapentin and vigabatrin, are eliminated predominantly through the kidneys, interactions at this level are likely to happen, but have not been reported to date.

Metabolically-based drug interactions

The most clinically important pharmacokinetic interactions of antiepileptic drugs occur at metabolic level as a result of enzyme inhibition or induction. Metabolic processes are necessary to convert a drug into one or more metabolites which are more water soluble than the parent drug, facilitating urinary excretion. The chemical reactions are catalysed by various enzyme systems and are divided into phase I (functionalization) and phase II (conjugation) biotransformations, which may occur in series. Phase I reactions include addition of a polar functional group (e.g. hydroxyl) or deletion of a non-polar alkyl group (e.g. *N*-demethylation) by oxidation, reduction or hydrolysis. Water solubility can be further increased by conjugation with endogenous compounds such as glucuronic acid, sulphate, acetate, glutathione or glycine. Although metabolic drug interactions may involve changes in the activity of any one of the numerous drug-metabolizing enzymes, the majority are associated with the cytochrome P450 mixed-function oxidases. Characterization of the major enzyme systems involved in the biotransformation of antiepileptics is essential for understanding the principles and mechanisms of metabolically-based drug interactions involving these drugs.

Major enzyme systems involved in the metabolism of antiepileptic drugs

Cytochrome P450 system (CYP)

The CYP system consists of a superfamily of isoenzymes located in the membranes of the smooth endoplasmic reticulum, mainly in the liver, but also in many extrahepatic tissues (e.g. intestinal mucosa, lung, kidney, brain, lymphocytes, placenta, etc.) [5,6]. These isoenzymes are haemoproteins which contain a single iron protoporphyrin IX prosthetic group. They are responsible for the oxidative metabolism of a number of drugs and other exogenous compounds, as well as many endogenous substrates such as prostaglandins, fatty acids and steroids. The multiple CYP enzymes are classified into families, subfamilies and isoenzymes according to a systematic nomenclature based on similarities in their amino acid sequences [7]. The first Arabic number designates the 'family' (>40% sequence identity within family members), the capital letter that follows indicates the 'subfamily' (>59% sequence identity within subfamily members), while the second Arabic number designates individual isoenzymes. The major CYP enzymes involved in drug metabolism in humans belong to families 1, 2 and 3, the specific isoforms being CYP1A2, CYP2C9, CYP2C19, CYP2D6, CYP2E1 and CYP3A4. Each CYP isoform is a specific gene product and possesses a characteristic broad spectrum of substrate specificity. The activity of these isoenzymes is genetically determined and may be profoundly influenced by environmental factors, such as concomitant administration of other drugs. A number of genes coding for CYP isoforms have variant alleles resulting from mutation. Mutation in the gene for a drug-metabolizing enzyme could result in enzyme variants with higher, lower or no activity, or result in the absence of the enzyme. The existence of these alleles in at least 1% of the population is referred to as genetic polymorphism [8]. The major polymorphisms of drug-metabolizing enzymes that have clinical implications are those related to the oxidation of drugs by CYP2D6, CYP2C9 and CYP2C19.

Over the past decade there have been great advances in our understanding of this system and the different substrates, inhibitors and inducers of these isozymes have been identified. As indicated in Table 10.1, the majority of commonly used antiepileptics are metabolized by CYP enzymes and some of these drugs may also inhibit or induce one or more of these isoforms [9]. It should be noted that any given drug may have several different metabolic pathways catalysed by different enzymes and that the same metabolic reaction can be mediated by two or more enzymes.

CYP1A2

CYP1A2 accounts for approximately 13% of total CYPs expressed in human liver [10]. There is increasing awareness of the importance of CYP1A2 in human hepatic drug metabolism. It is the primary enzyme responsible for the metabolism of phenacetin, paracetamol, tacrine, theophylline, caffeine, clozapine and olanzapine. To date, none of the compounds used for the treatment of epilepsy appears to be metabolized to a significant extent by CYP1A2. There is a wide interindividual variability in CYP1A2 activity, but the impact of the genetic polymorphism on the CYP1A2 metabolic capacity is controversial. The activity of this isoform may be inhibited by fluvoxamine and ciprofloxacin. Inducers of CYP1A2 include cigarette smoking, rifampicin, omeprazole and, possibly, the antiepileptic agents phenobarbital, phenytoin and carbamazepine.

CYP2C subfamily: CYP2C9 and CYP2C19

The human CYP2C subfamily, which represents approximately 20% of total hepatic CYP, consists of at least four isoforms, 2C8, 2C9, 2C18 and 2C19, the genes for which are located together on chromosome 10. Of these isoforms, CYP2C9 and CYP2C19 seem to be the most important for drug metabolism. On the other hand, it has been reported that CYP2C8 plays a major role in the metabolism of carbamazepine. CYP2C9 and CYP2C19 show a 91% identity in amino acid sequence. Thus, most substrates of CYP2C9 are metabolized by CYP2C19 as well.

CYP2C9, the most abundant among human CYP2C isoforms, metabolizes a number of therapeutically important drugs including phenytoin, tolbutamide, S-warfarin, losartan and many nonsteroidal anti-inflammatory agents such as ibuprofen, diclofenac and piroxicam. CYP2C9 is polymorphically expressed in humans. To date, three different allelic variants have been found that code for enzymes with different catalytic activity. People carrying two detrimental alleles lack almost completely CYP2C9 activity and, therefore, are unable to metabolize 2C9 substrates such as phenytoin [11]. CYP2C9 inhibitors include sulfaphenazole, amiodarone and fluconazole. Among antiepileptics, only valproic acid acts as an inhibitor of this isoform.

CYP2C19 is responsible for the 4-hydroxylation of the S-enantiomer of the anticonvulsant mephenytoin, and contributes to the clearance of diazepam, omeprazole, proguanil, citalopram and tricyclic antidepressants (demethylation reactions). CYP2C19 also exhibits genetic polymorphism. The frequency of the poor metabolizer phenotype varies in populations of different racial origin, being approximately 2–6% of individuals in Caucasian populations, and 12–25% in Asian populations. Inhibitors of CYP2C19 include ticlopidine, omeprazole and the antiepileptic agents felbamate and topiramate.

The activity of CYP2C isoforms is induced by administration of rifampicin, barbiturates, phenytoin and carbamazepine.

CYP2D6

CYP2D6 represents an average of 2% of hepatic CYP content. The gene encoding its synthesis is located on the long arm of chromosome 22. Although expressed at rather low levels compared with other human CYPs, this isoform plays an important role in drug metabolism, being partially or entirely responsible for the oxidative biotransformation of a variety of psychopharmacological and cardiovascular drugs. Apparently, this isoform is not involved in the biotransformation of any of the currently available antiepileptics. CYP2D6 exhibits a common genetic polymorphism that divides the populations into two phenotypes, extensive metabolizers and poor metabolizers. Approximately 3–10% of individuals in Caucasians are of the poor metabolizer phenotype, but only 1–2% of Asians. Quinidine is a potent and selective inhibitor of this isoform. Fluoxetine, paroxetine and different phenothizines are also potent inhibitors. In contrast to all other CYPs involved in drug metabolism, CYP2D6 is not inducible.

Table 10.1 Substrates, inhibitors and inducers of the major cytochrome P450 isoforms involved in drug metabolism

Enzymes	Substrates	Inhibitors	Inducers
CYP1A2	Antidepressants: amitriptyline,[1] clomipramine,[1] imipramine,[1] fluvoxamine, mirtazapine Antipsychoticis: clozapine, olanzapine, haloperidol Metilxantines: theophylline, caffeine Miscellaneous: paracetamol, phenacetin, tacrine, R-warfarin	Fluvoxamine Ciprofloxacin	Smoking Rifampicin Omeprazole Barbiturates Phenytoin Carbamazepine
CYP2C9	NSAIDs: diclofenac, ibuprofen, naproxen, piroxicam Antiepileptics: phenytoin, phenobarbital, valproic acid Miscellaneous: S-warfarin, tolbutamide, losartan, torasemide	Sulfaphenazole Amiodarone Phenylbutazone Fluconazole Miconazole Valproic acid Fluoxetine Fluvoxamine	Rifampicin Barbiturates Phenytoin Carbamazepine
CYP2C19	Antidepressants: amitriptyline,[1] clomipramine,[1] imipramine,[1] citalopram, moclobemide Miscellaneous: phenytoin, diazepam, omeprazole, propranolol, proguanil, S-mephenytoin, R-warfarin	Omeprazole Ticlopidine Fluvoxamine Fluoxetine Felbamate Topiramate	Rifampicin Barbiturates Phenytoin Carbamazepine
CYP2D6	Antidepressants: amitriptyline,[1] clomipramine,[1] imipramine,[1] desipramine,[2] nortriptyline,[2] fluoxetine, paroxetine, fluvoxamine, citalopram, venlafaxine, mianserin, mirtazapine Antipsychotics: thioridazine, perphenazine, zuclopenthixol, haloperidol, risperidone, clozapine, olanzapine, sertindole Opiates: codeine, destromethorphan, tramadol β-blockers: alprenolol, bufuralol, metoprolol, propanolol, timolol, pindolol Antiarrhythmics: encainide, flecainide, propafenone Miscellaneous: debrisoquine, sparteine, phenformin	Quinidine Propafenone Thioridazine Perphenazine Fluoxetine Paroxetine	None known
CYP2E1	Ethanol, halotane, dapsone, isoniazid, felbamate	Disulfiram	Ethanol Isoniazid
CYP3A4	Antidepressants: amitriptyline,[1] clomipramine,[1] imipramine,[1] sertraline, nefazodone, mirtazapine Antipsychotics: haloperidol, clozapine, risperidone, quetiapine, ziprasidone, sertindole Benzodiazepines: alprazolam, midazolam, triazolam Antiepileptics: carbamazepine, felbamate, tiagabine, zonisamide Calcium antagonists: diltiazem, felodipine, nifedipine, verapamil Steroids: cortisol, ethinyloestradiol, levonorgestrel Immunosuppressants: cyclosporin, tacrolimus Miscellaneous: cisapride, terfenadine, astemizole, erythromocyn, clarytromicin, tamoxifen, amiodarone, quinidine	Ketoconazole Itraconazole Fluconazole Erythromycin Troleandomycin Ritonavir Indinavir Saquinavir Fluvoxamine Nefazodone Grapefruit juice	Rifampicin Barbiturates Phenytoin Carbamazepine Hypericum Oxcarbazepine* Topiramate* Felbamate*

[1] Demethylation.
[2] Hydroxylation.
* Weaker enzymatic inducers as compared to previous ones.

CYP2E1. CYP2E1 accounts for an average of 7% of total human hepatic CYPs and is of greater importance to toxicant metabolism than drug metabolism. This isoform is responsible for the metabolism of ethanol, halothane and dapsone, and plays a minor role in the oxidative biotransformation of the anticonvulsant felbamate. CYP2E1 is inhibited by acute administration of ethanol and disulfiram and is induced by long-term ethanol consumption and by isoniazid.

CYP3A4. The human CYP3A subfamily is composed of three isoforms, 3A4, 3A5 and 3A7, encoded by genes located on chromosome 7. These CYP3A isoforms are the most abundant in human liver, accounting for approximately 30% of total CYP content. CYP3A4 is the predominant isoform of CYP3A subfamily in adult humans and is present both in liver and in small intestine. This isoform catalyses, at least in part, the biotransformation of an amazingly large number of structurally diverse drugs and endogenous compounds. Examples of drugs that are primarily metabolized by CYP3A4 include the immunosuppressants ciclosporin (cyclosporin) and tacrolimus, triazolobenzodiazepines (e.g. alprazolam, midazolam and triazolam), the non-sedating antihistamines (e.g. terfenadine and astemizole), the calcium antagonists diltiazem, nifedipine and verapamil, the antiarrhythmics amiodarone and quinidine, and several steroids (e.g. cortisol, ethinyloestradiol and levonogestrel). In addition, CYP3A4 is the primary enzyme responsible for the metabolism of carbamazepine and also plays a role in the biotransformation of other antiepileptic drugs such as ethosuximide, tiagabine and zonisamide. The hepatic and enteric location of CYP3A4 makes it well suited to play a significant role in first-pass (or presystemic) drug metabolism. It should be noted that many drugs metabolized by CYP3A4 are also substrates for P-glycoprotein, a transmembrane adenosine triphosphate-dependent active transport protein found in a number of organs including the gut, brain, liver and kidney. Although CYP3A4 drug-metabolizing activity has been reported to vary more than 20-fold widely among individuals, it has a unimodal distribution in the population and does not appear to be subject to genetic polymorphism as seen for other CYP isoforms (2C9, 2C19, 2D6). The wide interindividual variability is likely, in part, to be caused by ethnic or cultural differences, presumably related to an interaction between race and diet. In addition to interindividual differences related to constitutive expression of these isoenzymes, there can be wide swings in the metabolic clearance of CYP3A substrates as a result of enzyme induction and inhibition. There are many different compounds that may inhibit CYP3A4 activity. The most potent include azole antimycotics, macrolide antibiotics, human immunodeficiency virus (HIV) protease inhibitors (ritonavir, indinavir and saquinavir), nefazodone and grapefruit juice. The hepatic and possibly intestinal CYP3A4 isoform is induced by rifampicin, dexamethasone and by the anticonvulsants phenobarbital, phenytoin and carbamazepine. The new antiepileptics felbamate, oxcarbazepine and topiramate appear to selectively induce this isoform.

Epoxide hydrolases (EHs)

Epoxide hydrolases are a family of enzymes that function to hydrate simple epoxides to vicinal diols and arene oxides to trans-dihydrodiols [12]. They belong to the broad group of hydrolytic enzymes, which include esterases, proteases, dehalogenases and lipases. The epoxide intermediates are frequently generated in situ through oxidative metabolic processes involving xenobiotics and endogenous substances. These intermediates may function as critical initiators of cellular damage including protein and RNA adduction with the epoxide as well as genetic mutation. Therefore, EHs are usually implicated in detoxification processes, although in certain instances they may be involved in bioactivation reactions. Of the five classes of EHs that have been characterized, the microsomal form is involved in the metabolism of xenobiotics. Microsomal EH exhibits a broad substrate specificity and, in particular, plays an important role in the metabolism of some anticonvulsant medications. Antiepileptic agents such as phenobarbital, phenytoin and carbamazepine are oxidatively metabolized through the CYP system to epoxide intermediates. These intermediates have been implicated in teratogenic events and other developmental abnormalities in offspring whose mothers were treated with these agents during pregnancy. In addition, they may have a role in the occurrence of hypersensitivity reactions, characterized by fever, rash, lymphoadenopathy and hepatitis, associated with the above-mentioned anticonvulsants. As the epoxide metabolites of these antiepileptics are substrate for microsomal EH, whose activity is subject to large interindividual variation, it has been hypothesized that the EH enzymatic status might be a potential risk factor for drug-induced congenital malformations and hypersensitivity reactions [13]. Based on in vitro and in vivo drug interactions with carbamazepine-10,11-epoxide, it has been documented that valpromide and, to a lesser extent, valproic acid, inhibit microsomal EH [14]. A modest induction of microsomal EH may occur after administration of phenobarbital and carbamazepine.

Uridine diphosphate glucuronosyltransferases (UGTs)

Glucuronidation is a phase II metabolic process and represents the most common metabolic pathway in the formation of hydrophilic drug metabolites which are more readily excreted by renal or biliary routes. These reactions are catalysed by UGTs. These enzymes catalyse the glucuronidation of a large number of endobiotics and xenobiotics, and are located in the endoplasmic reticulum of cells of the liver, kidney, intestine, skin, lung, spleen, prostate and brain [15]. Quantitatively, hepatic glucuronidation is the most important. Identification and classification of various UGTs has been accomplished in recent years. Thirty-three families of UGTs have been defined in vitro so far, and a specific nomenclature, similar to that used for the CYP system, has been established and recently refined [16]. Three families of UGTs have been identified in humans, of which the UGT1 and the UGT2 families seem to be the most important in drug metabolism. Among the isoforms of the UGT1 family, UGT1A1 is the major enzyme responsible for the glucuronidation of bilirubin and is inducible by phenobarbital. With regard to anticonvulsants, UGT1A3 is involved in the O-glucuronidation of valproic acid and UGT1A4 has been found to be the major isoform responsible for the N-glucuronidation of lamotrigine and retigabine. Among the isoforms of the UGT2 family, the UGT2B7 variant appears to contribute to O-glucuronidation of valproic acid. In contrast to extensive documentation for CYP-mediated drug interactions, there are fewer data on drug–drug interactions involving glucuronidation. Any substrate of UGT has the potential to competitively inhibit glucuronidation of other substrates metabolized by the same enzyme. Unlike the CYP system, no specific inhibitors of individual UGT isoforms have been identified. Valproic acid has been reported to inhibit several glucuronidation reactions, while phenobarbital, phenytoin and carbamazepine were found to act as inducers.

Enzyme inhibition

A large number of compounds have the ability to interact with drug-metabolizing enzymes, in particular with CYPs, thereby temporarily blocking their activity and usually resulting in a decrease in the rate of metabolism of the affected drug. Clinically, this can be associated with increased plasma concentrations. Enzyme inhibition occurs by mechanisms that range from rapidly reversible, to slowly reversible, to irreversible [17,18]. Reversible enzyme inhibition is transient, and the normal function of the enzyme is restored after the inhibitor has been eliminated from the body. In contrast, the loss of enzyme activity caused by irreversible inactivation persists even after the elimination of the inhibitor, and *de novo* biosynthesis of new enzyme is the only means by which activity can be regenerated.

Reversible inhibition. This type of enzyme inhibition is probably the most common mechanism responsible for the documented drug interactions. Kinetically, reversible inhibition can be divided further into competitive, non-competitive and uncompetitive. Competitive inhibition involves a mutually exclusive competition between the substrate and the inhibitor for the binding to the catalytic site of the enzyme. Usually, competitive inhibitors are alternative substrates of the enzyme with higher binding affinity. The binding of the inhibitor prevents the substrate binding to the active site of the enzyme and therefore the substrate cannot be metabolized. This inhibition can be reversed by increasing the concentrations of the substrate. In the case of non-competitive inhibition, the inhibitor binds to another site of the enzyme and the inhibitor has no effect on binding of substrate, but the enzyme–substrate–inhibitor complex is non-productive. Uncompetitive inhibition occurs when the inhibitor does not bind to the enzyme, but to the enzyme–substrate complex, and again the enzyme–substrate–inhibitor is non-productive.

Competitive inhibition of drug metabolism is typically a rapid and dose-dependent process. The initial effect of hepatic enzyme inhibition usually occurs within 24 h from the addition of the inhibitor. The time to maximal inhibition will depend on the elimination half-life of the affected drug and the inhibiting agent. When the inhibitor is withdrawn, the time course of de-inhibition is dependent on the rate of the elimination of the inhibitor from the liver.

Inhibitors of drug metabolism usually interfere with only a limited number of isoenzymes and therefore may be used as discriminators between different enzymatic forms. Compounds acting as inhibitors of different CYPs are listed in Table 10.1. Potent inhibitors of a given enzyme are usually substrates of the same enzyme. However this is not always true. For example quinidine is a potent inhibitor of CYP2D6 in humans, but is metabolized by CYP3A4. Inhibition of non-oxidative phase I and conjugating phase II enzymes has also been documented.

Among antiepileptic drugs, valproic acid, felbamate and topiramate have been associated with inhibitory drug interactions. Valproic acid is considered a broad-spectrum inhibitor of drug-metabolizing enzymes as it may cause inhibition of CYP2C9, UGTs and microsomal EH. Conversely, felbamate and topiramate selectively inhibit CYP2C19. However, it must be emphasized that other antiepileptics, though not clearly behaving as inhibitors of drug metabolism, may compete with drugs metabolized by the same enzymes, decreasing their metabolic clearance. Moreover, as most antiepileptics undergo extensive biotransformation in the liver, their metabolism is vulnerable to inhibition by competitive substrates or specific inhibitors.

Slowly reversible or quasi-irreversible inhibition. Several drugs including macrolide antibiotics and hydrazines undergo metabolic activation by CYP enzymes to form inhibitory metabolites. These metabolites can form stable complexes with the prosthetic haem of CYPs, called metabolic intermediate (MI) complex, so that the CYP isoform is sequestered in a functionally inactive state. While *in vitro* MI complexation can be reversed, in *in vivo* situations, the MI complex is usually so stable that the CYP involved in the complex is not available for drug metabolism, and the activity can be restored only after synthesis of new enzymes. The effect of this inhibition may therefore persist well after the elimination of the precursor. Troleandomycin and erythromycin are probably the best known macrolide antibiotics involved in the formation of MI complexes. These two agents are associated with a clinically significant inhibition of CYP3A4-mediated metabolism of carbamazepine. Hydrazine derivatives represent another class of compounds that may form stable complexes with the haem of CYP enzymes and make them inactive. Among these agents, isoniazid may cause a significant inhibition of phenytoin metabolism probably through MI complexation with CYP enzymes involved in its biotransformation.

Irreversible inhibition. Drugs containing certain functional groups can be oxidized by CYPs to reactive intermediates that cause irreversible inactivation of the enzyme. As metabolic activation is required for enzyme inactivation, these drugs are classified as mechanism-based inactivators or suicide inhibitors. This inactivation of CYPs may result from irreversible alteration of haem or protein, or a combination of both. The furanocoumarins contained in grapefruit juice cause irreversible suicide inhibition of CYP3A4.

Enzyme induction

The activity of drug-metabolizing enzymes in the liver and/or other organs may be increased ('induced') by prolonged administration of several exogenous agents including drugs, alcohol, components in the diet and cigarette smoke, as well as by endogenous factors. The inducing phenomenon involves predominantly CYP isoenzymes, but induction of other drug-metabolizing enzymes including microsomal EH and UGTs has also been documented. Interestingly, within the CYP system, some, but not all, isoforms appear to be inducible.

From the biological point of view, induction is an adaptive response that protects the cells from toxic xenobiotics by increasing the detoxification activity. Although the process of enzyme induction has been known for more than four decades, only in recent years have the molecular mechanisms involved started to be elucidated. Typically, enzyme induction is the consequence of an increase in the concentration of the enzyme protein [17,18]. In most cases, this occurs because of an enhanced protein synthesis resulting from an increase in gene transcription, usually mediated by intracellular receptors. However, enzyme induction may also occur by an inducer-mediated decrease in the rate of enzyme degradation, mainly by protein stabilization, as in the case of the ethanol-type of induction. Each inducer has its own pattern of induction of drug-metabolizing enzymes and several mechanisms of induction are often activated by a single agent, but to a different extent. While some compounds selectively induce only members of a specific family of enzymes (monofunctional inducers), others act on more than one enzyme system (multifunctional inducers) [19].

Currently, different mechanisms of enzyme induction have been discovered, but an exhaustive description is beyond the scope of this chapter [20]. The two best known examples of induction are the polycyclic aromatic hydrocarbon type and the phenobarbital type.

Polycyclic aromatic hydrocarbons such as benzo(a)pyrene and 3-methylcholanthrene are environmental contaminants which are formed by incomplete combustion of organic matter. These agents selectively induce few specific CYP enzymes, namely CYP1A1 and CYP1A2, but the concentrations of additional enzymes including UGTs are also increased. The mechanism of this type of induction involves the initial binding of the inducer to an intracellular aryl hydrocarbon (Ah) receptor. The co-induction of phase I and phase II enzymes appears to decrease the risk caused by CYP induction alone.

Phenobarbital is the prototype of a class of agents known to induce hepatic drug metabolism. Many other compounds including the antiepileptic drugs phenytoin, primidone and carbamazepine, and the antitubercular agent rifampicin, also stimulate drug-metabolizing enzymes with induction patterns which overlap, at least in part, that of barbiturates. The cluster of enzymes induced by phenobarbital and related agents appears to include several CYPs such as CYP2B6, CYP2C8, CYP2C9, CYP2C19, CYP3A4, CYP1A2, but not CYP2D6, some UGTs and microsomal EH. Thus, the drugs metabolized by enzymes subject to phenobarbital-type induction include a major fraction of all drugs undergoing biotransformation. The spectrum of substrates is not limited to drugs but extends to endogenous compounds such as cortisol, testosterone and vitamin D_3. Until a few years ago no receptor for phenobarbital or other chemicals causing the same pattern of change in protein expression had been found, but new findings suggest that the orphan receptor CAR (constitutive androstane receptor) is the molecular target and mediator of phenobarbital-type induction [21]. It should be pointed out that the molecular mechanism of phenobarbital-type induction often shows partial overlap with that of the PXR (pregnane X receptor), which mediates CYP3A4 induction by rifampicin and glucocorticoids.

Unlike enzyme inhibition, which is an almost immediate response, enzyme induction is a slow regulatory process, usually dose- and time-dependent. The amount of enzyme induction is generally proportional to the dose of the inducing agent. As enzyme induction usually requires synthesis of new enzymes, it occurs with some delay after the exposure to the inducing agent. Therefore, the time required for induction depends on both the time to reach the steady-state of the inducing agent (approximately 5 elimination half-lives) and the rate of synthesis of new enzymes. Similarly, the time course of de-induction is usually gradual and depends on the rate of degradation of the enzyme and the time required to eliminate the inducing drug. The rate-limiting step is usually the elimination half-life of the inducing agent.

Enzyme induction may have a profound impact on the pharmacokinetics of drugs metabolized by the susceptible enzyme. Elevated enzyme concentrations in an eliminating organ generally results in an increase in the rate of metabolism of the affected drug, leading to a decrease in serum concentrations of a parent drug, and possibly a loss of clinical efficacy. If the affected drug has an active metabolite, induction increases metabolite concentrations and enhances toxicity.

There are three different situations where enzyme induction plays a role in therapeutic decision-making:
• addition of a medication when an inducer is already present
• addition of an inducer to an existing therapy
• removal of an inducer from chronic therapy.
In the first two cases a higher dose of the affected drug will be needed to achieve or maintain clinical efficacy, while a reduction of the dose of the affected drug may be necessary to prevent toxicity after removal of the inducer. The magnitude and timing of these interactions are critical to allow clinicians to adjust dosages in order to maintain therapeutic effects and prevent toxicity.

In addition to classical enzyme-inducing antiepileptics, among newer agents, felbamate, oxcarbazepine and topiramate are the only drugs that appear to cause substantial enzyme induction.

Predictability of metabolic drug interactions

Because of the potential for adverse effects, metabolically-based drug interactions have always been an important aspect to consider during the development of new drugs. In the past, most drug interaction studies were performed relatively late in phase II and III clinical studies, using a strategy based on the therapeutic indices of drugs and the likelihood of their concurrent use. Since drug–drug interaction is usually considered to be an undesirable property of a drug, the information on the potential for enzyme inhibition or induction ideally should be obtained already in the preclinical phase. Over the last decade, a great deal of information on human CYPs at the molecular level has become available. With the availability of human tissues including liver microsomes and slices, and recombinant human CYP enzymes, *in vitro* systems have been used in recent years as screening tools to predict the potential *in vivo* drug interaction at a much earlier stage, before the drug reaches the clinical phases of development.

For a correct prediction of the potential for drug interactions it is essential to identify the CYP isoforms (or the other drug-metabolizing enzymes) responsible for the biotransformation of a given drug. In addition, to assess the possible clinical relevance, it is important to determine the relative contribution of the metabolic pathway(s) being inhibited or induced to the overall elimination of the drug. Identification of the individual CYP isoforms responsible for oxidative metabolism of various drugs and evaluation of their relative contribution to the overall drug elimination can be accomplished by the use of a general *in vitro* strategy [17] involving: (a) use of selective inhibitors; (b) immunoinhibition with monoclonal or polyclonal antibodies against the various CYP isoforms; (c) catalytic activity in cDNA-based vector systems; (d) catalytic activity in purified enzymes; and (e) metabolic correlation of activity with markers for known CYP isoforms. Each approach has its advantages and disadvantages, and a combination of approaches is usually required to accurately identify the CYP involved in the biotransformation of a given drug.

In vitro knowledge of the isoform(s) that catalyse(s) the major metabolic pathway of a particular drug may allow predictions *in vivo*. With regard to antiepileptics, typical examples of the utility of this approach have been achieved with carbamazepine and phenytoin [22]. Identification of CYP3A4 as the primary catalytic enzyme for the main clearance pathway of carbamazepine has allowed the understanding of the effects of several drugs on its plasma concentrations. In fact, most of the drug interactions with carbamazepine that have been documented in clinical practice involve CYP3A4 inhibitors or inducers. Similarly, identification of CYP2C9 and CYP2C19 as the major enzymes involved in the metabolism of phenytoin provides an explanation for many inhibitory interactions occuring with this compound. This knowledge on the isoenzymes involved in the metabolism of carbamazepine and phenytoin also allows a prediction of competitive inhibition with other substrates for the same enzymes.

The same approach may also be used for the evaluation of the enzyme-inhibiting properties of a given drug. The potential for any drugs to inhibit the various CYPs can be assessed initially *in vitro* by using probes (i.e. specific substrates) for those isoforms. If the new drug inhibits one isoform at therapeutic concentrations, we can predict that it will interact with any substrate of that isoform. In this respect, a good correlation was found between *in vitro* findings concerning the ability of the new antiepileptic agents felbamate and topiramate to inhibit various CYPs and their *in vivo* inhibitory interaction profile. On the other hand, assessment of the enzyme-inducing properties of a drug cannot be easily achieved. However, new *in vitro* techniques using cultures of primary human hepatocytes have been recently developed to evaluate CYP enzyme induction [23].

Although it is relatively easy to assess *in vitro* a drug interaction, the correct prediction and extrapolation of *in vitro* interaction data to *in vivo* situations requires a good understanding of pharmacokinetic principles. In addition, the proper interpretation of *in vitro* interaction studies can be complicated by various factors and results cannot be easily extrapolated to *in vivo* situations. For more detailed information on these aspects, the reader is referred elsewhere [17,24,25].

Extent and clinical relevance of metabolically-based drug interactions

Drugs undergoing extensive hepatic biotransformation, as most antiepileptics, have a high potential for metabolic interactions with a variety of other agents. The available knowledge of the various drug-metabolizing enzyme systems and their different substrates, inhibitors and inducers may help the physician to predict and eventually avoid potential interactions. In fact, coadministration of two substrates of the same enzyme, or coadministration of a substrate with an inhibitor or an inducer, entails the possibility of a drug interaction. As a consequence, plasma concentrations of the coadministered drugs may be increased or decreased, possibly resulting in clinical toxicity or diminished therapeutic effect. Dosage adjustments may be then required to avoid adverse effects or clinical failure. Obviously, the opposite will be true after discontinuation of enzyme inhibitors or inducers. However, not all theoretically possible interactions are clinically relevant and several factors must be considered when evaluating the magnitude and clinical significance of a potential interaction [26] (Table 10.2). Some of these factors need to be briefly discussed.

Therapeutic index of the substrate
The therapeutic index of a drug is the ratio of the average toxic dose divided by the average effective dose. (Concentrations can be substituted for doses.) The greater the difference between the doses that

Table 10.2 Factors to be considered when evaluating the clinical significance of a potential metabolic drug interaction

Drug-related factors	Therapeutic index of the substrate
	Extent of metabolism of the substrate through the affected enzyme (versus alternative metabolic routes)
	Presence of active or toxic metabolites
	Nature of activity at the enzyme site (substrate, inhibitor, inducer)
	Potency of the inhibitor/inducer
	Concentration of the inhibitor/inducer at the enzyme site
Patient-related factors	Individual inherent enzyme activity
	Level of risk for toxicity
Epidemiological factors	Probability of concurrent use

are beneficial versus those that cause adverse effects, the higher and better the drug's therapeutic index. Although discussed infrequently in recent years, the therapeutic index is a time-tested gauge of a drug's general usefulness. Patients receiving older antiepileptics, anticoagulants, some antidepressants or cardiovascular drugs are at a much greater risk than patients treated with other kinds of agents because of their narrow therapeutic index. In fact, as a consequence of the same degree of inhibition or induction, plasma levels of a given substrate are more likely to reach toxic or subtherapeutic values if the substrate has a narrow therapeutic index, while this is less likely with compounds with a broader therapeutic index, as illustrated in Fig. 10.1.

Extent of metabolism of the substrate through the affected enzyme
A clinically relevant metabolic interaction is likely to occur if the affected enzyme is the major responsible for the elimination of a given substrate. By contrast, as most drugs have several metabolic pathways, the inhibition of an enzyme contributing less than 20–30% to the overall clearance of a given drug may have a limited impact on its disposition, presumably resulting only in a minimal increase in plasma concentrations, since another isoform may provide sufficient secondary metabolic pathways. On the other hand, coadministration of an inducer of a minor pathway of drug elimination might produce more relevant consequences. In this case, the elimination of the drug might be significantly affected and that minor pathway might become the major responsible for drug clearance, causing a relevant decrease in its plasma levels. The different susceptibility of felbamate and topiramate to the action of inhibitors and inducers of their metabolism provide a typical example of this situation, as will be further discussed.

Presence of active or toxic metabolites
If a drug has a pharmacologically active metabolite, then the impact of an inhibitor or an inducer may be reduced. This may vary again depending on the subsequent metabolism of the metabolites. If a pathway that leads to a formation of a toxic metabolite is induced, adverse effects may increase without an elevation in plasma concentrations of the parent drug compound.

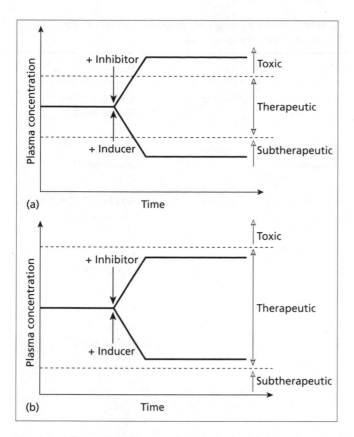

Fig. 10.1 Different clinical impact of an enzyme inhibitor or inducer on plasma concentrations of drugs with low (a) or wide (b) therapeutic index.

Nature of activity at the enzyme site (substrate, inhibitor or inducer)

Enzyme induction and inhibition are not mutually exclusive and may occur at the same time. The ability of a given compound to act as an inducer and inhibitor at the same time provides an explanation for the inconsistent and apparently contradictory nature of certain drug interactions. Phenobarbital, for example, may either decrease or increase the serum concentration of phenytoin depending on whether induction or inhibition of phenytoin metabolism prevails in an individual patient. Even more complex is the interaction between phenytoin and warfarin. When phenytoin is started in a patient stabilized on warfarin therapy, phenytoin initially may competitively inhibit the metabolism of warfarin because both phenytoin and S-warfarin are substrates for CYP2C9. After the initial increased effect of S-warfarin, plasma concentrations may decline within 1–2 weeks because of CYP2C9 induction. Therefore, warfarin dosage should be initially decreased and then increased to keep the anticoagulant effect desired.

Individual inherent enzyme activity

There is a large intersubject variability in the extent of a metabolic drug interaction, partially resulting from the enzyme status of an individual. In patients receiving drugs metabolized by a polymorphic enzyme, the effects of inhibitors or inducers may vary between different phenotypes/genotypes. In this respect, extensive metabolizers are more susceptible to enzyme inhibition or induction than poor metabolizers. For example, poor metabolizers for CYP2C19,

which plays a role in the metabolism of phenytoin, will not be subject to interactions with a selective inhibitor of that isoform such as felbamate. Similarly, it can be speculated that subjects carrying two detrimental alleles for CYP2C9, the primary enzyme responsible for phenytoin metabolism, are not likely to be affected by CYP2C9 inducers or inhibitors. Moreover, the interindividual differences in both hepatic and enteric CYP3A4 content, possibly dependent on genetic and/or environmental factors, may provide an explanation to the variability in the extent of pharmacokinetic interactions involving CYP3A4 inhibitors or inducers.

Level of risk for toxicity

The individual's level of risk to experience adverse effects should be taken into account when evaluating the clinical relevance of a potential metabolic drug interaction. Elderly patients are in general more prone to adverse drug interactions, since they are more likely to be on several drugs and because dosage requirements may be reduced, even in the absence of interactions, due to renal or hepatic disease or to changes in target organ responsiveness. On the other hand, elderly patients appear to be less susceptible than younger patients to inducers. The reason for such an age-dependent response to inducers is not fully understood and remains to be investigated.

Protein binding displacement interactions

Drugs are found in plasma either bound to serum protein or free (unbound). The principal proteins involved are albumin and α_1-acid glycoprotein. Generally, acid drugs bind predominantly to albumin, but not necessarily to the same site, while basic and neutral drugs may bind to various sites on α_1-acid glycoprotein in addition to albumin. The fraction of drug not bound to proteins is equal to the ratio of the concentration of unbound drug to total drug (bound plus unbound drug) and is designated as the free fraction. Plasma protein binding interactions result in the displacement of one drug that has less affinity for the protein by another with greater affinity. This will cause a rise in the fraction of free or unbound drug in plasma or tissue, and thus the potential for an increased effect of the displaced drug. If the displacing drug is withdrawn the reverse will occur. However, such interactions are only likely to be clinically significant if two criteria are fulfilled: (a) the displaced drug must be highly protein bound (usually greater than 90%); and (b) it must have a low apparent volume of distribution. In fact, if the displaced drug is less highly bound the amount displaced (which is usually of the order of a few per cent) will make little impact on the circulating unbound concentration, and if it is widely distributed to the tissues any increase in the free concentration will be diluted by further distribution. The important drugs which fulfil these criteria and may therefore be object drugs in protein binding displacement interactions include warfarin, phenytoin and tolbutamide. The commonest displacers from protein binding sites include sulfonamides, salicylates, chloral hydrate and some of its congeners (because of their metabolite trichloracetic acid), phenylbutazone and valproic acid.

The relevance of protein binding displacement interactions has been overestimated and such interactions are often of no clinical significance. For highly protein-bound drugs eliminated by low extraction hepatic metabolism, like phenytoin, the initial displacement may result in transient increase in free (or pharmaco-

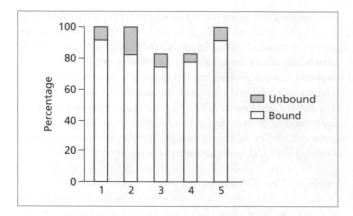

Fig. 10.2 Hypothetical events following displacement of a drug from its binding sites on plasma protein. (1) The drug has a protein binding of 90%. (2) Displacement of the drug leads to an increase in the unbound fraction from 10% to 20%. The unbound concentration is increased and the pharmacological effect is enhanced. (3) If the drug has a low extraction rate its total clearance is proportional to the unbound fraction and the clearance increases. The total concentration may decrease, so that although the unbound fraction is still increased, the unbound concentration is the same as it was before displacement occurred. (4) When the displacer is removed the reverse occurs. The unbound drug occupies the binding sites previously taken by the displacer. The unbound fraction and the unbound concentration are decreased, while the total concentration is still the same. (5) As the drug clearance decreases, the predisplacement situation is gradually re-established.

logically active) drug concentrations. However, the increased unbound drug is metabolized by the hepatic enzymes and a new steady-state occurs. This results in an increased free fraction, decreased total drug concentration, but no change in the unbound plasma concentrations of the displaced drug [27,28]. Therefore, total drug concentrations no longer reflect unbound plasma concentrations and unbound drug concentrations may need to be monitored. The hypothetical events following displacement of a drug with a low hepatic extraction from its binding sites on plasma proteins are illustrated in Fig. 10.2. The picture is more complex if the displacer also interferes with the metabolism of the affected drug. Valproate and phenytoin are the only antiepileptics involved in clinically important protein binding interactions.

Potential for pharmacokinetic interactions of antiepileptics

In this section we will examine the potential for pharmacokinetic interactions of the currently available antiepileptics by using a mechanistic approach and providing examples of specific clinically important interactions.

Effects of antiepileptics on the pharmacokinetics of other drugs

Antiepileptic drugs may influence the pharmacokinetics of other drugs by mechanisms of enzyme inhibition, enzyme induction or protein binding displacement. The effect of antiepileptics on the most common drug-metabolizing enzyme systems is reported in Table 10.3.

Table 10.3 Effects of antiepileptic drugs on the most common drug-metabolizing enzyme systems

Drug	Effect	Enzymes involved
Phenytoin	Inducer	CYP2C, CYP3A Microsomal EH UGT
Phenobarbital/primidone	Inducer	CYP2C, CYP3A Microsomal EH UGT
Carbamazepine	Inducer	CYP2C, CYP3A, CYP1A2 Microsomal EH UGT
Valproic acid	Inhibitor	CYP2C9 Microsomal EH UGT
Ethosuximide	None	
Felbamate	Inhibitor Inducer	CYP2C19 β-oxidation CYP3A4
Gabapentin	None	
Lamotrigine	None or weak inducer	UGT
Levetiracetam	None	
Oxcarbazepine	Weak inducer Weak inducer	CYP3A4 UGT
Tiagabine	None	
Topiramate	Weak inhibitor Weak inducer	CYP2C19 CYP3A4 β-oxidation
Vigabatrin	None	
Zonisamide	None	

Antiepileptics as inhibitors of metabolic enzymes

Valproic acid

Valproic acid is a broad-spectrum inhibitor of the major drug-metabolizing enzymes including not only CYP isoforms, but also microsomal EH and UGT enzymes. As a consequence, valproic acid may decrease the metabolic clearance of drugs metabolized by the aforementioned enzymes.

The effect of valproic acid on the activity of different human CYP isoforms has been recently investigated in vitro in human liver microsomes [29,30]. Valproic acid was found to competitively inhibit CYP2C9 activity at clinically relevant concentrations, while it was only a weak inhibitor of CYP2C19 and CYP3A4, and had no appreciable effect on CYP2D6 and CYP2E1 activities. These results are in agreement with previous clinical studies documenting that valproic acid may significantly increase plasma concentrations of substrates of the CYP2C9 isoform, such as phenytoin and phenobarbital [31]. On the other hand, valproic acid does not affect plasma concentrations of oral contraceptives or ciclosporin, which are substrates of CYP3A4.

Studies in human liver microsomes have indicated that valproic acid may inhibit EH activity [14]. Consistent with this *in vitro* evidence, clinical investigations have demonstrated that valproic acid may cause an increase in plasma concentrations of carbamazepine-10,11-epoxide, presumably through inhibition of the EH catalysed formation of carbamazepine *trans*-dihydrodiol.

Valproic acid also has an important inhibitory effect on drugs metabolized by the UGTs. Although no data are available on the effect of valproic acid on these enzymes in human liver microsomes, clinical studies have indicated that valproic acid significantly inhibits the glucuronide conjugation of lamotrigine, lorazepam and zidovudine as well as the *N*-glucosidation of phenobarbital. The specific UGT isoform involved in these metabolic reactions is known only for lamotrigine whose glucuronidation is metabolized by UGT1A4. With regard to this interaction, half-life and serum concentrations of lamotrigine have been reported to double after addition of valproate and this may contribute to the increased risk for mild or serious rashes when lamotrigine is added to valproate [32].

Felbamate

The inhibitory effects of felbamate towards seven CYP isoforms were investigated *in vitro* by incubating probes specific for each isoform in human liver microsomes [33]. The only isoform inhibited by concentrations of felbamate within the therapeutic range was CYP2C19. This is consistent with clinical experience indicating that felbamate may reduce the clearance of phenytoin and increase its plasma concentrations [34]. This effect may be attributed to inhibition of the *para*-hydroxylation of phenytoin by felbamate with specific inhibition of the formation of the R-hydroxy derivative, which is mediated by CYP2C19. Moreover, coadministration of felbamate with phenobarbital has been reported to increase by 20–30% plasma phenobarbital concentrations [35]. These changes were due to reduced *para*-hydroxylation of phenobarbital, suggesting that CYP2C19 may also be involved in this metabolic reaction. Felbamate can also significantly reduce the clearance of valproic acid, presumably via inhibition of its mitochondrial β-oxidation [36].

Topiramate

In vitro studies with human liver microsomes indicated that topiramate moderately inhibits the activity of CYP2C19, but not that of CYP1A2, CYP2C9, CYP2D6, CYP2E1 and CYP3A4 [37]. These findings suggest that topiramate may decrease the clearance of CYP2C19 substrates such as phenytoin, diazepam and omeprazole. Consistent with this, increased plasma phenytoin concentrations were observed in half of patients on phenytoin after addition of topiramate [38]. The intersubject difference in the phenytoin–topiramate interaction probably reflects the interindividual variability in the fraction of phenytoin metabolized by CYP2C9 versus CYP2C19. The inhibitory effect of topiramate towards phenytoin metabolism might become apparent only at higher plasma phenytoin concentrations, when CYP2C9 becomes saturated and CYP2C19 is likely to play a more prominent role in phenytoin elimination.

Antiepileptics as inducers of metabolic enzymes

Phenobarbital, phenytoin, carbamazepine

Phenobarbital is the prototypical inducer of a class of compounds with different chemical structures, including also phenytoin and carbamazepine. These agents induce several drug-metabolizing enzymes including CYPs, microsomal EH and UGTs, with associated proliferation of smooth endoplasmic reticulum in the liver [39]. Early *in vitro* investigations conducted in human liver microsomes obtained from individuals exposed to phenobarbital and in primary cultures of human hepatocytes had documented the ability of phenobarbital to induce P450s, but the specific isoforms induced could not be identified. More recently, with the improvement in culture techniques and the development of isoform-specific reagents, it has been possible to demonstrate that phenobarbital, phenytoin and carbamazepine induce CYP3A4 and CYP2C subfamily members. The possibility of induction of CYP1A2 by carbamazepine is supported by the evidence that this agent increases the metabolic clearance of substrates of this isoform such as olanzapine and R-warfarin and increases the percentage of labelled caffeine exhaled as carbon dioxide, a method used to assess CYP1A2 activity *in vivo* [40]. *In vivo* studies in healthy volunteers and patients with epilepsy have confirmed the *in vitro* evidence. Phenobarbital, phenytoin and carbamazepine have been reported to increase the clearance of antipyrine, a general probe of cytochrome P450 activity, and the urinary ratio of 6β-hydroxycortisol to cortisol, a marker of CYP3A activity. Phenytoin and carbamazepine appear to be less potent inducers than phenobarbital at doses used in clinical practice [41]. Though these agents also induce microsomal EH and phase II UGTs, almost all clinically significant drug interactions involve CYP enzymes.

The time course of induction and de-induction for phenobarbital is primarily dependent on its long elimination half-life. Therefore, induction usually begins in approximately 1 week, with maximal effect occurring after 2–3 weeks after initiation of phenobarbital therapy. The de-induction follows a similar time course, as plasma concentrations of phenobarbital decline over 2–3 weeks after therapy withdrawal [27,28]. With phenytoin, maximal induction or deinduction occurs approximately 1–2 weeks after initiation or removal of phenytoin therapy [27,28]. Carbamazepine is the only antiepileptic agent which significantly induces its own metabolism during long-term therapy (autoinduction). The plasma clearance of carbamazepine more than doubles during the initial weeks of therapy. The time course of the autoinduction process appears to be complex, discontinuous and prolonged. This usually occurs within 1 week of initiation of carbamazepine therapy and should be completed within approximately 3–5 weeks of treatment [27,28].

Consistent with their enzyme-inducing properties, phenobarbital, phenytoin and carbamazepine have been reported to increase the clearance or reduce the therapeutic efficacy of many different compounds including other antiepileptics. As a general rule they will induce the metabolism of any drug that is primarily dependent upon CYP3A4 activity and possibly CYP2C9, CYP2C19 and CYP1A2 (Table 10.1). Because the induction profiles of phenobarbital, phenytoin and carbamazepine are not fully overlapping, stimulation of the metabolism of all drugs listed in Table 10.1 may not necessarily be observed with each of these antiepileptics.

Clinically relevant drug interactions may occur when enzyme-inducing antiepileptics are coadministered with drugs with a low therapeutic index [28]. Concurrent administration of phenobarbital and warfarin may cause a decrease in plasma concentrations of warfarin and in its anticoagulant effects. Another clinically important interaction with enzyme-inducing antiepileptics involves the concomitant administration of oral contraceptives, which has been reported to result in menstrual disturbance and unplanned pregnancies. The increased metabolism of both oestrogenic and progesteronic components of oral contraceptives is believed to be the underlying mechanism. Enzyme-inducing antiepileptics may also accelerate the CYP3A4-mediated metabolism of ciclosporin, resulting in low blood concentrations of the immunosuppressive agent. The subtherapeutic blood concentrations of ciclosporin may cause acute allograft rejection.

When active metabolites are formed, enzyme induction may result in potentiation of therapeutic and/or toxic effects. For example, the enhanced hepatotoxicity of valproic acid in children concurrently treated with enzyme inducers could be explained by accelerated formation of a reactive oxidative product [42].

Induction of the metabolism of endogenous substrates may also be important. Increased metabolism of vitamin D_3 is probably responsible for the development of anticonvulsant-induced osteomalacia [43]. A possible role of enzyme induction has been hypothesized also in the development of anticonvulsant-induced folate deficiency and in the pathogenesis of the vitamin K-responsive haemorrhagic disorder in neonates born to drug-treated epileptic mothers.

Felbamate

Though no *in vitro* studies have examined the induction potential of felbamate on CYP enzymes, there is strong clinical evidence that this agent may induce the activity of CYP3A4 [33]. In fact, felbamate has been consistently shown to reduce plasma concentrations of carbamazepine and to increase levels of its active metabolite, carbamazepine-10,11-epoxide [34]. As CYP3A4 is the primary enzyme responsible for the epoxidation of carbamazepine, it is likely that these changes might be explained by an inducing effect of felbamate on this isoform. In agreement with this, felbamate has also been reported to cause a significant decrease in the plasma concentrations of other substrates of CYP3A4 such as the oral contraceptives ethinyl oestradiol and gestodene, thereby reducing the efficacy of the contraceptive pill [44].

Oxcarbazepine

Unlike carbamazepine, oxcarbazepine does not induce significantly hepatic metabolism and its metabolism is not subject to autoinduction. Among people with epilepsy receiving monotherapy with carbamazepine, valproic acid or phenytoin, additional treatment with oxcarbazepine did not modify steady-state plasma concentrations of these antiepileptics, indicating that oxcarbazepine does not interfere with their metabolism [45]. On the other hand, it has been suggested that oxcarbazepine, even if not inducing the CYP system in general, could selectively induce the specific isoforms of the CYP3A group involved in the metabolism of oral contraceptives and dihydropyridine calcium antagonists. In fact, oxcarbazepine has been reported to reduce significantly the plasma concentrations of ethinyloestradiol and levonorgestrel and those of the calcium an-

tagonist felodipine that are primarily metabolized by this isoenzyme [46–48]. Oxcarbazepine may also cause a significant inducing effect on lamotrigine, although less pronounced than that of carbamazepine [49]. This suggests that oxcarbazepine probably induces UGTs. The low induction capacity of oxcarbazepine should be taken into account if the drug is substituted for a more potent inducer, such as carbamazepine. Therefore, if patients are to be switched from carbamazepine to oxcarbazepine, reduction of concomitant drug dosage regimen might be necessary in order to avoid toxicity.

Topiramate

Topiramate is a weak inducer of CYP3A4. It has been reported to reduce plasma concentrations of ethinyloestradiol, which may result in decreased efficacy of the contraceptive pill [50]. Topiramate has no meaningful effects on plasma concentrations of carbamazepine and phenobarbital, while it may cause a slight but clinically unimportant decrease in plasma concentrations of valproic acid [51]. This effect has been attributed to induction of the β-oxidation of valproate.

Antiepileptics as protein binding displacers

Valproic acid

Valproic acid is highly protein bound to albumin. Because of the high molar concentrations of valproate obtained clinically, valproic acid is able to displace other antiepileptic drugs such as phenytoin and carbamazepine from albumin binding sites [31]. The effect of valproic acid on phenytoin pharmacokinetics is complex, being a combination of protein binding displacement and enzyme inhibition. Valproic acid displaces phenytoin from plasma proteins, increasing its unbound fraction, and inhibits phenytoin metabolism, reducing its intrinsic clearance. Overall, the result is that the increased unbound fraction cannot be completely counterbalanced by a proportional reduction in total concentration, and unbound concentrations cannot return to baseline values but may remain higher. Total phenytoin concentrations may be reduced, unchanged or even increased. The magnitude of the increase in unbound concentrations is thus widely variable with unpredictable clinical consequences. Whatever the outcome of the interaction, total serum phenytoin will not provide a reliable guideline to clinical management in the presence of valproic acid. Valproic acid has also been reported to displace carbamazepine from plasma binding sites, but the magnitude of this interaction is generally small and without clinical significance.

Effects of other drugs on the pharmacokinetics of antiepileptics

Antiepileptics as a target of pharmacokinetic interactions

The pharmacokinetics of antiepileptic drugs may be affected by concomitant administration of several drugs including other antiepileptics and medications used to treat comorbid disorders. Identification of the specific enzyme(s) involved in their metabolism may be of help in rational understanding, prediction and avoidance of drug–drug interactions. Antiepileptics that are not metabolized through the liver, like gabapentin and vigabatrin, are typically free

Table 10.4 Elimination pathways and protein binding for antiepileptic drugs. Average values are given for patients on monotherapy. CYP isoforms at least partially involved are shown in parentheses

Drug	Proportion of drug eliminated (%) by:				Protein binding (% bound)
	CYP	UGT	Other metabolism	Renal	
Phenytoin	90 (CYP2C9, CYP2C19)	No	Negligible	<5	90
Phenobarbital	30 (CYP2C9, CYP2C19)	Negligible	20 (N-glucosidation)	25	50
Carbamazepine	65 (CYP3A4, CYP2C8, CYP1A2)	15	Negligible	<5	75
Valproic acid	10 (CYP2C9)	40	35 (β-oxidation)	<5	90
Ethosuximide	70 (CYP3A4)	No	Negligible	20	0
Felbamate	15 (CYP3A4, CYP2E1)	10	25 (hydrolysis)	50	30
Gabapentin	No	No	No	100	0
Lamotrigine	No	65	Negligible	10	55
Levetiracetam	No	No	Hydrolysis	66	<10
Oxcarbazepine[a]	<5	45%	No	45	40
Tiagabine	>30 (CYP3A4)	No	Not identified	<2	96
Topiramate	10	No	No	60	15
Vigabatrin	No	No	No	100	0
Zonisamide	>20 (CYP3A4)	Negligible	Acetylation	30	40–60

Based on [1,28].

[a] Data refer to monohydroxy-carbazepine, the active metabolite.

of significant interactions. The elimination pathways and protein binding for antiepileptic drugs are shown in Table 10.4.

Phenytoin

Phenytoin is almost completely eliminated by hepatic metabolism with less than 5% of a dose excreted unchanged. The main metabolic pathway is the *para*-hydroxylation to form *para*-hydroxyphenytoin, which is then glucuronidated and excreted in urine. CYP2C9 has been identified as the primary isoform involved in this reaction, with CYP2C19 playing a minor role [52]. The first phenytoin metabolic step exhibits non-linear, saturable pharmacokinetics at therapeutic plasma concentrations and even minor metabolic interferences may cause clinically significant interactions. As CYP2C9 and CYP2C19 both participate in the metabolism of phenytoin, it can be anticipated that coadministration of any drug that inhibits these two isoforms will decrease the clearance of phenytoin and increase its plasma concentrations [53,54]. Interactions consistent with inhibition of CYP2C9 may be caused for example by amiodarone, phenylbutazone, fluconazole, miconazole and valproic acid. As previously stated the effect of valproic acid on phenytoin is a combination of a protein binding displacement and enzyme inhibition. Interactions consistent with inhibition of CYP2C19 are those caused by ticlopidine, omeprazole, felbamate and topiramate. Isoniazid non-competitively inhibits the metabolism of phenytoin, but it is not clear which CYP enzyme is involved.

Other enzyme-inducing anticonvulsants such as phenobarbital and carbamazepine have limited effects on plasma phenytoin concentrations as they can also inhibit its metabolism.

Phenytoin is highly bound to plasma proteins (about 90%). A large number of agents have been shown to displace phenytoin from plasma binding sites, leading to an increased phenytoin unbound fraction. As previously discussed, displacement will have no effect on steady-state unbound concentration of phenytoin in plasma and,

therefore, clinical response is unlikely to be altered. However, the total phenytoin concentration will be reduced.

Phenobarbital

Phenobarbital is eliminated both by hepatic metabolism and by renal excretion. The major metabolic route is the aromatic hydroxylation to form *para*-hydroxyphenobarbital, which is subsequently conjugated with glucuronic acid and excreted into the urine. Another metabolic pathway is the N-glucosidation to form phenobarbital-glucoside. The enzymes involved in the biotransformation of phenobarbital have not been fully characterized. However, *in vitro* studies with human liver preparations or expressed enzymes suggest that CYP2C9 and CYP2C19 are the major isoforms responsible for the *para*-hydroxylation of phenobarbital [28]. As each phenobarbital metabolic pathway contributes for no more than 20–30% of its total clearance, it can be expected that only broad-spectrum inhibitors could produce clinically relevant effects on phenobarbital elimination. In line with this prediction, valproic acid may cause an up to two-fold increase in phenobarbital concentrations, presumably by inhibiting at the same time the CYP2C9-mediated *para*-hydroxylation and the UGT-mediated N-glucosidation [55].

Potent enzyme-inducing anticonvulsants such as carbamazepine and phenytoin have limited effects on phenobarbital metabolism and usually do not modify its plasma concentrations.

Primidone

Primidone therapy results in the formation of two active metabolites, phenobarbital and phenylethylmalonamide. Therefore, the interaction profile described for phenobarbital also relates to the administration of primidone [55].

Carbamazepine

Carbamazepine is almost completely eliminated by metabolism

with less than 5% of a dose excreted unchanged in urine. The main metabolic pathway of carbamazepine is epoxidation of the 10,11 double bond to form carbamazepine-10,11-epoxide. This reaction is catalysed by CYP3A4 and, to a lesser extent, CYP2C8 [56]. The epoxide is subsequently hydrated to a *trans*-dihydrodiol by microsomal EH. Other routes of carbamazepine metabolism include aromatic hydroxylation, mediated by CYP1A2, and direct conjugation with glucuronic acid catalysed by UGT.

Although all enzyme systems responsible for carbamazepine metabolism may be inhibited, the most important type of inhibitory interactions occur with drugs that bind to CYP3A4, the primary enzyme responsible for the epoxidation of carbamazepine. As this reaction accounts for 30–50% of total carbamazepine clearance, impairment of this pathway may potentially increase plasma carbamazepine levels into the toxic range. In line with this prediction, different compounds known to inhibit CYP3A4 activity such as the calcium channel blockers diltiazem and verapamil, the macrolide antibiotics troleandomycin and erythromycin, the antidepressants viloxazine and nefazodone, the antifungal ketoconazole and fluconazole and various other compounds including cimetidine, propoxyphene, danazol, ritonavir, etc. have been reported to cause clinically significant elevation of plasma concentrations of carbamazepine [57].

A second type of inhibitory drug interaction is mediated by inhibition of microsomal EH, the enzyme responsible for the conversion of carbamazepine epoxide to inactive diol. These interactions typically result in increased levels of the epoxide metabolite which may explain the clinical signs of toxicity in the absence of any change in parent drug concentrations. The most notable interactions mediated through this pathway occur with valpromide, the amide derivative of valproic acid, and its isomer valnoctamide, an over-the-counter tranquillizer. Valproic acid also causes some inhibition of microsomal EH and increases plasma levels of carbamazepine epoxide, but the magnitude of this effect is less pronounced as compared with valpromide or valnoctamide.

The metabolism of carbamazepine is highly inducible, most probably through induction of CYP3A4. Plasma carbamazepine concentrations are reduced by concomitant administration of other anticonvulsants including barbiturates, phenytoin and felbamate.

Valproic acid

Valproic acid is almost completely eliminated by hepatic metabolism, with less than 5% of the dose excreted unchanged in the urine. The metabolism of valproic acid involves a variety of processes including direct glucuronide conjugation, mediated by UGT, mitochondrial β-oxidation and minor CYP-dependent oxidation, mainly mediated by CYP2C9 [28]. Because of the multiplicity of pathways of valproic acid metabolism, drug interactions resulting in increased plasma concentrations are complex and often multifactorial. The new antiepileptic felbamate may significantly decrease the clearance of valproic acid and therefore increase its plasma concentrations, presumably by inhibition of the β-oxidation pathway [36]. On the other hand, valproate plasma concentrations are decreased in the presence of CYP2C9- and UGT-inducing drugs such as the anticonvulsants phenytoin, phenobarbital and carbamazepine.

Ethosuximide

Ethosuximide is eliminated by hepatic enzymes (70–80%) to one or two primary oxidative metabolites, which are subsequently excreted into urine as their respective glucuronide conjugates, and partly unchanged by renal excretion (about 20%) [58]. Experimental studies in isolated rat liver microsomes indicate that the oxidative metabolism of ethosuximide is primarily carried out by CYP3A4, with minor metabolism by isoforms of the CYP2E, CYP2B and CYP2C subfamilies [59]. At this time the relative contribution of each subfamily in human metabolism has not been definitively characterized, and it is not possible to accurately extrapolate animal data to humans. Because ethosuximide is eliminated predominantly by oxidative biotransformation, its rate of metabolism would be expected to be accelerated by concomitant administration of enzyme-inducing anticonvulsants such as phenobarbital, phenytoin and carbamazepine. In line with this prediction, these metabolic inducers have been reported to increase the clearance of ethosuximide and to reduce its half-life. Conversely, valproic acid and isoniazid have been reported to inhibit the metabolism of ethosuximide and cause a small increase in its plasma concentrations. The negligible protein binding of ethosuximide eliminates the potential for protein binding interactions.

Felbamate

Felbamate is partially eliminated unchanged by the renal route (about 50%) and partially by different hepatic metabolic pathways including carbamate chain hydrolysis (about 25%) with wide further oxidation, direct N-glucuronidation (about 10%), *p*-hydroxylation (about 10%) and 2-hydroxylation (about 5%). The last two pathways seem to be dependent, at least in part, on CYP3A4 and CYP2E1, while the enzymes responsible for the chain hydrolysis have not been identified [33]. As CYP3A4 plays a minor role in the metabolism of felbamate, inhibitors of this isoform appear to have only minimal effects on the overall clearance of this drug. Consistent with this, felbamate pharmacokinetics were not significantly affected by coadministration of erythromycin, a potent inhibitor of CYP3A4. On the other hand, the clearance of felbamate is significantly increased and its plasma concentrations decreased by concomitant treatment with the enzyme-inducing antiepileptic drugs phenytoin, phenobarbital and carbamazepine. Induction of CYP3A4 is the most likely mechanism of these interactions. The sensitivity of felbamate to interaction with CYP3A4 inducers and the lack of effects of CYP3A4 inhibitors should not be viewed as a contradiction. As previously stated, this behaviour is expected and explained by the fact that the pathways controlled by this enzyme represent less than 20% of the overall felbamate clearance. Even if these pathways were appreciably inhibited, increases in plasma felbamate concentrations would be barely measurable. By contrast, there is no such limit on increases of clearance of a small pathway if induction occurs.

Gabapentin

The new antiepileptic agent gabapentin is not metabolized and is excreted mostly unchanged in urine. Consequently, it is unlikely that this compound might be involved in metabolically-based drug interactions [60]. In agreement with this, standard antiepileptic drugs did not affect the pharmacokinetics of gabapentin. The lack of protein binding of vigabatrin also makes protein binding interactions unlikely.

Lamotrigine

Lamotrigine is extensively metabolized by N-glucuronidation with only minor renal elimination. Therefore lamotrigine pharmacokinetics should not be affected by concomitant administration of CYP inhibitors. On the other hand, the rate of elimination of lamotrigine may be significantly modified by other drugs interfering with the UGT-dependent lamotrigine glucuronidation. Consistent with this, valproic acid may cause a significant increase in plasma concentrations of lamotrigine, by competitively inhibiting its glucuronidation [32]. Conversely, the clearance of lamotrigine is increased substantially in patients receiving traditional enzyme-inducing antiepileptics, an effect attributable to induction of UGT [60]. Oxcarbazepine has also been reported to induce lamotrigine metabolism, but such an effect is lower than that of the other anticonvulsants [49].

Levetiracetam

The new antiepileptic drug levetiracetam is not protein bound (< 10%) and is mainly excreted unchanged in urine (66%). Its major metabolic pathway, the enzymatic hydrolysis of the acetamide group to the inactive carboxylic derivative, does not seem to be mediated by CYPs or UGTs. As a consequence, the elimination of levetiracetam is unlikely to be affected by inhibitors or inducers of these enzymes [61,62]. In addition, in vitro studies in human liver microsomes have indicated that levetiracetam and its metabolite have no influence on the activity of different CYPs, enzymes, EH and UGTs [63]. These findings are consistent with a lack of clinically significant drug interactions involving this agent.

Oxcarbazepine

Oxcarbazepine is chemically and structurally related to carbamazepine, but has a different metabolic fate. Oxcarbazepine is essentially a prodrug that is rapidly and extensively reduced (more than 70% of a dose) by the action of hepatic cytosolic, noninducible, arylketone reductase to form the major active metabolite monohydroxy-carbazepine. The metabolite is partly excreted unchanged in the urine, partly eliminated through glucuronide conjugation, with a minor amount oxidized to carbamazepine-diol (less than 5%). Other minor routes of oxcarbazepine metabolism include direct N-glucuronidation and sulphation. Because oxcarbazepine and its metabolite are eliminated primarily through non-oxidative pathways, significant interactions resulting from metabolic inhibition seem to be unlikely [60]. Consistent with this, none of the known inhibitors of carbamazepine metabolism (e.g. erythromycin, dextropropoxyphene, verapamil, cimetidine) has been reported to interfere significantly with the elimination of oxcarbazepine. Although the metabolism of oxcarbazepine to its active metabolite is mediated by a non-inducible reductase, enzyme-inducing anticonvulsants are expected to increase the elimination of the active metabolite monohydroxycarbazepine through the glucuronide and/or diol pathways. In this respect, phenobarbital, phenytoin and carbamazepine have been reported to accelerate the catabolism of monohydroxycarbazepine and reduce its plasma concentrations. However, the magnitude of the effect is small and unlikely to be clinically significant. For this reason, the potential for interactions with enzyme-inducing anticonvulsants is in general lower during oxcarbazepine therapy compared with carbamazepine treatment.

Tiagabine

Tiagabine is extensively metabolized with only 1–2% excreted unchanged in the urine. The major metabolic pathway is the oxidation of the thiophene ring, forming two 5-oxo-tiogabine isomers, which accounts for approximately 22% of the total dose [64], a reaction that appears to be mediated by CYP3A4. Consequently, it may be anticipated that inhibitors of CYP3A4 may interact with tiagabine by decreasing its clearance and increasing plasma concentrations. However, coadministration of erythromycin, a potent CYP3A4 inhibitor, did not significantly affect the pharmacokinetics of tiagabine [65]. The rate of elimination of tiagabine may be markedly accelerated by inducing agents. In a study in patients with epilepsy, concomitant treatment with enzyme-inducing anticonvulsants has been reported to decrease plasma tiagabine concentrations to one-half to one-third as compared to those observed in patients not comedicated [66]. Tiagabine is highly bound to plasma proteins (96%) and protein–binding interactions are theoretically possible. In vitro, it is displaced from plasma protein binding sites by naproxen, salicylates and valproic acid, but these displacement interactions are clinically insignificant.

Topiramate

Topiramate is predominantly eliminated unchanged through the kidneys (60–70%). It is also metabolized by hydroxylation and hydrolysis, but the isoenzymes involved have not yet been identified. Because metabolism is of minor importance in the overall clearance of topiramate, significant interactions resulting from inhibition are unlikely. On the other hand, metabolic elimination possibly becomes the major determinant of topiramate disposition in patients treated with inducing drugs. In this respect, concurrent use of enzyme-inducing antiepileptic drugs has been reported to reduce plasma topiramate concentrations by approximately 40–50% [51].

Vigabatrin

Vigabatrin is eliminated almost completely unchanged by the kidneys. As is predictable from the fact that vigabatrin is not metabolized, coadministration of metabolic inhibitors or inducers does not modify its pharmacokinetics [60]. Also, because vigabatrin is not bound to plasma proteins, interactions due to competition with other drugs for protein binding are circumvented.

Zonisamide

Zonisamide is a sulfonamide derivative that is chemically and structurally unrelated to other anticonvulsants. It is partly eliminated unchanged in urine and partly metabolized by acetylation and by cleavage of the isoxazole ring followed by conjugation with glucuronic acid. Studies with human liver microsomes suggest that CYP3A4 is involved in cleavage of the isoxazole ring [67]. Therefore, it can be anticipated that inducers of CYP3A4 might stimulate zonisamide elimination. Consistent with this, enzyme-inducing anticonvulsants such as carbamazepine, phenytoin and phenobarbital were all reported to enhance the clearance of zonisamide and to decrease its plasma concentrations [68]. On the other hand, there is no evidence that inhibitors of the CYP3A4 isoform may decrease zonisamide clearance.

Pharmacodynamic interactions

Pharmacodynamic interactions may occur when two drugs act at the same or interrelated receptor sites. These interactions may be additive, synergistic or antagonistic and may be beneficial or associated with increased toxicity. Pharmacodynamic interactions of antiepileptic drugs have been well documented in animal studies [69], but limited information is available on the occurrence and magnitude of these interactions in man, as they are often uncovered during clinical trials or are reported anecdotally. Moreover, in many situations the clinical picture is complicated by concomitant pharmacokinetic modifications. Combinations of antiepileptic drugs may result in increased efficacy, but also a higher risk for toxic effects [70]. The mode of action of licensed anticonvulsants involves different mechanisms including sodium channel blockade, calcium channel blockade, inhibition of GABAergic transmission and potentiation of glutamatergic transmission. Theoretically, older antiepileptics which act by a combination of these mechanisms are at higher risk as compared to newer drugs that, with the exception of topiramate and gabapentin, are reputed to have a single, well-defined mode of action. Polypharmacy with antiepileptics is believed to be responsible for an increased frequency of adverse events and teratogenesis, in addition to pharmacokinetic interactions.

There are many examples of undesirable potentiation of toxic effects that can occur when antiepileptics are given in combination due to pharmacodynamic interactions. Combinations of drugs that enhance GABAergic inhibition, such as valproic acid and phenobarbital, may result in profound sedation that cannot be explained by a pharmacokinetic interaction [71]. Concomitant administration of valproic acid with lamotrigine may produce disabling tremor [72]. Carbamazepine and lamotrigine have been particularly noted to enhance each other's side-effect profile, with possible occurrence of diplopia, dizziness, nausea and vomiting. As plasma concentrations of both carbamazepine (including the epoxide metabolite) and lamotrigine were not significantly affected following addition of either agent, these effects appear to be the result of a pharmacodynamic interaction [73].

It has been hypothesized that concomitant administration of different anticonvulsants to pregnant women with epilepsy may increase the risk of congenital malformations in newborns. In general, the overall rate of malformations is 11.1% in offspring of epileptic mothers taking antiepileptics, while it is 5.7% in offspring of untreated epileptic mothers and 4.8% in those of the general population. It has been observed that the incidence of these malformations increases with increasing number of antiepileptic agents administered during the first trimester of pregnancy [74]. Therefore, antiepileptic polypharmacy is clearly related to the risk of teratogenicity and the incidence of malformations is remarkably high with some combinations. As the mechanism of teratogenesis may involve the production of epoxide or other toxic metabolite intermediates, it is difficult to differentiate the relative contribution of pharmacokinetic and pharmacodynamic factors in the occurrence of a teratogenic interaction.

Increased toxicity may also occur as a consequence of a pharmacodynamic interaction between antiepileptics and other drugs. Concomitant administration of antiepileptics with central nervous system depressants such as alcohol, antihistamines, and phenothiazines may enhance central nervous system depression, thereby impairing psychomotor and cognitive function, especially in an elderly population. A number of antiepileptics, particularly carbamazepine, valproic acid and lamotrigine, are increasingly used in the management of psychiatric disorders and often in combination with antidepressants, lithium or antipsychotics. There is some evidence that the combination of lithium and carbamazepine may lead to an increased incidence of neurotoxicity. The mechanism of interaction appears to be mainly pharmacodynamic [75]. Concurrent treatment with lithium and valproate has been associated with additive adverse reactions such as weight gain, sedation, gastrointestinal complaints and tremor. On the other hand, the combination of carbamazepine and clozapine is generally contraindicated due to concerns about potential additive adverse haematological side-effects [76].

Conclusions

Drug interactions represent a frequent complication in patients treated with antiepileptic drugs. The most common interactions involving antiepileptics are pharmacokinetic and occur through metabolic inhibition or induction and, less frequently, from protein binding displacement. It should be emphasized that only a few drug interactions have clinical implications. In general, the clinician should expect a clinically significant interaction when a drug with a low therapeutic index is coadministered with a potent inhibitor or inducer of the major pathway of its metabolism. Based on the available evidence, many of the new antiepileptic agents appear to have a lower potential for drug interactions than older agents. Information about the specific enzymes responsible for the metabolism of individual antiepileptic drugs and about the effects of these compounds on the activity of the various metabolic enzymes may help in predicting and avoiding clinically significant interactions. Apart from careful clinical observation, monitoring of plasma concentrations of the relevant drugs may be useful in determining the need for dosage adjustments in individual cases.

References

1 Riva R, Albani F, Contin M, Baruzzi A. Pharmacokinetic interactions between antiepileptic drugs: clinical considerations. *Clin Pharmacokinet* 1996; 31: 470–93.
2 Patsalos PN, Duncan JS. Antiepileptic drugs: A review of clinically significant drug interactions. *Drug Saf* 1993; 9: 156–84.
3 French JA, Gidal BE. Antiepileptic drug interactions. *Epilepsia* 2000; 41 (Suppl. 8): S30–S36.
4 Perucca, E. The new generation of antiepileptic drugs: Advantages and disadvantages. *Br J Clin Pharmacol* 1996; 42: 531–43.
5 Gonzalez FJ. Human cytochrome P450: Problem and prospects. *Trend Pharmacol Sci Rev* 1992; 13: 346–52.
6 Guengerich FP. Role of cytochrome P450 enzymes in drug–drug interactions. *Adv Pharmacol* 1997; 43: 7–35.
7 Nelson DR, Koymans L, Kamataki T *et al.* P450 superfamily: update on new sequences, gene mapping, accession numbers and nomenclature. *Pharmacogenetics* 1996; 6: 1–42.
8 Meyer UA. The molecular basis of genetic polymorphism of drug metabolism. *J Pharm* 1994; 46: 409–15.
9 Rendic S, Di Carlo FJ. Human cytochrome P450 enzymes: a status report summarizing their reactions, substrates, inducers, and inhibitors. *Drug Metab Rev* 1997; 29: 413–580.
10 Shimada T, Yamazaki H, Mimura M, Inui Y, Guengerich FP. Interindividual variations in human liver cytochrome P450 enzymes involved in oxidation of drugs, carcinogens, and toxic chemicals: studies with human liver

microsomes of 30 Japanese and 30 Caucasians. *J Pharmacol Exp Ther* 1994; 270: 414–23.

11 Brandolese R, Scordo MG, Spina E, Gusella M, Padrini R. Severe phenytoin intoxication in a subject homozygous for CYP2C9*3. *Clin Pharmacol Ther* 2001; 70: 391–4.

12 Omcienski CJ. Epoxide hydrolases. In: Levy RH, Thummel KE, Trager WF, Hansten PD, Eichelbaum M, eds. *Metabolic Drug Interactions*. Philadelphia: Lippincott Williams & Wilkins, 2000: 205–14.

13 Lindhout D. Pharmacogenetics and drug interactions: role in antiepileptic drug-induced teratogenesis. *Neurology* 1992; 42: 43–7.

14 Kerr BM, Rettie AE, Eddy AC *et al*. Inhibition of human liver microsomal epoxide hydrolase by valproate and valpromide: in vitro/in vivo correlation. *Clin Pharmacol Ther* 1989; 46: 82–93.

15 Liston HL, Markowitz JS, Devane L. Drug glucuronidation in clinical psychopharmacology. *J Clin Psychopharmacol* 2001; 21: 500–15.

16 Mackenzie PI, Owens IS, Burchell B *et al*. The UDP glycosyltransferase gene superfamily: recommended nomenclature update based on evolutionary divergence. *Pharmacogenetics* 1997; 7: 255–69.

17 Lin JH, Lu AYH. Inhibition and induction of cytochrome P450 and the clinical implications. *Clin Pharmacokinet* 1998; 35: 361–90.

18 Thummel KE, Kunze KL, Shen DD. Metabolically-based drug–drug interactions: principles and mechanisms. In: Levy RH, Thummel KE, Trager WF, Hansten PD, Eichelbaum M, eds. *Metabolic Drug Interactions*. Philadelphia: Lippincott Williams & Wilkins, 2000, 3–19.

19 Park BK, Kitteringham NR, Pirmohamed M, Tucker GT. Relevance of induction of human drug-metabolizing enzymes: pharmacological and toxicological implications. *Br J Clin Pharmacol* 1996; 41: 477–91.

20 Fuhr U. Induction of drug metabolising enzymes: pharmacokinetic and toxicological consequences in humans. *Clin Pharmacokinet* 2000; 38: 493–504.

21 Sueyoshi T, Kawamoto T, Zelko I, Honkakoski P, Negishi M. The repressed nuclear receptor CAR respond to phenobarbital in activating the human CYP2B6 gene. *J Biol Chem* 1999; 274: 6043–6.

22 Levy RH. Cytochrome P450 isozymes and antiepileptic drug interactions. *Epilepsia* 1995; 36 (Suppl. 5): S8–S13.

23 Li AP, Maurel P, Gomez-Lechon MJ, Cheng LC, Jurima-Romet M. Preclinical evaluation of drug–drug interaction potential: present status of the application of primary human hepatocytes in the evaluation of cytochrome P450 induction. *Chem Biol Interact* 1997; 107: 5–16.

24 Bertz RJ, Granneman GR. Use of in vitro and in vivo data to estimate the likelihood of metabolic pharmacokinetic interactions. *Clin Pharmacokinet* 1997; 32: 210–58.

25 Levy RH, Trager WF. From *in vitro* to *in vivo*: an academic perspective. In: Levy RH, Thummel KE, Trager WF, Hansten PD, Eichelbaum M, eds. *Metabolic Drug Interactions*. Philadelphia: Lippincott Williams & Wilkins, 2000, 21–7.

26 Sproule BA, Naranjo CA, Bremner KE, Hassan PC. Selective serotonin reuptake inhibitors and CNS drug interactions: A critical review of the evidence. *Clin Pharmacokinet* 1997; 33: 454–71.

27 Anderson GD, Graves NM. Drug interactions with antiepileptic agents: prevention and management. *CNS Drugs* 1994; 2: 268–79.

28 Anderson GD. A mechanistic approach to antiepileptic drug interactions. *Ann Pharmacother* 1998; 32: 554–63.

29 Hurst SI, Labroo R, Carlson SP, Mather GG, Levy RH. In vitro inhibition profile of valproic acid for cytochrome P450 (abstract). *Int Soc Xenobiotics Proc* 1997; 12: 64.

30 Wen X, Wang JS, Kivisto KT, Neuvonen PJ, Backman JT. In vitro evaluation of valproic acid as an inhibitor of human cytochrome P450 isoforms: preferential inhibition of cytochrome P450 2C9 (CYP2C9). *Br J Clin Pharmacol* 2001; 52: 547–53.

31 Scheyer RD, Mattson RH. Valproic acid: interactions with other drugs. In: Levy RH, Thummel KE, Trager WF, Hansten PD, Eichelbaum M, eds. *Antiepileptic Drugs*. New York: Raven Press 1995: 621–31.

32 Yuen AW, Land G, Weatherley BC, Peck AW. Sodium valproate acutely inhibits lamotrigine metabolism. *Br J Clin Pharmacol* 1992; 33: 511–13.

33 Glue P, Banfield CR, Perhach JL, Mather GG, Racha JK, Levy RH. Pharmacokinetic interactions with felbamate: in vitro–in vivo correlation. *Clin Pharmacokinet* 1997; 33: 214–24.

34 Fuerst RH, Graves NM, Leppik IE, Brundage RC, Holmes GB, Remmel

RP. Felbamate increases phenytoin but decreases carbamazepine concentrations. *Epilepsia* 1988; 29: 488–91.

35 Gidal BE, Zupanc ML. Potential pharmacokinetic interaction between felbamate and phenobarbital. *Ann Pharmacother* 1994; 28: 455–8.

36 Hooper WD, Franklin ME, Glue P *et al*. Effect of felbamate on valproic acid disposition in healthy volunteers: inhibition of beta-oxidation. *Epilepsia* 1996; 37: 91–7.

37 Levy RH, Bishop F, Streeter AJ *et al*. Explanation and prediction of drug interactions with topiramate using a CYP450 inhibition spectrum. *Epilepsia* 1995; 36 (Suppl. 4): 47.

38 Gisclon LG, Curtin CR, Sachdeo RC, Levy RH. The steady-state (SS) pharmacokinetics (PK) of phenytoin (Dilantin) and topiramate (Topamax) in epileptic patients on monotherapy, and during combination therapy. *Epilepsia* 1994; 35 (Suppl. 8): 54.

39 Abdel-Rahman SM, Leeder JS. Phenobarbital, phenytoin, and carbamazepine. In: Levy RH, Thummel KE, Trager WF, Hansten PD, Eichelbaum M, eds. *Metabolic Drug Interactions*. Philadelphia: Lippincott Williams & Wilkins, 2000: 673–89.

40 Parker AC, Pritchard P, Preston T, Choonara I. Induction of CYP1A2 activity by carbamazepine in children using the caffeine breath test. *Br J Clin Pharmacol* 1998; 45: 176–8.

41 Shaw PN, Houston JB, Rowland M *et al*. Antipyrine metabolite kinetics in healthy human volunteers during multiple dosing of phenytoin and carbamazepine. *Br J Clin Pharmacol* 1985; 20: 611–18.

42 Kondo T, Otani K, Hirano T, Kaneko S, Fukushima Y. The effects of phenytoin and carbamazepine in serum concentrations of mono-unsaturated metabolites of valproic acid. *Br J Clin Pharmacol* 1990; 29: 116–19.

43 Perucca E, Richens A. Biotransformation. In: Levy RH, Mattson RH, Meldrum B, eds. *Antiepileptic Drugs*, 4th edn. New York: Raven Press, 1995, 31–50.

44 Saano V, Glue P, Benfield CR *et al*. Effects of felbamate on the pharmacokinetics of a low-dose combination oral contraceptive. *Clin Pharmacol Ther* 1995; 58: 523–31.

45 McKee PJW, Blacklaw J, Forrest G *et al*. A double-blind, placebo-controlled interaction study between oxcarbazepine and carbamazepine, sodium valproate and phenytoin in epileptic patients. *Br J Clin Pharmacol* 1994; 37: 27–32.

46 Klosterkov Jensen P, Saano V, Haring P, Svenstrup B, Menge GP. Possible interaction between oxcarbazepine and an oral contraceptive. *Epilepsia* 1992; 33: 1149–52.

47 Fattore C, Cipolla G, Gatti G *et al*. Induction of ethinylestradiol and levonorgestrel metabolism by oxcarbazepine in healthy women. *Epilepsia* 1999; 40: 783–7.

48 Zaccara G, Gangemi PF, Bendoni L, Menge GP, Schwabe S, Monza GC. Influence of single and repeated doses of oxcarbazepine on the pharmacokinetics profile of felodipine. *Ther Drug Monit* 1993; 15: 39–42.

49 May TW, Rambeck B, Jurgens U. Influence of oxcarbazepine and methsuximide on lamotrigine concentrations in epileptic patients with and without valproic acid co-medication: results of a retrospective study. *Ther Drug Monit* 1999; 21: 175–81.

50 Rosenfeld WE, Doose DR, Walker SA, Nayak RK. Effect of topiramate on the pharmacokinetics of an oral contraceptive containing norethindrone and ethinyl estradiol in patients with epilepsy. *Epilepsia* 1997; 38: 317–23.

51 Johannesen SI. Pharmacokinetics and interaction profile of topiramate. Review and comparison with other newer antiepileptic drugs. *Epilepsia* 1997; 38 (Suppl. 1): S18–S23.

52 Bajpai M, Roskos LK, Shen DD, Levy RH. Roles of cytochrome P4502C9 and cytochrome P4502C19 in stereoselective metabolism of phenytoin to its major metabolite. *Drug Metab Dispos* 1996; 24: 1401–3.

53 Kutt H. Phenytoin: interactions with other drugs. Part 1. Clinical aspects. In: Levy RH, Mattson RH, Meldrum BS, eds. *Antiepileptic Drugs*. New York: Raven Press, 1995: 315–28.

54 Levy RH, Bajpai M. Phenytoin: interactions with other drugs. Part 2. Mechanistic aspects. In: Levy RH, Mattson RH, Meldrum BS, eds. *Antiepileptic Drugs*. New York: Raven Press, 1995: 329–44.

55 Bernus I, Dickinson G, Hooper WD, Eadie MJ. Inhibition of phenobarbital N-glucosidation by valproate. *Br J Clin Pharmacol* 1994; 38: 411–16.

56 Kerr BM, Thummel KE, Wurden CJ *et al*. Human liver carbamazepine metabolism: role of CYP3A4 and CYP2C8 in the 10,11-epoxide formation. *Biochem Pharmacol* 1994; 47: 1969–79.

57 Spina E, Pisani F, Perucca E. Clinically significant pharmacokinetic drug interactions with carbamazepine: an update. *Clin Pharmacokinet* 1996; 3: 198–214.

58 Bialer M, Xiaodong S, Perucca E. Ethosuximide: absorption, distribution and excretion. In: Levy RH, Mattson RH, Meldrum BS, eds. *Antiepileptic Drugs*. New York: Raven Press, 1995: 659–65.

59 Sarver JG, Bachmann KA, Zhu D, Klis WA. Ethosuximide is primarily metabolized by CYP3A when incubated with isolated rat liver microsomes. *Drug Metab Dispos* 1998; 26: 78–82.

60 Rambeck B, Specht U, Wolf P. Pharmacokinetic interactions of the new antiepileptic drugs. *Clin Pharmacokinet* 1996; 31: 309–24.

61 Patsalos PN. Pharmacokinetic profile of levetiracetam: towards ideal characteristics. *Pharmacol Ther* 2000; 85: 77–85.

62 Strolin Benedetti M. Enzyme induction and inhibition by new antiepileptic drugs: a review of human studies. *Fundam Clin Pharmacol* 2000; 14: 301–19.

63 Nicolas JM, Collart P, Gerin B *et al*. In vitro evaluation of potential drug interactions with levetiracetam, a new antiepileptic agent. *Drug Metab Dispos* 1999; 27: 250–4.

64 Adkins JC, Noble S. Tiagabine: a review of its pharmacodynamic and pharmacokinetic properties and therapeutic potential in the management of epilepsy. *Drugs* 1998; 55: 437–60.

65 Thomsen MS, Groes L, Agerso H, Kruse T. Lack of pharmacokinetic interaction between tiagabine and erythromycin. *J Clin Pharmacol* 1998; 38: 1051–6.

66 So EL, Wolff D, Graves NM *et al*. Pharmacokinetics of tiagabine as add-on therapy in patients taking antiepilepsy drugs. *Epilepsy Res* 1995; 22: 221–6.

67 Nakasa H, Komiya M, Ohmori S, Rikihisa T, Kiuchi M, Kitada M. Characterization of human liver microsomal cytochrome P450 involved in the reductive metabolism of zonisamide. *Mol Pharmacol* 1993; 44: 218–21.

68 Shinoda M, Akita M, Hasegawa M, Hasegawa T, Nabeshima T. The necessity of adjusting the dosage of zonisamide when coadministered with other anti-epileptic drugs. *Biol Pharm Bull* 1996; 19: 1090–2.

69 Bourgeois BF. Anticonvulsant potency and neurotoxicity of valproate alone or in combination with carbamazepine or phenobarbital. *Clin Neuropharmacol* 1988; 11: 348–59.

70 Leach JP. Polypharmacy with anticonvulsants: focus on synergism. *CNS Drugs* 1997; 8: 366–75.

71 Kutt H. Phenobarbital: interactions with other drugs. In: Levy RH, Mattson RH, Meldrum BS, eds. *Antiepileptic Drugs*. New York: Raven Press, 1995: 389–99.

72 Reutens DC, Duncan JS, Patsalos PN. Disabling tremor after lamotrigine and sodium valproate. *Lancet* 1993; 342: 185–6.

73 Besag FMC, Berry DJ, Pool F, Newbery JE, Subel B. Carbamazepine toxicity with lamotrigine: pharmacokinetic or pharmacodynamic interaction? *Epilepsia* 1998; 39: 183–7.

74 Kaneko S, Kondo T. Antiepileptic agents and birth defects: incidence, mechanisms and prevention. *CNS Drugs* 1995; 3: 41–55.

75 Freeman MP, Stoll AL. Mood stabilizer combinations: a review of safety and efficacy. *Am J Psychiatry* 1998; 155: 12–21.

76 Junghan U, Albers M, Woggon B. Increased risk of hematological side-effects in psychiatric patients treated with clozapine and carbamazepine? *Pharmacopsychiatry* 1993; 26: 262.

Section 2
Principles of Medical Treatment

11 General Principles of Medical Treatment

E. Perucca

Although the medical treatment of epilepsy almost invariably involves prescription of anticonvulsant drugs, rational management necessitates much more than a good knowledge of clinical pharmacology. First, the decision on whether treatment is indicated requires careful consideration of the risk to benefit equation in the individual patient, which, in turn, is influenced not only by the type and the frequency of seizures, but also by age, sex, presence of associated medical conditions and the prospected impact of potential side-effects on the patient's quality of life. A thorough diagnostic evaluation is essential in this process because the type of treatment, its anticipated duration and long-term prognosis are dependent upon a correct identification of the epilepsy syndrome and, possibly, even its aetiology. Although achieving seizure control is usually the most important objective of medical management, seizures are not the only cause for concern for patients with epilepsy. Associated neurological, intellectual, psychological and social handicaps need to be equally addressed. Patients and their caregivers need to be informed about the nature of the disease, its prognostic implications, the objectives of therapy, the risks and benefits of treatment (including the risks associated with poor compliance and with abrupt discontinuation of therapy) and the existence of alternative therapeutic strategies (including epilepsy surgery) should the initial treatment fail to produce the desired response. Medical management should also involve a discussion of factors that could impact negatively on seizure control, without placing undue restrictions on the patient's lifestyle. Counselling about marriage, reproduction, driving regulations and other legal matters may be indicated. Even in affluent societies, epilepsy is still associated with stigma, and affected patients may suffer more from prejudice and discrimination than from the actual manifestations of the disease. As a result, psychological and social support is often required and represents a major component of clinical management in individual cases.

The purpose of the present chapter is to review the general principles which should guide medical management. Specific therapeutic strategies to be adopted in relation to the stage of the disease and to the individual patient's characteristics, including age, sex, associated learning disability, pychiatric disorders and other concomitant medical conditions, are discussed in greater detail in the following chapters.

Aims of treatment

The primary goal of epilepsy treatment is to ensure the best possible quality of life that is compatible with the nature of the patient's seizure disorder and with any associated mental or physical disabilities [1]. To achieve this general goal, various objectives need to be addressed whenever relevant or feasible.

Complete seizure control

If exception is made for the control of ongoing seizures and status epilepticus, the treatment of epilepsy is primarily prophylactic, e.g. aimed at preventing seizure recurrence. Prospective studies have demonstrated that there is a world of difference for the patient's quality of life between a state of complete seizure freedom and even rare seizures separated by long intervals. Therefore, the primary objective of treatment should be complete seizure control. This, however, should not be achieved at all costs. Antiepileptic drugs may produce severe side-effects, particularly when they are administered at high dosages or in combination, and the situation should never arise where a patient is made to suffer more from the side-effects of treatment than from the symptoms of the underlying disease. Whenever complete seizure freedom proves to be a non-realistic goal, optimal treatment results from a compromise between the desire to minimize seizure frequency and the need to maintain side-effects within acceptable limits.

Reduction of seizure severity

In patients whose seizures cannot be controlled completely by anticonvulsant medication at maximally tolerated dosages, a secondary important aim is to suppress or to reduce the frequency of those seizures which have the worst impact on the patient's quality of life. For example, in patients with Lennox–Gastaut syndrome control of drop attacks may produce far greater clinical benefits than suppression of associated partial or atypical absence seizures. Likewise, a treatment that will prevent secondary generalization would be expected to have a major impact on the quality of life of a patient with simple sensory partial seizures. Antiepileptic drugs may have a range of effects on the components of ictal events by suppressing or modifying the type or the duration of auras, convulsive manifestations, associated autonomic features and postictal events [2]. Assessing the most disabling seizure types may require assistance from an external observer, but the patient's perceptions are more important. A seizure component that may appear trivial or negligible to an observer may be perceived as extremely distressing by the patient. Unfortunately, how antiepileptic drugs modify seizure components has been little studied, but in individual patients this aspect has an important impact on clinical management.

Avoidance of side-effects

As discussed above, prescription of antiepileptic medication entails a significant risk of side-effects. Choice of drugs, titration rate and dosage need to be tailored to the needs of the individual patient. In many patients with recently diagnosed epilepsy, it is realistic to expect that complete seizure control be achieved at dosages that produce no detectable toxicity. Patients with severe types of epilepsy, on the other hand, may have to pay a significant price in terms of side-effects to avoid or minimize the risk of seizure recurrence. Occasionally, patients are encountered in whom available medications do not seem to have any significant effect on the frequency of their seizures. These patients are only harmed by prescription of antiepileptic drugs, and physicians should be prepared to accept that the best management in such cases is not to prescribe any drug at all. Treatment may also not be indicated in patients with very infrequent seizures, especially when these occur only at night or in relation to predictable precipitating events, such as severe sleep deprivation, or have no important impact on the patient's psychological, social or professional conditions.

Suppression of subclinical epileptic activity

Antiepileptic drug therapy as a rule should be aimed at suppressing the clinical manifestations of seizures, and normalization of the EEG generally is neither a primary nor an attainable objective. In certain situations, however, suppression of epileptiform EEG abnormalities becomes a justifiable therapeutic goal. This is the case when there is a close correlate between clinical seizures and EEG paroxysms, and seizures are not easily quantifiable clinically, as in childhood absence epilepsy or some photosensitive epilepsies. In infants and children with severe epileptiform EEG abnormalities coexisting with brain dysfunction, the extent of EEG-related dysfunction should be determined and vigorous treatment may be needed to abate its effects (see Chapter 14). In other cases, intermittent and short-lived epileptiform discharges in the EEG may lead to subtle functional impairment, which is only detectable at careful cognitive testing, especially in children with generalized epilepsies. While monitoring the EEG response in these patients can be useful in optimizing treatment, it is important to document that suppression of the EEG discharges does result in significant functional improvement. In fact, there is a risk that any improvement secondary to suppression of such discharges be overshadowed by direct negative effects of drug treatment on cognitive function or behaviour.

Reduction of mortality and morbidity

In certain cases where seizures are triggered by a treatable cause, such as a brain tumour, removal of the latter is essential to reduce any related morbidity and mortality. In recent years, however, evidence has accumulated that seizures *per se* are associated with an increased mortality, partly in relation to accidents which may occur during a seizure and partly in relation to the risk of sudden unexpected death in epilepsy (SUDEP) [3]. In patients with frequent convulsive seizures, the incidence of SUDEP may be as high as 1 per 100 or 200 patient years. Seizures are also associated with an increased risk of physical injuries, particularly burns, head trauma and bone fractures. An effective antiepileptic drug treatment would be expected to reduce mortality and morbidity, even though this has not been adequately investigated.

Avoidance of adverse drug interactions

In patients requiring therapy with a combination of antiepileptic drugs, there is a risk of adverse drug interactions, either at pharmacokinetic or pharmacodynamic level. Additionally, interactions may occur between antiepileptic drugs and medications taken for contraception, or for the management of concomitant medical conditions. Physicians should be aware of this, and take all necessary steps to minimize the adverse consequences that may result from drug interactions. In most cases, drug interactions can be predicted based on current knowledge of the influence of antiepileptic drugs on liver cytochrome P450 isoenzymes (see Chapter 10), and they can be safely managed through appropriate dosage adjustment and monitoring of plasma drug concentrations.

Avoidance of obstruction to patient's life

Even in the presence of adequate pharmacological treatment, therapeutic outcome may be influenced by the patient's ability to identify and avoid situations which could adversely affect susceptibility to seizures, such as excessive sleep deprivation, or—in some photosensitive epilepsies—exposure to intermittent flashing lights or certain video games. While these risk factors need to be discussed and appropriate counselling given, it is equally important to avoid imposing undue restrictions on the patient's lifestyle. For example, alcohol abuse should be actively discouraged, but there is no reason to prohibit one glass of beer or wine at meal times. In general, patients should be encouraged to live a normal life, while avoiding extreme deviations from what would be considered a regular lifestyle. Prescription of medication should also be aimed at minimizing interference with daily activities. Antiepileptic drugs which can be given once or twice daily are less likely to obstruct daily routines and to cause psychosocial embarrassment, and they are associated with a better compliance. For drugs which can be given once or twice daily but do not have a very long half-life, a twice daily schedule may be preferable because it minimizes the adverse consequences of missing one dose. In general, once daily dosing does not entail better compliance than twice daily dosing, but it may have psychological advantages, particularly in patients who are seizure free and perceive each pill-taking as the only unpleasant reminder of their disease.

Prevention of epileptogenesis

Experiments in animal models suggest that some antiepileptic drugs not only exert a symptomatic effect by raising seizure threshold, but they may also antagonize the process of epileptogenesis, i.e. the mechanisms through which an epileptic condition becomes established [4]. The suggestion has been made that recurrence of clinical seizures could also cause irreversible neuroanatomical changes, which may render the disease more difficult to control, but evidence for this is controversial [5,6], as illustrated by the unsolved debate on whether hippocampal sclerosis is a cause or a consequence of temporal lobe seizures [3,7]. If uncontrolled seizure activity leads to chronicization of the disorder, a case could be made for early and aggressive treatment, and for preferential use of drugs which antagonize putative epileptogenic processes. Available clinical studies, however, suggest that in most epilepsy syndromes antiepileptic drugs exert merely a symptomatic effect and do not affect the natural course of the disease [8,9]. Admittedly, special conditions may exist in which early effective treatment may improve the ultimate prognosis, possible examples being West's syndrome and other early childhood myoclonic encephalopathies associated with progressive cognitive decline. In the latter conditions, however, the benefits of early seizure control seem to relate more to cognitive outcome than to the history of epilepsy *per se* [9].

When to start treatment

As discussed in greater detail in Chapter 12, a correct diagnosis should be formulated before rational treatment can be instituted. Differentiation between epileptic and non-epileptic attacks (e.g. psychogenic seizures or syncopal episodes) is not always obvious, and appropriate investigations are required to establish the nature of the disorder. In addition, every effort should be made to identify as early as possible seizure type and syndromic form, because these are important in determining drug selection and prognosis. Although it is acknowledged that a syndromic diagnosis is not always easy at outset, a recent study in children has shown that experienced physicians can identify correctly the vast majority of epilepsy syndromes at the very beginning [10]. Indeed, less than 10% of initial diagnoses had to be rectified at reassessment 2 years later, and most of these rectifications involved syndromes that represented incomplete classifications in the first place.

Institution of antiepileptic drug treatment is indicated whenever the expected benefits outweigh potential risks. The risk to benefit equation, in turn, is determined by many factors, including the type of epilepsy, the frequency and severity of the seizures, the age and the occupation of the patient, associated medical conditions, the characteristics of the drug(s) being considered and the presumed influence of treatment on the patient's wellbeing and aspirations [3]. In many situations, the decision on whether to start treatment or to withhold it will involve no uncertainty, but grey areas exist where the optimal therapeutic strategy is uncertain. In any case, the patient should be involved in the therapeutic decision, because his/her attitude towards the possibility of recurrence of seizures and towards the risks of antiepileptic drug treatment represents an important consideration in establishing the indications for treatment. The actual decision must be based on consideration of individual factors, and a number of different scenarios will be briefly discussed.

Patients with a single seizure

Since epilepsy by definition is characterized by recurrent paroxysmal episodes, occurrence of a single seizure does not allow the diagnosis of epilepsy to be made, and generally it does not warrant institution of treatment [11]. However, there may be situations where treatment may be considered even after a single seizure.

The most common situation where a physician faces a therapeutic dilemma is when a patient experiences a single unprovoked tonic-clonic seizure whose nature is considered to be probably epileptic. Because many such patients will not have a recurrence when left untreated [12], and because treatment after a first seizure does not improve long-term prognosis [13], indiscriminate prescription of antiepileptic drugs after a first tonic-clonic seizure, whilst effective in reducing the risk of relapse [14], will expose many patients unnecessarily to adverse effects. Therefore, drug therapy

should generally be deferred until a second seizure occurs. Treatment after a first seizure, however, may be considered when specific prognostic factors indicate a high risk of recurrence (in particular, when the EEG shows interictal epileptiform abnormalities, and/or there is an identified persisting cause for the seizures, such as MRI-documented cortical dysplasia), or when it is felt that the physical or psychosocial consequences of a seizure recurrence outweigh the risks associated with drug treatment [15].

Patients with a history of two or more unprovoked seizures

Provided that the epileptic nature of the seizures has been established, patients with recurrent seizures generally require antiepileptic drug therapy. Exceptions may be represented by patients with rare seizures, particularly when these are mild, brief or occur only during sleep, and they do not interfere with the patient's psychological state, daily activities, occupation and social integration. Additionally, pharmacological treatment is generally not indicated in some benign childhood epilepsies with a self-remitting course, when the side-effects of antiepileptic drugs are expected to affect quality of life to a greater extent than the seizures themselves. The best example is represented by children with benign partial epilepsy with centrotemporal spikes (rolandic epilepsy), where treatment is usually indicated only in the few cases in whom seizures are frequent, severe and occur during daytime.

Patients with seizures precipitated by specific triggers

When seizures are precipitated by specific triggers, avoidance of the latter may be sufficient. Some forms of photosensitive epilepsy for example, can be managed by prescribing appropriate lenses, or by instructing the patient on how to avoid exposure to the offending light frequencies. Continuous pharmacological prophylaxis is also not indicated in most children with febrile seizures who are older than 1 year [16].

Other situations

Occasionally, treatment may be justified without a clear-cut diagnosis of epilepsy. When even intensive monitoring techniques fail to provide differentiation between epileptic seizures and pseudoseizures, a therapeutic trial may be indicated. Lack of response to treatment suggests a non-epileptic nature of the attacks, but it should not be regarded as a conclusive proof for this. Conversely, improvement or even disappearance of seizures after treatment does not prove that the attacks were epileptic in origin. Apart from the possibility of a placebo response or a spontaneous change in the natural history of the disorder, it should be remembered that antiepileptic drugs are not fully specific in their action and may influence a wide array of symptoms and signs, including some originating from psychiatric and cardiac diseases. Interpretation of response to treatment is also complicated by the fact that epileptic seizures and pseudoseizures may coexist.

It has been argued that under certain circumstances prophylactic treatment may be justified even in the absence of any previous seizure. For example, it has been suggested that in infants with tuberous sclerosis early antiepileptic drug therapy may prevent the occurrence of infantile spasms and, possibly, associated neurological deterioration [3]. Patients in whom antiepileptic drugs are at times prescribed prophylactically in the absence of a history of seizures are those who had a severe head trauma, or those who underwent supratentorial brain surgery. While phenytoin has been found to reduce the risk of early post-traumatic seizures (i.e. seizures occurring in the first 7 days after head trauma), it has not been found to be of value in the long-term management of patients with head trauma or brain surgery [4,17]. In fact, the vast majority of these patients will not develop seizures in the long term and, more importantly, no antiepileptic drug has been found to be effective in reducing the incidence of late post-traumatic or postoperative epilepsy [4,18,19].

Which drug?

In the past, there was a belief that prescription of several drugs in small doses could result in greater efficacy and improved tolerability compared with a single drug given at a full dosage. This assumption, however, has not been found to be correct, and several studies have demonstrated that most patients with newly diagnosed epilepsy are best treated with a single antiepileptic drug [20]. Use of a single medication minimizes toxicity, eliminates the risk of drug interactions, facilitates assessment of the effects of individual drugs and may improve patient compliance (Table 11.1). Up to 60–70% of patients with partial seizures and up to 70–80% of those with primarily generalized tonic-clonic seizures achieve complete seizure control on the initially prescribed drug [21–27]. Even greater response rates are achieved in children with absence epilepsy, whereas most symptomatic generalized epilepsies tend to be at least partly refractory to drug treatment [11].

None of the available antiepileptic drugs can be recommended as the treatment of choice in all patients, irrespective of clinical features. Rational prescribing requires selecting drugs on a case-by-case basis, taking into consideration a combination of factors such as seizure type, syndromic form, other patient characteristics, medical expertise, regulatory aspects and cost considerations. A detailed discussion of criteria used in selecting antiepileptic drugs is provided in Chapter 26, and only some major variables are considered below.

Seizure type and epilepsy syndrome

The efficacy of individual antiepileptic drugs varies considerably in relation to seizure type (Table 11.2). Because of this, a correct classification of the seizures which occur in an individual patient represents the most valuable piece of information in choosing the drug to be prescribed. Additionally, all efforts should be made to establish as early as possible a correct syndromic diagnosis. In fact, if the

Table 11.1 Advantages of monotherapy

High efficacy (complete seizure control in the majority of patients)
Better tolerated than multiple drug therapy
Easy management (efficacy and safety of individual drugs can be evaluated separately)
Simple (possibly better compliance)
No adverse drug interactions
Cost effective

Table 11.2 Efficacy spectrum of antiepileptic drugs in different seizure types

Effective or possibly effective against all seizure types	Effective against all seizure types except absences	Effective against partial and generalized tonic-clonic seizures	Effective against absence seizures
Valproic acid	Phenobarbital	Carbamazepine[f]	Ethosuximide[h]
Lamotrigine[a]	Primidone	Phenytoin[f]	
Benzodiazepines[b]		Oxcarbazepine[f]	
Topiramate[c]		Gabapentin[f]	
Zonisamide[d]		Tiagabine[f]	
Levetiracetam[e] (?)		Vigabatrin[f,g]	
Felbamate[d]			

Modified from [41].

[a] Lamotrigine may aggravate severe myoclonic epilepsy of infancy. Efficacy is best documented for partial and secondarily generalized tonic-clonic seizures, primarily generalized tonic-clonic seizures absence seizures and drop attacks associated with the Lennox–Gastaut syndrome.

[b] Benzodiazepines occasionally exacerbate tonic seizures, particularly after intravenous use in patients with Lennox–Gastaut syndrome or West syndrome.

[c] Efficacy against absence seizures has not been clearly documented. Topiramate efficacy is best documented for partial and secondarily generalized tonic-clonic seizures, primarily generalized tonic-clonic seizures, and drop attacks associated with the Lennox–Gastaut syndrome.

[d] Evidence of efficacy against some generalized seizure types is preliminary. Efficacy is best documented for partial and secondarily generalized tonic-clonic seizures. With felbamate, efficacy is also well documented in drop attacks associated with the Lennox-Gastaut syndrome.

[e] Tentative classification. Broad-spectrum efficacy is suggested by findings in animal models but adequately controlled clinical studies have been completed only in partial and secondarily generalized tonic-clonic seizures.

[f] Carbamazepine, phenytoin, vigabatrin, tiagabine and oxcarbazepine may exacerbate myoclonic jerks and absence seizures. Gabapentin may exacerbate myoclonic jerks/seizures. Carbamazepine may be effective against tonic seizures associated with the Lennox–Gastaut syndrome.

[g] Vigabatrin is also effective against infantile spasms.

[h] Ethosuximide may also be effective against myoclonic seizures.

epilepsy syndrome has been identified, drug choice can be made more rationally through prediction of additional seizure types which might occur as part of the natural history of the disorder. For example, the fact that tonic-clonic seizures develop later in life in many children with absence epilepsy can be used as an argument for prescribing in these children a medication effective against both these seizure types (e.g. valproate or lamotrigine) instead of one effective against absence seizures only (ethosuximide). The epilepsy classification also provides a useful insight into the probability of a favourable response to treatment, since within each seizure type responsiveness to drugs may vary depending on the syndromic form: for example, myoclonic jerks associated with juvenile myoclonic epilepsy are much more easily controlled than myoclonic seizures associated with the Lennox–Gastaut syndrome. Finally, knowledge of the epilepsy syndrome allows the best prediction of the probability of the patient's achieving spontaneous remission. This is of crucial importance in determining whether drug treatment should be administered for life, as is usually the case in juvenile myoclonic epilepsy, or whether discontinuation of therapy is feasible following an adequate interval of freedom from seizures [11].

A correct identification of seizure type and syndromic form is also important because some antiepileptic drugs may paradoxically precipitate or aggravate seizures when given to patients with certain epilepsy syndromes [28]. The most common example of this is the precipitation of absence seizures and myoclonic jerks following prescription of carbamazepine in patients with juvenile myoclonic epilepsy, a syndrome which is often misdiagnosed and, therefore, incorrectly treated. Carbamazepine may precipitate myoclonic and absence (or absence-like) seizures in other types of epilepsies, par-

ticularly in patients known to have bursts of generalized bilateral spike-and-wave discharges in their EEG. Other seizure types, such as tonic and atonic seizures, may also be aggravated by carbamazepine. Oxcarbazepine, tiagabine and vigabatrin may trigger or worsen myoclonic and absence seizures, gabapentin may precipitate or worsen myoclonus, barbiturates may aggravate absence seizures, and lamotrigine may aggravate severe myoclonic epilepsy of infancy [28,29]. Even status epilepticus, particularly nonconvulsive status, can be precipitated by antiepileptic drugs, particularly when an agent has been chosen which is inappropriate against the seizure types associated with a specific epilepsy syndrome.

Among available anticonvulsants, valproic acid shows possibly the broadest spectrum of activity, being effective against virtually all seizure types, irrespective of syndromic form. However, while most neurologists consider valproic acid as the drug of choice for the treatment of generalized epilepsies, in most countries there is a tendency to prefer carbamazepine or phenytoin in patients with partial epilepsies (Fig. 11.1). This strategy is usually based on the assumption that the latter drugs have greater efficacy than valproic acid against partial seizures, even though there is little evidence for this. In fact, while one large trial found carbamazepine to be slightly more effective than valproic acid in controlling complex partial seizures [22], other randomized controlled trials failed to identify significant differences in efficacy between these drugs in patients with newly diagnosed tonic-clonic or partial seizures [23–26]. Of the newer drugs, only oxcarbazepine, lamotrigine, vigabatrin, gabapentin and topiramate have undergone relatively extensive evaluation in randomized monotherapy trials in patients with

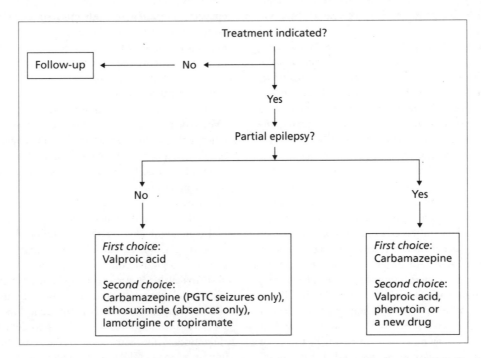

Fig. 11.1 The two-drug approach to the treatment of epilepsy. In this algorithm, which is commonly used, valproic acid is utilized as first choice in generalized epilepsies, whereas carbamazepine is used preferentially in partial epilepsies. Phenytoin may be used as an alternative to carbamazepine as second choice in patients with primarily generalized tonic-clonic (PGTC) seizures only. Neither carbamazepine nor phenytoin are a recommended second choice in patients with PGTC seizures associated with idiopathic generalized epilepsies, due to the risk of precipitating other seizure types such as absence or myoclonic seizures. Topiramate is not a recommended second choice in patients with absence seizures. Some rare syndromes may require different treatments (e.g. vigabatrin or ACTH for West syndrome).

newly diagnosed epilepsy. In partial epilepsy, oxcarbazepine, lamotrigine and topiramate were found to be similarly effective to carbamazepine or valproate, whereas vigabatrin and gabapentin showed lower efficacy than carbamazepine [30]. Vigabatrin, on the other hand, was more efficacious than hydrocortisone against infantile spasms associated with tuberous sclerosis [31], but tended to be less efficacious, though better tolerated, than adrenocorticotropic hormone (ACTH) in spasms associated with other conditions [32].

While differences in efficacy among drugs effective in a given seizure type seem to be relatively modest, there are important differences in toxicity profiles between these drugs, and it is generally the latter which determines the final selection in the individual patient (see below). Based on this background, it is no surprise that drug prescribing is based more on subjective perceptions of individual practitioners than on scientific evidence of superiority of one treatment over another.

Aetiology of epilepsy

Definition of the aetiology of epilepsy is important in excluding conditions which require specific treatments, e.g. surgery for a brain tumour. Based on current knowledge, identification of the aetiology of epilepsy has relatively little impact on drug selection, but the situation may change in the future as our understanding of the pathophysiology of the epilepsies and mechanisms of drug action will progressively improve. The best example of how information on aetiological factors could influence drug choice is provided by the already mentioned observations suggesting that symptomatic infantile spasms secondary to tuberous sclerosis may respond better to vigabatrin than to hydrocortisone [31], whereas cryptogenic spasms or symptomatic spasms secondary to other aetiologies may respond better to ACTH than to vigabatrin [32]. Unfortunately, vigabatrin, steroids and ACTH have not been compared in the same trial, and there have been no randomized comparisons of vigabatrin vs. ACTH in spasms associated with tuberous sclerosis. Evidence from controlled studies of a preferential drug response in relation to underlying aetiology in other epilepsy syndromes is lacking, although there have been anecdotal reports of potentially useful associations. For example, in preliminary studies, seizures associated with glial tumours have been found to respond particularly well to tiagabine [33].

Aetiology is related to syndromic classification, and therefore it is no surprise that aetiological factors are valuable in predicting response to treatment. In a hospital-based observational survey in a total of 2200 patients, 1-year remission rates following institution of drug treatment were 82% in patients who had idiopathic generalized epilepsy, 45% in those with cryptogenic partial epilepsy, 35% in those with symptomatic partial epilepsy and only 11% in those with partial epilepsy associated with hippocampal sclerosis [34]. Patients with hippocampal sclerosis and another lesion had only 3% probability of achieving seizure freedom. In the same study, patients with temporal lobe epilepsy responded more poorly to treatment compared with patients with extratemporal foci.

EEG features

Like aetiological factors, EEG features are important for differen-

tial diagnosis and prognostic considerations, and therefore they have an indirect influence on the process leading to drug selection. Whether specific EEG features can be useful to predict responses to different antiepileptic drugs in a given epilepsy syndrome has been little investigated, but it is plausible to assume that this may be the case. As discussed above, for example, patients with a history of generalized spike-and-wave paroxysms in the EEG may be at special risk of developing absence seizures and even non-convulsive status when treated with carbamazepine [28]. It has been suggested that patients with a left-sided focus tend to respond better to carbamazepine compared with patients with a right-sided focus, although this has not been a consistent finding.

If exception is made for patients with absence seizures (in whom there is a good correlation between clinical response and suppression of EEG abnormalities), the EEG is generally of little or no value in assessing therapeutic response. It is the amelioration in seizure control and not the modification in EEG activity which is important, and in some cases marked clinical improvement may occur despite an unchanged or even deteriorated EEG. As discussed above, however, there are patients in whom epileptiform EEG discharges can cause functional impairment, particularly in cognitive performance, and suppression of such discharges may then become a therapeutic goal. The presence or appearance of paroxysmal EEG activity in patients in remission may also provide a useful predictor of the risk of seizure recurrence when therapy is discontinued (Chapter 13).

Side-effect profiles vs. patient's characteristics

When two or more drugs have similar efficacy in a given type of epilepsy, the agent whose side-effect profile is least likely to interfere with patient's wellbeing should be used preferentially. The relative importance of any potential adverse effect varies depending on patient's age, sex, profession and presence of associated medical conditions. A few examples will illustrate how these principles apply to practical situations.

The toxicity of many antiepileptic drugs is age dependent [35]. The incidence of valproic acid-induced liver toxicity, for example, is much higher in children below 2 years of age, particularly in those receiving concomitant enzyme-inducing anticonvulsants, than in adults (1 : 600 vs. 1 : 30 000), an observation which has a major influence in deciding whether valproic acid should or should not be prescribed in an individual patient. The incidence of lamotrigine-induced serious skin rashes, including Stevens–Johnson syndrome, is also greater in children than in adults (about 1 : 100 vs. 1 : 1000, respectively). While benzodiazepines and barbiturates may affect adversely cognitive function in any age group, children are more likely to develop hyperactivity and other behavioural disturbances, and overall they tend to tolerate these drugs poorly compared with adults. Phenytoin is known to cause acne, hirsutism, gum hyperplasia and coarsening of facial features, particularly when taken during childhood. While many of these effects would be of relatively little importance to a middle-aged or elderly male, their potential impact is a consideration against the first-line use of phenytoin in children and young females. At the other extreme of age, the elderly, there may be similar alterations in sensitivity to the adverse effects of individual drugs: in a recent double-blind study in elderly patients with newly diagnosed epilepsy, 42% of those randomized to receive carbamazepine dropped out due to adverse effects, compared with 18% of those randomized to lamotrigine [36]. At the end of the 16-week follow-up period, more patients continued on treatment with lamotrigine than with carbamazepine (71% vs. 42%), suggesting that lamotrigine may be a better choice for treating epilepsy with onset in old age.

In women of childbearing potential, interactions with steroid oral contraceptives are a consideration in drug selection. Valproic acid, benzodiazepines, lamotrigine, gabapentin, tiagabine and vigabatrin have no influence on the kinetics of the contraceptive pill, whereas carbamazepine, phenytoin, phenobarbital, primidone, oxcarbazepine, topiramate (at doses ≥ 200 mg/day) and felbamate stimulate the metabolism of contraceptive steroids, thereby reducing their efficacy [37]. In fertile women, adverse effects of drugs on the developing embryo and fetus are of even greater concern. While it is known that old generation anticonvulsants increase 2- to 3-fold the risk of major fetal malformations compared with the general population rate (Chapter 23), the risk associated with the newer drugs has not been ascertained due to limited exposure to date. As far as comparative risks related to specific anticonvulsants are concerned, valproate, particularly when used at dosages ≥ 1000 mg/day, has been associated with an overall risk of fetal malformations (including a 1–3% risk of neural tube defects) which may be higher than that reported for other older generation drugs.

Many other patient's characteristics influence drug selection [3]. For example, topiramate, which causes weight loss, may be a rational choice in patients who are overweight. Since many anticonvulsants have indications outside epilepsy, comorbidities influence drug selection. In a patient who suffers from epilepsy and migraine, for example, valproate would be a reasonable choice because it has the potential for producing beneficial effects in both conditions. Likewise, gabapentin could be useful in a patient with partial epilepsy and neuropathic pain. Some drugs have the potential for aggravating comorbidity: vigabatrin and tiagabine, for example, may cause depression and other psychiatric disturbances, and may not be the preferred choice in patients with a history of mood or behavioural disorders. In patients with acute intermittent porphyria, gabapentin appears to be one of the few anticonvulsants which does not precipitate porphyric attacks [37,38]. Drugs with a low interaction potential, such as gabapentin and levetiracetam, may also be preferentially used in patients who require concomitant pharmacotherapy for the management of associated conditions.

Medical expertise and availability of ancillary services

The treatment of epilepsy varies widely in different parts of the world. Although in most European countries epilepsy is usually managed by specialists, in some other places it is the primary care physician who is mainly involved in diagnosis and therapy. These differences in management may justify differential approaches to treatment. For example, in 1993 Richens and Perucca [74] proposed a 'non-expert' approach to the treatment of epilepsy based on the use of valproic acid as initial treatment irrespective of seizure type and syndromic form (Fig. 11.2). As discussed above, valproic acid is effective in all seizure types, and it would be expected to control the majority of cases. Only patients failing on valproic acid would need referral to a specialist for re-evaluation. This approach has the advantage of minimizing costs of specialist care and may work well in those countries where epilepsy is managed at the primary care level. Of course, physicians should be competent in making a correct diagnosis, in excluding aetiologies requiring specific treatment and in identifying conditions contraindicating the use of valproic acid. A disadvantage of this approach is that the precise nature of the epileptic syndrome may never be correctly identified, with its inherent drawbacks in determining prognosis and risk of relapse following discontinuation of treatment.

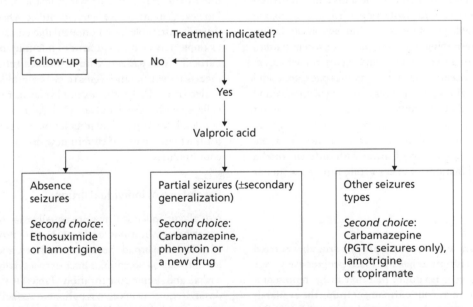

Fig. 11.2 The one-drug approach to the treatment of epilepsy. In this algorithm, which exploits the broad-spectrum activity of valproic acid, valproate is utilized as the treatment of choice in both partial and generalized epilepsies. Phenytoin may be used as an alternative to carbamazepine as second choice in patients with primarily generalized tonic-clonic (PGTC) seizures only. Neither carbamazepine nor phenytoin are a recommended second choice in patients with PGTC seizures associated with idiopathic generalized epilepsies, due to the risk of precipitating other seizure types such as absence or myoclonic seizures. Some rare syndromes may require different treatments (e.g. vigabatrin or ACTH for West syndrome).

The availability of ancillary services also has an influence on drug selection. Due to the occurrence of saturation kinetics, phenytoin is a difficult drug to use, particularly when individualization of dosage cannot be assisted by monitoring of plasma drug concentrations [39]. Lack of availability of a drug monitoring service is an argument for preferring a drug which is easier to use, such as carbamazepine or valproate.

Is the mechanism of anticonvulsant action important in choosing a drug in the clinic?

It may sound heretical to state that knowledge of mechanisms of drug action has little relevance for selecting a drug in the clinic, but this is the way antiepileptic drugs are prescribed at present. In fact, our understanding of the pathophysiology of the epilepsies and of the modes of action of individual drugs is still too fragmentary to allow mechanism-driven rational drug selection. Although a number of primary modes of actions have been described for most anti-convulsants, additional mechanisms have been identified and it is difficult to predict what their relative contribution is in an individual patient. Lamotrigine, for example, is often referred to as a selective blocker of voltage-dependent sodium channels, but it has also been found to inhibit N-type, L-type and P-type calcium channels, to increase brain γ-aminobutyric acid (GABA) levels, to increase potassium conductance, to stimulate taurine-mediated neurotransmission and to act as an antagonist or negative modulator at the 5-hydroxytryptamine 1A ($5HT_{1A}$) receptor [37].

In time, research on the relationship between specific modes of drug action and clinical response in well-defined epilepsy syndromes or subsyndromes could yield important clues for rational treatment: for example, it might be possible in the future to determine which drug produces the best response in a patient whose epilepsy is caused by a specific channelopathy, a mutation in an excitatory amino acid receptor, or an impairment in central GABAergic transmission. Evidence is already starting to accumulate that in certain conditions knowledge of modes of drug action can be important for rational prescribing. For example, a consistent pattern is emerging whereby drugs like tiagabine and vigabatrin, which act by increasing GABA concentration in the synaptic space, are useful in controlling partial seizures but can be aggravating in absence and myoclonic seizures. Mechanistic considerations are also important in selecting drugs for adjunctive therapy in difficult-to-treat patients, as it has been suggested that refractory seizures are more likely to respond to combinations of drugs with different modes of action than to combinations of drugs acting through a similar mechanism [40].

Old vs. new drugs

Over the last decade, a new wave of antiepileptic drugs has entered the market, and their utilization has increased progressively over time [37,41]. While there is no doubt that new drugs represent a welcome addition to the therapeutic armamentarium, the availability of over 15 drugs to treat epilepsy has made rational drug selection increasingly complicated. As many physicians may not be fully familiar with the indications, contraindications, drug interactions and precautions of use of so many agents, there is a danger that some of these drugs be used suboptimally, with consequent risks in

terms of adverse effects. This situation is further compounded by intense marketing pressures, as manufacturers of individual drugs struggle to support claims that their product offers advantages over those produced by their competitors.

At present, the major use of the new drugs is as adjunctive therapy for the management of seizures that are not fully controlled by old generation agents. However, new drugs are being used increasingly early in the treatment algorithm, and in some countries they are not uncommonly prescribed as first line. When old and new generation drugs have been compared in randomized monotherapy trials in newly diagnosed patients, new drugs have been found to be no more effective, but usually better tolerated than older agents [30]. However, a critical evaluation of these studies reveals that at times the trial design had bias in favour of the new agent. For example, in a trial comparing lamotrigine with carbamazepine, both drugs were administered on a twice daily basis [42], which is appropriate for lamotrigine but may lead to suboptimal tolerability for carbamazepine, whose plasma levels may fluctuate excessively on this schedule [43]. Likewise, in a trial comparing vigabatrin with carbamazepine, the dosage of the latter could be increased up to the level at which side-effects occurred, whereas vigabatrin could not exceed a predetermined dosage irrespective of side-effects [44]: this may explain not only the better tolerability of vigabatrin in this study, but also possibly its lower efficacy compared with carbamazepine. Vigabatrin's example is also illustrative of how difficult it is to draw definite conclusions about a new drug's safety. It took 8 years after the introduction of vigabatrin in the market, and an exposure of over 100 000 patients, to discover the occurrence of irreversible visual field defects, despite the fact that these develop in about one-third of patients treated with the drug [45].

At the present time, the precise role of new antiepileptic drugs in the treatment of different epilepsy syndromes has not been determined, due to the paucity of well-controlled studies in conditions other than cryptogenic or symptomatic partial epilepsies [30,46]. However, situations are being identified where first-line use of new drugs is justifiable based on available efficacy or safety data. One example may be the treatment of infantile spasms with vigabatrin, particularly in patients with associated tuberous sclerosis, where the risk to benefit ratio seems to be favourable despite the risk of visual toxicity [3]. Another example may be the use of lamotrigine in epilepsy with onset in old age [36]. As discussed above, differences in tolerability profile and interaction potential provide a rationale for the first-line use of certain new drugs in patients with specific comorbidities.

Ease of use of individual drugs

Not all antiepileptic drugs are equally easy to use, a consideration which has implications for drug selection. Properties favouring ease of use include broad spectrum of efficacy, good tolerability profile, low interaction potential, a once or twice daily dosing schedule, and a rapid and simple dose titration (Table 11.3). A small variability in dosage requirements across patients also facilitates clinical use.

In general, dosage adjustments are easier for drugs with linear kinetics, i.e. drugs whose plasma concentration is linearly related to dose. Several anticonvulsants exhibit non-linear kinetics: in the case of phenytoin, in particular, saturation of the enzymes responsible for its metabolism lead to a curvilinear and increasingly steep rela-

Table 11.3 Ideal properties for an easy-to-use antiepileptic drug

Broad spectrum of activity against all seizure types
High efficacy
Good tolerability
No risk of allergic or idiosyncratic reactions (including teratogenicity)
Low interaction potential
Low variability in dosage requirements
Favourable pharmacokinetics (linear kinetics, half-life compatible with
    once or twice daily dosing)
Fast and easy dose escalation rate
No tolerance to antiepileptic effects
No withdrawal seizures
No need for intensive laboratory monitoring
Availability of convenient formulations (including paediatric dosage
    forms and a parenteral formulation)
Low cost

Table 11.4 Medication cost for 1 year of treatment with individual antiepileptic drugs at the indicated dosages. Costs are based on 2001 retail prices in Italy, using the lowest-cost formulations

Drug	Daily dosage (mg)	Cost (Euro)
Phenobarbital	150	41
Primidone	750	53
Phenytoin	300	68
Clobazam	20	126
Carbamazepine	800	128
Ethosuximide	750	133
Valproate	1000	172
Oxcarbazepine	1200	513
Vigabatrin	2500	1425
Tiagabine	30	1519
Lamotrigine	300	1623
Gabapentin	2400	2179
Topiramate	300	2264
Levetiracetam	2000	2697
Felbamate	2400	3864

tionship between dosage and steady-state plasma concentration. As a result, small changes in dosage can produce a disproportionate change in plasma phenytoin concentration and associated clinical response. In the case of carbamazepine and gabapentin, the relationship between daily dosage and steady-state plasma concentration flattens at high dosages, due to dose-dependent autoinduction and dose-dependent decrease in oral bioavailability, respectively.

Some drugs, most notably benzodiazepines, may be associated with the development of tolerance to their antiepileptic effects, and a risk of withdrawal seizures upon their discontinuation, which may complicate clinical management. For other drugs, ease of use may be affected adversely by the need to perform repeated safety tests, such as visual field examinations with vigabatrin or haematology and liver function tests with felbamate.

Availability of convenient formulations is a factor which plays an important role in drug selection, particularly in children. Many antiepileptic drugs are not available in palatable, user-friendly formulations suitable for use in small children. For most drugs, a parenteral formulation is not available, and this could also cause problems.

Cost of treatment

In 28 countries, which contain over 40% of the world population, the per capita annual gross national product barely suffices to buy a year's supply of carbamazepine or valproate for one or two patients (Table 11.4). Therefore, it is no surprise that in many regions of the world cost is a major consideration not only in deciding which drug to use, but also in determining whether drug treatment is feasible at all. This problem is aggravated by the fact that in many developing countries the price of antiepileptic drugs is considerably higher than in Europe and the US. For most patients living in these countries, only phenobarbital, phenytoin and ethosuximide may be available at prices affordable by the general population, and many of the newer drugs may not be available at all. Figure 11.3 provides an example of a therapeutic algorithm which may be used when drugs have to be chosen preferentially on the basis of their comparative cost.

Cost considerations have a significant impact on prescribing even in affluent societies. This is especially true for the most recently licensed drugs, which are far more expensive than conventional agents (Table 11.4). In some countries, reimbursability by national health service or insurance schemes is only permitted for certain drugs, special diagnostic categories or patients within predefined income limits.

Route of administration and drug formulations

When an immediate effect is required, such as in the treatment of status epilepticus, the intravenous route should be used. Intramuscular administration of drugs such as phenytoin, phenobarbital and diazepam is generally not recommended, because absorption may be slow and poorly predictable. Midazolam and fosphenytoin, on the other hand, are absorbed efficiently when given intramuscularly. In the case of diazepam, the rectal route provides rapid and efficient absorption when solutions, gels or rectal capsules are used, and can be utilized by non-medical personnel in selected situations, for example to prevent or terminate a seizure in a febrile child. With midazolam, the buccal and the intranasal routes may also provide a means for ensuring rapid absorption, and have been used for rescue therapy in seizure patients [47]. Alternative formulations for patients unable to take a medicine orally are not available for all drugs. This may complicate management, for example when there is a need to provide therapeutic cover for a patient undergoing abdominal surgery. In some cases, the availability of a parenteral formulation is a factor to be taken into consideration in deciding which drug should be preferentially prescribed.

For long-term oral treatment, tablets or capsules should be preferred to syrups, whenever possible, because they allow more precise dosing, avoid the effect of tooth damaging ingredients such as sucrose and minimize the risk of adverse effects associated with excessively rapid absorption, which may be a problem particularly

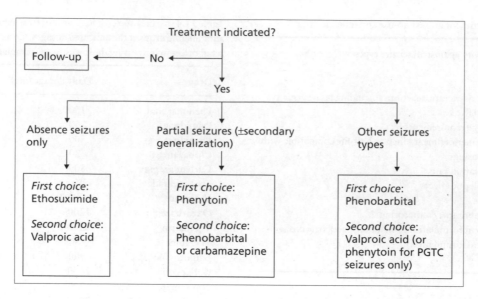

Fig. 11.3 The low-budget approach to the treatment of epilepsy. In this algorithm, cost is the primary determinant in drug selection. In some countries, carbamazepine may be preferable to phenytoin on a cost basis. Neither phenytoin nor carbamazepine are a recommended second choice in patients with primarily generalized tonic-clonic (PGTC) seizures associated with idiopathic generalized epilepsies, due to the risk of precipitating other seizure types such as absence or myoclonic seizures. Some rare syndromes may require different treatments (e.g. ACTH for West syndrome).

Table 11.5 Suggested initial target dosages, maintenance dosages, frequency of administration and titration rates for the main AEDs in adults. This information reflects the authors' experience and may differ from information reported in data sheets in individual countries. Some patients will require dosages, titration rates and dosing regimens different from those given in this table

Drug	Usual initial target dosage (mg/day)	Usual maintenance dosage (mg/day)	Frequency of administration	Suggested titration rate
Carbamazepine	400–600[a]	400–1600	2 to 3 times/day (twice daily with controlled-release formulations)	Start with 100 or 200 mg/day and increase to target dosage over 1–4 weeks
Clobazam	10	10–30	Once or twice daily	Start with 10 mg/day. If indicated, increase to 20 mg/day after 1–2 weeks
Ethosuximide	500–750[a]	500–1500	2 to 3 times/day	Start with 250 mg/day and increase to target dosage over 1–3 weeks
Felbamate	1800–2400	1800–3600	3 or 4 times /day	Start with 600–1200 mg/day and increase to target dosage over 10–21 days
Gabapentin	900–1800	900–3600	2 or 3 times /day	Start with 300–900 mg/day and increase to target dosage over 5–10 days
Lamotrigine	50–100 (monotherapy) 50–100 mg (patients on valproate) 200–300 (patients on enzyme inducing comedication)	50–200 (monotherapy or patients on valproate) 200–500 (patients on enzyme inducing comedication)	Twice daily (once daily possible with monotherapy and valproate comedication)	• Monotherapy: Start with 25 mg/day for 2 weeks, then increase to 50 mg/day for 2 weeks. Further increases by 50 mg/day every 2 weeks • Valproate comedication: Start with 25 mg on alternate days for 2 weeks, then 25 mg/day for 2 weeks. Further increases by 25–50 mg/day every 2 weeks • Enzyme-inducing comedication: Start with 25 or 50 mg/day for 2 weeks, then increase to 50 or 100 mg/day for 2 weeks. Further increases by 50–100 mg/day every 2 weeks

Continued.

Table 11.5 *Continued*

Drug	Usual initial target dosage (mg/day)	Usual maintenance dosage (mg/day)	Frequency of administration	Suggested titration rate
Levetiracetam	1000–2000	1000–3000	Twice daily	Start with 500 or 1000 mg/day and increase, if indicated, after 2 weeks
Oxcarbazepine	600–900[a]	600–3000	2 or 3 times/day	Start with 300 mg/day and increase to target dosage over 1–3 weeks
Phenobarbital	50–100[a]	50–200	Once daily	Start with 30–50 mg at bedtime and increase, if indicated, after 10–15 days
Phenytoin	200–300[a]	200–400	Once or twice/day	Start with 100 mg/day and increase to target dosage over 3–7 days
Primidone	500–750[a]	500–1500	2 or 3 times/day	Start with 62.5 mg/day and increase to target dosage over about 3 weeks. In patients on enzyme-inducing comedication a faster titration may be used
Tiagabine	30 (patients on enzyme inducers) 15 (patients not receiving enzyme inducers)	30–50 (patients on enzyme inducers) 15–30 (patients not receiving enzyme inducers)	2 to 4 times/day	Start with 5 mg/day and increase by 5 mg/day increments at weekly intervals
Topiramate	100	100–400	Twice daily	Start with 25 mg/day and increase by 25 or 50 mg/day increments every 2 weeks
Valproic acid	500–1000[a]	500–2500	2 or 3 times/day (once or twice daily with controlled-release formulations)	Start with 500 mg/day and increase, if indicated, after about 1 week
Vigabatrin	1000	1000–3000	Once or twice daily	Start with 250 or 500 mg/day and increase to target dosage over 1–2 weeks
Zonisamide	200	200–500	Twice daily	Start with 100 mg/day and increase to target dosage after 2 weeks

From [52].

[a] Suggested target dosage for initial monotherapy in patients with newly diagnosed epilepsy. For some AEDs, larger target dosages may be appropriate in refractory patients.

with carbamazepine. Nearly all children above the age of 5 years can cope with solid dosage forms. The type of formulation influences the rate of drug delivery to the bloodstream and, hence, to the site of action. Enteric-coated tablets, such as those utilized in some valproate formulations, can only be absorbed after the tablet reaches the intestine, and therefore absorption shows a lag-time related to the rate of gastric emptying. Typically, the passage of enteric-coated tablets to the intestine is delayed by the concomitant ingestion of food, and therefore drug absorption from these formulations may not take place for up to several hours after the ingestion [48].

In some countries, similar formulations of the same drug may be available, including generic preparations. Although regulations have been introduced to ensure that similar products on the market be comparable in terms of rate and extent of absorption, physicians should be aware that at least in some countries differences in bioavailability may exist between apparently equivalent formulations. While in most situations generic drugs provide the most cost-

effective therapy [49], problems with side-effects or breakthrough seizures have been reported when patients were switched from one formulation to another which was subsequently found not to have equivalent bioavailability. Even switching to formulations which meet regulatory requirements for bioequivalence can be occasionally problematic [50], presumably because in some patients even a minor change in steady-state plasma drug concentration may be sufficient to cause an alteration in clinical response. In view of these considerations, monitoring plasma concentrations is recommended when switching a patient from one formulation to another.

For drugs which are absorbed and eliminated rapidly, sustained-release preparations have been developed which are designed to prolong the absorption and to allow less frequent dosing [51]. Such modified-release products are available for carbamazepine, valproic acid and phenytoin. Some of these formulations may differ from conventional formulations not only in rate, but also in extent of absorption.

Individualization of dosage

One of the major advances which has been made in the treatment of epilepsy is the rejection of the 'standard dosage' approach, and recognition that dose requirements vary greatly from one patient to another. This variability results to some extent from pharmacokinetic differences between individuals, but pharmacodynamic variation may be equally important. If therapeutic success has to be achieved, tailoring dosage to meet individual needs is more important than drug selection itself [52]. Optimizing dosage is a complex process, and different aspects need to be addressed.

Rate of dose escalation

When a full therapeutic effect is required immediately, as in the management of status epilepticus or frequently recurring seizures, treatment can be started with a loading dose, followed by an adequate maintenance dosage. In most situations, however, this aggressive approach is neither necessary nor desirable, and treatment should be initiated with a small dose and increased gradually to a target maintenance level. Gradual dose escalation has several advantages:

1 With most antiepileptic drugs, adaptation (tolerance) to adverse central nervous system and, sometimes, gastrointestinal side-effects occurs slowly after initiation of treatment, and immediate prescription of a full maintenance dosage could cause major tolerability problems. Drugs which are most likely to produce central nervous system side-effects when started at doses close to the maintenance dosage include primidone, benzodiazepines, topiramate, tiagabine, valproic acid, vigabatrin and zonisamide. Primidone may cause a particularly marked transient intolerance reaction in patients not previously exposed to barbiturates [22], and it should be started at a dose (62.5 mg/day in adults) which is only about one-tenth of the usual maintenance dosage.

2 Despite common belief, allergic and idiosyncratic reactions are often dependent on starting dose and rate of dose escalation. Skin rashes requiring drug withdrawal when treatment is initiated at too high doses are especially frequent with carbamazepine, phenytoin and lamotrigine. The risk of allergic reactions to lamotrigine is greatly increased when the drug is added on to pre-existing treatment with valproic acid, and in these patients it is essential to use a particularly slow rate of escalation [53].

3 Some patients can be optimally controlled even at doses below the initial target maintenance dosage. When there is no need to minimize rapidly the risk of seizure recurrence, and when seizure frequency is sufficiently high to permit a meaningful assessment of therapeutic response over a short period, slow dose escalation may allow identification of the lowest dose regimen at which patients respond. Conversely, some patients are unusually sensitive to adverse effects, and slow dose escalation will prevent them from being exposed to dosages larger than those tolerated.

Unfortunately, for most anticonvulsants, starting dose and guidelines for dose escalation are poorly defined in the literature. The optimal dosage titration is seldom investigated adequately in regulatory clinical trials and, therefore, it is mostly established through clinical experience [3]. As shown in Table 11.5, phenytoin, levetiracetam and gabapentin are among the drugs which are best tolerated when started from the beginning at full dosage, which is an advantage when there is a need to minimize the latency to the onset of a full therapeutic action. Phenobarbital may similarly be started at a 'therapeutic' dosage, but because of the long half-life of this compound, pharmacological action is influenced by the slow accumulation of the drug in plasma, a process which may require several weeks. The escalation schemes given in Table 11.5 are only intended for general orientation, and deviations from these recommendations may be indicated as new information becomes available. Children, elderly patients and patients with certain comorbidities may require doses and titration rates different from those given in the table. The rate of dose escalation is also partly dependent on the treatment setting: a patient with frequent seizures, for example, may require a more rapid dose escalation than a patient with infrequent seizures.

Initial target maintenance dosage

The initial target maintenance dosage is defined as the dosage at which the physician aims to stabilize the patient at the end of the initial escalation phase [52]. In general, this corresponds to the lowest daily dosage which is expected to produce seizure control in that individual patient. This approach is justified by the desire to minimize the probability of imposing long-term treatment with dosages higher than necessary.

While a range of initial maintenance dosages is proposed in Table 11.5, the actual target dosage should be individualized based on the physician's expectations about the patient's responsiveness to the drug. Many idiopathic generalized epilepsies respond well to treatment, and it may be justified in these patients to aim at initial maintenance dosages and plasma drug levels in the low range. For example, the dosage of valproic acid required to control primary generalized tonic-clonic seizures has been found to be about 30% lower than that required to control partial seizures [23]. A high seizure frequency before starting therapy, symptomatic epilepsy, partial seizures, multiple seizure types, associated neurological handicaps and an unfavourable response to previous antiepileptic drug therapy may all influence the prognosis negatively [27,54], and patients with these features are expected to require comparatively higher doses and plasma drug levels. Other factors affecting choice of the initial maintenance dosage include the presence of physiological or pathological conditions leading to altered drug disposition, and any comedication expected to interact pharmacokinetically or pharmacodynamically with the administered anticonvulsant.

The patient's attitude should also be considered. A higher maintenance dosage is justifiable wherever recurrence of seizures is expected to have a particularly severe psychological or social impact on the individual's life. Some neurologists also favour the use of relatively high initial maintenance dosages out of fear that a delay in achieving complete seizure control may increase the probability of the epilepsy becoming intractable. However, as discussed earlier in this chapter, at least for most of the epilepsy syndromes there is no evidence that this is the case.

Frequency of administration

For most antiepileptic drugs, attainment of an adequate response is dependent on the persistence of stable drug concentrations at the site of action in the brain. Because the concentration at the site of action is in equilibrium with the concentration in plasma, a dosing scheme should be used which is adequate to maintain relatively stable plasma drug concentrations throughout a 24-h period [48]. The degree of fluctuation in plasma concentration is dependent on the interval between doses, the rate of absorption of the drug and its elimination half-life. With rapidly absorbed compounds, it is a good general rule to choose a dosing interval which is no greater than the half-life of the drug.

Drugs with a slow elimination rate such as phenobarbital may be given once daily at bedtime, but most other anticonvulsants need to be given two or three times daily. The optimal frequency of administration may also vary depending on pharmacokinetic pattern in different patient groups. For example, the half-life of phenytoin is usually compatible with once daily dosing in adults, but it is considerably shorter in children, who therefore require more frequent dosing (unless a modified release formulation is used). Likewise, lamotrigine should be given twice daily in patients taking concomitant enzyme-inducing anticonvulsants (due its relatively short half-life in these patients), but it can be given once daily in adults receiving no comedication, or in those comedicated with valproic acid.

For short half-life compounds such as carbamazepine and tiagabine, more than two daily administrations may be required to minimize excessive fluctuations in plasma concentration. This is especially important for patients with half-lives at the shorter end of the spectrum, such as children and patients comedicated with enzyme inducers. With these drugs, intermittent side-effects are not uncommon at the time of peak drug concentration, whereas breakthrough seizures may occur when plasma drug levels fall below a critical threshold. Multiple daily doses are similarly required for gabapentin, which has a short half-life and is absorbed from the intestine by a saturable transport mechanism: particularly in patients receiving high dosages of gabapentin, utilizing multiple daily administrations is a useful strategy to improve oral absorption and, consequently, bioavailability. To minimize the inconvenience of multiple daily dosing and to improve compliance, modified-release formulations have been developed for carbamazepine, valproic acid and phenytoin.

In occasional patients, even drugs with a very short half-life such as gabapentin and tiagabine may still produce adequate responses with a twice daily schedule. This may be explained at least in part by pharmacodynamic variability, i.e. by the fact that some patients may tolerate well high peak plasma drug levels or, conversely, maintain a good response at low trough concentrations. For some drugs, there is also evidence that a dissociation may exist between their plasma concentration profile and the duration of effect. For example, levetiracetam is recommended for use on a twice daily schedule despite a plasma half-life of about 7h. In the case of vigabatrin, which also has a plasma half-life of about 7h, once daily dosing is appropriate due to the fact that its action involves irreversible inhibition of GABA-transaminase, and therefore its duration of effect is dependent more on the turnover rate of the enzyme than on the chemical half-life of the drug in plasma [37,38]. There is some evidence that valproic acid also has a longer duration of action than expected from its half-life, and once daily dosing of this drug is feasible in many patients. Once daily valproic acid, however, is contraindicated in women with childbearing potential, because the risk of

teratogenicity may be increased by excessive fluctuations in plasma drug levels (Chapter 23).

Dosage adjustments in patients not responding to the target dosage

According to pharmacokinetic principles, about five half-lives are required to reach steady-state plasma concentrations after stabilizing the patient on a given dosage. Response to treatment cannot be fully evaluated before this period, and this should be taken into account in determining the minimum interval which should elapse before assessing the need for dosage adjustments. For drugs such as valproic acid and carbamazepine, which have relatively short half-lives, steady-state conditions are achieved within a few days (Table 11.6), whereas for phenytoin and phenobarbital it may take weeks for the plasma concentration to stabilize following a dose change. There are reports of patients who have been discharged from clinical observation too soon after a dose increment and became subsequently intoxicated as a result of progressive drug accumulation.

In patients who continue to have seizures after stabilization at the initial target dose, dosage should be increased stepwise within the recommended range until seizures are controlled or until intolerable side-effects appear. The magnitude of dosage increments should be determined by the steepness of the dose–response relationship, which varies between drugs, and by the patient's response at the previously assessed dose. Particular care should be taken when adjusting phenytoin dosage, because small increments can result in disproportionate elevations in plasma drug levels. Although most physicians are aware of the need for careful individualization of dosage, inadequate dosing remains a major determinant of inability to achieve seizure control. In a recent study of 74 consecutive patients referred for epilepsy surgery to a tertiary level centre in Germany due to 'medical intractability', careful evaluation of medical history revealed that these patients had not been exposed to maximally tolerated doses of carbamazepine, phenytoin, or barbiturates [55]. When the patients were rechallenged with appropriate doses of one or more of these drugs, seven (9.5%) showed such a major improvement in seizure control that their surgery programme had to be cancelled. Admittedly, it may be difficult to reach consensus on what is a maximally tolerated dosage in an individual patient, as this is influenced by both the physician's and the patient's perceptions. In particular, the acceptability of side-effects depends on the patient's lifestyle priorities: for example, age and occupation will influence a patient's reaction to the modest cognitive impairment or verbal slowness which can be associated with some treatments. If individual preferences are not addressed adequately, the patient may find it difficult to adhere to the prescribed dosing regimen.

The efficacy of antiepileptic drugs does not necessarily increase with increasing dosage. Too large dosages, or simultaneous prescription of too many drugs, may lead to a paradoxical increase in seizure frequency [28]. The physician should be aware of this possibility, because failure to recognize drug-induced seizure aggravation may lead to further dosage increases and consequent worsening of the patient's condition.

Monitoring plasma drug concentrations can be useful in deciding the need and magnitude of dosage adjustments. However, as discussed below, dose adjustments should be based primarily on

Table 11.6 Elimination half-lives of antiepileptic drugs and time to reach steady-state plasma drug concentrations in adults. Half-lives may be longer in newborns and shorter in infants and children

Drug	Half-life		Time to reach steady-state (days)	Comments
	Patients not taking enzyme inducers[a]	Patients taking enzyme inducers[a]		
Clobazam	10–30 h	8–16 h	2–6 days	Active demethylated metabolite with longer half-life requires about 10 days to reach steady-state
Clonazepam	20–60 h	10–30 h	2–10 days	
Carbamazepine	15–25 h	5–15 h	2–7 days	Due to autoinduction, plasma drug levels may decline after about 14 days following initiation of treatment
Ethosuximide	40–60 h	20–40 h	4–10 days	
Felbamate	14–23 h	10–18 h	2–4 days	
Gabapentin	5–7 h	5–7 h	2 days	
Lamotrigine	15–35 h	8–20 h	2–6 days	In patients comedicated with valproate half-life is longer (40–80 h) and steady-state may not be reached until 7 to 15 days
Levetiracetam	6–8 h	4–8 h	2 days	
Oxcarbazepine	8–15 h	7–12 h	2–4 days	Data refer to the metabolite mono-hydroxycarbazepine, for which oxcarbazepine can be considered a prodrug
Phenobarbital	50–170 h	50–170 h	8–30 days	
Phenytoin	10–80 h	10–80 h	3–15 days	Half-life and time to reach steady-state increase with increasing dosage
Primidone	10–20 h	5–10 h	2–4 days	Most of the pharmacological effects are mediated by the metabolite phenobarbital, which may require 8–30 days to reach steady-state
Tiagabine	4–13 h	2–3 h	2 days	
Topiramate	20–30 h	10–15 h	2–5 days	
Valproic acid	12–18 h	6–12 h	2–4 days	
Vigabatrin	5–8 h	5–8 h	2 days	
Zonisamide	50–70 h	25–35 h	5–12 days	

[a] Enzyme inducers include carbamazepine, phenytoin, phenobarbital and primidone.

clinical response and patients who are seizure free at 'suboptimal' plasma drug concentrations should not have their dosage increased. Conversely, since some patients may tolerate and indeed require plasma drug concentrations above the upper limit of the optimal range, no patient should be considered drug resistant unless seizures continue at the maximal tolerated dosage (within the clinically used dose range), irrespective of plasma drug concentrations.

Dose optimization in special situations

The rate of dose titration used in children is usually comparable to that applied to adults, although some severe conditions, such as West syndrome, may dictate more aggressive treatment with rapid dose escalation. Since drug clearance for most anticonvulsants is higher in infants and in children than in adults, dosage requirements on a milligram per kilogram basis are also higher in pediatric patients than in adults (Table 11.7). Conversely, newborns, especially when born prematurely, often show a reduced drug clearance and therefore may require lower dosages. During chronic treatment, dosage is rarely modified based on body weight changes alone, and dose adjustments usually are necessary only if the child experiences

relapse or worsening of seizures [52]. Compared with adults, children are more often treated with liquid dosage forms, which are associated with faster rates of absorption compared with tablets or capsules. Coupled with the shorter half-life of many drugs in children, this results in amplified fluctuations in plasma drug levels, often necessitating multiple daily dosing to avoid intermittent side-effects.

At the other extreme of age, in the elderly, dosage may need to be adjusted to compensate for ageing-related changes in renal and hepatic drug clearance. Binding of drugs to plasma proteins may be altered in the elderly with hypoalbuminaemia, and consequently total plasma drug concentrations may underestimate the levels of unbound, pharmacologically active drug. In general, epilepsy in the elderly tends to respond to lower drug dosages compared with those used in younger patients, but the elderly may also show an increased susceptibility to adverse effects [56].

Associated diseases, particularly those affecting the liver and the kidney, may alter dosage requirements to a major extent. Patients with associated diseases are also more likely to take concomitant medications, with the attendant risk of drug interactions (Chapter 10).

Table 11.7 Suggested maintenance dosages of AEDs in infants and children. This information reflects the authors' experience and may differ from information reported in data sheets in individual countries. Some patients will require dosages different from those given in this table

Drug	Maintenance dosage for infants (mg/kg/day)	Maintenance dosage for children (mg/kg/day)
Carbamazepine	10–40[a]	5–30
Clobazam	0.5–1	0.25–0.75
Clonazepam	0.1–0.2	0.05–0.1
Ethosuximide	20–40	15–45
Felbamate	20–60	15–45
Gabapentin	ND	10–30
Lamotrigine	ND	1–5 (valproate comedication)
		5–15 (enzyme-inducing comedication)
Levetiracetam	ND	ND
Oxcarbazepine	15–60	10–50
Phenobarbital	3–5	2–4
Phenytoin	5–15[a]	5–9
Primidone	ND	5–25
Tiagabine	ND	ND
Topiramate	ND	1–5
Valproic acid	20–40[b]	10–30[b]
Vigabatrin	80–150	40–80
Zonisamide	ND	4–12

Modified from [52].

[a] Bioavailability may be poor in infants.

[b] Higher dosages may be needed in patients comedicated with enzyme inducers.

ND, no adequate data available or not approved in this age group.

Assessing clinical response

Under usual circumstances, assessment of therapeutic response is based on direct observation of seizures. Patients or their relatives should be provided with a diary and instructed to record carefully all seizures, utilizing simple codes which allow differentiation by seizure type. In addition to dates on which seizures occur, it may be useful to include in the diary information on the actual timing of the seizures (e.g. nocturnal, awakening or diurnal seizures) and events potentially affecting seizure susceptibility, i.e. menstrual periods, situations leading to sleep deprivation, and days where medication was missed or taken incorrectly. When assessing the effect of therapy on seizure frequency, consideration should be given to whether plasma drug levels had reached steady-state conditions after a change in dosage. Baseline seizure frequency also needs to be considered: if at baseline the patient experienced only one seizure every 2 or 3 months, it may take up to 1 year to determine with reasonable confidence whether a change in drug therapy led to seizure freedom. As discussed earlier in this chapter, efficacy should not be established by assessing changes in the EEG: however, EEG recordings may be useful or even required to assess drug response in special situations, e.g. in status epilepticus (particularly when anaesthesia has been applied and there is no other method to determine ongoing

electrical activity in the brain), in patients with absence seizures and wherever subclinical EEG paroxysms cause functional impairment.

It is essential that the patient be monitored carefully not only for seizure activity, but also for potential adverse effects [57]. While this can be done by interviews and examinations at appropriate intervals, it is equally important to inform the patient and the family about side-effects that may be anticipated and any action that may need to be taken, particularly with respect to early signs of serious toxicity. Routine haematology and blood chemistry tests should be obtained before starting treatment, and repeated at least once during treatment and when another anticonvulsant is added or substituted. While more frequent laboratory safety monitoring may be recommended for certain drugs (most notably for felbamate), for detection of serious adverse effects it is much more important to alert the patient about the need to recognize immediately any warning symptoms. In particular, bleeding, bruising and infections may be early manifestations of a blood dyscrasia, whereas profound asthenia, marked sedation, vomiting, fever and an increase in seizure frequency in a patient treated with valproic acid should alert one to the possibility of liver toxicity. Specialized safety tests may be required in special circumstances: patients started on vigabatrin, for example, should have their visual fields tested regularly by Goldman perimetry. The value of monitoring plasma drug concentrations as an aid to improve efficacy and safety is discussed later in this chapter.

What next when treatment fails?

When seizures continue at the maximally tolerated dosage, the patient should be reviewed to confirm that the diagnosis was correct, that the initial treatment was appropriate and that there are no removable causes of inadequate response (e.g. poor compliance, sleep deprivation, alcohol abuse). After excluding these sources of poor response, the best strategy is usually to substitute the first drug with a second, also given as monotherapy. As discussed below, monotherapy with an alternative drug will produce seizure control in an appreciable number of patients, and is likely to be better tolerated than combination therapy. When sequential monotherapies with two or more drugs fail to control seizures, however, a trial of combination therapy is justified. Early consideration should also be given to the feasibility of epilepsy surgery.

Alternative monotherapy

The first formal trial comparing alternative monotherapy with combination therapy was conducted by Hakkarainen [58], who randomized 100 patients with newly diagnosed convulsive seizures to either carbamazepine or phenytoin. The 50 patients who continued to have seizures after 1 year on the allocated treatment were switched to monotherapy with the alternative drug and, of these, 17 (34%) became seizure free. On the other hand, of the 33 patients who were refractory to *both* phenytoin and carbamazepine as monotherapy, only five (15%) could be controlled when the two drugs were given together. While the value of combination therapy in this trial may have been underestimated due to the fact that carbamazepine and phenytoin, sharing similar mechanisms of action and side-effect profiles, are probably not the best drugs to use together, the study clearly showed that alternative monotherapy is a valuable option in patients refractory to initial treatment. These re-sults have been confirmed repeatedly. For example, in a trial com-paring vigabatrin and carbamazepine in newly diagnosed partial epilepsy, 11 of 25 (44%) patients who did not respond to the initial monotherapy became seizure free when switched to the alternative drug, and only five of the 14 remaining refractory patients were con-trolled when the same drugs were used in combination [59]. In a large observational study in which a variety of drugs were used, 67 of 248 patients (27%) refractory to initial monotherapy were ren-dered seizure free with a second or third drug used as monotherapy, and only 12 were controlled by combination therapy [27]. In other studies where patients refractory to initial treatment were switched to combination therapy, response rates have been comparable to those described for patients managed with alternative mono-therapy, but it was also noted that the burden of side-effects was greater when more than one drug was used [21].

Based on the above evidence, switching to an alternative monotherapy seems to be the most rational strategy in patients un-responsive to initial treatment. While it could be argued that addi-tion (rather than substitution) of a second drug will allow more rapid achievement of seizure control in those few patients who do require combination therapy, such a policy has the drawback of ex-posing to a greater burden of side-effects many patients who can be managed with a single drug. In practice, to minimize the risk of withdrawal seizures, it is preferable to avoid abrupt discontinua-tion of pre-existing medication when switching to an alternative drug. Many physicians prefer to titrate the dosage of the second agent up to the maintenance level before starting the gradual with-drawal of the initial medication. This procedure offers the advan-tage of minimizing the risk of withdrawal seizures, although there is a drawback in that the patient may be exposed to a greater risk of potentially adverse drug interactions during the addition or discon-tinuation phase. An alternative strategy is to decrease gradually the dosage of the initial drug whilst substitution therapy is being intro-duced, but this may involve a greater risk of seizures during the switch-over process. Some drugs, particularly benzodiazepines, carbamazepine, barbiturates, phenytoin and vigabatrin, should be withdrawn with special caution, taking into consideration previous duration of treatment and pre-existing dosage, with at least 2–3 months being usually necessary to complete the withdrawal.

A therapeutic strategy which is intermediate between alternative monotherapy and combination therapy involves adding initially a second drug, stabilizing the patient for a period sufficient to assess the response to combination therapy, and then proceeding with gradual removal of the initial drug if a good response has been achieved. If the patient needs the drug combination to remain seizure free, this will become readily apparent and the withdrawal procedure can be rapidly reversed. While apparently attractive, this procedure has major drawbacks in that it may expose the patient to adverse drug interactions and to the side-effects of prolonged poly-therapy. Moreover, many patients who become seizure free will be unwilling to take any risks associated with a treatment change, and may therefore elect to continue to take a pharmacological load which is possibly greater than necessary.

Combination therapy

As discussed above, combination therapy should be reserved for patients refractory to two or more sequential monotherapies, even though earlier, more aggressive utilization of polypharmacy may be justified in occasional cases, for example in severe and notoriously refractory epilepsy syndromes. The usefulness of adding a second and, sometimes, even a third drug in patients with refractory epilep-sy is well documented by long-standing clinical experience and by the results of many placebo-controlled add-on trials [46], even though it cannot be excluded that in some of those trials an im-provement in seizure frequency could have been obtained simply by increasing the dosage of baseline medication. In general, between 20% and 50% of patients with chronic refractory epilepsies are expected to benefit from addition of a second or third drug [37,38], although the actual proportion who will achieve seizure freedom will be considerably smaller (less than 20%). When another drug is added on, pharmacokinetic and/or pharmacodynamic interactions may occur, leading to the need for dosage adjustments (Chapter 10). For example, valproic acid inhibits the metabolism of lamotrigine and phenobarbital, and a reduction in the dosage of the latter drugs is usually indicated when valproic acid is added on [60]. Most phar-macokinetic interactions can be identified and managed by moni-toring plasma drug concentrations, but measurement of drug levels is of no value when the mechanism of the interaction is pharma-codynamic. One example of an adverse pharmacodynamic inter-action is provided by the appearance of side-effects suggestive of carbamazepine intoxication after addition of lamotrigine in patients stabilized on carbamazepine. These symptoms may not be associated with any change in the plasma concentration of carbamazepine or carbamazepine-10,11-epoxide, though they usu-ally disappear after a reduction in carbamazepine dosage [61].

While the value of combination therapy in selected patients cannot be questioned, it is important to emphasize that the risk of overtreatment is significant. Concomitant administration of more than one drug, especially when high dosages are used, involves a greater burden in terms of adverse effects, and the overall impact on the patient's quality of life needs to be closely scrutinized. It should also be remembered that in patients with chronic refractory epilep-sy, any beneficial effects following a change in treatment may be more apparent than real. In fact, these patients typically show wide fluctuations in seizure frequency over time, and it is not uncommon for an antiepileptic drug to be added on during a period of sponta-neous exacerbation: under these conditions, the subsequent improvement in seizure frequency may be related to spontaneous amelioration (the so-called phenomenon of regression to the mean) rather than to the effect of the added drug [43]. Because of this, the need for maintaining combination therapy should be reassessed at regular intervals, and monotherapy should be reinstituted whenever appropriate. As discussed above, an excessive drug burden created by drug combinations may lead to a paradoxical deterioration in seizure control. In many patients who fail to achieve sustained benefit from an added drug, restoration of monotherapy often leads to relief from side-effects without deterio-ration, and sometimes even with improvement, in seizure control.

Are some drug combinations more useful than others?

The possibility exists that two antiepileptic drugs interact pharma-codynamically by potentiating their respective seizure-suppressing effects, without necessarily potentiating their toxicity. In animal experiments, some antiepileptic drug combinations show a better therapeutic index than others, but the clinical relevance of these findings is difficult to assess [62]. Although the suggestion has been made that combining drugs with different mechanisms of action should be beneficial [40], in practice our knowledge of the modes of action of the various drugs, most of which have more than one primary action, is too incomplete to allow a rational application of this approach [37]. Therefore, drugs are usually combined on empirical grounds, taking into consideration a number of simple rules, the most important of which relate to the obvious practice of preferring combinations of drugs with different (or possibly, even antagonistic) side-effects and avoiding drugs associated with major adverse interactions.

Clinical evidence does indicate that some drug combinations are more advantageous than others. The best examples of useful combinations are valproic acid plus ethosuximide in the management of refractory absence seizures [63] and valproic acid plus lamotrigine in a variety of refractory seizure types [40,64,65]. The latter combination is also advantageous in pharmacoeconomic terms, because valproic acid inhibits lamotrigine metabolism and reduces the dosage requirements (and associated cost) of the latter. In a recent trial, four of 13 patients with refractory complex partial seizures who had failed to respond to maximally tolerated dosages of either valproic acid or lamotrigine given separately became seizure free when the two drugs were given together, and an additional four experienced seizure reductions of 62–78% [65]. Although addition of valproic acid to lamotrigine produced initially an increase in plasma lamotrigine levels, the appearance of side-effects, particularly tremor, required reduction in the dosage of both medications, and seizure control was finally achieved at plasma drug concentrations which were lower than those achieved before using combination therapy. There have been several reports on other potentially useful drug combinations, though evidence for these is mostly anecdotal.

Monitoring plasma drug concentrations (therapeutic drug monitoring) as a guide to dosage adjustments

The pharmacokinetics of most antiepileptic drugs exhibits remarkable interindividual variation, resulting in wide differences in plasma drug concentrations at steady-state among patients receiving the same dose. Since the concentration of a drug in plasma is in equilibrium with that in the brain, this variability will affect the degree of pharmacological response achieved at any given dosage, and therapeutic and toxic effects would be expected to correlate better with the drug concentration in plasma than with the prescribed daily dose [66]. Based on these considerations, monitoring plasma drug concentrations (therapeutic drug monitoring) has been found to provide a useful guide to adjusting dosage of many anticonvulsants [39].

In practice, the use of therapeutic drug monitoring requires considerable interpretative skills [67], and the physician should always adhere to the principle that therapeutic decisions must be based primarily on direct evaluation of clinical response rather than drug measurements alone. The basic principles for a rational use of plasma drug levels are outlined below.

When should blood samples be taken?

In general, blood samples for drug measurements should be taken at steady-state, i.e. when at least five half-lives have elapsed since the last dose change. For drugs with a long half-life, such as phenobarbital, the daily fluctuation in plasma concentration is negligible and the exact time of sampling is unimportant. With other compounds, it is preferable to collect the sample in the morning before the first daily dose, when the concentration is usually at its trough. For drugs exhibiting significant variation in plasma concentration during the dosing interval, namely carbamazepine and valproic acid, it is sometimes useful to obtain a second sample at the time of the expected peak concentration, in order to estimate the degree of fluctuation as a potential cause of intermittent side-effects.

The concept of 'therapeutic range'

Although 'therapeutic ranges' of drug concentrations have been described for many anticonvulsants (Table 11.8), it would be incorrect to suggest that all patients should have their dosage adjusted in order to produce plasma concentrations within the indicated limits. These ranges are simply representative of the plasma concentrations at which most patients respond. There may be a large variation in the degree of response at any given plasma drug level, and many patients achieve control at concentrations which are below or above the therapeutic ranges quoted in the literature [66]. If a patient is well controlled at 'subtherapeutic' concentrations there is no need for the dosage to be increased.

Several factors are responsible for the differences in clinical response observed at any drug concentration, and many of these are incompletely understood. It is clear, however, that one of the main sources of variability is represented by differences in the pathophysiology of the disease. Because epilepsies encompass a variety of disorders characterized by high heterogeneity in aetiology, mechanisms subserving seizure spread and generation, type of structural damage (if present) and clinical manifestations, it is no surprise that the type and severity of epilepsy are important factors affecting the response to any given plasma drug concentration. Patients with easily manageable forms of epilepsy tend to be controlled at plasma drug concentrations below the lower limit of the 'therapeutic range', whereas patients with epilepsies more difficult to control (e.g. symptomatic partial epilepsies) tend to require higher levels. In a representative study, Schmidt and Haenel [54] assessed the plasma concentration required to achieve optimal seizure control in patients with different seizure types treated with monotherapy. Among 40 well-controlled patients with generalized tonic-clonic seizures, 26 achieved freedom from seizures at plasma drug concentrations below the mid-portion of the 'therapeutic range'. Conversely, among 19 well-controlled patients with both generalized tonic-clonic and complex partial seizures, only three were controlled at plasma drug levels in the lower range. The median number of seizures during the first year of epilepsy was five for the patients who were controlled at lower concentrations compared with 29 for those who required higher concentrations. The fact that the 'therapeutic ranges' quoted in Table 11.8 have been established mostly in relatively severe forms of epilepsy provides an explanation for the observation that in newly diagnosed patients optimal responses are not infrequently seen at concentrations lower than

Table 11.8 Optimal ranges of plasma concentrations for commonly used antiepileptic drugs

Drug	Optimal range	Comments
Phenytoin	10–20 µg/ml (40–80 µmol/l)	Plasma drug level monitoring very useful because of saturation kinetics
Carbamazepine	4–11 µg/ml (17–46 µmol/l)	Plasma drug level monitoring useful, though often dosage adjustment can be based solely on clinical response
Ethosuximide	40–100 µg/ml (284–710 µmol/l)	Plasma drug level monitoring useful, though often dosage adjustments can be based solely on clinical response
Phenobarbital	10–40 µg/ml (43–172 µmol/l)	Imprecise upper limit due to tolerance to the sedative effects
Primidone	4–12 µg/ml (18–55 µmol/l)	Plasma drug level monitoring of unchanged primidone seldom required. It is more relevant to measure the levels of metabolically derived phenobarbital
Valproic acid	50–100 µg/ml (350–700 µmol/l)	Usefulness of plasma drug level monitoring limited in most cases
Zonisamide	7–30 µg/ml (33–140 µmol/l)	Optimal range not clearly established. Some patients may tolerate higher concentrations
Benzodiazepines		Plasma drug level monitoring not indicated. No consistent relationship between plasma drug concentration and effect
Felbamate		Usefulness of plasma drug level monitoring not demonstrated
Gabapentin		Usefulness of plasma drug level monitoring not demonstrated
Levetiracetam		Usefulness of plasma drug level monitoring not demonstrated
Lamotrigine		Usefulness of plasma drug level monitoring not demonstrated
Oxcarbazepine		Effect mediated by 10-hydroxy-metabolite. Usefulness of plasma drug level monitoring not demonstrated
Tiagabine		Usefulness of plasma drug level monitoring not demonstrated
Topiramate		Usefulness of plasma drug level monitoring not demonstrated
Vigabatrin		Plasma drug level monitoring not indicated due to irreversible (hit-and-run) mode of action

these. Based on this, Perucca and Richens [68] proposed that the lower limits of the commonly quoted 'therapeutic ranges' should be disregarded altogether, and that any concentration up to the upper limit of these ranges should be considered as potentially therapeutic.

Response at any given plasma drug concentration may vary over time within the same patient. For some drugs, therapeutic and/or toxic effects may decrease gradually over time, due to 'adaptation' mechanisms at the site of action, despite persistence of stable drug concentrations in blood. This phenomenon, known as pharmacodynamic tolerance, is seen most frequently with benzodiazepines and barbiturates. Because of the development of tolerance to the sedative effects of these drugs, patients treated chronically with benzodiazepines or barbiturates may tolerate well plasma drug concentrations which would be very toxic and even cause coma in acutely exposed subjects [68]. With phenobarbital, tolerance to sedative effects usually does not entail a simultaneous loss of anticonvulsant activity. This is not always the case for benzodiazepines, whose therapeutic value during chronic treatment is often limited by full or partial loss of efficacy.

Apart from the heterogenicity of the disease and adaptive changes at the site of drug action, other factors contribute to variability in the relationship between plasma drug concentration and response. These include alterations in the degree of drug binding to plasma proteins (see the section below on monitoring unbound drug concentrations) and the confounding effects caused by active metabolites and by pharmacodynamic interactions with concomi-

tant medications. Plasma concentrations of the active metabolites of some anticonvulsants are not routinely measured, and therapeutic errors may arise when concentrations of the parent drug are interpreted without taking into account the potential contribution of these metabolites [66]. For example, addition of valpromide, a valproic acid derivative, to the regimen of patients stabilized on carbamazepine causes a marked increase in the plasma concentration of the active metabolite carbamazepine-10,11-epoxide, resulting frequently in signs of intoxication (Fig. 11.4). Since the plasma concentration of the parent drug is not affected by this interaction, monitoring plasma carbamazepine concentration provides no clue to the mechanism of interaction. A similar situation arises in the presence of other drugs which interact at pharmacodynamic levels. Since the adverse central nervous system effects of different anticonvulsants may be additive, it is not uncommon for patients on multiple drug therapy to develop clinical signs of toxicity despite 'therapeutic' or even 'subtherapeutic' concentrations of individual drugs.

Individualized therapeutic drug concentrations

As discussed above, the marked interindividual variability in the response seen at any drug concentration complicates considerably the interpretation of therapeutic drug monitoring data. However, the fact that the therapeutic concentration of an anticonvulsant varies from patient to patient does not eliminate the value of measuring drug concentrations. In clinical practice, it is often feasible, and

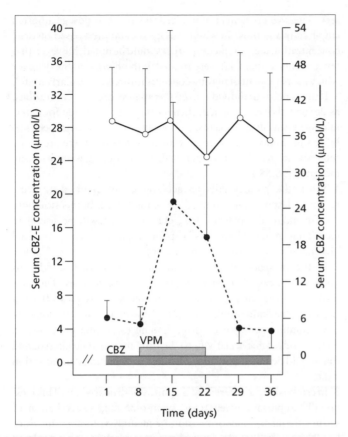

Fig. 11.4 Effect of valpromide (VPM, 1200 mg/day for 2 weeks), the amide derivative of valproic acid, on the serum concentration of carbamazepine (CBZ) and its active 10,11-epoxide metabolite (CBZ-E) in six patients stabilized on a constant dosage of carbamazepine. Values are means ± SEM. Note the marked elevation in the concentration of carbamazepine-10,11-epoxide after addition of valpromide, an inhibitor of the enzyme responsible for the conversion of the epoxide to the corresponding diol. The apparent decrease in the concentration of carbamazepine-10,11-epoxide on day 14 of combined therapy (compared with day 7) is due to exclusion of two patients with very high concentrations of the metabolite, who required discontinuation of valpromide because of side-effects. Data from [73].

even desirable, to establish empirically the plasma concentration at which an individual patient exhibits the best therapeutic response [66,69]. Because seizures occur unpredictably and often at long intervals, optimizing dosage on the basis of clinical response requires considerable skills and may take a long time. Once such an optimal dosage has been identified on empirical grounds, measurement of the steady-state drug concentration at that dosage may provide valuable information which can be exploited during subsequent management. For example, if a few years later the patient experiences a seizure breakthrough, a second measurement of the plasma drug concentration may give useful clues as to possible causes, such as a change in compliance or a change in drug disposition under the influence of developmental factors, disease states or drug interactions. Moreover, knowledge of the plasma concentration at which that patient responded in the past (the so-called 'individualized therapeutic drug concentration') will provide a useful reference in making dosage adjustments [66].

Even the concept of 'individualized therapeutic drug concentra-

tion', however, needs to be interpreted flexibly because the patient's sensitivity to a given drug concentration may change over time. This may be due to alterations in the pathophysiology of the seizure disorder, particularly during the period of brain maturation, to the occurrence of a pharmacodynamic interaction with concomitant medication, or to a modification in drug binding to plasma proteins due to disease or to displacement by an interacting drug.

Value of therapeutic drug monitoring for individual anticonvulsants

The value of therapeutic drug monitoring is greatest for phenytoin, for which the relationship between plasma concentration and effect is relatively consistent (Table 11.8). Since the enzymes responsible for phenytoin metabolism become easily saturated, small modifications in phenytoin dosage can produce unpredictably large changes in plasma drug concentration. Knowledge of plasma phenytoin concentration is particularly important in deciding the magnitude of dosage adjustments: in particular, when the steady-state concentration approaches the lower limit of the therapeutic range, dose increments should be very small to minimize the risk of intoxication [39,66].

A relatively good relationship between plasma concentration and response is also observed for ethosuximide and carbamazepine, but the dosage of these drugs can be individualized more easily on the basis of clinical response [68]. In the case of phenobarbital, as discussed above, interpretation of plasma drug concentrations is complicated by the development of tolerance, which causes a large variation in the levels at which toxicity occurs. For valproic acid, the relationship between concentration and response is rather variable and there is little value in monitoring the plasma levels of this drug in patients who are treated with usual dosages and show no obvious signs of toxicity. However, some adverse effects of valproic acid, such as tremor, certain encephalopathic symptoms and changes in platelet function, may be related to high plasma valproic acid concentrations, and monitoring plasma valproic acid levels may be of value when toxicity is suspected or in patients receiving high dosages.

In the case of vigabatrin, measuring plasma drug levels is not indicated because of its irreversible mode of action and the lack of a temporal relationship between plasma drug concentration and intensity of pharmacological effect. Well-defined therapeutic ranges have not been identified for other new generation anticonvulsants, and routine monitoring of their concentration is equally not indicated [69]. However, some of the newer drugs, particularly lamotrigine, topiramate, gabapentin, tiagabine, zonisamide and felbamate, show a marked pharmacokinetic variability which is likely to contribute to differences in dosage requirements. The concept outlined above of an 'individualized therapeutic drug concentration' may be usefully applied to some of these drugs.

Monitoring unbound drug concentrations

Although routine analytical methods measure the total concentration of the drug in plasma, it is only the free, non-protein bound fraction which is available to equilibrate with receptor sites and to produce pharmacological effects. When the unbound fraction is increased, the total concentration in plasma may underestimate the amount of drug which is pharmacologically active, and this should be taken into account when interpreting the plasma concentration of highly protein-bound drugs such as phenytoin and valproic acid. An increased unbound fraction of these drugs is observed in several conditions associated with hypoalbuminaemia (e.g. neonatal age, advanced pregnancy, old age, chronic liver disease, nephrotic syndrome) or with accumulation of endogenous displacing agents (e.g. uraemia). An increase in unbound fraction may also be caused by drug interactions: valproic acid, for example, increases the unbound fraction of phenytoin by displacing phenytoin molecules from protein binding sites. In all these conditions, therapeutic and toxic effects may be observed at total drug concentrations lower than usual, and failure to recognize this may mislead the clinician into making inappropriate dosage adjustments [48]. The suggestion has been made that in the presence of altered binding to plasma proteins it would be preferable to monitor directly the unbound drug concentration. In practice, however, this is not always necessary because often the increase in unbound fraction may be predicted on the basis of other parameters such as plasma albumin or, in uraemic patients, plasma creatinine concentration. In addition, unbound plasma drug concentrations are not always easy to measure, and results may be variable depending on the assay technique, and the possibility of analytical error.

With certain drugs such as carbamazepine and phenytoin, the concentration in saliva correlates relatively well with the unbound concentration in plasma. Therefore, salivary concentrations have been proposed for monitoring purposes, particularly in children who find venepunctures distressing. However, the use of salivary samples is not without problems because leakage of exudate (e.g. due to gingivitis) or dose residuates in the mouth may lead to erroneous results. Moreover, as mentioned above, measuring drug concentrations is subject to error, particularly when laboratories do not apply rigorous quality control measures, and such errors are more likely to occur with salivary samples, partly due to the fact that for some drugs the concentration in saliva is lower than in plasma. It should be stressed that the relationship between unbound drug concentration in plasma and drug concentration in saliva is not the same for all drugs. In the case of phenobarbital, the concentration in saliva is dependent upon salivary pH and cannot be used as a measure of free concentration in plasma unless calculations are made to account for differences in pH. For valproic acid, measuring salivary concentrations is meaningless because the drug concentration in saliva bears no consistent relationship with the concentration in plasma.

When should drug concentrations be measured?

The practice of monitoring plasma drug concentrations has played a major role in improving the quality of epilepsy care. It is thanks to therapeutic drug monitoring that many drug interactions have been discovered, and plasma drug level measurements have contributed greatly to stimulating physicians' awareness about the need to tailor dosage to the characteristics of the individual patient [66]. As a result of these advances in knowledge, however, physicians have also acquired skills in utilizing antiepileptic drugs correctly even without the aid of plasma drug concentration measurements. Antiepileptic drug therapy can often be optimized on purely clinical grounds, as shown in a recent trial where no differences in outcome were observed between patients randomized to have their dosage adjusted empirically and those in whom dosage was tailored based on drug concentration measurements [70]. It should be noted, however, that few patients in that trial were treated with phenytoin, the drug for which measurement of plasma concentrations is particularly useful.

If the concept of individualized therapeutic drug concentrations, as defined above, is applied, then a case could be made for determining plasma drug concentrations in any patient who has been stabilized on a satisfactory drug regimen. However, there are many other situations where therapeutic drug monitoring is more clearly indicated [66,68]:

1 When the patient fails to achieve an adequate therapeutic response despite an apparently adequate dosage. In this situation, assessment of the plasma drug concentration will be useful in identifying potential sources of poor response, such as unusual pharmacokinetic patterns or poor compliance.

2 In the presence of physiological or pathological conditions known to be associated with pharmacokinetic changes. These include paediatric age, pregnancy, old age and diseases affecting the liver, the kidney and the gastrointestinal tract. In some of these conditions, however, drug binding to plasma proteins and pharmacodynamic sensitivity to the drug may also be altered, and this should be taken into account when interpreting concentration data.

3 In establishing a differential diagnosis of drug toxicity. This is especially important when toxic symptoms (e.g. exacerbation of seizure frequency, incoordination or mental symptoms) may not be differentiated easily from those of underlying or associated diseases.

4 To minimize the difficulties in dosage adjustments caused by dose-dependent pharmacokinetics, particularly with phenytoin.

5 In patients receiving multiple drug therapy, in order to identify and to minimize the consequences of adverse drug interactions. When seizure control is unsatisfactory or toxic signs develop in patients on polytherapy, measuring the concentration of individual drugs may also assist in identifying the agent whose dosage should be preferentially adjusted.

6 When a drug formulation has been changed, to assess the possibility of a clinically significant change in bioavailability.

7 When poor compliance is suspected. Compliance problems are suggested by unusually low and variable concentrations, which increase following supervision of drug intake.

While the value of therapeutic drug monitoring cannot be questioned, it has also been pointed out that drug concentrations are often measured unnecessarily or interpreted incorrectly [71]. These determinations should be requested only when there is a sound indication, and dosage adjustments should be made only when there is a clinical need, irrespective of the drug level in blood. Physicians must always remember that the primary aim of therapy is to treat a patient and not a laboratory value.

How long should treatment be continued?

Since many epilepsies are prone to undergo spontaneous remission, the possibility of discontinuing antiepileptic medication after an adequate period of seizure freedom should be considered. This is especially important in children who show a higher prevalence of self-remitting syndromes and in whom the psychosocial consequences of seizure relapse are less severe than in adults. The option of discontinuing treatment should be discussed with the patient and the family, taking into consideration not only the probability of relapse, but also any side-effects of treatment, the patient's attitude to continuation of treatment and to the possibility of seizure recurrence and legal implications with special reference to driving regulations.

Because stopping antiepileptic drugs abruptly carries a serious risk of withdrawal seizures and even status epilepticus, discontinuation of medications should be carried out gradually, to allow assessment of response at each dose level and to minimize risks. The proportion of patients whose seizures recur within 2 years following discontinuation of therapy is on average about 30% [72], but this figure in itself has little meaning because relapse rates range from close to zero to over 90% depending on the characteristics of the population. Predictors associated with an increased risk of relapse include increasing age, symptomatic epilepsy, an abnormal EEG and a longer duration of active disease prior to seizure control [11]. The most important prognostic factor is, however, the epilepsy syndrome, with relapse rates being very rare in rolandic epilepsy, relatively rare (5–25%) in childhood absence epilepsy, intermediate (25–75%) in cryptogenic or symptomatic partial epilepsies and high (85–95%) in juvenile myoclonic epilepsy [11]. A detailed discussion of clinical management of patients in remission is given in Chapter 13.

References

1 Perucca E. Principles of pharmacotherapy of the epilepsies. In: Asbury AK, McKhann G, McDonald WI *et al.*, eds. *Diseases of the Nervous System: Clinical Neuroscience and Therapeutic Principles.* Cambridge: Cambridge University Press, 2002; 2: 1301–12.

2 Smith D, Baker GB, Davies G *et al.* Outcomes of add-on treatment with lamotrigine in partial epilepsy. *Epilepsia* 1993; 34: 312–22.

3 Perucca E, Beghi E, Dulac O *et al.* Assessing risk to benefit ratio in antiepileptic drug therapy. *Epilepsy Res* 2000; 41: 107–39.

4 Temkin NR. Antiepileptogenesis and seizure prevention trials with antiepileptic drugs: Metanalysis of controlled trials. *Epilepsia* 2001; 42: 515–24.

5 Chadwick D. Do anticonvulsants alter the natural course of epilepsy? Case for early treatment is not established. *Brit Med J* 1995; 310: 177–8.

6 Reynolds EH. Do anticonvulsants alter the natural course of epilepsy? Treatment should be started as early as possible. *Brit Med J* 1995; 310: 176–7.

7 Jefferys JG. Hippocampal sclerosis and temporal lobe epilepsy: cause or consequence? *Brain* 1999; 122, 1007–8.

8 Camfield C, Camfield P, Gordon K, Dooley J. Does the number of seizures before treatment influence ease of control or remission of childhood epilepsy? Not if the number is 10 or less. *Neurology* 1996; 46: 41–4.

9 Shinnar S, Berg AT. Does antiepileptic drug therapy prevent the development of 'chronic' epilepsy? *Epilepsia* 1996; 37: 701–8.

10 Berg AT, Shinnar S, Levy SR *et al.* How well can epilepsy syndromes be identified at diagnosis? A reassessment 2 years after initial diagnosis. *Epilepsia* 2000; 41: 1269–75.

11 Beghi E, Perucca E. The management of epilepsy in the 1990s: Acquisitions, uncertainties, and perspectives for future research. *Drugs* 1995; 49: 680–94.

12 Berg AT, Shinnar S. The risk of seizure recurrence after a first unprovoked seizure: a quantitative review. *Neurology* 1991; 41: 965–72.

13 Musicco M, Beghi E, Solari A *et al.* Treatment of first tonic-clonic seizure does not improve the prognosis of epilepsy. *Neurology* 1997; 49: 991–8.

14 First Seizure Trial Group. Randomized clinical trial of the efficacy of antiepileptic drugs in reducing the risk of relapse after first unprovoked tonic-clonic seizure. *Neurology* 1993; 43: 478–83.

15 Hirtz D, Berg A, Bettis D *et al.* Practice parameter: treatment of the child with a first unprovoked seizure. Report of the Quality Standards Subcommittee of the American Academy of Neurology and the Practice Committee of the Child Neurology Society. *Neurology* 2003; 60: 166–75.

16 American Academy of Pediatrics. Committee on Quality Improvement, Subcommittee on Febrile Seizures. Practice parameter: Long-term treatment of the child with simple febrile seizures. *Pediatrics* 1999; 103: 1307–9.

17 Temkin NR, Dikmen SS, Wilensky AJ *et al.* A randomized, double-blind study of phenytoin for the prevention of posttraumatic seizures. *N Engl J Med* 1990; 323: 497–502.

18 Foy PM, Chadwick DW, Rajgopalan N *et al.* Do prophylactic anticonvulsant drugs alter the pattern of seizures after craniotomy? *J Neurol Neurosurg Psych* 1992; 55: 753–7.

19 Temkin NR, Dikmen SS, Anderson GD *et al.* Valproate therapy for prevention of post-traumatic seizures: A randomized trial. *J Neurosurgery* 1999; 91: 593–600.

20 Shorvon SD, Chadwick D, Galbraith AW, Reynolds EH. One drug for epilepsy. *Brit Med J* 1978; 1: 474–6.

21 Mattson RH, Cramer JA, Collins JF *et al.* Comparison of carbamazepine, phenobarbital, phenytoin, and primidone in partial and secondarily generalized tonic-clonic seizures. *N Engl J Med* 1985; 13: 145–51.

22 Mattson RH, Cramer JA, Collins JF, and the Department of the Veteran Affairs Epilepsy Cooperative Study Group. A comparison of valproate with carbamazepine for the treatment of complex partial sezures and secondarily generalized tonic-clonic seizures in adults. *N Engl J Med* 1992; 327: 765–71.

23 Richens A., Davidson DLW, Cartlidge NEF, Easter DJ. A multicentre comparative trial of sodium valproate and carbamazepine in adult-onset epilepsy. *J Neurol Neurosurg Psychiatr* 1994; 57: 682–7.

24 Heller AJ, Chesterman P, Elwes RDC *et al.* Phenobarbitone, phenytoin, carbamazepine, or sodium valproate for newly diagnosed adult epilepsy: a randomized comparative monotherapy trial. *J Neurol Neurosurg Psychiatr* 1995; 58: 44–50.

25 Verity CM, Hosking G, Easter DJ, on behalf of the Pediatric EPITEG Collaborative Group. A multicentre comparative trial of sodium valproate and carbamazepine in paediatric epilepsy. *Dev Med Child Neurol* 1995; 37, 97–108.

26 De Silva M, MacArdle B, McGowan M *et al.* Randomized comparative monotherapy trial of phenobarbitone, phenytoin, carbamazepine, or sodium valproate for newly diagnosed childhood epilepsy. *Lancet* 1996; 347: 709–13.

27 Kwan P, Brodie MJ. Early identification of refractory epilepsy. *N Engl J Med* 2000; 342: 314–19.

28 Perucca E, Gram L, Avanzini G, Dulac O. Antiepileptic drugs as a cause of worsening of seizures. *Epilepsia* 1998; 39: 5–17.

29 Guerrini R, Dravet C, Genton P *et al.* Lamotrigine and seizure aggravation in severe myoclonic epilepsy. *Epilepsia* 1998; 39: 508–12.

30 Perucca E, Tomson T. Monotherapy trials with the new antiepileptic drugs: study designs, practical relevance and ethical implications. *Epilepsy Res* 1999; 32: 247–62.

31 Chiron C, Dumas C, Jambaqué I *et al.* Randomized trial comparing vigabatrin and hydrocortisone in infantile spasms due to tuberous sclerosis. *Epilepsy Res* 1997; 26: 389–95.

32 Vigevano F, Cilio MR. Vigabatrin versus ACTH as first-line treatment for infantile spasms. A randomized prospective study. *Epilepsia* 1997; 38: 1270–74.

33 Dean AC, Gosey C, Matsuo F. Utility of tiagabine in epilepsy patients with glial tumors. *Epilepsia* 1998; 39 (Suppl. 6): 57.

34 Semah F, Picot MC, Adam C *et al.* Is the underlying cause of epilepsy a major prognostic factor for recurrence? *Neurology* 1998; 51: 1256–62.

35 Battino D, Dukes MNG, Perucca E. Anticonvulsants. In: Dukes MNG, Aronson JK, eds. *Meyler's Side-Effects of Drugs*, 14th edn. Amsterdam: Elsevier Science BV, 2000: 83–95.

36 Brodie MJ, Overstall PW, Giorgi L. Multicentre, double-blind randomised comparison between Lamotrigine and carbamazepine in elderly patients

with newly diagnosed epilepsy. The UK Lamotrigine Elderly Study Group. *Epilepsy Res* 1999; 37: 81–7.

37 Perucca E. Clinical pharmacology and therapeutic use of the new antiepileptic drugs. *Fund Clin Pharmacol* 2001; 15: 405–17.

38 Perucca E. The new generation of antiepileptic drugs: Advantages and disadvantages. *Brit J Clin Pharmacol* 1996; 42: 531–43.

39 Eadie MJ. The role of therapeutic drug monitoring in improving the cost-effectiveness of anticonvulsant therapy. *Clin Pharmacokinet* 1995; 29: 29–35.

40 Brodie MJ, Yuen AWC, and 105 Study Group. Lamotrigine substitution study: Evidence for synergism with sodium valproate. *Epilepsy Res* 1997; 26: 423–32.

41 Gatti G, Bonomi I, Jannuzzi G, Perucca E. The new antiepileptic drugs: pharmacological and clinical aspects. *Curr Pharmacol Design* 2000; 6: 617–38.

42 Brodie MJ, Richens A, Yuen AW. Double-blind comparison of lamotrigine and carbamazepine in newly diagnosed epilepsy: *Lancet* 1995; 345: 476–9.

43 Perucca E. What can we learn from clinical trials of new anticonvulsant drugs in epilepsy? *Eur J Pain* 2002; 6 (Suppl. A): 35–44.

44 Kälviäinen R, Aikia M, Saukkonen AM *et al*. Vigabatrin versus carbamazepine monotherapy in patients with newly diagnosed epilepsy: A randomized controlled study. *Arch Neurol* 1995; 52: 989–96.

45 Kälviäinen R, Nousiainen I. Visual field defects with vigabatrin: Epidemiology and therapeutic implications. *CNS Drugs* 2001; 15: 217–30.

46 Cramer JA, Fisher R, Ben-Menachem E *et al*. New antiepileptic drugs: Comparison of key clinical trials. *Epilepsia* 1999; 40: 590–600.

47 Scheepers M, Scheepers B, Clarke M *et al*. Is intranasal midazolam an effective rescue medication in adolescents and adults with severe epilepsy? *Seizure* 2000; 9: 417–22.

48 Perucca E. Pharmacokinetics. In: Engel J, Jr and Pedley TA, eds. *Epilepsy— A Comprehensive Textbook*. New York: Raven Press, 1997: 1131–53.

49 Richens A. Impact of generic substitution of anticonvulsants on the treatment of epilepsy. *CNS Drugs* 1997; 8: 124–33.

50 Mayer TH, May TW, Altenmuller DM *et al*. Comparison of sustained release formulations of carbamazepine. *Clin Drug Invest* 1999; 18: 17–26.

51 Collins RJ, Garnett WR. Extended release formulations of anticonvulsant medications, clinical pharmacokinetics and therapeutic advantages. *CNS Drugs* 2000; 14: 203–12.

52 Perucca E, Dulac O, Shorvon S, Tomson T. Harnessing the clinical potential of antiepileptic drug therapy: Dosage optimisation. *CNS Drugs* 2001; 15: 609–21.

53 Besag FMC. Approaches to reducing the incidence of lamotrigine-induced rash. *CNS Drugs* 2000; 13: 21–3.

54 Schmidt D, Haenel F. Therapeutic plasma levels of phenytoin, phenobarbital and carbamazepine: individual variation in relation to seizure type. *Neurology* 1984; 34: 1252–3.

55 Hermanns G, Noachtar S, Taxhorn I *et al*. Systematic testing of medical intractability for carbamazepine, phenytoin and phenobarbital or primidone in monotherapy for patients considered for epilepsy surgery. *Epilepsia* 1996; 37: 675–9.

56 Krämer G, ed. *Epilepsy in the Elderly*. Stuttgart: Thieme, 1999: 69–124.

57 Harden CL. Therapeutic safety monitoring: What to look for and when to look for it. *Epilepsia* 2000; 41 (Suppl. 8): S37–S44.

58 Hakkarainen H. Carbamazepine vs diphenylhydantoin vs their combination in adult epilepsy. *Neurology* 1980; 30: 354.

59 Tanganelli P, Regesta G. Vigabatrin vs carbamazepine monotherapy in newly diagnosed focal epilepsy: A randomized response conditional crossover study. *Epilepsy Res* 1996; 25: 257–62.

60 Patsalos PV, Perucca E. Clinically important drug interactions in epilepsy: general features and interactions between antiepileptic drugs. *Lancet Neurol* 2003; 2: 347–56.

61 Besag FMC, Berry DJ, Pool F *et al*. Carbamazepine toxicity with lamotrigine: Pharmacokinetic or pharmacodynamic interaction? *Epilepsia* 1998; 39: 183–7.

62 Deckers CLP, Czuczwar SJ, Hekster YA *et al*. Selection of antiepileptic drug polytherapy based on mechanisms of action: The evidence reviewed. *Epilepsia* 2000; 41: 1364–74.

63 Rowan AJ, Meijer JWA, de Beer-Pawlikowski N, van der Geest P. Valproate ethosuximide combination therapy for refractory absence seizures. *Arch Neurol* 1983; 40: 797–802.

64 Panayiotopoulos CP, Ferrie CD, Knott C, Robinson RO. Interaction of lamotrigine with sodium valproate. *Lancet* 1993; 341: 445.

65 Pisani F, Oteri G, Russo R *et al*. The efficacy of valproate-lamotrigine comedication in refractory complex partial seizures: Evidence for a pharmacodynamic interaction. *Epilepsia* 1999; 40: 1141–6.

66 Glauser TA, Pippenger CE. Controversies in blood-level monitoring: Reexamining its role in the treatment of epilepsy. *Epilepsia* 2000; 41 (Suppl. 8): S6–S15.

67 Beardsley RS, Freeman JM, Appel FA. Anticonvulsant serum levels are useful only if the physician appropriately uses them: An assessment of the impact of providing serum level data to physicians. *Epilepsia* 1983; 24: 330–5.

68 Perucca E, Richens A. Antiepileptic drugs. Clinical aspects. In: Richens A, Marks V, eds. *Therapeutic Drug Monitoring*. Edinburgh: Churchill-Livingstone, 1983: 320–48.

69 Perucca E. Is there a role for therapeutic drug monitoring of new anticonvulsants? *Clin Pharmacokinet* 2000; 38: 191–204.

70 Jannuzzi G. Cian P, Fattore C *et al*. A multicenter randomized controlled trial on the clinical impact of therapeutic drug monitoring in patients with newly diagnosed epilepsy. *Epilepsia* 2000; 41, 222–30.

71 Chadwick DW. Overuse of monitoring of blood concentrations of antiepileptic drugs. *Brit Med J* 1987; 294: 723–4.

72 Berg AT, Shinnar S. Relapse following discontinuation of antiepileptic drugs: A meta-analysis. *Neurology* 1994; 44: 601–8.

73 Pisani F, Fazio A, Oteri G *et al*. Sodium valproate and valpromide: Potential interactions with carbamazepine in epileptic patients. *Epilepsia* 1986; 27: 548–52.

74 Richens A, Perucca E. Clinical pharmacology and medical treatment. In: Laidlaw J, Richens A, Chadwick DW, eds. *A Textbook of Epilepsy*. Edinburgh: Churchill-Livingstone, 1993: 495–559.

12 Management of Newly Diagnosed Epilepsy

Y.M. Hart

The implications of newly diagnosed epilepsy

The diagnosis of epilepsy has important medical and social implications. First, the seizures themselves may cause accident or injury, as well as embarrassment at the associated lack of control. Secondly, there may be anxiety about the underlying cause, with fear of a brain tumour being common. Thirdly, the secondary effects of seizures may affect many aspects of everyday life. The loss of the driving licence is often particularly distressing, causing loss of independence, with consequences for employment, finance and even housing, if a mortgage is involved or if the patient lives in an isolated area. Leisure activities may be affected, and for children, epilepsy may disrupt education if seizures are frequent or if the child is sent home from school on a regular basis. The need for regular medication may cause adverse effects or, for women, worries about teratogenicity and breastfeeding. Finally, parents may worry that their children will inherit the epileptic tendency. For all these reasons, it is essential both to ensure that the diagnosis is correct before considering treatment, and to provide the patient with adequate education and information about the condition.

The diagnosis of epilepsy

Epilepsy has been defined as 'the tendency to recurrent unprovoked seizures'. A complete diagnosis involves not only confirmation of the fact that the person is having seizures, but also classification of the seizure type, which will guide the choice of antiepileptic drug, if required, and epilepsy syndrome, which may give an indication of the likely prognosis. The International Classification of Epileptic Seizures and International Classification of Epilepsies and Epileptic Syndromes produced by the International League against Epilepsy [1,2] are commonly used for this purpose. An attempt should also be made to identify the underlying cause.

The differential diagnosis of epilepsy is wide (Table 12.1), with syncope and non-epileptic seizures of psychological origin being the most frequently encountered. Except in the rare situation where the patient has a seizure while undergoing recording of an EEG, the diagnosis of epilepsy is made on the basis of the clinical history, taken both from the patient and from someone who has observed the seizures. Particularly where consciousness is lost during the attack, it may be impossible to make the diagnosis with certainty in the absence of such an eye-witness description. The duration of the attack, presence of precipitating factors and the duration and severity of the postictal phase are often the most discriminating factors in differentiating seizures from syncope. Rigidity and sometimes jerking may occur in syncope [3], as may incontinence and automatisms, although the latter are uncommon. In addition to the description of the attack, information regarding the presence or absence of precipitating factors, family history of epilepsy, other medical history indicating a possible predisposition towards seizures or other paroxysmal conditions (for example, prolonged febrile seizure, head injury, somatization disorder), drug history and alcohol intake, should be sought.

Even where a good eye-witness account is available, neurologists may differ in their opinion regarding diagnosis, as shown by van Donselaar *et al.* [4], who examined interrater variability of seizure diagnosis and concluded that a committee approach was desirable. Unfortunately, once made, an inappropriate diagnosis of epilepsy is often difficult to correct, and in one study [5] it was found that up to 20% of patients admitted to a psychiatric hospital with refractory epilepsy, did not have this disorder.

The routine EEG is of low sensitivity in making the diagnosis of epilepsy. Only about 35% of patients with epilepsy consistently show epileptic abnormalities on their EEG [6], though the yield is increased by repeated recordings, particularly with sleep deprivation [7]: in patients presenting with a suspected single seizure, the proportion with epileptic abnormalities may be as low as 21% [8]. However, the presence of epileptic abnormalities in circumstances suggestive of a seizure is helpful in confirming the diagnosis, since only around 0.5–2% of people without epilepsy exhibit them [9–11]. The EEG may be helpful in classifying the seizure type, particularly in the case of generalized tonic-clonic seizures where it is not clear if they are due to idiopathic generalized epilepsy or are secondarily generalized.

An attempt should also be made to classify the epilepsy syndrome, which may have implications both for prognosis and treatment; for example, benign epilepsy of childhood with centrotemporal spikes confers a good prognosis, with remission by the age of 16, while juvenile myoclonic epilepsy is associated with a very high risk of relapse without medication [12]. There has been debate as to the extent to which it is possible to identify the syndrome precisely at the time of initial diagnosis of epilepsy. King *et al.* [13] studied 300 consecutive adults and children over the age of 5 years presenting with unexplained seizures, systematically collecting clinical data from patients and witnesses. Although the intention was to study patients presenting with a first generalized tonic-clonic seizure, 17% were found to have had previous similar events and 28% had experienced other epileptic symptoms such as absences, myoclonus or temporal lobe auras. An EEG was performed within 24 h of the seizure where possible, and MRI scanning was also performed electively. The authors were able to diagnose a generalized or partial epilepsy syndrome clinically in 141 patients (47%), with only three of these clinical diagnoses later being proved incorrect: after EEG and MRI, it was possible to diagnose 81% of patients as having a generalized epilepsy (23%) or partial epilepsy (58%). Nineteen per cent had unclassified seizures. A study of 1942 patients presenting with unprovoked seizures, of whom 47.7% had had a single seizure and 52.3% more than one seizure at initial presentation, was carried out by Jallon *et al.* [14]. All but 17 patients had EEGs, and 73.0% underwent neuroimaging. In the group presenting after a single seizure, partial seizures were diagnosed in 46.2%, generalized seizures in 31.9% and the seizures were unclassified in 21.9%. Amongst those in whom two seizures had already occurred at the time of initial presentation, the first seizure type was partial in 48.1% of the group, generalized in 39.9% and unclassified in 12%. An epilepsy syndrome could be assigned in 98.6% of this group of patients. In contrast, Manford *et al.* [15], commenting on the results of a community-based study, noted that it was possible to assign a specific classification to only 33.6% of patients with newly diagnosed epilepsy, the remainder falling into various poorly characterized categories (cryptogenic localization-related epilepsies, seizures without unequivocal focal or generalized features and situation-related epilepsies, including isolated seizures). In this study, which was carried out a decade earlier than those of King *et al.* [13]

and Jallon *et al.* [14], few patients underwent MRI and EEG data were not available in all cases.

Rationale for treatment

As indicated above, the diagnosis of epilepsy has important medical and social implications. The decision whether to start medication depends on the likelihood of recurrence and an evaluation of the risk of harmful consequences from the seizures themselves (including injury, death, psychosocial morbidity and any adverse effect of recurrent seizures on long-term prognosis), weighed against the adverse effects of medication, both physical and in terms of reinforcing the concept of illness.

Risk of recurrence after a first seizure

Estimates of the risk of recurrence following a first seizure have varied widely from 27% by 3 years [16] to 84% after a variable period of follow-up [17]. Table 12.2 shows the risk of recurrence estimated in various studies. The enormous differences between the results can be largely explained on the basis of variations in study design. The time of entry into the study after the first seizure is particularly important: the risk of recurrence is greatest in the first few weeks after the first seizure [18] (Fig. 12.1), and in those studies in which there is a significant delay between the seizure occurrence and the time to review in clinic, the recurrence rate may be artificially low due to the exclusion of those patients who have already experienced a second seizure [19]. A further problem in assessing recurrence is the difficulty in making the diagnosis in the early stages, particularly if the initial seizure was not witnessed, or if earlier seizures have been mild (for example, absences, myoclonus or simple partial seizures), a fact illustrated by the Rochester study of Hauser *et al.* [20], who found that the time from the first afebrile seizure to diagnosis was longer than 6 months in 50% of patients, and greater than 2 years in more than 30%. Similarly, Shorvon [21], in a hospital-based study of 106 patients with newly diagnosed tonic-clonic and/or partial seizures, found that the median number of seizures experienced by patients prior to referral was four (three, range 1–36, for tonic-clonic seizures and six, range 1–180, for partial seizures). Other important issues in methodology are the use of

Table 12.1 Conditions which may be confused with seizures

Vasovagal syncope
Cardiac dysrhythmias
Non-epileptic seizures (of psychological
　origin)
Panic attacks
Migraine
Breath-holding attacks (in children)
Sleep terrors and other parasomnias
Other paroxysmal movement disorders (e.g.
　paroxysmal kinesigenic choreoathetosis)
Narcolepsy/cataplexy
Vertigo
Hypoglycaemia
Other metabolic disorders
Alcohol/substance abuse

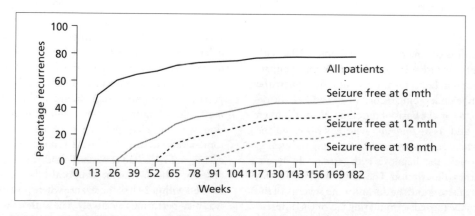

Fig. 12.1 National General Practice Study of Epilepsy: actuarial percentage of recurrence after first seizure. A study of 564 patients followed prospectively from the time of diagnosis. Within 3 years of their first seizure, 78% of patients had a recurrence of their attacks. If attacks had not recurred within 6, 12 or 18 months, the chance of recurrence was substantially reduced, falling to 44, 32 and 17%, respectively. From [18].

Table 12.2 Studies of recurrence following a first seizure

Study	Patient sample	Prospective/ Retrospective	Number of patients	Age of patients	Total follow-up	Recurrence		
						By 1 yr	By 3 yrs	Total
Thomas, 1959	Patients attending for EEG	Retrospective	48	2–66 y	3.5–8.5 y			27%
Costeff, 1965	Children attending paediatric clinic	Retrospective	500	0–5 y	33–60 mo			50%
Saunders and Marshall, 1975	Patients attending for EEG	Retrospective	33 (+ 6 lost to f/u)	15–57 y	10–52 mo			33%
Blom et al, 1978	Children attending paediatric clinic	Prospective	73	0–15 y	3 y			59%
Cleland et al, 1981	Patients attending neurological clinic	Retrospective	70 (+ 14 lost to f/u)	16–65 y	3–10 y			39%
Hauser et al, 1982	Patients identified at 4 Minnesota hospitals	Prospective	244 (+ 34 lost to f/u)	All	6–55 mo	16%	27%	
Goodridge and Shorvon, 1983	Patients identified from GP records	Retrospective	122	All	0–>15 y			81%
Elwes et al, 1985	Patients attending hospital at median of 1 day after 1st tonic clonic seizure	Prospective	133	2–74 y	1–69 mo	62%	71%	
Camfield et al, 1985a	Children attending for EEG after 1st seizure	Retrospective	168 (+ 9 lost to f/u)	0.1–16 y	Mean 31.4 mo	40%		52%
Annegers et al, 1986	Cases identified through record linkage system	Retrospective	424	All	Up to 10 y	36%	48%	56%
Hopkins et al, 1988	Patients attending hospital clinic with seizures in absence of prior neurological disease	Prospective	408	≥16 y	Up to 3 y	39%	52%	
Hart et al, 1990	Patients attending general practitioners	Mainly prospective	564	>1 mo	2–4 y	67%	78%	
First Seizure Trial Group, 1993	Patients seen in any of 35 hospitals within 1 week of first unprovoked tonic-clonic seizure	Prospective	397	≥2 y	Up to 3 y	51% (untreated) 25% (treated)		

f/u, follow-up.

crude figures versus actuarial analysis when estimating recurrence, the former being liable to distortion through incomplete follow-up, and bias occurring as a result of retrospective study design.

Several studies have attempted to identify the factors affecting the risk of recurrence. The influence of aetiology, seizure type, age of the patient, EEG abnormalities, timing of first seizure (during sleep or while awake) and coexistence of mental retardation or other neurological abnormalities is controversial. Van Donselaar et al. [22], studying patients with idiopathic first seizures, found that the strongest predictor of recurrence was the EEG, with a cumulative risk of recurrence at 2 years of 81% (95% CI 66–97%) in patients with epileptic discharges on a standard or partial sleep deprivation

EEG, 39% (27–51%) in patients with other EEG abnormalities and 12% (3–21%) in patients with normal EEGs. Other factors increasing the risk of recurrence were younger age, occurrence of first seizure during sleep or on awakening and tongue biting, while family history, provocative circumstances and gender had no effect. The First Seizure Trial Group [23] found a 1.7 times increase in the risk in patients with epileptiform abnormalities on their EEG. Hauser et al. [16] also found the EEG to be of use in predicting prognosis among patients with idiopathic seizures, those with a generalized spike and wave pattern having a significantly higher rate of recurrence than those with normal or non-specific tracings (50% compared with 14% at 24 months). However, those with focal slowing or spikes did not have a significantly different rate of recurrence from those with normal or non-specifically abnormal tracings. Other adverse factors in this study included a known remote aetiology for a first seizure, a Todd's paresis following the first seizure and a history of acute symptomatic seizures. EEG abnormalities were similarly found to be predictive of recurrence among idiopathic cases by Annegers et al. [24], but other studies have not found them to be helpful [25,26]. In the study by Gilad et al. [26] in univariate analysis, the only clinical variable associated with recurrence was the time of day at which the initial seizure occurred, the risk of relapse being higher if the first seizure occurred between the hours of midnight and breakfast time. An increased risk of seizure recurrence following a first seizure in sleep in children, particularly those with idiopathic seizures, was similarly found by Shinnar et al. [27].

Age less than 16 years was found to be a significant predictive factor for recurrence in the FIRST seizure study by Musicco et al. [28], who reported 419 patients over the age of 2 years seen within 7 days of their first witnessed, unprovoked, primary or secondarily generalized seizure, and randomized to receive treatment immediately or only if they had a recurrence of seizures. This study also found the presence of epileptic abnormalities on EEG (as noted above) and remote aetiological factors to be predictive of relapse, whereas acute treatment of the initial seizure with benzodiazepines was associated with a lower subsequent relapse rate.

The National General Practice Study of Epilepsy [18] found that the aetiology of the seizures was of prognostic importance. Recurrence after a first seizure was significantly lower in patients experiencing acute symptomatic seizures (seizures occurring in the context of an acute insult to the brain, such as stroke, head injury or encephalitis, or as a result of drugs or metabolic disturbance) than those with idiopathic seizures or seizures due to a remote symptomatic cause. Seizures associated with a neurological deficit presumed present at birth had the highest rate of recurrence (100% by 18 months). Other factors predisposing to an increased risk of recurrence in this study included age (the highest risk being for patients under the age of 16 or over the age of 59) and seizure type, recurrence being considerably higher in patients with simple or complex partial seizures. The influence of EEG was not examined in this study.

A meta-analysis of 16 studies examining the risk of recurrence after a first seizure was carried out by Berg and Shinnar [29], who concluded that the seizure aetiology and the EEG were the strongest predictors of recurrence.

Effect of repeated seizures on risk of recurrence

The risk of recurrence appears to be higher in patients who have a second or third seizure. Hauser et al. [30] studied 204 patients (70% of them male) with a first unprovoked seizure, prospectively from the day of the initial seizure for 5 years or until the time of the third seizure. The overall recurrence rate was lower than in many other studies, the risk of a second unprovoked seizure within 5 years of the first being 33% (95% CI 26–40%). Among the 63 patients who had a second seizure the risk of further unprovoked seizures was 32% by 3 months, increasing to 73% at 4 years. Of the 37 patients classified as having idiopathic or cryptogenic epilepsy who had a second seizure, the risk of a third seizure was 64% at 5 years, compared with 87% in those with remote symptomatic epilepsy. Of note in

this study is that 432 patients were excluded through having had multiple seizures before their first medical evaluation, emphasizing the late presentation of many patients with epilepsy: similarly in the National General Practice Study of Epilepsy [18] only 44.7% of patients were registered at the time of their first seizure, and in the CAROLE study (Coordination Active du Réseau Observatoire Longitudinal de l'Epilepsie [14]) 52.3% of patients had already had two or more seizures at the time of presentation.

Elwes et al. [31], in a study of patients presenting with untreated tonic-clonic seizures, examined the time intervals between consecutive seizures. They found that the median interval between the first two seizures was 12 weeks (95% CI 10–18 weeks), between the second and third seizure, 8 weeks (4–12), between the third and fourth, 4 weeks (2–20), and between the fourth and fifth, 3 weeks (1–4). They deduced that in many patients there is an accelerating disease process in the early stages of epilepsy.

Effect of treatment after a first seizure on risk of recurrence

In several of the studies quoted above, assessment of the recurrence rate has been confounded by the fact that a proportion of the patients were treated following their first seizure. Usually this has not been on a random basis, in that treatment was started in those patients deemed to be at higher risk of recurrence and because of this, such patients were retained within the study to avoid bias due to their exclusion. The effect of medication on recurrence as determined in these studies has been confusing, probably because they were the high-risk patients: in the National General Practice Study of Epilepsy [18] patients starting medication after a first seizure had a lower risk of recurrence (50% (95% CI 40–61%) by 1 year), while other trials [16,25,32–34] have found no difference in the risk of recurrence between treated and untreated patients.

In the three studies in which patients have been randomized to immediate or delayed treatment following a single seizure, however, a clear reduction in the risk of seizure recurrence has been shown. The largest such study was carried out by the First Seizure Trial Group [23]. This was a multicentre study of 397 patients ranging in age from 2 to 70 years, presenting within 7 days of a first generalized tonic-clonic seizure and randomized to immediate treatment with carbamazepine, phenytoin, phenobarbital or sodium valproate, according to the preference of the physician, or to treatment with the same drugs only after seizure recurrence. The dose was increased to be within the therapeutic range within 1 month of entry into the study. Patients with acute symptomatic seizures or progressive neurological disorders were excluded, as were those whose seizures were related to metabolic disorders or alcohol addiction. Twenty per cent of patients assigned to immediate treatment discontinued the antiepileptic drug at some time during follow-up, though all but two restarted after visiting the treatment centre: analysis was on an intention to treat basis. Among the treated group, the probability of recurrence was 4% by 1 month, 7% by 3 months, 9% by 6 months, 17% by 1 year and 25% by 2 years: the corresponding figures for the untreated subjects were 8%, 18%, 41% and 45%. The hazard ratio of relapse for untreated subjects, estimated by the Cox proportional hazard model adjusting simultaneously for the prognostic predictors, was 2.8 (95% CI 1.9–4.2). The effect of treatment was even greater in those compliant with medication: among the 20% allocated to treatment who discontinued it at some time, 27% had a relapse, compared with only 15% in whom compliance was good. However, it is notable that even among the group not receiving treatment, fewer than 50% had a recurrence within 2 years.

Gilad *et al.* [26] studied the effect of early versus delayed treatment of 91 patients aged between 18 and 50 years presenting to the emergency department within 24 h of a single generalized tonic-clonic seizure: again patients with acute symptomatic seizures and progressive neurological disorders were excluded. Patients receiving treatment were given carbamazepine, which was changed to valproic acid if adverse effects were experienced: follow-up continued for 36 months. The risk of recurrence in the untreated group, calculated using actuarial analysis, was 33% at 12 months, 62% at 24 months and 77% at 36 months, while the corresponding figures for the treated group were 10%, 20% and 40%.

A randomized study of carbamazepine versus no medication after a first unprovoked seizure, this time in 31 children, was undertaken by Camfield *et al.* [35]. Once again patients presenting with acute symptomatic seizures or progressive neurological disorder were excluded, but in this study, children with any seizure type except akinetic-atonic, generalized absence and myoclonic seizures were eligible. Eighteen of the children had generalized tonic-clonic seizures while 13 had focal seizures with or without secondary generalization. Fourteen children were randomized to treatment with carbamazepine. Follow-up was continued for 1 year. Overall, two of the 14 children treated with carbamazepine and nine of the 17 not receiving treatment had a recurrent unprovoked seizure within 1 year: one of the two treated children with a recurrence had stopped the carbamazepine 5 days before the second seizure. The incidence of adverse effects from the carbamazepine was significant, however, and only six of the 14 patients taking carbamazepine completed the study year without significant side-effects or seizures of any kind.

Effect of treatment on long-term prognosis

There has for many years been debate about the effect of treatment on the long-term prognosis of epilepsy [36–38]. Gowers' view was that the occurrence of seizures facilitated the development of further seizures. This standpoint has been endorsed by Reynolds [39], arguing on the basis of studies of patients with newly diagnosed epilepsy treated with antiepileptic drugs, in which the most important influence on prognosis was the number of seizures prior to starting treatment, and also on the basis of Elwes' work [31] (of which he was coauthor) of a declining interval between seizures, suggesting an accelerating process in the development of epilepsy.

Others have argued that the hypothesis that early antiepileptic drug treatment improves the prognosis of epilepsy has not been proven. Chadwick [38] pointed out that the prognosis for certain types of epilepsy is consistent regardless of treatment. Hence benign epilepsy of childhood with centrotemporal spikes almost invariably remits by puberty, while the prognosis for relapse in juvenile myoclonic epilepsy is very high after withdrawal of treatment, regardless of how early it was introduced and how few seizures had occurred at that time. O'Donoghue and Sander [40] noted the importance of other factors such as aetiology on prognosis, with remission rates for those with neurological deficits present since birth being considerably worse than those seen in idiopathic or cryptogenic epilepsy.

Several studies have suggested that the latter view may be correct. The FIRST Seizure Trial Group [28] found no significant difference in longer-term outcome between patients randomized to treatment immediately after a first unprovoked seizure and those in whom treatment was delayed, despite the fact that early recurrences were more common in the latter group. Eighty-seven per cent of patients randomized to immediate treatment had no seizures for 1 year, and 86% had no seizures for 2 years, compared with 83% and 60%, respectively, in the group randomized to delayed treatment. Indirect evidence is provided by a study carried out by Feksi *et al.* [41], who established a primary health-care antiepileptic drug treatment programme in rural and semi-urban Kenya. Of 302 patients with active seizures recruited and randomized to treatment with either carbamazepine or phenobarbital, 249 completed the study, 53% became seizure free in the second 6 months of therapy (the two drugs being equally effective) and a further 26% had a reduction in their seizures of greater than 50% compared to their pretreatment frequency. The effect of therapy was not influenced by the duration of epilepsy (more or less than 5 years) prior to treatment, nor by the lifetime number of seizures before treatment.

Two surveys of people with epilepsy who remained untreated also indicate that epilepsy may run a benign course in many people. In a community-based survey undertaken in Ecuador [42], 44% of all patients who were identified as having had epilepsy had been free of seizures for at least 12 months, even though nearly two-thirds of these had never received treatment with antiepileptic drugs. Similarly, in a survey of all people who had had at least two unprovoked non-febrile seizures living in the Kuopio University Hospital district in Finland, 50 patients (4.1%) had never had their seizures treated. Of 33 followed for at least 2 years, the probability of remission was 42% at 10 years and 52% at 20 years after the onset of epilepsy [43].

The question also arises as to whether seizures cause intellectual deterioration which might be prevented by antiepileptic drug treatment. On occasion falls due to seizures cause significant head injury, which might be expected to cause cognitive problems as a result [44]. However, with respect to seizures in general, no significant deterioration was found in the Collaborative Perinatal Project of the National Institute of Neurological and Communicative Disorders and Stroke [45], in which a cohort of children studied from birth to the age of 7, who developed seizures between the ages of 4 and 7 years, were compared with age- and sex-matched controls of the same socioeconomic level and with the same IQ score at the age of 4 years. Half of the children in the study group had had at least three seizures. There was no significant difference in IQ from the control group at the age of 7 years. However, in a small study of 17 children (mean age 10.2 years) and 17 adults (mean age 24.4 years), all with refractory epilepsy, undergoing repeat IQ testing at mean intervals of 3.5 years for the children and 6.0 years for the adults, a significant difference was found between the children and the adults regarding IQ testing, the mean IQ declining in the children but increasing in the adults [46]. Further studies are required to assess the significance of these results.

Risk of mortality in early epilepsy

Until relatively recently the entity of sudden unexplained death in epilepsy and the associated increase in mortality were poorly appreciated [47,48]. Measurement of excess mortality is difficult for several reasons, particularly poor documentation of epilepsy on death certificates, with misclassification of the cause of death almost certainly being common in addition. It is now recognized, however, that the standardized mortality ratio (SMR) in people with epilepsy is of the order of 2–3. It is higher in the first few years after diagnosis and in males, those with learning disabilities, those with symptomatic (rather than idiopathic or cryptogenic) epilepsy, those with convulsive seizures and younger age groups [49]. Causes of this excess mortality include accidental death or drowning due to seizures, death due to the underlying cause, suicide, aspiration, status epilepticus, death due to complications of treatment and sudden unexplained death in epilepsy. The risk of the latter has been estimated at between 1 in 500 and 1 in 1000 per year, but is higher in those with severe epilepsy, reaching around 1 in 100 per year in those rejected for epilepsy surgery or in whom epilepsy surgery is not successful [50]. Data about death early after the onset of epilepsy are sparse. However, Loiseau et al. [51] examined the short-term mortality of epilepsy after a first epileptic seizure. One hundred and forty-nine of the 804 patients had died by the end of the first year of follow-up (compared with 16 expected, SMR 9.3 (95% CI 7.9–10.9)). In nine patients death occurred during a seizure, and in a further 14 the cause of death was unknown (in this group patients died suddenly, sometimes without witnesses and without postmortem, but with a history of other disease). Ninety-six patients died of underlying disease, and 30 of causes thought to be unrelated to seizures. Overall, the SMR was 0.0 for patients with idiopathic epilepsy, 1.6 (95% CI 0.4–4.1) for those with cryptogenic epilepsy and 19.8 (95% CI 14.0–27.3) for symptomatic seizures in progressive conditions. Further studies will be required to confirm the incidence of preventable death after a first seizure, and indicate whether the approach commonly taken currently of withholding treatment until the occurrence of a second seizure, on the assumption that death following a single seizure is uncommon, is justified.

Risk of injury

Accidental injury is common as a result of seizures, though generally poorly documented in epidemiological terms. Almost all studies are retrospective, so it is likely that some injuries will have been forgotten. In one community-based study in which questionnaires were mailed to an unselected population of patients, 24% of patients suffering at least one seizure during the previous year had had a head injury, 16% a burn or scald, 10% a dental injury and 6% some other fracture [52]. The authors identified key predictors for each of these injuries: seizure frequency, seizure severity and sex were predictors of burns or scalds; seizure severity was a key predictor for dental injury, and seizure severity and type were predictors for head injury. One clinic-based survey of 244 patients reported that 25 had had at least one seizure-related burn requiring medical attention, 12 of these requiring hospitalization [53]. All patients with seizure-related burns had alteration of consciousness during most seizures: other predictive factors were the lifetime total number of seizures, the presence of interictal neurological impairment and gender. Such a study may be biased to the extent that it is clinic-based and therefore likely to include patients with more severe epilepsy (if those whose epilepsy is well-controlled are discharged or default from the clinic). A similar clinic-based questionnaire

(again retrospective) by Neufeld et al. [54] found that 30% (91 of 298 patients) reported trauma at some time, with a total of 185 events of which 61 were severe. However, this translated to a surprisingly low rate of injury, one seizure-related injury every 21 patient-years and a serious injury once every 64 patient-years. Head injury was the most common (55% of events). Patients with seizure-related injury had an earlier onset of epilepsy, and more commonly had tonic-clonic seizures which were generalized from the onset, complex partial, myoclonic or absence seizures. The risk was less in those patients having partial seizures with secondary generalization. Even children with typical absence epilepsy, sometimes considered one of the 'milder' types of epilepsy, are prone to injury, with 16 of 59 patients (27%) in one study [55] having experienced an accidental injury at some time during an absence seizure, the risk of injury being 9% per person-year of absence epilepsy. It is notable that the majority of these injuries (81%) occurred during the course of treatment. This fact, in conjunction with the relatively low risk of injury per patient-year found by Neufeld et al. [54], means that although the risk of accident due to seizures needs to be weighed in the balance with other factors when the decision to start antiepileptic drugs is taken, it should probably have only a minor impact in early epilepsy.

Psychosocial morbidity

In addition to the physical aspects of the seizures themselves, a diagnosis of epilepsy carries with it considerable psychosocial morbidity. Patients with newly diagnosed epilepsy recruited into the National General Practice Study of Epilepsy [56] had difficulty accepting the diagnosis and had significant fears about future seizures and about the effect of stigma due to the epilepsy on employment. Other studies have produced similar results. In a study of quality of life data from more than 5000 people with epilepsy living in 15 countries in Europe, almost half (48%) said they worried a lot or some about their epilepsy, and a similar proportion felt that it substantially affected their plans and ambitions for the future [57]. Other areas affected were their feelings about themselves, and their social life. The difficulties experienced seem to be related to the severity of the epilepsy: in a Dutch study, inpatients with epilepsy had serious problems in emotional, interpersonal and vocational adjustment, adjustment to seizures and overall psychosocial functioning, while seizure-free outpatients experienced significant problems only in the emotional adjustment area [58]. Jacoby et al. [59], in a UK community-based study, similarly found patients with active seizures were more likely to be anxious or depressed, and to feel that their lives were significantly affected by the epilepsy: they were also less likely to be married and more likely to be unemployed or registered 'permanently sick'.

Adverse effects of drugs

Balanced against the benefits of antiepileptic drugs is their propensity to cause adverse effects, which affect a significant minority of patients (the exact incidence being difficult to determine, as indicated by the frequency with which possible side-effects occur in those patients randomized in placebo-controlled studies to receive placebo). They range from being mild, and of nuisance value only, to being life-threatening. At the very least, they are likely adversely to affect compliance. They include symptoms of acute toxicity (such as the ataxia and blurred vision which occur in association with an excessive dose of carbamazepine, phenytoin or lamotrigine); chronic toxic symptoms (for example, gingival hyperplasia occurring in about one-third of patients taking phenytoin); idiosyncratic reactions, an example of which is the rash which may be seen with such drugs as phenytoin, carbamazepine and lamotrigine; and teratogenicity.

The systems mainly involved by adverse antiepileptic drug reactions are the central nervous system, liver, skin and bone marrow [60]. The central nervous system is frequently symptomatic, particularly in dose-related acute toxicity, sedation, lethargy and dizziness being common symptoms. Other central nervous system manifestations of adverse effects include the psychosis sometimes seen with vigabatrin [61] and certain other antiepileptic drugs, and mood or behavioural changes, for example those sometimes seen with phenobarbital therapy. Phenytoin, carbamazepine and phenobarbital induce the hepatic microsomal enzymes, and elevations of alkaline phosphatase and γ-glutamyltransferase commonly seen in patients taking these drugs are usually of no clinical significance. Severe, sometimes fatal hepatotoxicity, occasionally occurs in association with valproate use, mainly in children under the age of 2 years receiving polytherapy [62]. Haematological abnormalities may be clinically unimportant, as is often the case with the mild leukopenia seen in 12% of people receiving carbamazepine therapy [60], but also include such life-threatening conditions as aplastic anaemia. Valproate not infrequently causes a dose-related thrombocytopenia, usually mild. Dermatological adverse effects are sometimes severe, and include Stevens–Johnson syndrome and exfoliative dermatitis.

Finally, it is important to remember that antiepileptic therapy only produces complete seizure control in around 70–80% of patients with epilepsy. In many not fully controlled patients antiepileptic drugs remain beneficial, for example by reducing the severity of seizures (perhaps preventing secondary generalization), or the seizure frequency. Where seizure control is not achieved, however, it is important to minimize adverse effects by reducing the amount of medication to that required to produce the benefit. This is particularly the case where multiple drugs have been introduced, when the risk of toxicity is increased considerably.

When to start medication

The adverse effects mentioned above mean that certain criteria should be fulfilled before antiepileptic medication is started (Table 12.3). It is essential that the diagnosis (based on the descriptions of a patient and an eye-witness) is definite before medication is started,

Table 12.3 Criteria for starting antiepileptic drugs

Diagnosis of epilepsy must be firm
Risk of recurrence and nature of seizures must justify treatment
Good compliance must be likely
The patient should be fully counselled
The patient's wishes should be taken into account

particularly since treatment almost invariably continues for several years. Despite the frustrations caused for both patient and physician when the diagnosis remains uncertain, 'trials of treatment' should be avoided. It is uncommon for them to clarify the situation, and they may introduce additional complications, including adverse drug reactions. The risks of seizure recurrence should be discussed with the patient, bearing in mind the effect of the time elapsing since the last seizure [18]. The severity and frequency of the seizures may influence the decision: it may be deemed reasonable not to treat those which have a relatively mild effect on day-to-day life (such as some simple partial seizures) or occur only rarely. Where the seizures are more severe, however, the risk of injury or sudden unexplained death in epilepsy (SUDEP) becomes more significant. In the UK, it is usual not to treat patients until the occurrence of a second seizure, unless there is a specific factor which makes recurrence more likely (such as the presence of a cerebral tumour, or the presence of clear epileptic abnormalities in the interictal EEG). In the USA, on the other hand, it was until recently commonplace for patients to be treated after a single seizure [16], possible reasons for this being the issue of driving or a difference in the medicolegal approach, although it may also have been based on concerns about epilepsy being a progressive condition. Although the decision must depend on an appreciation by the patient of all the risks and benefits of medication, it seems likely that in the absence of a progressive underlying condition, for most people it will be appropriate to delay treatment until a second seizure has occurred. As noted below, the epilepsy syndrome is also important in determining prognosis and, as such, will affect the decision to start or withhold treatment.

Wishes of the patient

Patients differ considerably in their views about epilepsy and drug treatment. For some, particularly those for whom driving is important or where seizures are likely to cause difficulties with employment, and those suffering significant psychosocial morbidity as a result of the seizures, the desire to minimize the risk of further events is of paramount importance. Others have concerns about the concept of long-term medication and would prefer to risk an occasional seizure, particularly if their attacks do not inconvenience them unduly. Although there are some patients (such as those with recurrent injuries due to seizures, or a tendency to status epilepticus) in whom one would strongly recommend treatment, and others in whom the benefits of treatment are more doubtful, the cooperation of the patient is essential in all instances to ensure compliance.

Regardless of their wishes or expectations, it is important to discuss the purpose and limitations of antiepileptic drugs with people developing epilepsy. It is common, for example, for patients to expect that their seizures will be completely controlled as soon as treatment is commenced, or when a 'therapeutic' drug level is reached, whereas in practice, in 20–30% of patients, seizures may be refractory to treatment. The need for taking medication regularly, and guidance on what to do if a dose is missed, should also be discussed. In addition, the likely duration of treatment should be explained. Patients should also be alerted to the more common possible adverse effects of medication, particularly skin rash: frequently serious skin reactions can be averted by withdrawing medication at the first indication of their development.

Likelihood of compliance

Antiepileptic drugs must be taken reliably and regularly to maximize their efficacy and minimize the risk of withdrawal seizures due to omission of medication. Compliance with antiepileptic medication is often poor [63], but may be improved by providing adequate explanation about the nature of epilepsy, the rationale for treatment, and the risk of withdrawal seizures; by the use of drugs with a low incidence of adverse effects; and by simplifying the treatment regime as far as possible. This may be achieved by the use of a single drug given in the lowest effective dose, in a once or twice daily regime if possible. Adverse effects experienced early are especially likely to cause dissatisfaction, and care should be taken to build up the dose of such drugs as carbamazepine sufficiently slowly to avoid this complication. Alcohol may be another reason for poor compliance, either because of patients' concern about 'mixing' it with antiepileptic drugs, or as a result of the effects of alcohol abuse itself.

Type of epilepsy seizures or syndrome

In addition to ensuring that the diagnosis of epilepsy is certain, it is important to characterize the seizure type (according to the classification of the Commission on Classification and Terminology of the International League against Epilepsy [1]) and the epileptic syndrome (Commission on Classification and Terminology of the International League against Epilepsy [2]). As indicated below, the choice of drug will be influenced by the seizure type. The syndromic classification is also important when considering the necessity for any medication. Some types of epilepsy, such as benign childhood epilepsy with centrotemporal spikes, confer a benign prognosis. Although generalized tonic-clonic seizures may occur in this syndrome, often the attacks take the form of simple partial seizures occurring during sleep, and treatment may well not be required. In contrast, in other epilepsy syndromes (such as Lennox–Gastaut syndrome), the chance of complete seizure control may be small. Juvenile myoclonic epilepsy, which is characterized by the presence of myoclonic jerks and, usually, generalized tonic-clonic seizures, commonly responds well to medication (valproate commonly being used as drug of first choice), but carries a very high risk of relapse (of the order of 90%) if medication is withdrawn.

A knowledge of the seizure type also informs the choice of drug for treatment (see below). Thus while carbamazepine is a useful drug in the treatment of generalized tonic-clonic seizures, it is usually avoided where these form part of a generalized epilepsy syndrome which also includes absence seizures and myoclonic jerks, since these may be exacerbated by carbamazepine (and also by phenytoin). The three seizure types commonly occurring in idiopathic generalized epilepsy (generalized tonic-clonic seizures, myoclonic jerks and absence seizures) are all commonly responsive to sodium valproate, while ethosuximide is effective only against generalized absence seizures. For these reasons, every effort should be made to classify the epilepsy by seizure type and syndrome, if possible.

Which drug to use

Until recently there has been a dearth of randomized controlled trials of medication, and possibly as a result of this, there has been con-siderable variation between different countries in the customs and guidelines influencing treatment. With regard to choice of drug, phenytoin is the most commonly used antiepileptic drug in North America [64], but in the UK carbamazepine is popular and has been recommended as the drug of choice for seizures of partial onset [65,66]. In Italy, the drug most frequently prescribed in the FIRST study [28] following a first generalized tonic-clonic seizure was phenobarbital, which was given to 50% of the treated patients.

A detailed discussion of factors to be considered in drug selection in patients with newly diagnosed epilepsy can be found in Chapter 11.

Valproate has traditionally been used as the drug of choice in idiopathic generalized epilepsies. It is effective against all the seizure types characterizing these syndromes (including generalized tonic-clonic seizures, myoclonic jerks and absences), and in the short term, is often well tolerated. In the longer term, weight gain may be unacceptable in some patients, while hair loss and dose-related tremor may also be problematic. The issue of teratogenicity is currently being researched: some studies have suggested a higher rate of fetal malformations (particularly neural tube defects) in women taking valproate compared with those taking other drugs. Several pregnancy and epilepsy registers are currently underway and should provide further information regarding the relative safety of the various antiepileptic drugs in women of childbearing age. Lamotrigine also appears to be effective in many people with idiopathic generalized epilepsy and may be tried as an alternative to valproate, although experience with this drug in pregnancy is as yet limited. In children with absence seizures as their sole seizure type, ethosuximide may be used. Carbamazepine and phenytoin, as noted above, are effective in the treatment of generalized tonic-clonic seizures but may worsen absence seizures and myoclonic jerks and as such may be best avoided in idiopathic generalized epilepsy. Topiramate is also licensed for the treatment of primary generalized tonic-clonic seizures.

With regard to seizures of partial onset, carbamazepine is commonly used as drug of first choice in the UK and some other European countries, while as noted above, phenytoin remains popular in the USA. The effects of carbamazepine, phenobarbital, phenytoin and primidone were compared in a randomized double-blind study of 622 adults with partial and secondarily generalized tonic-clonic seizures carried out by Mattson et al. [67]. The retention rate was highest with carbamazepine and phenytoin, with primidone having the worst retention rate, mainly due to adverse effects (particularly acute adverse reactions occurring at the onset of treatment). At 12 months, control of secondarily generalized tonic-clonic seizures was similar for all drugs at about 45%. However, carbamazepine was reported to provide significantly better total control of partial seizures (43%) than phenobarbital (16%) or primidone (16%), with phenytoin providing intermediate control (26%). A later study by Mattson et al. [68] compared valproate with carbamazepine for the treatment of complex partial and secondarily generalized tonic-clonic seizures in adults. The two drugs were shown to have comparable efficacy in the treatment of tonic-clonic seizures, but carbamazepine gave better results for four of the five outcome measures for complex partial seizures, and was also the preferred drug when adverse effects were included in the analysis. On the other hand, in two prospective randomized studies in patients with newly diagnosed partial or primarily generalized tonic-clonic seizures carried out in the UK, one in adults [69] and one in children [70], valproate and carbamazepine were found to have virtually equivalent efficacy, a finding which applied to both subgroups of patients with partial and with generalized epilepsy, respectively. Likewise, in a smaller randomized comparative UK study of phenobarbital, phenytoin, carbamazepine or sodium valproate in adults with newly diagnosed epilepsy with tonic-clonic or partial seizures (with or without secondary generalization), no difference in efficacy was found. However, phenobarbital was considerably more likely to be withdrawn on account of adverse effects. In another study carried out in children [71], phenobarbital caused unacceptable adverse effects in six of the first 10 children assigned to this drug: no further children were allocated to this arm. Of the other three drugs, phenytoin was withdrawn due to adverse effects in 9%, compared with 4% of those randomized to take carbamazepine or sodium valproate: these differences were not statistically significant.

The place of the more modern drugs in patients newly presenting with epilepsy remains unclear, and a large multicentre study of standard and new antiepileptic drugs, in which patients with newly diagnosed epilepsy are randomized to valproate, carbamazepine, or one of the newer antiepileptic drugs (lamotrigine, gabapentin, topiramate, or oxcarbazepine) has been set up to try to address this issue. An earlier randomized, double-blind comparison of lamotrigine with carbamazepine in 260 patients with newly diagnosed epilepsy showed the two drugs to be similarly effective in controlling seizures, but found that fewer patients on lamotrigine withdrew as a result of adverse effects [72]. This study has been criticized because the titration of carbamazepine was carried out more quickly than recommended by many neurologists, and this would be expected to increase the number of adverse events. Use of an immediate release formulation of carbamazepine on a twice daily administration schedule may also have impacted adversely on the tolerability profile of carbamazepine. A further study compared lamotrigine with phenytoin in the treatment of patients with newly diagnosed untreated partial seizures or generalized tonic-clonic seizures (whether primary or secondarily generalized) [73]. In this study, the starting dose of lamotrigine was 100 mg/day, and that of phenytoin, 200 mg/day. No significant difference was found in the percentages of patients remaining on each treatment and seizure free during the last 24 and 40 weeks of the study, nor in the time to first seizure after the first 6 weeks of treatment. Adverse events were the cause of discontinuation in 19% of the patients receiving phenytoin and 15% of those receiving lamotrigine, skin rash being more common in the lamotrigine group (possibly due to an excessively high starting dose), and central nervous system effects in the phenytoin group.

Oxcarbazepine has been compared with sodium valproate, carbamazepine and phenytoin in separate studies of adults with newly diagnosed epilepsy. There was no statistically significant difference in efficacy between oxcarbazepine and any of the other three drugs. Comparison with carbamazepine [74] showed that oxcarbazepine caused fewer 'severe' side-effects than carbamazepine (although again, titration of the latter was carried out relatively quickly). In the comparison of oxcarbazepine with valproate [75], there was no significant difference between the two drugs with regard to either efficacy or adverse effects. The study comparing oxcarbazepine with phenytoin [76] showed no difference between the groups with respect to the total number of premature discontinuations, but with

regard to those due to adverse effects, there was a statistically significant difference in favour of oxcarbazepine. Oxcarbazepine also showed superior tolerability when compared with phenytoin in a randomized trial in children and adolescents [77].

Vigabatrin has been compared with carbamazepine in the treatment of newly diagnosed epilepsy [78]. There were fewer withdrawals in the vigabatrin group, vigabatrin being better tolerated than carbamazepine, although psychiatric symptoms and weight gain were more common in the vigabatrin group. With regard to efficacy, however, all efficacy outcomes favoured carbamazepine. Since the recognition that visual field defects may occur in a high proportion (around 30–40%) of patients treated with vigabatrin [79,80], this drug cannot be recommended as a first-line treatment in the management of adult epilepsy.

Newer drugs are invariably more costly than the older agents available, and where health resources are limited, they must justify their use by clear benefits. It will become easier to define their place in treatment with greater experience in using them, and as a result of the trials currently underway. Although the issues of teratogenicity, weight gain and possibly polycystic ovaries may lead to lamotrigine (or another new drug) being used as an alternative to valproate in women of childbearing age, valproate remains the drug of choice in idiopathic generalized epilepsy in other circumstances, while carbamazepine is an appropriate choice in people with epilepsy of partial onset.

Women's issues

Epilepsy has specific implications for women, both on account of the effects of epilepsy and antiepileptic drugs on the reproductive cycle and on the unborn child, and because of the effects of pregnancy and hormonal changes on the epilepsy. The issue of teratogenicity has received considerable attention. It is accepted that the risk of major congenital malformations, usually estimated at around 2–3% in the general population, doubles or trebles in women taking antiepileptic drugs during the first trimester of pregnancy, the risk being probably greater in women taking polytherapy than in those taking a single drug (Chapter 23). Such malformations include cleft lip and palate, cardiac malformations and neural tube defects, the latter occurring in 1–2% of children of women treated with valproate. However, as yet the relative risks of the different antiepileptic drugs remain undetermined. The appearance of several new antiepileptic drugs over the last decade or so has increased the urgency for obtaining more information about the teratogenicity of all such medications, and the various 'pregnancy and epilepsy' registers currently underway should provide this.

The fact that antiepileptic drugs can reduce the efficacy of the oral contraceptive pill due to induction of the hepatic cytochrome P450 system is also now widely recognized. The drugs involved include carbamazepine, oxcarbazepine, phenytoin, phenobarbital, primidone and, at doses >200 mg/day, also topiramate. The chance of an unwanted pregnancy can be reduced by the use of a combined oral contraceptive pill containing at least 50 µg oestrogen (a higher dose may be required if breakthrough bleeding occurs).

Some reports have suggested that there may be an increased incidence of polycystic ovaries in women with epilepsy taking sodium valproate [81]. At the time of writing there remains considerable debate about the general applicability of these findings. However, if proven, they may influence the future choice of antiepileptic drug in women with epilepsy, as would any difference in rates of teratogenicity between antiepileptic drugs. In the event of this occurring, it would affect the choice of drug in all women of childbearing age, including adolescents, since a high proportion of pregnancies are unplanned (56% in the community-based study of Fairgrieve *et al.* [82] of women with epilepsy).

How to start medication

In the past two to three decades it has been shown that in the majority of people with epilepsy, satisfactory control is achieved with a single antiepileptic drug, with only 10–15% of patients benefiting from polytherapy [83]. A drug appropriate to the seizure type should be chosen (Tables 12.4 and 12.5), giving preference to an agent whose adverse effect profile is least likely to interfere with the quality of life of the patient. Both the dosage required to obtain a particular level of the drug in the blood, and the level required to achieve control of the seizures, vary considerably from person to person, as does the level at which symptoms of toxicity are experienced (Chapter 11). In order to minimize adverse effects, particu-

Table 12.4 Choosing medication for generalized seizures

First-line drugs
Valproate
Carbamazepine: generalized tonic-clonic seizures (may exacerbate absence seizures and myoclonic jerks)
Phenytoin: generalized tonic-clonic seizures (may exacerbate absence seizures and myoclonic jerks)[a]
Ethosuximide: absence seizures only
Lamotrigine

Second-line drugs
Clobazam: all seizure types
Topiramate: all seizure types except absence seizures
Clonazepam: myoclonic seizures
Phenobarbital: all seizure types except absence seizures
Primidone: all seizure types except absence seizures

[a] Considered by some to be second-line drug.

Table 12.5 Choosing medication for partial onset seizures

First-line drugs	Second-line drugs
Carbamazepine	Clobazam
Phenytoin[a]	Clonazepam
Valproate	Gabapentin
	Lamotrigine[b]
	Levetiracetam
	Oxcarbazepine[b]
	Phenobarbital
	Primidone
	Tiagabine
	Topiramate
	Zonisamide

[a] Considered by some to be second-line drug.
[b] Considered by some to be first-line drug.

larly acute idiosyncratic reactions and symptoms of toxicity, it is recommended that a single first-line drug for the seizure type be given in a small dose, the dose being gradually increased until either complete control of seizures is obtained, or until symptoms of toxicity occur (Table 12.6). In practice, if the seizures are infrequent, such a strategy may mean prolonging the titration phase excessively, and in such circumstances it may be reasonable to increase the dose of medication to an 'average' dose regardless of the occurrence of seizures. For example, most adults with initially diagnosed epilepsy will respond to dosages of 400–600 mg/day of carbamazepine, or 600–1000 mg/day of sodium valproate [84]. Measurement of serum drug levels is helpful as a guide to dosage in the case of phenytoin, which has non-linear pharmacokinetics. Drug level measurements approaching the therapeutic range are an indication that any increase in dosage of phenytoin must be by very small increments (for example, by increasing the total daily dose by 25 mg and checking the blood level again at a suitable interval). Drug level monitoring is occasionally helpful in the case of carbamazepine, phenobarbital and ethosuximide, but is usually unhelpful in the case of valproate and the newer antiepileptic drugs.

If the patient's seizures fail to be controlled by a single antiepileptic drug, the diagnosis should be reviewed. The possibility of a progressive underlying aetiology should also be considered, and further neuroimaging may be warranted. If the diagnosis is confirmed, a second first-line antiepileptic drug for the seizure type should be added and the original drug gradually withdrawn. Many physicians prefer to complete the titration of the new drug before beginning withdrawal of the original medication, so that any adverse effects of the drug change can be correctly attributed (although, in some cases, tolerability problems may result from drug interactions), and to avoid the situation in which the patient is receiving two drugs, both at suboptimal doses. Others, however, initiate the tapering off of the original drug whilst the second medication is being gradually introduced. Only if two first-line drugs given individually fail should the use of polytherapy be contemplated as a longer-term measure.

Provoking factors for seizures

Some people with epilepsy have seizures which are caused by specific precipitating factors. Where the seizures are consistently due to such factors, it may be possible to control them without medication by avoiding the relevant stimuli. Other patients will have some spontaneous seizures in addition to the provoked events, and will therefore require antiepileptic drug treatment.

Table 12.6 How to start antiepileptic drugs

Use a first-line drug for the seizure type
Start at a low dose
Gradually increase until seizures stop or adverse effects develop
If seizures remain uncontrolled, review the diagnosis and underlying aetiology
Substitute gradually another first-line drug for the seizure type and increase dosage until seizures stop or adverse effects develop
If necessary, try drug combinations

Excess alcohol intake (or its abrupt withdrawal) was thought to be the cause of seizures in 6% of patients registered with the National General Practice Study of Epilepsy [85], and was particularly common in people between the ages of 30 and 39 years, in whom it was responsible for 27% of cases. These patients may be particularly difficult to treat if formal detoxification fails and drug treatment is attempted: compliance is likely to be poor and there may be concern about the combined adverse effects on the liver of the alcohol and antiepileptic drugs. Sleep deprivation may also be a precipitating factor for seizures in susceptible individuals, and is often a contributory factor in those abusing alcohol. Stress, fever or other illness, sleep, heat, flashing lights and, in women, menstruation, were identified as seizure precipitants by patients undertaking a survey at a tertiary care centre [86]. Certain drugs, including most antidepressants and other psychotropic agents, lower the seizure threshold: however, although this may influence choice of drug it is important that mental health disorders are treated appropriately despite the epilepsy. Withdrawal of benzodiazepines and other sedatives should be undertaken slowly to avoid withdrawal seizures.

Photosensitivity, in which generalized epileptic discharges occur in response to intermittent photic stimulation, occurs in about 5% of people with epilepsy. It is seen particularly in people with idiopathic generalized epilepsy (often developing in childhood or adolescence), but also occurs in some people with occipital epilepsy. The risk of seizures occurring as a result of photosensitivity may be reduced by using a small television screen and increasing the viewing distance, using a remote control to change channels, closing one eye or using polarized spectacles and reducing the screen contrast and brightness.

Other counselling

Education of the person developing epilepsy is a major part of the initial management (Table 12.7 provides an example of a counselling checklist) and in this respect epilepsy nurse practitioners, and also epilepsy societies, may be helpful in reinforcing the information provided by the physician, and providing written information. The diagnosis of epilepsy carries significant implications for work and leisure, as discussed above, but is also a frightening experience leading to loss of confidence, and often a reluctance to undertake normal daily activities.

Table 12.7 Counselling check-list for people developing epilepsy

Nature of epilepsy
First aid management of seizures
Avoidance of precipitating factors, including alcohol and sleep deprivation
Purpose of medication, and likely duration
Nature of common adverse effects of medication
Need to take medication regularly
Risks of seizures and advice regarding common hazards
Laws regarding driving
Interaction with other drugs, especially oral contraceptive pill (where relevant)
Possibility of teratogenicity, where relevant

Information provided to the patient should explain the nature of epilepsy, its causes and the purpose of the various investigations performed (many patients are confused, for example, by the fact that they are diagnosed as having epilepsy despite having a normal EEG). First aid measures for treating seizures should be discussed with the patient and those relatives and friends for whom they deem it appropriate. The risks of seizures (including SUDEP) should be addressed in a sensitive manner, and measures to discuss injury (such as the avoidance of unguarded heights, unguarded fires, swimming alone) in the event of a further seizure discussed. Driving laws vary from country to country, and the patient must be educated about the relevant regulations, and of the need to inform the driving authorities, where it is incumbent on them to do so. The need to lead as normal a life as possible within the confines of taking reasonable care, however, should be emphasized: most sports are possible, though some, such as boxing, wrestling, pot-holing and scuba diving should be avoided.

The issues relating to drugs mentioned above should be discussed. In some countries patients with epilepsy are eligible to receive free medication. The possibility of interactions with other drugs, especially the oral contraceptive pill, is of particular importance. Patients should be advised to avoid excess alcohol, sleep deprivation and other factors likely to precipitate seizures: on the other hand, they should be reassured where, for example, photosensitivity is *not* an issue. Women should be informed of the risk of teratogenicity, and of the importance of planning any pregnancy, reviewing their medication beforehand and taking folic acid 5 mg daily prior to any pregnancy and for the first trimester.

Some occupations, particularly those requiring a driving licence, or those where the person with epilepsy has sole responsibility for the safety of another, may not be possible. However, many occupations can continue to be safely performed, particularly with education of the employer. It is important that children with epilepsy be treated in a similar manner to other children, except for simple safety measures to avoid injury: the morbidity attributable to overprotection and underexpectation of such children is often considerably greater than the effect of the seizures themselves. Adequate schooling is also important: it is usually possible for children suffering seizures to rejoin their class after a short recovery period, rather than being sent home on each occasion. On the other hand, teachers and parents should be alert to the possible effects of ongoing epileptic discharges and of antiepileptic drugs on cognition, with appropriate action being taken if these occur.

References

1 Commission on Classification and Terminology of the International League Against Epilepsy. Proposal for revised clinical and electroencephalographic classification of epileptic seizures. *Epilepsia* 1981; 30: 389–99.

2 Commission on Classification and Terminology of the International League Against Epilepsy. Proposal for revised classification of epilepsies and epileptic syndromes. *Epilepsia* 1989; 30: 389–99.

3 Lempert T, Bauer M, Schmidt D. Syncope: a videometric analysis of 56 episodes of transient cerebral hypoxia. *Ann Neurol* 1994; 36: 233–7.

4 Van Donselaar CA, Geerts AT, Meulstee J, Habbema JDF, Staal A. Reliability of the diagnosis of a first seizure. *Neurology* 1989; 39: 267–71.

5 Betts TA. Psychiatry and epilepsy. In: Laidlaw J, Richens A, eds. *A Textbook of Epilepsy*. Edinburgh: Churchill Livingstone, 1983, 145–84.

6 Marsan CA, Zivin LS. Factors related to the occurrence of typical paroxys-

mal abnormalities in the EEG records of epileptic patients. *Epilepsia* 1970; 11: 361–81.

7 Salinsky M, Kanter R, Dashieff RM. Effectiveness of multiple EEGs in supporting the diagnosis of epilepsy: an operational curve. *Epilepsia* 1987; 28: 331–4.

8 Neufeld MY, Chistik V, Vishne TH, Korczyn AD. The diagnostic aid of routine EEG findings in patients presenting with a presumed first-ever unprovoked seizure. *Epilepsy Res* 2000; 42: 197–202.

9 Zivin L, Marsan CA. Incidence and prognostic significance of 'epileptiform' activity in the EEG of non-epileptic subjects. *Brain* 1968; 91: 751–78.

10 Gregory RP, Oates T, Merry T. Electroencephalogram epileptiform abnormalities in candidates for aircrew training. *Electroencephalogr Clin Neurophysiol* 1993; 86: 75–7.

11 Goodin DS, Aminoff MJ. Does the interictal EEG have a role in the diagnosis of epilepsy? *Lancet* 1984; 1: 837–8.

12 Delgado-Escueta AV, Enrile-Bacsal F. Juvenile myoclonic epilepsy of Janz. *Neurology* 1984; 34: 285–94.

13 King MA, Newton MR, Jackson GD *et al.* Epileptology of the first-seizure presentation: a clinical, electroencephalographic, and magnetic resonance imaging study of 300 consecutive patients. *Lancet* 1998; 352: 1007–11.

14 Jallon P, Loiseau P, Loiseau J, on behalf of Groupe CAROLE (Coordination Active du Réseau Observatoire Longitudinal de l'Epilepsie). Newly diagnosed unprovoked epileptic seizures: presentation at diagnosis in CAROLE study. *Epilepsia* 2001; 42: 464–75.

15 Manford M, Hart YM, Sander JWAS, Shorvon SD. The National General Practice Study of Epilepsy. The Syndromic classification of the International League against Epilepsy applied to epilepsy in a general population. *Arch Neurol* 1992; 49: 801–8.

16 Hauser WA, Anderson VE, Loewenson RB, McRoberts SM. Seizure recurrence after a first unprovoked seizure. *N Engl J Med* 1982; 307: 522–8.

17 Goodridge DMG, Shorvon SD. Epileptic seizures in a population of 6000. II Treatment and prognosis. *Br Med J* 1983; 287: 645–7.

18 Hart YM, Sander JWAS, Johnson AL, Shorvon SD, for the NGPSE (National General Practice Study of Epilepsy). Recurrence after a first seizure. *Lancet* 1990; 336: 1271–4.

19 Cleland PG, Mosquera I, Steward WP, Foster JB. Prognosis of isolated seizures in adult life. *Br Med J* 1981; 283: 1364.

20 Hauser WA, Kurland LT. The epidemiology of epilepsy in Rochester, Minnesota, 1935 through 1967. *Epilepsia* 1975; 16: 1–66.

21 Shorvon SD. The drug treatment of epilepsy. University of Cambridge MD thesis, 1982.

22 Van Donselaar CA, Geerts AT, Schimsheimer R-J. Idiopathic first seizure in adult life: who should be treated? *Br Med J* 1991; 302: 620–3.

23 First Seizure Trial Group. Randomized clinical trial on the efficacy of antiepileptic drugs in reducing the risk of relapse after a first unprovoked tonic clonic seizure. *Neurology* 1993; 43: 478–83.

24 Annegers JF, Shirts SB, Hauser WA, Kurland LT. Risk of recurrence after an initial unprovoked seizure. *Epilepsia* 1986; 27: 43–50.

25 Hopkins A, Garman A, Clarke C. The first seizure in adult life: value of clinical features, electroencephalography, and computerised tomographic scanning in prediction of seizure recurrence. *Lancet* 1988; i: 721–6.

26 Gilad R, Lampl Y, Gabbay U, Eshel Y, Sarova-Pinhas I. Early treatment of a single generalized tonic-clonic seizure to prevent recurrence. *Arch Neurol* 1996; 53: 1149–52.

27 Shinnar S, Berg AT, Ptachewich Y, Alemany M. Sleep state and the risk of seizure recurrence following a first unprovoked seizure in childhood. *Neurology* 1993; 43: 701–6.

28 Musicco M, Beghi E, Solair A, Viani F, for the First Seizure Trial Group (FIRST Group). Treatment of first tonic-clonic seizure does not improve the prognosis of epilepsy. *Neurology* 1997; 49: 991–8.

29 Berg AT, Shinnar S. The risk of seizure recurrence following a first unprovoked seizure. A quantitative review. *Neurology* 1991; 41: 965–72.

30 Hauser WA, Rich SS, Lee JR-J, Annegers JF, Anderson VE. Risk of recurrent seizures after two unprovoked seizures. *N Engl J Med* 1998; 338: 429–34.

31 Elwes RDC, Johnson AL, Reynolds EH. The course of untreated epilepsy. *Br Med J* 1988; 297: 948–50.

32 Hirtz DG, Ellenberg JH, Nelson KB. The risk of recurrence of non-febrile seizures in children. *Neurology* 1984; 34: 637–41.

33 Camfield PR, Camfield CS, Dooley JM, Tibbles JAE, Fung T, Garner B. Epilepsy after a first unprovoked seizure in childhood. *Neurology* 1985; 35: 722–5.

34 Boulloche J, Leloup P, Mallet E, Parain D, Tron P. Risk of recurrence after a single, unprovoked, generalized tonic-clonic seizure. *Dev Med Child Neurol* 1989; 31: 626–32.

35 Camfield P, Camfield C, Dooley J, Smith E, Garner B. A randomised study of carbamazepine versus no medication after a first unprovoked seizure in childhood. *Neurology* 1989; 39: 851–2.

36 Gowers W. *Epilepsy and Other Chronic Convulsive Diseases*. London: Churchill, 1881.

37 Reynolds EH. Do anticonvulsants alter the natural course of epilepsy? Treatment should be started as early as possible. *Br Med J* 1995; 310: 176–7.

38 Chadwick D. Do anticonvulsants alter the natural course of epilepsy? Case for early treatment is not established. *Br Med J* 1995; 310: 177–8.

39 Reynolds EH, Heller AJ, Elwes RDC *et al.* Factors influencing prognosis of newly diagnosed epilepsy. *Epilepsia* 1989; 30: 648.

40 O'Donoghue M, Sander JWAS. Does early anti-epileptic drug treatment alter the prognosis for remission of the epilepsies? *J R Soc Med* 1996; 89: 245–8.

41 Feksi AT, Kaamugisha J, Sander JWAS, Gatiti S, Shorvon SD, for ICBERG (International Community-based Epilepsy Research Group). Comprehensive primary health care antiepileptic drug treatment programme in rural and semi-urban Kenya. *Lancet* 1991; 337: 406–9.

42 Placencia M, Sander JWAS, Roman M *et al.* The characteristics of epilepsy in a largely untreated population in rural Ecuador. *J Neurol Neurosurg Psychiatry* 1994; 57: 320–5.

43 Keränen T, Riekkinen P. Remission of seizures in untreated epilepsy. *Br Med J* 1993; 307: 483.

44 Zwimpfer RJ, Brown J, Sullivan I, Moulton RJ. Head injuries due to falls caused by seizures: a group at high risk for traumatic intracranial haematomas. *J Neurosurg* 1997; 86: 433–7.

45 Ellenberg JH, Hirtz DG, Nelson KB. Do seizures in children cause intellectual deterioration? *N Engl J Med* 1986; 314: 1085–8.

46 Bjornaes H, Stabell K, Henriksen O, Loyning Y. The effects of refractory epilepsy on intellectual functioning in children and adults. A longitudinal study. *Seizure* 2001; 10: 250–9.

47 Schwade ED, Otto O. Mortality of epilepsy. *JAMA* 1954; 156: 1526–8.

48 Alström CH. A study of epilepsy in its clinical, social and genetic aspects. *Acta Psychiatry Neurol Scand* 1950; (Suppl. 53): 1–284.

49 O'Donoghue MF, Sander JWAS. The mortality associated with epilepsy, with particular reference to sudden unexpected death: a review. *Epilepsia* 1997; 38 (Suppl. 11): S15–S19.

50 Dashieff RM. Sudden unexpected death in epilepsy: a series from an epilepsy surgery program and speculation on the relationship to sudden cardiac death. *J Clin Neurophsyiol* 1991; 8: 216–22.

51 Loiseau J, Picot M-C, Loiseau P. Short-term mortality after a first epileptic seizure: a population-based study. *Epilepsia* 1999; 40: 1388–92.

52 Buck D, Baker GA, Jacoby A, Smith DF, Chadwick DW. Patients' experiences of injury as a result of epilepsy. *Epilepsia* 1997; 38: 439–44.

53 Spitz MC, Towbin JA, Shantz D, Adler LE. Risk factors for burns as a consequence of seizures in persons with epilepsy. *Epilepsia* 1994; 35: 764–7.

54 Neufeld MY, Vishne T, Chistik V, Korczyn AD. Life-long history of injuries related to seizures. *Epilepsy Res* 1999; 34: 123–7.

55 Wirrell EC, Camfield PR, Camfield CS, Dooley JM, Gordon KE. Accidental injury is a serious risk in children with typical absence epilepsy. *Arch Neurol* 1996; 53: 929–32.

56 Chaplin JE, Yepez Lasso R, Shorvon SD, Floyd M. National General practice study of epilepsy: the social and psychological effects of a recent diagnosis of epilepsy. *Br Med J* 1992; 304: 1416–18.

57 Baker GA, Jacoby A, Buck D, Stalgis C, Monnet D. Quality of life of people with epilepsy: A European study. *Epilepsia* 1997; 38: 353–62.

58 Swinkels WAM, Shackleton DP, Kasteleijn-Nolst T, Tremite D. Psychosocial impact of epileptic seizures in a Dutch epilepsy population: a compara-

tive Washington Psychosocial Seizure Inventory study. *Epilepsia* 2000; 41: 1335–41.

59 Jacoby A, Baker GA, Steen N, Potts P, Chadwick DW. The clinical course of epilepsy and its psychosocial correlates: findings from a UK community study. *Epilepsia* 1996; 37: 148–61.

60 Plaa GL, Willmore LJ. General principles: toxicology. In: Levy RH, Mattson RH, Meldrum BS, eds. *Antiepileptic Drugs*, 4th edn. New York: Raven Press, 1995: 51–60.

61 Sander JWAS, Hart YM, Trimble M, Shorvon SD. Vigabatrin and psychosis. *J Neurol Neurosurg Psychiatry* 1991; 54: 435–9.

62 Dreifuss FE, Santilli N, Langer DH, Sweeney KP, Moline KA, Menander KB. Valproic acid hepatic fatalities: a retrospective review. *Neurology* 1987; 37: 379–85.

63 Reynolds EH. Early treatment and prognosis of epilepsy. *Epilepsia* 1987; 26: 97–106.

64 Wilder BJ. Phenytoin. Clinical use. In: Levy RH, Mattson RH, Meldrum BS, eds. *Antiepileptic Drugs*, 4th edn. New York: Raven Press, 1995: 339.

65 Wallace H, Shorvon SD, Hopkins A, O'Donoghue M. *Adults with Poorly Controlled Epilepsy*. London: Royal College of Physicians, 1997.

66 Scottish Intercollegiate Guidelines Network. *Diagnosis and Management of Epilepsy in Adults. A national clinical guideline recommended for use in Scotland*. Edinburgh: Royal College of Physicians of Edinburgh, 1997: 14.

67 Mattson RH, Cramer JA, Collins JF *et al*. Comparison of carbamazepine, phenobarbital, phenytoin, and primidone in partial and secondarily generalised tonic-clonic seizures. *N Engl J Med* 1985; 313: 145–51.

68 Mattson RH, Cramer JA, Collins JF, and the Department of Veterans Affairs Epilepsy Cooperative Study No 264 Group. A comparison of valproate with carbamazepine for the treatment of complex partial seizures and secondarily generalized tonic-clonic seizures in adults. *N Engl J Med* 1992; 327: 765–71.

69 Richens A, Davidson DLW, Cartlidge NEF, Easter DJ. A multicentre trial of sodium valproate and carbamazepine in adult-onset epilepsy. *J Neurol Neurosurg Psych* 1994; 57: 682–7.

70 Verity CM, Hosking G, Easter DJ on behalf of the Pediatric EPITEG Collaborative Group. A multicentre comparative trial of sodium valproate and carbamazepine in pediatric epilepsy. *Dev Med Child Neurol* 1995; 37: 97–108.

71 De Silva M, MacArdle B, McGowan M *et al*. Randomised comparative monotherapy trial of phenobarbitone, phenytoin, carbamazepine or sodium valproate for newly diagnosed childhood epilepsy. *Lancet* 1996; 347: 709–13.

72 Brodie MJ, Richens A, Yuen AWC, for UK Lamotrigine/Carbamazepine Monotherapy Trial Group. Double-blind comparison of lamotrigine and carbamazepine in newly diagnosed epilepsy. *Lancet* 1995; 345: 476–9.

73 Steiner TJ, Dellaportas CI, Findley LJ *et al*. Lamotrigine monotherapy in newly diagnosed untreated epilepsy: a double-blind comparison with phenytoin. *Epilepsia* 1999; 40: 601–7.

74 Dam M, Ekberg R, Løyninb Y, Waltimo O, Jakobsen K (the Scandinavian Oxcarbazepine Study Group). A double-blind study comparing oxcarbazepine and carbamazepine in patients with newly diagnosed, previously untreated epilepsy. *Epilepsy Res* 1989; 3: 70–6.

75 Christe W, Kramer G, Vigonius H, Steinhoff B, Brodie M, Moore A. A double-blind controlled clinical trial: oxcarbazepine versus sodium valproate in adults with newly diagnosed epilepsy. *Epilepsy Res* 1997; 26: 451–60.

76 Bill PA, Vigonius U, Pohlmann H *et al*. A double-blind controlled clinical trial of oxcarbazepine versus phenytoin in adults with previously untreated epilepsy. *Epilepsy Res* 1997; 27: 195–204.

77 Guerreiro MM, Vigonius U, Pohlmann H *et al*. A double-blind controlled clinical trial of oxcarbazepine versus phenytoin in children and adolescents with epilepsy. *Epilepsy Res* 1997; 27: 205–13.

78 Chadwick D, for the Vigabatrin European Monotherapy Study Group. Safety and efficacy of vigabatrin and carbamazepine in newly diagnosed epilepsy: a multicentre randomised double-blind study. *Lancet* 1999; 354: 13–19.

79 Lawden MC, Eke T, Degg C, Harding GFA, Wild JM. Visual field defects associated with vigabatrin therapy. *J Neurol Neurosurg Psychiatry* 1999; 67: 716–22.

80 Kalviainen R, Nousiainen I. Visual field defects with vigabatrin: epidemiology and therapeutic implications. *CNS Drugs* 2001; 15: 217–30.

81 Isojarvi JIT, Laatikainen TJ, Pakarinen AJ *et al*. Polycystic ovaries and hyperandrogenism in women taking valproate for epilepsy. *N Engl J Med* 1993; 329: 1383–8.

82 Fairgrieve SD, Jackson M, Jonas P *et al*. Population based, prospective study of the care of women with epilepsy in pregnancy. *Br Med J* 2000; 321: 674–5.

83 Shorvon SD, Chadwick D, Galbraith AW, Reynolds EH. One drug for epilepsy. *Br Med J* 1978; 1: 474–6.

84 Kwan P, Brodie MJ. Effectiveness of first antiepileptic drug. *Epilepsia* 2001; 42: 1255–60.

85 Sander JWAS, Hart YM, Johnson AL, Shorvon SD, for the NGPSE. National General Practice Study of Epilepsy: newly diagnosed epileptic seizures in a general population. *Lancet* 1990; 336: 1267–71.

86 Frucht MM, Quigg M, Schwaner C, Fountain NB. Distribution of seizure precipitants among epilepsy syndromes. *Epilepsia* 2000; 41: 1534–9.

87 Thomas MH. The single seizure: its study and management. *JAMA* 1959; 169: 457–9.

88 Costeff H. Convulsions in childhood: their natural history and indications for treatment. *N Engl J Med* 1965; 273: 1410–13.

89 Saunders M, Marshall C. Isolated seizures: an EEG and clinical assessment. *Epilepsy* 1975; 16: 731–3.

90 Blom S, Heijbel J, Bergfors PG. Incidence of epilepsy in children: a follow-up study three years after the first seizure. *Epilepsia* 1978; 19: 343–50.

91 Elwes RDC, Chesterman P, Reynolds EH. Prognosis after a first untreated tonic clonic seizure. *Lancet* 1985; ii: 752–3.

13 Management of Epilepsy in Remission

D. Chadwick

Population and cohort studies have shown that 70–80% of patients diagnosed and treated for epilepsy will attain long-term remission in excess of 2 or more years [1,2]. Most of those who enter remission do so immediately or shortly after beginning therapy. It is for this group of subjects that decision-making about whether or not to continue with antiepileptic drugs (AED) is critical and potentially most difficult. For adults, the penalties for seizure recurrence are high, but on the other hand there may be real or perceived adverse effects of AED on concentration and cognitive function, as well as unwanted complications of drugs on contraception and pregnancy for women.

The difficulty of the decision arises from a lack of understanding of the way in which AED treatment may or may not interact with the natural history of epilepsy. Are people with a significant period without seizures now cured (i.e. their seizure freedom is no longer dependent on treatment) of the condition, or are they simply controlled by ongoing treatment? If some are cured is this due to the treatment they received or would their susceptibility to seizures have remitted in any event?

How long seizure free?

Most commonly, periods of 2 years or more are generally considered necessary before consideration of withdrawal. Recently, paediatricians have advocated treatment for shorter periods of time (see below). It is usually suggested that longer seizure-free periods result in a lower risk of recurrence. This is most likely to be due to selection bias rather than any treatment effect, patients who relapse while still on medication after short periods of time being excluded from estimates of risk. In the Medical Research Council's (MRC) randomized controlled trial (RCT) the most influential prognostic factor for recurrence was the period of time seizure free; however, this applied both to patients continuing their treatment as well as to those stopping it [3].

An RCT has supported this view by comparing policies of differing lengths of treatment prior to stopping medication. Peters *et al.* [4] randomized children who entered remission within 2 months of starting treatment to stop medication after 6 months or 12 months. Six months after the first follow-up, 22% still on AED had relapsed despite treatment, compared to 37% who had been withdrawn from their drugs. However, by 24 months after randomization the risk of relapse was 49% and 48%, respectively. This study shows higher rates of seizure recurrence than would usually be expected in children staying on treatment for 2 or more years (29% by 2 years after withdrawal [5]). Braathen *et al.* [6] came to somewhat different conclusions. They randomized 244 children to treatment for either 1 or 3 years. Randomization took place before treatment was

commenced. Drugs were withdrawn in each group only in those patients who were seizure free for at least 6 months at the end of 1 and 3 years, respectively. The primary study outcome was reinstitution of medications, not seizure recurrence as in most studies. One hundred and sixty-one children commenced withdrawal, 77 after 1 year's treatment and 84 after 3 year's treatment. The report gives no information about the median period seizure free in the two groups withdrawing treatment, but the probabilities of reinstitution of treatment were generally higher than might be expected from studies demanding remission of 2 years: a 30% probability in patients treated for 3 years compared to a 50% probability in the group treated for 1 year. The observed outcome is consistent with the effect of longer periods of remission having better outcomes and probably does not indicate a true treatment benefit for 3 years of therapy compared to 1 year.

Relevant to the question of whether longer periods of treatment increase the true chance of cure, there are a number of studies from developing countries where individuals with a diagnosis of epilepsy remained untreated. One study found 55% of untreated patients achieved spontaneous remission [7]. This is not dissimilar from rates of remission in the developed world where approximately 70% become seizure free on medication, of whom 60–70% can successfully withdraw therapy. This, again, suggests that, regardless of length of treatment or indeed of treatment at all, half of all cases of epilepsy spontaneously remit.

The shape of the relationship between the time elapsed seizure free and the risk of seizures in the following year on treatment is illustrated in Fig. 13.1 using data from the MRC study [8,9]. This uses data from those patients who had a recurrence of seizures during the course of the study, all of whom were on treatment after such a seizure, and all those patients randomized to continue treatment at the outset of the study. The risk of a seizure in the next year is about 50% immediately after a seizure and approximately 20% after 1-year seizure free. By 4–5 years, the risk of a seizure in the next year falls to about 10%. The risk for seizures after this time changes relatively little so that a policy of considering discontinuation of AED after 2–5 years in adults and after only 1 or more years in children seems reasonable.

This topic has been the subject of a Cochrane systematic review [10].

Estimates of risk of relapse

Studies that include a broad mix of patients and that require 2 years seizure remission before stopping treatment on average show a risk of relapse of 25% in the first year and 29% after 2 years [5]. Of all recurrences 80% occur within the first year and 90% within the first

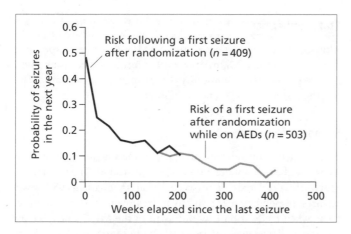

Fig. 13.1 The probability of a further seizure in a following year while on drug therapy and its relationship to the passage of time. Data is derived from the MRC study of AED withdrawal. Early risk is calculated from those patients who experienced a seizure following randomization, and who were thereafter treated. Later risk is calculated from the group of patients randomized to continued therapy whose median duration of remission was 3 years.

Table 13.1 Some factors which have been reported to adversely affect the risk of seizure relapse after discontinuation of AED in patients with epilepsy in remission

---

Short duration of seizure freedom prior to drug withdrawal
Age above 16 years
Epilepsy with onset in adolescence or adulthood
Juvenile myoclonic epilepsy
Remote symptomatic epilepsy
History of myoclonic seizures
History of multiple seizure types
History of primary or secondarily generalized tonic-clonic seizures
History of atypical febrile seizures (in children)
Prolonged period before achieving seizure control
Seizures while on treatment
Seizure control requiring multiple drug therapy
Abnormal EEG
Learning disability
Associated neurological handicaps
Previous failed attempts to stop medication

---

2 years. These estimates are derived from a meta-analysis across several studies and the great majority of these provide individual estimates within about 10% of the summary estimate. They may, however, represent an overoptimistic picture of the results of AED withdrawal. Because the majority of patients in remission have a history of relatively few attacks, there may be greater uncertainty about the initial diagnosis of epilepsy than is often the case. If the error rate for misdiagnosis is high one would expect the true relapse rate to be higher than that observed.

Many factors have been identified that appear to influence the degree of risk (Table 13.1).

Electroclinical syndrome

Epilepsy syndromes can be used to define both the prognosis for response to treatment and to treatment withdrawal. The international classification of the epilepsies was first approved after a number of revisions in 1989 [11]. Syndromes are identified by age at onset, seizure type, EEG characteristics, the presence or absence of underlying aetiology and diurnal pattern of seizure occurrence. Some syndromes are very clearly associated with particular risk of relapse after stopping treatment. Benign rolandic epilepsy (BRE) has been shown by a number of investigators to have an excellent long-term prognosis, and relapse is almost unknown when medications are stopped. Outcome seems entirely unrelated to treatment [12,13]. Childhood absence epilepsy has a more uncertain prognosis for remission. Although in the short term, most of these children become seizure free on treatment, about 25% relapse when medications are withdrawn [14,15]. Juvenile myoclonic epilepsy (JME) has an excellent response to treatment; however, relapses occur in almost all patients when medications are stopped [16]. Other symptomatic or cryptogenic partial epilepsies are less well defined with respect to both response to treatment and the prognosis following withdrawal.

Epilepsy syndromes are most easily identified in patients with fre-

quent and varied seizures, many of whom will never enter remission. They may be difficult to identify with confidence in patients with mild epilepsies characterized by only a few seizures responding immediately to treatment.

Seizure type

Most studies have examined the outcome of particular types of seizures rather than syndromes. Because a single seizure type may be a characteristic of very differing syndromes, the results of such analyses are in some conflict. Thus, tonic-clonic seizures may occur in JME, BRE, juvenile absence epilepsy and many other syndromes. Similarly, simple partial seizures occur in both BRE as well as the more refractory types of temporal lobe epilepsy. Having multiple as compared to single seizure types has been associated with a higher risk of relapse in several studies. An equal number of studies, however, failed to find such an effect [17]. As a number of epilepsy syndromes are characterized by multiple seizure types, it is likely that the underlying epilepsy syndrome may better account for the likelihood of relapsing after stopping AED.

Age at onset

Most studies find a favourable prognosis in epilepsy with onset in childhood, which is likely to be due at least in part to the occurrence of many benign epilepsy syndromes in this age group. Studies including both childhood and adolescent onset epilepsy usually find a substantially increased risk of relapse in those with adolescent onset. Childhood onset of epilepsy is usually associated with a risk of relapse of approximately 20% compared to 35–40% for adolescent onset epilepsy. Adult onset epilepsy, on the other hand, is about 30% more likely to relapse than childhood onset epilepsy [5]. Some confusion exists in this literature because of a common failure to differentiate between the age of onset of epilepsy and the age at which discontinuation is considered. The former is a function of the underlying biology of the epilepsy, while the latter is a function not only of age of onset but also of the period of time that it took for the epilepsy to come under control.

Underlying aetiology

If exception is made for JME, individuals with an identifiable aetiology associated with their epilepsy (remote symptomatic epilepsy) are less likely to enter remission than those with idiopathic or cryptogenic epilepsy. Once in remission, patients with remote symptomatic epilepsy are about 50% more likely to relapse if medication is stopped [5]. Learning disability, at least in children, may be a stronger predictor of relapse than motor impairments or other neurological disorders that are not associated with impairment of cognitive function [18]. The impact of remote symptomatic epilepsy on prognosis for adult onset epilepsy is rather less dramatic and was not found to be an important factor in the MRC Withdrawal Study, which was essentially a study of adults in remission [8].

EEG

There is considerable controversy over the value of the EEG in predicting the prognosis for relapse after stopping treatment. Some studies have examined the amount of 'improvement' in the EEG from starting treatment to the time of its cessation. Most studies examine the correlation between an EEG immediately prior to withdrawal and relapse. Different studies have focused on different types of EEG abnormalities. In one study [19], children with normal EEGs had an extremely low risk of relapse, those with either epileptiform abnormalities or slowing had a moderate risk and those with both epileptiform abnormalities and slowing had almost a 100% risk of relapse. Mastropaolo *et al.* [20] reported high rates of relapse in patients with photoconvulsive responses on EEG. The appearance or worsening of EEG abnormalities during the AED discontinuation period might also be a separate important prognostic factor. Overall, data suggest that the EEG is of greater prognostic significance in children than in adults. It is uncertain to what degree EEG abnormalities are independent prognostic variables and to what degree EEG abnormalities are simply more common in individuals already identified as high risk by clinical factors such as having a symptomatic epilepsy or other adverse clinical prognostic factors. Because of considerable variation amongst the studies, we cannot say with any certainty which aspects of the EEG are most important. Certainly, in a multivariate model predicting outcomes, the EEG added little to other more important clinical factors [3].

Severity of epilepsy

A number of different clinical features that may reflect the severity of epilepsy have been studied and reported in the literature. They include a history of status epilepticus, the duration of epilepsy, the number of seizures before remission, the duration of treatment, the requirement for two or more AED for remission and previous failed attempts to stop medication. Most studies indicate that these surrogate measures of severity all adversely affect the risk of recurrence [17]. However, no single indicator or set of indicators is clearly superior to the others as a marker of prognosis after stopping AED.

Status epilepticus

Although status epilepticus is associated with poorer response to drug treatment [21,22], patients with a history of status and who become seizure free do not seem to have a higher risk of relapse. This was the case in adults [8] and in children [18].

Response to treatment

Factors such as the duration of epilepsy and the duration of treatment have been examined by a number of studies. The two factors are clearly correlated. There is a consensus that patients with fewer seizures, responding more rapidly to treatment, have a better outcome when medication is withdrawn. In the MRC study, having seizures whilst on drug treatment and requiring two or more drugs for remission have both been associated with an increased risk of relapse.

In both children [18] and adults [8] a previous failed attempt to stop treatment has not been found, by itself, to be associated with an increased risk of relapse, although the power of these studies to detect an effect is poor, given that relatively few patients will be keen to undertake a second attempt of withdrawal.

Influence of individual drugs

It is often suggested that the risk of seizure recurrence may differ depending on the drug that is to be withdrawn. Withdrawal seizures are particularly said to occur with the discontinuation of benzodiazepines and phenobarbital. The subject has rarely been exposed to systematic study. There were large subgroups of patients receiving monotherapy with carbamazepine, valproate, phenytoin and barbiturate drugs (phenobarbital and primidone) in the MRC Withdrawal Study [23]. The temporal pattern of seizure recurrence was similar in the barbiturate group and the other groups. Surprisingly, the withdrawal of carbamazepine was associated with a lower relative risk of seizure recurrence on withdrawal than were other drugs even after adjustment for other predictors of outcome. The significance of these findings is uncertain. One explanation is that carbamazepine may in some way influence the natural history in the patients in which it was prescribed, leading to higher 'cure rate'. Alternatively, the observation may have arisen because of a difficult-to-identify difference in patients who are treated with one drug versus another.

Models for prediction of relapse

The MRC AED Withdrawal Study [3], was sufficiently large to develop and test a predictive model for relapse in patients continuing or stopping their medication. The model gives decreasing weight to the following factors: whether or not treatment is withdrawn, period of time seizure free, taking two or more AED, being 16 or older at the time of withdrawal, having myoclonic seizures and having tonic-clonic seizures of any type. The final factor was an abnormal EEG. While the model does not include the presence of remote symptomatic epilepsy, factors retained in the model may, singly or in combination, provide surrogate measures for symptomatic epilepsy and capture those aspects of remote symptomatic epilepsy that are most associated with an increased risk of relapse. In addition, as the MRC study was largely in adults, it is possible that the types of underlying aetiologies present in adult onset epilepsy do not carry the same risk for relatively poor prognosis as those factors associated with childhood onset epilepsy. Because of the methods and inclusion criteria, the MRC study was able to recruit a large number of patients from a general population who were highly representative of relevant patients in the population with respect to clinical prognostic factors. Consequently, this model should have good generalizability outside the study population from which it was derived, though this has never formally been tested. The resulting predictive equation was well calibrated for risks between 10% and 80% and would correctly identify JME as having a high risk of relapse. Table 13.2 outlines the use of this model.

Two groups of investigators have developed relatively simple models to predict relapse in children. Dooley *et al.* [24] developed a model derived from a study of 97 children in whom drugs were withdrawn after 12 months of remission. A point scoring system was devised in which subjects were allocated 1 point for being female; 1 for seizure onset after 10 years, the presence of neurological abnormality and generalized seizures; and 2 points for partial seizures (other than those of BRE). No subjects with 0 points relapsed (they had BRE by definition). Ninety-five per cent of patients with 1 point, 80% with 2 points, 45% with 3 points and 5% with 4 points remained seizure free. Shinnar *et al.* [18] determined risk of relapse 2 years after stopping AED in 264 children as a function of the number of risk factors for relapse that a child had, between 0 and 3. This was done separately for those with cryptogenic/idiopathic versus remote symptomatic epilepsy. In the idiopathic group, predictors of relapse were age at onset > 12 years, family history of

epilepsy, slowing on the EEG and atypical febrile seizures. The risk of relapse after 2 years was 12%, 46% and 71% in children with 0, 1 and 2 of these factors, respectively. No child had more than 2 factors. In remote symptomatic cases, predictors were age of onset > 12 years, mental retardation, absence seizures and atypical febrile seizures. The risk of relapse after 2 years was 11%, 35%, 51% and 78% in children with 0, 1, 2 and 3 risk factors, respectively. No child had all four risk factors. Of note, the lowest risk stratum in the remote symptomatic group had virtually the same risk as the lowest risk stratum in the cryptogenic/idiopathic group. The lowest risk stratum represented only 10% (9/99) of the remote symptomatic group, whereas it comprised 59% (97/165) of the cryptogenic/idiopathic group.

When discussing the risk of relapse when medication is withdrawn it is important to recognize that continued treatment with AED is not a guarantee of freedom from seizures. Data from the MRC study indicated a risk of 10% per annum in patients who had a median of 3 years seizure free at the point of randomization and who continued to take medication (Fig. 13.1).

Prognosis after relapse

Most evidence indicates that the majority of patients who relapse when medication is stopped will regain acceptable control when treatment is reintroduced. In the MRC Study, 95% of those who relapsed experienced at least a 1-year remission within 3 years of the initial relapse. By 5 years, 90% had experienced a remission of at least 2 years' duration. Factors associated with a poorer outcome after relapse were having a partial seizure at the time of relapse, having a previous history of seizures whilst on medication and shorter duration of seizure freedom prior to the relapse. All patients who had further seizures were analysed regardless of whether they had been randomized to stop or continue treatment. The outcome was the same following seizure recurrence regardless of whether a patient had discontinued or remained on treatment prior to the recurrence [9].

Psychosocial consequences of withdrawal and continued treatment

In the MRC Study the impact of the two randomized policies (continued treatment or withdrawal) on psychosocial outcomes was assessed [25]. There was good evidence that seizure recurrence had an adverse effect on psychosocial outcomes but that this was very much counterbalanced by the effects of continuing to take medication in the group randomized to do so. Thus, even though the group randomized to withdrawal experienced more seizures, psychosocial outcome was similar between the two groups. This indicates that there are significant benefits to the successful withdrawal of AED that may relate to the removal of the stigma of diagnosis of epilepsy and the daily burden of taking AED, when treatment is stopped.

For these reasons the decision to withdraw AED will be influenced both by the risk of further seizures and also by a personal view of the impact of further seizures on the individual's expectations and the risk of continued AED treatment. These issues demand careful consideration and discussion, and ultimately the decision can only be made by the patient. Personal circumstances may play a

Table 13.2 Factors for the calculation of a prognostic index for seizure recurrence by 1 and 2 years following continued treatment or slow withdrawal of AED, in patients with a minimum remission of seizures lasting for 2 years while on treatment

	Factor value to be added to score
1 Starting score for all patients	−175
Age > 16 years	45
Taking more than 1 AED	50
Seizures occuring after the start of treatment	35
History of any tonic-clonic seizure (generalized or partial in onset)	35
History of myoclonic seizures	50
EEG while in remission	
not done	15
abnormal	20
Duration of seizure-free period (years) = D	200/D
2 Total score	T
3 Exponentiate T/100 ($Z = e^{T/100}$)	Z

Probability of seizure recurrence	*by 1 year*	*by 2 years*
On continued treatment	$1-0.89^Z$	$1-0.79^Z$
On slow withdrawal of treatment	$1-0.69^Z$	$1-0.60^Z$

very important role. For example, a 25-year-old man whose job is dependent on holding a driving licence might well feel that a 40% risk of seizure recurrence on drug withdrawal was unacceptable. However, a similar risk in his 25-year-old wife might be acceptable if it allowed a drug-free pregnancy.

The complexity of these issues is further highlighted by studies of patients' views. Jacoby et al. [26] found that 43% of subjects with their epilepsy in remission were undecided what to do after a period in remission. This number was considerably reduced (to 9%) by the use of a predictive model, which presented the risk of seizure recurrence for policies of continued treatment and withdrawal. The latter policy consistently predicted greater risks of relapse than did the former. Only 10% of subjects (almost entirely adults) decided to withdraw treatment after reviewing the results of the model. In children, Gordon et al. [27] found parents' views of acceptable risk of withdrawal corresponded very poorly with those of their physicians, and in a way that was not easily predicted by clinical factors in the children.

If a decision is taken to withdraw treatment, clear advice should be offered about the speed of withdrawal and the steps to take if seizures recur. Tennison et al. [28] found no evidence of difference in recurrence rates when AED were tapered over 6 weeks as opposed to 9 months. From a practical point of view, it seems reasonable to taper most regimes gradually over a 2–3-month period, though for patients taking high dosages or multiple drug therapy, and for those taking drugs such as barbiturates and benzodiazepines, many physicians will favour a slower withdrawal. For children in remission, occasional seizures while remaining off treatment may be acceptable under some circumstances, but for many adults a seizure recurrence will usually require the prompt re-institution of the AED that was previously successful, though often seizure control can be achieved at dosages lower than those used before tapering.

Remission following epilepsy surgery

Surgery for epilepsy is increasingly practised and most series indicate that temporal lobe surgery will render approximately 70% of subjects seizure free for significant periods [29]. For many the question of whether to withdraw some or all of their treatment will arise. Unfortunately, in contrast to pharmacologically induced remission there are no RCT to inform patients or guide practice.

Studies show that anywhere between 25% and 67% of patients may stop AED treatment after epilepsy surgery. There is little doubt that withdrawal greatly increases risk of seizure recurrence from 7% to 36% at 5 years in one study [30]. In the absence of satisfactorily designed prospective studies it is impossible to quantify the magnitude of the excess risk (vs. continuing AED treatment) and the factors that influence it, although absence of defined pathology in the preoperative MR scan may be important. This is an area that demands further study.

Conclusions

The decision to stop the drug treatment of epilepsy requires a careful assessment of individual risk of both seizures and continuing treatment (Table 13.3). The physician's role is to provide satisfactory information for the individual patient and their family to

Table 13.3 Factors influencing a decision to continue or discontinue AED treatment in patients with epilepsy in remission

Reliable prediction of risk of seizure recurrence
Presence or absence of adverse drug effects
Patient's attitude towards implications of seizure recurrence
Patient's attitude towards implications of continuation of therapy
Patient's age and social/professional status

make a decision. In adults treatment should usually be continued until there has been a remission of between 2 and 5 years, but in children shorter remission periods of 12 months may be adequate. The benefits of stopping medications in children certainly seem to outweigh their risks in most circumstances. In adults, by contrast, the risks and consequences associated with a relapse are such that the decision to stop medications is more complicated. Overall, the clinical risks of relapse may be largely counterbalanced by the psychosocial benefits of discontinuing treatment. Predictive models can be satisfactorily used to identify risks of further seizures. There is no evidence from RCT to indicate that withdrawal of treatment and seizure recurrence adversely affects future responsiveness to AED therapy.

References

1 Annegers JF, Hauser WA, Elverback LR. Remission of seizures and relapse in patients with epilepsy. *Epilepsia* 1979; 20: 729–37.
2 Cockerell OC, Johnson AL, Sander JWAS, Shorvon SD. Prognosis of epilepsy: A review and further analysis of the first nine years of the British National General Practice Study of Epilepsy, a prospective population-based study. *Epilepsia* 1997; 38: 31–46.
3 Medical Research Council Antiepileptic Drug Withdrawal Study Group. Prognostic index for recurrence of seizures after remission of epilepsy. *Br Med J* 1993; 306: 1374–8.
4 Peters ACB, Brouwer OF, Geerts AT et al. Randomised prospective study of early discontinuation of antiepileptic drugs in children with epilepsy: Dutch study of epilepsy in childhood. *Neurology* 1998.
5 Berg AT, Shinnar S. Relapse following discontinuation of antiepileptic drugs: A meta-analysis. *Neurology* 1994; 44: 601–8.
6 Braathen G, Andersson T, Gylje H et al. Comparison between one and three years of treatment in uncomplicated childhood epilepsy: a prospective study. I. Outcome in different seizure types. *Epilepsia* 1996; 37 (9): 822–32.
7 Placencia M, Shorvon S, Paredes V et al. Epileptic seizures in an Andean region of Ecuador: Incidence and prevalence and regional variation. *Brain* 1992; 115: 771–82.
8 Medical Research Council Antiepileptic Drug Withdrawal Study Group (D. Chadwick CC). Randomized study of antiepileptic drug withdrawal in patients in remission. *Lancet* 1991; 337: 1175–80.
9 Chadwick D, Taylor J, Johnson T. Outcomes after seizure recurrence in people with well-controlled epilepsy and the factors that influence it. The MRC Antiepileptic Drug Withdrawal Group. *Epilepsia* 1996; 37 (11): 1043–50.
10 Sirven JI, Sperling M, Wingerchuk DM. Early versus late withdrawal for people with epilepsy in remission. *The Cochrane Library* 2001.
11 Commission on Classification and Terminology of the International League Against Epilepsy. Proposal for revised classification of epilepsies and epileptic syndromes. *Epilepsia* 1989; 30: 389–99.
12 Ambrosetto G, Tassinari CA. Antiepileptic drug treatment of benign childhood epilepsy with rolandic spikes: is it necessary? *Epilepsia* 1990; 31: 802–5.
13 Peters JM, Camfield CS, Camfield PR. Population study of benign rolandic epilepsy: Is treatment needed? *Neurology* 2001; 57: 537–9.

14 Wolfe P, Inoue Y. Therapeutic response of absence seizures in patients of an epilepsy clinic for adolescents and adults. *J Neurol* 1984; 231: 225–9.

15 Bouma PA, Westendorp RG, van Dijk JG, Peters AC, Brouwer O. The outcome of absence epilepsy: a meta-analysis. *Neurology* 1996; 47: 802–8.

16 Delgado-Escueta AV, Enrile-Bacsal F. Juvenile myoclonic epilepsy of Janz. *Neurology* 1984; 34: 285–94.

17 Berg AT, Shinnar S, Chadwick D. Discontinuing antiepileptic drugs. In: Engel J, Pedley TA, eds. *Epilepsy: a Comprehensive Text*. New York: Lippincott-Raven, 1998: 1275–84.

18 Shinnar S, Berg AT, Moshe SL *et al*. Discontinuing antiepileptic drugs in children with epilepsy: A prospective study. *Ann Neurol* 1994; 35: 534–45.

19 Shinnar S, Vining EPG, Mellits ED *et al*. Discontinuing antiepileptic medication in children with epilepsy after two years without seizures. *N Engl J Med* 1985; 31: 976–80.

20 Mastropaolo T, Tondi C, Carboni F, Manca S, Zoroddu F. Prognosis after therapy discontinuation in children with epilepsy. *Eur Neurol* 1992; 32: 141–5.

21 Berg AT, Levy SR, Novotny EJ, Shinnar S. Predictors of intractable epilepsy in childhood: A case-control study. *Epilepsia* 1996; 37: 24–30.

22 Sillanpaa M. Remission of seizures and prediction of intractability in long-term follow-up. *Epilepsia* 1993; 34: 930–6.

23 Chadwick D. Does withdrawal of different antiepileptic drugs have different effects on seizure recurrence? Further results from the MRC Antiepileptic Drug Withdrawal Study. *Brain* 1999; 122 (Pt 3): 441–8.

24 Dooley J, Gordon K, Camfield P, Camfield C, Smith E. Discontinuation of anticonvulsant therapy in children free of seizures for 1 year: A prospective study. *Neurology* 1996; 46: 969–74.

25 Jacoby A, Johnson A, Chadwick D. Psychosocial outcomes of antiepileptic drug discontinuation. *Epilepsia* 1992; 33: 1123–31.

26 Jacoby A, Baker G, Chadwick D, Johnson A. The impact of counselling with a practical statistical model on patients' decision-making about treatment for epilepsy: findings from a pilot study. *Epilepsy Res* 1993; 16: 207–14.

27 Gordon K, MacSween J, Dooley J *et al*. Families are content to discontinue antiepileptic drugs at different risks than their physicians. *Epilepsia* 1996; 37: 557–62.

28 Tennison M, Greenwood R, Lewis D, Thorn M. Discontinuing antiepileptic drugs in children with epilepsy. A comparison of a six-week and a nine-month taper period. *N Engl J Med* 1994; 300: 1407–10.

29 Engel J Jr. Surgery for seizures. *N Engl J Med* 1996; 334: 647–52.

30 Schiller Y, Cascino GD, So EL, Marsh WR. Discontinuation of antiepileptic drugs after successful epilepsy surgery. *Neurology* 2000; 54: 346–9.

14 Management of Epilepsy in Infants

C. Chiron

Infancy is defined as the age range that occurs between the neonatal period (the first month of life) and childhood (from 2 years of age). The population of infants therefore excludes neonates and school-age children. As in later life, the management of epilepsy in infants includes medical and/or surgical treatment options, as well as appropriate rehabilitation. As in the other age ranges, the choice of antiepileptic drugs (AEDs) is highly dependent on the type of epilepsy syndrome and limited by tolerability. However, because of various age-related characteristics, management of epilepsy is quite specific in infancy. The specificity concerns age-related properties of AEDs, the epilepsy itself and the effects of the drugs on the epilepsy. We shall review these peculiarities and then detail the management of the main infantile epilepsy syndromes.

Infancy-specific issues in the management of epilepsy

Age-dependent pharmacokinetics and pharmacodynamics

The pharmacokinetics of AEDs varies according to maturational stage, being different in neonates, infants and older children, and this has important implications in determining dose requirements in these age groups. Specific pharmacokinetic features in infants compared to children and adults may include slower gastrointestinal absorption rates, higher volumes of distribution, higher apparent clearance values and shorter half-lives (Fig. 14.1). As a result, dose requirements (normalized for body weight) are higher in infants than in older children, and the intervals between doses may need to be shortened. Equally important, intra- and interindividual variability in pharmacokinetics and dose requirement is more marked in infants than in older children.

Pharmacokinetic parameters in infants are known for most established AEDs [1]. Valproic acid and phenobarbital exhibit relatively favourable pharmacokinetics in infants, whereas carbamazepine and phenytoin have less favourable pharmacokinetic features in this population. Carbamazepine daily dosages in infants need to be increased up to mean values of 30–50 mg/kg compared with 15–25 mg/kg for older children, and in infants t.i.d. administration is usually required while in older age groups b.i.d. dosing may be feasible. The use of phenytoin is even more problematic because of non-linear pharmacokinetics, and an adequate dose of phenytoin is particularly difficult to determine in infants. In a retrospective series of 82 infants with epilepsy who received phenytoin, 55% were controlled when the drug was administered i.v., but only 9% were controlled with oral administration and it was difficult to obtain adequate plasma phenytoin concentrations in 69% of the patients receiving oral chronic treatment [2].

As far as new AEDs are concerned, pharmacokinetic data are still scarce in infants. The pharmacologically active S(+)-enantiomer of vigabatrin has age-dependent kinetics: its absorption is significantly slower in infants ($t_{max} = 2.9$ h) compared with children ($t_{max} = 1.4$ h) and adults ($t_{max} = 0.8$ h), and its area under the curve and its elimination half-life increase linearly with age [3]. As for lamotrigine, apparent clearance also increases during the first year of life, from the age of 2 months [4]. Preliminary data also suggest that infants have lower concentrations of topiramate than older children and adults [5].

Tolerability profiles may differ in infants compared with other age groups. The risk of hepatic failure with valproate is an obvious example. Although the overall incidence is very low (1/37 000), the risk is small in adults and is greatly increased below the age of 2 years, especially in infants who had been recently started on the drug and are treated with high doses, in polytherapy and in the presence of an associated psychomotor delay [6]. Some of these patients may suffer from an undiagnosed inherited metabolic disease decompensated by valproate, such as carnitine deficiency or Alpers' disease. By contrast, in infants, phenobarbital induces very frequently behavioural side-effects which limit its use in this age group: about one-third of phenobarbital-treated children develop hyperexcitability and insomnia, and the IQ has been reported to be significantly reduced in children who received 2 years of treatment with phenobarbital as prophylaxis against recurrence of febrile seizures [7]. As far as phenytoin is concerned, overdosing is not an uncommon cause of side-effects in infants [2]. Benzodiazepines induce a paradoxical hyperexcitation, with sleep disorders rather than somnolence, in infants. When infantile spasms are treated with clonazepam, more than half of the infants experience severe side-effects such as increased secretion of saliva, difficulty in swallowing and mucous obstruction of the bronchi. With nitrazepam, a mortality rate of 25% among infants with spasms has been reported after administration of doses above 0.8 mg/kg/day [8]. Hypotonia and somnolence have been specifically reported in infants treated with vigabatrin [9]. The risk for visual field defects due to vigabatrin is not evaluable at this age, although recent reports suggest that retinal toxicity may be lower in children than in adults [10]. Adverse events were reported to be similar in infants and older children taking lamotrigine as add-on therapy [4]. By contrast, metabolic acidosis induced by topiramate may be more frequent in infants than in adults.

Available formulations of many AEDs are highly unsatisfactory for use in infants. The liquid form of valproate has an unpleasant taste. Carbamazepine and valproate lack a controlled-release formulation suitable for low daily dosages. Phenytoin and clobazam also do not have a formulation suitable for infants. Similarly, there has been little or no investment of the pharmaceutical industry to-

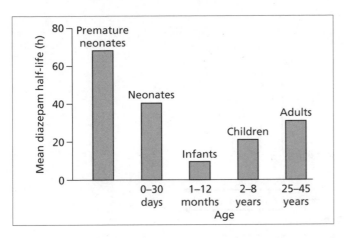

Fig. 14.1 The mean half-life of diazepam as a function of age. As with most other AEDs, the longest values are found in premature neonates, while the shortest are found in infants. Inter- and intraindividual variation may be considerable, especially in the youngest age groups.

wards development of formulations of new AEDs which would be appropriate for use in infants.

Characteristics of infantile epilepsies

The distinction between partial and generalized epilepsies, which is considered crucial to determine drug choice in children and adults, is not easily applicable to infants. Generalized epilepsy syndromes may be difficult to identify at onset because their initial manifestations may involve partial seizures, as clearly seen in severe myoclonic epilepsy in infancy (Dravet's syndrome), where the first seizures frequently involve one hemisoma. In addition, there can be rapid changes in epilepsy syndromes during infancy, eventually mixing the characteristics of both partial and generalized epilepsy, as in the case of infantile spasms progressing to partial epilepsy.

The incidence of epilepsy is higher in infancy than in childhood, possibly due to active maturational phenomena, and infancy is therefore a critical period for epileptogenesis. For the same reasons, epilepsy carries major associated risks in this age group, including a risk for altered motor function, as in the hemiplegia–hemiconvulsion syndrome, and a risk for cognitive deterioration, as in epileptic encephalopathies. Epileptic encephalopathies are conditions in which neurological deterioration results mainly from epileptic activity. Cognitive deterioration can be due to very frequent or severe seizures, or to subcontinuous paroxysmal 'interictal' activity. The former situation is seen mainly in severe myoclonic epilepsy in infancy, in which patients exhibit severe convulsive seizures from the middle of the first year of life with repeated episodes of status epilepticus, and in migrating partial epilepsy in infancy in which, from the first trimester of life, partial seizures affect various areas of the cortex randomly and in a subcontinuous fashion. Cognitive deterioration related to subcontinuous paroxysmal interictal activity is seen in infants with suppression bursts, as in Ohtahara's syndrome, and in infants with infantile spasms.

Effects of AEDs on infantile epilepsies

The efficacy of AEDs is known to be partly determined by the type of epilepsy syndrome being treated. Some syndromes may be improved by certain drugs, whereas others may be worsened. Identification of paradoxical reactions is especially important in infantile epilepsies. For example, carbamazepine may worsen infantile spasms and myoclonic epilepsies [11], lamotrigine may worsen severe myoclonic epilepsy in infancy [12] and vigabatrin may aggravate myoclonic epilepsies [13].

The management of infantile epilepsy syndromes

Severe epilepsies are highly prominent in infancy, whereas 'benign' or idiopathic epilepsies are very rare in this age group (Fig. 14.2) [14]. Except for some cases of symptomatic partial epilepsy associated with a normal mental development, most infants with generalized or partial epilepsies experience refractoriness to conventional AEDs and a severe impairment of their neurological status. The so-called 'catastrophic epilepsies' constitute a heterogeneous group, but they share several common characteristics, including a high seizure frequency, intractability and stagnation or regression of development. The causes of intractability may be multiple, including structural brain abnormalities, genetic background, secondary epileptogenic foci and maturational phenomena. The causes of mental impairment are also multiple, and may involve the original structural lesion, secondary lesions due to status epilepticus and continuous and diffuse interictal EEG abnormalities, all of which may result in epileptic encephalopathies.

Epileptic encephalopathies

Epileptic encephalopathies comprise a series of age-related generalized epilepsy syndromes (Fig. 14.2) which in infancy include, in order of decreasing frequency, infantile spasms, severe myoclonic epilepsy in infancy and myoclonic epilepsy in non-progressive encephalopathy, which mostly occur between 3 and 9 months, infantile epileptic encephalopathy with suppression bursts (Ohtahara's syndrome) and infantile epilepsy with migrating partial seizures [15], which occur in very young babies, at a mean age of 3 months. The latter two conditions are so intractable that no therapeutic strategy has provided valuable improvement to date. The reverse is true for infantile spasms, severe myoclonic epilepsy in infancy and myoclonic epilepsy in non-progressive encephalopathy, which do carry high refractoriness overall, but can be improved by specific treatment algorithms. Population-based studies of patients with epilepsy covering all ages show no evidence that early AED therapy can prevent the development of chronic epilepsy and that AED choice makes any difference for long-term outcome. However, in infantile epilepsies the situation may be different, and early choice of an appropriate treatment could make a world of difference, especially with respect to cognitive outcome [16].

Infantile spasms (West's syndrome)

The syndrome of infantile spasms (West's syndrome) was named after Dr W.J. West who in 1841 first reported observations of epileptic spasms occurring in his son. It was only a century later that introduction of the EEG allowed the definition of the characteristic pattern of hypsarrhythmia. West's syndrome is an epileptic en-

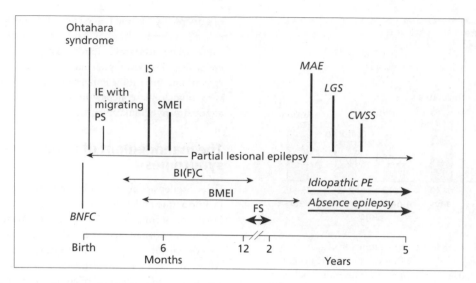

Fig. 14.2 Epilepsy syndromes as a function of their age of onset in the first 5 years of life. Syndromes with onset in childhood (beyond 2 years of age) are shown in italics. Severe epilepsy syndromes (epileptic encephalopathies) are listed above, while 'benign' or idiopathic syndromes are listed below. The thickness of the bars reflects the frequency of the syndrome. BI(F)C, benign infantile (familial) convulsions; BMEI, benign myoclonic epilepsy in infancy; BNFC, benign neonatal familial convulsions; CWSS, continuous slow waves during slow sleep; FS, febrile seizures; IE, infantile epilepsy; IS, infantile spasms; LGS, Lennox–Gastaut syndrome; MAE, myoclono-astatic epilepsy; PE, partial epilepsy; PS, partial seizures; SMEI, severe myoclonic epilepsy in infancy (Dravet's syndrome).

cephalopathy characterized by the triad of infantile spasms, arrest or regression of psychomotor development and a characteristic interictal EEG pattern (hypsarrhythmia), all occurring mainly during the first year of life. However, atypical features such as other associated seizure types (mainly partial seizures), lack of hypsarrhythmia or atypical hypsarrhythmia, normal development and onset after 1 year, are frequent and should not delay the diagnosis.

Infantile spasms have traditionally been classified into flexor, extensor or mixed flexor–extensor type, based on the pattern of the muscle contraction. However, this classification does not aid in establishing aetiology, therapeutic decisions or prognosis. What must be emphasized is the need for careful review and observation for the presence of any asymmetric spasms and/or concomitant partial onset seizures that point towards a symptomatic form of the syndrome.

The syndrome is classified as symptomatic when the aetiology has been identified, with evidence of abnormal psychomotor development, abnormal neurological signs and/or cerebral lesions or cortical atrophy identified by neuroimaging studies. Symptomatic cases are further subdivided according to prenatal, perinatal or postnatal causes. The prenatal group includes isolated cerebral malformations such as corpus callosal agenesis, sometimes associated with Aicardi's syndrome, septal aplasia and schizencephaly. This group also includes neuronal migrational disorders such as lissencephaly, particularly in the Miller–Dieker syndrome with 17p13 chromosomal deletion, focal cortical dysplasia, hemimegalencephaly, agyria–pachygyria, laminar heterotopias, bilateral perisylvian microgyria, porencephaly and microdysgenesis. Cerebral malformations associated with West's syndrome can also occur as part of neurocutaneous syndromes, such as tuberous sclerosis, neurofibromatosis type I and sebaceous naevi of Jadassohn and Sturge–Weber syndrome. Prenatal brain injury from intrauterine infections due to rubella, cytomegalovirus, toxoplasmosis and

syphilis can also lead to the development of West's syndrome. Infantile spasms occur in 1–3% of cases of Down's syndrome.

Perinatal brain injuries, including hypoxic–ischaemic encephalopathy, intraventricular and intracranial haemorrhages, and neonatal hypoglycaemia can be responsible for the subsequent development of West's syndrome. In full-term infants who survive severe hypoxic–ischaemic encephalopathy, the gradual evolution of serial EEGs has some predictive value for the later occurrence of hypsarrhythmia and West's syndrome. In addition, two-thirds of preterm infants who have cystic periventricular leukomalacia and electrographic features of irregular polyspike-wave discharges in the parietooccipital regions in early infancy develop West's syndrome.

Postnatal brain insults that may lead to West's syndrome include sudden anoxic–ischaemic events, traumatic intracranial injuries, intracranial infections, such as bacterial meningitis, abscesses and viral encephalitis, and rarely cerebral tumours. Although various inborn errors of metabolism have been associated with occurrence of West's syndrome, the most common ones are phenylketonuria, Leigh's syndrome, non-ketotic hyperglycinaemia and pyridoxine dependency. As for many other neuropsychiatric disorders in paediatrics, immunization has also been implicated in the development of West's syndrome. Nevertheless, the causal association has been disproved, as vaccination may only trigger West's syndrome in infants in whom the condition is going to develop anyway [17].

In the past, up to a third of patients who developed West's syndrome had normal neurodevelopment prior to the onset of infantile spasms, without demonstrable brain lesions at neuroimaging investigations available at the time. These cases were then classified as 'cryptogenic' by Gastaut et al., or as 'idiopathic' by Jeavons and Bower. According to the definition adopted in the 1989 classification of epilepsies and epileptic syndromes, these terms are not synonymous. Cryptogenic implies that the lesion is hidden and suspected but not demonstrable yet, whereas idiopathic implies that no known cause is expected to be responsible for the syndrome. With advances in neuroimaging techniques, the proportion of cryptogenic cases has progressively decreased. However, subtle cortical dysplasia may still be missed by MRI unless cerebral maturation and myelination is sufficient to allow clear differentiation of the grey and white matter, usually after 2 years of age. The recent availability of functional neuroimaging using PET of glucose utilization allows up to 95% of cases initially thought to be cryptogenic to be correctly classified as symptomatic. The majority of cases with unifocal or multifocal abnormalities on PET are believed to represent dysplastic cerebral lesions. This is of importance as about 20% of infants with these lesions on PET could be candidates for epilepsy surgery if they remain refractory to medical treatment.

The term 'idiopathic West's syndrome' has been used to describe the condition in some patients who recover spontaneously following a brief course of infantile spasms. Some of the more reliable features for the diagnosis of idiopathic West's syndrome include: (a) normal psychomotor development with preserved visual contact and tracking at the onset of the infantile spasm; (b) symmetric hypsarrhythmia with absence of focal EEG abnormalities (spike-and-slow-wave focus) after intravenous diazepam; and (c) reappearance of hypsarrhythmia between successive spasms in a cluster in an ictal record. Long-term follow-up of patients with idiopathic West's syndrome indicate that these infants show no adverse effects in terms of cognition, behaviour and seizure recurrence. Probably less than 5% of patients with West's syndrome have the truly idiopathic form.

West's syndrome takes a special place among childhood epilepsies because of the severe prognosis in terms of seizure recurrence and mental development, rapid deterioration of psychomotor status concomitantly with onset of the epilepsy, usual resistance to conventional AEDs, and unsatisfactory and poorly tolerated reference treatments (steroids or adrenocorticotropic hormone (ACTH)). There is evidence for some efficacy of a new compound, vigabatrin, but there are controversial guidelines on its indications because of safety issues.

Epilepsy adds its own severity to the condition, not only because of frequent seizures, but also because of interictal paroxysmal EEG activity which interferes with normal activity and impairs cognitive development. Between 35% and 85% of the patients develop mental retardation. The treatment of infantile spasms should therefore have two goals, i.e. the control of both the seizures and the hypsarrhythmia. Complete cessation of spasms is a necessary prerequisite.

Conventional AEDs and new AEDs other than vigabatrin

Infantile spasms are one of the most resistant epilepsy syndromes. In one study, 25% of the patients experienced spontaneous remission after a 1-year course of therapy that did not include hormones, but 90% of the cases remained mentally delayed [18]. Conventional AEDs are usually ineffective except for a limited number of cases. Valproate and clonazepam control about one-quarter and one-third of the cases, respectively, but relapse rate is very high [19]. Nitrazepam was as effective as ACTH in a randomized study, but there were life-threatening side-effects [8]. High-dose pyridoxine has been proposed [20], while initial promising reports with immunoglobulins were not confirmed in later studies. Worsening has been observed using carbamazepine [11].

Preliminary data suggest some improvement with lamotrigine used as add-on therapy [4]. Prolonged control of spasms was found in four out of 11 patients with refractory infantile spasms treated with add-on topiramate at very high dose, but none of these patients had received vigabatrin before [21]. Felbamate, zonisamide, the ketogenic diet and thyrotropin-releasing hormone may be occasionally helpful in refractory cases.

ACTH and corticosteroids

ACTH and corticosteroids have been considered for many years as reference treatments for infantile spasms around the world. However, tolerability is unanimously recognized as poor and there is no controlled study comparing these compounds with placebo. Efficacy of ACTH and steroids is also difficult to assess retrospectively because of differences in treatment schedules: there is no consensus about the dose, duration or type of compound (ACTH vs. steroids) in order to provide the best benefit/risk profile. Response seems to be very different according to the aetiology of spasms, but the various causes of infantile spasms are rarely specified in the published studies. The level of relapse seems to be relatively high, but long-term surveys are scarce and the benefit in terms of cognitive outcome from the control of spasms during the initial phase of the disease remains uncertain.

ACTH has been the first and most extensively studied. In the review made by Dulac and Schlumberger [22], the often recommended daily dose of 40 IU (3–6 IU/kg) controlled seizures initially in about 75% of the patients. A lower dose (20 IU) was less efficacious, while higher doses (150 IU) were more efficacious initially, even though because of relapse long-term response rates did not show significant differences between the 40 IU and 150 IU dosage regimens. A long duration of treatment (more than 5 months) at 40 IU/day in one series seemed to be more efficient than a duration of less than 1 month in another. Relapse rates ranged from 33% to 56%. Although relapse rates according to treatment duration were not reported, the lowest relapse rates were observed in patients receiving prolonged high-dose treatment. After a first relapse, a second course of therapy produced a 74% response rate. The incidence of adverse events was very high, reaching almost 100% if one considers Cushing-like effects. Other common adverse effects include infections, increased arterial blood pressure, gastritis and hyperexcitability. These are often reported as severe, with a mortality rate between 2% and 5%. Tetracosactrin (synthetic corticotropin) seems to be even less well tolerated than ACTH [23].

Oral steroids are less extensively prescribed, although they seem to be better tolerated than ACTH. With hydrocortisone, reported adverse effects rates are in the order of 17%. In a prospective, randomized, blinded study, the efficacy of prednisone (2 mg/kg/day) was inferior to that of ACTH (150 IU/day) given for 2 weeks, but no differences were found when ACTH was administered at lower doses [24,25]. There are no controlled studies comparing hydrocortisone with ACTH, but a prospective study including 94 infants, treated for 2 weeks with 15 mg/kg/day of hydrocortisone and given tetracosactrin for another 2 weeks if spasms persisted, showed that 74% of patients benefited from low doses of oral steroids, with a relapse rate of 18%. Among the 10 infants treated secondarily with tetracosactrin, nine ceased having spasms [23].

Rates for favourable cognitive outcome range from 14% to 58%, being higher in cryptogenic than in symptomatic cases. In a large series of 214 Finnish children with symptomatic infantile spasms, about 90 had normal intelligence and socioeconomic status at 20–35 years follow-up [26]. They represented 64% of the surviving patients (one-third died before 3 years of age, mostly because of infection). All patients in this report had received ACTH. This provides an important argument in favour of the prescription of this form of treatment, even in symptomatic cases.

Vigabatrin

The development of vigabatrin has totally modified the approach to the treatment of infantile spasms in recent years. Because vigabatrin provided a clear improvement over steroids or ACTH in terms of similar or even superior efficacy, better tolerability and more rapid effect, it rapidly became the drug of first choice for infantile spasms in most European centres and in most countries in which this drug was approved. Controlled data have now confirmed that this approach is justified for some aetiologies like tuberous sclerosis, but the superiority of vigabatrin over steroids or ACTH is not well established for spasms secondary to other aetiologies. Long-term data on vigabatrin efficacy as well as tolerability are still scarce, especially with respect to monotherapy use. The most alarming side-effect came to light a few years ago when vigabatrin was reported to cause visual field constriction. Although this condition is asymptomatic in more than 90% of cases, it seems to be frequent (about 30% in adults), irreversible even after stopping the drug and partly related to cumulative dose exposure. Prevalence of vigabatrin-induced visual field defects may be lower in children (19%) [10], but there are no reliable means to detect such defects before the age of 6–8 years. The efficacy data on vigabatrin should therefore be scrutinized very carefully.

Shortly after an initial add-on open study showed a complete control of spasms in 43% of 70 patients with refractory West's syndrome [27], vigabatrin was advocated for first-line monotherapy. While extensive experience in routine clinical practice appeared to confirm its efficacy as first-line treatment [28,29], four randomized studies provided more various results. One of these studies, conducted in 40 infants with infantile spasms (none of whom had tuberous sclerosis), just failed to demonstrate a significant superiority of vigabatrin over placebo ($P = 0.06$) [30]. In another randomized trial restricted to 22 infants with infantile spasms associated with tuberous sclerosis [31], vigabatrin was more efficacious than oral hydrocortisone, and it acted more rapidly and produced less side-effects compared with hydrocortisone or ACTH. On the other hand, vigabatrin was less efficacious than ACTH in a series of 42 infants with infantile spasms of various aetiology [32]. A recent study confirmed the rapid effect and the significantly higher response in tuberous sclerosis than in other aetiologies, and proved that high doses (100–150 mg/kg/day) produced the best results [33]. Asian authors reported constant relapse at doses under 60 mg/kg/day [34].

Vigabatrin-induced seizure control appears to be associated with improved intellectual outcome. In one study, control of spasms in infants with tuberous sclerosis led to a significant improvement of cognitive functions in the following 7 years [35]. Developmental quotient (DQ) significantly rose in six of the seven patients by 10 to over 45 DQ points, and autistic behaviour disappeared in five of the

six patients who manifested such behaviour. Although patients were left with visuospatial disabilities, verbal performances returned to normal. In comparison, patients in whom spasms persisted had much worse cognitive outcome, including a high incidence of autistic features.

In view of these results and the potential retinal toxicity, three points need to be addressed: (a) for which aetiologies, in addition to tuberous sclerosis, do infants benefit from vigabatrin? (b) At which point is it possible to determine that vigabatrin has been successful, or that a switch to steroids or ACTH is indicated? (c) How long should vigabatrin treatment be continued? Only incomplete answers can be drawn from the literature. With respect to the first question, in open studies vigabatrin has been reported to be more efficacious in infants with cryptogenic spasms than in those with symptomatic spasms (50% to 71% vs. 19% to 38% responder rates, respectively) [29,36]. Adding steroids or ACTH to patients not responding to vigabatrin has produced spasm-free rates of up to 100% for cryptogenic cases [29,36]. In one study, all five patients with focal cortical dysplasia treated with vigabatrin had their spasms controlled [37]. In patients with psychomotor delay before appearance of the spasms but without overt aetiology, including a negative MRI, the response is poor to both vigabatrin and steroid/ACTH monotherapy, but a few respond to a combination of these agents, provided that steroids (or ACTH) are given for more than 3 months in order to prevent relapse [29]. As for the definition of a successful response, in a series of 34 infants receiving vigabatrin as first-line monotherapy, spasms became subtle before disappearing and the disappearance of spasms preceded the disappearance of the hypsarrhythmia [38]. Hypsarrhythmia changed to multifocal spikes before complete disappearance. Therefore, definition of a successful response should require demonstration not only of disappearance of spasms, but also of disappearance of EEG spikes. This usually occurs within the first 2 weeks of vigabatrin treatment. Persistence of spikes after 2 weeks should be considered as a failed response, and the patient should be switched to steroids or ACTH. Finally, there is no consensus on the optimal duration of vigabatrin treatment. Occasional cases of relapse have been reported following vigabatrin withdrawal after more than 3 years without spasms. By contrast, five infants with infantile spasms associated with Down's syndrome were recently reported in whom vigabatrin could be stopped at the age of 15 months without relapse [39].

Proposals for the management of infantile spasms

In addition to varying availability of drugs (vigabatrin is not approved in the USA or Japan, whereas oral hydrocortisone is not available in most countries), habits play a non-rational role in the choice of the first-line treatment for infantile spasms. Vigabatrin tends to be used as first-line drug in most countries of Europe, South America and Asia, as well as in Canada. ACTH is preferred in the USA and in Japan, as well as by some European physicians because of concerns about the toxicity of vigabatrin on the retina. In some countries, steroids are only prescribed as second line after pyridoxine or high-dose valproate. Some physicians are even reluctant to administer ACTH to patients with a clear cerebral lesion, because they consider that the disadvantages related to side-effects outweigh the probability of a reasonably favourable mental outcome. The latter concern, however, does not apply to hydrocortisone [40].

Most effective drugs do have side-effects, and response to treatment is often unpredictable as a sizeable proportion of spasms are difficult to treat whereas some respond easily. Therefore, a graded therapeutic strategy should be considered, provided that it takes place within less than a month. The endpoint in treating this syndrome is clearly the cessation of spasms and the disappearence of spikes on the EEG. Vigabatrin has been shown to be efficacious not only in tuberous sclerosis, where it is the drug of choice and leads to improved cognitive functions, but also in focal cortical dysplasia and in cryptogenic cases, conditions where close to 100% of cases are controlled after vigabatrin treatment, supplemented, if necessary, with steroids or ACTH. We recommend to begin with vigabatrin 100 mg/kg/day for 1 week, and in the case of lack of or incomplete response we suggest an increase of the dosage to 150 mg/kg/day for 1 week. If there is still an incomplete response, we add hydrocortisone 15 mg/kg/day to 100 mg/kg/day vigabatrin for 2 weeks, and finally if this is still insufficient we replace hydrocortisone with ACTH.

The duration of vigabatrin treatment in controlled patients should be determined by the balance between the risk of visual field defects and the risk of relapse of seizures. On one hand, no case of visual field defect has been reported in children after less than 15 months of vigabatrin exposure [10]. On the other hand, the persistence of spikes on the EEG seems to be the best predictor of relapse of spasms, particularly in infants and in the case of cerebral lesions [38]. It is therefore reasonable to stop vigabatrin monotherapy at around 2 years of age if the EEG is normal. This practice remains questionable in children with focal malformations of cortical development, who carry the risk of suddenly developing refractory partial epilepsy when vigabatrin is discontinued (personal data).

Severe myoclonic epilepsy in infancy (Dravet's syndrome)

Among the severe childhood epilepsies listed in the classification of the International League Against Epilepsy (1989), severe myoclonic epilepsy in infancy is one of the most deleterious. Mutations in a sodium channel subunit gene, *SCN1A*, have been recently identified in some patients with this syndrome. The remarkably stereotyped clinical characteristics make this syndrome nosologically homogeneous and diagnosis is usually feasible early in the course of the disorder [42]. The first seizures always occur during the first year of life, between 2 and 9 months of age. These are convulsive tonic-clonic or clonic seizures, either generalized or affecting alternatively each side of the body. The initial seizures are often prolonged, resulting in recurrent convulsive status epilepticus lasting over 30 min. Seizures are often provoked by fever, although only a moderate increase of the temperature may be observed. Afebrile seizures also occur. Children typically have a normal perinatal history and the MRI is normal. In the initial stages of the disorder, affected patients present with normal psychomotor development, normal neurological examination and a normal EEG between seizures. This pattern changes from the second year: tonic-clonic or clonic seizures persist with the same characteristics, but additional myoclonic manifestations, atypical absences and partial seizures occur, and generalized spike and waves are observed during sleep. In addition, patients develop ataxia, hyperactivity and mental retardation.

Severe myoclonic epilepsy in infancy is one of the few epilepsy syndromes whose refractoriness is truly predictable from the onset [16,42]. Moreover mental prognosis is always poor, with an early and severe deterioration even in patients who were normal before the onset of the seizures [43]. The age of onset of mental deterioration and its magnitude are related to the frequency and the duration of seizures [43]. Therefore, AEDs that could impact positively on seizure activity would also be expected to affect favourably cognitive prognosis.

Most authors agree that the response to conventional AEDs is generally disappointing. Valproate and benzodiazepines may decrease the frequency and duration of afebrile convulsive seizures, but their effect is modest. Some investigators associate phenobarbital, phenytoin or ethosuximide with poor outcome [42]. Paradoxically, some AEDs can aggravate the seizures and should be avoided. In one study, lamotrigine induced worsening of seizures in 80% of 20 patients recruited at three epilepsy centres, generalized tonic-clonic seizures being more often exacerbated (40%) compared with myoclonic seizures (33%) [12]. Clear-cut worsening appeared within 3 months in most patients, but the worsening was insidious in some cases, resulting in stopping lamotrigine after a mean of 14 months of treatment. Improvement followed withdrawal in 95% of cases. Potential aggravation of seizures has been also described with carbamazepine and vigabatrin [11,13]. In a personal series of 46 patients, 67% of those who received lamotrigine experienced a worsening of seizures, compared with 64% of those who received vigabatrin and 61% of those who received carbamazepine [44].

Two new drugs, stiripentol and topiramate, could be helpful in some patients. Stiripentol is an investigational compound whose main action, when given as add-on therapy, consists in inhibiting the cytochrome P450 system in the liver, resulting in increased plasma concentration of concomitant AEDs, particularly clobazam. The efficacy and tolerability of stiripentol as add-on therapy in children with refractory epilepsy were first assessed in more than 200 patients in an open trial [45]. Of the 20 children with severe myoclonic epilepsy in infancy included in this trial, 10 experienced a more than 50% decrease in seizure frequency when stiripentol was used in combination with valproate and clobazam. To confirm these results, 41 children with severe myoclonic epilepsy in infancy were included in a randomized placebo-controlled trial of stiripentol at a mean dosage of 50 mg/kg/day added to valproate and clobazam [46]. Fifteen (71%) patients on stiripentol were responders for tonic-clonic seizures (including nine who became seizure free), whereas there was only one partial responder (5%) on placebo. The percentage of change in seizure frequency from baseline was higher on stiripentol (–69%) than on placebo (+7%). Twenty-one patients had moderate side-effects (drowsiness, loss of appetite) on stiripentol compared with eight on placebo. Most of these side-effects were related to a significant increase in the plasma concentration of valproic acid, clobazam and norclobazam after adding stiripentol, and disappeared when the dose of comedication was decreased. This controlled trial demonstrated the short-term value of add-on stiripentol in this difficult-to-treat syndrome. To study its long-term usefulness, we assessed retrospectively our cohort of 46 patients with severe myoclonic epilepsy in infancy treated with stiripentol in combination with valproate and clobazam [44]. None of the patients remained seizure free after a median follow-up of 3 years; however, the frequency and the duration of seizures was significantly reduced, as was the number of episodes of convulsive status epilepticus. Ten patients were dramatically improved (seizures significantly decreased in number and duration, with disappearance of episodes of status epilepticus), 20 were moderately improved (seizures significantly decreased in duration, and less frequent status epilepticus), four had no response and efficacy could not be evaluated in 12 mainly because of adverse effects. Response appeared to be better in younger patients. The most frequent adverse effects were loss of appetite and loss of weight. These were so severe in patients over 12 years that stiripentol dosage could not be increased to 50 mg/kg/day. Overall, these results suggest that stiripentol maintains its long-term efficacy, and that it should be introduced in polypharmacy as early as possible in order to prevent convulsive status epilepticus.

Topiramate has not been as extensively studied in severe myoclonic epilepsy in infancy. In two open studies conducted each in 18 patients, add-on topiramate was given at maximum dosages of 6–8 mg/kg/day and 12 mg/kg/day, respectively [47,48]. After a mean 1-year follow-up, 55% of the patients from both studies experienced a more than 50% seizure decrease and three were seizure free. No patient was aggravated, and side-effects were observed in nine and four patients, respectively. These were generally mild and transient, and related to rapid dosage titration. Adverse effects usually attributed to valproate, such as apathy and elevated blood ammonia levels, have been recently reported in patients receiving a combination of topiramate and valproate, possibly due to an interaction between these drugs. In the French and Italian experience, topiramate has been administered in 27 children with severe myoclonic epilepsy in infancy at a mean age of 12 years and added to valproate in 22, to benzodiazepines in 23 and to stiripentol in 11 [49]. Eighty-five per cent of patients were responders for generalized tonic-clonic seizures, including five who became seizure free, at a dose over 3 mg/kg/day. Behaviour improved in six patients and tolerability was acceptable, although eight patients lost weight due to loss of appetite.

In conclusion, for the treatment of severe myoclonic epilepsy in infancy we recommend to avoid carbamazepine, phenobarbital, phenytoin, vigabatrin and lamotrigine. Because of the remarkably stereotyped clinical manifestations at onset, diagnosing severe myoclonic epilepsy in infancy is usually feasible early in the course of the disorder. The diagnosis should be suspected in any infant experiencing recurrent prolonged seizures with only moderate fever (so-called 'complex febrile seizures') and can usually be confirmed as soon as afebrile seizures occur. We therefore suggest the use of AED treatment as soon as a first complex febrile seizure occurs in a young infant, as well as intermittent prophylaxis with diazepam in case of fever. Considering the risk of exacerbating seizures with phenobarbital, we recommend valproate as the first-choice drug in this context. The association of clobazam and stiripentol clearly adds benefit after the first prolonged seizure or repeated seizures, by decreasing seizure duration significantly. Topiramate may also be helpful in combination with valproate and benzodiazepines. Differential responses to AEDs in patients with severe myoclonic epilepsy in infancy could be related to the existence, in this condition, of defects affecting a sodium channel gene. This could theoretically explain why AEDs which act mainly by blocking sodium channels (carbamazepine, phenytoin and lamotrigine) do not appear to be effective and may even worsen seizures, whereas broad-spectrum

AEDs like valproate, benzodiazepines and topiramate may confer some benefit.

Myoclonic epilepsy in non-progressive encephalopathy

Non-progressive encephalopathies represent a group of conditions with various aetiologies which include pre- and perinatal anoxia–ischaemia, fetopathies and chromosome abnormality syndromes such as Angelman's syndrome. Myoclonic manifestations are one of the most usual seizure types experienced by these patients during infancy, usually very early in life. In addition to massive myoclonic manifestations as a cause of drop attacks, erratic myoclonic manifestations are frequent and often misdiagnosed [50]. They can be associated with non-convulsive status epilepticus, and they may be prolonged for weeks or months before being diagnosed on the EEG [51]. As a result, patients experience psychomotor and neurological deterioration, which simulates the deterioration typical of a progressive encephalopathy [51]. Because of the major myoclonic components, carbamazepine, phenytoin and vigabatrin carry a high risk of worsening the epileptic condition [11,13]. Valproate is usually the first-choice agent, followed by benzodiazepines. Lamotrigine has unpredictable effects, since it may be most useful in some cases and it may precipitate myoclonus in others. Piracetam provides benefit in Angelman's syndrome, due to its antimyoclonic effects, but the high doses required are difficult to administer to infants [50].

Symptomatic partial epilepsies

Diagnosing focal seizures and focal lesions is more difficult in infants than in later life. Because of the lack of subjective feedback from the patient, focal ictal symptoms are usually missed when they do not include any motor component. Because of myelinic immaturity, focal cortical dysplasia may be undetectable on MRI. As a result, pure focal epilepsies are likely to be strongly underestimated in infancy: for example, frontal epilepsy was thought to be non-existent in infants until the first video-EEG studies were performed [52]. Moreover, a large proportion of infants with partial seizures develop infantile spasms during the first year of life. Choice of AED should therefore take into account the potential risk of spasms being facilitated by administration of carbamazepine, and carbamazepine should be avoided if a close follow-up of clinical signs and EEG changes cannot be performed. Valproate should be preferred as a first-line agent, although it is often ineffective in infants with symptomatic partial epilepsy. Phenytoin and benzodiazepines are not recommended because of unfavourable pharmacokinetic and/or safety profiles in infants [2]. None of the new AEDs is approved in this age range, except for vigabatrin which can be very useful in this indication.

Partial seizures in infants are usually highly refractory and therefore surgical treatment is being considered at increasingly earlier stages. Half of the cases of partial symptomatic epilepsy in children are due to focal malformations of cortical development and low-grade tumours. In focal cortical dysplasia, intrinsic epileptogenicity sustains intractability, but 60% of the children become seizure free after surgery, provided that the entire epileptogenic area has been removed [53]. In hemimegalencephaly, except for some rare cases that are easily controlled, seizures are generally refractory and there is a risk for the contralateral hemisphere to become functionally impaired: disconnecting the malformed hemisphere should therefore be indicated as early as possible. Operating on the patients before 3 years of age leads to seizure control in 62% of cases of catastrophic epilepsies [53].

Sturge–Weber syndrome has a special place among symptomatic partial epilepsies in infancy. It is a rare condition where epilepsy can be predicted before occurrence of the first seizure based on recognition of a facial angioma located in the V1 area: more than 75% of the patients develop epilepsy, 50% of them during the first year of life. These infantile seizures often result in convulsive status epilepticus and carry great risks for motor and mental development. Starting preventive treatment has therefore been proposed. We compared 37 children with Sturge–Weber disease, of whom 16 were treated with phenobarbital before the occurrence of the first seizure and 21 were treated after the first seizures [54]. Whereas prophylactic treatment did not significantly prevent the incidence of seizures and motor deficits, it decreased the number of episodes of status epilepticus, and mental development was found to be better in the group given prophylactic treatment (44% were mentally delayed in the latter group, compared with 76% in patients started on treatment after the appearance of seizures). Although a randomized prospective study is necessary to confirm these results, Sturge–Weber disease constitutes a possible model for the study of disease modification in severe epilepsy.

Idiopathic epilepsies

Compared with catastrophic epilepsies, idiopathic (i.e. 'benign') epilepsies are very rare in infants. Infancy corresponds to a kind of hollow of their incidence, after the initial incidence peak represented by benign neonatal convulsions (whose onset is limited to the neonatal period) and before the second incidence peak related to the onset of idiopathic partial epilepsies such as benign partial epilepsy with centrotemporal spikes or idiopathic generalized epilepsies such as absence-epilepsy, which manifest themselves after 2 years of age (Fig. 14.2).

Two benign epilepsy syndromes identified during infancy, for which less than 100 patients have been reported, include benign infantile convulsions, either sporadic or familial [55,56] and benign myoclonic epilepsy in infancy [41]. All these patients fulfil the criteria of benign epilepsy, including a normal development prior to onset, no underlying disorders, no neurological abnormalities and normal interictal EEG. Seizures are easily and completely controlled by treatment, usually valproate given in monotherapy. These patients usually show a normal developmental outcome, although some learning difficulties have been reported occasionally on long-term follow-up of patients with benign myoclonic epilepsy in infancy.

Febrile seizures

Onset of febrile seizures is in infancy and young childhood, at a median age of 18 months. Most febrile seizures are simple in type, e.g. they are brief (generally < 10 or 15 min), generalized in onset and occurring only once during an illness episode. Up to a third of febrile seizures may have one or more complex features (prolonged, focal onset, multiple seizures within a single illness episode). Between 30 and 40% of children who have febrile seizures experience recurrent febrile seizures, but the vast majority encounter no substantial long-term consequences. Intellectual, educational and behavioural outcomes appear to be unaffected by the seizures [57,58].

The management of febrile seizures is discussed in detail in Chapter 15. As a general rule, continuous prophylactic treatment with phenobarbital or valproate is not indicated in children with simple febrile seizures, though intermittent rectal diazepam given at the time of the fever, or immediately after seizure onset, may be used in individual cases. Special situations when continuous prophylaxis is considered indicated include complex febrile seizures, particularly those occurring before the age of 1 year, in order to reduce the risk of febrile status epilepticus [59] and further epilepsy such as severe myoclonic epilepsy in infancy, with valproate having possibly the best benefit/risk ratio.

Initiation of treatment in infantile epilepsies

The decision to start treatment in infantile epilepsies depends to a large extent on whether the syndrome is identified, because drug choice varies depending on the syndromic form. Thus, vigabatrin is usually preferred in infantile spasms or symptomatic focal epilepsies before 6 months of age, valproate is often the first choice in generalized or focal convulsive epilepsies, including severe myoclonic epilepsy in infancy, and carbamazepine can be given in symptomatic partial epilepsies after the age of 6 months (to minimize the risk of the occurrence of spasms, which is considerable in younger age groups). If the syndrome is not identified, treatment with valproate is preferred. If there is any suspicion of an inborn error of metabolism, which represents a contraindication to the use of valproate (e.g. Alpers' disease), clobazam should be considered.

In conclusion, the prognosis of infantile epilepsies partly depends on a timely and appropriate AED choice. Diagnosis of the epilepsy syndrome is crucial in this process, since inappropriate medication can worsen the condition. There is place for the use of some new compounds as agents of first choice in this age range.

Acknowledgements

I thank Olivier Dulac and Gerard Pons for their friendly collaboration.

References

1 Morselli G, Baruzzi A. Serum levels and pharmacokinetics of anticonvulsants in the management of seizure disorders. In: Mirkin B ed. *Clinical Pharmacological Therapy*. Chicago: Yearbook Medical Publisher, 1978: 89–106.
2 Sicca F, Contaldo A, Rey E, Dulac O. Phenytoin administration in the newborn and infant. *Brain Dev* 2000; 22: 35–40.
3 Rey E, Pons G, Richard MO et al. Pharmacokinetics of the individual enantiomers of vigabatrin (gamma-vinyl GABA) in epileptic children. *Br J Clin Pharmacol* 1990; 30: 253–7.
4 Mikati MA, Fayad M, Koleilat M et al. Efficacy, tolerability, and kinetics of lamotrigine in infants. *J Pediatr* 2002; 141: 31–5.
5 Schwabe MJ, Wheless JW. Clinical experience with topiramate dosing and serum levels in children 12 years or under with epilepsy. *J Child Neurol* 2001; 16: 806–8.

6 Dreifuss F, Santili N, Langer DH *et al*. Valproic acid hepatic fatalities: a retrospective review. *Neurology* 1987; 37: 379–85.

7 Farwell JR, Lee YJ, Hirtz DG *et al*. Phenobarbital for febrile seizures—effects on intelligence and on seizure recurrence. *N Engl J Med* 1990; 322: 364–9.

8 Dreifuss F, Farwell J, Holmes G *et al*. Infantile spasms. Comparative trial of nitrazepam and corticotropin. *Arch Neurol* 1986; 43: 1107–10.

9 Aicardi J, Mumford JP, Dumas C, Wood S. Vigabatrin as initial therapy for infantile spasms: a European retrospective survey. Sabril IS, Investigator and Peer Review Groups. *Epilepsia* 1996; 37: 638–42.

10 Vanhatalo S, Nousiainen I, Eriksson K *et al*. Visual field constriction in 91 Finnish children treated with vigabatrin. *Epilepsia* 2002; 43: 748–56.

11 Talwar D, Arora MS, Sher PK. EEG changes and seizure exacerbation in young children treated with carbamazepine. *Epilepsia* 1994; 35: 1154–9.

12 Guerrini R, Dravet C, Genton, P. *et al*. Lamotrigine and seizure aggravation in severe myoclonic epilepsy. *Epilepsia* 1998; 39: 508–12.

13 Lortie A, Chiron C, Mumford J, Dulac O. The potential for increasing seizure frequency, relapse, and appearance of new seizure types with vigabatrin. *Neurology* 1993; 43 (Suppl. 5): S24–S27.

14 Commission on Classification and Terminology of the International League Against Epilepsy. Proposal for revised classification of epilepsies and epileptic syndromes. *Epilepsia* 1989; 30: 389–99.

15 Coppola G, Plouin P, Chiron C, Robain O, Dulac O., Migrating partial seizures in infancy: a malignant disorder with developmental arrest. *Epilepsia* 1995; 36: 1017–24.

16 Arroyo S, Brodie MJ, Avanzini G *et al*. Is refractory epilepsy preventable? *Epilepsia* 2002; 43: 437–44.

17 Bellman MH Ross EM, Miller DL. Infantile spasms and pertussis immunization. *Lancet* 1983; 1: 1031–4.

18 Hrachovy RA, Glaze DG, Frost JD Jr. A retrospective study of spontaneous remission and long-term outcome in patients with infantile spasms. *Epilepsia* 1991; 32: 212–14.

19 Siemes H, Spohr HL, Michael T, Nau H. Therapy of infantile spasms with valproate: results of a prospective study. *Epilepsia* 1988; 29: 553–60.

20 Takuma Y. ACTH therapy for infantile spasms: a combination therapy with high-dose pyridoxal phosphate and low-dose ACTH. *Epilepsia* 1998; 39 (Suppl. 5): 42–5.

21 Glauser TA, Clark PO, McGee K. Long-term response to topiramate in patients with West syndrome. *Epilepsia* 2000; 41 (Suppl. 1): S91–S94.

22 Dulac O, Schlumberger E. Treatment of West syndrome. In: Wyllie E, ed. *The Treatment of Epilepsy: principles and practice*. Philadelphia: Lea and Febiger, 1993: 595–604.

23 Schlumberger E, Dulac O. A simple, effective and well-tolerated treatment regime for West syndrome. *Dev Med Child Neurol* 1994; 36: 863–72.

24 Baram TZ, Mitchell WG, Tournay A *et al*. High-dose corticotropin (ACTH) versus prednisone for infantile spasms: a prospective, randomized, blinded study. *Pediatrics* 1996; 97: 375–9.

25 Hrachovy RA, Frost JD Jr, Kellaway P, Zion TE. Double-blind study of ACTH vs prednisone therapy in infantile spasms. *J Pediatr* 1983; 103: 641–5.

26 Riikonen R. Long-term outcome of patients with West syndrome. *Brain Dev* 2001; 23: 683–7.

27 Chiron C, Dulac O, Beaumont D, Palacios L, Pajot N, Mumford J. Therapeutic trial of vigabatrin in refractory infantile spasms. *J Child Neurol* 1991; (Suppl. 2): S52–S59.

28 Fejerman N, Cersosimo R, Caraballo R *et al*. Vigabatrin as a first-choice drug in the treatment of West syndrome. *J Child Neurol* 2000; 15: 161–5.

29 Villeneuve N, Soufflet C, Plouin P, Chiron C, Dulac O. Treatment of infantile spasms with vigabatrin as first-line therapy and in monotherapy: apropos of 70 infants. *Arch Pediatr* 1998; 5: 731–8.

30 Appleton RE, Peters AC, Mumford JP, Shaw DE. Randomised, placebo-controlled study of vigabatrin as first-line treatment of infantile spasms. *Epilepsia* 1999; 40: 1627–33.

31 Chiron C, Dumas C, Jambaque I, Mumford J, Dulac O. Randomized trial comparing vigabatrin and hydrocortisone in infantile spasms due to tuberous sclerosis. *Epilepsy Res* 1997; 26: 389–95.

32 Vigevano F, Cilio MR. Vigabatrin versus ACTH as first-line treatment for infantile spasms: a randomized, prospective study. *Epilepsia* 1997; 38: 1270–4.

33 Elterman RD, Shields WD, Mansfield KA, Nakagawa J. Randomized trial of vigabatrin in patients with infantile spasms. *Neurology* 2001; 57: 1416–21.

34 Tay SK, Ong HT, Low PS. The use of vigabatrin in infantile spasms in Asian children. *Ann Acad Med Singapore* 2001; 30: 26–31.

35 Jambaque I, Chiron C, Dumas C, Mumford J, Dulac O. Mental and behavioural outcome of infantile epilepsy treated by vigabatrin in tuberous sclerosis patients. *Epilepsy Res* 2000; 38: 151–60.

36 Granstrom ML, Gaily E, Liukkonen E. Treatment of infantile spasms: results of a population-based study with vigabatrin as the first drug for spasms. *Epilepsia* 1999; 40: 950–7.

37 Lortie A, Plouin P, Chiron C, Delalande O, Dulac O. Characteristics of epilepsy in focal cortical dysplasia in infancy. *Epilepsy Res* 2002; 51: 133–45.

38 Gaily E, Liukkonen E, Paetau R, Rekola R, Granstrom ML. Infantile spasms: diagnosis and assessment of treatment response by video-EEG. *Dev Med Child Neurol* 2001; 43: 658–67.

39 Nabbout R, Melki I, Gerbaka B, Dulac O, Akatcherian C. Infantile spasms in Down syndrome: good response to a short course of vigabatrin. *Epilepsia* 2001; 42: 1580–3.

40 Velez A, Dulac O, Plouin P. Prognosis for seizure control in infantile spasms preceded by other seizures. *Brain Dev* 1990; 12: 306–9.

41 Dravet C, Bureau M, Genton P. Benign myoclonic epilepsy of infancy: electroclinical symptomatology and differential diagnosis from the other types of generalized epilepsy of infancy. *Epilepsy Res* 1992; 6 (Suppl.): 131–5.

42 Dravet C, Bureau M, Guerrini R, Giraud N, Roger J. Severe myoclonic epilepsy in infants. In: Roger J *et al*. eds. *Epileptic Syndromes in Infancy, Children and Adolescence*, 2nd edn. London: John Libbey & Company, 1992: 75–88.

43 Casse-Perrot C, Wolf M, Dravet C. Neuropsychological aspects of severe myoclonic epilepsy in infancy. In: Jambaque I, Lassonde M, Dulac O, eds. *Neuropsychology of Childhood Epilepsy*. New York: Kluwer Academic/Plenum Publishers, 2001: 131–40.

44 Nguyen Thanh T, Chiron C, Dellatolas G, Rey E, Pons G, Vincent J, Dulac O. Long term efficacy and tolerability of stiripentol in severe myoclonic epilepsy of infancy (Dravet syndrome). *Arch Pediatr* 2002; 9: 1120–7.

45 Perez J, Chiron C, Musial C *et al*. Stiripentol: efficacy and tolerability in children with epilepsy. *Epilepsia* 1999; 40: 1618–26.

46 Chiron C, Marchand MC, Tran A *et al*. Stiripentol in severe myoclonic epilepsy in infancy: a randomised placebo-controlled syndrome-dedicated trial. STICLO study group. *Lancet* 2000; 356: 1638–42.

47 Coppola G, Capovilla G, Montagnini A *et al*. Topiramate as add-on drug in severe myoclonic epilepsy in infancy: an Italian multicenter open trial. *Epilepsy Res* 2002; 49: 45–8.

48 Nieto-Barrera M, Candau R, Nieto-Jimenez M, Correa A, del Portal LR. Topiramate in the treatment of severe myoclonic epilepsy in infancy. *Seizure* 2000; 9: 590–4.

49 Villeneuve N, Portilla P, Ferrari AR, Dulac O, Chauvel P, Dravet C. Topiramate (TPM) in severe myoclonic epilepsy in infancy (SMEI): study of 27 patients. *Epilepsia* 2002; 43: 155.

50 Guerrini R, De Lorey TM, Bonanni P *et al*. Cortical myoclonus in Angelman syndrome. *Ann Neurol* 1996; 40: 39–48.

51 Dalla Bernardina, B, Fontana E, Sgro V, Colamaria V, Elia M. Myoclonic epilepsy ('myoclonic status epilepticus') in the non progressive encephalopathies. In: Roger J *et al*. eds. *Epileptic Syndromes in Infancy, Children and Adolescence*, 2nd edn. London: John Libbey & Company, 1992: 89–96.

52 Rathgeb JP, Plouin P, Soufflet C, Cieuta C, Chiron C, Dulac O. Le cas particulier des crises partielles du nourrisson: sémiologie clinique. In: Bureau M, Kahane P, Munari C, eds. *Epilepsies Partielles Graves Pharmaco-résistantes de l'Enfant*. London: John Libbey Eurotext, 1998: 122–34.

53 Duchowny M, Jayakar P, Resnick T *et al*. Epilepsy surgery in the first three years of life. *Epilepsia* 1998; 39: 737–43.

54 Ville D, Enjolras O, Chiron C, Dulac O. Prophylactic antiepileptic treatment in Sturge-Weber disease. *Seizure* 2002; 11: 145–50.

55 Vigevano F, Fusco L, Di Capua M, Ricci S, Sebastianelli R, Lucchini P. Benign infantile familial convulsions. *Eur J Pediatr* 1992; 151: 608–12.

56 Watanabe K, Yamamoto N, Negoro T, Takahashi I, Aso K, Maehara M. Benign infantile epilepsy with complex partial seizures. *J Clin Neurophysiol* 1990; 7: 409–16.

57 Annegers JF, Hauser WA, Shirts SB, Kurland LT. Factors prognostic of unprovoked seizures after febrile convulsions. *N Engl J Med* 1987; 316: 493–8.

58 Ellenberg JH, Nelson KB. Sample selection and the natural history of disease. Studies of febrile seizures. *JAMA* 1980; 243: 1337–40.

59 Nelson KB, Ellenberg JH. Predictors of epilepsy in children who have experienced febrile seizures. *N Engl J Med* 1976; 295: 1029–3.

15 Management of Epilepsy in Children

W.-L. Lee and H.-T. Ong

Infancy and early childhood are high incidence periods for epilepsy. Aetiologies, clinical features and response to treatment of epilepsies in this age group differ significantly from those observed in adult epilepsies. Paediatric patients may respond differently to antiepileptic drugs (AEDs) both pharmacodynamically and pharmacokinetically. Finally, both seizures and AEDs may affect behaviour, learning, schooling, social and emotional development. Although the general rules of epilepsy treatment outlined in other chapters in this book generally apply to children, especially those with epilepsies of relatively late onset, these rules may require considerable modifications in younger patients or in individual syndromes (Table 15.1).

The clinical manifestations of certain paediatric epilepsies differ greatly from those observed in adults. Such differences are probably due to immaturity of brain development and function. In some cases, they may reflect fundamental differences in epileptogenic mechanisms. This is probably the case in syndromes such as infantile spasms and other epileptic encephalopathies that respond to unconventional therapies such as adrenocorticotropic hormone or corticosteroids.

The causes of epilepsies of early onset often differ from those in adults. Specifically, diffuse brain damage of prenatal or early postnatal origin is more common than acquired lesions. Hence, assessment of young children with epilepsy will require special attention to overall mental and neurological development. Approximately 20–30% of children with epilepsy have mental retardation and/or learning problems. In many cases, intellectual impairment is a more important problem than seizures. Careful psychological assessment is essential to define the patient's strengths and weaknesses and enable tailoring of the educational programme. On the other hand, many childhood epilepsies are idiopathic, age related and benign, associated with normal neurodevelopmental status and eventual total remission. In such patients, an optimistic prognosis, avoidance of overmedication and minimal restrictions will ensure the best possible psychosocial outcome.

The impact of having epilepsy on the life of children is very different from that in adults. Growing up with seizures may affect personality development and will interfere with many aspects of everyday life, schooling and choice of career. Sociopsychological support for the child and family is an important part of management, as is sensible counselling about the risk from seizures and the manner of dealing with it. Although factual information in this regard is limited in children, common sense indicates that patients with epilepsy should lead a lifestyle that is as normal as possible. Small increases in risk are to be preferred to extensive prohibitions. This should be discussed fully with the patient and family. Certain types of childhood epilepsy, such as the Lennox–Gastaut syndrome

and other syndromes associated with drop attacks, however, require special precautions because of repeated falls, and these epilepsies inevitably interfere with daily activities. Special schooling may be required for such patients and protection of the head and face by wearing an adequate helmet is an essential measure. In all cases, a confident relationship between the physician and family is essential. Adequate time should be devoted to explaining the aims and shortcomings of therapy, probable duration of treatment and problems that may arise upon discontinuation of therapy.

Drug regimens in young patients often have to be different from those in adults, not just because of differences in body weight but because of changes in pharmacokinetics with age. Absorption of AEDs is usually faster in infants and young children than in adults, partly due to more frequent use of liquid formulations in the younger age groups. The half-lives of most AEDs are quite prolonged in the first 1–3 weeks of life and drastically shorten thereafter. High metabolic rates are maintained during the first years of life until a marked slowing to adult values occurs at adolescence. The high metabolic rates account for higher doses per unit of weight required by children, and abrupt changes in drug clearance explain the therapeutic difficulties encountered in the neonatal period and at adolescence. The above facts are generalizations and the pattern of change in pharmacokinetics varies from one AED to another. The pharmacokinetics of phenytoin in very young patients is particularly unpredictable and makes its usage in this age group difficult. In neonates and young children, phenytoin absorption is often incomplete and erratic, and the metabolism of phenytoin is much faster in children than in adults, with half-lives of 5–18 h and 10–34 h, respectively. Hence, paediatric patients often require very large oral doses of phenytoin to achieve therapeutic levels, and because of Michaelis–Menten kinetics slight changes in dosage may result in subtherapeutic levels or drug toxicity.

The pharmacodynamic effects of AEDs may not be the same in infants and children compared with adults. A classic example is the paradoxical effect of barbiturates and benzodiazepines, which often cause excitation rather than sedation in young subjects. Moreover, toxicity of AEDs is difficult to recognize in young infants and retarded children, so these groups may require special surveillance. Some AEDs may be more toxic in young patients than in adults. For example, the risk of valproate-induced liver failure is much greater in patients aged less than 2 years than in older patients. The possible effects of some AEDs on intellectual development are also of concern [1,2] although there is no agreement on the magnitude of such effects [3].

The factors which determine when to start AED therapy in children differ somewhat from those in adults. Epilepsy is not a homogeneous disease. There are many seizure types and epilepsy syndromes with different aetiologies, consequences and prognoses, each of which may have different implications for individual patients. Hence indications for treatment also vary. The consequences of the seizures depend on the type and timing of the attacks, the age and condition of the patient, the patient's daily activities and the reaction of the patient and the family to the seizures. Hence, each patient must be considered individually and the impact of further seizures weighed against the potential side-effects of treatment. The younger the patient, the less likely he or she would be unsupervised or in a potentially dangerous situation if seizures were to occur. Hence, the need to start AED after a first seizure is less pressing. Ultimately, the decision whether or not to start AED rests with the patient and the family.

In children, administration of AEDs in more than two daily doses is best avoided, as a midday dose has often to be taken at school. This is difficult to control and may cause embarrassment for the child. Slow-release preparations of carbamazepine and sodium valproate have made it possible to maintain adequate plasma levels with twice daily dosing.

The use of the newly marketed AEDs in paediatrics has not been as extensively studied as in adults and these drugs should seldom, if ever, be used as first-line AEDs in paediatric patients, except for special situations (e.g. vigabatrin in West's syndrome associated with tuberous sclerosis). The choice of AEDs in children may be more dependent on the epilepsy syndrome than is the case in adult epilepsies (Table 15.2).

Table 15.1 Specific aspects which explain why the treatment of epilepsy in childhood differs from that in adult life

Different spectrum of aetiologies
Different paediatric epilepsy syndromes
Different seizure manifestations (due to immature brain development)
Evolution of clinical manifestations may occur in young patients (as the brain matures)
Greater impact of psychosocial factors
Distinctive AED pharmacokinetics
Distinctive AED pharmacodynamics
Specific therapies (corticotropins, corticosteroids, ketogenic diet)

Treatment of the major epilepsies of childhood will be discussed below.

Febrile seizures

Febrile seizures represent the most common and benign of all the epilepsy syndromes. A febrile seizure is a seizure event which occurs in infancy or childhood, usually between 3 months and 5 years of age, and is associated with fever without evidence of intracranial infection or other defined cause. Seizures with fever in children who have suffered a previous non-febrile seizure are excluded. Most febrile seizures are brief, generalized convulsions. Features of febrile seizures which have been found to be correlated with an increased risk for epilepsy [4,5] include: (a) a duration longer than 15–30 min; (b) more than one seizure in 24 h; and (c) seizures with focal features or followed by Todd's paralysis. Whilst a third of the patients will have a second febrile seizure, only 2–4% subsequently will develop epilepsy [4,5].

Acute management

Any child admitted with ongoing febrile seizures should be promptly treated. The use of rectal liquid diazepam has been documented in several uncontrolled studies [6,7]. The efficacy of rectal diazepam gel in terminating seizures has also been demonstrated in several small randomized open studies comparing it with intravenous diazepam in the prehospital treatment of children with status epilepticus of all types [8]. Thus, firm pharmacological and clinical evidence suggests that rectal diazepam in solution or gel effectively treats ongoing seizures and is a rational alternative to intravenous treatment. Diazepam suppository absorption through the rectal mucosa is slow, taking at least 15–20 min or more to reach anticonvulsant levels; whilst intramuscular diazepam has erratic and often slow absorption. Hence suppositories and intramuscular administration of diazepam are not suitable for treatment of ongoing seizures. The dose of rectal diazepam is 0.5 mg/kg/dose. If the seizure continues for more than 5 min, the same dose is repeated. In a prehospital setting, a maximum of two doses should be given. The risk of adverse events with this regime is minimal. If the seizures continue or recur, the child should be referred to a hospital. In a

Table 15.2 Drugs of choice for some common paediatric epilepsy syndromes

Epilepsy syndrome	Drugs of choice
Febrile seizures	Intermittent rectal diazepam[a]
West's syndrome	Vigabatrin, ACTH
Lennox–Gastaut syndrome	Valproate, lamotrigine, topiramate, clobazam
Benign epilepsy of childhood with centrotemporal spikes	Carbamazepine, valproate[a]
Early onset benign occipital seizures	Intermittent rectal diazepam[a]
Late onset childhood idiopathic occipital seizures	Carbamazepine
Childhood absence epilepsy	Valproate, ethosuximide, lamotrigine
Juvenile absence epilepsy	Valproate, ethosuximide, lamotrigine
Juvenile myoclonic epilepsy	Valproate, lamotrigine
Cryptogenic and symptomatic partial epilepsies	Carbamazepine, valproate

[a] No treatment may be preferable in many patients.

hospital setting diazepam is given intravenously 0.2–0.5 mg/kg up to a total (rectal plus intravenous dose) of 2–3 mg/kg over 30 min. A total dose of 20–30 mg diazepam is often required, but higher doses are usually not helpful.

Diazepam-resistant seizures should be treated with standard treatment protocols for convulsive status epilepticus [9,10]. A full discussion of this topic is outside the scope of this chapter. Note, however, that drugs such as phenytoin or phosphenytoin, which are ineffective in preventing recurrent febrile seizures, are effective in the treatment of all forms of convulsive status epilepticus, including febrile status epilepticus [9,10].

Long-term management

A rationale approach to long-term management needs to be based on the prognosis for the patient, which is usually excellent, as well as family circumstances.

Parental counselling

This is the most important but often neglected aspect of long-term management. The parents should be reassured that brain damage is highly unlikely after febrile seizures and that the risk of epilepsy is very small. However, the risk of subsequent febrile seizures is significant and parents should be told to stay calm, to place the child on the side, not to force anything between the teeth and, if appropriate, to administer rectal diazepam. If the seizure lasts more than 10 min, then the child should be brought immediately to the nearest medical facility.

Management of fever

There is no evidence that antipyretics prevent febrile seizures. A British study found that children with an initial febrile seizure had received an appropriate dose of antipyretics within an hour or two of the seizure [11]. A Canadian study found no clear benefits with regards to recurrence risk from intensive antipyretic instructions to parents [12]. A Finnish study randomized children to receive placebo or paracetamol at the time of illness for 2 years following a febrile seizure [13]. Again, there was no effect on recurrence of febrile seizures.

At present, the only apparent effect of antipyretics on febrile seizures may be to increase 'fever phobia'. This may be contrasted with the increasing evidence of beneficial effects of fever during recovery from infections. The compulsive use of antipyretics cannot be recommended, other than to make the patient more comfortable. Because sponging the child is ineffective to reduce body temperature and is uncomfortable, it should be abandoned [14].

Continuous prophylaxis vs. intermittent treatment of febrile seizures with anticonvulsants

Although studies have not been designed to answer this question directly, some data are available from studies designed to determine whether AEDs prevent recurrent febrile seizures. These studies find that prophylactic anticonvulsants, while reducing the risk of recurrent febrile seizure, do not prevent the occurrence of subsequent unprovoked seizures [15]. There are case reports of children

adequately treated with AEDs who went on to develop epilepsy [16].

Some studies have reported that continuous daily treatment with phenobarbital or valproate decreases the risk of recurrent febrile seizures [17,18]. Most of these studies have excluded from analysis patients with poor compliance or low serum drug levels. Other studies have questioned the efficacy of treatment, and a pooled data analysis from Great Britain [19] found that the odds of experiencing a recurrent febrile seizure in children prescribed either phenobarbital or valproate was not significantly lower than those for the untreated control groups. Two randomized trials [1,20] which examined selected populations of children with febrile seizures at increased risk for subsequent seizures, analysed according to intention to treat, also failed to demonstrate efficacy of phenobarbital or valproate in preventing recurrence of the seizures.

Phenobarbital is widely used in children with febrile seizures, in spite of its well-documented behavioural side-effects. There has also been concern about possible cognitive side-effects, although this has been less well documented. Farwell et al. [1] in 1990 studied 217 children between 8 and 36 months of age who had had at least one febrile seizure and were at increased risk of further seizures (early, complex or repeated febrile seizures). They compared the IQs of a group randomly assigned to daily doses of phenobarbital (4–5 mg/kg/day) with the IQs of a group randomly assigned to placebo. After 2 years, the mean IQ was 7.03 (corrected) points lower in the group assigned to phenobarbital than in the placebo group ($P=0.006$). Six months later, after phenobarbital had been tapered and discontinued, the mean IQ was 4.3 points lower in the group assigned to phenobarbital ($P=0.092$). The proportion of children remaining free of subsequent seizures did not differ significantly between the treatment groups. This study, however, has been criticized for methodological flaws, and the slightly lower IQ scores 6 months after discontinuation of phenobarbital compared to the placebo group did not reach statistical significance [2]. Therefore, doubts still remain about the effect of long-term phenobarbital on cognitive function.

Valproate has been found to be effective in the prevention of febrile seizure recurrence by McKinlay and Newton [20], and the incidence of side-effects with this drug is very low. However, rare but life-threatening complications such as pancreatitis and acute liver failure have been reported and make valproate an inappropriate medication in a relatively benign disorder such as febrile seizures. Carbamazepine [21] and phenytoin [22] are both ineffective in preventing the recurrence of febrile seizures.

Based on the findings summarized above, continuous pharmacological prophylaxis should generally be avoided in children with febrile seizures (an exception to this rule may be represented by complex febrile seizures, particularly those occurring before the age of 1 year, as discussed in Chapter 14). Instead, consideration should be given to the possibility of prescribing a rapidly acting drug only when the child becomes febrile. A French randomized study of oral diazepam at the time of illness after a first febrile seizure, however, found the drug ineffective [23] and a larger study found a modest reduction in recurrence of febrile seizures with intermittent oral diazepam, 0.33 mg/kg every 8 h during illness (recurrence rate for treated patients 21% compared with 31% for placebo). Forty per cent of children experienced significant side-effects, which included lethargy, ataxia and irritability [24]. A Finnish study also failed to find any benefit from intermittent oral diazepam at doses of 0.2 mg/kg, given every 8 h when the child was febrile, during the 2 years after a first febrile seizure [13]. In one large American study, 30% of children with a febrile seizure were not recognized as being febrile before the convulsion; in these cases, seizures cannot be prevented by intermittent prophylactic treatment [25].

Intermittent rectal diazepam is more effective than oral diazepam as a preventive treatment against the recurrence of febrile seizures. Rectal diazepam is rapidly absorbed and can produce effective anticonvulsant serum levels within minutes. When used as prophylaxis against febrile seizures, diazepam solution or rectal capsules can be administered rectally every 12 h when the child has a fever (38.5°C). Intermittent diazepam prophylaxis by way of a few doses each year reduces the recurrence rate by one-half or two-thirds [6]. Transient apnoea may occur, but serious side-effects are remarkably rare [26].

Because a brief febrile seizure does not pose any risk, an alternative and more practical strategy is home treatment with rectal diazepam as soon as a seizure begins. This approach will prevent prolonged seizures and eliminates the unnecessary administration of the drug for febrile illnesses which do not cause seizures. Parents should be advised not to administer rectal diazepam if the seizure has already stopped.

A recent study from Israel [27] suggested that intranasal midazolam at 0.2 mg/kg was as effective as intravenous diazepam in arresting febrile seizures. Because of the extra time required to set up an intravenous line in a seizing child, the interval between arriving at the emergency department seizing and the time of termination of the seizure was shorter in the intranasal midazolam group compared to the intravenous diazepam group. If these findings are replicated, intranasal midazolam may become the treatment of choice for the therapy of febrile seizures.

There does not seem to be any compelling reason to treat children with drugs on a daily or intermittent basis after a first or second febrile seizure, because the potential side-effects of the drugs outweigh their benefits. Even most children with multiple recurrent febrile seizures do not require drug treatment. If treatment is to be offered, the use of liquid rectal diazepam to be given at home at the time of an actual seizure is recommended, the benefit being prevention of a prolonged seizure. Alternatively, intermittent rectal diazepam at the time of illness might be considered. This treatment is appropriate for a well-organized family with only a few individuals caring for the child.

West's syndrome

The presentation and management of West's syndrome are discussed in detail in Chapter 14.

Lennox–Gastaut syndrome

Lennox–Gastaut syndrome is an age-dependent epileptic encephalopathy occurring in childhood, with devastating and intractable seizures associated with developmental regression or arrest. The characteristic features of the syndrome include: (a) polymorphic epileptic seizures, including tonic seizures, atypical absences and astatic seizures (drop attacks); (b) EEG abnormalities consisting of diffuse slow-spike-wave discharges in the presence of an abnormal background, and paroxysms of fast rhythms at 10–12 Hz, which may be associated with a tonic seizure; and (c) cognitive dysfunction and/or personality disorders.

With regards to symptomatology, Gastaut et al. in 1966 emphasized the occurrence of tonic seizures in wakefulness but most often during slow-wave sleep, when they are not recognized or are subclinical. Tonic seizures are reported in up to 75% of patients with Lennox–Gastaut syndrome. During these seizures, complete loss of consciousness may not always occur. The ictal EEG during tonic seizures often shows bursts of fast rhythmic spike discharges, or a sudden flattening of the background, or a combination of the two sometimes preceded by generalized spike-and-wave discharges. Atypical absences are also a common clinical feature but they are difficult to detect because the onset and termination are gradual, with incomplete impairment of consciousness that may allow the patient to continue with some voluntary activity. Runs of diffuse slow-spike-wave discharges could be interictal, or ictal when they correlate with clinical atypical absences. The presence of diffuse slow-spike-wave discharges alone is an insufficient criterion to diagnose Lennox–Gastaut syndrome, as these can also occur in other severe symptomatic epilepsies, and in partial epilepsies with secondary bilateral synchrony, without the presence of typical tonic seizures. In Lennox–Gastaut syndrome, the presentation may also include epileptic 'falls' or 'drop attacks' that could be the result of astatic, tonic or myoclonic seizures. The EEG correlates for these seizure types are less precise and could include slow-spike-waves, slow-polyspike-waves and diffuse electrodecremental response. Besides these seizure types, partial onset seizures, generalized tonic-clonic seizures or generalized clonic seizures could also be present but they are not an essential part of the syndrome. In addition to the high seizure frequency, about 50–97% of patients experience status epilepticus, either as non-convulsive status epilepticus with fluctuating confusional states lasting up to weeks or as tonic status epilepticus.

Based on the absence or presence of an aetiological diagnosis and/or evidence of neurological abnormalities prior to the onset of Lennox–Gastaut syndrome, patients can be classified as cryptogenic or symptomatic. This is a useful classification because cryptogenic cases have a better prognosis. Cryptogenic Lennox–Gastaut syndrome occurs in a previously normal child, usually between the age of 1 and 8 years, without any evidence of neurological abnormality and with normal neuroimaging studies. Cryptogenic cases account for up to 30% of all patients who develop Lennox–Gastaut syndrome. Symptomatic Lennox–Gastaut syndrome occurs in patients who had prior cerebral abnormalities and/or neurological insults, and the age of onset of these cases could extend up to 15 years. For symptomatic cases with onset in late infancy, the syndrome usually represents an evolution of West's syndrome, and almost 50% of infants with symptomatic West's syndrome go on to develop Lennox–Gastaut syndrome [28]. This can occur in two ways, i.e. the infantile spasms continue without remission and are gradually replaced by tonic seizures, or the infantile spasms disappear with EEG resolution of hypsarrhythmia, associated with improvement in psychomotor development for a period of time before the onset of Lennox–Gastaut syndrome. Lennox–Gastaut syndrome could also develop in patients with a previous diagnosis of symptomatic partial epilepsy.

The causes underlying symptomatic Lennox–Gastaut syndrome are similar to those underlying symptomatic West's syndrome.

These include the broad categories of cerebral malformations or dysgenesis, with the exception of Aicardi's syndrome and lissencephaly, neurocutaneous syndromes, particularly tuberous sclerosis and hypoxic–ischaemic brain injury, central nervous system infection, traumatic brain injury, brain tumour and rarely mitochondrial cytopathies. The onset of Lennox–Gastaut syndrome in patients with Down's syndrome tends to be late, beyond 10 years of age.

Cognitive dysfunction or decline may not be evident at the onset or in the initial stages of Lennox–Gastaut syndrome. However, psychomotor retardation is detected eventually in up to 96% of patients. Adverse prognostic factors for intellectual deterioration include the development of Lennox–Gastaut syndrome prior to 3 years of age, frequent seizures and/or status epilepticus and a symptomatic classification, especially in infants with a previous diagnosis of West's syndrome. This could be compounded by the adverse effects of polypharmacy or rapid escalation of doses in an attempt to control the seizures. In older children, behavioural and personality disorders such as short attention span, aggressiveness and disinhibition make the implementation of specialized education and social integration difficult.

Effective treatment of Lennox–Gastaut syndrome remains one of the greatest challenges of paediatric epileptology. Although monotherapy is preferred, the intractability of this syndrome together with the multiple seizure types often necessitate polytherapy. Based on its broad spectrum of activity, especially against myoclonic seizures, atypical absences and astatic seizures, valproic acid is the mainstay of treatment for most patients. This drug, however, should be prescribed with caution in patients below 3 years of age, especially when an underlying inborn error of metabolism contraindicating its use has not been excluded, due to the risk of fatal hepatic failure. Prior to the availability of the newer AEDs, the addition of a benzodiazepine when valproic acid proved ineffective was usual. Although both clonazepam and nitrazepam have been extensively used in Lennox–Gastaut syndrome, there is some evidence that clobazam is associated with much less sedation [29,30], which is advantageous because drowsiness could activate tonic seizures. Nevertheless, the efficacy of clobazam is limited by the development of tolerance in up to 40% of patients [31]. For some of these, withdrawing the drug for 2–3 weeks may allow successful control of seizures with subsequent reintroduction of treatment [29]. The efficacy of other first-generation AEDs, such as phenytoin, carbamazepine and barbiturates, has not been demonstrated in controlled trials, and in general these drugs produce little benefit. Carbamazepine, though useful for partial onset and tonic seizures, could in itself precipitate generalized seizures. Barbiturates increase the hyperactivity and behavioural disorders often present in children with Lennox–Gastaut syndrome, and their sedative effects could also precipitate further tonic seizures. Phenytoin is useful against tonic seizures and tonic status epilepticus, but is not effective in controlling astatic seizures and atypical absences.

Great enthusiasm and hope followed the report that the new AED felbamate was also effective in treating Lennox–Gastaut syndrome, reducing seizure frequency, in particular atonic and tonic-clonic seizures, as well as improving global evaluation scores [32]. Its long-term efficacy was also documented by a 12-month open-label follow-up [33]. However, initial enthusiasms were dampened considerably when reports of severe adverse effects appeared, including

fatalities from aplastic anaemia [34] and hepatotoxicity [35]. Based on the combined risk for both of these complications of about 1 in 4600 patients, and risk of fatality of 1 in 9300 [35], a consensus recommendation soon followed limiting the use of felbamate in Lennox–Gastaut syndrome to patients not responding to other appropriate AEDs [36]. This effectively excluded consideration of felbamate as either the first- or second-line AED in the management of Lennox–Gastaut syndrome.

At about the time felbamate began to fall out of favour, two clinical trials showed that another new AED, lamotrigine, was effective in patients with Lennox–Gastaut syndrome [37], as well as in a group of paediatric patients with refractory generalized epilepsies which also included Lennox–Gastaut syndrome in two-thirds of cases [38]. Besides the occurrence of drug-induced rash, and the rare but potentially fatal risk of Stevens–Johnson syndrome, lamotrigine is well tolerated. The incidence of rash can be minimized by a very slow dose titration schedule, especially in children comedicated with valproic acid. Lamotrigine use in children with Lennox–Gastaut syndrome and brain damage has been also associated with improvement in global functioning and quality of life scores [39]. Thus, lamotrigine can be considered as one of the most important tools for the treatment of childhood epileptic encephalopathies.

An open-label adjunctive therapy study of topiramate in Lennox–Gastaut syndrome showed a 50% seizure reduction in 75% of the patients who tolerated the drug [40]. This led to a double-blind placebo-controlled trial which confirmed its efficacy. The addition of topiramate at a target maintenance dose of 6 mg/kg/day resulted in at least 50% reduction in seizure frequency in 33% of patients, with a median reduction in the frequency of drop attacks of 14.8% [41]. There were no serious adverse events. Common side-effects were central nervous system related and could be minimized by a slow escalation starting with a low dose of 0.5–1 mg/kg/day. Behavioural difficulties, loss of appetite and sleep-related problems can be seen in children treated with topiramate [42]. An open-label extension to the double-blind placebo-controlled trial using a mean topiramate dosage of 10 mg/kg/day showed even better seizure control [28]. There was a reduction of drop attacks by at least 50% in 55% of the patients, and 15% of the patients had no drop attacks for at least 6 months. Based on its efficacy and safety profile, topiramate has become an important agent for the treatment of Lennox–Gastaut syndrome.

Other new AEDs that have been reported to have some efficacy against Lennox–Gastaut syndrome in uncontrolled studies include vigabatrin and zonisamide. Vigabatrin is effective for some children with Lennox–Gastaut syndrome, but it may aggravate myoclonic seizures [43]. Due to the recent reports of concentric visual field defects associated with vigabatrin use, the role of this drug in the management of Lennox–Gastaut syndrome is going to be minimal. Zonisamide has a broad spectrum of antiepileptic activity, and it was effective in decreasing seizure frequency by at least 50% in half of the patients with Lennox–Gastaut syndrome included in a small open-label study from Japan [44]. Among other new AEDs, gabapentin is probably contraindicated as it may worsen seizures in Lennox–Gastaut syndrome [45].

Open-label studies have shown that ACTH at doses of 30–40 IU/day is effective if started early, especially in patients with cryptogenic Lennox–Gastaut syndrome [46]. As seizure control with

ACTH may only be achieved after 6 weeks of treatment, complications of prolonged therapy are likely. Thus, the only definite role for steroids is during periods of severe seizure exacerbation or nonconvulsive status epilepticus.

The ketogenic diet is an important non-pharmacological treatment for children with refractory symptomatic generalized epilepsies, including the Lennox–Gastaut syndrome, but evidence for its efficacy in controlled trials remains scanty, except for one preliminary double-blind study confirming its effects [47]. Besides the practical difficulties in implementing the diet and ensuring compliance, the ketogenic diet is associated with possible adverse effects related to various metabolic disturbances. Other adjunctive treatments tried with limited success include imipramine, amantadine, bromide, allopurinol and flunarizine.

In view of the poor response of Lennox–Gastaut syndrome to AEDs, at least four studies [48] including 4–10 patients each assessed the potential value of vagus nerve stimulation in this syndrome. One additional report focused on the results of vagus nerve stimulation in 13 patients [49]. Most of the studies reported seizure reduction rates of between 34% and 60% compared with baseline. One of the studies with six patients reported that five patients had more than 90% reduction in seizure frequency [49]. On average, a 55% seizure reduction rate has been described over 18 months of treatment with vagus nerve stimulation, with only minor side-effects such as hoarseness of voice, irritation in the throat or excessive coughing [50].

As most patients with Lennox–Gastaut syndrome have multiple or diffuse lesions or abnormalities in their brain, resective surgery is often not possible. However, corpus callosotomy may be a useful option to decrease secondarily generalized seizures and drop attacks [51], though total remission is not to be expected. Use of a helmet should be considered for all patients with frequent drop attacks.

The long-term prognosis for children with Lennox–Gastaut syndrome remains guarded despite the increase in available therapeutic options. The need for special educational assistance and social support must not be overlooked.

Idiopathic partial epilepsies of childhood

The idiopathic partial epilepsies of childhood are classified among the 'age and localization-related idiopathic epilepsies' and comprise one-quarter of epilepsies with onset between 1 and 13 years. They are age related in that they only occur in children, and they are idiopathic because physical, mental and laboratory examinations other than the EEG are normal. The prognosis is usually excellent.

Benign childhood epilepsy with centrotemporal spikes and childhood epilepsy with occipital paroxysms are the only syndromes currently recognized by the Commission on Classification and Terminology of the International League Against Epilepsy (ILAE). Panayiotopoulos [52], however, pointed out that the definition of childhood epilepsy with occipital paroxysms requires major revision to recognize the distinction between early onset benign childhood occipital seizures (EBOS) and late onset childhood idiopathic occipital epilepsy (LOE).

Benign partial epilepsy with centrotemporal spikes (BECTS)

This is a common childhood epilepsy syndrome with onset between 3 and 12 years of age. The patients are neurologically and intellectually normal. The seizures usually occur in sleep, affecting preferentially the facial and oropharyngeal muscles. The patient often remains fully conscious but unable to talk because of involvement of oropharyngeal muscles in the seizure. The EEG shows sharp waves with a typical morphology, most commonly over the central and mid-temporal areas and normal background. The sharp waves are further activated by sleep. Patients with typical clinical features and EEG findings do not need further investigations. The seizures are usually brief, infrequent and invariably stop by the late teens. AEDs do not alter the natural history of this epileptic syndrome.

Although BECTS resolves spontaneously without treatment, some patients have many seizures or have seizures for several years prior to remission. Hence, three questions may be asked: Who should be treated? What treatment should be prescribed? How long should the patient be treated for?

AED treatment is unnecessary after a first or even a second seizure, unless the seizure is generalized, occurs during waking or the child or family are very frightened about the seizure. Even frequently recurrent seizures, when they are always focal and/or only occur in sleep, do not need AED treatment if the parents and child are not disturbed by the seizures. Because the seizures are benign and the epilepsy invariably remits regardless of treatment, AED therapy, if initiated, must be chosen with careful consideration for possible side-effects. Polypharmacy should be preferably avoided even if seizures are not fully controlled because the adverse effects of multiple drugs far outweigh the danger of seizures in BECTS. The drugs of choice are carbamazepine and valproate. Phenobarbital should be avoided because of its cognitive and behavioural side-effects, whereas phenytoin should be avoided because of its unfavourable pharmacokinetics in the paediatric age group and its cosmetic effects. The newer AEDs such as lamotrigine and gabapentin may not be justified in this very benign condition. Although seizures are usually very easily controlled in BECTS, a few patients may be highly resistant. Even these patients, however, have an excellent long-term outcome, which is not affected by recurrent seizures. Hence it is better to continue monotherapy at moderate doses and to tolerate occasional seizure recurrences.

AEDs can be tapered and discontinued after 1–2 years of seizure control, even before EEG normalization. Lerman and Kivity [53] found that psychosocial problems associated with epilepsy do not arise when the family and teachers are educated about the benign nature of the syndrome, and this is probably the most important aspect of medical management. If adequate counselling is not provided, parents may overreact to the diagnosis of epilepsy with feelings of apprehension, shame and despair. Likewise, the child may become overprotected and spoiled and excessive restrictions and prohibitions may be imposed, leading to the child becoming emotionally immature, overly dependent on the parents, demanding and antisocial. All this can be avoided if the parents are told from the beginning that the child will recover in several years and should be brought up normally, with the same rights and responsibilities as a healthy child, without overprotection or unnecessary restrictions.

Early onset benign childhood occipital seizures (EBOS)

This is the commonest childhood epilepsy syndrome after BECTS. Seizures are infrequent, often single, partial seizures manifested with deviation of the eyes and vomiting, frequently evolving to hemi- or generalized convulsions. Ictal behaviour changes, irritability, pallor, and rarely cyanosis, and eyes wide open are frequent. Retching, coughing, aphaemia, oropharyngeal movements and incontinence may occur. Consciousness is usually impaired or lost, either from the onset or in the course of the seizures, but in a few children it may be preserved. Seizure duration varies from a few minutes to hours (partial status epilepticus), and the seizures are usually nocturnal. Onset is between 1 and 12 years with a peak at 5 years. One-third of children have a single seizure, the median total number of seizures is two to three, and the prognosis is invariably excellent, with remission usually occurring within 1 year from the onset. A few children may develop rolandic or other benign partial seizures. The likelihood of having seizures after age 12 years is exceptional and lower than the likelihood associated with febrile seizures. The EEG shows occipital paroxysms demonstrating fixation-off sensitivity, but random occipital spikes, occipital spikes in sleep EEG alone or a normal EEG may be observed. Centrotemporal and other spike foci may appear in the same or in subsequent EEGs, but the EEG does not reflect the clinical course and severity [52].

EBOS may not need long-term AED treatment because the natural course may involve only one seizure. Rectal diazepam may be prescribed as for febrile seizures. There is no evidence of differences in outcome amongst monotherapy with phenobarbital, carbamazepine, valproate or no treatment [54]. However, some children may need a 1- to 2-year course, probably with carbamazepine.

Late onset childhood idiopathic occipital epilepsy (LOE)

Although rare, less well defined and of uncertain prognosis, LOE is, questionably, the only occipital syndrome which is recognized and defined by the current ILAE classification. LOE is a rare idiopathic partial epilepsy of childhood, whose cardinal clinical features are visual seizures with mainly elementary visual hallucinations, blindness or both. Seizures are usually frequent, brief and diurnal. Elementary visual hallucinations are often the first and frequently the only seizure manifestation, which may progress and coexist with other occipital symptoms such as sensory illusions of ocular movements and ocular pain, tonic deviation of the eyes, eyelid fluttering or repetitive eye closures. Complex visual hallucinations, visual illusions and other symptoms from more anterior ictal spreading rarely occur from the beginning or from seizure progression and may terminate with hemiconvulsions or generalized convulsions. Ictal blindness, appearing from the beginning or less commonly after other occipital seizure manifestations, usually lasts for 3–5 min. Symptoms suggestive of spreading of the seizure to the temporal lobe are exceptional and may indicate a symptomatic cause. Consciousness is intact during the visual symptoms but may be disturbed or lost if the seizures progress to other symptoms or convulsions. Postictal headache, sometimes indistinguishable from migraine, occurs in one-third of patients. Headaches, mainly orbital, may occasionally be ictal. The EEG abnormalities are similar to those observed in EBOS [52].

The age of onset of LOS is from 3 to 16 years, with a mean of about 8 years. Prognosis may be relatively good with remission often occurring within 2–4 years from onset for 50–60% and a very good response to treatment, mainly with carbamazepine, in >90%. However, 30–40% of patients may continue to have visual seizures and infrequent secondarily generalized tonic-clonic convulsions, particularly if not appropriately treated with carbamazepine [52].

Childhood absence epilepsy and juvenile absence epilepsy

Typical absences, by definition, are epileptic seizures manifested with impairment of consciousness and 2.5- to 4-Hz generalized spike-and-slow-wave discharges. Impairment of consciousness may be mild, requiring special testing, or severe and may be associated with other clinical manifestations, such as automatisms, myoclonia and autonomic disturbances. Four epileptic syndromes with typical absences are recognized by the current ILAE classification: childhood absence epilepsy, juvenile absence epilepsy, juvenile myoclonic epilepsy and myoclonic absence epilepsy. The first three syndromes have been well studied and documented and are considered idiopathic generalized epilepsies. The fourth, myoclonic absence epilepsy, is rare and less well studied and it will not be discussed further in this chapter.

Childhood absence epilepsy in most cases begins between the ages of 4 and 8 years with typical absence seizures which are very frequent, up to hundreds of times a day. Tonic-clonic seizures occur in approximately 40% of patients but are infrequent and easily controlled. They often begin near puberty but they can also occur in the first decade or, rarely, in early adult life. Myoclonic seizures usually are not seen in childhood absence epilepsy. Patients may have some degree of clonic or myoclonic twitching as part of their absences, but distinct myoclonic jerks without impairment of consciousness are uncommon, occurring mainly in those patients in whom absences persist during the teens.

Childhood absence epilepsy is one of the relatively benign childhood epilepsies. Absence seizures persisting into adult life are rare, but occasional cases have continued into old age. Tonic-clonic seizures are the seizure type most likely to persist but they are nearly always easy to control.

Juvenile absence epilepsy usually begins near or after puberty, between 10 and 17 years of age. Absences occur in all patients but, unlike the multiple cluster patterns seen in childhood absence epilepsy, which may involve hundreds of seizures per day, absences in juvenile absence epilepsy are relatively infrequent, with only one or a few episodes daily. Tonic-clonic seizures are considerably more frequent in juvenile absence epilepsy than in childhood absence epilepsy, occurring in about 80% of patients. Myoclonic seizures occur in about 15% of patients. Unlike childhood absence epilepsy, in which most patients eventually become seizure free, the long-term evolution of juvenile absence epilepsy has not yet been properly characterized.

Both ethosuximide and valproate suppress absence seizures in more than 80% of patients [55–57]. As valproate was introduced more recently and has been associated with rare hepatotoxic reactions, ethosuximide has been proposed by some authors as the first-choice drug for younger children. This recommendation, however, is questionable. Valproate is at least as effective as ethosuximide, it produces less frequently neurotoxic side-effects and hepatotoxicity is not a major issue in patients in this age group. In addition, ethosuximide is ineffective against tonic-clonic seizures, whereas valproate is highly effective. In patients with both absences and tonic-clonic seizures, valproate is clearly the drug of choice and it is rapidly becoming so also in patients who have absences alone, because of its better tolerability and its ability to prevent tonic-clonic seizures that may manifest at a later time in these patients.

Patients with refractory absences are rare. Valproate and ethosuximide should be tried sequentially and then in combination. Lamotrigine may be tried as second-line therapy. Low dosages of lamotrigine added to valproic acid may have a dramatic beneficial effect [58,59]. Clonazepam, particularly in absences with myoclonic components, and acetazolamide may be useful adjuncts. Zonisamide may also be useful in absence epilepsy. Carbamazepine, oxcarbazepine, phenytoin, barbiturates and vigabatrin are contraindicated because there is clinical and experimental evidence that they exacerbate absences [59]. Tiagabine may induce absence status epilepticus [59].

Seizure control should be monitored with EEG recordings. Persisting generalized spike-wave discharges, even if subclinical, may impair attention and learning, and attempts should be made to suppress them.

In seizure-free patients, a minimum seizure-free interval of 2 years must be achieved before tapering AED treatment. EEG findings may help guide the decision to discontinue drug treatment, but the presence of occasional brief epileptiform discharges should not preclude tapering AEDs in the seizure-free patient.

Juvenile myoclonic epilepsy

Juvenile myoclonic epilepsy is a genetically determined syndrome included among the idiopathic generalized epilepsies. The main characteristic manifestation is sudden, mild to moderate myoclonic jerks of the shoulders and arms that occur usually after awakening; 90% of patients also have generalized tonic-clonic or clonic-tonic-clonic seizures, and a third also have absences. Common precipitating factors are sleep deprivation, alcohol intake and fatigue. Seizures typically start at ages 14–15 years, but onset may range from ages 8 to 23 years. In almost half of the patients, myoclonic jerks precede the onset of generalized tonic-clonic seizures. Myoclonic jerks are often mistaken for nervousness until a generalized convulsion mandates medical help. Intelligence is normal, and neurological examination and brain imaging studies show no abnormality. Interictal EEGs in untreated patients show generalized, symmetrical, synchronous, 3.5–6 Hz polyspike-and-wave discharges and about 30% of patients are photosensitive.

Management of patients with juvenile myoclonic epilepsy should include not only AEDs but also control of precipitating factors. Patients should be educated about avoiding sleep deprivation, alcohol intake, excessive fatigue and those with known photosensitivity should avoid flickering lights.

Valproic acid is effective in up to 90% of patients and is the drug of choice [59]. Valproic acid is the AED that most consistently stops myoclonic jerks, generalized convulsions and absence seizures without significant side-effects. Lamotrigine controls generalized tonic-clonic seizures and absences but at times it may worsen myoclonic jerks [58,59]. The risks of valproate-induced terato-

genicity and weight gain are potentially unacceptable in young women of childbearing age, making lamotrigine an attractive alternative. However, not enough data exists on the safety of lamotrigine in pregnancy. In clinical practice, topiramate is being increasingly used as monotherapy for juvenile myoclonic epilepsy; many patients appreciate the accompanying weight loss seen with topiramate, but the drug has potentially troubling side-effects, has not been well studied as monotherapy for juvenile myoclonic epilepsy and its safety in pregnancy has yet to be established. Zonisamide may be potentially of value in some patients. Phenytoin, carbamazepine and oxcarbazepine may worsen myoclonus and absence seizures when used alone, but they may have a role as add-on treatment to valproate or lamotrigine, especially when generalized tonic-clonic seizures are not controlled [59]. Phenobarbital and primidone may also be useful as add-on treatment, but often they have unacceptable side-effects. Clonazepam may be useful as adjunctive treatment for resistant myoclonic jerks but it is not highly effective against generalized tonic-clonic seizures. Used alone, clonazepam may suppress the jerks that herald a generalized tonic-clonic seizure, and may not allow the patient to prepare for this type of attack. Vigabatrin and gabapentin may worsen myoclonic jerks and absences in juvenile myoclonic epilepsy [59].

Juvenile myoclonic epilepsy carries an excellent prognosis because AEDs will control seizures in the majority of patients. However, AED should be continued for life, as there is a 90% relapse rate after withdrawal of medication.

Symptomatic and cryptogenic partial epilepsies

Partial epilepsy associated with cerebral lesions and mesial temporal sclerosis is the most common group of medically intractable epilepsies seen in adults, and it is also an important cause of intractable seizures in children. There is a strong correlation between the site of the lesion and the site of the epileptogenic zone. The identification of an epileptogenic lesion on MRI is predictive of a poor response to AED [60], but these patients are more likely to become seizure free postoperatively than those in whom no structural abnormality is found. Nevertheless, surgical options are still an underutilized alternative to medical therapy in these patients.

Although clinical history and ictal behaviour may give a clue to the site of the underlying epileptogenic lesion, there is large overlap in the ictal symptomatology produced by lesions at different cortical locations. Lesions at any site may result in either simple partial, complex partial or secondarily generalized seizures. Complex partial seizures are commonly thought to indicate temporal lobe seizures, but in a study of high-resolution MRI in 129 consecutive patients with video-EEG proven complex partial seizures, discrete neocortical lesions were only detected in 58 (45%), of which 22 were extratemporal (O'Brien *et al.* personal communication). Boon *et al.* [61], in 51 patients with lesions, found that although patients with temporal lesions had complex partial seizures, 74% of patients with extratemporal lesions also had complex partial seizures. This study also found that although visual auras may give a clue to the presence of an occipital lesion, the nature of the aura was not otherwise useful in predicting the location of the lesion. Clinical features, including seizure type, age of patient at onset and duration of epilepsy, response to AEDs and findings on neurological examination are also not useful in predicting the nature of the underlying lesion. Studies using MRI suggest that before the age of 12 years, lesional epilepsy, particularly gangliogliomas and disorders of cortical development such as focal cortical dysplasia, may be more common, and mesial temporal sclerosis less common. The structural lesions revealed by high-resolution MRI are low-grade tumours (34.1%), disorders of cortical development (36.8%), vascular malformations (23.9%) and focal encephalomalacia (17.1%) [62].

Before the advent of high-resolution MRI, the term cryptogenic temporal lobe epilepsy had been frequently used to describe the condition of patients with the characteristic features of temporal lobe epilepsy but no obvious lesions on structural imaging. Pathological studies of mesial temporal lobe tissue resected from patients with cryptogenic temporal lobe epilepsy revealed mesial temporal sclerosis in most, so that the adjective cryptogenic, as opposed to lesional or symptomatic, was used tacitly to denote a subtype of temporal lobe epilepsy that has now been more clearly defined in most patients as the syndrome of mesial temporal lobe epilepsy.

Ammon's horn sclerosis and mesial temporal sclerosis are the two most common pathological terms that have been used more or less synonymously with hippocampal sclerosis, although strictly speaking they imply different degrees of anatomical involvement. The term hippocampal sclerosis refers to a specific type of hippocampal cell loss involving the CA1 and hilar neurones most and CA2 neurones least, which distinguishes this entity from non-specific cell loss from other causes. Other characteristic features, such as mossy fibre sprouting and selective loss of somatostatin and neuropeptide Y-containing hilar neurones, also help to identify this distinct pathological entity.

In surgical series of patients with medically refractory temporal lobe epilepsy, careful pathological analysis of hippocampal specimens, including cell counts and special staining procedures, reveals that 70% have hippocampal sclerosis. Because the syndrome of mesial temporal lobe epilepsy has only recently been clearly defined, and because only the medically refractory forms of this disorder referred to epilepsy surgery centres are usually identified, no epidemiological information is available. Nevertheless, in view of the prevalence of temporal lobe epilepsy and the high prevalence of hippocampal sclerosis among patients with this diagnosis who undergo surgery, it is quite likely that mesial temporal lobe epilepsy is the most common human epileptic syndrome.

Current information on the clinical features of mesial temporal lobe epilepsy is derived almost exclusively from patients with medically intractable seizures who are evaluated for surgical intervention. Many patients have early risk factors, especially prolonged febrile convulsions and a variety of other early insults, such as head injury, meningitis or encephalitis, which are often associated with acute seizures. The onset of recurrent seizures typically occurs towards the end of the first decade of life, and seizures may initially respond well to AEDs. Characteristically, patients do well for several years, but seizures may return in adolescence or early adulthood and become refractory to AEDs.

The seizures in mesial temporal lobe epilepsy often begin with an aura. The most common aura is a rising epigastric sensation. Fear as an aura is far less common. Other frequently described auras, such as déjà vu, jamai vu, micropsia, macropsia, olfactory hallucinations and feeling of depersonalization are uncommon. Some aural symp-

toms may not have a counterpart in human experience and cannot be described. Auras can occur as the first manifestation of a complex partial seizure, or they can occur in isolation as simple partial seizures. If auras evolve into complex partial seizures, consciousness is impaired. In complex partial seizures, there is often motor arrest, staring and pupillary dilatation. The seizure may not progress beyond this point, but more often, semi-purposeful coordinated motor activities (automatisms) follow. Oral-alimentary automatisms are highly characteristic of mesial temporal lobe epilepsy. Stereotyped automatisms that consist of fumbling, picking and gesticulating movements, or automatisms suggesting reactions to environmental objects or situations, are also common in mesial temporal lobe epilepsy. Head and eye deviation, unilateral tonic or dystonic posturing and language disturbances may have lateralizing significance. Mesial temporal lobe seizures are typically followed by postictal dysfunction of variable duration, as opposed to some extratemporal seizures with minimal or no postictal phase.

The most important procedure in the diagnostic evaluation of patients with symptomatic or cryptogenic partial epilepsy is a high-resolution MRI. This will detect almost all tumours, vascular malformations, a high percentage of cases of mesial temporal sclerosis and some cases of disorders of cortical development. The findings on routine EEG and even video-EEG are often variable and non-diagnostic.

Whilst many patients with partial seizures due to structural lesions in the brain or mesial temporal sclerosis have intractable seizures which are poorly controlled by AEDs, nevertheless, almost all patients should have a trial of AEDs before proceeding to surgery. This is especially necessary when the epileptogenic focus is in an eloquent area of the brain. The exceptions would be patients with brain tumours, arteriovenous malformations or other lesions which have indications for surgical resection even if they had not caused epilepsy.

Carbamazepine is considered by most as the first-line therapy for children with partial seizures on the basis of two adult Veterans Administration (VA) studies, open-labelled controlled paediatric studies and clinical experience. Phenytoin may also be used, but its cosmetic side-effects argue against its first-line prescription in children, particularly girls. In the first VA study [63], carbamazepine and phenytoin were more effective and had greater tolerability over time compared to primidone and phenobarbital in the treatment of complex partial seizures. All four AEDs were equally effective as monotherapy for secondarily generalized tonic-clonic seizures. In the second VA cooperative study [64], carbamazepine was superior to valproate in the treatment of complex partial seizures but was equivalent to valproate in the management of secondarily generalized tonic-clonic seizures. Some investigators consider valproate as a possible first-line therapy for partial onset seizures based on the results of other recent randomized, double-blind controlled trials in adults and children [65–68].

Although many new AEDs have demonstrated efficacy in controlled trials in adults and children with partial seizures, additional issues must be examined before these new AEDs can be considered as first-line therapy for paediatric patients. Among new AEDs which are candidates for first-line therapy, oxcarbazepine has demonstrated efficacy in monotherapy and adjunctive therapy in paediatric partial seizures, along with good tolerability [69]. Topiramate has also demonstrated efficacy and tolerability in paediatric partial seizures, but it needs to be titrated more slowly compared with oxcarbazepine. Gabapentin can be considered as first-line therapy for paediatric seizures if preliminary favourable results of a monotherapy trial are confirmed. There is not yet enough data on efficacy and tolerability to support consideration of lamotrigine, tiagabine, levetiracetam or zonisamide as first-line therapy for paediatric seizures.

Many patients with lesional epilepsy or mesial temporal sclerosis continue to have poorly controlled seizures despite treatment with AEDs [60], and they should not be subjected to too many prolonged unsuccessful trials of multiple different drugs and polypharmacy before epilepsy surgery is considered.

Conclusions

The clinical presentation and course of epilepsy in infancy and childhood vary widely, from the epileptic encephalopathies with severe neurodevelopmental compromise to the benign epilepsy syndromes that hardly warrant therapy. Precise diagnosis of the epilepsy syndrome is essential for both prognostic and therapeutic purposes, especially as some of the epilepsies in this age range require unconventional treatments such as ACTH or corticosteroids.

There is need for further research in the treatment of epilepsies in young patients using both medical and surgical approaches. Only in recent years has research primarily targeted at this patient population been carried out. It is hoped that this will lead to better management strategies resulting in improved long-term outcome.

References

1 Farwell JR, Lee YJ, Hirtz DG, Sulzbacher SI, Ellenberg JH, Nelson KB. Phenobarbital for febrile seizures—Effects on intelligence and on seizure recurrence. *N Engl J Med* 1990; 322: 364–9.

2 Farwell JR, Lee YJ, Hirtz DG, Sulzbacher SI, Ellenberg JH, Nelson KB. Phenobarbital for febrile seizures—Effects on intelligence and on seizure recurrence. (Published erratum appears in *N Engl J Med* 1992; 326(2): 144.)

3 Dodrill CB, Wilensky AJ. Neuropsychological abilities before and after 5 years of stable antiepileptic drug therapy. *Epilepsia* 1992; 33: 327–34.

4 Nelson KB, Ellenberg JH. Predictors of epilepsy in children who have experienced febrile seizures. *N Engl J Med* 1976; 295: 1029–33.

5 Annegers JF, Hauser WA, Shirto S *et al.* Factors prognostic of unprovoked seizures after febrile convulsions. *N Engl J Med* 1987; 316: 493–8.

6 Knudsen FU. Rectal administration of diazepam in solution in the acute treatment of convulsions in infants in children. Anticonvulsant and side effects. *Arch Dis Child* 1979; 54: 855–7.

7 Camfield CS, Camfield PR, Smith E, Dooley JM. Home use of rectal diazepam to prevent status epilepticus in children with convulsive disorders. *J Child Neurol* 1989; 4: 125–6.

8 Alldredge BK, Wall DB, Ferriero DM. Effect of prehospital treatment on the outcome of status epilepticus in children. *Pediatr Neurol* 1995; 12: 213–16.

9 Dodson WE, DeLorenzo RJ, Pedley TA, Shinnar S, Treiman DB, Wannamaker BB. The treatment of convulsive status epilepticus: Recommendations of the Epilepsy Foundation of America's working group on status epilepticus. *JAMA* 1993; 270: 854–9.

10 Maytal J, Shinnar S. Status epilepticus in children. In: Shinnar S, Amir N, Branski D, eds. *Childhood Seizure.* Karger: Switzerland; 1995: 111–22.

11 Rutter N, Metcalfe DH. Febrile convulsions—what do parents do? *Br Med J* 1978; 2: 1345–6.

12 Camfield PR, Camfield CS, Shapiro S *et al.* The first febrile seizure-antipyretic instructions plus either phenobarbital or placebo to prevent recurrence. *J Pediatr* 1980; 97: 16–21.

13 Rantala H, Uhari M, Vainionpää L, Kurttila R. Ineffectiveness of aceta-

14 Newman J. Evaluation of sponging to reduce body temperature in febrile children. *Can Med Assoc J* 1985; 132: 641–2.

15 Knudsen FU. Febrile seizures—Treatment and outcome. *Brain Dev* 1996; 18: 438–99.

16 Hirata Y, Mizuno Y, Nakano M, Sohmiya K. Epilepsy following febrile convulsions. *Brain Dev* 1985; 7: 1–75.

17 Wolf SM, Carr A, Davis DC *et al.* The value of phenobarbital in the child who has had a single febrile seizure: A controlled, prospective study. *Pediatrics* 1977; 59: 378–85.

18 Lee K, Melchior JC. Sodium valproate versus phenobarbital in the prophylactic treatment of febrile convulsions in childhood. *Eur J Pediatr* 1981; 137: 151–3.

19 Newton RW. Randomized controlled trials of phenobarbitone and valproate in febrile convulsions. *Arch Dis Child* 1988; 63: 1189–91.

20 McKinlay I, Newton R. Intention to treat febrile convulsions with rectal diazepam, valproate, or phenobarbitone. *Dev Med Child Neurol* 1989; 31: 617–25.

21 Antony JH, Hawke SHB. Phenobarbital compared with carbamazepine in prevention of recurrent febrile convulsions. *Am J Dis Child* 1983; 137: 842–95.

22 Melchior JD, Buchthal F, Lennox-Buchthal M. The ineffectiveness of diphenylhydantoin in preventing febrile convulsions in the age of greatest risk, under three years. *Epilepsia* 1971; 12: 55–62.

23 Autret E, Billard C, Bertrand P *et al.* Double-blind randomized trial of diazepam versus placebo for prevention of recurrence of febrile seizures. *J Pediatr* 1990; 117: 490–5.

24 Rosman NP, Colton T, Labazzo RNC *et al.* A controlled trial of diazepam administration during febrile illnesses to prevent recurrences of febrile seizures. *N Engl J Med* 1993; 329: 79–84.

25 Wolf SM, Forsythe A. Behavior disturbance, phenobarbital and febrile seizures. *Pediatrics* 1978; May 61(5): 728–31.

26 Knudsen FU. Intermittent diazepam prophylaxis in febrile convulsions. Pros and cons. *Acta Neurol Scand* 1991; 135 (Suppl.): 1–24.

27 Lahat E, Goldman M, Barr J, Bistritzer T, Berkovitch M. Comparison of intranasal midazolam with intravenous diazepam for treating febrile seizures in children: prospective randomised study. *BMJ* 2000; 321: 83–6.

28 Glauser TA, Levisohn PM, Ritter F, Sachdeo RC, and the Topiramate YL Study Group. Topiramate in Lennox–Gastaut syndrome: open-label treatment of patients completing a randomised controlled trial. *Epilepsia* 2000; 41 (Suppl. 1): S86–90.

29 Gastaut H, Low MD. Antiepileptic properties of clobazam, a 1,5-benzodiazepine, in man. *Epilepsia* 1979; 20: 437–46.

30 Shimizu H, Abe J, Futagi Y *et al.* Antiepileptic effects of clobazam in children. *Brain Dev* 1982; 4: 57–62.

31 Koeppen D. A review of clobazam studies in epilepsy. In: Hindmarch I, Stonier PD, Trimble MR, eds. *Clobazam: human psychopharmacology and clinical applications.* International congress and symposium series, no. 74. London: Royal Society of Medicine, 1985: 201–15.

32 Felbamate Study Group in Lennox–Gastaut Syndrome. Efficacy of felbamate in childhood epileptic encephalopathy (Lennox–Gastaut syndrome). *N Engl J Med* 1993; 328: 29–33.

33 Dodson WE. Felbamate in the treatment of Lennox–Gastaut syndrome: results of a 12-month open-label study following a randomized clinical trial. *Epilepsia* 1993; 34 (Suppl. 7): S18–S24.

34 Kaufman D, Kelly J, Anderson T *et al.* Evaluation of case reports of aplastic anaemia among patients treated with felbamate. *Epilepsia* 1997; 38: 1265–69.

35 O'Neil M, Perdun C, Wilson M *et al.* Felbamate-associated fatal hepatic necrosis. *Neurology* 1996; 46: 1457–59.

36 French J, Smith M, Faught E *et al.* Practice advisory: the use of felbamate in the treatment of patients with intractable epilepsy. Report of the Quality Standards Subcommittee of the American Academy of Neurology and the American Epilepsy Society. *Neurology* 1999; 52: 1540–5.

37 Motte J, Trevathan E, Arvidsson JF *et al.* Lamotrigine for generalized seizures associated with the Lennox–Gastaut syndrome. Lamictal Lennox-Gastaut Study Group. *N Engl J Med* 1997; 337: 1807–12.

38 Eriksson AS, Nergardh A, Hoppu K. The efficacy of lamotrigine in children

and adolescents with refractory generalised epilepsy: a randomised, double-blind crossover study. *Epilepsia* 1998; 39: 495–501.

39 Buchanan N. Lamotrigine: clinical experience in 93 patients with epilepsy. *Acta Neurol Scand* 1995; 92: 28–32.

40 French JA, Bourgeois BFD, Dreifuss FE *et al*. An open-label multi-centre study of topiramate in patients with the Lennox–Gastaut syndrome. *Neurology* 1995; 4 (Suppl.): A250 (abstract).

41 Sachdeo RC, Glauser TA, Ritter FJ, Reife R, Lim P, Pledger G, and the Topiramate YL Study Group. A double-blind, randomised trial of topiramate in Lennox–Gastaut syndrome. *Neurology* 1999; 52: 1882–7.

42 Glauser TA. Preliminary observations on topiramate in pediatric epilepsies. *Epilepsia* 1997; 38 (Suppl. 1): S37–S41.

43 Dulac O, Chiron C, Luna D *et al*. Vigabatrin in childhood epilepsy. *J Child Neurol* 1991; 6 (Suppl. 2): S30–S37.

44 Yamatogi Y, Ohtahara S. Current topics of treatment. In: Ohtahara S, Roger J, eds. *Proceedings of the International Symposium, New Trends in Pediatric Epileptology*. Okayama, Japan: Department of Child Neurology, Okayama University Medical School. 1991: 136–48.

45 Vossler DG. Exacerbation of seizures in Lennox–Gastaut syndrome by gabapentin. *Neurology* 1996; 46: 852–3.

46 Yamatogi Y, Ohtsuka Y, Ishida T *et al*. Treatment of the Lennox–Gastaut syndrome with ACTH: a clinical and electroencephalographic study. *Brain Dev* 1979; 1: 267–76.

47 Freeman JM, Vining PG. Seizures decrease rapidly after fasting. Preliminary studies of the ketogenic diet. *Arch Pediatr Adolesc Med* 1999; 153: 946–9.

48 Hosain S, Nikalov B, Harden C, Li M, Fraser R, Labar D. Vagus nerve stimulation for Lennox–Gastaut syndrome. *J Child Neurol* 2000; 15: 509–12.

49 Hornig GW, Murphy JV, Schallert G *et al*. Vagus nerve stimulation in children with refractory epilepsy: an update. *South Med J* 1997; 90: 484–8.

50 Schmidt D, Bourgeois B. A risk-benefit assessment of therapies for Lennox–Gastaut syndrome. *Drug Safety* 2000; 22: 467–77.

51 Wyllie E. Corpus callosotomy for intractable generalized epilepsy. *J Pediatr* 1988; 113: 255–61.

52 Panayiotopoulos CP. Early-onset benign childhood occipital seizure susceptibility syndrome: a syndrome to recognize. *Epilepsia* 1999; 40: 621–30.

53 Lerman P, Kivity S. Benign focal epilepsy of childhood. A follow-up of 100 recovered patients. *Arch Neurol* 1975; 32: 261–4.

54 Ferrie CD, Beaumanoir A, Guerrini R *et al*. Early-onset benign occipital susceptibility syndrome. *Epilepsia* 1997; 38: 285–93.

55 Sato S, White BG, Penry JK *et al*. Valproic acid versus ethosuximide in the treatment of absence seizures. *Neurology* 1982; 32: 157–63.

56 Aicardi J. *Epilepsy in Children*, 2nd edn. New York: Raven Press, 1994: 94–117.

57 Loiseau P, Duche B, Pedespan J-M. Absence epilepsies. *Epilepsia* 1995; 36: 1182–7.

58 Panayiotopoulos CP. Treatment of typical absence seizures and related epileptic syndrome. *Pediatr Drugs* 2001; 3: 379–403.

59 Murphy K, Delanty N. Primary generalized epilepsies. *Curr Treat Options Neurol* 2000; 2: 527–42.

60 Engel J Jr, Shewmon DA. Who should be considered a surgical candidate? In: Engel J Jr, ed. *Surgical Treatment of the Epilepsies*. New York: Raven Press; 1993: 23–34.

61 Boon PA, Williamson PD, Fried I *et al*. Intracranial, intraaxial, space-occupying lesions in patients with intractable partial seizures: an anatomo-clinical, neuropsychological and surgical correlation. *Epilepsia* 1991; 32: 467–76.

62 Li LM, Fish DR, Sisodiya SM, Shorvon SD, Alsanjari N, Stevens JM. High resolution magnetic resonance imaging in adults with partial or secondarily generalized epilepsy attending a tertiary referral unit. *J Neurol Neurosurg Psychiatry* 1995; 59: 384–7.

63 Mattson RH, Cramer JA, Collins JF *et al*. Comparison of carbamazepine, phenobarbital, phenytoin, and primidone in partial and secondarily generalized tonic-clonic seizures. *N Engl J Med* 1985; 313: 145–51.

64 Mattson RH, Cramer JA, Collins JF *et al*. A comparison of valproate with carbamazepine for the treatment of complex partial seizures and secondarily generalized tonic-clonic seizures in adults. *N Engl J Med* 1992; 327: 765–71.

65 Willmore LJ, Shu V, Wallin B. Efficacy and safety of add-on divalproex sodium in the treatment of complex partial seizures. The M88-194 Study Group. *Neurology* 1996; 46: 49–53.

66 Richens A., Davidson DLW, Cartlidge NEF, Easter DJ. A multicentre comparative trial of sodium valproate and carbamazepine in adult-onset epilepsy. *J Neurol Neurosurg Psychiatr* 1994; 57: 682–7.

67 Verity CM, Hosking G, Easter DJ, on behalf of the Pediatric EPITEG Collaborative Group. A multicentre comparative trial of sodium valproate and carbamazepine in paediatric epilepsy. *Dev Med Child Neurol* 1995; 37: 97–108.

68 Beydoun A, Sackellares JC, Shu V. Safety and efficacy of divalproex sodium monotherapy in partial epilepsy: a double-blind, concentration-response design clinical trial. Depakote Monotherapy for Partial Seizures Study Group. *Neurology* 1997; 48 (Suppl. 1): S182–S188.

69 Glauser TA. Expanding first-line therapy options for children with partial seizures. *Epilepsia* 2000; 55 (Suppl. 3): S30–S37.

16 Management of Epilepsy in the Elderly Person

R.C. Tallis

The importance of epilepsy and epileptic seizures in the elderly population has dawned only slowly on the medical profession. There may be several reasons for this. First is perhaps the assumption that elderly onset seizures are uncommon. Secondly, there is the belief that seizures in old age may be less important than in young people. Finally, clinicians seem to assume that findings in middle-aged and younger people with epilepsy can be extrapolated directly to the older population obviating the need for separate studies. Recent textbooks on epilepsy and epileptic seizures in old age [1,2] may mark the end of this era of neglect. Nevertheless, it is worth addressing each of these assumptions at the outset of the chapter.

Epidemiology

Twenty-five years ago, Hauser and Kurland [3] reported a rise in the prevalence of epilepsy above the age of 50 years and an even steeper rise in incidence—from 12/100 000 in the 40–59 age range to 82/100 000—in those over 60 [3]. This rise has been confirmed in their more recent studies [4]. The incidence given in their 1975 paper is close to that of Luhdorf *et al.* [5] of 77/100 000 in subjects over 60 years. The UK National General Practice Survey of Epilepsy (NGPSE), a prospective community-based study, found that 24% of new cases of definite epilepsy were in subjects over the age of 60 years [6]. Tallis *et al.* [7] examined a primary care database covering 82 practices and nearly 370 000 patients, 62 000 of whom were over the age of 65 years. They found that, whereas the incidence for the overall population was 69/100 000, in the 65–69 age group it was 87/100 000; in the 70s 147/100 000; and in the 80s 159/100 000. Perhaps most significantly, over one-third of all incident cases placed on anticonvulsant treatment were individuals over the age of 60 years. Analysis of an expanded database of over 2 000 000 subjects has generated very similar findings [8]. Loiseau [9] found an annual incidence for all seizures (single and recurrent) of 127 in subjects over 60 years, and the over 60s accounted for 28% of cases of confirmed epilepsy (two or more unprovoked seizures) and 52% of acute symptomatic seizures. Hauser *et al.* [4] also found that both single unprovoked seizures and definite epilepsy increased sharply with age.

If elderly onset seizures are numerically very important at present, demographic trends, with a very sharp rise in the older old and the oldest old, indicate that they will be even more important in the future, especially since cerebrovascular disease is the most common cause of elderly onset seizures (see below) and has an exponential relationship with age. The Rochester surveys [4] reveal that in the period of 1935–84, while the incidence of seizures in children under the age of 10 years decreased significantly (by about 40%), this was more than compensated for by a near doubling of the incidence of epilepsy in the elderly population in the same 50-year period. The upward time trend for a single unprovoked seizure is even more dramatic.

The impact of seizures in old age

Nothing could be further from the truth than the suggestion that seizures in old age somehow matter less than in younger people. First and foremost, there is the actual experience of the seizures, the unpleasantness of which is self-evident. Secondly, in older people, postictal states may be prolonged: 14% of subjects in one series suffered a confusional state lasting more than 24 h and in some cases it persisted as long as 1 week [10]. Todd's phenomena are also common, especially postictal hemiparesis. This may lead to misdiagnosis of stroke; indeed, in one series, this was the most common non-stroke cause of referral to a stroke unit [11]. This is particularly likely to happen where fits occur against a background of known cerebrovascular disease, and a recurrence of stroke may be incorrectly diagnosed.

Although no adequate prospective studies have been undertaken, one might anticipate that seizures more often lead to injury and these are more likely to be serious in older people, osteoporotic bones being easier to fracture.

Seizures may have wider and more chronic consequences. Studies of falls (reviewed in [12]) have repeatedly confirmed how a fall may mark a watershed in an older patient's life, after which there is a sharp decline in functional independence. In some instances, this decline will be due to the disease underlying the fall but in many more it will be due to loss of confidence. The well-known three 'Fs' (fear of further falls) that may cause an elderly person to become effectively semi-housebound must surely have its analogue in 'fear of further fits'. Moreover, the terrifying experience of a seizure may seem like a harbinger of death. This fear may be greater in elderly people not only because they may have known a contemporary who has died after 'a funny turn' but also because they may have distant memories of childhood when epilepsy was stigmatized, poorly controlled, very much an affair of the street or the institution and often, partly due to the adverse effects of toxic but useless drugs, associated with severe chronic impairment of mental function.

The impact of seizures will also include their effect on the attitudes of others, including friends, relatives and carers, to the patient: decreased activity, more exclusion from normal activity in decision-making processes, less grandparental involvement in child rearing, more susceptibility to interference in their affairs by others; in summary, marginalization, disempowerment and a shrinkage of life space. So, although the diagnosis of seizures will not have the effects on employment and education that it may have in a younger person, the impact on interpersonal relationships may be no less important. Elderly people may be more dependent on motorized transport for mobility; if the individual who has the fit is the only licence holder, the consequent ban on driving may mean that two people are housebound.

How patients with elderly onset seizures differ from the general population of people with epilepsy

The paucity of separate studies of epilepsy in old age in part reflects, as already indicated, the erroneous belief that what we have learned about seizures and treatment of seizures in younger patients can be extrapolated to older individuals. In fact, information about the effect of pharmacological treatment in the elderly is especially scanty, due to the fact that the elderly are usually excluded from Phase I and Phase II antiepileptic drug (AED) trials, and even Phase III studies are rarely performed in this population. Therefore, it is worthwhile spelling out the ways in which older patients with epilepsy may be different from the overall adult population of people with seizures and why AED trials should be conducted in older people (Table 16.1):

1 The underlying causes will be different, more often being symptomatic and frequently related to focal cerebral lesions, in particular cerebrovascular disease.

2 Seizures may present differently (often without an adequate history) and the problem of a diagnosis (in particular, that of separating cardiac from cerebral causes of episodic loss of consciousness) can be especially difficult.

3 There will frequently be concurrent pathologies unrelated to the seizures and the patient will often be on medication other than AEDs. 'Multiple pathology' is one of the characteristic features of illness in old age.

4 Since elderly patients may be close to the threshold of functional failure, seizures and the adverse effects of their treatment may be more likely to cause loss of confidence and even of independence, as noted earlier.

5 Finally, there will be differences in drug kinetics and dynamics due in part to age but also (and more importantly) to concurrent illness.

This is not to imply that elderly people with epilepsy form a homogeneous group. Despite the special problems listed above, not all older people with seizures can be characterized by all of these features. Old age is less a period of predictable change than of increased variance between individuals. Some of this variance will be due to biological ageing—a 90-year-old is going to be more biologically aged than a 60-year-old—and some will be due to concurrent disease. The latter will be a much more important sources of variance than the former.

The complexity of the situation may be illustrated by a specific example. The changes in the pharmacokinetics of AEDs associated with ageing are often presented as the differences between the mean values for young and elderly groups. Detailed examination typically reveals wide variation within an age group and substantial overlap between groups [13]; age alone explains only a small proportion of the total variance. For example, only about 25% of the interindividual variation in the maximum rate of phenytoin clearance is attributable to age [14]. Moreover, when one is considering the impact of seizures and the treatment of seizures on cognitive function and quality of life, other sources of variance—current and past life experience, education, social class, etc.—increase the heterogeneity of elderly people [15].

The management of epilepsy at all ages extends far beyond drug treatment. This is particularly true of older patients in whom seizures may have complex physical, psychological and social effects. Nevertheless, the major elements of the management of epileptic seizures in old age are the same as in younger patients (Table 16.2).

Diagnosis of seizures

Three key issues are involved in diagnosis:
1 Determining that the events are seizures and not, for instance, syncope or other causes of episodic 'funny turns'.
2 Determining the type of seizures.
3 Identifying the aetiology and precipitating factors.

There is an abundance of causes of 'funny turns' in older people (Table 16.3). These include syncope, hypoglycaemia, transient ischaemic attacks, transient global amnesia, episodic vertigo and non-specific episodes of dizziness, which may affect up to 10% of older populations [16]. As in younger people, the most powerful diagnostic tool is an accurate history of the onset, evolution of and recovery from the episode. As many people live alone, this is frequently lacking.

The greatest challenge is to differentiate seizures from syncopal attacks, as the causes of the latter in elderly people are legion; most notably, cardiac arrhythmias, carotid sinus syncope [17,18] and

Table 16.1 Some important aspects to be considered in diagnosing and managing epilepsy in old age

Distinctive range of causes of epilepsy
Distinctive differential diagnosis (especially syncope)
Frequency of concurrent pathologies, unrelated to epilepsy
Pharmacokinetic differences (e.g. differences in effective drug dose and dosing regimens, occurrence of interactions and complications of polytherapy)
Pharmacodynamic differences (differences in sensitivity to side-effects and dosage requirements)
Distinctive psychological or social effects
Danger of precipitating failure in daily functioning

Table 16.2 Key elements for a correct management of seizure disorders in old age

Accurate diagnosis of the nature, cause and precipitating factors of the episodes
General advice and reassurance
Treatment with AEDs if indicated
Monitoring the response to treatment and side-effects of medication
Looking for emergent clues as to the cause of the seizures if this is not apparent at first
Ensuring that epilepsy intrudes as little as possible upon the life of the patient

Table 16.3 Some conditions, particularly common in the elderly, that need to be considered in the differential diagnosis of epileptic seizures

Syncope
Hypoglycaemia
Transient ischaemic attacks
Transient global amnesia
Episodic vertigo
Non-specific episodes of dizziness
Non-specific confusional states
Functional psychiatric illness

postural hypotension, often due to drugs. Even where there is a reasonably good history, this still may not differentiate seizures from faints as sharply as it does in younger adults. Of all the discriminating features, the rapidity of recovery after syncope compared with a seizure is often thought to be the most useful. However, a seizure may take the form of a brief absence whereas syncope associated with an arrhythmia may be prolonged. Postevent confusion, typically prolonged with seizures and brief with faints, may also be prolonged in cerebral anoxia due to syncope associated with a serious cardiac arrhythmia. Cardiogenic or neurocardiogenic syncope may be associated with brief myoclonic jerks, head turning, automatisms (lipsmacking, chewing) and upward deviation of the eyes and vocalizations may occur [19]. If the anoxic episode itself triggers a full-blown seizure, the situation becomes even more complicated. Typically, faints are infrequent but in an elderly patient with postural hypotension this may not be the case. Faints may be associated with incontinence in old age. In short, one could list all the most useful discriminators between seizures and faints and find them to be less powerful in elderly people.

Diagnosis is especially difficult where there are coexisting conditions that predispose to syncope and, in elderly patients with features suggestive of cerebrovascular disease and of cardiac disease, it may prove impossible to determine whether or not transient symptoms are cardiac or cerebral in origin. Non-specific abnormalities on an EEG, or cardiac arrhythmias recorded on a 24-h tape unrelated to the symptoms, may add to the confusion. It has been suggested that head-up tilt testing may be useful in differentiating convulsive syncope from epilepsy [20] and Kenny and Dey [18] have extended this to include carotid sinus massage before and after atropine in prolonged head-up tilt, as cardioneurogenic syncope secondary to carotid sinus hypersensitivity is common in older people [17].

The presentation of seizures in older people may be particularly misleading [10]. In all age groups, complex partial seizures with or without automatisms, may be labelled as non-specific confusional states or even, where there are affective or cognitive features or hallucinations, as manifestations of functional psychiatric illness [21–23]. Older patients with non-convulsive status epilepticus may present with acute behavioural changes: withdrawal, mutism, delusional ideas, paranoia, vivid hallucinations and fugue states. Fluctuating mental impairment may easily be attributed to other causes of recurrent confusional states or even misread as part of a dementing process.

It may be necessary, after a careful history, examination and appropriate investigations, simply to wait and see. A 'therapeutic trial' of anticonvulsants as a diagnostic test is to be recommended even less frequently than in younger patients: unless events are happening very frequently for a therapeutic response to be assessed quickly, it will rarely produce a decisive answer and only add the burden of unnecessary drug treatment to the patient's problems. After a clear history, the second most powerful diagnostic tool is probably the passage of time.

Identification of an underlying cause

There are two reasons for wanting to determine why a patient is having seizures: the underlying cause may warrant treatment in its own right and this may lead to remission of seizures; and the patient will wish to have some explanation of the seizures.

The most common cause of elderly onset seizures is cerebrovascular disease, accounting for between 30 and 50% of cases in different series [9,24,25]. It accounts for an even higher proportion—nearly 75% [6]—of those cases in which a definite cause is found. The more carefully cerebrovascular disease is sought in late onset epileptic patients, the more frequently it is identified [26]. This observation may have to be treated with some caution. The presence of areas of ischaemia on a CT scan may not mean that these are the cause of the seizures. However, Sander et al. [6] argue that their estimate of the proportion of elderly onset seizures due to cerebrovascular disease may be an underestimate rather than an overestimate. Seizures commonly follow an overt stroke with about 4% of cases having early seizures [27] and poststroke seizures occurring in about 10% of ischaemic strokes within 5 years [28]. Haemorrhagic stroke in the Oxford series and that of Lancman [29] was particularly associated with seizures. Finally, seizures may be the first manifestation of hitherto silent cerebrovascular disease. Shinton et al. [30] found an excess of previous seizures of patients admitted to hospital with an acute stroke compared with controls, suggesting that clinically undetectable cerebrovascular disease may present with seizures and that an otherwise unexplained elderly onset seizure may warn of future stroke. A more recent study derived from a very large primary care database confirms that an elderly onset seizure predicts a greatly increased incidence of stroke subsequently [31].

Clinicians are often concerned that late onset epilepsy may indicate a cerebral tumour. Most series indicate that this applies to only a minority of cases—between 5 and 15% in most series [6,24,25]. The exception to this was the large study from southwest France [9] where 22% of cases of recurrent unprovoked seizures were associated with cerebral tumours. In the reported series, tumours were either metastatic or due to (inoperable) gliomas, although a few meningiomas were found. Until, however, there is information on an adequately documented, adequately investigated and sufficiently large population-based series, one cannot be certain what proportion of very late onset epilepsy is due to treatable and non-treatable tumours. At any rate, the proportion of seizures due to tumours without any pointers to the underlying cause—such as progressive neurological signs or features suggestive of raised intracranial pressure—will be smaller still.

Epidemiological studies (e.g. see [24]) have underlined the importance of toxic and metabolic causes of seizures in old age, accounting for about 10% of cases. Alcohol is important at any age and it must also be remembered that pyrexia and other acute conditions may precipitate seizures in older people [9] and that pneumonia, which in the biologically aged may be more likely to cause hypoxia, may predispose to seizures or precipitate them in an individual who has otherwise well-controlled epilepsy. Many drugs cause confusion and convulsions [32]. Drug-induced seizures are particularly likely when blood levels are high; this is often the case in patients with impaired drug clearance—a category which will include many elderly people.

Much uncertainty surrounds the relationship between non-vascular dementia and epileptic seizures and there has never, in my opinion, been a series in which the diagnosis of Alzheimer's disease has been sufficiently precise to rule out either the alternative diagnosis of multi-infarct dementia or mixed vascular and non-vascular dementia, to sustain the suggestions that Alzheimer's dementia *per se* is associated with an overall increase in seizures [33]. However, there is a specific form of myoclonic epilepsy that occurs in Alzheimer's disease [34] and is amenable to treatment with valproic acid.

Investigations

What has been said already underlines the importance of as full a history as possible and comprehensive examination in all cases. Some investigations, which should be regarded as routine, may yield helpful clues. These should include a full blood count, erythrocyte sedimentation rate (ESR), urea and electrolytes, blood glucose, chest X-ray and an ECG. Biochemical tests should include an estimate of γ-glutamyl transferase as a marker of recent alcohol consumption, and the threshold for carrying out thyroid function tests should be low, as myxoedema, which is associated with seizures, is common in older people and may present atypically. Other investigations, such as serological testing for syphilis, will be influenced by the history and examination.

Many investigations will be directed towards ruling out non-epileptic causes of loss of consciousness. Often, even after extensive cerebral and cardiovascular investigation (including ECG, 24-h ambulatory ECG monitoring and tilt-table testing with and without carotid sinus massage), the clinician will remain uncertain whether the patient's episodes are cardiac or cerebral in origin. Given that cardiac disease (for example a malignant arrhythmia) is more likely to be more life-threatening, in cases of uncertainty, the protocol for diagnosing syncope should be followed in the first instance. The protocols recommended by Kenny and Dey [18] for pursuing the diagnosis of and the underlying cause of syncope should be followed.

The value of special investigations, in particular EEG and neuroimaging, is sometimes overestimated [35]. Excessive reliance on EEG to make or refute a diagnosis of epilepsy is as dangerous in this group of patients as in younger patients. A routine EEG may support the diagnosis of epilepsy, especially if clear-cut epileptogenic or ictal discharges are observed. The absence of such activity on a routine recording does not, however, rule out the diagnosis. The range of normal increases with age, so that discriminating normal from abnormal becomes more difficult and non-specific or unrelated abnormalities are common [36]. Recently, there has been a trend back to the belief that clear-cut epileptogenic activity on an EEG should influence the decision to treat a single unprovoked seizure [37]. However, in the elderly onset patient, there may be special reasons

Table 16.4 Findings which may be regarded as special indications for CT or MRI in elderly onset seizures

Unexplained focal neurological signs
Progressive or new neurological signs or symptoms
Poor control of seizures not attributable to poor compliance with AEDs or continued exposure to precipitants such as alcohol
Clear-cut, stereotyped focal seizures
Persistent marked slow-wave abnormality on the EEG

to suspect that the EEG alone cannot determine the need for treatment in a newly diagnosed case, establish the adequacy of treatment or predict the safety of discontinuing therapy. Ictal or profuse interictal discharges may be useful in diagnosing non-convulsive status epilepticus, or epilepsy presenting with recurrent behavioural disturbance or other neuropsychiatric manifestations [22]. This may be particularly difficult to diagnose in a patient with mental impairment due to cerebrovascular disease.

CT will yield positive findings in as many as 60% of very late onset patients [38]. This, however, would be an argument for routine scanning only if identification of such lesions influenced management—as in the case of a space-occupying lesion amenable to neurosurgical removal. However, in only a minority of patients with elderly onset epilepsy is a neoplasm or subdural haematoma the cause, and in only a small proportion of tumour cases would neurosurgical intervention be appropriate. In the light of this, arguable indications for CT scanning or MRI are set out in Table 16.4. MRI has an increased diagnostic yield compared with CT, but it remains to be seen how often the information obtained would alter management of elderly onset seizures [39].

Some authors (e.g. [2]) have strongly argued for routine neuroimaging in all cases. The more positive attitude towards active management of cerebrovascular disease should probably lower the threshold for scanning as revealing otherwise occult ischaemic areas will influence management.

General aspects of management

The general principle that the management of patients with epilepsy goes far beyond AED treatment applies with particular force to older people (Table 16.5). Reassurance, education and support are crucial. Reassurance is of overriding importance: (a) that, in the vast majority of cases, seizures do not indicate serious brain damage; (b) that they do not imply psychiatric disease or dementia; (c) that they can be controlled by medication; and (d) that medication itself does not cause cumulative damage (a frequent worry with elderly people). Patients may want to know whether seizures are brought on by any particular activity and whether, for this reason, they should lead restricted lives. The advice in this age group is the same as that given to any patient: avoid only those activities that would mean immediate danger if a seizure occurred.

Management often involves a multidisciplinary team. A patient who has a seizure may suffer loss of confidence and, in the case of individuals who already have locomotor or other disability, this may lead not only to voluntary restriction of activities and a shrinkage of 'life space' but be the beginning of a progressive descent into a vicious spiral of reduced mobility. In such patients, restoration of

Table 16.5 Principles of epilepsy management in the elderly

Establish diagnosis. Give appropriate reassurance and counselling. Determine if medication is indicated

If treatment is indicated, inform patient, and sometimes relative or caregiver, about expected risks (side-effects) and benefits

Give appropriate instructions about need to take medication regularly

Start with a low dose and increase it gradually according to clinical response (unless special circumstances dictate otherwise)

Obtain careful recording of seizures and adverse experiences

Monitor blood levels of medication, if indicated. Adjust dosage only if seizures are uncontrolled or side-effects occur

If seizures recur at maximally tolerated dosage, reassess diagnosis and switch to alternative monotherapy. If seizures remain uncontrolled, try combination therapy

Monitor regularly clinical response and assess need for dosage adjustments and/or possibility of drug discontinuation

mobility, the assessment of the need for walking or other aids and a review of the patient's home circumstances and need for social support services will require input from remedial therapists and social workers. A home visit by an occupational therapist to look for potential sources of dangers—unguarded fires for example—may be helpful. In the case of frequent seizures, especially where there is a warning (aura), the patient may wish to be provided with a personal alarm.

Factors that are known to precipitate seizures, such as inadequate sleep or excess alcohol, should be avoided. Patients should be warned that alcohol will increase the side-effects of medication and that other drugs may have a convulsant effect or interact with anticonvulsants. They should be advised to remind their doctors that they have epilepsy when they are seen about other conditions for which they may receive prescriptions.

As with younger people, elderly patients should be given appropriate written advice and contact numbers for the relevant epilepsy associations, although they may find the age range of the other members rather young. The nature of seizures should be explained. Spouses, relatives, caring neighbours and other carers should be advised as to how to manage seizures if they occur. Standard advice about driving should be given.

When should AED treatment be started?

Epilepsy is defined as a tendency to recurring seizures, and treatment with AEDs presupposes that a patient does have such a tendency [40]. A single seizure—especially if it has an obvious precipitating cause such as fever or alcohol—does not, just as in younger people, count as epilepsy, the assumption being that it does not necessarily imply an underlying tendency to recurrence. Here the correct approach is not to prescribe a drug but to remove the cause. Where there is a single apparently unprovoked seizure, the decision whether or not to treat with AEDs is more difficult. It will be influenced by several considerations:

1 The clinician's view as to the likelihood of recurrence.

2 The estimate of the risks, such as injury, associated with a recurrent seizure.

3 The severity of the index seizure.

4 The estimated hazards of AEDs.

5 The credibility one gives to the notion that 'fits breed fits' such that early treatment may prevent epilepsy becoming chronic or intractable.

At present, we seem to have inadequate information to make rational decisions as to whether one should or should not treat a single unprovoked seizure in an older person. Age itself is not a consistent predictor of recurrence, although the presence of a clear-cut aetiological factor, such as a focal lesion, is. The relative dangers of non-treatment (injury due to recurrence) and of treatment (adverse effects of medication) have never been assessed in a systematic population-based, prospective manner. Until this has been done—and we have the results of the long-term outcome of suitable trials—the decision whether or not a single unprovoked seizure should be treated is a matter of personal prejudice, albeit dignified by the term 'clinical judgement'. It is encouraging that the UK Medical Research Council-funded study of early versus late treatment of seizures has proposed to recruit sufficient numbers of elderly people to permit conclusions to be drawn about elderly onset seizures.

My own practice is to treat a single unprovoked seizure if it is prolonged, especially if it has a clear-cut underlying cause, such as a previous stroke or a cerebral tumour. Where there is no such cause, and the seizure has not been prolonged, the decision is more difficult. In the case of a short-duration generalized convulsive seizure or a partial or non-convulsive seizure, I tend to wait. A patient whose driving licence is important may prefer to be treated after a single seizure. In a patient who has had a single seizure, it is important to emphasize prompt treatment of conditions, such as chest infections, that might lead to hypoxia and so precipitate further seizures.

The choice of AED

Since the last edition of this textbook, there has been a significant increase in the information available to prescribers about AEDs and, although not all this can be extrapolated from the rather young population that tends to predominate in AED trials, some of it is highly relevant. Moreover, there has been a modest increase in the number of trials specifically looking at AEDs in older patients. Of even greater importance has been the establishment of the Cochrane Collaboration, which over the last few years has produced high-quality systematic reviews of the information made available in randomized controlled trials. The problems of pooling the data have been addressed by sophisticated methodologies including accessing, as far as possible, individual patient data made available by the trialists. This has been of particular importance for assessing the relevance of the data to older patients. Ironically, one of the messages that has come through most clearly from the findings of the Cochrane Collaboration has been the lack of adequate information to support the therapeutic choices that we have to make. Another development since the last edition has been a further proliferation of the new-generation AEDs available to prescribers although there is little information about their role in the treatment of older patients.

Perhaps not unsurprisingly, the widening knowledge base and the increased range of therapeutic choices have made life more difficult for the thoughtful prescriber for older patients. Rational prescribing may become easier in the future when the respective merits of older- and newer-generation AEDs will hopefully be clarified by the result of the ongoing SANAD Trial (Standard and New Antiepileptic Drugs, National Health Service) in the UK and the VA Elderly Antiepileptic Drug Trial in the US. Any recommendations in this chapter must, therefore, be regarded as provisional.

Standard (old generation) AEDs

The majority of patients with either primary or secondary generalized seizures or partial seizures can be controlled with a single standard AED, and 70% of these patients can expect a 5-year remission.

For a long time, phenytoin, carbamazepine and valproic acid were considered to be equally effective as first-line AEDs for partial or generalized tonic-clonic seizures [41,42]. More recently, however, the findings of the Cochrane Collaboration lent partial support to the belief, held by some physicians, that carbamazepine may have some edge over valproic acid in the treatment of partial and secondarily generalized seizures, an important observation since most epilepsies with onset in old age are localization related [43]. In an analysis of individual data from 1265 patients from five trials [44], there was a trend for carbamazepine to be superior to valproic acid for all efficacy endpoints tested (time to withdrawal from the allocated treatment, time to 12-month remission, time to 6-month remission and time to first seizure), although based on confidence limits a statistically significant difference was found only for time to first seizure, a parameter which is of questionable clinical significance as it is influenced by the somewhat arbitrary choice of the starting dosage. Interestingly, the trend for carbamazepine to be superior to valproic acid in partial epilepsies was more evident with increasing age of the patient. For primary generalized tonic-clonic seizures, efficacy endpoints tended to favour valproic acid, but again confidence limits were too wide to allow detection of statistically significant differences. The authors commented that analysis of data for generalized epilepsies could have been confounded by the fact that at least in some patients secondarily generalized seizures were probably misclassified as primarily generalized.

In the light of the above findings, carbamazepine would be a reasonable first-line drug for the treatment of epilepsy with onset in old age, at least in those patients (the vast majority) for whom there is evidence of a focal onset. If carbamazepine is chosen, a sustained-release preparation is probably preferable to a standard (immediate-release) formulation. As discussed above, a small minority of seizures in older people are generalized in origin and these may benefit from valproic acid rather than carbamazepine: this is especially true for myoclonic seizures in patients with Alzheimer's disease, and late onset idiopathic primary generalized seizures. Some clinicians, moreover, have the impression that carbamazepine is less well tolerated than valproic acid in very old patients and recommend valproic acid as the first choice in the majority of patients. It is uncertain how valid this impression is.

In addition to valproic acid, alternative choices may be represented by phenytoin or, as discussed below in this section, a newer AED such as lamotrigine. Barbiturates were a popular choice in the past, but their propensity to cause sedation, cognitive disturbances and other side-effects, including shoulder–hand syndrome, make them less desirable for first-line treatment in this population.

If carbamazepine (or a new drug) is not used, there is little evidence-based data on whether valproic acid or phenytoin should be preferred. In the Cochrane meta-analysis that included 669 patients with partial and primarily or secondarily tonic-clonic seizures

treated with either phenytoin or valproic acid, no overall difference was found between the two drugs for the main efficacy outcomes examined [45]. Moreover, a multicentre comparative trial of efficacy in 150 elderly patients showed both valproic acid and phenytoin to be useful first-line AEDs in elderly onset seizures [46]. There were no significant differences in efficacy nor, surprisingly, in overall tolerability, between the two drugs. Interestingly, actuarial analysis suggested that 6-month remission by 12-month follow-up would be enjoyed by 78% of the patients on valproic acid and 76% of patients on phenytoin—very similar to the findings from monotherapy studies in the general adult population.

Adverse effects are of paramount importance in choosing an AED, and there are significant differences in the spectrum of acute dose-related, acute idiosyncratic and chronic toxic effects caused by individual agents. These adverse effects are summarized elsewhere in this textbook. It is important to appreciate, however, that they may present rather subtly in an older patient who may have preexisting pathology impairing either cognitive function or mobility.

Effects on cognitive function are of particular relevance to older people, whose seizures may take place against the background of existing cerebrovascular disease. Earlier studies suggested that, of the commonly used standard AEDs, the maximum adverse impact was seen with phenytoin, and lesser effects were seen with valproic acid and carbamazepine [47]. Interestingly, however, this difference has not been found in elderly patients. A detailed comparison of the impact of valproic acid and phenytoin on various aspects of cognitive function, including attention, concentration, psychomotor speed and memory, in elderly people failed to show major differences between the two drugs [48]. This is in keeping with more recent literature which also failed to demonstrate significant differences in the cognitive effects of AEDs in the general adult population [49]. It is probable that, if the dose of AEDs is kept at the minimum effective level, differences in adverse cognitive effects are less important even in older people. However, neurological or neuropsychiatric side-effects—for example, unsteadiness and tiredness (including the frustration of repeatedly falling asleep during one's favourite TV soap)—may be significant and there may be important differences in the frequency and severity of these. Studies from the US indicate that elderly patients are more vulnerable to develop AED-induced impairment of gait, as well as action and postural tremor [2]. However, we know little about subtle adverse neurological and other effects of AEDs in older people.

As far as less commonly used AEDs are concerned, the risks associated with inappropriate use of benzodiazepines should be mentioned. Elderly patients are very sensitive to the adverse effects of these drugs on cognition, and may experience prolonged confusion and an increased tendency to falls and injuries after intake of doses of benzodiazepines which are usually well tolerated in younger people.

Of the many non-neurological side-effects, osteomalacia [50] may be especially relevant since this is more likely to occur in older people whose poor dietary intake of vitamin D and reduced exposure to sunlight already puts them at risk. Carbamazepine, phenytoin and barbiturates, in particular, induce enzymes in the liver that accelerate the metabolism of vitamin D, and there may be a case for routine vitamin supplementation in patients on these AEDs. A recent report suggested that valproic acid, which is not an enzyme inducer, may also cause a decrease in bone mineral density [51].

Carbamazepine-induced hyponatraemia increases significantly with age [52] and may occur at very low doses. The risk of hyponatraemia, which may be even greater with oxcarbazepine (see below), is especially important in patients on diuretics—particularly potassium-sparing, sodium-losing diuretics—or in patients who are prone to hyponatraemia from other causes, such as recurrent chest infections. Disturbances in cardiac rhythm or conduction may also be more common with carbamazepine than with other drugs, particularly in patients with pre-existing heart disease. Another problem not infrequently encountered with carbamazepine and phenytoin are skin rashes, which may be occasionally severe.

Many other factors, in addition to efficacy and adverse effects, need to be taken into account in choosing a first-line AED. One is ease of use by the patient. Phenytoin can be used once daily, which is an advantage in the case of patients requiring help from others with their medication. Though sustained-release valproic acid has been used by some once daily, it is still usually given twice daily and the same is true of sustained-release carbamazepine. Ease of use by the physician is also important. Phenytoin is unusual in exhibiting saturation kinetics near the therapeutic range, so that a small change in the dose may be associated with a disproportionately large change in serum drug concentration, with the risk of a switch from subtherapeutic to toxic levels. This makes phenytoin potentially problematic in inexperienced hands. There is also the question of drug–drug and drug–disease interactions. Finally, cost is an issue, although the difference in price between the older-generation AEDs is small compared with the difference in price between older and newer AEDs.

Monotherapy is always preferable to polytherapy, particularly in patients who are likely already to be on one or more medications. When monotherapy is unsuccessful, this is often due to poor compliance, or it is sometimes related to the presence of a serious underlying cerebral condition. In compliant patients not responding adequately to initial monotherapy, an alternative monotherapy with another AED is usually the best course of action (Table 16.5). Adding a second drug sometimes contributes only additional side-effects, and in some patients who are on more than one drug, withdrawal of the second or third drug may actually improve control. Though monotherapy should be the aim, there will be a proportion of patients who will require two AEDs, but before embarking on this the advice of an expert should be sought.

In summary, among standard AEDs there may be a case for preferring carbamazepine as the first choice in partial epilepsies, though some would prefer valproic acid or phenytoin. At any rate, there should be no blanket recommendation for the 'elderly'. There may be individual drugs that are more suited to individual patients. Whatever drug is chosen, the prescribing physician should be familiar with its kinetics, dosing requirements, efficacy profile and side-effects.

New-generation AEDs

We have little clear evidence about the comparative advantages and disadvantages of old- and new-generation AEDs. There are general characteristics of some new AEDs that make them very attractive to physicians caring for older people with seizures. In trials of the general adult population, these drugs have shown comparable efficacy, but—at times—fewer side-effects than the older agents. Moreover, some of the newer AEDs have simpler pharmacokinetics and they are less prone to cause drug interactions. Against this, two important considerations should weigh against a wholesale switch in prescribing habits. First of all, new-generation drugs are much more expensive than the older ones and, since epilepsy is a chronic illness affecting large numbers of patients, this has significant implications for the national drug budget. Secondly, these drugs remain relatively untried compared with the standard drugs and unexpected adverse effects may still emerge. This has been dramatically illustrated in the case of vigabatrin, which looked very promising indeed but is no longer recommended because it causes serious irreversible visual field loss which might be especially difficult to pick up in older patients [53]. The following brief notes should therefore be regarded as provisional reports from a rapidly changing situation.

Lamotrigine

Lamotrigine is the only new AED which has been tested relatively extensively in the elderly. Indeed, a recent multicentre, double-blind randomized monotherapy comparison in elderly patients with new onset epilepsy found advantages for lamotrigine over carbamazepine [54]. The main difference between the drugs was the rate of drop out due to adverse events (lamotrigine 18% vs. carbamazepine 42%): this was partly due to a lower rash rate with lamotrigine, but lamotrigine patients also complained less frequently of somnolence. Although there was no difference between the two drugs in time to first seizure, a greater percentage of lamotrigine-treated patients remained seizure free during the last 16 weeks of treatment. Overall, more patients continued on treatment with lamotrigine than carbamazepine (71% and 42%, respectively) for the duration of study. The median daily doses of lamotrigine and carbamazepine in the patients completing the trial were 100 mg (range 75–300 mg) and 400 mg (range 200–800 mg), respectively. The authors concluded that lamotrigine could be regarded as an acceptable choice of initial treatment for elderly patients with newly diagnosed epilepsy. A combination of lamotrigine with valproic acid can reduce seizures in refractory cases, but this combination should be used cautiously because the risk of skin rashes (and other adverse effects) from lamotrigine is markedly increased in patients taking valproic acid. In these patients, lamotrigine should be started at reduced dosages and escalated very slowly.

Oxcarbazepine

Oxcarbazepine is an analogue of carbamazepine, developed in an effort to retain the therapeutic effects of the latter while offering improved tolerability [55]. It has a lower allergenic potential than carbamazepine and, although it retains some enzyme-inducing activity, it causes fewer drug interactions. Given these advantages, it could be a useful alternative to carbamazepine for older people. There is, however, insufficient information in large numbers of elderly people and there is concern about hyponatraemia, though how important this is remains a matter of controversy [56]. Personal experience indicates that one has to be as careful when introducing oxcarbazepine as carbamazepine, despite theoretical reasons for thinking that it will be better tolerated in the early stages of titration. When substituting carbamazepine with oxcarbazepine, it should be remembered that the enzyme-inducing effect of the former will wear off, and dosage of comedication may need to be adjusted.

Gabapentin

Gabapentin is a relatively easy drug to use because it is excreted unchanged in the kidney, has a wide therapeutic window and it has no interactions with other drugs. For these reasons, it is another potentially attractive first-line drug for older patients with partial epilepsy, particularly as it appears to be relatively free from side-effects [57]. There is, however, insufficient evidence to determine its place in monotherapy [58]. As with other new drugs, research is needed into long-term use: studies have tended to focus on its short-term effects. There is certainly a case for more studies comparing gabapentin with other AEDs as monotherapy in partial epilepsy with onset in old age.

Topiramate

Topiramate has relatively simple pharmacokinetics, is excreted mostly unchanged in the kidney (at least when it is not associated with enzyme-inducing AEDs) and appears to have few significant interactions. The incidence of central nervous system side-effects can be reduced with a slow dose titration. Most studies with topiramate have been conducted in adjunctive use in patients with drug-resistant epilepsy, where it has been found to have a broad spectrum of activity [59]. There are few data for monotherapy, and little data on its use in elderly patients.

Levetiracetam

Levetiracetam is the most recently introduced AED, and it has been found to be effective in the adjunctive therapy of patients with drug refractory partial epilepsy [60]. Levetiracetam is administered twice daily, and it shows simple pharmacokinetics, renal elimination mostly in unchanged form, good tolerability and lack of clinically significant drug interactions. These properties make levetiracetam an attractive drug for the treatment of epilepsy in old age, particularly in patients receiving complex comedications. On the other hand, there are no adequate data on its value when given as monotherapy, and clinical experience in the elderly has been very limited so far.

Tiagabine

Tiagabine is a γ-aminobutyric acid (GABA) uptake inhibitor which has been found effective in improving seizure frequency following add-on use in patients with refractory partial epilepsy [61]. Current information is insufficient to determine its usefulness when used as monotherapy, and there are no adequate data concerning its use in the elderly. A disadvantage of tiagabine is its short half-life necessitating 2–4 times daily administration, which is a consideration in elderly patients.

Zonisamide

Zonisamide has been available in Japan for over a decade, and it has recently been introduced in the US. There is, as yet, relatively little experience with this drug. Zonisamide has been studied most extensively in patients with drug-resistant partial epilepsy, but other studies suggest a broader spectrum efficacy [62]. As with other newer AEDs, experience in monotherapy and in the elderly has been very limited.

Vigabatrin

Vigabatrin has been found to be quite useful in the management of refractory partial seizures, but its prescriptions have been drastically curtailed following discovery of irreversible visual field defects associated with its use [53]. In pharmacokinetic studies, considerable central nervous system side-effects were observed when elderly patients were given vigabatrin doses which were well tolerated in young subjects [63]. This could be explained, at least in part, by an age-related reduction in the clearance of this renally excreted drug.

In summary, some new AEDs have promise for the treatment of seizure disorders in the elderly, mainly due to improved tolerability and/or reduced potential for drug interactions. However, in view of the fact that they are much more expensive, and that few have been specifically evaluated in an elderly population, it would be premature to consider these drugs as first choice for elderly patients, with the possible exception of lamotrigine. As discussed in a recent review [64] 'At present, the main use of the new agents is in patients refractory to first-line drugs . . . and further studies are required to characterize their activity spectrum as well as their potential value in monotherapy. In most patients, new drugs cannot be recommended for first-line use until evidence is obtained that potential advantages in tolerability or ease of use outweigh the drawback of their high cost.' Marson *et al.* [65] suggest that, if add-on treatment is required with the drugs discussed above, gabapentin and lamotrigine offer the best option for patients with drug intolerance but adequate seizure control, while in patients with poor seizure control in whom potency is the main issue, topiramate might be an optimal choice.

As discussed above, lamotrigine is currently the only new AED where a case could be made for its first-line use in the elderly. Indeed, this drug has been formally tested and found to be efficacious and well tolerated when used as monotherapy in patients with onset of epilepsy in old age. A useful feature of lamotrigine is the lack of enzyme-inducing properties, which is advantageous when an AED has to be used in patients receiving medications for unrelated medical conditions.

Prescribing strategies

As discussed above, treatment should be started with a single drug, and dosage increased gradually according to clinical response (Table 16.5). If, despite adequate dosage and good compliance, there is poor control, then a second first-line AED should be tried as an alternative monotherapy. In a small minority of patients it may be necessary to use more than one AED at a time, but such patients should be referred to a physician with special expertise.

Some patients may not be fully controlled even with optimal AED treatment. This should not prompt ever-increasing, toxic doses of multiple drugs, but a more modest goal: a reduction in seizure frequency to tolerable levels without unacceptable side-effects. Feeling continually wretched from the adverse effects of AEDs may be even worse than suffering the intermittent unpleasantness of a seizure.

Dosages

The dosages recommended for the general adult population may be inappropriate for elderly patients, due to a number of factors (Table 16.6). There is considerable evidence to support an age-related increase in pharmacodynamic sensitivity to certain AEDs [2,13]. For example, a study of carbamazepine found that a 400-mg dose caused a greater effect on body sway in the elderly than in the young, despite the absence of differences in blood levels of the drug between the two groups. In many cases, pharmacokinetic changes contribute to the greater susceptibility of elderly patients to side-effects. In particular, old age is associated with a physiological reduction in renal function, resulting in reduced clearance of AEDs which are eliminated extensively in unchanged form by the kidney. These include, among others, primidone, gabapentin, vigabatrin and levetiracetam. Metabolic drug clearance may also be reduced in old age: for example, the metabolic clearance of unbound valproic acid and phenytoin is lower in the elderly than in the young.

Because albumin concentrations tend to be lower in elderly people, the total serum drug concentration of drugs which are highly bound to plasma proteins may underestimate the concentration of unbound, pharmacologically active drug. This has been demonstrated for phenytoin, valproic acid and certain benzodiazepines. Prolongation of the half-life of some AEDs, due to changes in drug clearance and/or volume of distribution, should also be considered as it may cause a prolongation in the time required to reach steady-state conditions after initiation of therapy or dosage adjustment.

It should be emphasized that present knowledge of age-related changes in pharmacodynamics or pharmacokinetics may not find easy applicability to an individual patient. As already noted, so-called age changes are often derived by comparing mean values for groups of young and old subjects, but differences within these groups may be at least as important. In the case of phenytoin, for example, only 20% of the interindividual variation noted in one series was attributable to age alone [66]. In this context, as so often in clinical geriatrics, age is more important as a source of unpredictable variability than of predictable change.

Other sources of unpredictability arise from concurrent diseases, particularly those that affect pharmacokinetics through hepatic metabolism or those, such as cerebral disease, which affect pharmacodynamic sensitivity. Moreover, multiple pathology associated with old age will often mean multiple medications, and many drugs interact with AEDs and they interact with one another. The British National Formulary [67], which is updated 3-monthly, is a good reference for clinically important interactions. Among these, interactions between AEDs such as phenytoin and anticoagulants are of particular importance in view of their potential seriousness and the escalating number of elderly patients who may benefit from anticoagulant prophylaxis against cardiovascular disease. This may direct the clinician towards those of the newer AEDs that do not interact with anticoagulants.

In the light of the considerations made above, to suggest specific doses 'for the elderly' is misconceived. All that can be recommended is a general strategy, i.e. 'start low and go slow', and be prepared to find that the response, either in terms of adverse effects or efficacy, is not precisely what one had expected or hoped for. Overall, epilepsy with onset in old age tends to respond very favourably to AED treatment in terms of seizure control, even at low dosages, even though susceptibility to adverse effects may also be increased [2]. There is now sufficient evidence to suggest that the initial dose of phenytoin in an elderly person should not be more than 200 mg, possibly lower. Most patients will be controlled on 150–250 mg daily. Cau-

Table 16.6 Factors leading to altered responsiveness to antiepileptic drugs (AEDs) in old age

Factor	Consequences	Implications
Altered pharmacodynamic sensitivity	Generally, increased susceptibility to adverse effects. Suggestive evidence of good seizure control at lower dosages	Risk of toxicity. Reduced AED dose requirements
Reduced glomerular filtration rate	Reduced clearance of AEDs eliminated predominantly in unchanged form in urine (e.g. primidone, gabapentin, levetiracetam, vigabatrin, topiramate)	Risk of toxicity. Reduced AED dose requirements
Reduced drug metabolizing capacity	Reduced metabolic clearance of some drugs (e.g. valproic acid, phenytoin, carbamazepine, oxcarbazepine)	Risk of toxicity. Reduced AED dose requirements
Hypoalbuminemia	Reduced plasma protein binding of highly albumin-bound drugs (e.g. phenytoin, valproic acid)	Altered relationship between total serum AED concentration and response (therapeutic and toxic effects observed at lower total drug concentrations)
Increased body fat/lean mass ratio	Increased volume of distribution of lipid soluble drugs. Prolongation of half-life (reduced clearance may contribute to this)	Longer time to reach steady-state following initiation of treatment of dosage adjustments
Comorbidity	Alterations in AED pharmacokinetics and/or pharmacodynamics	Risk of toxicity. Altered AED dose requirements
Comedication	Drug interactions (especially enzyme induction and enzyme inhibition)	Risk of toxicity (enzyme inhibition) or loss of therapeutic response (enzyme induction) for either AEDs or comedications.

tion in dosage alteration is particularly important with phenytoin where, as already noted, near the therapeutic range, an increment of as little as 25 mg may cause a marked rise in blood levels. For carbamazepine, it would seem reasonable to commence at 100–200 mg total daily dose, with a maintenance between about 400 mg and 800 mg daily. Valproic acid should be started at 400 mg total daily dose, increasing to about 1–1.2 g total daily dose if necessary. Except where seizures are frequent and control is a matter of urgency, dosage increases should be gradual.

As for the newer drugs, the 'start low, go slow' principle is even more relevant given the limited published information about their use in older people. At any rate, it is difficult in view of the lack of clinical experience to make more specific dosage recommendations with these drugs. Identifying the optimal procedure for substituting one drug for another may be complex, though in some cases, as in the replacement of valproic acid by lamotrigine, there is useful guidance from the manufacturers.

Therapeutic drug monitoring

The long-term management of patients with epilepsy was helped by the introduction in the 1970s of the practice of monitoring serum AED concentrations (Chapter 11). Therapeutic drug monitoring may be useful where: seizures are not controlled by average doses of drugs; there are doubts about compliance; there are signs of intoxication, or odd neuropsychiatric symptoms; there is a sudden loss of seizure control; new interacting drugs are introduced; there are other diseases that may complicate treatment; and before withdrawing therapy. The poor predictability of pharmacokinetic changes in the elderly makes AED monitoring particularly appropriate in this age group.

It must be appreciated, however, that the most important part of patient monitoring is not measurement of AED levels, but the use of information derived from history and examination [68]. The patient or relative should keep a record of seizures. Moreover, the patient should always be accompanied by a well-informed relative, neighbour or caretaker to ensure that an accurate account of events is obtained. Independent witnesses may also help the physician to pick up adverse effects that may be subtle in elderly people and, if not actively looked for, missed. Some attempt should be made to assess compliance and this should always be discussed with the patient. Increasing the dose because poor control due to variable compliance has been misinterpreted as implying insufficient dosage may lead to disaster. It is vital to emphasize the need to take medication consistently and indefinitely, as some elderly patients may be under the erroneous impression that AEDs need to be taken only when seizures occur or as a 'course'. Finally, doctors should be aware that generic substitution may be associated with changes in serum drug levels and consequent alteration in seizure control and/or an increase in side-effects. This is particularly important with phenytoin, due to its dose-dependent pharmacokinetics.

Serum AED levels are most helpful when they are used to answer a particular question. Measuring drug concentration tends to be more useful with phenytoin, because of its non-linear relationship between dose and blood level, its propensity to produce adverse neuropsychiatric effects that may present non-specifically or be lost in the noise of other neurological and non-neurological pathology and its marked pharmacokinetic variability. Moreover, for phenytoin there is a relatively close correlation, at least at the population level, between serum drug concentration and clinical effect. It should be remembered, however, that in the presence of hypoalbuminaemia, renal insufficiency or concomitant administration of displacing drugs (e.g. salicylates), the total serum phenytoin concentration may underestimate the unbound drug concentration, i.e. therapeutic and toxic effects may be seen at total concentrations lower than usual.

The place of anticonvulsant monitoring is less well defined for carbamazepine, phenobarbital and valproic acid. Values given for the therapeutic range should be interpreted with caution especially in elderly people: seizure control may be achieved throughout a very wide range of concentrations. Moreover, for carbamazepine and valproic acid, a single measurement may give misleading information because of large fluctuations in serum concentration during a dosage interval. The monitoring of these drugs, however, may help to rationalize treatment in patients on polypharmacy and to identify the cause for treatment failure when a patient is on an apparently adequate dose. Except for phenobarbital, which shows negligible fluctuations during a dosing interval, samples should be taken at a standard time in relation to doses.

Overdoing or overinterpreting AED levels may lead to mismanagement [68]. As already indicated, levels are only a small part of the clinical assessment and the results obtained from the laboratory must be interpreted in the light of the larger picture. Therapeutic ranges defined on general adult populations may not apply to the elderly population, and certainly will not necessarily apply to any individual elderly patient. Doses should not be adjusted in seizure-free non-toxic patients simply to bring the levels into the 'therapeutic range'. Conversely, a patient with symptoms suggestive of intoxication should not be required to continue on the same dose simply because the values from the laboratory fall within the notional therapeutic range. It must be remembered that laboratory results may be incorrect for all sorts of technical reasons, ranging from the time the specimen was taken, through the labelling of the specimen, to the method used in the measurement.

Improving compliance

People of all age groups tend to comply poorly with AED treatment—which is not surprising in view of the chronicity of treatment, the purely prophylactic nature of the benefit and the frequency of side-effects. There is little evidence that non-cognitively impaired elderly patients are much less compliant than younger people [69]. Nevertheless, poor or variable compliance will be another reason for the lack of a predictable relationship between prescribed dose and plasma drug level, and between the doctor's action and the patient's response. Moreover, there are special problems for an older patient who may be on several drugs in addition to AEDs. A number of ways in which compliance may be assisted are listed in Table 16.7.

Prognosis

Seizure control

There is little information on the proportion of elderly onset patients who are satisfactorily controlled on AEDs. A report from the

Table 16.7 Strategies which may be used to optimize compliance in the elderly patient

Simplifying regimes
Giving clear instructions, both orally and written
Making sure that medication is clearly labelled
Making sure that medication is accessible (childproof bottles and
  blister packs may defeat the patient)
Coopting the help of caretakers, relatives and others where appropriate
Using compliance aids, such as dosette containers
Adopting a non-adversarial approach to compliance
Trying to determine the reason for non-compliance if it is detected
Home visits or telephone contact by a specialist nurse

NGPSE found that 9 years after the index seizure, 68% of subjects with definite epilepsy had had a 5-year remission and that age was not relevant [70]. In a comparative study of phenytoin and valproic acid [46], failure due to unacceptable seizure control was found in only 2% of patients on valproic acid and 4% of those on phenytoin, though 10% and 14%, respectively, withdrew due to adverse effects. Larger-scale studies are required to confirm these estimates, and to determine whether the newer AEDs will improve this picture. As already noted, lamotrigine seems to have the edge over carbamazepine in terms of patients' acceptability.

Can AEDs be withdrawn?

There is little data on which to guide decisions about the possibility of withdrawing AED treatment in the elderly. Studies looking at outcome after drug withdrawal [71,72] assessed much younger populations, and the same is true for a recent study [73] where the number of patients over 55 (hardly elderly from a geriatrician's perspective!) scarcely exceeded double figures. A review of slow AED withdrawal in over 1000 people who had been seizure free for at least 2 years found that 78% of patients on continuing treatment remained seizure free, compared with 59% of those taken off AEDs. Clinical predictors of relapse after drug withdrawal include age, syndrome, seizure type, number of AEDs being taken, occurrence of seizures after AEDs were started and duration of remission before drug withdrawal. Because late onset epilepsy, partial and secondarily generalized seizures (which are, of course, more common in the elderly) and presence of known cerebral pathology (also more common in elderly epileptic patients) are associated with an increased rate of relapse, one may have to reluctantly concede that withdrawal of therapy should not be attempted in most elderly patients who have had a good reason to be placed on AEDs in the first place. However, this does not preclude attempting withdrawal in a patient who has a strong desire to be taken off AEDs, provided the decision is taken after a full discussion with the patient of risks and benefits, and implications for driving if seizures recur.

Mortality

Mortality is increased in people with epilepsy, even though the relative increase (the standard mortality ratio) may be less marked in those diagnosed over 60 years of age than in those diagnosed in youth or middle age. Hauser *et al.* [74] found that the death rate from cardiac disease was increased in patients with elderly onset epilepsy, but that the incidence of sudden cardiac death was increased only in patients with symptomatic epilepsy in whom cerebrovascular disease was the attributed cause. Luhdorf *et al.* [75] followed 251 patients for a minimum period of 2 years. Although survival at 6 years was 60% of what was expected, most deaths were related to cerebrovascular disease or tumours, and when patients with tumours or overt cerebrovascular disease were excluded, mortality was no higher than that of the age-matched population. The bulk of the little evidence we have suggests that, in the absence of serious progressive disease, the prognosis both for control of seizures and for survival is good in elderly onset cases. However, more prospective long-term studies are required, particularly because a report from Alabama [76] suggested a high death rate (4%) in elderly patients discharged from hospital with a primary diagnosis of convulsions.

Services for patients with epilepsy

The challenge presented by an elderly patient whose symptoms suggest seizures is formidable. Making a correct differential diagnosis may require a good deal of clinical acumen and, sometimes, access to sophisticated investigative tools. Beyond this, there is the task of ensuring that patients are fully informed about their condition and its implications, and that the necessary reassurance, education and counselling are given. Finally, there is the challenge of ensuring that the appropriate medication is prescribed, and that a correct dosage is taken over many years in a patient who may have or develop other illnesses influencing the response to AED therapy.

The nature of these challenges argues for the development of specialist services. Perhaps these should not be addressed specifically to patients with epilepsy but should be open to patients who suffer from paroxysmal disorders of all kinds. Disease-specific clinics, such as clinics for epilepsy or clinics for syncopal episodes, tend to prejudge diagnoses. My own epilepsy clinic operates in close partnership with a colleague's syncope clinic: there is only a 'semi-permeable membrane' between the two services. If such specialist services are developed, a crucial element is specific diagnostic facilities, because often the most difficult challenge is arriving at a robust diagnosis of seizures.

At present, there is little experience of such specialist services for older people. Elderly people with seizures may fall between two stools, between specialist geriatrics services that have little expertise in epilepsy and specialist epilepsy services that have little expertise in the medical problems of old age. Ideally, specialist clinics should be the hub of a population-based service crossing the divide between hospital and primary care. At the least, the clinic should reach out to the wider geriatric medical services and to community services. There should be clear definition of the respective roles of general practitioners and specialists in what will, inevitably in a chronic disease, be 'shared care'.

A crucial role in the services may be played by the specialist epilepsy nurse, who can be cost-effective in supporting patients with epilepsy in the long term, meeting their needs for information, education, counselling and monitoring [77]. More recent overviews, however, failed to provide convincing evidence that specialist epilepsy nurses improve outcome for people with epilepsy overall [78,79]. Seizure frequency, psychosocial functioning,

Table 16.8 Areas for future research in geriatric epileptology

Better definition of underlying aetiologies
Evaluation of physical and psychosocial implications of seizures
Indications for early vs. deferred drug treatment
Evaluation of the comparative efficacy and safety of traditional AEDs
Evaluation of the comparative value of newer-generation AEDs
Evaluation of optimal structure and cost-effectiveness of specialist
    services

knowledge of epilepsy, general health status, work days lost, depression and anxiety scores showed no significant improvement. The latter findings, however, should be interpreted cautiously. First of all, lack of evidence of benefit was not evidence of lack of benefit, and the authors emphasize the need for further research. Moreover, nurses enable an overstretched service to reach out to more patients who would otherwise be overlooked and would not even be included in studies. Finally, these studies did not look at older patients who might be expected to be more in need of support, for example over management of their medication. Our ignorance of the potential benefits of specialist clinics is even more profound, as to date there have been no controlled trials of suitable quality comparing specialist with non-specialist clinics.

Areas for research

It is evident from the foregoing that, despite recent interest, geriatric epileptology is a relatively underdeveloped and underresearched field. These are some of the areas that urgently require investigation (Table 16.8).

Causes of seizures

Although it is now clear that cerebrovascular disease is the most common cause of seizures in old age, the relation may be overestimated because of the frequency of CT scan evidence of vascular disease in the general elderly population. More studies are needed to determine the frequency and type of cerebral tumors as a cause.

The physical impact of seizures

Seizures might be expected to have more adverse physical effects in the elderly. Studies are required to test whether this the case. It is unclear, in particular, how common seizure-related fractures and other significant injuries are in old people.

The psychosocial impact of seizures

Jacoby *et al.* [80] emphasized how the 'impact of a chronic illness is experienced not only through its physical symptoms, but also as a result of its effect on psychosocial functioning. In the case of an illness such as epilepsy, where the physical manifestations are transient, the psychosocial consequences may, with time, come to be of greater concern'. We know little or nothing about this in older people. We need to gain an understanding of what they think about seizures, what misconceptions or fears they have and how much these contribute to inducing dependency and shrinking life space. It

is important to assess what the information needs are of these patients, and how those needs can be best met. A small start in trying to assess quality of life in older people with seizures has been made [81].

When to use AEDs

Studies are required to determine whether, and when, one should treat a single unprovoked tonic-clonic seizure in old age. Additional unsolved questions concern the chances of recurrence where there is no overt cause for the seizure, and how easy seizures are to control in old age.

The role of newer-generation AEDs

Prospective studies are needed to assess the place of monotherapy with new-generation AEDs in the *de novo* treatment of elderly onset seizures. These studies should focus not simply on the traditional endpoints such as seizure control, but also on the feasibility of reducing subtle adverse effects on, for example, gait and mobility, which in a frail elderly person can translate into significant dysfunction.

The organization of epilepsy services

Issues to be addressed include how best we can provide a service for elderly people with seizures, what are the elements of an optimal overall comprehensive service, who should provide it and how it could be evaluated.

If we had answers to these questions our management of seizures in old age would be considerably better than it is now.

References

1 Rowan AJ, Ramsay GR. *Seizures and Epilepsy in the Elderly*. Boston: Butterworth-Heinemann, 1997.
2 Kramer G. *Epilepsy in the Elderly: Clinical Aspects and Pharmacotherapy*. Stuttgart: Georg Thieme Verlag, 1999.
3 Hauser WA, Kurland LT. The epidemiology of epilepsy in Rochester, Minnesota, 1935 through 1967. *Epilepsia* 1975; 16: 1–66.
4 Hauser WA, Annegers JF, Kurland LT. Incidence of epilepsy and unprovoked seizures in Rochester Minnesota: 1935–1984. *Epilepsia* 1993; 34: 453–68.
5 Luhdorf K, Jensen LK, Plesner AM. Epilepsy in the elderly: incidence, social function, and disability. *Epilepsia* 1986; 27: 135–41.
6 Sander JWAS, Hart YM, Johnson AL, Shorvon SD. National General Practice Study of Epilepsy: newly diagnosed epileptic seizures in general population. *Lancet* 1990; 336: 1267–70.
7 Tallis RC, Craig I, Hall G, Dean A. How common are epileptic seizures in old age? *Age Ageing* 1991; 20: 442–8.
8 Wallace H, Shorvon S, Tallis RC. Age-specific incidence and prevalence rate of treated epilepsy in an unselected population of 2,052,922 and age-specific fertility rates of women with epilepsy. *Lancet* 1998; 352: 1970–3.
9 Loiseau J, Loiseau P, Duche B, Guyot M, Dartigues J-F, Aublot B. A survey of epileptic disorders in southwest France: seizures in elderly patients. *Ann Neurol* 1996; 27: 232–7.
10 Godfrey JW. Misleading presentation of epilepsy in elderly people. *Age Ageing* 1989; 18: 17–20.
11 Norris JW, Hachinski VC. Mis-diagnosis of stroke. *Lancet* 1982; i: 328–31.
12 Downton JH. *Falls in the Elderly*. London: Edward Arnold, 1993.

13 Mawer G. Specific pharmacokinetic and pharmacodynamic problems of anticonvulsant drugs in the elderly. In: Tallis RC, ed. *Epilepsy and the Elderly*. London: Royal Society of Medicine Services, 1988: 21–30.

14 Bauer LA, Blouin RA. Age and phenytoin kinetics in adult epileptics. *Clin Pharmacol Ther* 1982; 31: 301–4.

15 Tallis RC, Baker G. Epilepsy in old age: quality of life issues. In: Baker G, Jacoby A, eds. *Quality of Life in Epilepsy*. London: Harwood, 2000: 135–45.

16 Colledge NR, Wilson LA, Macintyre CCA, Maclennan WJ. The prevalence and characteristics of dizziness in an elderly community. *Age Ageing* 1993; 23: 121–6.

17 McIntosh S, DaCosta D, Kenny RA. Outcome of an integrated approach to the investigation of dizziness, falls and syncope in elderly patients referred to a 'syncope' clinic. *Age Ageing* 1993; 22: 53–8.

18 Kenny RA, Dey S. Syncope. In: Tallis R, Fillett H, eds. *Brocklehurst's Textbook of Geriatric Medicine and Gerontology*, 6th edn. London: Harcourt, 2002.

19 Lempert T, Bauer M, Schmidt D. Syncope: a videometric analysis of 56 episodes of transient cerebral anoxia. *Ann Neurol* 1994; 36: 233–8.

20 Grubb BP. Differentiation of convulsive syncope and epilepsy with head-up tilt testing. *Ann Intern Med* 1991; 115: 871–6.

21 Ellis JM, Lee SI. Acute prolonged confusion in later life as an ictal state. *Epilepsia* 1978; 19: 119–28.

22 Jamal GA, Fowler CJ, Leslei K, Prior PF, Gawler J. Non-convulsive status epilepticus as a cause of acute confusional state in the over-60 age group. *J Neurol Neurosurg Psychiatry* 1988; 51: 738.

23 Blumer D. Epilepsy and disorders of mood. *Adv Neurol* 1991; 55: 185–95.

24 Luhdorf K, Jensen LK, Plesner A. Etiology of seizures in the elderly. *Epilepsia* 1986; 27: 458–63.

25 Sung C-Y, Chu N-S. Epileptic seizures in elderly people: aetiology and seizure type. *Age Ageing* 1990; 19: 25–30.

26 Shorvon SD, Gilliatt RW, Cox TCS, Yu YL. Evidence of vascular disease from CT scanning in late-onset epilepsy. *J Neurol Neurosurg Psychiatry* 1984; 47: 225–30.

27 Kilpatrick CJ Davis SM, Tress BM, Rossitor SC, Hopper JL, Vandendriesen ML. Epileptic seizures in acute stroke. *Arch Neurol* 1990; 47: 157–60.

28 Burn JM, Dennis M, Bamford J, Sandercock P, Wade D, Warlow C. Epileptic seizures after a first stroke in the Oxford Community Stroke Project. *Br Med J* 1997; 315: 1582–7.

29 Lancman ME, Golimstok A, Norscini J, Granillo R. Risk factors for developing seizures after stroke. *Epilepsia* 1993; 34(1): 141–3.

30 Shinton RA, Gill JS, Melnick SC, Gupta AK, Beevers DG. The frequency, characteristics and prognosis of epileptic seizures at the onset of stroke. *J Neurol Neurosurg Psychiatry* 1988; 51: 273–6.

31 Cleary P, Tallis R, Shorvon S. Late-onset seizures as a prediction of subsequent stroke. *Age Ageing* 2003; 32 (Suppl. 1): 15.

32 Schachter SC. Iatrogenic seizures. *Neurol Clin North Am* 1998; 16: 157–70.

33 Mcareavey BJ, Ballinger BR, Fenton GW. Epileptic seizures in elderly patients with dementia. *Epilepsia* 1991; 33: 657–60.

34 Hauser WA, Morris ML, Heston LL, Anderson VE. Seizures and myoclonus in patients with Alzheimer's disease. *Neurology* 1986; 36: 1226–30.

35 Dam AM. Late-onset epilepsy, etiologies, types of seizure and value of clinical investigation, EEG and CT scan. *Epilepsia* 1985; 26: 227–31.

36 Smith J. Clinical neurophysiology in the elderly. In: Tallis RC, ed. *The Clinical Neurology of Old Age*. Chichester: John Wiley, 1989: 89–97.

37 Beghi E, Ciccione A and the First Seizure Trial Group (FIRST). Recurrence after a first unprovoked seizure. Is it still a controversial issue? *Seizure* 1993; 2: 5–10.

38 Ramirez-Lassepas M, Cipolle RJ, Morrillo LR, Gumnit RJ. Value of computed tomography scan in the evaluation of adult patients after their first seizure. *Ann Neurol* 1984; 15(6): 436–43.

39 Kilpatrick CJ, Tress BM, O'Donnell C, Rossitor C, Hopper JL. Magnetic resonance imaging and late-onset epilepsy. *Epilepsia* 1991; 32: 358–64.

40 Berg AT, Shinnar S. The risk of seizure recurrence following a first unprovoked seizure: a quantitative review. *Neurology* 1991; 41: 965–72.

41 Callaghan N, Kenny RA, O'Neill B, Crowley M, Goggin T. A prospective study between carbamazepine, phenytoin and sodium valproate as monotherapy in previously untreated and recently diagnosed patients with epilepsy. *J Neurol Neurosurg Psychiatry* 1985; 48: 639–44.

42 Treiman DM. Efficacy and safety of antiepileptic drugs: a review of controlled trials. *Epilepsia* 1987; 28 (Suppl. 3): S1–S8.

43 Jallon P, Loiseau P. Epileptic seizures and epilepsy in the elderly. Sanofi, Winthrop, SCIP, Vincenne, 1995.

44 Marson AG, Williamson PR, Hutton JL, Clough ME, Chadwick DW. Carbamazepine versus valproate monotherapy for epilepsy. (Cochrane Review) In: *The Cochrane Library*, 1. Oxford: Oxford Update Software, 2000.

45 Tudor Smith C, Marson AG, Williamson PR. Phenytoin versus valproate monotherapy for partial onset seizures and generalized onset tonic-clonic seizures (Cochrane Review). In: *The Cochrane Library*, Issue 3. Oxford: Oxford Update Software, 2000.

46 Tallis RC, Easter D, Craig I. Multicentre trial of sodium Valproate and phenytoin in elderly patients with newly diagnosed epilepsy. *Age Ageing* 1994; 23 (Suppl. 2): 5 pp (abstract).

47 Trimble MR. Anticonvulsant drugs and cognitive function: a review of the literature. *Epilepsia* 1987; 28 (Suppl. 3): 37–S45.

48 Craig I, Tallis R. The impact of sodium valproate and phenytoin on cognitive function in elderly patients: results of a single-blind randomised comparative study. *Epilepsia* 1994; 35: 381–90.

49 Meador KM, Loring DW, Huh K, Gallagher BB, King DW. Comparative cognitive effects of anticonvulsants. *Neurology* 1990; 40: 391–4.

50 Gough H, Goggin T, Bissessar A, Baker M, Crowley M, Callaghan N. A comparative study of the relative influence of different anticonvulsants, UV exposure and diet on vitamin D and calcium metabolism in out-patients with epilepsy. *Q J Med* 1986; 55: 569–77.

51 Sato Y, Kondo I, Ishida S *et al*. Decreased bone mass and increased bone turnover with valproate therapy in adults with epilepsy. *Neurology* 2001; 57: 445–9.

52 Lahr MB. Hyponatraemia during carbamazepine therapy. *Clin Pharmacol Ther* 1985; 37: 693–6.

53 Kalviainen R, Nousiainen I, Mantyjarvi M *et al*. Vigabatrin, a gabaergic antiepileptic drug, causes concentric field defects. *Neurology* 1999; 53: 922–60.

54 Brodie M, Overstall P, Giorgi L. The UK Lamotrigine Elderly Study Group. Multicentre, double blind, randomised comparison between lamotrigine and carbamazepine in elderly patients with newly diagnosed epilepsy. *Epilepsy Res* 1999; 37: 871–6.

55 Lott RS, Helmboldt K. Oxcarbazepine. A carbamazepine analogue for partial seizures in adults and children with epilepsy. *Formulary* 2000; 35: 219–30.

56 Van Amelsvoort T, Bakshi R, Devaux CB, Schwabe S. Hyponatraemia associated with carbamazepine and oxcarbazepine therapy: a review. *Epilepsia* 1994; 35: 181–8.

57 Chadwick DW, Anhut H, Greuner MJ *et al*. A double blind trial of gabapentin monotherapy for newly diagnosed partial seizures. International Gabapentin Monotherapy Study Group 945–77. *Neurology* 1998; 51: 1282–8.

58 Marson AG, Chadwick DW. New drug treatment for epilepsy. *J Neurol Neurosurg Psychiatry* 2001; 70: 143–8.

59 Langtry HD, Gillis JC, Davis R. Topiramate. A review of its pharmacodynamic and pharmacokinetic properties, and clinical efficacy in the management of epilepsy. *Drugs* 1997; 94: 752–73.

60 Dooley M, Plosker GI. Levetiracetam. A review of its adjunctive use in the management of partial seizures. *Drugs* 2000; 60: 871–930.

61 Adkins JC, Noble S. Tiagabine. A review of its pharmacodynamic and pharmacokinetic properties and therapeutic potential in the management of epilepsy. *Drugs* 1998; 55(3): 437–60.

62 Peters DH, Sorkin EM. Zonisamide. A review of its pharmacodynamic and pharmacokinetic properties, and therapeutic potential in epilepsy. *Drugs* 1993; 45: 760–87.

63 Haegele KD, Huebert ND, Ebel M, Tell GP, Schechter PJ. Pharmacokinetics of vigabatrin: Implications of creatinine clearance. *Clin Pharmacol Ther* 1988; 44: 558–65.

64 Perucca E. The new generation of antiepileptic drugs: advantages and disadvantages. *Br J Clin Pharmacol* 1996; 42: 531–43.

65 Marson AG, Kadir ZA, Chadwick DW. New antiepileptic drugs: a systematic review of their efficacy and tolerability. *Br Med J* 1996; 313: 1169–74.

66 Bauer LA, Blouin RA. Age and phenytoin kinetics in adult epileptics. *Clin Pharmacol Ther* 1982; 31: 301–4.

67 *British National Formulary*, 19 (June). London: British Medical Association and the Royal Pharmaceutical Society of Great Britain, 2001.

68 Chadwick DW. Overuse of monitoring of blood concentrations of antiepileptic drugs. *Br Med J* 1987; 294: 723–4.

69 Weintraub M. *Compliance in the Elderly. Clinics in Geriatric Medicine.* Philadelphia: WB Saunders, 1990.

70 Cockerell OC, Johnson AL, Sander JWAS, Hart YM, Shorvon SD. Remission of epilepsy: results from the National General Practice Study of Epilepsy. *Lancet* 1995; 346: 140–4.

71 Medical Research Council Antiepileptic Withdrawal Study Group. A randomised study of antiepileptic drug withdrawal in patients in remission of epilepsy. *N Engl J Med* 1991; 337: 1175–80.

72 Berg AT, Shinnar S. Relapse following discontinuation of antiepileptic drugs. *Neurology* 1994; 44: 601–8.

73 Specchio LM *et al.* Discontinuing anti-epileptic drugs in patients who are seizure free on monotherapy. *J Neurol Neurosurg Psychiatry* 2002; 72: 22–5.

74 Hauser WA, Annegers JF, Elveback LR. Mortality in patients with epilepsy. *Epilepsia* 1980; 21: 399–412.

75 Luhdorf K, Jensen LK, Plessner AM. Epilepsy in the elderly: life expectancy and causes of death. *Acta Neurol Scand* 1987; 76: 183–90.

76 Geyer J, Kuzniecky R, Faught E. Admission and mortality rates for convulsive seizures in patients aged 65 years and older. *Epilepsia* 1995; 36 (Suppl. 4): 148.

77 Hartshorn JC. A nurse-managed clinic for individuals with epilepsy. *Epilepsia* 1995; 36 (Suppl. 4; abstract) 99.

78 Bradley P, Lindsay B. Specialist epilepsy nurses for treating epilepsy. (Cochrane Review) In: *The Cochrane Library* 1. Oxford: Oxford Update Software, 2001.

79 Bradley P, Lindsay B. Epilepsy clinics versus general 'neurology or medical clinics'. (Cochrane Review) In: *The Cochrane Library* 1, 2001. Oxford: Oxford Update Software.

80 Jacoby A, Baker G, Smith D *et al.* Measuring the impact of epilepsy: the development of a novel scale. *Epilepsy Res* 1993; 16: 83–8.

81 Baker GA, Jacoby A, Buck D, Brooks J, Potts P, Chadwick DW. The quality of life of older people with epilepsy: findings from a UK community study. *Seizure* 2001; 10(2): 92–9.

17 Management of Epilepsy in People with Learning Disability

E. Brodtkorb

The same disorder that causes seizures may in many patients also have the potential to limit intellectual development. Mental retardation is present in more than 20% of adult individuals with epilepsy [1]. The risk of developing a seizure disorder increases with the severity of cognitive deficit. People with learning disabilities represent an important subgroup within the population of patients with epilepsy. Here we are faced with many of the most refractory patients. The general principles in the management of epilepsy are no different for these people than for any other patients. Nevertheless, the coexistence of intellectual deficits and behavioural abnormalities may substantially interfere with the medical assessment of seizures. Adverse drug reactions may remain unrecognized and may be more harmful than the seizures themselves. Particular care should be taken to avoid overmedication in this group. During a lifetime, these patients belong to some of the most drug-exposed groups in society. The treatment objective must not necessarily be a seizure-free state, but improvements in seizure control, alertness, mood and behaviour.

Previously, textbooks often conveyed the impression that the combined occurrence of epilepsy and learning disabilities is predominantly confined to the younger age groups. However, numerically, this problem is certainly not restricted to childhood. Figure 17.1 illustrates that adult patients far outnumber children [2]. Comprehensive medical follow-up of this patient category must continue beyond the end of adolescence. This chapter will highlight some particular medical problems and complications which accumulate in patients with learning disabilities and associated handicaps.

Comprehensive epilepsy service

The multidisciplinary approach

The cognitive deficits expressed via IQ level are certainly not the only factor for disability in the large and heterogeneous group of individuals with learning disabilities. The total social handicap largely depends on concomitant neurological handicaps, such as epilepsy, various motor deficits, sensory impairments and behaviour abnormalities, including autistic features. Many problems are augmented in the paediatric age group, but several continue and some arise in adulthood. Patients with learning disabilities represent a particular challenge to the epileptologist. Investigation and treatment are often hampered by contact problems. These people usually have reduced abilities to express their own wishes and requests. Carers have to be relied upon, and a multidisciplinary and comprehensive approach is needed [3–5]. Attention should be focused on several factors other than just the seizures, such as behaviour, alertness, mood, communication, cooperation, appetite and sleep pattern. The scope of a comprehensive epilepsy service is the prevention, detection and reduction of all epilepsy-related handicapping factors, and its aim is to (re-)habilitate the patient to his full potential. Comprehensive epilepsy service may be divided into three overlapping fields: the medical, the psychological and the social and educational (Table 17.1). A strong awareness of the need for these different approaches is mandatory for an optimal management of patients with learning disabilities [6]. However, in the global assessment of these patients, care should be taken that the pure medical needs are not overshadowed by other aspects.

The medical aspects

From a medical point of view, there has in the past been a tendency to consider the mentally retarded more or less as a uniform group. In large parts of the world, patients with epilepsy and severe intellectual deficits previously tended to cluster in centralized institutions, where health services were often provided separately from the general population. Lack of expertise in these large, 'custodial'-like institutions sometimes contributed to a kind of 'collective' medical practice. However, the awareness of the fact that these patients are very heterogeneous regarding the pathogenetic mechanisms and clinical manifestations of their brain dysfunction has been progressing. During recent years, there has been an increasing trend in many countries to integrate this group of citizens into their original local communities and, consequently, they have been incorporated into the general epilepsy service. As reflected in this chapter, clinical experience derived from particular problems accumulated or exaggerated in the management of this demanding population undoubtedly has contributed to a better understanding of epilepsy *per se* and to an improvement of epilepsy care in general.

Nevertheless, myths and prejudices about people with learning disabilities are still present, despite the practice of modern medicine. Even in the most developed countries it may still be questioned whether this group receives epilepsy service of equal quality to that of other patients. EEG recordings may be impossible to perform. The presented history is often inaccurate. The key to a precise evaluation is the detailed observation and description of seizures and behaviour by carers and family members. The fundamental importance of detailed anamnestic data, including those from good informants, must be emphasized. To improve diagnostic accuracy, home video recordings may be helpful. Non-epileptic, seizure-like behaviour is common in the severely learning disabled. The differential diagnosis is often difficult, and these patients may be more prone to inadequate, long-term antiepileptic drug (AED) treatment than other patients. Inappropriate epilepsy service often starts with

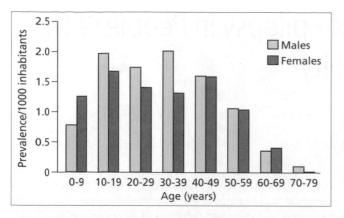

Fig. 17.1 Prevalence rates by age and sex of 299 persons with epilepsy and learning disability in the county of Västerbotten, Sweden. Redrawn from [2] with permission from Elsevier Science.

Table 17.1 The three overlapping fields of comprehensive epilepsy service to people with learning disabilities

Medical	The need for continuous access to current developments in diagnosis and treatment throughout all age groups
Psychological	The need to consider the symptoms and the treatment in relation to psychological and intellectual functioning
Social	The need for social and educational support, and for information and supervision not only for the sufferer but also for the family and the carers

an insufficient history, particularly in adult patients who are accompanied by caregivers with a limited knowledge of their clients. Information about the individual's past and current health status is the basis of clinical decision making. Optimal medical management of these patients is often very time consuming. Meeting these challenges may demand new attitudes and additional resources in many neurological departments. A specialist epilepsy nurse may play a key role in the service of these patients, providing supervision of the carers and warranting the availability and continuity of high-quality medical care. The best seizure control often requires specialist management at the highest competence level.

The psychological and cognitive aspects

The symptoms and their treatment should be considered in relation to psychological and cognitive functioning. Central nervous side-effects of AEDs may be masked by the intellectual handicap. Drowsiness, mood change and behavioural problems may be signs of toxicity. Adverse reactions, neurodeficits, seizure effects and social, educational and behavioural problems often merge. The various factors may sometimes be difficult to identify and they may interact in different ways in different patients (Fig. 17.2) [7]. In particular, it is important to distinguish between permanent learning disability on the one hand and state-dependent learning disability (pseudo-retardation) on the other [8]. Both forms often occur to-

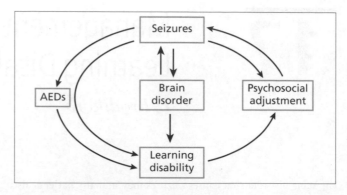

Fig. 17.2 In people with learning disability, overtreatment with AEDs may enhance cognitive dysfunction, impair psychosocial adjustment and increase behavioural problems. The various factors may be difficult to identify and may interact in different ways in different patients. Adapted from [7] with permission from Wrightson Biomedical Publishing.

gether. State-dependent learning disability is reversible and potentially treatable, but is unfortunately often unrecognized. In patients with epilepsy, it may be of two kinds; either drug induced or seizure related due to epileptiform discharges, subtle or 'subclinical' seizures or postictal effects. When treating patients with learning disabilities, it is imperative to bear in mind the complex interrelationship between cognitive function and epilepsy-related factors (Fig. 17.2).

The social and educational aspects

Frequently, there is a continuous need for social and educational support, not only for the sufferer but also for the family and other persons in the patient's environment. The transfer of competence to the community caregivers should be given high priority. Specialist epilepsy nurses should be assigned the responsibility for providing counselling and relevant information under the supervision of an epileptologist, and for ensuring that each patient has the possibility of taking full advantage of all available services. Close cooperation and coordination between the various professions throughout the organizational levels of health care are essential parts of a well-organized comprehensive treatment programme [3,4,6]. The quality of these services should be equally distributed without regard to age, intellectual level or geography. Meaningful occupation and activities may improve wellbeing, enhance psychosocial adjustment and contribute to improved seizure control. Epilepsy management needs to be integrated into the larger context of comprehensive quality care, in which services to the mentally retarded and patients with acquired cognitive deficits form an essential part.

Prophylactic AED treatment

Compliance

A prerequisite for the successful therapy of epilepsy is drug compliance that ensures a stable effect of the medication. People with intellectual disability do not always accept taking tablets, especially if these are large. In multiply-handicapped individuals additional impairments in the form of swallowing problems and/or behavioural

Table 17.2 Measures supporting drug compliance in handicapped patients with swallowing difficulties or cooperation problems

Severe multiple handicaps
Alternative drug formulations:
   liquid (carbamazepine, valproate)
   soluble tablets (carbamazepine, lamotrigine)
   powder (vigabatrin)
   sprinkle (topiramate, valproate)

Mild cognitive deficits
Drug dispenser
Alarm wristwatch
Simple dosing tailored to individual habits
Social support with regular nurse visits

Table 17.3 Adverse reactions of traditional AEDs causing particular concern in patients with learning disabilities

Phenobarbital	Somnolence, mood disturbances, behaviour disorders, including hyperactivity
Phenytoin	Cognitive impairment and cerebellar symptoms (phenytoin encephalopathy) after long-term use. Gingival hyperplasia, particularly in patients with poor oral hygiene
Carbamazepine	Seizure aggravation in symptomatic generalized epilepsies
Valproate	Severe hepatotoxicity, particularly in developmentally delayed young children on polytherapy. Tremor. Weight gain

abnormalities may interfere with the oral intake of solid formulations. Drugs that are available as liquid, soluble, powder or granular formulations for children may be useful in the mentally retarded adult (Table 17.2). To maintain adequate prophylactic treatment, the rectal route may sometimes be necessary. Suppositories of carbamazepine and valproate are available. When intravenous administration is impossible or inconvenient, the liquid peroral form may in exceptional situations be given rectally. Patients with severe nutritional problems requiring tube feeding and percutaneous gastrostomy also need drugs in fluid or soluble forms. Gabapentin is at present only delivered in capsules, which can be opened and administered by tube. However, the powder cannot be taken orally due to its very bitter taste. The caregivers are extremely important partners in the treatment of this patient category. The need for education and guidance concerning the goals of therapy and the importance of adherence to the prescribed regimen is obvious.

Patients with only mild intellectual deficits who live partly independently but have an irregular behaviour may need various other measures to enhance drug compliance, including drug dispensers, alarm wristwatches and a social support system which may include regular nurse visits at medication times. Dosing should be kept as simple as possible and the drug intake tailored to their individual habits (Table 17.2). In training for autonomy and independent living, self-medication should not be given early priority. When memory is reduced and the understanding of the need for medication inadequate, close supervision is necessary to maintain sufficient treatment. Non-compliance is a significant problem in intractable epilepsy, and may in particular be prevalent in people who have impaired abilities to express their views and discuss their feelings about the drugs and their effects.

Old drugs

The traditional medications, including phenobarbital, phenytoin, carbamazepine and valproate, still form the backbone of epilepsy therapy. They are all effective in controlling seizures, but their utility is hampered by adverse effect profiles and unwanted drug interactions. In patients with intellectual disabilities, some specific issues concerning these drugs need to be taken into account (Table 17.3).
• Phenobarbital is not considered a first-line agent due to its associ-

ation with somnolence, irritability and mood disturbances. The most consistent problems in patients with learning disabilities are the exacerbation of behaviour disorders, mostly hyperactivity, as well as sleep disorders and depression [9].
• Phenytoin is also not recommended as a first-choice drug due to its potential adverse effects. Patients with severe brain damage who are receiving multiple AEDs are particularly susceptible to the toxic effects of phenytoin, even at low plasma concentrations. Phenytoin encephalopathy is a rare complication, manifested as cognitive impairment and cerebellar symptoms, which may be partly related to the dose-dependent kinetics of the drug, individual differences in drug metabolism and polytherapy. The long-term use of phenytoin is not recommended for patients with loss of locomotion, marked cognitive impairment, or symptoms and signs of cerebellar disease. Phenytoin encephalopathy may become progressive if exposure to the drug continues [10].
• Carbamazepine is still one of the most commonly prescribed drugs for partial epilepsy. It is also indicated in the treatment of neuralgias and manic depressive disorders. Because of its minimal unwanted effects on cognition and behaviour, carbamazepine is an excellent drug for the treatment of people with learning disability and epilepsy. Nevertheless, one should bear in mind that patients with cognitive impairment may have a particularly low threshold for neurotoxicity and that carbamazepine may sometimes have a seizure-inducing effect in these patients, especially in those with symptomatic generalized epilepsies.
• Valproate is a first-line drug in the treatment of primarily generalized seizures, but also has effect in other seizure types. It has been the most frequently used drug in the treatment of the Lennox–Gastaut syndrome because it is effective against multiple seizure types [11]. Particularly in the area of intellectual disability severe hepatotoxicity is an important but rare idiosyncratic adverse reaction. A frequency of hepatic fatalities of about 1:30 000 treated individuals has been estimated. Developmental delay or other evidence of brain injury seem to be a predisposing factor. Other risk factors include young age, polytherapy and metabolic disorders. Patients less than 2 years of age on polytherapy are at the greatest risk (1:600). Decreased alertness, jaundice, vomiting, haemorrhage, increased

seizures, anorexia and oedema are the most common presenting signs [12].

New drugs

The newer AEDs broaden the therapeutic options in patients with refractory epilepsy. Several of these drugs have obtained a particular place in the treatment of patients with learning disabilities and associated handicaps. All of them may have strengths as well as drawbacks in this large and heterogeneous patient group (Table 17.4). Most studies on the treatment of these patients are postmarketing surveillances, but two epilepsy syndromes which are strongly associated with learning disabilities have recently been the subject of several drug trials: infantile spasms and the Lennox–Gastaut syndrome [13–18] (Table 17.5).

• Vigabatrin now appears to be an advance in the treatment of infantile spasms, particularly when due to tuberous sclerosis or other brain lesions [13–15]. The potential adverse reaction in the form of constricted visual fields may be difficult to assess in this group. The manufacturer recommends perimetric follow-up every 6 months [19], but visual field examinations require a mental level corresponding to at least 9 years. Psychiatric (depression, psychosis) and behavioural side-effects may also be difficult to identify in patients with learning disabilities [20].

• Lamotrigine is effective in partial seizures and a wide range of generalized seizures. Tolerability is usually excellent. There is evidence of a synergistic effect with valproate in some patients. However, valproate-induced tremor, an occasional side-effect, may be enhanced by lamotrigine, particularly in neurologically impaired individuals. Low starting and maintenance lamotrigine doses and slower rates of dose escalation are also required to minimize the risk of skin rashes when lamotrigine is added on to patients receiving therapy with valproate. Lamotrigine has shown efficacy in patients with symptomatic generalized epilepsies, including the Lennox–Gastaut syndrome [17]. Benefits on behaviour have been demonstrated in learning disabled patients [21,22]. It is usually not sedative and may increase attention and alertness, particularly in children with developmental problems [23]. Improved social engagement has been reported. On the other hand, aggravated hyperactivity and irritability have occasionally also been attributed to lamotrigine [24]. The exacerbation of myoclonic seizures has been noted along with the appearance of tics [23].

• Felbamate is a potent drug with efficacy across a range of seizure types. It has a documented beneficial effect in the Lennox–Gastaut syndrome, particularly in atonic seizures [16], but the use of felbamate is restricted due to potential toxicity in the bone marrow and liver. Liver function tests and blood counts every 2 weeks are recommended by the manufacturer for the first year of treatment [25],

Table 17.4 Strengths and drawbacks of commonly used new AEDs in treatment of patients with learning disabilities

Drug	Strengths	Drawbacks
Vigabatrin	Effective in infantile spasms	Visual field defects Psychiatric side-effects Weight gain
Lamotrigine	Broad spectrum Effective in Lennox–Gastaut syndrome Non-sedating Increased attention and alertness	Behaviour problems in some Sometimes exacerbation of myoclonic seizures Skin rashes
Felbamate	Broad spectrum Effective in Lennox–Gastaut syndrome Non-sedating Increased alertness	Bone marrow and liver toxicity Regular laboratory monitoring Insomnia Behaviour problems Anorexia, weight loss
Topiramate	Broad spectrum Effective in Lennox–Gastaut syndrome	Potential cognitive side-effects Anorexia, weight loss
Gabapentin	May ameliorate tremor, spasticity and anxiety ?Psychotropic effects	Narrow spectrum (partial epilepsy) Behaviour problems in some Weight gain
Oxcarbazepine	Less interactions and improved tolerability compared with carbamazepine	Hyponatraemia Potential seizure aggravation in symptomatic generalized epilepsies
Tiagabine	May improve spasticity	Narrow spectrum (partial epilepsy) Dizziness, asthenia, tremor, depression
Levetiracetam	Good tolerability	Limited experience Behaviour problems in some
Zonisamide	Efficacy in some myoclonic epilepsies	Central nervous system side-effects

Table 17.5 Randomized trials with new AEDs in epilepsy syndromes associated with learning disabilities

Syndrome	Drug	Control drug	Design	Number of patients	Reference
Infantile spasms	Vigabatrin	Hydrocortisone	Open, monotherapy	22	Chiron et al., 1997 [13]
Infantile spasms	Vigabatrin	ACTH	Open, monotherapy	42	Vigevano & Cilio, 1997 [14]
Infantile spasms	Vigabatrin	Placebo	Double blind, monotherapy	40	Appleton et al., 1999 [15]
Lennox–Gastaut	Felbamate	Placebo	Double blind, add-on	73	The Felbamate Study Group, 1993 [16]
Lennox–Gastaut	Lamotrigine	Placebo	Double blind, add-on	169	Motte et al., 1997 [17]
Lennox–Gastaut	Topiramate	Placebo	Double blind, add-on	98	Sachdeo et al., 1999 [18]

a safety procedure which may be difficult to perform in some patients. Insomnia, anorexia and weight loss are common side-effects. As with other non-sedating AEDs brightening and improvement of alertness may occur. However, hyperactivity and aggressiveness have also been noted [23]. Of particular concern is the effect of felbamate on behaviour in the developmentally delayed population. Pharmacokinetic interactions complicate its use in combination therapy.

• Topiramate is a potent broad-spectrum drug which is also effective in primarily generalized seizures. It has documented effect in the Lennox–Gastaut syndrome and may particularly be of benefit in myoclonic seizures [18]. In a subgroup of patients treatment has been associated with cognitive complaints such as mental slowing and speech problems in the form of reduced verbal fluency, particularly when the drug is used in polytherapy. Behavioural disturbances may at times be caused by topiramate. Nevertheless, many patients with learning disabilities seem to tolerate the drug well. In a study examining the retention of topiramate in patients with chronic epilepsy, the presence of learning disability and early onset seizures were among the factors that were likely to result in continuation of treatment [26].

• Gabapentin is indicated for partial and secondarily generalized seizures. It may also be effective in tremor [27] as well as in spasticity [28], important issues to bear in mind when treating patients with organic brain disorders. This drug has a favourable side-effect profile and may reduce anxiety. In learning disabled patients the drug has been shown to improve rating scales on a range of behavioural parameters, including cooperation, restlessness and challenging behaviour [22]. However, adverse reactions in the form of aggression, hyperexcitability and tantrums have also been reported. This is more common in patients with pre-existing behavioural difficulties and developmental delay [23]. Even rare cases of involuntary choreiform movements and myoclonus have been reported in neurologically impaired patients [29], an unusual reaction that gabapentin may share with several other AEDs, particularly phenytoin.

• Oxcarbazepine is similar to carbamazepine in its mechanism of action. It exerts its antiepileptic effect through its monohydroxy derivative and is not metabolized into an epoxide. Compared with carbamazepine, it has fewer pharmacokinetic interactions and improved tolerability. Hyponatraemia may be more common than with carbamazepine and is probably caused by influence on the secretion of antidiuretic hormone. Usually it is mild and asymptomatic. In the multiply handicapped, this side-effect may be more pronounced due to cerebral regulatory dysfunction and altered fluid intake patterns [23].

• Tiagabine is also effective in partial seizures and has little impact on cognition. Dizziness, asthenia, tremor and depression are among its side-effects. In contrast to vigabatrin, which increases γ-aminobutyric acid (GABA) by inhibiting GABA transaminase, tiagabine increases GABA in the synaptic cleft by reuptake inhibition. According to preliminary reports, it does not seem to share the same retinotoxic effect with vigabatrin [30], but long-term follow-up of more patients on tiagabine with visual field examination is called for. There is some evidence that this drug also may improve spasticity [31], making it suitable for treatment in patients with epilepsy and cerebral palsy. However, controlled studies are needed in these patients.

• Piracetam is an antimyoclonic agent and is effective against cortical myoclonus. Controlled trials have shown improvement in patients with progressive myoclonic epilepsy [32].

• Levetiracetam is chemically related to piracetam. It has documented efficacy in partial epilepsy but, according to preliminary clinical experience, it may have a broader efficacy spectrum. Its side-effect profile is mild. Systematic exposure to special populations is as yet quite limited. It is a promising drug in patients with encephalopathies and multiple seizure types. Behavioural side-effects may occur in some, usually in the form of invisibility and restlessness, and particularly in learning disabled patients.

• Zonisamide is at present only marketed in a limited part of the world. It is effective in partial as well as generalized seizure types, but has a potential for problematic side-effects. Of particular interest are the reports of efficacy against myoclonus. Responses have been seen in patients belonging to the group of progressive myoclonus epilepsies [23].

Future AED treatment may be tailored according to neurobiological findings in specific epilepsy disorders. In the pathogenesis of Rett's syndrome, for example, an excess of glutamate is thought to play an important role [33]. From a mechanistic view, compounds with antiglutaminergic properties may be tried in this condition. Lamotrigine, by blocking sodium channels, inhibits glutamate release and has shown beneficial effects in Rett's syndrome patients [34]. Angelman's syndrome involves a defect in the DNA coding for subunits of the GABA-A receptor. Carbamazepine and phenytoin are typically not effective and may result in worsening of seizures. A paradoxical effect of vigabatrin may be caused by an excessive stimulation of GABA-B receptors. Topiramate has multiple mechanisms of action, including effect on GABA-A receptors. Promising results with this drug have been found in Angelman's syndrome [35].

We still need better drugs with lower potential for adverse reactions and known modes of action. More rational drug combinations consisting of agents with complementary mechanisms and with marginal central nervous depressant effects may further improve the quality of life for patients with intractable epilepsy, in particular for those with pre-existing cognitive deficits. A pitfall in the evaluation of better tolerated treatments in the severely retarded patient lies in the fact that increased alertness and self-assertion may be misinterpreted as behavioural side-effects. A more demanding behaviour should not be invariably considered as a sign of toxicity. Such symptoms should be analysed carefully before a new treatment is abandoned. Environmental support and activity programme adjustments may be needed to meet new requirements of more attentive patients.

Further prospective studies comparing efficacy and tolerability, including rating scales on behaviour parameters and other measures adapted for people with intellectual deficits, should be performed to collect systematic clinical experience in these patients [22]. High-quality randomized trials in learning disabled patients are currently called for [36]. However, in this patient category, severe difficulties in trial methods exist due to the heterogeneity of aetiologies and comorbidities, the frequently limited number of patients within one specific subgroup, as well as particular ethical issues.

Central nervous system side-effects

Difficulties in achieving a satisfactory balance between seizure control and adverse drug effects may be pronounced in people with learning disabilities. These patients are often unable to report the early symptoms of toxicity, such as sedation, blurred vision and ataxia. Subtle cognitive adverse reactions may occur unnoticed by the carers. Side-effects may also sometimes manifest themselves indirectly as behavioural problems [37] (Fig. 17.2). The four previous front-line AEDs, phenobarbital, phenytoin, carbamazepine and valproate, have all been reported to be associated with dose-related cognitive side-effects, first in the form of slowing of central information processing. These are definitely large for phenobarbital and possibly larger for phenytoin than for carbamazepine and valproate [38]. Patients with intellectual deficits and severe brain lesions who are on multiple AED therapy may have a predisposition for a chronic phenytoin encephalopathy, causing cognitive and cerebellar dysfunction, even with plasma levels within the accepted range [10]. Some of the new drugs seem to have favourable cognitive profiles [39], but available data are sparse in this group of patients. As mentioned, topiramate may have a risk for cognitive impairment, which frequently may be overcome by gradual initial titration. However, a subgroup of patients does not tolerate the drug. Mood effects may occur with some of the new drugs, secondarily also affecting cognitive performance [38].

Although the severity of cognitive side-effects is considered to be mild for most of the AEDs when therapeutic serum concentrations are considered, their clinical impact may be significant when treating specific populations. Clinical experience suggests that patients with learning disabilities are often more vulnerable to cognitive side-effects than other patients. However, the subgroup of patients with severe intellectual handicaps is excluded from the ordinary 'pencil and paper' tests of cognitive functions and mood. Nevertheless, in lesional epilepsy, there is evidence that cognitive abilities may be affected in a circumscribed manner for those functions that are represented by the area of the seizure focus (e.g. language functions) [40,41]. In tests of memory following monotherapy with carbamazepine and valproate, a subgroup of patients with evidence of significant brain lesions performed more poorly than other patients [42]. The existence and extent of underlying brain damage both seem to influence the adverse cognitive effects of a particular drug.

Many patients with learning disabilities have an inappropriate and excessive medication load which impairs their quality of life. Reduction of undue polytherapy should always be aimed at in these patients. It has repeatedly been emphasized that AED therapy should not exclusively focus on seizure freedom. Patients who for reasons other than their epilepsy cannot achieve independent living and driving abilities may tolerate incomplete seizure control better than others.

Paradoxical effects

Some AEDs occasionally have a paradoxical effect in the form of increased frequency or severity of seizures. This may occur as a nonspecific manifestation of overdosage or as a relatively specific effect in some seizure types or epilepsy syndromes [43]. A range of predisposing factors are related to conditions which are associated with learning disabilities (Table 17.6). More frequent seizures may be a part of the clinical picture of insidious phenytoin encephalopathy [10]. There is also evidence that carbamazepine may aggravate seizures, particularly 'minor' generalized seizures, and in some patients even generalized tonic-clonic seizures. In symptomatic generalized epilepsies several seizure types that respond differently to treatment may be present. In the Lennox–Gastaut syndrome, carbamazepine may be effective for tonic seizures, but may aggravate atypical absences and myoclonic or atonic seizures. Benzodiazepines may cause an increase of tonic seizures in the same disorder [43]. Vigabatrin may aggravate generalized seizures (particularly absence, tonic and myoclonic seizures, and even generalized tonic-clonic seizures), possibly due to disinhibition from activation of GABA-B receptors. Other GABAergic drugs may share this mechanism. Lamotrigine [20], as well as levetiracetam, may also increase seizure frequency. Lamotrigine may in particular have a negative effect in severe myoclonic epilepsy of infancy [44]. The clinician should not forget that seizure aggravation may occur as part of the rare valproate hepatotoxicity, which particularly may occur in young children with metabolic disorders associated with developmental delay [12]. Increased seizure frequency may also occur within the context of a toxic valproate encephalopathy, not necessarily associated with high drug plasma levels, often accompanied by confusion, lethargy, ataxia and hyperammonia. Drug-induced drowsiness and inactivity alone may probably contribute to seizure

Table 17.6 Factors predisposing to paradoxical AED-induced aggravation of seizures

Young age
Multiple seizure types
Prominent epileptiform EEG activity
Learning disabilities and behavioural disorders
Polytherapy
Drug-induced drowsiness

induction in some multiply-handicapped patients. The use of sedative drugs, in particular phenobarbital, should be minimized in this patient category. Not surprisingly, a reduction of polytherapy may sometimes lead to improved seizure control.

These paradoxical pharmacodynamic effects have recently received increased attention [43,45,46]. Young patients with polytherapy and encephalopathies comprising intellectual deficits, multiple seizure types and prominent epileptiform EEG activity seem to be particularly prone to develop paradoxical effects [45]. This problem is probably widely underestimated in patients with intractable epilepsy, particularly in patients with intellectual deficits who cannot themselves express their opinions about the prescribed treatment. It is often overlooked by the non-specialist, and even by the carers, as the history is often insufficient due to a lack in the continuity of information sharing. Appropriate follow-up is imperative when prescribing new drugs to these patients.

Can AEDs alter the disease process?

The traditional AEDs have a proven symptomatic antiseizure effect. There is little scientific clinical evidence to support their having an effect on the development or on the prognosis of underlying disorders in epilepsy patients [47]. Animal studies have shown that several of the new AEDs may act as neuroprotective agents [39]. Neuroprotection is an important field in modern neurology, but its relevance in epilepsy remains to be proven in the clinical setting. An agent which could not only prevent symptomatic seizures but also lower the likelihood of developing epilepsy after a brain injury would be very valuable. It is believed that a neuroprotective effect might block further seizure-induced damage in the brain and associated functional alterations, which may possibly include seizure-promoting factors. In prolonged febrile seizures, excitotoxic cell death in epileptogenic regions like the hippocampus seems to be responsible for future spontaneous seizures and sometimes for neurological deficits, such as in the hemiconvulsion hemiplegia epilepsy (HHE) syndrome [48].

In most children with epilepsy and learning disabilities, a structural or a metabolic underlying abnormality is the cause of the seizures as well as the cognitive problems. However, in some children, the development of an additional encephalopathy seems to be secondary to the seizure activity. The so-called catastrophic epilepsies of childhood have their onset in patients younger than 5–6 years of age. This period is critical for brain maturation and includes developmental plasticity. Frequent seizures and/or abundant epileptiform activity may in some patients apparently induce or further consolidate a dysfunctional state in the brain. By this mechanism, harmful neuronal reorganization in the form of abnormal synaptic connections with deleterious consequences for cognitive development may be generated. In the catastrophic epilepsies of childhood, several reports suggest that controlling seizures does alter the outcome of intellectual functioning. In patients with a history of infantile spasms, the patients who quickly became spasm free are those who are developmentally normal. In children with tuberous sclerosis, the occurrence of autistic regression is often clearly linked to the onset and presence of seizures. In Sturge–Weber syndrome, intellectual deficits inevitably ensue, if the seizures are poorly controlled [49].

In infantile spasms, early treatment with adrenocorticotropic hormone (ACTH) or hydrocortisone has been considered to improve the overall prognosis. These medications are believed to suppress seizures as well as to ameliorate or protect against the development of the associated encephalopathy. The effects of these treatments seem to be syndrome and age specific. They have also been used in other forms of childhood epilepsy encephalopathies, such as the Landau–Kleffner syndrome and the Lennox–Gastaut syndrome [47]. Due to potential severe side-effects, these agents are restricted to limited courses. As already mentioned, vigabatrin is now established as an effective treatment in suppressing infantile spasms [15]. Preliminary follow-up indicates that controlling secondary generalization induced by infantile spasms in tuberous sclerosis represents a key factor for mental and behavioural development [50]. Further long-term, prospective studies including the outcome of mental and visual status in patients treated with vigabatrin are anticipated. We may hope for the development of newer effective compounds with antiepileptogenic and neuroprotective effects which can alter the natural course of the epileptic disorders and prevent the development of refractory epilepsy, and hopefully also the progressive cognitive decline, particularly that associated with the catastrophic epilepsies of childhood, including infantile spasms and the Lennox–Gastaut syndrome.

Can AEDs have a harmful effect on the underlying disorder? It has been speculated that phenytoin may have a potential to decrease free radical scavenger capacity [51,52], an effect that in some patients possibly may have clinical significance. In progressive myoclonus epilepsy of Baltic type, phenytoin has been believed to accelerate the disease process, an effect which has in part been reversible after switching to valproate [10]. Similar mechanisms may be implicated in the chronic phenytoin encephalopathy seen in other patients. Beneficial effects from antioxidant treatment have been described in preliminary case reports in progressive myoclonus epilepsy [53] as well as in other neurodegenerative conditions where excessive free radical activity may contribute to disease progression, e.g. in juvenile ceroid lipofuscinosis (Spielmeyer–Vogt), which is associated with seizures, visual loss and neurological deterioration [51].

Non-pharmacological treatment

Epilepsy surgery

Also for patients with learning disabilities, one should bear in mind that modern epilepsy treatment now includes methods other than drug treatment. Cognitive deficits are no longer considered a contraindication for epilepsy surgery [54]. However, mental retardation is a poor prognostic sign for localized cortical resection because it usually indicates more diffuse cerebral dysfunction and the likelihood of widespread or multifocal epileptogenic regions. Nevertheless, a large retrospective survey including more than 1000 temporal lobectomies suggested that preoperative IQ scores alone are not good predictors of seizure outcome and should not be used to exclude patients as potential surgical candidates [55]. In infants and young children with catastrophic epilepsies, developmental delay can be reversed with successful resection of a dysfunctional and epileptogenic cortical area [49]. Disconnective surgery, such as corpus callosotomy, may be beneficial in symptomatic and cryptogenic generalized seizures, first of all in the Lennox–Gastaut syndrome, where it may reduce the number of generalized tonic-clonic seizures, by preventing their generalization from partial onset, and decrease drop attacks, including atonic seizures [11]. Other options include hemispherectomy and multiple subpial transections (Chapters 66 and 68).

Vagus nerve stimulation

Vagus nerve stimulation may benefit patients with refractory partial epilepsy and learning disabilities. Promising results are reported also in children and adults with symptomatic generalized epilepsy. Vagal nerve stimulation appears to be free from cognitive adverse effects; however, increased alertness and energy have been reported in mentally retarded children [56]. Recent data also suggest that it has a potential as an antidepressant therapy. Data from open-label treatment suggest that vagal nerve stimulation may also be an effective and safe adjunctive therapy in the Lennox–Gastaut syndrome [11,57]. In some patients with cognitive deficits the full compliance ensured by this form of therapy may represent a particular advantage. On the other hand, patients with learning disability might be at an increased risk for certain rare complications such as aspiration pneumonia.

The ketogenic diet

This option has had a variable number of advocates through several decades. The diet is high in fat and low in carbohydrate and protein. It has mainly been employed in children with significant neurological handicaps, particularly in the Lennox–Gastaut syndrome (Chapter 21). Palatability problems may be pronounced. Thus, it requires strict supervision and has serious limitations. In patients with cognitive or behavioural problems implementation may be difficult [11].

Acute seizure treatment with diazepam

Clusters of seizures, prolonged seizures and status epilepticus are more commonly seen in the developmentally delayed population and require special attention in the comprehensive approach to these patients. Impending status epilepticus needs swift and effective action. The rectal administration of diazepam is now widely employed in the acute treatment of all kinds of epileptic seizures. It is given by parents, teachers and care staff without medical or nursing training. This route may provide therapeutic levels within a few minutes. Tolerance and dependence may develop during long-term treatment. Withdrawal symptoms, including seizures, may occur if the drug is stopped after regular intake.

The rectal route of diazepam has definitely granted a safer existence to many patients with refractory epilepsy and learning disabilities. However, in individuals with poor seizure control, problems from excessive and too frequent administration of diazepam may occur, particularly when the carers are insecure and insufficiently trained. Intermittent, large and frequent rectal diazepam doses administered at will may cause fluctuations in the plasma drug levels which by themselves may be seizure inducing. Toxic effects, withdrawal manifestations and epileptic symptoms may be intermingled and difficult to manage. The combination of high bolus doses and an enhanced drug clearance due to enzyme in-

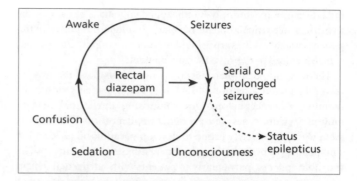

Fig. 17.3 The vicious circle of excessive rectal diazepam treatment in refractory epilepsy. A pattern of cyclic reappearance of prolonged seizures every 3–5 days, interrupted by diazepam and followed by sedation and gradual awakening may be characteristic for this complication. Adapted from [7] with permission from Wrightson Biomedical Publishing.

duction by underlying AEDs may increase the risk for rebound reactions. Some patients, after longstanding practice of this procedure, may enter a vicious circle, which cannot be broken before the use of the drug is restricted. A cyclic reappearance of prolonged seizures every 3–5 days, interrupted by diazepam, and followed by sedation and gradual awakening, is a characteristic pattern [58] (Fig. 17.3). Non-convulsive status epilepticus may sometimes occur in such patients [59]. An appropriate balance of diazepam treatment may sometimes be difficult to achieve. When restricting intermittent diazepam intake, seizures, wakefulness and behavioural problems may improve. If this strategy proves difficult, oral benzodiazepines in low doses may be another option to abort this vicious circle. Either a stable prophylactic regimen or a gradual tapering off may be chosen.

Diazepam is a very potent drug, and adequate counselling and medically appropriate, written directions for its rectal administration are mandatory both for patient security and for the legal position of caregivers. Counselling and education of family members and personnel should be given high priority. The correct and successful use of rectal diazepam depends to a great extent on the competence of the caregiver. These problems underline the need for highly qualified epilepsy nurses. One of their responsibilities should be to provide such information and follow-up for these patients. This is an important part of a comprehensive epilepsy service. The frequency of rectal administration of diazepam should not approach twice weekly for prolonged periods, and it should not be routinely used in short, non-life-threatening seizures lasting less than 2–4 min.

Buccal and nasal delivery of midazolam has recently been suggested as a more convenient and socially acceptable route of administration in the acute treatment of seizures [60].

Concomitant psychopharmacological treatment

Maladaptive, violent or self-injurious behaviour is not unusual in individuals with intellectual disabilities. Autistic behaviour is particularly common in retarded children with epilepsy [61]. An exact psychiatric diagnosis is usually difficult to obtain in the severely retarded, but patients with severe learning disabilities or brain lesions often need concomitant antiepileptic and antipsychotic treatment. A range of pharmacodynamic or pharmacokinetic interactions may occur. High doses of antipsychotic drugs may provoke seizures, particularly in patients with organic brain dysfunction [62]. AEDs may induce or aggravate behavioural problems [20,24,37], which may lead to the prescription of antipsychotic drugs. These drugs may also have cognitive side-effects, which can add to those of the AEDs. On the other hand, enzyme-inducing AEDs, such as carbamazepine, phenytoin and phenobarbital, may lower the plasma levels of antipsychotic drugs.

Among traditional typical antipsychotic drugs, the propensity to induce seizures seems partly linked with their sedative properties and is less pronounced when extrapyramidal side-effects are prominent. Chlorpromazine was previously regarded as the most proconvulsant antipsychotic, but it is now probably surpassed by clozapine. Other phenothiazines, such as perphenazine and thioridazine, have been regarded as having less effect on the seizure threshold, whereas haloperidol has been considered to have the least propensity to cause seizures [62,63]. The new atypical antipsychotics, such as risperidone and olanzapine which are similar to clozapine in having little extrapyramidal effects, do not seem to share the same degree of seizure-inducing properties. However, there is as yet limited experience with these drugs in patients with epilepsy. Several anecdotal observations of seizures during olanzapine treatment have been reported [64]. The ranking of the tendencies to precipitate seizures of antipsychotic drugs (Table 17.7) is not based on accurate data, as doses, comedication and risk factors for seizures vary among patients.

The seizure-inducing properties of antipsychotic drugs at small to standard doses should not be overestimated. In some patients low doses may probably improve seizure control, possibly by suppressing emotional seizure-inducing factors. However, high doses, or an abrupt large dose increase, should be used with caution, especially with antipsychotic drugs with known tendencies to lower the seizure threshold [62].

Polypharmacy with various drugs having the potential to influence seizure threshold is common in patients with learning disabilities or encephalopathies. Tricyclic antidepressants, and even selective serotonin reuptake inhibitors, may also induce seizures [63]. The introduction of antipsychotics or antidepressants during the tapering off and discontinuation of drugs with anticonvulsant activity, such as benzodiazepines and AEDs, may increase greatly the risk of seizures, sometimes even in the absence of epilepsy. A detailed account of all current medications, even PRN prescriptions, is of utmost importance in the evaluation of seizures in this population.

Table 17.7 Seizure-inducing properties of some antipsychotic drugs

High	Clozapine
	Chorpromazine
Moderate	Other phenothiazines, such as perphenazine and thioridazine
Low	Haloperidol
	New atypical antipsychotics, such as risperidone

Prognosis of epilepsy in learning disabled patients

Overall prognosis

In about 25% of patients with newly diagnosed epilepsy, seizure control is not possible with the presently available AEDs. However, in prevalence studies, the proportion of uncontrolled epilepsy is larger; 57% had experienced seizures during the last year in a large Swedish study, and the mean yearly seizure frequency was higher in persons with mental retardation than in others [1]. Severe epilepsy is significantly related to early onset in this patient group [65]. In prospective studies, associated neurological or cognitive handicaps have consistently been reported to have an adverse effect on the outcome of epilepsy [66]. Malformations of cortical development are often associated with refractory seizures. These conditions range from the extreme example of lissencephaly, with a smooth cortex and severely affected brain function, to less distinct syndromes with nodular heterotopias and localized cortical dysgenesis with mild clinical symptomatology. In recent studies correlating aetiology and treatment response in partial epilepsy, cortical dysgenesis had the second worst prognosis after mesial temporal sclerosis [67]. In the catastrophic epilepsies of childhood, the overall prognosis is generally very poor. A high seizure activity is associated with developmental stagnation or regression in these conditions [49]. Nevertheless, multiply handicapped patients sometimes have a favourable prognosis [65,68]. There is evidence that patients with severe intellectual deficits have an increased tendency to develop generalized tonic-clonic seizures in adult life even in the absence of prior epilepsy or a diagnosis of Down's syndrome. When late onset epilepsy occurs in such patients without the presence of overt recent or current brain damage, the outlook is usually good [65]. The spectrum of seizure disorders in individuals with learning disabilities is wide, and spans from the most intractable epilepsies to disorders with only isolated attacks, an important fact to bear in mind.

It has recently been better recognized that the diagnosis of specific syndromes is relevant for the prognosis of the seizure disorders, even in adulthood. Some examples follow.
• Down's syndrome: with advancing age, an increased incidence of epilepsy has been demonstrated in this condition, in one study reaching 46% in those over 50 years [69]. This has essentially been explained as an associated development of rapidly progressing Alzheimer dementia. The majority of these patients have primarily generalized seizures [70]. The neurological deterioration is also frequently accompanied by myoclonus. The generalized tonic-clonic seizures seem to respond well to antiepileptic treatment in the early stages, but the tendency to seizures usually progresses. The myoclonus may be intractable. AEDs often cause marked side-effects even at plasma levels well within the 'therapeutic' range [71]. This relatively common complication of Down's syndrome has received surprisingly little scientific attention.
• Rett's syndrome: most girls with this syndrome (80–90%) have epilepsy usually starting somewhere between 3 and 5 years. The seizures are of various types; many are partial, a remarkable finding in a generalized neurodevelopmental disorder. In adulthood, their seizure situation often improves considerably and sometimes they may stop having seizures. Many of these profoundly retarded females tend to react adversely to standard antiepileptic regimens

[72]. Withdrawal of AEDs should thus always be considered in seizure-free women with Rett's syndrome.

• Angelman's syndrome: epileptic seizures occur in 80% of these patients with a mean age of onset at 2–3 years. A diversity of seizure types can be seen, generalized tonic-clonic seizures, atypical absences, myoclonic seizures and tonic seizures. The seizures seem more difficult to control in patients with a chromosomal deletion. Some authors have suggested a decreasing seizure frequency with age, but according to recent reports few patients become seizure free. In adulthood, atypical absences and/or myoclonic seizures are most common [73].

• Fragile X syndrome: epilepsy is present in about 20% of mentally retarded patients with this chromosomal abnormality, usually with onset in childhood. The most common seizure type is complex partial. The characteristic EEG pattern may resemble the typical findings of benign epilepsy of childhood with centrotemporal spikes. However, the course of the epilepsy is variable and continuous AED treatment in adult life is often needed. Seizures are usually easy to control and may remit [74].

Prognosis after withdrawal of AEDs

It was previously felt by many physicians that epilepsy is a permanent condition when it occurs in the mentally retarded. The risk of seizure recurrence after AED withdrawal has been shown to correlate with the severity of intellectual disabilities in children [75]. Nevertheless, many patients with intellectual deficits may have a self-limiting seizure disorder. One important study showed that almost half of the adult, mentally retarded patients who had been seizure free for at least 2 years had no recurrences when AEDs were withdrawn [68]. This study refers to patients with a 'diagnosis of epilepsy' rather than 'patients with epilepsy'. This reflects common clinical problems. Epilepsy may be overdiagnosed in severely retarded patients. Other studies of patients with learning disability and controlled epilepsy confirm the possibility of successful discontinuation of AED treatment, in adults [65], as well as in children [76]. In a large, multicentre AED withdrawal study in patients in remission, the risk of seizure recurrence in patients with delayed development/special schooling was not significantly increased compared to other patients [77]. Withdrawal of AEDs may also be tried in patients with cerebral palsy. It has been found that spastic hemiparesis is more likely to be associated with seizure recurrence than other forms of cerebral palsy, but the presence of mental subnormality does not seem to have prognostic value [78,79].

Learning disabled patients with longstanding remission of seizures should not be withheld from the benefit of discontinuing AEDs. Recurrence of seizures in the severely retarded and multiply handicapped group usually implies fewer hazards and social consequences as these patients are usually surrounded by carers at all times.

Conclusion

The management of epilepsy in people with learning disabilities represents a particular challenge. A substantial proportion of these patients develop refractory seizures in early life. Epilepsy-related factors often impair intellectual performance and limit mental development. As outlined in this chapter, numerous aspects need to be appreciated when treating this patient category. The threshold for central nervous side-effects of AEDs may be lower in this group and the adverse drug effects may be masked by pre-existing neurodeficits. The ultimate goal of AED therapy should not only include complete seizure control but also improvements of cognition, mood and social functioning. The prevention of further epileptogenesis as well as the prevention of the influence of seizures on intellectual and behavioural development should also be considered. Simple medical measures may contribute to substantial improvement in the overall quality of life of these patients and consequently have a beneficial impact on the situation of their family and carers. At any age, these patients should be given access to the highest specialist competence. Compared to others, they need a more comprehensive and individually tailored approach to achieve an adequate level of epilepsy service. The appointment of specially trained epilepsy nurses is recommended. The transfer of competence to community care should be one of their commitments.

Patients with epilepsy and cognitive deficits should not be needlessly subjected to sedation or the risk of side-effects. Polytherapy and overmedication are frequent in this group. A restricted approach in the use of all medications which potentially affect adaptive functioning and learning (particularly AEDs, antipsychotics and benzodiazepines) is warranted.

References

1 Forsgren L. Prevalence of epilepsy in adults in Northern Sweden. *Epilepsia* 1992; 33: 450–8.

2 Forsgren L, Edvinsson, S-O, Blomquist HK, Heijbel J, Sidenvall, R. Epilepsy in a population of mentally retarded children and adults. *Epilepsy Res* 1990; 6: 234–48.

3 Coulter DL. Comprehensive management of epilepsy in persons with mental retardation. *Epilepsia* 1997; 38 (Suppl. 4): 24–31.

4 Hannah JA, Brodie MJ. Epilepsy and learning disabilities—a challenge for the next millennium? *Seizure* 1998; 7: 3–13.

5 Bowley C, Kerr M. Epilepsy and intellectual disability. *J Intellect Disabil Res* 2000; 44: 529–43.

6 Nakken KO, Brodtkorb E. Epilepsy services for the patient with mental retardation in Norway. In: Sillanpää M, Gram L, Johannessen SI, Tomson T, eds. *Epilepsy and Mental Retardation*. Petersfield: Wrightson Biomedical Publishing, 1999.

7 Brodtkorb E. Treatment of epilepsy in patients with intellectual disabilities: general principles and particular problems. In: Sillanpää M, Gram L, Johannessen SI, Tomson T, eds. *Epilepsy and Mental Retardation*. Petersfield: Wrightson Biomedical Publishing, 1999.

8 Besag, FMC. Treatment of state-dependent learning disability. *Epilepsia* 2001; 42 (Suppl. 1): 52–4.

9 Alvarez N. Barbiturates in the treatment of epilepsy in people with intellectual disability. *J Intellect Disabil Res* 1998; 42 (Suppl. 1): 16–23.

10 Iivanainen M. Phenytoin: effective but insidious therapy for epilepsy in people with intellectual disability. *J Intellect Disabil Res* 1998; 42 (Suppl. 1): 24–31.

11 Schmidt D, Bourgeois B. A risk-benefit assessment of therapies for Lennox–Gastaut syndrome. *Drug Saf* 2000; 22: 467–77.

12 Bryant AE, Dreifuss FE. Valproic acid hepatic fatalities III. US experience since 1986. *Neurology* 1996; 46: 465–9.

13 Chiron C, Dumas C, Jambaque I, Mumford J, Dulac O. Randomized trial comparing vigabatrin and hydrocortisone in infantile spasms due to tuberous sclerosis. *Epilepsy Res* 1997; 26: 389–95.

14 Vigevano F, Cilio MR. Vigabatrin versus ACTH as first-line treatment for infantile spasms: A randomized, prospective study. *Epilepsia* 1997; 38: 1270–4.

15 Appleton RE, Peters AC, Mumford JP, Shaw DE. Randomised, placebo-controlled study of vigabatrin as first-line treatment of infantile spasms. *Epilepsia* 1999; 40: 1627–33.

16 The Felbamate Study Group in Lennox–Gastaut Syndrome. Efficacy of felbamate in childhood epileptic encephalopathy (Lennox–Gastaut syndrome). *N Engl J Med* 1993; 328: 29–33.

17 Motte J, Trevathan E, Arvidsson JFV *et al*. Lamotrigine for generalized seizures associated with the Lennox–Gastaut syndrome. *N Engl J Med* 1997; 337: 1807–12.

18 Sachdeo RC, Glauser TA, Ritter F, Reife R, Lim P, Pledger G. A double blind trial of topiramate in Lennox–Gastaut syndrome. *Neurology* 1999; 52: 1882–7.

19 Kälviäinen, R, Nousiainen I. Visual field defects with vigabatrin: epidemiology and therapeutic implications. *CNS Drugs* 2001; 15: 217–30.

20 Bhaumik S, Branford D, Duggirala C, Ismail IA. A naturalistic study of the use of vigabatrin, lamotrigine and gabapentin in adults with learning disabilities. *Seizure* 1997; 6: 127–33.

21 Eriksson A-S, Nergårdh A, Hoppu K. The efficacy of lamotrigine in children and adolescents with refractory generalized epilepsy: A randomized, double-blind, cross-over study. *Epilepsia* 1998; 39: 495–501.

22 Crawford P, Brown S, Kerr M *et al*. A randomized open-label study of gabapentin and lamotrigine in adults with learning disability and resistant epilepsy. *Seizure* 2001; 10: 107–15.

23 Pellock JM, Morton LD. Treatment of epilepsy in the multiply handicapped. *Ment Retard Dev Disabil Res Rev* 2000; 6: 309–23.

24 Ettinger AB, Weisbrot DM, Saracco J, Dhoon A, Kanner A, Devinsky O. Positive and negative psychotropic effects of lamotrigine in patients with epilepsy and mental retardation. *Epilepsia* 1998; 39: 874–7.

25 French J, Smith M, Faught E, Brown L. Practice advisory: The use of felbamate in the treatment of patients with intractable epilepsy. *Neurology* 1999; 52: 1540–5.

26 Lhatoo SD, Wong ICK, Sander JWAS. Prognostic factors affecting long-term retention of topiramate in patients with chronic epilepsy. *Epilepsia* 2000; 41: 338–41.

27 Gironell A, Kulisevsky J, Barbanoj M, Lopez-Villegas D, Hernandez G, Pasqual-Sedano, B. A randomized placebo-controlled comparative trial of gabapentin and propranolol in essential tremor. *Arch Neurol* 1999; 56: 475–80.

28 Cutter NC, Scott DD, Johnson JC, Whiteneck G. Gabapentin effect on spasticity in multiple sclerosis: a placebo-controlled, randomized, trial. *Arch Phys Med Rehabil* 2000; 81: 164–9.

29 Chudnow RS, Dewey RB, Lawson CR. Choreoathetosis as a side effect of gabapentin therapy in severely neurologically impaired patients. *Arch Neurol* 1997; 54: 910–12.

30 Nousiainen I, Mäntyjärvi M, Kälviäinen R. Visual function in patients treated with the GABAergic anticonvulsant tiagabine. *Clin Drug Invest* 2000; 20: 393–400.

31 Holden KR, Titus MO. The effect of tiagabine on spasticity in children with intractable epilepsy: a pilot study. *Pediatr Neurol* 1999; 21: 728–30.

32 Koskiniemi M, Van Vleymen B, Hakamies L, Lamusuo S, Taalas J. Piracetam relieves symptoms in progressive myoclonus epilepsy: a multicentre, randomised, double blind, crossover study comparing the efficacy and safety of three dosages of oral piracetam with placebo. *J Neurol Neurosurg Psychiatry* 1998; 64: 344–8.

33 Lappalainen R, Riikonen RS. High levels of cerebrospinal fluid glutamate in Rett syndrome. *Pediatr Neurol* 1996; 15: 213–16.

34 Stenbom Y, Tonnby B, Hagberg B. Lamotrigine in Rett syndrome: treatment experience from a pilot study. *Eur Child Adolesc Psychiatry* 1998; 7: 49–52.

35 Franz DN, Glauser TA, Tudor C, Williams S. Topiramate therapy of epilepsy associated with Angelman's syndrome. *Neurology* 2000; 54: 1185–8.

36 Kerr M, Bowley C. Evidence-based prescribing in adults with learning disability and epilepsy. *Epilepsia* 2001; 42 (Suppl. 1): 44–5.

37 Devinsky, O. Cognitive and behavioral effects of antiepileptic drugs. *Epilepsia* 1995; 36 (Suppl. 2): 46–65.

38 Aldenkamp AP. Effects of antiepileptic drugs on cognition. *Epilepsia* 2001; 42 (Suppl. 1): 46–9.

39 Kälviäinen R, Äikiä M, Riekkinen PJ. Cognitive adverse effects of antiepileptic drugs. Incidence, mechanisms and therapeutic implications. *CNS Drugs* 1996; 5: 358–68.

40 Durwen HF, Elger CE, Helmstaedter C, Penin, F. Circumscribed improvement of cognitive performance in temporal lobe epilepsy patients with in-tractable seizures following reduction of anticonvulsant medication. *J Epilepsy* 1989; 2: 147–53.

41 Durwen HF, Elger CE. Verbal learning differences in epileptic patients with left and right temporal lobe foci—a pharmacologically induced phenomenon. *Acta Neurol Scand* 1993; 87: 1–8.

42 Helmstaedter C, Wagner G, Elger CE. Differential effects of first antiepileptic drug application on cognition in lesional and non-lesional patients with epilepsy. *Seizure* 1993; 2: 125–30.

43 Perucca E, Gram L, Avanzini G, Dulac O. Antiepileptic drugs as a cause of worsening seizures. *Epilepsia* 1998; 39: 5–17.

44 Guerrini R, Dravet C, Genton P, Belmonte A., Kaminska A, Dulac, O. Lamotrigine and seizure aggravation in severe myoclonic epilepsy. *Epilepsia* 1998; 39: 508–12.

45 Bauer J. Seizure-inducing effects of antiepileptic drugs: a review. *Acta Neurol Scand* 1996; 94: 367–77.

46 Genton P. When antiepileptic drugs aggravate epilepsy. *Brain Dev* 2000; 22: 75–80.

47 Shinnar, S, Berg AT. Does antiepileptic therapy prevent the development of 'chronic' epilepsy? *Epilepsia* 1996; 37: 701–8.

48 Salih, MA, Kabiraj M, Al-Jarallah AS, El Desouki M, Othman S, Palar VA. Hemiconvulsion–hemiplegia–epilepsy syndrome. A clinical, electroencephalographic and neuroradiological study. *Child Nerv Syst* 1997; 13: 257–63.

49 Shields D. Catastrophic epilepsy in childhood. *Epilepsia* 2000; 41 (Suppl. 2): 2–6.

50 Jambaque I, Chiron C, Dumas C, Mumford J, Dulac O. Mental and behavioural outcome of infantile epilepsy treated with vigabatrin in tuberous sclerosis patients. *Epilepsy Res* 2000; 38: 151–60.

51 Maertens P, Dyken P, Graf W, Pippenger C, Chronister R, Shah A. Free radicals, anticonvulsants, and the neuronal ceroid-lipofuscinoses. *Am J Med Genet* 1995; 57: 225–8.

52 Liu CS, Wu HM, Kao SH, Wei YH. Serum trace elements, glutathione, copper/zink superoxide, and lipid peroxidation in epileptic patients with phenytoin or carbamazepine monotherapy. *Clin Neuropharmacol* 1998; 21: 62–4.

53 Hurd RW, Wilder BJ, Helveston WR, Uthman BM. Treatment of four siblings with progressive myoclonus epilepsy of the Unverricht-Lundborg type with N-acetylcysteine. *Neurology* 1996; 47: 1264–8.

54 Levisohn PM. Epilepsy surgery in children with developmental disabilities. *Semin Pediatr Neurol* 2000; 7: 194–203.

55 Chelune GJ, Naugle RI, Hermann BP *et al*. Does presurgical IQ predict seizure outcome after temporal lobectomy? Evidence from the Bozeman epilepsy consortium. *Epilepsia* 1998; 39: 314–18.

56 Lundgren J, Åmark P, Blennow G, Strömblad, LG, Wallstedt, L. Vagus nerve stimulation in 16 children with refractory epilepsy. *Epilepsia* 1998; 39: 809–13.

57 Hosain S, Nikalov B, Harden C, Li M, Fraser R, Labar, D. Vagus nerve stimulation treatment for Lennox–Gastaut syndrome. *J Child Neurol* 2000; 15: 509–12.

58 Brodtkorb E, Aamo T, Henriksen O, Lossius, R. Rectal diazepam: pitfalls of excessive use in refractory epilepsy *Epilepsy Res* 1999; 35: 123–33.

59 Brodtkorb E, Sand T, Kristiansen A, Torbergsen T. Non-convulsive status epilepticus in the adult mentally retarded. Classification and role of benzodiazepines. *Seizure* 1993; 2: 115–23.

60 Scott RC, Besag FM, Neville BG. Buccal midazolam and rectal diazepam for treatment of prolonged seizures in childhood and adolescence. *Lancet* 1999; 353: 623–6.

61 Steffenburg S, Gillberg C, Steffenburg U. Psychiatric disorders in children and adolescents with mental retardation and active epilepsy. *Arch Neurol* 1996; 53: 904–12.

62 Brodtkorb E, Sand T, Strandjord RE. Neuroleptic and antiepileptic treatment in the mentally retarded. *Seizure* 1993; 2: 205–11.

63 Stimmel GL, Dopheide JA. Psychotropic drug-induced reductions in seizure threshold. Incidence and consequences. *CNS Drugs* 1996; 5: 37–50.

64 Pillmann F, Schlote K, Broich K, Marneros A. Electroencephalogram alterations during treatment with olanzapine. *Psychopharmacology* 2000; 150: 216–19.

65 Brodtkorb, E. The diversity of epilepsy in adults with severe developmental

disabilities: age at seizure onset and other prognostic factors. *Seizure* 1994; 3: 277–85.

66 Sillanpää M, Jalava M, Kaleva O, Shinnar, S. Long-term prognosis of seizures with onset in childhood. *N Engl J Med* 1998; 338: 1715–22.

67 Stephen LJ, Kwan P, Brodie MJ. Does the cause of localisation-related epilepsy influence the response to antiepileptic drug treatment? *Epilepsia* 2001; 42: 357–62.

68 Alvarez N. Discontinuance of antiepileptic medications in patients with developmental disability and diagnosis of epilepsy. *Am J Ment Ret* 1989; 93: 593–9.

69 McVicker RW, Shanks OE, McClelland RJ. Prevalence and associated features of Down's syndrome. *Br J Psychiatr* 1994; 164: 528–32.

70 Johannsen P, Christensen JEJ, Goldstein H, Nielsen VK, Mai, J. Epilepsy in Down syndrome—prevalence in three age groups. *Seizure* 1996; 5: 121–5.

71 Evenhuis HM. The natural history of dementia in Down's syndrome. *Arch Neurol* 1990; 47: 263–7.

72 Steffenburg U, Hagberg G, Hagberg B. Epilepsy in a representative series of Rett syndrome. *Acta Paediatr* 2001; 90: 34–9.

73 Laan LA, v Haeringen A, Brouwer OF. Angelman syndrome: a review of clinical and genetic aspects. *Clin Neurol Neurosurg* 1999; 101: 161–70.

74 Musumeci SA, Hagerman RJ, Ferri R *et al*. Epilepsy and EEG findings in males with fragile X syndrome. *Epilepsia* 1999; 40: 1092–9.

75 Shinnar S, Berg AT, Moshe SL *et al*. Discontinuing antiepileptic drugs in children with epilepsy: A prospective study. *Ann Neurol* 1994; 35: 534–45.

76 Marcus JC. Stopping antiepileptic therapy in mentally-retarded, epileptic children. *Neuropediatrics* 1998; 29: 26–8.

77 Medical Research Council Antiepileptic Drug Withdrawal Study Group. Prognostic index for recurrence of seizures after remission of epilepsy. *BMJ* 1993; 306: 1374–8.

78 Delgado MR, Riela AR., Mills J, Pitt A, Browne R. Discontinuation of antiepileptic drug treatment after two seizure-free years in children with cerebral palsy. *Pediatrics* 1996; 97: 192–7.

79 Zafeiriou DI, Kontopoulos EE, Tsikoulas I. Characteristics and prognosis of epilepsy in children with cerebral palsy. *J Child Neurol* 1999; 14: 289–94.

18 Emergency Treatment of Seizures and Status Epilepticus

M.C. Walker and S.D. Shorvon

Introduction

Epilepsy is, for the most part, self-terminating. On occasions, however, seizures of any type can continue unabated and they are then considered as a separate entity—status epilepticus. One of the earliest references to status epilepticus can be found in a Babylonian treatise on epilepsy from the middle of the first millennium BC, in which the grave prognosis of this condition was described: 'If the possessing demon possesses him many times during the middle watch of the night, and at the time of his possession his hands and feet are cold, he is much darkened, keeps opening and closing his mouth, is brown and yellow as to the eyes. . . . It may go on for some time, but he will die' [1]. There were, however, few references to status epilepticus in the ensuing years. Why this may be so is a matter of speculation; Hunter [2] noted that status epilepticus was rare before the advent of powerful antiepileptic drugs, and the consequent risk of drug withdrawal [2]. This is undoubtedly an important cause of status epilepticus, but cannot account for the large number of drug-naive patients presenting with status epilepticus in present times. In the 19th century the entity of status epilepticus was first clearly distinguished amongst the epilepsies. Calmeil [3] used the term 'etat de mal' and later the term status epilepticus appeared in Bazire's translation of Trousseau's lectures on clinical medicine [4]. From that time status epilepticus was, on the whole, a term used to describe solely convulsive status epilepticus. It was not until the Marseilles conference in 1962 that status epilepticus was generally recognized to include all seizure types and that the definition was based solely on the persistence of the seizure rather than its form [5]. This is of great importance as it is now apparent that a persistent seizure may result in neuronal damage irrespective of any systemic metabolic compromise. Although the length of time that a seizure or series of seizures have to continue before being classified as status epilepticus has been a matter of debate and is to an extent arbitrary, most would accept a limit of 30 min [6]. Treatment, however, should begin before this period (see below). The necessity of differentiating status epilepticus from other seizure conditions relates to its high morbidity and mortality.

The term status epilepticus, as used by Gastaut and colleagues, included three entities: generalized status epilepticus, partial status epilepticus and unilateral status epilepticus [7]. This classification is, however, both incomplete and too broad to be clinically useful, and recently more detailed classifications have been proposed [6] (Table 18.1).

Estimates of the overall incidence of status epilepticus have varied from 10 to 60 per 100 000 person-years, depending on the population studied and the definitions used [8–11]. Some studies are likely to have underestimated incidence due to incomplete case ascertainment. The incidence also varies in different ethnic groups; status epilepticus is commoner in Afro-Americans than Caucasians, and it is not clear to what extent this difference is due to genetic or socioeconomic factors. Status epilepticus is also more frequently associated with mental handicap, and with structural cerebral pathology (especially in the frontal areas). In established epilepsy, status epilepticus can be precipitated by drug withdrawal, intercurrent illness or metabolic disturbance, or the progression of the underlying disease, and is more common in symptomatic than in idiopathic epilepsy. About 5% of all epileptic adult clinic patients will have at least one episode of status epilepticus in the course of their epilepsy [6,12], and in children the proportion is higher (10–25%) [6,12,13]. Most status epilepticus episodes, however, do not develop in patients with a previous diagnosis of epilepsy, and are often due to an acute cerebral disturbance [8–10], emphasizing the importance of identifying and treating the acute precipitant. Infections with fever are a common cause of status epilepticus in children, whilst in adults cerebrovascular accidents (CVAs), hypoxia, metabolic causes and alcohol are the main acute causes [9]. Although the prognosis of status epilepticus is related to aetiology, the prognosis of certain conditions such as stroke may be worse if associated with status epilepticus [13]. The overall mortality for status epilepticus is about 20%, most patients dying of the underlying condition, rather than the status epilepticus itself [9,14]. The mortality is age related, and is much lower in children and higher in the elderly [9]. Permanent neurological and mental deterioration can result from status epilepticus, particularly in young children; the risks of morbidity are greatly increased the longer the duration of the status epilepticus episode [13,15]. Furthermore status epilepticus can result in chronic epilepsy, and indeed, 43% of those with acute symptomatic status epilepticus have a subsequent unprovoked seizure compared to 13% of those with acute symptomatic seizures [16].

Before describing the particular treatment of the various forms of status epilepticus, it is necessary to have an understanding of status-induced neuronal damage, and drug pharmacokinetics and pharmacodynamics during status epilepticus.

Status epilepticus and neuronal damage

The association of neuronal damage with status epilepticus had been noted in the 19th century. In more recent times, postmortem studies of individuals who died during status epilepticus have revealed extensive neuronal damage in the temporal lobes [17–19]. Furthermore, levels of neurone-specific enolase, a marker of neuronal injury, are elevated immediately following status epilepticus [15], and there have been case reports describing the development of hippocampal atrophy in patients followed with neuroimaging after an episode of status epilepticus [20–22]. The interpretation of

Table 18.1 Revised classification of status epilepticus

Status epilepticus confined to early childhood
Neonatal status epilepticus
Status epilepticus in specific neonatal epilepsy syndromes
Infantile spasms

Status epilepticus confined to later childhood
Febrile status epilepticus
Status in childhood partial epilepsy syndromes
Status epilepticus in myoclonic-astatic epilepsy
Electrical status epilepticus during slow-wave sleep
Landau–Kleffner syndrome

Status epilepticus occurring in childhood and adult life
Tonic-clonic status epilepticus
Absence status epilepticus
Epilepsia partialis continua
Status epilepticus in coma (subtle generalized tonic-clonic seizure)
Specific forms of status epilepticus in mental retardation
Syndromes of myoclonic status epilepticus
Non-convulsive simple partial status epilepticus
Complex partial status epilepticus

Status epilepticus confined to adult life
De novo absence status of late onset

After [6].

the human data is, however, confounded by other factors such as aetiology, metabolic compromise and treatment. Animal experiments have thus provided a greater insight into neuronal damage associated with status epilepticus [23]. Initial experiments demonstrated that convulsive status epilepticus resulted in neuronal damage, and that neuronal damage occurred even if the systemic and metabolic compromise that occurs in convulsive status epilepticus was controlled. This led to the concept that it was the presence of on-going electrographic seizure activity that itself resulted in neuronal damage (excitotoxic neuronal damage [24]). Animal studies of non-convulsive status have shown similar changes [25]. Importantly this neuronal damage is time dependent, and as such stopping the status epilepticus as soon as possible will prevent much of the damage from occurring.

Status epilepticus can, thus, undoubtedly cause neuronal damage, but does it inevitably cause such damage? It is important to realize that the animal models were developed to explore excitotoxicity, and caution is needed in extrapolating these findings to the human condition. The animal models used generally involve induction of status epilepticus in a non-epileptic animal with either powerful chemoconvulsants or prolonged high-frequency repetitive stimulation [25–27]. There are rare occurrences of comparable precipitants in humans, such as domoic acid poisoning from mussels in which pathological changes occurred that are similar to the animal models [20], but these are exceptional. Complex partial status epilepticus in humans, in particular, is very different from that in animal models. Complex partial status epilepticus in humans tends to have lower frequency discharges, which if reproduced in animal models produces substantially less neuronal damage [28–30]. It is still not clear to what extent complex partial status results in neu-

ronal damage in humans. There have been reports of prolonged memory problems, hemiparesis and death occurring following complex partial status epilepticus, although, in many of these cases, the outcome relates to the underlying aetiology [31–33]. In one study, only 10 patients were identified with significant morbidity from complex partial status epilepticus over a 10-year period (this almost certainly represents a small fraction of all patients with complex partial status epilepticus during this period) [34]. Furthermore, in seven of these patients, coincident conditions undoubtedly contributed significantly to this morbidity. In many reported cases, aggressive treatment with intravenous therapy and, on occasions, barbiturate anaesthesia could also contribute to the consequent morbidity. Importantly, there have also been large case series of prolonged complex partial status epilepticus with no neurological sequelae [35,36]. Ceiling effects (damage only in the early episodes) in patients with repeated episodes of status also complicate assessment.

One postmortem study has reported substantial neuronal damage following partial status epilepticus in three patients [19]. The aetiology of the status epilepticus is unclear in two cases and the aetiology in the third case was related to carcinomatous meningitis. It is thus difficult to know if the damage is due to the status epilepticus or some unknown pathogenic process such as viral encephalitis.

Rises in serum neurone-specific enolase have also been used as an argument that complex partial status epilepticus results in neuronal damage [37,38]. These rises could be partially the result of a breakdown in the blood–brain barrier rather than an increase in neuronal death, and cerebrospinal fluid neurone-specific enolase would be a more accurate predictor [39]. The degree to which serum neurone-specific enolase correlates with neurological and cognitive disability in complex partial status epilepticus is especially unclear, since some patients with very high serum neuronal enolase have a good outcome. Neuroimaging in complex partial status has largely also been inconclusive; reversible changes do occur and in some selected patients mild atrophy can be associated with complex partial status epilepticus [40].

Animal evidence also suggests that there may be certain groups who are less prone to neuronal damage from status epilepticus; epileptic animals, animals pretreated with antiepileptic drugs and young animals are all resistant to chemoconvulsant-induced neuronal damage [41–46]. Thus young age, antiepileptic drugs and prior history of epilepsy may all confer neuroprotection.

What is the relationship of this neuronal damage to the subsequent morbidity of status epilepticus? It appears that the neuronal damage that occurs during status epilepticus is not necessary for epileptogenesis [47,48]. Indeed, damaging the hippocampus through severe hypoxic injury seems to inhibit epileptogenesis [49]. The neuronal damage probably more closely relates to other pathologies post-status epilepticus such as memory and behavioural problems [47,50].

The main epileptogenic changes following status epilepticus have yet to be clearly defined. Changes have been reported in intrinsic properties of neurones [51], rate of neurogenesis [52], receptor function [53], inhibitory interneurones [54], synaptic arrangements [55] and the extracellular space. All of these could be epileptogenic; however, it has been difficult to identify one critical or necessary process.

Drug pharmacokinetics and pharmacodynamics

In the rational drug treatment of status epilepticus, an understanding of the pharmacokinetics of acutely administered drugs is needed. In particular it is important to realize three fundamental points:

1 The pharmacokinetics of a drug administered acutely may greatly differ from that of the drug administered chronically.

2 The pharmacokinetics of a drug may be different in an animal that is seizing.

3 The longer seizures continue the more difficult they are to treat.

Acute drug pharmacokinetics

Fast drug absorption is essential in the treatment of status epilepticus, and thus almost all drugs need to be administered intravenously. Paraldehyde and midazolam, however, may be given intramuscularly, and diazepam and paraldehyde rectally. Other drugs are less commonly given rectally, and midazolam is given by buccal instillation.

In order to act rapidly, the drugs need to cross the blood–brain barrier readily. Drugs achieve this either by being lipid soluble or by having an active transport mechanism. Thus the drugs that are effective in status epilepticus usually have a high lipid solubility. This leads to them having a large volume of distribution.

During intravenous administration, a drug directly enters the central compartment (blood and extracellular fluid of highly perfused organs) from where it is distributed to peripheral compartments, in particular fat and muscle. Since most of the drugs with which we are concerned are highly lipid soluble, they are rapidly redistributed into the peripheral compartment from the central compartment. This leads to an initial drop in plasma concentrations, which can be quantified as a distribution half-life. In addition the drug may be eliminated from the central compartment either through renal excretion, hepatic metabolism (the major route of elimination for the majority of antiepileptic drugs) or exhalation, and the efficiency of this process is reflected in the elimination half-life. The antiepileptic drugs used in status epilepticus often have a much shorter distribution half-life than elimination half-life (see

Fig. 18.1). For highly lipid-bound drugs following acute administration, there is a rapid initial fall in plasma levels and brain levels (Fig. 18.1), and thus loss of effect. This has led to the practice of repeat boluses and infusions in order to maintain adequate plasma levels. However, with persistent administration there is accumulation of the drug within the peripheral compartment, and this results in two important effects [6,56]:

1 Higher peak levels with subsequent boluses or with continued infusions.

2 Clearance of the drug from the central compartment becomes dependent on the elimination half-life and therefore it occurs much more slowly (Fig. 18.2).

These two effects are potentially dangerous, and some of the mortality and morbidity of status epilepticus is due to injudicious use of repeated boluses or continuous infusions of lipid-soluble drugs.

Kinetics of drugs during seizures

Seizures (especially convulsive seizures) can affect both peripheral and central pharmacokinetics of drugs. During convulsive seizures, there is a fall in the pH of the blood resulting in a change in the degree of ionization (and thus lipid solubility) of drugs in plasma. This will affect the distribution half-lives, the ability to cross the blood–brain barrier and the protein binding. In addition, the pH in blood decreases to a greater degree than in brain; this pH gradient facilitates the movement of a weakly acid drug from blood to brain. This effect can be seen, for instance, with phenobarbital [57,58]. Other peripheral pharmacokinetic effects are also apparent during status epilepticus. These may result from increased blood flow to muscle, and hepatic and renal compromise (often resulting in a prolongation of the elimination half-life of anticonvulsant drugs). In addition to these peripheral effects, there is also a direct effect of status epilepticus on the brain compartment. There is a breakdown in the blood–brain barrier during convulsive seizures, which again results in more effective brain penetration of anticonvulsant drugs. During seizures there is increased blood flow to seizing brain; thus drugs in which the cortical blood flow determines the rate at which

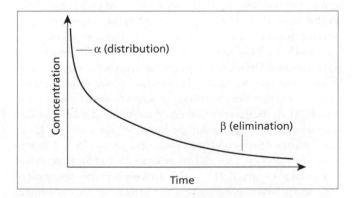

Fig. 18.1 Concentration–time profile of acutely administered drugs showing two phases: a rapid distribution phase (α), in which drug is distributed from the blood compartment to fat and muscle, a slower elimination phase (β).

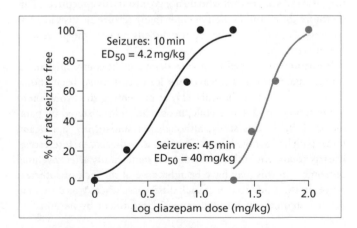

Fig. 18.2 Diazepam was effective in controlling brief (10 min) seizures but lost potency after prolonged (45 min) seizures in a lithium–pilocarpine rat model of status epilepticus. From [59].

the drug crosses the blood–brain barrier (e.g. phenobarbital) may concentrate in foci of seizure activity in the brain.

Drug responsiveness

As status epilepticus progresses it becomes more difficult to treat, probably largely because of changes in brain receptors with continued seizure activity [59–62]. Many of the treatments that are successful in the initial stages are ineffective later. Indeed, the potency of benzodiazepines decreases as status epilepticus progresses, although their efficacy remains (Fig. 18.2) [59]; the decrease in their potency is associated with a decrease in the sensitivity of γ-aminobutyric acid (GABA) receptors to benzodiazepines [59].

Serial seizures (premonitory phase)

It has been noted that the development of status epilepticus is preceded by an increasing frequency of seizures (a premonitory phase) [6]. Furthermore, animal data suggest that treatment at this early stage has a much higher chance of success than treatment of established status epilepticus [62]. Treatment at this stage also prevents neuronal damage. Serial seizures and prolonged seizures do not, however, necessarily result in status epilepticus, and in one study of seizures lasting 10–29 min, half the seizures terminated without treatment (whether some of the other episodes that were treated would have terminated without treatment is unknown) [63]. Similarly a study of new onset seizures in children found that half the children had seizures lasting longer than 5 min, and 92% of the seizures stopped spontaneously; indeed, approximately three-quarters of the seizures lasting longer than 5 min stopped spontaneously [64]. This introduces two notes of caution: first that status epilepticus is not an inevitable consequence of prolonged seizures, and that treatment studies based on seizures that last less than 30 min may overestimate treatment effects due to spontaneous seizure cessation.

Randomized control studies have established the efficacy of oral and rectal diazepam and buccal midazolam in the treatment of serial seizures [65–68]. Most of these studies, however, consider episodes in patient groups (often institutionalized) who have a history of serial seizures but who do not go into status epilepticus. Furthermore these studies often include many seizure clusters in a few patients. Thus these studies do not directly address the prevention of status epilepticus.

With more prolonged seizures (> 10 min) in the community, intravenous diazepam and intravenous lorazepam have been shown to be more effective than placebo at preventing the evolution to or continuation of status epilepticus when administered by paramedics [69]. In this study, although not statistically significant, lorazepam had a more impressive effect than diazepam. Interestingly early treatment in this study did not significantly affect eventual outcome, but this may have been because of the lack of sufficient power in the study to detect such differences (there was a trend to better outcomes for those given active treatment by paramedics) [69].

Rectal paraldehyde has been proposed as an alternative, especially in children. Paraldehyde is, however, difficult to use and administer, and its use should be perhaps reserved for those in whom a rectal benzodiazepine has failed [70,71].

Convulsive status epilepticus

Diagnosis

Non-epileptic attacks are frequently prolonged and can be confused with status epilepticus. In an audit of patients transferred to a specialist neurological intensive care unit for further treatment of their status epilepticus, approximately half the patients transferred were not in status epilepticus, and were either in pseudostatus or in drug-induced coma (usually secondary to large amounts of chlormethiazole) [72]. The inadequacy of diagnosis from most referring centres was partly due to absent or insufficient EEG services available at those centres [72]. As has been found in another study [73], many patients with pseudostatus had a previous diagnosis of epilepsy that may have confounded the diagnosis. Pseudostatus is often misdiagnosed as true status epilepticus and is often refractory to initial therapy (leading to general anaesthesia and mechanical ventilation) [72,73]. Failure by admitting doctors to recognize the possibility of pseudostatus was common. It should thus be emphasized that pseudostatus must be considered if an episode of status epilepticus does not respond promptly to initial therapy (especially if the seizures are in any way atypical).

EEG patterns have also been proposed to be a means of staging the status epilepticus. From experimental models, a progression of EEG changes have been suggested from discrete seizures, to merging seizures, to continuous seizure activity and then eventually PLEDs (periodic lateralized epileptiform discharges) or PBEDs (periodic bilateral epileptiform discharges) [74]. This progression has been proposed to mirror increasing drug resistance and a worsening prognosis [62]. In humans this clear EEG sequence is not usually found [75]. Although patients with PLEDs generally fare less well, outcome is probably more related to age and aetiology than to specific ictal EEG patterns [75].

Medical management and complications

Convulsive status epilepticus is a medical emergency because of the significant potential for excitotoxic cerebral damage, other forms of cerebral damage and associated medical complications. In the early phase, cerebral autoregulation and homeostasis are largely preserved. The systemic effects of convulsive status epilepticus can be divided into early and late stages. The initial consequence of a prolonged convulsion is a massive release of plasma catecholamines [76], which results in an increase in heart rate, blood pressure and plasma glucose. During this stage cardiac arrhythmias are frequently seen, and may be fatal [77]. Cerebral blood flow is greatly increased and thus glucose delivery to active cerebral tissue is maintained [78]. As the seizure continues, there is a steady rise in the core body temperature, and prolonged hyperthermia above 40°C can cause cerebral damage and has a poorer prognosis [79–81]. Acidosis also commonly occurs, and in one series 25% of the patients had an arterial pH below 7.0 [81]. This acidosis is mainly the result of lactic acid production, but there is also a rise in carbon dioxide tension that can, in itself, result in life-threatening narcosis [81]. The acidosis can increase the likelihood of life-threatening cardiac arrhythmias, hypotension and in conjunction with the cardiovascular compromise may result in severe pulmonary oedema [82].

The status epilepticus may then enter a second late phase in which cerebral and systemic protective measures progressively fail. The main characteristics of this phase are: a fall in blood pressure; a loss of cerebral autoregulation resulting in the dependence of cerebral blood flow on systemic blood pressure and hypoglycaemia due to the exhaustion of glycogen stores and the increased neurogenic insulin secretion [76,83,84]. Intracranial pressure may rise precipitously in status epilepticus. The combined effects of systemic hypotension and intracranial hypertension can result in a compromised cerebral circulation and cerebral oedema, particularly in children [85]. Further complications may occur including rhabdomyolysis leading to acute tubular necrosis, hyperkalaemia and hyponatraemia [86]. Hepatic compromise is not uncommon, and rarely there may be disseminated intravascular coagulation with its subsequent complications [87]. Because of these medical complications, status epilepticus that has lasted an hour or more (and sometimes earlier) should be managed in the intensive care unit, where there is adequate monitoring and treatment of these potential complications.

Thus for the new patient presenting as an emergency in status epilepticus, it is helpful to plan therapy in a series of progressive phases.

First stage (0–10 min)

Oxygen and cardiorespiratory resuscitation

It is first essential to assess cardiorespiratory function, to secure the airway and to resuscitate where necessary. Oxygen should always be administered, as hypoxia is often unexpectedly severe.

Second stage (1–60 min)

Monitoring

Regular neurological observations and measurements of pulse, blood pressure, ECG and temperature should be initiated. Metabolic abnormalities may cause status epilepticus, or develop during its course, and biochemical, blood gas, pH, clotting and haematological measures should be monitored.

Emergency anticonvulsant therapy

This should be started (see below).

Intravenous lines

These should be set up for fluid replacement and drug administration (preferably with 0.9% sodium chloride (normal or physiological saline) rather than 5% glucose solutions). Drugs should not be mixed and, if two antiepileptic drugs are needed (for example, phenytoin and diazepam), two intravenous lines should be sited. The lines should be in large veins, as many antiepileptic drugs cause phlebitis and thrombosis at the site of infusion. Arterial lines must never be used for drug administration.

Emergency investigations

Blood should be drawn for the emergency measurement of blood gases, sugar, renal and liver function, calcium and magnesium levels, full haematological screen (including platelets), blood clotting measures and anticonvulsant levels. Fifty millilitres of serum should also be saved for future analysis especially if the cause of the status epilepticus is uncertain. Other investigations depend on the clinical circumstances.

Intravenous glucose and thiamine

Fifty millilitres of a 50% glucose solution should be given immediately by intravenous injection if hypoglycaemia is suspected. If there is a history of alcoholism, or other compromised nutritional states, 250 mg of thiamine (for example, as the high-potency intravenous formulation of Pabrinex, 10 mL of which contains 250 mg) should also be given intravenously. This is particularly important if glucose has been administered, as a glucose infusion increases the risk of Wernicke's encephalopathy in susceptible patients. Intravenous high-dosage thiamine should be given slowly (for example, 10 mL of high-potency Pabrinex over 10 min), with facilities for treating the anaphylaxis which is a potentially serious side-effect of Pabrinex infusions. Routine glucose administration in non-hypoglycaemic patients should be avoided as there is some evidence that this can aggravate neuronal damage.

Acidosis

If acidosis is severe, the administration of bicarbonate has been advocated in the hope of preventing shock, and mitigating the effects of hypotension and low cerebral blood flow. In most cases, however, this is unnecessary and more effective is the rapid control of respiration and abolition of motor seizure activity.

Third stage (0–60/90 min)

Establish aetiology

The causes of status epilepticus differ with age, and in the presence or absence of established epilepsy. The investigations required depend on clinical circumstances. CT or MRI and cerebrospinal fluid examination are often necessary—the latter should be carried out only with facilities for resuscitation available as intracranial pressure is often elevated in status epilepticus.

If the status epilepticus has been precipitated by drug withdrawal, the immediate restitution of the withdrawn drug, even at lower doses, will usually rapidly terminate the status epilepticus. Pyridoxine should also be given intravenously to children under the age of 3 years, who have a prior history of epilepsy, and to all neonates.

Physiological changes and medical complications

The physiological changes of uncompensated status epilepticus, listed above, may need specific therapy. Active treatment is most commonly required for: hypoxia, hypotension, raised intracranial pressure, pulmonary oedema and hypertension, cardiac arrhythmias, cardiac failure, lactic acidosis, hyperpyrexia, hypoglycaemia, electrolyte disturbance, acute hepatic or renal failure, rhabdomyolysis or disseminated intravascular coagulation.

Pressor therapy

Dopamine is the most commonly used pressor agent, given by continuous intravenous infusion. The dose should be titrated to the desired haemodynamic and renal responses (usually initially between 2 and 5 µg/kg/min, but this can be increased to over 20 µg/kg/min in severe hypotension). Dopamine should be given into a large vein as extravasation causes tissue necrosis. ECG monitoring is required, as conduction defects may occur, and particular care is needed in dosing in the presence of cardiac failure.

Fourth stage (30–90 min)

Intensive care

If seizures are continuing in spite of the measures taken above, the patient must be transferred to an intensive care environment, and the usual measures instituted.

Intensive care monitoring

In severe established status epilepticus, intensive monitoring may be required, including intra-arterial blood pressure, oximetry, central venous pressure and pulmonary artery pressure monitoring.

Although magnesium is effective at preventing eclampsia, there is no evidence to suggest that increasing magnesium serum concentrations to supranormal levels has any benefit in status epilepticus. Indeed, such a policy can result in motor paralysis, difficulty in detecting clinical seizure activity and hypotension [88]. However, serum magnesium can be low in alcoholics and patients with acquired immune deficiency syndrome (AIDS) [89,90], and in these patients intravenous loading with 2–4 g of magnesium sulphate over 20 min may help with seizure control and prevention of arrhythmias.

Seizure and EEG monitoring

In prolonged status epilepticus, or in comatose ventilated patients, motor activity can be barely visible. In this situation, continuous EEG monitoring using a full EEG or a cerebral function monitor is necessary, and at the very least intermittent daily EEGs should be recorded. The latter must be calibrated individually, and then can register both burst suppression and seizure activity. Burst suppression provides an arbitrary physiological target for the titration of barbiturate or anaesthetic therapy. Drug dosing is commonly set at a level that will produce burst suppression with interburst intervals of between 2 and 30 s.

Intracranial pressure monitoring and cerebral oedema

Continuous intracranial pressure monitoring is advisable, especially in children in the presence of persisting, severe or progressive elevated intracranial pressure. The need for active therapy is usually determined by the underlying cause rather than the status epilepticus. Intermittent positive pressure ventilation, high-dose corticosteroid therapy (4 mg dexamethasone every 6 h), or mannitol infusion may be used (the latter is usually reserved for temporary respite for patients in danger of tentorial coning). Neurosurgical decompression is occasionally required.

Long-term anticonvulsant therapy

Long-term, maintenance, anticonvulsant therapy must be given in tandem with emergency treatment. The choice of drug depends on previous therapy, the type of epilepsy and the clinical setting. If phenytoin or phenobarbital has been used in emergency treatment, maintenance doses can be continued orally (through a nasogastric tube) guided by serum level monitoring. Other maintenance antiepileptic drugs can be started also by giving oral loading doses.

Drug treatment

The doses of drugs commonly used in status epilepticus are contained in Table 18.2. There have been six randomized studies of intravenous drug treatment in status epilepticus [91–96]. These studies are beset by methodological problems. They use different definitions of status epilepticus, most do not take adequate precautions to exclude patients with pseudostatus epilepticus, and they use different doses of drugs. Also there are problems of rapid randomization and of defining outcome. These studies compared lidocaine against placebo [95], lorazepam against diazepam [91,93], phenobarbital against diazepam and phenytoin [94], intramuscular midazolam against intravenous diazepam [92] and four different intravenous treatment regimes (lorazepam, phenytoin alone, diazepam and phenytoin, and phenobarbital) [96].

Certain conclusions can be drawn from these studies: (a) lidocaine is effective in the treatment of status epilepticus [95]; (b) lorazepam and diazepam are equally effective although more patients required additional antiepileptic drugs if given diazepam [91,93]; (c) lorazepam is more effective than phenytoin alone [96]; (d) intramuscular midazolam is as effective as initial intravenous diazepam and may be an alternative if intravenous access is difficult in children [92]; (e) phenobarbital alone is as effective as other regimens [94,96]; (f) lorazepam is faster to administer than other drugs [96]; and (g) no particular drug or drug combination has significantly more side-effects including respiratory depression (importantly phenytoin alone was not significantly superior to regimens containing benzodiazepines) [96]. Overall drug choice is perhaps not as important as having a protocol so that satisfactory doses of reasonable drugs are given rapidly; indeed, retrospective studies have found that approximately 70% of patients in status epilepticus are given inadequate doses of antiepileptic medication [72,97]. It seems sensible to stage treatment, with less intensive initial therapy requiring less support.

Early treatment

Benzodiazepines are widely accepted as the drugs of choice for initial therapy (Table 18.2). Of these, intravenous lorazepam is now generally preferred over diazepam as first-line therapy in established status epilepticus [96,98]. The disadvantage of diazepam is its short redistribution half-life (less than 1 h) and large volume of distribution (1–2 L/kg) [99]. These properties mean that serum and brain concentrations rapidly fall after initial intravenous dosing,

Table 18.2 Drugs used in the initial management of convulsive status epilepticus

Drug	Route	Adult dose	Paediatric dose
Diazepam at 2–5 mg/min[a]	IV bolus	10–20 mg at 2–5 mg/min[a]	0.25–0.5 mg/kg
	Rectal administration	10–30 mg[a]	0.5–0.75 mg/kg[a]
Midazolam	IM or rectally	5–10 mg[a]	0.15–0.3 mg/kg[a]
	IV bolus	0.1–0.3 mg/kg at 4 mg/min[a]	
	IV infusion	0.05–0.4 mg/kg/h	
Paraldehyde	Rectally or IM	5–10 mL (approx 1 g/mL) in equal vol. of water[a]	0.07–0.35 mL/kg[a]
	IV	5–10 mL/h as a 5% solution in 5% dextrose	
Chlormethiazole	IV infusion of 0.8% solution	40–100 mL at 5–15 mL/min, then 0.5–20 mL/min	0.1 mL/kg/min increasing every 2–4 h
Clonazepam	IV bolus	1–2 mg at 2 mg/min[a]	250–500 µg
Fosphenytoin	IV bolus	15–20 mg PE/kg at 150 mg PE/min	
Lignocaine	IV bolus	1.5–2.0 mg/kg at 50 mg/min[a]	
	IV infusion	3–4 mg/kg/h	
Lorazepam	Rectally		0.05–0.1 mg/kg
	IV bolus	0.07 mg/kg (usually 4 mg)[a]	0.1 mg/kg
Phenytoin	IV bolus/infusion	15–20 mg/kg at 50 mg/min	20 mg/kg at 25 mg/min
Phenobarbital	IV bolus	10–20 mg/kg at 100 mg/min	15–20 mg/kg
Valproate	IV bolus	15–30 mg/kg	20–40 mg/kg

After [148].

[a] May be repeated. IM, intramuscular; IV, intravenous; PE, phenytoin equivalents.

leading to potentially high rates of seizure recurrence. Within 2 h of successful treatment with diazepam, over half the patients with status epilepticus relapse [100]. Repeat boluses of diazepam can lead to significant accumulation, prolongation of action and progressively greater peak levels [101]. This may result in cardiorespiratory arrest, and so cannot be recommended. Clonazepam shares many of the pharmacokinetic features of diazepam. It has a similarly rapid brain penetration, short distribution half-life and long elimination half-life. Lorazepam, on the other hand, has a lesser volume of distribution and is less lipid soluble. It enters the brain more slowly, taking up to 30 min to reach peak levels. Its distribution half-life is much longer, 2–3 h, and its elimination half-life is shorter, approximately 10–12 h. Its effects therefore are longer lasting than are those of diazepam, and for this reason lorazepam is the benzodiazepine of choice in status epilepticus [91,98,99]. Lorazepam should be given as a bolus that can be repeated once after 10 min at which time phenytoin should be administered. Lidocaine as a bolus followed by an infusion has been recommended as an alternative to benzodiazepines in those in whom respiratory depression is a concern [102].

Established status epilepticus

If initial benzodiazepine therapy is ineffective, then the patient can be considered to be in established status epilepticus. Phenobarbital or phenytoin (or fosphenytoin) are the drugs of choice in this situation (Table 18.3). Phenobarbitone is easier to use, and possibly more effective, but phenytoin may have a lower risk of respiratory depression. Controlled studies have not however been carried out, and the relative merits of the two therapies are unclear. Intravenous valproate has also been proposed as an alternative, but there are, at present, inadequate data to justify its use before phenytoin.

Table 18.3 The intravenous (IV) antiepileptic drug treatment of convulsive status epilepticus in adults

Stage of early status
Lorazepam 4 mg IV bolus (can be repeated once)
If seizures continue after 30 min →

Stage of established status
Phenobarbital IV infusion of 10 mg/kg at a rate of 100 mg/min, or
Phenytoin IV infusion of 15 mg/kg at a rate of 50 mg/min, or
Fosphenytoin IV infusion of 15 mg PE/kg at a rate of 100 mg PE/min
If seizures continue after 30 min →

Stage of refractory status
General anaesthesia should be induced with either:
Propofol: IV bolus of 2 mg/kg, repeated if necessary, and then followed by a continuous infusion of 5–10 mg/kg/h initially reducing to a dose sufficient to maintain a burst suppression pattern on the EEG (usually 1–3 mg/kg/h)
When seizures have been controlled for 12 h, the drug dosage should be slowly reduced over a further 12 h *or*
Thiopental: IV bolus of 100–250 mg given over 20 s with further 50 mg boluses every 2–3 min until seizures are controlled, followed by a continuous IV infusion at a dose sufficient to maintain a burst suppression pattern on the EEG (usually 3–5 mg/kg/h).
When seizures have been controlled for 12 h, the drug dosage should be slowly reduced over a further 12 h *or*
Midazolam: IV bolus of 0.1–0.3 mg/kg at a rate not exceeding 4 mg/min initially, followed by a continuous IV infusion at a dose sufficient to maintain a burst suppression pattern on the EEG (usually 0.05–0.4 mg/kg/h).
When seizures have been controlled for 12 h, the drug dosage should be slowly reduced over a further 12 h
If seizures recur, the general anaesthesic agent should be given again for a further 12 h, and then withdrawal attempted again. This cycle may need to be repeated until seizure control is achieved

Table 18.4 Anaesthetics for refractory status epilepticus

Drug	Adult dose	Comments
Midazolam	0.1–0.3 mg/kg at 4 mg/min bolus followed by infusion at 0.05–0.4 mg/kg/h	Elimination half-life of 1.5 h, but accumulates with prolonged use. Tolerance and rebound seizures can be problematic
Thiopentone	100–250 mg bolus over 20 s then further 50 mg boluses every 2–3 min until seizures are controlled. Then infusion to maintain burst suppression (3–5 mg/kg/h)	Complicated by hypotension. It has saturable pharmacokinetics, and a strong tendency to accumulate. Metabolized to pentobarbital. Can also cause pancreatitis, hepatic disturbance and hypersensitivity reaction
Pentobarbital	10–20 mg/kg at 25 mg/min then 0.5–1 mg/kg/h increasing to 1–3 mg/kg/h	As above
Propofol	2 mg/kg then 5–10 mg/kg/h	Large volume of distribution and short half-life. Rapid recovery. Can be complicated by lipaemia, acidosis and rhabdomyolysis especially in children. Rebound seizures with abrupt withdrawal

Phenytoin is relatively insoluble in water, and its parental formulation has a high PH; it consequently has a number of side-effects related to its physiochemical properties. It may crystallize and precipitate in solutions; it may cause thrombophlebitis (particularly with extravasation); its vehicle, propylene glycol, can cause hypotension; and phenytoin is poorly and erratically absorbed after intramuscular injection. Fosphenytoin (3-phosphoryloxymethyl phenytoin disodium) is a water-soluble phenytoin prodrug, which has some potential advantages over phenytoin [103]. Fosphenytoin is itself inactive, but is metabolized to phenytoin with a half-life of 8–15 min [103]. It can be administered 2–3 times faster than phenytoin and achieves similar serum concentrations. Cardiac monitoring is still required with fosphenytoin, and the dosing units of the drug are confusing. There are no controlled trials of fosphenytoin in status epilepticus, and it is not clear if the potential advantages of fosphenytoin result in better outcome than that achieved by phenytoin.

Refractory status epilepticus

In most cases of convulsive status epilepticus (over 80%), therapy with benzodiazepine and phenobarbital or phenytoin will control the seizures rapidly. If the seizures are continuing, however, there is a risk of physiological compromise, neuronal damage and progressive drug resistance. This is the stage of refractory status epilepticus, and transfer to an intensive care unit is required [104]. In many emergency situations (for example, postoperative status epilepticus, severe or complicated convulsive status epilepticus, patients already in intensive care), anaesthesia should be introduced earlier. Chlormethiazole infusions, which were commonly used at this stage, cannot be recommended except in the intensive care unit [6]. The prognosis of status epilepticus at this stage is less good; in one meta-analysis, the mortality at this stage was estimated to be as high as 48% with only 29% returning to their premorbid functional baseline [105]. This mortality is greater in older patients, those with longer seizure duration, those in a poorer medical condition and those with acute brain injury.

Anaesthesia can be induced by barbiturate or non-barbiturate drugs (Table 18.4). A number of anaesthetics have been recommended [104,106]. The most commonly used anaesthetics are the intravenous barbiturates thiopentone or pentobarbital, the intravenous non-barbiturate infusional anaesthetic propofol or continuous midazolam infusion [104,106]. There have been no randomized control studies comparing these treatment options. A meta-analysis of reports of these different treatment regimes suggests that there is no difference between these anaesthetics in terms of mortality, but that pentobarbitone was perhaps more effective than midazolam at the expense of greater hypotension [106]. These data, however, need to be interpreted with caution, as the studies compared were non-randomized, had different outcome measures and were subject to considerable reporting bias (the reports are mostly retrospective). Propofol and midazolam have pharmacokinetic advantages over the barbiturates, which readily accumulate. In addition to anaesthesia, it is important that antiepileptic drug treatment should continue.

It is imperative at this stage to have EEG monitoring of the patient, as a patient may enter a drug-induced coma with little outward sign of convulsions yet have on-going electrographic epileptic activity [106,107]. In addition, patients with prolonged convulsive status epilepticus can enter a stage of subtle generalized convulsive status epilepticus characterized by profound coma, bilateral EEG ictal discharges and only subtle motor activity, regardless of the presence or absence of sedating drugs or paralysing agents [108].

The electrographic endpoint for anaesthetic titration is controversial as there is sparse published data on the subject. The titration of the dose of anaesthetic agents in their use in status is commonly based upon burst suppression on the EEG or cerebral function monitor (CFM) with interburst intervals of 2–30s as an acceptable endpoint [109–111]. Burst suppression supposedly represents disconnection of cerebral grey matter from underlying white matter. Burst suppression can be difficult to achieve, because the degree of anaesthesia required commonly leads to hypotension. Aiming for a more realistic endpoint such as seizure suppression, although more difficult to define, may be more acceptable [72]. EEG monitoring should either be continuous or occur at least every 24 h.

Once the patient has been free of seizures for 12–24 h and provided that there are adequate plasma levels of concomitant antiepileptic medication, then the anaesthetic can be slowly tapered. If one anaesthetic agent is ineffective then it should be substituted by another. There are some data to suggest that those who are loaded with

Table 18.5 Treatment of non-convulsive status epilepticus

Type	Treatment choice	Other
Typical absence status epilepticus	IV or oral benzodiazepines	Intravenous acetazolamide, valproate or chlormethiazole
Complex partial status epilepticus	Oral clobazam	Intravenous lorazepam and phenytoin (fosphenytoin) or phenobarbital
Atypical absence status epilepticus	Oral valproate	Oral benzodiazepines (with caution), lamotrigine, topiramate
Tonic status epilepticus	Oral lamotrigine	Methylphenidate, steroids
Non-convulsive status epilepticus in coma	IV phenytoin (fosphenytoin) or phenobarbital	Concomitant anaesthesia with thiopentone, pentobarbital, propofol or midazolam

phenobarbital do better than those who are not [12]. If seizures recur, anaesthesia should be re-established. In severe cases, anaesthesia may be required for weeks or even months.

Non-convulsive status epilepticus

The advent of more widely accessible EEG and, in particular, the availability of EEG on intensive care units has led to the recognition that non-convulsive status epilepticus is a much more common condition than previously recognized. Indeed, indirect estimates for the incidence of non-convulsive status epilepticus have been as high as 14–24 per 100 000 population per year (the majority of these are non-convulsive status epilepticus in the setting of learning difficulties) [6]. Population studies have demonstrated that non-convulsive status epilepticus comprises at least one-third of all cases of status epilepticus [9]. Non-convulsive status epilepticus can be subdivided into typical absence status epilepticus, complex partial status epilepticus, non-convulsive status epilepticus in coma and specific forms of status epilepticus in patients with learning difficulties, including tonic status epilepticus and atypical absences status epilepticus [6,113]. The treatment of these is considered in Table 18.5. Electrical status epilepticus during slow-wave sleep and Landau–Kleffner are considered elsewhere (Chapter 15).

Diagnosis

The diagnosis of non-convulsive status epilepticus is critically dependent on EEG. In patients with a previous diagnosis of epilepsy, any prolonged change in personality, prolonged postictal confusion (greater than 30 min) or recent onset psychosis should be investigated with EEG as these can all be presentations of non-convulsive status epilepticus [114–116]. If new onset developmental delay occurs in the setting of epilepsy then a sleep EEG should be considered to identify status epilepticus during slow-wave sleep. In non-comatose patients with no history of epilepsy, non-convulsive status epilepticus can present as confusion or personality change, but almost invariably in the setting of a metabolic derangement, encephalitis or other acute precipitant. Rarely, non-convulsive status epilepticus can present as autism and if suspicions are raised (usually a fluctuating course) then EEG is indicated [117,118].

Non-convulsive status epilepticus can result from convulsive status epilepticus, and is an important, treatable cause of persistent coma following convulsive status epilepticus [114,119]. This and status epilepticus with subtle manifestations such as twitching of the limbs, or facial muscles or nystagmoid eye jerking, which can re-

sult from hypoxic brain damage, are often collectively referred to as subtle motor status epilepticus [108]. Up to 8% of patients in coma who have no outward signs of seizure activity are in non-convulsive status epilepticus, thus emphasizing the importance of EEG in the investigation of comatose patients [120]. Similarly, non-convulsive status epilepticus is underdiagnosed in the confused elderly in whom the confusion is frequently blamed on other causes [121,122].

Although EEG interpretation is usually straightforward with regular repetitive discharges occurring in some patients in a cyclical fashion, difficulties can occur in differentiating non-convulsive status epilepticus from an encephalopathy of other cause [123]. Triphasic waves due to metabolic encephalopathies (particularly hepatic or hyperammonaemic) can be frequent and occasionally sharpened, leading to confusion. Thus definitions of non-convulsive status epilepticus should include either: (a) unequivocal electrographic seizure activity; (b) periodic epileptiform discharges or rhythmic discharge with clinical seizure activity; and (c) rhythmic discharge with either clinical or electrographic response to treatment [123]. Although these definitions are helpful, difficulties can still arise; triphasic waves can respond to treatment with benzodiazepines, and thus response to treatment is not a definitive indication of an epileptic cause [124]. There is also uncertainty about the relevance of PLEDs [125]. This is most notable following severe encephalitis or hypoxic injury in which discharges can occur with such periodicity so as to be confused with periodic discharges seen following prolonged status epilepticus. Some have argued that such discharges represent on-going seizure activity, and should be treated thus. The general consensus, however, is that a multitude of aetiologies can underlie PLEDs, and that they should only be treated as epileptic if there is other evidence of ictal activity [125].

Treatment

Typical absence status epilepticus

This entity needs to be distinguished from complex partial status epilepticus and atypical absences seen in patients with learning difficulties.

This term should perhaps be reserved for prolonged absence attacks with continuous or discontinuous 3 Hz spike and wave occurring in patients with primary generalized epilepsy [6]. The EEG, however, may include irregular spike/wave, prolonged bursts of spike activity, sharp wave or polyspike and wave, and whether to include such cases as absence status epilepticus is uncertain.

Although absence epilepsy has its peak in childhood and commonly remits in adolescence, absence status epilepticus not uncommonly occurs in later life [126]. Absence status epilepticus can be divided into childhood absence status epilepticus (those usually already receiving treatment), late onset absence status epilepticus with a history of primary generalized history (often a history of absences in childhood) and late onset absence status epilepticus developing *de novo* (usually following drug or alcohol withdrawal) [127].

There is no evidence that absence status induces neuronal damage, and thus aggressive treatment is not warranted [6,128]. Treatment can either be intravenous or oral (Table 18.5). Absence status epilepticus responds rapidly to intravenous benzodiazepines; there is no good evidence to favour one benzodiazepine over another. Sodium valproate is one of the alternative.

Complex partial status epilepticus

Complex partial status epilepticus has to be differentiated from other forms of non-convulsive status epilepticus, from postictal states and from other neurological and psychiatric conditions. EEG may be helpful, but the scalp EEG changes can be non-specific and the diagnosis has to be largely clinical [6,31]. The definition as 'a prolonged epileptic episode in which focal fluctuating or frequently recurring electrographic epileptic discharges, arising in temporal or extratemporal regions, result in a confusional state with variable clinical symptoms' is suitably vague and is necessary to emphasize that complex partial status epilepticus can originate in any cortical region and can fluctuate in a cyclical fashion [6]. A further factor that could be included in this definition is the absence of coma; electrographic status epilepticus in coma is considered separately below, partly because of its poor prognosis. The differentiation of complex partial status epilepticus from generalized non-convulsive status epilepticus can be difficult, as rapid generalization can occur despite an initial focus that may only become apparent after treatment [30,129].

How aggressively complex partial status epilepticus needs to be treated depends upon: (a) the prognosis of the condition; and (b) if treatment improves the prognosis. As in all epilepsies the prognosis relates partly to the prognosis of the underlying aetiology and any concomitant medical conditions. Indeed, complex partial status epilepticus in someone with epilepsy is a more benign condition than complex status epilepticus resulting from an acute cerebral event, and should perhaps be treated thus [35]. There is no good evidence that aggressive treatment improves prognosis in this condition; it is important to note that intravenous medication can result in hypotension, respiratory depression and occasionally cardiorespiratory arrest. This is more so with rapid intravenous administration with its resultant high serum drug levels. Indeed, in one series of non-convulsive status epilepticus in the elderly, aggressive treatment carried a worse prognosis than no treatment [122]. At present, early recognition of the condition and treatment with oral or rectal benzodiazepines can be effective. In patients who have repetitive attacks of complex partial status epilepticus (a common occurrence), oral clobazam over a period of 2–3 days given early at home can usually abort the status epilepticus, and such strategies should be discussed with the patient and carers [130,131]. Early recognition is a critical goal, as the delay in treatment comes not from therapeutic strategy, but from failure to diagnose the condition in the first place. For more persistent or resistant complex partial status epilepticus intravenous therapy should perhaps be used (see Table 18.5), and lorazepam followed by phenytoin (or fosphenytoin) are the drugs of choice [132]. In contrast to absence status epilepticus, the response to benzodiazepines can be disappointing, and often there is a resolution of the electrographic status epilepticus without concomitant clinical improvement (possibly due to postictal effects) [35]. Whether general anaesthesia is ever justified remains a matter for speculation. Since most complex partial status epilepticus is self-terminating usually without any serious neurological sequelae, then such aggressive therapy should, in most instances, be avoided. Treatment of the underlying cause (e.g. encephalitis or metabolic derangement) is of course paramount.

Non-convulsive status epilepticus in coma

Electrographic status epilepticus in coma is not uncommon and is seen in up to 8% of patients in coma with no clinical evidence of seizure activity [120]. Misdiagnosis is common, and burst suppression patterns, periodic discharges and encephalopathic triphasic patterns are often taken to represent electrographic status epilepticus, but in fact probably simply indicate underlying widespread cortical damage or dysfunction (see above). Non-convulsive status epilepticus in coma consists of three groups: those who had convulsive status epilepticus, those who have subtle clinical signs of seizure activity and those with no clinical signs [133]. Convulsive status epilepticus has, as part of its evolution, subtle status epilepticus in which there is minimal or no motor activity but on-going electrical activity [114,119]. This condition should be treated aggressively with deep anaesthesia and concomitant antiepileptic drugs (see Table 18.5). The association of electrographic status epilepticus with subtle motor activity often follows hypoxic brain activity and has a poor prognosis. Aggressive therapy may be justified, although there is little evidence that such treatment improves prognosis [133]. Electrographic status epilepticus with no overt clinical signs is difficult to interpret—does it represent status epilepticus or widespread cortical damage? Since these patients have a poor prognosis, aggressive treatment is recommended in the hope that it may improve outcome. There is also a group of patients in whom there are clinical signs of repetitive movements, but no electrographic seizure activity. The movements are usually not epileptic in nature, and aggressive sedation is not recommended [133].

Atypical absence status epilepticus

Atypical absence status epilepticus is associated with the epileptic encephalopathies such as Lennox–Gastaut syndrome [6]. This entity can be difficult to diagnose, but should be considered if there is change in behaviour, personality, cognition or increased confusion in a patient with one of these epilepsies. The EEG characteristics are usually that of continuous or frequent slow (<2.5 Hz) spike and wave. This condition is usually poorly responsive to intravenous benzodiazepines, which should, in any case, be given cautiously, as they can induce tonic status epilepticus in susceptible patients [134]. Oral rather than intravenous treatment is usually more appropriate, and the drugs of choice are valproate, lamotrigine, clonazepam, clobazam and topiramate (see Table 18.5). Sedating medication, carbamazepine and vigabatrin have been reported to worsen atypical absences.

Tonic status epilepticus

Tonic status epilepticus is not uncommon in patients with syndromes such as Lennox–Gastaut. Tonic status epilepticus can also rarely occur in the setting of normal premorbid intelligence [135]. The tonic seizures may not necessarily be clinically apparent; the EEG, however, demonstrates bursts of paroxysmal, generalized fast discharges [135,136]. Tonic status epilepticus is poorly responsive to conventional treatment. It can be worsened with benzodiazepines, which should be used with care [134]. Sedating medication can worsen all seizure types in the Lennox–Gastaut syndrome, and thus should be avoided. Conversely stimulants such as methylphenidate can be effective. There has also been a case report of the effective termination of tonic status epilepticus with oral lamotrigine [137]. In Lennox–Gastaut, both adrenocorticotropic hormone (ACTH) and corticosteroids are helpful in the emergency treatment of status epilepticus of all types.

Epilepsia partialis continua

This can be considered the status equivalent of simple partial motor seizures, and can be defined as regular or irregular clonic muscular twitching affecting a limited part of the body, occurring for a minimum of 1 h, and recurring at intervals of no more than 10 s [138]. It needs to be differentiated from myoclonic dystonia and brainstem myoclonus. Additionally status epilepticus occurring in coma may have some features of epilepsia partialis continua. Diagnosis can be difficult; the EEG may show focal abnormalities, but can be normal [138,139]. Epilepsia partialis continua can result from structural abnormalities such as stroke, trauma, cerebral infarction, cerebral abscess, neuronal migration disorders and vascular malformation [138–141]. In approximately 50% of cases, the MRI is normal [139]. Epilepsia partialis continua can be associated with a variety of encephalitides, commonly Rasmussen's encephalitis, but also subacute panencephalitis and Creutzfeldt–Jakob disease [139,141]. Metabolic causes have also been described including importantly hyponatraemia, and hyperglycaemia, although the majority of such patients also have a focal cortical lesion [142]. Treatment is best targeted at the underlying cause. Antiepileptic drugs may prevent seizure spread into complex partial and secondary generalized seizures, but are usually only partially effective in treating the epilepsia partialis continua [139]. Oral corticosteroid therapy and immunosuppression can be of benefit to patients with chronic inflammatory conditions (e.g. Rasmussen's encephalitis), and nimodipine has been reported to have been successful in two cases of epilepsia partialis continua following an acute cerebral event [143]. Neurosurgical resection should be considered in refractory cases.

Myoclonic status epilepticus in coma

Myoclonic status epilepticus is a well-recognized complication of cardiorespiratory arrest, and is characterized by spontaneous and stimulus-sensitive myoclonus usually occurring within 24 h of the coma [144]. These patients generally have burst suppression EEGs, cerebral oedema and a poor prognosis [144]. There are instances, however, of survival of such patients, especially if the initial insult was primarily hypoxia related [145], and thus the presence of such myoclonus is not necessarily an agonal event. Survivors are usually left with Lance–Adams type action myoclonus, which in itself can have a good prognosis [146]. To what extent this myoclonic status epilepticus in coma should be treated is unknown, and since survival is likely to correlate with the damage due to the causative insult rather than the myoclonus, aggressive treatment with anaesthesia is not warranted [147]. Nevertheless the myoclonus can respond to clonazepam, valproate, piracetam or levetiracetam.

Other forms of myoclonic status epilepticus

Myoclonic status in the progressive myoclonic epilepsies and in primary generalized epilepsy do not usually require intravenous therapy, although if needed an intravenous benzodiazepine can be given. The preferred therapy is with oral valproate, clonazepam or piracetam.

Drugs most commonly used in status epilepticus (see also Tables 18.2 and 18.4)

Diazepam

Diazepam is useful in the premonitory or early stages of status. There is extensive clinical experience in adults, children and the newborn; the drug has well-proved efficacy in many types of status, a rapid onset of action, and well-studied pharmacology and pharmacokinetics. It can be given by rectal administration, and the rectal tubule is a convenient rectal preparation. Diazepam has two important disadvantages, however, which limit its usefulness in status. First, although it has a rapid onset of action, it is highly lipid soluble and thus has a short duration of action after a single injection. This means that there is a strong tendency for seizures to relapse after initial control. Secondly, diazepam accumulates on repeated injections or after continuous infusion, and this accumulation carries a high risk of sudden respiratory depression, sedation and hypotension. Other disadvantages are its dependency on hepatic metabolism and the formation of an active metabolite, which can complicate prolonged therapy. Diazepam has a tendency to precipitate from concentrated solutions and to interact with other drugs, and is absorbed onto plastic on prolonged contact.

Usual preparations

IV formulation

Diazepam solution, 2 mL ampoule containing 5 mg/mL *or* diazepam emulsion (Diazemuls®), 1 mL ampoule containing 5 mg/mL.

Rectal formulation

2.5 mL rectal tube (Stesolid® containing 2 mg/mL) or, alternatively, the same solution utilized for IV administration (2 mL ampoule containing 5 mg/mL).

Usual dosage

IV bolus (undiluted) 10–20 mg (adults) or 0.25–0.5 mg/kg (children), at a rate not exceeding 2–5 mg/min. The bolus dosing can be repeated. Rectal administration 10–30 mg (adults) or 0.5–0.75 mg/kg (children), and this can be repeated.

Fosphenytoin

Fosphenytoin is a prodrug of phenytoin. It is converted in the plasma into phenytoin by widely distributed phosphatase enzymes. The half-life of conversion is about 15 min, and conversion is not affected by age, hepatic status or by the presence of other drugs. Fosphenytoin is water soluble and prepared in a TRIS buffer; it thus causes less thrombophlebitis when given intravenously. It can also be administered intramuscularly. Fosphenytoin itself is inert, and its action in status is entirely due to the derived phenytoin. When fosphenytoin is infused at 100–150 mg phenytoin equivalents (PE)/min, the rate at which free phenytoin levels are reached in the serum is similar to that achieved by a phenytoin infusion of 50 mg/min (PE — 15 mg PE of fosphenytoin is the same as 15 mg of phenytoin). Fosphenytoin can therefore be administered three times faster than phenytoin, with equivalent risks of hypotension, cardiac arrhythmias and respiratory depression. Its rate of antiepileptic action is also similar. The lower incidence of local side-effects is an advantage over phenytoin, but in other ways the two drugs are equivalent and fosphenytoin is more expensive.

Usual preparation

Fosphenytoin is formulated in a TRIS buffer at physiological pH. Phials of 50 mg PE are available for mixture with dextrose or saline.

Usual dosage

Fosphenytoin is given at a dose of between 15 mg PE/kg at a rate of 100–150 mg PE/min (an average adult dose of 1000 mg PE in 10 min).

Ligocaine

Ligocaine is a second-line drug for use in early status only. It is given as a bolus injection or short IV infusion. The clinical effects and pharmacokinetics have been extensively studied in patients of all ages, and the drug is highly effective. The main disadvantage of ligocaine is that its antiepileptic effects are short-lived and seizures are controlled for a matter of hours only. Ligocaine is thus useful only while more definitive antiepileptic drug treatment is administered. The risk of drug accumulation is low, and the incidence of respiratory or cerebral depression and hypotension is lower than with other antiepileptics. The drug may be particularly valuable in patients with respiratory disease. Other disadvantages include a possible proconvulsant effect at high levels, an active metabolite which may accumulate on prolonged therapy, the need for cardiac monitoring as cardiac rhythm disturbances are common, and the dependency of the clearance of ligocaine on hepatic blood flow.

Usual preparations

5 mL ready-prepared syringe containing ligocaine 20 mg/mL (2%) or 10 mL ready-prepared syringe containing ligocaine 10 mg/mL (1%) (i.e. both syringes containing 100 mg). Ligocaine is also available as a 5-mL phial containing 20 mg/mL (i.e. 100 mg) of ligocaine (2%) or a 5-mL phial containing 200 mg/mL (i.e. 1000 mg) of ligocaine (20%), and as ready made 0.1% (1 mg/mL) and 0.2% (2 mg/mL) infusions (in 500-mL containers in 5% dextrose).

Usual dosage

Intravenous bolus injections 1.5–2.0 mg/kg (usually 100 mg in adults), at a rate of injection not exceeding 50 mg/min. The bolus injection can be repeated once if necessary. A continuous infusion can be given at a rate of 3–4 mg/kg/h (usually of 0.2% solution in 5% dextrose, for no more than 12 h) or 3–6 mg/kg/h (neonates).

Lorazepam

Lorazepam is the drug of choice in the early stage of status, given by IV bolus injection. A single injection is highly effective, and the drug has a longer initial duration of action and a smaller risk of cardiorespiratory depression than diazepam. There is little risk of drug accumulation, and also a lower risk of hypotension. The main disadvantage of lorazepam is a stronger tendency for tolerance to develop, the drug being usually effective for about 12 h only. It is thus usable only as initial therapy, and longer-term maintenance antiepileptic drugs must be given in addition. There is a large clinical experience in adults, children and the newborn, with well-proven efficacy in tonic-clonic and partial status, and the pharmacology and pharmacokinetics of the drug are well characterized. Lorazepam is a stable compound which is not likely to precipitate in solution, and is relatively unaffected by hepatic or renal disease.

Usual preparation

1 mL ampoule containing 4 mg/mL for IV injection.

Usual dosage

IV bolus of 0.07 mg/kg (usually 4 mg), repeated after 10 min if necessary (adults); bolus of 0.1 mg/kg (children). The rate of injection is not crucial.

Midazolam

Midazolam is another benzodiazepine which can be used in the premonitory or early stages of status. It is a water-soluble compound whose ring structure closes when in contact with serum to convert it into a highly lipophilic structure. Its water solubility provides one major advantage over diazepam, and in that it can be rapidly absorbed by IM injection or by intranasal or buccal administration. It is therefore useful in situations in which IV administration is difficult or ill-advised. Blinded comparisons with diazepam after IM and buccal administration show it to be equivalent in efficacy and speed of action. Although there is a danger of accumulation on prolonged or repeated therapy, this tendency is less than with diazepam. There is however only limited published experience in adults or children with status. Occasionally severe cardiorespiratory depression occurs after IM administration, and other adverse effects include hypotension, apnoea, sedation and thrombophlebitis. Like diazepam, the drug is short acting, and there is a strong tendency for seizures to relapse after initial control, and as with diazepam its metabolism is altered by hepatic disease. Its half-life is prolonged in hepatic disease or in the elderly. There are also encouraging reports of the use of IV infusions of midazolam as an anaesthetic in the refractory stage of status, and midazolam is probably the only benzodiazepine which should be used as a continuous infusion. With more experience, IV midazolam may become the drug of choice for anaesthesia in refractory status.

Usual preparation

5 mL ampoule containing 2 mg/mL midazolam hydrochloride.

Usual dosage

IM or rectally 5–10 mg (adults); 0.15–0.3 mg/kg (children). This can be repeated once after 15 min. IV bolus of 0.1–0.3 mg/kg, may be given at a rate not to exceed 4 mg/min, which can be repeated once after 15 min. An IV infusion can be given at a rate of 0.05–0.4 mg/kg/h. Buccal instillation of 10 mg can be given by a syringe and catheter in children or adults.

Phenobarbital

Phenobarbital is one of the drugs of choice in the stage of established status. It is a reliable antiepileptic drug, with well-proven effectiveness in tonic-clonic and partial status and there is extensive clinical experience in adults, children and in neonates. Phenobarbital has a stronger anticonvulsant action than other barbiturates and an additional potential cerebral protective action. It has a rapid onset and long-lasting action, and can be administered much faster than can phenytoin. Its safety at high doses has been established, and the drug can be continued as chronic therapy. The disadvantages of the drug relate to prolonged use, where because of the long elimination half-life, there is a risk of drug accumulation and inevitable sedation, respiratory depression and hypotension. Marked autoinduction may also occur.

Usual preparation

1 mL ampoule containing phenobarbital sodium 200 mg/mL in propylene glycol 90% and water for injection 10%.

Usual dosage

IV loading dose in adults is 10 mg/kg at rate of 100 mg/min (usual adult dose 600–800 mg), followed by maintenance dose of 1–4 mg/kg (adults). For neonates and children, the IV loading dose of 15–20 mg/kg, followed by maintenance dose of 3–4 mg/kg. Higher doses can be given, with monitoring of blood concentrations.

Phenytoin

Phenytoin is a drug of choice and a highly effective medication for the stage of established status. Extensive clinical experience has been gained in adults, children and neonates, and phenytoin has proven efficacy in tonic-clonic and partial status. The drug has a prolonged action, with a relatively small risk of respiratory or cerebral depression and no tendency for tachyphylaxis. Its main disadvantage is the time necessary to infuse the drug and its delayed onset of action. However, the phenytoin pro-drug fosphenytoin (see above) can be administered more quickly. The pharmacokinetics of phenytoin are problematic, with Michaelis–Menten kinetics at conventional dosages and wide variation between individuals. Toxic side-effects include cardiac rhythm disturbances, thrombophlebitis and hypotension. The risk of cardiac side-effects is greatly increased if the recommended rate of injection is exceeded, and cardiac monitoring is advisable during phenytoin infusion. There is a risk of precipitation if phenytoin is diluted in other solutions than 0.9% saline or if mixed with other drugs.

Usual preparations

5 mL ampoule containing 250 mg stabilized in propylene glycol, ethanol and water (alternatives exist: e.g. phenytoin in TRIS buffer or in infusion bottles containing 750 mg in 500 mL of osmotic saline).

Usual dosage

In adults, a 15–18 mg/kg IV infusion can be given via the side arm of a drip or preferably directly via an infusion pump at a rate not exceeding 50 mg/min (20 mg/min in the elderly). In children, a 20 mg/kg IV infusion is usually given, at a rate not exceeding 25 mg/min. The drug should never be given by IM injection.

Propofol

Propofol is the anaesthetic agent of choice for non-barbiturate infusional anaesthesia in status. It is an excellent anaesthetic with very good pharmacokinetic properties. In status, it has a very rapid onset of action and rapid recovery. There are few haemodynamic side-effects, and the drug has been used at all ages. There is however only limited published experience of its use in status, or indeed of prolonged infusions. Unlike isoflurane, it is metabolized in the liver and affected by severe hepatic disease. As with all anaesthetics, its use requires assisted ventilation, intensive care and intensive care monitoring. It causes lipaemia and acidosis which may complicate its use, especially on long-term therapy and in infants. Involuntary movements (without EEG change) can occur, and should not be confused with seizure activity. Rebound seizures are a problem when it is discontinued too rapidly, and a decremental rate of 1 mg/kg every 2 h is recommended when the drug is to be withdrawn.

Usual preparation

20 mL ampoule containing 10 mg/mL (i.e. 200 mg) as an emulsion.

Usual dosage

2 mg/kg bolus, repeated if necessary, and then followed by a continuous infusion of 5–10 mg/kg/h initially, reducing to 1–3 mg/kg/h. When seizures have been controlled for 12 h, drug dosages should be slowly tapered over 12 h.

Thiopentone/pentobarbital

Thiopentone is in most countries the usual choice for barbiturate anaesthesia. It is a highly effective antiepileptic drug, with additional potential cerebral protective action It reduces intracranial pressure and cerebral blood flow, has a very rapid onset of action, and there is wide experience of its use. The drug has a number of pharmacokinetic disadvantages including saturable kinetics, a strong tendency to accumulate and a prolonged recovery time after anaesthesia is withdrawn. Serum concentration monitoring of the parent drug and its active metabolite (pentobarbital) is advisable on prolonged therapy. There is often some tachyphylaxis to its sedative and to a lesser extent its anticonvulsant properties. Respiratory depression and sedation is inevitable, and hypotension is common. Other less common side-effects include pancreatitis, hepatic dysfunction and spasm at the injection site. Full intensive care facilities with artificial ventilatory support and intensive EEG and cardiovascular monitoring are needed. It can react with comedication, and with plastic giving sets, and is unstable when exposed to air. Autoinduction occurs, and hepatic disease prolongs its elimination.

Usual preparations

Injection of thiopentone sodium 2.5 g diluted in 100 mL, and 5 g in 200 mL diluent, to make 100 and 200 mL of a 2.5% solution. Thiopentone sodium is also available as 500 mg and 1 g phials to make 2.5% solutions.

Usual dosage

100–250 mg IV bolus given over 20 s, with further 50 mg boluses every 2–3 min until seizures are controlled, followed by a continuous IV infusion to maintain a burst suppression pattern on the EEG (usually 3–5 mg/kg/h). The dose should be lowered if systolic blood pressure falls below 90 mmHg despite cardiovascular support. Thiopentone should be slowly withdrawn 12 h after the last seizure.

References

1 Wilson JV, Reynolds EH. Texts and documents. Translation and analysis of a cuneiform text forming part of a Babylonian treatise on epilepsy. *Med Hist* 1990; 34, 185–98.

2 Hunter RA. Status epilepticus: history, incidence and problems. *Epilepsia* 1959; 1: 162–88.

3 Calmeil LF. De l'épilepsie, étudiée sous le rapport de son siège et de son influence sur la production de l'aliénation mentale. Université de Paris, Thesis/Dissertation, 1824.

4 Trosseau A. *Lectures in Clinical Medicine* (translated by P.V. Bazire). London: New Sydenham Society, 1868.

5 Gastaut H, Roger, J, Lob, H. *Les États de Mal Épileptiques*. Paris: Masson, 1967.

6 Shorvon S. *Status Epilepticus: its clinical features and treatment in children and adults*. Cambridge: Cambridge University Press, 1994.

7 Gastaut H. Classification of status epilepticus. *Adv Neurol* 1983; 34: 15–35.

8 Coeytaux A, Jallon P, Galobardes B, Morabia A. Incidence of status epilepticus in French-speaking Switzerland: (EPISTAR). *Neurology* 2000; 55: 693–7.

9 DeLorenzo RJ, Hauser WA, Towne AR *et al.* A prospective, population-based epidemiologic study of status epilepticus in Richmond, Virginia. *Neurology* 1996; 46: 1029–35.

10 Hesdorffer DC, Logroscino G, Cascino G, Annegers JF, Hauser WA. Incidence of status epilepticus in Rochester, Minnesota, 1965–1984. *Neurology* 1998; 50: 735–41.

11 Knake S, Rosenow F, Vescovi M *et al.* Incidence of status epilepticus in adults in Germany: a prospective, population-based study. *Epilepsia* 2001; 42: 714–18.

12 Hauser W.A. Status epilepticus: epidemiologic considerations. *Neurology* 1990; 40: 9–13.

13 Aicardi J, Chevrie JJ. Convulsive status epilepticus in infants and children. A study of 239 cases. *Epilepsia* 1970; 11: 187–97.

13 Rumbach L, Sablot D, Berger E, Tatu L, Vuillier F, Moulin T. Status epilepticus in stroke: report on a hospital-based stroke cohort. *Neurology* 2000; 54: 350–4.

14 Logroscino G, Hesdorffer DC, Cascino G, Annegers F, Hauser WA. Short-term mortality after a first episode of status epilepticus. *Epilepsia* 1997; 38: 1344–9.

15 DeGiorgio CM, Correale JD, Gott PS *et al.* Serum neuron-specific enolase in human status epilepticus [see comments]. *Neurology* 1995; 45: 1134–7.

16 Hesdorffer DC, Logroscino G, Cascino G, Annegers JF, Hauser WA. Risk of unprovoked seizure after acute symptomatic seizure: effect of status epilepticus. *Ann Neurol* 1998; 44: 908–12.

17 Corsellis JA, Bruton CJ. Neuropathology of status epilepticus in humans. *Adv Neurol* 1983; 34: 129–39.

18 DeGiorgio CM, Tomiyasu U, Gott PS, Treiman DM. Hippocampal pyramidal cell loss in human status epilepticus. *Epilepsia* 1992; 33: 23–7.

19 Fujikawa DG, Itabashi HH, Wu A, Shinmei SS. Status epilepticus-induced neuronal loss in humans without systemic complications or epilepsy. *Epilepsia* 2000; 41: 981–91.

20 Cendés F, Hermann F, Carpenter S, Zatorre RJ, Cashman NR. Temporal lobe epilepsy caused by domoic acid intoxication: evidence for glutamate receptor-mediated excitotoxicity in humans. *Ann Neurol* 1995; 37: 123–6.

21 Meierkord H, Wieshmann U, Niehaus L, Lehmann R. Structural consequences of status epilepticus demonstrated with serial magnetic resonance imaging. *Acta Neurol Scand* 1997; 96: 127–32.

22 Wieshmann UC, Woermann FG, Lemieux L *et al.* Development of hippocampal atrophy: A serial magnetic resonance imaging study in a patient who developed epilepsy after generalized status epilepticus. *Epilepsia* 1997; 38: 1238–41.

23 Meldrum B. Excitotoxicity and epileptic brain damage. *Epilepsy Res* 1991; 10: 55–61.

24 Olney JW, Collins RC, Sloviter RS. Excitotoxic mechanisms of epileptic brain damage. *Adv Neurol* 1986; 44: 857–77.

25 Ben-Ari Y. Limbic seizure and brain damage produced by kainic acid: mechanisms and relevance to human temporal lobe epilepsy. *Neuroscience* 1985; 14: 375–403.

26 Lothman EW, Bertram EH, Bekenstein JW, Perlin JB. Self-sustaining limbic status epilepticus induced by 'continuous' hippocampal stimulation: electrographic and behavioral characteristics. *Epilepsy Res* 1989; 3: 107–19.

27 Sloviter RS. Decreased hippocampal inhibition and a selective loss of interneurons in experimental epilepsy. *Science* 1987; 235: 73–6.

28 Krsek P, Mikulecka A, Druga R, Hlinak Z, Kubova H, Mares P. An animal model of nonconvulsive status epilepticus: a contribution to clinical controversies. *Epilepsia* 2001; 42: 171–80.

29 Drislane FW. Evidence against permanent neurologic damage from nonconvulsive status epilepticus. *J Clin Neurophysiol* 1999; 16: 323–31.

30 Granner MA, Lee SI. Nonconvulsive status epilepticus: EEG analysis in a large series. *Epilepsia* 1994; 35: 42–7.

31 Cascino GD. Nonconvulsive status epilepticus in adults and children. *Epilepsia* 1993; 34 (Suppl. 1): S21–S28.

32 Treiman DM, Delgado EA. Complex partial status epilepticus. *Adv Neurol* 1983; 34: 69–81.

33 Engel J, Ludwig BI, Fetell M. Prolonged partial complex status epilepticus: EEG and behavioral observations. *Neurology* 1978; 28: 863–9.

34 Krumholz A, Sung GY, Fisher RS, Barry E, Bergey GK, Grattan LM. Complex partial status epilepticus accompanied by serious morbidity and mortality [see comments]. *Neurology* 1995; 45: 1499–504.

35 Cockerell OC, Walker MC, Sander JW, Shorvon SD. Complex partial status epilepticus: a recurrent problem. *J Neurol Neurosurg Psychiatry* 1994; 57: 835–7.

36 Williamson PD, Spencer DD, Spencer SS, Novelly RA, Mattson RH. Complex partial status epilepticus: a depth-electrode study. *Ann Neurol* 1985; 18: 647–54.

37 DeGiorgio CM, Gott PS, Rabinowicz AL, Heck CN, Smith TD, Correale JD. Neuron-specific enolase, a marker of acute neuronal injury, is increased in complex partial status epilepticus. *Epilepsia* 1996; 37: 606–9.

38 DeGiorgio CM, Heck CN *et al.* Serum neuron-specific enolase in the major subtypes of status epilepticus. *Neurology* 1999; 52: 746–9.

39 Correale J, Rabinowicz AL, Heck CN, Smith TD, Loskota WJ, DeGiorgio CM. Status epilepticus increases CSF levels of neuron-specific enolase and alters the blood–brain barrier. *Neurology* 1998; 50: 1388–91.

40 Lansberg MG, O'Brien MW, Norbash AM *et al.* MRI abnormalities associated with partial status epilepticus. *Neurology* 1999; 52: 1021–7.

41 Kelly ME, McIntyre DC. Hippocampal kindling protects several structures from the neuronal damage resulting from kainic acid-induced status epilepticus. *Brain Res* 1994; 634: 245–56.

42 Pitkanen A, Nissinen J, Jolkkonen E, Tuunanen J, Halonen T. Effects of vigabatrin treatment on status epilepticus-induced neuronal damage and mossy fiber sprouting in the rat hippocampus. *Epilepsy Res* 1999; 33: 67–85.

43 Albala BJ, Moshe SL, Okada R. Kainic-acid-induced seizures: a developmental study. *Brain Res* 1984; 315: 139–48.

44 Sperber EF, Haas KZ, Stanton PK, Moshe SL. Resistance of the immature hippocampus to seizure-induced synaptic reorganization. *Brain Res Dev Brain Res* 1991; 60: 88–93.

45 Wozniak DF, Stewart GR, Miller JP, Olney JW. Age-related sensitivity to kainate neurotoxicity. *Exp Neurol* 1991; 114: 250–3.

46 Najm IM, Hadam J, Ckakraverty D *et al.* A short episode of seizure activity protects from status epilepticus-induced neuronal damage in rat brain. *Brain Res* 1998; 810: 72–5.

47 Zhang X, Cui SS, Wallace AE *et al.* Relations between brain pathology and temporal lobe epilepsy. *J Neurosci* 2002; 22: 6052–61.

48 Andre V, Ferrandon A, Marescaux C, Nehlig A. Vigabatrin protects against hippocampal damage but is not antiepileptogenic in the lithium-pilocarpine model of temporal lobe epilepsy. *Epilepsy Res* 2001; 47: 99–117.

49 Milward AJ, Meldrum BS, Mellanby JH. Forebrain ischaemia with CA1 cell loss impairs epileptogenesis in the tetanus toxin limbic seizure model. *Brain* 1999; 122 (Pt 6): 1009–16.

50 Stafstrom CE, Chronopoulos A, Thurber S, Thompson JL, Holmes GL. Age-dependent cognitive and behavioral deficits after kainic acid seizures *Epilepsia* 1993; 34: 420–2.

51 Sanabria ER, Su H, Yaari Y. Initiation of network bursts by Ca^{2+}-dependent intrinsic bursting in the rat pilocarpine model of temporal lobe epilepsy. *J Physiol* 2001; 532: 205–16.

52 Parent JM, Yu TW, Leibowitz RT, Geschwind DH, Sloviter RS, Lowenstein DH. Dentate granule cell neurogenesis is increased by seizures and contributes to aberrant network reorganization in the adult rat hippocampus. *J Neurosci* 1997; 17: 3727–38.

53 Brooks-Kayal AR, Shumate MD, Jin H, Rikhter TY, Coulter DA. Selective changes in single cell GABA(A) receptor subunit expression and function in temporal lobe epilepsy. *Nat Med* 1998; 4: 1166–72.

54 Cossart R, Dinocourt C, Hirsch JC *et al.* Dendritic but not somatic GABAergic inhibition is decreased in experimental epilepsy. *Nat Neurosci* 2001; 4: 52–62.

55 Okazaki MM, Evenson DA, Nadler JV. Hippocampal mossy fiber sprouting and synapse formation after status epilepticus in rats: visualization after retrograde transport of biocytin. *J Comp Neurol* 1995; 352: 515–34.

56 Walker MC, Tong X, Brown S, Shorvon SD, Patsalos PN. Comparison of single- and repeated-dose pharmacokinetics of diazepam. *Epilepsia* 1998; 39: 283–9.

57 Simon RP, Copeland JR, Benowitz NL, Jacob P, Bronstein J. Brain phenobarbital uptake during prolonged status epilepticus. *J Cereb Blood Flow Metab* 1987; 7: 783–8.

58 Walton NY, Treiman DM. Phenobarbital treatment of status epilepticus in a rodent model. *Epilepsy Res* 1989; 4: 216–21.

59 Kapur J, Macdonald RL. Rapid seizure-induced reduction of benzodiazepine and Zn^{2+} sensitivity of hippocampal dentate granule cell GABAA receptors. *J Neurosci* 1997; 17: 7532–40.

60 Mazarati AM, Baldwin RA, Sankar R, Wasterlain CG. Time-dependent decrease in the effectiveness of antiepileptic drugs during the course of self-sustaining status epilepticus. *Brain Res* 1998; 814: 179–85.

61 Holtkamp M, Tong X, Walker MC. Propofol in subanesthetic doses terminates status epilepticus in a rodent model. *Ann Neurol* 2001; 49: 260–3.

62 Walton NY, Treiman DM. Response of status epilepticus induced by lithium and pilocarpine to treatment with diazepam. *Exp Neurol* 1988; 101: 267–75.

63 DeLorenzo RJ, Garnett LK, Towne AR *et al.* Comparison of status epilepticus with prolonged seizure episodes lasting from 10 to 29 minutes. *Epilepsia* 1999; 40: 164–9.

64 Shinnar S, Berg AT, Moshe SL, Shinnar R. How long do new-onset seizures in children last? *Ann Neurol* 2001; 49: 659–64.

65 Scott RC, Besag FM, Neville BG. Buccal midazolam and rectal diazepam for treatment of prolonged seizures in childhood and adolescence: a randomised trial [see comments]. *Lancet* 1999; 353: 623–6.

66 Cereghino JJ, Mitchell WG, Murphy J, Kriel RL, Rosenfeld WE, Trevathan E. Treating repetitive seizures with a rectal diazepam formulation: a randomized study. The North American Diastat Study Group. *Neurology* 1998; 51: 1274–82.

67 Dreifuss FE, Rosman NP, Lloyd JC *et al.* A comparison of rectal diazepam gel and placebo for acute repetitive seizures. *N Engl J Med* 1998; 338: 1869–75.

68 Milligan NM, Dhillon S, Griffiths A, Oxley J, Richens A. A clinical trial of single dose rectal and oral administration of diazepam for the prevention of serial seizures in adult epileptic patients. *J Neurol Neurosurg Psychiatry* 1984; 47: 235–40.

69 Alldredge BK, Gelb AM, Isaacs SM *et al.* A comparison of lorazepam, diazepam, placebo for the treatment of out-of-hospital status epilepticus. *N Engl J Med* 2001; 345: 631–7.

70 Browne TR. Paraldehyde, chlormethiazole, lidocaine for treatment of status epilepticus. *Adv Neurol* 1983; 34: 509–17.

71 Garr RE, Appleton RE, Robson WJ, Molyneux EM. Children presenting with convulsions (including status epilepticus) to a paediatric accident and emergency department: an audit of a treatment protocol. *Dev Med Child Neurol* 1999; 41: 44–7.

72 Walker MC, Howard RS, Smith SJ, Miller DH, Shorvon SD, Hirsch NP. Diagnosis and treatment of status epilepticus on a neurological intensive care unit. *QJM* 1996; 89: 913–20.

73 Howell SJ, Owen L, Chadwick DW. Pseudostatus epilepticus [see comments]. *Q J Med* 1989; 71: 507–19.

74 Treiman DM, Walton NY, Kendrick C. A progressive sequence of electroencephalographic changes during generalized convulsive status epilepticus. *Epilepsy Res* 1990; 5: 49–60.

75 Garzon E, Fernandes RMF, Sakamoto AC. Serial EEG during human status epilepticus. Evidence for PLED as an ictal pattern. *Neurology* 2001; 57: 1175–83.

76 Benowitz NL, Simon RP, Copeland JR. Status epilepticus: divergence of sympathetic activity and cardiovascular response. *Ann Neurol* 1986; 19: 197–9.

77 Boggs G, Painter JA, DeLorenzo RJ. Analysis of electrocardiographic changes in status epilepticus. *Epilepsy Res* 1993; 14: 87–94.

78 Ingvar M, Siesjo BK. Cerebral oxygen consumption and glucose consumption during status epilepticus. *Eur Neurol* 1981; 20: 219–20.

79 Meldrum BS, Vigouroux RA, Brierley JB. Systemic factors and epileptic brain damage. Prolonged seizures in paralyzed, artificially ventilated baboons. *Arch Neurol* 1973; 29: 82–7.

80 Meldrum BS, Brierley JB. Prolonged epileptic seizures in primates.

Ischemic cell change and its relation to ictal physiological events. *Arch Neurol* 1973; 28: 10–17.

81 Aminoff MJ, Simon RP. Status epilepticus. Causes, clinical features and consequences in 98 patients. *Am J Med* 1980; 69: 657–66.

82 Simon RP. Physiologic consequences of status epilepticus. *Epilepsia* 1985; 26 (Suppl. 1), S58–S66.

83 Meldrum BS, Horton RW. Physiology of status epilepticus in primates. *Arch Neurol* 1973; 28: 1–9.

84 Meldrum BS. Endocrine consequences of status epilepticus. *Adv Neurol* 1983; 34, 399–403.

85 Brown JK, Hussain IH. Status epilepticus. I: Pathogenesis [see comments]. *Dev Med Child Neurol* 1991; 33: 3–17.

86 Singhal PC, Chugh KS, Gulati DR. Myoglobinuria and renal failure after status epilepticus. *Neurology* 1978; 28: 200–1.

87 Fischer SP, Lee J, Zatuchni J, Greenberg J. Disseminated intravascular coagulation in status epilepticus. *Thromb Haemost* 1977; 38: 909–13.

88 Walker MC, Smith SJ, Shorvon SD. The intensive care treatment of convulsive status epilepticus in the UK. Results of a national survey and recommendations [see comments]. *Anaesthesia* 1995; 50: 130–5.

89 Alldredge BK, Lowenstein DH. Status epilepticus related to alcohol abuse. *Epilepsia* 1993; 34: 1033–7.

90 van-Paesschen W, Bodian C, Maker H. Metabolic abnormalities and new-onset seizures in human immunodeficiency virus-seropositive patients. *Epilepsia* 1995; 36: 146–50.

91 Appleton R, Sweeney A, Choonara I, Robson J, Molyneux E. Lorazepam versus diazepam in the acute treatment of epileptic seizures and status epilepticus. *Dev Med Child Neurol* 1995; 37: 682–8.

92 Chamberlain JM, Altieri MA, Futterman C, Young GM, Ochsenschlager DW, Waisman Y. A prospective, randomized study comparing intramuscular midazolam with intravenous diazepam for the treatment of seizures in children [see comments]. *Pediatr Emerg Care* 1997; 13: 92–4.

93 Leppik IE, Derivan AT, Homan RW, Walker J, Ramsay RE, Patrick B. Double-blind study of lorazepam and diazepam in status epilepticus. *JAMA* 1983; 249: 1452–4.

94 Shaner DM, McCurdy SA, Herring MO, Gabor AJ. Treatment of status epilepticus: a prospective comparison of diazepam and phenytoin versus phenobarbital and optional phenytoin. *Neurology* 1988; 38: 202–7.

95 Taverner D, Bain WA. Intravenous lidocaine as an anticonvulsant in status epilepticus and serial seizures. *Lancet* 1958; 2: 1145–7.

96 Treiman DM, Meyers PD, Walton NY *et al.* A comparison of four treatments for generalized convulsive status epilepticus. Veterans Affairs Status Epilepticus Cooperative Study Group. *N Engl J Med* 1998; 339: 792–8.

97 Cascino GD, Hesdorffer D, Logroscino G, Hauser WA. Treatment of non-febrile status epilepticus in Rochester, Minn, from 1965 through 1984. *Mayo Clin Proc* 2001; 76: 39–41.

98 Cock HR, Schapira AH. A comparison of lorazepam and diazepam as initial therapy in convulsive status epilepticus. *QJM* 2002; 95: 225–31.

99 Walker MC, Sander JW. Benzodiazepines in status epilepticus. In: Trimble MR, Hindmarch I, eds. *Benzodiazepines*. Petersfield: Wrightson Biomedical, 2000: 73–85.

100 Prensky AL, Raff MC, Moore MJ, Schwab R.S. Intravenous diazepam in the treatment of prolonged seizure activity. *N Engl J Med* 1967; 276: 779–84.

101 Walker MC, Tong X, Brown S, Shorvon SD, Patsalos PN. Comparison of single- and repeated-dose pharmacokinetics of diazepam. *Epilepsia* 1998; 39: 283–9.

102 Pascual J, Ciudad J, Berciano J. Role of lidocaine (lignocaine) in managing status epilepticus. *J Neurol Neurosurg Psychiatry* 1992; 55: 49–51.

103 Browne TR. Fosphenytoin Cerebyx. *Clin Neuropharmacol* 1997; 20: 1–12.

104 Walker MC, Smith SJ, Shorvon SD. The intensive care treatment of convulsive status epilepticus in the UK. Results of a national survey and recommendations. *Anaesthesia* 1995; 50: 130–5.

105 Mayer SA, Claassen J, Lokin J, Mendelsohn F, Dennis LJ, Fitzsimmons BF. Refractory status epilepticus: frequency, risk factors, impact on outcome. *Arch Neurol* 2002; 59: 205–10.

106 Claassen J, Hirsch LJ, Emerson RG, Mayer SA. Treatment of refractory status epilepticus with pentobarbital, propofol, or midazolam: a systematic review. *Epilepsia* 2002; 43: 146–53.

107 DeLorenzo RJ, Waterhouse EJ, Towne AR *et al.* Persistent nonconvulsive status epilepticus after the control of convulsive status epilepticus. *Epilepsia* 1998; 39: 833–40.

108 Treiman DM. Generalized convulsive status epilepticus in the adult. *Epilepsia* 1993; 34 (Suppl. 1): S2–11.

109 Rashkin MC, Youngs C, Penovich P. Pentobarbital treatment of refractory status epilepticus. *Neurology* 1987; 37: 500–3.

110 Lowenstein DH, Aminoff MJ, Simon RP. Barbiturate anesthesia in the treatment of status epilepticus: clinical experience with 14 patients. *Neurology* 1988; 38: 395–400.

111 Van-Ness PC. Pentobarbital and EEG burst suppression in treatment of status epilepticus refractory to benzodiazepines and phenytoin. *Epilepsia* 1990; 31: 61–7.

112 Yaffe K, Lowenstein DH. Prognostic factors of pentobarbital therapy for refractory generalized status epilepticus [see comments]. *Neurology* 1993; 43: 895–900.

113 Walker MC. Diagnosis and treatment of nonconvulsive status epilepticus. *CNS Drugs* 2001; 15: 931–9.

114 Fagan KJ, Lee SI. Prolonged confusion following convulsions due to generalized nonconvulsive status epilepticus. *Neurology* 1990; 40: 1689–94.

115 Tomson T, Lindbom U, Nilsson BY. Nonconvulsive status epilepticus in adults: thirty-two consecutive patients from a general hospital population. *Epilepsia* 1992; 33: 829–35.

116 Kaplan PW. Nonconvulsive status epilepticus in the emergency room. *Epilepsia* 1996; 37: 643–50.

117 Walker MC, Cockerell OC, Sander JW. Non-convulsive status epilepticus presenting as a psychiatric condition. *J R Soc Med* 1996; 89: 91–2.

118 Rapin I. Autistic regression and disintegrative disorder: how important the role of epilepsy? *Semin Pediatr Neurol* 1995; 2: 278–85.

119 DeLorenzo RJ, Waterhouse EJ, Towne AR *et al.* Persistent nonconvulsive status epilepticus after the control of convulsive status epilepticus. *Epilepsia* 1998; 39: 833–40.

120 Towne AR, Waterhouse EJ, Boggs JG *et al.* Prevalence of nonconvulsive status epilepticus in comatose patients. *Neurology* 2000; 54: 340–5.

121 Thomas RJ. Seizures and epilepsy in the elderly [see comments]. *Arch Intern Med* 1997; 157: 605–17.

122 Litt B, Wityk RJ, Hertz SH *et al.* Nonconvulsive status epilepticus in the critically ill elderly. *Epilepsia* 1998; 39: 1194–202.

123 Husain AM, Mebust KA, Radtke RA. Generalized periodic epileptiform discharges: etiologies, relationship to status epilepticus, prognosis. *J Clin Neurophysiol* 1999; 16: 51–8.

124 Kaplan PW. Prognosis in nonconvulsive status epilepticus. *Epileptic Dis* 2000; 2: 185–93.

125 Pohlmann-Eden B, Hoch DB, Cochius JI, Chiappa KH. Periodic lateralized epileptiform discharges—a critical review. *J Clin Neurophysiol* 1996; 13: 519–30.

126 Agathonikou A, Panayiotopoulos CP, Giannakodimos S, Koutroumanidis M. Typical absence status in adults: diagnostic and syndromic considerations. *Epilepsia* 1998; 39: 1265–76.

127 Thomas P, Lebrun C, Chatel M. De novo absence status epilepticus as a benzodiazepine withdrawal syndrome. *Epilepsia* 1993; 34: 355–8.

128 Porter RJ, Penry JK. Petit mal status. *Adv Neurol* 1983; 34: 61–7.

129 Tomson T, Svanborg E, Wedlund JE. Nonconvulsive status epilepticus: high incidence of complex partial status. *Epilepsia* 1986; 27: 276–85.

130 Corman C, Guberman A, Benavente O. Clobazam in partial status epilepticus. *Seizure* 1998; 7: 243–7.

131 Tinuper P, Aguglia U, Gastaut H. Use of clobazam in certain forms of status epilepticus and in startle-induced epileptic seizures. *Epilepsia* 1986; 27 (Suppl. 1): S18–S26.

132 Treiman DM. Status epilepticus. *Bailliere Res Clin Neurol* 1996; 5: 821–39.

133 Lowenstein DH, Aminoff MJ. Clinical and EEG features of status epilepticus in comatose patients. *Neurology* 1992; 42: 100–4.

134 Tassinari CA, Dravet C, Roger J, Cano JP, Gastaut H. Tonic status epilepticus precipitated by intravenous benzodiazepine in five patients with Lennox–Gastaut syndrome. *Epilepsia* 1972; 13: 421–35.

135 Somerville ER, Bruni J. Tonic status epilepticus presenting as confusional state. *Ann Neurol* 1983; 13: 549–51.

136 Brenner RP, Atkinson R. Generalized paroxysmal fast activity: electroencephalographic and clinical features. *Ann Neurol* 1982; 11: 386–90.

137 Pisani F, Gallitto G, Di-Perri R. Could lamotrigine be useful in status epilepticus? A case report [letter]. *J Neurol Neurosurg Psychiatry* 1991; 54: 845–6.

138 Thomas JE, Reagan TJ, Klass DW. Epilepsia partialis continua. A review of 32 cases. *Arch Neurol* 1977; 34: 266–75.

139 Cockerell OC, Rothwell J, Thompson PD, Marsden CD, Shorvon SD. Clinical and physiological features of epilepsia partialis continua. Cases ascertained in the UK. *Brain* 1996; 119 (Pt 2): 393–407.

140 Desbiens R, Berkovic SF, Dubeau F *et al.* Life-threatening focal status epilepticus due to occult cortical dysplasia. *Arch Neurol* 1993; 50: 695–700.

141 Gurer G, Saygi S, Ciger A. Epilepsia partialis continua: clinical and electrophysiological features of adult patients. *Clin Electroencephalogr* 2001; 32: 1–9.

142 Singh BM, Strobos RJ. Epilepsia partialis continua associated with non-ketotic hyperglycemia: clinical and biochemical profile of 21 patients. *Ann Neurol* 1980; 8: 155–60.

143 Brandt L, Saveland H, Ljunggren B, Andersson KE. Control of epilepsy partialis continuans with intravenous nimodipine. Report of two cases. *J Neurosurg* 1988; 69(6): 949–50.

144 Wijdicks EF, Young GB. Myoclonus status in comatose patients after cardiac arrest [letter]. *Lancet* 1994; 343: 1642–3.

145 Morris HR, Howard RS, Brown P. Early myoclonic status and outcome after cardiorespiratory arrest. *J Neurol Neurosurg Psychiatry* 1998; 64: 267–8.

146 Werhahn KJ, Brown P, Thompson PD, Marsden CD. The clinical features and prognosis of chronic posthypoxic myoclonus. *Mov Disord* 1997; 12: 216–20.

147 Young GB, Gilbert JJ, Zochodne DW. The significance of myoclonic status epilepticus in postanoxic coma. *Neurology* 1990; 40: 1843–8.

148 Shorvon SD. In: *Handbook of Epilepsy Treatment.* Blackwell Science Ltd. Oxford, 2000.

19 Treatment of Epilepsy in General Medical Conditions

J.M. Parent and M.J. Aminoff

Epileptic seizures occur in a variety of general medical contexts. Seizures during the acute phase of metabolic or electrolyte disturbances or with acute systemic infections in patients without any prior history of epilepsy do not generally require chronic anticonvulsant drug treatment. Instead, attention should be directed at the treatment of the underlying medical disorder. Seizures also occur in non-epileptic patients as a consequence of medication prescribed for therapeutic purposes, for example tricyclic antidepressant drugs or theophylline. In such circumstances, the seizures do not require anticonvulsant medication for their control; rather, the offending medication should be withdrawn and the underlying medical condition managed by alternative therapeutic strategies. In patients with pre-existing epilepsy, seizure frequency can be increased by intercurrent metabolic or infective disorders, but will usually revert to its previous level once the exacerbating medical disorder is treated appropriately. In such circumstances, it is usually unnecessary to adjust the anticonvulsant drug regime if this previously provided good control of seizures. Patients presenting in status epilepticus, however, require urgent treatment with intravenous anticonvulsant drugs regardless of the precipitating cause.

In this chapter, attention is directed primarily at certain common medical conditions that may either produce recurrent seizures or exacerbate an existing seizure disorder. Attention is also directed at the treatment of epilepsy in patients with medical conditions that might complicate management.

Treatment of post-traumatic epilepsy

Civilian head trauma, most often from road accidents, falls or recreational injuries, is a significant cause of recurrent seizures in the general population. It is estimated that between 2 and 12% of all cases of epilepsy result from traumatic brain injury [1] and that approximately 5% of patients requiring hospitalization for head trauma will develop seizures [2]. Post-traumatic epilepsy is more frequent after penetrating trauma or severe, closed head injuries, with an incidence as high as 53% after combat missile injuries [3]. Although most seizures occur within the first year after cerebral injury, an increased risk is present for 5 years or more [2–4].

Seizures occurring after cerebral trauma are commonly divided into early and late categories. Early seizures occur within 1 week of trauma, are more common in young children [1] and have an incidence of 2–6% [2,4]. They may consist of generalized convulsions or of partial seizures without generalization; complex partial seizures occur only rarely [1]. Seizures occurring immediately do not necessarily imply a risk of recurrence. However, seizures developing more than 1 h after injury convey an increased risk of late seizures [2,4]. Other risk factors for late seizures include focal lesions (haematoma, contusion), focal neurological signs, depressed skull fracture with dural laceration, and prolonged coma or amnesia [1,2,4,5]. With penetrating missile injuries, the risk of seizures also increases with the volume of brain tissue destroyed, with lesions located centroparietally, and if metal fragments are retained [3]. The risk of late epilepsy remains high in these different circumstances, even if early seizures do not occur [1]. The seizures that occur in patients with late epilepsy are either generalized convulsions (sometimes with a focal onset) or—in about one-third of cases—simple or complex partial seizures.

The EEG is disappointing as a predictor of the risk of developing post-traumatic epilepsy. Approximately 20% of patients with normal EEGs at 3 months developed epilepsy in one study [2]. In a more recent investigation, EEGs recorded at 1 month were normal in 8.3% of patients with partial seizures and 27.3% of patients with generalized seizures after head injury [6].

Although some physicians often prescribe long-term anticonvulsant prophylaxis in patients at risk of seizures after severe head trauma, there is no evidence that such treatment is effective in preventing the formation of an epileptic focus and the subsequent development of epilepsy [7,8].

Early reports suggesting a decreased incidence of seizures after cerebral trauma in patients who received long-term prophylaxis with one or two anticonvulsants, usually phenytoin alone or combined with phenobarbital [9–11], have been difficult to interpret because of lack of randomization, therapeutic monitoring and adequate control subjects. In fact, subsequent prospective trials failed to show any protective effect of long-term prophylactic antiepileptic medication, using again phenytoin alone, carbamazepine alone, or phenytoin combined with phenobarbital [12–16]. While most of the above studies had methodological shortcomings, with special reference to inadequate statistical power due to small sample size, the ability of anticonvulsant medication to prevent post-traumatic seizures was examined more definitely in two large randomized, double-blind studies by Temkin *et al.* [17,18]. The first of these studies compared the efficacy of phenytoin with placebo for seizure prophylaxis in 404 patients with severe head trauma. An intravenous loading dose of phenytoin was given within 24 h of trauma, treatment was continued for 1 year and serum phenytoin levels were maintained within the optimum therapeutic range in most patients. Patients were followed up for 2 years. Phenytoin was effective in preventing early (acute) seizures in the first week after cerebral injury, but it was no better than placebo in protecting against seizures during the remainder of the study period. Moreover, reduction in post-traumatic seizures during the first week was not associated with a reduction in mortality rate [19]. The second study examined the potential protective effects of 1–6-

month valproic acid prophylaxis in comparison with 1-week phenytoin in 384 patients with traumatic brain injury. One hundred and thirty-two patients were randomized to receive a 1-week course of phenytoin, 120 were assigned to receive a 1-month course of valproate, and 127 were assigned to receive a 6-month course of valproate. Follow-up was 2 years for all patients. Rates of early seizures were low in all groups (1.5% in the phenytoin arm compared with 4.5% in the valproate arms combined, a non-statistically significant difference), while the incidence of late seizures did not differ across groups, being 15% in the patients who received short-term phenytoin compared with 16% and 24% in those who received 1- and 6-month courses of valproate, respectively. There was a trend for mortality rates being higher in the valproate groups than in the phenytoin group (13.4% vs 7.2%, respectively). It was concluded that valproate confers no benefit over short-term phenytoin for the prevention of early post-traumatic seizures, and is ineffective in preventing the subsequent development of post-traumatic epilepsy. The latter finding is particularly disappointing in view of the evidence that valproic acid, unlike phenytoin, has been reported to inhibit epileptogenesis in some animal models [8].

A meta-analysis of controlled studies of anticonvulsant drugs given as prophylaxis after severe head trauma has been published recently [20]. This analysis concluded that both phenytoin and carbamazepine are efficacious in preventing seizures occurring during the first week after brain trauma, relative risk being 0.12 for phenytoin (95% confidence intervals 0.04–0.40) and 0.39 (95% confidence intervals 0.17–0.92) for carbamazepine. However, phenytoin, phenobarbital, carbamazepine and valproate were not found to be effective in protecting against the appearance of late unprovoked seizures.

Based on the above findings, it is reasonable to recommend that, because of the toxicity of antiepileptic medications in this setting [21], pharmacological prophylaxis, if instituted, should only be limited to the early use of phenytoin for the first 7–14 days after severe head trauma. The drug should then be discontinued unless further seizures occur. Long-term administration of antiepileptic drugs is not routinely indicated in most of these patients, although it remains to be clarified whether long-term prophylaxis could be of value in special subgroups, with special reference to those patients who develop epileptiform abnormalities in their EEG. It has in fact been shown that, in a minority of patients, cerebral trauma induces a sequence of events which results in the emergence of an epileptic focus. Mechanisms underlying these events are not well understood, but may relate to the extravasation of blood, haemolysis, deposition of haem-containing compounds and subsequent oxidative reactions in brain tissue leading to the generation of free radicals. The existence of a genetic predisposition to post-traumatic epilepsy has been proposed, but remains unproved [3]. Further investigation remains to be undertaken to determine the efficacy of other antiepileptic drugs or other agents, such as antioxidants, antiperoxidants, corticosteroids and chelators, which may prevent the development of post-traumatic epilepsy [8].

Postneurosurgical seizures

The risk of developing seizures and epilepsy after supratentorial neurosurgical procedures is similar in many respects to that after head injury. As with cerebral trauma, the risk of seizures after neurosurgical intervention relates to the extent and location of damage. It is important to define risk factors and the utility of prophylactic treatment for both conditions. However, difficulties unique to the investigation of postoperative seizures complicate the interpretation of published studies.

In the first place, the cerebral pathology that necessitated the surgical intervention may itself lead to seizures. Even if patients with preoperative seizures are excluded, it is usually still not possible to eliminate an underlying pathological process which may cause postoperative seizures. Secondly, most studies of this topic are retrospective and uncontrolled, lack uniformity of prophylactic anticonvulsant treatment and involve patients with differing cerebral pathology, thereby confounding accurate analysis. Nevertheless, certain conclusions can be drawn from the available data.

The incidence of seizures after supratentorial neurosurgical procedures for non-traumatic pathology varies according to the underlying disease process. A large retrospective study by Foy et al. [22] found an overall incidence of 17% for postoperative seizures in 877 consecutive patients undergoing supratentorial neurosurgery for non-traumatic conditions. Patients had no prior history of epilepsy, and the minimum follow-up was 5 years in surviving patients. Details of prophylactic anticonvulsant therapy were not given. The incidence of seizures ranged from 4% in patients undergoing miscellaneous procedures (midline explorations, Frazier's operations, stereotaxic procedures and external ventricular drainage) to 92% for surgically treated cerebral abscesses. Among the patients developing postoperative seizures, 37% did so during the first postoperative week, 77% within the first year and 92% by 2 years. Of patients with early seizures (i.e. occurring in the first week), 41% developed late recurrent seizures. Single seizures occurred in 21% of the seizure group and were most often early seizures.

Keränen et al. [23] retrospectively analysed a series of 177 patients who underwent surgery for ruptured supratentorial aneurysms and were followed up for a mean of 3.4 years (whether or not preoperative seizures occurred was not stated). All patients received phenytoin treatment for at least 2 months. Late seizures, defined as those after the first postoperative week, occurred in 25 patients (14%), in all cases within 2 years of surgery, and were recurrent in 21 patients (12%). Only two patients had early seizures. Risks factors for seizure occurrence included poor preoperative grade, aneurysm involving the middle cerebral artery, large intracerebral haematoma, fixed neurological deficit, and perioperative complications such as hydrocephalus and vasospasm with infarction. Many of these risk factors overlap, but parenchymal brain injury from the underlying disease process is clearly important as a risk factor for seizures. In another retrospective study, Ukkola and Heikkinen [24] also found a higher risk of seizures after surgery for ruptured aneurysm if there was perioperative vasospasm or ischaemia, and with aneurysms of the middle cerebral artery. The presence of intraparenchymal haematoma did not increase seizure risk in this group, in contrast to the findings of Foy et al. [25]. Although the above studies suggest a rather high incidence of seizures after aneurysm surgery, other investigators have failed to confirm this, with incidence rates of 3–4.5% [26,27].

Rabinowicz et al. [28] examined the incidence of seizures following surgery for unruptured intracranial aneurysm. They retrospectively analysed only 21 patients followed for a mean of 2 years (range 2–68 months), but found that seizures developed in three of 19 previously seizure-free patients (15.7%) between 2 days and 13 months after surgery. All three patients had perioperative complications, including transient hemiparesis, transient dysphasia and meningitis, and two had temporal lobe retraction intraoperatively. Only four of 16 patients without postoperative seizures experienced perioperative complications.

Several studies have looked at the incidence of seizures after ventricular shunt procedures. Dan and Wade [29] found a 9.4% incidence of postoperative seizures in 180 patients without prior attacks who received shunt placement for a variety of conditions, including trauma and subarachnoid haemorrhage. No convulsions occurred in the first 7 days after surgery. The risk of subsequent seizures increased with the number of shunt revisions, and for parietal as compared with frontal shunt placement (54.5 versus 6.6%). Follow-up was for a minimum of 2 years unless death occurred in the second year after surgery. Of the patients with seizures, 52.9% had onset within the first postoperative year, and 23.6% did not experience seizures until after the second year. Foy *et al.* [25] reported that 12 of 55 patients (22%) developed seizures after ventricular shunt placement, five during the first week, three in the first month and the remaining four patients between 9 months and 3 years after the surgical procedure.

The literature on the prophylactic use of anticonvulsants after neurosurgical procedures is sparse. Most studies have been retrospective and of small numbers of patients, and were not designed specifically to evaluate the prophylactic efficacy of anticonvulsants. In many, serum drug levels were not monitored to evaluate compliance and ensure the adequacy of treatment. One retrospective study of 100 consecutive survivors of supratentorial surgery for intracranial aneurysm compared the incidence of seizures in the first 67 patients, who were treated with phenytoin, with that of the subsequent 33 patients, who received no antiepileptic medication [27,30]. There was no difference between groups in the incidence of seizures during the treatment phase of at least 1 year. However, only three patients experienced seizures in this small sample, and two of these had a prior history of epilepsy.

A prospective investigation by Foy *et al.* [31] also found no effect of prophylactic anticonvulsant therapy in a group of 276 consecutive adult patients undergoing supratentorial neurosurgery and estimated to have a high risk for developing postoperative seizures from non-traumatic conditions such as abscess, vascular lesions, meningiomas and other benign tumours. Follow-up was 3–8 years in survivors (median, 4 years). The first 102 patients were randomized to treatment with carbamazepine or phenytoin for 6 or 24 months. When no effect was found compared with historical controls, subsequent patients were randomized equally to either an untreated group, a group receiving phenytoin or a group receiving carbamazepine. Early seizures (within the first week) did not increase the risk of later seizures. There was no significant difference in effectiveness between the two treatment groups and the no-treatment group, with respect to seizure prophylaxis. However, barely half of the patients had at least one serum anticonvulsant level in the optimal therapeutic range during the study, and in many cases serum levels were either not checked or were always suboptimal. There was also no effect of anticonvulsant treatment in the first postoperative week. The authors concluded that prophylactic anticonvulsant therapy was not indicated even in high-risk patients after supratentorial neurosurgical procedures.

A somewhat different conclusion was reached in an earlier prospective, randomized, placebo-controlled study of phenytoin for seizure prophylaxis among 281 patients after supratentorial neurosurgery [32]. Patients received placebo (141 patients) or phenytoin (140 patients) in the immediate postoperative period and for the year following surgery, which was for various conditions including head trauma. Patients with preoperative epilepsy or prior anticonvulsant treatment were excluded. Follow-up was for 1 year. In the first postoperative week, there appeared to be a disproportionate benefit among the group receiving phenytoin, although this did not reach statistical significance because of the small numbers of seizures that occurred. There was a clearly significant beneficial effect of phenytoin when the cumulative number of seizures was analysed from the end of the first week up to the tenth postoperative week. The early prophylactic effect might have been greater if loading doses of phenytoin had been used to achieve therapeutic blood levels in the immediate postoperative period.

Evidence that phenytoin may be effective in protecting against early postoperative seizures is reinforced by the findings of Lee *et al.* [33], who treated 189 patients with intravenous phenytoin for 3 consecutive days after supratentorial surgery. During the 3-day observation period, only two phenytoin-treated patients experienced seizures, compared with nine of 185 patients randomized to placebo. A more recent randomized trial in a total of 200 patients, on the other hand, failed to detect even a trend for a protective effect of phenytoin against seizures occurring within 7 days after craniotomy [34]. In the latter study, however, phenytoin was mostly used in addition to pre-existing treatment with carbamazepine or phenobarbital, and the control group also received medication with other anticonvulsants.

A meta-analysis of randomized controlled trials exploring the potential value of anticonvulsant prophylaxis following brain surgery has been completed recently [20]. This analysis suggested that phenytoin does protect against the risk of early seizures, i.e. seizures occurring within 7 days after craniotomy (relative risk 0.42, 95% confidence intervals 0.25–0.71). However, there was no evidence that long-term treatment with phenytoin or carbamazepine can protect against the appearance of late spontaneous seizures.

The results of anticonvulsant prophylaxis following neurosurgical procedures thus parallel those for cerebral trauma. All therapies assessed to date seem to have no effect on the development of an epileptic focus. Prospective studies with other therapeutic agents are needed to explore the potential protective effects against epileptogenesis in patients with well-defined risk factors. In the meantime, although prophylactic anticonvulsant drugs are commonly prescribed for several months or more after supratentorial neurosurgical procedures penetrating the dura, it may be more appropriate to prescribe them for no more than 4 weeks and then gradually withdraw them unless further seizures occur.

Seizures and renal failure

Seizures are a manifestation of uraemic encephalopathy and occur in about 35% of patients with acute or chronic renal failure. In acute uraemia, seizures are usually of the generalized tonic-clonic variety and are often multiple; they are commonly associated with a severe encephalopathy, typically developing between 7 and 10 days after the onset of renal failure, in the anuric or oliguric stages [35]. Focal seizures may also occur, including epilepsia partialis continua [36]. However, the onset of seizures, especially if focal, in the uraemic patient should prompt investigations to exclude a structural cerebral lesion.

Uraemic convulsions due to chronic renal failure usually occur with advanced disease, commonly in the setting of a significant encephalopathy or as a preterminal event [35,36]. The incidence of seizures in chronic renal insufficiency has declined to less than 10% of cases because of earlier, more aggressive treatment of renal failure and its complications (including hypertensive encephalopathy, and fluid and electrolyte disturbances), and more cautious use of proconvulsant medications such as penicillin [36].

Seizures in patients with chronic renal failure are typically generalized tonic-clonic, although focal motor and generalized myoclonic seizures may also occur [35,36]. Treatment should be directed at correcting any identified metabolic abnormalities and the associated renal failure; often no specific cause of the convulsions can be identified and anticonvulsant treatment is necessary [35]. Phenytoin is commonly used, but phenobarbital and valproic acid are also effective [35–37]. Status epilepticus is a rare manifestation of chronic renal failure, and should be managed in the same manner as status epilepticus from other causes [36].

Seizures sometimes result from the treatment of renal failure. The dialysis disequilibrium syndrome has been associated with generalized convulsions, typically during the late stages of haemodialysis or several hours after a session. Such seizures have been attributed to fluid shifts resulting in cerebral oedema due to the increased brain osmolality in the uraemic state [38]. With the advent of more recent dialysis techniques, severe complications such as seizures and coma are no longer common [38].

Dialysis encephalopathy is a progressive and frequently fatal syndrome associated with chronic haemodialysis. It is characterized by a distinctive speech abnormality, psychiatric disturbances, dementia, asterixis and myoclonus, gait ataxia and seizures. The EEG may show paroxysmal bursts of frontally predominant high-voltage delta or spike-wave activity prior to the initial symptoms [39]. The syndrome usually occurs after dialysis has been given for several years and has been attributed to aluminium intoxication, with increased aluminium levels in the brain [40]. The aluminium may be derived from the water used in the dialysate, although its oral ingestion in phosphate-binding compounds may play a role; the incidence of the disorder has been declining with treatment of the dialysate to remove aluminium [38–40]. Seizures occur in approximately 60% of patients with dialysis encephalopathy, and commonly during or immediately after dialysis. They are usually generalized tonic-clonic seizures, although myoclonic, simple partial and complex partial seizures can also occur [35]. Convulsions may be controlled initially by diazepam, phenytoin or carbamazepine, but become increasingly difficult to control with disease progression [35,39].

A common clinical issue relates to the use of anticonvulsants in patients with pre-existing renal disease. Uraemia complicates therapy with anticonvulsants because of changes in pharmacokinetics as a result of altered protein binding and renal excretion; dialysis may also lead to removal of anticonvulsant agents.

The pharmacokinetics of phenytoin are altered in uraemic patients, even though it is metabolized almost exclusively by the liver. Phenytoin is 90% protein bound, and less than 5% is excreted unchanged in the urine [41]. In patients with severe renal failure, protein binding of phenytoin decreases by as much as 20%, due to the accumulation of endogenous displacing agents and hypoalbuminaemia. This may lead to a greater volume of distribution and reduced total serum phenytoin concentrations [37]. However, because the proportion of pharmacologically active, unbound phenytoin increases, the benefit of a given dose will be maintained. Thus, in advanced renal disease the therapeutic range decreases from the usual 10–20 µg/mL to approximately 5–10 µg/mL [41]. Measurement of free phenytoin levels is the best way to monitor therapy in the uraemic patient, with the therapeutic range remaining 1–2 µg/mL. It is not necessary to decrease the total daily dose as accumulation of phenytoin is unlikely if hepatic function is preserved. The half-life of phenytoin may be decreased in uraemic patients [42], leading some to discourage the prescription of a single daily dose [37]. Supplemental doses are not required in patients undergoing dialysis because phenytoin is not removed to any significant extent [41].

Valproic acid may be particularly effective in treating myoclonic and generalized tonic-clonic seizures in uraemic patients [37]. It undergoes pharmacokinetic changes similar to those of phenytoin in the setting of renal insufficiency. Plasma protein binding decreases, but the free concentration remains constant [41]. Thus, the therapeutic range of valproic acid may be decreased, and careful clinical and laboratory monitoring is necessary in patients with severe renal failure. Additional doses are not required after dialysis.

Plasma levels of phenobarbital may accumulate in the setting of uraemia [41]. Lower maintenance doses should be used when phenobarbital is given chronically to patients with severe renal insufficiency [37]. Phenobarbital is 40–60% protein bound and thus may be partially removed by haemodialysis, making supplemental doses necessary after dialysis in some patients [41]. Primidone and its metabolites may also accumulate and clinical toxicity has been reported in patients with renal insufficiency [37]. Serum levels of carbamazepine are unchanged in uraemic patients and dose adjustments are unnecessary [41]. Ethosuximide levels are significantly reduced by haemodialysis, and supplementation after dialysis is necessary [41].

Experience with newer anticonvulsants in the setting of kidney disease is more limited. Patients with impaired renal function show a reduced rate of elimination of gabapentin [43], levetiracetam [44], topiramate [45], vigabatrin [46], felbamate [47], oxcarbazepine and the active oxcarbazepine metabolite monohydroxycarbazepine [48]. These drugs should be used with caution and at reduced dosages in these patients. When gabapentin is used in patients on haemodialysis, it should be given as a single 200–300 mg dose after each 4 h of dialysis. With levetiracetam, a 250–500 mg supplemental dose is required after dialysis [44]. Topiramate [45] and vigabatrin [49] are also removed to a significant extent during haemodialysis.

The pharmacokinetics of lamotrigine [50] and tiagabine [51] do not appear to be markedly altered by moderate or severe renal insufficiency, and dosage adjustment for these agents is usually not necessary. With lamotrigine, however, some prolongation of the half-life may occur in severe renal impairment, while a faster elimination is observed during haemodialysis [52]. Although preliminary data suggest that zonisamide pharmacokinetics is not affected to a major extent by impaired renal function [53], prescribing information for this drug contraindicates its use in patients with a glomerular filtration rate below 50 mL/min, due to inadequate experience concerning drug dosing and toxicity.

Seizures and liver disease

Hepatic disease is associated with seizures less frequently than is uraemia. Early reports suggested that convulsions occurred in up to one-third of patients with acute hepatic encephalopathy, but Plum and Posner [54] found a much lower incidence and suggested that many of the seizures in prior reports were related to alcohol withdrawal and were not a manifestation of liver disease. Seizures may be generalized or focal, and are typically seen in stage 3 hepatic encephalopathy [55]. Treatment should be directed at the cause of the hepatic dysfunction and at ameliorating the hepatic encephalopathy with protein restriction and agents such as lactulose. Anticonvulsant therapy is usually not necessary unless there is an underlying cause of epilepsy such as prior cerebral trauma or intracranial haemorrhage.

Chronic liver disease is rarely the cause of convulsions [56]. When seizures do occur in alcoholics with hepatic cirrhosis, they are usually due to prior trauma, intracranial haemorrhage or alcohol withdrawal. Seizures are common in the acute hepatic failure associated with Reye's syndrome [57], and are infrequently encountered in Wilson's disease [55]. Convulsions in the setting of acute hepatic necrosis are frequently associated with severe hypoglycaemia.

Most anticonvulsant agents are metabolized by the liver and have been associated with hepatic toxicity, although they rarely lead to fatal hepatic dysfunction. Hepatic toxicity due to anticonvulsants are discussed in the chapters on individual drugs.

Because of the large reserve capacity of the liver, the effect of liver disease on anticonvulsant pharmacokinetics is usually not clinically significant until hepatic dysfunction is severe. Little experience is available to guide anticonvulsant dosing in patients with liver disease. Phenytoin and valproic acid exhibit decreased protein binding in patients with hepatic disease, and this correlates well with levels of serum albumin and bilirubin [37,41]. However, intoxication from accumulation of drug is not likely unless liver disease is severe. Dosages of phenytoin and valproic acid may need to be decreased in these situations, and serum drug concentrations should be determined frequently and interpreted cautiously, taking into account the fact that, due to decreased protein binding, therapeutic and toxic effects may be seen at concentrations lower than usual. Valproic acid should be used with extreme caution in patients with liver disease because of its known hepatic toxicity [37].

Phenobarbital, benzodiazepines and other sedatives can precipitate hepatic encephalopathy in patients with otherwise compensated liver disease [57]. These agents should therefore be used cautiously in the setting of hepatic dysfunction; because decreased hepatic metabolism may lead to drug accumulation, it may be necessary to lower the dosages prescribed [41]. Carbamazepine exhibits slightly decreased protein binding in patients with liver disease, but this is not clinically significant [37].

As far as newer antiepileptic drugs are concerned, lamotrigine may require dosage reduction when significant hepatic dysfunction is present [58]. Lamotrigine clearance has also been found to be re-duced by approximately 35% in subjects with Gilbert's syndrome (unconjugated hyperbilirubinaemia) compared with normal controls, and therefore a need for moderately lower dose requirements can be anticipated in these subjects [59].

Moderate or severe hepatic insufficiency reduces tiagabine clearance such that the dosage should be reduced or dosing intervals increased [60]. For topiramate, a modest reduction in drug clearance has been reported in five patients with moderate or severe stable liver impairment (Child-Pugh score 5–9) after a single dose, but this was not considered to be of great clinical significance [45]. Gabapentin is not metabolized to any significant extent by the liver, and dosage adjustments in this setting are unnecessary as long as normal renal function is preserved. Levetiracetam is also eliminated to a large extent by the kidney, and a reduction in the clearance of this drug has been described in liver disease patients showing a concomitant impairment in renal function [44]. Felbamate is best avoided in patients with pre-existing hepatic dysfunction due to the probably increased risk of felbamate-induced hepatic failure.

Hepatic porphyrias

The hepatic porphyrias are a group of disorders characterized by a partial defect in the haem biosynthetic pathway of the liver. Acute intermittent porphyria, hereditary coproporphyria and variegate porphyria are the three autosomal dominant forms of the disease that produce neurological manifestations, and the latter two forms also cause cutaneous photosensitivity. The partially deficient enzyme in acute intermittent porphyria is porphobilinogen deaminase, resulting in a build-up of δ-aminolaevulinic acid and porphobilinogen, which are excreted in excess quantities in the urine. Hereditary coproporphyria and variegate porphyria are caused by partial deficiencies of enzymes in the same porphyrin synthetic pathway—coproporphyrinogen oxidase and protoporphyrinogen oxidase, respectively.

The neurological manifestations of each of the acute hepatic porphyrias are similar and include peripheral neuropathy, autonomic dysfunction and neuropsychiatric disturbance. Seizures occur in 10–20% of patients with acute intermittent porphyria and occasionally are the presenting feature of the disorder [61]. Convulsions may be partial or generalized [62,63], and status epilepticus has also been reported [63]. The aetiology of brain dysfunction in porphyria is unknown but may relate to γ-aminobutyric acid receptor binding by δ-aminolaevulinic acid, which has been shown to cause seizures when infused directly into rat brain [61]. Moreover, defects in hepatic haem synthesis can lead to alterations of the levels of neurotransmitter substrate in the central nervous system (CNS), such as tryptophan [61]. In addition to the effects of defective porphyrin synthesis on the CNS, patients with acute porphyric attacks may also have seizures due to fluid and electrolyte disturbances, usually from excessive vomiting and inappropriate antidiuretic hormone secretion. Although seizures are typically a manifestation of acute attacks, porphyria may also coexist with idiopathic or symptomatic epilepsy [64–66]. Thus, anticonvulsant treatment is sometimes needed in both the acute and chronic setting in patients with hepatic porphyria.

Anticonvulsant therapy poses a dilemma in the management of the porphyric patient. Acute attacks may be precipitated by hormonal influences, by dietary changes and by numerous medications. Almost all antiepileptic agents have been implicated in exacerbating hepatic porphyria by stimulating hepatic δ-aminolaevulinic acid synthase activity, either in humans, animal models or *in vitro* assays. The list includes phenobarbital, phenytoin and other hydantoins, primidone, carbamazepine, valproic acid, succinimides, oxazolidiones and benzodiazepines [62–70]. Clonazepam and paraldehyde have had mixed results using *in vivo* and *in vitro* studies [68,69]. Bromides and magnesium sulphate do not have this enzyme-stimulating effect and may be safe to use in patients with porphyria [62,66,67,69]. As far as the new antiepileptic drugs are concerned, studies conducted *in vitro* and/or in animal models suggest that felbamate, lamotrigine, topiramate and tiagabine may be porphyrogenic [71,72], and lamotrigine in particular has been implicated in causing a porphyric attack in one patient who developed multiorgan failure on the drug [73]. Although oxcarbazepine was used safely in one patient with porphyria cutanea tarda [74], this carbamazepine derivative retains some enzyme-inducing properties and extreme caution should be exercised when prescribing it in patients with porphyria. On the other hand, the renally eliminated anticonvulsants gabapentin and vigabatrin have not shown porphyrogenic activity in experimental models [71], and gabapentin's safety in porphyric patients has been documented in preliminary case reports [75–77].

The treatment of seizures during acute attacks of porphyria should be directed at the underlying porphyrinogenic metabolic defect. This includes intravenous carbohydrate, usually in the form of a 10% dextrose solution, infusions of haematin or haem-arginate [61] and correction of associated metabolic abnormalities such as hyponatraemia. If seizures persist or if status epilepticus occurs, therapeutic options are limited because almost all standard anticonvulsants may worsen the acute porphyric episode. Alternatively, magnesium sulphate has been recommended, given as an intravenous infusion to keep serum magnesium concentrations between 2.5 and 7.5 mmol/L [63,69]. Others believe that the acute use of paraldehyde or intravenous benzodiazepines is safe [67], but this remains controversial [69].

Chronic therapy of recurrent seizures either coexistent with or due to hepatic porphyria is also difficult. Bromides have been recommended most commonly, despite their significant toxicity and narrow therapeutic index [62,64,67,69]. Serum bromide concentrations should be monitored closely and kept below 90 mg/dL [69]. Additionally, although both clinical and experimental evidence indicates that clonazepam is porphyrinogenic [62,67], many reports suggest that low-dose clonazepam may be safe in the chronic treatment of patients with hepatic porphyria [62,64,66,69]. The modern treatment of choice is probably with gabapentin, although published experience is limited. Levels of urinary δ-aminolaevulinic acid and porphobilinogen should be followed closely during therapy. If seizures are not controlled, cautious empirical therapy with standard anticonvulsants may be necessary. Finally, between attacks of acute porphyria, patients must maintain an adequate nutritional intake, avoid the use of porphyrinogenic drugs and obtain prompt treatment of intercurrent illnesses and infections.

Seizures and connective tissue diseases

Seizures occur in a variety of connective tissue diseases, usually because of a cerebral vasculitis or vasculopathy. Patients with Sjögren's or Behçet's syndrome occasionally have convulsions that are associated with a flare of disease activity, and seizures may rarely reflect cerebral involvement in rheumatoid arthritis, scleroderma and mixed connective tissue disease [78]. Both systemic and isolated CNS vasculitides may lead to seizures in association with focal or diffuse cerebral abnormalities. In many of these disorders, seizures also arise from the effects of the underlying disease on other organs, such as the kidneys, or from complications of therapy, especially with immunosuppressive agents, which predispose to CNS infections and which may also be inherently epileptogenic.

The connective tissue disease with probably the highest incidence of seizures and other neurological manifestations is systemic lupus erythematosus (SLE). Epilepsy and psychiatric abnormalities are the most frequently observed neurological symptoms of lupus [79], and these two manifestations frequently coexist. The published incidence of seizures in SLE ranges from 10 to 54% [79–81]. Generalized convulsions are most common, but simple partial, complex partial, absence and akinetic seizures may also occur, as may status epilepticus [80]. Seizures and other neurological abnormalities are uncommonly the initial feature of SLE and may precede systemic manifestations by many years.

Cerebral microinfarcts and, less frequently, subarachnoid and intracerebral haemorrhages are the major pathological findings in patients with SLE and seizures. They are believed to result usually from an immunologically mediated vasculopathy [82]. Convulsions may also arise indirectly from various complications of lupus, such as infections related to immunosuppressive therapy, uraemia from lupus nephritis, hypertensive encephalopathy, and as a terminal event [79,81]. Evaluation of seizures in patients with SLE must therefore include brain imaging, cerebrospinal fluid (CSF) examination and a thorough search for metabolic abnormalities and systemic disease activity.

The treatment of seizures or epilepsy in patients with SLE depends on the aetiology of the seizures, and the associated disease processes that are active. Convulsions that are a result of a flare of cerebral lupus are frequently isolated, self-limited events that do not require anticonvulsant therapy; if several seizures occur in a period exceeding 24–48 h, however, anticonvulsant medications should be prescribed for a limited interval (e.g. 3 months), depending on response to treatment of the underlying SLE. In more severe cases of cerebral lupus associated with recurrent seizures and other neurological or systemic manifestations, immunosuppression with corticosteroids is indicated. Other immunosuppressive agents, such as cyclophosphamide and azathioprine, have also been used [80]. Although the prognosis is poorer when there are neuropsychiatric manifestations, the presence of seizures or psychosis without other neurological features or significant renal disease does not affect survival adversely [80].

Anticonvulsant drug therapy in patients with SLE is complicated by the fact that many anticonvulsants are associated with the phenomenon of drug-induced lupus. This can be caused by the hydantoins, trimethadione and ethosuximide [83,84]. Rare cases of an SLE-like syndrome have also been reported in association with primidone [83], carbamazepine [85], valproate [86] and lamotrigine [87].

Symptoms of drug-induced SLE typically occur many months after initiation of anticonvulsant therapy and usually remit days to weeks after its discontinuation, although they may persist for several months. Renal and CNS involvement are uncommon, and laboratory findings differ from those of idiopathic SLE in that complement levels are usually normal and antibodies to native DNA are rarely present [83]. Despite this association of lupus and anticonvulsant therapy, there is no evidence that antiepileptics exacerbate idiopathic SLE [88]. Therefore, appropriate therapy should not be withheld from patients with seizures due to SLE or with coexistent epilepsy and lupus.

Epilepsy and cardiac disease

Cardiac disease may lead to recurrent seizures due to focal or global cerebral ischaemia. The former usually occurs in the setting of cardiogenic cerebral embolism, and the latter as a consequence of cardiac arrest, which not infrequently results in convulsive or myoclonic seizures and occasionally in status epilepticus.

Because of its high prevalence, heart disease and epilepsy frequently coexist, especially in the elderly. The treatment of acute seizures and status epilepticus in patients with heart disease is complicated by the increased risk of adverse effects from anticonvulsant drugs. Although intravenous phenytoin, in conjunction with benzodiazepines, remains the mainstay of therapy for acute life-threatening convulsions and status epilepticus, it must be used with care in patients with underlying cardiac dysfunction because it may cause hypotension and cardiac arrhythmias. These effects depend to a great extent on the rate of drug delivery and may be due to the toxicity of the diluent, propylene glycol, although direct cardiac effects of phenytoin also contribute [89,90]. Advanced age and underlying cardiovascular disease increase the risk of significant and life-threatening hypotension and cardiac arrhythmias from phenytoin infusion [91,92]. In patients with cardiovascular disease, intravenous phenytoin should be administered at 25 mg/min rather than 50 mg/min and is best given diluted in normal saline via an infusion pump, with continuous ECG monitoring and frequent blood pressure measurements [89,90]. Transient hypotension or arrhythmias typically respond to temporary discontinuation of the infusion, but the rate may need to be further decreased to 10 mg/min or less when the phenytoin is reintroduced.

Fosphenytoin is a water-soluble prodrug of phenytoin. It does not require propylene glycol as a diluent and it may therefore have a lower risk of producing hypotension or cardiac arrhythmias than parenteral phenytoin [93]. Although the advantages related to cardiovascular adverse effects of this more expensive agent remain to be firmly established, the risk of local adverse effects at the site of infusion is clearly reduced by using this water-soluble phenytoin prodrug preparation.

Chronic administration of anticonvulsant drugs is rarely associated with significant cardiovascular complications. However, there are reports of conduction heart defects and/or symptomatic arrhythmias developing in patients receiving carbamazepine in dosages associated with plasma levels in the optimal therapeutic range, usually in patients with underlying cardiac abnormalities [94,95]. Carbamazepine should only be prescribed after critical risk-to-benefit appraisal in patients with a history of cardiac disease. It is also prudent to obtain routine ECGs in patients with a history of cardiac disease who receive either carbamazepine or phenytoin as long-term anticonvulsant therapy, and to bear in mind

that events associated with loss of consciousness may result from arrhythmia as well as seizures in such patients.

Anticonvulsant agents can also exhibit pharmacokinetic or pharmacodynamic interactions with certain cardiac medications. In particular, enzyme-inducing anticonvulsants such as phenytoin, carbamazepine and barbiturates can stimulate the metabolism and reduce the clinical efficacy of several cardiovascular drugs, including, for example, quinidine, digoxin, dihydropyridine calcium channel antagonists, and mexiletine [96]. Amiodarone can lead to increased serum phenytoin levels, while verapamil and diltiazem can increase serum carbamazepine concentrations. Thus, in complicated patients with coexisting epilepsy and cardiac dysfunction, it is often necessary to measure serum levels of anticonvulsant drugs at frequent intervals and to monitor cardiovascular function carefully when initiating or adjusting both antiepileptic and cardiac medications.

Seizures in the transplant patient

Seizures are a frequent complication of solid-organ and bone marrow transplantation. Transplant patients are at risk for seizures because of the nature of their underlying illness, prior treatments such as radiation and chemotherapy and perioperative metabolic abnormalities and complications such as cerebral ischaemia; in the postoperative period, the effects of immunosuppression, drugs and rejection are also important. The incidence of seizures after transplant procedures depends on the type of transplant, the methods used and the age and nature of the patient population under study. Children generally appear to be at greater risk for post-transplant seizures [97–99].

The aetiology of seizures in transplant patients is often multifactorial. Immunosuppressive agents have themselves been associated with seizures. This is especially true of ciclosporin A, which is commonly used for immunosuppression after all forms of transplantation. Neurological complications due to ciclosporin A occur in between 10 and 25% of patients treated with the drug; in addition to seizures, these include tremor, ataxia, leucoencephalopathy, cortical blindness, neuropathy, quadriparesis and dysaesthesias. Seizures attributed to ciclosporin A occur in 1.5% of renal transplant patients and 5.5% of bone marrow recipients [100]. Other studies have suggested higher incidences, especially after liver transplantation [101,102] and in children [97].

Although patients with ciclosporin A-induced seizures frequently have serum levels exceeding the therapeutic range, levels are within the therapeutic range in some instances. It has been suggested that a ciclosporin A metabolite is responsible for the occurrence of seizures [103]. Various metabolic and systemic abnormalities and other therapeutic agents have been implicated as potentiators of ciclosporin A-related seizures and neurotoxicity, including concomitant methylprednisolone therapy [104], hypertension [105], hypomagnesaemia [102,106], hypocholesterolaemia [101], microangiopathic haemolytic anaemia [107] and (in renal transplant patients) aluminium overload [108]. However, these conditions do not necessarily lead to seizures, and many patients with suspected ciclosporin A-induced seizures are without any of the above abnormalities.

Other immunosuppressive agents have also been implicated in the aetiology of post-transplant seizures. Tacrolimus is a newer agent that has neurological complications similar to those of ciclosporin A, including seizures and encephalopathy [109]. The antirejection agent OKT3 can cause seizures as one of the manifestations of a cytokine encephalopathy [110]. Finally, in bone marrow recipients, busulphan or the combination of busulphan and cytoxan can cause seizures [111,112].

Seizures in transplant patients commonly result from CNS infections. Seizures can also be a manifestation of non-infectious structural and metabolic lesions, some of which require specific treatment. These lesions include cerebral ischaemia or haemorrhage, hyponatraemia with central pontine myelinolysis, hyperosmolar states, hypoglycaemia, delayed malignancy related to prior treatment and multiorgan system failure [97]. Finally, transplant rejection has been associated with an encephalopathic syndrome that includes seizures [97,113]. This syndrome is important to recognize as it may be the first manifestation of rejection [114].

The incidence (Table 19.1) and aetiology of post-transplant seizures also vary according to the type of transplant performed. Bone marrow recipients are susceptible to seizures due to prior irradiation, the effects of intrathecal or systemic chemotherapy, associated systemic complications such as thrombocytopenia and disease relapse in certain conditions such as leukaemia. Renal transplant patients may be predisposed to seizures because of the effects of uraemia, associated metabolic abnormalities and post-transplant cerebral reticuloendothelial tumours [97]. Cardiac, lung and liver transplant patients are much more likely to have early postoperative seizures due to focal or global cerebral ischaemia than are patients undergoing renal or bone marrow transplants.

Seizures are a symptom of an underlying cerebral abnormality in all patients, and therefore require thorough evaluation to exclude the different aetiological factors referred to earlier. The type and time of the seizure may be a useful guide. Early postoperative focal seizures in cardiac or hepatic transplant recipients frequently suggest a perioperative cerebral ischaemia event [97].

Metabolic screening tests, determination of blood levels of immunosuppressive agents, examination of the CSF, EEG and cerebral imaging studies (preferably MRI) are often required.

The neurological management of transplant patients with seizures is difficult. First, it must be determined whether antiepileptic medications are required. If seizures are self-limited and are due to correctable abnormalities with low recurrence risk, anticonvulsant therapy is probably not needed. Seizures that are prolonged or place the patient at high risk of complications should be termi-

nated with benzodiazepines. When seizures are recurrent, chronic anticonvulsant therapy is indicated. Second, the choice of anticonvulsant agents depends upon several important factors, including the type of transplant procedure undergone by the patient and the nature of the immunosuppressive drugs being taken. Certain anticonvulsants are contraindicated, depending on the tissue that has been transplanted. Valproic acid should not be used in liver recipients because it may cause irreversible hepatic toxicity. Similarly, carbamazepine should be avoided in bone marrow recipients because of its myelosuppressive effects. Bone marrow engraftment occurs 2–6 weeks after transplantation, and during this time it is prudent also to avoid the use of phenytoin and valproic acid. Phenobarbital has been suggested as an alternative therapy [97].

The enzyme-inducing anticonvulsants have an effect on immunosuppressive agents which are metabolized by the liver. Thus, phenobarbital, phenytoin and carbamazepine have been shown to increase the clearance of ciclosporin A and corticosteroids [97,115,116]. The decreased graft survival in renal transplant patients has been attributed to this effect [117]. If such agents are used, it is necessary to increase the dosage of corticosteroids by 25–30% and to increase ciclosporin A doses, with close monitoring of serum ciclosporin A levels [97]. Enzyme-inducing anticonvulsants may also increase the clearance of tacrolimus [118]. Some authors have suggested using valproic acid to avoid pharmacokinetic interactions [115]. Although bromides have been suggested as an alternative therapy because of their renal clearance, their significant toxicity limits their clinical utility. Experience with the newer antiepileptics is limited, but the lack of hepatic enzyme-inducing activity of lamotrigine, gabapentin, levetiracetam, tiagabine and vigabatrin, for instance, implies that they may be useful in this situation.

References

1 Pagni CA. Posttraumatic epilepsy: incidence and prophylaxis. *Acta Neurochirurg* 1990; Suppl. 50: 38–47.
2 Jennett B. *Epilepsy After Non-missile Head Injuries*, 2nd edn. Chicago: Year Book Medical, 1975.
3 Salazar AM, Jabbari B, Vance SC, Grafman J, Amin D, Dillon JD. Epilepsy after penetrating head injury. I. Clinical correlates: a report of the Vietnam Head Injury Study. *Neurology* 1985; 35: 1406–14.
4 Annegers JF, Grabow JD, Groover RV, Laws ER, Elveback LR, Kurland LT. Seizures after head trauma: a population study. *Neurology* 1980; 30: 683–9.
5 Martins da Silva A, Vaz AR, Ribeiro I, Melo AR, Nune B, Correia M. Controversies in posttraumatic epilepsy. *Acta Neurochirurg* 1990; Suppl. 50: 48–51.
6 Martins da Silva A, Nunes B, Vaz AR, Mendonca D. Posttraumatic epilepsy in civilians: clinical and electroencephalographic studies. *Acta Neurochirurg* 1992; Suppl. 55: 56–63.
7 Iudice A, Murri L. Pharmacological prophylaxis of post-traumatic epilepsy. *Drugs* 2000; 59: 1091–9.
8 Temkin NR, Jarell AD, Anderson GD. Antiepileptogenic agents: How close are we? *Drugs* 2001; 61: 1045–55.
9 Wohns RNW, Wyler AR. Prophylactic phenytoin in severe head injuries. *J Neurosurg* 1979; 51: 507–9.
10 Young B, Rapp R, Brooks WH, Madauss W, Norton JA. Posttraumatic epilepsy prophylaxis. *Epilepsia* 1979; 20: 671–81.
11 Servit Z, Musil F. Prophylactic treatment of posttraumatic epilepsy: results of a long-term follow-up in Czechoslovakia. *Epilepsia* 1981; 22: 315–20.
12 Penry JK, White BG, Brackett CE. A controlled prospective study of the pharmacologic prophylaxis of posttraumatic epilepsy. *Neurology* 1979; 29: 601–2.

Table 19.1 Incidence of seizures after transplantation procedures

Transplanted organ	Incidence of seizures (%)	Reference
Bone marrow	3–11.5	[119]
		[107]
Kidney	1.5–5	[108]
		[100]
Liver	17–25	[106]
		[102]
Heart	15	[120]
Lung	3.7–22	[121]
		[122]

13 Glotzner FL, Haubitz I, Miltner F, Kapp G, Pflughaupt KW. Anfallspro-phylaxe mit Carbamazepin nach schweren Schadelhirnverletzungen. *Neurochirurgia (Stuttgart)* 1983; 26: 66–79.

14 McQueen JK, Blackwood DHR, Harris P, Kalbag RM, Johnson AL. Low risk of late post-traumatic seizures following severe head injury: implications for clinical trials of prophylaxis. *J Neurol Neurosurg Psychiatry* 1983; 46: 899–904.

15 Young B, Rapp RP, Norton JA, Haack D, Tibbs PA, Bean JR. Failure of prophylactically administered phenytoin to prevent late posttraumatic seizures. *J Neurosurg* 1983; 58: 236–41.

16 Manaka S. Cooperative prospective study on posttraumatic epilepsy: Risk factors and the effect of prophylactic anticonvulsants. *J Psychiatry Neurol* 1992; 46: 311.

17 Temkin NR, Dikmen SS, Wilensky AJ, Keihm J, Chabal S, Winn HR. A randomized, double-blind study of phenytoin for the prevention of post-traumatic seizures. *N Engl J Med* 1990; 323: 497–502.

18 Temkin NR, Dikmen SS, Anderson GD *et al.* Valproate therapy for prevention of post-traumatic seizures: A randomized trial. *J Neurosurg* 1999; 91: 593–600.

19 Haltiner AM, Newell DW, Temkin NR, Dikmen SS, Winn HR. Side effects and mortality associated with use of phenytoin for early posttraumatic seizure prophylaxis. *J Neurosurg* 1999; 91: 588–92.

20 Temkin NR. Antiepileptogenesis and seizure prevention trials with antiepileptic drugs: Metanalysis of controlled trials. *Epilepsia* 2001; 42: 515–24.

21 Dikmen SS, Temkin NR, Miller B *et al.* Neurobehavioural effects of phenytoin prophylaxis for posttraumatic seizures. *JAMA* 1991; 265: 1271–7.

22 Foy PM, Copeland GP, Shaw MDM. The natural history of postoperative seizures. *Acta Neurochirur* 1981; 57: 15–22.

23 Keränen T, Tapaninaho A, Hernesniemi J, Vapalahti M. Late epilepsy after aneurysm operations. *Neurosurgery* 1985; 17: 897–900.

24 Ukkola V, Heikkinen ER. Epilepsy after operative treatment of ruptured cerebral aneurysms. *Acta Neurochirur* 1990; 106: 115–18.

25 Foy PM, Copeland GP, Shaw MDM. The incidence of postoperative seizures. *Acta Neurochirur* 1981; 55: 253–64.

26 Fabinyi GCA, Artiola-Fortuny L. Epilepsy after craniotomy for intracranial aneurysm. *Lancet* 1980; i: 1299–300.

27 Sbeih I, Tamas LB, O'Laoire SA. Epilepsy after operation for aneurysm. *Neurosurgery* 1986; 19: 784–8.

28 Rabinowicz AL, Ginsburg DL, DeGiorgio CM, Gott PS, Giannotta SL. Unruptured intracranial aneurysm: seizures and antiepileptic drug treatment following surgery. *J Neurosurg* 1991; 75: 371–3.

29 Dan NG, Wade MJ. The incidence of epilepsy after ventricular shunting procedures. *J Neurosurg* 1986; 65: 19–21.

30 O'Laoire SA. Epilepsy following neurosurgical intervention. *Acta Neurochirur* 1990; Suppl. 50: 52–4.

31 Foy PM, Chadwick DW, Rajgopalan N, Johnson AL, Shaw MDM. Do prophylactic anticonvulsant drugs alter the pattern of seizures after craniotomy? *J Neurol Neurosurg Psychiatry* 1992; 55: 753–7.

32 North JB, Penhall RK, Hanieh A, Frewin DB, Taylor WB. Phenytoin and postoperative epilepsy. *J Neurosurg* 1983; 58: 672–7.

33 Lee ST, Lui TN, Chang CN *et al.* Prophylactic anticonvulsants for prevention of immediate and early postcraniotomy seizures. *Surg Neurol* 1989; 31: 361–4.

34 De Santis A, Villani R, Sinisi M, Stocchetti N, Perucca E. Add-on phenytoin fails to prevent early seizures following surgery for supratentorial brain tumors: A randomized controlled study. *Epilepsia* 2002; (in press).

35 Bolton CF, Young GB. *Neurological Complications of Renal Disease.* Boston: Butterworths, 1990.

36 Raskin NH, Fishman RA. Neurologic disorders in renal failure. *N Engl J Med* 1976; 294: 143–8, 204–10.

37 Asconapé JJ, Penry JK. Use of antiepileptic drugs in the presence of liver and kidney diseases: a review. *Epilepsia* 1982; 23: S65–79.

38 Fraser CL, Arieff AI. Nervous system complications in uremia. *Ann Intern Med* 1988; 109: 143–53.

39 O'Hare JA, Callaghan NM, Murnaghan DJ. Dialysis encephalopathy: clinical, electroencephalographic and interventional aspects. *Medicine* 1983; 62: 129–41.

40 Arieff AI, Cooper FD, Armstrong D, Lazarowitz VC. Dementia, renal failure, and brain aluminum. *Ann Intern Med* 1979; 90: 741–7.

41 Lauer RM, Flaherty JF, Gambertoglio JG. Neuropsychiatric drugs. In: Schrier RW, Gambertoglio JG, eds. *Handbook of Drug Therapy in Liver and Kidney Disease.* Boston: Little, Brown, 1991: 207–41.

42 Letteri JM, Mellk H, Louis S, Kutt H, Durante P, Glazko A. Diphenylhy-dantoin metabolism in uremia. *N Engl J Med* 1971; 285: 648–52.

43 Blum RA, Comstock TJ, Sica DA *et al.* Pharmacokinetics of gabapentin in subjects with various degrees of renal function. *Clin Pharmacol Ther* 1994; 56: 154–9.

44 Dooley M, Plosker GL. Levetiracetam. A review of its adjunctive use in the management of partial onset seizures. *Drugs* 2000; 60: 871–93.

45 Langtry HD, Gillis JC, Davis R. Topiramate. A review of its pharmacodynamic and pharmacokinetic properties and clinical efficacy in the management of epilepsy. *Drugs* 1997: 54: 752–73.

46 Haegele KD, Huebert ND, Ebel M, Tell GP, Schechter PJ. Pharmacokinetics of vigabatrin: Implications of creatinine clearance. *Clin Pharmacol Ther* 1988; 44: 558–65.

47 Glue P, Sulowicz W, Colucci R *et al.* Single-dose pharmacokinetics of felbamate in patients with renal dysfunction. *Brit J Clin Pharmacol* 1997; 44: 91–3.

48 Rouan MC, Lecaillon JB, Godbillon J *et al.* The effect of renal impairment on the pharmacokinetics of oxcarbazepine and its metabolites. *Eur J Clin Pharmacol* 1994; 47: 161–7.

49 Bachmann D, Ritz R, Wad N, Haefely WE. Vigabatrin dosing during hemodialysis. *Seizure* 1996; 5: 239–42.

50 Wootton R, Soul-Lawton J, Rolan PE, Sheung CT, Cooper JD, Posner J. Comparison of the pharmacokinetics of lamotrigine in patients with chronic renal failure and healthy volunteers. *Br J Clin Pharmacol* 1997; 43: 23–7.

51 Cato A, Gustavson LE, Qian J, El-Shourbagy T, Kelly EA. Effect of renal impairment on the pharmacokinetics and tolerability of tiagabine. *Epilepsia* 1998; 39: 43–7.

52 Fillastre JP, Taburet AM, Fialaire A, Etienne I, Bidault R, Sinlas E. Pharmacokinetics of lamotrigine in patients with renal impairment: Influence of hemodialysis. *Drugs Exp Clin Res* 1993: 19: 25–32.

53 Schentag JJ, Gengo FM, Wilton JH *et al.* Influence of phenobarbital, cimetidine, and renal disease on zonisamide pharmacokinetics. *Pharm Res* 1987; 4 (Suppl.): 79.

54 Plum F, Posner JB. *The Diagnosis of Stupor and Coma,* 3rd edn. Philadelphia: F.A. Davis, 1980: 224–5.

55 Rothstein JD, Herlong HF. Neurologic manifestations of hepatic disease. *Neurol Clin* 1989; 7: 563–78.

56 Lockwood AH. Hepatic encephalopathy. In: Arieff AI, Griggs RC, eds. *Metabolic Brain Dysfunction in Systemic Disorders.* Boston: Little, Brown, 1992: 167–82.

57 Plum F, Hindfelt B. The neurological complications of liver disease. In: Vinken PH, Bruyn GW, eds. *Handbook of Clinical Neurology,* Vol. 27, *Metabolic and Deficiency Diseases of the Nervous System,* Part I. Amsterdam: Elsevier, 1976: 349–77.

58 Marcellin P, De Bony F, Garret C *et al.* Influence of cirrhosis on lamotrigine pharmacokinetics. *Br J Clin Pharmacol* 2001; 51: 410–14.

59 Posner J, Cohen AF, Land G, Winton C, Peek AW. The pharmacokinetics of lamotrigine (BW430C) in healthy subjects with unconjugated hyperbilirubinemia (Gilbert's syndrome). *Br J Clin Pharmacol* 1989; 28: 117–20.

60 Lau AH, Gustavson LE, Sperelakis R *et al.* Pharmacokinetics and safety of tiagabine in subjects with various degrees of hepatic function. *Epilepsia* 1997; 38: 445–51.

61 Kappas A, Sassa S, Galbraith RA, Nordmann Y. The porphyrias. In: Scriver CR, Beauder AL, Sly WS, Valle D, eds. *The Metabolic Basis of Inherited Disease.* New York: McGraw Hill, 1989: 1305–55.

62 Bonkowsky HL, Sinclair PR, Emery S, Sinclair JF. Seizure management in acute hepatic porphyria: risks of valproate and clonazepam. *Neurology* 1980; 30: 588–92.

63 Sadeh M, Martonovits G, Karni A, Goldhammer V. Treatment of porphyric convulsions with magnesium sulfate. *Epilepsia* 1991; 32: 712–15.

64 Garcia-Merino JA, Lopez-Lozano JJ. Risks of valproate in porphyria. *Lancet* 1980; ii: 856.

65 Herrick AL, McColl KEL, Moore MR, Brodie MJ, Adamson AR, Goldberg A. Acute intermittent porphyria in two patients on anticonvulsant therapy and with normal erythrocyte porphobilinogen deaminase activity. *Br J Clin Pharmacol* 1989; 27: 491–7.

66 Suzuki A, Aso K, Ariyoshi C, Ishimaru M. Acute intermittent porphyria and epilepsy: safety of clonazepam. *Epilepsia* 1992; 33: 108–11.

67 Reynolds NC, Miska RM. Safety of anticonvulsants in hepatic porphyrias. *Neurology* 1981; 31: 480–4.

68 Reynolds NC. Seizure management and hepatic porphyrias. *Neurology* 1982; 32: 1409–10.

69 Shedlofsky SI, Bonkowsky HL. Seizure management in the hepatic porphyrias: results from a cell-culture model of porphyria. *Neurology* 1984; 34: 399.

70 McGuire GM, MacPhee GJA, Thompson GG, Moore MR, Brodie MJ. Effects of sodium valproate on haem biosynthesis in man: implications for seizure management in the porphyric patient. *Eur J Clin Invest* 1988; 18: 29–32.

71 Hahn M, Gilderneister OS, Krauss GL *et al*. Effects of new anticonvulsant medications on porphyrin synthesis in cultured liver cells: Potential implications for patients with acute porphyrias. *Neurology* 1997; 49: 97–106.

72 Krijt J, Krijtova H, Sanitrak J. Effect of tiagabine and topiramate on porphyrin metabolism in an in vivo model of porphyria. *Pharmacol Toxicol* 2001; 89: 15–22.

73 Gregersen H, Niclsen JS, Peterslund NA. Acute porphyria and multiorgan failure during treatment with lamotrigine. *Ugeskr Laeger* 1996; 158: 4091–2.

74 Gaida-Hommernick B, Rieck K, Runge U. Oxcarbazepine in focal epilepsy and hepatic porphyria: A case report. *Epilepsia* 2001; 42: 793–5.

75 Krauss GL, Simmons-O'Brien E, Campbell M. Successful treatment of seizures and porphyria with gabapentin. *Neurology* 1995; 45: 594–5.

76 Tatum WO, Zachariah SB. Gabapentin treatment of seizures in acute intermittent porphyria. *Neurology* 1995; 45: 1216–17.

77 Zadra M, Grandi R, Erli LC, Mirabile D, Brambilla A. Treatment of seizures in acute intermittent porphyria: Safety and efficacy of gabapentin. *Seizure* 1998; 7: 415–16.

78 Messing OR, Simon RP. Seizures as a manifestation of systemic disease. *Neurol Clin* 1986; 4: 563–84.

79 Futrell N, Schultz LR, Millikan C. Central nervous system disease in patients with systemic lupus erythematosus. *Neurology* 1992; 42: 1649–57.

80 Brown MM, Swash M. Systemic lupus erythematosus. In: Toole JF, ed. *Handbook of Clinical Neurology*, Vol. 55. Amsterdam: Elsevier, 1989: 369–85.

81 Wong KL, Woo EKW, Yu YL, Wong RWS. Neurological manifestations of systemic lupus erythematosus: a prospective study. *Quart J Med* 1991; 81: 857–70.

82 Hanly JG, Walsh NMG, Sangalang V. Brain pathology in systemic lupus erythematosus. *J Rheumatol* 1992; 19: 732–41.

83 Weinstein A. Drug-induced systemic lupus erythematosus. *Prog Clin Immunol* 1980; 4: 1–21.

84 Harmon CE, Portanova JP. Drug-induced lupus: clinical and serological studies. *Clin Rheum Dis* 1982; 8: 121–35.

85 Drory VE, Yust I, Korczyn AD. Carbamazepine-induced systemic lupus erythematosus. *Clin Neuropharmacol* 1989; 12: 115–18.

86 Park-Matsumoto YC, Tazawa T. Valproate induced lupus-like syndrome. *J Neurol Sci* 1996; 143: 185–6.

87 Sarzi-Puttini P, Panni B, Cazzola M, Muzzupappa S, Turiel M. Lamotrigine-induced lupus. *Lupus* 2000; 9: 555–7.

88 Hughes GRV. The treatment of SLE: the case for conservative management. *Clin Rheum Dis* 1982; 8: 299–313.

89 Cloyd JC, Gumnit RJ, McLain LW. Status epilepticus: the role of intravenous phenytoin. *JAMA* 1980; 244: 1479–81.

90 Dreifuss FE. Anticonvulsant agents. *Crit Care Clin* 1991; 7: 521–32.

91 Earnest MP, Marx JA, Drury LR. Complications of intravenous phenytoin for acute treatment of seizures: recommendations for usage. *JAMA* 1983: 249: 762–5.

92 Donovan PJ, Cline D. Phenytoin administration by constant intravenous infusion: selective rates of administration. *Ann Emerg Med* 1991; 20: 139–42.

93 DeToledo JC, Ramsay RE. Fosphenytoin and phenytoin in patients with status epilepticus: improved tolerability versus increased costs. *Drug Safety* 2000; 22: 459–66.

94 Benassi E, Bo G-P, Cocito L, Maffini M, Loeb C. Carbamazepine and cardiac conduction disturbances. *Ann Neurol* 1987; 22: 280–1.

95 Kennebäck G, Bergfeldt L, Vallin H, Tomson T, Edhag O. Electrophysiologic effects and clinical hazards of carbamazepine treatment for neurologic disorders in patients with abnormalities of the cardiac conduction system. *Am Heart J* 1991; 121: 1421–9.

96 French JA, Gidal BE. Antiepileptic drug interactions. *Epilepsia* 2000; 41 (suppl. 8): 30–6.

97 Gilmore RL. Seizures and antiepileptic drug use in transplant patients. *Neurol Clin* 1988; 6: 279–96.

98 McEnery PT, Nathan J, Bates SR, Daniels SR. Convulsions in children undergoing renal transplantation. *J Pediatr* 1989; 115: 532–6.

99 Martin AB, Bricker JT, Fishman M *et al*. Neurologic complications of heart transplantation in children. *J Heart Lung Transpl* 1992; 11: 933–42.

100 O'Sullivan DP. Convulsions associated with cyclosporin A. *Br Med J* 1985; 290: 858.

101 De Groen PC, Aksamit AJ, Rakela J, Forbes GS, Krom RAF. Central nervous system toxicity after liver transplantation: the role of cyclosporine and cholesterol. *Engl J Med* 1987; 317: 861–6.

102 Grant D, Wall W, Duff J, Stiller C, Ghent C, Keown P. Adverse effects of cyclosporine therapy following liver transplantation. *Transpl Proc* 1987; 19: 3463–5.

103 Cilio MR, Danhaive O, Gadisseux JF, Otte JB, Sokal EM. Unusual cyclosporin related neurological complications in recipients of liver transplants. *Arch Dis Child* 1993; 68: 405–7.

104 Durrant S, Chipping PM, Palmer S, Gordon-Smith EC. Cyclosporin A, methylprednisolone, and convulsions. *Lancet* 1982; ii: 829–30.

105 Joss DV, Barrett AJ, Kendra JR, Lucas CF, Desai S. Hypertension and convulsions in children receiving cyclosporin A. *Lancet* 1982; i: 906.

106 Adams DH, Ponsford S, Gunson B *et al*. Neurological complications following liver transplantation. *Lancet* 1987; i: 949–51.

107 Ghany AM, Tutschka PJ, McGhee RB *et al*. Cyclosporine-associated seizures in bone marrow transplant recipients given busulfan and cyclophosphamide preparative therapy. *Transplantation* 1991; 52: 310–15.

108 Nordal KP, Talseth T, Dahl E *et al*. Aluminium overload, a predisposing condition for epileptic seizures in renal-transplant patients treated with cyclosporin? *Lancet* 1985; ii: 153–4.

109 Schneck FX, Jordon ML, Jensen CWB. Pediatric renal transplantation under FK-506 immunosuppression. *J Urol* 1992; 147: 1585–7.

110 Shihab F, Barry JM, Bennett WM, Meyer MM, Norman DJ. Cytokine-related encephalopathy induced by OKT3: incidence and predisposing factors. *Transpl Proc* 1993; 25: 564–5.

111 De La Camara R, Tomas JF, Figuera A, Berberana M, Fernandez-Rañada JM. High dose busulfan and seizures. *Bone Marrow Transpl* 1991; 7: 363–4.

112 Tiberghien P, Flesch M, Paintaud G, Cahn J-Y. Isolated/primary CNS relapse in women in remission after ABMT for metastatic breast cancer. *Bone Marrow Transpl* 1992; 9: 147–9.

113 Gross MLP, Pearson RM, Kennedy J, Moorhead JF, Sweny P. Rejection encephalopathy. *Lancet* 1982; ii: 1217.

114 Gross MLP, Pearson RM, Sweny P, Moorhead JF. Convulsions associated with cyclosporin A in renal transplant recipients. *Br Med J* 1985; 290: 555.

115 Hillebrand G, Castro LA, van Scheidt W, Beukelmann D, Land W, Schmidt D. Valproate for epilepsy in renal transplant recipients receiving cyclosporine. *Transplantation* 1987; 43: 915–16.

116 Alvarez JS, Del Castillo JAS, Ortiz MJA. Effect of carbamazepine on ciclosporin blood level. *Nephron* 1991; 58: 235–6.

117 Wassner SJ, Malekzadeh MH, Pennisi AJ, Ettenger RB, Uittenbogaart CH, Fine RN. Allograft survival in patients receiving anticonvulsant medications. *Clin Nephrol* 1977; 8: 293–7.

118 Karasu Z, Gurakar A, Carlson J et al. Acute tacrolimus overdose and treatment with phenytoin in liver transplant recipients. *J Okla State Med Assoc* 2001; 94: 121–3.

119 Patchell RA, White CL, Clark AW, Beschorner WE, Santos GW. Neurologic complications of bone marrow transplantation. *Neurology* 1985; 35: 300–6.

120 Grigg MM, Constanzo-Nordin MR, Celesia GG et al. Cyclosporine-induced seizures following cardiac transplantation: fact or fiction? *Epilepsia* 1987; 28: 626.

121 Vaughn BV, Ali II, Olivier KN et al. Seizures in lung transplant recipients. *Epilepsia* 1996; 37: 1175–9.

122 Lee J, Raps EC. Neurologic complications of transplantation. *Neurol Clin* 1998; 16: 21–33.

20 Treatment of Psychiatric Disorders in Epilepsy

E.S. Krishnamoorthy

The interface between epilepsy and psychiatric disorders has a long and chequered history. Beginning in the 19th century, neurologists and psychiatrists have expended great effort in researching various aspects of psychopathology in epilepsy. However, the treatment of psychiatric disorders in epilepsy has received little attention, and remains poorly researched and controversial. Thus, while considerable progress has been made in several areas of this interface [1], the literature on psychiatric management techniques in epilepsy remains largely 'opinion led'. Evidence from randomized controlled trials is relatively scanty, and few systematic investigations have been conducted in this specific area.

There are several controversies that further complicate matters (Table 20.1). First, the relationship between epilepsy and psychopathology is by itself controversial. Epilepsy has been reported to either facilitate [2] or to inhibit [3] the development of psychopathology, and it is likely that both types of relationships exist in different individuals and possibly at different times in the same individual.

Second, psychopathology in epilepsy can apparently be provoked by a number of factors, many of which are related to treatment. The seizures themselves [4], the drugs used to treat seizures [5], the withdrawal of anticonvulsant drugs [6], other treatments, with special reference to epilepsy surgery [7], and the social consequences of epilepsy [8] have all been linked to the development of psychopathology.

Third, psychotropic treatments may be proconvulsant; in particular, antipsychotics and antidepressants can lower seizure threshold, and can provoke seizures in those with no past history of seizures [5]. On the other hand, many anticonvulsant drugs have psychotropic properties, with carbamazepine, sodium valproate and lamotrigine being some of the most widely used mood stabilizers [9].

Fourth, there is renewed interest in questions such as the role of seizure cessation in the development of psychopathology. It is also interesting that electroconvulsive therapy (ECT), i.e. the use of seizures to treat psychiatric disorders, can by increasing the seizure threshold result in a cessation of seizures, at least transiently [10].

In this chapter, the psychiatric disorders associated with epilepsy (Table 20.2) will be briefly outlined, based on a discussion document currently in circulation within the International League Against Epilepsy (ILAE) Commission on Epilepsy and Psychobiology, Sub-commission on Classification, and the management of these disorders will be discussed in some detail. In the absence of hard evidence from randomized controlled trials, anecdotal experience and the opinion of experts have been relied upon in making these recommendations. Further, the complexities of the relationship between epilepsy and psychopathology outlined above have to be taken into account. The discerning reader is advised to consider the recommendations made herein in this light.

Overview of therapeutic tools

The management tools available to the psychiatrist can be broadly classified into those that are biological and those that are psychological. Of the biological treatments, antidepressants, anxiolytics, antipsychotics and mood stabilizers are employed extensively. ECT, although an important tool in mainstream psychiatry, is rather infrequently employed in subjects with epilepsy, and this too largely in specialist settings. However, new treatments that may have beneficial effects on both seizures and psychopathology have emerged in the past decade, vagus nerve stimulation and transcranial magnetic stimulation being important examples of such development.

A number of psychological treatments are also available, ranging from counselling that is widely available in developed nations like the UK, even in primary care, to the more sophisticated brief psychotherapeutic techniques that have in many cases replaced conventional psychotherapy. By far the most popular psychological technique today is cognitive behaviour therapy, a technique that can be adapted to address specific conditions such as epilepsy, and one that also lends itself to scientific testing through randomized controlled trials.

The discussion below will focus on biological treatments; psychological treatments and novel therapies will be outlined briefly. As a general principle, the combination of biological and psychological treatments is superior to either treatment alone, and the vast majority of experts effectively deploy both forms of treatment individually, in tandem or sequentially, depending on the complexity of the clinical situation they are faced with.

Organic mental disorders

Presentation

Psychiatric symptoms are often a feature of the seizure itself (Table 20.3). Auras encountered in simple partial seizures, in particular, may include psychiatric symptoms like anxiety, dysphoric mood and panic, agitation and irritability, hallucinations in various modalities and even transient abnormal beliefs. Abnormal (sometimes bizarre) behaviour can also characterize partial seizures arising from the frontal and temporal lobes that do not always generalize. Subclinical seizure activity and non-convulsive status can also present with catatonic features, and with other neuropsychiatric manifestations like apathy and aggression [11]. Ictal states presenting in this way include the following:

Table 20.1 Issues to be considered when assessing the relationship between epilepsy and psychopathology

Relationship between psychiatric manifestations and seizure activity
Psychiatric side-effects of antiepileptic drugs (and other therapeutic interventions, including epilepsy surgery)
Favourable effects of some antiepileptic drugs on psychopathology (e.g. mood stabilization)
Effects of psychotropic medications on seizure threshold
Role of social factors
Unrelated psychiatric comorbidities

Table 20.2 Psychiatric disorders most commonly described in patients with epilepsy

Organic mental disorders
Psychosis
Mood disorders
Personality disorders

Table 20.3 Organic mental disorders in epilepsy

Seizure-related manifestations
• complex partial seizures (and complex partial status)
• simple partial seizures (and simple partial status)
• absence status
Drug-induced encephalopathies
Other metabolic encephalopathies
Catatonic states

• Complex partial seizure status (associated with impaired awareness).
• Simple partial seizure status (aura continua, associated with intact awareness).
• Absence status (spike-wave stupor, presenting as a stuporous state, at times associated with minor myoclonic manifestations).

As far as non-ictal conditions are concerned, the drugs employed to treat refractory epilepsy with their associated side-effects (valproate encephalopathy or valproate-induced pseudodementia [12], for example) and medical comorbidities with resulting metabolic complications can all result in encephalopathic states. The manifestations of these encephalopathies may include delirium, characterized primarily by a significant impairment in attention, but also agitation, restlessness, hallucinations and bizarre behaviour [13]. Often the development of delirium is closely associated with a change in drug therapy, and a good history is helpful. Chronic delirium may be misdiagnosed as dementia, and the reversible nature of delirium makes the differentiation an important one to make.

Catatonic states are also a feature in patients with intractable epilepsy, especially those living in institutions. Catatonia is a syndrome with several medical causes, many of which are reversible [14]. This author has experience of repeated episodes of catatonia (periodic catatonia) [15] accompanying seizure cessation in an institutionalized male. It is noteworthy that both in such catatonic states and in valproate encephalopathy, routine metabolic parameters including liver function tests may be normal. At times, there is

an abnormality in blood ammonia, that may be raised several-fold. The EEG is an important investigation here, and can provide valuable diagnostic clues, thus aiding management [16].

Treatment

Management requires identification and correction of the primary cause. The EEG will help in the differential diagnosis between subclinical status and encephalopathy, particularly metabolic encephalopathy, and other haematological and biochemical tests will support the diagnosis. If the psychiatric manifestations are due to subclinical seizure activity, achieving better seizure control would be the cornerstone of treatment. If on the other hand a metabolic disturbance, intercurrent infection or a drug-induced state were the prime cause of the mental disorder, identification and correction of these is necessary. For example, the offending drug may be withdrawn gradually, intercurrent infections can be treated with antibiotics and metabolic disturbances can be corrected appropriately.

As in other conditions characterized by delirium, there can also be a role for the use of benzodiazepines or antipsychotics in small doses, especially when agitation or aggression pose a major management problem by placing the patient or others in his environment at serious risk. Benzodiazepines, especially lorazepam, clobazam and clonazepam, can be very effective adjunctive agents, leading to the resolution of the psychopathology, while helping to maintain or indeed to improve seizure control. Benzodiazepines such as lorazepam and clonazepam are widely recognized as effective agents in psychiatric emergencies [17], and in this author's experience can be useful in dealing with the agitated or violent patient with encephalopathy. In catatonic syndromes, benzodiazepines such as lorazepam and clonazepam are indeed the drugs of choice, and have been found to be effective in a number of studies [18].

When there is severe agitation and/or psychotic features, small doses of haloperidol or a newer antipsychotic such as sulpiride, risperidone, olanzapine and quetiapine may be appropriate. However, as many of these drugs can potentiate seizure activity and may worsen the primary condition, a thoughtful decision by an expert is called for. Droperidol is the antipsychotic of choice for parenteral administration in an emergency situation [17].

In choosing the appropriate dose, a useful rule of thumb is to begin with one half the dose recommended for a psychiatric emergency in someone with an organic brain syndrome. In the elderly, frail, learning disabled or demented patient, even greater caution must be exercised, and a third to a quarter of the standard recommended dose can be a useful starting point. Oral preparations are generally preferable to parenteral ones, unless the clinical condition warrants otherwise. The risk of complications such as neuroleptic malignant syndrome cannot be underestimated in these individuals.

Psychoses

Presentation

The classification of psychoses in patients with epilepsy is most often linked to their relationship with seizures (Table 20.4). The following presentations are most commonly encountered.

Table 20.4 Epilepsy-related psychoses

Interictal psychosis
Alternative psychosis (including forced EEG normalization)
Postictal psychosis

Interictal psychosis

This is a paranoid psychosis, with a strong affective component, whose features may include command hallucinations, third-person auditory hallucinations and other first-rank symptoms. There can be a preoccupation with religious themes. Personality and affect tend to be well preserved, unlike in other forms of schizophrenic psychosis. The psychosis is usually independent of the epilepsy, and is not affected by seizure activity (see [11] for review). Interictal psychosis has also been referred to as schizophrenia-like psychosis of epilepsy and, more recently, as psychosis of epilepsy [19].

Alternative psychosis

In alternative psychosis, the patient alternates between periods of clinically manifest seizures and normal behaviour, and other periods of seizure freedom accompanied by a behavioural disturbance. The behavioural disturbance, which is often accompanied by paradoxical normalization of the EEG (forced normalization) [3], is polymorphic, with paranoid and affective features. Depression, anxiety, depersonalization, derealization and even hysteria have been reported as presenting manifestations [20]. The diagnosis of alternative psychosis [21] may be made in the absence of the EEG, but if EEG confirmation is available the diagnosis should be qualified by indicating whether there is a 'forced normalization of the EEG'. (For a recent comprehensive review and diagnostic criteria, see [22].)

Postictal psychosis

In this condition, the psychosis follows clusters of seizures (rarely single seizures), usually after a 24–48-h period of relative calm (the lucid interval). These episodes can last from a few days to a month, but they usually subside in 1 or 2 weeks. Confusion and memory loss may be present. The content of thought is paranoid and visual and auditory hallucinations may be present. Manifestations are often polymorphic with affective features and with a strong religious theme. For a psychosis to be classified as postictal, the first manifestation of abnormal behaviour should occur within a 7-day period from the last seizure [23].

Treatment

The mainstays of treatment are antipsychotic drugs. Evidence from randomized controlled trials is lacking, and drug choice is based primarily on side-effect profile. Of the older agents, haloperidol remains by far the safest drug to use in epilepsy [24]. The newer agents, with the exception of clozapine [25], have generally a lower potential to reduce seizure threshold. Sulpiride and risperidone are in this author's experience relatively safe and effective, and this view is shared by other authors [24]. More recently, olanzapine has

emerged as a useful alternative, although opinion is divided about its seizure-facilitating effects. Quetiapine is another new drug with fewer side-effects and a reasonable safety profile, and it was in a recent study the only antipsychotic that did not cause EEG changes in 323 hospitalized psychiatric patients [26]. However, it should be emphasized that data about the comparative efficacy and safety of antipsychotic drugs in epilepsy-related psychoses is lacking, and practice is largely opinion-led and individualized, taking into consideration the classification of the psychosis as outlined above.

Interictal psychosis

The antipsychotic agent sulpiride has significant anxiolytic effects, and it is very suitable for the grumbling interictal psychosis often seen in epilepsy, with subtle psychotic features, but manifest irritability, anxiety and dysphoria. In this author's experience it may be used in low doses to reduce the anxiety, agitation and emotional lability that are manifest in this condition. However, sulpiride may not be sufficiently effective during acute exacerbations of psychotic behaviour, and risperidone, olanzapine or quetiapine may become necessary. Sometimes, exacerbations of interictal psychosis are prolonged and non-responsive to treatment. In this situation, clozapine may need to be introduced, but this requires special caution because clozapine may precipitate seizures and may induce a fall in white cell count. Therefore admission to hospital is advisable for the initial period of clozapine treatment. Close monitoring of blood counts is necessary, and withdrawal of other drugs such as carbamazepine, which can also reduce white cell counts, should be considered. A series of patients with intractable psychosis of epilepsy treated with clozapine has recently been reported [27].

Although acute interictal psychosis usually responds to clozapine, the use of ECT may become necessary in some patients, and referral to a specialist setting served by both neurologists and psychiatrists is recommended in this situation. Both exacerbation of seizure activity and psychotic states are known complications of ECT, and the consultation with a neuropsychiatrist with expertise in epilepsy is recommended before such therapy is embarked upon. Particular attention should also be given to safety issues, including access to emergency medical support in the event of ECT-induced status epilepticus.

Alternative psychosis and forced normalization

Although the behavioural disturbance associated with alternative psychosis cannot go unnoticed, a correct diagnosis of this condition is not infrequently missed. Moreover, in the absence of EEG recordings on and off the period of behavioural disturbance, forced normalization (which is an EEG diagnosis) cannot be diagnosed. The diagnostic challenge is complicated by the fact that alternative psychoses occur with a myriad of presentations, some with psychotic features, others encompassing the breadth of all psychopathologies seen in epilepsy [22]. Gradual withdrawal of the offending agent, such as a newer antiepileptic drug, can in many cases lead to resolution of the psychopathology but at times this may also involve reappearance of seizures. Antipsychotics, antidepressants and anxiolytic drugs, as appropriate, may also be employed to treat these episodes, but again the return of seizures (possibly provoked by the introduction of the psychotropic agent) often heralds a return to normal behaviour. In these individuals, one should perhaps accept the concept that the ideal of seizure freedom is not a panacea for all ills. As Landolt rather crudely put it, 'there would seem to be epileptics who must have a pathological EEG in order to be mentally sane' [3].

Postictal psychosis

Postictal psychosis is often preceded by a period of relative calm (lucid interval), and this provides a therapeutic window for prevention. While episodes of postictal psychosis may occur in the average person with epilepsy due to discontinuation of drugs (e.g. due to non-compliance), they sometimes occur in a repetitive and predictable fashion in certain individuals. In these individuals with recurrent episodes, preventive therapy with loading doses of clobazam may be useful after a second seizure has occurred, and in some patients with frequent or serious episodes clobazam may be given even after a first seizure. The practice followed by this author is to give 10 mg of clobazam every 6 h for a few days, and then to taper slowly and stop over 7–10 days. Continuous use of clobazam is not recommended, as the development of tolerance is known to complicate its prolonged administration [28].

To treat the acute psychotic episode, antipsychotic drugs and lorazepam may be used. Patients with postictal psychosis can show violent and destructive behaviour, and episodes of self-mutilation, attempted suicide and significant aggression have been observed in specialist units. Admission to hospital, close observation and the appropriate use of benzodiazepines and antipsychotics is therefore important and essential. A breakthrough seizure may in many cases lead to resolution of the behavioural symptoms. A few subjects fail to return to normal behaviour, and progress to a grumbling interictal psychotic state.

Depression and anxiety disorders

Presentation

Conventional mood disorders are encountered in a number of patients with epilepsy [29]. Anxiety is also a frequent manifestation, and it may lead to diagnostic uncertainty because panic and anxiety symptoms may represent a feature of seizure activity in the temporal lobe as well as a comorbid disorder [30]. The symptoms of major depression, dysthymia, generalized anxiety, panic disorder and mixed anxiety disorder are well described elsewhere [29,30], and will not be detailed herein. However, patients with epilepsy may suffer from specific mood disorders that are paroxysmal, relatively short lasting and often unrecognized. Although brief, these episodes are recurring, resulting in many workdays lost, and they are a source of considerable disability. These epilepsy-specific mood and anxiety disorders are described in some detail below, and their treatment is also discussed.

Intermittent affective-somatoform symptoms are frequently present in chronic epilepsy and include irritability, depressive moods, anergia, insomnia, atypical pains, anxiety, phobic fears and euphoric moods. These occur at various intervals and tend to last from hours to 2 or 3 days. Some of the symptoms may be present continually but their intensity will show considerable fluctuations. The presence of at least three symptoms generally is associated with

Table 20.5 Seizure- and epilepsy-related mood disorders

Interictal dysphoric disorder
Prodromal dysphoric disorder
Postictal dysphoric disorder
Specific phobic disorders (fear of seizures, agoraphobia and social phobia)

significant disability [31]. Similar affective-somatoform symptoms may also occur during the prodromal phase before a seizure, or in the postictal phase. The seizure-related disorders (Table 20.5) include the following conditions:
• Interictal dysphoric disorder: this consists of intermittent dysphoric symptoms (at least three symptoms among those described above), each occurring to a troublesome degree. In women, the disorder may become manifest or accentuated during the premenstrual phase.
• Prodromal dysphoric disorder: in this condition, irritability or other dysphoric symptoms may precede a seizure by hours to days and cause significant disability.
• Postictal dysphoric disorder: this includes symptoms of anergia or headaches, as well as depressed mood, irritability or anxiety, which may develop after a seizure and be prolonged or exceptionally severe.
• Specific phobic fears such as fear of seizures [32], agoraphobia and social phobia: these phobic symptoms may occur in patients with recurrent seizures and may either occur alone or be part of an interictal dysphoric disorder. In the latter case, a diagnosis of interictal dysphoric disorder is preferred. Unlike the symptoms associated with comorbid phobic anxiety disorder, the phobic fears revolve around epilepsy, and the fear of the situation and the subsequent avoidance are linked to the fear of having a seizure in a specific situation, and of the consequences involved.

Treatment

Both depression and anxiety in epilepsy respond to antidepressant drugs. In a randomized double-blind comparison of nomifensine and amitriptyline, Robertson and Trimble [33] showed that all patients improved at 6 weeks, though the nomifensine group had a greater improvement at 12 weeks. These studies in epilepsy are rare, and therapeutic recommendations are mostly derived from general clinical experience, including anecdotal or indirect evidence.

There is general agreement that the selective serotoninergic reuptake inhibitors (SSRIs) are safe to use in epilepsy [24]. Fluoxetine is probably the drug most widely prescribed, although it has the drawback of inhibiting the metabolism of some antiepileptic drugs, particularly phenytoin and carbamazepine, and it has been occasionally implicated in the provocation of seizures in patients without a history of epilepsy. Other SSRIs commonly used in patients with epilepsy include paroxetine and citalopram. Paroxetine is advantageous in that it does not interact with common antiepileptic drugs [34] and it has a relatively short half-life compared with fluoxetine. Therefore, its withdrawal should lead to rapid recovery should deterioration of seizures occur after institution of treatment. In any case, paroxetine is considered to have a low seizure-inducing potential and there are actually patients in whom its introduction seems to improve seizure control (Trimble, personal communication). Citalopram is another SSRI that is being used to treat depression in epilepsy, and may be particularly beneficial in the subgroup of patients with mixed anxiety and depression [29].

It is a common practice to add an anxiolytic drug during the initial phase of treatment, before the antidepressant can produce its full therapeutic effects. The anxiolytic drug is slowly withdrawn when the action antidepressant becomes fully manifest, which may take between 4 and 6 weeks. This practice is particularly helpful because during the initial phases of therapy many antidepressants may provoke rather than control anxiety. In epilepsy, however, the use of anxiolytic agents such as benzodiazepines has to be tempered by knowledge that their withdrawal could result in deterioration of seizure control. Therefore, the use of benzodiazepines, particularly those with strong anxiolytic properties but limited anticonvulsant properties (alprazolam being a case in point), must be cautious. Drugs such as clobazam and lorazepam can be useful adjuncts in patients with acute anxiety and agitation, or in those with profound withdrawal and apathy (catatonic depression). The use of ECT may become necessary in some patients with unremitting major depression not responsive to drug treatment, but this should be undertaken with special precautions as discussed above.

As far as the treatment of paroxysmal dysphoric disorder is concerned, Blumer [31] advocates the prophylactic use of antidepressant drugs. While preference has been expressed for conventional tricyclic antidepressants, these are known to have significant seizure-potentiating effects. In this author's opinion, SSRIs are as efficacious as tricyclic antidepressants, but they have a lower potential of precipitating seizures and therefore may be a preferable choice in this setting.

Prodromal dysphoric disorders tend to appear a few hours before a seizure and to be short lived. Clobazam may be used to prevent seizures in this setting, but this approach may not be easy to apply in practical terms, except for those patients where the clinical pattern is so stereotyped as to predict reliably the occurrence of a seizure sufficiently in advance. Postictal dysphoria is similarly short-lived, and it is usually described as a self-remitting period of 'black mood' following a seizure. This condition may have several psychological and psychodynamic explanations, and it is seen by many as an understandable reaction to an adverse life event. However, the sudden onset, the intensity and the often sudden disappearance of the symptom, which may be witnessed repeatedly (for example, in the setting of a seizure monitoring unit), are so distinct as to suggest the intervention of specific pathogenetic factors.

A separate dysphoric disorder is observed in young women with epilepsy around the time of their menstrual periods. In this catamenial disorder, a triad of symptoms including dysphoria, cluster of seizures and menses occur every month, starting a few days before onset of the menstrual period and resolving with the completion of menses. This pattern is repeated month after month and can be a source of significant distress. A parallel exists in the widely recognized premenstrual dysphoric disorder [35], except that in women with epilepsy seizures complicate the situation further. The intermittent use of clobazam, starting in the week before the onset of menses, may be helpful in breaking this cycle. In some individuals, continuous prophylaxis with an antidepressant drug may be required.

Personality disorders

Presentation

Historically, patients with chronic epilepsy have been reported to show an increased prevalence of certain personality changes. In particular, based on initial work by Geschwind, temporal lobe epilepsy has been associated with a triad of disorders consisting of changes in sexual behaviour (hyposexuality, or a decreased interest in sexual matters), hypergraphia (compulsive writing) and hyper-religiosity (an expansive interest in religious matters). Bear and Fedio [36] developed an instrument sensitive to detection of these personality changes.

Interestingly, laterality differences have been described. Patients with left-sided epileptogenic foci have been reported as being more ideative (i.e. to have philosophical interests, sense of personal destiny), with a tendency to tarnish their own image (i.e. to have a poorer opinion about themselves compared with reports from their spouses), whereas persons with right-sided foci have been described as being more emotional, with a tendency to alternate between periods of sadness and elation, and to polish their own image (i.e. to have a better opinion of themselves than that reported by their spouses) [37]. This so-called syndrome of temporal hyperconnection [38] appears to contrast with the Kluver–Bucy syndrome of disconnection, which is associated with hypermetamorphosis (as opposed to viscosity and attention to detail), inappropriate hypersexuality (as opposed to hyposexuality) and placidity (as opposed to emotional intensity).

It has been pointed out that the personality traits described in temporal lobe epilepsy usually manifest in a mild form, and have positive implications in that they make these persons honest, reliable, dependable and upstanding members of the community they live in. It is only when the above manifestations are very prominent, and interfere with normal social functioning, that problems are encountered [1].

In contrast with patients with temporal lobe epilepsy, patients with juvenile myoclonic epilepsy have been reported as having a tendency to show lability of mood and emotion, and immaturity (referred to as eternal adolescence). This impulsive trait has been claimed to result potentially in socially inappropriate behaviour, and occasionally in dyscontrol phenomena [39].

Treatment

Some antiepileptic drugs have a thymoleptic effect and therefore they may help in achieving some control and stabilization of behaviour. There have been elegant proposals recently that have called for rationalization of drug therapy based on the cognitive and behavioural side-effects of the drugs concerned (i.e. activating vs. sedating agents) [40]. According to this approach, choice of the correct drug could prevent or minimize disruption due to intermittent behavioural instability.

In subjects who suffer from paroxysmal affective-somatoform symptoms, the use of antidepressants has been recommended. The implications of antidepressant therapy in a patient with personality disorder are no different from those discussed earlier in this chapter with respect to the use of the same drugs in other psychopathologies. However, there is a caveat in that the differential diagnosis between the behavioural manifestation of a personality disorder (for example, irritability) and the manifestations of a comorbid affective-somatoform disorder can be difficult even for the most experienced clinician. Therefore, caution is necessary when psychotropic agents are prescribed. Antipsychotic agents may also be required from time to time, especially in patients prone to significant irritability, outbursts of temper and bouts of aggression. A low potency antipsychotic such as sulpiride, administered continuously in divided daily doses, can be a useful adjunctive therapy, and may help to prevent behavioural exacerbations in some individuals. As in all other personality disorders, long-term management strategy should rely on psychological treatment aimed at helping the individual and those in his environment to identify and to cope with the specific problem areas.

Novel treatments for epilepsy-associated neuropsychology

Vagal nerve stimulation has in recent times been increasingly used in the treatment of patients with partial seizures that are refractory to antiepileptic drugs and unsuitable for epilepsy surgery. Vagal nerve stimulation is claimed to be relatively safe and well tolerated, and to reduce seizure frequency by 50% or more in up to 50% of patients. In some patients, vagal nerve stimulation has been reported to reduce seizure severity, to abort seizures with on-demand stimulation and to improve mood and alertness [41].

While the mechanisms underlying the therapeutic effect of vagal nerve stimulation are not known, the possibility of this treatment having favourable effects on mood have stimulated considerable interest, and there are a number of on-going trials to explore this further. The advantage of vagal nerve stimulation in patients with epilepsy and comorbid depression is that the treatment might have a beneficial effect in both disorders [42,43]. Recent research is also focusing on the potential value of other stimulation techniques such as transcranial magnetic stimulation for the treatment of epilepsy and neuropsychiatric disorder. These techniques, however, are still in their infancy, and extensive reasearch is required to define their potential value [44].

There have also been reports suggesting that in some patients these innovative treatments, including vagal nerve stimulation, may lead to the emergence of psychopathology and accompanying EEG changes [45]. These observations reinforce our inability to clearly understand the mechanisms underlying the relationship between epilepsy and psychopathology, and the mechanisms by which available treatments exert their effects.

Psychological therapies

A recent meta-analysis of psychological therapies in epilepsy concluded that 'in view of the methodological deficiencies and limited number of patients studied, we have found no reliable evidence to support the use of these treatments and further trials are needed' [46]. The techniques reviewed in this study included relaxation therapy, cognitive behaviour therapy, EEG biofeedback and educational interventions. The caveat of course, was that very few studies were randomized or quasi-randomized, and the vast majority of studies were thus excluded from the analysis.

However, if one accepts that useful data can be derived from stud-ies other than randomized trials and meta-analysis, there is some evidence that psychological interventions may have a role in the management of patients with epilepsy. Indeed, in epilepsy units privileged enough to have dedicated psychological support, there is a common belief that these methods significantly contribute to effective patient management.

Several models of cognitive behaviour therapy have been applied in epilepsy, ranging from more generic applications of cognitive behaviour theory [47] to rather more specific models based on original research in patients with epilepsy or non-epileptic attack disorder (see [48] for a review). Cognitive behaviour therapy as a technique is amenable to testing in randomized controlled trials, and it could be adapted to an epilepsy-focused treatment. Many teams in specialist centres in the UK have successfully developed in-house approaches based on the cognitive behaviour therapy model, and use these to some effect.

The brief form of psychotherapy is another technique frequently used by psychologists. This is usually directed at more psychologically minded individuals, especially those with difficult backgrounds and past emotional trauma, issues that the skilled therapist is able to address. The role of specialist epilepsy nurses must not be underestimated, and there is emerging evidence of success with such nurse practitioner interventions [49,50]. Group psychotherapy or patient support groups, family therapy and counselling (often by trained lay counsellors) may all be helpful in the management of patients with epilepsy. There have also been efforts recently to develop neurobehavioural treatments specific to epilepsy [51], and the results of formal trials with such therapies are awaited. Undoubtedly, as the authors of the meta-analysis conclude, randomized controlled trials that meet current scientific standards need to be carried out [46].

Conclusions

The treatment of psychiatric disorders in epilepsy remains largely opinion-led, and not based on evidence from modern clinical trials. In most units, the choice of treatment is still based on existing clinical practice, availability of resources, access to such resources and cost. Since paradoxically many antiepileptic drugs can either stabilize mood or induce psychopathology, the first step in treatment is to optimize drug therapy.

The most widely used therapeutic tools include antidepressants, antipsychotics and anxiolytics, depending on the characteristics of the disorder being managed. Among these drug classes, drug choice is driven by consideration of side-effect profiles, with special reference to the risk of drug-induced seizure aggravation, and the potential for interactions with underlying medication. ECT is used only in the most severe cases in specialized units with good facilities and back-up.

A range of psychological therapies are currently employed, and while it is difficult to choose between them in the absence of hard evidence, cognitive behavioural approaches are finding favour, both because they lend themselves to clinical testing, and because they can be adapted to address specific issues in epilepsy. Novel treatments such as vagal nerve stimulation and transcranial magnetic stimulation have the potential to improve both epilepsy and behavioural disorder, and may well gain greater popularity in the future.

References

1 Krishnamoorthy ES. Psychiatric issues in epilepsy. *Curr Opin Neurol* 2001; 14: 217–24.

2 Slater E, Beard AW. The schizophrenia like psychosis of epilepsy. *Br J Psychiatr* 1963; 109: 95–112.

3 Landolt H. Serial electroencephalographic investigations during psychotic episodes in epileptic patients and during schizophrenic attacks. In: Lorentz de Haas AM, ed. *Lectures on Epilepsy*. Amsterdam: Elsevier, 1958: 91–133.

4 Lancman M. Psychosis and peri-ictal confusional states. *Neurology* 1999; 53 (Suppl. 2): S33–S38.

5 Trimble MR. New antiepileptic drugs and psychopathology. *Neuropsychobiology* 1998: 38(3); 149–51.

6 Ketter TA, Malow BA, Flamini R, White SR, Post RM, Theodore WH. Anticonvulsant withdrawal-emergent psychopathology. *Neurology* 1994; 44(1): 55–61.

7 Anhoury S, Brown RJ, Krishnamoorthy ES, Trimble MR. Psychiatric outcome following temporal lobectomy: A predictive study. *Epilepsia* 2000; 41(12): 1608–15.

8 Fisher RS, Vickrey BG, Gibson P *et al.* The impact of epilepsy from the patient's perspective I. Descriptions and subjective perceptions. *Epilepsy Res* 2000; 41: 39–51.

9 Post RM, Ketter TA, Denicoff K *et al.* The place of anticonvulsant therapy in bipolar illness. *Psychopharmacology (Berl)* 1996; 128(2): 115–29.

10 Kellner CH, Bernstein HJ. ECT as a treatment for neurologic illness. In: Coffey CE, ed. *The Clinical Science of Electroconvulsive Therapy*, series ed. Spiegel D. *Progress in Psychiatry*, Number 38, Washington, DC: American Psychiatric Press, 1993: 183–212.

11 Trimble MR. *The Psychoses of Epilepsy*. New York: Raven Press, 1991.

12 Guerrini R, Belmonte A, Campichi R, Casalini C, Perucca E. Reversible pseudo-atrophy of the brain and mental deterioration associated with valproate treatment. *Epilepsia* 1998; 39: 27–32.

13 Strub RL, Black FW. *The Mental Status Examination in Neurology*. Philadelphia: FA Davis Company, 1985: 15–17.

14 Gelenberg AJ. The catatonic syndrome. *Lancet* 1976; 19, 1 (7973): 1339–41.

15 Gjessing LR. A review of periodic catatonia. *Biol Psychiatry* 1974; 8(1): 23–45.

16 Kifune A, Kubota F, Shibata N, Akata T, Kikuchi S. Valproic acid-induced hyperammonemic encephalopathy with triphasic waves. *Epilepsia* 2000; 41(7): 909–12.

17 Allen MH, Currier GW, Hughes DH, Reyes-Harde M, Docherty JP; The Expert Consensus Panel for Behavioural Emergencies. The Expert Consensus Guideline Series. Treatment of behavioural emergencies. *Postgrad Med* 2001; (Spec No): 1–88.

18 Lee JW, Schwartz DL, Hallmayer J. Catatonia in a psychiatric intensive care facility: incidence and response to benzodiazepines. *Ann Clin Psychiatr* 2000; 12(2): 89–96.

19 Kanner AM. Psychosis of epilepsy: a neurologist's perspective. *Epilepsy Behav* 2000; 1: 219–27.

20 Wolf P. Acute behavioural symptomatology at disappearance of epileptiform EEG abnormality: paradoxical or forced normalisation. In: Smith D, Trieman D and Trimble MR, eds. *Neurobehavioral Problems in Epilepsy*. New York: Raven Press, 1991: 127–42.

21 Tellenbach H. Epilepsiaals Anfallsleiden und Als Psychose. *Nervenartz* 1965; 36: 190–202.

22 Krishnamoorthy ES, Trimble MR. Forced normalisation—clinical and therapeutic relevance. *Epilepsia* 1999; 40 (Suppl. 10): S57–S64.

23 Logsdail SJ, Toone BK. Post-ictal psychoses. A clinical and phenomenological description. *Br J Psych* 1988; 152: 246–52.

24 McConnell HW, Duncan D. Treatment of psychiatric co-morbidity in epilepsy. In: McConnell HW, Snyder PJ, eds. *Psychiatric Co-morbidity in Epilepsy: Basic Mechanisms, Diagnosis, and Treatment*. Arlington, VA: American Psychiatric Press, 1998.

25 Miller DD. Review and management of clozapine side effects. *J Clin Psychiatr* 2000; 61 (Suppl. 8): 14–17.

26 Centorrino F, Price BH, Tuttle M *et al.* EEG abnormalities during treatment with typical and atypical antipsychotics. *Am J Psychiatr* 2002; 159 (1): 109–15.

27 Langosch JM, Trimble MR. Epilepsy, psychosis and clozapine. *Human Psychopharmacol* 2002; 17(2): 115–19.

28 Satishchandra P, Trimble MR. On being seizure free. *Epilepsy Behav* 2001; 2: 4–7.

29 Lambert M, Robertson MM. Depression in epilepsy: etiology, phenomenology, and treatment. *Epilepsia* 1999; 40 (Suppl. 10): S21–S47.

30 Goldstein MA, Harden CL. Epilepsy and anxiety. *Epilepsy Behav* 2000; 1: 228–34.

31 Blumer D. Dysphoric disorders and paroxysmal effects: recognition and treatment of epilepsy-related psychiatric disorders. *Harvard Rev Psychiatr* 2000; 8(1): 8–17.

32 Newsom-Davis I, Goldstein LH, Fitzpatrick D. Fear of seizures—an investigation and treatment. *Seizure* 1998; 7: 101–6.

33 Robertson MM, Trimble MR. The treatment of depression in patients with epilepsy. A double-blind trial. *J Affect Disord* 1985; 9(2): 127–36.

34 Andersen BB, Mikkelsen M, Vesterager A *et al.* No influence of the antidepressant paroxetine on carbamazepine, valproate and phenytoin. *Epilepsy Res* 1991; 10(2–3): 201–4.

35 Endicott J. History, evolution, and diagnosis of premenstrual dysphoric disorder. *J Clin Psychtr* 2000; 61 (Suppl. 12): 5–8.

36 Bear DM, Fedio P. Quantitative analysis of interictal behaviour in temporal lobe epilepsy. *Arch Neurol* 1977; 34: 454–67.

37 Blumer D. Personality disorders in epilepsy. In: Ratey JJ, ed. *Neuropsychiatry of Personality Disorders*. Boston: Blackwell Science, 1995: 230–63.

38 Bear DM. Temporal lobe epilepsy—a syndrome of hyperconnection. *Cortex* 1979; 15: 357–84.

39 Trimble M. Cognitive and personality profiles in patients with juvenile myoclonic epilepsy. In: Schmitz B, Sander T, eds. *Juvenile Myoclonic Epilepsy—The Janz Syndrome*. Petersfield: Wrightson Biomedical Publishing, 2000: 101–11.

40 Ketter TA, Post RM, Theodore WH. Positive and negative psychiatric effects of antiepileptic drugs in patients with seizure disorders. *Neurology* 1999; 53 (Suppl. 2): S53–S67.

41 Schmidt D. Vagus nerve stimulation for the treatment of epilepsy. *Epilepsy Behav* 2001; 2: S1–S5.

42 Harden CL, Pulver MC, Ravdin LD, Nikolov B, Halper JP, Labar DR. A pilot study of mood in epilepsy patients treated with vagus nerve stimulation. *Epilepsy Behav* 2000; 1: 93–9.

43 Elger G, Hoppe C, Falkai P, Rush AJ, Elger CE. Vagus nerve stimulation is associated with mood improvements in epilepsy patients. *Epilepsy Res* 2000; 42 (2–3): 203–10.

44 George MS. Summary and future directions of therapeutic brain stimulation: neurostimulation and neuropsychiatric disorders. *Epilepsy Behav* 2001; 2: S95–S100.

45 Gatzonis SD, Stamboulis E, Siafakas A. Acute psychosis and EEG normalisation after vagus nerve stimulation. *Lett J Neurol Neurosurg Psych* 2000; 69: 278–9.

46 Ramaratnam S, Baker GA, Goldstein L. Psychological treatments for epilepsy (Cochrane Review). *Cochrane Database Syst Rev* 2001; 4: CD002029.

47 Beck AT. Cognitive therapy: past, present, and future. *J Consult Clin Psychol* 1993; 61(2): 194–8.

48 Goldstein LH. Behavioural and cognitive-behavioural treatments for epilepsy: a progress review. *Br J Clin Psychol* 1990; 29 (Pt 3): 257–69.

49 Ridsdale L, Kwan I, Cryer C. The effect of a special nurse on patients' knowledge of epilepsy and their emotional state. Epilepsy Evaluation Care Group. *Br J Gen Pract* 1999; 49: 285–9.

50 Ridsdale L, Kwan I, Cryer C. Newly diagnosed epilepsy: can nurse specialists help? A randomised controlled trial. Epilepsy Care Evaluation Group. *Epilepsia* 2000; 41 (8): 1014–19.

51 Andrews DJ, Reiter JM, Schonfeld W, Kastl A, Denning P. A neurobehavioral treatment for unilateral complex partial disorders: A comparison of right- and left-hemisphere patients. *Seizure* 2000; 9: 189–91.

The Ketogenic Diet

E.H. Kossoff and E.P.G. Vining

The ketogenic diet is a high-fat, adequate protein, low-carbohydrate diet that has been used for the treatment of intractable childhood epilepsy since the 1920s. The diet mimics the biochemical changes associated with starvation that have been well documented to reduce seizures. Although less well utilized in the decades to follow due to the increased availability of anticonvulsants such as phenytoin and carbamazepine, it has re-emerged as a viable therapeutic option. Whereas only a decade ago the ketogenic diet was seen as a last resort, it has become more frequently used in academic centres throughout the world even early in the course of epilepsies. Advances in research have helped to elaborate on the mechanisms by which the ketogenic diet reduces seizures, identify new indications for the diet, and clarify issues regarding side-effects.

History

The history of the ketogenic diet has been described in great detail [1]. The use of diet manipulation to control seizures has its origins in biblical times, with descriptions of Jesus curing 'possessed' patients with prayer and fasting. In 1911, Guelpa and Marie [2] reported the use of fasting to improve epilepsy in the French population. Interest in the USA originates with Geyelin [3], who reported at the 1921 American Medical Association convention the successful use of 3 weeks of fasting for 26 patients with severe epilepsy. Much of his protocol was based on the work of Conklin [4], an osteopathic physician from Michigan who treated a 10-year-old boy with the help of a faith healer, Bernarr Macfadden, and a 'water diet'.

Research into the effectiveness of the ketogenic diet soon followed as the word of this successful advance in epilepsy spread. Gamble and Howland subsequently investigated the ketogenic diet at the Johns Hopkins Hospital [5]. Early research indicated a potential role of acidosis, dehydration and ketosis [6–8]. Wilder [8] from the Mayo Clinic first proposed attempting an actual diet. This ketogenic diet mimicked starvation by providing a regimen of 1 g/kg protein, 10–15 g of carbohydrate and the remaining calories per day as fat [9]. A ratio of fats to carbohydrates and protein of at least 2 : 1 was required to maintain ketosis. Calories were based on the basal metabolic rate plus 50%. This is quite similar to the ketogenic diet still in use today.

Further reports of efficacy followed [10] but were later overshadowed by the discovery of phenytoin in 1938. As the era of new anticonvulsants began, the ketogenic diet was viewed as rigid and restrictive. A medium-chain triglyceride (MCT) oil containing diet was developed to make the diet easier to use [11]. A study comparing the classical ketogenic diet, the MCT oil diet and a modified MCT oil diet revealed similar efficacies, with 81% of patients on both diets having a greater than 50% reduction in seizures [12].

As new anticonvulsants continued to become available, many epileptologists felt the diet was not useful. However, several centres continued to use the diet actively [13]. In 1992, a 2-year-old boy named Charlie was brought to the Johns Hopkins Hospital due to intractable epilepsy [14]. After his son responded extremely well to the ketogenic diet, Charlie's father created the Charlie Foundation that has helped inform patients and physicians about the ketogenic diet. Since then, many medical centres have started using the ketogenic diet and several large studies have demonstrated its effectiveness [15–17]. The ketogenic diet is now well established in the medical community and even reimbursed by insurance companies including Blue Cross/Blue Shield [18].

Mechanisms of action

The ketogenic diet mimics the starvation state by utilizing a high-fat, adequate protein, low-carbohydrate diet. The actual mechanism by which the ketogenic diet helps suppress epilepsy remains unclear despite decades of research [19]. Initial research theorized that acidosis, dehydration and hyperlipidaemia reduced seizures, but these have been abandoned in favour of ketone bodies [1].

Ketone bodies (acetoacetate and α-hydroxybutyrate) are formed in the liver, often preferentially when the body is forced to use stored fats for energy (Fig. 21.1) [1]. Long-chain fatty acids are released from adipose tissue in a starvation state, transported via plasma to the liver cytosolic membrane, and then enter mitochondria via the carnitine acyltransferase system [20]. Once inside the mitochondria, α-fatty acid oxidation converts the fatty acids to acetyl coenzyme A (CoA). Acetyl CoA is then converted to ketone bodies. Medium-chain fatty acids are also converted to acetyl CoA via acyl-CoA synthetase, but are able to bypass the carnitine acyltransferase system.

Ketone bodies are utilized efficiently by the body, and can provide 65% of the brain's energy requirements in starvation states [21]. Ketone bodies are transported into the brain after being synthesized in the liver via a monocarboxylic acid transporter [22]. Once there, they are both metabolized via the tricarboxylic acid (TCA) cycle into energy and converted into cholesterol, lipids and fatty acids [1]. Elevated levels of ketone bodies also inhibit glucose metabolism in the brain, returning the glucose to the liver for gluconeogenesis as lactate and pyruvate [23].

The exact mechanism by which elevated ketone bodies in the brain reduce seizures is less clear. Uhlemann and Neims [24] developed the first animal model of the ketogenic diet in 1972. Mice were made ketotic using a diet and were then tested for protection against

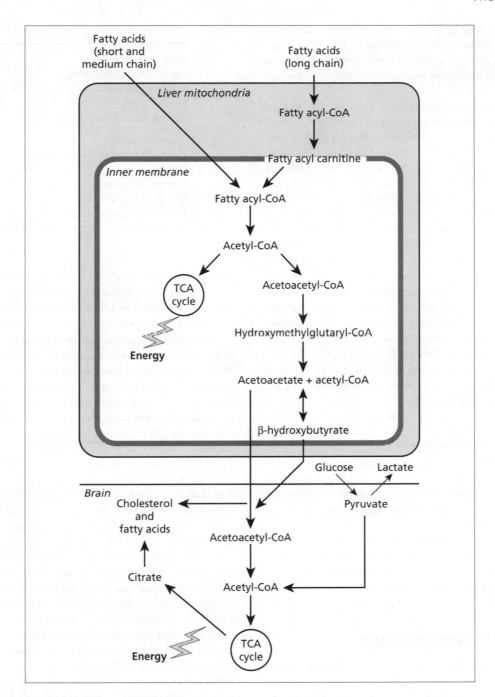

Fig. 21.1 Fatty acid metabolism in the liver and brain.

electroshock- and bicuculline-induced seizures. Ketonaemia protected the mice against both methods of seizure induction, with loss of this protection within 3.5 h of diet discontinuation [24]. In addition, younger mice (16 days old) were able to produce higher ketonaemia and thus longer seizure protection than older mice (40 days old). Other studies of rats have reproduced this protective effect [25,26]. A more recent study [27] showed effectiveness in the more standard models of pentylenetetrazole- and electroshock-induced seizures.

More recent research has attempted to elucidate the mechanisms by which ketone bodies affect seizure thresholds. There has been some suggestion that ketone bodies are structurally similar to γ-aminobutyric acid (GABA) and may act as anticonvulsants in themselves [19,28]. Thio *et al.* [29], however, recently demonstrated that direct application of ketone bodies to rat hippocampus failed to affect directly synaptic transmission. Another study [30] in epileptic mutant mice found that the ketogenic diet increased glial fibrillary acidic protein (GFAP) expression in the dentate gyrus of the hippocampus, suggesting that protection against seizures may involve a depressive effect on synaptic reorganization.

Outcomes

Many retrospective studies of the ketogenic diet's efficacy have been performed. Initial findings by Peterman in 1925 [31] showed that 95% of children on the ketogenic diet had more than 50% reduction in their seizures. Reports of results from the 1980s also showed efficacy, with 67% of children showing greater than 50% improvement in their seizures [17].

Two prospective uncontrolled studies in 1998 [15,16] brought the ketogenic diet's usefulness for intractable epilepsy to the medical mainstream. A multicentre study from seven sites enrolled 51 children aged 1–8 years on a 4:1 ketogenic diet. At 3 months, 54% had a greater than 50% reduction in seizures, compared with 55% at 6 months, and 40% at 1 year [15]. In addition, side-effects were uncommon, and 47% stayed on the diet to 1 year.

The Johns Hopkins Pediatric Epilepsy Center published their experience with 150 children that same year [16]. These children were of similar ages and had intractable epilepsy (mean 410 seizures/month, 6.2 prior anticonvulsants). Efficacy was similar to the multicentre study, with 50% having greater than 50% seizure reduction at 1 year and 27% having greater than 90% seizure reduction. This original 150 patient cohort was subsequently followed for 3–6 years [32]. Families were surveyed and 142 responded. Of these children, 44% were still more than 50% improved several years later, and 78% of those who remained on the diet at least 12 months were more than 50% improved. Of these parents, 50% were moderately to extremely satisfied with the ketogenic diet and 50% reduced their child's anticonvulsants.

A study is underway to address prospectively the efficacy of the ketogenic diet in a randomized, placebo-controlled manner at the Johns Hopkins Pediatric Epilepsy Center. Children are being started on a ketogenic diet but then are provided with a solution to take orally daily of either placebo or glucose. After 5 days, each subject is crossed over to restart the ketogenic diet with the alternative solution. EEGs, clinical seizure activity and ketones are being monitored to assess efficacy.

A possible additional benefit of the ketogenic diet is a reduction in medication costs. In one study [33], 74% of patients had their medications reduced with a cost reduction of 70%. The average estimated cost reduction per child per year was $530 (US) in this report.

Indications for the ketogenic diet (Table 21.1)

Use of the ketogenic diet is restricted mainly to the treatment of refractory paediatric epilepsies. Intractability is the main reason that children are placed on the ketogenic diet, as many clinicians are aware of the difficulty in controlling seizures after two anticonvulsants have failed. There is no question that children who have cognitive or behavioural side-effects from multiple anticonvulsants can have improvement on the ketogenic diet in combination with a reduction in medications [34]. In addition, the ability to exercise control over their child's epilepsy makes the ketogenic diet attractive to many parents [34]. Children with gastrostomy tubes are also a population that is likely to be compliant with good efficacy (La Vega-Talbott, unpublished observations, 2001). Some important contraindications for the ketogenic diet are listed in Table 21.1.

Many researchers have sought to identify predictive factors for maximal benefit from the ketogenic diet. Age of the child does not seem to be a factor in predicting effectiveness, with several studies showing no difference in outcome [15,16]. Certainly infants can

Table 21.1 Indications and contraindications of the ketogenic diet

Indications
Intractable epilepsy (children)
Epilepsy with intolerable anticonvulsant side-effects
Glucose transporter protein deficiency (GLUT-1)
Pyruvate decarboxylase deficiency
Contraindications
Pyruvate carboxylase deficiency
Porphyria
Carnitine deficiency
Mitochondrial disorders
Fatty acid oxidation defects

tolerate and derive significant benefit from the ketogenic diet if followed carefully [35]. Infants can do extremely well, especially as the diet can be provided as a liquid formula using Ross Carbohydrate Free (RCF), microlipids (Mead Johnson) and polycose. In addition, a commercially available, powder form, ketogenic diet quite similar in appearance to our prescribed liquid diet has now been produced (SHS International, Ltd, Rockville, Maryland).

Seizure type and EEG pattern also does not seem to be predictive [15–17]. In the multicentre trial [15], there was no difference in outcome between seizure types although a small decreased efficacy was seen for those children with multifocal spikes on EEG at 3 months ($P=0.04$). A common conception is that children with Lennox–Gastaut-type seizure disorders will have better improvement on the ketogenic diet, but at least one study looking at that issue found no statistically significant difference [16]. Seizure frequency also has not been shown to be predictive [16].

A retrospective study of 23 infants placed on the ketogenic diet for difficult-to-control infantile spasms revealed 38% with greater than 90% seizure reduction at 3 months and 46% at 12 months with greater than 90% seizure reduction [36]. Of these infants, 57% had their medications reduced and the same number had developmental progression, which was correlated with seizure control ($P=0.03$). Even in this age range, in which some children were as young as 5 months, tolerability was high.

Special indications for the ketogenic diet do exist in paediatric epilepsy. Children with glucose transporter protein deficiency (GLUT-1) and pyruvate dehydrogenase deficiency should be treated with the ketogenic diet as first-line [37,38]. In both cases, the utilization of alternative sources to glucose for brain metabolism can prevent seizures by providing acetyl CoA directly into the TCA cycle without prior glycolysis.

Some centres have attempted to use the ketogenic diet in adults [39]. In one study [39], 10 adults were placed on a 4:1 ketogenic diet as adjunctive therapy for predominantly partial epilepsy. All 10 patients had greater than 50% improvement, but two had to stop the diet due to intolerability.

Calculation of the ketogenic diet

The ketogenic diet is calculated individually for each patient and can be quite variable at times. In general, certain guidelines do apply for deciding on the ratio, calories and fluid requirements for a given child. The ratio of fats to carbohydrates and protein is based on the age, size, weight and activity level of the patient. A young child or infant often receives a 3 : 1 diet to provide additional protein. Older children will receive a 4 : 1 diet with the exception of obese children (3 : 1). Adolescents will often be started on a 3 : 1 diet to also provide the extra protein necessary during this age period and because it is slightly less restrictive.

Calories have historically been targeted at 75% of the recommended daily intake for age; however, at our institution it is more variable than this. Parents are asked to provide a 3-day menu of typical foods for the child and we then assess current body weight. Significantly overweight children may be given only 25–30% of the recommended calories until they approach their ideal body weight.

Fluids are targeted at 80% of daily needs, with instructions given to parents to provide as much clear, non-carbohydrate containing fluids as necessary during illnesses. If a child has a family history of renal calculi or is also receiving topiramate, acetazolamide or zonisamide, fluids are increased to 100%.

Initiation of the ketogenic diet (Table 21.2)

For 1–2 days before the child is fasted, the family provides less carbohydrates to the child. The child begins to fast after dinner of the evening prior to admission. Occasionally small children will be fasted for 24 h, but this shortening of the fast is often unnecessary. Several centres have preliminary data reporting excellent ketosis within a similar number of days in children not fasted; however the rapid reduction of seizures that can be seen with earlier ketosis is often very reassuring for family members [40,41].

On Day 1 of hospitalization, the child is admitted. Fluids are restricted to 60–75 mL/kg and children often need to be encouraged

Table 21.2 Ketogenic diet protocol (see text for more details)

Before diet
Less carbohydrates for 1–2 days
Fasting starts the night before admission

Day 1
Admitted to the hospital
Fasting continues
Fluids restricted to 60–75 cm³/kg
Blood glucose monitored every 6 h
Use carbohydrate-free medication

Day 2
Dinner given as 1/3 of calculated diet meal as eggnog
Blood glucose checks discontinued after dinner

Day 3
Breakfast and lunch given as 1/3 of diet
Dinner increased to 2/3 (still eggnog)

Day 4
Breakfast and lunch given as 2/3 of diet allowance
Dinner is first full ketogenic meal (not eggnog)

Day 5
Full ketogenic diet breakfast given
Child discharged to home

to drink secondary to the effects of ketosis on thirst. Blood glucose is monitored with finger dextrosticks every 6 h unless it falls below 40 mg/dL, after which it is checked every 2 h. If the child has symptoms of hypoglycaemia or the glucose level falls below 25 mg/dL, 30 mL of orange juice is provided and the glucose is checked 1 h later. Even small children tolerate the fast well, with rare symptomatic hypoglycaemia. Daily urine ketones are checked as well. Ketosis can begin during the fasting period, and the resultant nausea and vomiting can occasionally require intravenous hydration using non-dextrose containing fluids.

Anticonvulsant medications are continued during the fasting period at their previous doses. Phenobarbital is one exception as its serum level often rises during ketosis and its daily dose may need to be reduced, often by about 30%, particularly in children with high baseline serum phenobarbital concentrations and/or pre-existing side-effects from phenobarbital. All medications are carefully examined for carbohydrate content and formulations changed when necessary.

On Day 2, fasting continues until dinner when one-third of the calculated diet is provided as an 'eggnog' which looks and tastes like a milk shake and can be sipped, frozen as ice cream or cooked as scrambled eggs. Excess ketosis at this time that causes nausea and vomiting can be relieved with a small amount of orange juice. Once the child begins eating, serum glucose checks are unnecessary and discontinued.

Breakfast and lunch remain at one-third of the calculated calories as eggnog on Day 3, but dinner increases to two-thirds of the usual allowance (still eggnog). On Day 4, breakfast and lunch are also increased to two-thirds of allowance, and dinner is then given as the first full ketogenic diet meal (with actual foods provided). On hospital Day 5, the child receives a full ketogenic breakfast and is discharged to home. All children are sent home with prescriptions for urine ketosticks, additional calcium and a sugar-free, fat-soluble vitamin and mineral supplement. Medications are left unchanged and follow-up is arranged.

Throughout the 5-day hospital stay, classes are held with physicians, nurses and dietitians to teach the family about the rationale of the ketogenic diet, calculation of meals, nutrition label reading and management of their children during illnesses. This is just as important to achieving a favourable outcome as the actual logistics of the diet initiation. Examples of typical ketogenic meals are given in Table 21.3.

After discharge parents are instructed to check urine ketones daily and the diet is individually adjusted after consultation by telephone to maximize seizure control. Another option is to use commercially available blood ketone meters that measure α-hydroxybutyrate levels (range 0–4 mmol/L) (Polymer Technology Systems, Inc., Indianapolis). The advantages of these meters over urine ketones remains to be determined, but in many cases the urine ketones may measure 4+ (maximum) while serum will only be 2 mmol/L, with additional seizure control gained when the level increases above 4 mmol/L [42].

Serum glucose or electrolytes are not routinely monitored after discharge. Weight is monitored by the parents and reported if significantly changed. Periodic laboratory measures are obtained to monitor for side-effects (lipid profile, electrolytes, anticonvulsant levels, urine calcium/creatinine). Urine alkalinization is accomplished with the use of Polycitra K should the urine calcium to crea-

Table 21.3 Examples of typical 'attractive' ketogenic meals (3:1 ratio, 349 calories each)

Breakfast
23 g 36% heavy cream
49 g fresh egg
9 g moderate carbohydrate vegetable (carrots, broccoli, tomato)
20 g butter
9 g cooked bacon

Lunch
40 g 36% heavy cream
34 g chunk albacore tuna fish (in water)
8 g moderate carbohydrate vegetable
20 g butter

Table 21.4 Major side-effects reported with the ketogenic diet

Constipation
Exacerbation of gastrooesophageal reflux
Water-soluble vitamin deficiency
Elevated serum cholesterol and LDL
Renal stones (5–8%)
Growth inhibition
Worsening of acidosis with illnesses

tinine ratio exceed 0.2. Medications may be tapered and discontinued in an individual and non-systematic manner as early as 2–3 months after diet initiation.

Handling increased seizures

Parents and physicians not familiar with the ketogenic diet are often very uncomfortable handling increased seizures. Certain basic management options apply to help improve seizure control. First, we always try to ensure that no new medications have been added that might contain carbohydrate (e.g. antibiotics, anticonvulsants). Occasionally, topical ointments and lotions (e.g. sunscreen, hair gels) contain sorbitol, which can be systemically absorbed, especially in very young children. Many food additives are described as 'sugar-free' but contain carbohydrate-containing chemicals such as maltodextrin, sorbitol, starch and fructose. Secondly, the family should check urine ketones to ensure adequate ketosis. If ketones are not 4+, the child can be fasted with clear liquids for 24 h to improve ketosis rapidly. Periodic oral or rectal benzodiazepines can be useful for seizure exacerbations as well.

Discontinuation of the ketogenic diet

The issue of when to discontinue the ketogenic diet is a difficult one. Many families are reluctant to discontinue a therapy that has been effective for years and risk restarting the anticonvulsants that were either ineffective in the past or caused side-effects [43]. With potential long-term effects of the diet on lipids and growth, after several years on the diet one is somewhat inclined to try and discontinue it. Similarly to anticonvulsants, the diet is tapered slowly over 3–6 months by gradually lowering the fat to protein and carbohydrate ratio, then relaxing the weighing of ingredients and lastly adding new carbohydrate foods over weeks while keeping calories constant. If the child is having significant difficulty with the ketogenic diet, it can be discontinued immediately, however, without dramatic increase in seizures in many cases.

In the rare patient who has remained on the diet for as long as 15 years, no major side-effects have been seen. An outcome study of 150 children [32], questioned 3–6 years after starting the diet, revealed that 10% were still on the ketogenic diet after more than 4 years with no cardiac complications. Discontinuation during the first year of therapy was often secondary to perceived ineffectiveness or restrictiveness. After 1 year, significantly fewer children were discontinued for these reasons and comparatively more had the diet stopped for being seizure free (often greater than 2 years) or intercurrent illness.

Side-effects

The ketogenic diet is not without side-effects. Just as with any medical therapy for seizures, benefits need to be balanced with risks (Table 21.4). Side-effects were recently well summarized in an editorial by Wheless [44].

During the initiation of the ketogenic diet, the fast itself can cause vomiting, dehydration and food refusal. These are usually transitory and easily treated; however, if the child has an underlying metabolic disorder the fast and ketogenic diet can be dangerous. All children, especially infants, need to have a thorough history, physical examination and often screening tests (lactate, pyruvate, urine organic acids and serum amino acids) performed prior to initiating the diet. Diseases that could potentially deteriorate on the ketogenic diet include pyruvate carboxylase deficiency, porphyria, carnitine deficiency, mitochondrial disorders and fatty acid oxidation defects (Table 21.1) [44].

Some of the more common side-effects include constipation, exacerbation of gastrooesophageal reflux, acidosis with illnesses, growth difficulties, renal stones and hyperlipidaemia. Constipation and gastrooesophageal reflux disease are common and likely secondary to the low roughage component of the ketogenic diet. Both can be effectively treated with increased fluids, stool softeners and laxatives when necessary. The use of MCT oil in the diet can often be helpful. Acidosis, not only during the initiation of the diet but also during acute illnesses, is a true concern and needs to be discussed at length with the family. At the time of diet initiation, parents should be taught the signs of acidosis and how to hydrate with non-sugar containing fluids.

Growth is often of concern for parents, and they need to understand that weight gain is not important with the ketogenic diet. Recent review of the diet in 237 children revealed that the rate of weight gain decreased (more so in children above the average median weight) at 3 months but then remained constant for up to 3 years [45]. The rate of height increase remained similar to the national average for the first 6 months of the diet; however it then dropped over the next 18 months, especially in those children above the median to start. There were also significant differences between age groups for height and weight, with younger children growing less well.

Renal stones occur in 5–8% of patients and tend to be either uric acid or calcium oxalate stones [46,47]. Children with a family history of kidney stones (even calcium stones) and those on carbonic anhydrase inhibitors (topiramate, zonisamide, acetazolamide) may be at higher risk for renal calculi and should be hydrated more aggressively and their urine alkalinized [48]. Renal ultrasound should be performed in any child with haematuria or pain upon urination. Periodic spot urine calcium to creatinine ratios can also help screen for this condition. If the ratio is > 0.2, potassium citrate should be started to help alkalinize the urine in children. Lithotripsy or occasionally surgical removal can be performed successfully in patients and the diet continued.

Hypercholesterolaemia does occur on the ketogenic diet. Unpublished data demonstrated that children had an increase in their cholesterol and low-density lipoprotein (LDL) levels from the 75th to the 99th percentiles after 3 months. Cholesterol levels can routinely increase to 200 mg/dL. The increase in cholesterol may be due to a ketogenic diet induced decrease in apolipoprotein B (apoB), the major serum carrier of cholesterol [49]. Triglycerides also increased in this study, but then later normalized. The long-term effects of the ketogenic diet on atherosclerosis remain to be determined. Adjustments to the diet can be made in children with significantly elevated triglycerides and cholesterol to avoid complications. Children should be screened with a serum cholesterol level if physical examination findings (such as cholesterol deposits in skin or retina) or a family history of early atherosclerosis indicates a potential case of familial hypercholesterolaemia.

More uncommon complications attributed in the literature to the diet have been reported [50–54]. They include cardiomyopathy, pancreatitis, bruising and vitamin deficiency. Most were case reports and do not conclusively prove that these problems were diet related. Four of five patients reported by Ballaban-Gil [50] had severe hypoproteinaemia, Fanconi's renal tubular acidosis and increased liver function tests potentially in combination with valproate. The correlation of these complications with the ketogenic diet is unclear, but the authors propose a possible additive effect with valproate interfering with carnitine function and fatty acid oxidation. In a study by Best et al. [51], prolonged QT interval (QTc) was discovered in three of 20 patients, but this has not been reported elsewhere. No child at our institution has ever had arrhythmias or cardiomyopathy attributable to the ketogenic diet. Increased tendency for bruising was seen in a recent study in 16 of 51 children reported by Berry-Kravis et al. [52]. A single report [53] of a child with pancreatitis did not show direct evidence of a relationship to the ketogenic diet. Vitamin deficiency is rare [54]; however it can be appropriately avoided using supplementation. Routine administration of magnesium, zinc, vitamin D, vitamin C, B complex vitamins and additional calcium is recommended.

Summary

The ketogenic diet requires skill and commitment to initiate and to maintain, especially in older children. A well-trained team of physicians and dietitians is required. Results can be quite dramatic, even in children with epilepsy who failed multiple anticonvulsants. Efficacy has been established in both retrospective and prospective studies and further studies are underway to examine its utility in specific syndromes. Side-effects, especially growth failure, hyperlipidaemia, renal calculi, constipation and acidosis, do occur, but they are expected and they are treatable.

References

1 Swink TD, Vining EPG, Freeman JM. The ketogenic diet: 1997. *Adv Pediatr* 1997; 44: 297–329.

2 Guelpa G, Marie A. La lutte contre l'epilepsie par la desintoxication et par la reeducation alimentaire. *Rev Ther Med-Chirurg* 1911; 78: 8–13.

3 Geyelin HR. Fasting as a method for treating epilepsy. *Med Record* 1921; 99: 1037–9.

4 Conklin HW. Cause and treatment of epilepsy. *J Am Osteopathic Assoc* 1922; 26: 11–14.

5 Gamble JL, Ross GS, Tisdall FF. The metabolism of fixed base during fasting. *J Biol Chem* 1923; 57: 633–95.

6 Lennox WG. Ketogenic diet in treatment of epilepsy. *N Engl J Med* 1928; 199: 74.

7 McQuarrie I. Epilepsy in children: The relationship of water balance to the occurrence of seizures. *Am J Dis Child* 1929; 38: 451–67.

8 Wilder RM. The effect of ketonemia on the course of epilepsy. *Mayo Clin Bull* 1921; 2: 307–8.

9 Peterman MG. The ketogenic diet in the treatment of epilepsy: A preliminary report. *Am J Dis Child* 1924; 28: 28–33.

10 Talbot FB, Metcalf KM, Moriarty ME. Epilepsy, chemical investigation of rational treatment by production of ketosis. *Am J Dis Child* 1927; 33: 218–25.

11 Huttenlocher PR, Wilbourn AJ, Signore JM. Medium-chain triglycerides as a therapy for intractable childhood epilepsy. *Neurology* 1971; 21: 1097–103.

12 Schwartz RH, Eaton J, Bower BD et al. Ketogenic diets in the treatment of epilepsy: Short-term clinical effects. *Dev Med Child Neurol* 1989; 31: 145–51.

13 DeVivo DC. How to use other drugs (steroids) and the ketogenic diet. In: Morselli PL, Pippenger CE, Penry JK, eds. *Antiepileptic Drug Therapy in Pediatrics*. New York: Raven Press, 1983: 283–92.

14 Abrahams J. *An Introduction to the Ketogenic Diet: A treatment for pediatric epilepsy* (videotape). The Charlie Foundation, Santa Monica, California.

15 Vining EPG, Freeman JM, Ballaban-Gil K et al. A multicenter study of the efficacy of the ketogenic diet. *Arch Neurol* 1998; 55: 1433–7.

16 Freeman JM, Vining EPG, Pillas DJ, Pyzik PL, Casey JC, Kelly MT. The efficacy of the ketogenic diet – 1998: a prospective evaluation of intervention in 150 children. *Pediatrics* 1998; 102: 1358–63.

17 Kinsman SL, Vining EP, Quaskey SA, Mellits D, Freeman JM. Efficacy of the ketogenic diet for intractable seizure disorders: review of 58 cases. *Epilepsia* 1992; 33: 1132–6.

18 Lefevre F, Aronson N. Ketogenic diet for the treatment of refractory epilepsy in children: a systematic review of efficacy. *Pediatrics* 2000; 105: E46.

19 Stafstrom CE, Spencer S. The ketogenic diet: a therapy in search of an explanation. *Neurology* 2000; 54: 282–3.

20 Williamson DH. Ketone body production and metabolism in the fetus and newborn. In: Polin RA, Fox WW, eds. *Fetal and Neonatal Physiology*. Philadelphia: W.B. Saunders, 1992: 330–40.

21 Owen OE, Morgan AP, Kepm HG et al. Brain metabolism during fasting. *J Clin Invest* 1967; 46: 1589–95.

22 Moore TJ, Lione AP, Sugden MC et al. α-hydroxybutyrate transport in rat brain: Developmental and dietary modulations. *Am J Physiol* 1976; 230: 619–30.

23 DeVivo DC, Leckie MP, Ferrendelli JS, McDougal DB. Chronic ketosis and cerebral metabolism. *Ann Neurol* 1978; 3: 331–7.

24 Uhlemann ER, Neims AH. Anticonvulsant properties of the ketogenic diet in mice. *J Pharmacol Exp Ther* 1972; 180: 231–8.

25 Appleton DB, DeVivo DC. An animal model for the ketogenic diet. *Epilepsia* 1974; 15: 211–27.

26 DeVivo DC, Malas KL, Leckie MP. Starvation and seizures. *Arch Neurol* 1975; 32: 755–60.

27 Bough KJ, Eagles DA. A ketogenic diet increases the resistance to pentylenetetrazole-induced seizures in the rat. *Epilepsia* 1999; 40: 138–43.

28 Erecinska M, Nelson D, Daikhin Y, Yudkoff M. Regulation of GABA level in rat brain synaptosomes: fluxes through enzymes of the GABA shunt and effects of glutamate, calcium, and ketone bodies. *J Neurochem* 1996; 67: 2325–34.

29 Thio LL, Wong M, Yamada KA. Ketone bodies do not directly alter excita-

tory or inhibitory hippocampal synaptic transmission. *Neurology* 2000; 54: 325–31.

30 Rho JM, Robbins CA, Wenzel J, Tempel BL, Schwartzkroin PA. An experimental ketogenic diet promotes long-term survival and reduces synaptic reorganization in the hippocampus of epileptic KV1.1 null mutant mice. *Epilepsia* 2000; 41 (Suppl. 7), 34.

31 Peterman MG. The ketogenic diet in epilepsy. *J Am Med Assoc* 1925; 84: 1979–83.

32 Hemingway C, Freeman JM, Pillas DJ, Pyzik PL. The ketogenic diet: A 3–6 year follow-up of 150 children enrolled prospectively. *Pediatrics* 2001; 108: 898–905.

33 Gilbert DL, Pyzik PL, Vining EP, Freeman JM. Medication cost reduction in children on the ketogenic diet: data from a prospective study. *J Child Neurol* 1999; 14: 469–71.

34 Wheless JW. The ketogenic diet: fa(c)t or fiction. *J Child Neurol* 1995; 10: 419–23.

35 Nordli DR Jr, Kuroda MM, Carroll J *et al.* Experience with the ketogenic diet in infants. *Pediatrics* 2001; 108: 129–33.

36 Kossoff EH, Pyzik PL, McGrogan JR, Vining EP, Freeman JM. Efficacy of the ketogenic diet for infantile spasms. *Pediatrics* 2002; 109: 780–3.

37 DeVivo DC, Trifiletti RR, Jacobson RI *et al.* Glucose transport across the blood–brain barrier as a cause of persistent hypoglycorrhachia, seizures, and developmental delay. *N Engl J Med* 1991; 325: 703–9.

38 Wexler ID, Hemalatha SG, McConnell J *et al.* Outcome of pyruvate dehydrogenase deficiency treated with ketogenic diets. Studies in patients with identical mutations. *Neurology* 1997; 49: 1655–61.

39 Sirven JI, Liporace JD, O'Dwyer JL *et al.* A prospective trial of the ketogenic diet as add-on therapy in adults: preliminary results (abstract). *Epilepsia* 1998; 39: 195.

40 Wirrell EC, Darwish HZ, Williams-Dyjur C, Blackman M, Lange V. Is a fast necessary when initiating the ketogenic diet? *J Child Neurol* 2002; 17: 179–82.

41 Freeman JM, Vining EPG. Seizures decrease rapidly after fasting: preliminary studies of the ketogenic diet. *Arch Pediatr Adolesc Med* 1999; 153: 946–9.

42 Gilbert DL, Pyzik PL, Freeman JM. The ketogenic diet: seizure control correlates better with serum α-hydroxybutyrate than with urine ketones. *J Child Neurol* 2000; 15: 787–90.

43 Vining EPG. Clinical efficacy of the ketogenic diet. *Epilepsy Res* 1999; 37: 181–90.

44 Wheless JW. The ketogenic diet: An effective medical therapy with side effects. *J Child Neurol* 2001; 16: 633–5.

45 Vining EP, Pyzik P, McGrogan J *et al.* Growth of children on the ketogenic diet. *Dev Med Child Neurol* 2002; 44: 796–802.

46 Furth SL, Casey JC, Pyzik PL *et al.* Risk factors for urolithiasis in children on the ketogenic diet. *Pediatr Nephrol* 2000; 15: 125–8.

47 Herzberg GZ, Fivush BA, Kinsman SL, Gearhart JP. Urolithiasis associated with the ketogenic diet. *J Pediatr* 1990; 117: 743–5.

48 Kossoff EH, Pyzik PL, Furth SL, Hladky HD, Freeman JM, Vining EP. Kidney stones, carbonic anhydrase inhibitors, and the ketogenic diet. *Epilepsia* 2002; 43: 1168–71.

49 Kwiterovich PO, Vining EPG, Pyzik PL, Skolasky R, Freeman JM. The effect of a high fat, ketogenic diet on the plasma levels of lipids, lipoproteins, and apolipoproteins in children: a prospective study. *JAMA* under final review.

50 Ballaban-Gil K, Callahan C, O'Dell C, Pappo M, Moshe S, Shinnar S. Complications of the ketogenic diet. *Epilepsia* 1998; 39: 744–8.

51 Best TH, Franz DN, Gilbert DL, Nelson DP, Epstein MR. Cardiac complications in pediatric patients on the ketogenic diet. *Neurology* 2000; 54: 2328–30.

52 Berry-Kravis E, Booth G, Taylor A, Valentino LA. Bruising and the ketogenic diet: Evidence for diet-induced changes in platelet function. *Ann Neurol* 2001; 49: 98–103.

53 Stewart WA, Gordon K, Camfield P. Acute pancreatitis causing death in a child on the ketogenic diet. *J Child Neurol* 2001; 16: 682.

54 Hahn TJ, Halstead LR, DeVivo DC. Disordered mineral metabolism produced by ketogenic diet therapy. *Calcif Tissue Int* 1979; 28: 17–22.

22 Complementary and Alternative Treatments in Epilepsy

T.E. Whitmarsh

Most general reviews of treatment for epilepsy concentrate entirely on the pharmacological agents on offer. When non-pharmacological treatments are discussed, almost without exception these include only surgical interventions, vagal nerve stimulation and the ketogenic diet [1,2]. This chapter is about other treatments which have been tried and which continue to be used by a large number of people with neurological illness and epilepsy. One survey of 230 neurological outpatients found that 30% had used a non-conventional treatment in the past year [3]. The rising tide of concern amongst patients in the Western world about the side-effects of conventional pharmaceuticals has been considered one reason for the rapid rise in popularity of many forms of unconventional medicine [4]. Nowhere is this concern more likely to be felt than amongst sufferers of epilepsy and their families, where a predominantly youthful population have to take such agents daily for many years. Any techniques or treatments which could be applied to reduce the need for conventional medication in even a small proportion of sufferers are worth noting by all those who care for people with epilepsy.

Some of these techniques, such as EEG biofeedback, psychotherapy, relaxation and hypnosis verge on the mainstream, but most of them are more commonly viewed under the complementary and alternative medicine (CAM) banner. CAM refers to 'those forms of treatment which are not widely in use by orthodox healthcare professionals' [5]. A more recent definition of complementary medicine is 'diagnosis, treatment and/or prevention which complements mainstream medicine by contributing to a common whole, by satisfying a demand not met by orthodoxy, or by diversifying the conceptual frameworks of medicine' [6]. I feel that there is an unfortunate tendency to lump all non-conventional practices together as 'alternative' and label them all as either 'good' or 'bad', depending on one's preference. Viewed more holistically, there are approaches on both sides of a notional dividing line which bring health benefits to particular individuals. There is little to guide us in knowing in advance which sufferers will benefit from which therapy. It is perhaps one of the tasks of medicine over the next few decades to integrate CAM therapies into treatment pathways, the prime goal being to alleviate suffering and promote health. Some such attempts are available as case reports [7,8].

What evidence is already available to help in this task and what might be the most promising lines for future research to take? This chapter aims to help answer these questions.

Experience from the developing world suggests that people with epilepsy are extremely pragmatic in their approach to potential therapies, continuing to use anything which they perceive as helpful and quickly rejecting anything perceived as unhelpful. For example in a neurology outpatient setting in Lagos, Nigeria, it has been found that many people with epilepsy develop a personal care strategy which may combine elements of 'conventional' (pharmaceutical) and 'complementary' (traditional remedies and/or spiritual healing) medicine [9]. Similarly, this approach is widely adopted in the developed world [10]. Hence, it is vital for those who care for people affected by epilepsy to have at least a basic familiarity with the more commonly used CAM treatments. This should enable appreciation of any safety issues, such as potential drug interactions, enhance the understanding relationship between health professional and patient and even allow the occasional referral for appropriate, effective non-conventional treatments.

There are a number of unconventional and CAM therapeutic approaches which are sometimes helpful in the treatment of epilepsy in addition to conventional pharmacology. There are some studies which help to indicate which individual patients might benefit, but since there has been relatively very little funding of research in CAM and there are few well-established research networks, case reports and individual clinical experience have a strong role.

Therapies with varying levels of evidence of efficacy in epilepsy include behavioural/psychological therapies such as psychotherapy, cognitive therapy, hypnosis, meditation, EEG biofeedback and relaxation, herbal medicine, low antigen diets, dietary supplements, music therapy, exercise, homeopathy, acupuncture, transcranial magnetic stimulation and chiropractic therapy.

Psychological treatments

Many different therapies which could come under the 'psychological' or 'behavioural' tags have been tried in epilepsy. Much of the literature reports single cases or very small studies and it has been extensively reviewed by Fenwick [11] and, more recently, by Goldstein [12]. The reader is directed to these authors for further detail, but broadly, psychotherapy, individual counselling and cognitive behavioural therapy may help the psychological problems associated with epilepsy, and there is a suggestion of reduction in seizure frequency with some of these techniques. Operant or classical conditioning is reported to decrease seizure frequency and to be particularly helpful in control of the reflex epilepsies (seizures reliably triggered by a specific sensory stimulus, such as music or strong smells). Cases have also been reported of the beneficial effect of changing arousal levels in response to cues indicative of the onset of a seizure. Such 'countermeasures' are individually designed, according to the seizure cues and many patients soon discover what action is effective for them to abort a threatened seizure.

Hypnosis

Hypnosis is a technique by which general arousal levels can be changed. A report on just two patients suggests that it can be effective in control of seizures [13]. An impressive case report gives great detail of the hypnotic processes learned by a woman with jacksonian seizures due to a benign, but inoperable, frontotemporal tumour. She reduced her seizure frequency from 35 to 5 per week over the course of hypnotic treatment lasting 16 months [14].

Meditation and yoga

In a well-conducted study, 11 adults with drug-resistant epilepsy were taught meditation (of classical Indian word-repetition, non-religious type) and followed up for a year of practice (20 min daily) [15]. They were compared with a waiting list control group of nine subjects, well-matched for age, duration of illness and seizure type. Both groups received the same professional attention except that the control group did not practise meditation. The meditation group showed a reduction in attack frequency and duration after 6 months' practice compared to the 6-month period pretreatment (baseline), which became highly significant with a further 6 months' treatment. The meditators also demonstrated normalization of EEG recordings with prolonged treatment, with a reduction in mean spectral intensity of the 0.7–7.7 Hz segment and an increment in intensity of the 8–12 Hz segment. There were no changes in the controls. The authors discuss the rationale for the study in terms of eliciting the 'relaxation response' of Benson et al. [16] and suggest that this might be a common link towards understanding the mode of action of all of these psychological techniques.

Yoga teaches a combination of physical postures, breathing exercises, relaxation and meditation to attain optimal physical and mental health. A number of documented clinical and physiological effects are relevant to epilepsy [17]. There are many different schools of yoga practice, some emphasizing control over the physical body, some control over the breathing and some specifically using meditative practices to calm the mind and achieve 'union of the individual energy ("prana") with the universal energy ("Brahman")'. Most of the reports of yoga as treatment for epilepsy have been concerned with the directly meditative forms (specifically Sahaja yoga) and so should be considered along with meditation as an intervention. A Cochrane review of yoga in epilepsy [18] identified five studies, but only considered data from one of them in detail. Interestingly, one of the excluded studies in this review of 'yoga' is that of meditation considered in detail above and does not in fact mention yoga at all [15].

The study included by the Cochrane reviewers randomized 32 uncontrolled epileptic patients to three groups [19]. Group I ($n=10$) was the yoga group, who practised Sahaja yoga meditation under guidance of an instructor twice daily for 20–30 min for the 6-month duration of the study. Group II ($n=10$) practised mimicking exercises in the same environment as group I and were provided with the same attention. Group III ($n=12$) was a control group, just being followed up in outpatients.

Four out of 10 patients in the active group became seizure free after 6 months of practice, compared with none out of 22 in the controls. Nine in the active group had more than a 50% reduction in seizure frequency compared to just one among the 22 controls. These differences are significant and suggest that further research in this area is justified, with larger group sizes. Whether any changes are specific to a form of meditation called yogic or indeed to any

form of deep relaxation and whether similar effects might be obtained with other, more familiar, physical forms of yoga remains to be elucidated.

EEG biofeedback

Biofeedback in general involves the use of electronic displays to collect and show physiological processes to the patient, with the goal of increasing the patient's control over the internal processes and changing them at will. It has been extensively studied in a variety of neurological conditions. For example, thermal biofeedback (in which control of the skin temperature of a finger is learned) and EMG biofeedback (in which control is learned over the tension in a muscle, such as temporalis) are well established as treatments for migraine and tension-type headache, respectively, at least in the USA [20,21]. In EEG biofeedback, also referred to as EEG operant conditioning or neurotherapy, the subject learns to voluntarily control a chosen EEG rhythm which has been associated with suppressing seizure activity and thereby gain control over the seizures themselves. Initial work was done on the sensory-motor rhythm (SMR) over the somatosensory cortex and it is this rhythm which has been most studied. Biofeedback reinforcement of other rhythms such as the α rhythm and also the suppression of slow-wave and spike activity have also been investigated and found to be effective in some studies. There is much debate in the literature about which rhythms are likely to be most useful for biofeedback for which conditions.

Sterman and Friar first observed protection against drug-induced seizures in cats following operant conditioning of 11–15 Hz sensorimotor EEG rhythm to produce a sustained increase in the rhythm. They used the technique to successfully treat a 23-year-old woman with a 7-year history of generalized major tonic-clonic seizures of unknown origin, occurring at least twice monthly. The seizures had proved resistant to many drug regimes. With 3 months of twice-weekly biofeedback training enhancing 11–15 Hz activity, she became seizure free [22].

In a comprehensive review of the literature from the first case report in 1972 up to 1996, Sterman [23] collected the results on a total of 174 patients with intractable epilepsy treated with sensorimotor EEG operant conditioning, in 18 studies from many different authors. One hundred and forty-two (82%) of these showed 'clinical improvement'—that is, reductions in seizure frequency of at least 30%. The average value of reduction of seizure frequency was above 50% and many of the studies reported reductions in seizure severity. Approximately 5% of this difficult subset of epileptic patients experienced complete control of seizures for up to 1 year. Not all studies reported EEG findings, but of those that did, 66% of reported cases (in 13 studies) showed 'EEG improvement'. Most of the studies are of very small groups of under 10 patients and many of them report individual patient characteristics and outcomes, often using the patients as their own controls in pretreatment vs. post-treatment comparisons of frequency and severity. Two larger studies [24,25] report on groups of 23 and 83 patients and find significant beneficial effects on seizure frequency.

Sterman [23] comments that 'the consensus arising (from the studies) is that most epileptic patients who show clinical improvement with EEG biofeedback also show contingency-related EEG changes and a shift towards EEG normalisation. However not all patients who respond to this treatment show EEG changes and a few patients who show EEG changes experience little clinical improvement'.

Advocates of EEG biofeedback point to an accumulation of evidence of positive effects in neurophysiological and clinical studies over the past 25 years. They lament the lack of interest in its potential usefulness for a most difficult-to-help group of patients in the wider neurological community and specifically that the technique should still be regarded as 'experimental' [23]. Sceptics may acknowledge that there are 'adequate data to suggest that EEG biofeedback can work in some clinical conditions' [26], but clearly, a lot more work needs to be done to satisfy the demands of non-enthusiasts before EEG biofeedback can take its place as a generally available option for people with intractable seizures. For the individual strong-responding patients who have been able to come off all anticonvulsants and return to work [27] or be issued with a driving licence for the first time [22], this view may seem a little narrow.

It is undoubtedly a rather lengthy and expensive treatment in terms of laboratory, technician and patient time and there is as yet no way of determining in advance which patients will benefit.

Relaxation

Relaxation has been investigated as a possible treatment for epilepsy in at least four controlled studies. The particular form of relaxation generally used has been progressive muscular relaxation (PMR), as codified by Bernstein and Borkovec [28]. An early report was that of Snyder [29], who recruited 16 patients with mostly 'mixed' seizures. Only four practised relaxation on 15 or more days each month, but of these three reported a decrease in seizure frequency. Rousseau *et al.* performed a controlled study [30] and placed eight subjects into two groups on a sequential, alternating basis. Group I underwent a training session in PMR and were then asked to practise the exercise twice daily for the next 3 weeks. Group II were initially trained in a sham treatment and sat quietly for 20 min twice daily relaxing as best as they could. Baseline seizure frequency was recorded for the 3 weeks before training and both groups continued to record seizure frequency through the first 3 weeks of the study. At the end of 3 weeks, group II were taught PMR and practised twice daily for the next 3 weeks, recording seizure in frequency. There was a significant decrease in seizure frequency after PMR training (by 43–100%) compared to after the sham (0–51%), although two subjects also did well with the sham.

Whitman *et al.* [31] trained 12 patients in PMR who had at least six seizures in an 8-week baseline period and followed them up for 6 months, but did not include a control group. The mean reduction from baseline in seizure frequency at 6 months was 54%. Puskarich *et al.* [32] enrolled 24 subjects with at least six seizures in a baseline period of 8 weeks. They were randomized in alternating blocks of five to a group which received six sessions of training in PMR ($n = 13$) and a control 'quiet sitting' (QS) group ($n = 11$) which attended six times for 30 min of non-directive conversation, followed by 15 min of sitting alone in a reclining chair in a darkened room. This training period lasted 8 weeks. The groups were then followed up for 8 weeks. In the PMR group, 11 subjects had a decrease in frequency of seizures from baseline to follow-up ($P < 0.01$) and in the QS group, seven had a decrease ($P < 0.05$). The mean decrease in seizure frequency was 29% (from 17.0 at baseline to 12.1 during

follow-up) for the PMR group and 3% for the QS group (from 10.3 at baseline to 10.0 during follow-up). Subject numbers and study quality have risen with each new report and there is increasing evidence for a worthwhile effect on seizure frequency of this simple psychological intervention.

There is also evidence that adults with resistant seizures can learn early signs of cortical dysrhythmias and apply relaxation acutely to inhibit the seizure [33].

Psychiatric interventions

One study reviewed experience with 37 patients with uncontrolled seizures, whose seizures seemed to be precipitated by emotional stress [34]. Each received psychiatric intervention on at least two occasions (range 2–70, median 7.5). The intervention consisted of 'individual and family assessment, followed by the formulation of a treatment strategy geared toward alleviating possible psychogenic contributants to the patient's seizures'. It should be noted that in an appreciable proportion of these cases, 'hysterical' seizures were rated as being probably (19 of 37) or definitely (three of 37) present. After 2–36 months follow-up (median = 6.5 months), nine of 37 patients became seizure free and 12 additional patients showed a marked improvement (at least 2/3 decrease in seizure frequency). Patients with partial seizures were more likely to respond than those with generalized seizures and those with non-epileptic ('hysterical') seizures were especially responsive. Hypnotizability and having an IQ within the average range were also positively associated with a favourable outcome.

An analysis of 70 case studies in psychological approaches for prevention of nocturnal seizures encompasses extremely heterogeneous groups of patients and treatments [35]. Its author is unable to draw any firm conclusions, specifically about factors which might predict good response to a particular therapy. Most provocatively, it is suggested that freedom from seizures as a consequence of psychological treatment of epilepsy is most often achieved in these 70 cases when antiepileptic drugs are withdrawn.

In conclusion, there are a number of psychological/behavioural interventions which have been well studied and considered to be helpful as additional therapy for even the most drug-resistant epileptic patients. Choice of intervention probably depends mostly on local availability and patient preference and motivation, as there are as yet few indications of which technique is most likely to be helpful in an individual.

Exercise

There has been a reluctance to allow normal participation by epileptic patients in physical activity and sport, generally due to fear of injury or concern about exercise-induced seizures. In fact there appears to be no generalized increase in seizure frequency with physical exercise [36], although there is considerable individual variation and exercise has been studied as a possible means of reducing seizures in drug-resistant epilepsy. Eriksen *et al.* [37] gave 15 women with drug-resistant epilepsy (median 2.9 seizures per week) physical exercise sessions twice per week for 15 weeks. The exercise sessions lasted 1 h and consisted of a warm up, 30 min of aerobic dancing, a cool down, 15 min strength training and 5 min relaxation, all accompanied by music. Seven subjects had a total of 27 seizures during the 30 exercise sessions, mostly during the aerobic dancing or cool down periods. Self-reported seizure rate was significantly reduced during the 15 weeks of the intervention (from 2.9 seizures/week at baseline to 1.7/week during exercise) and there was also a reduced level of other health complaints, such as muscle pains, sleep problems and fatigue. The positive effects did not, however, last through a follow-up period of 3 months, when most subjects were unable to continue exercise on their own. The authors feel that 15 weeks is not long enough to effect a complete lifestyle change towards regular, hard physical activity. They believe that the benefits of increased fitness, decreased overall health complaints and reduction in total number of seizures more than balance the relatively few seizures during exercise that occurred in half of the subjects. Accordingly, they recommend that physical activity such as aerobic dance can be recommended to epileptic patients, its most important effect being 'the normalization of the life situation for severely affected hypoactive and understimulated epileptic patients'.

Music

The 'Mozart effect' was first reported as an enhancement of spatiotemporal reasoning after listening to Mozart sonata for two pianos (K448) for 10 min [38]. Later, EEG changes such as enhanced synchrony of the firing pattern of the right frontal and left temporoparietal areas, persisting for 12 min, were demonstrated. In 23 of 29 epileptic patients with focal discharges, there was a significant normalization of the EEG after listening to Mozart's music and one case report describes an 8-year-old girl with Lennox–Gastaut syndrome and intractable, frequent seizures (about two per hour) who achieved a very significant reduction in attacks by the playing of the Mozart sonata for 10 min each hour of her waking time. These studies and the probability that this effect is not specific to Mozart's music are considered by Jenkins [39].

The effect of another form of music—'medical resonance therapy music'—has been studied in 34 patients in an epilepsy hospital in Minsk, Belarus [40]. Subjects listened to the music daily for 1 h for 6–16 sessions. The author claims a 75% reduction in seizure frequency and a significant improvement in psychological state. Unfortunately, the report is very unclear, with no actual numbers of seizures given, just percentage improvements on undefined scales. The kind of music is not well described, but appears to be a rhythmical, computer-generated creation. Since there are no formal studies of more conventional music (Mozart K448, for example) with which to compare it, this study stands as the only one of its type in epilepsy. The field looks ripe for experimentation.

Herbal medicine

A large number of plants are traditionally used throughout the world for the treatment of epilepsy. One review of the literature found around 150 plants or other natural substances from traditional medicines which have been tested for their *in vivo/in vitro* anticonvulsant activities in the last 30 years [41]. The authors felt that 10 of these warrant further study. It should be remembered that many herbal preparations have very significant interactions with commonly prescribed conventional drugs [42,43] and use of these preparations should always be specifically enquired about, as it is

known that approximately 60% of users of non-conventional treatments do not reveal their use to their physician [10].

One herbal mixture which has been quite extensively studied and which is sometimes recommended as add-on treatment for epilepsy is the Chinese mixture Saiko-Keishi-To (SK). This is made up of parts of nine plants. One study gave SK to 24 poorly controlled epileptic patients daily for at least 10 months, as add-on treatment, keeping the conventional antiepileptic drug regimes constant. Six became seizure free and 13 improved in seizure frequency or severity [44].

Another study found a greater than 25% reduction in seizure numbers in eight of 24 patients with drug-resistant partial epilepsy after 8 weeks daily treatment with SK. There were corresponding cognitive improvements [45]. Neither of these studies was adequately controlled, but the results are suggestive of a useful action of SK in drug-resistant epilepsy and there has been an extensive experimental research on the cellular actions of this preparation [46].

Interestingly, it appears that only the crude mixture of plants which is SK possesses activity, at least in *in vitro* models [47]. Attempts to refine the preparation too far looking for the pharmacologically active agent may prove fruitless. This is very much in line with herbalists the world over, who believe that 'the whole is more than the sum of its parts', holding that plants act synergistically within such mixtures and also that the balance of compounds within a single plant acting in concert is likely to be responsible in large part for its actions [48].

Dietary measures

Food sensitivity

Oligoantigenic diets and avoidance of foods to which the patient is sensitive appear to be effective in children with epilepsy and migraine, although not those with epilepsy alone [49]. There is evidence that seizures can be precipitated in some adult subjects by eating certain foods to which they have an allergic response. One study used double-blinded food challenge in a 19-year-old woman with frequent seizures, a history of allergies to dust, pollen and mould, a strong family history of allergies and an eosinophilia, discovered by elimination diet to be sensitive to beef. Seizures occurred soon after taking capsules containing beef, but not chicken, and she remained seizure free long term by avoiding any beef products, having stopped anticonvulsant medication [50]. Particularly in those epileptic patients who have a strong family or personal history of allergy (asthma, allergic rhinitis or other allergy) or an eosinophilia, it is recommended to look for food sensitivities by means of exclusion diet and phased reintroduction.

Nutritional supplements

Anticonvulsant actions have been claimed in clinical trials for vitamins E and D, the trace elements selenium, manganese and zinc and the amino acid taurine. Vitamin E in particular has been used relatively widely [8] for its presumed anticonvulsant activity.

One trial randomized 24 subjects aged 5–18 years with various types of seizures and at least four seizures per month to receive either 294 mg (400 IU) of vitamin E (*n*=12) or matching placebo (*n* =12) daily for 3 months in addition to their usual antiepileptic drugs

[51]. Ten of the patients in the active group were considered 're-sponders', that is their seizure frequency declined by at least 60%, and the two non-responders were actually non-compliant (by blood levels of vitamin E). There were no responders in the placebo group. This difference in response rate (83% vs. 0%) was significant at $P < 0.05$. Blood levels of standard antiepileptic drugs were not altered during the study and it was concluded that vitamin E may be a useful antiepileptic agent, at least in a paediatric population with drug-resistant epilepsy. Unfortunately no further studies seem to have been conducted to confirm these promising preliminary results.

A single study [52] supplemented the diet of 23 adult epileptic patients with various seizure types, who stayed on their standard antiepileptic drugs, with vitamin D, 4000–16000 IU daily. Seizure frequency declined by about 30% only whilst taking vitamin D, not on placebo, and the result was discussed in terms of the possible effects of antiepileptic drugs on calcium and magnesium metabolism. The authors concluded that it might be advisable for all patients taking antiepileptic drugs to receive prophylactic vitamin D. Again, this result has not been taken forward.

Low levels of serum magnesium [53], manganese and zinc [54] have been reported in epileptic patients and supplementation has been reported to be sometimes helpful with seizure control.

Selenium is a widely used antioxidant supplement. Its use in epilepsy is based on findings of low selenium levels in the serum of some patients, and rare case reports suggesting potential clinical usefulness. Four children with intractable seizures since birth were found to have glutathione peroxidase deficiency, likely due to a primary deficiency in two and to defective selenium resorption or transport, as this enzyme has selenium at its active centre [55]. Supplementation with selenium and discontinuation of antiepileptic drugs led to clinical improvement in all four.

The amino acid taurine has been extensively studied for its anticonvulsant properties. It appears to have only a moderate effect in general, but there are case reports of complete effectiveness in previously severe drug-resistant epilepsies [56].

Naturopathy

Naturopaths use a wide range of techniques in people with epilepsy, with the aim of allowing or stimulating the body to 'heal itself'. Any or all of the therapies discussed in this chapter can be brought to bear on the problem, but this is especially true for dietary, nutritional and homeopathic interventions [57].

Despite the wide range of evidence, there seems to be little current general enthusiasm for utilizing or researching these non-pharmacological, dietary methods of seizure control. Particularly in paediatric epilepsy, however, some of these approaches might bring worthwhile benefit.

Homoeopathy

Homoeopathy is a complementary medical system which uses preparations of substances whose effects when administered to healthy subjects produce the manifestations of the disorder seen in the individual patient. It was developed by Samuel Hahnemann (1755–1843) and is now practised throughout the world [58]. This 'like heals like' method of prescribing and the use of extremely diluted substances are the most contentious aspects of homoeopathy.

Recent large-scale meta-analyses of randomized controlled clinical trials of homoeopathy [59,60] provided some evidence of activity over placebo in a wide range of conditions, even though the strength of the evidence was considered to be low because of the poor methodological quality of the trials. Evidence for activity of homoeopathy is considered in detail elsewhere [61,62].

There are five homoeopathic hospitals within the NHS in the UK. There are no clinical trials of homoeopathy as add-on treatment in epilepsy, but there are uncontrolled case series which report improvements in seizure control [63,64]. The homoeopathic approach lends itself to management of complex cases with extensive psychosocial overlay. An individualized prescription is made, so that it is not possible to exactly list homoeopathic drugs for epilepsy, as each patient will have a different prescription (of one of approximately 2500 available remedies). Experience from the Department of Developmental Neurology, Hospital for Sick Children, Glasgow suggests that previously uncontrolled epileptic children, with seizures arising from congenital defects, birth injury, infections or other usually intractable causes, can gain improvement at the hands of a skilled homoeopathic doctor (Dr R. Leckridge, personal communication).

Acupuncture

In its oldest form, acupuncture is a part of traditional Chinese medicine (TCM). In traditional Chinese physiology, energy ('Qi') runs in meridians which are said to course just below the surface of the skin over the whole body. TCM encompasses an enormous range of practices including Chinese herbal medicine, Chinese acupressure and massage, dietary therapy and mind–body exercise such as QiGong and T'ai chi. It is a major established health-care system used by millions of people throughout the world for every medical condition. In TCM acupuncture, the insertion of very fine needles into the meridians at predefined points is held to rebalance blocked or excessive energy flow and so cure symptoms. It has been used for thousands of years as part of TCM treatment of epilepsy [65]. It is complex to learn this sort of approach and Western scientists have seen the theoretical structure as off-putting. In epilepsy treatment, the acupuncture literature has been largely confined to speculative articles and single case reports, but there are also some indications of efficacy from case series.

Good results in long-term reduction of seizures [66] and even status epilepticus [67] have been reported, but nearly always in uncontrolled fashion or in retrospective case series. Different forms of acupuncture have been employed, but a lot of the work has been done using electroacupuncture, i.e. stimulation of the needles by electric impulses or just stimulation of the acupuncture points by surface electrodes. One study [66] reports on 98 cases of drug-resistant epilepsy treated with courses of scalp electroacupuncture, 30 min of electrical stimulation at 2–3.5 Hz through needles placed under the scalp, given daily for 15 days and repeated with a week-long break between courses. In this uncontrolled study, 89% of cases experienced a worthwhile reduction in seizure frequency and severity after a mean follow-up of 4 years.

The anticonvulsant action of acupuncture has been demonstrated in animal models and its mechanism investigated. Acupuncture can significantly change levels of some neurotransmitters responsible for inhibition of seizures at specific brain sites [68].

In contrast to the vast Chinese experience, many Western practitioners learn a form of acupuncture which makes fewer therapeutic claims. This 'medical acupuncture' assumes that one day it will be possible to explain all the undoubted clinical effects of acupuncture scientifically. So far, it has been most used and studied in painful conditions with good evidence of efficacy [69]. It is now a widely used therapeutic modality in, for example, physiotherapy departments and pain clinics.

It has been much more difficult to demonstrate the claimed efficacy of TCM acupuncture in systemic illness according to conventionally acceptable scientific methodology. One study which aimed to do this in chronic intractable epilepsy was that of Kloster et al. [70]. They recruited 39 patients with partial or generalized epilepsy with a duration of at least 2 years and a seizure frequency of one or more per week. Five withdrew in the 8-week baseline period. For the 8-week treatment period, they were divided into two groups by four-block randomization. One group ($n=18$) received acupuncture and the second group ($n=16$) acted as controls. The patients in the acupuncture group were all needled in a standard set of acupuncture points, with the possibility of one or more extra points being treated, chosen according to their TCM diagnosis. Stimulation was applied either manually or electrically (3 Hz, 3–20 mA), and all TCM diagnoses were made and the acupuncture treatments were given by two professors from the Shanghai University of TCM. The control group were given 'sham' acupuncture, that is standardized, bilateral, shallow needling of three points chosen for their minimum expected effect. Treatment time in both groups was 30 min and there were three treatment sessions per week for 7.5 weeks, with a 4-day break in the middle. Assessment of outcome was done weekly by neurologists, blind to the allocation of the subjects.

The groups were comparable in baseline characteristics, although it is a strange omission that details on use of antiepileptic drugs was not reported. There was a non-significant reduction in seizure frequency in both groups, and an increase in the number of seizure-free weeks, which reached significance in the 'sham' group. There were no EEG changes of significance throughout the study and no factors could be identified which correlated with response to treatment, including age, age of onset of epilepsy, duration of epilepsy, educational level, IQ or TCM diagnosis. A subsequent paper documents the inability to detect an effect of acupuncture on health-related quality of life within this study [71]. The authors concluded that they have been unable to prove a beneficial effect of acupuncture in chronic epilepsy. The trial is certainly the study that conforms closest to the conventional norms of scientific investigation and will no doubt be taken as convincing evidence against the use of acupuncture, but it can be criticized. The lack of information on baseline antiepileptic drugs is potentially important, as the two groups could have been imbalanced by this, which is presumably at least as important a factor in 'severity' as frequency of seizures. Moreover, the study was small and the patients had a mean duration of epilepsy of 26–28 years so that the findings may not be representative for more benign epilepsies. Another important problem is the control used, and the question of just what is the most appropriate control condition in acupuncture research has been much discussed. Generally, it is accepted that sham acupuncture cannot be considered a placebo, as it has measurable physiological and clinical effects [72]. If the control condition has a positive clinical effect and if the specific effect size of the active intervention is not large, then very large groups would be needed to detect a significant difference between groups. It would therefore be overhasty to conclude that acupuncture does not 'work' in epilepsy, and more research in this area would be justified.

Transcranial magnetic stimulation

One brief report [73] describes an open pilot study in which nine patients with refractory, very frequent partial and secondary generalized seizures were treated with low-frequency, repetitive transcranial magnetic stimulation (rTMS). The subjects had experienced, on average, more than seven seizures per week in the 6 months before the study. rTMS was done on 5 consecutive days, using a coil placed over the vertex. Five hundred pulses at 0.33 Hz were delivered twice each study day. In the 4 weeks after the study, seizure frequency was reduced from a mean of 10.3/week in the 4 weeks prior to the study, to a mean of 5.8/week. The mean reduction in seizures per week was 36.6% ($P=0.017$). Further studies are needed, but rTMS may turn out to be a non-invasive option to add to antiepileptic drugs in the control of intractable epilepsy.

Chiropractic treatment

Chiropractic therapy is a form of manipulation of the joints, particularly those of the vertebral column. As originally formulated by Daniel David Palmer, all illness stems from entrapment of spinal nerves by subluxations of the vertebrae and so all illness can be removed by manipulating these vertebral subluxations back into proper alignment. This rather rough view has been gradually replaced with a sophisticated diagnostic system and a steadily enlarging research base, which largely supports the use of chiropractic treatment in many areas, most (but not all) of which are related to the musculoskeletal system [74,75].

The effects of chiropractic care on the progress of epilepsy in adults remain largely unreported, but Pistolese [76] reviews 17 case reports of children with epilepsy who received chiropractic treatment. Fourteen of these were receiving antiepileptic drugs which had not been successful in controlling their seizures. 'Upper cervical care to correct vertebral subluxation' was administered to 15 patients and all reported positive outcomes in terms of decreased seizure activity. The critical predictor of a favourable outcome seemed to be the finding of a cervical spine malalignment in chiropractic terms. This is undoubtedly a more subtle phenomenon than most clinicians are accustomed to detecting. The analysis goes no further than this and the author suggests that further investigations into the potential value of chiropractic care in paediatric epilepsy would be justified. Some of the cases detailed are truly impressive. For example, a 6-year-old girl experiencing 20–25 absence seizures per day had 'upper cervical specific adjustments to correct the atlas subluxation complex', weekly for an (unfortunately) unspecified number of weeks. There was an immediate reduction in attack frequency after the first treatment and by the end of the treatment course, she was experiencing one attack per week or fewer.

Alcantara et al. [77] report on a 21-year-old woman who had epilepsy since childhood and now suffered a generalized tonic-clonic seizure every 3 h, lasting 10 s to 30 min. Examination revealed very extensive abnormalities (in a chiropractic sense) in the cervical spine and specific adjustments were administered. The seizure rate dropped to one per day by the fifth treatment session, when the treatment technique was changed. A marked increase in seizure rate followed and in fact she had a seizure during the sixth session. Rapid chiropractic adjustment at the C6–C7 level aborted the seizure immediately. Subsequent examinations showed no evidence of recurrence of the subluxation complex and all seizure activity had ceased. At 12 and 18 month follow-up, she reported minor seizures of short duration about once per month, but had experienced up to 2 months seizure free. Interestingly in this case, the subject realized that many of her seizures were preceded by neck pain, and this is the only report of successful acute treatment of an epileptic seizure by chiropractic manipulation. The authors discuss models of how upper spine malalignment might lower seizure threshold, invoking concepts of seizure triggering by sensory input to the brain and aberrant sensory impulses from a disordered cervical spine. Again, they call for more research.

These case reports are well-written and document apparent beneficial effects of chiropractic care in some patients with epilepsy at least as well as in many case reports for the psychological treatments mentioned earlier. There are a number of controlled studies demonstrating specific effects of chiropractic care in different clinical conditions against a variety of inventive placebo conditions. Controlled trials may be justified in those patients with epilepsy who have cervical spine disorders demonstrable by chiropractic techniques.

Conclusions

Most of the studies and case reports discussed in this chapter are based on uncontrolled observations, and therefore claims of therapeutic success should be interpreted with caution. In randomized trials, many patients with epilepsy may respond well to placebo, which may be explained by emotional influences on seizure activity and also by the phenomenon of the regression to the mean (i.e. the tendency of patients to seek medical attention during periods of seizure exacerbation, which tend to be naturally followed by a spontaneous decline of seizure frequency towards its average value). While these limitations should be kept in mind, the evidence discussed in this chapter does suggest that some of the CAM approaches reviewed above may have worthwhile efficacy, and high-quality research should be supported in the more suggestive areas. In particular, there appears to have been a peculiar blindness to the benefits which can be obtained from behavioural techniques such as EEG biofeedback and dietary measures such as oligoantigenic diets. Patients are already using many of these treatments, often without divulging this fact to their medical attendants, with all that this implies. An effective way to select patients and advise them about particular treatments should be the aim.

Love it or loath it, patients with epilepsy will continue along their pragmatic therapeutic paths. It would be of benefit to all if their caregivers could, if not walk with them, guide them safely.

Acknowledgement

I am extremely grateful to Sandra Davies of the British Homeopathic Library, Glasgow Homeopathic Hospital, for literature searches.

References

1 Ben-Menachem E. New antiepileptic drugs and non-pharmacological treatments. *Curr Opin Neurol* 2000; 13(2): 165–70.
2 Thiele EA, Gonzalez-Heydrich J, Riviello JJ Jr. Epilepsy in children and adolescents. *Child Adolesc Psychiatr Clin N Am* 1999; 8(4): 671–94.
3 Freeman JW, Landis J. Alternative/complementary therapies. *S Dakota J Med* 1997; 50(2): 36–42.
4 Whorton JC. The history of complementary and alternative medicine. In: Jonas WB, Levin JS, eds. *Essentials of Complementary and Alternative Medicine*. Philadelphia: Lippincott, Williams and Wilkins: 1999.
5 British Medical Association. *Complementary Medicine. New approaches to good practice.* Oxford: Oxford University Press, 1993.
6 Ernst E, Mills S *et al.* Complementary medicine—a definition (letter). *Br J Gen Pract* 1995; 48: 506.
7 Richard A. Integrating mind, brain, body, and spirit in treating epilepsy. *Advances* 1992; 8(4): 7–20.
8 Caspi O, Greenfield RH, Gurgevich S. Case report in integrative medicine: a 24-year-old male with medically intractable seizures. *Integrative Med* 1998; 1 (4): 173–6.
9 Danesi MA, Adetunji JB. Use of alternative medicine by patients with epilepsy: A survey of 265 epileptic patients in a developing country. *Epilepsia* 1994; 35(2): 344–51.
10 Eisenberg DM, Davis RB, Ettner SL *et al.* Trends in alternative medicine use in the United States, 1990–1997. *JAMA* 1998; 280: 1569–74.
11 Fenwick P. The behavioral treatment of epilepsy generation and inhibition of seizures. *Neurol Clin* 1994; 12(1): 175–202.
12 Goldstein LH. Effectiveness of psychological interventions for people with poorly controlled epilepsy. *J Neurol Neurosurg Psychiatr* 1997; 63(2): 137–42.
13 Szupera Z, Rudisch T, Boncz I. The effect of cue-controlled modification of the level of vigilance on the intentional inhibition of seizures in patients with partial epilepsy. *Austral J Clin Exp Hypnosis* 1995; 16: 34–45.
14 Campbell A. Hypnotic control of epileptic seizures. *Austral J Clin Exp Hypnosis* 1997; 25(2): 135–46.
15 Deepak KK, Manchanda SK, Maheshwari MC. Meditation improves clinicoelectroencephalographic measures in drug-resistant epileptics. *Biofeedback Self Reg* 1994; 19(1): 25–40.
16 Benson H, Beary JF, Carol MP. The relaxation response. *Psychiatry* 1974; 37: 37–46.
17 Yardi N. Yoga for control of epilepsy. *Seizure* 2001; 10(1): 7–12.
18 Ramaratnam S, Sridharan K. Yoga for epilepsy. (Cochrane Review). In: *The Cochrane Library*, Issue 2, 2001. Oxford: Update Software.
19 Panjwani U, Selvamurthy W, Singh SH, Gupta HL, Thakur L, Rai UC. Effect of sahaja yoga practice on seizure control and EEG changes in patients with epilepsy. *Ind J Med Res* 1996; 103: 165–72.
20 Gauthier JG, Carrier S. Longterm effects of biofeedback on migraine headache: a prospective follow-up study. *Headache* 1991; 31: 605–12.
21 Bogaards MC, ter Kuile MM. Treatment of recurrent tension headache: a meta-analytic review. *Clin J Pain* 1994; 10: 174–90.
22 Sterman MB, Friar L. Suppression of seizures in epileptics following sensorimotor EEG feedback training. *Electroencephalogr Clin Neurophysiol* 1972; 33: 89–95.
23 Sterman MB. Basic concepts and clinical findings in the treatment of seizure disorders with EEG operant conditioning. *Clin Electroencephalogr* 2000; 31(1): 45–55.
24 Engle J, Troupin MD, Crandall PH, Sterman MB, Wasterlain CG. Recent developments in the diagnosis and therapy of epilepsy. *Ann Int Med* 1982; 97: 584–98.
25 Lantz D, Sterman MB. Neuropsychological assessment of subjects with uncontrolled epilepsy: effects of biofeedback training. *Epilepsia* 1988; 29(2): 163–71.
26 Duffy FH. The state of EEG biofeedback therapy (EEG operant conditioning) in 2000: an editor's opinion. *Clin Electroencephalogr* 2000; 31(1): V–VII.
27 Tozzo CA, Elfner LF, May JG. EEG biofeedback and relaxation training in the control of epileptic seizures. *Int J Psychophysiol* 1988; 6(3): 185–94.
28 Bernstein DA, Borkovec TD. *Progressive Relaxation Training*. Champaign, IL: Research Press, 1973.

29 Synder M. Effect of relaxation on psychosocial functioning in persons with epilepsy. *J Neurosurg Nurs* 1983; 15(4): 250–4.

30 Rousseau A, Hermann B, Whitman S. Effects of progressive relaxation on epilepsy; analysis of a series of cases. *Psychol Rep* 1985; 57(3 pt 2): 1203–12.

31 Whitman S, Dell J, Legion V, Eibhlyn A, Statsinger J. Progressive relaxation for seizure reduction. *J Epilepsy* 1990; 3: 17–22.

32 Puskarich CA, Whitman S, Dell J, Hughes JR, Rosen AJ, Hermann BP. Controlled examination of effects of progressive relaxation training on seizure reduction. *Epilepsia* 1992; 33(4): 675–80.

33 Dahl J, Melin L, Lund L. Effects of a contingent relaxation treatment program on adults with refractory epileptic seizures. *Epilepsia* 1987; 28(2): 125–32.

34 Williams DT, Gold AP, Shrout P, Shaffer D, Adams D. The impact of psychiatric intervention on patients with uncontrolled seizures. *J Nerv Ment Dis* 1979; 167 (10): 626–31.

35 Muller B. Psychological approaches to the prevention and inhibition of nocturnal epileptic seizures: a meta-analysis of 70 case studies. *Seizure* 2001; 10(1): 13–33.

36 Nakken KO, Bjorholt PG, Johannessen SI, Loyning T, Lind E. Effect of physical training on aerobic capacity, seizure occurrence, and serum level of antiepileptic drugs in adults with epilepsy. *Epilepsia* 1990; 31: 88–94.

37 Eriksen HR, Ellertsen B, Gronningsaeter H, Nakken KO, Loyning Y, Ursin H. Physical exercise in women with intractable epilepsy. *Epilepsia* 1994; 35(6): 1246–64.

38 Rauscher FH, Shaw GL, Ky KN. Music and spatial task performance. *Nature* 1993; 365: 611.

39 Jenkins J S. The Mozart effect. *J Roy Soc Med* 2001; 94(4): 170–2.

40 Sidorenko VN. Effects of the Medical Resonance Therapy Music in the complex treatment of epileptic patients. *Integrative Physiol Behav Sci* 2000; 35(3): 212–17.

41 Nsour WM, Lau CB, Wong IC. Review on phytotherapy in epilepsy. *Seizure* 2000; 9(2): 96–107.

42 Kshirsagar NA, Dalvi SS, Joshi MV *et al.* Phenytoin and ayurvedic preparation—clinically important interaction in epileptic patients. *J Assoc Phys Ind* 1992; 40(5): 354–5.

43 De Smet PAGM, D'Arcy PF. Drug interactions with herbal and other non-orthodox drugs. In: Wellington PJ, D'Arcy PF, eds. *Drug Interactions*. Heidleberg: Springer-Verlag, 1996.

44 Narita Y, Satowa H, Kokubu T, Sugaya E. Treatment of epileptic patients with the Chinese herbal medicine 'saiko-keishi-to' (SK). *IRCS Med Sci* 1982; 10: 88–9.

45 Nagakubo S, Niwa S, Kumagai N *et al.* Effects of TJ-960 on Sternberg's paradigm results in epileptic patients. *Jpn J Psychiatr Neurol* 1993; 47: 609–20.

46 Sugaya E, Sugaya A, Kajiwara K *et al.* Nervous diseases and Kampo (Japanese herbal) medicine: a new paradigm of therapy against intractable nervous diseases. *Brain Dev* 1997; 19: 93–103.

47 Sugaya A, Tsuda T, Yasuda K, Sugaya E, Onozuka M. Effect of Chinese herbal medicine 'saiko-keishi-to' on intracellular calcium and protein behavior during pentylenetetrazole-induced bursting activity in snail neurons. *Planta Medica* 1985: 2–6.

48 Low Dog T. Phytomedicine. In: Jonas WB, Levin JS, eds. *Essentials of Complementary and Alternative Medicine*. Philadelphia: Lipincott, Williams and Wilkins, 1999.

49 Egger J, Carter CM, Soothill JF, Wilson J. Oligoantigenic diet treatment of children with epilepsy and migraine. *J Pediatr* 1989; 114: 51–8.

50 Crayton JW, Stone T, Stein G. Epilepsy precipitated by food sensitivity: report of a case with double-blind placebo-controlled assessment. *Clin Encephalogr* 1981; 12(4): 192–8.

51 Ogunmekan AO, Hwang PA. A randomized, double-blind, placebo-controlled, clinical trial of D-alpha-tocopheryl acetate (vitamin E), as add-on therapy, for epilepsy in children. *Epilepsia* 1989; 30(1): 84–9.

52 Christiansen C, Rodbro P, Sjo O. 'Anticonvulsant action' of vitamin D in epileptic patients? A controlled pilot study. *BMJ* 1974; 2: 258–9.

53 Pfeiffer C, *Mental and Elemental Nutrients*. New Canaan, CT: Keats.

54 Pfeiffer C, LaMola S. Zinc and manganese in the schizophrenias. *J Orthomol Psych* 1983; 12: 215–34.

55 Weber GF, Maertens P, Meng X, Pippenger CE. Glutathione peroxidase deficiency and childhood seizures. *Lancet* 1991; 337: 1443–4.

56 Fukuyama Y, Ochiai Y. Therapeutic trial by taurine for intractable childhood epilepsies. *Brain Dev* 1982; 4(1): 63–9.

57 Morello G. Epilepsy. In: Pizzorno JE, Murray MT, eds. *Textbook of Natural Medicine*, 2nd edn. Edinburgh: Churchill Livingstone, 1999.

58 Boyd H. *Introduction to Homoeopathic Medicine*, 2nd edn. Beaconsfield: Beaconsfield Publishers, 1989.

59 Linde K, Clausius N, Ramirez G *et al.* Are the clinical effects of homoeopathy placebo effects? A meta-analysis of placebo-controlled trials. *Lancet* 1997; 350: 34–43.

60 Cucherat M, Haugh MC, Gooch M, Boissel J-P. Evidence of clinical efficacy of homoeopathy. A meta-analysis of clinical trials. *Eur J Clin Pharmacol* 2000; 56(1); 27–33.

61 Walach H, Jonas WB. Homeopathy. In: Lewith G, Jonas WB, Walach H, eds. *Clinical Research in Complementary Therapies. Principles, problems and solutions*. Edinburgh: Churchill Livingstone, 2002.

62 Whitmarsh TE. The nature of evidence in complementary and alternative medicine: ideas from trials of homeopathy in headache. In: Callahan D, ed. *The Role of Complementary and Alternative Medicine*. Washington, D.C.: Georgetown University Press, 2002.

63 Hamilton J. A survey of fourteen epileptic cases. *Br Homoeopathic J* 1946; 36: 59–75.

64 Herscu P. Thoughts on the treatment of seizure disorders with case examples. *N Engl J Homeopath* 1998; 7(2): 61–80.

65 Lai CW, Lai YH. History of epilepsy in Chinese traditional medicine. *Epilepsia* 1991; 32(3): 299–302.

66 Shi Z, Gong B, Jia Y, Huo Z. The efficacy of electro-acupuncture on 98 cases of epilepsy. *J Trad Chin Med* 1987; 7(1): 21–2.

67 Yang J. Treatment of status epilepticus with acupuncture. *J Trad Chin Med* 1990; 10(2): 101–2.

68 Wu D. Acupuncture and neurophysiology. *Clin Neurol Neurosurg* 1990; 92(1): 13–25.

69 Filshie J, White A, eds. *Medical Acupuncture. A Western scientific approach*. Edinburgh: Churchill Livingstone, 1998.

70 Kloster R, Larsson P G, Lossius R *et al.* The effect of acupuncture in chronic intractable epilepsy. *Seizure* 1999; 8(3): 170–4.

71 Stavem K, Kloster R, Rossberg E *et al.* Acupuncture in intractable epilepsy: lack of effect on health-related quality of life. *Seizure* 2000; 9(6): 422–6.

72 Lewith GT, Vincent CA. The clinical evaluation of acupuncture. In: Filshie J, White A, eds. *Medical Acupuncture. A Western scientific approach*. Edinburgh: Churchill Livingstone, 1998.

73 Tergau F, Naumann U, Paulus W, Steinhoff B. Low-frequency repetitive transcranial magnetic stimulation improves intractable epilepsy. *Lancet* 1999; 1353: 2209.

74 Meade TW, Dyer S, Browne W, Townsend J, Frank AO. Low back pain of mechanical origin: randomised comparison of chiropractic and hospital outpatient treatment. *BMJ* 1990; 300: 1431–7.

75 Nilsson N, Christensen HW, Hartvigsen J. The effect of spinal manipulation in the treatment of cervicogenic headache. *J Manipulative Physiol Ther* 1997; 20: 326–30.

76 Pistolese RA. Epilepsy and seizure disorders: a review of literature relative to chiropractic care of children. *J Manip Physiol Therap* 2001; 24(3): 199–205.

77 Alcantara J, Heschong R, Plaugher G, Alcantara J. Chiropractic management of a patient with subluxations, low back pain and epileptic seizures. *J Manip Physiol Therap* 1998; 21(6): 410–18.

23 Reproductive Aspects of Epilepsy Treatment

T. Tomson

The reproductive aspects of epilepsy and of antiepileptic drug treatment are major concerns for patients with epilepsy. A few decades ago, people with epilepsy in many parts of the world were often denied the fundamental right to form a family, due to prejudiced legislation and public attitudes. Fortunately, this situation has changed radically due to improvements in diagnosis and therapy, as well as changes in social attitudes. Today, more and more women with epilepsy become pregnant and have children and it has been estimated that 0.3–0.4% of all children today are born to mothers with epilepsy.

While reproductive health is regarded as one of the most important health issues for women with epilepsy, surveys in different countries have repeatedly revealed marked deficiencies in the provision of health care and advice on this issue. Only a minority of women with epilepsy who plan to have children have any pre-pregnancy counselling and knowledge among health-care providers about the reproductive health of women with epilepsy is often inadequate. To be worthwhile, counselling should ideally be provided long before pregnancy in order to allow for adequate treatment measures which reduce risks. Reproduction may be more complicated for people with epilepsy for a number of reasons related to epilepsy and to its treatment. Although most women with epilepsy will be able to give birth to perfectly normal children, a number of questions are raised when they consider becoming pregnant and these need to be addressed early in the pregnancy planning.

Fertility may be altered, and the efficacy of steroid oral contraceptives may be reduced by certain antiepileptic drugs. Epilepsy might affect the outcome of pregnancy and there may be increased risks of obstetric complications. Seizure control may change during pregnancy and treatment may need to be adjusted because of altered pharmacokinetics of antiepileptic drugs. Fetal risks associated with uncontrolled seizures during pregnancy need to be weighed against the teratogenic effects and other potential developmental toxicity of antiepileptic drugs. The possibility for a woman on antiepileptic drugs to nurse her child also needs to be discussed. These and other related issues will be addressed in this chapter.

Fertility

There are several studies suggesting that the fertility rate in people with epilepsy is lower than in the general population [1–5]. One large population-based register study from the UK reported the rate of live births in a population of women under treatment for epilepsy. This study showed that fertility rates in the general population were 33% higher than among women with epilepsy [5]. On the other hand, a smaller population-based retrospective cohort study from Iceland found no evidence of altered fertility among people

with epilepsy with the exception of those with mental retardation and cerebral palsy [6]. The study from Iceland was a 30-year follow-up of patients diagnosed in the early 1960s, and, in contrast to the UK study, a substantial proportion of the patients from Iceland were in remission at follow-up. Thus, according to available data, it is likely that there is a reduced fertility rate in women with active epilepsy. Fertility may also be decreased in men with epilepsy [1,3,4].

There are many possible causes for reduced fertility rates among people with epilepsy. Social isolation and stigmatization may contribute, which also explain why marriage rates are reported to be lower. Concurrent disabilities may be another reason as suggested by the study from Iceland. Women may also refrain from pregnancy because of fears of deterioration in their epilepsy or risks to the fetus incurred by seizures or the drug treatment. The lesion causing epilepsy and the epileptic activity as such may also induce endocrine dysfunction that could affect fertility. Finally, treatment with antiepileptic drugs can contribute to lower fertility.

Reproductive dysfunction

Reproductive dysfunction and endocrine disorders are common among both men and women with epilepsy. In men, this will manifest itself as hyposexuality and reduced potency and in women by menstrual dysfunction. Men with epilepsy have a reduced likelihood of fathering a child [4], in particular those with complex partial seizures of early onset. In some studies, between 40 and 70% report decreased potency and hyposexuality, but this apparently high figure needs to be related to the proportion among control populations [7]. Duncan *et al.* [8] compared 118 men with epilepsy treated with antiepileptic drugs with 32 untreated men with epilepsy and 34 healthy controls and found no indication of hyposexuality among those with epilepsy who had a partner. In a more recent study, Rättyä *et al.* [9] evaluated sexual function, including libido, potency, satisfaction with erection and orgasm in 90 men, 18–50 years of age, under treatment with an antiepileptic drug in monotherapy. Of the men 77% were considered to have a normal sexual function compared with 88% among 25 healthy age-matched controls.

Herzog *et al.* [10] observed reproductive endocrine disorders (hypogonadotropic hypogonadism, hypergonadotropic hypogonadism, hyperprolactinaemia) in nine of 20 patients with temporal lobe epilepsy. Some of these abnormalities are also seen in men with untreated epilepsy, suggesting that epilepsy plays a role in the development of these disorders. It has been suggested that epileptiform discharges may promote the development of reproductive endocrine disorders by disruption of normal temporolimbic modulation of hypothalamopituitary function [11]. This is supported by the observation that successful temporal lobe epilepsy surgery may lead to a normalization of low preoperative serum androgen concentrations in men with epilepsy despite unchanged drug treatment [12].

Treatment with antiepileptic drugs can also contribute to reproductive dysfunction. Enzyme-inducing drugs such as carbamazepine, phenytoin and phenobarbital may increase the concentration of sex hormone binding globulin (SHBG) and may reduce the unbound, biologically active concentrations of testosterone [8]. In a cross-sectional study [9], monotherapy with carbamazepine was associated with decreased serum androgen levels and high SHBG concentrations in men with predominantly partial seizures. Oxcarbazepine treatment in doses of at least 900 mg/day was associated with similar endocrine effects. In contrast, serum androgen levels were increased in 12 out of 21 men treated with valproic acid for generalized or partial seizures [9].

Infertility in men may also be related to impaired spermatogenesis or sperm function. Poor sperm motility was noted in epileptic patients with long-term antiepileptic drug treatment and *in vitro* studies suggest a direct effect of phenytoin, carbamazepine and valproic acid on sperm membrane function [13]. However, large-scale studies comparing effects on sperm function of different antiepileptic drugs, including the newer products, are lacking.

Epileptic discharges in temporal and limbic structure may also affect hypothalamic regulation of pituitary secretion in women. Endocrine disorders occur in women with generalized epilepsy [14] as well as partial epilepsies [10]. Abnormal luteinizing hormone (LH) secretion has been reported in both treated and untreated women with epilepsy, and the pattern of LH pulse frequency seems to depend on the side of the EEG focus [15]. Hence, the epilepsy and the epileptic activity play a role in reproductive endocrine disorders in women and men.

Polycystic ovary syndrome (PCOS), epilepsy and antiepileptic drugs

The discussion on reproductive endocrine disorders in women with epilepsy has focused on polycystic ovaries (PCO) and PCOS. PCO, which is normally a diagnosis made on ultrasound examination and which may be asymptomatic, is a common condition with an estimated prevalence of about 20% in the general population. PCOS has been defined as ovulatory dysfunction with clinical evidence of hyperandrogenism and/or hyperandrogenaemia in the absence of identifiable adrenal or pituitary pathology, although criteria vary between researchers [16]. PCOS is a syndrome with multiple aetiologies and a prevalence ranging from about 4% up to 18% in the general female population, depending on the criteria and the population studied [17]. Genetic as well as environmental factors can contribute to the development of this syndrome. PCOS has been reported to occur in 20–25% of patients with complex partial seizures of temporal lobe origin [10]. In these early studies, which were small and probably used selected cohorts, PCOS was found to be more frequent among unmedicated compared to medicated women with epilepsy [10]. Subsequent studies have indicated that PCOS [14], menstrual disorders and PCO [18] occur at similar frequencies in patients with primary generalized and localization-related epilepsies.

Taken together, these observations seem to indicate that the higher prevalence of PCOS among women with epilepsy may be unrelated to the drug treatment. However, a series of reports from Finland has indicated that PCO and hyperandrogenism in women with epilepsy is related to the drug treatment and specifically to treatment with valproic acid [19–21]. In these cross-sectional studies, Isojärvi *et al.* [19] reported a high incidence of PCO, hyperandrogenism and menstrual disorders among women treated with valproic acid for their epilepsy. Among the 238 women with epilepsy under investigation, 43% of those on valproic acid and 22% of those taking carbamazepine had PCO and hyperandrogenism, compared with 18% of the healthy control women. Menstrual disturbances were reported in 45% of women on valproic acid, in 19% of those taking carbamazepine and in 16% of the controls. In a subsequent analysis of a subset of this cohort, valproic acid related abnormalities were shown to be associated with obesity, hyperinsulinaemia and altered serum lipids [20]. An attempt was made to switch drug therapy for 16 women with PCO and hyperandrogenism whilst on valproic acid to lamotrigine. It was possible to complete the change in therapy in 12 patients who during a 12-month follow-up on lamotrigine experienced a normalization of endocrine function [21]. This observation provides strong evidence for the opinion that PCO and the hyperandrogenism that occurs during valproic acid treatment may be related to the drug treatment and that this effect is reversible. However, it is biased as comparison between valproic acid and lamotrigine, since patients were selected primarily for having PCO and hyperandrogenism while on valproic acid. In a study from Italy, Murialdo *et al.* [22] reported higher androgen levels and more ovulatory dysfunction in women treated with valproic acid than in those on carbamazepine or phenobarbital or among normal controls although the incidence of PCO and hirsutism was similar.

Although these observations suggest an important role for antiepileptic drugs and in particular for valproic acid for reproductive endocrine disorders such as PCOS, the interpretation is still under debate [16,17,23,24]. A recent German study found similar rates of PCOS among women treated with valproic acid and carbamazepine and in untreated patients with epilepsy [25].

Based on their observations of a high incidence of PCOS also in untreated women with epilepsy, Herzog and Schachter [17] discussed the possibility that epilepsy in itself may promote the development of PCOS, and that enzyme-inducing antiepileptic drugs may counteract such abnormalities whereas valproic acid, devoid of inducing effects, does not. Although this hypothesis is somewhat speculative, such mechanisms might explain the high incidence in untreated women as well as in women on valproic acid.

There are several potential explanations for the apparently conflicting observations with respect to the role of antiepileptic drugs in PCOS. First, investigators use different criteria. Second, the populations being studied vary, the cohorts exposed to specific drugs are generally small, and sometimes highly selected. Third, prospective studies assessing women with epilepsy before and after initiation of treatment are lacking. Ideally, this issue should be addressed in prospective controlled trials comparing reproductive function in women randomized to treatment with different antiepileptic drugs.

Two cross-sectional studies from Finland assessed endocrine function in a younger population with epilepsy [26,27]. A cohort of 77 girls, 8–18 years of age, under treatment with valproic acid (*n*= 40), carbamazepine (*n*=19) or oxcarbazepine (*n*=18) were compared with 49 healthy age-matched controls. No difference was observed in linear growth and sexual maturation [26]. When 41 girls on valproic acid were compared with 54 healthy controls, hyperandrogenism was observed more frequently among the valproic acid exposed girls, but the incidence of PCO or menstrual disturbances was not increased [27].

Choice of antiepileptic drugs

Given the lack of conclusive evidence concerning the association between valproic acid and reproductive dysfunction, and the excellent effectiveness of this drug particularly in idiopathic generalized epilepsies, valproic acid is still a reasonable first choice also in young women with these types of epilepsy. However, based on the intriguing observations discussed above, the patients should be monitored closely. If adverse effects such as considerable weight gain or menstrual disturbances occur, a change in drug therapy should be considered. Although prospective, randomized controlled trials are lacking, the potential role of antiepileptic drugs always needs to be considered in women and men with epilepsy with reproductive dysfunction, and in such cases, it may be necessary to reassess the choice of treatment.

Birth control

Enzyme-inducing antiepileptic drugs may reduce the effectiveness of steroid oral contraceptives by inducing the metabolism of the oestrogen and progestogen components, and possibly also by increasing the hepatic synthesis of SHBG, thus decreasing the unbound, active concentration of progestogen. A number of unexpected pregnancies in women taking oral contraceptives and antiepileptic drugs have been reported and the contraceptive failure rate has been estimated to be several times higher among women on antiepileptic drugs than expected in the general population [28]. At the time of the report from Coulam and Annegers [28], oral contraceptives contained 50–100 µg of oestrogen. Since then, the oestrogen content has been reduced gradually in order to decrease the risks of adverse effects. The risk of failure is thus likely to be higher with the low-dose pills most commonly used today. Contraceptive failure may have particularly serious consequences for women taking antiepileptic drugs considering the increased risks of birth defects and other possible pregnancy complications. Hence, effective family planning is particularly important for women with epilepsy. Breakthrough bleeding may indicate insufficient dosage of hormones and should be regarded as a sign of reduced contraceptive effectiveness. However, failure may occur without preceding breakthrough bleedings. Antiepileptic drugs with and without known inducing effects on oral contraceptives are listed in Table 23.1, which is based on data from Guberman [29] and Perucca [30].

Injectable medroxyprogesterone given every 2–3 months is an alternative hormonal contraceptive, which is affected by enzyme-inducing drugs to a lesser extent. However, trials comparing the effectiveness of medroxyprogesterone and oral contraceptives in women with epilepsy are lacking [31].

Oestrogens are proconvulsant in experimental studies, which may raise a concern as to the use of oral contraceptives in women with epilepsy. However, there are no data suggesting an oestrogen-

Table 23.1 Effects of antiepileptic drugs on the pharmacokinetics of steroid oral contraceptives

Drugs which increase the clearance of oral contraceptives	Drugs which do not affect the clearance of oral contraceptives
Phenobarbital	Valproate
Phenytoin	Gabapentin
Carbamazepine	Vigabatrin
Felbamate	Tiagabine
Topiramate	Lamotrigine
Oxcarbazepine	Levetiracetam
Ethosuximide (?)	Benzodiazepines

induced deterioration in seizure control in women with epilepsy taking oral contraceptives. Some reports of worsened seizure control following prescription of oral contraceptives to women with epilepsy stabilized on lamotrigine has been ascribed to a reduction in serum lamotrigine levels caused by oral contraceptives [32].

In conclusion, enzyme-inducing properties should be taken into account when choosing an antiepileptic drug for a woman on oral contraceptives. Given the choice of two drugs similar in all other important respects (which is seldom the case), it is reasonable to select a drug known not to interact with oral contraceptives. Patients treated with inducing antiepileptic drugs should be prescribed oral contraceptives with an oestrogen content of at least 50 µg. Women should be given information that breakthrough bleeding may indicate an increased risk of failure but also that absence of such bleeding is no guarantee against unwanted pregnancies. The possibility of using complementary or alternative contraceptive methods should also be discussed, and it should be stressed that the effectiveness of many contraceptive methods other than the intrauterine device may actually be lower than that of an oral contraceptive taken together with enzyme-inducing drugs.

Pregnancy in women with epilepsy

In the treatment of epilepsy during pregnancy, maternal and fetal risks associated with uncontrolled seizures need to be weighed against the increased risk of adverse outcomes in the offspring due to maternal use of antiepileptic drugs.

Effects of maternal seizures on the fetus

Epileptic seizures in a pregnant woman may have adverse effects on the fetus in addition to the risks for the woman. With respect to the risks to the fetus, effects of generalized tonic-clonic seizures are probably different from effects of other types of seizures. Tonic-clonic seizures are associated with transient lactic acidosis, which is likely to be transferred to the fetus. Prolonged decrease in fetal heart rate, which is a common response to acidosis, has been reported after maternal tonic-clonic seizures [33,34]. Furthermore, generalized tonic-clonic seizures induce alterations in blood pressure and blood flow, but it is presently not known to what extent this affects uterine blood flow and thus the fetus. Seizure-related maternal abdominal trauma could also theoretically cause injury to the fetus or placental abruption. Despite these effects, intrauterine fetal death as a result of a single seizure appears to be rare and only a few such reports have been published. In contrast, prolonged seizure activity, such as status epilepticus, is a serious threat to the fetus as well as to the woman. In a review, Teramo and Hiilesmaa [35] reported fetal death in about 50% of cases with status epilepticus during pregnancy, and in 30% of the mothers.

Other types of seizures are rarely associated with secondary circulatory or metabolic effects and are thus in general unlikely to affect the fetus unless they lead to a secondarily generalized tonic-clonic seizure. However, they may cause some risks if the seizure results in injury or trauma.

Generalized tonic-clonic seizures during labour can cause fetal asphyxia [33]. Observations from a single case also suggest that complex partial seizures during labour can be associated with significant fetal heart rate decelerations and prolonged uterine contractions [36]. Partial seizures that impair consciousness may also impose risks since the mother's ability to cooperate during the delivery is lost. In such situations, caesarean delivery should be considered.

According to most prospective studies, seizures during early pregnancy are not associated with an increased risk of birth defects. However, occasional reports have indicated an increased risk for cognitive dysfunction in the offspring of women who have had convulsive as well as non-convulsive seizures during pregnancy [37], although conclusive evidence for a causative role of the seizures is lacking.

In conclusion, our knowledge concerning fetal risks associated with maternal seizures is based on case reports rather than systematic studies and we lack quantitative risk estimates. Nevertheless, there is a general consensus among physicians that in particular generalized tonic-clonic seizures should be avoided during pregnancy for the sake of the wellbeing of the fetus as well as the mother.

Seizure control during pregnancy and delivery

Early studies mainly from specialized epilepsy centres indicated that approximately one-third of women with epilepsy will experience an increase in seizures during pregnancy. Prospective studies of less selected women with epilepsy suggest that the proportion of women who deteriorate is smaller [38–40]. Among these women with closely monitored treatment throughout pregnancy, the majority will have an unchanged seizure control as compared with before pregnancy and some may even improve (Table 23.2).

It appears that women with mild or well-controlled epilepsy are overrepresented among those who become pregnant and most of them will remain seizure free throughout pregnancy. Although increases and decreases in seizure frequency during pregnancy to some extent reflect normal fluctuations in seizure control, some

periods of pregnancy are associated with a significant increase in seizures. A generalized tonic-clonic seizure occurs during labour in about 1–2% and within 24 h after delivery in another 1–2% [38]. This has been estimated to be nine times higher than the average probability of tonic-clonic seizures during pregnancy. Taking all seizure types together, roughly 5% of women with epilepsy will experience seizures during labour, delivery or immediately thereafter [41].

Status epilepticus occurs in less than 1% of all pregnancies of women with epilepsy and does not seem to occur more frequently during pregnancy than in other periods of life [41]. Most studies report that patients with a satisfactory seizure control before pregnancy are less likely to deteriorate than patients with uncontrolled epilepsy. Others suggest that localization-related epilepsy is more likely to get worse although there are conflicting results. There are observations suggesting that those women who fail to have pre-pregnancy counselling are most at risk to deteriorate during pregnancy. This agrees with several reports indicating that poor compliance with the drug treatment, often due to fear of the teratogenic effects, is the major cause for loss of seizure control during pregnancy [41].

Some women may experience onset of a seizure disorder during pregnancy, and they should be investigated according to the same general principles as non-pregnant patients with new onset epilepsy, although there are some causes of seizures that need to be considered more specifically. If seizures occur for the first time during the last 20 weeks of pregnancy, eclampsia needs to be excluded. Stroke and cerebral venous thrombosis also occur at a higher frequency during pregnancy. The general principles for initiation and choice of antiepileptic drug treatment also apply for women in pregnancy, although treatment is often withheld during the first trimester unless the risk is high for recurrent tonic-clonic seizures.

Pharmacokinetics of antiepileptic drugs during pregnancy

The aim of antiepileptic drug treatment during pregnancy is to maintain seizure control with the lowest effective dose and serum drug concentration, in order to avoid the harm from seizures and from drugs both to the mother and the fetus. Pregnancy-related alterations in the pharmacokinetics of antiepileptic drugs have been discussed as a factor contributing to a change in seizure control. The pharmacokinetics of many drugs undergoes significant changes during pregnancy [42]. At constant drug dosages, serum levels of most of the older antiepileptic drugs tend to decrease during pregnancy, and return to pre-pregnant levels within the first month or two after delivery. This appears to be due mainly to a decrease in drug binding to plasma proteins and/or an increase in drug metabo-

Table 23.2 Prospective population-based studies of seizure control during pregnancy compared with pre-pregnancy period

Reference	Country	Number of pregnancies	Unchanged %	Improved %	Worse %
Bardy [38]	Finland	154	54	14	32
Gjerde et al. [39]	Norway	78	67	17	17
Tomson et al. [40]	Sweden	93	61	34	15

lism and elimination. A decrease in protein binding will result in lower total drug levels but leave unchanged the unbound, active concentration of the drug.

By the end of pregnancy, total and unbound concentrations of phenobarbital decline by up to 50% [43]. Total concentrations of carbamazepine decline to a lesser extent and the changes in unbound concentrations are insignificant [40,43]. Marked decreases in total phenytoin concentrations to about 40% of pre-pregnancy levels have been reported [40,43], whereas free concentration decreased to a much lesser extent. For valproic acid, no significant changes were noted in unbound concentrations despite a fairly marked decrease in total concentrations [43]. Hence, for highly protein bound drugs such as valproic acid and phenytoin, total plasma concentrations may be misleading during pregnancy, underestimating the pharmacological effects of the drugs.

Much less is known about the pharmacokinetics of newer antiepileptic drugs during pregnancy. However, a pronounced decrease in total serum concentration of lamotrigine has been reported in late pregnancy with normalization within a few weeks postpartum [44].

The figures quoted above represent average changes for groups of patients. It is important to understand that the effect of pregnancy varies between individuals. The decline in plasma concentration may be insignificant in some patients and pronounced in others, prompting dosage adjustments to maintain seizure control. Monitoring drug levels is therefore recommended during pregnancy. For highly protein bound antiepileptic drugs such as valproic acid and phenytoin, unbound drug levels should ideally be measured. A single drug level is of limited value since the optimal concentration is individual. When pregnancy is planned in advance, it is therefore advisable to obtain serum drug concentrations before pregnancy, when seizure control is optimal, in order to establish a baseline to be used for comparison purposes.

Complications during pregnancy and delivery

The literature on complication rates in pregnant women with epilepsy is somewhat conflicting although the risk of some complications seems to be increased [45]. The pathogenesis is likely to be multifactorial including socioeconomic and genetic factors, drug treatment and possibly the epileptic disorder and the seizures. Preeclampsia has been reported to be up to twice as common among women with epilepsy in some studies, although there are reports

that find no difference [45,46]. Earlier studies suggest that induction of labour and instrumental deliveries are more frequent in women with epilepsy [46]. This may be a consequence of fear of seizures and unfamiliarity with epilepsy among obstetricians rather than a reflection of an increased rate of obstetric complications. Some more recent studies have not reported higher rates of instrumental deliveries [45]. It is difficult to obtain accurate estimates of the rate of spontaneous abortions, but this is probably not significantly increased in epilepsy.

Finally, perinatal mortality has consistently been reported to be 2–3 times higher in infants of women with epilepsy than in the general population [45], although the cause for this is unclear. For the reasons summarized above, pregnant women with epilepsy should be counselled by obstetricians who are familiar with epilepsy-related problems and delivery should take place in well-equipped obstetric units.

Developmental toxicity of antiepileptic drugs

The first reports of adverse effects of antiepileptic drugs on the fetus were published in the 1960s. Since then all of the major old generation antiepileptic drugs such as phenobarbital, phenytoin, valproic acid and carbamazepine, have been shown to be teratogenic. Adverse effects reported in exposed infants include major congenital malformations, minor anomalies and dysmorphism, growth retardation and impaired psychomotor development. Although the pathogenesis is likely to be multifactorial, including genetic predisposition, socioeconomic circumstances, seizures and epilepsy, the available data strongly suggest that antiepileptic drugs are the major cause for the increased risks.

Major congenital malformations

A large number of retrospective and prospective cohort studies have confirmed an increased frequency of major malformations in offspring of women treated with antiepileptic drugs. Some of the more recent large-scale studies [47–52] are summarized in Table 23.3. The incidence of major congenital malformations has ranged from 4 to 10%, corresponding to a two- to four-fold increase compared to the expected incidence. Differences in treatment strategy, study populations, controls and criteria for malformations can account for the variation in outcome. Some studies have included untreated women with epilepsy as additional controls. In general, such studies

Table 23.3 Recent cohort studies of major congenital malformations among infants exposed to antiepileptic drugs *in utero*

Reference	Study design	Number exposed	Number malformed (%)	Controls (% malformed)	Relative risk (95% CI)
Samrén *et al.* [47]	International multicentre prospective	1221	108 (9%)	Non-epileptic[a]	2.3 (1.2–4.7)
Samrén *et al.* [48]	Multicentre retrospective	1411	52 (3.7%)	Non-epileptic (1.5%)	2.5
Canger *et al.* [49]	Prospective	452	44 (9.7%)	Eurocat (2.3%)	4.2
Kaneko *et al.* [50]	International multicentre prospective	885	80 (9%)	Untreated patients with epilepsy (3.2%)	2.9
Wide [51]	Prospective and retrospective	977	47 (4.8%)	General population (3.2%)	1.5 (1.1–2.0)
Holmes *et al.* [52]	Retrospective	316	18 (5.7%)	Non-epilepsy (1.8%)	3.3 (0.9–8.3)

[a] Comparison with controls made for a subset of the cohort.

have not found an increased malformation rate among children of mothers with untreated epilepsy [52], suggesting that the increased risk for major malformations in the offspring of women taking antiepileptic drugs is due to the drug therapy rather than the epilepsy. However, untreated women with epilepsy are probably different in many other respects from those who are under treatment during pregnancy.

Although all major old generation antiepileptic drugs have been shown beyond doubt to be teratogenic, published data have so far not revealed any major differences between them in overall teratogenic potential. The number of pregnant women on each individual drug as monotherapy has been too small to allow a meaningful comparison even in the largest cohort studies so far. Pregnancies need to be collected over several years in order to obtain reasonably large cohorts of children exposed to antiepileptic drugs *in utero*. Therefore, even the more recently published studies assess outcomes of treatment sometimes spanning the past 20–25 years, and their results may perhaps not accurately reflect outcome of pregnancies managed according to present guidelines. For obvious reasons these studies include very few exposures to the newer antiepileptic drugs. Although pharmaceutical companies and independent research groups have established pregnancy registries to collect such data prospectively, the clinical experience is at present too limited to determine whether the newer generation antiepileptic drugs are teratogenic or not and how they compare in this respect with the older drugs. However, preliminary data from such registries suggest that valproic acid may be associated with a higher risk for birth defects than other standard drugs such as carbamazepine [53].

While conclusive evidence for differences in overall teratogenic potential is still lacking, and no malformation is specific for a given drug, the pattern of birth defects differs between drugs. Orofacial clefts, congenital heart defects and distal digital defects are more common in children exposed to phenytoin and barbiturates [54]. Valproic acid exposure has been associated with an increased risk of neural tube defects, reported to occur in 1–2% of exposed infants [55]. Valproic acid has also been associated with skeletal abnormalities including radial aplasia [56]. A risk of neural tube defects of 0.5–1% has also been reported after carbamazepine exposure [57,58]. Carbamazepine is also associated with an increased risk of congenital heart defects.

A dose–effect relationship has been demonstrated for valproic acid, with significantly higher risks for birth defects with doses exceeding 1000 mg/day [48–50], but not for other antiepileptic drugs. Polytherapy has consistently been associated with a higher risk for major congenital malformations than monotherapy (Table 23.4) [47,48,50,52]. A shift in therapeutic strategy from polytherapy to monotherapy during pregnancy has been paralleled by a decrease in the incidence of major malformations [59].

Minor anomalies and fetal antiepileptic drug syndromes

Minor anomalies can also occur, including structural variations that are visible at birth but without medical, surgical or cosmetic importance. Such anomalies frequently occur in normal unexposed infants but combinations of several anomalies are less common and can form a pattern, or a dysmorphic syndrome, which may indicate a more severe underlying dysfunction. Minor anomalies and dysmorphic syndromes have been reported to occur more frequently in infants of mothers treated for epilepsy during pregnancy. Facial features such as hypertelorism, depressed nasal bridge, low set ears, micrognathia and distal digital hypoplasia sometimes in combination with growth retardation and developmental delay were first reported in association with exposure to phenytoin [60]. Subsequently, however, similar patterns have been associated with exposure to carbamazepine [61]. Valproic acid exposure has been claimed to cause a somewhat different dysmorphic syndrome characterized by high forehead, a small and flat nose, long philtrum and long digits. However, there is a considerable overlap in the various dysmorphisms and their drug specificity has been questioned. A more general term, fetal or prenatal antiepileptic drug syndrome, has therefore been suggested [31]. In addition, the pathogenesis is still somewhat controversial and Gaily *et al.* [62] attributed most of the minor anomalies to genetic factors rather than drug exposure. However, a recent study examined physical features of infants born to women with a history of epilepsy but not taking antiepileptic drugs in pregnancy [63]. No infants were found to have features of the fetal antiepileptic drug syndrome, suggesting that such features indeed are related to drug exposure. Finally, it should be underlined that minor anomalies are much more difficult to assess objectively than major malformations, and that the incidence of minor anomalies in exposed infants varies markedly between studies.

Growth retardation

Several studies have reported that exposure to antiepileptic drugs is associated with an impaired intrauterine growth. Reduced birth weight, body length and head circumference in the offspring of women treated with phenytoin was reported as early as the 1970s [60]. Reductions in body dimensions, in particular head circumference, have been confirmed in several subsequent studies of larger cohorts [64–68]. Most studies report a more pronounced effect in infants exposed to polytherapy [64,65,67,68]. However, the association with specific antiepileptic drugs in monotherapy varies. Some

Table 23.4 Risk of major malformations in relation to number of antiepileptic drugs taken during pregnancy

	Samrén *et al.* [47]	Samrén *et al.* [48]	Kaneko *et al.* [50]	Holmes *et al.* [52]
Healthy controls		1.5%		1.8%
Untreated epilepsy			3.1%	0
Monotherapy	8.6%	3.3%	7.8%	4.5%
Polytherapy	12.0%	4.8%	10.6%	8.6%

investigators found an association with phenobarbital and primidone, whereas others report carbamazepine to be more strongly associated with a small head circumference. In a recent publication, Wide et al. [67] studied body dimensions in infants exposed to antiepileptic drugs in utero in a Swedish population over a period of 25 years comparing data to the general population. There was a clear trend towards normalization of the head circumference over the time period in parallel with a shift from polytherapy towards monotherapy despite an increasing use of carbamazepine. The reason for being interested in small head circumference, or microcephalia, is that it might signal a functional deficit. However, a recent study failed to find an association between a small head circumference in children exposed to antiepileptic drugs and cognitive functioning in adulthood [68].

Psychomotor development

One of the most important issues is whether exposure to antiepileptic drugs in utero could adversely affect postnatal psychomotor development. Long-term follow-up studies of large cohorts of exposed individuals are necessary in order to address this issue. Such studies are difficult to perform and also complicated to interpret since environmental factors become more important with increasing age of the child. Only a few studies have been published in this area, all with fairly small cohorts and the results are conflicting. In one of the largest controlled prospective studies, Gaily et al. [69] found no influence on global IQ, and the observed cognitive dysfunction in exposed children was attributed to maternal seizures and the educational level of the parents rather than to the treatment [70]. The children in this study were assessed at 5.5 years of age, and had been exposed in most cases to low doses of phenytoin and carbamazepine as monotherapy. Only a few were exposed to phenobarbital or valproate prenatally. In a German study, 67 young people, representing 41% from a prospective study of children born to mothers with epilepsy, were reassessed at school age and adolescence [71]. Of those, 13 were unexposed to antiepileptic drugs during pregnancy, 31 were exposed to monotherapy, in most cases phenytoin or primidone, and 23 to polytherapy. In contrast to exposure to monotherapy, polytherapy was associated with significantly lower IQ scores compared to the controls. Reinisch et al. [72] found lower verbal intelligence than expected among adult men who had been exposed prenatally to phenobarbital, mainly for reasons other than maternal epilepsy. Although other risk factors, such as low socioeconomic status, were identified, last trimester exposure to phenobarbital was the most detrimental. Dessens et al. [68] reported normal intellectual capacity, assessed in adulthood, in most of 147 individuals exposed to phenobarbital and/or phenytoin in utero, but 12% of the exposed subjects versus 1% of unexposed controls had learning problems persisting into adulthood. A recent retrospective survey from England found that additional educational needs were considerably more frequent among children who had been exposed to valproate monotherapy than in those exposed to carbamazepine or in unexposed children [73]. The authors, however, conclude that their results need to be interpreted with caution due to the retrospective nature of the study. Holmes et al. [63] assessed children of mothers with untreated epilepsy and found normal intelligence suggesting that epilepsy as such does not imply an increased risk for cognitive dysfunction in the offspring.

Taken together the available information on potential adverse effects of antiepileptic drug exposure on long-term development is sparse and at present inconclusive. More prospective studies on larger cohorts are urgently needed.

Mechanisms of teratogenic effects of antiepileptic drugs

Better understanding of the mechanisms behind the developmental toxicity of antiepileptic drugs is essential for a more rational approach to the treatment of women with epilepsy of childbearing potential. The structural defects, and the retardation of growth and development observed in children exposed to antiepileptic drugs in utero, have been reproduced in various animal species [74] demonstrating the importance of the antiepileptic drugs in their pathogenesis. In animal models, as in humans, the pattern of birth defects is to some extent different for different antiepileptic drugs, which indicates that multiple mechanisms are involved.

The earliest hypothesis suggests that the teratogenic effects of antiepileptic drugs are related to their interference with folate metabolism. In animal studies, a folate-deficient diet has resulted in an increased incidence of malformations in the offspring. Some antiepileptic drugs are known to reduce folate levels, and some clinical studies [75,76] have reported an association between low maternal serum folate levels and adverse pregnancy outcome including malformations. The latter observation, however, is controversial since other studies have failed to confirm this finding. Pretreatment with folinic acid reduced valproic acid induced malformations in mouse models [77]. In humans, extra periconceptional supplementation with folate has been demonstrated to reduce the risk of neural tube defects [78] and also the risk of their recurrence in high-risk groups [79]. These clinical studies however did not study the prevention of neural tube defects in women with epilepsy or under treatment with antiepileptic drugs.

Although phenytoin and phenobarbital are the antiepileptic drugs that decrease folate levels the most, these drugs have been linked to neural tube defects to a lesser extent than valproic acid and carbamazepine, which have less prominent effects on folate levels. Nevertheless, the available experimental data suggest that interference with embryonic folate metabolism may be involved in some aspects of drug-induced teratogenesis, particularly that associated with valproic acid. Genetic factors related to folate metabolism may explain differences in susceptibility observed between different strains of animals [76].

A prevailing hypothesis in recent years is that antiepileptic drugs are metabolized to toxic reactive intermediates that are responsible for the teratogenic effects [74]. The toxic intermediate could be an epoxide produced during oxidation of phenytoin, carbamazepine or phenobarbital. In general, epoxides are highly reactive and may bind to fetal macromolecules in the embryo and thus cause teratogenic effects. Such epoxides are metabolized by the enzyme epoxide hydrolase, and may accumulate and react if the rate of formation of the epoxide exceeds the elimination by epoxide hydrolase. The balance between enzyme activities catalysing the formation and the elimination of reactive epoxides may be genetically determined and also affected by interactions with antiepileptic drugs. Interestingly, some specific combinations of antiepileptic drugs, notably carbamazepine, phenobarbital and valproic acid, have been associated with a particularly high rate of malformations [80]. Hypothetically, the inducing effects of carbamazepine and phenobarbital on the formation of epoxides and the inhibitory effect of valproic acid on epoxide hydrolase could explain this particularly high risk. However, some of the teratogenic antiepileptic drugs lack the premises to form epoxides. A proposed alternative bioactivating pathway is cooxidation to free radical intermediates that may cause oxidative stress resulting in birth defects [74].

A more recent hypothesis suggests that many antiepileptic drugs, such as phenytoin, trimethadione, carbamazepine and phenobarbital, are exerting their developmental adverse effects by inducing episodes of embryonic cardiac arrhythmia during restricted periods of embryonic development [81]. According to this hypothesis, embryonic hypoxia is followed by reoxygenation and generation of reactive oxygen species, which will cause tissue damage (Fig. 23.1). All typical malformations such as orofacial clefts, heart defects, distal digital defects and growth retardation can be induced in experimental studies by hypoxia, and antiepileptic drugs have been shown to affect the embryonic heart in animal models. Hence, the embryonic heart appears to be more sensitive than the adult heart to effects of antiepileptic drugs.

In conclusion the mechanisms behind developmental toxicity of antiepileptic drugs are presently far from completely understood and are likely to be multiple and also differ between drugs.

Sensitive periods

Sensitive periods in embryonic development with reference to some of the more important major malformations associated with antiepileptic drugs are summarized in Table 23.5. Obviously, adverse effects of this type occur early, often before the woman is aware that she is pregnant. In contrast, drugs may affect growth and psychomotor development throughout pregnancy.

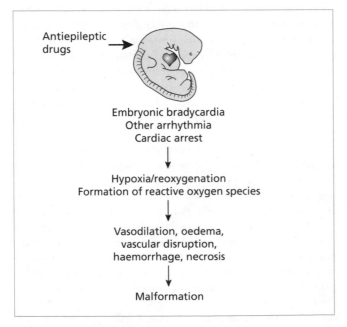

Antiepileptic drugs

→

Embryonic bradycardia
Other arrhythmia
Cardiac arrest

↓

Hypoxia/reoxygenation
Formation of reactive oxygen species

↓

Vasodilation, oedema,
vascular disruption,
haemorrhage, necrosis

↓

Malformation

Fig. 23.1 Series of events which, according to the hypoxia–reoxygenation hypothesis, could lead to teratogenic effects of some antiepileptic drugs.

Breastfeeding

Most drugs pass from maternal plasma to breast milk and are transferred to the nursed infant. In general, the amounts thus transferred are much smaller than those transferred via the placenta during pregnancy. The amount that the infant will be exposed to through breastfeeding depends on the maternal plasma concentration, the extent of transfer to breast milk and the amount of milk intake by the infant. Drug exposure of the suckling infant is also dependent on the infant's absorption, distribution, metabolism and elimination of the drug. In particular metabolism and excretion may be markedly different in the infant compared with children and adults and also vary with the drug in question. Relevant pharmacokinetic information, based on data from Vinge [82], Hägg and Spigset [83] and Öhman *et al.* [44] is summarized in Table 23.6.

It should be emphasized that data on the new generation antiepileptics are scarce. No information is available concerning levetiracetam, tiagabine, topiramate or zonisamide. Information on oxcarbazepine, gabapentin and vigabatrin is limited to a few cases whereas data on lamotrigine are accumulating.

For phenytoin, carbamazepine, oxcarbazepine and valproic acid, only small amounts are transferred and serum levels in suckling infants are generally so low that pharmacological effects are unlikely to occur. For ethosuximide and lamotrigine infant serum concentrations may occasionally reach levels at which pharmacological effects can be seen. However, so far there is no clear evidence for the occurrence of adverse effects in nursed infants. Phenobarbital, and phenobarbital as a metabolite of primidone, can accumulate in the suckling infant and sedation and poor suckling have been reported. Similarly sedation may occur due to exposure to benzodiazepines such as diazepam, clonazepam and possibly clobazam if taken chronically by the nursing mother. However, such adverse effects do not occur in all nursed infants.

The benefits of breastfeeding in general are unquestionable. These must be weighed against the possible risks to the infant induced by drug exposure. Taking this into account, women with epilepsy should in general be encouraged to nurse their infants and the risk for adverse effects due to drug exposure through breast milk is in most cases negligible.

Women who nurse while taking phenobarbital, primidone, benzodiazepines and perhaps also ethosuximide and the new antiepileptic drugs should be encouraged to monitor their infant for side-effects such as sedation or poor suckling, rather than being advised not to nurse. If suspicion of pharmacological effects arises, this could be confirmed or rejected by measuring serum drug levels in the infant.

Table 23.5 Gestation periods sensitive to specific congenital malformations

Malformation	Approximate sensitive period (gestational weeks)
Neural tube defects	3–4
Congenital heart defects	4–8
Orofacial clefts	6–10

Table 23.6 Antiepileptic drugs in breast milk and in the suckling infant

Antiepileptic drug	Milk/maternal plasma concentration ratio	Highest serum drug concentration in the suckling infant (μmol/L)
Carbamazepine	0.1–0.3	20
Clobazam	0.1–0.3	Data not available
Clonazepam	0.3–0.4	0.06
Ethosuximide	0.8–1.0	285
Gabapentin	0.7–0.8	Data not available
Lamotrigine	0.4–0.8	11
Oxcarbazepine	0.5[a]	Data not available
Phenobarbital	0.3–0.5	39
Phenytoin	0.1–0.6	<1
Valproate	0.01–0.1	28

Data from [44,82,83].
[a] Mono-hydroxy derivative of oxcarbazepine

Folate supplementation

As discussed previously, low folate intake has been associated with an increased risk of congenital malformations, in particular neural tube defects, in animal studies and in humans. Periconceptional consumption of folic acid supplements reduces the risk of giving birth to a child with a neural tube defect [78,79,84]. In a randomized study of more than 7000 Hungarian women planning pregnancy, supplementation with 0.8 mg folic acid reduced the risk of neural tube defects significantly [78]. This study demonstrated the effectiveness of folate for prevention of first occurrence of neural tube defects. A randomized British study [79] assessed the effect of folic acid supplementation on the risk of recurrence of neural tube defects in high-risk pregnancies. More than 1000 pregnancies were included and 4.0 mg/day folate reduced the recurrence risk by 72%. Periconceptional intake of 0.4 mg of folic acid daily has also been shown to reduce the risk of neural tube defects in a public health campaign in China [84]. Unfortunately, no study has specifically assessed the effectiveness of folic acid supplementation in women with epilepsy. In fact, such patients were excluded from the study in the UK [79]. The reason was a concern that the high-dose folic acid might be seizure provoking in women with epilepsy, but evidence for such adverse effects is insubstantial. A general concern, related also to low-dose supplementation, has been a suggestion that folate intake may be associated with an increased risk for miscarriage, but this has not been confirmed in a large study from China [85].

In the absence of data specific for women with epilepsy, recommendations have to be drawn from studies based on the general population. In general, women of childbearing potential are recommended a daily intake of 0.4 mg folic acid daily and the most practical way of achieving that is as a daily supplementation. It is reasonable to suggest this also to all women with epilepsy. A higher dose, 4 mg/day, is recommended for secondary prevention to women with a previous history of giving birth to a child with neural tube defects or with a family history of such malformations. The risk of giving birth to a child with a neural tube defect is in the same order among women taking valproic acid and carbamazepine as in these women. It may therefore seem reasonable to recommend a supplementation of 4 mg/day also to women with epilepsy on these antiepileptic drugs, although evidence for the effectiveness of such supplementation is lacking in this population. Consequently, it is essential to inform the patient that it is uncertain whether folate supplementation will reduce this risk and pregnancy monitoring with prenatal diagnoses should be offered in the same way whether high-dose folate is prescribed or not.

Vitamin K supplementation and neonatal haemorrhage

Vitamin K deficiency can cause early neonatal haemorrhage and neonates of mothers treated with enzyme-inducing antiepileptic drugs during pregnancy may have an increased risk [86]. Decreased levels of vitamin K dependent clotting factors are found in cord blood of newborns of women taking enzyme-inducing antiepileptic drugs and supplementation with 10 mg/day of vitamin K orally for the last month of pregnancy has been shown to normalize these levels [87]. It remains to be shown that prenatal oral vitamin K supplementation also reduces the risk of neonatal haemorrhage. The issue is thus controversial. Hey [88] studied prospectively cord blood prothrombin time in 137 babies born to women on phenobarbital, phenytoin or carbamazepine. Only 14 of the babies had prolonged prothrombin time and none an overt bleeding tendency. The abnormality was corrected within 2 h by 1 mg of parenteral vitamin K. Based on these observations, Hey concluded that evidence is lacking for a particular early form of neonatal haemorrhage related to use of anticonvulsants and that oral vitamin K supplementation during late pregnancy is unjustified. However, 137 babies is too small a cohort to exclude an increased risk for uncommon events such as neonatal haemorrhage. Since there are no significant risks associated, oral vitamin K supplementation (10–20 mg/day) is often recommended from the 36th week to women on enzyme-inducing antiepileptic drugs. Additionally, 1 mg vitamin K should be given i.m. to the newborn at birth as is done routinely for all neonates in many countries.

Preconception counselling

Several surveys have revealed that women with epilepsy often receive insufficient and even inaccurate information concerning issues related to reproductive function. Clinical practical guidelines for the care of women with epilepsy of childbearing age have been published in many countries and also by the International League Against Epilepsy [89–91]. Unfortunately, many important questions are still unanswered, and many of the recommendations build on rather weak evidence, from observational studies rather than randomized trials. This is reflected in the slight differences found in the different guidelines. Nevertheless, they provide useful tools and need to be brought to the attention of health-care providers and utilized in their counselling of women with epilepsy. An optimal management of pregnancy depends largely on considerations that have to be made, and measures that have to be taken, before conception. Pre-pregnancy counselling is therefore essential and it is an important challenge to change the present situation where such counselling seems to be offered in only a minority of women with epilepsy. Preconceptional counselling should cover the issues listed below.

• Contraception and fertility. The potential of enzyme-inducing antiepileptic drugs to interact with oral contraceptives should be discussed when relevant. The possibility that drug treatment may induce endocrine dysfunction affecting fertility should also be addressed.

• Genetic counselling with respect to the risk of giving birth to a child who will develop epilepsy and with respect to birth defects.

• Risks associated with seizures during pregnancy, and information that such risks to the fetus probably outweigh the risks incurred by an optimized treatment with antiepileptic drugs.

• Risks of adverse effects of antiepileptic drugs to the fetus, including a two- to four-fold increase in the incidence of major malformations.

• The option of prenatal diagnosis of birth defects including possibilities and risks with the different methods.

• General principles of antiepileptic drug use in pregnancy and the importance of optimizing seizure control and making any major change in drug therapy before pregnancy. The importance of medication compliance during pregnancy and the risks associated with abrupt withdrawal need to be underlined.

• Recommendations concerning folate supplementation, including information on the lack of evidence for its effectiveness in preventing birth defects related to antiepileptic drug exposure.

• Risk of seizures at delivery and the recommendation that delivery should take place in well-equipped obstetric units.

• Risk for deterioration in seizure control due to sleep deprivation after delivery.

• Feasibility of breastfeeding.

In conclusion, although there are specific risks and problems associated with pregnancy in women with epilepsy, counselling should focus on the feasibility of reducing risks and on the fact that more than 90% of women with epilepsy can look forward to an uneventful pregnancy and to giving birth to a normal and healthy child.

Some of the issues discussed above, e.g. genetic counselling and the risk for deterioration in seizure control due to sleep deprivation, are also relevant for men with epilepsy who are considering having children, although this is often completely neglected.

Management during pregnancy

Antiepileptic drug treatment during pregnancy

The optimal management of a woman with epilepsy during pregnancy relies on a close collaboration with exchange of information between the physician responsible for epilepsy care and the obstetrician. Treatment with antiepileptic drugs should be optimized before conception, with the objective to use monotherapy at the lowest effective dosage. Since conclusive evidence is lacking with regard to differences in overall teratogenic potential between most antiepileptic drugs, including the newly licensed ones, it is reasonable to select the antiepileptic drug that is most likely to control seizures, i.e. the appropriate first-line drug for seizure type and epilepsy syndrome. However, accumulating data suggest that valproic acid should be avoided if other suitable treatment options are available. Valproic acid and carbamazepine are best avoided when there is a family history of neural tube defects. For valproic acid, experimental studies suggest that the risk of birth defects is related to peak concentrations rather than daily dosage. Although this has not

Table 23.7 Strategies for treatment with antiepileptic drugs during pregnancy

All major changes in treatment should be accomplished before conception

Use the appropriate drug for the patient's seizures or epilepsy syndrome but avoid valproic acid if possible

Aim at monotherapy with the lowest effective dose/serum concentration

Monitor the patient clinically and with serum drug concentration measurements each trimester, more frequently in patients with poor seizure control

Adjust dosage on clinical indications, utilizing information on changes in serum drug levels compared with preconceptional optimal concentrations

Stress the importance of compliance with medication and in particular the need for regular intake also during labour

been demonstrated clinically, a slow-release formulation given 2–3 times daily is often advocated during pregnancy (Table 23.7).

Treatment should aim at complete control of, in particular, generalized tonic-clonic seizures. Other seizure types are probably less hazardous but may in some patients signal an increased risk also for tonic-clonic seizures. Complex partial seizures may also compromise maternal cooperation at delivery.

An attempt to withdraw treatment should be considered in women who plan pregnancy and who have been seizure free for 2 years or more. However this needs to be assessed individually based on the estimated risk of recurrence and potential consequences thereof. In case of polytherapy, conversion to monotherapy should be considered, and an attempt to titrate the lowest effective dosage be made. All such major changes should ideally be completed several months before conception to allow a reasonable observation period before pregnancy. It may be useful to document the optimal serum drug level before pregnancy to facilitate interpretation of serum concentration measurements during pregnancy.

Conversion from polytherapy to monotherapy, or changes between antiepileptic drugs, for the purpose of reducing teratogenic risks, should not be attempted during pregnancy. At this stage of pregnancy the potential gain is minor compared to the risks associated with such procedures.

The treatment should be monitored more closely during pregnancy than otherwise. This too needs to be tailored to the individual but in most cases an assessment each trimester, with a last visit at week 34–36, will suffice. This should include clinical evaluation and drug level monitoring where appropriate. Where phenytoin and valproic acid are used, monitoring the unbound levels is preferred. A decrease in serum levels of antiepileptic drugs alone does not generally justify an increase in dosage. The overall clinical state should be assessed and the individual patient's optimal drug concentration and sensitivity to changes in drug levels documented before pregnancy should be taken into account. If a dosage increment was made during pregnancy, serum drug levels should be monitored during the first 4–6 weeks after delivery since a dose reduction may be necessary.

Prenatal diagnosis

Women on antiepileptic drugs should be offered the possibility of prenatal testing if elective termination of pregnancy is acceptable. A malformation directed ultrasound investigation at 16–20 weeks of gestation has a high sensitivity and specificity in the detection of major malformations, including more than 90% of neural tube defects, and a high proportion of cardiac malformations, skeletal defects and orofacial clefts. An ultrasound examination is often offered also at week 33–34 for assessment of intrauterine growth retardation. Amniocentesis for amniotic fluid α-fetoprotein may also be considered when appropriate. This method however carries 0.5–1.0% risk of abortion.

Vitamin supplementation

Women with epilepsy considering pregnancy should be prescribed supplementation with folic acid, 0.4 mg/day from before conception. A higher dose, 4 mg/day, should be given to those who have a family history of neural tube defects and may be considered also for women on valproic acid or carbamazepine. Vitamin K, 10 mg/day orally during the last month of pregnancy, could be considered for women on enzyme-inducing antiepileptic drugs.

Delivery and labour

In general, labour and delivery do not imply any particular obstetric measures. However delivery should take place in a well-equipped obstetric unit in view of the increased risk of seizures during labour and delivery and the increased risk of neonatal death.

Hiilesmaa [92] has listed the following epilepsy-related indications for elective caesarean section: (a) substantial neurological or mental deficit causing reduced cooperation in labour; (b) very poor seizure control in late pregnancy (i.e. daily complex partial seizures or weekly tonic-clonic seizures); and (c) prior knowledge of the occurrence of severe seizures during heavy physical or mental stress.

Emergency caesarean delivery is indicated during labour in cases where seizures induce fetal asphyxia or cause poor maternal cooperation. Intravenous benzodiazepines to the mother are also indicated in such cases.

Puerperium

Stress and sleep deprivation in the puerperium may sometimes adversely affect seizure control. Furthermore, the new responsibilities of the care of the newborn may necessitate special considerations and precautions at home. It is recommended that the mother with epilepsy is given extra support from her partner or others during the first weeks at home, in particular if she is sensitive to sleep deprivation where seizures are likely to occur. In order to minimize risks to the infant, care for the child including breastfeeding is best carried out on the floor, and another person should supervise bathing of the newborn.

Implications for the treatment of women of childbearing age

The rate of unplanned pregnancies in the general population is high and the first contact with health-care providers is frequently late. These factors are true for women with epilepsy as they are for anyone else. Therefore, issues related to management during pregnancy will have implications for the treatment of women with epilepsy of childbearing potential in general. Furthermore, the potential adverse effects of epilepsy and drug therapy on reproductive function, pharmacokinetic interactions with oral contraceptives as well as developmental toxicity of antiepileptic drugs, need to be included in the overall risk–benefit equation which should be the basis for decisions on when and how to treat epilepsy in young women. Thus, it is sometimes reasonable to withhold treatment in new onset seizures if the indication is weak or ambiguous. If treatment is indicated, it is particularly important in this patient group to aim at monotherapy with the lowest effective dosage. When treatment is initiated in a woman of childbearing potential, information must be given concerning drug effects on oral contraceptives, when appropriate, as well as potential adverse effects on endocrine reproductive function and implications in relation to pregnancy. The benefits of planning pregnancy should be emphasized. Because of the high rate of unplanned pregnancies, supplementation with folic acid (0.4 mg/day) is reasonable to all women of childbearing potential who take antiepileptic drugs. Counselling needs to be iterated at regular intervals. It is also important to inform, at an appropriate age, those women who had onset of their epilepsy as young girls but continue on antiepileptic drugs beyond puberty.

Based on the considerations above, it is essential to identify young women with epilepsy who are likely to be able to withdraw their treatment without seizure recurrence, and to support them in attempts to taper treatment before they consider pregnancy. Likewise, suitable candidates for epilepsy surgery have the prospect of becoming seizure free, eventually without medication, after a successful operation. Hence it is of particular value to avoid unnecessary delay in assessment for epilepsy surgery in women of childbearing potential.

Potential adverse effects on reproductive function should be considered along with all other relevant properties when selecting an antiepileptic drug for a woman with epilepsy. The most important property of an antiepileptic drug is its effectiveness in preventing seizures, and for women of childbearing potential, the best choice is the drug that is most appropriate for the seizure type or syndrome. However, the patient should be closely monitored for possible adverse effects on reproductive endocrine function and the treatment reassessed should such side-effects occur. It should also be remembered that drug preferences are likely to change as we gain more information on adverse effects on endocrine function from randomized clinical trials and comparative data on teratogenic effects of different antiepileptic drugs from pregnancy registries.

References

1 Webber MP, Hauser WA, Ottman R, Annegers JF. Fertility in persons with epilepsy: 1935–1974. *Epilepsia* 1986; 27: 746–52.
2 Dansky LV, Andermann E, Andermann F. Marriage and fertility in epileptic patients. *Epilepsia* 1980; 21: 261–71.
3 Schupf N, Ottman R. Likelihood of pregnancy in individuals with idiopathic/cryptogenic epilepsy: social and biologic influences. *Epilepsia* 1994; 35: 750–6.
4 Schupf N, Ottman R. Reproduction among individuals with idiopathic/cryptogenic epilepsy: risk factors for reduced fertility in marriage. *Epilepsia* 1996; 37: 833–40.
5 Wallace H, Shorvon S, Tallis R. Age-specific incidence and prevalence rates of treated epilepsy in an unselected population of 2,052,922 and age-specific fertility rates of women with epilepsy. *Lancet* 1998; 352: 1970–3.

6 Olafsson E, Hauser WA, Gudmundsson G. Fertility in patients with epilepsy: a population-based study. *Neurology* 1998; 51: 71–3.

7 Penovich PE. The effects of epilepsy and its treatment on sexual and reproductive function. *Epilepsia* 2000; 41 (Suppl. 2): S53–S61.

8 Duncan S, Blacklaw J, Beastall GH, Brodie MJ. Antiepileptic drug therapy and sexual function in men with epilepsy. *Epilepsia* 1999; 40: 197–204.

9 Rättyä J, Turkka J, Pakarinen AJ *et al.* Reproductive effects of valproate, carbamazepine, and oxcarbazepine in men with epilepsy. *Neurology* 2001; 56: 31–6.

10 Herzog AG, Seibel MM, Schomer DL, Vaitukaitis JL, Geschwind N. Reproductive endocrine disorders in men with partial seizures of temporal lobe origin. *Arch Neurol* 1986; 43: 347–50.

11 Herzog AG. A hypothesis to integrate partial seizures of temporal lobe origin and reproductive endocrine disorders. *Epilepsy Res* 1989; 3: 151–9.

12 Bauer J, Stoffel-Wagner B, Flugel D *et al.* Serum androgens return to normal after temporal lobe epilepsy surgery in men. *Neurology* 2000; 55: 820–4.

13 Chen SS, Shen MR, Chen TJ, Lai SL. Effects of antiepileptic drugs on sperm motility of normal controls and epileptic patients with long-term therapy. *Epilepsia* 33: 149–53.

14 Bilo L, Meo R, Nappi C *et al.* Reproductive endocrine disorders in women with primary generalized epilepsy. *Epilepsia* 1988; 29: 612–19.

15 Drislane FW, Coleman AE, Schomer DL *et al.* Altered pulsatile secretion of luteinizing hormone in women with epilepsy. *Neurology* 1994; 44: 306–10.

16 Duncan S. Polycystic ovarian syndrome in women with epilepsy: a review. *Epilepsia* 2001; 42 (Suppl. 3): 60–5.

17 Herzog AG, Schachter SC. Valproate and the polycystic ovarian syndrome: final thoughts. *Epilepsia* 2001; 42: 311–15.

18 Murialdo G, Galimberti CA, Magri F *et al.* Menstrual cycle and ovary alterations in women with epilepsy on antiepileptic therapy. *J Endocrinol Invest* 1997; 20: 519–26.

19 Isojärvi JI, Laatikainen TJ, Pakarinen AJ, Juntunen KT, Myllyla VV. Polycystic ovaries and hyperandrogenism in women taking valproate for epilepsy. *N Engl J Med* 1993; 329: 1383–8.

20 Isojärvi JI, Laatikainen TJ, Knip M, Pakarinen AJ, Juntunen KT, Myllyla VV. Obesity and endocrine disorders in women taking valproate for epilepsy. *Ann Neurol* 1996; 39: 579–84.

21 Isojärvi JI, Rättya J, Myllyla VV *et al.* Valproate, lamotrigine, and insulin-mediated risks in women with epilepsy. *Ann Neurol* 1998; 43: 446–51.

22 Murialdo G, Galimberti CA, Gianelli MV *et al.* Effects of valproate, phenobarbital, and carbamazepine on sex steroid setup in women with epilepsy. *Clin Neuropharmacol* 1998; 21: 52–8.

23 Genton P, Bauer J, Duncan S *et al.* On the association between valproate and polycystic ovary syndrome. *Epilepsia* 2001; 42: 295–304.

24 Isojärvi JI, Tauböll E, Tapanainen JS *et al.* On the association between valproate and polycystic ovary syndrome: a response and an alternative view. *Epilepsia* 2001; 42: 305–10.

25 Bauer J, Jarre A, Klingmuller D, Elger CE. Polycystic ovary syndrome in patients with focal epilepsy: a study in 93 women. *Epilepsy Res* 2000; 41: 163–7.

26 Rättyä J, Vainionpää L, Knip M, Lanning P, Isojärvi JI. The effects of valproate, carbamazepine, and oxcarbazepine on growth and sexual maturation in girls with epilepsy. *Pediatrics* 1999; 103: 588–93.

27 Vainionpää L, Rättyä J, Knip M *et al.* Valproate induced hyperandrogenism during pubertal maturation in girls with epilepsy. *Ann Neurol* 1999; 45: 444–50.

28 Coulam CB, Annegers JF. Do anticonvulsants reduce the efficacy of oral contraceptives? *Epilepsia* 1979; 20: 519–25.

29 Guberman A. Hormonal contraception and epilepsy. *Neurology* 1999; 53 (Suppl. 1): S38–S40.

30 Perucca E. The clinical pharmacokinetics of the new antiepileptic drugs. *Epilepsia* 1999; 40 (Suppl. 9): S7–S13.

31 Zahn CA, Morrell MJ, Collins SD, Labiner DM, Yerby MS. Management issues for women with epilepsy: a review of the literature. *Neurology* 1998; 51: 949–16.

32 Sabers A, Buchholt JM, Uldall P, Hansen EL. Lamotrigine plasma levels reduced by oral contraceptives. *Epilepsy Res* 2001; 47: 151–4.

33 Teramo K, Hiilesmaa V, Bardy A, Saarikoski S. Fetal heart rate during a maternal grand mal epileptic seizure. *J Perinatal Med* 1979; 7: 3–6.

34 Hiilesmaa VK, Bardy A, Teramo K. Obstetric outcome in women with epilepsy. *Am J Obstet Gynecol* 1985; 152: 499–504.

35 Teramo K, Hiilesmaa VK. Pregnancy and fetal complications in epileptic pregnancies. In: Janz D, Dam M, Richens A, Bossi L, Helge H, Schmidt D, eds. *Epilepsy, Pregnancy and the Child.* New York: Raven Press, 1982: 53–9.

36 Nei M, Daly S, Liporace J. A maternal complex partial seizure in labor can affect fetal heart rate. *Neurology* 1998; 51: 904–6.

37 Gaily E, Kantola-Sorsa E, Granström M-L. Specific cognitive dysfunction in children with epileptic mothers. *Dev Med Child Neurol* 1990; 32: 403–14.

38 Bardy AH. Incidence of seizures during pregnancy, labor and puerperium in epileptic women: a prospective study. *Acta Neurol Scand* 1987; 75: 356–60.

39 Gjerde IO, Strandjord RE, Ulstein M. The course of epilepsy during pregnancy: a study of 78 cases. *Acta Neurol Scand* 1988; 78: 198–205.

40 Tomson T, Lindbom U, Ekqvist B, Sundqvist A. Epilepsy and pregnancy: a prospective study of seizure control in relation to free and total plasma concentrations of carbamazepine and phenytoin. *Epilepsia* 1994; 35: 122–30.

41 Tomson T. Seizure control during pregnancy and delivery. In: Tomson T, Gram L, Sillanpää M, Johannessen SI, eds. *Epilepsy and Pregnancy.* Petersfield: Wrightson Biomedical Publishing Ltd, 1997: 113–23.

42 Perucca E. Drug metabolism in pregnancy, infancy and childhood. *Pharmacol Ther* 1987; 34: 129–43.

43 Yerby MS. Friel PN. McCormick K. Antiepileptic drug disposition during pregnancy. *Neurology* 1992; 42 (Suppl. 5): 12–16.

44 Öhman I, Vitols S, Tomson T. Lamotrigine in pregnancy: pharmacokinetics during delivery, in the neonate, and during lactation. *Epilepsia* 2000; 4: 709–13.

45 Sabers A. Complications during pregnancy and delivery. In: Tomson T, Gram L, Sillanpää M, Johannessen SI, eds. *Epilepsy and Pregnancy.* Petersfield: Wrightson Biomedical Publishing Ltd, 1997: 105–11.

46 Yerby M, Koepsell T, Daling J. Pregnancy complications and outcomes in a cohort of women with epilepsy. *Epilepsia* 1985; 26: 631–5.

47 Samrén B, van Duijn C, Koch S *et al.* Maternal use of antiepileptic drugs and the risk of major congenital malformations: A joint European prospective study of human teratogenesis associated with maternal epilepsy. *Epilepsia* 1997; 38: 981–90.

48 Samrén B, van Duijn C, Christiaens GC, Hofman A, Lindhout D. Antiepileptic drug regimens and major congenital abnormalities in the offspring. *Ann Neurol* 1999; 46: 739–46.

49 Canger R, Battino D, Canevini MP *et al.* Malformations in offspring of women with epilepsy: a prospective study. *Epilepsia* 1999; 40: 1231–6.

50 Kaneko S, Battino D, Andermann E *et al.* Congenital malformations due to antiepileptic drugs. *Epilepsy Res* 1999; 33: 145–58.

51 Wide K. Children exposed to antiepileptic drugs in utero. Clinical and epidemiological aspects on growth, development and occurrence of malformations. Thesis, Karolinska Institutet, Stockholm, 2000.

52 Holmes LB, Harvey EA, Coull BA *et al.* The teratogenicity of anticonvulsant drugs. *N Engl J Med* 2001; 344: 1132–8.

53 Craig J, Russell A, Parsons L *et al.* The UK Epilepsy and Pregnancy Register: update of results 1996–2002. Abstract. *Epilepsia* 2002; 43 (Suppl. 8): 56.

54 Källen B, Robert E, Mastroiacovo P, Martinez-Frias ML, Castilla EE, Cocchi G. Anticonvulsant drugs and malformations: is there a drug specificity? *Eur J Epidemiol* 1989; 5: 31–6.

55 Lindhout D, Schmidt D. In-utero exposure to valproate and neural tube defects. *Lancet* 1986; 1: 1392–3.

56 Verloes A, Frikiche A, Gremillet C *et al.* Proximal phocomelia and radial ray aplasia in fetal valproic syndrome. *Eur J Pediatr* 1990; 149: 266–7.

57 Rosa FW. Spina bifida in infants of women treated with carbamazepine during pregnancy. *N Engl J Med* 1991; 324: 674–7.

58 Källen AJ. Maternal carbamazepine and infant spina bifida. *Reprod Toxicol* 1994; 8: 203–5.

59 Lindhout D, Meinardi H, Meijer JW, Nau H. Antiepileptic drugs and teratogenesis in two consecutive cohorts: changes in prescription policy paralleled by changes in pattern of malformations. *Neurology* 1992; 42 (Suppl. 5): 94–110.

60 Hanson JW, Smith DW. The fetal hydantoin syndrome. *J Pediatr* 1975; 87: 285–90.

61 Jones KL, Lacro RV, Johnsson KA, Adams J. Pattern of malformations in the children of mothers treated with carbamazepine during pregnancy. *N Engl J Med* 1989; 320: 1661–6.

62 Gaily E. Minor anomalies and effects on psychomotor development associated with maternal use of antiepileptic drugs. In: Tomson T, Gram L, Sillanpää M, Johannessen SI, eds. *Epilepsy and Pregnancy*. Petersfield: Wrightson Biomedical Publishing Ltd, 1997: 63–70.

63 Holmes LB, Rosenberger PB, Harvey EA, Khoshbin S, Ryan L. Intelligence and physical features of children of women with epilepsy. *Teratology* 2000; 61: 196–202.

64 Hiilesmaa VK, Teramo K, Granstrom ML, Bardy AH. Fetal head growth retardation associated with maternal antiepileptic drugs. *Lancet* 1981; 2: 165–7.

65 Battino D, Kaneko S, Andermann E *et al*. Intrauterine growth in the offspring of epileptic women: a prospective multicenter study. *Epilepsy Res* 1999; 36: 53–60.

66 Steegers-Theunissen RP, Renier WO, Borm GF et al. Factors influencing the risk of abnormal pregnancy outcome in epileptic women: a multi-centre prospective study. *Epilepsy Res* 1994; 18: 261–9.

67 Wide K, Winbladh B, Tomson T, Källen B. Body dimensions of infants exposed to antiepileptic drugs in utero: observations spanning 25 years. *Epilepsia* 2000; 41: 854–61.

68 Dessens A, Cohen-Kettins P, Mellenbergh G, van de Poll N, Koppe J, Boer K. Association of prenatal phenobarbital and phenytoin exposure with small head size at birth and with learning problems. *Acta Paediatr* 2000; 89: 533–41.

69 Gaily E, Kantola-Sorsa E, Granström M-L. Intelligence of children of epileptic mothers. *J Pediatr* 1988; 113: 677–84.

70 Gaily E, Kantola-Sorsa E, Granström ML. Specific cognitive dysfunction in children with epileptic mothers. *Dev Med Child Neurol* 1990; 32: 403–14.

71 Koch S, Titzke K, Zimmermann RB, Schroeder M, Lehmkuhl U, Rauh H. Long-term neuropsychological consequences of maternal epilepsy and anticonvulsant treatment during pregnancy for school-age children and adolescents. *Epilepsia* 1999; 40: 1237–43.

72 Reinisch JM, Sanders SA, Mortensen EL, Rubin DB. In utero exposure to phenobarbital and intelligence deficits in adult men. *J Am Med Ass* 1995; 274: 1518–25.

73 Adab N, Jacoby A, Smith D, Chadwick D. Additional educational needs in children born to mothers with epilepsy. *J Neurol Neurosurg Psychiatry* 2001; 70: 15–21.

74 Finnell RH, Dansky LV. Parental epilepsy, anticonvulsant drugs, and reproductive outcome: epidemiologic and experimental findings spanning three decades; 1: Animal studies. *Reprod Toxicol* 1991; 5: 281–99.

75 Dansky LV, Andermann E, Rosenblatt D, Sherwin AL, Andermann F. Anticonvulsants, folate levels, and pregnancy outcome: a prospective study. *Ann Neurol* 1987; 21: 176–82.

76 Ogawa Y, Kaneko S, Otani K, Fukushima Y. Serum folic acid levels in epileptic mothers and their relationship to congenital malformations. *Epilepsy Res* 1991; 8: 75–8.

77 Nau H. Towards the mechanism of valproic acid induced neural tube defects. In: Tomson T, Gram L, Sillanpää M, Johannessen SI, eds. *Epilepsy and Pregnancy*. Petersfield: Wrightson Biomedical Publishing Ltd, 1997: 35–42.

78 Czeizel AE, Dudas I. Prevention of the first occurrence of neural-tube defects by periconceptional vitamin supplementation. *N Engl J Med* 1992; 327: 1832–5.

79 MRC Vitamin Study Research Group. Prevention of neural tube defects: results of the Medical Research Council Vitamin Study. *Lancet* 1991; 338: 131–7.

80 Lindhout D, Höppener RJ, Meinardi H. Teratogenicity of antiepileptic drug combinations with special emphasis on epoxidation (of carbamazepine). *Epilepsia* 1984; 25: 77–83.

81 Danielsson BR, Sköld AC, Azarbayjani F. Class III antiarrhythmics and phenytoin: teratogenicity due to embryonic cardiac dysrhythmia and reoxygenation damage. *Curr Pharmaceut Design* 2001; 7: 787–802.

82 Vinge E. Breast-feeding and antiepileptic drugs. In: Tomson T, Gram L, Sillanpää M, Johannessen SI, eds. *Epilepsy and Pregnancy*. Petersfield: Wrightson Biomedical Publishing Ltd, 1997: 93–103.

83 Hägg S, Spigset O. Anticonvulsant use during lactation. *Drug Safety* 2000; 22: 425–40.

84 Berry RJ, Li Z, Erickson JD *et al*. Prevention of neural-tube defects with folic acid in China. China–US Collaborative Project for Neural Tube Defect Prevention. *N Engl J Med* 1999; 341: 1485–90.

85 Gindler J, Zhu L, Berry RJ *et al*. Folic acid supplements during pregnancy and risk of miscarriage. *Lancet* 2001; 358: 796–800.

86 Mountain KR, Hirsh J, Gallus AS. Neonatal coagulation defect due to anticonvulsant drug treatment in pregnancy. *Lancet* 1970; 1: 265–8.

87 Cornelissen M, Steegers-Theunissen R, Kollee L, Eskes T, Motohara K, Monnens L. Supplementation of vitamin K in pregnant women receiving anticonvulsant therapy prevents neonatal vitamin K deficiency. *Am J Obstetr Gynecol* 1993; 168: 884–8.

88 Hey E. Effect of maternal anticonvulsant treatment on neonatal blood coagulation. *Arch Dis Child* 1999; 81: F208–10.

89 Anonymous. Guidelines for the care of women of childbearing age with epilepsy. Commission on Genetics, Pregnancy, and the Child, International League Against Epilepsy. *Epilepsia* 1993; 34: 588–9.

90 Crawford P, Appleton R, Betts T, Duncan J, Guthrie E, Morrow J. Best practice guidelines for the management of women with epilepsy. The Women with Epilepsy Guidelines Development Group. *Seizure* 1999; 8: 201–17.

91 Morrell MJ. Guidelines for the care of women with epilepsy. *Neurology* 1998; 51 (5 Suppl. 4): S21–S7.

92 Hiilesmaa VK. Pregnancy and birth in women with epilepsy. *Neurology* 1992; 42 (Suppl. 5): 8–11.

24 Genetic Counselling in Epilepsy

F. Zara

Recent advances in the genetics of epilepsy indicate that the aetiology of many different epileptic phenotypes will be clarified in the near future. Although most of the work towards this goal still lies ahead, current knowledge provides important clues to the pathogenesis and mode of inheritance of various epileptic syndromes. An important issue facing epileptology, and medicine in general, is the management of genetic data on hereditary disorders. Central to this process is the way patients and their families are dealt with, which is commonly referred to as genetic counselling. The American Society of Human Genetics has defined genetic counselling as a communication process dealing with human problems associated with the occurrence, or risk of recurrence, of a genetic disorder in a family [1]. Genetic counselling is hence aimed at helping patients and families to:

1 Comprehend medical data, the diagnosis, the probable course of the disease and the treatment available.

2 Understand how hereditary factors contribute to the disorder and the risk of recurrence in specific relatives.

3 Choose the appropriate course of action in view of their risks, goals and personal morality.

Genetic counselling therefore involves a diagnostic task, risk assessment and a communicative process.

The pedigree as a diagnostic tool

Accurate genetic counselling is based on reliable diagnoses, and the principal task for clinicians is to reach as firm a diagnosis as possible.

As familial recurrence is the distinctive feature of most hereditary disorders, the first step towards an accurate diagnosis is to review the patient's family history. The medical history of the family can be rapidly gathered by drawing up the family pedigree. The family tree is a powerful tool which provides the clinician with essential clinical and biological information and constitutes a permanent and concise record that can be widely interpreted. Pedigrees are drawn by using a universal language that includes symbols indicating sex, disease status and relationships (Fig. 24.1). The pedigree may be used (a) to decide on testing strategies; (b) to distinguish genetic from non-genetic aetiology; (c) to establish the pattern of inheritance and to calculate risks; and (d) to decide on medical screening for unaffected individuals.

The collection of family data should include basic clinical details of both sides of the family for three or four generations. It is advisable to examine personally family members that may be affected or at risk. Unexpected findings may often emerge from families of patients with apparently negative history. A clear diagnosis may be difficult to establish in family members who are deceased. However, detailed information may be obtained by interviewing close relatives, and the exclusion of specific disorders may often be possible. Home visits may be considered in selected cases. When collecting family data, it is also important to enquire about consanguinity as a clue to autosomal recessive inheritance. The ethnic and geographical origins of family members should also be carefully investigated in order to detect hidden consanguinity. Unacknowledged paternity (e.g. adoption) should be considered in puzzling situations, as this may exert a confounding effect on segregation of the disease.

In medical genetics the most distinctive tool for establishing a diagnosis is genetic testing. A genetic test is defined as a laboratory analysis aimed at detecting the alteration of a gene, chromosomal abnormality and DNA variation associated with a genetic disorder. Genetic tests may focus on the analysis of the DNA structure (chromosomes or specific DNA segments) or of gene products (e.g. biochemical assays). Although genetic testing is a very promising and attractive diagnostic tool, its use is not a panacea for clinicians. Indeed, population screening is recommended for very few genetic disorders, and genetic tests are usually performed on the basis of precise clinical indications. Moreover, as genetic tests have not yet been developed for most genetic disorders, the accurate analysis of clinical data is the only means of establishing a diagnosis.

Risk assessment

Once a hereditary disorder has been diagnosed, it is possible to estimate any family member's risk of developing the disease. However, as the genetics of most hereditary disorders have not yet been discovered nor appropriate tests devised, the risk of recurrence cannot be calculated exactly and, for many hereditary disorders, will be estimated on the basis of probability. Risk assessment therefore mainly depends on the information available.

Empirical risks are based on observed data collected through epidemiological studies; these usually provide an acceptable approximation and are widely used for several poorly understood genetic conditions. Population-based estimates are, however, strongly influenced by worldwide variability in incidence and aetiology and may therefore not be applicable to all populations. Moreover, empirical risks may be frequently revised in accordance with the current definition of phenotypes and more accurate genotype–phenotype correlations.

By contrast, genetic risks are defined when the mode of inheritance of the disease is known. To date, such risks may be calculated for disorders that are caused by mutations in a single gene and segregate throughout populations according to mendelian laws. Family members may be classified into clear-cut categories: no risk (i.e. offspring of healthy sibs in autosomal dominant disorders), low risk

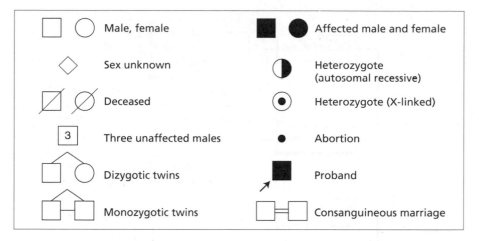

Fig. 24.1 Most common symbols used for drawing a pedigree.

(i.e. offspring of a potential carrier of autosomal recessive disease) and high risk (i.e. offspring of individuals affected by an autosomal dominant disorder).

Communication

Genetic counselling is not just a communication process aimed at informing patients of the risk of recurrence in specific relatives. It should also support patients in taking decisions (e.g. on reproduction) in accordance with their view of life. To this end, genetic counselling should help the patient to understand medical data and clarify any misconceptions.

Diagnosing a specific genetic disorder often implies the involvement of many family members who have been unaware of being at risk. Whether or not to contact members of extended families should be carefully discussed with patients and, if this is deemed necessary, an *ad hoc* strategy should be planned.

The evolution of genetic counselling into a process that involves an entire family requires extreme caution. A central principle of genetic counselling is that a non-directive attitude should be adopted. Non-directiveness implies that patients are fully aware of the genetic risks and their consequences and are therefore able to make their own decisions. A totally neutral approach to genetic counselling cannot realistically be achieved; nevertheless, it must be emphasized that counsellors should not provide solutions to critical questions concerning patients' lives.

Mode of inheritance of genetic disorders

It has long been known that the phenotypic characteristics of many living beings are transmitted according to Mendel's laws. In Mendel's model, genetic factors segregate from parents to offspring as independent and unaltered units, and phenotypes result from the interaction of variants (alleles) of these discrete units according to hierarchical relationships (dominant vs. recessive).

Mendel can be acknowledged for providing a valid exemplifying model of the transmission of phenotypic traits just by observing peas in a garden. However, it was subsequently realized that mendelian laws were too simple and that the segregation of pheno-

types in humans was far more complicated. We now know that Mendel's units (genes) lie along chromosomes in close proximity and that DNA is transmitted in segments containing tens to hundreds of genes. Genes are not, therefore, always independently transmitted. We have learned that genes sometimes undergo mutations during transmission (i.e. *de novo* mutations and dynamic mutations due to trinucleotide repeat expansions) instead of being maintained unaltered. Moreover, most molecular pathways and cellular functions are regulated by very complex systems that may involve hundreds of genes. Thus, most cellular, physiological and clinical phenotypes frequently result from the interaction of several genes and not from single genes. The presence of genes along the X chromosome and maternally inherited mitochondrial DNA constitutes a further variant in the transmission of clinical phenotypes.

In accordance with the above considerations, we may class inheritance patterns as: (a) chromosomal inheritance; (b) single-gene mendelian inheritance; (c) X-linked inheritance; (d) mitochondrial inheritance; and (e) complex inheritance (Fig. 24.2). Moreover, it should be stressed that a genetic disorder is not always a transmitted condition. Although several cellular mechanisms strive to maintain DNA structure and sequence unaltered during the cell cycle, mutations and chromosomal anomalies may take place during gametogenesis (so-called *de novo* mutations). When *de novo* mutations occur, clinical phenotypes manifest as sporadic events in families with unremarkable history, and no increased risk of recurrence is found. *De novo* mutations are usually associated with severe phenotypes and represent a persisting reserve of otherwise selectively eliminated conditions.

Chromosomal inheritance

The correct segregation of genes through meiotic division is a critical step for the survival of a species. In humans, this function is carried out by 23 pairs of chromosomes (22 autosomal pairs and two sex chromosomes) each harbouring tens to thousands of genes. In chromosomal disorders, chromosome segments are missing from or added to the normal set, leading to the absence or duplication of various genes and to composite phenotypes. Most common clinical

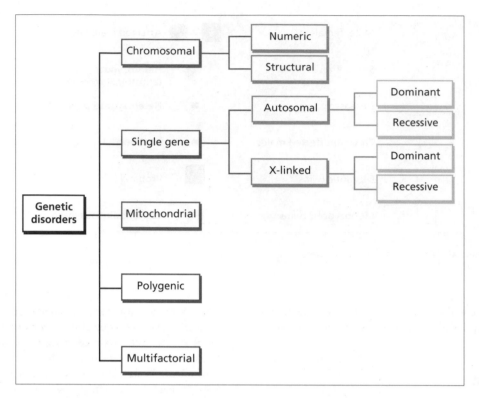

Fig. 24.2 Classification of genetic disorders.

signs of chromosomal disorders are dysmorphic features and mental retardation, resulting from an unbalanced dosage of different genes. The severity of the phenotype may however vary according to the type and number of genes involved.

Most chromosomal disorders are associated with chromosomal abnormalities occurring *de novo* and thus the occurrence of the clinical phenotype is a sporadic manifestation. More rarely, chromosomal disorders (e.g. balanced translocations) arise from healthy carriers of balanced and phenotypically silent rearrangements. The presence of multiple miscarriages and/or mental retardation in a family may be suggestive of such parental rearrangements. The recurrence risk mainly depends on the type and size of the rearrangement, the chromosome involved and the sex of the carrier (the father being at increased risk) (Table 24.1).

Mendelian inheritance

Mendelian inheritance applies when mutations in a single autosomal gene are sufficient to determine a clinical phenotype. According to the type of genes and mutations implicated, we find autosomal recessive disorders, in which both copies of the disease gene have to be mutated in order to express a phenotype, and autosomal dominant disorders, in which a single copy of the gene is mutated.

• Autosomal recessive disorders are characterized by healthy carriers who are heterozygous for a mutated allele and affected individuals who have inherited two mutated alleles from carriers. Affected individuals may be homozygous or compound heterozygous according to whether alleles bear the same or different mutations. Autosomal recessive inheritance usually manifests as a sporadic event within pedigrees in which carriers are phenotypically normal. At conception, the sibs of probands have a 25% chance of inheriting both disease-causing alleles and being affected, a 50% chance of inheriting one disease-causing allele and being a carrier, and a 25% chance of inheriting both normal alleles and being unaffected. The normal sibs of a proband have a 2/3 chance of being a carrier. The offsprings of a proband are all obligate heterozygotes (Table 24.1). Consanguinity may significantly increase the risk of an autosomal recessive disorder being expressed, since a single ancestral mutation could be transmitted along both paternal and maternal lineages (Fig. 24.3).

• Autosomal dominant disorders are characterized by vertical transmission of the disease through generations. Affected individuals present a 50% risk of transmitting the phenotype to their offspring (Table 24.1). Autosomal dominant inheritance is typically recognized in large multigenerational pedigrees showing a high density of affected cases (Fig. 24.3).

By definition, single-gene mendelian disorders are homogenous traits; transmission of the disease is defined by Mendel's laws and phenotypes show little variability among affected individuals.

However, it is well known that several disorders classified as mendelian—mostly in the autosomal dominant category—show a certain degree of variability in expression of clinical features, resulting in incomplete penetrance (defined as the proportion of individuals carrying the mutation/s who do not manifest the phenotype), variable onset of clinical symptoms and variation in the severity of the phenotype (Fig. 24.3). Recent advances in genetic research have

Table 24.1 Risk for relatives of proband for different disease modes of inheritance

Inheritance	Risk to family members of a proband			
	Parents	Sibs	Offspring	Other family members
Chromosomal	Relative risks depend upon specific chromosomal rearrangement			
Autosomal recessive (AR)	Obligate heterozygotes. Heterozygotes are asymptomatic	At conception: • 25% chance of inheriting both disease alleles and being affected • 50% chance of inheriting one disease-causing allele and being a carrier • 25% chance of inheriting both normal alleles and being unaffected Normal sibs: • 2/3 chance of being a carrier	>99% probability of being heterozygotes (healthy carriers) • Very rare probability of being homozygous, i.e. affected by the disease (only if husband/wife is heterozygous or affected)	Maternal and paternal relatives are at risk of being carriers
Autosomal dominant (AD)	One parent of the proband has the same disease-causing allele as the proband; that parent may or may not have symptoms depending on the penetrance of the disease allele	• 50% risk of inheriting the disease allele • 50% risk of developing the disease for fully penetrant genes • <50% risk to develop the disease for incomplete penetrant disease allele ($0.5 \times$ penetrance rate). A proportion of sibs [$0.5 \times (1 - \text{penetrance rate})$] may carry disease allele without expressing the phenotype	• 50% risk of inheriting the disease allele • 50% risk of developing the disease for fully penetrant disease alleles • <50% risk to develop the disease for incomplete penetrant disease alleles ($0.5 \times$ penetrance rate). A proportion of offspring [$0.5 \times (1 - \text{penetrance rate})$] may carry the disease allele without expressing the phenotype	
X-linked recessive	Mothers are obligate carriers. Mild symptoms of the disease may manifest	• Males: 50% chance of inheriting the disease allele and to be affected • Females: 50% change of being carriers with no or mild symptoms, 50% chance of not inheriting the disease allele and being normal	• All daughters will be carriers • All sons will not inherit the mutant allele, will not have the disease and will not pass it on to their offspring	Maternal aunts and their offspring may be at risk of being carriers or affected depending upon their gender
Mitochondrial	mtDNA deletions generally occur *de novo* and thus cause sporadic disease with no significant risk to other family members. mtDNA point mutations and duplications may be transmitted through the maternal line • Mother of a proband usually has the mtDNA mutation and may or may not have symptoms • Father of a proband is not at risk of having the disease-causing mtDNA mutation	The risk to the sibs depends upon the genetic status of the mother. If the mother has the mtDNA mutation, all sibs are at risk of inheriting it	A male does not transmit the mtDNA mutation to his offspring • A female harbouring a mtDNA mutation may transmit a variable amount of mutant mtDNA to her offspring, resulting in a clinical variability amongst sibs within the same nuclear family	The proband's grandmother and their descendants are at risk
Complex	Empirical risks should be deduced from disease-specific epidemiological studies			

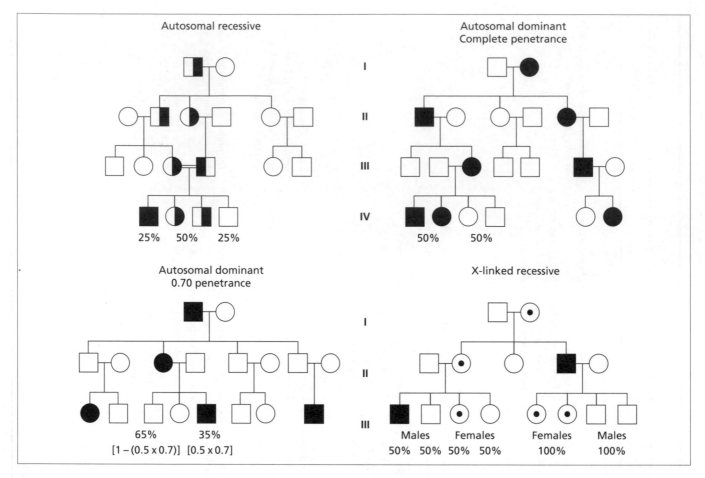

Fig. 24.3 Pedigrees showing different single-gene patterns of inheritance and relative risks for offspring.

revealed that the variability in expressivity found in some single-gene mendelian traits is definitively influenced by other genes. Since the phenotype is mostly determined by mutations in a single gene, we may define these traits as major-gene disorders. For the sake of simplicity, these are included in the single-gene disorder category, as the pattern of inheritance (so-called pseudomendelian inheritance) overlaps to a great extent with mendelian inheritance.

X-linked inheritance

When mutations occur in genes lying on the X chromosome, a peculiar mode of inheritance is found because of the difference in gene dosage between males and females. X-linked mutations are usually transmitted from heterozygous healthy females (carriers) to 50% of their offspring. Male offspring will develop the disease, since they lack the second normal copy of the gene (hemizygosity), whereas females will be healthy carriers. A distinctive feature of X-linked inheritance is the absence of male-to-male transmission of the disease (since the Y chromosome is always transmitted). Since the disease is transmitted by normal carriers, we may define most X-linked disorders as recessive traits (Table 24.1, Fig. 24.3).

It should, however, be stressed that the recessive/dominant dichotomy should be used with caution, as female carriers may show a variable phenotype, usually mild, that is the expression of the random inactivation of one X chromosome. Moreover, some X-linked genes show a clear dominant effect and heterozygous females express the full phenotype. Furthermore, in rare X-linked dominant syndromes, hemizygosity is lethal in males.

It is noteworthy that the counterpart of X-linked inheritance does not exist in practice, since no genes responsible for serious diseases are known to be mapped on chromosome Y. For those rare disease genes that are mapped on both sex chromosomes (within the so-called pseudoautosomal regions) the pattern of inheritance is typically mendelian.

Mitochondrial inheritance

In human cells about 1% of the DNA is contained within mitochondria as small circular genomes. The mitochondrial DNA (mtDNA) of each individual is known to derive from maternal mitochondria (in humans, sperm does not contribute to the initial set of mitochondria) and to replicate independently from nuclear DNA.

mtDNA harbours 37 genes encoding for tRNA and proteins that are involved in mitochondrial function. Mitochondrial genes undergo a variety of mutations leading to disorders that typically affect the central nervous system, heart, skeletal muscle, endocrine glands and kidneys; transmission is always from females, no trans-

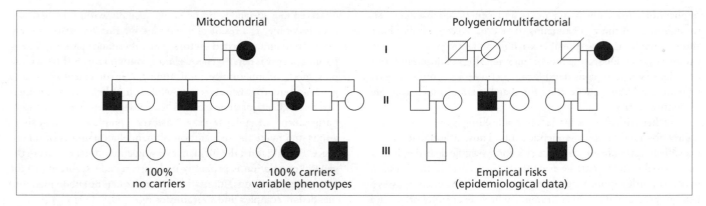

Fig. 24.4 Pedigrees showing complex patterns of inheritance.

mission being observed from males (Table 24.1). Because of the maternal origin of mtDNA, a peculiar inheritance pattern is found (Fig. 24.4).

A further distinctive feature of these disorders is phenotypic variability in both the severity and progression of disease and the age of onset. Furthermore, individuals with no clinical manifestations may transmit the disease. The biological basis for clinical heterogeneity is provided by the observation that the proportion of mutated mtDNA varies among different cells; in some cells all mitochondria carry the mutated mtDNA (homoplasmy), while in others only a fraction of mtDNA is mutated (heteroplasmy). Thus, the variable expression of the disease is strongly influenced by the amount and the tissue distribution of mutated mtDNA. The proportion of offspring possibly affected is therefore variable and cannot be determined by any rule.

Since several genes involved in mitochondrial function are localized in nuclear DNA, it should be emphasized that mitochondrial inheritance does not apply to all mitochondrial disorders.

Complex inheritance

Most common disorders show a complex aetiology that includes multiple genetic and environmental factors. In these disorders, a single gene is not sufficient to cause the disease by itself, but increases the risk. The disease may develop when other genes (polygenic disorders) or environmental factors (multifactorial disorders) are superimposed on a genetic predisposition. As a result, these conditions may show a familial tendency but do not fit into a clear inheritance pattern (Fig. 24.4).

Distinctive epidemiological features of genetically complex disorders are: (a) increased clinical concordance among monozygous twins; (b) increased risk for close relatives of affected individuals, rapidly decreasing for more distant relatives; and (c) pedigrees showing a sparse aggregation of affected cases. Recurrence risks are usually based on empirical data indicating the risk for relatives of affected individuals as a function of the degree of relationship and of the presence of multiple affected cases in the family (Table 24.1). For many complex disorders, large and dense pedigrees have been reported, suggesting that a subset of affected cases may be determined by the effect of rare major genes. Recognizing these mendelian subsets is crucial to identifying high-risk individuals.

Genetic counselling in epilepsy: approaching a heterogeneous disorder

Epilepsy is a very heterogeneous disorder which is manifested in a variety of clinical signs and as a consequence of multiple causes. Generally speaking, humans may have a seizure or develop epilepsy as a result of acquired and/or genetic causes.

In symptomatic epilepsies, unprovoked seizures are determined by prior neurological damage. These conditions are commonly acquired during postnatal life as a result of head injury, cerebrovascular disease, central nervous system infections, brain tumours or degenerative disorders, and are therefore little influenced by the genetic background. In rare cases, symptomatic epilepsy may arise from structural brain lesions or altered metabolic states that are associated with specific inherited disorders (e.g. tuberous sclerosis, neuronal ceroid lipofuscinoses or NCLs).

By contrast, individuals with idiopathic epilepsies suffer recurrent unprovoked seizures without any detectable neurological or metabolic abnormality. Epidemiological studies have shown that genetic factors strongly contribute to the aetiology of idiopathic epilepsies. The mode of inheritance of idiopathic epilepsy is however highly variable and includes mendelian, polygenic and multifactorial traits [2].

In recent decades, a great effort has been made to narrow down phenotypes according to clinical details such as age of onset, type of seizures and EEG findings. Epileptic syndromes have been defined according to unique clusters of signs and symptoms, and then grouped into extended classifications [3,4]. On this basis, epidemiological studies have been undertaken in an attempt to provide empirical estimates of recurrence risks for each phenotypic trait. In epilepsy, most of the available data for genetic counselling are derived from this exhaustive work-up. Although many patients may not fit any proposed phenotypic class, and clinical classification may have little aetiological value, it is important to approach the current classification as a diagnostic scheme on which empirical risks for recurrence have been calculated. Thus, by definition, relatives of probands affected by idiopathic generalized epilepsy show an increased risk of developing generalized epilepsy. By contrast, relatives of individuals showing temporal lobe epilepsy with hippocampal sclerosis are not considered to be at increased risk.

The classification of many genetically determined forms of epilepsy is likely to undergo extensive reappraisal, with significant implications for clinical diagnosis and genetic counselling. Although most of the work remains to be done, recent studies have shown that it is now possible to link epileptic phenotypes to causative genes. Dissecting the complex aetiology of different forms of epilepsy will have considerable impact on genetic counselling by providing reliable genetic tests for diagnosis and more accurate estimation of risks.

A further critical issue for genetic counselling is the clinical variability observed for many epileptic traits. Thus, although it is often possible to estimate a recurrence risk for a specific disorder, it may be impossible to estimate severity of the disease. While the question may be of little significance when clinical variability encompasses a benign spectrum, it becomes dramatic where severe phenotypes are concerned. A deeper knowledge of the aetiological factors involved in such disorders and the development of appropriate tests are again crucial to address this issue.

Idiopathic epilepsies

In epilepsy, the term idiopathic refers to clinical conditions in which seizures manifest as unique symptoms in the absence of structural brain lesions or other neurological dysfunctions. Historically, a strong genetic contribution was assumed for generalized idiopathic epilepsies. Recent studies, however, have shown that several focal forms of epilepsy are also genetically determined [5]. A distinctive feature of most idiopathic forms is the age dependency of clinical manifestations, in that seizures and EEG abnormalities can be observed in a specific window of age, usually within the first two decades of life, as a result of a complex interaction between brain maturation and inherited factors. The inheritance pattern of idiopathic epilepsy is heterogeneous; most common forms show a complex mode of inheritance, indicating the involvement of several genes and environmental factors, while some phenotypes are inherited as single/major-gene traits. The age dependency of most idiopathic forms of epilepsy may, however, complicate diagnosis in adults and make the recognition of mendelian patterns of inheritance difficult; thus, the incidence of single/major-gene traits in the general population is probably underestimated. According to the above considerations, idiopathic epilepsies can be subdivided into mendelian, complex and sporadic forms.

Mendelian epilepsies

Five syndromes have so far been identified as having mendelian inheritance: benign familial neonatal seizures (BFNS), benign familial infantile seizures (BFIS), autosomal dominant nocturnal frontal lobe epilepsy (ADNFLE), benign familial adult myoclonic epilepsy (BFAME) and generalized epilepsy and febrile seizures plus (GEFS+) syndrome (Table 24.2).

BFNS

Seizures are the most frequent neurological events in newborns. In most cases, seizures are determined by acute acquired conditions

Table 24.2 Mendelian epilepsies

Disease	Age of onset	Suggestive clinical and EEG features	Genetics	DNA test
Benign familial neonatal seizures	2–4 days	Tonic posture, ocular signs, apnoea evolving into clonic movements and motor automatisms. Ictal EEG: bilateral flattening of the EEG followed by bilateral discharge of slow waves and spikes	AD 0.85 penetrance	KCNQ2, KCNQ3
Benign familial infantile seizures	4–7 months	Seizures usually in clusters: psychomotor arrest, slow deviation of the head and eyes, diffuse tonic contraction, cyanosis and limb jerks. Ictal EEG: fast activity in occipitoparietal areas and secondary generalization	AD high penetrance	—
Autosomal dominant nocturnal frontal lobe epilepsy	1–55 years (mean 14)	Nocturnal motor seizures: moans, extension and abduction of arms, axial rocking, grabbing, oral automatisms, aura. Ictal EEG: fast bifrontal rhythm	AD 0.80 penetrance	CHRNA4, CHRNB2
Benign familial adult myoclonic epilepsy	18-45 years (mean 30)	Tremulous finger movements and/or myoclonus of the extremities and rare generalized tonic-clonic seizures. Photic sensitivity. Enhanced long-loop C reflex. Ictal EEG: generalized spikes or polyspikes and slow-wave complexes	AD	—
Generalized epilepsy and febrile seizures plus (GEFS+) syndrome	1-9 years (mean 1.5)	Very frequent febrile seizures lasting beyond 6 years and/or followed by generalized tonic-clonic seizures. Occasional recurrence of afebrile generalized myoclonic, absence and atonic seizures	AD 0.80 penetrance	SCN1A, SCN1B, GABRG2

and do not involve a diagnosis of epilepsy. By contrast, neonatal seizures showing no obvious precipitating factors, benign prognosis and significant familial recurrence may indicate a genetic syndrome defined as BFNS. Peculiar clinical features of BFNS include brief focal or generalized seizures with onset between 2 and 4 days of life, which spontaneously remit within a few weeks. Seizures usually start with a tonic posture, ocular signs (staring, blinking or gaze deviation) and apnoea and progress to clonic movements and motor automatism [6]. The ictal EEG usually shows a characteristic sequence of bilateral flattening for 1–5 s, followed by bilateral discharges of slow waves and spikes lasting 1–2 min. The cortical spread may vary between left and right among seizures, resulting in asymmetric motor signs. BFNS was originally classified as a generalized epilepsy but it has been recently included among the partial epilepsies [4]. In view of the immaturity of the brain in newborns, however, its classification into a rigid scheme may be inappropriate. Seizures are usually controlled by phenobarbital; phenytoin and valproate are occasionally used in non-responsive patients. Psychomotor development is normal, although about 10–15% of patients will develop febrile or non-febrile seizures later in childhood or adolescence [7]. The pattern of inheritance is typically autosomal dominant with high penetrance (around 85%), indicating involvement of a single gene.

Mutations in the voltage-gated potassium channel α subunit genes *KCNQ2* and *KCNQ3* have been identified as responsible for BFNS, and several mutations have so far been described which result in either a truncated or altered protein [8,9].

Genetic testing for BFNS includes the mutational screening of *KCNQ2* and *KCNQ3* by using genomic DNA from patients. This is costly and should be undertaken when the clinical diagnosis is highly suggestive. Familial clustering of neonatal seizures constitutes a distinctive marker of the syndrome, although it may not be easily recognized because of the absence of clinical and EEG signs in adult individuals. For genetic counselling, the risk estimate is that typical of any autosomal dominant single-gene disorder with high penetrance, with a 50% risk of transmission for offspring or siblings of affected individuals.

BFIS

BFIS was described in 1992 as an autosomal dominant disorder characterized by partial seizures occurring between 4 and 7 months and spontaneously remitting at about 18 months, and benign outcome [10]. Seizures are brief (usually less than 1 min), occur mainly in clusters of 4–10 per day and last for a period of 2–4 days. Isolated seizures may sporadically precede clusters. Clinically, seizures are highly stereotyped among patients, and include psychomotor arrest, slow deviation of the head and eyes to one side, diffuse tonic contraction, cyanosis and limb jerks starting unilaterally and evolving into synchronous or asynchronous bilateral manifestations. Depending on the seizure, the head and eyes may be turned to either the right or left side. Ictal EEG shows a fast activity originating in the occipitoparietal areas of one hemisphere and then spreading over the entire brain and increasing in amplitude. Phenobarbital therapy is usually effective and brings seizures under control within 2 days. Interictal EEG and psychomotor development are normal and no increased risk of developing febrile or non-febrile seizures is observed in later life.

The mode of inheritance of BFIS is typically autosomal dominant, although occasionally the disease is transmitted from apparently healthy individuals. It is not clear whether this is due to incomplete penetrance or difficulties in collecting a reliable history from adult individuals.

Non-familial cases with idiopathic seizures with onset within the first year of age, spontaneously remitting and showing overlapping clinical features with BFIS, have been described [11]. Clinical dissection of benign infantile seizures has been attempted in order to identify any phenotypic variants that may underlie the observed difference in inheritance pattern. In some (but not all) sporadic cases, EEG recordings have demonstrated a temporal lobe onset, suggesting a different pathogenesis.

Extensive family studies led to the localization of two different BFIS genes on chromosomes 19q and 2q. Genetic heterogeneity is further emphasized by families in which the disease is not linked to either 19q or 2q, thus suggesting the presence of at least a third BFIS gene [12–14]. The complexity of the BFIS syndrome is, moreover, highlighted by recent reports of familial cases of infantile seizures and paroxysmal choreoathetosis (ISCA syndrome) [15]. In ISCA, typical epileptic manifestations of BFIS are associated with involuntary movements that occur spontaneously (dystonic type) or are induced by movement (kinesiogenic type), exertion or anxiety. In familial ISCA, both choreoathetosis and seizures show reduced penetrance and thus the disorder may manifest as an epileptic, choreoathetotic or combined phenotype. Whether BFIS and ISCA constitute different clinical manifestations of the same genetic defects is unclear. The ISCA phenotype has been associated with a specific locus on chromosome 16p, suggesting a different genetic aetiology for ISCA and BFIS [15]. More recently, however, BFIS has been linked to chromosome 16p in some families, suggesting a genetic overlap that varies from one family to another [16].

Since no BFIS or ISCA genes have yet been identified, the genetic aetiology of both disorders is unknown, thus making genotype–phenotype correlations unreliable. Indirect methods may be applied to compare segregation of the disease with segregation of candidate loci within families (linkage analysis). However, in the presence of genetic heterogeneity, this approach can only be adopted when extended pedigrees are available, which makes its application difficult in clinical practice. For genetic counselling, diagnosis has to rely on identification of the typical clinical and EEG findings.

ADNFLE

Frequently misdiagnosed as sleep disorder, ADNFLE is characterized by clusters of brief nocturnal motor seizures that begin at different ages—usually in childhood—and may persist throughout adult life [17]. Seizures are brief—usually between 30 and 40 s— and occur in clusters of up to 20 attacks during light sleep. Clinical manifestations include moans, extension and abduction of arms, axial rocking, grabbing at people or objects and oral automatisms. Individuals may experience an aura associated with tonic and hyperkinetic motor activity. The ictal EEG shows generalized high-voltage slow and sharp activity, followed by fast bifrontal rhythm and then by a burst of polyspikes and slow waves with sudden cessation. Intrafamilial variability in the severity of symptoms is frequently observed. Interictal and psychomotor development are normal. Carbamazepine is usually effective in controlling seizures.

The mode of inheritance of ADNFLE is autosomal dominant with 80% penetrance, though seizures may be difficult to detect through the generations. Nocturnal motor manifestations are frequently misdiagnosed as sleep disorders such as nightmares, hysteria and paroxysmal dystonia, and clinical heterogeneity further complicates clinical diagnosis. The presence of non-familial cases suggests a composite aetiology for nocturnal frontal lobe epilepsy. Mutations in the neuronal acetylcholine receptor α_4 and β_2 subunit genes (CHRNA4 and CHRNB2) have been identified in ADNFLE patients [18,19]. A third ADNFLE locus has been mapped on chromosome 15q, indicating a highly heterogeneous genetic aetiology [20]. Analysis of ADNFLE genes demonstrated a de novo mutation in only one of several patients affected by non-familial nocturnal frontal lobe epilepsy, thus suggesting that other factors are involved in sporadic nocturnal frontal lobe epilepsy [21].

In ADNFLE, as in mendelian forms of epilepsy, genetic counselling should first focus on clinical diagnosis and the recognition of familial clustering. The screening of CHRNA4 and CHRNB2 may then be attempted when the transmission pattern supports autosomal dominant inheritance. Current data do not suggest extending the test to sporadic cases.

BFAME

BFAME or (BAFME) has been described so far only in Japanese families and constitutes a very rare phenotype. Its clinical features include tremulous finger movements and/or myoclonus of the extremities and rare generalized tonic-clonic seizures. Myoclonus is easily precipitated by photic stimuli and sporadically by insomnia and fatigue. Peculiar electrophysiological findings are generalized spikes or polyspikes and slow-wave complexes in the EEG, enlarged cortical components of somatosensory-evoked potential and enhanced long-loop C reflex [22]. As for other mendelian idiopathic forms of epilepsy, no neurological degeneration, dementia or ataxia are found in BFAME patients. Myoclonic jerks and tremulous finger movements typically begin around the third or fourth decade of life. This late age of onset is one of the most distinctive signs of BFAME. Clonazepam or sodium valproate is usually effective in treating the disorder, though the tremulous finger movements may not disappear with therapy.

Family studies indicate that BFAME is an autosomal dominant trait showing high/complete penetrance. A BFAME gene has been localized on chromosome 8q24 [23,24]; so far, no evidence of genetic heterogeneity has been observed. Since the gene has not yet been identified, no genetic tests are available other than linkage analysis of the chromosome 8q24 locus and informative extended pedigrees. The accurate analysis of clinical and electroclinical findings and the pattern of inheritance can yield critical clues to establishing a diagnosis and providing genetic counselling.

GEFS+ syndrome

The GEFS+ syndrome was originally described in Australia and then reported worldwide as an autosomal dominant epileptic trait [25]. Clinical features include febrile seizures (FS) and various forms of idiopathic generalized epilepsy. FS last beyond 6 years of age (hence the term febrile seizure plus) and are frequently followed by generalized non-febrile seizures of various types, such as my-oclonic, absence and atonic seizures. In GEFS+ families, however, about 40% of affected individuals show typical FS, which indicates a variable expression of the disease.

The pattern of transmission is typically autosomal dominant and a single major gene is thought to determine the phenotype. Incomplete penetrance and variable expression of the disease suggest that minor alleles might influence the phenotype. So far, three major genes have been associated with the GEFS+ syndrome: voltage-gated sodium channel subunits α_1 and β_1 genes (SCN1A and SCN1B, respectively) [26,27] and the GABA-A receptor subunit γ gene (GABRG2) [28]. A third voltage-gated sodium channel subunit gene (SCN2A) has been found to be mutated in a single nuclear pedigree showing FS and generalized idiopathic epilepsy, resembling the GEFS+ phenotype [29].

GEFS+ can be difficult to distinguish from FS or common forms of idiopathic generalized epilepsy if the familial clustering is missed. The occurrence of FS plus is an important diagnostic clue. Genetic counselling should take into account the variability of the disease which may be manifested with severe (i.e. myoclonic astatic epilepsy) or mild phenotypes [30]. Incomplete penetrance (about 80%) lowers the risk for relatives of probands compared to fully penetrant traits. The fact that the GEFS+ genes so far identified account for about 20% of the GEFS+ phenotypes indicates that other genes are involved. The screening of GEFS+ genes is a costly task and should only be undertaken to confirm diagnosis when febrile plus seizures are consistently found in different family members.

Despite considerable clinical and electroclinical diversity, the mendelian idiopathic forms of epilepsy so far described share important genetic features:
- Mendelian idiopathic forms segregate with autosomal dominant inheritance and are mostly determined by mutant neuronal ion-channel genes.
- Different genes are involved in the same phenotype, thus indicating genetic heterogeneity. A single gene has been identified for BFAME only, but further data are required to determine whether this disorder is restricted to the Japanese population as a genetically homogeneous trait.
- Sporadic cases of mendelian forms are occasionally found, whose significance is not fully understood. Possible explanations include failure to recognize familial clustering, de novo mutations arising from non-carrier individuals and inadequate differential diagnosis from other epileptic conditions.
- Genetic tests for mendelian idiopathic forms of epilepsy are not yet available or are very costly (e.g. mutational screening of different genes).

In the light of the above considerations, genetic counselling in cases of mendelian epilepsy should rely on careful analysis of clinical signs in patients and family members and on recognition of a clear pattern of transmission. When available, genetic testing may be undertaken to confirm the diagnosis and to better estimate recurrence risks in relatives of affected individuals.

Complex epilepsies

In human genetics, the term complex refers to conditions arising from multiple concomitant factors of either genetic (polygenic inheritance) or genetic and environmental origin (multifactorial inheritance). In mendelian disorders, the mode of inheritance may easily be deduced from the analysis of transmission patterns within pedigrees. In complex disorders, segregation of the disease does not fit a precise pattern and more exhaustive epidemiological studies are needed in order to define the mode of inheritance. In genetic epidemiology, important indexes are defined in terms of the clinical concordance of monozygotic twins and the risk of recurrence for different degree relatives of affected individuals. The first index indicates the heritability of a disorder; the second indicates the complexity of the genetic component. The higher the concordance rate among monozygotic twins, the stronger the contribution of genetic factors to the disorder. The lower the risk for relatives of probands, the higher is the number of genetic factors involved. Many forms of epilepsy show a complex inheritance, and epidemiological data are the only available tools for genetic counselling.

Idiopathic generalized epilepsies (IGE)

IGE cover the most common forms of idiopathic epilepsy and includes childhood absence epilepsy (CAE), juvenile absence epilepsy (JAE), juvenile myoclonic epilepsy (JME) and epilepsy with generalized tonic-clonic seizures only (EGTCS), as defined by the 1989 International Classification of Epileptic Syndromes and further modifications [3,4].

Several epidemiological studies have been conducted in recent decades in order to dissect the genetic aetiology of IGE. Although different methodological approaches have been adopted, results agree on a concordance rate of about 70–80% in monozygotic twins, increasing up to 90% when epileptiform EEG changes are considered [31–33], and a risk of developing IGE for first-degree relatives of probands of about 5–15% (compared with a cumulative incidence of about 0.5% in the general population) [34,35]. The recurrence risk for first-degree relatives is significantly lower in IGE

than in single-gene disorders; when second-degree or more distant relatives are considered, the risk is close to that of the general population.

When considered together, the high concordance rate in monozygotic twins and the rapid decrease in risks for more distant relatives indicate a strong but complex genetic aetiology [36]. The involvement of multiple interacting susceptibility genes would result in low familial clustering and the absence of a recognizable pattern of inheritance. On the other hand, large and dense pedigrees are rarely found, thus suggesting mendelian inheritance for a subset of IGE cases (Table 24.3).

The Rochester study has drawn up various clinical parameters in order to further refine recurrence risks for relatives of affected individuals [34,35].

1 Risk for siblings: when all forms of epilepsy are considered, the risk of developing epilepsy for a sibling of a proband is about 4%. This increases to 6% when the IGE subgroup is considered and to 8% if photosensitivity is found in the proband or if a parent has epilepsy. The risk of developing generalized epilepsy for a sibling rises to 12% when a parent also shows generalized EEG abnormalities and to 15% when the sibling shows a generalized EEG trait.

2 Risk for offspring: for all forms of epilepsy, the risk of recurrence for offspring of affected individuals is about 4–6%. A striking difference is seen between the offspring of affected females (8.7%) and those of affected males (2.5%) but why this is so is not yet understood. If the IGE subgroup is considered, the risk for offspring increases to about 9%.

Interestingly, if EEG abnormalities are considered, a recurrence rate of about 25–30% is found for specific traits (e.g. generalized spike-wave 3 Hz or generalized polyspike EEGs) in first-degree relatives of probands [37,38]. Clinical variability among family members provides further epidemiological evidence. A study of 74 families with at least three members affected by IGE showed that

Table 24.3 Complex epilepsies

Disease	Mode of inheritance and empiric risks for first-degree relatives	Mendelian subsets	Mode of inheritance
Idiopathic generalized epilepsies (childhood absence epilepsy, juvenile absence epilepsy, juvenile myoclonic epilepsy, epilepsy with generalized tonic-clonic seizures only)	Polygenic/multifactorial Risk for first-degree relatives: • seizures 5–15% • generalized spike-wave EEG trait 20–30%	Juvenile myoclonic epilepsy Familial infantile myoclonic epilepsy Childhood absence epilepsy with tonic-clonic seizures	AD (penetrance 0.7) AR AD (penetrance 0.8)
Rolandic epilepsy	Polygenic/multifactorial Risk for first-degree relatives: • seizures: 10% • centrotemporal spikes: 20–30%	Rolandic epilepsy and speech dyspraxia Rolandic epilepsy and exercise induced dystonia and writer's cramp	AD AR
Temporal lobe epilepsy	Acquired factors Sporadic conditions: No increased risk for relatives	Familial temporal lobe epilepsy with auditory symptoms Familial partial epilepsy with variable foci Familial temporal lobe epilepsy with febrile convulsions	AD AD Digenic

only 25% of the families were concordant for a specific IGE syndrome, whereas 75% of families segregated at least two IGE syndromes [39]. These data reinforce the hypothesis that IGE might represent a clinical continuum which is determined by a cohort of susceptibility genes.

Efforts have been made to identify both susceptibility alleles for common forms of IGE and major genes involved in rare mendelian subsets. In various studies, putative susceptibility loci have been localized on chromosome 3p [40] and on chromosomes 6p, 8p, 8q, 5p and 5q [41,42]. Although the genetic background may vary among different family samples, discordant results suggest caution in interpreting these data. So far, however, no genes or genetic variations have been associated with genetic susceptibility to IGE. Moreover, genes for rare autosomal dominant subsets have been mapped or identified for CAE (chromosome 8q) and for JME (chromosome 6p and GABRA1 gene on chromosome 5q) [43–45].

In clinical practice, the estimation of recurrence risks for relatives of individuals affected by IGE is, in most situations, based on epidemiological data. A possible methodological approach to the estimation of risks for IGE has been proposed above.

Idiopathic partial epilepsies

Different forms of partial epilepsy have been described as having a genetic origin (Table 24.3).

Benign childhood epilepsy with centrotemporal spikes (rolandic epilepsy)

Rolandic epilepsy is a common disorder characterized by brief, focal, hemifacial motor seizures usually manifesting during sleep and frequently evolving into generalized tonic-clonic seizures. The seizures typically begin between 3 and 13 years of age, and abate by the age of 16 years. The EEG hallmark of the syndrome is peculiar age-dependent centrotemporal spikes. The genetics of rolandic epilepsy is quite complex and controversial. Although the rate of clinical concordance in monozygotic twins varies from 0 to 100% in different studies, it is widely accepted that genetic factors are involved in the aetiology of rolandic epilepsy [33,46,47]. A 15% risk of developing rolandic epilepsy has been reported for first-degree relatives of probands; this rises to about 30% if centrotemporal EEG abnormalities are considered [48]. In view of this, polygenic and multifactorial inheritance have each been proposed for seizures, and a pseudodominant mode of inheritance for rolandic discharges. So far, however, the mode of inheritance is somewhat unclear. Rolandic epilepsy has also been found to segregate in association with other neurological conditions, thus defining very rare mendelian phenotypes such as autosomal dominant rolandic epilepsy and speech dyspraxia [49], and autosomal recessive rolandic epilepsy with paroxysmal exercise-induced dystonia and writer's cramp [50].

Familial temporal lobe epilepsy

Temporal lobe epilepsy has so far been considered to be of lesional origin although a positive family history has been long recognized [51]. In recent years, however, different familial forms of temporal epilepsy have been described. Most of these represent rare phenotypes observed in one or a few pedigrees. Autosomal dominant temporal lobe epilepsy with auditory/visual symptoms has been described in different pedigrees worldwide and associated to mutations within the LGI1 gene on chromosome 10q [52]. Temporal lobe epilepsy has, furthermore, been found to segregate in familial partial epilepsy with variable foci (FPEVF) and a gene has been mapped on chromosome 22q [53]. Familial temporal lobe epilepsy was also found to segregate with FS in one large pedigree, and two loci have been mapped on chromosomes 18q and 1q, thus suggesting digenic inheritance [54]. The recognition of rare mendelian phenotypes through the analysis of specific clinical and familial data is critical to identifying high-risk pedigrees.

Sporadic epileptic syndromes

For some epilepsies, neither hereditary nor environmental/lesional causes have unequivocally been identified. Most of these are complex and usually severe phenotypes with onset in infancy or early childhood, such as West's syndrome, Lennox–Gastaut syndrome, epilepsy with myoclonic-astatic seizures and severe myoclonic epilepsy in infancy. A recent study which identified mutations within the neuronal sodium channel gene SCN1A in patients with severe myoclonic epilepsy of infancy yielded important insight into the genetics of severe sporadic epileptic conditions [55].

Severe myoclonic epilepsy of infancy (SMEI)

SMEI manifests itself within the first year of life with tonic, clonic or tonic-clonic seizures. Seizures are frequent and prolonged and are frequently associated with fever. Later in life, patients develop atypical absence, myoclonic, generalized tonic-clonic and partial seizures. Psychomotor development is normal at onset but development stagnation and progressive ataxia occur after the second year. Seizures are usually refractory to drug therapy [56].

Although a positive familial history of FS has been described, SMEI manifests itself as a sporadic condition [57]. SMEI appears to be related to sporadic mutations in the neuronal sodium channel gene SCN1A which occur during gametogenesis, thus explaining the lack of familial clustering [55]. From this standpoint SMEI is a genetic disorder even though it is not hereditary. Interestingly, SCN1A is also involved in GEFS+ syndrome, a milder phenotype sharing important clinical features with SMEI. The observed differences in severity are probably due to the different effects of mutations on SCN1A function: in SMEI, channel activity is heavily impaired, whereas in GEFS+ a residual activity is maintained. Although most patients so far reported showed a mutated SCN1A, the genetic basis of the disorder may be heterogenous. However the screening of SCN1A is a very promising diagnostic tool. The identification of de novo mutations leads us to exclude any increased risks of recurrence for relatives of probands.

Febrile seizures (FS)

The most common precipitant of seizures is fever and 3% of the population experience FS during childhood. Although febrile illnesses are acquired, pre-existing inherited factors determining a low threshold for FS are indicated by the high rate of familial clustering.

FS have been long observed to occur in pedigrees. In monozygotic twins, clinical concordance has been found to be increased by 35–70% depending on ascertainment strategy [58,59]. Epidemiological studies have reported an increased risk for first-degree relatives of probands ranging from 8% in whites to up to 20% in Japanese, in comparison with rates of 3% and 7%, respectively, in the general population [60,61]. The mode of inheritance is by definition multifactorial, since an environmental condition is needed to trigger seizures. By contrast, the mode of transmission of genetic susceptibility is controversial. Polygenic inheritance has been proposed as most common, whereas pseudodominant inheritance has been suggested for rare large pedigrees [62]. A clinical approach has attempted to differentiate high-risk families segregating high penetrant genes from the general population. Whether the number of seizures occurring in patients and EEG abnormalities correlate with higher recurrence risk is controversial.

A major epidemiological finding is the 2–10-fold increased risk for FS probands of developing afebrile seizures later in life. A possible scenario includes both developmental and genetic factors. On the basis of retrospective studies, it has been proposed that prolonged FS frequently observed in the history of patients with temporal lobe epilepsy may lead to mesial temporal sclerosis [63,64]. On the other hand, genetic factors underlying FS could also confer liability to epilepsy [30].

Recent studies provided important clues to the mode of inheritance of FS and their relationship with epilepsy. Genotype–phenotype correlations in GEFS+ families demonstrate that about 90% of individuals carrying mutations on *SCN1A*, *SCN2A*, *SCN1B* and *GABRG2* genes show FS and about half of these develop idiopathic generalized epilepsy [26–29]. Thus, early epidemiological data indicating autosomal dominant inheritance in a subset of FS cases and a common genetic aetiology for FS and epilepsy found strong support from biological evidence. On the other hand, other studies on families showing multiple cases of typical FS alone failed to detect mutations in *SCN1A* and *SCN1B*, and confirmed that the genetics of most common forms of FS is complex. The lack of data on pure FS provides an indirect confirmation of this genetic complexity. Although FS is the most common seizure disorder in humans, no genes have been found that specifically correlate with it and only a locus on chromosome 19p has been found to be linked in a single autosomal dominant FS pedigree [65].

Genetic counselling in FS relies on empirical epidemiological data. The recognition of occasional autosomal dominant subsets of FS (including GEFS+ syndrome) that may manifest as non-specific familial clustering of FS cases should, however, lead to caution when attempting to identify high-risk subjects.

Genetic syndromes including epilepsy as an important clinical feature

A variety of genetic syndromes include epilepsy as an important component (Table 24.4). The seizure disorders in these conditions usually consist in symptomatic generalized epilepsies associated with structural brain lesions and/or metabolic abnormalities of genetic origin. Malformational, metabolic, neurocutaneous and tumoral disorders showing chromosomal, single-gene and complex inheritance are included. Among these, progressive myoclonus epilepsies (PME) deserve special discussion.

Table 24.4 Genetic syndromes including epilepsy as important feature

Group	Name of disease
Neurocutaneous	Tuberous sclerosis
	Neurofibromatosis
	Sturge–Weber syndrome
Cortical malformations	Miller–Dieker syndrome
	X-linked lyssencephaly
	Subcortical band heterotopia
	Periventricular nodular heterotopia
Neurological	Dentatorubropallidoluysian atrophy
	Fragile X syndrome
	Angelman's syndrome
	Alzheimer's disease
	Huntington's disease
	Progressive encephalopathy with oedema, hypsarrhythmia and optic atrophy (PEHO) syndrome
	Retts' syndrome
Metabolic	Progressive myoclonic epilepsies (PME)
	Non-ketotic hyperglycinaemia
	D-glyceric acidaemia
	Propionic acidaemia
	Sulphite-oxidase deficiency
	Fructose 1–6 diphosphatase deficiency
	Piridoxine dependency
	Aminoacidopathies
	Urea cycle disorders
	Disorders of carbohydrate metabolism
	Disorders of biotin and folic acid metabolism
	Glucose transport protein deficiency
	Menkes' disease
	Glycogen storage disorders
	Krabbe's disease
	Fumarase deficiency
	Peroxisomal disorders
	Sanfilippo's syndrome
	Mitochondrial encephalopathy, lactic acidosis and stroke-like (MELAS) syndrome
	Pyruvate dehydrogenase deficiency
	Respiratory chain defects

Progressive myoclonus epilepsies

PME is a group of disorders characterized by myoclonic seizures, tonic-clonic seizures and progressive neurological dysfunction, in particular ataxia and dementia. Myoclonus is quite severe, with bilateral synchronous or multifocal asynchronous manifestations often affecting facial and bulbar muscles in addition to limbs. Convulsive seizures and neurological decline may predominate over myoclonic manifestations in some patients. Classical PME includes Unverricht–Lundborg disease, Lafora's disease, myoclonus epilepsy and red-ragged fibres (MERRF), sialidoses and NCLs. Although these conditions show substantial overlapping with other progressive encephalopathies (e.g. GM2 gangliosidosis) or progressive myoclonic ataxias (e.g. spinocerebellar ataxias), the strong contri-

Table 24.5 Progressive myoclonus epilepsies

Disease		Age of onset	Suggestive clinical features	Suggestive laboratory features	Genetics	DNA test
Unverricht–Lundborg disease		8–13 y	Severe myoclonus, mild dementia and ataxia	None identified	AR	*CSTB*
Lafora's disease		10–18 y	Severe myoclonus, occipital seizures, inexorable dementia, Lafora bodies	Lafora bodies in skin biopsies	AR	*EPM2A*
Myoclonus epilepsy and red-ragged fibres (MERRF)		Variable	Deafness, optic atrophy, myopathy, myoclonus	Ragged-red fibres, increased level of piruvate and lactate (blood)	Mt	*tRNA^{lys}*
Sialidoses	Type I	8–20 y	Severe myoclonus, tonic-clonic seizures, ataxia, cherry-red spots, visual failure	Elevated urinary sialyliloligosaccharides, deficiency of neuroaminidase in leukocytes and cultured skin fibroblasts	AR	*NEU*
	Type II	10–30 y	Severe myoclonus, ataxia, cherry-red spots, visual failure, dysmorphic features, hearing loss	Elevated urinary sialyliloligosaccharides, deficiency of neuroaminidase and β-galactosidase in leukocytes and cultured skin fibroblasts	AR	*PPGB*
Neuronal ceroid lipofuscinoses	CLN2	2.4–4 y	Myoclonic, tonic-clonic, atonic or atypical absence seizures, psychomotor delay and ataxia, visual failure	Curvilinear, rectilinear or fingerprint lipidic inclusions in skin biopsy at electron microscopy	AR	*TPP1*
	CLN3	5–10 y	Myoclonus and tonic-clonic seizures, macular degeneration, optic atrophy, dementia		AR	*CLN3*
	CLN4	15–50 y	Generalized seizures, myoclonic jerks, extrapyramidal symptoms		AR/AD	—

Mt, mitochondrial.

bution of the epileptic manifestations to the phenotype has led PME to be classified into epileptic disorders [3]. Autosomal recessive inheritance is always found except in MERRF, which is maternally transmitted through mitochondrial DNA (Table 24.5).

Unverricht–Lundborg disease

Initially described in Finland, Unverricht–Lundborg disease is a rare disorder subsequently recognized worldwide, whose clinical features include an onset at age 8–13 years with myoclonus or tonic-clonic seizures, mild progression to ataxia and dementia, and neuronal loss with no evidence of storage material [66]. Some individuals show slow disease progression and others a faster course, even within the same family. The typical course of the disease is, however, about 10–20 years. Improvement may be obtained with sodium valproate, whereas phenytoin can be deleterious [67].

The mutation causing Unverricht–Lundborg disease affects the gene encoding for cystatin B (*CSTB*), which is involved in the inhibition of a group of lysosomial proteases known as cathepsins [68]. The most common mutation is an expansion of an unstable dodecamer repeat in the 5′ untranslated region. In the general population, two or three repeats usually occur, whereas up to a

hundred repeats are found in patients. However, no correlation between clinical severity or age of onset and size of expansion has been observed [69]. Alleles in the range of 12–17 repeats have been found to be unstably transmitted to offspring. These alleles are not associated with clinical phenotypes and are therefore called 'premutational'. Most patients are homozygous for dodecamer expansion; point-mutations are occasionally found in compound heterozygotes.

Identification of the clinical features is the first step in diagnosing the disease. When suggestive indications are found, mutational analysis of *CSTB* may be attempted. Genetic testing is also a powerful tool for prenatal diagnosis and for the identification of carriers among at-risk individuals.

Lafora's disease

Lafora's disease is a rare disorder with onset between the ages of 10 and 18 years, characterized by progression to inexorable dementia, frequent occipital seizures, in addition to myoclonus and tonic-clonic seizures. Prognosis is poor, with death occurring 2–10 years after onset [70]. A distinctive feature of the disease is the occurrence of polyglucosan inclusions (Lafora's bodies) in neurones and in various other tissues [71]. In 1998 the gene involved in Lafora's disease

(*EPM2A*) was identified as the gene encoding for dual-specificity phosphatase (laforin) [72], a cytoplasmatic protein associated with polyribosomes and possibly involved in the translational regulation of glycogen metabolism. Microdeletions and point-mutations are observed in all four exons although *R241X* is found in about 40% of patients. In about 15% of families with typical Lafora's disease, the disorder is not due to laforin mutations, thus suggesting genetic heterogeneity [73].

Clinical diagnosis is not usually difficult when the disease is fully developed. Lafora bodies detected in skin biopsies constitute a unique marker. Although the screening of *EPM2A* for mutations can be carried out easily, the occurrence of genetic heterogeneity requires a search for Lafora bodies. Mutational screening of *EPM2A*, however, is of critical importance for prenatal diagnosis and carrier identification.

MERRF

MERRF is a mitochondrial disorder characterized by a broad clinical spectrum and intrafamilial variability in severity and age of onset. In addition to typical PME manifestations, patients may show deafness, optic atrophy and myopathy [74]. The pathological changes and other findings such as decreased metabolism for glucose and oxygen on PET and an increase in organic phosphate in resting muscle indicate a possible dysfunction in the mitochondrial respiratory chain. However, biochemical assays of mitochondrial respiratory enzymes may be normal and red-ragged fibres absent, suggesting a complex pathogenesis [75].

MERRF is inherited through the maternal line as a paradigmatic example of mitochondrial inheritance. Clinical variability is dependent on the amount of mutated mitochondrial DNA. In this perspective, MERRF may also manifest as a sporadic condition. A missense mutation (A8344G) affecting the tRNA^{lys}, and, consequently, the translation of all genes encoded by the mtDNA, has been described [76].

Although increased levels of piruvate, lactate and red-ragged fibres are often found, identification of clinical signs is crucial for diagnosis. In the presence of suggestive clinical data, the analysis of A8344G mutations is an excellent diagnostic tool. Genetic testing may also be used to perform prenatal diagnosis and to identify at-risk individuals.

Sialidoses

Sialidoses are very rare autosomal recessive lysosomial disorders characterized by complex phenotypes subgrouped into sialidosis type I and type II.

Occurring in the second decade of life, sialidosis type I presents with cherry-red macular spots, progressive severe myoclonus, gradual visual impairment, tonic-clonic seizures and ataxia without dementia [77]. Sialidosis type II includes complex phenotypes showing additional clinical symptoms such as coarse facies, corneal clouding, mental impairment and hearing loss, and may be subdivided into juvenile and infantile forms depending on the age of onset [78].

Neuronal lipidosis and vacuolated Kupffer cells are distinctive histological findings in sialidoses. Clinical diagnosis can be confirmed by documenting elevated urinary sialylil-oligosaccharides and a deficiency of α-*N*-acetylneuroaminidase in leukocytes and cultured skin fibroblasts [78]. In some cases of type II sialidosis—predominantly in Japanese cases of juvenile type II sialidosis—β-galactosidase deficiency is found in addition to neuroaminidase deficiency [78]. Complementation between neuroaminidase-deficient cells and combined neuroaminidase/β-galactosidase deficiency suggests different genetic aetiology and pathogenesis [79]. Thus, classification of sialidoses into type I and II has only a clinical value, whereas the definition of neuroaminidase deficiency and galactosialidosis best describes the aetiology and pathogenesis of sialidoses.

A direct implication of the neuroaminidase gene (*NEU*) on chromosome 6p has been detected in neuroaminidase deficiency [80]. In galactosialidosis mutations were found within the cathepsin A gene on chromosome 20q encoding a 32-kDa protein (PPGB, protective protein for β-galactosidase), which is required to protect galactosidase from degradation and to promote the catalytic action of neuroaminidase [81]. Genotype–phenotype correlations in neuroaminidase deficiency indicate that type I or type II sialidosis occurs depending on the residual activity of neuroaminidase resulting from different mutations.

Biochemical assays focus on measuring the activity levels of neuroaminidase and β-galactosidase. Mutational screening of the *NEU* and *PPGB* genes is a powerful tool for confirming the clinical diagnosis in probands and may be applied in prenatal diagnosis and carrier identification.

NCLs

NCLs are autosomal recessive neurodegenerative disorders characterized by accumulation of ceroid lipopigment of granular, curvilinear or fingerprint appearance in the lysosomes of various tissues. According to the age of onset and clinical variants, various NCLs have been described over the years, leading to a complex classification comprising at least seven different forms [82]. Among these, ceroid lipofuscinosis neuronal 2 (CLN2), CLN3 and CLN4 are most commonly involved in PME, whereas infantile neuronal ceroid lipofuscinosis (CLN1) does not manifest as PME. CLN5, CLN6 and CLN8 are very rare disorders restricted to specific geographical areas.

Neuronal ceroid lipofuscinosis late infantile type (CLN2)

Late infantile NCL displays myoclonic, tonic-clonic, atonic or atypical absence seizures between 2.5 and 4 years of age. Psychomotor delay and ataxia appear a few months later, whereas visual failure develops as the disease progresses. Prognosis is very poor, in that seizures are intractable, dementia is relentless and death usually occurs by the age of 5 years [83]. The gene has been localized on chromosome 11 and identified as encoding tripetidyl peptidase 1 (*TPP1*) [84]. Although affected individuals are sometimes clustered in specific areas (e.g. Newfoundland), cases have been reported worldwide and several different mutations reported.

In the past, electron microscopic detection of typical curvilinear lipidic inclusions was used to confirm the clinical diagnosis and to reach a prenatal diagnosis in uncultured amniocytes. The recent cloning of the gene has provided a further tool for the diagnosis of late infantile NCL.

Neuronal ceroid lipofuscinosis, juvenile type or Batten's disease (CLN3)

This disease usually appears between 5 and 10 years of age, with rapid deterioration of vision and progressive dementia. Macular degeneration, optic atrophy and attenuated vessels are revealed by fundoscopy. Seizures may be minor manifestations or major symptoms involving myoclonus and tonic-clonic seizures. Although the clinical course may vary among patients, death usually occurs within about 10–12 years of onset [85]. The Batten's disease gene encodes for an integral membrane protein (CLN3) that is primarily localized in the Golgi apparatus. More than 20 different mutations have so far been observed [86]. However, a 1-kb deletion is found in 70% of disease chromosomes, suggesting a strong founder effect.

Diagnosis may be established by electron microscopy examination of curvilinear and rectilinear bodies and fingerprint profiles in skin biopsies. The presence of inclusions in heterozygous carriers is controversial. Mutational screening of CLN3 may also be attempted for the molecular diagnosis of Batten's disease.

Neuronal ceroid lipofuscinosis, adult type (CLN4, Kufs' disease)

Kufs' disease is a very rare disorder characterized by generalized seizures with onset around 30 years of age and a subsequent cerebellar syndrome presenting with myoclonic jerks and extrapyramidal symptoms. Notably, fundoscopy examination is normal and blindness is absent. Death occurs within about 10–12 years of onset [87]. The pattern of inheritance is still unclear, in that both autosomal dominant and autosomal recessive inheritance have been described [88,89]. Since the Kufs' disease gene has not yet been localized or cloned, electron microscopy examination of muscle biopsies to detect curvilinear bodies is the only diagnostic test available.

Conclusions

Epilepsy is a complex phenotype with a complex aetiology. A variety of syndromes differing in clinical and physiological manifestations, pharmacological sensitivities and prognosis are influenced by multiple factors of acquired and genetic origin. Genetic aetiology is highly heterogeneous and autosomal dominant, autosomal recessive, polygenic, mitochondrial and multifactorial disorders are found. Genetic counselling in epilepsy therefore has to deal with a composite picture in which recurrent seizures may be the expression of individually acquired conditions and/or familial background. The genetics of several hereditary forms of epilepsy is still poorly understood and genetic counselling frequently has to rely on empirical data alone, as is the case for IGE, rolandic epilepsy or FS.

We should, however, be aware of the significant results obtained in recent times. Most genetic conditions underlying severe epileptic phenotypes such as PME have been successfully investigated. Genetic tests for the identification of at-risk carriers and for prenatal diagnosis are being developed and more accurate estimates of recurrence risks can be provided.

In idiopathic forms of epilepsy, different genes have been linked to mendelian phenotypes, and neuronal ion channels are promising candidates in investigating pathogenetic processes. The presence of several ion channel genes in the genome provides a promising working hypothesis for many idiopathic epileptic disorders of unknown genetic aetiology. A paradigmatic example is SCN1A, which was initially associated with the GEFS+ phenotype and was subsequently found to be mutated in SMEI. Mendelian subsets have also played an important role in proving genetic aetiology in apparently symptomatic forms of epilepsy such as temporal lobe epilepsy.

It will probably take a long time to dissect the complex aetiology of hereditary forms of epilepsy and before clinical practice and genetic counselling gain significant benefits. There is no doubt, however, that the journey has already begun.

References

1 ASHG Ad Hoc Committee on Genetic Counseling. Genetic counseling. *Am J Hum Genet* 1975; 27: 240–2.
2 Blandford M, Tsuboi T, Vogel F. Genetic counseling in the epilepsies. *Hum Genet* 1987; 76: 303–31.
3 Commission on Classification and Terminology of the International League against Epilepsy. Proposal for revised classification of epilepsies and epileptic syndromes. *Epilepsia* 1989; 30: 389–99.
4 Engel J Jr. A proposed diagnostic scheme for people with epileptic seizures and with epilepsy: report of the ILAE task force on classification and terminology. *Epilepsia* 2001; 42: 1–8.
5 Ottman R. Genetics of the partial epilepsies: a review. *Epilepsia* 1989; 30: 107–11.
6 Hirsch E, Velez A, Sellal F et al. Electroclinical signs of benign neonatal familial convulsions. *Ann Neurol* 1993; 34: 835–41.
7 Tibbles JAR. Dominant benign neonatal seizures. *Dev Med Child Neurol* 1980; 22: 664–7.
8 Singh NA, Charlier C, Stauffer D et al. A novel potassium channel gene, KCNQ2, is mutated in an inherited epilepsy of newborns. *Nature Genet* 1998; 18: 25–9.
9 Charlier C, Singh NA, Ryan SG et al. A pore mutation in a novel KQT-like potassium channel gene in an idiopathic epilepsy family. *Nature Genet* 1998; 18: 53–5.
10 Vigevano F, Fusco L, Di Capua M, Ricci S, Sebastianelli R, Lucchini P. Benign infantile familial convulsions. *Eur J Pediatr* 1992; 151: 608–12.
11 Gautier A, Pouplard F, Bednarek N et al. Benign infantile convulsions. French collaborative study. *Arch Pediatr* 1999; 6: 32–9.
12 Guipponi M, Rivier F, Vigevano F et al. Linkage mapping of benign familial infantile convulsions (BFIC) to chromosome 19q. *Hum Mol Genet* 1997; 6: 473–7.
13 Gennaro E, Malacarne M, Carbone I et al. No evidence of a major locus for benign familial infantile convulsions on chromosome 19q12-q13.1. *Epilepsia* 1999; 40: 1799–803.
14 Malacarne M, Gennaro E, Madia F et al. Benign familial infantile convulsions: mapping of a novel locus on chromosome 2q24 and evidence for genetic heterogeneity. *Am J Hum Genet* 2001; 68: 1521–6.
15 Szepetowski P, Rochette J, Berquin P, Piussan C, Lathrop GM, Monaco AP. Familial infantile convulsions and paroxysmal choreoathetosis: a new neurological syndrome linked to the pericentromeric region of human chromosome 16. *Am J Hum Genet* 1997; 61: 889–98.
16 Caraballo R, Pavek S, Lemainque A et al. Linkage of benign familial infantile convulsions to chromosome 16p12-q12 suggests allelism to infantile convulsions and choreoathetosis syndrome. *Am J Hum Genet* 2001; 68: 788–94.
17 Sheffer IE, Bhatia KP, Lopes-Cendes I et al. Autosomal dominant frontal epilepsy misdiagnosed as sleep disorder. *Lancet* 1994; 343: 515–17.
18 Steinlein OK, Mulley JC, Propping P et al. A missense mutation in the neuronal nicotinic acetylcholine receptor α4 subunit is associated with autosomal dominant nocturnal frontal lobe epilepsy. *Nature Genetics* 1995; 11: 201–3.
19 De Fusco M, Becchetti A, Patrignani A et al. The nicotinic receptor β2 subunit is mutant in nocturnal frontal lobe epilepsy. *Nature Genet* 2000; 26: 275–6.
20 Phillips HA, Scheffer IE, Crossland KM et al. Autosomal dominant noctur-

nal frontal-lobe epilepsy: genetic heterogeneity and evidence for a second locus at 15q24. *Am J Hum Genet* 1998; 63: 1108–16.

21 Phillips HA, Marini C, Scheffer IE, Sutherland GR, Mulley JC, Berkovic SF. A de novo mutation in sporadic nocturnal frontal lobe epilepsy. *Ann Neurol* 2000; 48: 264–7.

22 Yasuda T. Benign adult familial myoclonic epilepsy (BAFME). *Kawasaki Med J* 1991; 17: 1–13.

23 Plaster NM, Uyama E, Uchino M *et al.* Genetic localization of the familial adult myoclonic epilepsy (FAME) gene to chromosome 8q24. *Neurology* 1999; 53: 1180–3.

24 Mikami M, Yasuda T, Terao A *et al.* Localization of a gene for benign adult familial myoclonic epilepsy to chromosome 8q23.3-q24.1. *Am J Hum Genet* 1999; 65: 745–51.

25 Scheffer IE, Berkovic SF. Generalized epilepsy with febrile seizures plus. A genetic disorder with heterogeneous clinical phenotypes. *Brain* 1997; 120: 479–90.

26 Escayg A, MacDonald BT, Baulac S *et al.* Mutations of SCN1A, encoding a neuronal sodium channel, in two families with GEFS+. *Nature Genet* 2000; 24: 343–5.

27 Wallace RH, Wang DW, Singh R *et al.* Febrile seizures and generalized epilepsy associated with a mutation in the Na+-channel α1 subunit gene SCN1B. *Nature Genet* 1998; 19: 366–70.

28 Baulac S, Huberfeld G, Gourfinkel-An I *et al.* First genetic evidence of GABAA receptor dysfunction in epilepsy: a mutation in the γ2-subunit gene. *Nature Genet* 2001; 28: 46–8.

29 Sugawara T, Tsurubuchi Y, Agarwala KL *et al.* A missense mutation of the Na+ channel alpha II subunit gene Na(v)1.2 in a patient with febrile and afebrile seizures causes channel dysfunction. *Proc Natl Acad Sci USA* 2001; 98: 6384–9.

30 Singh R, Scheffer IE, Crossland K, Berkovic SF. Generalized epilepsy with febrile seizures plus: a common childhood-onset genetic epilepsy syndrome. *Ann Neurol* 1999; 45: 75–81.

31 Lennox WG, Lennox M. *Epilepsy and Related Disorders*. Boston: Little, Brown, 1960.

32 Italian League against Epilepsy Genetic Collaborative Group. The Italian series of twins with epilepsy. *Epilepsia* 1995; 36 (Suppl. 3): S7–S8.

33 Berkovic SF, Howell RA, Hay DA, Hopper JL. Epilepsies in twins: genetics of the major epilepsy syndromes. *Ann Neurol* 1998; 43: 435–45.

34 Annagers JF. The use of analytic epidemiologic methods in family studies of epilepsy In: Anderson VE, Hauser WA, Leppik IE, Noebels JL, Rich SS, eds. *Genetic Strategies in Epilepsy Research*. Amsterdam: Elsevier, 1991: 139–46.

35 Anderson VE, Rich SS, Hauser WA, Wilcox KJ. Family studies of epilepsy. In: Anderson VE, Hauser WA, Leppik IE, Noebels JL, Rich SS, eds. *Genetic Strategies in Epilepsy Research*. Amsterdam: Elsevier, 1991: 89–103.

36 Risch N. Linkage strategies for genetically complex traits. I. Multilocus models. *Am J Hum Genet* 1990; 46: 222–8.

37 Metrakos K, Metrakos JD. Genetics of convulsive disorders. II. Genetic and electroencephalographic studies in centroencephalic epilepsy. *Neurology* 1961; 11: 474–83.

38 Pedley TA. The use and role of EEG in the genetic analysis of epilepsy. In: Anderson VE, Hauser WA, Leppik IE, Noebels JL, Rich SS, eds. *Genetic Strategies in Epilepsy Research*. Amsterdam: Elsevier, 1991: 31–44.

39 Italian League Against Epilepsy Genetic Collaborative Group. Concordance of clinical forms of epilepsy in families with several affected members. *Epilepsia* 1993; 34: 819–26.

40 Sander T, Schulz H, Saar K *et al.* Genome search for susceptibility loci of common idiopathic generalised epilepsies. *Hum Mol Genet* 2000; 9: 1465–72.

41 Durner M, Zhou G, Fu D *et al.* Evidence for linkage of adolescent onset idiopathic generalized epilepsy to chromosome 8– and genetic heterogeneity. *Am J Hum Genet* 1999; 64: 1411–19.

42 Durner M, Keddache MA, Tomasini L *et al.* Genome scan of idiopathic generalized epilepsy: evidence for major susceptibility gene and modifying genes influencing the seizure type. *Ann Neurol* 2001 49: 328–35.

43 Fong GCY, Pravina US, Gee MN *et al.* Childhood absence epilepsy with tonic-clonic seizures and electroencephalogram 3–4 Hz spike and multi-spike-slow wave complexes: linkage to chromosome 8q24. *Am J Hum Genet* 1998; 63: 1117–29.

44 Liu AW, Delgado Escueta AV, Serratosa JM *et al.* Juvenile myoclonic epilep-

sy locus in chromosome 6p21.2-p11: linkage to convulsions and electroencephalography trait. *Am J Hum Genet* 1995; 57: 368–81.

45 Kalachikov S, Evgrafov O, Ross B *et al.* Mutations in LGI1 cause autosomal-dominant partial epilepsy with auditory features. *Nature Genet* 2002; 30: 335–41.

46 Doose H. Symptomatology in children with focal sharp waves of genetic origin. *Eur J Pediatr* 1989; 149: 210–15.

47 Kajitani T, Nakamura M, Ueoka K, Kobuchi S. Three pairs of monozygotic twins with rolandic discharges. In: Wada JA, Penry JK, eds *Advances in Epileptology: the Xth Epilepsy International Symposium*. New York: Raven Press, 1980: 171–5.

48 Heijbel J, Blom S, Rasmuson M. Benign epilepsy of childhood with centrotemporal EEG foci: a genetic study. *Epilepsia* 1975; 16: 285–93.

49 Sheffer IE, Jones L, Pozzebon M, Howell RA, Saling MM, Berkovic SF. Autosomal dominant rolandic epilepsy and speech dyspraxia: a new syndrome with anticipation. *Ann Neurol* 1995; 38: 633–42.

50 Guerrini R, Bonanni P, Nardocci N *et al.* Autosomal recessive rolandic epilepsy with paroxysmal exercise-induced dystonia and writer's cramp: delineation of the syndrome and gene mapping to chromosome 16p12–11.2. *Ann Neurol* 1999; 45: 344–52.

51 Rodin E, Gonzales S. Hereditary components in epileptic patients. *JAMA* 1966; 198: 221–5.

52 Cossette P, Liu L, Brisebois K *et al.* Mutation of GABRA1 in an autosomal dominant form of juvenile myoclonic epilepsy. *Nature Genet* 2002; 31: 184–9.

53 Xiong L, Labuda M, Li D *et al.* Mapping of a gene determining familial partial epilepsy with variable foci to chromosome 22q11-q12. *Am J Hum Genet* 1999; 65: 1698–710.

54 Baulac S, Picard F, Herman A *et al.* Evidence for digenic inheritance in a family with both febrile convulsions and temporal lobe epilepsy implicating chromosomes 18qter and 1q25-q31. *Ann Neurol* 2001; 49: 786–92.

55 Claes L, Del-Favero J, Ceulemans B, Lagae L, Van Broeckhoven C, De Jonghe. De novo mutations in the sodium-channel gene SCN1A cause severe myoclonic epilepsy of infancy. *Am J Hum Genet* 2001; 68: 1327–32.

56 Dravet C, Bureau M, Guerrini R, Giraud N, Roger J. Severe myoclonic epilepsy in infancy. In: Roger J, Bureau M, Dravet C, Dreifuss F, Perret A, Wolf P, eds *Epileptic Syndromes in Infancy, Childhood and Adoloscence*. London: John Libbey, 1992: 75–88.

57 Benlounis A, Nabbout R, Feingold J *et al.* Genetic predisposition to severe myoclonic epilepsy in infancy. *Epilepsia* 2001; 42: 204–9.

58 Corey LA, Berg K, Pellock JM, Solaas MH, Nance WE, DeLorenzo RJ. The occurrence of epilepsy and febrile seizures in Virginian and Norwegian twins. *Neurology* 1991; 41: 1433–6.

59 Tsuboi T, Endo S. Genetic studies of febrile convulsions: analysis of twin and family data. In: Anderson VE, Hauser WA, Leppik IE, Noebels JL, Rich SS, eds. *Genetic Strategies in Epilepsy Research*. Amsterdam: Elsevier, 1991: 119–28.

60 Frantzen E, Lennox-Buchthal M, Nygaard A, Stene J. A genetic study of febrile convulsions. *Neurology* 1970; 20: 909–17.

61 Tsuboi T. Febrile convulsions. In: Anderson VE, Hauser WA, Penry JK, Sing CF, eds. *Genetic Basis of the Epilepsies*. New York: Raven Press, 1982: 123–34.

62 Rich SS, Annagers JF, Hauser WA, Anderson VE. Complex segregation analysis of febrile convulsions. *Am J Hum Genet* 1987; 41: 249–57.

63 Maher J, McLachlan RS. Febrile convulsions. Is seizure duration the most important predictor of temporal lobe epilepsy? *Brain* 1995; 118: 1521–8.

64 Cendes F, Cook MJ, Watson C *et al.* Frequency and characteristics of dual pathology in patients with lesional epilepsy. *Neurology* 1995; 45: 2058–64.

65 Johnson EW, Dubovsky J, Rich SS *et al.* Evidence for a novel gene for familial febrile convulsions, FEB2, linked to chromosome 19p in an extended family from the Midwest. *Hum Mol Genet* 1998; 7: 63–7.

66 Koskiniemi M, Donner M, Majuri H, Haltia M, Norio R. Progressive myoclonus epilepsy: a clinical and histopathological study. *Acta Neurol Scand* 1974; 50: 307–32.

67 Iivanainen M, Himberg JJ. Valproate and clonazepam in the treatment of of severe progessive myoclonus epilepsy. *Arch Neurol* 1982; 39: 239.

68 Pennacchio LA, Lehesjoki A, Stone NE *et al.* Mutations in the gene encoding cystatin B in progressive myoclonus epilepsy (EPM1). *Science* 1996; 271: 1731–4.

69 Lalioti MD, Scott HS, Buresi C *et al.* Dodecamer repeat expansion in cystatin B gene in progressive myoclonus epilepsy. *Nature* 1997; 386: 767–9.

70 Schwarz GA, Yanoff M. Lafora's disease: distinct clinico-pathologic form of Unverricht's syndrome. *Arch Neurol* 1965; 12: 173–88.

71 Sakai M, Austin J, Witmer F, Trueb L. Studies in myoclonus epilepsy (Lafora body form); II. Polyglucans in the systemic deposits of myoclonus epilepsy and in corpora amylacea. *Neurology* 1970; 20: 160–76.

72 Minassian BA, Lee JR, Herbrick JA *et al.* Mutations in a gene encoding a novel protein tyrosine phosphatase cause progressive myoclonus epilepsy. *Nature Genet* 1998; 20: 171–4.

73 Gomez-Garre P, Sanz Y, Rodriguez de Cordoba S, Serratosa JM. Mutational spectrum of the EPM2A gene in progressive myoclonus epilepsy of Lafora: high degree of allelic heterogeneity and prevalence of deletions. *Eur J Hum Genet* 2000; 8: 946–54.

74 Rosing HS, Hopkins LC, Wallace DC, Epstein CM, Weidenheim K. Maternally inherited mitochondrial myopathy and myoclonic epilepsy. *Ann Neurol* 1985; 17: 228–37.

75 Berkovic SF, Carpenter S, Evans A *et al.* Myoclonus epilepsy and ragged-red fibres (MERRF). 1. A clinical, pathological, biochemical, magnetic resonance spectrographic and positron emission tomographic study. *Brain* 1989; 112: 1231–60.

76 Shoffner JM, Lott MT, Lezza AMS, Seibel P, Ballinger SW, Wallace DC. Myoclonic epilepsy and red-ragged fiber disease (MERRF) is associated with a mitochondrial DNA tRNA^{lys} mutation. *Cell* 1990; 61: 931–7.

77 Rapin I, Goldfischer S, Katzman R, Engel J Jr, O'Brien JS. The cherry-red spot–myoclonus syndrome. *Ann Neurol* 1978; 3: 234–42.

78 Lowden JA, O'Brien JS. Sialidosis: a review of human neuraminidase deficiency. *Am J Hum Genet* 1979; 31: 1–18.

79 D'Azzo A, Hoogeveen A, Reuser AJJ, Robinson D, Galjaard H. Molecular defect in combined β-galactosidase and neuroaminidase deficiency in man. *Procl Natl Acad Sci* USA 1982; 79: 4535–9.

80 Bonten E, van der Spoel A, Fornerod M, Grosveld G, d'Azzo A. Characterization of human lysosomal neuraminidase defines the molecular basis of the metabolic storage disorder sialidosis. *Genes Dev* 1996; 10: 3156–69.

81 Takano T, Shimmoto M, Fukuhara Y *et al.* Galactosialidosis: clinical and molecular analysis of 19 Japanese patients. *Brain Dysfunction* 1991; 4: 271–80.

82 Wisniewski KE, Kida E, Golabek AA, Kaczmarski W, Connell F, Zhong N. Neuronal ceroid lipofuscinoses: classification and diagnosis. *Adv Genet* 2001; 45: 1–34.

83 Berkovic SF, Andermann F. The progressive myoclonus epilepsies. In: Padley TA, Mledrum BS, eds. *Recent Advances in Epilepsy*. Edinburgh: Churchill Livingstone, 1986; 157–87.

84 Sleat DE, Donnelly RJ, Lackland H *et al.* Association of mutations in a lysosomal protein with classical late-infantile neuronal ceroid lipofuscinosis. *Science* 1997; 277: 1802–5.

85 Lake BD, Cavanagh NPC. Early-juvenile Batten's disease: a recognisable subgroup distinct from others of Batten's disease. *J Neurol Sci* 1978; 36: 265–71.

86 The International Batten Disease Consortium. Isolation of a novel gene underlying Batten disease, CLN3. *Cell* 1995; 82: 949–57.

87 Berkovic SF, Carpenter S, Andermann F, Andermann E, Wolfe SLS. Kufs' disease: a critical reappraisal. *Brain* 1988; 111: 27–62.

88 Boehme DH, Cottrell JC, Leonberg SC, Zeman W. A dominant form of neuronal ceroid-lipofuscinosis. *Brain* 1971; 94: 745–60.

89 Dom R, Brucher JM, Ceuterick C, Carton H, Martin JJ. Adult ceroid-lipofuscinosis (Kufs' disease) in two brothers. Retinal and visceral storage in one; diagnostic muscle biopsy in the other. *Acta Neuropath* 1979; 45: 67–72.

25 Diagnosis and Treatment of Non-Epileptic Seizures

J.R. Gates

Non-epileptic seizures have become a very significant issue for the physician treating epilepsy, because they occur in approximately 20% of patients admitted to epilepsy inpatient units and are easily confused with epileptic seizures [1]. Consequently, it is the neurologist/epileptologist who generally bears the brunt of the diagnostic clarification for this significant spectrum of disorders.

This chapter summarizes the current issues surrounding terminology and classification, epidemiology, cost of non-epileptic seizures, the diagnostic approach and subsequent treatment and outcome.

Terminology and classification

The terminology and classification of the spectrum of disorders listed under the rubric of non-epileptic seizures is quite confusing. Similarly, the epidemiology of non-epileptic seizures has not been adequately studied, and, at best, we have only gross estimates of the actual frequency of this spectrum of disorders. Also, the best diagnostic approaches remain to be elucidated, as are the optimal treatment strategies for psychogenic non-epileptic seizures. Nonetheless, there is a significant body of literature that this chapter will summarize to identify appropriate diagnostic and treatment strategies based upon the best available evidence.

Although there continues to be some controversy, the classification of non-epileptic seizures has been established. As summarized by Gates [1], there are two distinct sets of disorders. One includes the physiological spectrum of dysfunction, the other the psychogenic. The terms used to describe non-epileptic events, however, are not uniformly accepted. Many archaic terms such as 'hysteroepilepsy', 'hysterical pseudo-seizures' and 'hysterical epilepsy' [1] have been retired, but the term 'hysterical seizures' is still used. This is an anachronistic term, which was very specific in the old psychiatric literature in referring to a conversion disorder, which is only one of the disorders associated with non-epileptic seizures under the subcategory of psychogenic non-epileptic seizures. Consequently, using the term 'hysterical seizures' interchangeably with non-epileptic seizures is inaccurate and is much like calling all complex partial seizures 'temporal lobe seizures' and ignores the fact that such seizures may arise from extratemporal sites. Furthermore, the popular perception of 'hysteria' makes it one of the most pejorative terms still in use. Hysteria in lay terms implies 'out of control, beyond reason' and is replete with negative connotations. Similarly, the term 'pseudo-seizures' is also replete with pejorative overtones, especially in the American usage, which render it impractical for use in the communication with the patient with this spectrum of disorders.

Consequently, the term 'non-epileptic seizures', though not an ideal reference, in this author's opinion, is the least offensive and is preferred by most American clinicians in the field [2], including the members of the American Epilepsy Society.

International agreement in terminology has yet to be attained. For example, in the UK, Betts *et al.* [3] have suggested the term 'non-epileptic attack disorder' to refer to psychogenic non-epileptic seizures. The problem with this term is that many patients in the psychogenic category have a history of previous sexual abuse, generally at the hands of a trusted family member or close adult friend of the family. Consequently, the use of the word 'attack' would appear to be quite inadvisable. Very clearly, we need to adopt a consistent set of terms to move this field forward. These are proposed in Figs 25.1, 25.2 and 25.3, consistent with the current DSM-IV classification scheme for non-epileptic seizures of psychogenic origin and consistent with generally regarded terms for physiological non-epileptic events [4].

Physiological non-epileptic events

As summarized in Fig. 25.2, there is quite a spectrum of disorders with a physiological basis that can be confused with non-epileptic seizures. These include syncope, paroxysmal toxic phenomena, non-toxic organic hallucinosis, non-epileptic myoclonus, the spectrum of sleep disorders, paroxysmal movement disorders, paroxysmal endocrine disturbances, paroxysms of acute neurological insults and transient ischaemic cerebrovascular phenomena [5].

Syncope is one of the most challenging disorders that can be confused with epilepsy. For example, 5% of children under the age of 5 years can suffer breath-holding spells that are frequently associated with some myoclonic jerks, and with unresponsiveness that to the parent can appear to last for a very expanded length of time. The myoclonic jerks associated with this can also be misinterpreted by the uninitiated and concerned parent as the jerks of a clonic seizure or the tonic stiffening of a tonic seizure with breath-holding spells. Occasionally even urinary incontinence is seen. The brevity of the episodes and the prompt return of awareness without any significant postictal state, besides the appropriate age of onset in the history, is generally sufficient to make a clinical distinction, but sometimes the differential diagnosis can be very difficult [6]. The latter is particularly true when the hypoxaemia induced by the syncope is sufficient to induce a seizure. Separating out the physiological non-epileptic from the epileptic components in these particular cases can be very challenging.

Transient ischaemic cerebrovascular phenomena can also be quite chameleon in their appearance. Perhaps the most difficult patient presentations that result occasionally in admission to an epilepsy unit for investigation are migraine equivalents that are misinterpreted as simple partial seizures [7]. Similarly, transient ischaemic attacks in more elderly patients, resulting from atherosclerotic or embolic mechanisms, can appear as simple partial seizures, particularly when they involve symptoms of visual hallucinations or the visual aberration of a migraine attack. The important phenomenum from a clinical perspective is whether there is truly any positive phenomena that are experienced by the patient, specifically, in the jerking of the hand or a formed and moving visual hallucination. These latter phenomena are generally associated with seizures, whereas the deficits are the hallmark of ischaemic phe-

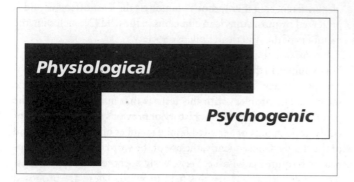

Fig. 25.1 Division of non-epileptic events into physiological and psychogenic.

nomena. For a given patient, however, the dysaesthesia that is sometimes induced by migraine or by a transient ischaemic attack can be very difficult to distinguish from a simple partial somatosensory seizure. Video-EEG monitoring may add significant assistance in such cases.

Paroxysmal toxic phenomena can include the transient effects of cocaine, the effects of other stimulants as well as scopolamine, the toxic effects of antiepileptic medications, and the effects of a full spectrum of toxic substances that can create paroxysmal brain phenomena that may be misinterpreted as seizures. A detailed history and appropriate urine or blood screen will help greatly in clarifying this confounding physiological non-epileptic diagnostic group [8].

Similarly, non-toxic organic hallucinosis, such as the spontaneous visual hallucinations of patients with advanced diabetic retinopathy or advanced polyneuropathy, can result in somatosensory aberrations. which can be misinterpreted as seizures. Not uncommonly, the visual hallucinations associated with advanced diabetic retinopathy and visual compromise can be quite an elaborate event taking the form of complex visual hallucinations. Generally, I have been struck by the lack of psychic significance to the hallucinations experienced by these patients, which often helps in distinguishing them from some form of paranoid organic hallucinosis. Nonetheless, I have seen formed visual hallucinations as a consequence of seizures. Some of the hallucinations of early schizophrenia can also be misinterpreted as epilepsy [7].

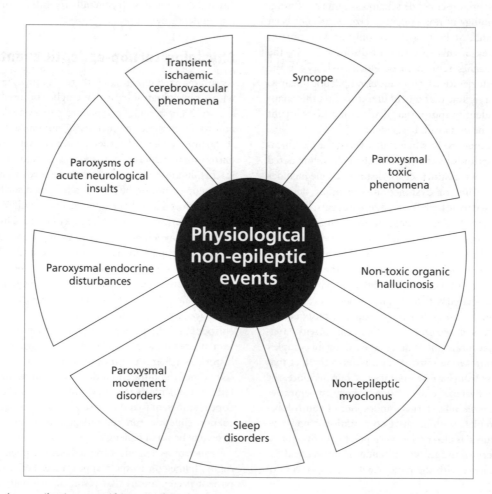

Fig. 25.2 Physiological non-epileptic events. Alternative diagnoses.

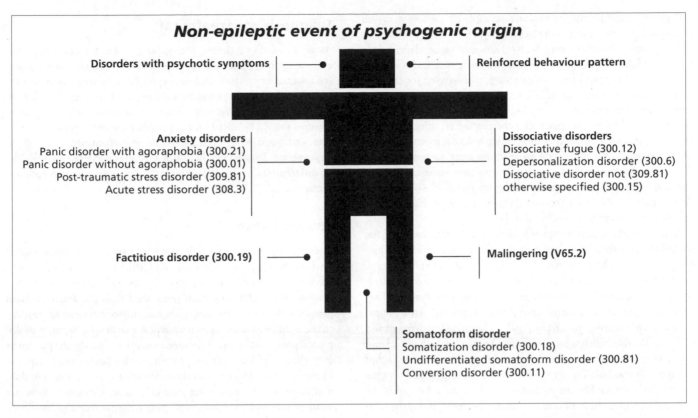

Fig. 25.3 General diagnostic categories that may be observed in patients with non-epileptic events. See the DSM-IV (Washington DC: American Psychiatric Association, 1994), for the meaning of the numbers in parentheses.

The paroxysms of acute neurological insults also provide a rich substrate for misinterpretation. For example, the rigors of decortization and cerebration in closed head injuries are not infrequently misinterpreted in intensive care units as seizures and treated aggressively with antiepileptic drugs before appropriate neurological consultation is obtained and appropriate clarification ensues. Patients can also develop, as a consequence of head injury or acute encephalitis, distorted visual perceptions that can be misinterpreted as partial simple seizures. Very often this can be clarified at the bedside by an experienced clinician, but not infrequently video-EEG monitoring is required as these patients show a significantly increased risk for seizures [1].

Endocrine disturbances that may cause non-epileptic seizures include phaeochromocytoma, with episodes of flushed redness associated with rapid heart rate and agitation, as well as carcinoid syndrome. Occasionally, these episodes can be misinterpreted as autonomic seizures [7].

Paroxysmal movement disorders such as kinesogenic choreoathetosis, the dyskinetic effects of parkinsonian medication, or acute movement disorders such as Huntington's chorea can also be misinterpreted as seizures. Patients with significant cognitive impairment not infrequently have paroxysmal movements that, by virtue of the fact that they often have epilepsy as well, are misinterpreted by care providers as an epileptic disorder. These episodes may also reflect merely self-stimulatory behaviour in individuals with very significant impairment of their perceptive apparatus. Not

infrequently, verification that these are not seizures in the inpatient environment of the long-term monitoring suite is required. Similarly, non-epileptic myoclonus can be so misinterpreted [1,5].

Other non-epileptic paroxysmal disorders include sleep disorders, specifically the REM behaviour disorder, which typically affect a middle-aged male effecting lack of inhibition of REM sleep. This results in acting out on his dreams, which often presents to the neurologist as a possible complex partial seizure disorder during sleep where, in fact, a distinctly different mechanism is going on and requires a different treatment strategy. Some of the other parasomnias similarly have been misinterpreted as epilepsy and require appropriate treatment, as discussed extensively by Mahowald and Schenck [9].

Psychogenic non-epileptic seizures

The spectrum of non-epileptic seizures of psychogenic origin is similarly broad. Anxiety disorders which represent a significant source of misdiagnosis include panic disorders with or without agoraphobia, post-traumatic stress disorder and acute stress disorder [1].

Factitious disorders such as Munchausen by proxy syndrome can similarly be a source of confusion as can somatoform disorders, most commonly conversion disorders, which constitute the majority of non-epileptic seizure patients and are most commonly due to some significant psychological or sexual abuse [10]. The multiple somatoform disorders constitute a significant group in which epilepsy-type symptoms are just one example of a whole array of symptoms affecting various organ systems [1].

Dissociative disorders, specifically dissociate fugue, depersonalization and dissociative disorders not otherwise specified represent another significant spectrum, as can frank malingering for the purpose of clear secondary gain. It is important to distinguish malingering from factitious disorders. Malingerers are often sorted out before referral to an epilepsy unit, whereas the factitious patients are not consciously mimicking their epilepsy-like symptomatology. This is particularly important to communicate to nursing staff during the diagnostic phase, so that a pejorative sense is not communicated to the patient prior to the opportunity to complete an evaluation and begin a treatment strategy that is not burdened by an alienation from the attending staff [1].

A particularly unique group of patients can be categorized in the so-called reinforced behaviour pattern. These are cognitively challenged patients who have unconsciously learned that epilepsy-type symptoms can result in a significant control of their environment. By having a seizure, considerable attention is paid to them and they gain an unconscious control of their environment. An example would be the patient with cerebral palsy, cognitive impairment and epilepsy secondary to a significant perinatal insult who has a seizure as the family is getting in the car to visit an aunt this patient is not particularly fond of. The trip to the aunt is cancelled and a vague awareness is realized by the patient that there is an opportunity the next time a trip to the aunt is anticipated. The next Sunday the family gets in the car. This time a different event with many features similar to an epileptic seizure occurs and it has the same effect: the trip to the aunt is cancelled and a paradoxical reinforcement has been given to this patient for the next potential visit to the aunt. There is no specific DSM category for this disorder, hence its designation as a reinforced behaviour pattern [1].

Epidemiology and the cost of non-epileptic seizures

The incidence of non-epileptic seizures is higher than most people realize. There is a significant coincidence of both epilepsy and non-epileptic seizures. This varies from different centres, but from studies in patients referred for long-term video-EEG monitoring, epilepsy and non-epileptic seizures appear to coexist in approximately 30% of inpatients. Patients with a diagnosis of non-epileptic seizures constitute 20% of overall referrals to epilepsy centres [1,11].

What is the total economic impact of non-epileptic seizures? Costs include the direct costs of diagnostic evaluation, intervention, blood tests, clinical office calls and visits, ineffective antiepileptic medications, inappropriate treatment, emergency room cost, hospitalizations in intensive care units, and death or complications for patients in non-epileptic status being aggressively treated with respiratory suppressants or being inappropriately intubated. The indirect costs of missed time from work for the patient and caretakers must also be considered. All this must be an enormous expense, but an economic impact study has never been done. We can only guess at this point, but those involved in the care of these patients know that the cost is enormous not just for the patients themselves but also for their families and society [12].

Diagnosis and treatment

As discussed above, there is a broad range of differential diagnostic issues and an approximate 30% probability of dual diagnosis, e.g. coexistence of epilepsy and non-epileptic seizures. Consequently, history and evaluation must proceed in a very organized and logical fashion. The diagnostic assessment for physiological non-epileptic seizures should be based on the patient's specific clinical presentation, and special investigations should be performed accordingly as appropriate. The sections below discuss in some detail the diagnostic differentiation between epileptic and psychogenic non-epileptic seizures.

Historical features

It is certainly common for a patient with psychogenic non-epileptic seizures to appear no different from his/her epileptic counterparts, having had seizures for many years, having been seen by several neurologists and having been prescribed multiple anticonvulsant medications. One of the more common historical elements leading to the initial suspicion of non-epileptic seizures, however, is multiple seizure types that are ill defined and ill described by the patient or even those who have witnessed them, with a paradoxical response to antiepileptic drugs, i.e. as the medications are increased in dose and number, the seizures actually get worse. Obviously there are some people with medically refractory epilepsy who can have such a history. However, multiple seizure types that are ill defined, with multiple medication failures and a paradoxical increase in the frequency of seizures as the drugs are increased, should be a potential red flag [7].

Not infrequently there is a lack of concern or an excessive emotional response to the seizures. Patients displaying a surprising lack of concern for a clearly intolerable seizure frequency, or patients with an excessive emotional reaction to a seizure, with exaggerated weeping, may indicate the possibility of non-epileptic seizures [7].

The history of repeated hospitalizations and emergency department visits is another potential warning sign that the seizures may be psychogenic/non-epileptic in origin. A history of a remarkable lack of injuries, despite repeated falls, should also suggest the possibility of non-epileptic seizures. Tongue biting in non-epileptic patients, when it occurs, generally involves the tip of the tongue, whereas in tonic-clonic seizures it is the sides of the tongue that are often bitten. Incontinence can be seen with non-epileptic seizures, but it is rare [1,7,8].

Associated psychiatric disorders such as depression, personality disorders or, in some cases, even psychosis, are more common in patients with psychogenic non-epileptic seizures. However, many patients with epilepsy or with a diagnosis of coexistent epilepsy and psychogenic seizures, can have psychiatric disorders as well. Therefore, this element is of very minor utility but, again, it should raise concern in association with other historical features [13].

Finally, a history of sexual abuse, especially in childhood, is very common, especially in adult females with conversion disorder non-epileptic seizures. The problem with this particular history is the remarkable commonality of sexual abuse in society at large. As reported by Finkelhor et al. [14], approximately 27% of women and 16% of men in the general population, when questioned in a large national survey, reported a history of some form of sexual abuse.

Paradoxically, in paediatric patients a history of sexual abuse is the exception, with other stressors being the more common predictors. These include family conflict, parental psychopathology, parental alcohol dependence, marital discord, school problems and peer relationship problems. There is also a below average IQ in a disproportionate number of female patients [15].

In a study in adults that included 35 women and 23 men [13], childhood sexual abuse contributed to non-epileptic seizures in one-half of the patients and childhood physical abuse in one-third. More commonly in men, there was a pattern of chronic repression of anger, followed by a series of adulthood frustrations. This was seen in eight of 23 men (35%) but in only two of 35 women, who more commonly manifest the reactivation of emotions about child abuse. This pattern was usually accompanied by a family history of dysfunctional handling of anger, personal denial of feeling or expressing anger, or distorted beliefs about anger [13].

Remote psychological and physical traumas apparently set the stage for non-epileptic seizures when the emotions they engender are not dealt with. As summarized by Bowman [13], 'like old volcanoes, the simmering emotions lay partially dormant until painful life context and immediate precipitants jolt them to life'.

Video-EEG monitoring

The gold standard for the diagnosis of non-epileptic seizures is to record multiple characteristic events on the video-EEG and to document apparent impairment of awareness in the absence of epileptiform EEG changes. As summarized by Rowan [7], there are cases of epileptic seizures, especially partial simple seizures, that do not generate sufficient EEG changes to confirm the diagnosis on surface EEG. However, in my experience, the strategy of recording multiple events, looking for a stereotypic pattern consistent with the established semiology of partial seizures (especially unusual frontal lobe seizures or seizures arising from various brain origins), has rarely failed to clarify which events are epileptic and which are not. When video-EEG is used in the context of a multidisciplinary team approach to the patient, involving nursing, neuropsychology, psychology and psychiatry as needed, definitive diagnosis will transpire.

Some clinical signs are often suggestive when they are observed on video-EEG, or when a history is obtained of the events, such as gradual onset and gradual cessation. Non-epileptic seizures tend to have a slower, more gradual beginning, becoming increasingly vigorous as the seizure progresses. As the seizure progresses, it often has a non-physiological progression. For example, generalized motor activity may precede loss of consciousness, or progressive involvement of body parts in a motor seizure may not follow the classic jacksonian march, consistent with the cortical homunculus. Nonetheless, unusual epileptic events, particularly those of frontal origin, can be quite bizarre in appearance. The key, again, is the remarkable stereotypic nature of multiple epileptic events that have been recorded [7].

In a classic paper from 1985 [16], out of phase motor activity, particularly out of phase arm and leg movements, high amplitude forward pelvic thrusting and lack of vocalization at the start of the event (as opposed to the transformation from the tonic to the clonic phase), were described as being suggestive features for distinguishing epileptic from non-epileptic seizures. As subsequent authors have demonstrated [17–19], a differentiation based on these features is not free from errors but can be highly effective in the clinical determination of epileptic and non-epileptic events. The ability of the examiner to modify the pattern of motor activity is also suggestive of a non-epileptic seizure. Such a modification is difficult, if not impossible, to achieve in events of epileptic origin.

Suggestion or provocation methods to induce non-epileptic seizures and thereby expedite the diagnostic process have been a hot topic in recent years [20]. Intravenous saline is the most commonly used technique. Schachter et al. [21] surveyed members of the American Epilepsy Society about their use of provocation techniques. Overall, 40% of the 426 respondents used provocation techniques, yet 23% of that group perceived ethical dilemmas in so doing [21]. At the Minnesota Epilepsy Group, we do not employ provocation techniques. We consider them potentially misleading, unethical and a hindrance to the therapeutic transition for our patients, especially those with conversion disorders, many of whom are young women whose faith in a trusted family or authority figure has been violated by sexual or physical abuse. It appears cognitively dissonant and counterproductive to begin a potential long-term therapeutic relationship of insight therapy or other treatment with an inherently deceptive practice. We appear to obtain a sufficient recording of events in a reasonable period of time without utilizing provocation techniques [12].

Neuropsychological testing

Neuropsychological assessment of non-epileptic seizures has been attempted by many investigators over the years. The findings from the literature summarized by Dodrill and Holmes [22] show that, like people with epilepsy, people with non-epileptic seizures fall into the lower quartile of the normal intellectual range. Consequently, differences in IQ are not particularly useful in differentiating epileptic from non-epileptic patients. In the area of adjustment, however, the Minnesota Multiphasic Personality Inventory (MMPI) has been the most commonly used measure and, though the test is not perfect, it does have a correct classification rate of 70% or slightly better with careful definition of subject groups. In particular, it shows the classic conversion V pattern, i.e. elevations in scale 1 (hypochondriasis) and scale 3 (hysteria), with a slightly elevated, or normal, depression scale. This obviously is not a foolproof diagnostic tool, but it is helpful.

Comprehensive neuropsychological test batteries fail to reveal a characteristic pattern for non-epileptic seizures, although, as with the epilepsy population, evidence of a pattern on neuropsychological testing consistent with post-brain injury is not uncommon. As suggested by Dodrill and Holmes [22], application of gender-specific rules to MMPI profiles could be explored as well as looking at the combination of personality variables.

Treatment of non-epileptic seizures

The treatment of physiological non-epileptic seizures is obviously determined by the underlying condition. As far as psychogenic non-epileptic seizures are concerned, despite our long-lasting awareness of the existence of 'hystero-epilepsy' (a term coined by Charcot in the second half of the 1880s), we have not had a clear treatment strategy for non-epileptic seizures that has been subject to appropriate prospective evaluation [23]. Charcot used ovarian compression. Gowers prescribed iron tonic to correct the presumed underlying anaemia and stated that 'water when poured on the head of the patient is often effectual, especially if the mouth is opened, however, a second gallon is often more effectual as the first may result in redoubled violence of the seizure' [24].

Nonetheless, based on over two decades of experience, there is a general consensus among epileptologists that non-epileptic seizures of psychogenic origin are a treatable condition. A multidisciplinary team approach appears to be most effective.

Diagnostic clarification by appropriate video-EEG recording, interviews with the psychologist and the social worker, and neuropsychological testing, with continued dialogue between the team members, can often result in appropriate treatment strategies.

As emphasized by Bowman [13]: (a) assessing for depression is critical. If major depression is present, treatment with antidepressants must be undertaken for at least 6 months. Psychotherapy of some form is often helpful, especially when it is targeted at incomplete bereavement, and depression is related to ongoing conflict or stress. (b) The possible presence of some form of panic disorder should be assessed. If a panic disorder coexists with depression, initial low doses of selective serotonin reuptake inhibitors (SSRIs) can be helpful. Benzodiazepines should be used carefully, but can be beneficial as supplements to SSRIs. Cognitive therapy to reduce and prevent panic attacks is essential to prevent relapse when antipanic medications are withdrawn. (c) It is important to assess any history of trauma, both in adulthood and in childhood, which can result in directed psychotherapy for verbal processing of the trauma and cognitive restructuring to reduce the impact. (d) The possibility of a dissociative disorder, including amnesia, fugue, depersonalization, derealization and identity alterations, should be evaluated. Again, these are usually related to a history of psychological trauma. In these patients, hypnosis may be helpful in assisting the person to assess the effect of the trauma. (e) Other life events or conflicts that may be causing non-epileptic seizures should be explored. (f) An effort should be made to identify complicated bereavements, family or marital conflict, or unexpressed anger and frustration (especially in males), and appropriate cognitive therapy should be implemented to address these issues. Finally, if the cause for non-epileptic seizures is not clear, hypnosis may be helpful in teaching the patient how to control the expression of seizures, as summarized by Barry and Atzmon [25].

In the inpatient environment, a supportive, non-judgmental attitude must be maintained. It is very easy for medical personnel who are trained to deal with life and death situations, to be intentionally or unintentionally pejorative about non-epileptic seizure expression. This is counterproductive and does not assist the patient in effecting an appropriate response. The Minnesota Epilepsy Group team approach includes an epileptologist, a clinical neuropsychologist, a social worker, dedicated nursing staff, EEG technologists and a consulting psychiatrist. This team performs a very thorough psychological assessment and examines the relative strengths and weaknesses of the patient and the environmental support system. Treatment guidelines are based on this evaluation. A great deal of attention is paid to the presentation of the diagnosis of non-epilep-

tic seizures to the patient and the family, in order to facilitate and set the stage for continued psychotherapy. This facilitates the patient's understanding of the nature of his/her condition and of its psychological causes, and sets the stage for successful transition of treatment to the outpatient environment. In a 27-month follow-up of 29 adult patients with highly intractable non-epileptic seizures managed by the Minnesota Epilepsy Group, 11 patients were free of seizures and 23 experienced at least a 75% decrease in seizure frequency as well as decreased severity [23]. In other studies, 25–87% of patients appropriately diagnosed with non-epileptic seizures ceased having events [26–32].

Patients tend to do better when they present with a shorter duration of non-epileptic seizures, especially less than 6 months [33]. Vigorous application of video-EEG diagnosis and a multidisciplinary approach should facilitate a better outcome than in previous years, when this technology was less available. Nonetheless, outcome studies are still quite limited. A few small case series suggest that children and adolescents have a better prognosis than adults. Clearly more work is needed to understand the efficacy of different therapeutic approaches and the best way of designing individual treatment plans.

Conclusions

We have made significant progress in the last 25 years, but much work remains to be done. We must agree on terminology and this chapter suggests that we are close to that consensus. Population-based epidemiological studies are required. The diagnostic evaluation of patients with psychogenic non-epileptic seizures requires further refinement. Controlled outcome studies must be standardized and then conducted at multiple epilepsy referral centres. Finally, the economic impact of non-epileptic seizures must be investigated since it will likely justify a more aggressive and comprehensive programme of research.

References

1 Gates JR. Epidemiology and classification of non-epileptic events. In: Gates JR, Rowan AJ, eds. *Non-Epileptic Seizures*, 2nd edn. Boston: Butterworth-Heinemann, 2000: 3–14.
2 Schachter SC, Fraser B, Rowan AJ. Provocative testing for nonepileptic seizures: Attitudes and practices in the United States among American Epilepsy Society members. *J Epilepsy* 1996; 9: 249–52.
3 Betts T, Duffy N. Treatment of non-epileptic attack disorder (pseudoseizures) in the community. In: Gram L, Johannessen SI, Osterman PO, Sillanpää M, eds. *Pseudo-Epileptic Seizures*. Briston, PA: Wrightson Biomedical, 1993: 109–21.
4 Gates JR, Rowan AJ, eds. *Non-Epileptic Seizures*, 2nd edn. Boston: Butterworth-Heinemann, 2000.
5 Andermann F. Non-epileptic paroxysmal neurologic events. In: Gates JR, Rowan AJ, eds. *Non-Epileptic Seizures*, 2nd edn. Boston: Butterworth-Heinemann, 2000: 51–69.
6 Ritter FJ, Prakash K. Non-epileptic paroxysmal neurologic events. In: Gates JR, Rowan AJ, eds. *Non-Epileptic Seizures*, 2nd edn. Boston: Butterworth-Heinemann, 2000: 95–110.
7 Rowan AJ. Diagnosis of non-epileptic seizures. In: Gates JR, Rowan AJ, eds. *Non-Epileptic Seizures*, 2nd edn. Boston: Butterworth-Heinemann, 2000: 15–30.
8 Devinsky O, Paraiso JO. Unusual epileptic events and non-epileptic seizures: differential diagnosis and coexistence. In: Gates JR, Rowan AJ, eds. *Non-Epileptic Seizures*, 2nd edn. Boston: Butterworth-Heinemann, 2000: 31–50.

9 Mahowald W, Schenck CH. Parasomnia purgatory: epileptic/non-epileptic parasomnia interface seizures. In: Gates JR, Rowan AJ, eds. *Non-Epileptic Seizures*, 2nd edn. Boston: Butterworth-Heinemann, 2000: 71–96.

10 Dreifuss FE, Gates JR. Manchausen syndrome by proxy and svengali syndrome. In: Gates JR, Rowan AJ, eds. *Non-Epileptic Seizures*, 2nd edn. Boston: Butterworth-Heinemann, 2000: 237–44.

11 Sigurdardottir KR, Olafsson E. Incidence of psychogenic seizures in adults: a population-based study in Iceland. *Epilepsia* 1998; 39: 749–52.

12 Gates JR. Nonepileptic seizures: time for progress. Editorial. *Epilepsy Behav* 2000; 1: 2–6.

13 Bowman ES. Relationship of remote and recent life events to the onset and course of non-epileptic seizures. In: Gates JR, Rowan AJ, eds. *Non-Epileptic Seizures*, 2nd edn. Boston: Butterworth-Heinemann, 2000: 269–83.

14 Finkelhor D, Hotaling G, Lewis IA, Smith C. Sexual abuse in a national survey of adult men and women: prevalence, characteristics and risk factors. *Child Abuse Neglect* 1990; 14: 19–28.

15 Hempel A. Cognitive features and predisposing factors in children with psychogenic seizures. In: Gates JR, Rowan AJ, eds. *Non-Epileptic Seizures*, 2nd edn. Boston: Butterworth-Heinemann, 2000: 185–95.

16 Gates JR, Ramani V, Whalens SM. Ictal characteristics of pseudoseizures. *Arch Neurol* 1985; 42: 1183–7.

17 Leis AA, Ross MA, Summers AK. Psychogenic seizures: ictal characteristics and diagnostic pitfalls. *Neurology* 1992; 42: 95.

18 Gulick TA, Spinks IP, King DW. Pseudoseizures: ictal phenomena. *Neurology* 1982; 32: 3440.

19 Kanner AM, Morris HH, Lüders H *et al*. Supplementary motor seizures mimicking pseudoseizures: some clinical differences. *Neurology* 1990; 40: 1404.

20 Burack JR, Back AL, Pearlman RA. Provoking nonepileptic seizures: the ethics of deceptive diagnostic testing. *Hastings Center Rep* 1997; 24(1): 24–33.

21 Schachter SC, Fraser B, Rowan AJ. Provocative testing for nonepileptic seizures: attitudes and practices in the United States among American Epilepsy Society members. *J Epilepsy* 1996; 9: 249–52.

22 Dodrill CB, Holmes MD. Part summary: psychological and neuropsychological evaluation of the patient with non-epileptic seizures. In: Gates JR, Rowan AJ, eds. *Non-Epileptic Seizures*, 2nd edn Boston: Butterworth-Heinemann, 2000: 169–81.

23 Ramani V. Treatment of the adult patient with non-epileptic seizures. In: Gates JR, Rowan AJ, eds. *Non-Epileptic Seizures*, 2nd edn. Boston: Butterworth-Heinemann, 2000: 311–16.

24 Gowers WR. *Epilepsy and Other Chronic Convulsive Disorders*. New York: William Wood & Co., 1995: 101.

25 Barry JJ, Atzmon O. Diagnosis of non-epileptic seizures. In: Gates JR, Rowan AJ, eds. *Non-Epileptic Seizures*, 2nd edn. Boston: Butterworth-Heinemann, 2000: 295–303.

26 Lancman ME, Brotherton TA, Asconape JJ, Penry JK. Psychogenic seizures in adults: a longitudinal analysis. *Seizure* 1993; 2: 281–6.

27 Kristensen O, Alving J. Pseudoseizures – risk factors and prognosis. *Acta Neurol Scand* 1992; 85: 177–80.

28 Meirkord H, Will B, Rish D, Shorvon S. The clinical features and prognosis of pseudoseizures diagnosed using video-EEG telemetry. *Neurology* 1991; 41: 1643–6.

29 Wyllie E, Friedman D, Luderse H *et al*. Outcome of psychogenic seizures in children and adolescents compared with adults. *Neurology* 1991; 41: 742–4.

30 Lempert T, Schmidt D. Natural history and outcome of psychogenic seizures: a clinical study in 50 patients. *J Neurol* 1990; 237: 35–8.

31 Krumholz A. Psychogenic seizures: a clinical study with follow-up data. *Neurology* 1983; 33: 498–502.

32 Ramani V, Gumnit RJ. Management of hysterical seizures in epileptic patients. *Arch Neurol* 1982; 39: 78–81.

33 Gates JR, Luciano D, Devinski O. The classification and treatment of nonepileptic events. In: Devinski O, Theodore WA, eds. *Epilepsy and Behavior*. New York: Wiley-Liss, 1991: 251–63.

Section 3
Drugs Used in the Treatment of Epilepsy

26 The Choice of Drugs and Approach to Drug Treatments in Partial Epilepsy

S. Shorvon

This chapter serves as an introduction to the chapters on the individual drugs in the rest of this section. In this introductory chapter, two specific areas will be considered.

1 The choice of drugs in patients with partial epilepsy. This will be considered in three parts. The first section is concerned with the analysis of data from randomized controlled trials (RCTs) of antiepileptic drugs (AEDs) in patients with established partial epilepsy and uncontrolled seizures. The second section is a consideration of other factors which enter into drug-choice decisions. The third section is concerned with the choice of initial drugs in newly diagnosed partial epilepsy.

2 The approach to treatment of patients with established partial epilepsy with active seizures. A protocol for therapy will be described.

It will be abundantly clear from the previous sections of this book that the treatment of epilepsy varies considerably in different clinical settings. A major aspect of therapy in all settings is of course the choice of drug. Choice is not easy, and many factors influence this decision (Table 26.1). Above all, treatment should be tailored to individual patients, and the relevance of any particular factor will vary from patient to patient. People differ, for instance, in their willingness to risk side-effects or to try new therapy. Patients' preferences regarding drug choice depend on age, gender or comorbidity, comedication, drug formulation and dosing frequencies, and such factors as risks in pregnancy and a whole range of social aspects. Doctors' preferences and prescribing patterns also vary, and are dependent on such factors as prior experience, marketing pressures, the medical system within which they work, reimbursement patterns and teaching and information sources. The problem of choice is furthermore complicated by the large number of drugs, at least 20 marketed worldwide, which have proven antiepileptic action—these drugs are considered in detail in the subsequent chapters of this section—and perhaps 15 with claim to be considered as first-line therapy. There is however only limited international consensus about drug choice. There are striking differences in the use of drugs in different countries. Phenytoin, for instance, is more widely prescribed in the USA than elsewhere, carbamazepine in Northern Europe and valproate in the Francophone world. The pattern of drug usage furthermore varies widely within countries and even within the same institution. The evidence base on which to formulate drug choice is largely based on data from RCTs, and these provide a good starting point for a consideration of the factors underlying drug choice.

Choice of drug: analysing data from RCTs

Whilst it is axiomatic that treatment needs to be tailored to the needs and preferences of an individual patient, it is also true that optimal therapy requires an understanding of the therapeutic properties and range of a drug. The priorities of the patient are not subject to objective analysis, but there is now a significant body of controlled evidence available for comparing the therapeutic range and properties of many drugs. In the following subsections, the methods which have been used to evaluate the efficacy of drugs will be examined. These methods are not perfect, and their limitations as well as their benefits will be highlighted.

I will restrict myself to the methodology of the clinical assessment of partial seizures, as this is where most studies have been carried out. Patients with partial epilepsy form the bulk of those with uncontrolled epilepsy. The seizures—partial, and secondarily generalized attacks—account for approximately two-thirds of all seizures numerically. This is also the pharmaceutical industry's battle ground, for these epilepsies are the usual material of the clinical trials used for drug registration. The definitive clinical trials of almost all the new AEDs which have been used for regulatory purposes have been carried out in populations of patients with partial seizures refractory to their previous medications. I will attempt to base this review where possible on sound and objective published evidence. Also, one might have anticipated that clear guidelines for clinical practice would exist; sadly this is far from the case and this is in part a reflection of the inadequacies of the clinical trial process.

Advantages of the RCT

There can be no doubt that the clinical evaluation of the effectiveness of AEDs has been greatly improved in the past two decades. The major reason for this improvement was the widespread adoption of the RCT, first introduced into medicine in 1948 and used extensively in the field of epilepsy since the 1980s. The standard of design and documentation of AED assessment prior to this was rather poor. An analysis of all published studies of phenytoin and carbamazepine prior to 1980, for instance, showed serious deficiencies in many aspects of trial methodology [1,2]. For instance, of the 155 published studies, only 3% had a placebo comparison, less than 5% had any type of blinding and only 14% had fixed periods of observation. Basic clinical features were often not stated in the published report, for instance, with only 77% documenting seizure type, 21% aetiology or 34% seizure frequency. Standards have improved since then. This is partly because of a better scientific awareness amongst doctors, but also because of a greatly strengthened regulatory framework. Three specific regulatory measures have had the greatest impact: (a) the requirement to conduct RCTs; (b) the requirement to use good clinical practice (GCP) standards in these RCTs; and (c) the requirement to standardize documentation, sta-

Table 26.1 Factors influencing choice of treatment regimen in epilepsy. This list illustrates the sort of factors which influence drug choice. It is not comprehensive, and the importance of factors will vary from individual to individual

---

Personal patient-related factors
Age and gender
Comorbidity (physical and mental)
Social circumstances (employment, education, domestic, etc.)
Emotional circumstances
Attitude to risk of seizures
Attitude to risk of side-effects

Factors related to the epilepsy
Syndrome and seizure type
Severity and chronicity
Aetiology (less important in chronic epilepsy)

Factors related to the drug
Mechanism of action
Strength of therapeutic effects
Strength and nature of side-effects
Formulation
Drug interactions and pharmacokinetic properties
Cost

---

tistical methods and inclusion criteria. These changes were in place when the wave of new AEDs (between 1983 and 2000) were ready for phase III trials and these new drugs have been evaluated using these methods, albeit with incremental strengthening of the regulatory requirements over the two decades. At the time of writing, there have been at least 26 parallel group RCTs and 10 crossover RCTs published for the eight new AEDs introduced in the past 15 years (gabapentin, lamotrigine, levetiracetam, oxcarbazepine, tiagabine, topiramate, vigabatrin, zonisamide) [3–41]. A cooperative effort between the Standards of Reporting Trials (SORT) and the Asilomar Working Group culminated in the Consolidated Standards of Reporting Trials (CONSORT), an easy-to-follow prescription for randomized drug trial design, and a checklist for authors of critical aspects of the trial report [42,43]. Regulatory agencies such as the Food and Drug Administration (FDA) and the European Medicines Evaluations Agency (EMEA) have insisted upon the adoption of stringent research guidelines, and amongst the statistical requirements is the use of a small number only of primary (and secondary) endpoints defined prior to the initiation of the study.

Limitations of the RCT

There is no doubt that the introduction of the RCT has greatly improved the quality and reliability of drug assessment. However, the data from RCTs have limitations. The RCT is essentially a regulatory tool, and the design of studies, the result of a negotiation between the pharmaceutical industry and the regulatory authority, is aimed at demonstrating whether or not the new compound has any antiepileptic action (and whether it has a short-term lack of toxicity). What the trials do not do is provide evidence of clinical utility—this is a related but essentially different attribute, which can only be determined by experimentation outside the constraints of regulatory RCTs. The scientific rigour of the studies themselves should not blind the physician to certain fundamental issues which limit their utility. These limitations include the following.

Lack of comparative data between AEDs

In almost all the RCTs in refractory epilepsies, the test drug is compared to placebo rather than to other standard therapies. This is largely because of the FDA requirement that, to obtain licensing approval, a new drug must prove superiority, not simply equivalence, of effect over its comparator in an RCT. As a result, there is a regrettable lack of head-to-head comparisons of a test drug with either standard therapy or another test drug in add-on therapy.

Primary efficacy measures of limited clinical value

The primary efficacy variable in most adjunctive-therapy RCTs is either: (a) the '50% responder rate', defined as the number of patients whose seizure frequency falls by 50% or more in the trial compared to baseline period; or (b) the per cent reduction in the number of seizures in the trial period compared to a prospectively controlled baseline. These two endpoints are not necessarily equivalent. These measures have been commonly criticized for having little relevance to patients. A 50% reduction in seizure frequency for most patients with severe epilepsy is an unsatisfactory endpoint, as demonstrated in a recent study [44] in which 50% seizure reductions produced minimal improvements in quality-of-life measures. More impressive would be the complete cessation of seizures, but this is seldom reported (or obtained) in studies. However, it should also be remembered that the 50% seizure-reduction rates reported in RCTs were achieved in patients with severe chronic epilepsy, and better results would be expected in less refractory cases. Furthermore, those drugs which have produced good 50% responder rates in RCTs have also turned out to be useful AEDs in routine clinical practice. Attempts to take a more holistic view of quality-of-life issues have resulted in the introduction of a number of secondary measures such as psychometric and quality-of-life scales. These, however, are essentially highly artificial in the context of a few weeks of clinical trial—what aspect of quality-of-life change can be measured meaningfully over such a short time?—and have proved of little value in assessing clinical utility.

The short duration of trials

Almost all of the adjunctive therapy regulatory trials are short term with treatment periods typically of 8–16 weeks. This is too short a time in the life of a patient with epilepsy to be meaningful particularly where seizures fluctuate due to environmental and emotional factors. High placebo response rates are also seen in many studies, presumably partly due to the statistical phenomenon of regression to the mean which is more prominent in short-term studies.

The inclusion of selected populations

Almost all the studies are conducted in adult patients with refractory partial epilepsy. Many are 'professional' trialists who have participated in previous studies. Such patients are highly unrepresentative of the generality of the epilepsy populations. Furthermore, almost all trials exclude key groups such as women of childbearing potential, the elderly, those with learning difficulty, children, pregnancy, patients with unquantifiable or unclassifiable seizures, those with progressive neurological disorders and those with concurrent illness. These patients make up perhaps more than 80% of patients with epilepsy. The RCTs also ignore other aspects of importance in clinical management, such as seizure severity or patient preference. The bias that this selectivity might cause has not been quantitated.

The inclusion of only partial seizures

The trials in refractory partial epilepsy usually exclude other types of seizures or epilepsy. There are many examples of drugs that have greater effects in generalized rather than partial epilepsy, for instance lamotrigine or valproate, yet these effects have often not been noticed nor subjected to formal evaluation for many years after the studies in partial epilepsy. A wider set of inclusion criteria would improve this unsatisfactory situation.

Fixed dosage

In RCTs, the dose of drugs is usually fixed. Surprisingly often, the dose chosen in the trials turns out not to be the dose most often used in clinical practice. Too high a dose, for instance, was used in trials of topiramate and vigabatrin, and too low a dose in those of gabapentin, lamotrigine and valproate. RCTs therefore have been a poor guide to dosage in routine practice, and indeed can be thoroughly misleading in this regard.

The artificiality of the clinical setting

The inclusion and exclusion criteria, the titration regimes and escape criteria and the logistics of follow-up result in a highly artificial clinical setting. Alternative 'pragmatic' trial designs would be possible, in which these aspects are not so rigidly controlled, but these have not found favour within the regulatory set-up. Pragmatic trials in the post-licensing phase, though, are urgently needed as only they can provide information for routine prescribing.

The recording of side-effects

The side-effects are usually recorded or coded according to predetermined dictionaries or checklists. These are interpreted differently by different investigators and are difficult to evaluate — the widely used dictionary term 'abnormal thinking', for instance, covers a variety of cognitive effects. Side-effects not listed in checklists may be overlooked, the visual field defects due to vigabatrin being an example. Rare side-effects also will be missed altogether. Felbamate, for instance, was grossly overmarketed as a safe drug until drug-induced aplastic anaemia and hepatic failure resulted in its withdrawal from use.

These considerations limit the value of RCTs. Furthermore, the utility of a drug in routine clinical practice depends on factors not considered in RCTs, examples being cost, patient preference, acceptability to patients and doctors, quality of life, the structure of health-care system and reimbursement policy. Finally, the difficulty in translating the findings of RCTs to routine practice have been exacerbated by the intense marketing of drugs, particularly in the immediate postregistration period. A period of post-licensing assessment in more open clinical settings would be very helpful to place a drug in its appropriate context. It is likely that regulatory authorities will attempt to introduce some such system, and this may improve clinical evaluation.

The primary efficacy endpoints in RCTs

The RCTs of AEDs, used in adjunctive therapy, have two conventional primary endpoints: (a) a comparison of seizure frequency reductions (mean or median); and (b) a comparison of responder rates. In monotherapy studies, survival analyses are increasingly used, as a third conventional measure. This insistence on one or two primary endpoints, predetermined before the initiation of the study, has been one of the fundamental improvements in trial design resulting from the more stringent regulatory environment. These endpoints are now used for licensing decisions, and are thus of extreme importance.

Seizure frequency reduction

Seizure counts are the most common primary outcome measure accepted by regulatory authorities, and are the most sensitive measure for assessing drug efficacy. The number of seizures is typically expressed as a mean or median seizure frequency (for normally and non-normally distributed data, respectively). The mean seizure reduction is a comparison of the number of seizures during experimental drug treatment vs. the number of seizures during a prospectively acquired baseline. Seizure frequency provides continuous data, and the mean with standard deviation, or median with quartiles can be displayed as a histogram or box plot. Statistical analysis of mean seizure frequency data can be conducted in the context of a generalized linear model (ANOVA, ANCOVA) or mixed model. Analysis of seizure frequencies can be complicated by the skewed distribution of seizure numbers. This is a particular problem in new patients who may have no seizures or very low seizure counts on therapy, or in severe chronic patients who may at times have very frequent seizures. Where data is not normally distributed, logarithmic transformation is appropriate and statistically valid. However, results presenting log transformed data can be difficult for non-statisticians to comprehend, and may not give clinicians a clear idea of the clinical magnitude of any drug effect. The results from the RCTs of levetiracetam, the most recently introduced AED, can be used as an example of the ways in which data can be presented. In Table 26.2, a comparison between logarithmically transformed and raw data in one levetiracetam clinical trial is shown. The logarithmic data (backtransformed mean) is more appropriate and robust, but the clinical relevance of the figures is far less comprehensible. The simple presentation of the raw seizure reduction data is clearer (see also Fig. 26.1), but open to statistical misinterpretation.

Seizure frequency remains the traditional primary measure for evaluating AED efficacy, and with good reason because this is a direct measure of the primary biological target action of AEDs. Focusing on seizure frequency as the sole measure of AED effect can be criticized, however, for ignoring other clinically relevant information, such as seizure severity, type, duration and expression pattern.

Table 26.2 Seizure count data for levetiracetam (LEV) in a multicentre trial [34]

	Baseline period			Treatment period		
	Placebo	LEV 1000 mg	LEV 2000 mg	Placebo	LEV 1000 mg	LEV 2000 mg
Mean	5.4	5.5	6.9	5.3	5.1	5.1
Backtransformed mean	3.2	3.4	3.8	3.1	2.6	2.7
Least-squares mean[a]	–	–	–	3.3	2.6	2.5
Median (quartile)	2.5 (1.3–4.9)	2.8 (1.8–4.4)	2.6 (1.5–6.3)	2.6 (1.3–5.2)	2.0 (1.2–4.1)	1.9 (0.9–5.6)

[a] Least-squares mean: adjusted mean over baseline obtained after analysis of covariance

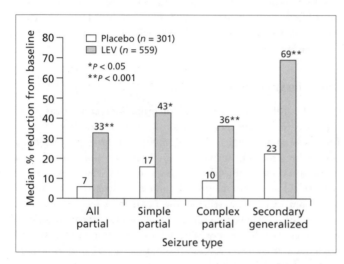

Fig. 26.1 Display of raw seizure data from placebo-controlled, adjunctive-therapy RCTs. Example from the three RCTs of levetiracetam (LEV) showing seizure reduction for different seizure types compared to placebo. From [94].

Furthermore, the measurement of short-term seizure frequency gives no indication of any antiepileptic (as opposed to antiseizure) properties of a drug.

Responder rates

The second classical measure of the efficacy of an AED is the evaluation of responder rates. The most commonly used index defines responders as those who achieve a 50% or greater reduction in seizure frequency. A 50% reduction is considered by the regulatory authorities to be the minimum reduction which has clinical value.

The results are clinically relevant, and easily understood and displayed (see Fig. 26.2 for the results from the clinical trials of levetiracetam). Statistical analysis is performed by a non-parametric test on a 2×2 table or logistic regression models, and statistical comparisons are usually made using chi-square statistics. The main statistical criticism of the 50% responder rate measure is that the division of data into a single (arbitrary) threshold results in an extreme of data reduction and is associated with a considerable loss of sensitivity. The use of this method may therefore miss important dif-

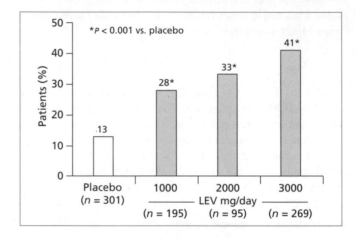

Fig. 26.2 Display of raw responder rate data from placebo-controlled, adjunctive-therapy RCTs. Example from the three RCTs of levetiracetam (LEV) showing 50% responder rate at different doses. From [94].

ferences between treatments that occur on either side of this threshold. It furthermore is not easy to extrapolate results to other groups of patients with lower seizure frequencies [45]. Theoretically, responder rates at different dosage could also be compared, but because of the inherent lack of power of the method, the numbers of patients in almost all (if not all) conventional RCTs, and the short duration of the RCTs, are insufficient to allow statistical differences to be demonstrated. Power could have been increased by increasing the numbers of patients, but as the responder rate was usually not the primary statistical endpoint required by the regulatory authority, this was seldom thought necessary.

One method of reducing data loss and increasing statistical sensitivity is to divide the data into response-rate bands, such as 0–25%, 26–50%, 51–75% and 76–100% reductions in seizure frequency. The use of multiple bands increases the information yield and produces results that are more likely to render visible the magnitude of an AED effect. Analysis is performed by a 2×C table (where C is the number of response categories) or by logistic regression or proportional odds models, and chi-square testing is used to test significance. The results can be displayed as bar charts (Fig. 26.3 shows, for instance, the results from the levetiracetam RCTs).

One frequently raised criticism of 50% responder rate calculations is that a 50% reduction of seizures is not important to patients,

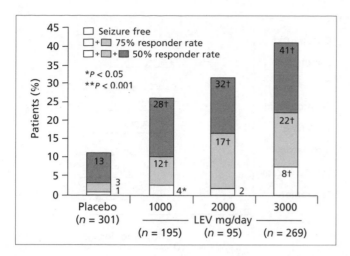

Fig. 26.3 Display of raw responder rate data from placebo-controlled, adjunctive-therapy RCTs. Example from the three RCTs of levetiracetam (LEV) showing 50%, 75% and 100% responder rates at different doses. From [93].

and that seizure freedom is a much more meaningful goal. Indeed, a recent study showed that there were few quality-of-life improvements in patients achieving 50% reductions [44]. However, as discussed above, drugs which had produced high 50% responder rates in RCTs have turned out to be useful AEDs in routine clinical practice, and to be associated with appreciable seizure freedom rates when used in populations of patients with less severe epilepsy.

Survival analyses and time to an event

Time-to-an-event analyses compare the time it takes for an event to occur on the trial drug compared to placebo or another drug. Typically, the event monitored is the first, or second, seizure recurrence. These analyses are used mainly in studies of monotherapy in newly diagnosed patients (e.g. [46]). Prolonged follow-up and precise dating of seizures are required. This method provides a solution to the problem of non-normally distributed and low seizure counts. The data are survival-type data, summarized as a percentage and displayed as per cent recurrence-free curves. The analysis is by log-rank testing or Cox proportional hazards regression modelling, and the significance testing is by methods such as that of Mantel–Cox, Breslow, Tarone–Ware; for Cox regression, Wald, score and likelihood ratio tests. Time-to-event analyses can also be used to analyse the time to withdrawal due to lack of efficacy or adverse events [47].

Survival analyses are statistically valid and robust, easily understood by clinicians, can be clearly displayed and have obvious clinical relevance. Sensitivity increases with the number of patients who reach the endpoint, and so time to first recurrence is a more sensitive outcome measure than is time to second recurrence [48]. This may be a disadvantage, however, in that information of events occurring after the first (or nth) recurrence is ignored, and the extent of a drug effect may therefore be obscured. The major disadvantage of such studies is the long duration required in newly diagnosed patients because of the mildness of their epilepsy. To overcome the problem of selection of what is the most appropriate recurrent event, statisticians are now developing survival analysis methods that could take several recurrent time points into consideration (e.g. in monotherapy studies of topiramate).

A variation of this method has been used in patients undergoing presurgical evaluation. Here conventional drugs are abruptly stopped or significantly reduced, and substituted by the trial drug or placebo (or 'active placebo', a low and suboptimum dose of a proven AED). These studies are very short term, lasting sometimes hours or days, and are so artificial as to render them meaningless for clinical purposes. The results can be obscured by the occurrence of withdrawal or rebound seizures and drug withdrawal effects, and the trials furthermore carry a level of risk which in many settings renders them ethically unacceptable.

Theoretically, a useful outcome measure would be the time until a certain period of seizure remission has been achieved. This is a standard measure in epidemiological and observational open studies of epilepsy. This would be a gold standard measure of obvious clinical relevance, but the long time required to observe treatment differences would be impractical in most RCTs, and therefore this endpoint has not been frequently used.

The use of RCT data to compare AEDs

Meta-analysis

In almost all RCTs of add-on AED therapy, the test drug has been compared with a placebo and not with an alternative medication. This is largely because of the regulatory requirement to show a difference in efficacy rather than equivalence. From the clinical (in contrast to the regulatory) perspective, however, this is a serious disadvantage. What the clinician requires is information about the relative benefits of individual drugs, in order to prescribe rationally. To meet this need, the methodology known as meta-analysis has been utilized. When applied to AEDs, meta-analyses allow a comparison of data on efficacy (and tolerability) of different AEDs from the independent add-on trials in which the same drugs were compared to placebo.

The first meta-analysis in medicine was published in 1977. Initially ignored, this method has became popular in the past decade, partly stimulated by the medicopolitical desire for evidence-based medicine and by the championship of the Cochrane Collaboration, with the aim of developing systematic reviews for all clinically relevant information [49]. The first meta-analysis of AEDs was carried out by Professor Chadwick and colleagues from Liverpool, and has become justly influential [50].

The apparent clinical utility of meta-analysis should not however detract from the fact that meta-analyses share (and perhaps magnify) the limitations of the RCT (listed above). Furthermore, they have additional problems and raise additional statistical concerns. The validity of any meta-analysis depends on the similarity (homogeneity) in the clinical trial design and patient populations of all the RCTs included in the analysis. The AED meta-analysis discussed below included all parallel group add-on trials (and crossover trials where the first period could be treated as a parallel trial) of partial epilepsy in which the treatment phase was at least 8 weeks long. The trial designs, however, and populations studied were not exactly equivalent. The criteria for entry to the study varied in relation to age, duration of epilepsy, permissible comedication and importantly the minimum number of baseline seizures (or the minimum baseline weekly frequency). The duration of the baseline period also varied between trials. The introduction of new AEDs over time also potentially reduced and changed the patient population eligible for selection into later studies. These variations render the analysis vulnerable to the charge of bias and lack of validity, but the extent to which these features have influenced the results in the AED studies has not yet been statistically scrutinized. In other therapeutic areas, these effects have been shown to be potentially significant. LeLorier *et al.*, for example, demonstrated the potential failure of meta-analyses to produce the same results as large randomized clinical trials [51]. They suggest that heterogeneities among trials limit the power of direct comparisons. Even small differences in trial parameters, such as inclusion and exclusion criteria, baseline requirements, drug doses, and number of coadministered drugs, can alter markedly trial outcome.

In other areas of medicine, bias has been introduced by the tendency of a meta-analysis to overlook negative trials because they are less likely to be published or to come to the attention of the investigators. Whether this bias exists in the epilepsy meta-analyses is unclear, but in the absence of a requirement to publish all epilepsy studies, one suspects that this bias occurs. The AED meta-analysis has also been criticized for using the 'odds ratio' as a measure of comparison between trials, and the validity of this has been the subject of statistical debate [51]. The odds ratio is attractive, because it can be used to compare trials with wide variations in numbers of events, but because it is not an absolute measure, its clinical relevance is difficult to evaluate.

For all these reasons, meta-analysis—although the best systematic comparison of drug trial results yet available—is no substitute for large-scale RCTs in which test drugs are compared head to head with each other (and not with placebo). These would be the gold-standard methods of analysis, but as yet few such studies have been published.

Meta-analysis of AED efficacy and tolerability

In the first AED meta-analysis, Chadwick and colleagues compared 13 published and 15 unpublished randomized clinical trials in which one of six new AEDs was tested against placebo as add-on treatment in patients with refractory partial epilepsy, allowing the efficacy and tolerability of these drugs to be compared for the first time [50]. Since then, new RCTs of these and also newer drugs have been published. In this chapter, the updated results from 36 RCTs will be discussed and the various methods of analysis described [3,6,8,9,11,15–17,19,21–24,31,35,36,38,40,41,49,52–54].

Odds ratios

Figure 26.4 shows the results of the meta-analysis using the methods published initially by Chadwick and colleagues, updated with data from newer trials. The meta-analysis plots the mean odds ratio with their 95% confidence intervals. In this analysis, the odds ratio is defined as the probability of a patient being a $\geq 50\%$ responder in the treated group divided by the probability of being a $\geq 50\%$ responder in the placebo group. An odds ratio of 1 (vertical line) indicates that there is an equal probability of being a $\geq 50\%$ responder with the test AED or with placebo. An odds ratio greater than 1 indicates that a patient is more likely to be a responder in the active

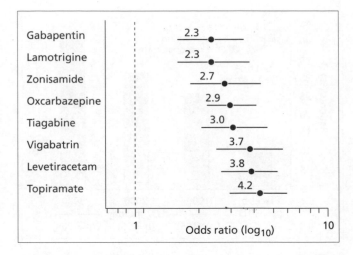

Fig. 26.4 Odds ratios for 50% responder rates from placebo-controlled, adjunctive-therapy RCTs of eight recently introduced AEDs. This figure shows the summary odds ratios (overall odds ratio and 95% confidence intervals) of the RCTs of eight newly introduced AEDs. Note that the horizontal scale is logarithmic and that there are marked differences between the mean odds ratios. However, as the confidence intervals overlap, there is no statistical difference. Note also that, as the confidence intervals are all to the right of the vertical line, all drugs are significantly more efficacious than placebo. Adapted from [50], with data added from studies of newer drugs—see text.

treatment group than in the placebo group. The more effective is the drug, the larger is the odds ratio and the farther the odds ratio is to the right in Fig. 26.4 (note too that the odds ratios are plotted on a logarithmic scale). As Fig. 26.4 shows, all drugs are statistically superior to placebo (i.e. the means and 95% confidence intervals are all greater than 1). Also, there are striking (nearly two-fold) differences between the mean odds ratios for different drugs, suggesting differences in efficacy but as the confidence intervals are wide and overlap, these differences are not statistically significant.

One criticism of this method of display is that drugs are being compared at the dosages used in the clinical trials, and that higher doses of the seemingly less effective drugs might produce better odds ratios. Analysis at different doses does certainly produce different mean values, and this effect is most clearly shown for topiramate and levetiracetam.

The rate of premature withdrawal from the RCT is a commonly used measure of tolerability in AED trials. Like all surrogate measures, this measure has limitations and for instance can be unduly influenced by transient initial side-effects, and dose escalation regimens. Nevertheless, it is a useful measure of overall tolerability and it is susceptible to meta-analysis using the same statistical treatment as for efficacy comparisons. Figure 26.5 illustrates the results of a meta-analysis of withdrawal rates of eight AEDs [50,55]. The mean odds ratios show a nearly four-fold difference in tolerability between AEDs (a greater difference than that in the efficacy analysis). Furthermore, the 95% confidence limits for three drugs (lamotrigine, gabapentin and levetiracetam) overlap the placebo response, indicating no significant difference in withdrawal rate between placebo and active therapy.

A good way of conveying the overall performance of drugs in RCTs is to display the odds ratio for efficacy and tolerability data on

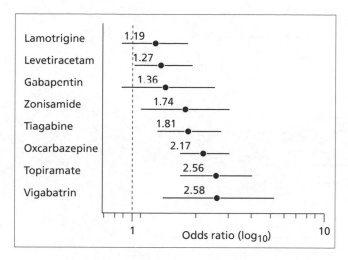

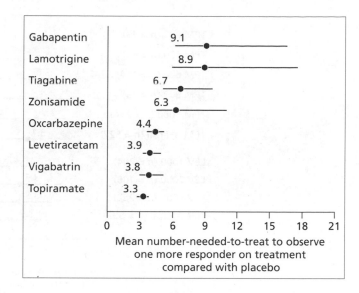

Fig. 26.5 Odds ratios for rates of premature withdrawal from published placebo-controlled, adjunctive-therapy RCTs of eight recently introduced AEDs. This figure shows the summary odds ratios (overall odds ratio and 95% confidence intervals) of the RCTs of eight newly introduced AEDs. Note that the horizontal scale is logarithmic and that there are marked differences between the mean odds ratios. However, as the confidence intervals overlap, there is no statistical difference. Adapted from [50,55,93].

Fig. 26.7 The mean 'number-needed-to-treat' analysis of data from the published placebo-controlled, adjunctive-therapy RCTs of eight recently introduced AEDs. See text for interpretation. From [60].

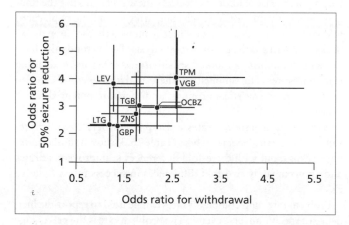

Fig. 26.6 A comparison of the odds ratio, with 95% confidence limits, for efficacy (responder rates) and tolerability (withdrawal rates) from published placebo-controlled, adjunctive-therapy RCTs of eight recently introduced AEDs. This is a useful way of graphically demonstrating the overall effectiveness of new AEDs based on placebo-controlled, adjunctive-therapy RCTs. Drugs in the upper left quadrant are relatively efficacious and well tolerated; drugs in the lower right quadrant are relatively inefficacious and poorly tolerated. From [93].

the same graph, as shown in Fig. 26.6. This is a novel method for summarizing efficacy and tolerability data and has the virtues of being easy to understand, clinically meaningful and simple to display. The closer a drug is to the top left-hand corner, the better the drug, since the odds ratio for seizure reduction is high and the odds ratio for withdrawal is low. This graph shows that there is a strong tendency for higher efficacy to be correlated with lower tolerability (levetiracetam is an exception, demonstrating relatively high mean efficacy and relatively low mean withdrawal rates).

Number-needed-to-treat (NNT) analysis

The NNT analysis is another method which can be used to compare data from RCTs. It was a statistic first introduced in the analysis of single trials [56] and then more recently applied to meta-analysis (Fig. 26.7; [57]). It has a number of advantages. It is one way of avoiding the statistical blunting introduced by varying placebo rates in individual trials and also is an easily understood and clinically relevant measure. The method provides an estimate of the number of patients needed to be treated by a drug in order to achieve one more responder than was achieved by placebo. The NNT is defined as the reciprocal of the absolute risk reduction and can range from 1 (or −1) to infinity (or −infinity). Positive numbers indicate the number of patients needed to treat for a beneficial outcome, while negative numbers indicate the number needed to treat for a negative outcome [57]. The sensitivity of this method is apparent from reinterpretations of a meta-analysis of eight AEDs in Fig. 26.7 [58–60]. In RCTs, three to four patients were treated before finding one responder more than with placebo when using vigabatrin, topiramate, levetiracetam or oxcarbazepine, compared with six to nine patients with gabapentin, lamotrigine, zonisamide or tiagabine. At least for vigabatrin, topiramate, levetiracetam, this difference is statistically significant, and this statistical difference was not seen in the odds ratio analysis method, using exactly the same dataset. The NNT analysis can also be used to compare drug dosages. As an example, an analysis for different doses of levetiracetam and topiramate are shown in Fig. 26.8, which suggests for instance that 2000–3000 mg/day of levetiracetam is approximately as efficacious as 400–600 mg/day of topiramate. It should be noted, however, that the apparently poor efficacy of lower doses of topiramate as shown in Fig. 26.8 are based on the results of a single small study, and a recent RCT re-evaluating low-dose adjunctive therapy topiramate in a more sizeable population of patients showed that responder rates at topiramate 200 mg/day were actually comparable to those previously reported at dosages of 400 mg/day or higher. This observation

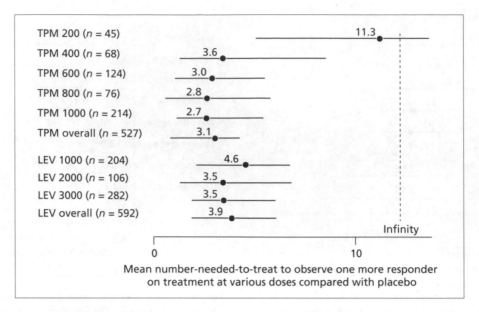

TPM 200 (*n* = 45) — 11.3
TPM 400 (*n* = 68) — 3.6
TPM 600 (*n* = 124) — 3.0
TPM 800 (*n* = 76) — 2.8
TPM 1000 (*n* = 214) — 2.7
TPM overall (*n* = 527) — 3.1

LEV 1000 (*n* = 204) — 4.6
LEV 2000 (*n* = 106) — 3.5
LEV 3000 (*n* = 282) — 3.5
LEV overall (*n* = 592) — 3.9

Infinity

0   10

Mean number-needed-to-treat to observe one more responder
on treatment at various doses compared with placebo

Fig. 26.8 The mean 'number-needed-to-treat' analysis of data at different doses: example from placebo-controlled, adjunctive-therapy RCTs of levetiracetam (LEV) and topiramate (TPM). From [59].

reinforces the concept that meta-analysis cannot be a substitute for high-quality RCTs [61].

It is worth noting that NNT calculations are simply an alternative way of presenting meta-analysis data, using the same dataset as for the more conventional odds ratio calculations. Moreover, a cautious approach should be taken to the intepretation of NNT statistical methods, especially as applied to meta-analysis [57]. Those evaluating NNT data should be aware that the results are estimates, subject to statistical variability and that the statistical properties are not classic. Potential problems in the statistical method are introduced by an awkward distribution of data, the possibly infinite population mean and variance, and the way in which confidence intervals are treated. The extrapolation of data between patients with different baseline risks, and the translation of clinical trial results to individual patients relies on the assumption of a constant risk reduction. It has been advised that, when combining NNT data from meta-analyses, to first combine absolute risk reduction data. The combined NNT can be calculated as the inverse of the combined absolute risk reduction, and 95% confidence intervals constructed by inverting and exchanging the limits of a 95% confidence interval for the absolute risk reduction.

Success rates, improvement rates, problem rates, complaint rates and summary complaint scores

Meta-analysis requires a sophisticated statistical treatment which, it can be argued, reduces clarity. In response to this concern, a variety of more simple methods have been employed to compare the results from individual RCTs. These include the following measures: success rates, improvement rates, problem rates, complaint rates and summary complaint scores, which attempt to remove the effects of varying placebo rates in different clinical trials by simple arithmetical means [45]. The success rate is the proportion of responders on treatment divided by the proportion of responders on placebo. The improvement rate is the success rate on the test drug

minus the success rate with placebo. These methods thus use simple calculations to remove the placebo effect in each trial and thus provide a pure measure of drug effect. As these measures use the findings from individual RCTs (each comparing a test drug to placebo) to compare active drugs, they suffer from exactly the same drawbacks and biases as the use of meta-analysis. The methods also have the same limitation (a blunted sensitivity) as other methods using responder rates. The simplicity of these analytical method can also be criticized on statistical grounds, and there are potential major biases.

A comparison of success rates and improvement rates with the results of the classical meta-analysis (Table 26.3) show a similar ranking of drugs, but with three-fold differences in improvement rates and approximately two-fold differences in success ratios (relative risk).

Problem rates and complaint rates can be used to report the incidence of specific adverse events. The problem rate is the percentage of patients that report an adverse event. The complaint rate for each adverse event is the problem rate reported during drug treatment minus the problem rate from patients receiving placebo. The summary complaint score is the sum of the complaint rates for each adverse events reported for an AED. Unfortunately, due to disparate definitions and reporting methods used to describe adverse events, data between trials often cannot be compared in any statistically valid way. These measures provide a simple but unfortunately statistically dubious format that allows clinicians and patients to make risk–benefit analysis decisions about potential treatment options.

Open extension phase of RCTs—retention rates and sustained efficacy measures

The maintenance treatment periods of all adjunctive-therapy RCTs reviewed here were between 4 and 12 weeks. This is of course too short a period to provide useful data on many aspects of clinical utility. In most studies, patients are then usually offered entry into an

Table 26.3 Improvement rates and success rates. Adapted from [45] — see text for definitions and interpretation

AED	Improvement rate (%) and 95% confidence interval	Success rate and 95% confidence interval
Gabapentin	11 (6; 16)	2.2 (1.5; 3.3)
Lamotrigine	11 (6; 17)	2.2 (1.4; 3.4)
Levetiracetam	26 (21; 31)	3.7 (2.6; 5.4)
Oxcarbazepine	23 (17; 29)	2.4 (1.8; 3.1)
Tiagabine	15 (10; 20)	3.4 (2.1; 5.6)
Topiramate	32 (26; 39)	3.8 (2.6; 5.6)
Vigabatrin	27 (19; 34)	2.9 (2.0; 4.2)
Zonisamide	16 (9; 23)	2.5 (1.6; 3.7)

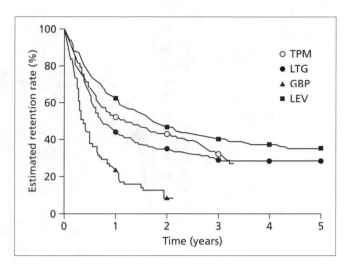

Fig. 26.9 Long-term retention rates on four new AEDs. The data are from two published studies of the four drugs. For interpretation, see text. From [48,95].

open extension phase during which the drug is given in an unblinded non-randomized fashion. Treatment in this phase approximates more to conventional practice, with dose changes allowed both of the test drug and concomitant medication. This phase has no predefined endpoints and there is no placebo control. The open extension phase is also less well audited than the blinded phase. For all these reasons, the findings are not taken into consideration by the regulatory agencies in their assessment of drug efficacy.

The open extension phase is subject to marked biases. Most important is the bias caused by the fact that patients are more likely to opt for continuing treatment if they had already responded in the RCT. There are also potential biases due to uncontrolled influences such as the changing treatment regimens over time and, not least in some centres, premature termination of therapy so that the individual can enter another clinical trial. Because of these biases, the data are more useful for assessing longer-term safety than efficacy. Two efficacy measures however have been derived from the open extension phase, retention rates and rates of sustained efficacy.

The retention rate of a test drug is defined as the percentage of patients continuing to take the drug at the end of a specified period. It is thus a summary statistic which reflects both drug efficacy and toxicity. It is an endpoint with clinical relevance, since it is a measure of the likelihood that a patient will continue and therefore potentially benefit from a given treatment. It is also an easily comprehended measure which mirrors normal practice to some extent, and this is its real value. The retention rate, however, often correlates poorly with effectiveness. Some patients prefer to continue therapy even if seizure frequency is not greatly altered, because of a reduction in seizure severity or a positive tolerability profile. Conversely, some patients will withdraw therapy even if there is a clear evidence of effectiveness because of perceived worsening in seizure severity or side-effects. Retention rates can be compared using Kaplan–Meier survival curves. The effects of different factors on retention rates can be examined using Cox regression analysis. The retention rates seen in clinical trials probably underestimate the rates in clinical practice because patients more readily withdraw from trials than from clinical treatment regimens, and because patients entering clinical trials are likely to have more severe epilepsy. A comparison of published retention rates for four drugs is shown in Fig. 26.9. The data shown in this figure should be interpreted cautiously, because allocation of patients to the various drugs was not randomized (hence, the populations treated with each drug may not be comparable) and treatment policies were likely to differ across centres.

The sustained efficacy rate is defined as the proportion of patients on a drug in whom efficacy is maintained over a specified period of time (e.g. patients who do not develop pharmacological tolerance). As such, it is a measure of the extent to which the effects of a drug wear off over time, although other factors, including the natural history of the seizure disorder and the influence of external factors can also influence apparent efficacy over time. As an example, Fig. 26.10 shows the data from the open extension phases of the RCTs of levetiracetam. The median per cent change in seizure frequency is compared to baseline. Each line shows the median per cent change in seizure frequency (compared to baseline) for patient groups followed for different lengths of time. This sort of analysis must be considered as an approximation only, as the data are subject to major potential bias. In particular, patients whose seizure rates worsen will tend to withdraw therapy and thus not be represented (each line represents only those patients continuing therapy), and there are only small numbers of patients in groups monitored for long periods of time. However, the data does provide limited evidence that there is no marked pharmacological tolerance of this drug.

Other drug-related factors which influence AED choice

There are other factors which usually are not adequately considered in RCTs but which are also of great importance in dictating drug choice. These can be conveniently divided into three categories: patient-related factors, disease-related factors and drug-related factors. Examples of each are listed in Table 26.1. Patient-related and epilepsy-related factors are discussed in previous sections and will not be described further here. The RCTs measure short-term efficacy and tolerability, but overlook various other drug-related effects. In this section, the most important of these will be

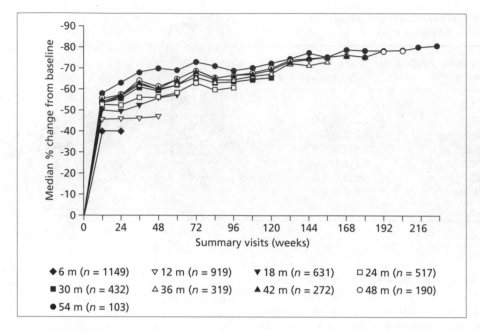

Fig. 26.10 Sustained efficacy rates. Example from the long-term extension phase that followed the RCTs of levetiracetam. Each line represents the mean percentage seizure frequency of populations of patients followed for different lengths of time (all patients in the long-term extension phase of the RCTs of levetiracetam). Note that the seizure frequency reductions are maintained over time and broadly similar whatever the period of follow-up. Although the data is uncontrolled, the fact that similar levels of responsiveness are recorded in patients followed for different periods of time suggests that tolerance to the effect of the drug does not develop.

described. A good review of how these factors can be considered from the risk–benefit perspective is provided by Perucca and colleagues [62].

The severe, irreversible and longer-term side-effects of AEDs

The side-effect profile reported in most clinical trials is largely confined to the common dose-related side-effects, many of which are transient and reversible. These side-effects are usually referable to the gastrointestinal tract (nausea, gastric disturbances) or central nervous system (drowsiness, behavioural or cognitive effects, ataxia, headache, etc.), and are usually mild, often transient and reversible. These largely determine the 'tolerability' reported in AED trials (see above).

Other side-effects also occur, however, which may not be recorded in short-term clinical trials, but which are in many ways more important. These are both the idiosyncratic and the longer-term effects often recorded only after prolonged periods of chronic therapy. These effects are often potentially serious. How to account for these risks in choosing a drug can be a difficult decision for the physician and patient.

The idiosyncratic effects are frequently life threatening. Severe haematological reactions can occur with many drugs (e.g. acetazolamide, carbamazepine, felbamate, phenytoin, lamotrigine, zonisamide) but these are usually rare. For carbamazepine, for instance, estimates of risk are about 1 : 200 000 for aplastic anaemia, 1 : 700 000 for agranulocytosis and 1 : 450 000 for death associated with these events [63]. Among major AEDs, felbamate is the only agent with a risk of bone marrow suppression high enough to limit

by regulation its clinical use. The incidence of aplastic anaemia with felbamate is probably about 1 : 4800–1 : 37 000 [64]. A number of AEDs can also cause fatal hepatotoxicity (e.g. acetazolamide, felbamate, phenytoin, carbamazepine, phenobarbital, primidone, valproate, lamotrigine and possibly topiramate). The drugs most commonly implicated are valproic acid and felbamate. At least 132 patients have died of valproate-induced liver failure and/or pancreatitis, the highest risk (1 : 600): being in children under 2 years of age with complex neurological disorders who are receiving AED polytherapy [65,66]. In older patients the incidence is about 1 : 37 000 for monotherapy and 1 : 12 000 for polytherapy, and fatalities beyond 20 years of age are rare. The incidence of fatal liver toxicity with felbamate is 1 : 26 000–1 : 34 000 [63]. The mortality rates of drug-induced hepatotoxicity are 10–38% with phenytoin and about 25% for carbamazepine [67].

The anticonvulsant hypersensitivity syndrome is a more common and potentially fatal reaction to arene oxide producing anticonvulsants such as phenytoin, carbamazepine and phenobarbital [68,69]. It occurs in 1 out of 1000–10 000 exposures and its main manifestations include fever, rash and lymphadenopathy accompanied by multiorgan system abnormalities. Cross reactivity between drugs is as high as 70%. The reaction is probably genetically determined and siblings of affected patients are at increased risk.

Stevens–Johnson syndrome and Lyell's syndrome are the main serious cutaneous reactions to AEDs. Lamotrigine, phenytoin, carbamazepine and barbiturates are most commonly involved. For Stevens–Johnson syndrome, the highest incidence (1 : 50 to 1 : 300), is observed in association with the use of lamotrigine in paediatric patients, particularly when a high starting dosage is used or the child is comedicated with valproate. In adults, the incidence of lamotrigine-induced Stevens–Johnson syndrome is in the order of 1 : 1000 [67,70]. Many other organs and systems can be affected by serious hypersensitivity reactions, but widespread organ involvement is rare.

Some life-threatening reactions are not mediated by hypersensitivity. These include neonatal haemorrhage in the offspring of mothers treated with certain AEDs during pregnancy [71], severe bradyarrhythmias after intravenous phenytoin [72], aspiration pneumonia with nitrazepam treatment in young children [73], and respiratory arrest following high-dose intravenous benzodiazepines [67].

Severe but not directly life-threatening side-effects due to chronic AED therapy are common. These vary from drug to drug, and are discussed in more detail in the individual drug chapters which follow in this section. These effects include cosmetic disorders with phenytoin (e.g. hirsutism, gum hyperplasia), shoulder–hand syndrome with barbiturates, various metabolic effects with phenytoin, weight gain with valproate and vigabatrin, nephrolithiasis with topiramate, visual field defects with vigabatrin, acute glaucoma with topiramate, cerebellar degeneration with phenytoin, and endocrine disturbances with many AEDs. These side-effects influence individual drug choice, often in a complex manner. An example is the use of topiramate, which tends to cause weight loss and may be relatively contraindicated in a thin, anorexic patient, while the reverse is true for valproic acid. Disturbances of the mental state, affective disorders and psychosis are also frequently seen with many drugs, although largely missed in the clinical trials.

It has been suggested that some of the newer AEDs are better tolerated than older agents, but this claim should be regarded cautiously because in many comparative studies the choice of titration schedules or dosing regimens were biased in favour of the innovative product [74]. Clinical exposure to the newer drugs is still relatively limited and experience shows that it may take many years for important adverse effects to be discovered (Table 26.4).

Teratogenicity

This topic is described in more detail in Chapter 23. Overall, the risk of major birth defects among babies born to drug-treated epileptic women is about 6–8% compared to 2–4% in the general population, and the difference is due in large measure to AED therapy. Minor anomalies such as hypertelorism, epicanthal folds and hy-

poplasia of distal digital phalangia also occur more frequently in children of mothers with epilepsy, although the incidence varies markedly between studies. Major effects are less common but include congenital heart defects, skeletal anomalies, gastrointestinal tract abnormalities, renal and urinary tract abnormalities, spina bifida, developmental abnormalities of the brain and possibly intellectual delay and behavioural disturbances. None of the major older anticonvulsants (phenytoin, carbamazepine, valproate and phenobarbital) is free from teratogenic potential, although recent evidence suggest the overall risks are generally greatest with valproate (e.g. for intellectual delay and behavioural disturbances in the offspring). Facial clefts and congenital heart defects are somewhat more common with phenytoin and barbiturates, whereas neural tube defects such as spina bifida are more common with valproic acid (2–3% risk) and carbamazepine (0.5–1% risk). It is likely that the incidence of fetal malformations increases with increasing dosages, number of drugs and, at least for valproic acid, increasing peak serum drug concentrations [75–78]. Although several of the newer AEDs have little or no teratogenic potential in animal models, the predictive value of these studies with respect to human safety is uncertain. There is currently insufficient clinical data for any of the AEDs introduced in the past 15 years to make clear statements about their safety in pregnancy [72,76].

Seizure-inducing effects of AEDs

Not often mentioned in the published results of drug trials is the occurrence of a paradoxical increase in seizures due to an AED; this phenomenon is usually hidden in the 'not improved' category. Sometimes this is an idiosyncratic effect, sometimes it is related to use of an incorrect drug for the particular syndrome or seizure type, and sometimes it is due to anticonvulsant intoxication or encephalopathy. Absence seizures can be precipitated by phenobarbital, carbamazepine, tiagabine and vigabatrin. Carbamazepine can precipitate focal, atonic, myoclonic and absence seizures especially in the Lennox–Gastaut syndrome, while intravenous benzodiazepines can at times precipitate tonic status in the same syndrome. Myoclonic seizures can be induced by carbamazepine, gabapentin, lamotrigine and vigabatrin. Phenytoin intoxication can markedly increase seizures and valproate can induce an epileptic encephalopathy with increased seizure frequency, at times associated with drug-induced hyperammonaemia.

Table 26.4 The delay in recognition of adverse side-effects to AEDs

Drug	Adverse reaction	Incidence	Year of introduction	Year of discovery
Phenobarbital	Shoulder–hand syndrome	Up to 12%	1912	1934
Phenytoin	Rickets and osteomalacia	Up to 5%	1938	1967
Folate deficiency	Folate deficiency	Over 50%	–	1964
Carbamazepine	Aplastic anaemia	1 : 200 000	1963	1964
Valproic acid	Hepatotoxicity	1 : 600 to 1 : 50 000	1967	1977
Vigabatrin	Visual field defects	40%	1989	1997

Adapted from [62].

Drug interactions, formulation and pharmacokinetic properties

A veritable industry has arisen around studies of drug interactions, and AEDs have been at the forefront. A large number of interactions have been described in recent years, reflecting the widespread availability of serum level monitoring. Many though are of little clinical importance, and others have significant consequences in only a small proportion of patients. Nevertheless, fatal outcomes do occur, for example, deaths resulting from haemorrhage in warfarin-treated patients when concomitant enzyme-inducing AEDs were discontinued without adjusting the dosage of the anticoagulant [79]. AED interactions with warfarin may indeed be more common than is generally recognized, and the risks are exacerbated by the danger of haemorrhage due to falling in epilepsy. To define the overall risk of clinically relevant interactions is more difficult than simply documenting the pharmacokinetics of these interactions. How these influence drug choice will obviously depend on individual circumstances. Drug interactions are described in detail in Chapter 10 and the individual drug sections.

Formulation and drug regimens can also be important. In children, sprinkle preparations can be better tolerated than tablets or syrup, and the need for frequent dosing can be a serious deterrent to compliance at all ages, but especially in adolescents and the elderly. The availability of an intravenous formulation is also valuable in those patients with a propensity to status epilepticus.

Rational polytherapy

There has been a recent vogue for recommending combination therapy with drugs that have different mechanisms of action. The proposition that combining drugs with different actions will have additive effects is superficially an attractive and reasonable one. There is, however, very little supportive clinical evidence and most studies in this area have been anecdotal, open and uncontrolled observations. Combinations that have been suggested for generalized epilepsy include mixtures of valproate, lamotrigine and ethosuximide. For partial epilepsy, combinations might include mixtures of GABAergic drugs (e.g. vigabatrin, benzodiazepines, phenobarbital), sodium channel blockers (e.g. phenytoin, carbamazepine, oxcarbazepine, lamotrigine), carbonic anhydrase inhibitors (e.g. acetazolamide), and/or drugs with other actions (e.g. levetiracetam, gabapentin). Topiramate is an example of a drug with several modes of action. There is limited experimental evidence to show synergistic effects of several drugs. In general, however, there is a striking lack of conclusive clinical evidence of any 'rationality' in combination prescribing, and treatment with a single drug remains the most appropriate therapy for most patients.

Cost

Cost is one issue which clearly differentiates the newer and older drugs. Figure 11.4 (p. 147) shows the unit costs of 1-year treatment with standard doses of different AEDs. Although these costs are only indicative and different purchasers can pay different prices, there is clearly a huge variation, with an approximately 100-fold difference between the highest and the lowest cost. The older and traditional medications such as carbamazepine, phenobarbital,

phenytoin or valproate are much cheaper than any of the newer drugs. Cost is of only limited interest unless related to outcome. A published study of total medical costs of prescribing carbamazepine, phenytoin, lamotrigine or valproate, using a cost-minimization mode, found that—assuming the same outcome—the overall costs of prescribing lamotrigine in newly diagnosed epilepsy were about four times those of the other three drugs. Other health economic studies of different drugs in different settings have reached broadly similar conclusions.

Choice of drug in newly diagnosed partial onset seizures

The principles of treatment in newly diagnosed cases are discussed extensively in Chapter 12, and only the choice of drug will be discussed here.

In most western countries, newly introduced AEDs require separate licences for use as monotherapy and for use as polytherapy (i.e. as add-on therapy in refractory epilepsy). Regulations require a new AED to show proof of efficacy and safety separately for monotherapy and polytherapy indications, in spite of the fact that there are few, if any, examples of an AED which is effective in combination but not as single drug therapy. It is difficult to escape the cynical conclusion that the purpose of these regulations, partially at least, is to erect a bureaucratic hurdle to prevent the widespread and costly use of the newer drugs as first-line treatment. These trials take time and are expensive and to date, of the newer AEDs, lamotrigine, oxcarbazepine, felbamate, gabapentin and topiramate have undergone sufficient monotherapy trials to have satisfied at least one of the major licensing authorities that monotherapy is appropriate. The older AEDs were introduced before this distinction between 'monotherapy' and 'polytherapy' licenses was made, and are licensed for both indications.

The landmark monotherapy study for traditional drugs was the double-blind multicentre comparison of phenytoin, carbamazepine, phenobarbital and primidone carried out by the American Veterans Administration collaborative network [80]. In this study, 622 patients were randomized to treatment with one of the four drugs and followed for 24 months or until toxicity or lack of seizure control required a treatment switch. The patients were adults, and a mixture of newly diagnosed drug-naïve patients and patients who had been previously undertreated. Overall treatment success was highest with carbamazepine or phenytoin, intermediate with phenobarbital, and lowest with primidone, but the proportion of patients rendered seizure free on the four drugs did not differ greatly (between 48 and 63%). Differences in failure rates were explained primarily by the fact that primidone caused more intolerable acute toxic effects, such as nausea, vomiting, dizziness and sedation. This study confirmed the widely held view that—in terms of antiepileptic efficacy—there was little to choose between the four drugs, and that the main differences among AEDs relate to side-effect profile. A follow-on study comparing carbamazepine and valproate in 480 adult patients showed no differences in control of secondarily generalized seizures, although carbamazepine was more effective in complex partial seizures. Two randomized open British studies, on the other hand, found no differences in efficacy when valproate and carbamazepine were compared in adults and children with newly diagnosed partial and/or generalized tonic-clonic seizures [81,82]. In two additional randomized studies, Heller *et al.* [83] and De Silva *et al.* [84] compared carbamazepine, valproate, phenytoin and phenobarbital as initial therapy in drug-naïve newly diagnosed children and adults. No differences in efficacy were noted, but phenobarbital was withdrawn more often in children because of side-effects. A similar comparative open monotherapy study in adults [85] found no significant differences between carbamazepine, phenytoin or valproate in efficacy or side-effects. Similarly, the efficacy of valproate against absence seizures was found to be similar to that of ethosuximide [85,86].

As far as newer drugs are concerned, monotherapy data (reviewed in subsequent chapters in this section) are limited. To date, the best studied drugs in this respect are lamotrigine and oxcarbazepine. There have been a number of randomized studies in adults comparing lamotrigine with carbamazepine [46,87,88] and phenytoin [89] and no major differences in efficacy were found, even though lamotrigine showed some tolerability advantages, particularly in the elderly. Oxcarbazepine has been compared with placebo or with a low-dose alternative AED in randomized double-blind monotherapy trials in various clinical settings [90]. While these studies showed that high-dosage oxcarbazepine is superior to placebo or a low-dose active control, no differences in efficacy were found when oxcarbazepine was compared in head-to-head trials with full dosages of carbamazepine, valproate and phenytoin, even though there were again tolerability trends favouring the innovative drug. Topiramate was evaluated as monotherapy in three double-blind dose-comparison studies, two of which were conducted in newly/recently diagnosed epilepsy [29,91], and results generally favoured the high-dose groups. In newly diagnosed epilepsy, topiramate 100 and 200 mg/day was found to be as effective as carbamazepine 600 mg/day or valproate 1250 mg/day. Monotherapy trials in which vigabatrin or gabapentin were compared with carbamazepine in patients with newly diagnosed epilepsy also failed to show any efficacy advantage in favour of the newer drugs and, if anything, there was a trend for seizure freedom rates to be higher in the groups assigned to carbamazepine [92].

The most striking finding from these studies is the similarity in responder rates among the various drugs, at least in patients with partial epilepsy. Because of this, choice in these patients will depend to a large extent on tolerability considerations and other factors. On cost grounds, carbamazepine or phenytoin are usually chosen as drugs of first choice in partial epilepsy, and in the author's practice, carbamazepine is the usual first choice. However, as emphasized above, patient's preference should be paramount. The relative merits of each drug should be carefully explained. Factors such as cost, tolerability, safety, potential for teratogenicity, comorbidity, convenience and ease of use are all important considerations which will vary from patient to patient. An informed choice can only be made by the patient on the basis of this information. The fact that the individual with newly diagnosed epilepsy is likely to stay for many years on the first AED chosen underlines the importance of adequate counselling and a carefully considered drug choice decision.

Approach to drug treatment in established epilepsy and continuing seizures

It is important to adopt a systematic approach when seizures persist

Table 26.5 Principles of treatment in a patient with established epilepsy and active seizures

Assessment
Review diagnosis and aetiology
    History, EEG, neuroimaging, other investigations
Classify seizure type and syndrome
Review compliance
Review drug history, by identifying
    Drugs which have been useful in the past
    Drugs which have not been useful in the past
    Drugs which have not been used in the past
    Dose and blood levels of drugs previously used
Review non-pharmacological factors

Treatment plan
Choose a sequence of drug changes (treatment trials)
    Medication to retain
    Sequence of drug withdrawal
    Sequence of drug addition
    Duration of treatment trials
    Serum level monitoring
Consider surgical therapy
Recognize limits to therapy

in spite of initial therapy. An assessment is needed and a treatment plan then formulated on the basis of this assessment. A checklist of factors to consider is given in Table 26.5.

Assessment

A reassessment of diagnosis and drug history should be carried out in all patients whose seizures continue despite AED therapy.

Diagnosis and aetiology

The following assessments should be made:

1 Review the diagnosis of epilepsy: an eye-witnessed account of the attacks should be obtained, and the previous medical records inspected. A series of normal EEG results should alert about the possibility that the attacks are non-epileptic (although this is not an infallible rule).

2 Establish aetiology: it is important at this stage to ascertain the cause of the epileptic attacks, and especially to exclude progressive pathology. This will usually require neuroimaging.

3 Classify seizure type using the ILAE scheme (Chapter 1): this is important to make decisions on which drugs should be used.

Previous treatment history

This is an essential step, often omitted. The response to an AED is generally relatively consistent over time. Find out which drugs have been previously tried, what was the response (effectiveness/side-effects), what was the maximum dose and the reasons for drug withdrawal. It is only on this basis that rational choices for future drug therapy can be made.

Review compliance

This may have been a reason for previously poor seizure control. Patient buy-in is necessary for good compliance. Therefore counselling and discussion about the role of drug therapy, the time course of effects, the limitations of therapy and the likely side-effects are essential. A drug wallet, filled up for the whole week, can be a great assistance for patients who often forget to take their medication. Other ways of improving compliance include the use of monotherapy and the simplification of the drug regimen, regular clinic follow-up, and the implementation of cues and aide-memoires.

Treatment plan

A treatment plan should be formulated on the basis of the assessment. The plan should take the form of therapeutic trials with individual drugs or drug combinations, each tried in turn. The treatment plan should establish the parameters for these trials (order of drugs, duration of treatment, outcome measure, etc.). The emphasis is to try each available AED in a reasonable dose singly or as two-drug therapy (or, more rarely, three-drug combinations). This will involve deciding upon which drugs to introduce, which drugs to withdraw and which drugs to retain. Decisions will also be needed about the duration of each treatment trial.

There is often a strange inertia in much of the treatment of chronic epilepsy which should be resisted, and an active and logical approach to therapy can prove very successful:

1 Choice of drug to introduce or retain: generally these should be drugs which are appropriate for the seizure type and which have either not been previously used in optimal doses or which have been used and did prove helpful. Rational choices depend on a well-documented history of previous drug therapy.

2 Choice of drug to withdraw: these should be drugs which have been given an adequate trial at optimal doses and which were either ineffective or caused unacceptable side-effects. There is obviously little point in continuing a drug which has had little effect, yet it is remarkable how often this is done.

3 Duration of treatment trial: this will depend on the baseline seizure rate. The trial should be long enough to have differentiated the effect of therapy from that of chance fluctuations in seizures.

4 It is usual to aim for therapy with either one or two suitable AEDs. If drugs are being withdrawn, it is wise to maintain one drug in good doses as an 'anchor' to cover the withdrawal period.

Choosing a drug in established epilepsy

Almost all RCTs discussed above were conducted in the setting of add-on therapy in patients with refractory partial epilepsy. This evidence base, although imperfect for all the reasons outlined above, provides the best objective data about the relative short-term efficacy and tolerability of the various drugs. The general consensus is that there is little to favour any of the mainline AEDs in terms either of efficacy or toxicity. However, as emphasized above, other factors are also important. The physician's role in this situation is to inform the patient adequately about the relative merits and disadvantages of any drug (including the cost), and make recommendations on this basis. The patient should be encouraged to make an informed choice as only the patient is in a position to weigh the relative

importance of individual factors. This is the art of prescribing and because of this, making inviolate recommendations is not advisable.

Monotherapy vs. combination therapy

Single drug therapy will provide optimal seizure control in about 80% of all patients with epilepsy, and should be chosen whenever possible. The advantages of monotherapy are:

1 Better tolerability and fewer side-effects.

2 Simpler and less intrusive regimen.

3 No potential for pharmacokinetic or pharmacodynamic interactions with other AEDs.

4 Less risk of teratogenicity.

Combination therapy is needed in about 20% of all those developing epilepsy, and in a much higher proportion of those whose epilepsy has remained uncontrolled despite initial monotherapy (chronic active epilepsy). The prognosis for seizure control in the latter patients, even in combination therapy, is far less good. Nevertheless, skilful combination therapy can make a substantial difference by optimising control of the epilepsy and minimising the side-effects of treatment. Patients need to be advised carefully about the implications of polytherapy in terms of drug interactions, teratogenesis and other potential adverse effects.

Withdrawing drugs

When adjusting drug therapy, drug withdrawal should be done cautiously. Withdrawal (or sudden reduction in dose) of AEDs can result in a severe worsening of seizures or in status epilepticus—even if the withdrawn drug was apparently not contributing much to seizure control. Why withdrawal seizures occur is not clear, although EEG-telemetry experience suggests that these seizures have electrophysiological features similar to the patient's habitual seizures. It is therefore customary, and wise, to withdraw medication slowly. This caution applies particularly to barbiturate drugs (phenobarbital, primidone), benzodiazepine drugs (clobazam, clonazepam, diazepam) and carbamazepine. As an example, suggested maximal decremental rates in an adult (expressed as magnitude of dose reduction every 4 weeks) could be in the order of 200 mg for carbamazepine, 250 mg for ethosuximide, 400 mg for gabapentin, 100 mg for lamotrigine, 500 mg for levetiracetam, 300 mg for oxcarbazepine, 30 mg for phenobarbital, 50 mg for phenytoin, 10 mg for tiagabine, 100 mg for topiramate, 200 mg for valproate and 500 mg for vigabatrin. In many situations even slower rates of withdrawal are safer. The magnitude of decrement will also depend on the initial dosage: for example, the suggested maximal 200 mg dose reduction for valproate would be appropriate in a patient taking 800 mg/day or less, but a larger decrement (e.g. 500 mg) may be appropriate in a patient taking 2500 mg/day or more. The only advantage of fast withdrawal is better compliance and faster establishment of the new drug regimen. Only one drug should be withdrawn at a time. If the withdrawal period is likely to be difficult, dangers can be reduced by covering the withdrawal with a benzodiazepine drug (usually clobazam 10 mg/day), given during the phase of active withdrawal. A benzodiazepine can also be given if clustering of seizures occurs following withdrawal. It is sometimes difficult to know whether seizures occurring during withdrawal are actual withdrawal seizures or simply reflect the background epilepsy, and whenever possible a long term view should be taken and overreaction in the short term avoided. Sometimes the simple withdrawal of a drug will result in improved seizure control simply by improving well being, assuring better compliance, and reducing interactions.

Adding drugs

New drugs added to a regimen should also be introduced slowly, at least in the routine clinical situation. This results in better tolerability, and is particularly important when adding lamotrigine, topiramate, carbamazepine, oxcarbazepine, primidone, tiagabine or benzodiazepines. Too fast an introduction of these drugs will almost invariably result in side-effects. It is usual to aim initially for a low maintenance dose. Absolute rules are difficult, and in severe epilepsy it is sometimes advisable to build up to high doses.

Concomitant medication

Changing the dose of one AED (either incrementally or decrementally) can influence the serum levels of other drugs, and the changing serum levels of concomitant medication may contribute to changing side-effects or indeed effectiveness. The serum levels or doses of concomitant AEDs may need to be monitored in this situation.

Limits to drug therapy

Generally speaking, the goal should be complete seizure control without side-effects. In some patients, it can take time to find the right medication, and seizure control may be possible only at the expense of side-effects. In about 30% of patients, this goal cannot be realized. In these patients, the epilepsy can be categorized as 'intractable' and the goal of therapy changes to defining the best compromise between inadequate seizure control and drug-induced side-effects. Individual patients will take very different views about where to strike this balance.

Intractability is inevitably an arbitrary classification. There are about 15 major AEDs, and far more combinations (with 15 major AEDs there are 105 different two-drug and 455 different three-drug combinations). All combinations can not therefore be tried. The chances of a new drug controlling seizures after five appropriate agents have failed to do so is small (less than 5%). At a pragmatic level, therefore, one can categorize an epilepsy as intractable when at least five of the major AEDs have proved ineffective in adequate doses. There will be occasional exceptions to this rule, however.

Acknowledgements

This chapter incorporates text in an expanded form from a paper submitted for publication, and presented in a lecture to the Singapore Neuroscience Society [93] and from the *Handbook of Epilepsy Treatment* [90].

References

1 Shorvon SD. Drug treatment of epilepsy. MD Thesis, University of Cambridge, 1982.

2 Shorvon SD, Johnson AL, Reynolds EH. Statistical and theoretical considerations in the design of anticonvulsant trials. In: Dam M, Gram L, Penry K, ed. *Advances in Epileptology*. XIIth Epilepsy International Symposium. New York: Raven Press, 1981: 123–34.

3 Anhut H, Ashman P, Feuerstein TJ, Sauermann W, Saunders M, Schmidt B. Gabapentin (Neurontin) as add-on therapy in patients with partial seizures: a double-blind, placebo-controlled study: the International Gabapentin Study Group. *Epilepsia* 1994; 35: 795–801.

4 Barcs G, Walker EB, D'Souza J et al. Oxcarbazepine placebo-controlled, dose ranging trial in refractory epilepsy. *Epilepsia* 2000; 41: 1597–607.

5 Ben-Menachem E, Henriksen O, Dam M et al. Double blind, placebo-controlled trial of topiramate as add-on therapy in patients with refractory partial seizures. *Epilepsia* 1996; 37: 539–43.

6 Ben-Menachem E, Falter U, for the European Levetiracetam Study Group. Efficacy and tolerability of levetiracetam 3000 mg/day in patients with refractory partial seizures: a multicenter, double-blind, responder-selected study evaluating monotherapy. *Epilepsia* 2000; 41: 1276–83.

7 Beran RC, Berkovic SF, Vajda F et al. A double blind placebo-controlled cross over study of vigabatrin 2 g/day and 3 g/day in uncontrolled partial seizures. *Seizure* 1996; 5: 259–65.

8 Betts T, Waegemans T, Crawford P. A multicentre, double-blind, randomized, parallel group study to evaluate the tolerability and efficacy of two oral doses of levetiracetam, 2000 mg daily and 4000 mg daily, without titration in patients with refractory epilepsy. *Seizure* 2000; 9: 80–7.

9 Binnie CD, Debets RM, Engelsman M et al. Double blind cross-over trial of lamotrigine (Lamictal) as add on therapy in intractable epilepsy. *Epilepsy Res* 1989; 4: 222–9.

10 Boas J, Dam M, Friis M et al. Controlled trial of lamotrigine (Lamictal) for treatment of resistant partial seizures. *Acta Neurol Scand* 1996; 94: 247–52.

11 Cereghino JJ, Biton V, Abou-Khalil B et al. Levetiracetam for partial seizures. Results of a double-blind, randomised clinical trial. *Neurology* 2000; 55: 236–42.

12 Chadwick DW, Marson T. Zonisamide add-on for drug resistant partial epilepsy (Cochrane Review). In: *The Cochrane Library*, Issue 4. Oxford: Oxford Update Software, 2002.

13 Dean C, Mosier M, Penry K. Dose response study of vigabatrin as add-on therapy in patients with uncontrolled complex partial seizures. *Epilepsia* 1999; 40: 74–82.

14 Faught E, Wilder BJ, Ramsey RE et al. Topiramate placebo controlled dose-ranging trial in refractory partial epilepsy using 200-, 400-, and 600-mg daily dosages. *Neurology* 1996; 46: 1684–90.

15 Faught E, Ayala R, Montouris G, Leppik IE. Randomized controlled trial of zonisamide for the treatment of refractory partial-onset seizures. *Neurology* 2001; 57: 1774–9

16 French JA, Mosier M, Walker S, Somerville K, Sussman N, and the Vigabatrin Protocol 024 Investigative Cohort. A double-blind, placebo controlled study of vigabatrin 3 g/day in patients with uncontrolled complex partial seizures. *Neurology* 1996; 46: 54–61.

17 Glauser TA, Migro M, D'Souza J et al. Adjunctive therapy with oxcarbazepine in children with partial seizures. *Neurology* 2000; 54: 2237–42.

18 Grunwald RA, Thompson PJ, Corcoran RS, Corden Z, Jackson G, Duncan JS. Effect of vigabatrin on partial seizures and cognitive function. *J Neurol Neurosurg Psychiatr* 1994; 57: 1057–63.

19 Jawad S, Richens A, Goodwin G, Yuen WC. Controlled trial of lamotrigine (Lamictal) for refractory partial seizures. *Epilepsia* 1989; 30: 356–63.

20 Kälviäinen R, Brodie MJ, Chadwick D et al. A double-blind, placebo-controlled trial of tiagabine given three-times daily as add-on therapy for refractory partial seizures. *Epilepsy Res* 1998; 30: 31–40.

21 Loiseau P, Yuen AW, Duche B, Menager T, Arne Bes MC. A randomised double blind placebo controlled cross-over add on trial of lamotrigine in patients with treatment resistant partial seizures. *Epilepsy Res* 1990; 7: 136–45.

22 Marson AG, Hutton JL, Leach JP et al. Levetiracetam, oxcarbazepine, remacemide and zonisamide for drug resistant localization-related epilepsy: a systematic review. *Epilepsy Res* 2001; 46: 259–70.

23 Matsuo F, Bergen D, Faught E et al. Placebo-controlled study of the efficacy and safety of lamotrigine in patients with partial seizures: U.S. Lamotrigine Protocol 0.5 Clinical Trial Group. *Neurology* 1993; 43: 2284–91.

24 Messenheimer J, Ramsay RE, Willmore LJ *et al*. Lamotrigine therapy for partial seizures: a multicenter, placebo-controlled, double-blind, cross-over trial. *Epilepsia* 1994; 35: 113–21.

25 Padgett CS, Ayala G, Montouris GD, Ascher S, Buchanan RA. Zonisamide efficacy and dose response. *Epilepsia* 1997; 38 (Suppl. 8): 107.

26 Privitera M, Fincham R, Penry J, Reife R, Kramer L, Pledger G. Topiramate placebo-controlled dose-ranging trial in refractory partial epilepsy using 600-, 800-, and 1000-mg daily dosages. *Neurology* 1996; 46: 1678–83.

27 Rosenfeld W, Abou-Khalil B, Reife R, Hegadus R, Pledger G, and Topiramate YF/YG study group. Placebo-controlled trial of topiramate as adjunctive therapy to carbamazepine or phenytoin for partial onset epilepsy. *Epilepsia* 1996; 37 (Suppl. 5): s153.

28 Sachdeo RC, Leroy R, Krauss G *et al*. Tiagabine therapy for complex partial seizures. A dose-frequency study. *Arch Neurol* 1997; 54: 595–601.

29 Sachdeo R, Reife R, Lim P, Pledger G. Topiramate monotherapy for partial onset seizures. *Epilepsia* 1997; 38: 294–300.

30 Schapel GJ, Beran RG, Vajda FJ *et al*. Double blind, placebo controlled, cross-over study of lamotrigine in treatment resistant partial seizures. *J Neurol Neurosurg Psychiatry* 1993; 56: 448–53.

31 Schmidt D, Jacob R, Loiseau P *et al*. Zonisamide for add on treatment of refractory partial epilepsy: a European double blind trial. *Epilepsy Res* 1993; 15: 67–73.

32 Schmidt D, Ried S, Rapp P. Add-on treatment with lamotrigine for intractable partial epilepsy: a placebo-controlled cross-over study. *Epilepsia* 1993; 34 (Suppl. 2): S66.

33 Sharief M, Viteri C, Ben-Menachem E, Weber M, Reife R. Double blind placebo-controlled study of topiramate in patients with refractory epilepsy. *Epilepsy Res* 1996; 25: 217–24.

34 Shorvon SD, Löwenthal A, Janz D, Bielen E, Loiseau P, for the European Levetiracetam Study Group. Multicenter double-blind, randomised, placebo-controlled trial of levetiracetam as add-on therapy in patients with refractory partial seizures. *Epilepsia* 2000; 41: 1179–86.

35 Silvenius J, Kalviainen R, Ylinen A, Riekkinen P. Double blind study of gabapentin in the treatment of partial seizures. *Epilepsia* 1991; 32: 539–42.

36 Smith D, Baker G, Davies G, Dewey M, Chadwick DW. Outcomes of add on treatment with lamotrigine in partial epilepsy. *Epilepsia* 1993; 34: 312–22.

37 Tassinari CA, Michelucci R, Chauvel P *et al*. Double blind, placebo-controlled trial of topiramate (600 mg daily) for the treatment of refractory partial epilepsy. *Epilepsia* 1996; 37: 763–8.

38 UK Gabapentin Study Group. Gabapentin in partial epilepsy. *Lancet* 1990; 335(8698): 1114–17.

39 Uthman B, Rowan J, Ahman PA *et al*. Tiagabine for complex partial seizures: a randomised, add-on, dose–response trial. *Arch Neurol* 1998; 55: 56–62.

40 US Gabapentin Study Group No. 5. Gabapentin as add-on therapy in refractory partial epilepsy: a double-blind, placebo-controlled, parallel-group study. *Neurology* 1993; 43: 2292–8.

41 Wilder BJ, Ramsay RE, Guterman A. *Double-blind Multicenter Placebo-controlled Study of the Efficacy and Safety of Zonisamide in the Treatment of Complex Partial Seizures in Medically Refractory Patients*. Japan: Internal report of the Dianippon Pharmaceutical Co., 1986.

42 Moher D, Schulz KF, Altman D, For the CONSORT Group. The CONSORT statement: revised recommendations for improving the quality of reports of parallel-group randomized trials. *JAMA* 2001; 285: 1987–91.

43 Rennie D. CONSORT revised–improving the reporting of randomized trials. *JAMA* 2001; 285: 2006–8.

44 Birbeck GL, Hays RD, Cui X, Vickrey BG. Seizure reduction and quality of life improvements in people with epilepsy. *Epilepsia* 2002; 43: 535–8.

45 Cramer JA, Fisher R, Ben-Menachem E, French J, Mattson RH. New antiepileptic drugs: comparison of key clinical trials. *Epilepsia* 1999; 40: 590–600.

46 Brodie MJ, Richens A, Yuen AWC, for UK Lamotrigine/Carbamazepine Monotherapy Trial Group. Double-blind comparison of lamotrigine and carbamazepine in newly diagnosed epilepsy. *Lancet* 1995; 345: 476–9.

47 Chadwick D. Safety and efficacy of vigabatrin and carbamazepine in newly diagnosed epilepsy: a multicentre randomized double-blind study. Vigabatrin European Monotherapy Study Group. *Lancet* 1999; 354: 13–19.

48 Lhatoo SD, Wong ICK, Sander JWAS. Prognostic factors affecting long-term retention of topiramate in patients with chronic epilepsy. *Epilepsia* 2000; 41: 338–41.

49 Marson A, Beghi E, Berg A, Chadwick D, Tonini C, on behalf of the Cochrane Epilepsy Network. The Cochrane Collaboration: systematic reviews and their relevance to epilepsy. The Cochrane Epilepsy Network. *Epilepsia* 1996; 37: 917–21.

50 Marson AG, Kadir ZA, Hutton JL, Chadwick DW. The new antiepileptic drugs: a systematic review of their efficacy and tolerability. *Epilepsia* 1997; 38: 859–80.

51 LeLorier J, Grégoire G, Benhaddad A, Lapierre J, Derderian F. Discrepancies between meta-analyses and subsequent large randomised, controlled trials. *N Engl J Med* 1997; 337: 536–42.

52 Castillo S, Schmidt DB, White S. *The Cochrane Library*, Issue 3. Oxford: Update Software, 2002.

53 Chaisewikul R, Privitera MD, Hutton JL, Marson AG. Levetiracetam add-on for drug-resistant localization related (partial) epilepsy (Cochrane Review). In: *The Cochrane Library*, Issue 2. Oxford: Update Software, 2002.

54 Halasz P, Walker EB, Elger CE *et al*. *Safety and Efficacy of Oxcarbazepine (Trileptal) in Refractory Epilepsy*. 51st American Academy of Neurology, Abstract, 17–24 April, 1999, Toronto, Canada.

55 Chadwick DW, Marson T, Kadir Z. Clinical administration of new antiepileptic drugs: an overview of safety and efficacy. *Epilepsia* 1996; 37 (Suppl. 6): S17–22.

56 Cook RJ, Sackett DL. The number needed to treat: a clinically useful measure of treatment effect. *BMJ* 1995; 310: 452–4 (published erratum *BMJ* 1005; 310: 1056).

57 Lesaffre E, Pledger G. A note on the number needed to treat. *Control Clin Trials* 1999; 20: 439–47.

58 Elferink AJA, van Zwieten-Boot BJ. Analysis based on number needed to treat shows differences between drugs studied, letter. *BMJ* 1997; 314: 603.

59 Lesaffre E, Boon P, Pledger GW. The value of the number-needed-to-treat method in antiepileptic drug trials. *Epilepsia* 2000; 41: 440–6.

60 Van Rijckevorsel K *et al*. The 'number needed to treat' with levetiracetam (LEV), comparison with the other new antiepileptic drugs (AEDs), letter. *Seizure* 2001; 10: 235–6.

61 Guberman A, Netop W, Gassmann-Mayer C. Low-dose topiramate in adults with treatment-resistant partial-onset seizures. *Acta Neurol Scand* 2002; 106: 183–9

62 Perucca E, Beghi E, Dulac O, Shorvon SD, Tomson T. Assessing risk to benefit ratio in antiepileptic drug therapy. *Epilepsy Res* 2000; 41: 107–39.

63 Pellock JM, Brodie MJ. Felbamate: 1997 update. *Epilepsia* 1997; 38: 1261–4.

64 Kaufman DW, Kelly JP, Anderson T, Harmon DC, Shapiro S. Evaluation of case reports of aplastic anemia among patients treated with felbamate. *Epilepsia* 1997; 38: 1265–9.

65 König SA, Siemes H, Blaker F *et al*. Severe hepatotoxicity during valproate therapy: An update and report of eight new fatalities. *Epilepsia* 1994; 35: 1005–15.

66 Bryant AE III, Dreifuss FE. Valproic acid hepatic fatalities. III. U.S. experience since 1986. *Neurology* 1996; 2: 465–9

67 Battino D, Dukes GMN, Perucca E. Antiepileptic Drugs. In: Aronson JK, Dukes GMN, eds. *Meyler's Side Effects of Drugs*. Amsterdam: Elsevier, 2000.

68 Vittorio CC, Muglia JJ. Anticonvulsant hypersensitivity syndrome. *Arch Int Med* 1995; 155: 2285–90.

69 Schlienger RG, Shear NH. Antiepileptic drug hypersensitivity syndrome. *Epilepsia* 1998; 39 (Suppl. 7): S3–S7.

70 Ruble J, Matsuo T. Anticonvulsant-induced cutaneous reactions. Incidence, mechanisms and management. *CNS Drugs* 1999; 12: 215–36.

71 Zahn CA, Morrell MJ, Collins SD *et al*. Management issues for women with epilepsy. A review of the literature. *Neurology* 1998; 51: 949–56.

72 Tomson T, Gram L, Sillanpää M, Johannessen SI. Recommendations for the management and care of pregnant women with epilepsy. In: Tomson T, Gram L, Sillanpää M, Johannessen SI, eds. *Epilepsy and Pregnancy*. Petersfield: Wrightson Biomedical, 1997: 201–8.

73 Rintahaka PJ, Nakagawa JA, Shewmon DA, Kyyronen P, Shields WD. Incidence of death in patients with intractable epilepsy during nitrazepam treatment. *Epilepsia* 1999; 40: 492–6.

74 Perucca E. The new generation of antiepileptic drugs: Advantages and disadvantages. *Br J Clin Pharmacol* 1996; 42: 531–43.

75 Battino D, Kaneko S, Andermann F. *et al.* Intrauterine growth in the offspring of epileptic women: a prospective multicenter study. *Epilepsy Res* 1999; 36: 53–60.

76 Lindhout D, Omtzight G. Teratogenic effects of antiepileptic drugs: Implications for management of epilepsy in women of childbearing age. *Epilepsia* 1994; 35 (Suppl. 4): S19–28.

77 Samren EB, van Duijn CM, Koch S *et al.* Maternal use of antiepileptic drugs and the risk of major congenital malformations: a joint European prospective study of human teratogenesis associated with maternal epilepsy. *Epilepsia* 1997; 38: 981–90.

78 Canger R, Battino D, Canevin MP. *et al.* Malformations in offspring of women with epilepsy: a prospective study. *Epilepsia* 1999; 40: 1231–6.

79 MacDonald MG, Robinson DS. Clinical observations of possible barbiturate interference with anticoagulation. *JAMA* 1968; 204: 97–9.

80 Mattson RH, Cramer JA, Collins JF *et al.* Comparison of carbamazepine, phenobarbital, phenytoin, and primidone in partial and secondarily generalized tonic-clonic seizures. *N Engl J Med* 1985; 313: 145–51.

81 Richens A, Davidson DLW, Cartlidge NEF, Easter DJ. A multicentre comparative trial of sodium valproate and carbamazepine in adult-onset epilepsy. *J Neurol Neurosurg Psychiatr* 1994; 57: 682–7.

82 Verity CM, Hosking G, Easter DJ. A multicentre comparative trial of sodium valproate and carbamazepine in paediatric epilepsy. The Paediatric EPITEG Collaborative Group. *Dev Med Child Neurol* 1995; 37: 97–108.

83 Heller AJ, Chesterman P, Elwes RD *et al.* Phenobarbitone, phenytoin, carbamazepine, or sodium valproate for newly diagnosed adult epilepsy: a randomized comparative monotherapy study. *J Neurol Neurosurg Psychiatry* 1995; 58: 44–50.

84 De Silva M, MacArdle B, McGowas M *et al.* Randomised comparative monotherapy trial of phenobarbitone, phenytoin, carbamazepine and sodium valproate for newly diagnosed childhood epilepsy. *Lancet* 1996; 347: 709–13.

85 Callaghan N, Kenny RA, O'Neill B *et al.* A prospective study between carbamazepine, phenytoin and sodium valproate as monotherapy in previously untreated and recently diagnosed patients with epilepsy. *J Neurol Neurosurg Psychiatr* 1985; 48: 639–44.

86 Sato S, White BG, Penry K *et al.* Valproate versus ethosucimide in the treatment of absence seizures. *Neurology* 1982; 32: 157–63.

87 Brodie MJ, Overstall PW, Giorgi L. Multicentre, double-blind, randomised comparison between lamotrigine and carbamazepine in elderly patients with newly diagnosed epilepsy. The UK Lamotrigine Elderly Study Group. *Epilepsy Res* 1999; 37: 81–7.

88 Reunanen OM, Dam M, Yuen AWC. A randomized open multicenter comparative trial of lamotrigine and carbamazepine as monotherapy in patients with newly diagnosed or recurrent epilepsy. *Epilepsy Res* 1996; 23: 149–55.

89 Steiner TJ, Dellaportas CI, Findley LJ *et al.* Lamotrigine monotherapy in newly diagnosed untreated epilepsy: a double-blind comparison with phenytoin. *Epilepsia* 1999; 40: 601–7.

90 Shorvon SD *Handbook of the Treatment of Epilepsy.* Oxford: Blackwell Science, 2000.

91 Arroyo, S., Squires, L, Twyman, R. Topiramate (TPM) monotherapy in newly diagnosed epilepsy: effectiveness in dose–response study. *Epilepsia* 2002: 43 (Suppl. 8): 47–8.

92 Perucca E, Tomson T. Monotherapy trials with the new antiepileptic drugs: Study designs, practical relevance and ethical implications. *Epilepsy Res* 1999; 33: 247–62.

93 Shorvon SD. Assessing antiepileptic drug efficacy: analytical methods of data from randomised controlled trials. (Submitted for publication.)

94 Shorvon SD, Van Rijckevorsal. A new antiepileptic drug. *J Neurol Neurosurg Psychiatr* 2002; 72: 2–5.

95 Krakow K, Walker M, Otoul C, Sander JWAS. Long term continuation of levetiracetam in patients with refractory epilepsy. *Neurology* 2001; 56: 1772–4.

27

Acetazolamide

M. Y. Neufeld

Primary indication	Adjunctive therapy in partial or generalized seizures (including absence) and myoclonus. Also Lennox–Gastaut syndrome. Intermittent therapy in catamenial epilepsy
Usual preparation	Tablets: 250 mg
Usual dosage	250–750 mg/day
Dosage intervals	2–3 times/day
Significant drug interactions	Salicylate, digitalis can increase acetazolamide levels. Acetazolamide can reduce carbamazepine levels
Serum level monitoring	Not useful
Target range	—
Common/important side-effects	Nausea, vomiting , diarrhoea, loss of appetite, paraesthesiae, headache, dizziness, flushing, fatigue, irritability, hyperventilation, depression, thirst, loss of libido, metabolic acidosis and electrolyte changes. Risk of renal calculi. Rarely severe haematological, dermatological or systemic idiosyncratic reactions
Main advantages	Useful adjunctive therapy and also as intermittent therapy, usually well tolerated
Main disadvantages	Risk of idiosyncratic reaction. High incidence of tolerance
Mechanism of action	Carbonic anhydrase inhibition
Oral bioavailability	>90%
Time to peak levels	1–3 h
Metabolism and excretion	No metabolism. Eliminated by the kidney, 20% by glomerular filtration and 80% by renal tubular excretion
Volume of distribution	1.8 L/kg
Elimination half-life	12–14 h
Plasma clearance	—
Protein binding	90–95%
Active metabolites	Nil
Comment	Useful broad-spectrum drug in adjunctive therapy for resistant epilepsy. Use limited by tolerance and risk of idiosyncratic reactions

(*Note*: this summary table was formulated by the lead editor.)

Acetazolamide (Diamox), 2-acetylamido-1,3,4-thiadiazole-5 sulfonamide, is a sulfonamide derivative with a chemical formula of $C_4H_6N_4O_3S_2$. A well-documented effect of the sulfonamide compounds is their specific inhibition of carbonic anhydrase, and this also confers antiepileptic activity [1]. Carbonic anhydrase is a widely distributed enzyme that has many different physiological functions [2,3]. Cohen and Cobb [4] were the first to identify antiepileptic activity in this chemical class. They found that azosulfamide, a vital dye, has an anticonvulsant action in experimental animals as well as in patients. They speculated that the effect produced by this drug, similar to the property of sulfanilamide [1], is due to the inhibition of carbonic anhydrase causing acid–base changes that are manifested by metabolic acidosis. Acetazolamide was first synthesized by Roblin and Clapp [5]. The acidifying effect of acetazolamide led Bergstrom et al. [6] to use it in treating epilepsy, although it was later shown [2,7,8] that its anticonvulsant effect is independent of the secondary metabolic acidosis and is correlated directly with the degree of inhibition of carbonic anhydrase in the brain. Because carbonic anhydrase is found in many tissues other than brain and it serves numerous functions, inhibition of carbonic anhydrase by acetazolamide is associated with diverse uses (Table 27.1). Acetazolamide decreases the secretion of aqueous humour by the ciliary process of the eye and results in a drop of intraocular pressure, a reaction that is exploited in the therapeutic use in glaucoma [9]. The drug was found to be effective in the promotion of diuresis [10], and the reduction of cerebrospinal fluid (CSF) pressure, for instance in pseudotumour cerebri [11]. It was found to be effective in patients with paroxysmal periodic ataxia [12], in patients with paroxysmal dystonia described with central demyelinating disease [13] and in valproate-induced tremor [14]. The drug was also discovered to be useful in hypokalaemic and hyperkalaemic periodic paralysis [15] as well as in myotonia [16]. It has been described as having prevented or ameliorated symptoms associated with acute mountain sickness [17].

The efficacy of acetazolamide in patients with epilepsy was reported mainly in the 1950s [8,18–30] and only occasional studies were performed several decades later [31–34]. However, as no well-controlled clinical trials were reported, the efficacy of this drug in different seizure types and syndromes, and specifications for appropriate management are neither well established nor well documented.

Mechanism of action

The anticonvulsant effect of acetazolamide was shown to be mediated through the inhibition of carbonic anhydrase [7,8] which catalyses the formation of H_2CO_3 in the equilibrium reaction $CO_2 +$

Table 27.1 Other therapeutic indications and uses of acetazolamide

Glaucoma
Diuresis
Pseudotumor cerebri
Paroxysmal ataxia
Paroxysmal dystonia
Periodic paralysis
Prevention of mountain sickness

$H_2O \leftrightarrow H_2CO_3$. The secondary reaction $H_2CO_3 \leftrightarrow H^+ + HCO_3^-$ is instantaneous causing spontaneous dissociation of the carbonic acid. Carbonic anhydrase is present in high concentration in erythrocytes, gastric mucosa, the renal cortex, and in the lens and retina [2,3]. It is located in the brain in the cytoplasm and the membrane of the glial cells and in the choroid plexus [35–37], as well as in the myelin derived from oligodendrocytes [37,38]. Also, oligodendrocytes have higher carbonic anhydrase activity than astrocytes [38]. Carbonic anhydrase in the brain has an important role in the neuron–glia metabolic relationship. It is involved in regulating ionic balance throughout the brain [39]. Specifically, it catalyses the hydration of CO_2 that is generated during neuronal activity. The results of this reaction are hydrogen and bicarbonate ions that are exchanged across the glial membrane for sodium and chloride, respectively [40]. Carbonic anhydrase is involved in the maintenance of Cl^- and K^+ concentrations in glial cells [41].

It was Mann and Keilin [1] who found that sulfanilamide had a specific and powerful inhibiting effect on the activity of carbonic anhydrase. A study of other sulfonamides revealed that acetazolamide was several hundred times more active than sulfanilamide as an inhibitor of carbonic anhydrase [5]. Acetazolamide has a wide spectrum of anticonvulsant activity, as demonstrated in several animal models. The drug exerts a depressant action in the spinal cord, highly selective for the monosynaptic pathway [42]. Acetazolamide was shown to abolish the tonic extensor component of maximal electroshock convulsions [7,42,43] thereby raising the electroshock seizure threshold [43], to protect against seizures caused by pentylenetetrazol [42] or CO_2 withdrawal [44], as well as against audiogenic seizures [45]. The anticonvulsant activity of acetazolamide was originally thought to be due to the acidifying effect of the drug, caused by inhibition of renal carbonic anhydrase—apparently resembling that of a ketogenic diet. However, by using the maximal electroshock seizure test in mice, Millichap et al. [7] demonstrated that acetazolamide has an anticonvulsant effect which is independent of its action on the kidney and which is correlated directly with the degree of inhibition of carbonic anhydrase in the brain. Subsequently, other investigators [8,46] have also demonstrated that the anticonvulsant action of carbonic anhydrase inhibitors was correlated with the inhibition of brain carbonic anhydrase and was independent of the inhibition of the erythrocyte enzyme or diuresis. In the brain, inhibition of glial carbonic anhydrase reduces the conversion of neuronally derived CO_2 to HCO_3, whereupon neuronal CO_2 accumulates and the pH of the glia is lowered [7,8,46,47]. The anticonvulsant action of carbonic anhydrase inhibition at the neuronal level may be related to the demonstrated effects of CO_2 on nerve sensitivity and propagation of nerve impulses [2,48]. Both CO_2 and acetazolamide increase the electroshock seizure threshold and abolish the tonic extensor phase in an animal model of maximal electroshock seizures [42,48]. In addition, the effects of acetazolamide on the maximal electroshock seizures and on the spinal cord synaptic transmission are potentiated by CO_2 [45]. The similarities between the effects of CO_2 and acetazolamide as anticonvulsants suggested that the relationship of carbonic anhydrase to seizure activity is mediated through the CO_2-buffering system [47,48]. Following administration of acetazolamide and inhibition of carbonic anhydrase, analysis of both the glial cells and myelin has shown elevation of CO_2 in the extracellular space surrounding the neurone cells and the axons, where it could inhibit the spread of neuronal activity or stabilize the axonal membrane [48]. Similar to CO_2, acetazolamide also increases γ-aminobutyric acid (GABA) levels in the brain [42] which may account for some of its anticonvulsant effects.

Pharmacokinetics

Acetazolamide is a weak acid with a pKa of 7.4. Absorption is affected by factors known to influence the absorption of weak acids, such as pH, lipid and water solubility and concentration in the gastrointestinal fluids [49]. Acetazolamide in oral doses of 5–10 mg/kg daily is completely absorbed from the gastrointestinal tract [50,51], whereas higher doses cause unpredictable levels in the plasma [51]. Following oral administration at normal doses, the bioavailability of acetazolamide is above 90%. Absorption begins in the stomach but occurs mainly in the duodenum and upper jejunum where the surface area is larger. The peak plasma concentrations (i.e. 10–18 µg/mL) were reached 1–3 h after oral ingestion of a single 250-mg dose, and the peak erythrocyte concentration that was reached 1 h later was 13–19 µg/mL [52]. Following administration of a single oral dose of 500 mg sustained release (SR), peak plasma concentration is obtained 3.5 h after dosing maintaining a value of about 10 µg/mL for 10 h [53]. Oral administration of SR form caused less fluctuation in plasma concentration of the drug [54]. Acetazolamide is extensively bound to plasma proteins (fraction bound 90–95%), and this binding is dose dependent and reduced in the elderly [50,55]. The free fraction of the drug increases with the elevation of the plasma level. One-half of the free fractions is an unionized form, and it is this part that penetrates into tissues and causes the inhibition of carbonic anhydrase [49]. When binding to tissue, carbonic anhydrase forms the enzyme–inhibitor (EI) complex and, after 24 h, almost all of the drug is present in the various tissues in this form, most of it being found in the erythrocytes, kidney and stomach. The plasma half-life has two components. The fast one represents the distribution of the unbound diffusible acetazolamide throughout the body and takes about 2 h [52]. The EI complex has a slow dissociation constant; the drug is released slowly from the tissues and is then excreted unchanged in the urine. The half-life of the second phase is 10–12 h [49]. The volume of distribution of acetazolamide in humans based on total plasma concentration is 0.2 L/kg, and it is 1.8 L/kg when calculated from the free level in the plasma [49,50]. Following penetration into tissues, the concentration of acetazolamide in these tissues is higher than in plasma, and highest in erythrocytes. Acetazolamide penetrates into the brain slowly where its concentration is lower than in plasma, but higher than in the CSF. The concentration of acetazolamide in the CSF can be increased more than that in plasma by high doses of the drug. This effect suggests that acetazolamide is actively carried out of the CSF, and that saturation of the transport system blocks this transfer thereby increasing the drug level in CSF [49].

The drug does not undergo metabolic alteration, and 20% of its elimination by urine is by glomerular filtration and 80% by renal tubular excretion [2,50,51]. This is restricted to the unbound fraction in plasma [55]. A single oral dose of acetazolamide is recovered in the urine in 24 h [51].

Drug interactions

Because acetazolamide reduces the production and flow rate of CSF, it may theoretically increase the concentration of other central nervous system active drugs. On the other hand, drugs that inhibit CSF production, such as digitalis, may increase the concentration of acetazolamide in the CSF and brain [49]. Since acetazolamide is highly bound to plasma proteins, it is likely to compete with other drugs that are bound to the same proteins. Salicylate appears to competitively inhibit the plasma protein binding of acetazolamide and to simultaneously inhibit its secretion by renal tubules [56]. This is the explanation that was offered in two cases of elderly patients with glaucoma who were treated with aspirin and acetazolamide and developed symptoms of lethargy and confusion with metabolic acidosis [56]. In another report, an undesirable interaction was shown in three patients in whom acetazolamide was reported to interfere with primidone absorption, causing decreased levels of primidone in the plasma and urine [57]. Acetazolamide was reported to increase the serum concentration of carbamazepine in children when given concomitantly [31]. The mechanism of this interaction remains obscure.

Finally, since acetazolamide is not metabolized by the liver, drugs that either induct or inhibit liver enzymes do not affect its level.

Clinical trials

In 1952, Bergstrom et al. [6] were the first to use acetazolamide in the treatment of patients with epilepsy. Given that the drug leads to failure of acid excretion by the kidney, causing metabolic acidosis, the authors speculated that it might be similarly effective in patients with epilepsy as the use of a ketogenic diet. They administered acetazolamide 10–30 mg/kg daily as an adjuvant to 42 patients with intractable epilepsy (neither their ages nor type of seizures was mentioned). Seizure control of 50–100% was achieved in eight of the 42 (20%) patients, and in none did the condition worsen.

In the published studies, the selection of patients, definition of seizure type, the method of treatment and the follow-up period have varied widely and results are therefore difficult to compare [6,18–34,49,58,59] (Table 27.2).

Most studies have found acetazolamide to be effective in refractory generalized and partial seizures. However, these reports were compiled prior to the adoption of the International Classification of Seizures and Epilepsies, and only a few studies classified seizures according to the present classification: Golla and Hodge [23] described the efficacy of acetazolamide in patients with petit mal only. Oles et al. [32] referred to patients with partial epilepsy, and Resor and Resor [33], treated patients with juvenile myoclonic epilepsy. Many papers were relatively short-term studies that followed the patients for several weeks [24,25] or months [22,23,26,28]. Only a few long-term studies were conducted [18,21,29,30]. All the trials except one [20] were open label, non-randomized and uncontrolled. The only double-blind placebo-controlled study was performed by Millichap [20] in a paediatric population. He examined 14 children with refractory seizures secondary to brain injury. Except for one child who had myoclonic jerks alone, major seizures occurred in all patients. Acetazolamide tablets and a control placebo were given alternatively to successive patients in a double-blind fashion as add-on to the existing medications. Initially, 375 mg was given daily and according to response the dose was increased at intervals of 2–4 weeks up to a maximum of 750 mg daily. After an adequate trial of the new therapy, which varied in duration according to the response, the alternative preparation was substituted. The anticonvulsant effect of acetazolamide was also compared with that of phenytoin in five patients. The follow-up period was 5–26 weeks. Acetazolamide was superior to placebo, and comparable to phenytoin. In eight of the 14 (57%) patients the maximal seizure reduction was more than 75%, and in five (36%) a similar control was obtained at the end of the trial period. However most patients became tolerant to the antiepileptic effect of the drug. Some studies have had more disappointing results. Livingston *et al.* [22] evaluated a series of 58 children with various types of seizures that were treated with acetazolamide. While there was a decrease in the frequency of seizures in a few patients, no patient became seizure free. Ross [28] conducted a study on 63 patients with idiopathic, temporal lobe and symptomatic epilepsy. Only two children with petit mal had a prolonged response over 1 year, and two patients (one with idiopathic epilepsy and one with temporal lobe epilepsy) had temporary reduction of seizures.

Absence seizures

The rate of control of absence seizures with acetazolamide varied extensively ranging from none [22] to 97% [23]. All the studies performed were uncontrolled. Acetazolamide was administered as monotherapy and as an add-on drug.

Lombroso *et al.* [18] examined 126 patients, among them 29 cases with petit mal only, 41 with petit mal and other seizures, and 56 patients had seizures other than petit mal. Patients with petit mal only reported a 90–100% reduction of seizures in more than one-third of the studied cases. Interestingly, the patients who improved the most were those whose EEG showed 3 per second spike and wave activity and had prominent slowing in the EEG during hyperventilation. Indeed, Saldias *et al.* [60] showed that intravenously administered acetazolamide abolished or decreased the paroxysmal slow-wave discharges provoked by hyperventilation. Better response to treatment with acetazolamide in patients whose EEG showed 3 per second spike and wave activity and had prominent slowing in the EEG during hyperventilation was substantiated by Chao and Plumb [30] but not by others [21,25,27]. Ansell and Clarke [21] evaluated 26 patients, five of whom had petit mal seizures. The response was excellent in three of these five. In a long-term follow-up study, Lombroso and Forsythe [29], described 91 (33%) patients who had petit mal seizures, 48 (53%) of whom were treated with acetazolamide alone. In 42% of patients 90–100% seizure control was observed for 3 months, in 25% for 1 year and in only 10% for 3 years. In 43 patients who had 50% control of their seizures acetazolamide was used adjunctively. Following the addition, 44% had 90–100% control for 3 months; this declined to 7% by 3 years. Golla and Hodge [23] treated 78 patients of different ages exclusively with petit mal seizures, with the addition of 250 mg acetazolamide to the previous therapy; only two failed to respond; 34 (44%) patients became seizure free and the others (54%) improved significantly. The partial tolerance that the majority of patients developed after 3 months was responsive to increased dosage (i.e. to 500 mg daily) of the drug. Holowach and Thurston [27] used acetazolamide in 56 children with different types of seizures. In 14

patients with petit mal, nine had complete remission of seizures and in five partial control was achieved. In contrast, Livingston *et al.* [22] found no improvement in 15 patients with absence seizures following treatment with acetazolamide and in the study conducted by Ross [28], only in one patient of 11 who had petit mal were the attacks abolished by acetazolamide.

Myoclonic seizures

Lombroso and Forsythe [29] described 15 paediatric patients aged 6 months to 7 years with massive myoclonus who were treated with acetazolamide monotherapy: 20% had 90–100% seizure control after 3 months. Long-term tolerance developed probably because no patient had maintained this degree of control by the second and third years of follow-up. Chao and Plumb [30] reported fair improvement in five of seven patients with massive spasm; however, on the contrary, Baird and Borofsky [26] noted no improvement in 16 children with infantile myoclonic seizures who received acetazolamide daily as monotherapy. In one case report study of acetazolamide as an add-on drug, a dramatic improvement of action myoclonus was recorded in two patients with progressive myoclonic epilepsy [61].

Acetazolamide, as monotherapy (dosage range 500–1750 mg daily) was evaluated in the treatment of patients with juvenile myoclonic epilepsy in a retrospective study by Resor and Resor [33]. Although initially all the patients reported complete control of myoclonus on a long-term basis, only four remained free of myoclonic jerks.

Generalized tonic-clonic seizures

Many studies that described patients with generalized seizures did not differentiate between primary and secondary generalized tonic-clonic seizures. Ansell and Clarke [21] described 26 patients, six of whom had major idiopathic epilepsy and were treated with acetazolamide as monotherapy. Excellent response was noted at the beginning in all patients, however only three patients remained seizure free for a follow-up of 18 months. In the study by Resor and Resor [33], 51 patients with juvenile myoclonic epilepsy were treated with acetazolamide monotherapy either because of a poor response to conventional antiepileptic drugs or to avoid valproate-associated side-effects. Fourteen out of 31 patients (45%) who had generalized tonic-clonic seizures became seizure free for 10–70 months. Holowach and Thurston [27] administered acetazolamide to four patients with grand mal seizures that had not been controlled on their previous medications, in three of them complete remission was noted. Of the 277 patients studied by Lombroso and Forsythe [29], 19 had grand mal seizures only. In 15 patients, acetazolamide was given as add-on treatment and as monotherapy to the remaining four. For 3 months, 90–100% seizure control was observed in 63% of all patients, in 37% for 1 year, 11% for 2 years and only 5% had maintained this degree of control at the end of 3 years.

In their study, Forsythe *et al.* [31] evaluated acetazolamide as an add-on treatment to carbamazepine in 54 children, 40 of whom had exclusively grand mal seizures. Twenty-four (60%) patients with generalized seizures had seizure frequency reduction of 50–100% at the 2-year follow-up. Relapse or no control after 2 years was noted in 16 children. Contrary to the above studies, Ross [28] and

Table 27.2 Clinical trials with acetazolamide

Reference	No. of evaluated pts	Age range	Diagnosis/seizure type	Therapeutic regimen	Follow-up period	Seizure decrease—no. (%) pts			Side-effects—no. (%) pts
						90–100%	>50%	No sig. effect	
Bergstrom et al. [6]	42		Refractory epilepsy	10–30 mg/kg	Not mentioned	4 (10)	4 (10)	34 (80)	Fatigue, flushing, polydipsia, hyperpnoea, paraesthesia, headache
Lombroso et al. [18]	126	82 pts <12 y, 24 pts 12–19 y, 20 pts >20 y	All seizures, 29 petit mal, 41 petit mal and other seizures, 56 non petit mal	8–30 mg/kg, 250–1500 mg/day, 63 pts mono, 63 pts add-on	3–36 m	46 (36), 8 (27), 19 (46), 20 (36)	22 (17), 4 (14), 8 (20), 9 (16)	58 (46), 17 (59), 14 (34), 27 (48)	Drowsiness 19 (15), anorexia 17 (13), irritability 11 (9), rash, tingling, dizziness, enuresis, vomiting, ataxia, hyperpnoea in 2–5 (2–4)
Merlis [19]	47	19–64 y	Chronic epilepsy with psychosis	500–1000 mg/day, 13 pts mono, 34 pts add-on	11 m	29 (62)	6 (13)	12 (25)	Transient flushing, headache, fatigue in 4 (9)
Millichap [20]	14	6 m–11 y	All seizures, 6 generalized, 7 focal, 1 myoclonic jerks	18–36 mg/kg, 750 mg/day, Double-blind placebo-controlled, 2 pts mono	5–26 w		5 (36)		Anorexia 5 (36), polyuria 5 (36), nocturnal enuresis 4 (28), drowsiness 3 (21), vomiting 1 (7), diarrhoea 1 (7)
Ansell and Clarke [21]	26	12–38 y	23 idiopathic generalized, 3 symptomatic	3–14 mg/kg, 9 pts mono, 17 pts add-on	1.5–20 m	8 (31)	6 (23)	12 (46)	5 (19) paraesthesia, 4 (15) drowsiness, 1 (4) depression
Livingston et al. [22]	58	8 m–14 y	25 major motor, 18 minor motor, 15 petit mal	"1250 mg/day, 14 pts mono, 44 pts add-on	2–6 m	Temporary decrease in the frequency of seizures in a few pts		25 (100), 18 (100), 15 (100)	
Golla and Hodge [23]	78	6–35 y	Petit mal	250 mg add on	3–10 m	76 (97)		2 (3)	Transient tingling of hands and feet, and somnolence
Minde et al. [24]	20	5–36 y	Symptomatic	12 mg/kg mono and add-on	50 days	12 (60)	5 (25), No improvement in pts on mono	3 (15)	Fatigue 3 (15), diarrhoea 2 (10), excitement 1 (5)
Wada et al. [25]	21	10 m–40 y	Convulsive group, petit mal group, psychomotor group	250–1000 mg/day, 5 pts mono, 16 pts add-on	8–85 days	6 (29)	6 (29)	9 (42)	Increased diuresis 6 (28)
Baird and Borofsky [26]	16	Children	Infantile spasm	1000 mg/day mono	1–3 m			16 (100)	
Holowach and Thurston [27]	56	3 m–16 y	All seizures, 4 grand mal, 14 petit mal, 20 focal (frontal and temporal), 11 massive myoclonic, 1 tonic, 6 mixed	250–1000 mg/day add-on	2–20 m	35 (63), 3 (75), 9 (64), 12 (60), 5 (47), 6 (100)	9 (16), 1 (25), 5 (36), 1 (5), 3 (27)	12 (21), 1 (25), 7 (35), 3 (27), 1 (100)	Drowsiness 2 (4), excitability 1 (2), numbness and tingling 2 (4), nocturnal enuresis 1 (2)

Study	No. of pts	Age	Seizure type (n)	Dose / treatment	Follow-up duration	Follow-up 3 m	3 y	At 2-year follow-up	Side effects
Ross [28]	63	17 children; 46 adults	11 petit mal only; 30 petit mal and grand mal; 12 temporal lobe; 10 miscellaneous	125–750 mg/day add-on	2–6 m	1 (9); 1 (3)		10 (90); 29 (97); 12 (100); 10 (100)	Nausea, dizziness, tingling in 5 (8)
Lombroso and Forsythe [29]	277	201 <12 y; 47 12–19 y; 29 >20 y	91 petit mal; 19 grand mal; 61 grand mal and petit mal; 24 psychomotor; 82 mixed	8–30 mg/kg; 250–1500 mg; >50% mono	3 y	38 (42); 12 (63)	9 (10); 1 (5)		Drowsiness, anorexia, irritability, nausea, vomiting, enuresis, paraesthesia, headache, dizziness, hyperventilation in 30 (11)
Chao and Plumb [30]	178	3 m–40 y	All seizures; 55 convulsive equivalent; 50 symptomatic; 20 temporal; 28 other focal; 18 generalized idiopathic; 7 massive spasm	15–30 mg/kg; 20 pts mono; 158 pts add-on	3 m–3 y	6 (26); 25 (30); 76 (43); 30 (55); 17 (34); 8 (40); 8 (29); 13 (72)	0 (0); 0 (0)	44 (25); 13 (24); 12 (24); 6 (30); 8 (29); 5 (71) — 55 (32); 12 (21); 21 (42); 6 (30); 12 (42); 5 (28); 2 (29)	Anorexia 27 (15), vomiting 10 (6), drowsiness 11 (6), irritability 8 (4), headache 7 (4), fatigue 6 (3), dizziness 5 (3), enuresis 5 (3), paraesthesia 4 (2); ataxia, depression, irregular respiration, polyuria, poor sleep, skin rash in 1
Forsythe et al. [31]	54	3–14 y	40 grand mal; 14 temporal lobe seizures	10–15 mg/kg add-on	2–5 y	16 (40); 7 (50)		8 (20), 16 (40); 2 (14), 5 (36)	Drowsiness 3 (5), ataxia 3 (5), nausea and vomiting 1 (2), paraesthesia 1 (2), school work deterioration 2 (4)
Oles et al. [32]	48	6–64 y	Partial seizures	3.8–22 mg/kg add-on	1–30 m	7 (15)		14 (29), 27 (56)	Lethargy 4 (8), paraesthesia 6 (12), anorexia 2 (4), nausea 3 (6), diarrhoea 2 (4), headache 1 (2), visual changes 1 (2)
Resor and Resor [33]	31		Juvenile myoclonic epilepsy; 31 GTCS; 31 myoclonus	500–1750 mg mono	10–70 m	14 (45); 4 (13)		17 (55)	Occasional paraesthesia, transient diuresis, weight loss 4 (13), renal calculi 6 (20)
Lim et al. [34]	20	16–43 y	Catamenial: 10 temporal; 8 extratemporal; 1 generalized; 1 not classified	125–750 mg add-on		8 (40)		8 (40)	Dizziness 3 (15), polyuria 3 (15)

pts: patients; Add-on, add-on treatment; GTCS, generalized tonic-clonic seizures; mono: monotherapy.

Livingstone *et al.* [22] found no improvement in patients with major motor seizures following treatment with acetazolamide.

Focal seizures

Lombroso and Forsythe [29] conducted a long-term follow-up study examining 24 patients with psychomotor seizures; six (26%) became seizure free after 3 months, only 10% were 90–100% seizure free for 1 and 2 years, and after 2 years none was seizure free. Chao and Plumb [30] evaluated retrospectively the value of acetazolamide in treating 178 patients of different ages, 48 of whom had temporal lobe or other focal seizures. In 16 (33%) of these patients, an 80–100% response was reported, and 14 (29%) had more than a 50% seizure reduction. Holowach and Thurston [27] used acetazolamide in 20 children with focal epilepsy who had not been controlled on their previous medications. In 12 (60%) of them over 90% seizure reduction was reported.

Forsythe *et al.* [31] evaluated long-term efficacy of acetazolamide as an add-on treatment to carbamazepine in 54 children of whom 14 had temporal lobe seizures only. Of these patients, nine (64%) had a reduction in seizure frequency of 70–100% at the 2-year follow-up; however, at the 3–5-year follow-up, six of the responders were found to have relapsed.

Oles *et al.* [32] identified, retrospectively, 48 children and adults with refractory partial seizures with acetazolamide as an adjunct to carbamazepine: 21 (44%) of them had a greater than 50% decrease in seizure frequency but only three became seizure free, while three patients lost response. Discouraging results were reported by Ross [28] who identified 12 patients with temporal lobe epilepsy only one of whom had a temporary reduction of seizures and no effect was apparent in the other 11.

Catamenial seizures

Body water content changes occur normally in women in the premenstrual phase. Gamble suggested that fluid balance has a role in the generation of seizures [62]. Excessive water ingestion was thought to produce seizures whereas dehydration was thought to have the opposite effect. Acetazolamide has a diuretic effect, which was thought to be part of its antiepileptic effect, and this was the rationale behind treatment with this drug in women with catamenial seizures. However, as pointed out by Ansell and Clarke [63], no significant differences in total body water were observed when comparing women with epilepsy and healthy controls or women with or without catamenial epilepsy treated with acetazolamide.

Although this mechanism of action was questioned [63], the exacerbation of the seizures during menstruation responded quite well without any side-effects to administration of acetazolamide in dosages of 250–500 mg daily for 5–7 days prior to the onset of the menstrual period and for its duration [64]. In three patients with catamenial exacerbation of generalized tonic-clonic or absence seizures, Ansell and Clarke [21] showed that only increasingly higher doses of the drug could maintain seizure control for a maximum follow-up of 4 months after the last period. The authors also described improvement for 3 months in two patients who were given acetazolamide only on the day before and the day of onset of menstruation; a prolonged follow-up, however, was not performed. Goetting [65] reported a case of postanoxic myoclonus severely ex-

acerbated premenstrually: 1000 mg acetazolamide given intermittently during 5 days starting at the onset of each exacerbation produced prompt and marked improvement. Ross [28], however, observed no response to acetazolamide in eight of the 25 menstruating females with epilepsy who reported having seizures related to their period.

In a retrospective study, Lim *et al.* [34] conducted a telephone questionnaire addressing the relationship of seizures and menstrual cycle. Twenty women were identified. The drug was given as an add-on drug in all patients but one. It was given continuously in 55% and intermittently in 45%. More than 59% decrease in seizure frequency was reported by 40% of the subjects, and the responses were similar in both focal and generalized seizures. There was no difference in effectiveness between continuous and intermittent dosing. Loss of efficacy was reported by 15% of patients over 6–24 months.

Dosage

The dosages by body weight used in different studies in children and adults with epilepsy varied from 3 to 36 mg/kg, whereas the total dose varied from 125 to 1750 mg.

The recommended dose for adults is 10–20 mg/kg, or 500–1000 mg/day, given 2–3 times daily [49,59]. Plasma levels with this dosage were reported to be 10–14 μg/mL [49]. The doses reported in children were 10–36 mg/kg [20,29,31]. Lombroso and Forsythe [29] noted that increasing doses above 750 mg was rarely effective and 500 mg/day was usually the maximal useful dose in children less than 7 years of age [29]. Monitoring plasma concentration is generally probably not helpful [32]. The starting dose should be in children 125 mg and in adults 250 mg twice daily, and it should be increased every week. The considerations of increasing dosage should be based on tolerance to adverse effects and seizure frequency. Slow discontinuation over several weeks is recommended to prevent withdrawal seizures [59]. Individuals at higher risk include older patients with reduced renal function who should have their dose reduced to avoid acidosis [66].

Tolerance

The use of acetazolamide has been limited by reports of development of tolerance to its effects; this loss of effect over time has proved to be a major consideration in the adoption of acetazolamide as therapy in epilepsy. On prolonged treatment, animals develop tolerance to the anti-maximal electro-shock (anti-MES) effects of acetazolamide [44,47,67,68]. Tolerance of acetazolamide is believed to develop due to increased amount and increased activity of carbonic anhydrase in glial cells, as well as proliferation of glial cells [44,67,68]. Patients with epilepsy were reported to develop tolerance after variable periods of time [18,20,21,29]. Loss of efficacy was noted in some studies after several weeks [20,21] and in other studies after months [18,23] or even years [29,31]. The development of tolerance was similar in patients with focal as well as generalized seizures. Once tolerance has developed, withdrawal of the drug for a period of time occasionally restored the antiepileptic effect [23].

Table 27.3 Adverse reactions

Potentially life-threatening effects
Blood disorders: aplastic anaemia, agranulocytosis,
  thrombocytopenia
Renal failure

Other adverse effects
Gastrointestinal symptoms: change in taste, abdominal discomfort,
  nausea, anorexia, diarrhoea
Paraesthesia of hands, feet and circumoral region
Increased diuresis
Drowsiness, dizziness, fatigue
Headache
Hyperpnoea, shortness of breath
Metabolic acidosis
Nephrolithiasis

Side-effects

Acetazolamide is a relatively safe drug. Most of the reported side-effects seem to be related to inhibition of carbonic anhydrase, with the exception of idiosyncratic reactions.

Idiosyncratic reaction (Table 27.3)

Isolated cases of acetazolamide-associated aplastic anaemia have been reported. A 73-year-old man who was treated with acetazolamide 250 mg daily because of oedema of the lower legs developed severe bone marrow depression, which resulted in death after 1 month of therapy [69]. Keisu *et al.* [70] reported 11 cases of acetazolamide-associated aplastic anaemia from voluntary recording over 17 years. Most of the patients were elderly and none was being treated for epilepsy. Since most of them were being treated with other drugs as well, Shapiro and Fraunfelder [71] had reservations about this relatively high incidence being attributed to the drug.

Allergic reactions to acetazolamide also include agranulocytosis that was described in a 66-year-old woman treated with 250 mg of the drug as an adjunct to digitalis and a low salt diet because of arteriosclerotic heart disease and peripheral oedema [72]. An 85-year-old man treated for congestive heart failure with acetazolamide 750 mg daily developed acute thrombocytopenia [73]. Acute renal failure has been described on rare occasions [74]. There are also a number of acute skin reactions attributed to acetazolamide, some of which can be very severe, and fatal cases of necrodermatolysis and Stevens–Johnson reactions have been reported. Cross-sensitivity to acetazolamide in patients allergic to sulfa drugs can occur [75].

Common symptomatic side-effects (Tables 27.2, 27.3)

Side-effects are encountered mainly upon drug initiation and most of them are transient. Patients with glaucoma, perhaps because of their age, have more difficulties in tolerating the drug [76], whereas patients with epilepsy tend to have fewer side-effects [29]. The most common side-effects include, drowsiness, fatigue, dizziness, paraesthesia of hands and feet, gastrointestinal symptoms such as nausea, vomiting and diarrhoea, loss of libido, diuresis, headache and hy-

perventilation [8,18–21,24,25,27–34,77]. In the largest study of 277 patients by Lombroso and Forsythe [29], 11% of patients reported the following side-effects in descending order of frequency: drowsiness, anorexia, irritability, nausea, vomiting, enuresis, headache, thirst, dizziness and hyperventilation. These side-effects were reported in 8–30% in most studies in patients with epilepsy [18–21,24,25,27–34]. Transient distortion of normal taste secondary to acetazolamide was described to carbonated and non-carbonated beverages and food, and was speculated to be due to altered taste receptors secondary to ingestion of carbonic anhydrase [78].

Interestingly enough, favourable effects were occasionally noted during treatment with acetazolamide manifested by improved behaviour and mental status [18,25].

Other side-effects

Metabolic acidosis

Acetazolamide has the potential risk of inducing metabolic acidosis by inhibiting carbonic anhydrase activity in the proximal tubular epithelium of the kidney which leads to diuresis, the excessive excretion of sodium and potassium ions, and alkaline urine. Although the metabolic acidosis which is produced is mild, it can sometimes be symptomatic, especially in elderly patients and in patients with renal failure [68,79].

In a study by Epstein and Grant [76], 44 of 92 (48%) patients treated with acetazolamide for chronic glaucoma complained of a symptom complex syndrome that included malaise, fatigue, weight loss, depression, anorexia and often the loss of libido. Patients with this syndrome were found to be significantly more acidotic. Although these symptoms are frequently associated with the development of mild metabolic acidosis and perhaps a subclinical respiratory acidosis, the central nature of these side-effects suggests that inhibition of brain carbonic anhydrase may also be important in their pathogenesis. These symptoms develop slowly and are often difficult to diagnose, especially in the elderly. The best documented treatment is the supplementation of sodium bicarbonate 56–70 mmol daily orally [76]. Sodium acetate administration has also been reported to be helpful [80].

The metabolic acidosis associated with acetazolamide was speculated to cause growth suppression in children when receiving it in combination with other antiepileptic drugs [81].

Increased incidence of kidney stones

This effect was described in association with acetazolamide intake. The mechanisms include induction of partial renal tubular acidosis with resultant hypercalciuria and hypocitraturia, both recognized risk factors for stone formation [82]. The occurrence of nephrolithiasis with acetazolamide was of special concern in patients treated with this drug for epilepsy [33] and glaucoma [83]. The frequency of stone formation varied among different reports: it was very rare in children treated for epilepsy (i.e. one of 277) [29]; however, six of 14 (43%) young adults with juvenile myoclonic epilepsy [33] were reported to have developed renal calculi without correlation to dosage. Kass *et al.* [83] reported a frequency as high as 12% in patients with glaucoma. Citrate supplementation and hydration may be effective in reducing stone formation [82].

Effect on bone

The data available on the effects of acetazolamide on bone are somewhat contradictory and the role of carbonic anhydrase in human bone resorption is not certain. Acetazolamide may accelerate osteomalacia through several mechanisms that include urinary calcium and phosphate excretion and systemic acidosis [84]. Mallette [84] described two patients with osteomalacia under treatment with acetazolamide, however both patients were also treated with barbiturates. In postmenopausal women with glaucoma, long-term (more than 4 years) carbonic anhydrase inhibitor use was associated with a bone-sparing effect, as judged by spinal bone mineral density [85]. This effect was absent in premenopausal women and in those who received acetazolamide for less than 2 years.

Effects on the fetus and newborn

Layton and Hallesy [86] reported that rats fed with acetazolamide in their diet during pregnancy gave birth to offspring in which about 36% had a defect confined mainly to the right forepaw. The plasma levels achieved were of the same order of magnitude as those generated in patients who receive 500–1500 mg acetazolamide. Similar susceptibility was also observed in mice and hamsters but not in monkeys [87]. Only one human case of multiple congenital malformations (glaucoma, microphthalmia and patent ductus arteriosus) was described in a letter from Lederle Laboratories in 1975, cited by Worsham *et al.* [88]. In a neonate of a 22-year-old patient treated with acetazolamide 750 mg daily because of glaucoma, sacrococcygeal teratoma was described [88].

There are no adequate and well-controlled studies in pregnant women and therefore the overall risk of fetal malformations associated with maternal treatment with acetazolamide has not been established.

A possible association between treatment for glaucoma throughout pregnancy with 500 mg acetazolamide and metabolic acidosis, hypocalcaemia and hypomagnesaemia was reported in a single preterm infant [89].

Soderam *et al.* [90] reported a very low dose of acetazolamide having been transferred to the child in breast milk: it was less than 0.7% of the dose per kilogram of body weight of the mother. Based on their findings, they speculated that it is unlikely that breastfeeding by an acetazolamide-treated mother would lead to any harmful effects upon the child.

Clinical therapeutics

Proof of efficacy studies of acetazolamide is restricted mainly to retrospective, uncontrolled studies. In the available papers (published mainly in the 1950s), the selection of patients, seizure type, method and duration of treatment, and definition of efficacy varied extensively, which makes it difficult to compare the investigated conditions with the seizures and syndromes as currently classified.

Most patients treated with acetazolamide were patients with refractory seizures who failed other antiepileptic treatment. Nonetheless, many studies define acetazolamide as an antiepileptic drug with a broad spectrum of action. Although some studies [22,28] failed to demonstrate its usefulness, efficacy in different types of seizures was shown in most of the published works. The best results

were reported with absence seizures [18,23,29], however good results have been observed in generalized tonic-clonic seizures [21,29,31,33], myoclonic seizures [29,30,33], as well as in partial seizures [29–32]. Viewed together, many of these studies suggest that acetazolamide is beneficial in reducing seizure frequency, and in some of the studies the patients had an initially spectacular effect. Thus, acetazolamide may be helpful mainly as an add-on drug in children and adults mainly with generalized seizures, particularly with absences, but in partial seizures as well. The lack of effect of acetazolamide on hepatic enzymes renders it valuable when drug interaction is a problem. The anticonvulsant effect of acetazolamide is prompt [27], and therefore the drug may be useful when rapid onset of effect is needed. The use of acetazolamide has been limited by reports of high development of tolerance. Loss of seizure control had been reported as early as several weeks after instituting treatment or after months and years, and occasionally elevated dosages were required to maintain equal effect. Since cyclical dosing may reduce the development of tolerance, acetazolamide has been proposed as an adjunct drug that is used intermittently in the therapy of catamenial epilepsy. However, controlled studies are warranted for documenting this type of effect before it can be recommended for use in regular practice. Other antiepileptic drugs are also well known to develop tolerance. For example, benzodiazepines that are used as adjuncts in partial seizures also have significant tolerance. Controlled studies designed to compare the development of tolerance of acetazolamide to benzodiazepines may be valuable.

Precautions and contraindications
(Tables 27.3, 27.4)

Experience with acetazolamide shows that it is a relatively safe agent, and that it can be used for long periods of time without serious side-effects.

Because of rare cases of aplastic anaemia, agranulocytosis and thrombocytopenia, obtaining a complete blood count before initiating treatment with the drug should be recommended. The usefulness of repeated tests is unknown. Patients with compromised renal function need a reduced dosage of acetazolamide because the ability to clear the drug correlates with creatinine clearance [55]. Liver disease is a contraindication to the systemic use of acetazolamide. Alkalinization of the urine diverts ammonia of renal origin from urine into the systemic circulation, causing hepatic encephalopathy [91]. Because of its tendency to cause potassium loss, acetazolamide is contraindicated in Addison's disease and adrenal insufficiency.

Whenever acetazolamide is given with carbamazepine, monitoring of serum sodium concentration may be indicated because both

Table 27.4 High-risk groups

Elderly patients
Concomitant disorders
  renal failure
  hepatic failure
  adrenal insufficiency
  conditions associated with sodium and potassium depletion
  sulfonamide hypersensitivity

drugs lower sodium [49], and carbamazepine levels should also be studied [31]. Also, special attention should be paid towards hydration when acetazolamide is given in combination with topiramate since both drugs are associated with development of renal calculi.

Acetazolamide is an animal teratogen [86,87]. In light of the two cases of possible teratogenicity related to acetazolamide that have been described [88], this effect should be taken into consideration when treating women of childbearing age.

In spite of the fact that we currently have an extensive choice of antiepileptic drugs, the inability of the current antiepileptic drugs to curtail seizure frequency in about 25% of patients underscores the fact that the 'magic bullet' remains elusive. When plowing through the articles reporting treatment with acetazolamide, it was apparent to the author that acetazolamide has been too quickly abandoned in favour of newer antiepileptic drugs without having undergone comprehensive evaluations for its potential therapeutic value, whether as an adjunct drug or as monotherapy in comparative studies. In some patients a dramatic effect has been observed, and a worthwhile effect is reported widely in many patients and in differing types of epilepsy. The major drawbacks to its usage are the potential for tolerance to develop and the risk of idiosyncratic reactions. The former though does not occur in all patients and the latter is rare. The drug is simple and easy to use and generally well tolerated. Even if its usefulness turns out to be limited, acetazolamide warrants re-evaluation using modern standards and appropriate controlled studies, as a drug of potentially considerable value in various forms of epilepsy.

References

1 Mann T, Keilin T. Sulphanilamide as a specific inhibitor of carbonic anhydrase. *Nature* 1940; 146: 164–65.
2 Maren TH. Carbonic anhydrase: chemistry, physiology, and inhibition. *Physiol Rev* 1967; 47: 595–765.
3 Carter MJ. Carbonic anhydrase: isoenzymes, properties, distribution and functional significance. *Biol Rev* 1972; 47: 465–513.
4 Cohen ME, Cobb S. Anticonvulsive action of azosulfamide in patients with epilepsy. *Arch Neurol Psychiatr* 1941; 46: 676–91.
5 Roblin RO, Clapp JW. The preparation of heterocyclic sulfonamides *J Am Chem Soc* 1950; 72: 4890–2.
6 Bergstrom WH, Carzoli RF, Lombroso C, Davidson DT, Wallace WM. Observations on the metabolic and clinical effects of carbonic-anhydrase inhibitors in epileptics. *Am J Dis Child* 1952; 84: 771–3.
7 Millichap JG, Woodbury DM, Goodman LS. Mechanism of the anticonvulsant action of acetazolamide, a carbonic anhydrase inhibitor. *J Pharmacol Exper Ther* 1955; 115: 251–8.
8 Gray WD, Maren TH, Sisson GM, Smith FH. Carbonic anhydrase inhibition VII. Carbonic anhydrase inhibition and anticonvulsant effect. *J Pharmacol Exp Ther* 1957; 121: 160–70.
9 Becker B. Decrease in intraocular pressure in man by a carbonic anhydrase inhibitor, diamox. *Am J Ophthalmol* 1954; 37: 13–15.
10 Belsky H. Use of new oral diuretic, Diamox in congestive heart disease. *N Engl J Med* 1953; 140: 249.
11 Ahlskog JE, O'neill BP. Pseudotumor Cerebri. *Ann Int Med* 1982; 97: 249–56.
12 Griggs RC, Moxley RT, Lafrance RA, McQuillen J. Hereditary paroxysmal ataxia: response to acetazolamide. *Neurology* 1978; 28: 1259–64.
13 Sethi KD, Hess DC, Huffnagle VH, Adams RJ. Acetazolamide treatment of paroxysmal dystonia in central demyelinating disease. *Neurology* 1992; 42: 919–21.
14 Lancman ME, Asconape JJ, Walker F. Acetazolamide appears effective in the management of valproic-induced tremor. *Mov Disord* 1994; 9: 369.
15 Riggs JE. Periodic paralysis. *Clin Neuropharmacol* 1989; 12: 249–57.
16 Griggs RC, Moxley RT, Riggs JE, Engel WK. Effects of acetazolamide on myotonia. *Ann Neurol* 1978; 3: 531–7.
17 Ellsworth AJ, Larson EB, Strickland D. A randomized trial of dexamethasone and acetazolamide for acute mountain sickness prophylaxis. *Am J Med* 1987; 83: 1024–9.
18 Lombroso CT, Davidson DT, Grossi-Bianchi ML. Further evaluation of acetazolamide (Diamox) in treatment of epilepsy. *JAMA* 1956; 160: 268–72.
19 Merlis S. Diamox: A carbonic anhydrase inhibitor: its use in epilepsy. *Neurology* 1956; 4: 863–8.
20 Millichap JG. Anticonvulsant action of diamox in children. *Neurology* 1956; 6: 552–9.
21 Ansell B, Clarke E. Acetazolamide in the treatment of epilepsy. *Br Med J* 1956; 1: 650–61.
22 Livingston S, Peterson D, Boks L. Ineffectiveness of diamox in the treatment of childhood epilepsy. *Pediatrics* 1956; 17: 541.
23 Golla F, Hodge SR. Control of petit mal by acetazolamide. *J Ment Sci* 1957; 103: 214–17.
24 Minde M, Garret GM, Cruise SE. Acetazolamide (Diamox) in the treatment of epilepsy. *S Afr Med J* 1957; 31: 563–6.
25 Wada T, Tokijiro S, Morita S. Diamox acetazolamide in the treatment of epilepsy. *Dis Nerv Syst* 1957; 18: 110–17.
26 Baird HW, Borofsky LG. Infantile myoclonic seizures. *J Pediatr* 1957; 50: 332–9.
27 Holowach J, Thurston DL. A clinical evaluation of acetazolamide (Diamox) in the treatment of epilepsy in children. *J Pediatr* 1958; 53: 160–71.
28 Ross IP. Acetazolamide therapy in epilepsy. *Lancet* 1958; 275: 1308–9.
29 Lombroso CT, Forsythe I. A long-term follow-up of acetazolamide (Diamox) in the treatment of epilepsy. *Epilepsia* 1960; 1: 493–500.
30 Chao DH, Plumb RL. Diamox in epilepsy. *J Pediatr* 1961; 58: 211–18.
31 Forsythe WI, Owens JR, Toothill C. Effectiveness of acetazolamide in the treatment of carbamazepine-resistant epilepsy in children. *Dev Med Child Neurol* 1981; 23: 761–9.
32 Oles KS, Penry JK, Cole DL, Howard G. Use of acetazolamide as an adjunct to carbamazepine in refractory partial seizures. *Epilepsia* 1989; 30: 74–8.
33 Resor SR, Resor LD. Chronic acetazolamide monotherapy in the treatment of juvenile myoclonic epilepsy. *Neurology* 1990; 40: 1677–81
34 Lim L, Foldvary N, Maschs E, Lee J. Acetazolamide in women with catamenial epilepsy. *Epilepsia* 2001; 42: 746–9
35 Giacobini E. A cytochemical study of the localization of carbonic anhydrase in the nervous system. *J Neurochem* 1962; 9: 169–77.
36 Rogers JH, Hunt SP. Carbonic anhydrase-II messenger RNA in neurons and glia of chick brain: Mapping by in situ hybridization. *Neuroscience* 1987; 23: 343–61.
37 Cammer W. Carbonic anhydrase in oligodendrocytes and myelin in the central nervous system. *Ann NY Acad Sci* 1984; 429: 494–7.
38 Roussel G, Delaunoy JP, Nussbaum JL, Mandel P. Demonstration of a specific localization of carbonic anhydrase C in the glial cells of rat CNS by an immunohistochemical method. *Brain Res* 1979; 160: 47–54.
39 Woodbury DM, Engstrom FL, White HS, Chen CF, Kemp JW, Chow SY. Ionic and acid-base regulation of neurons and glia during seizures. *Ann Neurol* 1984; 16 (Suppl.): S135–S144.
40 Maren TH. The general physiology of reactions catalyzed by carbonic anhydrase and their inhibition by sulfonamides. *Ann NY Acad Sci* 1984; 429: 568–79.
41 Woodbury DM. Antiepileptic drugs. Carbonic anhydrase inhibitors. In: Glaser GH, Penry JK, Woodbury DM, eds. *Antiepileptic Drugs: mechanism of action.* New York: Raven Press, 1980: 617–33.
42 Woodbury DM, Esplin DW. Neuropharmacology and neurochemistry of anticonvulsant drugs. *Proc Assoc Res Nerv Ment Dis* 1969; 37: 24–56.
43 Anderson RE, Howard RA, Woodbury DM. Correlation between effects of acute acetazolamide administration in mice on electroshock seizure pattern, and on carbonic anhydrase activity in subcellular fractions of the brain. *Epilepsia* 1986; 27: 504–9.
44 Engstrom FI, White HS, Kemp JW, Woodbury DM. Acute and chronic acetazolamide administration in DBA and C57 mice: effects of age. *Epilepsia* 1986; 27: 19–26.
45 Woodbury DM, Rollins LT, Gardner MD et al. Effects of carbon dioxide on brain excitability and electrolyte. *Am J Physiol* 1958; 192: 79–90.

46 Tanimukai H, Inui M, Hariguchi S, Kaneko Z. Antiepileptic property of inhibitors of carbonic anhydrase. *Biochem Pharmacol* 1965; 14: 961–70.

47 Koch A, Woodbury DM. Effects of carbonic anhydrase inhibition on brain excitability. *J Pharmacol Exp Ther* 1958; 122: 335–42.

48 Woodbury DM, Karler R. The role of carbon dioxide in the nervous system. *Anesthesiology* 1960; 21: 686–703.

49 Resor SR, Resor LD, Woodbury DM, Kemp JW. Other antiepileptic drugs. Acetazolamide. In: Levy RH, Mattson RH, Meldrum BS, eds. *Antiepileptic Drugs*, 4th edn. New York: Raven Press, 1995: 969–85.

50 Maren TH, Mayer E, Wadsworth BC. Carbonic anhydrase inhibitor. I. The pharmacology of Diamox (2-acetylamino-1,3,4-thiadiazole-5-sulfonamide). *Bull Johns Hopkins Hosp* 1954; 95: 199–243.

51 Maren TH, Robinson B. The pharmacology of acetazolamide as related to cerebrospinal fluid in the treatment of hydrocephalus. *Bull Johns Hopkins Hosp* 1960; 106: 1–24.

52 Wallace SM, Shah VP, Rigelman S. GLC analysis of acetazolamide in blood, plasma and saliva following oral administration to normal subjects. *J Pharm Sci* 1977; 66: 527–30.

53 Bayne WF, Rogers G, Crisologo N. Assay for acetazolamide in plasma. *J Pharm Sci* 1975; 64: 402–4.

54 Joyce PW, Mills KB, Richardson T, Mawer GE. Equivalence of conventional and sustained release oral dosage formulations of acetazolamide in primary open angle glaucoma. *Br J Clin Pharmacol* 1989; 27: 597–606.

55 Chapron DJ, Sweeney KR, Feig PU, Kramer PA. Influence of advanced age on the disposition of azetazolamide. *Br J Clin Pharmacol* 1985; 19: 363–71.

56 Sweeney KR, Chapron DJ, Brandt JL, Gomoling IH, Feig PU, Kramer PA. Toxic interaction between acetazolamide and salicylate: case reports and a pharmacokinetic explanation. *Clin Pharmacol Ther* 1986; 40: 518–24.

57 Syversen GB, Morgan JP, Weintraub M, Myers GJ. Acetazolamide-induced interference with primidone absorption. Case reports and metabolic studies. *Arch Neurol* 1977; 34: 80–4.

58 Ramsey RE, De Toledo J. Acetazolamide. In: Engel J, Pedley TA, eds. *Epilepsy: a comprehensive textbook.* Philadelphia: Lippincott-Raven Publishers, 1997: 1455–61.

59 Reiss WG, Oles KS. Acetazolamide in the treatment of seizures. *Ann Pharmacother* 1996; 30: 514–19.

60 Saldias C, Carbiese F, Eidelberg E. Electroencephalographic changes induced by the intravenous administration of acetazolamide (Diamox) in epileptic patients. *Electroencephalogr Clin Neurophysiol* 1957; 9: 333–6.

61 Vaamonde J, Legarda I, Jimenez J, Obeso JA. Acetazolamide improves action myoclonus in Ramsay Hunt syndrome. *Clin Neuropharmacol* 1992; 15: 392–6.

62 Gamble JL. Epilepsy: evidences of body fluid volume disturbance. *Arch Neurol Psychiatry* 1930; 23: 915–19.

63 Ansell B, Clarke E. Epilepsy and menstruation: the role of water retention. *Lancet* 1956; 2: 1232–5.

64 Poser CM. Modification of therapy for exacerbation of seizures during menstruation. *J Pediatr* 1974; 84: 779.

65 Goetting MG. Catamenial exacerbation of action myoclonus: successful treatment with acetazolamide. *J Neurol Neurosurg Psychiatr* 1985; 40: 1304–5.

66 Heller I, Halevy J, Cohen S, Theodor E. Significant metabolic acidosis induced by acetazolamide: not a rare complication. *Arch Intern Med* 1985; 145: 1815–17.

67 Banks DA, Anderson RE, Woodbury DM. Induction of new carbonic anhydrase II following treatment with acetazolamide in DBA and C57 mice. *Epilepsia* 1986; 27: 510–15.

68 Anderson RE, Chiu P, Woodbury DM. Mechanism of tolerance to the anticonvulsant effects of acetazolamide in mice: relation to the activity and amount of carbonic anhydrase in brain. *Epilepsia* 1989; 30: 208–16.

69 Underwood LC. Fatal bone marrow depression after treatment with acetazolamide (Diamox). *JAMA* 1956; 15: 1477–8.

70 Keisu M, Wihlom BE, Ost A, Mortimer O. Acetazolamide-associated aplastic anemia. *J Intern Med* 1990; 228: 627–32.

71 Shapiro S, Fraunfelder FT. Acetazolamide and aplastic anemia. *Am J Ophthalmol* 1992; 113: 328–30.

72 Pearson JR, Binder CI. Agranulocytosis following diamox therapy. *JAMA* 1955; 157: 339–41.

73 Reisner EH, Morgan MC. Thrombocytopenia following acetazolamide (Diamox) therapy. *JAMA* 1956; 160: 206–7.

74 Rossert J, Rondeau E, Jondeau G *et al.* Tamm-Horsfall protein accumulation in glomeruli during acetazolamide-induced acute renal failure. *Am J Nephrol* 1989; 9: 56–7.

75 Stock JG. Sulfonamide hypersensitivity and acetazolamide (Letter). *Arch Ophthalmol* 1990; 108: 634–5.

76 Epstein DL, Grant MW. Carbonic anhydrase inhibitor side effects. *Arch Ophthalmol* 1977; 95: 1378–82.

77 Wallace TR, Fraunfelder FT, Petursson GJ, Epstein DL. Decreased libido — a side effect of carbonic anhydrase inhibitor. *Ann Ophthalmol* 1979; 11: 1563–6.

78 Miller LG, Miller SM. Altered taste secondary to acetazolamide therapy. *J Fam Prac* 1990; 31: 199–200.

79 Maisey DN, Brown RD. Acetazolamide and symptomatic metabolic acidosis in mild renal failure. *BMJ* 1981; 283: 1527–8.

80 Arrigg CA, Epstein DL, Giovanoni R, Grant M. The influence of supplemental sodium acetate on carbonic anhydrase inhibitor-induced side effects. *Arch Ophthalmol* 1981; 99: 1969–72.

81 Futagi Y, Otani K, Abe J. Growth suppression in children receiving acetazolamide with antiepileptic drugs. *Pediatr Neurol* 1996; 15: 323–6.

82 Higashihara E, Natahara K, Takumi T, Nobuyuki S. Calcium metabolism in acidotic patients induced by carbonic anhydrase inhibitors: response to citrate. *J Urol* 1991; 145: 942–8.

83 Kass MA, Kolker AE, Gordon M, Goldberg I, Gieser DK, Krupin T, Becker B. Acetazolamide and urolithiasis. *Ophthalmology* 1981; 88: 261–5.

84 Mallette LE. Acetazolamide-accelerated anticonvulsant osteomalacia. *Arch Intern Med* 1977; 137: 1013–17.

85 Pierce WM, Nardin GF, Fuqua MF, Sabah-Mare E, Stern SH. Effect of chronic carbonic anhydrase inhibitor therapy on bone mineral density in white women. *J Bone Miner Res* 1991; 6: 347–54.

86 Layton WM, Hallesy DW. Deformity of forelimb in rats: association with high doses of acetazolamide. *Science* 1965; 149: 306–8.

87 Maren TH. Teratology and carbonic anhydrase inhibition. *Arch Ophthalmol* 1971; 85: 1–3.

88 Worsham GF, Beckman EN, Michell EH. Sacrococcygeal teratoma in a neonate: association with maternal use of acetazolamide. *JAMA* 1978; 240: 251–2.

89 Merlob P, Litwin A, Mor N. Possible association between acetazolamide administration during pregnancy and metabolic disorders in the newborn. *Eur J Obstet Gynecol Reprod Biol* 1990; 35: 85–8.

90 Soderam P, Hartwig P, Fagerlund C. Acetazolamide excretion in human breast milk. *Br J Clin Pharmacol* 1984; 17: 599–600.

91 Maren TH. Acetazolamide and advanced liver disease. *Am J Ophthalmol* 1986; 102: 672–3.

28 Carbamazepine

M. Sillanpää

Primary indications	First-line or adjunctive therapy in partial and generalized seizures (excluding absence and myoclonus). Also in Lennox–Gastaut syndrome and childhood epilepsy syndromes
Usual preparations	Tablets: 100, 200, 400 mg; chewtabs: 100, 200 mg; slow-release formulations: 200, 400 mg; liquid: 100 mg/5 mL; suppositories: 125, 250 mg
Usual dosages	Initial: 100 mg at night. Maintenance: 400–1600 mg/day (maximum 2400 mg). (Slow-release formulation, higher dosage.) Children: <1 year, 100–200 mg; 1–5 years, 200–400 mg; 5–10 years, 400–600 mg; 10–15 years, 600–1000 mg
Dosage intervals	2–3 times/day (2–4 times/day at higher doses or in children)
Significant drug interactions	Carbamazepine has a large number of interactions with antiepileptic and other drugs
Serum level monitoring	Useful
Target range	4–12 mg/L
Common/important side-effects	Drowsiness, fatigue, dizziness, ataxia, diplopia, blurring of vision, sedation, headache, insomnia, gastrointestinal disturbance, tremor, weight gain, impotence, effects on behaviour and mood, hepatic disturbance, rash and other skin reactions, bone marrow dyscrasia, leucopenia, hyponatraemia, water retention, endocrine effects
Main advantages	Highly effective and usually well-tolerated therapy
Main disadvantages	Transient adverse effects on initiating therapy. Occasional severe toxicity
Mechanisms of action	Action on neuronal sodium-channel conductance. Also action on monoamine, acetylcholine and NMDA receptors
Oral bioavailability	75–85%
Time to peak levels	4–8 h
Metabolism and excretion	Hepatic epoxidation and then conjugation
Volume of distribution	0.8–2 L/kg
Elimination half-life	5–26 h (but very variable)
Plasma clearance	0.133 L/kg/h (but very variable)
Protein binding	75%
Active metabolites	Carbamazepine epoxide
Comment	A drug of first choice in tonic-clonic and partial seizures in adults and children

(*Note*: this summary table was formulated by the lead editor.)

The origin of carbamazepine (CBZ) dates back to the year 1899, when Thiele and Holzinger [1] described iminodibenzyl and its efficacy profile. Besides local anaesthetic and antihistaminic properties, iminodibenzyl also showed a weak antiepileptic effect. This effect became substantially stronger when a carbamyl group was added at the 5 position of iminodibenzyl and then combined with iminostilbene making a double bond between the 10 and 11 positions and thus forming a tricyclic compound iminodibenzyl (10,11-dihydro-5H-dibenzo [b,f] azepine) or CBZ. In experimental animals, CBZ was found efficacious against maximal electroshock-induced seizures but the effect was minimal against pentylenetetrazol. Since the late 1950s, CBZ has been successfully used all over the world as one of the most important major antiepileptic drug. Coincident with its antiepileptic properties, CBZ was found effective against trigeminal neuralgia and, later on, its beneficial effect was found in certain psychiatric disorders and various pain syndromes.

Mechanism of action

The polycyclic chemical structure of CBZ is similar to that of certain psychotropic drugs, such as imipramine, chlorpromazine and maprotiline, and it shares some of the psychotropic effects and antipsychotic properties of this group. Its two-dimensional structure also shares features with antiepileptic drugs such as clonazepam, phenobarbital, phensuximide and phenytoin. These features include one saturated carbon atom, an amide group built into the heterocyclic ring and at least one aromatic ring twisted out of the plane of the heterocyclic ring. However, CBZ is differentiated from these compounds by lack of a saturated carbon atom, its tricyclic structure and the absence of an amide group in the heterocyclic ring. CBZ is virtually insoluble in water but soluble in absolute alcohol and benzene, chloroform, dichlormethane and other organic solvents. The major mechanism of action of CBZ is on neuronal sodium channel conductance by reducing high-frequency repetitive firing of action potentials. The effect is voltage dependent and use dependent. Although the mode of action is similar to that of phenytoin, CBZ has other effects, such as its beneficial effect on endogenous depression and on alcohol withdrawal seizures, which are not shared by phenytoin. Differences also exist in side-effects between the two drugs. This is possibly due to the fact that CBZ has other proposed actions on synaptic transmission and neurotransmitter receptors including purine, monoamine and N-acetyl-D-aspartate (NMDA) receptors.

Pharmacokinetics

Absorption and distribution in various tissues

The apparent volume of distribution varies reportedly from 0.8 to 2.0 L/kg in human adults. In neonates and infants it is 1.5-fold to 2-fold that of older children and adults. In consonance with its lower liposolubility, the active epoxy derivative of CBZ (CBZ-E) has a lower apparent volume of distribution, ranging from 0.6 to 1.5 L/kg.

Concentrations in solid tissues

In experimental animals, the brain tissue to plasma level ratio ranges from 0.9 to 1.5. The highest CBZ concentrations are noted in white matter and peripheral nerves. In humans, there is a significant positive relationship between the brain and plasma CBZ concentrations, with a ratio of 1.1 ± 0.1 for CBZ and 1.24–1.60 for CBZ-E. Brain concentrations have been reported to range from 2.2 to 14.5 for CBZ and 1.24–1.60 for CBZ-E. Brain tissue concentrations have been reported to rise slightly later than plasma levels and range from 2.2 to 14.5 μg/g [2]. Total and free plasma concentrations in epileptic brain tissue from postmortem specimens are similar to that of controls, in spite of the presence of gliosis and other consequential changes. The results argue for a non-specific binding of CBZ and CBZ-E to brain tissue constituents.

There is a close relationship between the daily dosage of CBZ, through plasma level and concentration in hair. Despite marked interindividual variation in plasma concentrations due to a wide range of daily dosages, a relatively small intraindividual variation over time and a close relationship between hair and plasma concentrations give a good additional tool for monitoring patient compliance. Higher CBZ levels have inconsistently been detected in black, untreated hair.

Plasma

In man, CBZ can only be administered orally (and rectally, but this route is seldom used). Though virtually water insoluble, CBZ can be dissolved in glycofurol and in aqueous CBZ solutions by complexing CBZ with 2-hydroxypropyl-β-cyclodextrin (HP-β-CD). Both solutions have been administered separately in mice with electrically induced generalized convulsive status epilepticus. An intravenous bolus of both solutions of CBZ rapidly suppressed seizures indicating association of rapid penetration into brain tissue. Glycoferol/CBZ solution caused marked sedation and motor impairment, but HP-β-CD/CBZ combination was well tolerated [3].

In human population studies, the relationship between oral dose and plasma level is largely linear, with smaller increments in plasma levels in relation to increases in oral dose of CBZ. In patients, after ingestion of CBZ, peak plasma levels of CBZ generally occur after 4–8 h, but several peaks may occur. The steady-state half-lives of CBZ and CBZ-E range from 5 to 26 h and 3 to 23 h, respectively. Marked intraindividual daily fluctuations may occur.

CBZ is highly bound to plasma proteins. In both volunteers and patients, albumin and other plasma protein binding was 75–80% of the total plasma concentration, although wide variation is found in children. Unbound plasma concentrations of CBZ are accordingly 20–25% of the total plasma concentrations of CBZ in treated patients. This is in line with the cerebrospinal fluid (CSF) concentrations of 17–31%. The unbound or free fraction is inversely correlated with serum α_1-acid glycoprotein concentration. Unbound CBZ-E fractions vary from 48% to 53%. Determinations of the active metabolite, CBZ-E, seem justified, because CBZ-E has antiepileptic properties comparable with CBZ and it also contributes to CBZ intoxication [4], especially in case of polytherapy.

Although oral dosages are largely related to plasma levels of CBZ, there are substantial interindividual and intraindividual variations in the clinical effects of the drug, and thus there is limited clinical utility in monitoring the CBZ level, especially when CBZ is taken with other antiepileptic drugs. CBZ-E concentrations follow the CBZ concentrations but fluctuations of CBZ-E concentrations are still larger than the CBZ concentrations (40–500% vs. 40–150%) and are probably further increased by age factors, autoinduction, comedication and variation in dosing schedules. Different formulations of the drug can also alter absorption and bioavailability.

Breast milk

There is a wide reported variation in milk to plasma CBZ concentration ratios ranging from 15% to 80%. Full-term neonates of normal birth weight (3000–3500 g) born to mothers on an appropriate daily CBZ medication have been estimated to receive a dose of 0.5–0.7 mg/kg. Breastfeeding of mother on CBZ medication is not contraindicated, but the effects of CBZ on newborns have so far not been investigated. Monitoring of newborn plasma levels is not compulsory but preferable. Two neonates with transient hepatic dysfunction have been reported.

Saliva and tears

Saliva concentrations of CBZ exceed the concentration of the free plasma fraction of the drug. In the first 2–3 h after oral drug intake, the determinations of saliva concentrations may be contaminated by retention of drug in the mouth if the mouth is not rinsed carefully before collection of saliva samples. Tear to plasma and tear to CSF ratios seem to be in a closer correlation than saliva to plasma and saliva to CSF ratios for CBZ and phenobarbital. Although tears and saliva are easily available, even in very young children, excessive evaporation, drooling, conjunctival irritation and infection may give erroneous and often too high values.

Dosage regimens

Greater fluctuations in plasma levels can be noted during once-daily dosing than during a multiple dose regimen. Controlled-release CBZ tablets have undoubtedly improved the tolerability of once or twice daily dosing regimes and lead to decreased fluctuation in plasma levels and improved patient compliance. In 48 patients followed for 8 months to 2 years, serum levels of CBZ and CBZ-E, taken 12 h after one daily evening dose of slow-release CBZ, correlated very well with the mean CBZ levels of the 24-h profile [5]. An acute oral loading of slow-release CBZ yields targeted plasma concentrations within the first 4 h after intake and is well tolerated by the patients.

Dosage forms

Dosage forms apparently do not significantly affect absorption or successive steady-state concentrations, efficacy, bioavailability or tolerability between conventional tablets, chewable tablets swallowed whole and chewable tablets chewed before swallowing. Bioavailablity varies between 75% and 85% and is virtually the same for tablets, suspension and syrup, but absorption of suspension is more rapid than that of tablets and needs to be considered in terms of lower and more frequent daily doses to avoid toxic symptoms. The bioavailability of the slow-release tablets is about 15%

lower than that of the other oral forms. Clinical experience has shown that dosage may therefore need to be increased when switching formulation. It is argued that generic forms of CBZ may not have similar absorption characteristics, and care may need to be taken when switching formulations.

Food

Food has not been shown to affect gastrointestinal absorption of CBZ significantly. CBZ absorption appears to be delayed in alcoholics, both after drinking and withdrawal. However, its bioavailability does not seem to be reduced. Single-dose studies in obese subjects showed a trend toward reduced CBZ clearance rate and shortening half-life following body weight reduction, compared with matched lean subjects. A linear correlation was found between apparent volume of distribution and body weight in both groups [6]. In lean subjects (<20 body mass index, BMI), plasma CBZ levels were significantly higher than in subjects of normal weight (20–25 BMI) and decreased with increasing total body weight. No significant difference in plasma levels has found between obese subjects and those of normal body weight.

Moistured tablets

Bioavailability is reduced up to 50% by storage of CBZ formulations in hot, humid conditions, which alter its form. Generalized convulsive status epilepticus has been reported in an adult male, who had ingested moisture-exposed swollen and enlarged CBZ tablets. A mean dissolution of 16% compared with more than 80% for fresh CBZ tablets has been demonstrated at 1 h but, after final dissolution, similar quantities of active drug could be detected both for moisture-exposed and fresh CBZ tablets. Reduced bioavailability can be caused by poor dissolution as a consequence of exposure to moisture. Consequently, CBZ tablets should be stored in a dry, cool and dark place.

Rectal administration

After rectal administration of CBZ mixture and sorbitol in water, absorption appears to be significantly slower than after oral administration, but total bioavailability is similar provided defaecation does not occur during the first 2 h. A defaecation effect elicited by sorbitol could be avoided using sorbitol-free CBZ gel in a patient who had refused to take oral medication for her complex partial seizures. In this case, CBZ powder, dissolved in alcohol, was mixed with methylhydroxyethyl-cellulose and administered three times per day. Both absorption and tolerability of CBZ rectal gel were good.

Determinants of plasma concentrations

CBZ plasma levels correlate relatively poorly with clinical reponse and so the concept of a CBZ 'therapeutic' range is of limited value (even for trough levels). Measurements of CBZ-E is seldom clinically indicated, except to explore the cause of symptoms of CBZ toxicity which occur with normal CBZ plasma levels. Measurements of free plasma levels are usually no better than determinations of total plasma concentrations, except in exceptional cases [7]. Causes of unpredictability are similar to those affecting the oral dose to plasma ratio. They include diurnal intraindividual variation, comedication (especially with valproate) and variability in protein binding of CBZ and CBZ-E. Again, tailoring of daily dosage and dosing in accordance with a clinical response, not with plasma levels, is necessary to obtain favourable therapeutic results.

Metabolism and elimination

In the first few weeks of therapy, autoinduction causes a shortened half-life resulting in falling plasma levels. After a single dose, the apparent elimination half-life varies between 20 and 65 h, but after multiple dosing for 10–20 days, it falls by approximately 50%. Clearance rates increase rapidly by the second day after the first dose. Because of autoinduction and decreasing plasma levels, increments in daily dosage are needed to maintain the plasma concentration at a target level. Autoinduction is dose dependent. CBZ-E metabolism is induced more than CBZ turnover. Independent of daily dosage, autoinduction is usually completed within 20–30 days. In the postinduced state, a new steady state after changes in drug dosages will be achieved within 3 days. CBZ and CBZ-E may also be heteroinduced.

CBZ is virtually completely metabolized in man. The main pathways of biotransformation are epoxidation, hydroxylation, glucuronidation and sulphuration. The main metabolite, CBZ-E, is hydrolysed to give trans-10,11-dihydroxy-CBZ. In the study of Faigle and Feldman [8], 72% of CBZ was detected in urine and 28% in faeces. CBZ-E is a biologically active metabolite which accumulates in clinically relevant concentrations and may contribute to intoxication after increase in daily CBZ dosage even in case of unchanged CBZ levels [4]. At similar plasma levels, the symptoms are less severe than the intoxication due to the parent compound, because of the relatively low reactivity of CBZ-E. The ratio of CBZ-E to CBZ is higher on polytherapy. However, the CBZ-E to CBZ ratio is not dose related [9], and hence the total CBZ plasma level does reflect the sum effect of CBZ and CBZ-E independent of daily dosage.

Pharmacokinetics in special groups

Pregnancy

During the first trimester, CBZ plasma levels are reportedly reduced, but the data are controversial and reasons for changes in concentrations still largely unknown. Total CBZ levels are lower toward the end of pregnancy, probably partly because of declining plasma proteins, but free CBZ fractions remain largely unchanged during late pregnancy, delivery and puerperium. Accordingly, probably no changes in daily dosage are needed.

The cord to maternal serum blood ratio of CBZ ranges from 0.5 to 0.8 and the breast milk to plasma ratio from 0.2 to 0.7. The fetal brain to plasma ratio is similar to that observed in adults, probably due to the fact that both CBZ and CBZ-E are easily transferred and evenly distributed in the fetal tissues [10]. The CBZ half-life of neonates of the mothers on continuing CBZ medication ranged from 8.2 to 27.7 h. Dosing in neonates should be proportionately lower than in older children.

Infants and children

Higher clearance rates occur in early childhood years, small body mass, and in males. However, there is a wide variation in the apparent half-life of CBZ, probably due to the child's age, comedication and duration of treatment. Similarly, there is a wide range of the CBZ-E to CBZ ratios, from 16% to 66%. The daily dosage to plasma level ratio of CBZ—but not CBZ-E—was noted to be higher on increasing dosages [11], and with increasing dosage and age. Increasing dose, but not increasing age, raised the CBZ-E concentration. The CBZ-E to CBZ ratio decreases progressively with age [12]. In children on continuing CBZ comedication, the CBZ level to daily dosage ratios were decreased, whereas the plasma CBZ-E concentrations were significantly increased, compared with the patients on CBZ monotherapy. The CBZ-E to CBZ ratios are also higher in polytherapy including CBZ, compared with CBZ monotherapy.

In infants and children, CBZ absorption can be greatly affected by malabsorption states, and protein energy malabsorption in particular. One-third of these children may have a lowered bioavailability of CBZ.

Drug interactions

In addition to autoinduction, CBZ has clinically relevant heteroinducing, inducible and inhibitory effects. CBZ is almost completely metabolized by liver and, consequently, its clearance is virtually equal to total body clearance. Cytochrome P450 3A4 (CYP3A4) is the main isoform which catalyses epoxidation, the main pathway of CBZ metabolism. CBZ increases the rate of synthesis of CYP3A4 and clearance of CBZ. Inhibition of this pathway by another drug has been estimated to result in 1.5–2-fold increases in steady-state plasma concentrations of CBZ.

Table 28.1 exhibits effects of CBZ on other antiepileptic drugs. The effects of CBZ on phenobarbital and primidone are somewhat controversial. CBZ increases phenobarbital levels in patients on primidone. The increase in phenobarbital concentrations is probably due to induction of phenobarbital-producing pathway of primidone metabolism rather than inhibition of phenobarbital clearance, because phenobarbital clearance remains unchanged in patients on both CBZ and phenobarbital. On the other hand, when phenobarbital is coadministered with CBZ, phenobarbital clearance decreases compared with that in monotherapy. The phenobarbital clearance in both monotherapy and CBZ cotherapy is highest

Table 28.1 Effects of carbamazepine on other antiepileptic drugs

Increasing	Decreasing	Variable	No effect
Flunarazine	Clobazam	Phenytoin	Gabapentin
Mephenytoin	Clonazepam	Phenobarbital	Lamictal
Phenobarbital	Ethosuximide	Primidone	Levetiracetam
(from primidone)	Felbamate		Piracetam
	Remacemide		Vigabatrin
	Tiagabine		
	Topiramate		
	Valproate		
	Zonisamide		

in the youngest children and decreases in weight-related fashion, approaching the rate of adults in older children.

The metabolism of several newer antiepileptic drugs is induced by CBZ, apparently via induction of the CYP3A4 enzyme system. These include felbamate, remacemide, tiagabine, topiramate, valproate and zonisamide.

In Table 28.2, the effects of other antiepileptic drugs on CBZ level are shown. The effects of valproate therapy on CBZ concentrations vary depending on the balance of induction, inhibition and protein binding displacement [13]. The free CBZ fraction in increased on valproate comedication. CBZ levels are lowered in combination therapy with phenobarbital, phenytoin, primidone and valproate. Induction of the cytochrome P450 system involved in the formation of CBZ-E or inhibition of the enzyme responsible for detoxification of CBZ-E, epoxide hydrolase, results in raised CBZ-E concentrations. CBZ-E concentrations (and CBZ-E to CBZ ratios) are higher on phenytoin, primidone, valproate and valproate–primidone bitherapy. In case of strong induction, for instance by felbamate, lamotrigine, phenobarbital, phenytoin, primidone, progabide and valnoctamide, the CBZ-E concentrations may reach toxic levels. However, in one study [14], CBZ oral clearance and CBZ-E to CBZ serum concentration ratios were not significantly affected by lamotrigine add-on. The role of felbamate cotherapy is interesting. While increasing phenytoin concentrations, it decreases CBZ levels. CBZ metabolism does not appear to be affected by gabapentin, levetiracetam, oxcarbazepine, tiagabine, topiramate, vigabatrin or zonisamide. A mutual interaction exists between remacemide and CBZ; while inhibited by remacemide, CBZ itself induces remacemide metabolism.

CBZ decreases plasma concentrations of concomitant alprazolam, clozapine, haloperidol, midazolam, olanzapine, tarazodone and the oral contraceptive (Table 28.3). Several psychotropic drug concentrations are raised by CBZ. These include lithium, monoamine oxidase inhibitors and perphenazine. Acenocoumarol, digitalis glycosides, furosemide, indinavir and isoniazid plasma concentrations were increased when CBZ was added on the therapy.

Because CBZ is a potent inducer of the cytochrome P450 (CYP)3A4 and other oxidative systems and may also increase glucuronyl transferase activity in liver, it can potentially induce the metabolism of many other drugs, such as tricyclic antidepressants, steroid oral contraceptives, glucocorticoids, oral anticoagulants, ciclosporin, theophylline and chemotherapeutic agents. Indeed, the metabolism of these drugs and chemotherapeutics has been shown

inducable by CBZ (Table 32.3). CBZ may also induce caffeine metabolism by inducing the cytochrome CYP1A2 pathway, the same isoenzyme that induces theophylline, imipramine and propranolol metabolism.

Many drugs other than antiepileptics also affect CBZ metabolism (Table 28.4). Loxapine is so far the only drug that decreases CBZ concentration, but the mechanism is unknown. CBZ concentrations have remained virtually unchanged during cotherapy with nortriptyline, phenelzine, ranitidine, sertraline and possibly thioridazine. Grapefruit inhibits CYP3A4 enzymes and accordingly increases plasma concentration of CBZ.

Effects of hepatic and renal diseases

A mild or moderate liver dysfunction does not affect CBZ metabolism. However, a marked decrease in protein binding may occur. More severe dysfunction may cause CBZ intoxication mainly due to decreased liver microsomal activity.

In patients with liver disease, no significant changes in CBZ pharmacokinetics have been noted. Free fraction might be decreased in renal liver disease because of lower serum levels of albumin and changes of binding in α-acid glycoprotein. A slight reduction in dose, if any, may be needed in renal disease. However, the risk of intoxication is low, because protein binding, total plasma concentration and plasma half-life are virtually unchanged. In heart failure, congestion of major vital organs, including liver, may result in abnormally slow absorption and metabolism. The haemodynamic disturbances may be further worsened by the tendency of CBZ to cause sodium and water retention.

Table 28.2 Effect of antiepileptic drugs on carbamazepine

Increasing	Decreasing	Variable	No effect
Acetazolamide	Felbamate	Clobazam	Flunarazine
Densimol	Lamotrigine	Clonazepam	Gabapentin
Remacemide	Phenobarbital	Ethosuximide	Levetiracetam
Stiripentol	Phenytoin	Valproate	Piracetam
Valnoctamide[a]	Primidone		Oxcarbazepine
Valpromide	Progabide		Vigabatrin
			Zonisamide

[a] Elevation of carbamazepine-epoxide.

Table 28.3 Effects of carbamazepine on other drugs

Increasing	Decreasing
Aceno-coumarol	Alprazolam
Chlorotiazides	Antipyrine
Digitalis glucosides	Clozapine
Lithium	Corticoteroids
Furosemide	Ciclosporin
Isoniazide	Desipramine
Monoamine oxidase inhibitors	Digitalis glucosides
Perphenazine	Doxycycline
	Fluphenazine
	Haloperidol
	Indinavir
	Itraconazole
	Midazolam
	Nicardipine
	Nifedipine
	Nortriptyline
	Oral steroid contraceptives
	Oxiacetam
	Praziquantel
	Propranolol
	Trazodone
	Theophylline
	Warfarin

Table 28.4 Effects of other drugs on carbamazepine

Increasing	Decreasing	No effect
Allopurinol	Loxapine	Azithromycin
Caffeine		Nifeditine
Cimetidine		Nortriptyline
Clarithromycin		Panthoprazole
Danazol		Paroxethine
Desipramine		Phenelzine
Dextropropoxyphene		Ranitidine
Diltiazem		Sertraline
Erythromycin		Thioridazine(?)
Fluoxetine		
Fluvoxamine		
Gemfibrozil		
Haloperidol		
Isoniazid		
Ketoconazole		
Miconazone		
Nefazodone		
Nicotinamide		
Omeprazole		
Propoxyphene		
Salicylate		
Terfenadine		
Triacetyloleandromycin		
Valnoctamide		
Verapamil		
Viloxazine		

Clinical efficacy

In addition to numerous open-label clinical trials, there are several randomized controlled studies on the clinical efficacy of CBZ compared with other antiepileptic drugs. The effects of CBZ depend in part on the type of epilepsy and seizures.

CBZ and lamotrigine again showed similar efficacy in a controlled multicentre monotherapy study of newly diagnosed seizures, even though patients treated with lamotrigine had slightly less side-effects and were more likely to continue with treatment [15].

A comparison between extended-release tablets twice a day and conventional CBZ tablets four times daily shows no significant difference in pharmacokinetics, and extended-release CBZ treatment controls seizures better than immediate-release CBZ therapy in adults and children.

Idiopathic generalized epilepsies

Primary generalized tonic-clonic seizures

Primary generalized epilepsies with tonic-clonic seizures are a major indication for CBZ.

In a double-blind, crossover trial [16], no significant differences were found between CBZ and phenytoin in efficacy against primary generalized, focal or secondary generalized seizures, or in acute side-effects.

One hundred and eighty-one newly diagnosed, untreated patients aged 4–72 years with epilepsy were prospectively randomized to monotherapy with CBZ, phenytoin or valproate. After follow-up of 4 months to 2 years, a decrease in seizure frequency of 51% to 100% was achieved in 75–81% of patients. Primary generalized tonic-clonic seizures were reduced 51–100% in 75% of CBZ-treated patients, 81% of phenytoin-treated patients and 78% of valproate-treated patients. Significantly more patients with generalized convulsive seizures became seizure free with phenytoin than with CBZ, but the efficacy of CBZ and valproate did not differ in patients with focal or generalized seizures [17]. This is the only report in the literature where phenytoin significantly better controlled seizures than CBZ.

Three hundred adults with newly diagnosed primary generalized, focal or secondary generalized seizures were randomized for either CBZ or sodium valproate in an open, multicentre study for long-term efficacy and safety [18]. Overall control of primary generalized, focal and secondary generalized seizures was good, but significantly more patients on valproate than on CBZ remained on randomized treatment (90% vs. 75%) for at least 6 months. Adverse effects were more common with CBZ therapy, but there was no more withdrawals because of poor control of any seizure type. A similar paediatric study was undertaken including 260 children randomized to CBZ and valproate groups [19]. CBZ and valproate showed equal efficacy in seizure control of both primary generalized and focal seizures with or without generalization. Adverse effects were mild and only few necessitated drug withdrawal.

Because clinical experience and several two-drug comparisons showed equal efficacy but different tolerability, multicomparisons of drugs were warranted. Heller *et al.* [20] undertook a prospective randomized comparative study of 243 adults with previously untreated tonic-clonic or partial with or without secondary generalized seizures. The patients were randomized to phenobarbital, phenytoin, CBZ or sodium valproate monotherapy. Time from onset of drug therapy to first seizure and time to enter 1-year remission defined efficacy. The overall outcome was favourable with a complete seizure control in 27% and 1-year remission until the end of 3-year follow-up in 75%. Adverse effects necessitating withdrawal were more common in phenobarbital-treated patients (22%) than patients with CBZ (11%), valproate (5%) or phenytoin (3%). A similar setting was used to examine efficacy and tolerability of major antiepileptic drugs in children [21]. One hundred and sixty-seven children aged 3–16 years, with tonic-clonic or partial seizures, with or without generalization, were randomly allocated to treatment with phenobarbital, phenytoin, and CBZ or sodium valproate. Efficacy was defined by time to first seizure after onset of therapy and time to achieving 1-year remission. One-fifth (20%) became seizure free and 73% had achieved a 1-year remission by 3 years of follow-up. Withdrawal of drug therapy was necessary in 9%. Of the first 10 withdrawals, six were randomized to phenobarbital, and thereafter no further children were randomized to the phenobarbital group. Of the remaining three drugs, phenytoin was more likely to result in withdrawal (9%) than CBZ (4%) or valproate (4%).

Symptomatic generalized epilepsies

It is well-known that infantile spasms are extremely drug resistant in 90% of cases. Trials with CBZ are unlikely to be successful if corticotropin, valproate or vigabatrin has failed. In symptomatic myoclonic-astatic seizures, CBZ has been recommended. In the author's experience, a few patients with symptomatic Lennox–Gastaut syndrome can achieve at least temporary seizure control with CBZ combined with benzodiazepine. Similar favourable results in some children with infantile spasms and symptomatic myoclonic-astatic seizures have been reported. Others have found CBZ to be ineffective against absence, myoclonus and atonic seizures and may even exacerbate them.

Localization-related epilepsies

If treatment of benign epilepsy with centrotemporal spikes is needed, CBZ is preferred to other major antiepileptic drugs. Although the efficacy is similar, other drugs produce cognitive, behavioural and sedative side-effects more frequently than CBZ.

CBZ is considered as a drug of choice for complex partial and secondary generalized seizures. Fifty-one patients with phenobarbital-resistant epilepsy were randomized to either CBZ or phenytoin. Patients who were administered CBZ showed greater improvement and less adverse effects than phenytoin but the global evaluation by physicians and patients found no significant differences in efficacy or tolerability. In a randomized, double-blind study of 236 children aged less than 6 years, 49% of the CBZ group and 47% of the phenytoin group remained seizure free for the 6-month study period. Side-effects were more common in the CBZ-treated group but the difference was not significant [22].

CBZ was as effective as valproate for the treatment of generalized tonic-clonic seizures but more effective than valproate in complex partial seizures and had fewer long-term side-effects [23].

Newly diagnosed or recurrent partial seizures with or without secondary generalization were randomized to open multicentre monotherapy study [24]. CBZ with daily dosage of 600 mg was compared with lamotrigine 100 mg/day and 200 mg/day. The efficacy measurements were comparable on all three treatments. However, side-effects and need for changing the dose were more common in CBZ therapy than in lamotrigine therapy. Adverse effects resulting in withdrawal were also more common in the CBZ group (10%) than in the two lamotrigine groups (4% and 5%).

In an open controlled study [25], 100 adult patients with newly diagnosed partial seizures, with or without secondary generalization, were randomized to CBZ or vigabatrin. Fifty-nine patients with a single epileptic seizure and no drug therapy served as controls for objective safety measurements. Remaining in the trial for more than 12 months of steady-state treatment was used as a parameter of success. CBZ was more effective than vigabatrin. Withdrawals were required because of side-effects in the CBZ group more often than in the vigabatrin group. In the latter, lack of efficacy was a more common cause of withdrawal than in the CBZ group. Another randomized study [26] included 230 patients with newly diagnosed, previously untreated patients with partial seizures. The patients were allocated to daily dosage of 600 mg CBZ, and 229 similar patients allocated to daily dosage of 2 g vigabatrin. The primary outcome was time to withdrawal because of lack of efficacy or adverse events. Secondary outcomes included efficacy determined as time to 6-month remission of seizures, and time to first seizure after initial dose stabilization. The primary outcome did not differ between the two monotherapies. Vigabatrin was better tolerated and necessitated fewer withdrawals but it was more frequently associated with psychiatric symptoms and weight gain. Both primary and secondary efficacy outcomes favoured CBZ and time to first seizure after the first 6 weeks from randomization showed CBZ to be significantly more effective than vigabatrin.

A multicentre, double-blind monotherapy study (CBZ vs. gabapentin) showed that the CBZ-treated group completed the study more often; the exit rate was lower but the withdrawal rate was higher with CBZ than with gabapentin [27].

Mattson *et al.* [28], in their multicentre double-blind study, randomized 622 adults with partial and secondary generalized seizures to CBZ phenobarbital, phenytoin or primidone to evaluate efficacy and tolerability. The follow-up period was 2 years or up to withdrawal for lack of efficacy or adverse effects. Overall success was reported highest with CBZ and phenytoin, intermediate with phenobarbital and lowest with primidone. Control of seizures was approximately equally good with all the four drugs but CBZ provided complete seizure control more often than primidone or phenobarbital. Primidone had the most severe adverse effects followed by phenytoin. The overall evaluation yields CBZ and phenytoin as drugs of first choice for adults with partial or generalized tonic-clonic seizures.

Febrile seizures

Febrile seizures are the most common seizure type in childhood. One hundred and six children with recurrent febrile seizures were randomized to either CBZ or phenobarbital. Although some children on CBZ had fewer side-effects, CBZ proved relatively ineffective and cannot be recommended against recurrent febrile seizures.

Combination therapy

A combination therapy with CBZ may be of benefit in some patients with partial seizures. Phenytoin combined with CBZ significantly decreased partial seizures resistant to CBZ monotherapy or phenytoin monotherapy and caused fewer side-effects. A combination of valproate to CBZ monotherapy gave substantially better results than CBZ monotherapy in 100 patients with partial seizures. In a multicentre, randomized double-blind study of 215 patients with partial seizures refractory to CBZ monotherapy, were allocated to either vigabatrin bitherapy or valproate bitherapy. A seizure freedom rate of 17% and 19%, respectively, was achieved [29].

Acetazolamide, combined to CBZ monotherapy, resulted in a complete seizure freedom in three of 48 patients and at least 50% decrease in frequency in a further 18 patients.

Side-effects

In comparison with many other major antiepileptic drugs, CBZ is less toxic, although nearly half the patients experience some kind of side-effects. However, most side-effects are mild, transient and reversible, and do not require discontinuation. Between 5 and 10% are severe enough to necessitate drug withdrawal because of adverse effects, mostly exanthema. Haematological and other adverse effects more commonly occur in association with polytherapy and in the elderly. Epoxidation of CBZ has been considered as an important factor in association with side-effects. However, in monotherapy, the relationship between epoxide concentrations and side-effects is controversial. In combination with liver enzyme inducers, the CBZ-E concentrations may rise to a subclinically or clinically toxic levels. In children, the spectrum of adverse effects is slightly different (e.g. skin reactions are fewer than in adults). A list of important side-effects is shown in Table 28.5.

Table 28.5 Side-effects of carbamazepine on different organ systems

Organ/organ system	Incidence[a]
Nervous system	Frequent
Drowsiness	Frequent
Dyskinesia/incoordination	Frequent
Vertigo and dizziness	Frequent
Ataxia	Less frequent
Diplopia	Less frequent
Sedation	Less frequent
Nystagmus	Less frequent
Tremor	Infrequent
Cognitive disturbance	Infrequent
Headache	Infrequent
Skin	Less frequent
Rash	Less frequent
Mucocutaneous syndrome	Rare
Serious dermatitis	Rare
Dermatomyositis	Rare
Haematological system	Rare
Transient leukopenia	Infrequent
Agranulocytosis	Rare
Thrombocytopenia	Rare
Immune reaction defect	Rare
Lymphadenopathia	Rare
Aplastic anaemia	Rare
Gastrointestinal system	Infrequent
Diarrhoea	Infrequent
Nausea	Infrequent
Colitis	Rare
Stomatitis	Rare
Liver	Infrequent
Elevation of liver enzymes	Less frequent
Endocrine system	Infrequent
Water and sodium balance	Infrequent
Hypothyroidism	Infrequent
Diabetes insipidus	Rare
Teratogenic effects	Infrequent
Cardiac effects	Rare
Other	
Skeletal system	Rare
Porphyria	Rare
Renal disorders	Rare

[a] Frequent ≥20%; less frequent 10–20%; infrequent 1–9%; and rare <1%.

Neurotoxicity

The most common side-effects that are dose related occur in the beginning of CBZ treatment and are reversible include drowsiness, dizziness, ataxia, dyskinesia and blurring of vision. Slow and gradual increase in dosage at the initiation of therapy minimizes these effects. With long-term administration, these effects generally subside.

In 622 patients, significantly more seizure-free patients and lower total toxicity battery scores were found in CBZ-treated patients than in patients treated with phenobarbital, phenytoin or primidone [30]. In another study, patients showed fewer side-effects with CBZ than with barbiturates, benzodiazepines, ethosuximide, phenytoin or valproate. Patients with valproate treatment experienced more long-term adverse side-effects than those with CBZ treatment, especially tremor and weight gain [23].

A significant decrease in interictal spike frequency with therapeutic, but not subtherapeutic, levels of CBZ or no changes may be found in EEG. On the other hand, abnormalities, such as background slowing or generalized epileptiform discharges without significant correlation with seizures can emerge during CBZ treatment. Similar abnormalities are found during CBZ treatment in patients who may experience an increase in seizure frequency and new seizure types, mostly absences.

Cognitive functions are consistently affected less by CBZ than do the other established major antiepileptic drugs. Withdrawal of CBZ, phenytoin or valproate resulted in faster motor performance in 58 patients compared with controls, but attention and concentration abilities improved significantly only after discontinuation of phenytoin [31]. CBZ produced no significant side-effects on cognition or behaviour during the first 6 months of treatment [32]. In a meta-analysis of the literature, improved behaviour was found in 18% and worsened behaviour in 1.7%. CBZ-related cognitive dysfunction is less common when CBZ and CBZ-E concentrations are lower, or when slow-release CBZ is used instead of conventional formulation.

Comparisons with newer antiepileptic drugs show slight differences in side-effect frequency. In one randomized controlled study, the efficacy of CBZ and lamotrigine was virtually the same. Side-effects were slightly more common on CBZ treatment than on lamotrigine treatment. With the exception of sleepiness, the differences were not significant. Skin rash was as common (19%) in the two treatments, but CBZ treatment lead to drug withdrawal more often (13% vs. 9%) [29]. In another study [24], side-effects and the need to change dose were more common in CBZ therapy than in lamotrigine therapy. Adverse effects resulting in withdrawal were also more common in the CBZ group (10%) than in the two lamotrigine groups (4% and 5%).

Vigabatrin has been found generally more tolerable than CBZ in both adults [25,26] and children [33], but visual field defects associated with vigabatrin, but not with CBZ [34], must be considered in the comparison. Similarly, in healthy senior adults [35], CBZ 800 mg daily, compared with gabapentin 2400 mg daily, resulted in more side-effects, but the magnitude of difference was modest, and self-reported mood was not significantly affected by either drug.

CBZ can occasionally interact with the changing seizure patterns to affect cognitive function. Two examples are given here. A 5-year-old boy with rare partial motor seizures and atypical 'absences', proved to experience important learning difficulties when starting to attend school. EEG became increasing active with an epileptic focus and continuous spike-waves during sleep (CSWS). On neurological examination, he had difficulties in speech fluency, word finding and naming, inattention and low IQ. CBZ was substituted by clobazam and later ethosuximide added on with rapid improvement in cognitive and linguistic performance and in behaviour. EEG was gradually normalized and he was able to follow regular school at an age-appropriate level. A similar anecdotal observation was made in a highly educated elderly man (77 years) who was on CBZ treatment for epilepsy following arterial hypertension and cerebral infarction. Mental deterioration occurred over 2 years on a conventional daily dose of CBZ with plasma concentration of 33 μmol/L (reference values 13–40 μmol/L). The patient was permanently institutionalized, bedridden and virtually uninterested in surroundings, but seizure free. Therefore, his medication was withdrawn. He rapidly became alert, became interested in communication, walking and reading. He had no seizure relapse, and he is periodically deinstitutionalized.

Dermatological and other hypersensitivity reactions

Skin rash occurs in about 10% but has been reported in up to 19% [29], but less than 1% of the reactions are serious or life threatening [36]. In children, rash is less common. The incidence of rash increases with age: from 5% at age 0–6 years to 15% at age 7 or older. In a literature review covering 1214 children, the most common side-effect was drowsiness (23%) followed by ataxia (10%), leucopenia (10%), visual disturbances (9%) and elevated values on liver function tests (9%). Laboratory screening for side-effects appeared to be of little benefit. CBZ hypersensitivity reactions may take the form of lymphadenopathy, hepatomegaly, splenomegaly, vasculitis, uveitis, pneumonitis, hypogammaglobulinaemia, aseptic meningitis, pseudolymphoma, myocarditis or interstitial nephritis. Single cases, ascribed to CBZ treatment, of hair loss, facial burns caused by a photocopier, photosensitivity reactions, colitis, stomatitis, gingivitis, pancreatitis and erythema multiforme have been reported.

Withdrawal of CBZ is followed by disappearance of hypersensitivity reactions. Patch testing may be diagnostic of CBZ hypersensitivity. Desensitization can be successfully carried out by means of slowly increasing doses of CBZ. Proliferation and activation of suppressor-cytotoxic subset of T cells, induced by CBZ, appear to be the mechanism underlying hypersensitivity.

Haematotoxicity

CBZ is rarely haematotoxic. Life-threatening events are in most cases idiosyncratic haematological reactions. The incidence has been estimated to be 1 in 200 000 CBZ exposures. During the first 25 years of clinical usage of CBZ, 31 cases of thrombocytopenia, 27 cases of aplastic anaemia, 10 cases of agranulocytosis and eight cases of pancytopenia had been reported. The prevalence of aplastic anaemia has been estimated less than 1/50 000 or even 5.1 per million and 1.4 per million for agranulocytosis. The overall risk for the general population is estimated to be 2 persons per million per year for aplastic anaemia and 4.7 persons per million per year for agranulocytosis.

A subclinical decrease in white cell count under 5000 cells/mm^3 can be found in about one-third of the CBZ-treated patients within the 6 first months of therapy. A leucopenia with decreasing number of cells needs consideration but is in most cases transient. In 2228 psychiatric patients, the white blood cell counts was less than 4000 cells/mm^3 in 2.05% in CBZ-treated and 0.32% in valproate-treated patients. The mean time of recovery from withdrawal of CBZ treatment is 3 days.

Hepatotoxicity

Levels of liver enzymes are elevated in 5–22% of patients on CBZ treatment, particularly γ-glutamyltransferase, alanine aminotransferase and aspartate aminotransferase. In most cases, the elevations are clinically insignificant and are rapidly normalized after discontinuation of CBZ treatment. CBZ appears to induce clinically significant liver pathology in two different ways. One is hypersensitivity-induced granulomatous hepatitis associated with cholestasis, and another, toxic type of hepatitis without cholestasis. Single cases of cholangitis and liver dysfunction associated with parkinsonian-like syndrome without toxic plasma CBZ levels have been reported. Children are at a lower risk of hepatotoxicity than adults. Only two fatal outcomes have been published.

Endocrinological effects

Antidiuretic hormone and hyponatraemia

Since the 1960s, CBZ has been known to have a vasopressin-like action in controlling polyuria in patients with diabetes mellitus resulting in water retention and hyponatraemia. This effect is accentuated by valproate or phenobarbital medication and counteracted by concurrent phenytoin, lithium or partially by demeclocycline administration. In addition to decrease in sodium levels, CBZ may cause low serum calcium and chloride levels with the highest risk in cases of low baseline sodium level, and high daily dosages and plasma levels of CBZ. However, hyponatraemia is not avoided by low daily dosages of CBZ. Interestingly, a pregnant mother who was administered CBZ for facial pain during the third semester, delivered a child with congenital adrenogenital syndrome of salt-losing type. The mechanism behind the antidiuretic action is unknown. A renal mechanism, a direct hypothalamic effect or increase in plasma cortisol level reflecting pituitary effect and a relative inefficacy of glucocorticoid negative feedback at the pituitary have been suggested.

Thyroid hormones

Serum thyroxine levels are lower during long-term CBZ therapy, compared with controls, and may result in clinical goitre. Decreased serum levels of total thyroxine, free thyroxine and free tri-iodothyronine have been found in children. The effect of CBZ may be accentuated by valproate cotherapy. Unaffected in CBZ monotherapy, valproate monotherapy and combination treatment are serum tri-iodothyronine and free tri-iodothyronine concentrations, thyroid-stimulating hormone levels, and the thyroid-stimulating hormone responses to the thyroid-releasing hormone. Serum thyroxine and free thyroxine concentrations are not affected by valproate monotherapy. Controversially, the thyroid-stimulating hormone levels were increased in the CBZ group, and particularly in the valproate group, compared with controls [37].

Contradictory results of the paradoxical situation between decreased serum free thyroxine and tri-iodothyronine concentrations and, on the other hand, euthyroid status and normal thyroid-stimulating hormone levels was addressed by Surks and DeFesi [38]. They showed that, measured from *in vitro* specimen, targeted levels of CBZ (and phenytoin) increased free thyroxine and tri-iodothyronine concentrations by displacing them in part from serum binding proteins. Thyroid-stimulating hormone levels were normal. In patients on CBZ, serum total thyroxine decreased significantly, but free thyroxine fraction increased significantly. Serum free tri-iodothyronine and thyroid-stimulating hormone levels were normal. Hence, in CBZ- (and phenytoin-) treated patients, increased free thyroxine and tri-iodothyronine levels offset the significant decrease in serum thyroxine and tri-iodothyronine resulting in normal free thyroxine and tri-iodothyronine and euthyroid status of the patient. The measurement of thyroid-stimulating hormone concentrations is the most reliable method to show the euthyroid status.

Sex hormones

The interrelationships between antiepileptic drugs, hormones (including testosterone, oestradiol, thyroid and gonadotropin) and different types of seizures is complex and reports arrive at contradictory conclusions. CBZ can affect sex hormone metabolisms in many ways. It may cause a rise in circulating sex hormone binding globulin, a continuous fall in dehydroepiandrosterone sulfate, and a transient fall in testosterone, free testosterone, and androstenedione. The increases in sex hormone binding globulin and sex hormone catabolism probably secondarily result from the activity of CBZ-induced hepatic mono-oxygenase enzyme. Sexual dysfunction, experienced by some patients with CBZ treatment might be derived from CBZ-related changes in sex hormone metabolism.

Hyposexuality and reproductive dysfunction are commonly considered as a result of decreased testosterone activity. However, testosterone administration gave a moderate effect only on restoration of sexual function. Conversion of testosterone to oestradiol is known to be enhanced by aromatase in the presence of antiepileptic medication. Oestradiol causes male hyposexuality and increases liability to seizures. The effect of oestradiol is inhibited by testolactone, an aromatase inhibitor. Administered to a man with low testosterone levels in the presence of CBZ, testolactone had a beneficial effect on both sexuality and seizures. In a man with impotence and other sexual dysfunctions, serum testosterone level was normal, but serum sex hormone binding globulin increased and free testosterone in relation to serum sex hormone binding globulin decreased during CBZ treatment. These changes were proposed as the cause of the sexual problems [39]. In another study of 37 males, eight of whom were impotent and two of whom had additional loss of libido, hyposexuality was related to decreased luteinizing hormone response to luteinizing hormone releasing hormone associated with imbalanced androgen to oestradiol ratio. No significant association with sexual dysfunction was found with several hormonal parameters: total and free testosterone, free dihydrotestos-

terone and oestradiol [40]. The effects of CBZ on sperm function are unclear.

Bone metabolism

CBZ may affect metabolism of bone calcium. Hypocalcaemia, hypophosphataemia, increased serum alkaline phosphatase and decreased serum 25-hydroxyvitamin D have been occasionally reported. In contrast to children treated with valproate, who had clear-cut decrease in calcium content associated with decreased bone density, the CBZ-treated patients had no demonstrable decrease in bone mineral density. However, two patients with CBZ-related osteomalacia on long-term treatment have been reported [41,42].

Teratogenic effects

Congenital malformations have been reported to occur at a rate between 5.7% and 7.5% [43,44]. The incidence of malformations on CBZ treatment (5.7%) was lower than with primidone (14.3%), valproate (11.1%), and phenytoin (9.1%) but slightly higher than with phenobarbital therapy (5.1%) [43]. The incidence increased with age and with increasing number of antiepileptic drugs and presence of malformations in siblings.

The relative risk of malformations was 2.24 compared with general controls [44]. A birth weight reduction of approximately 250 g was found after intrauterine exposure to CBZ.

In 8005 cases of malformations, 299 infants were exposed *in utero* to CBZ [45]. Of mothers of 299 infants, 46 (15.4%) had been on CBZ monotherapy during pregnancy. Among these infants, the only significant malformations were hypertelorism and localized skull defects, spina bifida on monotherapy and cardiac malformations on polytherapy. Spina bifida occurred in 8.7% and cardiac malformations in 17.4% of CBZ-exposed patients. The results may question the widely held belief that monotherapy is safer than polytherapy and demonstrates the need for further studies.

Minor malformations reported include facial dysmorphic features, fingernail hypoplasia and developmental delay. Their association with CBZ exposure is unclear.

Miscellaneous side-effects

The risk of increased cardiotoxic effects of CBZ treatment seems to increase with increasing duration of CBZ treatment and includes conduction disturbances with a predilection for bradycardia or Adams–Stokes attacks, aggravation of sick sinus syndrome, tachyarrhythmia and development of congestive heart failure. One mechanism may be CBZ-related hypothyroidism that increases the risk of cardiac disorders. Cardiac complications associated with CBZ treatment can be divided into two groups. One group develops sinus tachycardia and another group, comprising almost exclusively elderly women, have potentially life-threatening bradyarrhythmias of atrioventricular conduction delay. The latter group in particular must be considered in planning treatment with CBZ. Cardiac conduction defects can occur at the initiation of therapy, and the onset of syncopal symptoms in a patient on therapy requires urgent cardiological investigation.

Elevated cholesterol concentration may significantly decrease plasma CBZ concentration by enhancing total-body clearance of CBZ. On the other hand, cholesterol metabolism may be affected by CBZ, leading to elevations of high-density lipoprotein (HDL) cholesterol concentrations and HDL to total cholesterol ratio. Total cholesterol, HDL and low-density lipoprotein (LDL), and HDL cholesterol levels were significantly higher in CBZ-treated patients than in controls and significantly higher in women than in men [46]. Similarly, in children, these plasma levels were elevated. It is possible that high levels of LDL cholesterol levels associated with low apolipoprotein A-I levels during CBZ treatment increase risk of atherosclerosis.

Renal effects are rare and include proteinuria, haematuria, oliguria and renal failure. Acute renal failure has been described in a few patients on CBZ treatment, attributed to acute interstitial nephritis, acute tubular necrosis or membranous glomerulonephropathy. A few patients have also had interstitial nephritis and exfoliative dermatitis, nephrotic syndrome or a combination of nephropathy, haemolytic anaemia and thrombocytopenia.

CBZ monotherapy during pregnancy has in some cases resulted in a markedly increased abnormal form of prothrombin induced by the absence of vitamin K factor II (PIVKA-II), decreased total prothrombin levels in umbilical cord and subsequent vitamin K deficiency in the neonate.

Psychic disturbances are relatively few compared with other major antiepileptic drugs. They include asthenia, restlessness, insomnia, agitation, anxiety, mania and other psychoses.

Massive overdose and intoxication

In adults, on conventional CBZ treatment of adults, the lowest known lethal dose has been approximately 60 g. A 6-year-old has survived 10 g and a 3-year-old 5 g. However, the maximum tolerable dose varies within wide limits and depends on how much time has elapsed from ingestion. Several hundred patients with massive overdoses, fatalities included, have been reported.

Four clinical stages of CBZ intoxication can be identified [47]: (a) coma and seizures (CBZ level >25 mg/L (105.8 µmol/L)); (b) combativeness, hallucinations, choreiform movements (15–25 mg/L (63.5–105.8 µmol/L)); (c) drowsiness, ataxia (11–15 mg/L (46.5–63.5 µmol/L)); and (d) potentially catastrophic relapse (<11–15 mg/L (46.5 µmol/L)).

In adults, CBZ levels of ≥ 170 µmol/L were significantly associated with serious dysfunctions of several organ systems, including cardiac conduction disorders, respiratory failure, seizures and coma, and the authors emphasized the prognostic importance of blood levels in the evaluation of the severity of intoxication [48].

In children, the plasma levels of CBZ do not appear to predict accurately the severity of toxic reactions. CBZ half-life is prolonged, and CBZ-E level and CBZ-E to CBZ ratio is increased and CBZ-E level may be even higher than CBZ level [49]. In 30 children with CBZ overdoses, the most common effects were lethargy (in 93%) and ataxia (50%), followed by coma (27%), seizures (20%), need for intubation (20%), nystagmus (13%) and minor arrhythmias (10%).

In case of CBZ overdose, continuous EEG monitoring may be helpful in acute therapy and in the evaluation of follow-up after recovery (or worsening) and prognosis.

In addition to symptomatic therapy, CBZ intoxication should be managed with repeated gastric lavage and charcoal haemoperfusion. Forced diuresis, catharsics, peritoneal dialysis, plasmapheresis and haemodialysis have been reported to not be effective. Seizures should be treated with diazepam and phenytoin or fos-phenytoin.

Pharmacoeconomic aspects

During the 1990s, attention has been increasingly paid to the cost-effectiveness of the antiepileptic drugs in the treatment of epilepsy. One was a cost minimization study, conducted on the presumption that established and novel major antiepileptic drugs are similarly efficacious in controlling seizures. The study cohorts have been either hypothetical or various clinical sets of subjects differed from each other in terms of, for example, study design, age group, quality and severity of epilepsy, and setting of treatment and management.

In a US study, a 1-year cost of treatment with CBZ, phenytoin and valproate was estimated. Because seizure control was virtually similar with all the drugs, the costs consisted of the drug price and treatment of side-effects. The costs were $1220 for phenytoin, $1624 for CBZ and $2841 for valproate. In another study, the treatment period under estimation was 2 years and the patients were young adults with newly onset epilepsy. The expenses included in this study were seizure control, side-effects, retention rates, medical consultations, inpatient and emergency admissions, emergency costs, laboratory investigations and drug changes. The costs were estimated on the intention-to-treat basis and were £736–768 for phenytoin, £795–829 for CBZ, £868–884 for valproate and £1525–2076 for lamotrigine.

In a UK study, CBZ and lamotrigine were compared in monotherapy treatment in partial and/or generalized tonic-clonic seizures. A Delphi panel of clinicians advised treatment patterns for adverse events. The costs of CBZ therapy were about one-third of lamotrigine therapy (£179 for CBZ vs. £522 for lamotrigine).

Although the studies are defective and not so well comparable, they seem to show, in general, that CBZ and phenytoin are less expensive than valproate, while lamotrigine is much more expensive but no more effective.

Quality of life

In the treatment of patients with epilepsy, health-related quality of life is emerging as one of the most important aspects. Increasing emphasis is rightly put on a holistic view of the patient care. A European study, based on self-reported SF36 scale, confirmed the previous conception that minimization of side-effects and control of seizures, i.e. the effectiveness of drug therapy is the most important measure of the quality of life. Because all major antiepileptic drugs are virtually equally efficacious, the only difference is between side-effects and price paid by the patient. Despite numerous reports on quality of life in epilepsy, only a few have been associated with individual antiepileptic drugs. Gillham et al. [50] compared CBZ and lamotrigine in relation to quality of life using a modified side-effect and life satisfaction (SEALS) inventory divided into five subscales: worry, temper, cognition, dysphoria and tiredness. Two hundred and sixty patients with newly diagnosed epilepsy were randomized to 48 weeks of treatment with CBZ or lamotrigine. The only significant difference was at week 4. The result is in line with previous experiences on CBZ. The tolerability of CBZ improves after the first week of side-effects and is comparable to other major antiepileptic drugs in the long-term treatment.

However, the short-term measurement of the health-related quality of life will miss longer-term effects which may be highly significant, for instance the visual field defects associated with vigabatrin treatment.

Clinical therapeutics

CBZ is most effective against partial seizures with or without secondary generalization. Its effect against generalized convulsive seizures is also well-documented. CBZ has virtually no effect on absence seizures and may increase propensity to absence seizures and myoclonic seizures. CBZ has been successfully used in some psychiatric disorders and pain syndromes.

A gradual initiation of CBZ therapy is of importance to decrease the risk of dose-related side-effects. The initial daily dosage should usually be 5 mg/kg body weight for adults and 5–10 mg/kg for children, with subsequent increments according to individual clinical effects. The autoinduction phase is usually over within 2–3 weeks from the start-up of the therapy, which allows an increase in daily dosage. The dosing depends on the effectiveness: seizure control and tolerability, not on laboratory measurements.

A combination with another antiepileptic drug is often a second option. In combination treatment, one must consider the pharmacokinetic aspects of various antiepileptic drugs. Valproate often increases the total plasma concentration of CBZ by inhibiting its metabolism and CBZ-E concentration by displacing CBZ from protein binding. Erythromycin, propoxyphene and other drugs with inhibitory action to the metabolism of CBZ may cause toxic reactions. Liver enzyme-inducing drugs may decrease plasma total CBZ concentrations and increase CBZ-E plasma levels by accelerating the metabolism of CBZ. Plasma CBZ-E level may be especially decreased on combination treatment with CBZ, valproate and phenytoin or phenobarbital. Patients taking oral contraceptive, warfarin, ciclosporin or other drugs of non-antiepileptic but inducing effect should have higher daily dosage of CBZ than normally. Higher dosages should be administered if the interacting drug is withdrawn. A consistent formulation, whether registered trademark or generic, might be advisable to decrease variability in bioavailability.

Typical daily maintenance dosage ranges from 10 to 40 mg/kg for children and from 1000 to 2000 mg for adults. The elderly have a lower clearance rate and should have a more cautious increment of the dosage. Combination with other liver enzyme-inductive drugs in particular requires higher daily dosages.

The patient may have been on another drug treatment before CBZ therapy. A rapid switchover from phenytoin, phenobarbital or primidone to CBZ treatment can be safely made.

Measurements of plasma concentrations are advisable at the early stages of medication, e.g. for determining the effects of autoinduction, in polypharmacotherapy, in changes of seizure control or medication, in emergence of seizures of new type, and in case of toxic symptoms or signs. The elderly tolerate CBZ and other antiepileptic drugs less well than young adults and should particularly be considered. Measurements of serum sodium levels are especially indicated in patients with polydipsia, salt-restricted diet or diuretic therapy.

Plasma CBZ and CBZ-E measurements are helpful but are relatively poorly correlated with clinical effects. Diurnal interindividual and intraindividual variation, variability in plasma protein binding, comedication and other obvious factors affect plasma concentrations of CBZ and CBZ-E. Therefore, there is no distinct 'therapeutic' level of CBZ, although usual plasma concentrations are 5–14 µg/mL. Neither are determinations of free plasma levels more helpful than total plasma concentrations. Tailoring daily dosage in line with clinical response, not plasma levels, gives the best results. Slow-resease CBZ tablets on a twice daily basis are preferable to once a day regimes in maintenance therapy, to decrease diurnal fluctuation in blood levels and also improve patient compliance. A slow-release CBZ twice a day regimen appears to be bioequivalent to immediate-release CBZ four times a day.

References

1 Thiele J, Holzinger O. Ueber o-Diamidodibenzyl. *Justus Liebig's Ann Chem* 1899; 305: 96–102.
2 Bourgeois BFD, Awad IA, Pippenger CE *et al*. Brain concentrations of carbamazepine and carbamazepine epoxide in humans. *Epilepsia* 1990; 31: 603.
3 Loscher W, Honack D. Intravenous carbamazepine. comparison of different parental formulations in a mouse model of convulsive status epilepticus. *Epilepsia* 1997; 38: 106–13.
4 Dam M, Jensen A, Christiansen J. Plasma level and effect of carbamazepine in grand mal and psychomotor epilepsy. *Acta Neurol Scand* 1975; 78 (Suppl. 60): 33–8.
5 Stefan H, Schäfer H, Kuhnen C *et al*. Clinical monitoring during carbamazepine slow-release, once-daily monotherapy. *Epilepsia* 1988; 29: 571–7.
6 Caraco Y, Zylber-Katz E, Berry EM *et al*. Carbamazepine disposition in obesity. *Clin Pharmacol Ther* 1992; 51: 133.
7 Rambeck B, Salke-Treumann A, May T, Boenigh HE. Valproic acid-induced carbamazepine-10,11-epoxide toxicity in children and adolescents. *Eur Neurol* 1990; 30: 79–83.
8 Faigle JW, Feldman KF. Pharmacokinetic data of carbamazepine and its major metabolites in man. In: Schneider, H, Janz, D, Gardner-Thorpe, C, Meinardi, H, Shervin, AL, eds. *Clinical Pharmacology of Antiepileptic Drugs*. Berlin, Germany: Springer Verlag, 1975: 159–65.
9 Tomson T, Svensson JO, Hilton-Brown P. Relation of intraindividual dose to plasma concentration of carbamazepine: indication of dose-dependent induction of metabolism. *Ther Drug Monit* 1989; 11: 533–9.
10 Pynnönen S, Kanto J, Sillanpää M. Carbamazepine: placental transport, tissue concentrations in fetus and level in milk. *Acta Pharmacol Toxicol (Copenh)* 1977; 41: 244–53.
11 Hartley R, Lucock MD, Ng PC *et al*. Plasma level/dose ratios of carbamazepine in epileptic children. *Ther Drug Monit* 1990; 12: 438–44.
12 Altafullah I, Talwar D, Loewenson R *et al*. Factors influencing serum levels of carbamazepine and carbamazepine-10,11-epoxide in children. *Epilepsy Res* 1989; 4: 72–80.
13 Haidukewych D, Zielinski JJ, Rodin EA. Derivation and evaluation of an equation for prediction of free carbamazepine concentration in patients comedicated with valproic acid. *Ther Drug Monit* 1989; 11: 528–32.
14 Gidal BE, Rutecki P, Shaw R *et al*. Effect of lamotrigine on carbamazepine epoxide/carbamazepine serum concentration ratios in adult patients with epilepsy. *Epilepsy Res* 1997; 28: 207–11.
15 Brodie MJ, Richens A, Yuen AWC, for UK Lamotrigine/Carbamazepine Monotherapy Trial Group. Double-blind comparison of lamotrigine and carbamazepine in newly diagnosed epilepsy. *Lancet* 1995; 345: 476–9.
16 Kosteljanetz M, Christiansen J, Dam AM *et al*. Carbamazepine vs phenytoin. A controlled clinical trial in focal motor and generalized epilepsy. *Arch Neurol* 1979; 36: 22–4.
17 Callaghan N, Kenny RA, O'Neill B *et al*. A prospective study between

carbamazepine, phenytoin and sodium valproate as monotherapy in previously untreated and recently diagnosed patients with epilepsy. *J Neurol Neurosurg Psychiatr* 1985; 48: 639–44.

18 Richens A, Davidson DL, Cartlidge NE *et al*. A multicentre comparative trial of sodium valproate and carbamazepine in adult onset epilepsy. Adult EPITEG Collaborative Group. *J Neurol Neurosurg Psychiatry* 1994; 57: 682–7.

19 Verity CM, Hosking G, Easter DJ. A multicentre comparative trial of sodium valproate and carbamazepine in paediatric epilepsy. The Paediatric EPITEG Collaborative Group. *Dev Med Child Neurol* 1995; 37: 97–108.

20 Heller AJ, Chesterman P, Elwes RD *et al*. Phenobarbitone, phenytoin, carbamazepine, or sodium valproate for newly diagnosed adult epilepsy: a randomized comparative monotherapy study. *J Neurol Neurosurg Psychiatry* 1995; 58: 44–50.

21 De Silva M, MacArdle B, McGowas M *et al*. Randomised comparative monotherapy trial of phenobarbitone, phenytoin, carbamazepine and sodium valproate for newly diagnosed childhood epilepsy. *Lancet* 1996; 347: 709–13.

22 Stein J. CBZ vs phenytoin in young epileptic children. *Drug Ther* 1989; 19: 76–7.

23 Mattson RH, Cramer JA, Collins JF. A comparison of valproate with carbamazepine for the treatment of complex partial seizures and secondarily generalized tonic-clonic seizures in adults. The Department of Veterans Affairs Epilepsy Cooperative Study. *N Engl J Med* 1992; 327: 765–71.

24 Reunanen M, Dam M, Yuen AW. A randomized open multicentre comparative trial of lamotrigine and carbamazepine as monotherapy in patients with newly diagnosed or recurrent epilepsy. *Epilepsy Res* 1996; 23: 149–55.

25 Kälviäinen R, Äikiä M, Saukkonen AM *et al*. Vigabatrin vs carbamazepine monotherapy in patients with newly diagnosed epilepsy. A randomized controlled study. *Arch Neurol* 1995; 52: 989–96.

26 Chadwick D, Vigabatrin European Monotherapy Group. Vigabatrin vs. carbamazepine in newly diagnosed epilepsy. *Lancet* 1999; 354: 13–19.

27 Chadwick DW, Anhut H, Greiner MJ, International Gabapentin Monotherapy Study Group. Gabapentin vs. Carbamazepine in newly diagnosed partial epilepsy. *Epilepsia* 1998; 51: 1282–8.

28 Mattson RH, Cramer JA, Collins JF, The VA Epilepsy Cooperative Study Group. Connective tissue changes, hypersensitivity rash, and blood laboratory test changes associated with antiepileptic drug therapy. *Ann Neurol* 1986; 20: 119–20.

29 Brodie MJ, Mumford JP, 012 Study Group. Vigabatrin and valproate in carbamazepine-resistant partial epilepsy. *Epilepsy Res* 1999; 34: 199–205.

30 Smith DB, Mattson RH, Cramer JA *et al*. Results of a nationwide Veterans Administration Cooperative Study comparing the efficacy and toxicity of carbamazepine, phenobarbital, phenytoin, and primidone. *Epilepsia* 1987; 28 (Suppl. 3): 50–8.

31 Duncan JS, Shorvon SD, Trimple MR. Withdrawal symptoms from phenytoin, carbamazepine and sodium valproate. *J Neurol Neurosurg Psychiatr* 1988; 51: 924–8.

32 Williams J, Bates S, Griebel ML *et al*. Does short-term antiepileptic drug treatment result in cognitive or behavioral changes? *Epilepsia* 1998; 39: 1064–9.

33 Zamponi N, Cardinali C. Open comparative long-term study of vigabatrin vs carbamazepine in newly diagnosed partial seizures in children. *Arch Neurol* 1999; 56: 605–7.

34 Kälviäinen R, Nousiainen I. Visual field defects with vigabatrin. Epidemiology and therapeutic implications. *CNS Drugs* 2001; 15: 217–30.

35 Martin R, Meador K, Turrentine L *et al*. Comparative cognitive effects of carbamazepine and gabapentin in healthy senior adults. *Epilepsia* 2001; 42: 764–71.

36 Sillanpää M. Carbamazepine. Pharmacology and clinical uses. *Acta Neurol Scand* 1981; 88 (Suppl. 64): 1–202.

37 Eiris-Punal J, Del Rio-Garma M, Del Rio-Garma MC *et al*. Long-term treatment of children with epilepsy with valproate or carbamazepine may cause subclinical hypothyroidism. *Epilepsia* 1999; 40: 1761–6.

38 Surks MI, DeFesi CR. Serum free hormone concentrations on phenytoin or carbamazepine. *J Am Med Ass* 1996; 275: 1495–8.

39 Isojärvi JIT, Repo M, Pakarinen AJ *et al*. Carbamazepine, phenytoin, sex hormones, and sexual function in men with epilepsy. *Epilepsia* 1995; 36: 366–70.

40 Murialdo G, Calimberti CA, Fonzi S *et al*. Sex hormones and pituitary function in epileptic patients with normal or altered sexuality. *Epilepsia* 1995; 36: 360–5.

41 Schmidt D, Sheldon L. *Adverse Effects of Antiepileptic Drugs*. New York: Raven Press, 1982.

42 Feldkamp J, Becker A, Witte OW *et al*. Long-term anticonvulsant therapy leads to low bone mineral density—evidence for direct drug effects of phenytoin and carbamazepine on human osteoclast-like cells. *Exp Clin Endocrinol Diabetes* 2000; 108: 37–43.

43 Kaneko S, Battino D, Andermann E. Congenital malformations due to antiepileptic drugs. *Epilepsy Res* 1999; 33: 145–58.

44 Diav-Citrin O, Shechtman S, Arnon J *et al*. Is carbamazepine teratogenic? A prospective controlled study. *Neurology* 2001; 57: 321–4.

45 Arpino C, Brescianini S, Robert E *et al*. Teratogenic effects of antiepileptic drugs: use of an international database on malformations and drug exposure (MADRE). *Epilepsia* 2000; 41: 1436–43.

46 Sudhop T, Bauer J, Elger CE *et al*. Increased high-density lipoprotein cholesterol in patients with epilepsy treated with carbamazepine: a gender-related study. *Epilepsia* 1999; 40: 480–4.

47 Weaver DF, Camfield P, Fraser A. Massive carbamazepine overdose. clinical and pharmacologic observations. *Neurology* 1988; 38: 755–9.

48 Höjer J, Malmlund HO, Berg A. Clinical features in massive poisoning with carbamazepine. *J Toxicol Clin Toxicol* 1993; 31: 449–58.

49 De Groot G, van Heijst AN, Maes RA. Charcoal hemoperfusion in treatment of two cases of acute carbamazepine poisoning. *J Toxicol Clin Toxicol* 1984; 22: 349–62.

50 Gillham R, Kane K, Bryant-Comstock L *et al*. A double-blind comparison of lamotrigine and carbamazepine in newly diagnosed epilesy with health-related quality of life as an outcome measure. *Seizure* 2000; 9: 375–9.

29

Clobazam

M.A. Dalby

Primary indications	Adjunctive therapy for partial and generalized seizures. Also for intermittent therapy, one-off prophylactic therapy and non-convulsive status epilepticus
Usual preparations	Tablet, capsule: 10 mg
Usual dosages	10–20 mg/day (adults); higher doses can be used. Children aged 3–12 years, up to half adult dose
Dosage intervals	1–2 times/day
Significant drug interactions	Minor interactions are common, but usually not clinically significant
Serum level monitoring	Not useful
Target range	–
Common/important side-effects	Sedation, dizziness, weakness, blurring of vision, restlessness, ataxia, aggressiveness, behavioural disturbance, withdrawal symptoms
Main advantages	Highly effective in some patients with epilepsy resistant to first-line therapy. Less side-effects than with other benzodiazepines
Main disadvantages	Development of tolerance in as many as 50% of subjects within weeks or months
Mechanisms of action	$GABA_A$ receptor agonist. Also action on ion-channel conductance
Oral bioavailability	90%
Time to peak levels	1–4 h
Metabolism and excretion	Hepatic oxidation and then conjugation
Volume of distribution	–
Elimination half-life	10–77 h (clobazam); 50 h (*N*-desmethylclobazam)
Plasma clearance	–
Protein binding	83%
Active metabolites	*N*-desmethylclobazam
Comment	Excellent second-line therapy in some patients with resistant epilepsy

(*Note*: this summary table was formulated by the lead editor.)

Clobazam was synthesized in 1972 [1] by deliberate modification of the 1,4-diazepine structure (Fig. 29.1). The resulting 1,5 structure retained 20% of the the anxiolytic activity of diazepam, and only 10–15% of diazepam's sedative effects in animal studies. Clobazam is the only 1,5 benzodiazepine in wide clinical usage. Clobazam was introduced as an anti-anxiety agent about half as potent as diazepam and producing less psychomotor side-effects than diazepam. It was later found to have major antiepileptic effects in

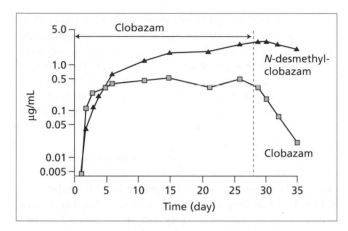

Fig. 29.1 Levels of clobazam and desmethylclobazam (norclobazam) in a single patient treated for 28 days with clobazam at a dose of 10 mg twice per day. Note that at steady state, the norclobazam levels are at least 10 fold higher than those of the parent drug [69].

mice and in animal studies [2]. The clinical potential as an antiepileptic drug was first reported in 1978 [3] and in 1979 [4]. Clobazam has been licensed in Europe since 1975, in Canada since 1988 and is still under investigation in the US. It was fully reported in *Antiepileptic Drugs* [5,6]. There have been at least two international symposia devoted to the antiepileptic uses of clobazam [7,8] and there is also a sizeable literature concerning its anxiolytic effects, relaxant and hypnotic properties.

Clobazam is a white hygroscopic powder with MW 300.73. It has a bitter taste, is relatively insoluble in water and cannot be given as intravenous or intramuscular injection. It is a weak organic acid and forms water-soluble salts at acidic pH. At physiological pH its lipid solubility is about 40% of that of diazepam [9].

Mode of action

Clobazam exerts its anxiolytic and anticonvulsant action at the benzodiazepine binding site of the γ-aminobutyric acid A (GABA-A) receptor complex by increasing the likelihood of opening of the ligand-gated Cl⁻ ion channel in response to a given concentration of GABA.

Clobazam enhances the current through the channel in a dose-dependent manner at concentrations up to 3 μmol. Above this level the enhancement is reduced. Concentrations of free clobazam and its active metabolite desmethylclobazam in the brain in patients with good therapeutic response range from 0.02 to 1.7 μmol and from 0.3 to 1.5 μmol, respectively [10]. These results point to a theoretical upper effective limit for the drug in the brain, achieved with 20–40 mg doses.

A number of subunits of the GABA-A receptor complex have now been cloned using recombinant techniques, demonstrating that the modulatory efficacy of drugs is dependent on receptor composition in different brain regions and developmental stages. Depending on their subunit composition, recombinant GABA-A receptors exhibit different benzodiazepine binding properties [11]. This may explain the differences in therapeutic action and side-effects between various 1,4 and 1,5 benzodiazepines, that could bind preferentially to different subgroups. The conformation of the vari-

ous benzodiazepine molecules and extent of receptor reserve among neurones could also contribute to the different pharmacological profiles of benzodiazepines.

Apart from the effect on the high-affinity GABA-A receptor there is also an action at a lower affinity membrane site which probably involves an increase in the population of sodium channels in the inactive state, limiting the repetitive firing of neurones. This is possibly directly reflected in the ability of benzodiazepines to reduce or terminate generalized epileptic activity in the EEG. A decrease of voltage-sensitive Ca(++) conductance is also observed, limiting Ca(++) entry presynaptically and decreasing neurotransmitter release [12].

In animal studies clobazam has been found effective against maximal electroshock seizures, pentetrazol seizures, kindled seizures and seizures in animals genetically prone to epilepsy [13–16]. Tolerance has also been described in animal models, albeit with marked interspecies differences. Clobazam differs from diazepam and other benzodiazepines in its broader antiepileptic spectrum and its better side-effect profile.

Pharmacokinetics

Clobazam is absorbed rapidly and almost completely. Mean absorption half-life is 20 min. It is unaffected by age or sex. The rate of absorption is reduced when the drug is taken with or after meals, but the extent of absorption is not affected by food intake [17]. The drug is highly lipophilic and, after absorption, is rapidly distributed in fat and cerebral grey matter. It is redistributed widely and has a large volume of distribution. Rectal absorption of the capsule and solution (but not suppository) is fast and complete. Peak levels obtained after rectal administration are similar to those obtained after oral therapy. On this basis, the rectal use of clobazam would be a promising alternative to diazepam, but this mode of administration has not gained wide clinical usage.

Maximal plasma concentration after a single dose is seen after 1–4 h and half-lives of the apparent elimination phase varies from 11 to 77 h in healthy subjects, with the longest half-life in the elderly [18]. The half-life of clobazam's major metabolite, *N*-desmethylclobazam is even longer, about 50 h [19]. However, when used in patients receiving other antiepileptic drugs, half-life is reduced to 12–13 h, though significantly longer in the elderly. This is also true for the major metabolite of clobazam, *N*-desmethylclobazam [20]. At clinical doses of 0.1–0.5 mg/kg the plasma concentration of the metabolite (300–3500 ng/mL) is usually 10-fold greater than clobazam concentrations (20–350 ng/mL) [21] (Fig. 29.1). There is a good correlation between plasma concentration and dose in the individual patient but large interindividual variations [22–24]. Measurements of serum levels, however, have not been found useful clinically.

Plasma protein binding of the benzodiazepines varies from nearly 99% for diazepam to 70% for alprazolam. Clobazam protein binding is 83%. The protein bound fraction is independent of plasma concentration of clobazam and is only changed by lowered protein content, which may be of importance in hepatic and renal diseases and other conditions with lowered protein, e.g. in the elderly.

Clobazam is distributed in the general circulation and to the brain in the first phase. It is assumed that the drug is later distributed to adipose tissue and bone. In cerebrospinal fluid clobazam and *N*-desmethylclobazam concentrations are lower than in serum [25]. The concentration in brain is proportional to the concentration of unbound clobazam in serum and is about 15% of total serum clobazam; brain distribution is determined by clobazam's lipid solubility rather than with specific receptor affinity [26]. Concentrations in saliva correlates with serum concentration [22].

Drug interactions

Clobazam has a complex pattern of interactions, with marked interindividual variability. However, these are usually not of clinical significance. Clobazam can cause an increase or decrease in the blood levels of phenobarbital, phenytoin or carbamazepine [27]. Phenytoin toxicity has been reported in patients on maximal tolerable phenytoin doses when clobazam was added [28], and levels of all enzyme-inducing antiepileptic drugs can alter in susceptible patients. The combination of valproate in doses of 1500–2000 mg and clobazam leads to an increase in serum valproate levels often with toxic-confusional states [29]. These rather unpredictable interactions may be the explanation for the aversion to clobazam shown by some patients with chronic epilepsy on antiepileptic polytherapy.

Clobazam levels are generally lower and norclobazam levels higher in patients who are comedicated with enzyme-inducing antiepileptic drugs. Comedication with carbamazepine seems to induce the epoxidation of this drug [30]. Conversely, it has also been reported that clobazam levels can be raised in bitherapy with phenobarbital, phenytoin and carbamazepine [31]. Concomitant administration of alcohol and cimetidine can also lead to a significant increase in clobazam levels.

Biotransformation

Clobazam is extensively metabolized with at least 12 different measurable metabolites. The initial biotransformation of clobazam is by oxidation in the liver to desmethylclobazam (norclobazam). This is an active metabolite. Norclobazam may be responsible for most of the effects of clobazam [32,33] as its serum concentrations are usually over 10-fold higher in chronic therapy than the parent drug. Studies in baboons have shown antiepileptic effects 5–6 h after IV infusion, by which time clobazam plasma concentrations have fallen to low levels. This suggests that the active metabolite is responsible for the antiepileptic properties of the drug. However, in humans, the lipophilicity of norclobazam is lower than that of clobazam, and the affinity for the benzodiazepine receptor is more than 10-fold lower than that of clobazam. It is thus unclear to what extent the parent drug and its metabolite contribute to the overall antiepileptic effect in human epilepsy [9]. Desmethylclobazam is further metabolized by conjugation and excreted in bile as glucuronate and in bile and urine as the sulphate [34].

Toxicity

The side-effects of clobazam have been extensively studied in patients taking the drug in psychiatric settings, as well as in patients with epilepsy. While sedation, development of tolerance and withdrawal symptoms can limit the use of 1,4 benzodiazepines in

chronic treatment of epilepsy, investigations have generally shown that clobazam has less detrimental effects on psychomotor performance than these drugs [35,36]. Impairment on a few cognitive tests, mainly retrieval processes and mental rapidity has been reported [37]. Muscle fatigue or weakness is an effect apparent in dynamic work situations where a disorderly recruitment of motor units is seen [38]. Clobazam like other benzodiazepines should not be given to myasthenic patients. The ventilatory response to CO_2 is unaffected by clobazam [39].

In clinical trials a number of side-effects are seen with increasing frequency as reports have become more formalized. Thus side-effects are reported in 20–85%, but only in 5–15% are they found of importance, leading to change of dose or termination of treatment [40,41]. Significant toxicity includes sedation, dizziness, headache, nausea, amnesia, ataxia and blurred vision or diplopia. With chronic institutionalized patient populations increased irritability, depression and disinhibition occurs [42] and behaviour disturbance may be seen. Koeppen [43] reviewed 23 open studies of clobazam (Table 29.1). Drowsiness and dizziness were the most common side-effects. In general however the side-effects were mild and transient, and in routine clinical practice the drug seems well tolerated. The plasma concentration of the metabolite norclobazam is increased significantly in polytherapy, and this may be the cause of some of the sedative side-effects [31].

Tolerance or 'escape' is usually measured as an increase of seizure frequency in the last half of a treatment period, and it has been noted in 0–77% usually appearing during the first months of treatment. Tolerance is increased by high doses, and decreased by intermittent treatment [44]. In patients with temporal lobe epilepsy tolerance was found to be increasing slowly from 3% after 1 month to 35% after 2 years and did not seem to increase further [45]. Used as monotherapy in childhood epilepsy, tolerance, i.e. a break through of seizures after a 3–6 months seizure-free period, was noted in

Table 29.1 Summary of reported side-effects to clobazam, diazepam and placebo in 70 double-blind studies of the anxiolytic effects of clobazam

	Clobazam ($n=1690$)	Diazepam ($n=1084$)	Placebo ($n=889$)
Drowsiness	25.8	45.5	9.9
Dizziness	7.0	12.0	2.8
Headache	2.1	3.2	2.9
Nausea	1.6	1.5	2.1
Dry mouth	3.0	2.3	0.9
Constipation	2.1	3.4	0.3
Diarrhoea	0.4	1.4	0.3
Blurred vision	0.6	1.3	0.0
Agitation	0.8	1.7	0.3
Confusion	1.0	1.2	0.0
Irritability	0.5	1.2	0.3
Depression	1.7	2.2	0.3
Insomnia	1.8	1.6	0.6
Ataxia	0.2	1.4	0.0
Amnesia	0.3	0.5	0.1

From [6,43].
Table shows the percentage of patients reporting side-effects.

7.5%, as compared to 4.3% for carbamazepine and 6.7% for phenytoin monotherapy [46]. This suggests that the development of tolerance has been overestimated in the past. Tolerance to sedation develops more quickly than tolerance to the anticonvulsant or anxiolytic effects [47,48].

The frequency of pretreatment interictal spiking was found significant for tolerance development and a poor outcome in the treatment of temporal lobe epilepsy [45]. Patients with Lennox–Gastaut syndrome may also benefit for long periods without tolerance setting in [49,50].

Withdrawal symptoms with irritability, restlessness and difficulty to concentrate appears in 5–10% during the first 14 days after termination of treatment. Tapering will in most cases prevent this. In the context of refractory epilepsy it is difficult to ascertain whether withdrawal seizures occur.

Antiepileptic effectiveness

Clobazam was first investigated as an antiepileptic in Marseilles in October 1977 by Gastaut *et al.* [4]. It was used first for a few days in 140 patients with frequent seizures and then continued in those patients showing a good response (at a dose of 0.5–1 mg/kg/day). Many clinical features of the drug were noted then and have been confirmed many times since. The drug was noted to have a rapid and potent effect in 76% of these patients although the effect was maintained in only 52% after a matter of months. Following this report, numerous studies have been carried out.

Clobazam was shown to be significantly better than placebo in nine double-blind trials with treatment periods of 2–6 months [41,42,51–56]. The drug has mostly been tried in patients with refractory epilepsy of long standing as an addition to other antiepileptic treatment. A number of patients have been freed from attacks, but some have recurrence when followed up later. A sizable number have attacks reduced considerably, which has made the treatment worthwhile. A large number of open studies have been carried out (Table 29.2). Twenty-two open studies of 880 patients published between 1979 and 1985 were reviewed by Koeppen *et al.* [43]. These studies were of patients aged between 0.6 months and 69 years with widely differing aetiologies and seizure types, 20 were of adjunctive therapy, and doses varied between 10 and 80 mg/day. A

Table 29.2 Summary of findings from 22 studies of clobazam in epilepsy

Reference	Number of patients	Daily dose	Efficacy (% improvement)	Number of patients seizure free	Incidence of tolerance (%)	Incidence of side-effects (%)	Length of study or F/U
[42]	52	10–30 mg	50	N/S	77	29	12 mo
[70]	35	0.5 mg/kg	74	N/S	43	N/S	1–12 mo
[71]	17	20–80 mg	82	2	43	24	6 mo
[72]	33	10–>40 mg	60	10 G (6 mo) 2 P (6 mo)	25	30	18 mo
[73]	86	0.1–1.2 mg/kg	51	17 (>3 mo)	N/S	N/S	3 mo
[50]	9	30–100 mg	78	5 (7 mo)	0	33	1–7 mo
[74]	34	1.27 mg/kg	68	4	65	47	27 mo
[64]	24	0.5–1 mg/kg	70	11	N/S	8	10 days–36 mo (mean, 9 mo)
[75]	10	60 mg	70	5	40	N/S	2
[76]	26	2–32 mg	50	2	N/S	12	N/S
[77]	23	0.5–2 mg/kg	70	11	21	52	6 mo (mean)
[63]	18	0.3–0.7 mg/kg	89	N/S	40	50	7–26 mo
[78]	140	0.5–1 mg/kg	76	35	33	33	7 days–14 mo >3 mo
[79]	54	0.1–0.75 mg/kg	75–80	27 (6 mo) 17 (>1 y)	25 25	19 19	48 mo 48 mo
[80]	48	0.1–0.75 mg/kg	75–80	13 (>2 y) 6 (4 y)			
[81]	35	0.5–1.5 mg/kg	83	11	11	69	1–4 mo
[49]	26	Up to 2.5 mg/kg	58	2 (1 y)	33	42	12 mo
[65]	15	0.5–1 mg/kg	87	6	23	N/S	12 mo
[82]	52	0.5–2 mg/kg	71	N/S	N/S	N/S	8 mo
[83]	60	20–40 mg	95	N/S	N/S	N/S	4–8 mo (12 pts)
[84]	36	0.2–1.82 mg/kg	50	9	N/S	47	12 mo
[85]	36	1.4 mg/kg	81	21	N/S	N/S	6 mo
[86]	34	10–130 mg	41	7	N/S	N/S	30–63 mo

G, generalized seizure; P, partial seizure.
Adapted from [6,43,87].

more recent retrospective study of 877 patients in Canada showed a greater than 50% response rate in 40% of patients and 10–30% became seizure free [40]. Only 4% discontinued the drug due to side-effects. These are excellent results, which can be matched by few other drugs. Patients of all ages, aetiologies and seizure types responded. Some authors consider partial seizures to do best, and others secondarily generalized attacks. It has been claimed that patients with symptomatic epilepsy, most often with partial seizures without secondary generalization and without mental retardation, respond best to clobazam [57], but this is an uncontrolled observation which has not been replicated [57]. In the largest double-blind study, no differences in efficacy between seizure types were observed [41].

The relation between serum level and seizure control is confused by the development of tolerance in many patients and an optimal range of serum levels in chronic users cannot be established [24].

Open studies have reported a beneficial and even astounding effect in non-convulsive status [58–61], in startle seizures [62], in Lennox–Gastaut syndrome [49] and in alcoholic withdrawal seizures [63], and in a few cases of continuous spike-waves during sleep (CSWS). Studies of clobazam used as monotherapy are very few. Clobazam has, however, been used in open studies as the only drug in benign childhood partial epilepsy and found of value even in carbamazepine-resistant cases [64,65].

Uncontrolled observations (as well as routine clinical experience) show good efficacy in acute epilepsy, in clusters, in serial seizures and as prophylaxis (e.g. on days when it is important to avoid a seizure such as when travelling, taking examinations, interviews, etc.). Clobazam is undoubtedly the drug of first choice for such intermittent therapy in the author's practice. Clobazam has a limited role also as intermittent therapy in catamenial epilepsy [44].

Dose and clinical therapeutics

Clobazam has been reportedly used at dosages between 5 and 140 mg/day. There is now general agreement that doses between 10 and 20 mg/day (in adults) are usually best, and few patients who continue to have seizures respond better to higher doses, nor does increasing the dose overcome tolerance. Dose adjustments are not usually needed in patients comedicated with other antiepileptic drugs. The frequency of side-effects increases sharply with higher doses (above 30 mg/day). The usual daily dose for acute prophylaxis is 10 mg. Clobazam withdrawal should be carried out slowly in a staged fashion. It is also advisable to observe the same general precautions in treatment with clobazam as with other benzodiazepines.

In summary clobazam is a useful adjunct in patients with most types of refractory epilepsy. On the basis of a large number of double-blind and retrospective investigations, clobazam appears to be more effective than implied from the early reports [66]. Its efficacy has been shown to be equivalent to that of other antiepileptic drugs as add-on for treatment of refractory seizures and it is well tolerated [67]. It has a wide spectrum of activity. The main drawback of the drug is the potential for tolerance to develop. It can also be used very effectively as a 'prophylactic' on special occasions, in clusters or serial seizures or to terminate acute seizures. The anxiolytic effects of clobazam is often of considerable value in chronic epileptic patients with interictal anxiety [68].

References

1 von Weber K, Bauer A, Hauptmann K.H. Benzodiazepine mit psychotroper Wirkung III. N-Aryl- und N-Heteroaryl-1H-1,5-benzodiazepin-2, 4-(3H,5H)-dione. *Liebigs Ann Chem* 1972; 756: 128–38.

2 Barzaghi F, Fournex R, Mantegazza P. Pharmacological and toxicological properties of Clobazam, a new psychotherapeutic agent. *Arzn Forsch* 1973; 23: 683–6.

3 Gastaut H. Proprietes antiepileptiques exceptionelles et meconnues d'un anxiolytique de commerce: le clobazam. *Concours Med* 1978; 100: 3697–701.

4 Gastaut H, Low MD. Anti-epileptic properties of clobazam, a 1,5-benzodiazepine, in man. *Epilepsia* 1979; 20: 437–46.

5 Shorvon SD. Clobazam. In: Levy R, Mattson R, Meldrum B, Penry JK, Dreifuss FE, eds. *Antiepileptic Drugs*, 3rd edn. New York: Raven Press, 1989: 821–40.

6 Shorvon SD. Clobazam. In: Levy R, Mattson R, Meldrum B, eds. *Antiepileptic Drugs*, 4th edn. New York: Raven Press, 1995: 763–78.

7 Hindmarch I, Stonier PD, eds. *Clobazam*. International Congress and Symposium Series no. 43. London: Royal Society of Medicine, 1981.

8 Hindmarch I, Stonier PD, Trimble M, eds. *Clobazam, Human Psychopharmacology and Clinical Applications*. International Congress and Symposium Series no. 74. London: Royal Society of Medicine, 1985.

9 Greenblatt DJ, Shader I. Pharmacokinetics of antianxiety agents. In: Meltzer HY, ed. *Psychopharmacology*. London: Raven Press, 1987.

10 Nakamura F, Suzuki S, Nishimura S, Yagi K, Seino M. Effects of clobazam and its active metabolite on GABA-activated currents in rat cerebral neurons in culture. *Epilepsia* 1996; 37(8): 728–35.

11 Sieghart W. GABAa receptors: ligand-gated CL⁻ ion channels modulated by multiple drug-binding sites. *TiPS* 1992; 131: 446–50.

12 Meldrum BS, Chapman AG. Benzodiazepine receptors and their relationship to the treatment of epilepsy. *Epilepsia* 1986; 27 (Suppl. 1): S3–S13.

13 Shenoy AK, Miyahara JT, Swinyard EA, Kupferberg HJ. Comparative anticonvulsant activity and neurotoxicity of clobazam, diazepam, phenobarbital and valproate in mice and rats. *Epilepsia* 1982; 23: 399–408.

14 Haigh JRM, Gent JP, Calvert R. Plasma concentrations of clobazam and its N-desmethyl metabolite; protection against pentetrazol-induced convulsions in mice. *J Pharm Pharmacol* 1984; 36: 636–8.

15 Teitz EL, Rosenberg HC, Chiu TH. A comparison of the anticonvulsant effects of 1,4- and 1,5-benzodiazepines in amygdala-kindled rats and their effects on motor functions. *Epilepsy Res* 1989; 3: 31–40.

16 Meldrum BS, Croucher MJ. Anticonvulsant action of clobazam and desmethylclobazam in reflex epilepsy in rodents and baboons. *Drug Dev Res* 1982; S1: 33–8.

17 Cenraud B, Guyot M, Levy RH *et al*. No effect of food intake on clobazam absorption. *Br J Pharmacol* 1983; 16/6: 728–30.

18 Greenblatt DJ, Divoll M, Puri SK *et al*. Clobazam kinetics in the elderly. *Br J Pharmacol* 1981; 12/5, 631–6.

19 Fielding S, Hoffmann I. Pharmacology of anti-anxiety drugs with special reference to clobazam. *Br J Clin Pharmacol* 1979; 7: 7s–15s.

20 Bun H, Coassolo P, Gouezo F, Cano JP, Dravet C, Roger J. Plasma levels and pharmacokinetics of clobazam and N-desmethylclobazam in epileptic patients. In: Hindmarch I, Stonier PD, Trimble MR, eds. *Clobazam, Human Psychopharmacology and Clinical Applications*. International Congress and Symposium Series, no 74. London: The Royal Society of Medicine, 1985.

21 Bun H, Monjanel-Mouterde S, Noel F, Durand A, Cano JP. Effects of age and antiepileptic drugs on plasma levels and kinetics of clobazam and N-desmethylclobazam. *Pharmacol Toxicol* 1990; 67(2): 136–40.

22 Bardy AH, Seppala T, Salokorpi T, Granstrom ML, Santavuori P. Monitoring concentrations of clobazam and norclobazam in serum and saliva of children with epilepsy. *Brain Dev* 1991; 13 (3): 174–9.

23 Guberman A, Couture M, Blaschuk K, Sherwin A. Add-on trial of clobazam in intractable adult epilepsy with plasma level correlations. *Canad J Neurol Sci* 1990; 17: 311–36.

24 Goggin T, Callaghan N. Blood levels of clobazam and its metabolites and therapeutic effect. In: Hindmarch I, Stonier PD, Trimble MR, eds. *Clobazam, Human Psychopharmacology and Clinical Applications*.

International Congress and Symposium Series, no 74. London: The Royal Society of Medicine, 1985.

25 Laux G, Koeppen D. Serum and cerebrospinal fluid concentrations of clobazam and N-desmethylclobazam. *Int J Clin Pharmacol Ther Toxicol* 1984; 22/7: 355–9.

26 Arendt RM, Greenblatt DJ, Liebisch DC, Luu MD, Paul SM. Determinants of benzodiazepine brain uptake: lipophilicity versus binding affinity. *Psychopharmacology* 1987; 93/1: 72–6.

27 Vakil SD, Critchley EMR, Cocks A, Hayward HW. The effect of clobazam on blood levels of phenobarbitone, phenytoin and carbamazepine. Preliminary report. In: Hindmarch I, Stonier PD, eds. *Clobazam*. International Congress and Symposium Series, no. 43. London: Royal Society of Medicine, 1981.

28 Zifkin B, Sherwin A, Andermann F. Phenytoin toxicity due to interaction with clobazam. *Neurology* 1991; 41 (2 Pt 1): 313–14.

29 Cocks A, Critchley EMR, Hayward HW, Thomas D. The effect of clobazam on the blood levels of sodium valproate. In: Hindmarch I, Stonier PD, Trimble MR, eds. *Clobazam, Human Psychopharmacology and Clinical Applications*. International Congress and Symposium Series, no 74. London: The Royal Society of Medicine, 1985.

30 Munoz JJ, De Salamanca RE, Diaz Obregon C, Timoneda FL. The effect of clobazam on steady state plasma concentrations of carbamazepine and its metabolites. *Br J Clin Pharmacol* 1990; 29 (6): 763–5.

31 Sennoune S, Mesdjian E, Bonneton J, Genton P, Dravet C, Roger J. Interactions between clobazam and standard antiepileptic drugs in patients with epilepsy. *Ther Drug Mon* 1992; 14(4): 269–74.

32 Caccia S, Guiso G, Garattini S. Brain concentrations of clobazam and N-desmethylclobazam and antileptazol activity. *J Pharm Pharmacol* 1980; 32/4: 295–6.

33 Haigh JRM, Pullar T, Gent JP *et al*. N-desmethylclobazam: a possible alternative to clobazam in the treatment of refractory epilepsy? *Br J Pharmacol* 1987; 23/2: 213–18.

34 Borel AG, Abbott FS. Metabolic profiling of clobazam, a 1,5-benzodiazepine in rats. *Drug Metab Dis Biol Fate Chem* 1993; 21 (3): 415–41.

35 Saletu B, Grunberger J, Berner P, Koeppen D. On differences between 1,5- and 1,4-benzodiazepines: Pharmaco-EEG and psychometric studies with clobazam and lorezepam. In: Hindmarch I, Stonier PD, Trimble MR, eds. *Clobazam, Human Psychopharmacology and Clinical Applications*. International Congress and Symposium Series, no 74. London: The Royal Society of Medicine, 1985.

36 Hindmarch I, Gudgeon AC. The effects of clobazam and lorazepam on aspects of psychomotor performance and car handling ability. *Br J Clin Pharmacol* 1980; 10/2: 145–50.

37 Cull CA, Trimble MR. Anticonvulsant benzodiazepines and performance. In: Hindmarch I, Stonier PD, Trimble MR, eds. *Clobazam, Human Psychopharmacology and Clinical Applications*. International Congress and Symposium Series, no 74. London: The Royal Society of Medicine, 1985.

38 Schaffle K, Rimkus A, Hirschmann K, Arnold H. The action of clobazam and diazepam on computer-assisted tests of muscle activity: dynamometric and myogenic effects. *Drug Dev Res* 1982; 2 (Suppl. 1): 177–82.

39 Wildin JD, Pleuvry BJ, Mawer GE, Onon T, Millington L. Respiratory and sedative effects of clobazam and clonazepam in volunteers. *Br J Clin Pharmacol* 1990; 29/2: 169–77.

40 Canadian Clobazam Cooperative Group. Clobazam in the treatment of refractory Epilepsy: The Canadian Experience. A retrospective survey. *Epilepsia* 1991; 32(3): 407–16.

41 Koeppen D, Baruzzi A, Capozza M *et al*. Clobazam in therapy-resistant patients with partial epilepsy: a double-blind placebo-controlled crossover study. *Epilepsia* 1987; 28(5): 495–506.

42 Allen JW, Oxley J, Robertson MM, Trimble M, Richens A, Jawad S. Clobazam as adjunctive treatment in refractory epilepsy. *Br Med J* 1983; 286: 1246–7.

43 Koeppen D. A review of clobazam studies in epilepsy. In: Hindmarch I, Stonier PD, Trimble MR, eds. *Clobazam, Human Psychopharmacology and Clinical Applications*. Internatinonal congress and symposium series: no 74. London: Royal Society of Medicine, 1985; 1207–15.

44 Feely M, Calvert R, Gibson J. Clobazam in catamenial epilepsy: a model for evaluating anticonvulsant. *Lancet* 1982; ii: 71–3.

45 Barcs G, Halàsz P. Effectivenss and tolerance of clobazam in temporal lobe epilepsy. *Acta Neurol Scand* 1996; 93: 88–93.

46 Canadian Study Group for Childhood Epilepsy. Clobazam has equivalent efficacy to carbamazepine and phenytoin as monotherapy for childhood epilepsy. *Epilepsia* 1998; 39 (9): 952–9.

47 Rosenberg HC, Tietz EI, Chiu TH. Differential tolerance to the antipentylenetetrazol activity of benzodiazepines in flurazepam treated rats. *Pharmacol Biochem Behav* 1991; July 39(3): 711–16.

48 File SE. Tolerance to the behavioral actions of benzodiazepines. *Neurosci Biobehav Rev* 1985; 9/1: 113–21.

49 Péchadre JC, Beudin P, Devoize JL, Gilbert J. Rapports sur les effects antiépileptiques dans le syndrome de Lennox et Gastaut. *L'Encéphale* 1981; 7: 181–90.

50 Dalby MA. Clobazam in resistant epilepsy. In: Hindmarch I, Stonier PD, Trimble MR, eds. *Clobazam, Human Psychopharmacology and Clinical Applications*. International Congress and Symposium Series, no 74. London: The Royal Society of Medicine, 1985.

51 Del Pesce M, Fua P, Guiliani G *et al*. *Clobazam as an Antiepileptic Drug. A controlled clinical trial of its efficacy, plasma and side-effects in partial and secondary generalized epilepsy*. Abstract 423. 11th Epilepsy International Symposium, Florence, Italy, 1979.

52 Critchley EMR, Vakil SD, Hayward HW *et al*. Double-blind clinical trial of clobazam in refractory epilepsy. In: Hindmarch I, Stonier PD, eds. *Clobazam*. International Congress and Symposium Series, no 43. Royal Society of Medicine. London: Academic Press, 1981: 159–63.

53 Dellaportas CI, Wilson A, Rose FC. Clobazam as adjunctive treatment in chronic epilepsy. In: Porter RJ, Mattson RH, Ward Jr AA, Dam M, eds. *Advances in Epileptology*. The XVth Epilepsy International Symposium. New York: Raven Press, 1984: 363–7.

54 Aucamp AK. Clobazam as adjunctive therapy in uncontrolled epileptic patients. *Curr Ther Res* 1985; 37: 1098–103.

55 Schmidt D, Rohde M, Wolf P, Roeder-Wanner U. Clobazam for refractory focal epilepsy. A controlled trial. *Arch Neurol* 1986; 43: 824–6.

56 Wilson A, Dellaportas CI, Rose CF. Low dose clobazam as adjunctive treatment in chronic epilepsy. In: Hindmarch I, Stonier PD, Trimble MR, eds. *Clobazam, Human Psychopharmacology and Clinical Applications*. International Congress and Symposium Series, no 74. London: The Royal Society of Medicine, 1985.

57 Heller AJ, Ring HA, Reynolds ER. Clobazam for refractory epilepsy. *Arch Neurol* 1987; 44: 578.

58 Manning DJ, Rosenbloom L. Nonconvulsive status epilepticus. *Arch Dis Child* 1987; 62/1: 37–40.

59 Tinuper P, Aguglia U, Gastaut H. Use of clobazam in certain forms of status epilepticus and in startle-induced seizures. *Epilepsia* 1986; 27 (Suppl. 1), S18–S26.

60 Gastaut H, Tinuper P, Aguglia U, Lugaresi E. Traitement de certains etats de mal par ingestion d'une dose unique de clobazam. *Rev EEG Neurophysiol Clin* 1984; 14/3: 203–6.

61 De Marco P. Electrical status epilepticus during slow sleep: one case with sensory aphasia. *Clin Electroencephalogr* 1988; 19(2): 111–13.

62 Aguglia U, Tinuper P, Gastaut H. Startle induced epileptic seizures. *Epilepsia* 1984; 25/6: 712–20.

63 Franceschi M, Ferrini-Strambi L, Mastrangelo M, Smirne S. Clobazam in drug-resistant and alcoholic withdrawal seizures. *Clin Trial J* 1983; 20/3: 119–25.

64 Dulac O, Figueroa D, Rey E, Arthuis M. Monotherapie par le clobazam dans les epilepsies de l'enfant. *Presse Med* 1983; 12/17: 1067–9.

65 Plouin P, Jalin C. EEG changes in epileptic children treated with clobazam as monotherapy. In: Hindmarch I, Stonier PD, Trimble MR, eds. *Clobazam, Human Psychopharmacology and Clinical Applications*. International Congress and Symposium Series, no 74. London: The Royal Society of Medicine, 1985.

66 Vajda FJ. New anticonvulsants. *Curr Opin Neurol Neurosurg* 1992; 5 (4): 519–25.

67 Montenegro MA, Cendes F, Noronha ALA *et al*. Efficacy of clobazam as add-on therapy in patients with refractory partial epilepsy. *Epilepsia* 2001; 42 (4): 539–42.

68 Judd FK, Burrows GD, Marriott PF, Norman TR. A short term open clinical trial of clobazam in the treatment of patients with panic attacks. *Int Clin Psychopharmacol* 1989; 4(4): 285–93.

69 Rupp W, Bandian M, Christ O *et al.* Pharmacokinetics of single and multiple doses of clobazam in humans. *Br J Pharmacol* 1979; 7 (Suppl. 1); S51–57.

70 Bianchi A, Bollea A, Sideri G. L'emploi du clobazam dans l'épilepsie; experience d'un an de traitement. *Boll Lega Italiana Epilepsia* 1980; 29–30: 215–18.

71 Bravaccio F, Tata MR, Ambrosio GD, De Rosa A, Volpe E. Sulle proprieta antiepilettiche di un diazepinico clobazam. *Acta Neurol* 1979; 39: 58–64.

72 Callaghan N, Goggin T. Clobazam as adjunctive treatment in drug resistant epilepsy—report on an open prospective study. *Ir Med J* 1984; 77: 240–4.

73 Cano JP, Bun H, Lliadis A, Dravet C, Roger J, Gastaut H. Influence of antiepileptic drugs on plasma levels of clobazam and desmethylclobazam: application of research on relations between doses, plasma levels and clinical efficacy. In: Hindmarch I, Stonier PD, eds. *Clobazam*. International Congress and Symposium Series, no. 43. London: Royal Society of Medicine, 1981: 169–74.

74 Dehnerdt M, Boenick HE, Rambeck B. Clobazam (Frisium) zur Behandlung komplizierter. In: Remschmidt H, Rentz R, Jungmann J, eds. *Epilepsien and Epilepsie*. Stuttgart: G. Thieme Verlag: 1980: 172–5.

75 Escobedo F, Otero E, Chaparro H, Flores T, Rubio DF. Experience with clobazam as another antiepileptic drug. *Rev Institute Nat Nerv* 1979; 13: 121–4.

76 Farrell K, Jan JE, Julian JV, Betts TA, Wong PK. Clobazam in children with intractable seizures. *Epilepsia* 1984; 25: 657.

77 Figueroa D, Adlerstein L, Manterola A. Clobazam in refractory epilepsies of children. *Rev Child Pediatr* 1984; 55(6): 401–5.

78 Gastaut H. The effects of benzodiazepines on chronic epilepsy in man (with particular reference to clobazam). In: Hindmarch I, Stonier PD, eds. *Clobazam*. International congress and symposium series, no. 43. London: Royal Society of Medicine, 1981: 141–50.

79 Martin AA. The antiepileptic effects of clobazam: a long term study in resistant epilepsy. In: Hindmarch I, Stonier PD, eds. *Clobazam*. International congress and symposium series, no. 43. London: Royal Society of Medicine, 1981; 151–7.

80 Martin AA. Clobazam in resistant epilepsy—a long term study. In: Hindmarch I, Stonier PD, Trimble MR, eds. *Clobazam: Human Psychopharmacology and Clinical Applications*. International congress and symposium series, no. 74. London: Royal Society of Medicine, 1985: 137–8.

81 Papini M, Pasquinelli A, Rossi L *et al.* Considerazioni preliminari sull attivita antiepilepttica del clobazam. *Riv Ital EEG Neurofis Clin* 1980; 3: 93–8.

82 Ramos PR, Diez-Cvervo A, Caro JS, Manrique M, Serrano JP, Coullant J. Pharmacological action of clobazam in serious epileptic patients. In: Struwe G, ed. *IIIrd World Congress of Biological Psychiatry* (Abstract F395). Stockholm: 1981.

83 Scott DF, Moffett AA. Clobazam as adjunctive therapy in chronic epilepsy: clinical, psychological and EEG assessment. In: Hindmarch I, Stonier PD, Trimble MR, eds. *Clobazam: Human Psychopharmacology and Clinical Applications*. International Congress and Symposium Series, no. 74. London: Royal Society of Medicine, 1985: 181–7.

84 Shimizu H, Abe J, Futagi Y *et al.* Antiepileptic effects of clobazam in children. *Brain Dev* 1982; 4(1): 57–62.

85 Tondi M, Mattu B, Monaco F, Masia G. Valutazione eletroclimica decli effetti antiepilepttici del clobazam nell 'eta evolutiva. *Riv Ital EEG Neurofis Clin* 1980; 3: 87–92.

86 Wolf P. Clobazam in drug-resistant patients with complex focal seizures—report of an open study. In: Hindmarch I, Stonier PD, Trimble MR, eds. *Clobazam: Human Psychopharmacology and Clinical Applications*. International Congress and Symposium Series, no. 74. London: Royal Society of Medicine, 1985: 167–71.

87 Robertson MM. Current status of 1,4 and 1,5 benzodiazepines in the treatment of epilepsy: the place of clobazam. *Epilepsia* 1986; 27 (Suppl. 1): S27–S41.

30

Clonazepam

S. Sato and E.A. Boudreau

Primary indications	Adjunctive therapy in partial and generalized seizures (including absence and myoclonus). Also, Lennox–Gastaut syndrome, neonatal seizures, Landau–Kleffner syndrome, infantile spasms and status epilepticus
Usual preparations	Tablets: 0.5, 1, 2 mg, liquid: 1 mg in 1 mL diluent
Usual dosages	Initial: 0.25 mg. Maintenance: 0.5–4 mg (adults); 1 mg (children under 1 year), 1–2 mg (children 1–5 years), 1–3 mg (children 5–12 years). Higher doses can be used
Dosage intervals	1–2 times/day
Significant drug interactions	Minor interactions are common, but usually not clinically significant
Serum level monitoring	Not useful
Target range	0.02–0.08 mg/L
Common/important side-effects	Sedation (common and may be severe), cognitive effects, drowsiness, ataxia, personality and behavioural changes, hyperactivity, restlessness, aggressiveness, psychotic reaction, seizure exacerbations, hypersalivation, leucopenia, withdrawal symptoms
Main advantages	Useful add-on action, especially in children. Wide spectrum of activity
Main disadvantages	Side-effects are sometimes prominent, particularly sedation, tolerance and a withdrawal syndrome
Mechanisms of action	$GABA_A$ receptor agonist. Also action on sodium-channel conductance
Oral bioavailability	>80%
Time to peak levels	1–4 h
Metabolism and excretion	Hepatic reduction and then acetylation
Volume of distribution	1.5–4.4 L/kg
Elimination of half-life	20–80 h
Plasma clearance	0.09 L/kg/h
Protein binding	86%
Active metabolites	None
Comment	A wide antiepileptic effect, use limited by side-effects, but helpful particularly in children with severe epilepsy

(*Note*: this summary table was formulated by the lead editor.)

Clonazepam (Klonopin) was approved for use as an antiepileptic drug in 1975. Apart from clobazam, it is the only benzodiazepine drug which is given as long-term therapy in chronic epilepsy, but today is rarely used as a first-line antiepileptic drug. Interestingly, its use in areas other than epilepsy has been expanding. It has been shown to be effective in conditions such as panic disorders and various psychiatric disorders [1–6], various movement disorders, including restless leg syndrome [7,8], familial startle disease [9], Tourette's syndrome [10,11], involuntary movements due to cobalamin deficiency [12], and sleep disorders such as REM sleep behaviour disorder [13].

Chemistry and metabolism

Clonazepam, α-5-(2-chlorophenol)-1,3,-dihydro-7-nitro-2H-1, 4-benzodiazepin-2-one, a chlorinated derivative of nitrazepam, belongs to a class of heterocyclic compounds, the benzodiazepines, that was synthesized by Dziewónski and Sternbach in 1933 [14].

Benzodiazepines are seven-membered hetero-ring compounds. The structure–activity relationship shows that electron-withdrawing substituents at the 7 position of ring A generally yield high activity, whereas electron-releasing groups decrease the activity. The character of the substituents is also important. Substituents at the 7 position of ring A with the electron-withdrawing properties of heavier halogens and particularly with some nitro- and trifluoromethyl groups, increase biological potency, e.g. activity against pentylenetetrazol-induced seizures. The substituent in the ortho position of ring C also plays an important role in biological activity. Fluorine or chlorine at this position has a strong positive effect. Clonazepam has a nitro substitution at the 7 position of ring A and a chlorine at the ortho position of ring C, which produces a strong positive effect [14].

Clonazepam is insoluble in water and is a light yellow crystalline powder with a molecular weight of 315.7 and pKa values of 1.5 and 10.5. The pKa of 1.5 corresponds to the removal of the proton of the protonated nitrogen in the 4 position of the molecule, and the pKa of 10.5 corresponds to the deprotonation of the nitrogen in the 1 position. Thus, the compound is virtually undissociated throughout the range of physiological pH [15]. The stability of the oral liquid (mixed with Ora-Sweet SF and Ora-Plus-Paddock Laboratories) format made from the clonazepam tablet is maintained for up to 60 days at 5 and 25°C [16].

The initial step in the metabolism of clonazepam is reduction of the nitro-group at position 7, yielding 7-amino-clonazepam. This is then transformed via acetylation into 7-acetamidoclonazepam. Neither metabolite appears to have clinically important pharmacological activity [17]. Hepatic cytochrome P450 3A4 had been implicated in the nitroreduction of clonazepam [18]. In a study of a single dosing interval in 10 paediatric patients on clonazepam therapy, Walson and Edge [19] presented preliminary evidence that N-reduction rates vary widely and that they may be under genetic control. Both the acetylation pathway for clonazepam and the clinical response may also be influenced by the patients' acetylator phenotype. Rapid acetylators are more likely to require higher doses of clonazepam, with the usual doses sometimes associated with seizure breakthrough and withdrawal symptoms [20].

Methods of determination

A time-consuming process of repeated extractions and acid hydrolysis was necessary in the earlier electron-capture chromatographic methods used for the determination of clonazepam [21]. Since then, other methods have been described. One study comparing underivatized gas–liquid chromatography (GLC), derivatized GLC, and high-performance liquid chromatography (HPLC), indicated that HPLC was the most precise method [22]. The use of HPLC with a solid-phase extraction column provided a simple, rapid and sensitive determination of serum clonazepam with a mean recovery of 99.9%, and a detection limit as high as approximately 2 ng/mL [23]. Improved selectivity for the HPLC determination of clonazepam was reported by using a synthetic silica-based stationary phase [24]. Song et al. have described a gas chromatographic-negative ion chemical ionization mass spectrometric (GC-NCI-MS) method using derivatized clonazepam that reached a detection limit of 0.1 ng/mL [25]. More recently, an HPLC method utilizing the column-switching technique for the simultaneous determination of frequently prescribed benzodiazepines has been described [26]. Recovery was 91% for clonazepam concentrations of 50 ng/mL and greater than 98% for concentrations of 100 ng/mL and higher. The newer techniques have increased the sensitivity of clonazepam detection. It is now possible to detect the major metabolite (7-aminoclonazepam) of clonazepam in hair, even after a single dose [27].

Pharmacokinetics

Absorption, distribution and excretion

Clonazepam is available as scored tablets containing 0.5 mg, 1 mg or 2 mg of clonazepam. Absorption of orally administered clonazepam is 80% or more [17], and the peak plasma level typically occurs within 1–4 h after oral administration, but may occur as late as 8 h [28]. Clonazepam administered orally in a solution of propylene glycol was absorbed completely, and micronization of clonazepam overcame the dissolution rate-limiting characteristics of the compound in the overall absorption of the drug [15]. After a dose of 1.5 mg of 2-[^{14}C] clonazepam [29], the absorption rate ranged from 81.2% to 98.1% of the dose, calculated from the total radioactivity and plasma concentration mean values of the radioactive compound. Clonazepam has also been given intranasally and buccally. One crossover study showed that intranasal absorption was comparable to buccal absorption but that the peak blood levels were not as high as with the IV formulation [30].

Benzodiazepines easily cross the blood–brain barrier and distribute rapidly in the brain [31]. Clonazepam appears to diffuse passively from the plasma into the brain, with a constant brain-to-plasma concentration ratio, and disappears in a parallel fashion from both brain and plasma, with no evidence of sequestration in brain tissue [17]. The distribution is rapid because of clonazepam's high lipid solubility [32]. Others [33] have reported that clonazepam has the lowest lipid solubility among the benzodiazepines, which implies slow distribution and slow onset of clinical effects. One study reported a range of volume distribution (Vd) between 1.5 and 4.4 L/kg in eight healthy adult volunteers [34]. Clonazepam is 86.5% protein bound [35].

Clearance of clonazepam is low, apparently less than 100 mL/min, and the bioavailability of an oral dose is 80% or more. Clearance is increased by the coadministration of carbamazepine, but clonazepam itself apparently does not have enzyme-inducing effects [17]. Less than 0.5% of clonazepam was recovered unchanged in the urine in a 24-h period [15], indicating extensive biotransformation or an alternative route of excretion. Total excretion of clonazepam and unconjugated 7-aminoclonazepam and 7-acetaminoclonazepam amounted to 5–20% of the dose given.

In a randomized study, Labbate et al. [36] described the relationship between the average daily dose of clonazepam and the approximated steady state concentrations of the drug. They found that for every added 1 mg/day dose there was an approximate 12 ng/mL increase in plasma levels, but with significant plasma drug concentration variability for a given dose. There have also been reported differences in bioavailability between brand and generic forms. Rapaport [37] reported two cases in which the generic form, which was being used to treat anxiety, increased sedation but showed better anxiolytic action than the brand form.

Plasma concentration, half-life and seizure control

In 10 adult males, a single 2-mg oral dose of clonazepam produced blood levels of 6.5–13 ng/mL with corresponding half-lives of 18.7–39.0 h, whereas 0.5 mg clonazepam given to epileptic patients twice daily for 15 days produced steady-state plasma levels of 4.6–12.0 ng/mL with plasma half-lives between 22 and 33 h. These levels were associated with a reduction in the frequency of absence seizures [38]. One study showed peak plasma levels 2–3 h after dosing in epileptic children [39]. Another study found no correlation between antiepileptic efficacy and plasma concentrations [28].

Clonazepam has also been associated with improvements in the EEG. In a study by Mitsudome et al. [40], 15 out of 20 patients with benign epilepsy in childhood with centrotemporal spikes (BECCT) taking clonazepam showed complete elimination of rolandic discharges on their EEG. In a double-blind, placebo-controlled, randomized study in 11 children, a single IM dose of 0.02 mg/kg of body weight, that produced median plasma concentrations of 18 to < 14 nmol/l, led to a significant decrease in the number of epileptiform discharges recorded on the EEG [41].

It has been stated that the population mean and variance of clonazepam half-life is not well defined, but its elimination half-life appears to fall in the range of 2–80 h [17]. The variability of plasma clonazepam concentrations in children with epilepsy is due to random sample collection after dosing, which contributes to the poor correlation between plasma concentrations and anticonvulsant or toxic effects [39]. In one study of 23 children, whose partial seizures were controlled for the first 12 months on clonazepam doses of 0.03–0.18 mg/kg, plasma levels were found to range between 13.8 and 67.9 ng/mL [42].

In eight newborns with convulsions, the slow intravenous infusion of 0.1 mg/kg clonazepam produced plasma levels of 28–117 ng/mL, and in 10 other newborns, 0.2 mg/kg clonazepam produced plasma levels of 99–380 ng/mL. The plasma half-life ranged from 20 to 43 h [43]. The long half-life is thought by some to allow the abrupt discontinuation of clonazepam therapy [20], but this conclusion is at variance with the usual clinical experience of adverse withdrawal side-effects, as described later.

Pharmacodynamics

Mechanisms of action

After GABAergic neurotransmission was determined to be enhanced by benzodiazepines, the benzodiazepine receptor was identified as part of the GABA-A complex [44]. GABA-evoked currents were found to be enhanced in the presence of benzodiazepines [45,46], with benzodiazepine binding increasing the affinity of GABA binding at the GABA-A receptor [47]. Specifically, benzodiazepines and GABA act through a chloride channel, which is part of the GABA-A receptor complex. Benzodiazepines increase the channel-opening frequency of the GABA-A receptor but do not increase the channel conductance or duration of channel opening [48]. The enhanced chloride uptake results in neuronal hyperpolarization. The endogenous neurosteroids have also been found to act selectively at GABA-A receptors [49,50]. Single-channel kinetic studies have shown that androsterone and pregnenolone enhance GABA-evoked currents by increasing both the channel opening frequency and the probability of channel opening [51].

Recent work has focused on GABA-A receptor subunit structure. GABA-A receptors are composed of five membrane proteins [52]. In mammals, seven classes of subunits have been identified, with most being composed of α, β and γ subunits [53]. The γ subunit seems to be especially important in benzodiazepine binding [54,55].

Clonazepam is unique in comparison to other benzodiazepine derivatives in terms of its relatively high-affinity binding [17]. There is also evidence for clonazepam specificity in binding to subgroups of GABA-A receptors. For example, in the rat spinal cord and striatum, clonazepam binds to receptors that do not bind diazepam or other benzodiazepines [56]. Rat cerebellum contains both clonazepam-sensitive and a considerable portion (20–25%) of clonazepam-insensitive receptors [57]. Clonazepam has also been implicated in reducing the serotonin turnover rate in rat hippocampi and downregulating $5HT_{1A}$ binding sites [58].

A subprotective dose of LY 300164, an antagonist of α-amino-3-hydroxy-5-methyl-4-isoazolepropionate (AMPA)/kainite receptors, significantly potentiated the anticonvulsant action of clonazepam against maximal electroshock, but not against pentylenetetrazol-induced convulsions in mice. Thus, the protective action of clonazepam depends upon the model of experimental seizures [59]. Clonazepam was one of the drugs found to be effective in controlling epileptiform discharges in an in vitro model of the primary generalized epilepsies [60].

Interactions with other drugs

The problem of drug interactions with clonazepam appears to be relatively small. Serum phenytoin levels following the administration of clonazepam may either rise [61], fall [62] or show no significant changes [63]. The addition of carbamazepine or phenobarbital lowers blood clonazepam levels [64], whereas the addition of lamotrigine reduces the plasma concentration [65].

Benzodiazepines are known to potentiate the action of central nervous system depressant drugs such as ethanol and barbiturates [66], or to produce nervous system depression and respiratory irregularities when given together with amphetamines or methylphenidate [67].

The antidepressant sertraline showed no significant pharmaco-kinetic or pharmacodynamic interaction with clonazepam [68], while fluoxetine, although not appearing to impair clonazepam clearance, did appear to increase the absorption rate [69]. Rella and Hoffman [70] reported a single case of possible serotonin syndrome in a 39-year-old female who had been on paroxitine and took a single dose of clonazepam. Another study reported slurred speech, confusion and walking difficulties in an elderly patient with hypothyroidism who was taking clonazepam with amiodarone [71].

Tolerance and withdrawal effects

The development of tolerance is a clinical problem with all benzo-diazepines. Clonazepam is probably not the most vulnerable drug in this respect. In a study in genetically epilepsy-prone rats, for instance, tolerance to clobazam developed rapidly, less rapidly to diazepam, and most slowly to clonazepam [72]. In another study, intermittent treatment with clonazepam was found to prevent the development of tolerance, as assessed by the ability of clonazepam to prevent pentylenetetrazol-induced clonic convulsions in mice [73]. Loscher *et al.* [74] examined the tolerance and withdrawal characteristics of four benzodiazepines (diazepam, clonazepam, clobazam and abecarnil) in various experimental seizure models. All four drugs lost their anticonvulsant activity during a 4-week treatment period with all approaches, although withdrawal symptoms (physical dependence) differed according to the model. L-Arginine (a donor of nitric oxide) administered with clonazepam may have the ability to inhibit the development of tolerance as well as withdrawal hyperexcitability, as shown in an electroshock seizure model using Wistar rats [75]. Cross-tolerance of clonazepam develops to diazepam-induced tolerance in bicuculline-induced convulsions in mice, and repeated abecarnil administration facilitated readaptation of receptors in the diazepam-free state [76].

Rebound seizures following clonazepam withdrawal have also been reported in a cobalt model of epilepsy. In this model, rats rendered epileptic by cobalt implantation initially experienced complete suppression of generalized seizure activity with clonazepam administration and without development of tolerance, but, 2 days after the last clonazepam injection, experienced significantly greater generalized seizure frequency as compared to untreated rats [77].

A literature review and study of children with treatment-resistant epilepsies [78] found that children with West's syndrome and Lennox–Gastaut syndrome developed the highest tolerance to clonazepam as compared to those children with isolated typical absence seizures. A negative therapeutic effect was described for all seizure types, especially generalized tonic-clonic and tonic seizures. Although this paradoxical effect is sometimes due to the interference of clonazepam with the action of other drugs during polytherapy [79], increased seizure frequency during clonazepam monotherapy has also been observed [80].

Clonazepam discontinuation has not only been associated with seizure exacerbation, but also with psychiatric reactions such as rebound insomnia, anxiety, tremor and psychosis [81,82]. Seizures associated with clonazepam withdrawal have also been reported in patients without a history of seizures, even during relatively slow taper rates, such as 3 mg/day reduced over 3 weeks [83].

The mechanisms of clonazepam tolerance and withdrawal remain unclear.

According to one study [84], clonazepam-induced tolerance does not appear to be related to pharmacokinetic factors, since no changes in clonazepam plasma or brain concentrations were observed during the study. The structure of the GABA-A receptor is increasingly targeted in studies of tolerance and withdrawal. Clonazepam treatment resulting in tolerance to its motor effects was associated with downregulation of the GABA-A receptor. Conversely, clonazepam discontinuation resulted in increased motor activity and GABA-A receptor upregulation [84]. The significance of these receptor alterations, however, remains unknown.

Treatment with clonazepam

Clonazepam is now rarely used as a primary antiepileptic drug despite its broad spectrum of efficacy. Sedation and development of tolerance were the prime reasons according to Brodie and Dicter [85] in a review of established antiepileptic drugs. Clonazepam is often used, however, as an adjunctive or last resort therapy when other antiepileptic drugs have failed. Since our last writing [86], there has been no large-scale trial of clonazepam as an antiepileptic drug. Most articles are case report studies documenting the excellent results achieved with clonazepam. On the other hand, clonazepam has been extensively used in the fields of psychiatry (panic disorder) and sleep disorder (REM behaviour disorder), and may be useful as adjunctive treatment for resistant myoclonic jerks [87].

In a randomized double-blind study involving 15 children with focal and generalized epilepsy, there was a statistically significant reduction of epileptiform discharges on a long-term EEG recording in response to a single intramuscular low dose of clonazepam (0.02 mg/kg). The concomitant plasma levels were also low, with median plasma concentrations of 18 to < 14 nmol/l [41]. There are special situations in which clonazepam may be especially useful. It was found to be one of the antiepileptic drugs effective in controlling cortical tremor and epilepsy in three families with these conditions [88]. In 18 patients with the northern epilepsy syndrome, an autosomal recessively inherited childhood onset epilepsy associated with mental deterioration, clonazepam proved to be the most effective antiepileptic drug [89]. Paradoxically, the discontinuation of clonazepam and primidone in a child on polytherapy was reported to result in a resolution of seizures [90].

Absence seizures

Clonazepam is a useful drug in treating absence seizures, as reported in both controlled and uncontrolled studies [38,91]. In combination with valproate, clonazepam improved absence seizure control in seven of eight patients [92]. It was also found to be a useful adjunct in treating absence seizures with myoclonic components [93]. Clonazepam combined with either valproate or ethosuximde had a good effect in stopping continuous spike-wave discharges during slow-wave sleep in children [94].

Tonic-clonic seizures

In general, phenytoin and carbamazepine are the drugs of choice in the treatment of generalized tonic-clonic seizures. Although intravenous clonazepam suppresses the EEG abnormality and can abolish generalized tonic-clonic status epilepticus, chronic administration of the drug has been found to be ineffective in this seizure type [95]. Futhermore, many reports have indicated that generalized tonic-clonic seizures are exacerbated by the addition of clonazepam to the regimen [96,97]. However, clonazepam combined with valproate was found to improve seizure control in three of 14 patients with intractable primary generalized tonic-clonic seizures [92]. The combination of clonazepam and carbamazepine was also shown to be effective in controlling a series of grand mal seizures following the use of the drug ecstasy (3,4-methylenedioxymetamphetamine) [98].

Lennox–Gastaut syndrome

Clonazepam has been found to have beneficial effects in many children with Lennox–Gastaut syndrome [80,99], and is conventionally considered a drug of importance in this syndrome. Comedication with valproate is often particularly effective [92], and continuous spike-and-wave activity during slow-wave sleep was also shown to disappear in five epileptic children when clonazepam was combined with either valproate or ethosuximde [94]. Other studies though have reported less favourable findings. No benefit or a negative therapeutic effect (decreased seizure frequency after discontinuation of clonazepam) was observed in 36 of 40 children with therapy-resistant epilepsies, including symptomatic focal epilepsy, West's syndrome, myoclonic-astatic seizures, Lennox–Gastaut syndrome and symptomatic generalized seizures by Specht et al. [78]. Also, a recent report suggests that clonazepam has limited usage in Lennox–Gastaut syndrome and is recommended it solely as a third-line treatment choice [100].

Partial seizures

The effectiveness of clonazepam against partial seizures has been shown in a number of case reports. One such study involving a rare case of temporal lobe epilepsy also reported improvement in the single photon emission CT scan [101]. Tonic seizures of frontal lobe origin occurred less frequently when clonazepam was used as an adjunctive therapy [102]. Rolandic discharges disappeared in 15 of 20 children with centrotemporal spikes, whereas only one of 10 responded to valproate [40]. A maintenance dose of clonazepam (0.03–0.18 mg/kg/day) alone or in combination with carbamazepine was reported to control carbamazepine-resistant partial seizures in 23 children, 3–15 years of age, producing only minor side-effects [42]. The combination of valproate and clonazepam improved seizures in 19 of 39 patients with intractable complex partial seizures [92]. Clonazepam is also effective in suppressing epilepsia partialis continua [103]. However, a literature analysis [104] concluded that clonazepam is not very effective in controlling simple and complex partial seizures.

Landau–Kleffner syndrome

There are no recent data supporting the use of clonazepam in Landau–Kleffner syndrome. An 8-year-old girl with this syndrome, who did not respond to valproate, clonazepam, prednisone or carbamazepine, did respond to intravenous γ-globulin [105].

Infantile spasms

Various studies have been performed to assess the effect of clonazepam in infantile spasm, with mixed results. The outcome of 25 patients following initial treatment with valproate sodium, clonazepam, and high doses of vitamin B_6 was reviewed by Suzuki et al. [106]. Five of nine cryptogenic cases (56%) and four of 16 symptomatic cases (25%) became seizure free. In the cryptogenic cases, clinical features alone could not predict outcome, whereas in the symptomatic cases, all had neurocutaneous syndromes (tuberous sclerosis or neurofibromatosis type I). Other authors have reported disappointing results [107], with the outcome of therapy ranging from no benefit or even a negative therapeutic effect [78]. Some success in controlling infantile spasms has been noted when benzodiazepines are combined with carbamazepine [108], although the usefulness is limited due to increased bronchial secretions and adverse effects on cognitive function. In a 5-month-old girl with West's syndrome, suppression of infantile spasms by adrenocorticotropic hormone was followed by induced microseizures characterized by irregular respiration, respiratory arrest, eye opening, mild extension of the neck and diffuse EEG fast activity. The EEG activity responded well to clonazepam [109].

Myoclonic seizures

Clonazepam is an effective treatment for myoclonus [110] which, having a variety of origins, has become a focus of recent research activity.

Clonazepam is useful in treating refractory myclonic seizures [85,111], juvenile myoclonic epilepsy [112], familiar myoclonus [113] and a rare epileptic syndrome with perioral myoclonia and absence seizures [114]. Severe myoclonic epilepsy of infants may show some response to zonisamide added to clonazepam [115], or to a combination of valproic acid, clonazepam and carbamazepine, as cited in one study of 10 patients [116]. Clonazepam is also effective in controlling segmental myoclonus [117,118]. A small amount of clonazepam proved very effective in controlling segmental myoclus due to brainstem infarction [118]. Propriospinal myoclonus, causing severe insomnia in three patients, improved with clonazepam [119]. However, palatal myoclonus may be either responsive [120] or refractory to clonazepam treatment [121]. Epileptic negative myoclonus responded dramatically to ethosuximide, but unpredictably to clonazepam and valproic acid [122]. Post-hypoxic myoclonus improved with clonazepam [123]. Clonazepam was markedly effective in both positive (production) and negative (suppression) myoclonus of cortical origin [124], as well as in cortical tremor, a variant of cortical relfex myoclonus [125]. Myoclonus coinciding with multiple sclerosis can also show a dramatic response to clonazepam [126].

Neonatal seizures

Infusions of diazepam or clonazepam controlled clinical and EEG seizures in eight neonates in one report [127]. Another study [43] suggested that a clonazepam dose of 0.1 mg/kg every 24 h, as opposed to every 12 h, was more efficacious in controlling seizures in the majority of patients. When both methylphenobarbital and phenytoin failed to control neonatal seizures, clonazepam with thiopentone was reported to increase the rate of cumulative control [128].

Reflex epilepsy

Clonazepam is effective not only in reducing the response to photic stimulation [129], but also in controlling the myoclonic jaw jerking evoked by reading [130] and the myoclonic contractions associated with high-dose opioid administration [131].

Status epilepticus

Although clonazepam is not typically used in the treatment of status epilepticus, its use in this setting has been reported in both children and adults [112,132]. A child with progressive neurological deficits and focal status epilepticus showed a remarkable response to clonazepam [133], as did another case of tiagabine-induced complex partial status epilepticus when clonazepam was given intravenously [134]. Clonazepam in combination with valproic acid or ethosuximide apparently stopped continuous spike-wave activity during slow-wave sleep in five children, who also improved clinically [94].

Adverse effects

The common side-effects of clonazepam include drowsiness, ataxia, incoordination, and behavioural and personality changes (hyperactivity, restlessness, short attention span, irritability, disruptiveness and aggressiveness). The other reported neurological side-effects include nystagmus, dizziness, dysarthria, hypotonia, blurred vision, diplopia and psychosis [28]. It is noteworthy that in hospitalized psychiatric patients, behavioural disinhibition (acts of self-injury, assaults on staff or other patients, need for seclusion or restraints, need for observation by hospital staff, need for decrease in patient privileges) was more common with clonazepam than with alprazolam or with no benozodiazepine [135]. Epileptic seizures and memory disturbance in an epileptic patient improved when carbamazepine was substituted for valproate and clonazepam [136]. One study reports intolerable burning mouth sensation with the use of clonazepam [137].

Clonazepam treatment may be associated with an increased frequency of various types of seizures [80,138] as well as the emergence of different seizure types [139,140]. Clonazepam has been associated with the precipitation of a tonic status epilepticus [141].

Hypersecretion and hypersalivation may be troublesome in children and infants who receive clonazepam [142]. Reasons for withdrawing clonazepam include freedom from seizures, lack of clinical effect, intolerable behaviour, personality changes, psychotic reactions, persistent drowsiness, leukopenia, increased seizure frequency and development of other types of seizures.

Withdrawal of benzodiazepines may be associated with acute onset of anxiety, agitation, insomnia, confusion, and severe and potentially life-threatening catatonia [143]. Furthermore, abrupt withdrawal may precipitate convulsions or status epilepticus [66,144].

Pregnancy

Limited information is available on the possible teratogenic effects of clonazepam. Laegrid et al. [145] reported preliminary findings from two studies on infants habitually exposed in utero to benzodiazepines. Seven of 37 infants showed intrauterine and extrauterine growth restriction, dysmorphism and malformations, and central nervous system dysfunction. A large retrospective cohort study done in The Netherlands by Samren et al. [146] found that clonazepam, when used in combination therapy with other antiepileptic medications, led to an increased relative risk of major congenital abnormalities. Clonazepam was also implicated in a case of paralytic ileus of the small bowel, reported in a woman who was also taking tegretol [147]. A more recent study, however, failed to show any direct relationship between clonazepam and obstetric complications or orofacial anomalies [148].

Summary

Clonazepam, a potent antiepileptic drug, is rarely used today as a primary drug for the control of epilepsy, but is used instead as an adjunct to other drugs or as a last resort, and although it has a wide spectrum of antiepileptic activity, it is rarely given to treat generalized tonic-clonic seizures. Clonazepam has a high incidence of adverse effects, such as behavioural and personality problems, psychotic reactions, leukopenia, persistent drowsiness and the emergence of different seizure types, which complicate its use. Interactions between clonazepam and other drugs are infrequent. The withdrawal of clonazepam, especially when done abruptly, typically results in adverse withdrawal symptoms, and requires close observation.

References

1 Santos AB, Morton WA. Use of benzodiazepines to improve management of manic agitation. *Hosp Commun Psychiatr* 1989; 40: 1069–1071.
2 Pols H, Zandbergen J, Lousberg H, de Loof C, Griez E. Low doses of clonazepam in the treatment of panic disorder. *Can J Psychiatry* 1991; 36: 302–3.
3 Hewlett WA, Vinogradow S, Agras WS. Clomipramine, clonazepam, and clonidine treatment of obsessive–compulsive disorder. *J Clin Psychopharmacol* 1992; 12: 420–30.
4 Ontiveros A, Fontaine R. Sodium valproate and clonazepam for treatment-resistant panic disorder. *J Psychiatr Neurosci* 1992; 17: 78–80.
5 Sonino N, Fava GA. Psychiatric disorders associated with Cushing's syndrome. Epidemiology, pathophysiology and treatment. *CNS Drugs* 2001; 15: 361–73.
6 Lerner AG, Skladman I, Kodesh A, Sigal M, Shufman E. LSD-induced hallucinogen persisting perception disorder treated with clonazepam: two case reports. *Isr J Psychiatr Rel Sci* 2001; 38: 133–6.
7 Horiguchi J, Inami Y, Sasaki A, Nishimatsu O, Sukegawa T. Periodic leg movements in sleep with restless legs syndrome: Effect of clonazepam treatment. *Jpn J Psychiatr* 1992; 46: 727–32.
8 Saletu M, Anderer P, Saletu-Zyhlarz G et al. Restless legs syndrome (RLS) and periodic limb movement disorder (PLMD): acute placebo-controlled sleep laboratory studies with clonazepam. *Eur Neuropsychopharmacol* 2001; 11: 153–61.
9 Ryan SG, Sherman SL, Terry JC et al. Startle disease, or hyperekplexia: response to clonazepam and assignment of the gene (STHE) to chromosome 5q by linkage analysis. *Ann Neurol* 1992; 31: 663–8.
10 Goetz CG. Clonidine and clonazepam in Tourette syndrome. *Adv Neurol* 1992; 58: 245–51.

11 Kossoff EH, Singer HS. Tourette syndrome: clinical characteristics and current management strategies. *Paediatr Drugs* 2001; 3: 355–63.

12 Ozer EA, Turker M, Bakiler AR, Yaprak I, Ozturk C. Involuntary movements in infantile cobalamin deficiency appearing after treatment. *Pediatr Neurol* 2001; 25: 81–3.

13 Silber MH. Sleep disorders. *Neurol Clin* 2001; 19: 173–86.

14 Sternbach LH. Chemistry of 1,4–benzodiazepines and some aspects of the structure–activity relationship. In: Garattini S, Mussini E, Randall LO, eds. *The Benzodiazepines*. New York: Raven Press, 1973; 1–26.

15 Kaplan SA, Alexander K, Jack ML *et al.* Pharmacokinetic profiles of clonazepam in dog and humans and of flunitrazepam in dog. *J Pharm Sci* 1974; 63: 527–532.

16 Allen LV Jr, Erickson MA III. Stability of acetazolamide, allopurinol, azathioprine, clonazepam, and flucytosine in extemporaneously compounded oral liquids. *Am J Health Syst Pharm* 1996; 53: 1944–9.

17 Greenblatt DJ, Miller LG, Shader RI. Clonazepam pharmacokinetics, brain uptake, and receptor interactions. *J Clin Psychiatr* 1987; 48: (Suppl.), 4–11.

18 Seree EJ, Pisano PJ, Placidi M, Rahmani R, Barra YA. Identification of the human and animal hepatic cytochromes P450 involved in clonazepam metabolism. *Fund Clin Pharmacol* 1993; 7: 69–75.

19 Walson PD, Edge JH. Clonazepam disposition in pediatric patients. *Ther Drug Monit* 1996; 18: 1–5.

20 DeVane CL, Ware MR, Lydiard RB. Pharmacokinetics, pharmacodynamics, and treatment issues of benzodiazepines: alprazolam, adinazolam, and clonazepam. *Psychopharmacol Bull* 1991; 27: 463–73.

21 De Silva JAF, Bekersky I, Puglisi CV, Brooks MA, Weinfeld RE. Determination of 1,4-benzodiazepines and -diazepine-2-ones in blood by electron-capture gas-liquid chromatography. *Analy Chem* 1976; 48: 10–19.

22 De Carvalho, D, Lanchote, V L. Measurement of plasma clonazepam for therapeutic control: A comparison of chromatographic methods. *Ther Drug Monit* 1991; 13: 55–63.

23 Furuno K, Gomita Y, Araki Y, Fukuda T. Clonazepam serum levels in epileptic patients determined simply and rapidly by high-performance liquid chromatography using a solid-phase extraction column. *Acta Med Okayama* 1991; 45: 123–7.

24 Le Guellec C, Gaudet ML, Breteau M. Improved selectivity for high-performance liquid chromatographic determination of clonazepam in plasma of epileptic patients. *J Chromatogr B Biomed Sci Appl* 1998; 719: 227–33.

25 Song D, Zhang S, Kohlhof K. Quantitative determination of clonazepam in plasma by gas chromatography-negative ion chemical ionization mass spectrometry. *J Chromatogr B Biomed Appl* 1996; 686: 199–204.

26 El Mahjoub A, Staub C. High-performance liquid chromatographic method for the determination of benzodiazepines in plasma or serum using the column-switching technique. *J Chromatogr B Biomed* 2000; 742: 381–90.

27 Negrusz A, Moore CM, Kern JL *et al.* Quantitation of clonazepam and its major metabolite 7-aminoclonazepam in hair. *J Anal Toxicol* 2000; 24: 614–20.

28 Sato S. Benzodiazepines: clonazepam. In Levy R, Mattson R, Meldrum B, Penry JK, Dreifuss FE, eds. *Antiepileptic Drugs*, 3rd edn. New York: Raven Press, 1989; 765–84.

29 Eschenhof E. Untersuchung uber das Schicksal des Antikonvulsivums Clonazepam in Organismus der Ratte, des Hundes und des menschen. *Arzneim Forsch* 1973; 23: 390–400.

30 Schols-Hendriks MW, Lohman JJ *et al.* Absorption of clonazepam after intranasal and buccal administration. *Br J Clin Pharmacol* 1995; 39: 449–51.

31 Garantti S, Mussini E, Marcucci F, Gauitam A. Metabolic studies on benzodiazepines in various animal species. In: Garantti S, Mussini E, Randall LO, eds. *The Benzodiazepines*. New York: Raven Press, 1973: 75–128.

32 Knopp HJ, van der Kleijn E, Edmunds LC. Pharmacokinetics of clonazepam in man and laboratory animals. In: Schneider H, Janz D, Gardner-Thorpe C, Meinardi H, Sherwin AL, eds. *Clinical Pharmacology of Antiepileptic Drugs*. Berlin: Springer-Verlag, 1975: 247–60.

33 Greenblatt DJ, Miller LG. Mechanism of the anticonvulsant action of benzodiazepines. *Cleve Clin J Med* 1990; 57 (Suppl.): 6–8.

34 Birket-Smith E, Lund M, Mikkelsen B, Vestermark D, Zander Olsen P, Holm P. A controlled trial on Ro 5–4023 (clonazepam) in the treatment of psychomotor epilepsy. *Acta Neurol Scand* 1973; 49: 18–25.

35 Benet LZ, Sheiner LB. Appendix II. Design and optimization of dosage regimens: pharmacokinetic data. In: Gilman AG, Goodman LS, Rall TW, Murad F, eds. *The Pharmacological Basis of Therapeutics*, 7th edn. New York: Macmillan, 1985: 1663–1733.

36 Labbate LA, Pollack MH, Otto MW, Tesar GM, Rosenbaum JF. The relationship of alprazolam and clonazepam dose to steady-state concentration in plasma. *J Clin Psychopharmacol* 1994; 14: 274–6.

37 Rapaport MH. Clinical differences between the generic and nongeneric forms of clonazepam. *J Clin Psychopharmacol* 1997; 17: 424.

38 Dreifuss FE, Penry JK, Rose SW, Kupferberg HJ, Dyken P, Sato S. Serum clonazepam concentrations in children with absence seizures. *Neurology (Minneap)* 1975; 23: 255–8.

39 Edge JH, Walson PD, Rane A. Clonazepam and 7-aminoclonazepam in human plasma. *Ther Drug Monit* 1991; 13: 363–8.

40 Mitsudome A, Ohfu M, Yasumoto S *et al.* The effectiveness of clonazepam on the Rolandic discharges. *Brain Dev* 1997; 19: 274–8.

41 Dahlin M, Knutsson E, Amark P, Nergardh A. Reduction of epileptiform activity in response to low-dose clonazepam in children with epilepsy: a randomized double-blind study. *Epilepsia* 2000; 4: 308–15.

42 Hosoda N, Miura H, Takanashi S, Shirai H, Sunaoshi W. The long-term effectiveness of clonazepam therapy in the control of partial seizures in children difficult to control with carbamazepine monotherapy. *Jpn J Psychiatry Neurol* 1991; 45: 471–3.

43 Andre M, Boutroy MJ, Bianchetti G, Vert P, Morselli PL. Clonazepam in neonatal seizures: dose regimens and therapeutic efficacy. *Eur J Clin Pharmacol* 1991; 40: 193–5.

44 Rogawski MA, Porter RJ. Antiepileptic drugs: pharmacological mechanisms and clinical efficacy with consideration of promising developmental stage compounds. *Pharmacol Rev* 1990; 42: 223–86.

45 Choi DW, Farb DH, Fischbach GD. Chlordiazepoxide selectively augments GABA action in spinal cord cell cultures. *Nature* 1977; 269: 342–4.

46 Macdonald R, Barker L. Benzodiazepines specifically modulate GABA-mediated postsynaptic inhibition in cultured mammalian neurones. *Nature* 1978; 271: 563–4.

47 Skerritt H, Willow M, Johnston GAR. Diazepam enhancement of low affinity GABA binding to rat brain membranes. *Neurosci Lett* 1982; 29: 63–6.

48 Twyman RE, Rogers CJ, Macdonald RL. Differential mechanisms for enhancement of GABA by diazepam and phenobarbital: a single channel study. *Ann Neurol* 1989; 25: 213–20.

49 Deutsch S, Mastropaolo J, Hitri A. GABA-active steroids: endogenous modulators of GABA-gated chloride ion conductance. *Clin Neuropharmacol* 1992; 15: 352–64.

50 Twyman R, Macdonald R. Neurosteroid regulation of GABAA receptor single-channel kinetic properties of mouse spinal cord neurons in culture. *J Physiol (Lond)* 1992; 456: 215–45.

51 Morrow AL, Pace JR, Purdy RH, Paul SM. Characterization of steroid interactions with gamma-aminobutyric acid receptor-gated chloride ion channels: evidence for multiple steroid recognition sites. *Mol Pharmacol* 1990; 37: 263–70.

52 Rudolph U, Crestani F, Mohler H. GABA(A) receptor subtypes: dissecting their pharmacological functions. *Trends Pharmacol Sci* 2001; 22: 188–94.

53 Barnard EA, Bateson AN, Darlison MG *et al.* Genes for the GABAA receptor subunit types and their expression. *Adv Biochem Psychopharmacol* 1992; 47: 17–27.

54 Gunther U, Benson J, Benke D *et al.* Benzodiazepine-insensitive mice generated by targeted disruption of the gamma 2 subunit gene of gamma-aminobutyric acid type A receptors. *Proc Natl Acad Sci USA* 1995; 92: 7749–53.

55 Smith GB, Olsen RW. Functional domains of GABAA receptors. *Trends Pharmacol Sci* 1995; 16: 162–8.

56 Massotti M, Schlichting JL, Antonacci MD *et al.* Gamma-aminobutyric acid A receptor heterogeneity in rat central nervous system: studies with clonazepam and other benzodiazepine liquids. *J Pharmacol Exp Ther* 1991; 256: 1154–60.

57 Khan ZU, Fernando LP, Escriba P *et al.* Antibodies to the human gamma subunit of the gamma-aminobutyric acidA/benzodiazepine receptor. *J Neurochem* 1993; 60: 961–71.

58 Lima L, Trejo E. Urbina M. Serotonin turnover rate {3H} paroxetine binding sites, and 5HT1A receptors in the hippocampus of rats synchronically treated with clonazepam. *Neuropharmacology* 1995; 34: 1327–33.

59 Borowicz KK, Luszczki J, Szadkowski M, Kleinrok Z, Czuczwar SJ. Influence of LY 300164, an antagonist of AMPA/kainate receptors, on the anticonvulsant activity of clonazepam. *Eur J Pharmacol* 1999; 380: 67–72.

60 Zhang YF, Gibbs JW III, Coulter DA. Anticonvulsant drug effects on spontaneous thalamocortical rhythms in vitro: valproic acid, clonazepam, and alpha-methyl-alpha-phenylsuccinimide. *Epilepsy Res* 1996; 23: 37–53.

61 Inami M, Hara T. The effects of clonazepam on the plasma diphenylhydantoin level in epileptic patients. *Electroencephalogr Clin Neurophysiol* 1977; 43: 497.

62 Saavedra IN, Aquilera LI, Faure E, Galdames DG. Phenytoin/clonazepam interaction. *Ther Drug Monit* 1985; 7: 481–4.

63 Sobaniec W. Certain aspects of interaction between sodium valproate and other anticonvulsant drugs in the therapy of epilepsy in children. *Mater Med Pol* 1992; 24: 115–19.

64 Lai A, Levy RH, Cutler RE. Time-course of interaction between carbamazepine and clonazepam in normal man. *Clin Pharmacol Ther* 1978; 24: 316–23.

65 Eriksson AS, Hoppu K, Nergardh A, Boreus L. Pharmacokinetic interactions between lamotrigine and other antiepileptic drugs in children with intractable epilepsy. *Epilepsia* 1996; 37: 769–73.

66 Rall TW, Schleifer LS. Drugs effective in the therapy of the epilepsies. In: Gilman AG, Goodman S, Rall TW, Murad F, eds. *The Pharmacological Basis of Therapeutics*, 7th edn. New York: Macmillan, 1985: 446–72.

67 Carson J, Gilden G. Treatment of minor motor seizures with clonazepam. *Dev Med Child Neurol* 1975; 17: 306–10.

68 Bonate PL, Kroboth PD, Smith RB, Suarez E, Oo C. Clonazepam and sertraline: absence of drug interaction in a multiple-dose study. *J Clin Psychopharmacol* 2000; 20: 19–27.

69 Greenblatt DJ, Preskorn SH, Cotreau MM, Horst WD, Harmatz JS. Fluoxetine impairs clearance of alprazolam but not of clonazepam. *Clin Pharmacol Ther* 1992; 52: 479–86.

70 Rella JG, Hoffman RS. Possible serotonin syndrome from paroxetine and clonazepam. *Clin Toxicol* 1998; 36: 257–8.

71 Witt DM, Ellsworth AJ, Leversee JH. Amiodarone–clonazepam interaction. *Ann Pharmacother* 1993; 27: 1463–4.

72 De Sarro G, Di Paola ED, Aguglia U, de Sarro A. Tolerance to anticonvulsant effects of some benzodiazepines in genetically epilepsy prone rats. *Pharmacol Biochem Behav.* 1996; 55: 39–48.

73 Suzuki Y, Edge J, Mimaki T, Walson PD. Intermittent clonazepam treatment prevents anticonvulsant tolerance in mice. *Epilepsy Res* 1993; 15: 15–20.

74 Loscher W, Rundfeldt C, Honack D, Ebert U. Long-term studies on anticonvulsant tolerance and withdrawal characteristics of benzodiazepine receptor ligands in different seizure models in mice. I. Comparison of diazepam, clonazepam, clobazam and abecarnil. *J Pharmacol Exp Ther* 1996; 279: 561–72.

75 Gupta N, Bhargava VK, Pandhi P. Tolerance and withdrawal to anticonvulsant action of clonazepam: role of nitric oxide. *Methods Find Exp Clin Pharmacol* 2000; 22: 229–35.

76 Zanotti A, Natolino F, Contarino A, Lipartiti M, Giusti P. Abecarnil enhances recovery from diazepam tolerance. *Neuropharmacology* 1999; 38: 1281–8.

77 Colasanti BK, Craig CR. Reduction of seizure frequency by clonazepam during cobalt experimental epilepsy. *Brain Res Bull* 1992; 28: 329–31.

78 Specht U, Boenigk HE, Wolf P. Discontinuation of clonazepam after long-term treatment. *Epilepsia* 1989; 30: 458–63.

79 Shorvon SD, Reynolds EH. Reduction in polypharmacy for epilepsy. *Br Med J* 1979; 2: 1023–5.

80 Sato S, Penry JK, Dreifuss FE, Dyken PR. Clonazepam in the treatment of absence seizures. *Neurology (Minneap)* 1977; 27: 371.

81 Sironi VA, Miserocchi G, DeRiu PL. Clonazepam withdrawal syndrome. *Acta Neurol* 1984; 6: 134–9.

82 Jaffe R, Gibson E. Clonazepam withdrawal psychosis. *J Clin Psychopharmacol* 1986; 6: 93.

83 Wong T, Tiessen E. Seizure in gradual clonazepam withdrawal. *Psychiatr J Univ Ottawa* 1989; 14: 484.

84 Galpern WR, Lumpkin M, Greenblatt DJ, Shader RI, Miller LG. Chronic benzodiazepine administration. *Psychopharmacology* 1991; 104: 225–30.

85 Brodie MJ, Dicter MA. Established antiepileptic drugs. *Seizure* 1997; 6: 159–74.

86 Sato S, Malow AB. Clonazepam. In: S Shorvon ed. *The Treatment of Epilepsy*. Australia: Blackwell Science, 1996: 378–90.

87 Murphy K, Delanty N. Primary generalized epilepsy. *Curr Treat Opt Neurol* 2000; 2: 527–42.

88 Okuma Y, Shimo Y, Shimura H *et al.* Familial cortical tremor with epilepsy: an underrecognized familial tremor. *Clin Neurol Neurosurg* 1998; 100: 75–8.

89 Lang AH, Hirvasniemi A, Siivola J. Neurophysiological findings in the northern epilepsy syndrome. *Acta Neurol Scand* 1997; 95: 1–8.

90 Borusiak P, Betterndorf U, Karenfort M, Korn-Merker E, Boenigk HE. Seizure-inducing paradoxical reaction to antiepileptic drugs. *Brain Dev* 2000; 22: 243–5.

91 Ishikawa A, Sakuma N, Nagashima T, Kohsaka S, Kajii N. Clonazepam monotherapy for epilepsy in childhood. *Brain Dev* 1985; 7: 610–13.

92 Mireles R, Leppik IL. Valproate and clonazepam comedication in patients with intractable epilepsy. *Epilepsia* 1985; 26: 122–6.

93 Panayiotopoulos CP. Treatment of typical absence seizures and related epileptic syndromes. *Paediatr Drugs* 2001; 3: 379–403.

94 Yasuhara A, Yoshida H, Hatanaka T, Sugimoto T, Kobayashi T, Dyken E. Epilepsy with continuous spikes-waves during slow sleep and its treatment. *Epilepsia* 1991; 32: 59–62.

95 Krue P, Blankenhorn V. Zusammenfassender Erfahrungsbericht uber die klinische Anwendung und Wirksamkeit von Ro 5–4023 (Clonazepam; auf verschiedene Formen epileptischer Anfalle). *Acta Neurol Scand* 1973; 49: 60–71.

96 Bladin PF. The use of clonazepam as an anticonvulsant—clinical evaluation. *Med J Aust* 1973; 1: 683–8.

97 Munthe-Kaas AW, Strandjord RE. Clonazepam in the treatment of epileptic seizures. *Acta Neurol Scand* 1973; 49: 97–102.

98 Theune M, Esser W, Druschky KF, Interschick E, Patscheke H. Gand mal series after Ecstasy abuse. *Nervenarzt* 1999; 70: 1094–7.

99 Moehler H, Okada, T. Benzodiazepine receptor: demonstration in the central nervous system. *Science* 1977; 198: 849–51.

100 Schmidt D, Bourgeois B. A risk–benefit assessment of therapies for Lennox–Gastaut syndrome. *Drug Saf* 2000; 22: 467–77.

101 Ide M, Mizukami K, Suzuki T, Shiraishi H. A case of temporal lobe epilepsy with improvement of clinical symptoms and single photon emission computed tomography findings after treatment with clonazepam. *Psychiatry Clin Neurosci* 2000; 54: 595–7.

102 Obeid T, Awada A, Sayes N, Mousali Y, Harris C. A unique effect of clonazepam on frontal lobe seizure control. Seizure 1999; 8: 431–3.

103 Scollo–Lavizzari G, Pralle W, de la Cruz N. Clinical experience with clonazepam (Rivotril) in the treatment of epilepsy in adults. *Eur Neurol* 1974; 11: 340–4.

104 Holmes, GL. The use of benzodiazepines in epilepsy and febrile seizures. *Cleve Clin J Med* 1990; 57 (Suppl.): 31–8.

105 Fayad MN, Choueiri R, Mikati M. Landau–Kleffner syndrome: consistent response to repeated intravenous gamma-globulin doses: a case report. *Epilepsia* 1997; 38: 489–94.

106 Suzuki Y, Kita T, Mano T *et al.* Outcome of initial treatment with high-dose vitamin B6, valproate sodium or clonazepam in West syndrome. *No to Hattatsu* 1996; 28: 398–402.

107 Wohlrab G, Boltshauser E, Schmitt B. Vigabatrin as a first-line drug in West syndrome: clinical and electroencephalographic outcome. *Neuropediatrics* 1998; 29: 133–6.

108 Tatzer G, Groh C, Muller R, Lischka A. Carbamazepine and benzodiazepines in combination—a possibility to improve the efficacy of treatment of patients with 'intractable' infantile spasms? *Brain Dev* 1987; 9: 415–17.

109 Otani K, Tagawa T, Futagi Y, Okamoto N, Yabuuchi H. Induced micro-seizures in West syndrome. Brain Dev 1991; 13: 196–9.

110 Greene P. Benzodiazepine in the treatment of movement disorders. Cleve Clin J Med 1990; 57 (Suppl.): 53.

111 Caviness JN. Myoclonus. Mayo Clin Proc 1997; 71: 679–88.

112 Alvarez N, Besag F, Iivanainen M. Use of antiepileptic drugs in the treatment of epilepsy in people with intellectual disability. J Intellect Disabil Res 1998; 42: 1–15.

113 Nagayama S, Kishikawa H, Yukitake M, Matsui M, Kuroda Y. A case of familial myoclonus showing extremely benign clinical course. Rinsho Shinkeigaku 1998; 38: 430–4.

114 Baykan BB, Gurses C, Gokyigit A. Perioral myoclonia with absence seizures: a rare epileptic syndrome. Epileptic Disord 2001; 3: 23–8.

115 Wallace SJ. Myoclonus and epilepsy in childhood: a review of treatment with valproate, ethosuximide, lamotrigine and zonisamide. Epilepsy Res 1998; 29: 147–54.

116 Wang PJ, Fan PC, Lee WT, Young C, Huang CC, Shen YZ. Severe myoclonic epilepsy in infancy: evolution of electroencephalographic and clinical features. Zhonghua Min Guo Xiao Er Ke Yi Xue Hui Za Zhi 1996; 37: 428–32.

117 Devetag Chalaupka F, Bernardi M. A case of segmental myoclonus in amputation stump: evidence for spinal generator and physiolopathogenetic hypothesis. Ital J Neurol Sci 1999; 20: 327–31.

118 Yoshikawa H, Takamori M. Benign segmental myoclonus: electrophysiological evidence of transient dysfunction in the brainstem. J Clin Neurosci 2000; 8: 54–6.

119 Montagna P, Provini F, Plazzi G, Liguori R, Lugaresi E. Propriospinal myoclonus upon relaxation and drowsiness: a cause of severe insomnia. Mov Disord 1997; 12: 66–72.

120 Fabiani G, Teive HA, Sa D et al. Palatal myoclonus: report of two cases. Arq Neuropsiquiatr 2000; 58: 901–4.

121 Chua HC, Tan AK, Venketasubramanian N, Tan CB, Tjia H. Palatal myoclonus—a case report. Ann Acd Med Singapore 1999; 28: 593–5.

122 Oguni H, Uehara T, Tanaka T, Sunahara M, Hara M, Osawa M. Dramatic effect of ethosuximide on epileptic negative myoclonus: implications for the neurophysiological mechanism. Neuropediatrics 1998; 29: 29–34.

123 Miro O, Chamorro A, del Mar Lluch M, Nadal P, Milla J, Urbano-Marquez A. Posthypoxic myoclonus in intensive care. Eur J Emerg Med 1994; 1: 120–2.

124 Yokota T, Tsukagoshi H. Cortical activity-associated negative myoclonus. J Neurol Sci 1992; 111: 77–81.

125 Ikeda A, Kakigi R, Funai N, Neshige R, Kuroda Y, Shibasaki H. Cortical tremor: a variant of cortical reflex myoclonus. Neurology 1992; 40: 1561–5.

126 Smith CR, Scheinberg L. Coincidence of myoclonus and multiple sclerosis: dramatic response to clonazapam. Neurology 1990; 40: 1633–4.

127 Hakeem VF, Wallace SJ. EEG monitoring of therapy for neonatal seizures. Dev Med Child Neurol 1990; 32: 858–64.

128 Fischer K, Baarsma R. Treatment of convulsions in newborn infants. Ned Tijdschr Geneeskd 1996; 140: 2146–7.

129 Ames FF, Enderstein O. Clinical and EEG response to clonazepam in four patients with self induced photosensitive epilepsy. S Afr Med J 1976; 50: 1432–34.

130 Yacubian EM, Castro LH, Grossmann RM, Marques-Assis L. Primary reading epilepsy: therapeutic efficacy of clonazepam in one case. Arq Neuropsiquiatri 1990; 48: 355–9.

131 Esele JH Jr, Grigsby EJ, Dea G. Clonazepam treatment of myoclonic contractions associated with high-dose opioids: case report. Pain 1992; 49: 231–2.

132 Bebin EM. Additional modalities for treating acute seizures in children: Overview. J Child Neurol 1998; (Suppl. 1): S23–6; Discussion S30–2.

133 Padma MV, Jain S, Maheshwari MC. Oral clonazepam sensitive focal status epilepticus (FSE). Indian J Pediatr 1997; 64: 424–7.

134 Trinka E, Moroder T, Nagler M, Staffen W, Loscher W, Ladurner G. Clinical and EEG findings in complex partial status epilepticus with tiagabine. Seizure 1999; 8: 41–4.

135 Rothschild AJ, Shindul-Rothschild, Viguera A, Murray M, Brewster S. Comparsion of the frequency of behavioral disinhibition on alprazolam, clonazepam, or no benozodiazepine in hospitalized psychiatric patients. J Clin Psychopharmacol 2000; 20: 7–11.

136 Terada T, Ishida S, Onuma T, Matsuda H, Muramatsu R. A patient with epilepsy manifesting reversible memory dysfunction—a neuropsychological, electroencephalographical and radiological study. No To Shinkei 1997; 49: 353–8.

137 Culhane NS, Hodle AD. Burning mouth syndrome after taking clonazepam. Ann Pharmacother 2001; 35: 874–6.

138 Browne TR. Clonazepam. A review of a new anticonvulsant drug. Arch Neurol 1976; 33: 326–32.

139 Yamauchi T, Hirabayashi Y, Kataoka N. A clinical study of clonazepam in the treatment of epilepsy Brain Nerve (Tokyo) 1978; 30: 107–16.

140 Iwakawa Y, Niwa T, Suzuki H. Clonazepam-induced tonic seizure. No To Hattatsu 1986; 18: 347–63.

141 Bittencourt PRM, Richens A. Anticonvulsant-induced status epilepticus in Lennox–Gastaut syndrome. Epilepsia 1981; 22: 129–34.

142 Pinder RM, Brogden RN, Speight TM, Avery GS. Clonazepam (Rivotril–Roche): an independent report. Curr Ther Res 1977; 18: 25–32.

143 Rosebuch PI, Mazurek MF. Catatonia after benzodiazepine withdrawal. J Clin Psychopharmacol 1996; 16: 315–19.

144 Gharisian AM, Gauthier S, Wong T. Convulsions in patients abruptly withdrawn from clonazepam while receiving neuroleptic medication. Am J Psychiatr 1987; 144: 686.

145 Laegrid L, Olegard R, Wahlstrom J, Conradi N. Abnormalities in children exposed to benzodiazepines in utero [letter]. Lancet 1987; (Jan 10): 108–9.

146 Samren, EB, van Duijn CM, Christiaens LM, Hofman A, Lindhout D. Antiepileptic drug regimens and major congenital abnormalities in the offspring. Ann Neurol 1999; 46: 739–46.

147 Haeusler MC, Hoellwarth ME, Holzer P. Paralytic ileus in a fetus–neonate after maternal intake of benzodiazepine. Prenat Diagn 1995; 15: 1165–7.

148 Weinstock L, Cohen LS, Bailey JW, Blatman R, Rosenbaum JF. Obstetrical and neonatal outcome following clonazepam use during pregnancy: a case series. Psychother Psychosom 2001; 70: 158–62.

Short-Acting and Other Benzodiazepines

L.J. Greenfield Jr and H.C. Rosenberg

Benzodiazepines (BZDs) are widely used in the management of epilepsy as well as other conditions including anxiety, insomnia and muscle spasms. Their major anticonvulsant role is in the treatment of status epilepticus (SE) and seizure clusters, for which they represent first-line therapy. They are well suited to this purpose because of their high lipophilicity, which enables rapid penetration of the blood–brain barrier [1]. The anticonvulsant properties of BZDs result from specific binding to γ-aminobutyric acid A (GABA-A) receptors (GABARs), where they augment inhibitory neurotransmission [2]. Despite generally long plasma half-lives, most BZDs are relatively 'short acting' after administration of a single dose, due to high plasma protein binding and rapid redistribution from brain to peripheral tissues [3,4]. For example, the elimination half-life of diazepam ranges from 20 to 54 h [5], but the duration of action after a single IV injection is often less than 1 h, with peak brain concentrations present for only 20–30 min [6]. These pharmacokinetic difficulties can easily be overcome by repeated dosing; however, the use of BZDs in the chronic management of epilepsy is generally limited by their sedative properties and the rapid development of tolerance to their anticonvulsant effects [7]. Sedation and tolerance limit the anticonvulsant use of BZDs primarily to the acute treatment of prolonged or serial seizures and SE.

Treatment of status epilepticus and seizure clusters (see also Chapter 18)

Status epilepticus is associated with significant morbidity and mortality [8,9], and requires emergent medical treatment to avoid neuronal damage and its neurological consequences [10,11]. The BZDs have become agents of choice for initial therapy of SE because of their rapid onset of action and proven efficacy [12,13]. The role of BZDs in SE has been confirmed in a number of well-controlled clinical trials. In a recent multicentre, double-blind study [14], patients presenting with SE were randomized to receive lorazepam (0.1 mg/kg), phenytoin (18 mg/kg), phenobarbital (15 mg/kg) or diazepam (0.15 mg/kg) followed by phenytoin (18 mg/kg). Lorazepam was effective as first-line treatment against generalized SE in 64.9% of patients, phenobarbital in 58.2%, diazepam/phenytoin in 55.8% and phenytoin in 43.6%; the difference was significant between lorazepam and phenytoin alone ($P < 0.001$). Efficacy against SE appeared to correlate with the rate at which therapeutic drug concentrations were achieved; lorazepam required the least time to infuse, while phenytoin required the longest ($P < 0.001$).

Both lorazepam and diazepam have been approved by the United States Food and Drug Administration (FDA) for treatment of SE in adults; diazepam has also been approved in children older than 30 days. Parenteral preparations of other BZDs, including midazolam,

flunitrazepam and clonazepam, expand the possibilities for BZD treatment of SE. However, parenteral clonazepam has very limited availability (primarily in Germany and the UK), and flunitrazepam is not available in the USA. Alternative routes of administration, including intramuscular injection and intranasal [15–18], buccal [19], endotracheal [20,21] or rectal [22–27] instillation, have also rapidly produced therapeutic levels and demonstrated efficacy against SE or seizure clusters.

The availability of parenteral and alternative methods of BZD administration increases the therapeutic options for acute treatment of SE and serial seizures, allowing treatment to be geared toward specific clinical situations. For example, repeated seizures in a patient rapidly tapered off anticonvulsants for inpatient epilepsy monitoring could be treated with diazepam (rather than lorazepam or longer-acting BZDs) since its shorter duration of action makes it less likely to suppress seizure activity on subsequent days of monitoring. In contrast, lorazepam may be a better choice for prehospital treatment of SE, where subsequent administration of phenytoin or phenobarbital is impractical. A large-scale clinical trial to evaluate this hypothesis is currently in progress [28]. In the case of serial seizures, the need for immediate high drug levels is less urgent, and ease of administration by family or allied health workers becomes important. Diazepam rectal gel is effective in preventing subsequent seizures during seizure clusters [24,26,27] and in paediatric SE [22] and can reduce the frequency of emergency department visits [23].

Although the use of BZDs in chronic treatment of epilepsy is limited by sedation and the development of tolerance, BZDs may have specific therapeutic indications in epilepsy, such as adjunctive treatment of myoclonic and other generalized seizure types, or in conjunction with comorbid anxiety disorders. Two of the more commonly used BZDs for chronic therapy, clobazam and clonazepam, are discussed in separate chapters (Chapters 29 and 30). This chapter will cover two of the BZDs less commonly used in chronic epilepsy treatment, clorazepate and nitrazepam, and also agents predominantly used for short-term therapy, diazepam, lorazepam and midazolam.

Mechanisms of action

Although only a few of the BZDs are routinely used in the management of epilepsy, almost all display anticonvulsant activity in experimental animal models [29], particularly against seizures induced by the chemical convulsants pentylenetetrazol (PTZ) and picrotoxin (PTX). The BZDs are less effective in the maximal electroshock model [30]. Diazepam [31] and clorazepate [32] have also been demonstrated to slow the development of kindling, an animal model in which repeated subconvulsive electrical stimulation produces increasingly severe seizure activity [33].

Early studies showed that BZDs enhanced inhibitory neurotransmission by increasing the amplitude of inhibitory postsynaptic potentials (IPSPs) mediated by GABA, the major inhibitory neurotransmitter of the mammalian brain [2]. Analysis of fluctuations in GABA-evoked membrane currents in the presence of diazepam suggested that the BZDs increased the opening frequency of a chloride channel opened by GABA [34]. This finding was later confirmed by direct single channel patch-clamp recordings of GABAR chloride channels [35]. Controversial evidence has suggested that diazepam may also increase the single-channel GABAR conductance, that is, the amount of current that flows through the open channel [36].

The discovery of BZD effects on inhibitory neurotransmission was accompanied by the demonstration of stereospecific, high-affinity, saturable BZD binding to receptors on central nervous system neuronal membranes [37,38]. The potency of binding for individual BZDs correlated with their clinical efficacy as sedative, anxiolytic or anticonvulsant agents [39]. Early binding studies demonstrated an association or 'coupling' between BZD binding and GABA binding, in which GABA enhanced the binding of [^{3}H]flunitrazepam [40]. This lead to the concept that BZDs act via a specific receptor associated with the bicuculline-sensitive GABA-A receptor to modulate its actions on a chloride channel. Affinity purification of the 'central BZD receptor' using a BZD-linked sepharose column yielded a 60-kDa protein (likely a mixture of the GABA-A receptor subunits) with a binding site for [^{3}H]muscimol, a GABA agonist [41,42]. These findings confirmed the concept of a 'GABA$_A$ receptor complex' incorporating binding sites for GABA, the BZDs and barbiturates with a ligand-gated chloride channel. Localization of the BZD and GABA sites on the same receptor complex helped to explain how BZDs increase the opening frequency of GABA-stimulated chloride channels.

In whole-cell recordings, 'coupling' between the BZD receptor and the GABA receptor results in a 'left shift' of the concentration–response curve for GABA in the presence of BZDs, that is, increased current amplitudes at lower GABA concentrations [43]. Single-channel recordings of GABAR currents suggested that the BZD effect on channel opening frequency occurs not by altering the kinetic properties of channel opening, but rather by increasing the apparent affinity for GABA at its binding site on the GABA-A receptor [35]. The BZDs thus increase the current produced by low GABA concentrations, but have no effect on maximal currents at high GABA concentrations. This has important implications for synaptic physiology, as studies of GABAergic inhibitory postsynaptic potentials have suggested that GABA is present in the synaptic cleft briefly (1–3 ms) at high concentrations (about 1 mmol/L) [44,45]. Thus, at individual synapses, BZDs do not increase the amplitude of miniature inhibitory postsynaptic currents (mIPSCs), but instead prolong the decay phase of mIPSCs [46,47] possibly by slowing the dissociation of GABA from the receptor [48,49]. Prolongation of the mIPSC increases the likelihood of temporal and spatial summation of multiple synaptic inputs, which in turn increases the amplitude of stimulus-evoked IPSCs. The BZDs thus increase the inhibitory 'tone' of GABAergic synapses, which prevents or limits the hypersynchronous firing of neurone populations that underlies seizure activity.

With a few caveats, the BZDs appear to derive their anticonvulsant properties from their specific binding interaction with GABARs. Several studies have noted that anticonvulsant efficacy of the BZDs cannot be fully accounted for by their high-affinity interactions with GABARs, as part of their anticonvulsant effect occurred at concentrations much higher than necessary to saturate the GABAR BZD binding site, was exponential rather than saturable and was not antagonized by flumazenil [50]. The explanation for these findings may be related to pharmacodynamic issues in BZD metabolism (see below) or other sites of action may be involved.

Molecular biology of GABARs

The GABARs are pharmacologically complex, with binding sites for a number of agents that modulate receptor function, including the barbiturates, neurosteroids, general anaesthetics, the novel anticonvulsant, loreclezole, and the convulsant toxins, picrotoxin and bicuculline. Recent advances in the molecular biology of GABARs have provided a detailed understanding of the mechanisms of BZD action.

GABARs are a member of the ligand-gated channel superfamily of receptors, which includes the nicotinic acetylcholine receptor, the glycine receptor and one type of serotonin receptor (5HT$_3$) [51]. GABARs are pentameric [52] transmembrane chloride channels assembled from combinations of protein subunits from several subunit families (Fig. 31.1). Four different families (α, β, γ, δ) have been studied extensively [53], and three others, π [54], ε [55] and θ [56] have been recently identified and characterized. In mammals, 16 subunit subtypes have been cloned, including α_1–α_6, β_1–β_3 and γ_1–γ_3 subtypes, single members of the π, δ, ε and θ families, as well as alternatively spliced variants of the β_2 and γ_2 subtypes. These subunits are highly homologous, with 30–40% homology between families and about 70% homology within families. Random combinations of subunits would produce tens of thousands of subunit compositions. However, GABAR subtypes are differentially expressed by central nervous system region and cell type [57] and developmentally regulated [58,59], reducing the total number of possible isoforms that can be assembled in specific brain regions and individual neurones. The most common GABA receptor conformation is composed of the α_1, β_2 and γ_2 subtypes, with presumed stoichiometry of two α, two β and a single γ subunit; the δ subunit may in some cases substitute for γ. The subunits are arranged around a central water-filled pore, which can open to conduct Cl$^-$ ions when GABA is bound (Fig. 31.1). Studies of recombinant receptors have shown that individual subunits and their subtypes confer different sensitivities to GABAR modulators including BZDs [60,61], loreclezole [62] and zinc ions [63].

GABAR subunit composition and BZD pharmacology

BZD augmentation of GABAR currents requires a γ subunit and is strongly influenced by which α subtype is present [53,64]. The effect of GABAR subunit composition on BZD binding has been well characterized by radioligand binding studies [65] and electrophysiology of the recombinant receptors expressed in fibroblasts [64]. Presence of the α_1 subtype results in a receptor with high affinity for the imidazopyridine hypnotic, zolpidem, defining the 'BZ-1' (or Ω_1) receptor type [65,66]. The α_2 and α_3 subtypes, combined with β and

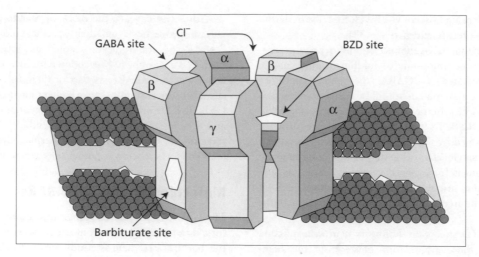

Fig. 31.1 Structural representation of the pentameric GABA-A receptor, with binding sites for GABA (between the α and β subunits), BZDs (between the α and γ subunits) and barbiturates. A central pore conducts chloride ions.

γ, result in receptors with moderate affinity for zolpidem, termed BZ-2 receptors. GABARs with an α_5 subunit and/or a γ_3 subunit are sensitive to diazepam, but have essentially no affinity for zolpidem, and are termed BZ-3 receptors. Subunit specificity is further defined by binding sensitivity of the triazolopyridazine, Cl 218,872. GABARs with α_4 or α_6 subunits are insensitive to most BZDs. Given the dependence of BZD binding and action on α and γ subunits, it is not surprising that the BZD binding site is located in a cleft between these two subunits [67]. Photoaffinity labelling and site-directed mutagenesis studies have shown that specific residues of the α_1 and γ subunits are involved in BZD binding and action [68–73].

GABARs and epilepsy

The anticonvulsant properties of BZDs are likely related to the prominent role of GABARs in epilepsy. The evidence linking epilepsy with dysfunction of GABAergic inhibition is substantial and growing. GABAR subunit expression is altered in the hippocampi of experimental animals with recurrent seizures [74] and in patients with temporal lobe epilepsy [75,76]. Angelman's syndrome, a neurodevelopmental disorder associated with severe mental retardation and epilepsy, is linked to a deletion mutation on chromosome 15q11–13 [77] in a region encoding the β_3 subunit [78] which may account for the epileptic phenotype. Reduction of γ_2 subunit expression using an antisense oligonucleotide in rats (to block translation of endogenous mRNA for that subunit) lead to spontaneous electrographic seizures that evolved into limbic SE [79], but increased the seizure threshold for the BZD inverse agonist, β-CCM [80]. Moreover, two mutations in the human γ_2 subunit, K289M [81] and R43Q [82] have been found in two large families with childhood absence epilepsy and febrile seizures, both producing loss of BZ sensitivity, which reinforces the association between epilepsy and defects in BZD sensitivity of GABARs.

GABAR α subunits and BZD effects

Specific GABAR α subunits appear to mediate the different clinical

properties of the BZDs. For example, a strain of 'alcohol-non-tolerant' rats was found to have a point mutation in the normally BZD-insensitive α_6 subunit (R100Q) that makes their α_6-containing GABARs (found mostly in the cerebellum) diazepam sensitive, likely accounting for their ethanol and BZD intolerance [83]. The BZD-sensitive α subunits have a histidine residue at this site, and are rendered BZD insensitive when the residue is mutated to arginine [71]. This finding has allowed investigation of the function of different BZD-sensitive α subunits by 'knock-in mutations' of BZD-insensitive α subunits in mice. In homozygous α_1(H101R) 'knock-in' mice, BZDs were not protective against pentylenetetrazol (PTZ)-induced convulsions and did not produce sedation or amnesia, suggesting that binding to the (wild type) α_1 subunit is responsible for sedative, amnestic and anticonvulsant actions [84]. Mice with this mutation displayed anxiolytic but not sedative responses to BZDs [85]. Moreover, the sedative-hypnotic, zolpidem, which binds with high affinity to α_1-containing GABARs and lower affinity to α_2 and α_3-containing GABARs, showed no sedative effect in α_1(H101R) mice [86]. Unfortunately, these findings underscore the association between sedative and anticonvulsant efficacy for the BZDs at α_1-containing GABARs. Other BZD-sensitive α subunits (α_2, α_3 or α_5) are likely responsible for anxiolytic, motor impairment and ethanol potentiation properties [84]. Corresponding 'knock-in' mutations of the α_2 and α_3 subtypes (α_2(H101R) and α_3(H126R)) suggested that anxiolytic [87] and myorelaxant [88] properties of BZDs derive from α_2- and (at higher BZD concentrations) α_3-containing GABARs.

While the majority of BZDs have similar clinical effects, there are significant quantitative differences in anticonvulsant potency compared to potency for sedation or motor impairment. For example, the dose of diazepam required to block PTZ-induced seizures is about 100-fold less than the dose required to cause loss of the righting reflex, while for clonazepam, the difference is more than 5000-fold [29]. The fact that GABARs with differing composition have varied sensitivity to specific BZDs, and that these receptors are expressed in specific brain regions or neurone populations, may partially explain the differences in anticonvulsant potency and efficacy relative to sedative and anxiolytic properties. It remains to be determined whether these varied clinical efficacies result from different binding affinities at receptors with the same GABAR subunit composition, or relative differences in affinities at GABARs with diverse α or γ subunits.

Antagonists, partial agonists, inverse agonists

An additional factor to consider is that BZDs and related compounds not only vary in their clinical potencies; antagonists and partial agonists at the BZD binding site have also been discovered. Preclinical and preliminary human data suggest that several of these compounds may be useful in the management of epilepsy.

Flumazenil

Flumazenil (RO15-1788, see structure diagram, Fig. 31.2) binds to the BZD site without causing any change in GABA site binding or GABA-evoked currents, thus meeting the pharmacological definition of an antagonist. This agent has been used primarily to reverse BZD-induced sedation [89,90], but may also have benefit in reversing hepatic coma [91,92] in patients who had no prior exposure to BZDs. The finding that a BZD antagonist benefits hepatic coma has been used to bolster arguments for an endogenous BZD ligand or 'endozapine', which could be displaced by flumazenil [91]. A 'diazepam binding inhibitor' peptide has been discovered and characterized [93], though its role in inhibitory neurotransmission remains unclear. Curiously, flumazenil has also shown efficacy as an anticonvulsant in some animal models, possibly due to partial agonism at high doses [94–96]. Flumazenil also reduces epileptiform discharges in hippocampal slices [97] and slows the development of

kindling [98,99]. Several small studies have suggested possible benefit in humans [100,101]. In nine of 11 previously untreated patients with epilepsy, oral flumazenil (10 mg once to three times daily) caused a 50–75% reduction in seizure frequency, and nine of 16 patients experienced 50–75% reduction in seizure frequency when flumazenil was added as an adjunctive anticonvulsant [102]. Flumazenil's ability to prevent interictal epileptiform discharges on EEG was similar to that of diazepam [103,104], suggesting that it may act as a partial agonist or block the action of an endogenous proconvulsant. However, flumazenil can also precipitate seizures in patients dependent on BZDs, particularly in the setting of hepatic encephalopathy or in patients who have ingested multiple agents in overdose (e.g. tricyclic antidepressants) [105]. The ability of flumazenil to induce seizures in patients previously treated with BZDs has been used to precipitate partial seizures during epilepsy monitoring to localize seizure onset [106]. In addition, [^{11}C]flumazenil has been used diagnostically in PET studies to demonstrate regions of neuronal loss associated with epilepsy [107,108], and may be useful in localizing the seizure focus in patients with dual pathology [109].

Partial and inverse BZD agonists

A number of 'partial agonists' at the BZD binding site have also been characterized, including abecarnil [110], imidazenil [111] and bretazenil [112]. Although less effective than full agonists like diazepam, these agents have demonstrated anticonvulsant efficacy in animal models and appear less prone to the development of tolerance [113–117]. Finally, a class of full and partial 'inverse agonists', including several β-carbolines, bind to the BZD site and inhibit

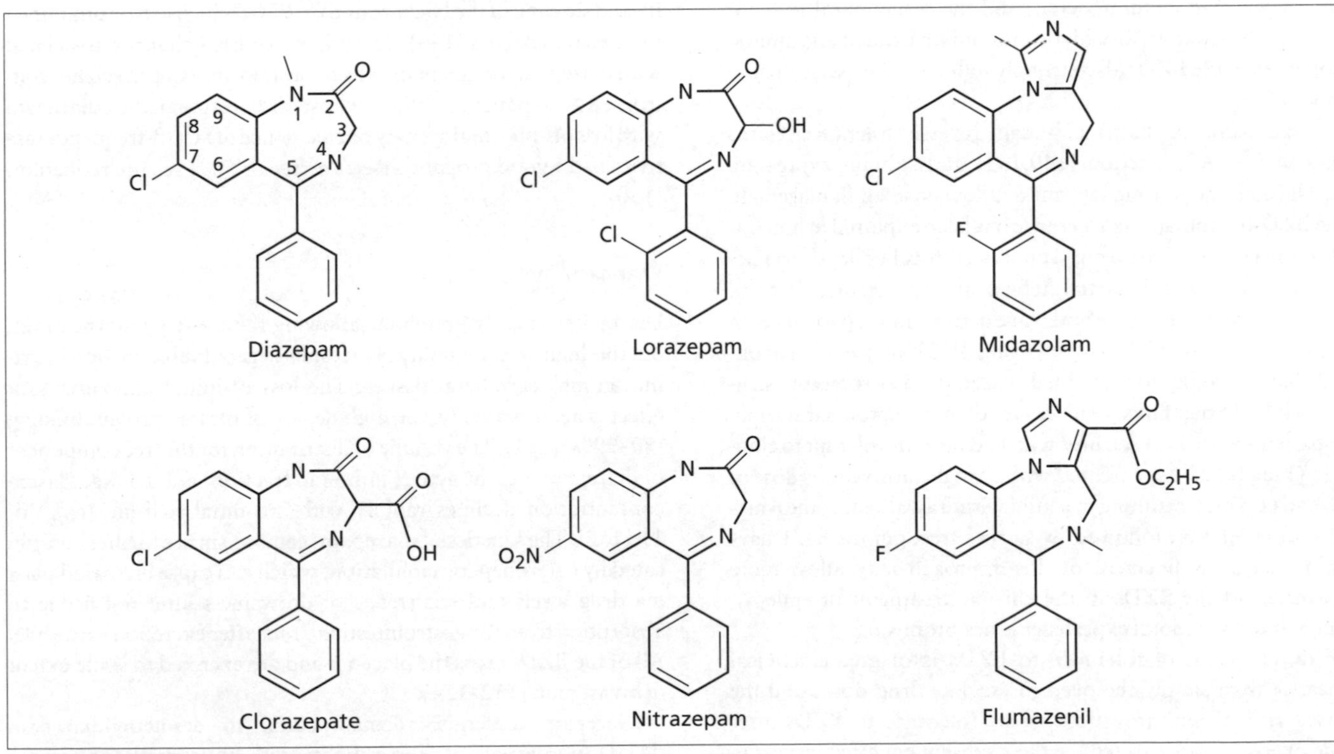

Fig. 31.2 Structures of the major BZD compounds presented in this chapter.

GABA binding or GABA-evoked currents. As one would expect, these agents can induce convulsions or anxiety [118,119]. They have been useful in characterizing GABAR function, but have no demonstrated clinical utility.

BZD tolerance and GABAR plasticity

Chronic BZD treatment is associated with tolerance, a decrease in sedative or anticonvulsant properties, and dependence, the need for continued drug to prevent a withdrawal syndrome [120]. Withdrawal symptoms are typically an exacerbation of initial symptoms (anxiety, insomnia or seizures) above the initial baseline, and are more common with short-acting than long-acting agents. Rebound symptoms typically return to baseline within 1–3 weeks after discontinuation of drug [121]. Tolerance develops proportionally to agonist efficacy. BZD partial agonists develop much less tolerance than full agonists, and the antagonist flumazenil causes no tolerance-related changes in receptor number or function [116]. Tolerance to one BZD with a particular regimen may not induce tolerance to a different BZD, suggesting drug-specific interactions at their receptors [122]. The duration of tolerance also varies between BZDs [123]. Chronic BZD-induced changes in GABAR subunit expression (decreased α_1, γ_{2L} and γ_{2S} and increased α_5) may underlie tolerance to BZD-induced cognitive dysfunction [124].

Experimental studies of tolerance have noted marked changes in GABAR subunit expression [125–134] as well as functional changes [135–138]; however, such changes are extremely dependent on the specifics of the model system. Such details as the drug, dosage, duration and method of drug administration, all contribute to the 'environment' of chronic BZD receptor occupancy that predisposes to tolerance. Moreover, the seizure model (PTZ, biculculine, pilocarpine, kindling, etc.), and the behavioural tests for tolerance to the sedative, anxiolytic, motor impairment and amnestic properties of the BZDs also strongly influence the assessment of tolerance [139].

Brief exposure to flumazenil can reverse tolerance-related changes in GABAR function [140,141] and subunit expression [142]. The concept of using intermittent low doses of flumazenil to reverse BZD anticonvulsant tolerance has been explored in humans [104]. Flumazenil (0.75–15 mg) suppressed focal epileptiform activity in six patients with partial (temporal lobe) seizures, but had no effect on generalized spike and wave activity in six patients with generalized seizures. PET studies using [11C]flumazenil demonstrated that a 1.5-mg dose resulted in about 55% receptor occupancy, while 15 mg flumazenil resulted in receptor saturation. Three patients with daily seizures who had become tolerant to clonazepam (1 mg b.i.d.) were treated with a single intravenous dose of flumazenil (1.5 mg), resulting in a mild withdrawal syndrome (shivering) lasting 30 min, followed by seizure freedom for 6–21 days (mean 13 days). Refinement of this approach may allow more extensive use of the BZDs in the chronic treatment of epilepsy, although initial anecdotal experience is not promising.

The development of tolerance to BZDs is of greater clinical significance than simply the need to escalate drug doses and the increased risk of withdrawal seizures. Tolerance to BZDs after chronic exposure can also reduce their subsequent effectiveness in acute conditions [143], rendering them ineffective for treatment of

SE. An additional difficulty is that prolonged seizures or SE itself can alter GABAR susceptibility to BZDs. Reduction in GABAR BZD sensitivity can occur within minutes in SE [144] and may be responsible in part for both the persistent epileptic state and its refractoriness to treatment. In an animal model of self-sustaining SE after perforant path stimulation, both diazepam and phenytoin showed decreased effectiveness for terminating seizures over time [145]. Refractoriness to diazepam may be mediated by N-methyl-D-aspartate (NMDA) receptor mechanisms, as NMDA antagonists improve the response to diazepam in late pilocarpine-induced SE [146]. Moreover, NMDA receptors are upregulated during BZD tolerance, and NMDA antagonists (e.g. MK801) can block BZD-withdrawal seizures [147]. These findings suggest a new strategy for treatment of late, BZD refractory SE with combinations of a BZD (e.g. intravenous midazolam) and an NMDA receptor antagonist such as the general anaesthetic, ketamine. Such approaches will require validation in controlled clinical trials.

Short-acting BZDs

Diazepam

Diazepam (Fig. 31.2) became the first BZD used for epilepsy when Gastaut et al. used intravenous diazepam to treat SE in 1965 [148]. Diazepam has subsequently become standard initial therapy for SE in adults and children, though its primary role may be usurped by lorazepam (see below). Diazepam is available in both oral and parenteral preparations. Rectal diazepam has been long used in Europe, and was classified as an orphan drug in 1993 in the US, allowing the development there of the rectal diazepam gel (Diastat) which has been used effectively in the treatment of serial seizures. Diazepam and other BZDs induce an increase in β-frequency activity and slowing of the background on EEG, which can be quantified by spectral analysis [149]. The pattern of EEG changes associated with diazepam treatment may be of prognostic value in seizure control; 88% of patients (29/33) whose EEG responded to diazepam with loss of abnormal activity or emergence of fast (β-frequency) activity had a good prognosis (seizure free or 50% seizure reduction) [150].

Pharmacokinetics

Diazepam is highly lipophilic, allowing rapid entry into the brain, but this high lipid solubility also results in rapid subsequent redistribution into peripheral tissues. The loss of initial anticonvulsant effect is accentuated by the high degree of plasma protein binding (90–99%) [151]. The volume of distribution for the free component of diazepam (i.e. the active, unbound fraction) is 1.1 L/kg. Plasma concentration declines rapidly with an initial half-life ($t_{1/2\alpha}$) of 1 h [152]. The kinetics of diazepam metabolism are further complicated by enterohepatic circulation, which can cause increased plasma drug levels and recurrence of drowsiness after 6–8 h due to absorption from the gastrointestinal tract after excretion in the bile. All of the BZDs cross the placenta and are excreted to some extent in breast milk [152–154].

Diazepam undergoes demethylation to desmethyldiazepam (DMD, nordiazepam), a metabolite with anticonvulsant activity and a long half-life (>20 h), followed by slow hydroxylation (at

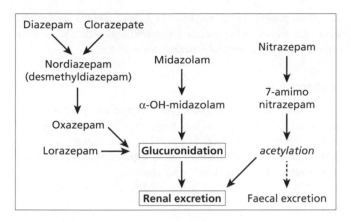

Fig. 31.3 Metabolic pathways for several BZDs.

position 3 of the diazepine ring) to oxazepam, which is also active (see Fig. 31.3) [155]. Both metabolites are conjugated with glucuronic acid in the liver [156] followed by renal excretion [155] with an elimination half-life ($t_{1/2\beta}$) of 24–48 h [152,157]. Diazepam treatment causes induction of cytochrome P450 type 2B (CYP2B) [158].

Adverse effects and drug interactions

Diazepam when given intravenously can produce respiratory depression [159], which may be exacerbated by postictal central nervous system depression and necessitate ventilatory support [160]. Rectal diazepam can also occasionally cause respiratory depression. Drowsiness, fatigue, amnesia, ataxia and falls can occur and are more prominent in the elderly. Intravenous diazepam can cause thrombophlebitis and lactic acidosis (due to the propylene glycol vehicle). Rarely, a paradoxical response to diazepam is observed in which diazepam increases seizure frequency, causes paradoxical muscle spasms or provokes SE [161]. An idiosyncratic allergic interstitial nephritis has also been reported [162]. Rare adverse events include cardiac arrhythmias, hepatotoxicity, gynaecomastia, blurred vision and diplopia, neutropenia or thrombocytopenia, rash and urticaria, and anaphylaxis [163]. There is significant potential for abuse, though it is rare in patients prescribed diazepam for appropriate indications [4]. The teratogenicity of diazepam is uncertain, but diazepam taken during the first trimester has been associated with oral clefts [164]. Diazepam may also amplify the teratogenic potential of valproic acid [165].

Diazepam enhances the elimination of phenobarbital [157], probably due to its ability to induce cytochrome P450 [158]. Valproic acid displaces diazepam bound to plasma proteins, leading to increased free diazepam and associated increased sedation [166].

Clinical applications

Status epilepticus (see also Chapter 18)

Diazepam is effective initial therapy in both convulsive and non-convulsive SE [14]. Diazepam may be particularly effective in gen-

eralized absence SE, with 93% of patients initially controlled [167]. In the same early study, diazepam also controlled 89% of generalized convulsions, 88% of simple motor seizures and 75% of complex partial SE. These numbers are higher than those observed in the VA Cooperative SE Trial [14], possibly due to differences in patient populations. When SE results from acute central nervous system disease or structural brain lesions, a single intravenous bolus of diazepam is likely to be ineffective due to its short duration of action [148,159,168]. Strategies to avoid this problem have included giving subsequent 5–10 mg intravenous doses every few hours, following diazepam with a longer-lasting anticonvulsant (e.g. phenytoin [14]), or continuous intravenous diazepam. Diazepam (100 mg in 500 mL of 5% dextrose in water) infused at 40 mL/h delivers 20 mg/h [169], and may be suitable to obtain a serum level in the range of 200–800 ng/mL, which has been reported as therapeutic [157,170]. Diazepam appears to be absorbed onto PVC bags, with a reduction in bioavailability of 50% after 8 h [171], which should be taken into account if a chronic infusion of diazepam for SE is contemplated.

Paediatric SE

The initial recommended intravenous diazepam dose in children is 0.1–0.3 mg/kg by slow bolus (< 5 mg/min) repeating every 15 min for 2 doses, with a maximum of 5 mg in infants and 15 mg in older children [172,173]. Continuous intravenous infusion of diazepam has also been used effectively in paediatric SE. Continuous diazepam infusion (0.01–0.03 mg/kg/min) controlled seizures in 86% of patients (49/57) within an average of 40 min [174]. Hypotension occurred in one patient (2%), respiratory depression in six patients (12%) and death in seven patients (14%). Patients who failed diazepam infusion were treated with thiopental, which controlled seizures in all patients but required ventilatory and haemodynamic support; four patients (44%) of this group died. A meta-analysis of 111 paediatric patients (aged 1 month to 18 years) with refractory generalized convulsive SE, treated with diazepam, midazolam, thiopental, pentobarbital or isoflurane, suggested that diazepam was less effective as continuous therapy than the other agents (86% vs. 100%) after stratifying for aetiology of SE [175]. However, all of the patients receiving diazepam were from one region (India), and none received continuous EEG monitoring, suggesting that differences in patient population, location or details of care may have been contributory. Mortality was 20% in symptomatic cases and 4% in idiopathic cases, and was less frequent in midazolam-treated patients.

Rectal diazepam in paediatric SE

Although intravenous administration is preferable, rectal administration of diazepam rapidly produces effective drug levels for treatment of paediatric SE [176] and safely aborts SE in paediatric patients [22,177]. In children found to be in electrographic SE during EEG monitoring, rectal administration of diazepam resulted in cessation of paroxysmal activity in 58% of cases [178]. Rectal diazepam was particularly effective in patients with electrical SE during sleep, and less effective in patients with hypsarrhythmia. Intraosseous injection (in children of suitable age) also produces rapid plasma levels comparable to intravenous administration

[179], and is a viable alternative when intravenous access is not available.

Febrile convulsions

Rectal diazepam is effective in aborting febrile and non-febrile seizures in the home setting [23]. While the concept of chronic prophylaxis for childhood febrile convulsions has long been in disrepute, it has not been clear whether there was benefit to short-term seizure prophylaxis during fever. A prospective trial randomized 289 children in Denmark to intermittent prophylaxis (diazepam at fever) or no prophylaxis (diazepam at seizure), and assessed neurological outcome, motor, cognitive and scholastic achievement 12 years later [180]. There were no differences in IQ scores, motor or scholastic test results, nor any difference between simple and complex febrile convulsions in neurological outcome (likelihood of future seizures), suggesting that short-term prophylaxis did not differ from abbreviation of febrile convulsions, and is probably not necessary. Moreover, the incidence of respiratory depression in children treated with intravenous and/or rectal diazepam is fairly high, with 11 of 122 patients (9%) showing a decrease in respiratory rate or oxygen saturation, eight of whom required short-term ventilatory support [160].

Serial seizures

In a large-scale multicentre open-label trial of rectal diazepam gel (Diastat) in 149 patients older than 2 years, treated with a total of 1578 drug administrations, 77% of administrations resulted in seizure freedom for the ensuing 12 h [27]. There was no difference in response rate between patients treated infrequently (2–7 administrations) and patients treated frequently (8–78 episodes), suggesting that tolerance did not reduce the effectiveness of diazepam under these conditions. Sedation occurred in 17%. Diazepam rectal gel was also useful against serial seizures in adult patients with refractory epilepsy [25,26], with 0.5 mg/kg found to be an effective dose [181].

Intramuscular diazepam injection may also be suitable for prophylaxis of serial seizures, but absorption is not rapid enough to be effective against SE. Intramuscular diazepam injection produced peak serum concentrations in 29 min in rhesus monkeys, with a volume of distribution of 1.5 L/kg and clearance rate of 19 mL/min/kg [182]. Intranasal administration of diazapam is another alternative in this setting. In healthy human volunteers, peak serum concentrations of diazepam (2 mg) after intranasal administration occurred after 18 ± 11 min with bioavailability of about 50% [18]. A pharmacodynamic effect was seen at 5 min. In rabbits, bioavailability of diazepam was 49–62% in the first 30 min after intranasal administration in a glycol solution, and a pharmacodynamic response occurred within 1.5 and 3.5 min [183].

Chronic epilepsies

In general diazepam is not useful as chronic therapy. However, periodic courses of diazepam can be considered for certain chronic conditions for which current alternatives are often inadequate, including West's syndrome, Lennox–Gastaut syndrome, Landau–Kleffner syndrome and electrical SE during sleep [184].

Oral diazepam (0.5–0.75 mg/kg/day) administered in cycles of 3 weeks duration were beneficial in interrupting electrical SE, and improved neuropsychological function in some cases.

Lorazepam

Lorazepam (Fig. 31.2) has greater potency and a longer duration of action than diazepam, and has frequently become the agent of choice for initial treatment of SE in adults [9]. Lorazepam is also less likely to produce significant respiratory depression [185]. It is available in both oral and parenteral preparations.

Pharmacokinetics

Lorazepam is rapidly absorbed but less bioavailable after oral than intravenous administration due to enterohepatic recirculation and first-pass biotransformation in the liver [186]. Peak plasma levels occur 90–120 min after oral dosing [187,188]. Lorazepam is about 90% protein bound, with CSF levels approximately equivalent to free serum levels, suggesting passive diffusion across the blood–brain barrier [189]. Clinical effects after intravenous lorazepam (sleep spindles in EEG recordings) were observed within 30 s to 4 min [6,190,191], though peak brain concentrations and maximal EEG effect did not occur until 30 min after lorazepam infusion [192,193]. After a single intravenous injection, plasma levels decrease initially due to tissue distribution with a half-life ($t_{1/2\alpha}$) of 2–3 h. The half-life for elimination ($t_{1/2\beta}$) is in the 8–25 h range, and is the same for oral administration [194,195]. The volume of distribution is about 1.8 L/kg [192]. Clinical effects of sedation, amnesia and anxiolysis occur at plasma levels between 10 and 30 ng/mL [187].

Lorazepam is metabolized via glucuronidation in the liver [196] and then excreted by the kidneys [197] (Fig. 31.3).

Adverse effects and drug interactions

Sedation, dizziness, vertigo, weakness and unsteadiness are relatively common, with disorientation, depression, headache, sleep disturbances, agitation or restlessness, emotional disturbances, hallucinations and delirium less common [191,197]. Impairment of psychomotor performance, dysarthria and anterograde amnesia have also been observed. Mild respiratory depression sometimes occurs, particularly with the first intravenous dose [198]. Rare adverse events include neutropenia. A paradoxical effect was observed in a patient with Lennox–Gastaut syndrome in which lorazepam precipitated tonic seizures [199]. Abuse liability is relatively low. Although lorazepam is in FDA pregnancy category D, of known teratogenic potential, short-term use in treatment of SE may be of life-saving benefit and likely to outweigh the uncertain risks. Sudden discontinuation after chronic use has caused withdrawal seizures [185].

Valproic acid increases plasma concentrations of lorazepam [200], and decreased lorazepam clearance by 40% [201], apparently by inhibiting hepatic glucuronidation, though lorazepam does not affect valproic acid levels [200]. Probenecid increased the half-life of lorazepam by inhibiting glucuronidation, resulting in toxicity in patients on long-term therapy [194].

Clinical applications

Status epilepticus (see also Chapter 18)

The recommended intravenous dose of lorazepam for SE is 0.1 mg/kg (up to a maximum of 4 mg) administered at 2 mg/min, with repeat doses after 10–15 min if necessary [14,185]. Although lorazepam is less lipophilic than diazepam, it appears to cross the blood–brain barrier readily, as onset of action occurred within 3 min in 37 cases of SE, and controlled seizures in 89% of episodes within 10 min [12]. In another early study, all 10 patients with generalized convulsive SE had seizures controlled with intravenous lorazepam (mean 4 mg), but nine of 11 patients with partial SE with decreased responsiveness experienced problems including respiratory depression, two of whom required entubation [202]. The VA Cooperative SE Trial demonstrated superiority of lorazepam (0.1 mg/kg) over phenytoin (18 mg/kg) in response rate to initial therapy (64.9% vs. 43.6% responders) [14]. The response rate was slightly better for lorazepam than diazepam (0.15 mg/kg) followed by phenytoin (18 mg/kg) (55.8% responders), but not significantly different. Intravenous lorazepam (4 mg) was effective against postanoxic myoclonic SE after cardiac arrest in six patients [203]. However, electroclinical dissociation was observed, hence continuous EEG monitoring during lorazepam treatment is advisable.

Paediatric SE

The usual intravenous lorazepam dose in paediatric SE is 0.05 mg/kg, repeated twice at intervals of 15–20 min [204]. In 31 children aged 2–18 presenting with SE, intravenous lorazepam (0.05 mg/kg, repeated up to 3 times at 15 min intervals) terminated seizure activity in 81% of patients [198]. A retrospective study found that lorazepam (0.1 mg/kg in children and 0.07 mg/kg in adolescents) was most effective in partial SE, terminating seizures in 90% of cases [143]. Prior treatment of SE with phenytoin, phenobarbital or diazepam did not alter the effectiveness of lorazepam, though chronic BZD treatment significantly reduced the effectiveness of lorazepam in SE [143], indicating tolerance. Respiratory depression, when observed, occurred after the first injection.

Lorazepam was effective in neonatal seizures refractory to phenobarbital and/or phenytoin in several small studies. In seven neonates (gestational ages 30–43 weeks) treated with intravenous lorazepam (0.05 mg/kg), seizures were controlled within 5 min in all seven patients, with no recurrence in 71.4% and at least 8 h of control in the remaining patients [205]. In a retrospective study of 13 neonates (gestational ages 25–43 weeks) treated with 0.04–0.1 mg/kg lorazepam, seizure control was obtained in 54% and partial benefit in another 23% [206]. No respiratory depression or other adverse effects were reported in either study.

Paediatric serial seizures

Sublingual lorazepam (1–4 mg) was effective against serial seizures in 80% (8/10) and partially effective in 20% (2/10) of children, with onset of clinical effect within 15 min in most cases [207].

Alcohol withdrawal seizures

Lorazepam (2 mg) administered after a witnessed ethanol withdrawal seizure prevented a second seizure better than placebo (3% recurrence in the lorazepam group vs. 24% in the placebo group, $P < 0.001$), and may be the agent of choice in this setting [208].

Chronic epilepsy

Lorazepam was effective as adjunctive treatment of complex partial seizures, with an optimal dose of 5 mg/day after slow upward titration from 1 mg twice daily [209]. Therapeutic levels were in the range or 20–30 ng/mL. However, long-term treatment with lorazepam is likely to result in tolerance, and is not generally recommended.

Midazolam

Midazolam is a water-soluble 1,4 benzodiazepine (Fig. 31.2) widely used for induction of anaesthesia or as a preanaesthetic agent. It is 3–4 times as potent as diazepam. Midazolam has gained popularity in acute treatment of SE by either intravenous or intramuscular use, though its short duration of action necessitates use of continuous intravenous maintenance or subsequent therapy with an additional anticonvulsant. Midazolam (10 mg) intramuscular injection caused a similar reduction in interictal spike frequency in EEG recordings as intravenous diazepam (20 mg) [210], and this route of administration provides a valuable alternative when intravenous access is unavailable.

Pharmacokinetics

Serum midazolam levels after intravenous administration were best fit by a two compartment model, with an initial tissue distribution phase ($t_{1/2\alpha}$ of 5.7 ± 2.4 min) and an elimination phase ($t_{1/2\beta}$ of 66 ± 37 min) [152]. After intravenous administration of 15–60 mg over 5 min in eight healthy adult volunteers, plasma concentrations for a half-maximal increase in β-frequency activity on EEG recording was 276 ± 64 μmol/L [204]. With an intramuscular injection, peak serum concentration occurred after 25 ± 23 min, and the half-life for elimination was 2.8 ± 1.7 h [211]. After oral administration, 44 ± 17% of the dose was bioavailable [152], while intranasal midazolam availability ranged from 50% [212] to 83% [213]. Bioavailability after rectal administration was 52% [214] and 74.5% after buccal administration [19]. Midazolam is 95 ± 2% protein bound, with a volume of distribution of 1.1 ± 0.6 L/kg and a half-life of 1.9 ± 0.6 h [152,215]. The clearance rate was 6.6 ± 1.8 mL/min/kg, with 56 ± 26% urinary excretion.

The pharmacokinetics of midazolam are altered in children and critically ill patients. In children aged 1–5 years, administration of midazolam (0.2 mg/kg) by intranasal or intravenous route resulted in a similar elimination half-life, 2.2 h for intranasal and 2.4 h for intravenous administration [216]. In critically ill neonates, the elimination half-life after intravenous administration was 12.0 h [217]. In adult patients in intensive care, the volume of distribution (3.1 L/kg) and elimination half-life (5.4 h) were significantly greater than in healthy volunteers (0.9 L/kg and 2.3 h, respectively) [218] though clearance was not significantly different (6.3 vs. 4.9 mL/min/kg for patients and volunteers, respectively).

Midazolam is metabolized rapidly by α-hydroxylation of the methyl group on the fused imidazo ring (Figs 31.2, 31.3) [219]. The α-hydroxylated compound is biologically active, but is eliminated with a half-life of about 1 h after hepatic conjugation with glucuronic acid [220].

Adverse effects and drug interactions

Dose-dependent sedation with midazolam may be prolonged after continuous infusion despite its short half-life [221]. Retrograde amnesia, euphoria, confusion and dysarthria also occur. Midazolam syrup has been associated with respiratory depression and arrest, and should only be given in a hospital setting or where resuscitative drugs, equipment and experienced personnel are immediately available. Paradoxical reactions (agitation, tremor, involuntary movements, hyperactivity, combativeness) occur in about 2%, seizures and nystagmus in about 1%. Nausea and vomiting occur with midazolam syrup in 8 and 4%, respectively, but are far less common with intravenous administration. Hypotension and decreased cardiac output likely result from peripheral vasodilatation [219,222]. Sudden discontinuation after long-term use can result in withdrawal seizures [223,224]. Midazolam is in FDA pregnancy risk category D.

Erythromycin may prolong the half-life of midazolam to 10–20 h [225]. Phenytoin and carbamazepine reduce the bioavailability of oral midazolam by inducing cytochrome P450, which enhances first-pass hepatic metabolism [226].

Clinical applications

Status epilepticus (see also Chapter 18)

For treatment of refractory SE, intravenous midazolam 0.2 mg/kg by slow bolus injection followed by 0.75–10 µg/kg/min maintenance infusion has been recommended [9,227]. In general, patients should be intubated, on ventilator and monitored by EEG and haemodynamic monitoring. Typically, infusion is maintained for 12 h and then slowly tapered during continuous EEG monitoring; if seizure activity returns, midazolam infusion is resumed for additional 12-h periods. Tolerance may develop, and doses up to 2 mg/kg/h have been required for seizure control [210]. Advantages of midazolam over other BZDs include rapid onset of action, ease of administration and titration (with the possibility of initial intramuscular injection), good efficacy and lack of serious adverse effects [228]. Continuous intravenous infusion of midazolam has been shown effective for treatment of refractory SE, terminating seizures within 100 s in seven of seven patients who had failed treatment with diazepam, lorazepam and phenytoin with or without phenobarbital [229]. Intramuscular midazolam has been used successfully for SE in several small series, with effective dose of 0.2 mg/kg [230,231].

Paediatric SE

Midazolam has also been demonstrated as safe and effective in paediatric SE. In 19 of 20 children (mean age 4 years) SE was controlled with midazolam (0.15 mg/kg bolus followed by 1–5 µg/kg/min infusion) alone or with concomitant phenytoin or phenobarbital [232]. In a series of eight paediatric patients (age 17 days to 16 years) with refractory SE treated with prolonged (>48 h) midazolam coma, the average dose for seizure cessation was 14 µg/kg/min and mean duration of therapy was 192 h; one patient could not be successfully weaned and died after 4 weeks [233]. In a similar series of 20 children (mean age 4 years), midazolam was well tolerated and stopped seizures in 95% of patients [234]. Intravenous midazolam was safe and effective as first-line therapy in 15 of 16 episodes of SE in 10 children (20 months to 16 years), using a loading dose of 0.1–0.3 mg/kg followed by average infusion of 2.7 µg/kg/min for 12 h to 6 days [235]. There was also benefit when midazolam was used as a second-, third- or fourth-line drug, with seizure control in 34 of 38 SE episodes. In neonates (1–9 days, 30–41 weeks gestational age) midazolam (0.1–0.4 mg/kg/h) controlled overt seizures refractory to high dose phenobarbital (with or without phenytoin) in six patients within 1 h [236]; electrographic seizures continued in two of the six for another 12 h. Midazolam was tolerated well by neonates, with no change in pulse or blood pressure and no adverse reactions.

Febrile seizures

In a prospective, randomized study of 47 children, intranasal midazolam was equally effective as intravenous diazepam for controlling prolonged febrile convulsions in children, with shorter mean time to starting treatment and shorter time for controlling seizures (3.5 vs. 5.5 min) [237].

Paediatric serial seizures

A study comparing intramuscular midazolam to intravenous diazepam in children with seizures lasting longer than 10 min found similar efficacy between these agents, though patients in the midazolam group received medication sooner and seizures ended sooner [238]. In 26 children in the home (11/26) or hospital (17/26) setting, intranasal midazolam stopped seizures in an average of 3.6 min, with 98% of seizures stopped within 10 min [239]. A randomized single-site trial in children (aged 5–19 years) with the Lennox–Gastaut syndrome or other symptomatic generalized epilepsies showed that midazolam (10 mg in 2 mL) administered around the buccal mucosa stopped 75% of 40 seizures in 14 patients, compared to 59% of 39 seizures in 14 patients stopped by rectal diazepam (10 mg) [240]. The time to end of seizure was not different between groups, and no cardiorespiratory adverse events occurred. Intrabuccal administration of midazolam is thus another viable route of administration in this patient population.

Other BZDs for chronic therapy

Clorazepate

Clorazepate is a benzodiazepine used in adjunctive treatment of seizure disorders, anxiety and alcohol withdrawal. Its role in epilepsy is limited to adjunctive therapy of refractory generalized or partial seizure disorders, particularly in the setting of comorbid anxiety disorders.

Pharmacokinetics

Clorazepate is a prodrug, available as a dipotassium salt, which is rapidly converted to nordiazepam (*N*-desmethyldiazepam, DMD), the same major active metabolite produced by diazepam (Fig. 31.3). Non-enzymatic decarboxylation at position 3 occurs at gastric pH, with 90% of clorazepate converted to DMD in less than 10 min. Conversion of absorbed clorazepate to DMD continues more slowly in the blood. DMD is clinically active and responsible for much of clorazepate's anticonvulsant effect. Clorazepate is 100% bioavailable by intramuscular route [241] and 91% by oral ingestion [242]. Clorazepate and DMD are 97–98% protein bound. The time to peak concentration is 0.7–1.5 h, with peak response in 1–2.5 h [243]. Volume of distribution ranged from 0.9 to 1.5 L/kg, and was greater in the elderly and in obese subjects [244]. The elimination half-life of clorazepate is 2.3 h, but the half-life of DMD is about 46 h [245], longer in elderly males and neonates [246], likely due to impaired oxidation of DMD. DMD is excreted predominantly by the kidney (62–67%) with renal clearance of 0.15–0.27 mL/min/kg [246]. DMD is further metabolized by hydroxylation to parahydroxy-DMD (oxazepam, Fig. 31.3), which is also clinically active [155], and then conjugated to glucuronic acid in the liver [156] and excreted by the kidneys with an elimination half-life of 1–2 days [157]. As with diazepam, drugs that alter hepatic metabolism can dramatically slow the metabolism and clearance of clorazepate, DMD and oxazepam.

Adverse effects and drug interactions

The major common side-effect of clorazepate is drowsiness, with dizziness, ataxia, nervousness and confusion less commonly seen. Paradoxical akathisia has been reported in two patients with history of head trauma and seizure disorders [247]. Personality changes with aggressive behaviour, irritability, rage or depression have been described [248–250], though some have attributed these changes to the suppression of epileptic activity in patients with temporal lobe epilepsy [251]. Hepatotoxicity and transient skin rashes have also been reported. Withdrawal symptoms after chronic use include nervousness, insomnia, irritability, diarrhoea, muscle aches and memory impairment. Clorazepate is in FDA pregnancy category D, and has been associated with major malformations in one infant born to a mother who took clorazepate during the first trimester [252].

Clinical applications

The recommended initial dose of clorazepate for adjunctive treatment of epilepsy is 7.5 mg three times daily, with slow increases as required, to a maximal daily dose of 90 mg. Rapid absorption and bioconversion to DMD requires b.i.d. to t.i.d. dosing to avoid toxicity, despite the long elimination half-life [253]. However, a sustained-release preparation is available which delivers 22.5 mg in a single daily dose (Tranxene-SD). Plasma DMD levels of 0.5–1.9 mg/mL may represent the therapeutic range [152].

In 61 patients, clorazepate adjunctive therapy produced a slight improvement in control of refractory seizures, with minimal adverse effects, but no improvement in the EEG [254]. In a double-blind, add-on study of clorazepate or phenobarbital to phenytoin, no difference in seizure control was noted, but patients preferred clorazepate [255]. Clorazepate was ineffective as monotherapy, but improved seizure control as adjunctive therapy in 59 patients with various seizure disorders [256]. Clorazepate controlled refractory generalized seizures in 11 children (age 3–17 years), either as adjunctive therapy with valproic acid (seven children) or alone (four children) [257]. However, seizures recurred in three patients, likely due to tolerance.

Nitrazepam

Nitrazepam is a benzodiazepine derivative with a nitro group at the 7 position of the benzodiazepine ring (Fig. 31.2). It has been used as a hypnotic and anticonvulsant, with benefit against infantile spasms and as adjunctive therapy for severe generalized epilepsies of childhood. Nitrazepam may be particularly effective against myoclonic seizures.

Pharmacokinetics

After oral ingestion, bioavailability is about 78% [258], with peak concentration occurring in 1.4 h [259]. Nitrazepam is 85–88% protein bound [258,260]. In the first 24 h after dosing, CSF levels were 8–11% of plasma levels, with a CSF elimination half-life ($t_{1/2\beta}$) of 68 h compared to 27 h in plasma [258,261,262]. Nitrazepam is metabolized in the liver by nitro reduction to the inactive aromatic amine (7-aminonitrazepam), followed by acetylation to 7-acetoamidonitrazepam (also inactive, see Fig. 31.3). [262–264]. Excretion occurs in both urine (45–65%) and faeces (14–20%), with the remainder bound in tissues for prolonged periods [265]. Metabolism is slowed in patients with hypothyroidism [264] and obesity [266].

Adverse effects and drug interactions

Like most BZDs, nitrazepam can produce central nervous system symptoms of disorientation, confusion and drowsiness, particularly in elderly patients [260,267,268]. Incoordination and driving difficulty have occurred [269], and generalized mental deterioration with dementia, inability to walk and incontinence was observed in a 75-year-old woman treated with nitrazepam; symptoms resolved upon discontinuation [267]. Vivid nightmares have occurred at the onset of therapy [270]. Drooling, impaired swallowing and aspiration have been observed in children [271,272]. Respiratory depression has occurred in elderly patients being treated for respiratory failure after single 5–10 mg oral doses of nitrazepam for sedation [273].

Nitrazepam is in FDA pregnancy category C, with teratogenic effects demonstrated in animals but no controlled studies in humans. Infants born to mothers on nitrazepam late in pregnancy have been somnolent, floppy, poorly responsive and required tube feeding, but recovered in several days [274].

Withdrawal symptoms have included delirium [275], involuntary movements, paraesthesias, confusion [276], persistent tinnitus and opisthotonus [277].

Nitrazepam therapy appears to increase the risk of death, particularly in young patients with intractable epilepsy. In a retrospective analysis of 302 patients treated for periods ranging from 3 days to 10 years, 21 patients died, 14 of whom were taking nitrazepam at time of death [278]. In patients younger than 3.4 years, the death rate was 3.98 per 100 patient-years, compared with 0.26 deaths per 100 patient-years in patients not taking nitrazepam. Nitrazepam had a slight protective effect (death rate of 0.50 vs. 0.86) in patients older than 3.4 years. Nitrazepam should therefore be used with extreme caution in children younger than 4 years.

Clinical applications

Initial doses of 1–6 mg daily, with gradual increases up to 60 mg daily, have been used in treatment of paediatric seizure disorders [279–281]. In 44 children under satisfactory seizure control, the average dose was 0.27 mg/kg/day, yielding a mean plasma concentration of 114 ng/mL [260]. Nitrazepam was particularly effective for myoclonic seizures [279,281,282]. In 36 infants and children (aged 3 months to 12 years) nitrazepam (1–6 mg daily initial dose followed by 0.3–1.1 mg/kg/day maintenance) produced a reduction in average daily seizure number from 17.7 to 7.2 [281]. In 31 mentally retarded children (aged 2 months to 15 years) with various seizure types, complete seizure control was obtained in seven patients and moderate control in 10, with best control in patients with myoclonic seizures [283].

Febrile convulsions

Nitrazepam (0.25–0.5 mg/kg/day, in t.i.d. dosing during fever) was effective in prophylaxis of febrile convulsions [284].

Infantile spasms and Lennox–Gastaut syndrome

In 52 patients (1–24 months) with infantile spasms and hypsarrhythmia on EEG, nitrazepam (0.2–0.4 mg/kg/day in two divided doses) and adrenocorticotropic hormone (ACTH, 40 U intramuscularly daily) were similar in efficacy and incidence of adverse effects [285]. Both regimens resulted in 75–100% reduction in seizure frequency in 50–60% of patients. Twenty children (4–28 months) with infantile spasms or early Lennox–Gastaut syndrome were treated with nitrazepam (0.5–3.5 mg/kg, median 1.5 mg/kg/day); of these, five had complete cessation of seizures, seven had greater than 50% seizure reduction and eight had no response [286]. Twelve children experienced pooling of oral secretions and six developed sedation, but no serious side-effects were reported.

Future directions: novel BZDs and novel uses

Partial BZD agonists (abecarnil, bretazanil, imidazenil) may retain anticonvulsant efficacy but be less prone to the development of tolerance. The utility of these agents in human epilepsy has not been adequately explored. Combination therapy using a full agonist with a partial agonist or antagonist (flumazenil) might also prevent the development of tolerance. Another novel approach involves using BZDs in a device capable of detecting seizure discharges and injecting the drug into the brain at the onset of seizure activity, either locally onto the epileptic focus or into the cerebral ventricles. A model for this type of device in rats showed a decrease in seizure frequency and duration when diazepam rather than vehicle was injected onto a bicuculline-created seizure focus [287]. Such approaches may increase the future role of BZDs in the treatment of SE, serial seizures and epilepsy.

References

1 Borea PA, Bonora D. Brain receptor binding and the lipophilic character of benzodiazepines. *Biochem Pharmacol* 1983; 32: 603–7.
2 Macdonald R, Barker JL. Benzodiazepines specifically modulate GABA-mediated postsynaptic inhibition in cultured mammalian neurones. *Nature* 1978; 271: 563–4.
3 Greenblatt DJ, Divoll M, Abernathy DR. Clinical pharmacokinetics of the newer benzodiazepines. *Clin Pharmacokinet* 1983; 8: 233–52.
4 Greenblatt DJ, Shader RI, Abernethy DR. Current status of benzodiazepines (first of two parts). *N Engl J Med* 1983; 309: 354–8.
5 Ochs HR, Greenblatt DJ, Divoll M. Diazepam kinetics in relation to age and sex. *Pharmacology* 1981; 23: 24–30.
6 Arendt RM, Greenblatt DJ, deJong RH *et al*. In vitro correlates of benzodiazepine cerebrospinal fluid uptake, pharmacodynamic action and peripheral distribution. *J Pharmacol Exp Ther* 1993; 277: 98–106.
7 Rosenberg HC, Tietz EI, Chiu TH. Tolerance to the anticonvulsant action of benzodiazepines. Relationship to decreased receptor density. *Neuropharmacology* 1985; 24: 639–44.
8 Towne AR, Pellock JM, Ko D, DeLorenzo RJ. Determinants of mortality in status epilepticus. *Epilepsia* 1994; 35: 27–34.
9 Lowenstein DH, Alldredge BK. Status epilepticus. *N Engl J Med* 1998; 338: 970–6.
10 Cavazos JE, Das I, Sutula TP. Neuronal loss induced in limbic pathways by kindling: evidence for induction of hippocampal sclerosis by repeated brief seizures. *J Neurosci* 1994; 14: 3106–21.
11 Lynch MW, Rutecki PA, Sutula TP. The effects of seizures on the brain. *Curr Opin Neurol Neurosurg* 1996; 9: 97–102.
12 Leppik IE, Derivan AT, Homan RW. Double-blind study of lorazepam and diazepam in status epilepticus. *JAMA* 1983; 249: 1452–4.
13 Treiman DM. The role of benzodiazepines in the management of status epilepticus. *Neurology* 1990; 40: 32–42.
14 Treiman DM, Meyers PD, Walton NY *et al*. A comparison of four treatments for generalized convulsive status epilepticus. Veterans Affairs Status Epilepticus Cooperative Study Group. *N Engl J Med* 1998; 339: 792–8.
15 Li L, Gorukanti S, Choi YM, Kim KH. Rapid-onset intranasal delivery of anticonvulsants: pharmacokinetic and pharmacodynamic evaluation in rabbits. *Int J Pharm* 2000; 199: 65–76.
16 Platt SR, Randell SC, Scott KC, Chrisman CL, Hill RC, Gronwall RR. Comparison of plasma benzodiazepine concentrations following intranasal and intravenous administration of diazepam to dogs. *Am J Vet Res* 2000; 61: 651–4.
17 Kendall JL, Reynolds M, Goldberg R. Intranasal midazolam in patients with status epilepticus. *Ann Emerg Med* 1997; 29: 415–17.
18 Gizurarson S, Gudbrandsson FK, Jonsson H, Bechgaard E. Intranasal administration of diazepam aiming at the treatment of acute seizures: clinical trials in healthy volunteers. *Biol Pharm Bull* 1999; 22: 425–7.
19 Schwagmeier R, Alincic S, Striebel HW. Midazolam pharmacokinetics following intravenous and buccal administration. *Br J Clin Pharmacol* 1998; 46: 203–6.
20 Pasternak SJ, Heller MB. Endotracheal diazepam in status epilepticus. *Ann Emerg Med* 1985; 14: 485.
21 Rusli M, Spivey WH, Bonner H. Endotracheal diazepam: absorption and pulmonary pathologic effects. *Ann Emerg Med* 1987; 16: 314.
22 Albano A, Reisdorff EJ, Wiegenstein JG. Rectal diazepam in pediatric status epilepticus. *Am J Emerg Med* 1989; 7: 168–72.
23 Camfield CS, Camfield PR, Smith E, Dooley JM. Home use of rectal diazepam to prevent status epilepticus in children with convulsive disorders. *J Child Neurol* 1989; 4: 125–6.
24 Seigler RS. The administration of rectal diazepam for acute management of seizures. *J Emerg Med* 1990; 8: 155–9.
25 Dreifuss FE, Rossman NP, Cloyd JC. A comparison of rectal diazepam gel and placebo for acute repetitive seizures. *N Engl J Med* 1998; 338: 1869–75.

26 Kriel RL, Cloyd JC, Pellock JM, Mitchell WG, Cereghino JJ, Rosman NP. Rectal diazepam gel for treatment of acute repetitive seizures. *N Am Diastat Study Group Pediatr Neurol* 1999; 20: 282–8.

27 Mitchell WG, Conry JA, Crumrine PK *et al.* An open-label study of repeated use of diazepam rectal gel (Diastat) for episodes of acute breakthrough seizures and clusters: safety, efficacy and tolerance. *North Am Diastat Group Epilepsia* 1999; 40: 1610–17.

28 Lowenstein DH, Alldredge BK, Allen F *et al.* The prehospital treatment of status epilepticus (PHTSE) study. *Design Method Control Clin Trials* 2001; 22: 290–309.

29 Randall LO, Kappell B. Pharmacological activity of some benzodiazepines and their metabolites. In: Garattini S, Mussini E, Randall LO, eds. *The Benzodiazepines*. New York: Raven Press, 1973: 27–51.

30 Swinyard EA, Castellion AW. Anticonvulsant properties of some benzodiazepines. *J Pharmacol Exp Ther* 1966; 151: 369–75.

31 Albertson TE, Stark LG, Derlet RW. Modification of amygdaloid kindling by diazepam in juvenile rats. *Brain Res Dev Brain Res* 1990; 51: 249–52.

32 Amano K, Takamatsu J, Ogata A *et al.* Effect of dipotassium clorazepate on amygdaloid-kindling and comparison between amygdaloid- and hippocampal-kindled seizures. *Eur J Pharmacol* 1999; 385: 111–17.

33 Goddard GV, McIntyre DC, Leech CK. A permanent change in brain function resulting from daily electrical stimulation. *Exp Neurol* 1969; 25: 295–330.

34 Study RE, Barker JL. Diazepam and pentobarbital: fluctuation analysis reveals different mechanisms for potentiation of γ-aminobutyric acid responses in cultured central neurons. *Proc Natl Acad Sci USA* 1981; 78: 7180–4.

35 Rogers CJ, Twyman RE, Macdonald RL. Benzodiazepine and beta-carboline regulation of single GABA$_A$ receptor channels of mouse spinal neurones in culture. *J Physiol (Lond)* 1994; 475: 69–82.

36 Eghbali M, Curmi JP, Birnir B, Gage PW. Hippocampal GABA$_A$ channel conductance increased by diazepam. *Nature* 1997; 388: 71–5.

37 Braestrup C, Squires RF. Specific benzodiazepine receptors in rat brain characterized by high-affinity [³H]diazepam binding. *Proc Natl Acad Sci USA* 1977; 74: 3805–9.

38 Mohler H, Okada T. Benzodiazepine receptor: demonstration in the central nervous system. *Science* 1977; 198: 849–51.

39 Braestrup C, Squires RF. Pharmacological characterization of benzodiazepine receptors in the brain. *Eur J Pharmacol* 1978; 48: 263–70.

40 Karobath M, Sperk G. Stimulation of benzodiazepine receptor binding by γ-aminobutyric acid. *Proc Natl Acad Sci USA* 1979; 76: 1004–6.

41 Siegel E, Mamalaki C, Barnard EA. Isolation of a GABA receptor from bovine brain using a benzodiazepine affinity column. *FEBS Lett* 1982; 147: 45–8.

42 Martini C, Rigacci T, Lucacchini A. [³H]Muscimol binding site on purified benzodiazepine receptor. *J Neurochem* 1983; 41: 1183–5.

43 Twyman RE, Rogers CJ, Macdonald RL. Differential regulation of γ-aminobutyric acid receptor channels by diazepam and phenobarbital. *Ann Neurol* 1989; 25: 213–20.

44 Maconochie DJ, Zempel JM, Steinbach JH. How quickly can GABA$_A$ receptors open? *Neuron* 1994; 12: 61–71.

45 Jones MV, Westbrook GL. Desensitized states prolong GABA$_A$ channel responses to brief agonist pulses. *Neuron* 1995; 15: 181–91.

46 Edwards FA, Konnerth A, Sakmann B. Quantal analysis of inhibitory synaptic transmission in the dentate gyrus of rat hippocampal slices: a patch-clamp study. *J Physiol (Lond)* 1990; 430: 213–49.

47 Puia G, Costa E, Vicini S. Functional diversity of GABA-activated Cl⁻ currents in purkinje versus granule neurons in rat cerebellar slices. *Neuron* 1994; 12: 117–26.

48 Otis TS, Mody I. Modulation of decay kinetics and frequency of GABA$_A$ receptor-mediated spontaneous inhibitory post-synaptic currents in hippocampal neurons. *Proc Natl Acad Sci USA* 1992; 78: 7180–4.

49 Mody I, De Doninck Y, Otis TS, Soltesz I. Bridging the cleft at GABA synapses in the brain. *Trends Neurosci* 1994; 17: 517–25.

50 Hoogerkamp A, Arends RH, Bomers AM, Mandema JW, Voskuyl RA, Danhof M. Pharmacokinetic/pharmacodynamic relationship of benzodiazepines in the direct cortical stimulation model of anticonvulsant effect. *J Pharmacol Exp Ther* 1996; 279: 803–12.

51 Schofield PR, Darlison MG, Fujita N *et al.* Sequence and functional expression of the GABA A receptor shows a ligand-gated receptor superfamily. *Nature* 1987; 328: 221–7.

52 Nayeem N, Green TP, Martin IL, Barnard EA. Quaternary structure of the native GABA$_A$ receptor determined by electron microscopic image analysis. *J Neurochem* 1994; 62: 815–18.

53 Macdonald RL, Olsen RW. GABA$_A$ receptor channels. *Ann Rev Neurosci* 1994; 17: 569–602.

54 Hedblom E, Kirkness EF. A novel class of GABA$_A$ receptor subunit in tissues of the reproductive system. *J Biol Chem* 1997; 272: 15346–50.

55 Davies PA, Hanna MC, Hales TG, Kirkness EF. Insensitivity to anesthetic agents conferred by a class of GABA$_A$ receptor subunit. *Nature* 1997; 385: 820–3.

56 Bonnert TP, McKernan RM, Le Bourdelles B *et al.* A novel γ-aminobutyric acid type A subunit. *Proc Natl Acad Sci USA* 1999; 96: 9891–6.

57 Wisden W, Laurie DJ, Monyer H, Seeburg PH. The distribution of 13 GABA$_A$ receptor subunit mRNAs in the rat brain. I. Telencephalon, diencephalon, mesencephalon. *J Neurosci* 1992; 12: 1040–62.

58 Brooks-Kayal AR, Pritchett DB. Developmental changes in human γ-aminobutyric acid$_A$ receptor subunit composition. *Ann Neurol* 1993; 34: 687–93.

59 Brooks-Kayal AR, Jin H, Price M, Dichter MA. Developmental expression of GABA$_A$ receptor subunit mRNAs in individual hippocampal neurons in vitro and in vivo. *J Neurochem* 1998; 70: 1017–28.

60 Pritchett DB, Sontheimer H, Shivers BD *et al.* Importance of a novel GABA$_A$ subunit for benzodiazepine pharmacology. *Nature* 1989; 338: 582–5.

61 Wieland HA, Luddens H, Seeburg PH. A single histidine in GABA$_A$ receptors is essential for benzodiazepine agonist binding. *J Biol Chem* 1992; 267: 1426–9.

62 Wingrove PB, Wafford KA, Bain C, Whiting PJ. The modulatory action of loreclezole at the γ-aminobutyric acid type A receptor is determined by a single amino acid in the β$_2$ and β$_3$ subunit. *Proc Natl Acad Sci USA* 1994; 91: 4569–73.

63 Draguhn A, Verdorn TA, Ewert M, Seeburg PH, Sakmann B. Functional and molecular distinction between recombinant rat GABA$_A$ receptor subtypes by Zn²⁺. *Neuron* 1990; 5: 781–8.

64 Verdoorn TA, Draguhn A, Ymer S, Seeburg PH, Sakmann B. Functional properties of recombinant rat GABA$_A$ receptors depend upon subunit composition. *Neuron* 1990; 4: 919–28.

65 Lüddens H, Korpi ER, Seeburg P. GABA$_A$/benzodizaepine receptor heterogeneity: neurophysiological implications. *Neuropharmacology* 1995; 34: 245–54.

66 Doble A, Martin IL. Multiple benzodiazepine receptors — no reason for anxiety. *Trends Pharmacol Sci* 1992; 13: 76–81.

67 Smith GB, Olsen RW. Functional domains of GABA$_A$ receptors. *Trends Pharmacol Sci* 1995; 16: 162–8.

68 Sigel E, Schaerer MT, Buhr A, Baur R. The benzodiazepine binding pocket of recombinant α1β2γ2 γ-aminobutyric acid$_A$ receptors: relative orientation of ligands and amino acid side chains. *Mol Pharmacol* 1998; 54: 1097–105.

69 McKernan RM, Farrar S, Collins I *et al.* Photoaffinity labelling of the benzodiazepine binding site of α1, β3, γ2, γ-aminobutyric acid$_A$ receptors with flunitrazepam identifies a subset of ligands that interact directly with His102 of the α subunit and predicts orientation of these within the benzodiazepine pharmacophore. *Mol Pharmacol* 1998; 54: 33–43.

70 Boileau AJ, Kucken AM, Evers AR, Czajkowski C. Molecular dissection of benzodiazepine binding and allosteric coupling using chimeric γ-aminobutyric acid$_A$ receptor subunits. *Mol Pharmacol* 1998; 53: 295–303.

71 Dunn SMJ, Davies M, Muntoni AL, Lambert JJ. Mutagenesis of the rat α1 subunit of the γ-aminobutyric acid$_a$ receptor reveals the importance of residue 101 in determining the allosteric effects of benzodiazepine site ligands. *Mol Pharmacol* 1999; 56: 768–74.

72 Boileau AJ, Czajkowski C. Identification of transduction elements for benzodiazepine modulation of the GABA$_A$ receptor: Three residues are required for allosteric coupling. *J Neurosci* 1999; 19 (23): 10213–20.

73 Kucken AM, Wagner DA, Ward PR, Teissere J, Boileau AJ, Czajkowski C. Identification of benzodiazepine binding site residues in the γ2 subunit of the γ-aminobutyric acid$_A$ receptor. *Mol Pharmacol* 2000; 57: 932–9.

74 Kokaia M, Pratt GD, Elmer E et al. Biphasic differential changes of GABA$_A$ receptor subunit mRNA levels in denate gyrus granule cells following recurrent kindling-induced seizures. Mol Brain Res 1994; 23: 323–32.

75 Brooks-Kayal AR, Shumate MD, Jin H, Rikhter TY, Coulter DA. Selective changes in single cell GABA$_A$ receptor subunit expression and function in temporal lobe epilepsy. Nature Med 1998; 4: 1166–72.

76 Loup F, Weiser HG, Yonekawa Y, Aguzzi A, Fritschy JM. Selective alterations in GABA$_A$ receptor subtypes in human temporal lobe epilepsy. J Neurosci 2000; 20: 5401–19.

77 Matsumoto A, Kumagai T, Miura K, Miyazaki S, Hayakawa C, Yamanaka T. Epilepsy in Angelman syndrome associated with chromosome 15q deletion. Epilepsia 1992; 33: 1083–90.

78 DeLorey TM, Handforth A, Anagnostaras SG et al. Mice lacking the β$_3$ subunit of the GABA$_A$ receptor have the epilepsy phenotype and many of the behavioral characteristics of Angelman syndrome. J Neurosci 1998; 18: 8505–14.

79 Karle J, Woldbye DP, Elster L et al. Antisense oligonucleotide to GABA$_A$ receptor γ2 subunit induces limbic status epilepticus. J Neurosci Res 1998; 54: 863–9.

80 Zhao TJ, Rosenberg HC, Chiu TH. Treatment with an antisense oligodeoxynucleotide to the GABA$_A$ receptor γ2 subunit increases convulsive threshold for β-CCM, a benzodiazepine 'inverse agonist', in rats. Eur J Pharmacol 1996; 306: 61–6.

81 Baulac S, Huberfeld G, Gourfinkel-An I et al. First genetic evidence of GABA$_A$ receptor dysfunction in epilepsy: a mutation in the γ2-subunit gene. Nat Genet 2001; 28: 46–8.

82 Wallace RH, Marini C, Petrou S et al. Mutant GABA$_A$ receptor γ2-subunit in childhood absence epilepsy and febrile seizures. Nat Genet 2001; 28: 49–52.

83 Korpi ER, Kleingoor C, Kettenmann H, Seeburg PH. Benzodiazepine-induced motor impairment linked to point mutation in cerebellar GABA$_A$ receptor. Nature 1993; 361: 356–9.

84 Rudolph U, Crestani F, Benke D et al. Benzodiazepine actions mediated by specific γ-aminobutyric acid$_A$ receptor subtypes. Nature 2000; 401: 796–800.

85 McKernan RM, Rosahl TW, Reynolds DS et al. Sedative but not anxiolytic properties of benzodiazepines are mediated by the GABA$_A$ receptor α1 subunit. Nature Neurosci 2000; 3: 529–30.

86 Crestani F, Martin JR, Mohler H, Rudolph U. Mechanism of action of the hypnotic zolpidem in vivo. Br J Pharmacol 2000; 131: 1251–4.

87 Low K, Crestani F, Keist R et al. Molecular and neuronal substrate for the selective attenuation of anxiety. Science 2000; 290: 131–4.

88 Crestani F, Low K, Keist R, Mandelli M, Mohler H, Rudolph U. Molecular targets for the myorelaxant action of diazepam. Mol Pharmacol 2001; 59: 442–5.

89 Gross JB, Blouin RT, Zandsberg S. Effect of flumazenil on ventilatory drive during sedation with midazolam and alfentanil. Anesthesiology 1996; 85: 713–20.

90 Shannon M, Albers G, Burkhardt K. Safety and efficacy of flumazenil in the reversal of benzodiazepine-induced conscious sedation. J Pediatr 1997; 131: 582–6.

91 Grimm G, Katzenschlager R, Holzner F et al. Effect of flumazenil in hepatic encephalopathy. Eur J Anaesthesiol 1988; 2 (Suppl.): 147–9.

92 Grimm G, Ferenci P, Katzenschlager R et al. Improvement of hepatic encephalopathy treated with flumazenil. Lancet 1988; 2: 1392–4.

93 Alho H, Costa E, Ferrero P, Fujimoto M, Cosenza-Murphy D, Guidotti A. Diazepam-binding inhibitor: a neuropeptide located in selected neuronal populations of rat brain. Science 1985; 229: 179–82.

94 Nutt DJ, Cowan PJ, Little HJ. Unusual interactions of benzodiazepine receptor antagonists. Nature 1982; 295: 436–8.

95 Vellucci SV, Webster RA. Is RO15-1788 a partial agonist at benzodiazepine receptors? Eur J Pharmacol 1983; 90: 263–8.

96 Polc P, Jahromi SS, Facciponte G, Pelletier MR, Zhang L, Carlen PL. Benzodiazepine antagonist flumazenil reduces hippocampal epileptiform activity. Neuroreport 1995; 6: 1549–52.

97 Polc P, Jahromi SS, Facciponte G, Pelletier MR, Zhang L, Carlen PL. Benzodiazepine antagonists reduce epileptiform discharges in rat hippocampal slices. Epilepsia 1996; 37: 1007–14.

98 Robertson HA, Riives ML. A benzodiazepine antagonist is an anti-convulsant in an animal model for limbic epilepsy. Brain Res 1983; 270: 380–2.

99 Morin AM. Ro 15–1788 suppresses the development of kindling through the benzodiazepine receptor. Brain Res 1986; 397: 259–64.

100 Scollo-Lavizzari G. The anticonvulsant effect of the benzodiazepine antagonist, Ro15–1788. An EEG study of 4 cases. Eur Neurol 1984; 23: 1–6.

101 Sharief MK, Sander JWAS, Shorvon S. The effects of oral flumazenil on interictal epileptic activity: results of a double-blind, placebo-controlled study. Epilepsy Res 1993; 15: 53–60.

102 Scollo-Lavizzari G. The clinical anticonvulsant effects of flumazenil, a benzodiazepine antagonist. Eur J Anaesthesiol 1988; Suppl. 2: 129–38.

103 Hart YM, Meinardi H, Sander JW, Nutt DJ, Shorvon SD. The effect of intravenous flumazenil on interictal electroencephalographic epileptic activity: results of a placebo-controlled study. J Neurol Neurosurg Psychiatr 1991; 54: 305–9.

104 Savic I, Widen L, Stone-Elander S. Feasibility of reversing benzodiazepine tolerance with flumazenil. Lancet 1991; 337: 133–7.

105 Spivey WH. Flumazenil and seizures. analysis of 43 cases. Clin Ther 1992; 14: 292–305.

106 Schulze-Bonhage A, Elger CE. Induction of partial epileptic seizures by flumazenil. Epilepsia 2000; 41 (2): 186–92.

107 Henry TR. Functional neuroimaging with positron emission tomography. Epilepsia 1996; 37: 1141–54.

108 Lamusuo S, Pitkanen A, Jutila L et al. [^{11}C]Flumazenil binding in the medial temporal lobe in patients with temporal lobe epilepsy: correlation with hippocampal MR volume try, T2 relaxometry and neuropathology. Neurol Res 2000; 17: 190–2.

109 Juhasz C, Nagy F, Muzik O, Watson C, Shah J, Chugani HT. [^{11}C]flumazenil PET in patients with epilepsy with dual pathology. Epilepsia 1999; 40: 566–74.

110 Turski L, Stephens DN, Jensen LH et al. Anticonvulsant action of the beta-carboline abecarnil: studies in rodents and baboon, Papio papio. J Pharmacol Exp Therap 1990; 253: 344–52.

111 Zanotti A, Mariot R, Contarino A, Lipartiti M, Giusti P. Lack of anticonvulsant tolerance and benzodiazepine receptor downregulation with imidazenil in rats. Br J Pharmacol 1996; 117: 647–52.

112 Rundfeldt C, WlaAP, Honack D, Loscher W. Anticonvulsant tolerance and withdrawal characteristics of benzodiazepine receptor ligands in different seizure models in mice. Comparison of diazepam, bretazenil and abecarnil. J Pharmacol Exp Ther 1995; 275: 693–702.

113 Loscher W, Honack D. Withdrawal precipitation by benzodiazepine receptor antagonists in dogs chronically treated with diazepam or the novel anxiolytic and anticonvulsant beta-carbolene abecarnil. Naunyn Schmiedebergs Arch Pharmacol 1992; 345: 452–60.

114 Serra M, Ghiani CA, Motzo C, Porceddu ML, Biggio G. Antagonism of isoniazid-induced convulsions by abecarnil in mice tolerant to diazepam. Pharmacol Biochem Behav 1995; 52: 249–54.

115 Natolino F, Zanotti A, Contarino A, Lipartiti M, Giusti P. Abecarnil, a beta-carboline derivative, does not exhibit anticonvulsant tolerance or withdrawal effects in mice. Naunyn Schmiedebergs Arch Pharmacol 1996; 354: 612–17.

116 Hernandez TD, Heninger C, Wilson MA, Gallager DW. Relationship of agonist efficacy to changes in GABA sensitivity and anticonvulsant tolerance following chronic benzodiazepine ligand exposure. Eur J Pharmacol 1989; 170: 145–55.

117 Zanotti A, Natolino F, Contarino A, Lipartiti M, Giusti P. Abecarnil enhances recovery from diazepam tolerance. Neuropharmacology 1999; 38: 1281–8.

118 Haefely W, Kyburz E, Gerecke M, Mohler H. Recent advances in the molecular pharmacology of benzodiazepine receptors and in the structure-activity relationships of their agonists and antagonists. Adv Drug Res 1985; 14: 165–322.

119 Polc P. Electrophysiology of benzodiazepine receptor ligands. Multiple mechanisms and sites of action. Prog Neurobiol 1988; 31: 349–423.

120 Lader M. Withdrawal reactions after stopping hypnotics in patients with insomnia. CNS Drugs 1998; 10: 425–40.

121 Schweitzer E, Rickels K. Benzodiazepine dependence and withdrawal: a

review of the syndrome and its clinical management. *Acta Psychiatr Scand* 1998; 98 (Suppl. 393): 95–101.

122 Ramsey-Williams VA, Wu Y, Rosenberg HC. Comparison of anticonvulsant tolerance, crosstolerance, and benzodiazepine receptor binding following chronic treatment with diazepam or midazolam. *Pharmacol Biochem Behav* 1994; 48: 765–72.

123 Rosenberg HC. Differential expression of benzodiazepine anticonvulsant cross-tolerance according to time following flurazepam or diazepam treatment. *Pharmacol Biochem Behav* 1995; 51: 363–8.

124 Longone P, Impagnatiello F, Guidotti A, Costa E. Reversible modification of GABA$_A$ receptor subunit mRNA expression during tolerance to diazepam-induced cognition dysfunction. *Neuropharmacology* 1999; 35 (9/10): 1465–73.

125 Heninger C, Saito N, Tallman JF, Garrett KM, Vitek MP, Duman RS, Gallager DW. Effects of continuous diazepam administration on GABA$_A$ subunit mRNA in rat brain. *Mol Neurosci* 1990; 2: 101–7.

126 Kang I, Miller LG. Decreased GABA$_A$ receptor mRNA concentrations following chronic lorazepam administration. *Br J Pharmacol* 1991; 103: 1285–7.

127 Primus RJ, Gallager DW. GABA$_A$ receptor subunit mRNA levels are differentially influenced by chronic FG7142 and diazepam exposure. *Eur J Pharmacol* 1992; 226: 21–8.

128 O'Donovan MC, Buckland PR, Spurlock G, McGuffin P. Bi-directional changes in the levels of messsenger RNA's encoding γ-aminobutyric acid$_A$ receptor α subunits after flurazepam treatment. *Eur J Pharmacol* 1992; 226: 335–41.

129 Zhao TJ, Chiu TH, Rosenberg HC. Reduced expression of γ-aminobutyric acid type A benzodiazepine receptor γ2 and α5 subunit mRNAs in brain regions of flurazepam-treated rats. *Mol Pharmacol* 1994; 45: 657–63.

130 Tietz EI, Huang X, Weng X, Rosenberg HC, Chiu TH. Expression of α1, α5, and γ2 GABA$_A$ receptor subunit mRNA's measured in *situ* in rat hippocampus and cortex following chronic flurazepam administration. *J Mol Neurosci* 1994; 4: 277–92.

131 Chen S, Huang X, Zeng XJ, Sieghart W, Tietz EI. Benzodiazepine-mediated regulation of α1, α2, β1–3, and γ2 GABA$_A$ receptor subunit proteins in the rat brain hippocampus and cortex. *Neuroscience* 1999; 93: 33–44.

132 Tietz EI, Huang X, Chen S, Ferencak WF. Temporal and regional regulation of α1, β2 and β3, but not α2, α4, α6, β1, or γ2 GABA$_A$ receptor subunit messenger RNAs following one week oral flurazepam administration. *Neuroscience* 1999; 91: 327–41.

133 Chen S, Sieghart W, Fritschy JM, Tietz EI. Differential temporal regulation of rat hippocampal GABA$_A$ receptor subunits (α1, α2, α4, α5, β1, β2, β3 and γ2) after discontinuation of chronic flurazepam treatment. *Soc Neurosci* 2000; 30: 237.

134 Li M, Szabo A, Rosenberg HC. Downregulation of benzodiazepine binding to α5 subunit-containing GABA $_A$ receptors in tolerant rat brain indicates particular involvement of the hippocampal CA1 region. *J Pharmacol Exp Therap* 2000; 295: 689–96.

135 Tietz EI, Rosenberg HC. Behavioral measurement of benzodiazepine tolerance and GABAergic subsensitivity in the substantia nigra pars reticulata. *Brain Res* 1988; 438: 41–51.

136 Xie XH, Tietz EI. Chronic benzodiazepine treatment of rats induces reduction of paired pulse inhibition in CA1 region of in vitro hippocampal slices. *Brain Res* 1991; 561: 69–76.

137 Zeng X, Xie XH, Tietz EI. Impairment of feedforward inhibition in CA1 region of hippocampus after chronic benzodiazepine treatment. *Neurosci Lett* 1994; 173: 40–4.

138 Zeng XJ, Tietz EI. Benzodiazepine tolerance at GABAergic synapses on hippocampal CA1 pyramidal cells. *Synapse* 1999; 31: 263–77.

139 Loscher W, Rundfeldt C, Honack D, Ebert U. Long-term studies on anticonvulsant tolerance and withdrawal characteristics of benzodiazepine receptor ligands in different seizure models in mice. 1. Comparison of diazepam, clonazepam, clobazam and abecarnil. *J Pharmacol Exp Ther* 1996; 279: 561–72.

140 Gonsalves SF, Gallager DW. Persistent reversal of tolerance to anticonvulsant effects and GABAergic subsensitivity by a single exposure to benzodiazepine antagonist during chronic benzodiazepine administration. *J Pharmacol Exp Therap* 1987; 244: 79–83.

141 Gonsalves SF, Gallager DW. Spontaneous and RO15-1788-induced reversal of subsensitivity to GABA following chronic benzodiazepines. *Eur J Pharmacol* 1985; 110: 163–70.

142 Tietz EI, Zeng X, Chen S, Lilly SM, Rosenberg HC, Kometiani P. Antagonist-induced reversal of functional and structural measures of hippocampal benzodiazepine tolerance. *J Pharmacol Exp Therap* 1999; 291: 932–42.

143 Crawford TO, Mitchell WG, Snodgrass SR. Lorazepam in childhood status epilepticus and serial seizures: effectiveness and tachyphylaxis. *Neurology* 1987; 37: 190–5.

144 Kapur J, Macdonald RL. Rapid seizure-induced reduction of benzodiazepine and Zn^{2+} sensitivity of hippocampal dentate granule cell GABA$_A$ receptors. *J Neurosci* 1999; 17: 7532–40.

145 Mazarati AM, Baldwin RA, Sankar R, Wasterlain CG. Time-dependent decrease in the effectiveness of antiepileptic drugs during the course of self-sustaining status epilepticus. *Brain Res* 1998; 814: 179–85.

146 Rice AC, DeLorenzo RJ. N-methyl-D-aspartate receptor activation regulates refractoriness of status epilepticus to diazepam. *Neuroscience* 1999; 93: 117–23.

147 Tsuda M, Shimizu N, Yajima Y, Misawa M. Hypersusceptibility to DMCM-induced seizures during diazepam withdrawal in mice. Evidence for upregulation of NMDA receptors. *Naunyn Schmiedebergs Arch Pharmacol* 1998; 357: 309–15.

148 Gastaut H, Naquet R, Poire R, Tassarini CH. Treatment of status epilepticus with diazepam (valium). *Epilepsia* 1965; 6: 167–82.

149 Huang ZC, Shen DL. Studies of quantitative beta activity in EEG background changes produced by intravenous diazepam. *Clin Electroencephalogr* 1997; 28: 172–8.

150 Huang ZC, Shen DL. The prognostic significance of diazepam-induced EEG changes in epilepsy: a follow-up study. *Clin Electroencephalogr* 1993; 24: 179–87.

151 Greenblatt DJ, Divoll M. Diazepam vs. lorazepam: relationship of drug distribution to duration of clinical action. In: Delgado-Escueta AV, Wasterlain C, Treiman DM, Porter RJ, eds. *Status Epilepticus: Mechanism of Brain Damage and Treatment*. New York: Raven Press, 1983: 487–90.

152 Thummel KE, Shen DD, Appendix II, Hardman JG, Limbird LE, Gilman AG, eds. *Goodman and Gilman's the Pharmacological Basis of Therapeutics*, 10th edn. New York: McGraw-Hill, 2001: 1917–2023.

153 Charney DS, Mihic SJ, Harris RA. Hypnotics and Sedatives. In: Hardman JG, Limbird LE, Gilman AG, eds. *Goodman and Gilman's the Pharmacological Basis of Therapeutics*, 10th edn. New York: McGraw-Hill, 2001: 399–427.

154 McNamara JO. Drugs effective in the therapy of the epilepsies. In: Hardman JG, Limbird LE, Gilman AG ed. *Goodman and Gilman's the Pharmacological Basis of Therapeutics*, 10th edn. New York: McGraw-Hill, 2001: 521–48.

155 Schwartz MA, Koechlin BA, Postma E, Palmer S, Krol G. Metabolism of diazepam in rat, dog and man. *J Pharmacol Exp Ther* 1965; 149: 423–35.

156 Klotz U, Antonin KH, Brügel H, Bieck JR. Disposition of diazepam and its major metabolite desmethyldiazepam in patients with liver disease. *Clin Pharmacol Ther* 1977; 21: 430–6.

157 Schmidt D. Benzodiazepines, diazepam. In: Levy RH, Dreifuss FE, Mattson RH, Meldrum BS, Penry JK, eds. *Antiepileptic Drugs*, 3rd edn. New York: Raven Press, 1989: 735–64.

158 Nims RW, Prough RA, Jones CR *et al.* In vivo induction and in vitro inhibition of hepatic cytochrome P450 activity by the benzodiazepine anticonvulsants clonazepam and diazepam. *Drug Metab Dispos* 1997; 25: 750–6.

159 Nichol CF, Tutton IC, Smith BH. Parenteral diazepam in status epilepticus. *Neurology* 1969; 19: 332–43.

160 Norris E, Marzouk O, Nunn A, McIntyre J, Choonara I. Respiratory depression in children receiving diazepam for acute seizures: a prospective study. *Dev Med Neurol* 1999; 41: 340–3.

161 Al Tahan A. Paradoxic response to diazepam in complex partial status epilepticus. *Arch Med* 2000; 31: 101–4.

162 Sadjadi SA, McLaughlin K, Shah RM. Allergic interstitial nephritis due to diazepam. *Arch Intern Med* 1987; 147: 579.

163 Haley CJ, Haun WM, Lin S *et al*. Diazepam. In: *Drugdex*. Greenwood Village, CO: Micromedix, Inc., 2001.

164 Saxén I, Saxén L. Association between maternal intake of diazepam and oral clefts. *Lancet* 1975; 2: 498.

165 Laegreid L, Kyllerman M, Headner R, Hagberg B, Viggedahl G. Benzodiazepine amplification of valproate teratogenic effects in children of mothers with absence epilepsy. *Neuropediatrics* 1993; 24: 88–92.

166 Dhillon S, Richens A. Valproic acid and diazepam interaction *in vivo*. *Br J Clin Pharmacol* 1982; 13: 553–60.

167 Browne R, Penry J. Benzodiazepines in the treatment of epilepsy. *Epilepsia* 1973; 14: 277–310.

168 Prensky AL, Raff MC, Moore MS, Schwab RS. Intravenous diazepam in the treatment of prolonged seizure activity. *N Engl J Med* 1967; 276: 779–86.

169 Delgado-Escueta AV, Wasterlain C, Treiman DM, Porter RJ. Current concepts in neurology: management of status epilepticus. *N Engl J Med* 1982; 306: 1337–40.

170 Ferngren HG. Diazepam treatment for acute convulsions in children. *Epilepsia* 1974; 15: 27–37.

171 Mahomed K, Nyamurera T, Tarumbwa A. PVC bags considerably reduce availability of diazepam. *Cent Afr J Med* 1998; 44: 172–3.

172 Phelps SJ, Cochran EB. Diazepam. American Society of Hospital Pharmacists. *Guidelines for Administration of Intravenous Medications to Pediatric Patients*, 4th edn. Bethesda, MD: Intelligence Publications, 1993.

173 Agurell S, Berlin A, Ferngren H, Hellström B. Plasma levels of diazepam after parenteral and rectal administration. *Epilepsia* 1975; 16: 277–83.

174 Singhi S, Banerjee S, Singhi P. Refractory status epilepticus in children: role of continuous diazepam infusion. *J Child Neurol* 1998; 13: 23–6.

175 Gilbert DL, Gartside PS, Glauser T. Efficacy and mortality in treatment of refractory generalized convulsive status epilepticus. *J Child Neurol* 1999; 14: 602–9.

176 Meberg A, Langslet A, Bredesen JE, Lunde PKM. Plasma concentration of diazepam and N-desmethyldiazepam in children after a single rectal or intramuscular dose. *Eur J Clin Pharmacol* 1978; 14: 273–6.

177 Dieckmann RA. Rectal diazepam for prehospital pediatric status epilepticus. *Ann Emerg Med* 1994; 23: 216–24.

178 De Negri M, Baglietto MG, Battaglia FM, Gaggero R, Pessagno A, Recanati L. Treatment of electrical status epilepticus by short diazepam (DZP) cycles after DZP rectal bolus test. *Brain Dev* 1995; 17: 330–3.

179 Lathers CM, Kam FJ, Spivey WH. A comparison of intraosseous and intravenous routes of administration for antiseizure agents. *Epilepsia* 1989; 30: 472–9.

180 Knudsen FU, Paerregaard A, Andersen R, Andersen J. Long term outcome of prophylaxis for febrile convulsions. *Arch Dis Child* 1996; 74: 13–18.

181 Remy C, Jourdil N, Villemain D, Favel P, Genton P. Intrarectal diazepam in epileptic adults. *Epilepsia* 1992; 33: 353–8.

182 Lukey BJ, Corcoran KD, Solana RP. Pharmacokinetics of diazepam intramuscularly administered to rhesus monkeys. *J Pharm Sci* 1991; 80: 918–21.

183 Bechgaard E, Gizurarson S, Hjortkjaer RK. Pharmacokinetic and pharmacodynamic response after intranasal administration of diazepam to rabbits. *J Pharmacol Exp Ther* 1997; 49: 747–50.

184 De Negri M, Baglietto MG, Biancheri R. Electrical status epilepticus in childhood: treatment with short cycles of high dosage benzodiazepine (preliminary note). *Brain Dev* 1993; 15: 311–12.

185 Appleton R, Sweeney A, Choonara I, Robson J, Molyneux E. Lorazepam versus diazepam in the acute treatment of epileptic seizures and status epilepticus. *Dev Med Child Neurol* 1995; 37: 682–8.

186 Herman RJ, Van Pham JD, Szakacs CB. Disposition of lorazepam in human beings: enterohepatic recirculation and first-pass effect. *Clin Pharmacol Ther* 1989; 46: 18–25.

187 Bradshaw EG, Ali AA, Mulley BA, Rye RM. Plasma concentrations and clinical effects of lorazepam after oral administration. *Br J Anaesth* 1981; 53: 517–21.

188 Bonati M, Kanto J, Tognomi G. Clinical pharmacokinetics of cerebrospinal fluid. *Clin Pharmacokinet* 1982; 7: 312–35.

189 Ochs HR, Greenblatt DJ, Eichelkraut W, LeDuc BW, Powers JF, Hahn N. Entry of lorazepam into cerebrospinal fluid. *Pharmacology* 1980; 42: 36–48.

190 Comer WH, Elliott HW, Nomof N. Pharmacology of parenterally administered lorazepam in man. *J Int Med* 1973; 1: 216–25.

191 Greenblatt DJ, Joyce KA, Comer WH, Elliott HW, Shader RI, Knowles JA. Clinical pharmacokinetics of lorazepam. III. Intravenous injection. Preliminary results. *J Clin Pharmacol* 1977; 17: 490–4.

192 Greenblatt DJ, Ehrenberg BL, Gunderman J *et al*. Kinetic and dynamic study of intravenous lorazepam: comparison with intravenous diazepam. *J Pharmacol Exp Ther* 1989; 250: 134–40.

193 Greenblatt DJ, von Moltke LL, Ehrenberg BL *et al*. Kinetics and dynamics of lorazepam during and after continuous intravenous infusion. *Crit Care Med* 2000; 28: 2750–7.

194 Dundee JW, Lilburn JK, Toner W, Howard PJ. Plasma lorazepam levels. *Anesthesia* 1978; 33: 15–19.

195 Greenblatt DJ, Shader RI, Franke K *et al*. Pharmacokinetics and bioavailability of intravenous, intramuscular, and oral lorazepam in humans. *J Pharm Sci* 1979; 68: 57–63.

196 Ochs HR, Greenblatt DJ, Eichelkraut W, LeDuc BW, Powers JF, Hahn N. Contribution of the gastrointestinal tract to lorazepam conjugation and clonazepam nitroreduction. *Pharmacology* 1991; 42: 36–48.

197 Greenblatt DJ, Schillings RT, Kyriakopoulos AA *et al*. Clinical pharmacokinetics of lorazepam. I. Absorption and disposition of oral ^{14}C-lorazepam. *Clin Pharmacol Ther* 1976; 20: 329–41.

198 Lacey DJ, Singer WD, Horwitz SJ, Gilmore H. Lorazepam therapy of status epilepticus in children and adolescents. *J Pediatr* 1986; 108: 771–4.

199 DiMario FJ Jr, Clancy RR. Paradoxical precipitation of tonic seizures by lorazepam in a child with atypical absence seizures. *Pediatr Neurol* 1988; 4: 249–51.

200 Samara EE, Granneman RG, Witt GF, Cavanaugh JH. Effect of valproate on the pharmacokinetics and pharmacodynamics of lorazepam. *J Clin Pharmacol* 1997; 37: 442–50.

201 Anderson GD, Gidal BE, Kantor ED, Wilensky AJ. Lorazepam–valproate interaction: studies in normal subjects and isolated perfused rat liver. *Epilepsia* 1994; 35: 221–5.

202 Levy RJ, Krall RL. Treatment of status epilepticus with lorazepam. *Arch Neurol* 1984; 41: 605–11.

203 Vincent FM, Vincent T. Lorazepam in myoclonic seizures after cardiac arrest [letter]. *Ann Intern Med* 1986; 104: 586.

204 Benitz WE, Tatro DS, eds. *The Pediatric Drug Handbook*, 2nd edn. Chicago, IL: Yearbook Medical Publishers, 1988.

205 Deshmukh A, Wittert W, Schnitzler E, Mangurten HH. Lorazepam in the treatment of refractory neonatal seizures: a pilot study. *Am J Dis Child* 1986; 140: 1042–4.

206 Roddy SM, McBride MC, Torres CF. Treatment of neonatal seizures with lorazepam (Abstract). *Ann Neurol* 1987; 22: 412.

207 Yager JY, Seshia SS. Sublingual lorazepam in childhood serial seizures. *Am J Dis Child* 1988; 142: 931–2.

208 D'Onofrio G, Rathlev NK, Ulrich AS, Fish SS, Freedland ES. Lorazepam for the prevention of recurrent seizures related to alcohol. *N Engl J Med* 1999; 340: 915–19.

209 Walker JE, Homan RW, Crawford IL. Lorazepam: a controlled trial in patients with intractable partial complex seizures. *Epilepsia* 1984; 25: 464–6.

210 Huff JS, Bleck TP. Propofol and midazolam in status epilepticus (letter). *Acad Emerg Med* 1996; 3: 179.

211 Bell DM, Richards G, Dhillon S, Oxley JR, Cromarty J, Sander JW, Patsalos PN. A comparative pharmacokinetic study of intravenous and intramuscular midazolam in patients with epilepsy. *Epilepsy Res* 1991; 10: 183–90.

212 Burstein AH, Modica R, Hatton M, Forrest A, Gengo FM. Pharmacokinetics and pharmacodynamics of midazolam after intranasal administration. *J Clin Pharmacol* 1997; 37: 711–18.

213 Bjorkman S, Rigemar G, Idvall J. Pharmacokinetics of midazolam given as an intranasal spray to adult surgical patients. *Br J Anaesth* 1997; 79: 575–80.

214 Clausen TG, Wolff J, Hansen PB, Larsen F, Rasmussen SN, Dixon JS, Crevoisier C. Pharmacokinetics of midazolam and α-hydroxy-midazolam following rectal and intravenous administration. *Br J Clin Pharmacol* 1988; 25: 457–63.

215 Thummel KE, O'Shea D, Paine MF *et al*. Oral first-pass elimination of

midazolam involves both gastrointestinal and hepatic CYP3A-mediated metabolism. *Clin Pharmacol Ther* 1996; 59: 491–502.

216 Rey E, Delaunay L, Pons G, Nurat I, Richard MO. Pharmacokinetics of midazolam in children: comparative study of intranasal and intravenous administration. *Eur J Clin Pharmacol* 1991; 41: 355–7.

217 Jacqz-Aigrain E, Oxley J, Wilson J, Richens A. Pharmacokinetics of midazolam during continuous infusion in critically ill neonates. *Eur J Clin Pharmacol* 1992; 42: 329–32.

218 Malacrida R, Fritz ME, Suter PM, Crevoisier C. Pharmacokinetics of midazolam administered by continuous intravenous infusion to intensive care patients. *Crit Care Med* 1992; 20: 1123–6.

219 Dundee JW, Halliday NJ, Harper KW, Brogden RN. Midazolam: a review of its pharmacological properties and therapeutic use. *Drugs* 1984; 28: 519–43.

220 Oldenhof H, de Jong M, Steenhoek A, Janknegt R. Clinical pharmacokinetics of midazolam in intensive care patients, a wide interpatient variability? *Clin Pharmacol Ther* 1988; 43: 263–9.

221 Caldwell CB, Gross JB. Physostigmine reversal of midazolam-induced sedation. *Anesthesiology* 1982; 57: 125–7.

222 Amrein R, Hetzel W, Bonetti EP, Gerecke M. Clinical pharmacology of dormicum (midazolam) and anexate (flumazenil). *Resuscitation* 1988; 16: S5–S27.

223 Hantson P, Clemessy JL, Baud FJ. Withdrawal syndrome following midazolam infusion. *Intensive Care Med* 1995; 21: 190–4.

224 Wijdicks EF, Sharbrough FW. New-onset seizures in critically ill patients. *Neurology* 1993; 43: 1042–4.

225 Olkkola KT, Aranko K, Luurila H et al. A potentially hazardous interaction between erythromycin and midazolam. *Clin Pharmacol Ther* 1993; 53: 298–305.

226 Backman JT, Olkkola KT, Ojala M, Laaksovirta H, Neuvonen PJ. Concentrations and effects of oral midazolam are greatly reduced in patients treated with carbamazepine or phenytoin. *Epilepsia* 1996; 37: 253–7.

227 Hanley FD, Kross JF. Use of midazolam in the treatment of refractory status epilepticus. *Clin Ther* 1998; 20: 1093–105.

228 Towne AR, DeLorenzo RJ. Use of intramuscular midazolam for status epilepticus. *J Emerg Med* 1999; 17: 323–8.

229 Kumar A, Bleck TP. Intravenous midazolam for the treatment of refractory status epilepticus. *Crit Care Med* 1992; 20 (4): 483–8.

230 Ghilain S, Van Rijckevorsel-Harmant K, Harmant J, de Barsy TH. Midazolam in the treatment of epileptic seizures (letter). *J Neurol Neurosurg Psychiatr* 1988; 51: 732.

231 Wroblewski BA, Joseph AB. The use of intramuscular midazolam for acute seizure cessation of behavioral emergencies in patients with traumatic brain injury. *Clin Neuropharmacol* 1992; 15: 44–9.

232 Koul RL, Raj AG, Chacko A, Joshi R, Seif EM. Continuous midazolam infusion as treatment of status epilepticus. *Arch Dis Child* 1997; 76: 445–8.

233 Igartua J, Silver P, Maytal J, Sagy M. Midazolam for refractory status epilepticus in children. *Crit Care Med* 1999; 27 (9): 1982–5.

234 Koul RL, Raj AG, Chacko A, Joshi R, Seif EM. Continuous midazolam infusion as treatment of status epilepticus. *Arch Dis Child* 1997; 76: 445–8.

235 Yoshikawa H, Yamazaki S, Abe T, Oda Y. Midazolam as a first-line agent for status epilepticus in children. *Brain Dev* 2000; 22: 239–42.

236 Sheth RD, Buckley DJ, Gingold M, Bodensteiner JB, Penney S. Midazolam in the treatment of refractory neonatal seizures. *Clin Neuropharmacol* 1996; 19: 165–70.

237 Lahat E, Goldman M, Barr J, Bistritzer T, Berkovitch M. Comparison of intranasal midazolam with intravenous diazepam for treating febrile seizures in children: prospective randomized study. *Br Med* 2000; 32: 183–6.

238 Chamberlain JM, Altieri MA, Futterman C, Young GM, Ochsenschlager DW, Waisman Y. A prospective, randomized study comparing intramuscular midazolam with intravenous diazepam for the treatment of seizures in children. *Pediatr Emerg Care* 1997; 13: 92–4.

239 Jeannet PY, Roulet E, Maeder-Ingvar M, Gehri M, Jutzi A, Deonna T. Home and hospital treatment of acute seizures in children with nasal midazolam. *Eur J Paediatr Neurol* 1999; 3: 73–7.

240 Scott RC, Besag FM, Neville BG. Buccal midazolam and rectal diazepam for treatment of prolonged seizures in childhood and adolescence: a randomized trial. *Lancet* 1999; 353: 623–6.

241 Bertler A, Lindgren S, Magnusson J-O, Malmgren H. Intramuscular bioavailability of clorazepate as compared to diazepam. *Eur J Clin Pharmacol* 1985; 28: 229–30.

242 Greenblatt DJ, Divoll MK, Soong MH, Boxenbaum HG, Harmatz JS, Shader RI. Desmethyldiazepam pharmacokinetics: studies following intravenous and oral desmethyldiazepam, oral clorazepate, and intravenous diazepam. *J Clin Pharmacol* 1988; 28: 853–9.

243 Greenblatt DJ, Shader RI, Harmatz JS, Georgotas A. Self-rated sedation and plasma concentrations of desmethyldiazepam following single doses of clorazepate. *Psychopharmacology (Berl)* 1979; 66: 289–90.

244 Abernethy DR, Greenblatt DJ, Divoll M, Shader RI. Prolongation of drug half-life due to obesity: studies of desmethyldiazepam (clorazepate). *J Pharm Sci* 1982; 71: 942–4.

245 Bertler A, Lindgren S, Magnusson J-O, Malmgren H. Pharmacokinetics of clorazepate after intravenous and intramuscular administration. *Psychopharmacol* 1983; 80: 236–9.

246 Shader RI, Greenblatt DJ, Ciraulo DA, Divoll M, Harmatz JS, Georgotas A. Effect of age and sex on disposition of desmethyldiazepam formed from its precursor clorazepate. *Psychopharmacol* 1981; 75: 193–7.

247 Joseph AB, Wroblewski BA. Paradoxical akathesia caused by clonazepam, clorazepate and lorazepam in patients with traumatic encephalopathy and seizure disorder. a subtype of benzodiazepine-induced disinhibition. *Behav Neurol* 1993; 6: 221–3.

248 Lion JR, Azcarate CL, Koepke HH. 'Paradoxical rage reactions' during psychotropic medication. *Dis Nervous System* 1975; 36: 557–8.

249 Feldman RG. Clorazepate in temporal lobe epilepsy. *JAMA* 1976; 236: 2603.

250 Karch FE. Rage reaction associated with clorazepate dipotassium. *Ann Intern Med* 1979; 91: 61–2.

251 Livingston S, Pauli LL, Pruce L. Clorazepate in epilepsy. *JAMA* 1977; 237: 1561.

252 Patel DA, Patel AR. Clorazepate and congenital malformations. *JAMA* 1980; 244: 135–6.

253 Wilensky AJ, Levy RH, Troupin AS, Moretti-Ojemann L. Clorazepate kinetics in treated epileptics. *Clin Pharmacol Ther* 1978; 24: 22–30.

254 Berchou RC, Odin EA, Russell ME. Clorazepate therapy for refractory seizures. *Neurology* 1981; 31: 1483–5.

255 Wilensky AJ, Ojemann LM, Temkin NR, Troupin AS, Dodrill CB. Clorazepate and phenobarbital as antiepileptic drugs: a double-blind study. *Neurology* 1981; 31: 1271–6.

256 Booker HE. Clorazepate dipotassium in the treatment of intractable epilepsy. *JAMA* 1974; 299: 552–5.

257 Naidu S, Gruener G, Brazis P. Excellent results with clorazepate in recalcitrant childhood epilepsies. *Pediatr Neurol* 1986; 2: 18–22.

258 Rieder J. Plasma levels and derived pharmacokinetic characteristics of unchanged nitrazepam in man. *Arzneimittelforschung* 1973; 23: 212–18.

259 Nicholson AN. Hypnotics: their place in therapeutics. *Drugs* 1986; 31: 164–76.

260 Kangas L, Iisalo E, Kanto J et al. Human pharmacokinetics of nitrazepam: effect of age and diseases. *Eur J Clin Pharmacol* 1979; 15: 163–70.

261 Kangas L, Kanto J, Siirtola T, Pekkarinen A. Cerebrospinal fluid concentrations of nitrazepam in man. *Acta Pharmacol Toxicol* 1977; 41: 74–9.

262 Breimer DD. Clinical pharmacokinetics of hypnotics. *Clin Pharmacokinet* 1977; 2: 93–109.

263 Breimer DD. Pharmacokinetics and metabolism of various benzodiazepines used as hypnotics. *Br J Clin Pharmacol* 1979; 8: 7S–13S.

264 Kenny RA, Kafetz K, Cox M, Timmers J, Impallomeni M. Impaired nitrazepam metabolism in hypothyroidism. *Postgrad Med* 1984; 60: 296–7.

265 Baruzzi A, Michelucci R, Tassinari CA. Benzodiazepines, nitrazepam. In: Levy RH, Dreifus FE, Mattson RH, Meldrum BS, Penry JK, eds. *Antiepileptic Drugs*. New York: Raven Press, 1989: 785–804.

266 Abernethy DR, Greenblatt DJ, Lockniskar A, Ochs HR, Harmatz JS, Shader RI. Obesity effects on nitrazepam disposition. *Br J Clin Pharmacol* 1986; 22: 551–7.

267 Evans JG, Jarvis EH. Nitrazepam and the elderly. *Br Med* 1972; 4: 487.

268 Linnoila M, Viukari M. Efficacy and side effects of nitrazepam and thioridazine as sleeping aids in psychiatric in-patients. *Br J Pharmacol* 1976; 128: 566–9.

269 Saario I, Linnoila M, Maki M. Interaction of drugs with alcohol and human psychomotor skills related to driving: effect on sleep deprivation of two weeks treatment with hypnotics. *J Clin Pharmacol* 1975; 15: 52–9.

270 Taylor F. Nitrazepam and the elderly. *Br Med* 1973; 1: 113–14.

271 Hagberg B. The chlordiazepoxide HCl (Librium®) analogue nitrazepam (Mogadon®) in the treatment of epilepsy in children. *Dev Med Neurol* 1968; 10: 302–8.

272 Wyllie E, Wyllie R, Cruse RP, Rothner AD, Erenberg G. The mechanism of nitrazepam-induced drooling and aspiration. *N Engl J Med* 1986; 314: 35–8.

273 Clark TJH, Collins JV, Tong D. Respiratory depression caused by nitrazepam in patients with respiratory failure. *Lancet* 1971; 2: 737–8.

274 Speight AN. Floppy infant syndrome and maternal diazepam and/or nitrazepam. *Lancet* 1977; 2: 878.

275 Darcy L. Delirium tremens following withdrawal from nitrazepam. *Med J Aust* 1972; 2: 450.

276 Busto U, Sellers EM, Naranjo CA *et al.* Withdrawal reaction after long-term therapeutic use of benzodiazepines. *N Engl J Med* 1986; 315: 854–9.

277 Speirs CJ, Navey FL, Brooks DJ, Impallomeni MG. Opisthotonos and benzodiazepine withdrawal in the elderly. *Lancet* 1986; 2: 1101.

278 Rintahaka PJ, Shewmon DA, Kyyronen P, Shields WD. Incidence of death in patients with intractable epilepsy during nitrazepam treatment. *Epilepsia* 1999; 40: 492–6.

279 Baldwin R, Kenny TJ, Segal J. The effectiveness of nitrazepam in a refractory epileptic population. *Curr Ther Res* 1969; 11: 413–16.

280 Peterson WG. Clinical study of Mogadon®, a new anticonvulsant. *Neurology* 1967; 17: 878–80.

281 Millichap JG, Ortiz WR. Nitrazepam in myoclonic epilepsies. *Am J Dis Child* 1966; 112: 242–8.

282 Snyder CH. Myoclonic epilepsy in children: short-term comparative study of two benzodiazepine derivatives in treatment. *South Med* 1968; 61: 17–20.

283 Jan JE, Riegel JA, Crichton JU, Dunn HG. Nitrazepam in the treatment of epilepsy in childhood. *Can Med Assoc J* 1971; 104: 571–5.

284 Vanasse M, Masson P, Geoffroy G, Larbrisseau A, David PC. Intermittent treatment of febrile convusions with nitrazepam. *Can J Neurol Sci* 1984; 11: 377–9.

285 Dreifus FE, Farwell J, Holmes GL *et al.* Infantile spasms: comparative trial of nitrazepam and corticotropin. *Arch Neurol* 1986; 43: 1107–10.

286 Chamberlain MC. Nitrazepam for refractory infantile spasms and the Lennox Gastaut syndrome. *J Child Neurol* 1996; 11: 31–4.

287 Stein AG, Eder HG, Blum DE, Drachev A, Fisher RS. An automated drug delivery system for focal epilepsy. *Epilepsy Res* 2000; 39: 103–14.

32 Ethosuximide

T.A. Glauser

Primary indications	First-line or adjunctive therapy in generalized absence seizures; also helpful in absence status epilepticus and some generalized epilepsies in childhood
Usual preparations	Capsules: 250 mg; syrup: 250 mg/5 mL
Usual dosages	Initial: 250 mg (adults): 10–15 mg/kg/day (children). Maintenance: 750–2000 mg/day (adults); 20–40 mg/kg/day (children)
Dosage intervals	2–3 times/day
Significant drug interactions	Ethosuximide levels are often increased by comedication with valproate and reduced by comedication with carbamazepine, phenytoin and phenobarbital
Serum level monitoring	Useful
Target range	40–100 mg/L
Common/important side-effects	Gastrointestinal symptoms, drowsiness, ataxia, diplopia, headache, dizziness, hiccups, sedation, behavioural disturbances, acute psychotic reactions, extrapyramidal symptoms, blood dyscrasia, rash, lupus-like syndrome, severe idiosyncratic reactions
Main advantages	Well-established treatment for absence epilepsy without the risk of hepatic toxicity carried by valproate
Main disadvantages	Side-effects common
Mechanisms of action	Effects on calcium T-channel conductance
Oral bioavailability	<100%
Time to peak levels	<4 h
Metabolism and excretion	hepatic oxidation, then conjugation
Volume of distribution	0.65 L/kg
Elimination half-life	30–60 h
Plasma clearance	0.010–0.015 L/kg/h
Protein binding	<10%
Active metabolites	None
Comment	Drug of first choice in absence seizures

(*Note*: this summary table was formulated by the lead editor.)

In the 1950s, ethosuximide was developed as an effective, safe and well-tolerated anticonvulsant for the treatment of absence seizures [1]. Trimethadione and its analogue paramethadione, introduced in the 1940s, were the first anticonvulsants to demonstrate efficacy against absence seizures but were associated with significant toxicity [2–5]. These toxicity issues prompted the discovery and testing in the 1950s of the succinimide family of anticonvulsants (ethosuximide, methsuximide and phensuximide) [5]. Among the members of the succinimide family, ethosuximide had the greatest efficacy against absence seizures and demonstrated the least toxicity [5]. Ethosuximide has since been considered as first-line therapy for absence seizures since its introduction in 1958 [6,7].

Ethosuximide (2-ethyl-2-methylsuccinimide, molecular weight 141.2) is a compound containing a five-member ring, two negatively charged carbonyl oxygen atoms with a ring nitrogen between them and one asymmetric carbon atom [8,9] (Fig. 32.1). It has a melting point of 64–65°C, along with a weakly acidic pKa of 9.3, and a partition coefficient of 9 (chloroform/water; pH 7) [9]. Ethosuximide is freely soluble in ethanol and water (solubility 190 mg/mL) [9]. A white crystalline material, ethosuximide is used clinically as a racemate and is commercially available in 250 mg capsules or 250 mg/mL syrup [6,8].

Mechanisms of action

Ethosuximide's presumed mechanism of action against absence seizures is reduction of low threshold T-type calcium currents in thalamic neurones [10,11]. The spontaneous pacemaker oscillatory activity of thalamocortical neurones involves low threshold T-type calcium currents [12]. These oscillatory currents are considered to be the generators of the 3 Hz spike-and-wave rhythms noted in patients with absence epilepsy [12]. Voltage-dependent blockade of the low threshold T-type calcium current was demonstrated at clinically relevant ethosuximide concentrations in thalamic neurones isolated from rats and guinea pigs [10,11,13]. Gating of these T-type Ca^{2+} channels is not altered by ethosuximide [5,11]. Based on these findings, it is proposed that ethosuximide's effect on low threshold T-type calcium currents in thalamocortical neurones prevent the 'synchronized firing associated with spike-wave discharges' [10].

There is no evidence to indicate ethosuximide exerts an anticonvulsant effect through other common mechanisms of action (e.g. postsynaptic enhancement of γ-aminobutyric acid (GABA) responses or action at voltage-dependent sodium channels) [5,14]. There is no alteration of brain GABA concentrations in mice following single-dose administration [15]. The anticonvulsant effects of ethosuximide's other actions in the brain (e.g. membrane transport processes, effects on brain enzyme physiology, and neurotransmitter processes [14]) are unclear. In cortical tissue ethosuximide inhibits Na^+,K^+-adenosine triphosphatase (ATPase) activity at ethosuximide concentrations significantly greater than those for anticonvulsant effect [14,16–18].

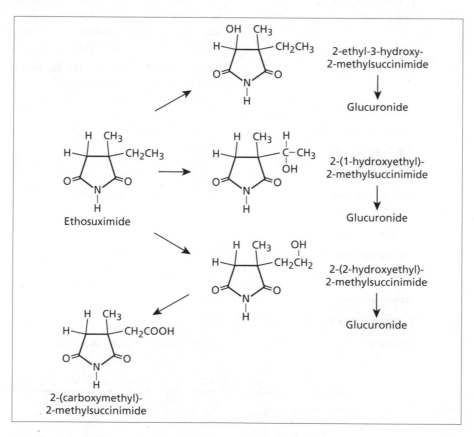

Fig. 32.1 Structure and biotransformation pathways of ethosuximide. Reprinted with permission from [9].

Experimental studies

Ethosuximide absorption and distribution in animals

In dogs, monkeys and rats the absorption of ethosuximide is rapid with nearly complete oral bioavailability in dogs of 88–95%, and monkeys of 93–97.5% [19–24]. In rats, ethosuximide distributes evenly to brain, plasma and other tissues except for adipose tissue (where steady-state ethosuximide concentrations are approximately one-third of those reached in plasma) [23]. Ethosuximide crosses the placenta in rats [24,25]. In both dog and rat studies, ethosuximide readily passed through the blood–brain barrier [19,24]. In dogs the plasma to cerebrospinal fluid (CSF) ratio was 1.01±0.15 with an estimated ethosuximide half-life of entry into the CSF at about 4–5 min [19,23,24,26]. In one study in rats, the whole brain to plasma ethosuximide concentrations was near unity while a second study in rats found ethosuximide was uniformly distributed in four discrete areas of the rat brain (cerebral cortex, cerebellum, midbrain and pons medulla) [22,24]. However a third study in rats receiving a single intraperitoneal dose of ethosuximide (50 mg/kg) found a decrease in brain to plasma ethosuximide concentrations over time suggesting ethosuximide may be actively transported out of the rat brain [23,27].

The apparent volume of distribution in rats, dogs and rhesus monkeys ranges from 0.7 to 0.8 L/kg [19,20,23,28]. Ethosuximide protein binding is 0–10% in dogs and rats [6,23,24]. Although ethosuximide is a racemic mixture, its disposition in rats is non-stereoselective [9].

Ethosuximide metabolism and elimination in animals

The main method of ethosuximide elimination in animals is metabolism. Unchanged ethosuximide accounts for only 12% of urinary recovery in rats [29]. In rhesus monkeys and rats, ethosuximide and its metabolites are excreted predominantly by the kidney with only a small proportion recovered in the faeces [23,25].

The major metabolite in rats and monkeys is 2-(1-hydroxyethyl)-2-methylsuccinimide with two other minor metabolites: 2-ethyl-3-hydroxy-2-methyl-succinimide and 2-(2-hydroxyethyl)-2- methylsuccinimide [23,30]. In rats, ethosuximide's biotransformation is catalysed predominantly by hepatic CYP450 3A isoenzymes with possible minor contributions by CYP450 2E, CYP450 2B and CYP450 2C isoenzymes [9,23,28,31,32]. These CYP450 enzymes are inducible and, in rats, autoinduction has been reported [23,28].

Ethosuximide's elimination appears to follow first-order kinetics in animals except in dogs where Michaelis–Menten kinetics may apply [19,23,30]. Studies of single and multiple dose ethosuximide administration in monkeys demonstrate comparable elimination half-life and total-body clearance [6,20,21]. In animals, there is a wide variation in ethosuximide elimination half-lives ranging from 1 h in mice to 9–26 h in rats and 11–25 h in dogs [19,23,30]. Steady-state ethosuximide plasma concentrations are significantly higher in the morning than the evening in rhesus monkeys receiving intravenous ethosuximide at a constant rate. It has been suggested that these fluctuations result from circadian changes in ethosuximide metabolizing enzymes [23,30,33].

Efficacy in animals

Ethosuximide exhibits very different efficacy profiles in the two major traditional animal models of epilepsy, the maximal electroshock test and the pentylenetetrazole seizure test. It is hypothesized that the maximal electroshock test identifies agents effective against partial onset and generalized tonic-clonic seizures and is used to identify agents that have the capacity to prevent the spread of seizures [5,34]. Ethosuximide was ineffective against maximal electroshock induced tonic seizures except at anaesthetic doses [5,34–36]. In contrast, ethosuximide blocked clonic seizures produced by subcutaneously administered pentylenetetrazole or biculline [5,34,36,37]. These chemically induced seizure models are said to identify agents which raise the seizure threshold and may be effective against absence seizures. This activity profile suggests that ethosuximide exerts its anticonvulsant effects by raising seizure threshold rather than by blocking the spread of seizures and predicts efficacy against absence rather than partial onset and generalized tonic-clonic seizures. In contrast to the complete protection by ethosuximide against pentylenetetrazole-induced clonic seizures in mice, ethosuximide's major metabolite, 2-(1-hydroxyethyl)-2-methylsuccinimide, demonstrated 'no significant anticonvulsant activity' [30].

Ethosuximide demonstrates activity against spontaneously occurring absence seizures in three other animal models (mutant tottering mice, Wistar rats, spontaneously epileptic rats) [38–40] along with activity against spike-wave seizures induced by systemic administration of γ-hydroxybutyrate [34,41–43].

Pharmacokinetics

Implications of racemic mixture

Ethosuximide is used as a racemate. It is theoretically possible that the two enantiomers could have different pharmacokinetic parameters or anticonvulsant effects. The enantiomer ratio was close to unity and there was little interindividual variability in plasma samples from 33 patients obtained for routine monitoring measured by chiral gas chromatographic analysis [44]. This implies the disposition of ethosuximide in humans is non-stereoselective and measurement of total ethosuximide for therapeutic monitoring is reasonable and appropriate [9,45]. The non-stereoselective disposition of ethosuximide was unaffected by pregnancy, placental transfer or passage into breast milk in a small study (three pregnancies in two women taking ethosuximide) [45].

Absorption

There is no intravenous formulation that can be used as a reference standard to determine absolute bioavailability in humans; nevertheless, absorption of ethosuximide is considered to be rapid and nearly complete in children and adults (90–95%) [1,23,46,47]. Absorption remains full after multiple administrations [23]. In two single-dose capsule administration studies (four healthy adults given 0.5 g oral dose and three volunteers given a single 1-g ethosuximide oral dose) peak ethosuximide plasma concentrations are reached between 1 and 4 h after drug administration [24,47,48].

In contrast a separate study in five institutionalized children comparing capsules and syrup formulations demonstrated peak plasma concentrations within 3–7h with either formulation [7,23,24,46,49]. The syrup had a faster absorption rate than the capsules but the two formulations were bioequivalent [6,7,23, 24,46,49].

Distribution

Ethosuximide homogeneously distributes throughout the body [6]. Ethosuximide concentrations in saliva, tears, and CSF are similar to plasma ethosuximide concentrations [23,24,50–55]. In three studies (involving six, 15 and 19 patients) the correlation between saliva and serum concentrations was $r=0.99$, $r=0.99$ and $r=0.74$, respectively [53–55]. A fourth study which examined ethosuximide concentrations in paired parotid saliva and plasma samples in 10 patients showed the average saliva to plasma ratio was 1.04 which appeared constant over the measured time intervals [52]. Based on these results, multiple studies have concluded saliva can be used in lieu of plasma for therapeutic monitoring of ethosuximide [24,50,52–54,56].

In humans, ethosuximide's apparent volume of distribution is 0.62–0.65 L/kg in adults and 0.69 L/kg in children, implying distribution through total body water [6,23,46,47,51]. Its protein binding is 0–10% [6,23,24].

Ethosuximide crosses the placenta in humans and has been detected in cord serum and amniotic fluid at concentrations of 104% and 111% of maternal serum concentrations, respectively [6,57]. Ethosuximide was detected in either the urine or plasma of a newborn infant of a woman receiving chronic ethosuximide therapy in two separate reports [24,58,59]. The newborn infant's ethosuximide serum concentration was similar to that observed in the mother [23,59].

Ethosuximide is also excreted through the breast milk of mothers on chronic ethosuximide therapy [23]. In multiple studies the average breast milk to maternal serum concentration ratio ranged from 0.8 to 0.94 [23,59–62] The ethosuximide serum concentration of breastfeeding infants of mothers on chronic ethosuximide therapy were 30–50% of their mother's ethosuximide serum concentration [23,61,62].

Metabolism and elimination

Metabolism is the main method of ethosuximide elimination in humans and animals. Ethosuximide undergoes extensive hepatic oxidative biotransformation (80–90%) to pharmacologically inactive metabolites. While most of the remaining ethosuximide is excreted unchanged in the urine, small amounts of unchanged ethosuximide can be recovered from bile and faeces [63]. Its oxidation is catalysed mainly by enzymes of the CYP3A subfamily [6].

The major metabolite recovered from human urine in patients receiving ethosuximide is 2-(1-hydroxyethyl)-2-methylsuccinimide, of which at least 40% is excreted as a glucuronide conjugate [9]. Two other ethosuximide metabolites recovered (often as a glucuronide conjugate) from human urine in patients receiving ethosuximide are 2-ethyl-3-hydroxy-2-methylsuccinimide and 2-(2-hydroxyethyl)-2-methylsuccinimide. This latter metabolite can undergo subsequent metabolism by the hepatic mixed-function ox-idase system to form the fourth major metabolite 2-carboxymethyl-2-methylsuccinimide [9,30] (Fig. 32.1).

In humans, ethosuximide's elimination follows first-order kinetics. Its total-body clearance in adults averages 0.01 L/kg/h [47] and in two children was 0.016 and 0.013 L/kg/h [46]. This is low when considering the rate of hepatic plasma flow (0.9 L/kg/h), implying ethosuximide does not undergo a significant first-pass effect and drug clearance is not blood flow limited [23,24]. Total-body clearance has been reported to decrease slightly after repeated dosing [23]. Ethosuximide does not induce hepatic microsomal CYP450 enzymes or the UDPGT (uridine diphosphate glucurono-syltransferase) system [64–66]. Autoinduction does not occur, unlike rats [66,67].

In general, ethosuximide has a long elimination half-life that varies with age. Ethosuximide's mean half-life in adults was reported to range from 40 to 60h compared with 30–40h in children [30,46–48,51,67–69]. There are large variations reported in ethosuximide's half-life (15–68h) in the paediatric studies [30,46,51,70]. The half-life of ethosuximide has been reported to be 32–41h in neonates [59,61]. The time to reach steady-state concentration following a dosage change is 6–7 days for children and 12 days for adults [6,71]. Clearance is reported to be lower in women than men [72]. Dose size and repeated dosing does not affect ethosuximide elimination half-life [51,70].

Drug interactions

Interactions with other antiepileptic medications

Ethosuximide has a low potential for drug interactions due to its lack of effect on either the hepatic microsomal CYP450 enzymes or the UDPGT system along with negligible protein binding [64,71]. Most authors conclude that ethosuximide therapy does not have a clinically significant effect on the pharmacokinetics of phenytoin, phenobarbital or carbamazepine; there are scattered reports of some changes in phenytoin or phenobarbital concentrations when ethosuximide is used in combination with phenytoin or primidone [6,73–80]. There is neither an alteration in the plasma protein binding of carbamazepine or phenytoin nor a change in the formation of phenobarbital from primidone when ethosuximide is used [81]. A recent study reported a significant decrease in valproic acid serum concentration following the addition of ethosuximide (120.0 ±20.1 μg/mL pre-ethosuximide vs. 87.0±13.1 μg/mL during co-therapy with ethosuximide, $P < 0.01$). Following cessation of ethosuximide, valproic acid levels rose by 36.7%. The mechanism underlying this observed effect of ethosuximide on valproic acid concentrations is unknown [82].

In contrast, concomitant therapy with enzyme inducing antiepileptic drugs (AEDs) can increase ethosuximide total clearance due to ethosuximide's extensive hepatic oxidative metabolism by CYP450 enzymes [80]. Ethosuximide's clearance is significantly accelerated (leading to a drop in the serum concentration) when ethosuximide is used concurrently with phenobarbital, phenytoin or carbamazepine [64,80,83–86]. Discontinuation of concomitant carbamazepine therapy in one study resulted in a 48% increase in ethosuximide plasma concentrations [87]. The magnitude of this effect varies considerably between patients [83]. The effect of valproic acid on the pharmacokinetics of ethosuximide is also variable, with different studies showing ethosuximide's clearance increased, decreased or remained unchanged when concomitant valproic acid therapy was employed [64,67,69,77,84,88–90]. Some authors postulate that valproic acid may inhibit the metabolism of ethosuximide resulting in an increase in the plasma ethosuximide concentration [91].

There have not been any formal pharmacokinetic interaction studies examining potential ethosuximide interactions with felbamate, gabapentin, lamotrigine, tiagabine, topiramate, oxcarbazepine, levetiracetam, vigabatrin or zonisamide.

Interactions with non-antiepileptic medications

The clearance of ethosuximide is substantially increased when used in combination with rifampin, an inducer of CYP450 3A isoenzymes [85]. In one report, use of ethosuximide and isoniazid, a potent inhibitor of CYP450 enzymes, resulted in increased ethosuximide serum concentrations and psychotic behaviour [92].

Liver and renal disease

The effects of liver and renal disease on ethosuximide elimination have not been formally studied [23]. Theoretically, liver disease should impair ethosuximide elimination due to the ethosuximide's substantial hepatic oxidative metabolism while the effect of renal disease on ethosuximide elimination would have much less impact [23]. Haemodialysis can readily remove ethosuximide. One report estimates approximately 50% of the body's ethosuximide was removed over a 6-h dialysis interval and that ethosuximide half-life dropped to 3–4 h during dialysis [23,93]. In a separate case report, peritoneal dialysis was able to decrease ethosuximide concentrations in a child taking both ethosuximide and phenobarbital [94].

Clinical efficacy

Although there are no double-blind controlled monotherapy trials rigorously proving ethosuximide is effective against typical absence seizures, two open studies conducted in the 1970s suggested a powerful effect [95,96]. As a result, ethosuximide is regarded as effective as first-line monotherapy against typical absence seizures.

Ethosuximide's efficacy against typical absence seizures has been examined in a study with well-constructed methodology for patient selection and assessment. In order to enrol, each patient's absence seizures were required (a) to meet a predetermined clinical definition of an absence seizure; and (b) be witnessed by the principal investigator. Seizure frequency was then assessed by five separate measures including (a) ward staff observation; (b) trained observer observation; (c) mother's observation; (d) physician observation (including during patient hyperventilation); and (e) standardized video-EEG recording. These five measures were combined into a 'seizure index' [95].

Thirty-seven patients enrolled. By the eighth week of ethosuximide treatment, 19% (7/37) were seizure free with a 100% reduction in seizure index. Overall, during ethosuximide therapy, 49% (18/37) demonstrated ≥ 90% reduction in seizures while 95% (35/37) exhibited a ≥50% reduction in seizures. The full antiabsence effect was noted rapidly (within a week) for any given etho-

suximide dose. Plasma ethosuximide concentrations ranged from 16.6 to 104.0 µg/mL (doses 6.5–36.7 mg/kg) and, based on the seizure index, the authors suggest the optimal ethosuximide plasma concentrations in this study was 40–100 µg/mL [95].

The second major study was a prospective longitudinal open label study of ethosuximide efficacy against absence seizures that investigated using therapeutic drug monitoring to maximize clinical response [96]. Seventy patients enrolled; the group was 54% (38/70) female with ages ranging from 4 to 28 years (median 12 years). Thirty-eight patients (54%) had only absence seizures while the remaining patients had either absence seizures with tonic-clonic seizures (30%) or absence seizures and one or more other generalized seizure types (16%). Approximately half the patients were on other AEDs in addition to ethosuximide. Patients received between 9.4 and 73.5 mg/kg/day and were evaluated at 6-month intervals. Introduction of ethosuximide therapy resulted in complete seizure control in 47% (33/70) of the patients. None of these patients had plasma ethosuximide concentrations below 30 µg/mL, only 9% were below 40 µg/mL [96].

During the next 2.5 years, attempts were made to achieve plasma ethosuximide concentrations above 40 µg/mL in the remaining patients (53%, 37/70) with uncontrolled absence seizures. Improved compliance and higher ethosuximide dosages led to significantly higher ethosuximide plasma concentrations in 19 patients; 10 of these 19 patients became seizure free. At the 2.5 years follow-up mark 61% (43/70) of the group was seizure free. In these patients, ethosuximide's effectiveness persisted over the next 2.5 years (total 5 years) of follow-up. In contrast ethosuximide was not able to control absence seizures in patients with absence seizures and tonic-clonic seizures on combination AED therapy [96].

Five controlled comparative trials have demonstrated that ethosuximide and valproic acid have similar efficacy against absence seizures [97–101] These studies utilized clinical observation only (n =2), video-EEG telemetry only (n=1) or both techniques (n=2) to assess response to therapy. Success was defined as 100% seizure control. In these five comparative trials, ethosuximide therapy resulted in 100% seizure reduction in 58% of patients utilizing clinical observation and 57% of patients using video-EEG telemetry; serum ethosuximide concentrations ranged from 26 to 114 µg/mL. In comparison, valproic acid therapy resulted in 100% seizure reduction in 63% of patients (using clinical observation) or 55% of patients (using video-EEG telemetry) with serum valproic acid concentrations ranging from 32 to 131 µg/mL.

One open label study in five patients examined ethosuximide and valproic acid combination therapy for absence seizures previously treated with ethosuximide or valproic acid monotherapy [102]. Subsequently, many authors have recommended ethosuximide and valproic acid combination therapy for patients with absence seizures resistant to monotherapy [7,49,71,103]. Similarly, ethosuximide therapy in patients with both absence and tonic-clonic seizures has been used in combination with another AED effective against tonic-clonic seizures such as valproic acid, carbamazepine or phenytoin [7,71,103]. Despite being reported as 'highly effective' against atypical absence seizures [71,103], ethosuximide is almost always used as part of combination therapy in patients with atypical absence seizures due to the high incidence of coexisting seizure types [7].

There is some evidence that ethosuximide is useful in the prevention and treatment of absence status epilepticus at serum concentrations greater than 120 µg/mL [104,105]. There are also reports of ethosuximide being effective in patients with severe myoclonic epilepsy in infancy [106], childhood epileptic encephalopathy (the Lennox–Gastaut syndrome) [4,107], juvenile myoclonic epilepsy [108,109], epilepsy with myoclonic absences [109], eyelid myoclonia with absences [109], epilepsy with continuous spike and wave during slow-wave sleep, photosensitive seizures [110] and gelastic seizures [49,111]. There are no controlled studies investigating ethosuximide's effectiveness against simple partial, complex partial or partial secondarily generalized tonic-clonic seizures. However recent reports suggest that ethosuximide is effective in the treatment of epileptic negative myoclonus associated with childhood partial epilepsy [112].

Side-effects

Ethosuximide's adverse events can be divided into four categories: (a) commonly observed; (b) infrequent but clinically relevant; (c) rare potentially life threatening; and (d) manifestations of overdose. Like most drugs [113,114], the most commonly observed adverse effects are directly related to the primary and secondary pharmacological effect of the drug, are usually predictable, dose dependent, host independent and resolve with dose reduction. The infrequent but clinically relevant adverse effects may result from multiple mechanisms including (a) dose-dependent, pharmacologically related side-effects; (b) effects of long-term therapy related to the cumulative dose; and (c) delayed effects of a drug (such as teratogenicity and carcinogenicity) that are dose independent but host dependent [113,114]. The rare potentially life-threatening adverse events, also called idiosyncratic drug reactions, cannot be predicted based upon the known pharmacological effect of the drug. These side-effects do not demonstrate a simple dose–response relationship, are host dependent, and can be serious and life threatening [115].

Commonly observed

Twelve large clinical trials (each involving over 50 patients) published between 1958 and 1966 detailed the spectrum of ethosuximide's adverse effects. Browne summarized these studies and found the overall incidence of ethosuximide-related adverse effects ranged from 26% to 46% (Table 32.1) [116–128]. In half of these large trials, 37% or more of the subjects experienced ethosuximide-related adverse effects [116].

Gastrointestinal

The most common ethosuximide concentration-dependent adverse effects involve the gastrointestinal system. These symptoms include nausea (the most common), abdominal discomfort, anorexia, vomiting and diarrhoea [1,7,49,129–131]. Symptoms usually occur at the onset of therapy, are considered mild in severity, affect 20–33% of children and resolve promptly to dose reduction [49,129–131]. In some patients the adverse effect is transient and no dose reduction is needed; in others dividing the total daily dosage and administering the smaller doses at mealtime helps lessen the symptoms

Table 32.1 Summary of adverse effect profiles noted in early studies involving 50 or more subjects receiving ethosuximide (12 reports, 1958–1966)

Adverse effect	Ethosuximide range (median, both in %)
Any adverse effect	26–46 (37)
Gastrointestinal disturbances (nausea, abdominal discomfort, anorexia, vomiting and diarrhoea)	4–29 (13)
Drowsiness	0–16 (7)
Rash	0–6 (0)
Ataxia	0–1 (0)
Dizziness	0–4 (1)
Hiccups	0–5 (0)
Irritability	0 (0)

Modified from [116] with permission, references [117–128].

[6,116]. Infrequently gastrointestinal symptoms are severe enough to cause discontinuation of ethosuximide [116].

Neurological

The second most common form of ethosuximide concentration-dependent adverse events is central nervous system related adverse events such as drowsiness [116]. Similar to the gastrointestinal side-effects, drowsiness usually occurs at the onset of therapy and resolves promptly when the ethosuximide dose is reduced [6,129–131].

Additional central nervous system related adverse events include insomnia, nervousness (12% of children), dizziness, hiccups, lethargy, fatigue, ataxia and behaviour changes (e.g. aggression, euphoria, irritability, hyperactivity) [7,131]. A direct relationship between these reported behavioural changes and ethosuximide therapy is not certain since poor study methodology make analysis of existing reports difficult at best. The lack of reliable methods for objectively measuring behaviour changes, the confounding variables of polypharmacy and the lack of serum AED concentrations during the studies are examples of these methodological concerns [129,130].

Headaches occur in approximately 14% of children taking ethosuximide. In contrast to the other neurological side-effects described above, these headaches do not appear to be concentration dependent, may not respond to dose reduction and may be persistent [6,129–132].

Assessing ethosuximide's effects on cognition is difficult. Few clinical trials have examined the issue in a controlled fashion accounting for confounding variables such as plasma concentrations, underlying mental retardation, concomitant AEDs or seizure type. Memory, speech and emotional disturbances were noted on psychometric testing in 25 children receiving ethosuximide for various seizure types in one early report [133]. However all the patients were also on barbiturates, 60% of the cohort had IQ scores below 83, no ethosuximide plasma concentrations were measured and no matched control group was used [133]. In contrast, ethosuximide therapy resulted in significant improvement in verbal and full scale IQ scores without change in motor performance or personality test scores in a cohort of children without epilepsy but with learning disorders and 14 and 6 per second positive spikes on EEG [134] Similarly, psychometric performance improved significantly over 8 weeks of ethosuximide therapy in 17 of 37 (46%) of children with absence seizures in a well-designed study [95]. This improvement was significantly different compared to a control group of patients tested in the same fashion over the same interval [95]. Only 25% of the study group had IQ scores less than 83 and only 32% were on other AEDs [95].

Infrequent but clinically relevant

Psychiatric

Some patients taking ethosuximide have developed episodes of psychotic behaviour manifested by anxiety, depression, visual hallucinations, auditory hallucinations and intermittent impairment of consciousness [119,129,135–137]. The patient's age (young adults in their teens or twenties) and a history of mental illness are risk factors for this adverse effect [6,116,129]. The acute psychotic episodes appeared following ethosuximide-induced seizure control with associated EEG improvement. The episodes resolved when ethosuximide was stopped and seizures returned, possibly illustrating the phenomena of 'forced normalization' [6,129]. Psychotic symptoms have recurred when ethosuximide was restarted in patients with previous ethosuximide-related psychotic episodes [129]. Among all antiabsence AEDs, this 'forced normalization' reaction occurs with highest frequency with ethosuximide and is not dose dependent [6,138]. This type of side-effect seldom occurs in young children with no previous history of psychiatric disease receiving ethosuximide for typical absence seizures [116].

Neurological

No evidence of ethosuximide-associated seizure exacerbation is found in most studies [95,121,126,128,129,139]. Exacerbation of myoclonic and absence seizures and transformation of absence into 'grand mal' seizures in patients receiving ethosuximide are reported in scattered reports [129,140,141]. Dreifuss considered this 'exacerbation' effect to be a consequence of the high incidence of generalized tonic-clonic seizures in patients with absence seizures coupled with ethosuximide's lack of efficacy against generalized tonic-clonic seizures [129].

Long-term cumulative dose ethosuximide side-effects are infrequent. Extrapyramidal reactions (e.g. severe bradykinesia, akasthesias, dyskinesias and parkinsonian syndrome) have been noted after several years of ethosuximide treatment [120,142].

Haematological

The incidence of ethosuximide-related granulocytopenia ranged from 0% to 7% in early studies [116]. This symptom has been considered probably dose dependent since it often resolved with dose reduction without requiring termination of ethosuximide therapy [129,130]. It is critical to distinguish between this probable dose-dependent haematological adverse event and ethosuximide-associated idiosyncratic bone marrow depression (see below). Careful clinical and laboratory monitoring is essential in making this distinction.

Other organ systems

Ethosuximide therapy is not reported to cause hepatotoxicity or serious endocrine adverse effects [116]. Ethosuximide can precipitate an attack of acute intermittent porphyria [131,143].

Little information is available about the overall risks maternal ethosuximide use poses to the fetus [129]. There is currently not enough data to assess accurately the teratogenic effect of ethosuximide in humans. There is one study that found two out of 13 newborns (born to 10 women with epilepsy taking ethosuximide) had major malformations (bilateral clefting, hare-lip). In addition, the cohort had a higher rate of minor abnormalities compared to a pair matched control group of newborns of women without epilepsy [61]. The mothers of these two seriously affected newborns were on ethosuximide in combination with phenobarbital in one mother and primidone in the other mother [61]. In another small series, one of five infants born to a mother taking ethosuximide was malformed [144].

Rare, potentially life threatening

Idiosyncratic drug reactions are serious, potentially, life-threatening adverse events that are unpredictable, dose-independent, host-dependent reactions that cannot be predicted based upon the known pharmacological effect of the drug [113,114]. In general, the skin is the most commonly affected site followed by the formed elements of the blood and the liver, and to a lesser extent the nervous system and kidneys [113,145]. These reactions can be very organ specific or present with generalized non-specific symptoms, such as lymphadenopathy, arthralgias, eosinophilia and fever [113,146]. Idiosyncratic reactions probably result from toxic metabolites that either directly or indirectly (by way of an immunological response or free radical mediated process) cause injury [115].

Ethosuximide has been associated (to varying degrees) with a wide variety of idiosyncratic reactions [129–131,147] including allergic dermatitis, rash, erythema multiforme, Stevens–Johnson syndrome [148], systemic lupus erythematosus [149–151], a lupus-like syndrome [129,152–154], blood dyscrasias (aplastic anaemia, agranulocytosis) [95,122,127,139,155–160], dyskinesia [161, 162], akathisia [161], autoimmune thyroiditis [163] and diminished renal allograft survival [164].

Dermatological

The most common idiosyncratic reactions associated with ethosuximide involve the skin. Allergic dermatitis and rash frequently resolve following ethosuximide withdrawal but some patients may require steroid therapy. Patients developing Stevens–Johnson syndrome, a potentially life-threatening condition, require hospitalization for more aggressive therapy.

Haematological

Ethosuximide-associated blood dyscrasias can involve any or all cell lines ranging from thrombocytopenia to pancytopenia and aplastic anaemia [95,122,127,139,155–159]. Only eight cases of ethosuximide-associated aplastic anaemia have been reported between 1958 and 1994 with onset 6 weeks to 8 months after ethosuximide initiation [158] Six patients were on polypharmacy, five taking either phenytoin or ethotoin in combination with ethosuximide [158]. Despite therapy, five of the eight patients died [95,122,127,139,155–159].

Other organ systems

The symptoms of the lupus-like syndrome are described as 'fever, malar rash, arthritis, lymphadenopathy, and, on occasion, pleural effusions, myocarditis, and pericarditis' [129]. Following ethosuximide discontinuation, patients with a lupus-like syndrome usually fully recover but recovery may be prolonged [129].

Manifestations of overdose

The manifestations of acute ethosuximide overdose include nausea, vomiting and symptoms of central nervous system depression including stupor and coma leading to respiratory depression. The management of an ethosuximide overdose involves life support measures, symptomatic treatment, procedures to decrease drug absorption and procedures to enhance drug elimination. Life support measures involve initial and immediate evaluation and stabilization of the patient's airway, breathing and circulation. Symptomatic treatment focuses on the subsequent care for each of the patient's overdose symptoms as they occur. No specific antidote exists for an ethosuximide overdose.

Methods to decrease absorption

Three potentially useful methods to decrease drug absorption following any overdose include induction of emesis, use of activated charcoal and use of gastric lavage. Since an ethosuximide overdose can rapidly lead to significant alteration of consciousness, induction of emesis is not recommended [165]. Administration of activated charcoal as an aqueous slurry may reduce absorption in conscious patients able to protect their airway. The effectiveness of activated charcoal is greatest if given within 1 h of an ethosuximide overdose [165]. The recommended dose of activated charcoal is 1 g/kg of weight for infants up to 1 year old, 25–50 g in children between 1 and 12 years old and 25–100 g in adults. The optimal dose has not been established [166]. If emesis or rapid deterioration of consciousness occurs or is impending, only personnel skilled in airway management should administer activated charcoal to minimize the potential for aspiration. The contraindications for the use of activated charcoal are a patient with an unprotected airway or if the therapy increases the risk or severity of aspiration [166].

Gastric lavage with a large-bore orogastric tube may be considered if a potentially life-threatening amount of succinimide has been ingested and the procedure can be performed within 1 h of the ingestion [167]. Gastric lavage should not be employed routinely in the management of patients following an overdose of ethosuximide due to the risk of significant morbidity associated with the procedure [167].

Methods to enhance drug elimination

Following a drug overdose, four potentially useful methods to enhance elimination are haemodialysis, haemoperfusion, exchange transfusion and forced diuresis. Haemodialysis may be useful in the treatment of an ethosuximide overdose. This is based an observed extraction efficiency of 61–100% in one study of four patients with chronic renal disease (supported by haemodialysis) who received a single dose of 500 mg of ethosuximide 4 h prior to dialysis. In this study the elimination half-life of ethosuximide was reduced by dialysis to an average of 3.5 h [168]. There have been no reports of haemoperfusion use in ethosuximide overdose. Both exchange transfusion and forced diuresis have little place in the treatment of ethosuximide overdose since ethosuximide has low protein binding and little of the parent ethosuximide compound is excreted unchanged in the urine.

Clinical therapeutics

Place in therapy

Ethosuximide and valproic acid are considered as 'treatment of choice' for first-line monotherapy against typical absence seizures in an expert consensus guideline [169]. Although ethosuximide may be the first choice in children less than 10 years old with absence epilepsy, as these children approach adolescence and the risk of generalized tonic-clonic seizures increases, many experts conclude valproic acid becomes the drug of choice [170].

Ethosuximide adjunctive therapy may be beneficial for (a) patients whose absence seizures are not controlled on valproic acid monotherapy; (b) patients with atypical absence seizures; and (c) patients with both absence and tonic-clonic seizures [7,49,71,103,170]. There is no evidence supporting a role for ethosuximide monotherapy or ethosuximide adjunctive therapy in patients with only simple partial, complex partial or partial secondarily generalized tonic-clonic seizures.

Additional clinical situations where ethosuximide may be useful include absence status epilepticus [104,105], severe myoclonic epilepsy in infancy [106], childhood epileptic encephalopathy (the Lennox–Gastaut syndrome) [4,107], juvenile myoclonic epilepsy [108,109], epilepsy with myoclonic absences [109], eyelid myoclonia with absences [109], epilepsy with continuous spike and wave during slow-wave sleep, photosensitive seizures [110], gelastic seizures [49,111] and epileptic negative myoclonus associated with childhood partial epilepsy [112].

Dose and titration rates

A common starting dose for children is 10–15 mg/kg/day; subsequent titration is performed according to the patient's clinical response [6,7]. Older children and adults often initiate ethosuximide at 250 mg/day and increase by 250 mg increments until the desired clinical response is reached. Ethosuximide can be administered either as once, twice or even thrice daily dosing (with meals) to maximize seizure control while minimizing adverse effects [6,7]. The interval between dosage changes for older children and adults varies from 3 days [7] to every 12–15 days [6].

In younger children, maintenance dosages frequently range from 15 to 40 mg/kg/day [71]. For older children and adults, common maintenance doses are 750–1500 mg/day [6,7]. When used in elderly patients, ethosuximide should be titrated using smaller increments with longer intervals between changes [7]. The time to reach steady-state concentration following a dosage change is 6–7 days for children and 12 days for adults [6,71].

If the clinical situation warrants discontinuing ethosuximide (e.g. intolerable side-effects without seizure control or ≥2 years free of absence seizures), then gradual reduction over 4–8 weeks is recommended [6,7]. If necessary, abrupt discontinuation is probably safe due to ethosuximide's long half-life [7].

Therapeutic ranges

Ethosuximide should always be titrated to clinical response (i.e. maximal seizure control with minimal side-effects). The generally accepted therapeutic range for ethosuximide is 40–100 µg/mL [6,7]. Some patients with refractory seizures or absence status may need serum concentrations up to 150 µg/mL [7]. Monitoring of ethosuximide serum concentration may aid in maximizing seizure control and is useful to identify non-compliance [96].

Laboratory monitoring

There is no evidence that laboratory monitoring of blood counts during ethosuximide therapy anticipates ethosuximide's idiosyncratic haematological reactions. Patient education is important; patients need to watch for fever, sore throat, and cutaneous or other haemorrhages, and alert their physician immediately if these symptoms occur [129]. However, one recommendation for blood monitoring has been that 'periodic blood counts be performed at no greater than monthly intervals for the duration of treatment with ethosuximide and that the dosage be reduced or the drug discontinued should the total white-blood-cell count fall below 3,500 or the proportion of granulocytes below 25% of the total white-blood-cell count' [129].

References

1 Brodie M, Dichter M. Established antiepileptic drugs. *Seizure* 1997; 6 (3): 159–74.
2 Lennox W. The petit mal epilepsies: their treatment with tridione. *JAMA* 1945; 129: 1069–74.
3 Lennox W. Tridione in the treatment of epilepsy. *JAMA* 1947; 134: 138–43.
4 Mattson RH. Efficacy and adverse effects of established and new antiepileptic drugs. *Epilepsia* 1995; 36 (Suppl. 2): S13–26.
5 Rogawski M, Porter R. Antiepileptic drugs. Pharmacological mechanisms and clinical efficacy with consideration of promising developmental state compounds. *Pharmacol Rev* 1990; 42: 223–86.
6 Sabers A, Dam M. Ethosuximide and Methsuximide. In: Shorvon S, Dreifuss F, Fish D, Thomas D , eds. *The Treatment of Epilepsy*. London: Blackwell Science, 1996: 414–20.
7 Bromfield E. Ethosuximide and other succinimides. In: Engel J, Pedley T, eds. *Epilepsy: a Comprehensive Textbook*. Philadelphia: Lippincott-Raven, 1997: 1503–8.
8 Millership JS, Mifsud J, Collier PS. The metabolism of ethosuximide. *Eur J Drug Metab Pharmacokin* 1993; 18 (4): 349–53.
9 Pisani F, Meir B. Ethosuximide. Chemistry and biotransformation. In: Levy R, Mattson R, Meldrum B, eds. *Antiepileptic Drugs*. New York: Raven Press Ltd, 1995: 655–8.
10 White HS. Comparative anticonvulsant and mechanistic profile of the established and newer antiepileptic drugs. *Epilepsia* 1999; 40 (Suppl. 5): S2–10.
11 Macdonald RL, Kelly KM. Antiepileptic drug mechanisms of action. *Epilepsia* 1993; 34 (Suppl. 5): S1–8.
12 Davies JA. Mechanisms of action of antiepileptic drugs. *Seizure* 1995; 4 (4): 267–71.
13 Coulter C, Huguenard J, Price D. Characterization of ethosuximide reduction of low-threshold calcium current in thalamic neurons. *Ann Neurol* 1989; 25: 582–93.
14 Ferrendelli J, Holland K. Ethosuximide, Mechanisms of Action. In: Levy R, Mattson, R, Meldrum B, Perry J, Dreifuss F, eds. *Antiepileptic Drugs*, 3rd edn. New York: Raven Press Ltd, 1989: 653–61.
15 Lin-Mitchell E, Chweh A. Effects of ethosuximide alone and in combination with gamma-aminobutyric acid receptor antagonists on brain gamma-aminobutyric acid concentration, anticonvulsant activity, and neurotoxicity in mice. *J Pharmacol Exp Ther* 1986; 237: 486–9.
16 Gilbert J, Buchan P, Scott A. Effects of anticonvulsant drug on monosaccharide transport and membrane ATPase activities of cerebral cortex. In: Harris, P, Mawdsley, C, eds. *Epilepsy*. Edinburgh: Churchill Livingstone, 1974: 98–104.
17 Gilbert J, Scott A, Wyllie M. Effects of ethosuximide on adenosine triphosphate activities of some subcellular fractions perpared from rat cerebral cortex. *Br J Pharmacol* 1974; 50: 452P–453P.
18 Gilbert J, Wyllie M. The effects of the anticonvulsant ethosuximide on adenosine triphosphatase activities of synaptosomes prepared from rat cerebral cortex. *Br J Pharmacol* 1974; 52: 139P–140P.
19 El-Sayed M, Loscher W, Frey H. Pharmacokinetics of ethosuximide in the dog. *Arch Int Pharmacodyn Ther* 1978; 234: 180–92.
20 Patel I, Levy R, Bauer T. Pharmacokinetic properties of ethosuximide in monkeys. Single dose intravenous and oral administration. *Epilepsia* 1975; 16: 705–16.
21 Patel I, Levy R. Pharmacokinetic properites of ethosuximide in monkeys. II. Chronic intravenous and oral administration. *Epilepsia* 1975; 16: 717–30.
22 Patel I, Levy R, Rapport R. Distribution characteristics of ethosuximide in discrete areas of rat brain. *Epilepsia* 1977; 18: 533–41.
23 Bialer M, Ziadong S, Perucca E. Ethosuximide: absorption, distribution, excretion. In: Levy R, Mattson R, Meldrum B, eds. *Antiepileptic Drugs*. New York: Raven Press, 1995: 659–65.
24 Chang T, Ethosuximide. Absorption, distribution, and excretion. In: Levy R, Mattson R, Meldrum B, Penry J, Dreifuss F, eds. *Antiepileptic Drugs*. New York: Raven Press, 1989: 671–8.
25 Chang T, Dill W, Glazko A, Ethosuximide. Absorption, distribution and excretion. In: Woodburg D, Penry J, Schmidt R, eds. *Antiepileptic Drugs*. New York: Raven Press, 1972: 417–23.
26 Loscher W, Frey H. Kinetics of penetration of common anticonvulsant drugs in serum of dog and man. *Epilepsia* 1984; 25: 346–52.
27 Aguilar-Veiga E, Sierra-Paredes G, Galan-Valiente J, Soto-Otero R, Mendez-Alvarez E, Sierra-Marcuno G. Correlations between ethosuximide brain levels measured by high performance liquid chromatography and its antiepileptic potential. *Res Comm Chem Pathol Pharmacol* 1991; 7: 351–64.
28 Bachmann K, Jahn D, Yang C, Schwartz J. Ethosuximide disposition kinetics in rats. *Xenobiotica* 1988; 18: 373–80.
29 Burkett A, Chang T, Glazko A. A hydroxylated metabolite of ethosuximide (Zarontin) in rat urine. *Fed Proc* 1971; 30: 391.
30 Chang T, Ethosuximide. Biotransformation. In: Levy R, Mattson R, Meldrum B, Penry J, Dreifuss F, eds. *Antiepileptic Drugs*. New York: Raven Press, 1989: 679–83.
31 Bachmann K. The use of single sample clearance estimates to probe hepatic drug metabolism in rats. IV A model for possible application to phenotyping xenobiotic influences on human drug metabolism. *Xenobiotica* 1989; 19: 1449–59.
32 Bachmann K, Chu C, Greear V. In vivo evidence that ethosuximide is a substrate for cytochrome P450IIIA. *Pharmacology* 1992; 45: 121–8.
33 Patel I, Levy R, Bauer T. Time dependent kinetics. II. Diurnal oscillations

in steady state plasma ethosuximide levels in rhesus monkeys. *J Pharm Sci* 1977; 66: 650–3.

34 White HS. Clinical significance of animal seizure models and mechanism of action studies of potential antiepileptic drugs. *Epilepsia* 1997; 38 (Suppl. 1): S9–17.

35 Reinhard J, Reinhard J. Experimental evaluation of anticonvulsants. In: Vida J, eds. *Anticonvulsants*. New York: Academic Press, 1977: 57–111.

36 Woodbury D. Applications to drug evaluations. In: Purpura P, Penry J, Tower D, Woodbury D, Walter R, eds. *Experimental Models of Epilepsy: a Manual for the Laboratory Worker*. New York: Raven Press, 1972: 557–83.

37 Swinyard E, Woodhead J, White H, Franklin M. General principles. Experimental selection, quantification and evaluation of anticonvulsants. In: Levy R, Mattson R, Meldrum B, Penry J, Dreifuss F, eds. *Antiepileptic Drugs*. New York: Raven Press, 1989: 85–102.

38 Heller A, Dichter M, Sidman R. Anticonvulsant sensitivity of absence seizures in the tottering mutant mouse. *Epilepsia* 1983; 25: 25–34.

39 Marescaux C, Micheletti G, Vergnes M, Depaulis A, Rumbach L, Warter J. A model of chronic spontaneous petit mal-like seizures in the rat: comparison with pentylenetetrazol-induced seizures. *Epilepsia* 1984; 25: 326–31.

40 Sasa M, Ohno Y, Ujihara H. Effects of antiepileptic drugs on absence-like and tonic seizures in the spontaneously epileptic rat, a double mutant rat. *Epilepsia* 1988; 29 (5): 505–13.

41 Godschalk M, Dzoljic M, Bonta I. Antagonism of gamma-hydroxybutyrate-induced hypersynchronization in the ECoG of the rat by anti-petit mal drugs. *Neurosci Lett* 1976; 3: 145–50.

42 Snead OI. Gamma-hydroxybutyrate in the monkey, II. Effect of chronic oral anticonvulsant drugs. *Neurology* 1978; 28: 643–8.

43 Snead OI. Gamma-hydroxybutyrate model of generalized absence seizures: further characterization and comparison with other absence models. *Epilepsia* 1988; 29: 361–8.

44 Villen T, Bertilsson L, Sjoqvist F. Nonstereoselective disposition of ethosuximide in humans. *Ther Drug Monit* 1990; 12: 514–16.

45 Tomson T, Villen T. Ethosuximide enantiomers in pregnancy and lactation. *Ther Drug Monit* 1994; 16 (6): 621–3.

46 Buchanan R, Fernandez L, Kinkel A. Absorption and elimination of ethosuximide in children. *J Clin Pharmacol* 1969; 7: 213–18.

47 Eadie M, Tyrer J, Smith J, McKauge L. Pharmacokinetics of drugs used for petit mal absence epilepsy. *Clin Exp Neurol* 1977; 14: 172–83.

48 Alvarez N, Besag F, Iivanainen M. Use of antiepileptic drugs in the treatment of epilepsy in people with intellectual disability. *J Intellect Disabil Res* 1998; 42 (Suppl. 1): 1–15.

49 Wallace SJ. Use of ethosuximide and valproate in the treatment of epilepsy. *Neurologic Clinics* 1986; 4 (3): 601–16.

50 Liu H, Al E. Therapeutic drug concentration monitoring using saliva samples. Focus on anticonvulsants. *Clin Pharmacokinet* 1999; 36 (6): 453–70.

51 Buchanan R, Kinkel A, Smith T. The absorption and excretion of ethosuximide. *Int J Clin Pharmacol* 1973; 7: 213–18.

52 Horning M, Brown L, Nowlin J, Lertratanangkoon K, Kellaway P, Zion T. Use of saliva in therapeutic drug monitoring. *Clin Chem* 1977; 23: 157–64.

53 Piredda S, Monaco F. Ethosuximide in tears, saliva and cerebral fluid. *Ther Drug Monit* 1981; 3: 321–3.

54 McAuliffe J, Sherwin A, Leppik I, Fayle S, Pippenger C. Salivary levels of anticonvulsants: a practical approach to drug monitoring. *Neurology (Minn)* 1977; 27: 409–13.

55 Van H. Comparative study of the levels of anticonvulsants and their free fraction in venous blood, saliva and capillary blood in man. *J Pharmacol* 1984; 15 (1): 27–35.

56 Bachmann K, Schwartz J, Sullivan T, Jauregui L. Single sample estimate of ethosuximide clearance. *Int J Clin Pharmacol Ther Toxicol* 1986; 24 (10): 546–50.

57 Meyer F, Quednow B, Potrafki A, Walther G. Pharmacokinetics of anticonvulsants in the perinatal period. *Gynakol* 1988; 110 (19): 1195–205.

58 Horning M, Stratton C, Nowlin J, Harvey D, Hill R. Metabolism of 2-ethyl-2-methylsuccinimide in the rat and human. *Drug Metab Dispos* 1973; 1: 569–76.

59 Koup J, Rose J, Cohen M. Ethosuximide pharmacokinetics in a pregnant patient and her newborn. *Epilepsia* 1978; 19: 535–9.

60 Kaneko S, Sato T, Suzuki K. The levels of anticonvulsants in breast milk. *Br J Clin Pharmacol* 1979; 7: 624–7.

61 Kuhnz W, Koch S, Hartmann A, Helge H, Nau N. Ethosuximide in epileptic women during pregnancy and lactation period. Placental transfer, serum concentrations in nursed infants and clinical status. *Br J Clin Pharmacol* 1984; 18: 671–7.

62 Rane A, Tunell R. Ethosuximide in human milk and in plasma of a mother and her nursed infant. *Br J Clin Pharmacol* 1981; 12: 855–8.

63 Eadie MJ. Formation of active metabolites of anticonvulsant drugs. A review of their pharmacokinetic and therapeutic significance. *Biomed Chromatogr* 1991; 5 (5): 212–15.

64 Tanaka E. Clinically significant pharmacokinetic drug interactions between antiepileptic drugs. *J Clin Pharm Ther* 1999; 24 (2): 87–92.

65 Gilbert J, Scott A, Galloway D, Petrie J, Ethosuximide. liver enzyme induction and D-glucaric acid excretion. *Br J Clin Pharmacol* 1974; 1: 249–52.

66 Glazko A. Antiepileptic drugs. biotransformation, metabolism, and serum half-life. *Epilepsia* 1975; 16: 376–91.

67 Bauer L, Harris C, Wilensky A, Raisys V, Levy R. Ethosuximide kinetics: possible interaction with valproic acid. *Clin Pharmacol Ther* 1982; 31: 741–5.

68 Dill W, Peterson L, Chang T, Glazko A. Physiologic disposition of alpha-methyl-alpha-ethyl succinimide (ethosuximide; Zarontin) in animals and in man. In: *149th National Meeting of the American Chemical Society*, 1965. Detroit, Michigan: American Chemical Society, 1965.

69 Pisani P, Narbone M, Trunfio C. Valproic acid–ethosuximide interaction: a pharmacokinetic study. *Epilepsia* 1984; 25: 229–33.

70 Buchanan R, Kinkel A, Turner J, Heffelfinger J. Ethosuximide dosage regimens. *Clin Pharmacol Ther* 1976; 19: 143–7.

71 Sherwin A. Ethosuximide: clinical use. In: Levy R, Mattson R, Meldrum B, eds. *Antiepileptic Drugs*. New York: Raven Press, 1995: 667–73.

72 Bachmann KA, Schwartz J, Jauregui L, Sullivan TJ, Martin M. Use of three probes to assess the influence of sex on hepatic drug metabolism. *Pharmacology* 1987; 35 (2): 88–93.

73 Browne T, Feldman R, Buchanan R. Methsuximide for complex seizures. efficacy, toxicity, clinical pharmacology, and drug interactions. *Neurology (Cleveland)* 1983; 33: 414–18.

74 Dawson G, Brown H, Clark B. Serum phenytoin after ethosuximide. *Ann Neurol* 1978; 4 (6): 583–4.

75 Frantzen E, Hansen J, Hansen O, Kristensen M. Phenytoin (Dilantin) Intoxication. *Acta Neurol Scand* 1967; 43 (4): 440–6.

76 Rambeck B. Pharmacological interactions of methsuximide with phenobarbital and phenytoin in hospitalized epileptic patients. *Epilepsia* 1979; 20 (2): 147–56.

77 Smith G, McKauge L, Dubetz D, Tyrer J, Werth B. Factors influencing plasma concentrations of ethosuximide. *Clin Pharmacokinet* 1979; 4 (1): 38–52.

78 Schmidt D. The effect of phenytoin and ethosuximide on primidone metabolism in patients with epilepsy. *J Neurol* 1975; 209 (2): 115–23.

79 Battino D, Avanzini G, Bossi L. Plasma levels of primidone and its metabolite phenobarbital: effect of age and associated therapy. *Ther Drug Monit* 1983; 5 (1): 73–9.

80 Riva R, Albani F, Contin M, Baruzzi A. Pharmacokinetic interactions between antiepileptic drugs. Clinical considerations. *Clin Pharmacokinet* 1996; 31 (6): 470–93.

81 Eadie M, Vajda F. *Antiepileptic Drugs. Pharmacology and Therapeutics*. Berlin: Springer-Verlag, 1999.

82 Salke-Kellermann R, May T, Boenigk H. Influence of ethosuximide on valproic acid serum concentrations. *Epilepsy Res* 1997; 26: 345–9.

83 Warren JJ, Benmaman J, Wannamaker B, Levy R. Kinetics of a carbamazepine–ethosuximide interaction. *Clin Pharmacol* 1980; 28: 646–51.

84 Battino D, Cusi C, Franceschetti S, Moise A, Spina S, Avanzini G. Ethosuximide plasma concentrations. Influence of age and associated concomitant therapy. *Clin Pharmacokinet* 1982; 7 (2): 176–80.

85 Bachmann K, Jauregui L. Use of single sample clearance estimates of cytochrome P450 substrates to characterize human hepatic CYP status in vivo. *Xenobiotica* 1993; 23 (3): 307–15.

86 Giaconne M, Bartoli A, Gatti G *et al.* Effect of enyzme inducing anticonvulsants on ethosuximide pharmacokinetics in epileptic patients. *Br J Clin Pharmacol* 1996; 41 (6): 575–9.

87 Duncan JS, Patsalos PN, Shorvon SD. Effects of discontinuation of phenytoin, carbamazepine, and valproate on concomitant antiepileptic medication. *Epilepsia* 1991; 32 (1): 101–15.

88 Bourgeois B. Pharmacologic interactions between valproate and other drugs. *Am J Med* 1988; 84 (1A): 28–33.

89 Gram L, Wulff K, Rasmussen K, Flachs H. Valproate sodium. A controlled clinical trial including monitoring of drug levels. *Epilepsia* 1977; 18 (2): 141–8.

90 Mattson R, Cramer J. Valproic acid and ethosuximide interaction. *Ann Neurol* 1980; 7 (6): 583–4.

91 Levy R, Koch K. Drug interactions with valproic acid. *Drugs* 1982; 24: 543–56.

92 van Wieringen A, Vrijlandt C. Ethosuximide intoxication caused by interaction with isoniazid. *Neurology* 1983; 33: 1227–8.

93 Marbury T, Lee C, Perchalski R. Hemodialysis clearance of ethosuximide in patients with chronic renal failure. *Am J Hosp Pharm* 1981; 38: 1757–60.

94 Marquardt E, Ishisaka D, Batra K, Chin B. Removal of ethosuximide and phenobarbital by peritoneal dialysis in a child. *Clin Pharm* 1992; 11 (12): 1030–1.

95 Browne TR, Dreifuss FE, Dyken PR *et al.* Ethosuximide in the treatment of absence (petit mal) seizures. *Neurology (Minneapolis)* 1975; 25 (6): 515–24.

96 Sherwin A, Robb P, Lechter M. Improved control of epilepsy by monitoring plasma ethosuximide. *Arch Neurol* 1973; 28: 178–81.

97 Callaghan N, Odriscoll D, Daley M. A comparative study between ethosuximide and sodium valproate in the treatment of petit mal epilepsy. In: *Royal Society of Medicine International Congress and Symposium, No. 30: the Place of Sodium Valproate in the Treatment of Epilepsy*. London: Academic Press, 1980: 47–52.

98 Callaghan N, Ohara J, Odriscoll D, Oneill B, Daly M. Comparative study of ethosuximide and sodium valproate in the treatment of typical absence seizures (petit mal). *Dev Med Child Neurol* 1982; 24: 830–6.

99 Martinovic Z. Comparison of ethosuximide with sodium valproate. In: Parsonage M, Grant R, Craig AAW Jr, eds. *Advances in Epileptology, XIVth Epilepsy International Symposium*. New York: Raven Press, 1983: 301–5.

100 Santavuori P. Absence seizures: Valproate or ethosuximide? *Acta Neurol Scand* 1983; 69 (9): 41–8.

101 Sato S, White BG, Penry JK, Dreifuss FE, Sackellares JC, Kupferberg HJ. Valproic acid versus ethosuximide in the treatment of absence seizures. *Neurology* 1982; 32 (2): 157–63.

102 Rowan A, Meijer J, Debeer-Pawlikowski N, Meinardi H. Valproate-ethosuximide combination therapy for refractory absence seizures. *Arch Neurol* 1983; 40: 797–802.

103 Sherwin A. Ethosuximide: clinical use. In: Levy R, Dreifus F, Mattson R, Medrum B, Penry J, eds. *Antiepileptic Drugs*. New York: Raven Press, 1989: 685–98.

104 Guberman A, Cantu-Reyna G, Stuss D, Broughton R. Nonconvulsive generalized status epilepticus. clinical features, neuropsychological testing, and long-term follow-up. *Neurology* 1986; 36: 1284–91.

105 Porter R, Penry J. Petit mal status. In: Delgado-Escueta A, Waterlain C, Treiman D, Porter R, eds. *Status Epilepticus Mechanisms of Brain Damage and Treatment*. New York: Raven Press, 1983: 61–7.

106 Roger J, Genton P, Bureau M, Dravet C. Less common epileptic syndromes. In: Wyllie E, ed. *The Treatment Of Epilepsy: Principles and Practice*. Philadelphia: Lea & Febiger, 1993: 624–35.

107 Farrell K. Secondary generalized epilepsy and Lennox–Gastaut syndrome. In: Wyllie E, ed. *The Treatment of Epilepsy: Principles and Practice*. Philadelphia: Lea & Febiger, 1993: 604–13.

108 Serratosa J, Delgado-Escueta A. Juvenile myoclonic epilepsy. In: Wyllie E, ed. *The Treatment of Epilepsy: Principles and Practice*. Philadelphia: Lea & Febiger, 1993: 552–70.

109 Wallace S. Myoclonus and epilepsy in childhood: a review of treatment with valproate, ethosuximide, lamotrigine and zonisamide. *Epilepsy Res* 1998; 29 (2): 147–54.

110 Zifkin B, Andermann F. Epilepsy with reflex seizures. In: Wyllie E, ed. *The Treatment of Epilepsy: Principles and Practice*. Philadelphia: Lea & Febiger, 1993: 614–23.

111 Ames F, Enderstein O. Ictal laughter. A case report with clinical, cinefilm, and EEG observations. *J Neurol Neurosurg Psychiatry* 1975; 38: 11–17.

112 Capovilla G, Al E. Ethosuximide is effective in the treatment of epileptic negative myoclonus in childhood partial epilepsy. *J Child Neurol* 1999; 14 (6): 395–400.

113 Park BK, Pirmohamed M, Kitteringham NR. Idiosyncratic drug reactions. A mechanistic evaluation of risk factors. *Br J Clin Pharmacol* 1992; 34 (5): 377–95.

114 Pirmohamed M, Kitteringham NR, Park BK. The role of active metabolites in drug toxicity. *Drug Saf* 1994; 11 (2): 114–44.

115 Glauser TA. Idiosyncratic reactions. new methods of identifying high-risk patients. *Epilepsia* 2000; 41 (Suppl. 8): S16–29.

116 Browne T. Ethosuximide (Zarontin) and Other Succinimides. In: Browne T, Feldman R, eds. *Epilepsy, Diagnosis and Management*. Boston: Little, Brown, 1983: 215–24.

117 Cohardon R, Loiseau P, Cohardon S. Results of treatment of certain forms of epilepsy of the petit mal type by ethosuximide. *Rev Neurol* 1964; 110: 201.

118 Dongier MS, Gastaut H, Roger J. Essai d'un nouvel anti-epileptique (PM671, alpha-ethyl-alpha-methyl-succinimide) chez l'enfant. *Rev Neurol (Paris)* 1961; 104: 441.

119 Fischer M, Korskjaer G, Pedersen E. Psychotic episodes in Zarontin treatment. Effects and side-effects in 105 patients. *Epilepsia* 1965; 6 (4): 325–34.

120 Goldensohn E, Hardie J, Borea E. Ethosuximide in the treatment of epilepsy. *JAMA* 1962; 180: 840–2.

121 Heathfield K, Jewesbury E. Treatment of petit mal with ethosuximide. *Br Med J* 1961; 2: 565.

122 Kiorboe E, Paludan J, Trolle E, Overvad E. Zarontin (ethosuximide) in the treatment of petit mal and related disorders. *Epilepsia* 1964; 5: 83–9.

123 Lorentz de Haas AM, Stoel LMK. Experiences with alpha-ethyl-alpha-methyl succinimide in the treatment of epilepsy. *Epilepsia* 1960; 1: 501.

124 Matthes A, Mallman-Muhlberger E. Erfahrungen bei der Behandlung kleiner epileptische Anfalle in Kindersalter mit Methyl-athyl-succinimid (MAS). *Munch Med Wochenschr* 1962; 104: 1095.

125 Spinner A. Indikation und Wirkung von Suxinutin bei Petit-mal-Epilepsien. *Munch Med Wochenschr* 1961; 103: 1110.

126 Vossen R. Uber die antikonvulsive Wirkung von Succinimiden. *Dtsch Med Wochenschr* 1958; 29: 1227–30.

127 Weinstein A, Allen R. Ethosuximide treatment of petit mal seizures. A study of 87 pediatric patients. *Am J Dis Child* 1966; 111: 63–7.

128 Zimmerman F, Bergemeister B. A new drug for petit mal epilepsy. *Neurology (Minneapolis)* 1958; 8: 769–76.

129 Dreifuss F. Ethosuximide: toxicity. In: Levy R, Mattson R, Meldrum B, eds. *Antiepileptic Drugs*. New York: Raven Press, 1995: 675–9.

130 Dreifuss F. Ethosuximide: toxicity. In: Levy R, Mattson R, Meldrum B, Penry J, Dreifuss F, eds. *Antiepileptic Drugs*. New York: Raven Press, 1989: 699–705.

131 Wallace SJ. A comparative review of the adverse effects of anticonvulsants in children with epilepsy. *Drug Saf* 1996; 15 (6): 378–93.

132 Abu-Arafeh I, Wallace S. Unwanted effects of antiepileptic drugs. *Dev Med Child Neurol* 1988; 30: 117–21.

133 Guey J, Charles C, Coquery C, Roger J, Soulayrol R. Study of psychological effects of ethosuximide (Zarontin) on 25 children suffering from petit mal epilepsy. *Epilepsia* 1967; 8: 129–41.

134 Smith L, Phillips M, Guard H. Psychometric study of children with learning problems and 14–6 positive spike EEG patterns, treated with ethosuximide (Zarontin) and placebo. *Arch Dis Child* 1968; 43: 616–19.

135 Cohadon F, Loiseau P, Cohadon S. Results of treatment of certain forms of epilepsy of the petit mal type by ethosuximide. *Rev Neurol* 1964; 110: 201–7.

136 Lairy C. Psychotic signs in epileptics during treatment with ethosuximide. *Rev Neurol* 1964; 110: 225–6.

137 Sato T, Kondo Y, Matsuo T, Iwata H, Okuyama Y, Aoki Y. Clinical experiences of ethosuximide (Zarontin) in therapy-resistant epileptics. *Brain Nerve (Toyko)* 1965; 17: 958–64.

138 Wolf P, Inoue Y, Roder-Wanner U-U, Tsai J-J. Psychiatric complications of absence therapy and their relation to alteration of sleep. *Epilepsia* 1984; 25 (Suppl. 1): S56–9.

139 Buchanan R. Ethosuximide: toxicity. In: Woodbury D, Penry J, Schmidt R, eds. *Antiepileptic Drugs*. New York: Raven Press, 1972: 449–54.

140 Gordon N. Treatment of epilepsy with O-ethyl-O-methylsuccinimide (P.M. 671). *Neurology (Minn)* 1961; 11: 266–8.

141 Todorov A, Lenn N, Gabor A. Exacerbation of generalized nonconvulsive seizures with ethosuximide therapy. *Arch Neurol* 1978; 35: 389–91.

142 Porter R, Penry J, Dreifuss F. Responsiveness at the onset of spike-wave bursts. *Electroencephalogr Clin Neurophysiol* 1973; 34: 239–45.

143 Reynolds NC Jr, Miska RM. Safety of anticonvulsants in hepatic porphyrias. *Neurology* 1981; 31 (4): 480–4.

144 Dansky L, Andermann E, Sherwin A. Maternal epilepsy and birth defects: a prospective study with monitoring of plasma anticonvulsant levels during pregnancy. In: Dam M, Gram L, Penry J, eds. *Advances in Epileptology: XIIth Epilepsy International Symposium*. New York: Raven Press, 1981: 607–12.

145 Uetrecht JP. The role of leukocyte-generated reactive metabolites in the pathogenesis of idiosyncratic drug reactions. *Drug Metab Rev* 1992; 24 (3): 299–366.

146 Gibaldi M. Adverse drug effect reactive metabolites and idiosyncratic drug reactions. *Ann Pharmacother* 1992; 26: 416–21.

147 Pellock JM. Standard approach to antiepileptic drug treatment in the United States. *Epilepsia* 1994; 35 (Suppl. 4): S11–18.

148 Taaffe A, O'Brien C. A case of Stevens–Johnson syndrome associated with the anti-convulsants sulthiame and ethosuximide. *Br Dent J* 1975; 138 (5): 172–4.

149 Dabbous IA, Idriss HM. Occurrence of systemic lupus erythematosus in association with ethosuccimide therapy. Case report. *J Pediatr* 1970; 76 (4): 617–20.

150 Alter BP. Systemic lupus erythematosus and ethosuccimide. *J Pediatr* 1970; 77 (6): 1093–5.

151 Ansell BM. Drug-induced systemic lupus erythematosus in a nine-year-old boy. *Lupus* 1993; 2 (3): 193–4.

152 Singsen B, Fishman L, Hanson V. Antinuclear antibodies and lupus-like syndromes in children receiving anticonvulsants. *Pediatrics* 1976; 57: 529–34.

153 Teoh PC, Chan HL. Lupus–scleroderma syndrome induced by ethosuximide. *Arch Dis Child* 1975; 50 (8): 658–61.

154 Takeda S, Koizumi F, Takazakura E. Ethosuximide-induced lupus-like syndrome with renal involvement. *Intern Med* 1996; 35 (7): 587–91.

155 Cohn R. A neuropathological study of a case of petit mal epilepsy. *Electroencephalogr Clin Neurophysiol* 1968; 24: 282.

156 Kousoulieris E. Granulopenia and thrombocytopenia after ethosuximide. *Lancet* 1967; 2: 310–11.

157 Spittler J. Agranulocytosis due to ethosuximide with a fatal outcome. *Klin Paediatr* 1974; 186: 364–6.

158 Massey GV, Dunn NL, Heckel JL, Myer EC, Russell EC. Aplastic anemia following therapy for absence seizures with ethosuximide. [Review]. *Pediatric Neurol* 1994; 11 (1): 59–61.

159 Mann L, Habenicht H. Fatal bone marrow aplasia associated with administration of ethosuximide (Zarontin) for petit mal epilepsy. *Bull Los Angeles Neurol Soc* 1962; 27: 173–6.

160 Seip M. Aplastic anemia during ethosuximide medication. Treatment with bolus-methylprednisolone. *Acta Paediatr Scand* 1983; 72 (6): 927–9.

161 Ehyai A, Kilroy A, Fenicheal G. Dyskinesia and akathisia induced by ethosuximide. *Am J Dis Child* 1978; 132: 527–8.

162 Kirschberg G. Dyskinesia—an unusual reaction to ethosuximide. *Arch Neurol* 1975; 32: 137–8.

163 Nishiyama J, Matsukura M, Fugimoto S, Matsuda I. Reports of 2 cases of autoimmune thyroiditis while receiving anticonvulsant therapy. *Eur J Pediatr* 1983; 140: 116–17.

164 Wassner S, Pennisi A, Malekzadeh M, Fine R. The adverse effect of anticonvulsant therapy on renal allograft survival. A preliminary report. *J Pediatr* 1976; 88: 134–7.

165 Anonymous. Succinimides—anticonvulsants. In: Toll L, Hurlbut K, eds. *Poisindex System*. Healthcare Series, Vol. 108 edn, expires June 2001. Greenwood Village, Colorado: Micromedex, Inc., 2001.

166 Chyka PA, Seger D. Position statement: single-dose activated charcoal. American Academy of Clinical Toxicology; European Association of Poisons Centres and Clinical Toxicologists. *J Toxicol Clin Toxicol* 1997; 35 (7): 721–41.

167 Vale JA. Position statement: gastric lavage. American Academy of Clinical Toxicology; European Association of Poisons Centres and Clinical Toxicologists. *J Toxicol Clin Toxicol* 1997; 35 (7): 711–19.

168 Marbury TC, Lee CS, Perchalski RJ, Wilder BJ. Hemodialysis clearance of ethosuximide in patients with chronic renal disease. *Am J Hosp Pharm* 1981; 38 (11): 1757–60.

169 Karceski S, Morrell M, Carpenter D. The Expert Consensus Guideline Series. Treatment of Epilepsy. *Epilepsy Behav* 2001; 2 (6): A1–50.

170 Bourgeois BFD. Antiepileptic drugs in pediatric practice. *Epilepsia* 1995; 36 (2): S34–45.

33

Felbamate

I.E. Leppik

Primary indications	Adjunctive therapy or monotherapy in refractory partial and secondarily generalized epilepsy. Also in Lennox–Gastaut syndrome
Usual preparations	Tablets: 400, 600 mg; syrup: 600 mg/5 mL
Usual dosages	Initial: 1200 mg/day (adults); 15 mg/kg/day (children). Maintenance: 1200–3600 mg/day (adults); 45–80 mg/kg/day (children)
Dosage intervals	3–4 times/day
Significant drug interactions	Felbamate increases the concentration of phenobarbital, phenytoin, carbamazepine epoxide and valproate. Felbamate lowers the concentration of carbamazepine. Phenytoin, phenobarbital and carbamazepine lower felbamate levels; valproate increases felbamate levels
Serum level monitoring	Useful
Target range	30–100 mg/L
Common/important side-effects	Severe hepatic disturbance and aplastic anaemia are rare but serious side-effects. Insomnia, weight loss, gastrointestinal symptoms, fatigue, dizziness, lethargy, behavioural change, ataxia, visual disturbance, mood change, psychotic reaction, rash, neurological symptoms
Main advantages	Highly effective novel antiepileptic drug for refractory patients
Main disadvantages	Severe hepatic and aplastic anaemia in occasional patients. Other side-effects also frequent on initial therapy, and in patients on polytherapy
Mechanisms of action	Probably by effect on NMDA receptor (glycine recognition site) and sodium-channel conductance
Oral bioavailability	90%
Time to peak levels	1–4 h
Metabolism and excretion	Hepatic hydroxylation and then conjugation (60%); renal excretion as unchanged drug (40%)
Volume of distribution	0.75 L/kg
Elimination half-life	20 h (13–30 h; lowest in patients comedicated with enzyme inducers)
Plasma clearance	0.027–0.032 L/kg/h (but variable)
Protein binding	20–25%
Active metabolites	None
Comment	Highly effective novel anticonvulsant in severe resistant epilepsy, but use limited by rare but severe hepatic and haematological toxicity

(*Note*: this summary table was formulated by the lead editor.)

Felbamate (2-phenyl-1,3-propanediol dicarbamate, Felbatol, FBM), was synthesized by Wallace Laboratories in the USA in 1954 [1]. The antiepileptic drug development (ADD) programme of the National Institutes of Health (NIH) identified FBM's potential for anticonvulsant activity in the 1980s [2]. Extensive clinical trials ensued, resulting in Food and Drug Administration (FDA) approval for use in the USA on 30 July 1993. FBM was approved for use as adjunctive and monotherapy in adults with partial seizures with or without generalization and as adjunctive therapy in children with the Lennox–Gastaut syndrome. The unexpected development of aplastic anaemia prompted the FDA and manufacturer, Carter Wallace, to issue a strong warning regarding continued use of FBM on 1 August 1994. Reports of FBM-associated hepatic failure also engendered further concern. As a result, FBM is not indicated as a first-line antiepileptic treatment; rather its use should be reserved for a few patients who respond inadequately to alternative treatments and whose epilepsy is severe enough that the risk of aplastic anaemia and/or liver failure is deemed acceptable by the patient compared to the benefits conferred by its use. Because of the effectiveness of this drug in many patients, FBM remains on the market in the USA and is available for limited use in other countries.

Mechanism of action

Although the specific mechanism by which FBM exerts its anticonvulsant activity is unknown, evidence exists for a number of possible mechanisms. The N-methyl-D-aspartate (NMDA) receptor is the site of action where FBM was found to be effective against NMDA-induced clonus in mice [3]. Inhibition of [^{3}H]5,7-dichlorokynurenic acid (a high-affinity glycine receptor antagonist) binding corresponding with peak plasma and brain concentrations of FBM has been demonstrated [4]. FBM may have dual actions in the brain, both inhibiting NMDA responses and potentiating γ-aminobutyric acid (GABA) action [5]. FBM has also been found to be effective in blocking sustained repetitive firing in mouse spinal cord neurones suggesting modulation of sodium channel conductance [3]. FBM has no effect on GABA or benzodiazepam receptor binding [2,6].

Animal model testing demonstrated a broad spectrum of activity against different seizure types, blocking seizures induced by maximal electroshock (MES), pentylenetetrazol (PTZ) and picrotoxin, but seizures induced by bicuculline and strychnine were not affected [2]. FBM is protective against epileptiform activity induced by the K$^+$ channel blocker 4-aminopyridine [7]. Thus, FBM seems to both increase seizure threshold and prevent seizure spread [2]. This profile in animal models would predict action against both partial and generalized (including absence) epilepsies in humans. FBM has also been found to be active in two rat models of status epilepticus [8,9]. It has also been found to be effective in preventing the expression of stage 5 kindled seizures in corneal-kindled rats [3].

The anticonvulsant effects of FBM against MES seizures may be enhanced in combination with non-protective doses of phenytoin (PHT), carbamazepine (CBZ), valproate (VPA) or phenobarbital (PB) in mice. This effect could not be accounted for by a pharmacokinetic mechanism and thus implies a pharmacodynamic interaction [10]. Also, a single subprotective dose of FBM combined with diazepam enhanced the effects of diazepam against seizures induced by MES, pentylenetetrazol and isoniazid [11]. In addition to its an-

Table 33.1 The protective index (median toxic dose/median effective dose) of FBM and standard AEDs in various animal models of seizures

Drug	MES	PTZ	PIC	NMDA	Kindling
Felbamate	16.3	5.51	5.2	146	35.8
Carbamazepine	8.1	NP	37.2	16	>17.3
Ethosuximide	NP	3.4	1.8	4	NP
Phenytoin	6.9	NP	NP	71	NP
Valproate	1.6	2.9	1.1	5.8	7.3

Adapted from [2,3,36].
NP, not protective.

ticonvulsant action, FBM has a neuroprotective effect in animal models [9,12,13]. FBM has a very favourable protective index in animals compared to other antiepileptic drugs (AEDs) (Table 33.1).

Absorption and distribution

FBM is rapidly and completely absorbed after oral administration in animals [14]. Over 90% relative bioavailability has been identified in humans [15]. Food does not interfere with the extent of absorption [16]. Time to peak plasma concentration in patients is 1–4 h postdose [17]. Tablets and suspension are bioequivalent [18].

It distributes rapidly into a number of animal tissues, including brain [14] and crosses the placenta in rats [19]. FBM extraction into brain in a single transcapillary passage was found to be 5–20% and it distributes relatively uniformly throughout the brain [20]. In humans, 20–25% of the total concentration is bound, primarily to serum albumin.

Biotransformation and excretion

FBM is extensively metabolized in the liver via hydroxylation and conjugation. A number of potentially pharmacoactive and toxic metabolites may be formed [21–23]. This hepatic metabolism sets the stage for drug interactions with concomitantly administered medications metabolized via similar pathways. In human volunteers, 40–49% of an FBM dose is recovered in the urine as the parent compound, with the rest as various metabolites [15]. Metabolites do not contribute significantly to activity in animal models of epilepsy [2]. However, in humans, FBM may be metabolized to lead to the formation of 2-phenylpropenal, an α,β-unsaturated aldehyde (atropaldehyde) which is a potent electrophile [24]. Atropaldehyde has been proposed to play a role in the development of toxicity during FBM therapy. It undergoes rapid conjugation with glutathione in most individuals. This has led to analysing urine samples from patients receiving FBM for two atropoldehyde-derived mercapturic acids as a possible method for monitoring patients [25].

Measurement

A number of methods have been developed to measure FBM and its metabolites in biological samples. An HPLC method for the simultaneous analysis of FBM, PHT, 5-(p-hydroxyphenyl)-5-

phenylhydantoin, CBZ, CBZ-10,11-epoxide and CBZ-10,11-diol in serum that could separate the compounds of interest and three internal standards in less than 15 min has been developed using a mobile phase optimization technique [26]. Some methods can measure FBM concentrations in as little as 0.1 mL of plasma [27]. Other methods can measure FBM and its three metabolites in brain and heart tissue homogenates [28].

Elimination

The half-life of FBM in normal male volunteers is approximately 20 h and ranges from 13 to 23 h as monotherapy [15,18] (Table 33.2). Multiple dosing does not appear to alter the elimination half-life. In patients with epilepsy receiving either PHT or CBZ, the half-life of FBM was shorter, approximately 13–14 h with a range of 11.4–19.6 h [17]. Conversely, when the PHT dose was decreased or the drug discontinued in patients on FBM receiving it, FBM concentrations increased and its apparent clearance decreased by 21%. Decreasing or eliminating CBZ in these patients led to an additional decrease of the apparent clearance by 16.5% [29,30]. Thus, PHT and CBZ increase the rate of FBM elimination. VPA has the opposite effect. Two studies have shown FBM concentration to be significantly higher than expected in the presence of VPA [18,31]. For example, 10 patients receiving only VPA in addition to FBM had a mean FBM level of 59.1 mg/L on a dose of 2.4 g/day. This can be compared to mean FBM concentrations of 32.4 mg/L for patients on the same FBM dose receiving PHT and CBZ [32].

As would be expected from a drug 40–50% eliminated unchanged in the urine, persons with renal failure will need lower doses of FBM, with urinary clearance representing only 9–22% of elimination in these patients [33].

The pharmacokinetics of FBM has not been as extensively studied in young animals or children with epilepsy. In studies of adult and paediatric beagles, the mean peak serum concentration

Table 33.2 Clinical characteristics of FBM

Half-life	13–30 h[a]
Usual daily dose	Adults 3600 mg (60 mg/kg for 60 kg person)
	Children 45 mg/kg (recommended but may need higher doses)[b]
Interaction	FBM increases concentrations of phenytoin, valproate and carbamazepine-10,11-epoxide
	FBM decreases concentrations of carbamazepine
	FBM concentrations decreased by PHT, CBZ, and PB.
Protein binding	20–25%
Elimination pathways	Hepatic (50–60%)
In humans	Renal (40–50%)
Absorption	Approximately 90%; not affected by food
Usually effective levels	30–100 μg/mL (lower range for adjunctive therapy; higher for monotherapy)

[a] Shorter in persons on inducing AEDs such as PHT; longest in persons receiving inhibitors such as valproate.
[b] [37].

and the mean elimination half-life were significantly lower in the younger group [14]. Further evaluation of this phenomenon revealed that the younger animals had higher rates of hydroxylation [34]. In a study of children using the non-linear mixed effects model (NONMEM) program for describing pharmacokinetics, the clearance of FBM was found to be 41.1 mL/h/kg, and increased by 49% and 40%, respectively, when used with CBZ and PHT. VPA and older age were found to decrease clearance [35]. Thus, children may need a higher dose per kilogram than adults.

FBM metabolism has not been well studied in the elderly, but it would be expected that with both decreased renal and hepatic functioning, doses on a milligram per kilogram basis would need to be lower in older persons.

Toxicity

Low toxicity was observed in animal models [36]. Studies of carcinogenicity after high doses have shown a statistically significant increase in hepatic cell adenomas in some rodents and an increase in benign interstitial cell tumours of the testes in male rats [37]. No teratogenic effects of FBM have been found in reproductive or teratology studies in rats and rabbits [37]. No evidence for bone marrow or hepatic toxicity was observed in any of the preclinical studies.

In human studies, FBM was better tolerated as monotherapy, adverse experiences being more common when FBM is used with other AEDs [38]. The most common side-effects of FBM as monotherapy were anorexia, vomiting, insomnia, nausea and headache. The most common adverse reactions in polytherapy trials include anorexia, vomiting, insomnia, nausea, dizziness, somnolence and headache [37,39]. In data provided by Carter Wallace, in clinical testing 12% (120 of 977 adults) discontinued FBM because of side-effects. In order of frequency greater than 1%, these were anorexia 1.6%, nausea 1.4%, rash 1.2%, weight decrease 1.1%, and various neurological symptoms 1.4% or psychological symptoms 2.2% [37]. In studies with children, 6% (22 of 357) had FBM discontinued, with symptoms leading to its discontinuance similar to those seen in adults. In one postmarketing use study, FBM was initiated in 132 persons with chronic, refractory epilepsy after its release. Three or more months after initiation, FBM had been discontinued in 24 patients because of side-effects. gastrointestinal symptoms were the most common single reason given, and dermatitis occurred in four patients [40].

In the clinical trials leading to FBM approval, there had been no significant changes in laboratory tests among patients on FBM, specifically white cell blood count, hematocrit and serum glutamate oxaloacetate transaminase (aspartate aminotransferase). However, as FBM came into wider use, reports of serious adverse events surfaced. Thrombocytopenia was described in one report [41]. Scattered cases of aplastic anaemia came to the attention of the FDA by mid-1994, and three cases were reported in July alone. This unexpectedly high rate in conjunction with increasing use led the FDA to issue a warning on 1 August 1994, with Dr Kessler stating 'Physicians should prescribe this drug only if it is absolutely necessary'. Information collected for the September 1994 FDA advisory panel meeting indicated that there had been 25 cases of aplastic anaemia reported, 24 in the USA and one in Spain [42]. In addition, 11 cases of hepatitis with four deaths had been reported. As of May 1995, Carter Wallace had evidence of 31 domestic postmarketing reports of aplastic anemia and 14 cases of hepatitis with eight deaths (Table 33.3).

A thorough review of aplastic anaemia was performed. Of the cases reported, 23 (74%) met all of the criteria of the International Agranulocytosis and Aplastic Anemia Study [43]. In 14, FBM was judged to be the only cause [3] or most likely [11]. Using a denominator of 110 000 persons exposed, the most 'probable incidence' was calculated to be 127 per million (lower limit 27; upper limit 209), with the general population rate for aplastic anaemia being 2 per million [43].

Patient history and demographics suggest several features that may identify the high-risk patient. A prior history of AED allergy or toxicity, especially rash, was observed in 52%; a history of prior cytopenia in 42%; and evidence of immune disease, especially lupus erythematosus in 33%. A case-by-case review of patients who developed aplastic anaemia revealed that an underlying immunological disease process was observed 34 times more frequently than expected, and if two of the above three factors were present, the patient's relative risk for aplastic anaemia quadrupled (Table 33.4). Only three patients had all three factors—cytopenia, allergy and an immunological process—within the entire aplastic anaemia and control groups available to the drug's manufacturer (Wallace), and all three developed aplastic anaemia. Only one paediatric patient (aged 18) was diagnosed with aplastic anaemia and she had a prior diagnosis of systemic lupus erythematosus [44].

Duration of therapy is also an important factor. Duration of therapy prior to aplastic anaemia ranged from 23 to 339 days (mean 173 days) [44]. No cases have occurred in persons treated more than 1 year.

Table 33.3 Haematological reactions reported for patients receiving FBM as of September 1994

Reaction	n	Serious	Died
Aplastic anaemia	25	25	6
Pancytopenia	15	14	3
Leukopenia	29	18	1
Thrombocytopenia	16	10	2
Anaemia	4	4	0
Two of above	14	11	1

Table 33.4 Associated conditions in persons developing aplastic anaemia while on FBM. A review of the 25 cases analysed by September, 1994

Previous history of bone marrow suppression	3
Previous history of blood dyscrasias	10
Previous history of drug allergy (not AEDs)	6
Previous history of autoimmune disease	5
Previous history of AED allergy	3
Current PHT use	16
Current clinical toxicity	3
Mental retardation	9
Taking drugs (not AEDs) associated with aplastic anaemia	12

A total of 18 cases of hepatic failure have been reported in patients receiving FBM. Evaluation of these reports indicates that 78% were female, 50% were aged 17 years or older, and the mean time to presentation was 217 days (25–939 days). A panel of hepatologists independently met to review the data on these cases and concluded that only seven had a likely association with FBM, whereas the others were complicated by status epilepticus, viral hepatitis, shock liver or acetaminophen toxicity [44]. Using all reported cases of hepatic failure, the estimated incidence would be 164 per million but using the numerator of 7, the incidence of hepatic failure would be estimated at 64 per million. Using the 130 000–170 000 exposed persons as a denominator and seven likely cases, the risk for hepatic failure is estimated at 1 per 18 500–25 000 exposures. Recently updated statistics regarding VPA reported hepatic-related fatality estimates of one case in 10 000–49 000 for the combined population and 1 in 500–800 cases in high-risk young children under the age of 2 years receiving VPA polypharmacy [45]. These data suggest that the hepatotoxicity associated with FBM is in the general range seen with VPA [44]. However, the age range differs markedly, with FBM safer in the paediatric population but worse in adults, with just the opposite for VPA. For both aplastic anaemia and hepatotoxicity, females are at much greater risk (67% and 78%, respectively).

FBM is excreted in the urine and one case of urolithiasis with an FBM stone in a 15-year-old boy has been reported [46]. One case of crystalluria and renal failure in an intentional overdose with FBM concentrations of 200 mg/mL has been observed [47]. Toxic epidermal necrolysis after initiation of FBM has also been reported [48].

Clinical efficacy

The first evidence that FBM may be effective in humans came from a study of the pharmacokinetics of this drug [17]. Since then, a number of controlled trials have been performed, some of which used novel study designs, including use of presurgical patients, monotherapy studies with 'active placebos', and a study using patients with the Lennox–Gastaut syndrome [49]. Many of these designs have been used subsequently in new AED development. The first pivotal study was an NIH-sponsored, double-blind, placebo-controlled, two-centre add-on trial [32]. The mean seizure frequencies during the 8-week analysis periods in the 56 patients completing the study were 34.9 for the FBM period and 40.2 during placebo period ($P = 0.007$). Another NIH-sponsored study involved a triple crossover of FBM and placebo while CBZ was maintained as the stable AED. Initial analysis showed no significant difference in seizure frequency between placebo and FBM periods, but when a correction was made for the lower CBZ level noted during FBM periods, the data suggested a strong antiseizure effect of FBM [50].

Additional open-label studies have demonstrated the effectiveness of FBM in drug-refractory partial epilepsy [51]. The first was an open pilot study of 15 patients with partial seizures. FBM was added rapidly after evaluation was completed. The first day dose was 1200 mg; the second day, it was increased to 2400 mg; and to 3600 mg the third day, if tolerated. Most patients tolerated this rapid titration with only mild nausea. During the evaluation phase, the mean number of seizures was 2.05/day; during FGM treatment the seizure rate decreased to 0.29/day, a statistically significant decrease ($P < 0.001$; [52]). Both of these studies were proof of principle studies to demonstrate the effectiveness of FBM in intractable patients. Some patient remained on other AEDs and this design was not intended to be used as a model of monotherapy, although it has been so used.

Two studies of FBM monotherapy using an 'active placebo' consisting of low-dose VPA have formed the basis of its recommended use as the sole AED in refractory patients [38,53]. Retention rate has also been favourable in a clinical setting, as in a postmarketing study, 91 of 132 refractory patients had enough clinical efficacy and lack of side-effects to warrant continuance of FBM 3 months or more after initiation [40].

Efficacy of FBM in the Lennox–Gastaut syndrome was evaluated in a double-blind add-on parallel study involving 73 patients, mostly in the paediatric age range. FBM or placebo was added to standard AEDs for 70 days. The dosage of FBM was titrated to a maximum of 45 mg/kg of body weight per day or 3600 mg/day, whichever was less. Patients treated with FBM had a 34% decrease in the frequency of atonic seizures ($P = 0.01$) and a 19% decrease in the frequency of all seizures ($P = 0.002$). A 'quality-of-life' measure, the global-evaluation scores, were significantly higher in the FBM group as compared to the placebo group [54]. The improvement that occurred in the double-blind study has been sustained for at least 12 months in subsequent open-label follow-up studies [55]. Additional open-label studies have confirmed the effectiveness of FBM in the Lennox–Gastaut syndrome [56].

In a practice advisory statement in the USA, FBM was classified as showing class I evidence efficacy for partial seizures in adult as adjunctive and monotherapy, and Lennox–Gastaut syndrome as adjunctive therapy. Class III evidence was found for primary generalized tonic-clonic seizures, absence seizures and partial seizures in children [57].

Drug interactions

In an evaluation of cytochrome P450 isoenzyme induction or inhibition using rats, phenobarbital resulted in a 150% increase and FBM a 65% increase at the highest tested doses [58]. After chronic administration, increased p-nitroanisole-O-demethylase activity was observed, indicative of some liver microsomal induction [59]. Although these animal studies would suggest that FBM is a mild inducer of metabolism of other drugs using the P450 pathways, clinical experience has not born this out. In humans, FBM is both an inhibitor of some drugs but an inducer of others. FBM significantly increases the concentrations of PHT, and dose decreases of about 20% were needed in the first major study of FBM as an add-on drug to maintain stable PHT concentrations [32,60,61]. This interaction may be due to competitive inhibition which may overcome the mild inductive effect of FBM [62,63]. CBZ concentrations are lowered by FBM; in one study CBZ concentrations decreased from 7.5 µg/mL during placebo treatment to 6.1 µg/mL during FBM treatment ($P < 0.05$), when used with FBM [64]. On the other hand, mean CBZ-10,11-epoxide concentrations increased from 1.8 µg/mL during placebo baseline periods to 2.4 µg/mL during FBM treatment [64]. The effect was evident after the first week of treatment and reached a plateau in 2–4 weeks [65]. FBM has been found to increase the serum concentrations of phenobarbital when added to an existing regimen [66,67].

Valproic acid levels are increased by FBM. In one study of 10 patients on VPA monotherapy, the VPA levels increased by 18% in the presence of 1200 mg FBM per day and by 31% with FBM doses of 2400 mg/day [68].

Although few studies are available regarding interactions with drugs other than AEDs, it can be anticipated that the elimination of other substances using the cytochrome P450 system will be either induced or inhibited. In addition, FBM metabolism may be influenced by other drugs as well. This may be of particular concern in the elderly who are taking many other drugs.

Laboratory testing

The FDA and Carter Wallace recommend full haematological evaluations prior to initiation of FBM therapy, frequently during therapy, and for a significant period of time after discontinuation of FBM. Liver function tests are recommended every 1–2 weeks while on FBM. It is not at all certain, however, that routine monitoring of haematological and hepatic parameters will be effective in detecting reactions. More important than laboratory testing is a careful review of the medical history and avoiding the use of FBM in patients who have a high-risk profile. Patients on FBM should be taught the warning signs of aplastic anaemia and have a complete blood cell count whenever any of these appear. These signs and symptoms include severe lethargy, nausea and vomiting, flu-like symptoms, easy bruising and unusual bleeding.

In the initial double-blind study, most serum levels ranged between 20 and 45 µg/mL [32]. However, in postmarketing experience, concentrations between 40 and 100 mg/mL are commonly found in persons responding favourably (Leppik, personal experience). Because there is a wide range of clearances for FBM resulting from comedication and individual genetic variability, concentrations are not readily predictable from the doses, and measurement of blood levels is useful to guide dosing.

Starting therapy

In adults, FBM can be initiated at 1200 mg/day in three or four divided doses, with increases to 2400 and 3600 mg/day in weekly or biweekly increments of 600 or 1200 mg steps, as tolerated, as outpatients (Table 33.2). In inpatient settings, FBM can be titrated over a few days, especially if the other AEDs have or are being eliminated or reduced [49]. In the outpatient environment, the doses of other AEDs should be reduced, generally by 20–33% upon initiation, and by further reductions as FBM dose is increased. Most side-effects can be eliminated by reducing doses of concomitant AEDs, especially if the goal is to attain monotherapy with FBM. Some patients have tolerated doses as high as 7200 mg/day as monotherapy. A useful method to determine more precise doses for titrating patients is to start at approximately 20 mg/kg, increase to 40 mg/kg and then 50 mg/kg, 60 mg/kg or higher as needed. Initiating FBM in the presence of other AEDs can be difficult because of the drug interactions and propensity to develop side-effects attributable to a greater total burden of AEDs. Nevertheless, careful attention to the general principle of reducing other AEDs vigorously in the presence of side-effects and increasing FBM doses if levels have not been increased to over 60 µg/mL will permit patients to have an adequate exposure to this drug. In a patient with refractory epilepsy with particularly intense seizures or a propensity for status epilepticus, it may be best to err on the side of less aggressive concomitant AED adjustments initially rather than decrease concomitant AEDs, as the patient develops signs and symptoms of concentration-related toxicity. In studies of adults, doses have ranged from 1800 to 4800 mg/day.

In children, recommended starting doses have been 15 mg/kg/day with weekly incremental increases to 45 mg/kg/day. Again, concomitant AEDs should be reduced by 20% or more upon initiation and reduced further as symptoms and blood levels indicate. It may be expected that doses for children may be larger than those for adults, and in our experience we have used doses of up to 80 mg/kg.

FBM is available as 400 mg tablets (scored, yellow, capsule shaped) useful for children; 600 mg tablets (peach-coloured scored, capsule shaped) and suspension, 600 mg per 5 mL.

Conclusions

After the first year of clinical experience, FBM came close to being withdrawn because of serious adverse events. In the subsequent years, however, FBM has been recognized to be a valuable drug for the treatment of intractable epilepsy in carefully selected patients. FBM should be reserved for consideration only in persons with intractable epilepsy under the care of a physician familiar with this drug and only in patients who have been well informed of the risks. Many patients have benefited significantly from FBM and have made a decision to remain on this drug at the presently known risk profile. Persons who have received FBM for more than 1 year and have had a normal urine screen for metabolites may not be at significant risk. The major challenge for FBM in the future is developing genomic tests to identify persons at risk for the idiosyncratic reactions and avoid FBM in these persons. The availability of these tests would greatly expand the number of persons with epilepsy for whom this potent AED could be used. A Felbatol registry, established in the USA in 1997, is gathering data on risk factors, and information on how to enter patients may be obtained by contacting the medical director of the manufacturer as listed in the most current *Physician's Desk Reference*.

Acknowledgements

The assistance of Liliane Dargis in manuscript preparation is gratefully acknowledged. Supported in part by P50 NS-16308.

References

1 Sofia RD, Kramer L, Perhach JL, Rosenberg A. Felbamate. *Epilepsy Res* 1991; 3 (Suppl.): 103–8.

2 Swinyard EA, Sofia RD, Kupferberg HJ. Comparative anticonvulsant activity and neurotoxicity of felbamate and four prototype antiepileptic drugs in mice and rats. *Epilepsia* 1986; 27: 27–34.

3 White HS, Wolf HH, Swinyard EA, Skeen GA, Sofia RD. A neuropharmacological evaluation of felbamate as a novel anticonvulsant. *Epilepsia* 1992; 33 (3): 564–72.

4 McCabe RT, Wasterlain CG, Kucharczyk N, Sofia RD, Vogel JR. Evidence for anticonvulsant and neuroprotectant action of felbamate mediated by strychnine-insensitive glycine receptors. *J Pharmacol Exp Ther* 1993; 264: 1248–52.

5 Rho JM, Donevan SD, Rogawski MA. Mechanism of action of the anticonvulsant felbamate: opposing effect on N-methyl-D-aspartate and gamma-aminobutyric acid A receptors. *Ann Neurol* 1994; 35 (2): 229–34.

6 Ticku MK, Kamatchi GL, Sofia RD. Effect of anticonvulsant felbamate on GABA receptor system. *Epilepsia* 1991; 32: 389–91.

7 Yamaguchi S, Rogawski MA. Effects of anticonvulsant drugs on 4-aminopyridine-induced seizures in mice. *Epilepsy Res* 1992; 11: 9–16.

8 Sofia RD, Gordon R, Gels M, Diamantis W. Effects of felbamate and other anticonvulsant drugs in two models of status epilepticus in the rat. *Res Commun Chem Pathol Pharmacol* 1993; 79: 335–41.

9 Chronopoulos A, Stafstrom C, Thurber S, Hyde P, Mikati M, Holmes GL. Neuroprotective effect of felbamate after kainic acid-induced status epilepticus. *Epilepsia* 1993; 34 (2): 359–66.

10 Gordon R, Gels M, Wichmann J, Diamantis W, Sofia RD. Interaction of felbamate with several other antiepileptic drugs against seizures induced by maximal electroshock in mice. *Epilepsia* 1993; 34 (2): 367–71.

11 Gordon R, Gels M, Diamantis W, Sofia RD. Interaction of felbamate and diazepam against maximal electroshock seizures and chemoconvulsants in mice. *Pharmacol Biochem Behav* 1991; 40 (1): 109–13.

12 Wallis RA, Panizzon KL. Glycine reversal of felbamate hypoxic protection. *Neuroreport (Endl)* 1993; 4 (7): 951–4.

13 Wasterlain CG, Adams LM, Hattori H, Schwartz PH. Felbamate reduces hypoxic-ischemic brain damage *in vivo*. *Eur J Pharmacol* 1992; 212: 275–8.

14 Adusumalli VE, Gilchrist JR, Wichmann JK, Kucharczyk N, Sofia RD. Pharmacokinetics of felbamate in paediatric and adult beagle dogs. Department of Biochemistry. *Epilepsia* 1992; 33: 955–60.

15 Shumaker RC, Fantel C, Kelton E, Wong K, Weliky I. Evaluation of the elimination of (14C) felbamate in healthy men (Abstract). *Epilepsia* 1990; 31: 642.

16 Gudipati RM, Raymond RH, Ward DI, Shumaker RC, Perhach JL. Effect of food on the absorption of felbamate in healthy male volunteers (Abstract). *Neurology* 1992; 42 (Suppl. 3): 332.

17 Wilensky AJ, Friel PN, Ojemann LM, Kupferberg HJ, Levy RH. Pharmacokinetics of W-554 (ADD03055) in epileptic patients. *Epilepsia* 1985; 26: 602–6.

18 Ward DL, Shumaker RD. Comparative bioavailability of felbamate in healthy men (Abstract). *Epilepsia* 1990; 31: 642.

19 Adusumalli VE, Wong KK, Kucharczyk N, Sofia RD. Felbamate in vitro metabolism by rat liver microsomes. *Drug Metab Dispos Biol Fate Chem* 1991; 19 (6): 1135–8.

20 Cornford EM, Young D, Paxton JW, Sofia RD. Blood–brain barrier penetration of felbamate. *Epilepsia*, 1992; 33 (5): 944–54.

21 Adusumalli VE, Yang JT, Wong KK, Kucharczyk N, Sofia RD. Felbamate pharmacokinetics in the rat, rabbit, and dog. *Drug Metab Dispos Biol Fate Chem* 1991; 19: 116–25.

22 Adusumalli VE, Choi YM, Romanyshyn LA *et al*. Isolation and identification of 3-carbamoyloxy-2-phenylpropionic acid as a major human urinary metabolite of felbamate. *Drug Metab Dispos Biol Fate Chem* 1993; 21: 710–16.

23 Yang JT, Adusumalli VE, Wong KK, Kucharczyk N, Sofia RD. Felbamate metabolism in the rat, rabbit, and dog. *Drug Metab Dispos Biol Fate Chem* 1991; 19 (6): 1126–34.

24 Thompson CD, Gulden PH, Macdonald TL. Identification of modified atropaldehyde mercapturic acids in rat and human urine after felbamate administration. *Chem Res Toxicol* 1997; 10 (4): 457–62.

25 Thompson CD, Barthen MT, Hopper DW *et al*. Quantification in patient urine samples of felbamate and three metabolites: acid carbamate and two mercapturic acids. *Epilepsia* 1999; 40 (6): 769–76.

26 Remmel RP, Miller SA, Graves NM. Simultaneous assay of felbamate plus carbamazepine, phenytoin, and their metabolites by liquid chromatography with mobile phase optimization. *Ther Drug Monit* 1990; 12 (1): 90–6.

27 Clark LA, Wichmann JK, Kucharczyk N, Sofia RD. Determination of the anticonvulsant felbamate in beagle dog plasma by high-performance liquid chromatography. *J Chromatogr* 1992; 573 (1): 113–19.

28 Jacala A, Adusumalli VE, Kucharczyk N, Sofia RD. Determination of the anticonvulsant felbamate and its three metabolites in brain and heart tissue of rats. *J Chromatogtr (Nether)*, 1993; 614 (2): 285–92.

29 Miller ML, Holmes GB, Marienau K, Graves NM, Leppik IE. Successful withdrawal of phenytoin in refractory patients with epilepsy (Abstract). *Neurology* 1989; 39: 120.

30 Wagner ML, Graves NM, Marienau K, Holmes GB, Remmel RP, Leppik

IE. Discontinuation of phenytoin and carbamazepine in patients receiving felbamate. *Epilepsia* 1991; 32: 398–406.

31 Ward DL, Wagner ML, Perhach JL *et al*. Felbamate steady-state pharmacokinetics during coadministration of valproate (Abstract). *Epilepsia* 1991; 32 (Suppl. 3): 8.

32 Leppik IE, Dreifuss FE, Pledger GW *et al*. Felbamate for partial seizures: results of a controlled clinical trial. *Neurology* 1991; 41 (11): 1785–9.

33 Glue P, Sulowicz W, Colucci R *et al*. Single-dose pharmacokinetics of felbamate in patients with renal dysfunction. *Br J Clin Pharmacol* 1997; 44 (1): 91–3.

34 Yang JT, Morris M, Wong KK, Kucharczyk N, Sofia RD. Felbamate metabolism in pediatric and adult beagle dogs. *Drug Metab Dispos Biol Fate Chem* 1992; 20: 84–8.

35 Kelley MT, Walson PD, Cox S, Dusci LJ. Population pharmacokinetics of felbamate in children. *Ther Drug Monit* 1997; 19 (1): 29–36.

36 Perhach JL, Weliky I, Newton JJ *et al*. Felbamate. In: Meldrum BS, Porter RJ, eds. *New Anticonvulsant Drugs*. London: John Libbey, 1986: 117–23.

37 *Physicians' Desk Reference*. Montvale, New Jersey: Medical Economic Company, 1994.

38 Sachdeo R, Kramer LD, Rosenberg A, Sachdeo S. Felbamate monotherapy: controlled trial in patients with partial onset seizures. *Ann Neurol* 1992; 32: 386–92.

39 Graves N. Felbamate. *Ann Pharmacother* 1993; 27: 1073–81.

40 Wolff DL, Kerrick JM, Rarick J, Leppik IE, Graves NM. Post-market felbamate use in the refractory epilepsy population. *Epilepsia* 1994; 35 (8): 32.

41 Ney GC, Schaul N, Loughlin J, Rai K, Chandra V. Thrombocytopenia in association with adjunctive felbamate use. *Neurology* 1994; 44 (5): 980–1.

42 FDA. *Memorandum. Postmarketing Safety Evaluator Reports Evaluation Branch, HFD-735* 9 September, 1994. Washington, DC: FDA.

43 Kaufman DW, Kelly JP, Anderson T, Harmon DC, Shapiro S. Evaluation of case reports of aplastic anemia among patients treated with felbamate. *Epilepsia* 1997; 38 (12): 1261–4.

44 Pellock JM. Felbamate. *Epilepsia* 1999; 40 (Suppl. 5): S57–62.

45 Bryant AE, Dreifuss FR. Valproic acid hepatic failures: US experience since 1986. *Neurology* 1996; 46: 465–8.

46 Sparagana SP, Strand WR, Adams RC. Felbamate urolithiasis. *Epilepsia* 2001; 42 (5): 682–5.

47 Rengstorff DS, Milestone AP, Seger DL, Meredith TJ. Felbamate overdose complicated by massive crystalluria and acute renal failure. *J Toxicol Clin Toxicol* 2000; 38 (6): 667–9.

48 Travaglini MT, Morrison RC, Ackerman BH, Haith LR Jr, Patton ML. Toxic epidermal necrolysis after initiation of felbamate. *Pharmacotherapy* 1995; 15 (2): 260–4.

49 Bourgeois B, Leppik IE, Sackellares JC *et al*. Felbamate: a double-blind controlled trial in patients undergoing presurgical evaluation of partial seizures. *Neurology* 1993; 43: 693–6.

50 Theodore WH, Raubertas RF, Porter RJ *et al*. Felbamate: a clinical trial for complex partial seizures. *Epilepsia* 1991; 32: 392–7.

51 Canger R, Vignoli A, Bonardi R, Guidolin L. Felbamate in refractory partial epilepsy. *Epilepsy Res* 1999; 34 (1): 43–8.

52 Leppik IE, Kramer LD, Bourgeois B, Graves NM, Campbell J, Cruz-Rodriguez R. Felbamate after withdrawal from other antiepileptic drugs (Abstract). *Neurology* 1990; 40: 158.

53 Faught E, Sachdeo RC, Remler MP *et al*. Felbamate monotherapy for partial-onset seizures: an active-control trial. *Neurology* 1993; 43: 688–92.

54 Felbamate Study Group in Lennox–Gastaut Syndrome. Efficacy of felbamate in childhood epileptic encephalopathy (Lennox–Gastaut syndrome). *N Engl J Med* 1993; 328: 29–33.

55 Dodson WE. Felbamate in the treatment of Lennox–Gastaut syndrome: results of a 12-month open-label study following a randomized clinical trial. *Epilepsia* 1993; 34 (Suppl. 7): S18–24.

56 Siegel H, Kelley K, Stertz B *et al*. The efficacy of felbamate as add-on therapy to valproic acid in Lennox–Gastaut syndrome. *Epilepsy Res* 1999; 34 (2–3): 91–7.

57 French J, Smith M, Faught E, Brown L. Practice advisory. The use of felbamate in the treatment of patients with intractable epilepsy. *Neurology* 1999; 52: 1540.

58 Segelman FH, Kelton E, Terzi RM, Kucharczyk N, Sofia RD. The comparative potency of phenobarbital and five 1.3-propanediol dicarbamazates for cytochrome p450 induction in rats. *Res Commun Chem Pathol Pharmacol* 1985; 48: 467–70.

59 Swinyard EA, Woodhead JH, Franklin MR, Sofia RD, Kupferberg HJ. The effect of chronic felbamate administration on anticonvulsant activity and hepatic drug-metabolizing enzymes in mice and rats. *Epilepsia* 1987; 28: 295–300.

60 Graves NM, Holmes GB, Leppik IE. Effect of felbamate on phenytoin and carbamazepine serum concentrations. *Epilepsia* 1989; 30: 225–9.

61 Graves NM, Ludden TM, Holmes GB, Fuerst RH, Leppik IE. Pharmacokinetics of felbamate, a novel antiepileptic drug: application of mixed-effect modeling to clinical trials. *Pharmacotherapy* 1989; 9: 372–6.

62 Fuerst RH, Graves NM, Leppik IE, Remmel RP, Rosenfeld WE, Sierzant TL. A preliminary report on alteration of carbamazepine and phenytoin metabolism by felbamate (Abstract) *Drug Intell Clin Pharm* 1986; 20: 465–6.

63 Fuerst RH, Graves NM, Leppik IE, Brundage RC, Holmes GB, Remmel RP. Felbamate increases phenytoin but decreases carbamazepine concentrations. *Epilepsia* 1988; 29: 488–91.

64 Wagner ML, Remmel RP, Graves NM, Leppik IE. Effect of felbamate on carbamazepine and its major metabolites. *Clin Pharmacol Ther* 1993; 53: 536–43.

65 Albani F, Theodore WH, Washington P *et al*. Effect of felbamate on plasma levels of carbamazepine and its metabolites. *Epilepsia* 1991; 32: 130–2.

66 Gidal BE, Zupanc ML. Potential pharmacokinetic interaction between felbamate and phenobarbital. *Ann Pharmacother* 1994; 28: 455–8.

67 Kerrick JM, Wolff DL, Risinger MW, Graves NM. Increased phenobarbital plasma concentrations after felbamate initiation (Abstract). *Epilepsia* 1994; 35 (8): 94.

68 Wagner ML, Graves NM, Leppik IE, Remmel RP, Ward DL, Shumaker RC. The effect of felbamate on valproate disposition (Abstract). *Epilepsia* 1991; 32: 15.

34 Fosphenytoin

R.E. Ramsay and F. Pryor

Primary indication	Status epilepticus and the treatment of acute seizures
Usual preparation	75 mg/mL (which equals 50 mgPE) in 10 ML for IV infusion
Usual dosage	50 mg PE/kg, at a rate of 100–150 mg PE/min
Target range	As for phenytoin
Common/important side-effects	As for IV phenytoin, but less reaction at injection site
Main advantages	Better tolerated than IV phenytoin
Main disadvantages	More expensive than IV phenytoin
Mechanism of action	It is a prodrug of phenytoin
Metabolism and excretion	It is metabolized in the plasma to phenytoin, which is the active agent
Half-life (conversion to phenytoin)	15 min
Active metabolites	Phenytoin
Comment	A useful alternative to IV phenytoin. It is better tolerated at the injection site as it has a more physiological pH than phenytoin, and has the same speed of action. However, it is more expensive and the dosing units (milligrams of phenytoin equivalents) can be confusing

(*Note*: this summary table was formulated by the lead editor.)

Background

Fosphenytoin is a phenytoin prodrug. It is the disodium phosphate ester of 3-hydroxymethyl-5,5-diphenylhydantoin. The phosphate moiety is rapidly and completely hydrolysed by phosphatases found in blood and vascularized tissue such as muscle (Fig. 34.1). There is some interindividual variability [1–10], but the conversion is not dependent on plasma fosphenytoin or phenytoin (PHT) concentrations [1,3,8,11,12] nor on age, race or gender [13]. It was originally formulated in the early 1970s, and has undergone recent clinical studies. It is proposed to be better tolerated than parenteral PHT [14] but equally effective. Fosphenytoin sodium (Cerebyx, Parke-Davis) was licensed in Europe and the US in the late 1990s and is marketed as a replacement for parenteral PHT [15].

Physical and chemical properties

Fosphenytoin has a molecular weight of 406.24 and consists of an off-white powder. Its water solubility at 37°C is 7.5×10^4 µg/mL

(compared to 20.5 µg/mL for PHT) [1]. Dosages of fosphenytoin are expressed as PHT equivalents (PE), which refers to the milligrams of active PHT converted by the hydrolysis of fosphenytoin. Thus, 150 mg of fosphenytoin is equivalent to 100 mg PE which is equivalent to 100 mg of parenteral PHT (Dilantin). Fosphenytoin is available as a ready-mixed solution of 50 mg PE/mL in water for injection (US Pharmacopeia or USP), tromethamine (USP) (Tris) buffer adjusted to pH 8.6–9.0 with either hydrochloric acid (National Formulary or NF) or sodium hydroxide (NF) [16]. In contrast to fosphenytoin, parenteral PHT requires a chemical vehicle consisting of 40% propylene glycol and 10% ethanol in water adjusted to pH 12 with sodium hydroxide. Local and systemic adverse effects of parenteral PHT have been attributed to the relatively high pH of its chemical vehicle [14,17–19]. The molecular structure of fosphenytoin consists of the attachment of a large phosphate ester to the central five-membered ring of PHT which changes its physical chemical properties and renders it water soluble [20]. It has a pH of 8.6–9.0 and does not require excipients such as propylene glycol or alcohol to remain in solution [20]. The increased water solubility of fosphenytoin obviates the need for the propylene glycol and alcohol which are required to make PHT water soluble. Upon entry into the vascular compartment, the phosphate molecule is removed by nonspecific tissue phosphatases thus converting fosphenytoin into active PHT. The only exception to this metabolic process has been described by Annesley *et al.* (2001) in which a unique immunoreactive oxymethylglucuronide metabolite was derived from fosphenytoin in uraemic patients [21]. This is of no clinical significance.

The half-life of conversion is 8–15 min and was the same regardless of dose or fosphenytoin concentration range achieved [3,22]. The plasma clearance of fosphenytoin is not dependent on dose administration and has been reported to be 19.8 ± 1.6 L/h. The conversion is rapid after an IV infusion and is essentially completed within 30–45 min [3].

Clinical pharmacology

Bioavailability

The bioavailability of PHT from fosphenytoin as compared to intravenously administered sodium PHT has been determined in healthy volunteers following IV and IM administration of fosphenytoin [11]. The mean absolute bioavailability of fosphenytoin was 0.992 after IV administration and 1.012 after IM injection. In one study, 12 healthy volunteers were randomized, in a double-blind, cross-over fashion to receive PHT sodium and fosphenytoin IV in 30 min [14]. The conversion half-life of fosphenytoin to PHT was 9.3 ± 2.7 min. More than 99% of fosphenytoin was converted to PHT and no fosphenytoin was detected in the urine. Fosphenytoin was shown to be bioequivalent to PHT and produced less irritation at the injection site than PHT. A pharmacokinetic study is underway to compare the bioavailability of IM stable-labelled fosphenytoin with IV stable-labelled PHT in adults and elderly patients and to determine if the two stable isotopes are kinetically equivalent [23]. The bioavailability of IM fosphenytoin is not affected by age.

Following IM injection, fosphenytoin is 100% bioavailable and rapidly metabolized. Fosphenytoin is undetectable in plasma 4 h after injection [1]. Two hours postadministration of 500 mg of fosphenytoin, the plasma PHT level is essentially the same following equivalent doses of IV Dilantin and IM Cerebyx (Fig. 34.1). Following a higher IM dose (20 mg/kg loading dose of fosphenytoin), blood levels above 10 μg/mL can be achieved within 45 min. Leppik *et al.* compared the maximum concentration (C_{max}) and time to maximum concentration (t_{max}) of fosphenytoin administered IM on a single site versus two sites [3]. For the single injection, the t_{max} was 0.97 ± 1.8 h compared with 0.32 ± 0.4 h. The C_{max} for a single site injection was 8.9 mg/L compared with 16.8 mg/L for two injection sites. Thus, more rapid and higher peaks are attained following injections at two sites. The tissue phosphatases responsible for the conversion of fosphenytoin to PHT are ubiquitous. Phosphatase activity is present at all ages and the activity is not altered by age, disease states or medications. Thus, the conversion should be similar in all patients.

Protein binding

The protein binding and pharmacokinetics of fosphenytoin, diazepam and PHT were evaluated in nine healthy male volunteers [24]. PHT-free fraction increased significantly with rising fosphenytoin concentrations, suggesting PHT displacement from its binding sites by fosphenytoin. Fosphenytoin is highly bound (95.7 ± 0.48%) to serum proteins, predominantly, albumin. Increased clearance of fosphenytoin may occur in hypoalbuminaemia [25]. Fosphenytoin competes with PHT for binding sites. With a 20 mg/kg loading dose of fosphenytoin, a higher unbound fraction is achieved using a faster infusion rate of 150 mg/min as compared to a slower rate of 50 mg/min [26]. However, PHT binding stabilizes as plasma fosphenytoin concentrations decline (30–60 min postinfusion).

Distribution

The volume of distribution of fosphenytoin has been evaluated in two pharmacokinetic studies. In the first, fosphenytoin was administered IV over 30 min using doses of 150, 300, 600 and 1200 mg to four different groups of volunteers [2]. The AUC was 10, 19, 43 and 55 mghr/L, respectively, and was proportional to dose. The clearance of fosphenytoin is 0.24 ± 0.08 L/kg/h. The volume of distribution is approximately 2.6 L, suggesting that most of the dose remains in plasma. In the second study, 10 patients (nine male and

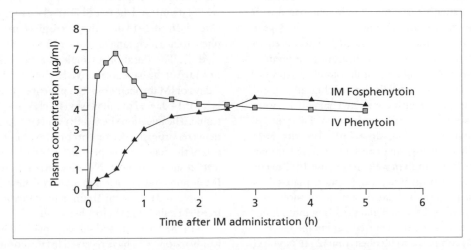

Fig. 34.1 Comparison of phenytoin levels following the administration of 500 mg of phenytoin IV or 500 mg of fosphenytoin IM.

one female) received a single IV dose of 100–200 mg PE and an equivalent IM dose was administered 1 week later [5]. The volume of distribution for IV dose was 0.040 ± 0.0084 L/kg with a conversion half-life of 8.0 ± 2.9 min. Mean clearance overall was 0.24 ± 0.080 L/kg/h in the 10 patients. The volume of distribution was 2.8 L in this group of patients, similar to that previously reported in healthy volunteers.

Chemical stability

A study of the chemical stability of fosphenytoin has been reported. Admixtures of fosphenytoin 1, 8 and 20 mg with NaCl 0.9% injection, dextrose 5% and 11 other IV solutions were prepared and stored at $-20°C$ in glass or PVC containers for 7 days [27]. Additionally, 63 syringes were filled with fosphenytoin sodium 50 mg PE/mL (undiluted) and stored at 25, 4 or $-20°C$. There were no discernible changes in colour or clarity in any of the fosphenytoin solutions throughout the study. No visible precipitation was observed. Fosphenytoin concentrations remained stable at each sampling, regardless of container, concentration, IV solution or storage temperature. Fosphenytoin remains stable for at least 30 days at room temperature, under refrigeration or frozen. Furthermore, solutions of fosphenytoin in a number of different IV fluids were stable for at least 7 days at room temperature. In another study, glass vials of fosphenytoin were placed in a water bath maintained at room temperature. Over a period of 12 months, assays were taken and analysed periodically to determine the extent of degradation of fosphenytoin. Results showed that there was no degradation of product over the 12 months. Findings from a subsequent study indicate that fosphenytoin remains physically stable for at least 2 years at $25°C$ in pH ranging from 7.4 to 8.0 [28].

Intravenous clinical trials

To compare the safety and tolerance of IV fosphenytoin, a single-dose, double-blind study was conducted in patients requiring a loading dose of PHT [29]. Fifty-two patients were randomized to receive either IV fosphenytoin ($n=39$) or IV Dilantin ($n=13$). Patients in the treatment group received similar doses of study drug (899 mg PE; 12.7 mg/kg) or Dilantin (879 mg; 11.3 mg/kg). However, the fosphenytoin was infused at nearly twice the rate of administration (82 mg PE/min; range 40–103 mg PE/min) compared with patients in the Dilantin group (42.4 mg/min). Despite the higher rate of infusion, fosphenytoin was well tolerated and produced no significant cardiac arrhythmias or changes in heart rate, respiration or diastolic blood pressure. A decline in systolic blood pressure occurred and was reported to be statistically but not clinically significant. A similar study was subsequently conducted but patients were given maintenance doses of IV fosphenytoin or IV Dilantin for 3–14 days after receiving a loading dose [30]. Patients were randomized to receive IV fosphenytoin ($n=88$, mean dose 1088 mg PE or 15.3 mg PE/kg) or IV Dilantin ($n=28$, mean dose 1082 mg or 15.0 mg/kg). Maintenance therapy was given for more than 4 days (fosphenytoin 4.3 days, Dilantin 4.7 days). Similar infusion rates were used (fosphenytoin 37 mg PE/min, Dilantin 33 mg/min). A significantly greater number of patients reported pain in the infusion site with Dilantin (17%) compared to fosphenytoin (2%). No ECG changes were found. Reduction in systolic and diastolic blood pressure was reported in five patients in both groups. However, symptomatic hypotension requiring reduction in infusion rates occurred four times more often with IV Dilantin ($n=4$, 17.9%). A subset of 10 patients had serial timed total and free plasma fosphenytoin and PHT levels drawn after the loading dose. At the first sample drawn at 1 h postinfusion, all patients had total PHT levels above 10 µg/mL and the mean concentrations were essentially the same for the two groups.

The pharmacokinetics, safety and tolerance of IV fosphenytoin has been investigated in 17 clinical studies. Of the 925 patients and subjects involved in the fosphenytoin clinical trials, 514 received IV injections. Nine clinical trials involving 136 healthy subjects were completed using doses of 100–1200 mg and infusion rates of 3.3–150 mg/min. Fosphenytoin, total PHT and free PHT concentrations and pharmacokinetic parameters were similar in patients and healthy subjects. Plasma fosphenytoin concentration increases with increasing dose and infusion rate, peaks at the end of infusion, and then declines with a half-life of approximately 0.25 h [22].

A total of 378 patients received fosphenytoin in doses ranging from 205 to 2280 mg (2.7–20.3 mg/kg) of PE and infusion rates of 3.3–167 mg PE/min. To investigate bioequivalence, 43 patients with chronic epilepsy were entered into an open-labelled, single-dose safety and pharmacokinetic study [3]. These patients had been treated with PHT with documented stable levels. Mean trough PHT levels were the same following oral Dilantin, IV fosphenytoin and IM fosphenytoin. Analysis of ECG revealed no significant change in RR, PR, QRS and QT intervals, and no disturbances of cardiac rhythms after IV administration of fosphenytoin. Minor and transient discomfort was reported with IV infusion 17% and IM injection (14%).

Intramuscular clinical trials

A prospective open-label study on safety, tolerance and pharmacokinetics was conducted in 118 patients [31]. Neurosurgical patients 12 years or older who were to be treated with PHT were included. Patients were given an IM loading dose of fosphenytoin (8–12 mg/kg) after which timed plasma samples were obtained for total and free fosphenytoin and PHT concentrations. The initial dose administered ranged from 480 to 1500 mg (8–22 mg/kg). By the time the first PHT sample was drawn at 1 h postdosing, the total level was 11 µg/mL and the free PHT level was approximately 1.5 µg/mL. Over the next 2–14 days they were given maintenance doses of fosphenytoin which ranged from 130 to 1250 mg/day (1.7–17.2 mg/kg/day). The duration of maintenance treatment varies: 98.8% ($n=116$) of the patients received 2 days and 14.4% ($n=17$) received 7 days of IM fosphenytoin. No patients received maintenance therapy for 14 days. Trough plasma levels were obtained and remained stable. The injection sites were evaluated daily with 96% of the patients reporting no discomfort or pain after the loading dose. At the end of the maintenance period, 98% of the patients reported no injection site discomfort. No adverse reactions were noted from the IM administration of fosphenytoin. These authors demonstrated the rapid and consistent attainment of therapeutic plasma total and free PHT following IM fosphenytoin.

Of the 882 patients and subjects involved in the clinical trials with fosphenytoin, 411 have received IM injections. These have included pharmacokinetics, dosage maintenance and loading dose studies.

In a double-blind parallel study, 240 patients were randomized to receive either oral Dilantin and IM placebo ($n=61$) or oral placebo and IM fosphenytoin ($n=179$) for 5 days [32]. This was conducted in patients receiving oral Dilantin once a day for the treatment of epilepsy or seizure prophylaxis following neurosurgery. The dose given to each patient remained constant throughout the study. The fosphenytoin dose for each patient provided an equivalent amount of PHT as the dose of Dilantin they had taken during the baseline period. The trough plasma levels remained the same during open baseline and the double-blind treatment phase. The injection sites were evaluated for pain, burning and itching after the loading and maintenance doses. The rating scale was none (score=0), mild (score=1), moderate (score=2) and severe (score=3). No severe reactions were reported. The average score 5 min postinjection was less than 0.3 for all measures except for pain in the IM placebo group which was 0.51. There was no difference in the scores for IM fosphenytoin and placebo for burning or itching. In a subset of 13 of the patients participating in this trial, serial timed plasma levels were drawn following oral Dilantin during baseline and on the last day of IM fosphenytoin administration during the blinded treatment period [10]. The average plasma level as measured by the AUC of the plasma level vs time was higher with IM fosphenytoin (AUC=418) than with oral Dilantin (AUC=400) but this was not a clinically significant difference. The trough plasma level at 24 h was the same for both groups.

The experience derived from these studies indicate that dosage adjustments are not usually necessary when converting from oral Dilantin to IM fosphenytoin for 1–2 weeks. The plasma total and free PHT concentrations were maintained in the therapeutic range following conversion from PO PHT to equimolar IM fosphenytoin. A 100-mg Dilantin capsule actually contains 92 mg of PHT while the IV preparation actually contains 100 mg of PHT per 1.0 mL of solution (50 mg/mL). Longer term maintenance on Cerebyx could result in some increase in the plasma level. The plasma level should be checked after 2 or more weeks of IM or IV Cerebyx therapy.

The rate and extent of absorption and the tolerability of IM fosphenytoin have been evaluated in an open-label, double-blind study [33]. Twenty-four patients, 12 males and 12 females, were enrolled. Patients selected required a loading dose of PHT for the treatment of epilepsy, seizure prophylaxis or volunteered to participate. Each patient received 10 mg/kg of fosphenytoin IM and a saline injection to compare tolerability. Half of the patients received a volume of saline equal to that of the fosphenytoin while the other half received only 2 cm^3 of saline. The group ranged in age from 19 to 60 years (mean, 35–10 SD years). Weight ranged from 49.1 to 97.3 kg (mean, 79.4–13.9 SD kg). Doses of fosphenytoin ranged from 491 to 973 mg PE which corresponded to injection volumes ranging from 9.8 to 19.5 mL. The accepted loading dose of fosphenytoin is 20 mg PE/kg which corresponds to injection volumes ranging from 20 to 40 mL. Typically, this full loading dose is divided into two injections of 10 mg/kg each. Since study participants would be receiving saline injections on the opposite side for tolerability comparison, a loading dose of 10 mg/kg was used to abide by standard clinical practice and avoid multiple injections of fosphenytoin. Therapeutic serum concentrations of PHT were achieved as early as 5 min after the IM administration of fosphenytoin in 14.3% of patients and in 26.3% after 10 min. By 20 min, 37% of the patients had achieved PHT serum concentrations greater than 10 μg/mL. More than half the patients had therapeutic serum concentrations at 30 min. Nearly 40% of patients had a free PHT level of 1.0 μg/mL or more by 40 min. At 50 min, 14 of 18 patients had achieved unbound PHT levels of 1.0 μg/mL or more (Fig. 34.2). There was a statistically significant difference in pain between the fosphenytoin and saline sides immediately postinjection and at 30 min ($\chi^2=$ 0.0386 and $\chi^2=0.0386$, respectively). However, there was no significant difference in pain at 60 min and thereafter. Fosphenytoin injections were slightly more uncomfortable than saline injections, however, volume did not appear to be the determining factor. These investigators demonstrated that IM administration of fosphenytoin produces therapeutic PHT serum concentrations very rapidly (as early as 5–20 min) and that it is well tolerated by most patients irrespective of injection volume.

The safety and tolerance of IM fosphenytoin have been tested in 60 patients (35 males, 25 females) requiring a loading dose of PHT [34]. The mean age of patients was 43 years (range 16–80 years); mean weight 79 kg (40–146 kg). Reasons justifying the use of a loading dose included non-compliance 18%; first-time PHT treatment 30%; decreased PHT serum levels 37%; other 15%. A dose of 20 mg/kg of PHT was given to patients with non-detectable plasma level. Those with a plasma level below 7.1 μg/mL were included in

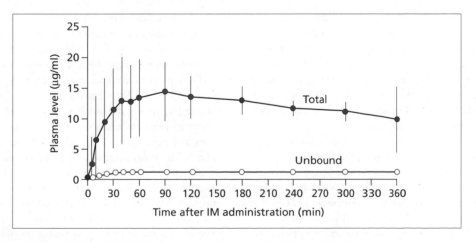

Fig. 34.2 Total phenytoin and unbound phenytoin levels after intramuscular injection of fosphenytoin.

the study and given a loading dose of 15 mg/kg. The mean loading dose administered was 17.7 mg/kg (range 5.4–30.3 mg/kg) for a mean total dose of 1359.8 mg (range 525–2250 mg). Most loading doses required 15–20 mL of fosphenytoin solution. Fosphenytoin was given as a single site injection in 29 cases, multiple injection sites were used in the remaining 31 cases. Site of administration was the gluteus in 58 cases and deltoid in two cases. Despite the relatively large volume of the IM injection, there was no unusual discomfort or side-effects with gluteal or deltoid injections. Local irritation at the site of injection occurred in 5% of cases and was considered mild in each case. No serious local adverse reactions were noted. The largest volume injected was 30 mL which was given into a single muscle site. This patient reported no pain, burning or discomfort, and attests to how well IM fosphenytoin is tolerated. Forty patients reported experiencing some adverse events (AEs) after the IM injection with the most frequent being nystagmus (47%), dizziness (17%) and ataxia (13%). Eighty-two per cent of the AEs reported were considered to be of mild intensity. It is important to note that the nature and frequency of side-effects reported after IM loading of fosphenytoin were similar to those experienced after IV PHT.

Fosphenytoin use in paediatric populations

In a retrospectic study, 52 paediatric patients who received fosphenytoin IV therapy for seizures were evaluated [35]. Age ranged from 4 days to 16 years of age. PHT serum levels were maintained within the therapeutic range (10–20 µg/mL). No infusion site complications were reported in any of the patients. Only one patient experienced cardiac arrhythmia from an accidental overdose. Eight neonates (1–146 days old) received IV fosphenytoin for the treatment of status epilepticus [36]. Six patients had failed to be treated with phenobarbital. Of these, two had received lorazepam as well. Loading doses of fosphenytoin PE ranged from 14.5 to 24.3 mg/kg. Seven of the eight patients achieved therapeutic PHT levels. Complete seizure control was obtained in 50%. No side-effects were observed in any of the patients.

Clinical efficacy

Acute seizures and status epilepticus

Intravenous Dilantin has been the mainstay in the treatment of status epilepticus. The above described studies used fosphenytoin infusion rates of approximately 100 mg PE/min. At this rate, the free PHT levels reached were less than that those achieved with 50 mg/min of Dilantin, a rate commonly employed in the treatment of SE. Fosphenytoin must be given at 150 mg PE/min to produce a free PHT level bioequivalent to that produced by 50 mg/min of PHT. Thus, additional clinical experience is needed in the area of status epilepticus and faster rates of infusion [37].

A double-blind parallel safety and tolerance study was conducted comparing IV fosphenytoin given at 150 mg PE/min vs. Dilantin at 50 mg/min [34]. Patients were randomized on a 4 : 1 basis to receive intravenous fosphenytoin (n=90) or Dilantin (n=22). Loading dose was either 20 mg/kg (patients with no detectable PHT in the plasma) or 15 mg/kg if plasma PHT level was 7 µg/mL or less. The most common reasons for patient inclusion were treatment of acute seizures, low PHT levels in patients with epilepsy or seizure prophy-

laxis in neurosurgical patients. Patient demographics were similar between the fosphenytoin and Dilantin groups. Infusions had to be slowed or discontinued significantly more often with IV Dilantin than with fosphenytoin. Adverse events with the two drugs were different, with pruritus, at times very uncomfortable, more common with fosphenytoin (48.9%) and pain at the site of infusion more frequently reported with Dilantin (63.6%). The other side-effects of dizziness, somnolence and ataxia are typical of PHT effect and were the same for both drugs. The pruritus with fosphenytoin typically occurred in the trunk, especially in the groin region, or the back of the head. Pruritus, when reported, presented soon after initiation of the infusion and abated rapidly when the infusion was discontinued. The occurrence and severity of the pruritus was a rate-dependent phenomenon as lowering the rate reduced or abolished the symptom. Changes in blood pressure were noted in both groups with a mean decline in systolic pressure of 13.7 mmHg with fosphenytoin and 5.9 mmHg with Dilantin. By this one measure, the decrease was statistically more common with fosphenytoin but it was not felt to be clinically significant. Direct cardiovascular effects in this study were difficult to compare as the duration of infusions were different (fosphenytoin, 13 min; Dilantin, 44 min). Blood pressure changes occurred 10–20 min after the initiation of the IV infusion. The decrease in systolic blood pressure was gradual and lasted for 10–15 min. Patients with pre-existing hypertension and under treatment with antihypertensives were at increased risk (13/16) for a systolic decline of 20 mmHg or more. There was no association between specific antihypertensive medication and a drop in systolic blood pressure. Patients with underlying ischaemic heart disease also seemed to be at increased risk for mild decline in BP (9/13). There were no cases in which the hypotension was judged to be severe enough to justify discontinuation of treatment although the IV infusion rate was reduced in a total of six patients—four on fosphenytoin (4.7%), two on Dilantin (9.1%). Several clinically unstable intensive care patients with neurosurgical, neurological or cardiac problems were included in the protocol. These patients tolerated the rapid infusions of IV fosphenytoin without clinically significant changes on blood pressure or cardiac arrhythmias.

The treatment for overt status epilepticus was evaluated in a Veterans Affairs Cooperative Study [38]. The highest treatment success rate was obtained with parenteral lorazepam (64.9%) followed by phenobarbital (58.2%), diazepam/PHT (55.8%) and PHT alone (43.6%). Based on these findings, the recommended first-line treatment for generalized convulsive status epilepticus is IV lorazepam. Fosphenytoin or PHT is still recommended as a second-line agent if SE is not controlled within 5–7 min [37].

An open-label, single-dose, safety, tolerance and pharmacokinetic trial of fosphenytoin was completed in 85 patients in convulsive status epilepticus [39]. Infusion rates of 100 mg/min were used in the first 10 patients and of 150 mg/min in the remaining 75 patients. Patients 5 years and older having two or more generalized convulsions without regaining consciousness between seizures were included. The study included 10 patients under the age of 16 years (mean 7.6 year) and 75 patients ranging from 18 to 82 years of age (mean 43.7 year). Applying the same criteria used in the VA Cooperative Study 265 on status epilepticus [38], seizures were controlled in 79 (92.9%) patients with fosphenytoin. Only two patients experienced seizure recurrence within the next 24 h. Three were not controlled and one was not evaluated because of the inadequate dose given (2 mg PE/kg). The mean dose administered was 967 mg PE (18.6 mg PE/kg) and ranged from 216 to 2000 mg PE (8.2–26.1 mg PE/kg). Mean rate of infusion was 2.6 mg/kg/min in children and 130 mg PE/min (36.4–218 mg PE/min) in the adults. The mean duration of the IV infusion was 11 min. No side-effects were encountered which required the infusion rate to be lowered. Hypotension, which has been a concern with high-dose high-rate infusion of IV Dilantin, was not encountered. Significantly higher free PHT levels were obtained in patient groups receiving fosphenytoin 20 mg/kg at 150 mg/min with more than half having free levels ranging from 5 to 20 µg/mL [40]. This is much higher than achieved using the same loading dose of parenteral Dilantin. Blood samples were drawn at the conclusion of the infusion. Free levels above 5 µg/mL were achieved in the majority of the fosphenytoin patients which is probably the reason for the greater efficacy found in this study. Free PHT levels ranged up to approximately 6 µg/mL when fosphenytoin was given at 100 mg PE/min [40]. Thus, greater efficacy would be expected with the more rapid infusion rate (150 mg PE/min). No cardiac arrhythmias were observed and no adjustments in infusion rates were required due to changes in vital signs. Some decline in blood pressure was observed during or after the infusion but was not judged to be clinically significant. At follow-up evaluation 24 h later, only 3% of the patients reported tenderness at the infusion site and no inflammation or phlebitis was found.

Medication errors

A case of acute intoxication with fosphenytoin has been reported by Presutti et al. (2000) in France [41]. A 74-year-old patient following surgery for a chronic subdural haematoma mistakenly received 10 times the prescribed dose of fosphenytoin as prophylaxis for epilepsy. The PHT blood level was 79 µg/mL. The patient was comatose for 5 days and required mechanical ventilation. No adverse cardiovascular event was noted. Within 8 days the PHT levels returned to normal. Twenty days after surgery, the patient was discharged from the hospital and suffered no further sequela from the acute fosphenytoin intoxication. The absence of cardiovascular complications suggests that even at very high doses fosphenytoin is safer than parenteral Dilantin.

Cardiac arrest was reported following fast intravenous infusion of PHT mistaken for fosphenytoin [42]. A 25-year-old woman admitted for status epilepticus was initially treated with 5 mg of lorazepam IV and later prescribed 1500 mg/PE of fosphenytoin to be administered intravenously at 150 PE/min. The patient developed acute sinus bradycardia (heart rate decreased to 34 over about 2 min) followed by a precipitous drop in blood pressure (45/0 mmHg). Asystole ensued and cardiopulmonary resuscitation was started. The patient recovered within 15 min. This report illustrates the importance of knowing which formulation of PHT is being administered. Rapid infusion of parenteral Dilantin as demonstrated here has been associated with serious adverse events including death [43,44].

Cost considerations

The cost-effectiveness of using parenteral fosphenytoin (Cerebyx) versus PHT (Dilantin) for the treatment of acute seizures and status

epilepticus remains a controversial issue. The cost per package for fosphenytoin (Cerebyx) is approximately 26 times greater than parenteral Dilantin (based on Parke-Davis catalogue prices) [45]. However, other factors must be considered in determining cost-effectiveness of a prescription. Marchetti et al. (1996) conducted a multicentre, double-blind, parallel group study to evaluate costs of administering IV fosphenytoin versus IV PHT in emergency departments [46]. A total of 52 patients were enrolled. Thirty-nine patients were randomized to the IV fosphenytoin group and 13 to IV PHT group. The acquisition cost per loading dose was significantly higher for fosphenytoin ($US90.00) compared with PHT ($US6.72). The average wholesale price for PHT was $US1.68 per package and $US45.00 per package for fosphenytoin (500-mg equivalent of PHT). Total adverse event monitoring costs were $US536.86 for IV PHT versus $US66.20 for IV fosphenytoin. The most common side-effects reported with the use of PHT were significant neurological toxicity (moderate to severe ataxia or vertigo), severe IV site reaction and symptomatic decrease in blood pressure (>20 mmHg systolic). Only the latter was reported with fosphenytoin. The adverse events resulted in higher utilization of resources. There was a significant cost savings of $US386.89 (11%) with IV fosphenytoin compared with IV PHT, primarily based on the less favourable side-effect profile of PHT.

Armstrong et al. (1999) developed a model of cost and clinical outcomes to compare the cost-effectiveness of parenteral PHT versus fosphenytoin [47]. The data were collected using a questionnaire. This model assumed that 50% of PHT would be replaced by fosphenytoin. They calculated mean cost-effectiveness ratios (defined as the cost to achieve the desired goal of administering a loading dose without complication) for PHT alone, fosphenytoin plus PHT (50% each) and fosphenytoin alone. The average cost of a loading dose of PHT ($US58) was less than the average cost of both 50% fosphenytoin/PHT ($US94) and fosphenytoin alone ($US130). However, the average cost-effectiveness ratios were $US225 for PHT, $US149 for the 50/50 option and $US130 for fosphenytoin alone. PHT-induced peripheral vascular failure (phlebitis-type effects) frequently required central line placement. In the PHT group, 62.3±43.4% of patients receiving loading doses and 74.0±32.9% receiving maintenance doses experienced venous irritation. In the fosphenytoin group, side-effects were uncommon (0.3±1.0%). These investigators concluded that institutions with comparable drug costs should consider replacing PHT with fosphenytoin for loading and maintenance doses primarily based on the reduction of side-effects. Further pharmacoeconomic studies are needed to better define the cost-effectiveness of replacing parenteral PHT with fosphenytoin. However, present information indicates that fosphenytoin is most cost-effective.

Clinical therapeutics

PHT is an effective parenteral anticonvulsant and despite the significant problems with its parenteral formulation, it has been the mainstay for the treatment of various forms of acute seizures and status epilepticus for almost 50 years. Amongst the disadvantages of parenteral Dilantin are the facts that it is formulated in propylene glycol and alcohol and has a pH of 14; both contribute to its toxicity. Fosphenytoin (Cerebyx) is water soluble and has a physiological pH, and these are the two main chemical advantages over the parent drug. It is also easier and quicker to administer, although the initially used rate of 150 mg PE/min carries some risk, and most authorities now administer the drug more slowly (100 mg PHT PE/min). PHT and fosphenytoin have similar but not identical therapeutic profiles. Both are of equal efficacy in acute epilepsy given IV, and probably in status epilepticus although there are no controlled or randomized trials in the latter indication. The good tolerability of IM fosphenytoin extends its use to other clinical situations where prompt administration of a non-depressing anticonvulsant is indicated but secure intravenous access and cardiac monitoring are not available. The units of administration are mg/PEs and this is a potentially confusing nomenclature which has lead to errors in prescribing; great care should be exercised in dosing. The manufacturers recommend that the drug should never be written in milligrams of fosphenytoin. The clinical therapeutics of status epilepticus are discussed in more detail in Chapter 18.

References

1 Browne TR, Szabo GK, McGovern J. Bioavailability studies of drugs with nonlinear pharmacokinetics. II. Absolute bioavailability of intravenous phenytoin prodrug at therapeutic phenytoin serum concentration determined by double stable isotope technique. *J Pharmacol Sci* 1993; 33: 89–94.

2 Gerber N, Mays DC, Donn KH. Safety, tolerance, and pharmacokinetics of intravenous doses of phosphate ester of 3-hydroxymethyl-5-diphenyl hydantoin: a new prodrug of phenytoin. *J Clin Pharm* 1988; 28: 1023–32.

3 Leppik IE, Boucher BA, Wilder BJ *et al.* Pharmacokinetics and safety of a phenytoin prodrug given IV in patients. *Neurology* 1990; 40: 456–60.

4 Browne TR, Le Duc B. Phenytoin and fosphenytoin: biotransformation. In: Levy RY, Mattson R, Meldrum BS, eds. *Antiepileptic Drugs*. New York: Raven, 1995: 283–300.

5 Boucher BA, Bombassaro A, Rasmussen SN *et al.* Phenytoin prodrug 3-phosphoryloxy-methyl phenytoin (ACC-9653): pharmacokinetics in patients following intravenous and intramuscular administration. *J Pharmacol Sci* 1989; 78: 929–32.

6 Eldon MA, Loewen GR, Voigtman RE, Holmes GB, Hunt TL, Sedman AJ. Safety, tolerance, and pharmacokinetics of intravenous fosphenytoin. *Clin Pharmacol Ther* 1993; 53: 212.

7 Aweeka F, Alldredge B, Boyer T, Warnock D, Gambertoglio J. Conversion of ACC-9653 to phenytoin in patients with renal or hepatic diseases. *Clin Pharmacol Ther* 1989; 45: 152.

8 Broumer K, Matier WL, Quon CY. Absolute bioavailability of phenytoin after IV 3-phosphoryloxymethyl phenytoin disodium. *Clin Pharmacol Ther* 1988; 43: 178.

9 Boucher BA, Kugler AR, Hess MM, Feler C. Pharmacokinetics of fosphenytoin, a phenytoin prodrug, following intramuscular administration in critically ill neurosurgery patients. *Crit Care Med* 1995; 23: A78.

10 Garnett WR, Kugler AR, O'Hara KA, Driscoll SM, Pellock JM. Pharmacokinetics of fosphenytoin following intramuscular administration of fosphenytoin substituted for oral phenytoin in epileptic patients. *Neurology* 1995; 45: A248.

11 Browne TR, Davoudi H, Donn KH *et al.* Bioavailability of ACC-9653 (phenytoin prodrug). *Epilepsia* 1989; 30: S27–S32.

12 Eldon MA, Loewen GR, Voigtman RE *et al.* Pharmacokinetics and tolerance of fosphenytoin and phenytoin administered intravenously to healthy subjects. *Can J Neurol Sci* 1993; 20: S180.

13 Kugler AR, Knapp LE, Eldon MA. Intravenous administration of fosphenytoin: Pharmacokinetics and dosing considerations in special populations. *Epilepsia* 1996; 37: 156.

14 Jamerson B. Venous irritation related to intravenous administration of phenytoin versus fosphenytoin. *Pharmacotherapy* 1994; 14: 47–52.

15 Stella VJ, Higuchi T. Esters of hydantoic acid as prodrugs of hydantoins. *J Pharmacol Sci* 1973; 62: 962.

16 Parke-Davis. Cerebyx injection (Parke-Davis). 1998.

17 Serrano EE, Roye DB, Hammer RH, Wilder BJ. Plasma diphenylhydantoin values after oral and intramuscular administration of diphenylhydantoin. *Neurology* 1973; 23: 311–17.

18 Wilder BJ, Ramsay RE, Serrano EE, Buchanan RA. A method for shifting from oral to intramuscular diphenylhydantoin administration. *Clin Pharm Ther* 1974; 16: 507–13.

19 Hanna DR. Purple glove syndrome: a complication of intravenous phenytoin. *J Neurosci Nurs* 1992; 24: 340–5.

20 Smith RD, Brown BS, Maher RW, Matier WL. Pharmacology of ACC-9653 (phenytoin prodrug). *Epilepsia* 1989; 30 (Suppl. 2): S15–S21.

21 Annesley TM, Kurzyniec S, Nordblom GD *et al.* Glucuronidation of prodrug reactive site: Isolation and characterization of oxymethylglucuronide metabolite of fosphenytoin. *Clin Chem* 2001; 47: 910–18.

22 Besserer J, Cook J, Eldon M. A randomized, double blind, placebo controlled, rising single dose study of the pharmacokinetic and tolerance profiles of intravenous fosphenytoin sodium (CI-982) administered at five different infusion rates to healthy subjects. Unpublished data, 1994.

23 Musib LC, Cloyd JC, Birnbaum AK *et al.* Pilot bioavailability study comparing intramuscularly administered stable-labeled fosphenytoin in adults and elderly patients. *Epilepsia* 2001; (Suppl. 7:90), Abst. 1.285.

24 Hussey EK, Dukes GE, Messenheimer JA *et al.* Evaluation of the pharmacokinetic interaction between diazepam and ACC-9653 (a phenytoin prodrug) in healthy male volunteers. *Pharmaceut Res* 1990; 7: 1172–6.

25 Lai CM, Moore P, Quon CY. Binding of fosphenytoin, phosphate ester pro drug of phenytoin, to human serum proteins and competitive binding with carbamazepine, diazepam, phenobarbital, phenylbutazone, phenytoin, valproic acid or warfarin. *Res Comm Mol Pathol Pharmacol* 1995; 88: 51–62.

26 Ramsay RE, Philbrook B, Fischer JH, Sloan EP, Allen FH, Runge JW, Smith MF, Kugler AR. Safety and pharmacokinetics of fosphenytoin (Cerebyx) compared with dilantin following rapid intravenous administration. *Neurology* 1996; 46(2): A245.

27 Fischer J, Cwik MJ, Luer MS, Sibley CB, Deyo KL. Stability of fosphenytoin sodium with intravenous solutions in glass bottles, polyvinyl chloride bags, and polypropylene syringes. *Ann Pharmacother* 1997; 31: 553–9.

28 Narisawa S, Stella VJ. Increased shelf-life of fosphenytoin: solubilization of a degradant, phenytoin, through complexation with (SBE) 7m-beta-CD. *J Pharmaceut Sci* 1998; 87: 926–30.

29 Fischer J, Turnbull T, Uthman BM, Wilder BJ, So EL, Cascino G. Safety, tolerance, pharmacokinetics of intravenous loading doses of fosphenytoin versus dilantin. *Neurology* 1995; 45 (Suppl. 4), A202.

30 Baron BA, Hankin S, Knapp LE. Advantages of intravenous fosphenytoin (Cerebyx) compared with IV phenytoin (Dilantin). *Neurology* 1995; 45: 248–9.

31 Dean JC, Smith KR, Boucher BA, Michie DD, Kugler AR, Marriott JG. Safety, tolerance and pharmacokinetics of intramuscular (IM) fosphenytoin, a phenytoin prodrug, in neurosurgery patients. *Epilepsia* 1993; 34: 111.

32 Wilder BJ, Ramsay RE, Marriott JG, Loewen G, Smith H. Safety and tolerance of intramuscular administration of fosphenytoin, a phenytoin prodrug, for 5 days in patients with epilepsy. *Neurology* 1993; 43 (Suppl. 2), A308.

33 Pryor FM, Ramsay RE, Gidal BE, Morgan RO. Fosphenytoin: Pharmacokinetics and tolerance of intramuscular loading doses. *Epilepsia* 2001; 42: 245–50.

34 Ramsay RE, Philbrook B, Martinez OA *et al.* A double-blinded, randomized safety comparison of rapidly infused intravenous loading doses of fosphenytoin vs. phenytoin. *Epilepsia* 1995; 36 (Suppl. 4): 52.

35 Morton LD, O'Hara KA, Meloche NM, Garnett WR, Pellock JM. Fosphenytoin experience in pediatric patients. *Epilepsia* 1999; 40: 131.

36 Gustafson MC, Ritter FJ, Minnesota Epilepsy Group PA. Fosphenytoin loading for status epilepticus in the neonate. *Epilepsia* 1999; 40: 124.

37 Bleck TP. Management approaches to prolonged seizures and status epilepticus. (Review). *Epilepsia* 1999; 40 (Suppl. 1): S59–S63.

38 Treiman DM, Meyers PD, Walton NY, Collins JF, Collings C, Rowan AJ *et al.* Treatment of generalized convulsive status epilepticus: a randomized double-blind comparison of four intravenous regimens. *N Engl J Med* 1998; 339 (Spe 17): 792–8.

39 Allen FH, Bunge JW, Legarda S *et al.* Safety, tolerance and pharmacokinetics of intravenous fosphenytoin (Cerebyx) in status epilepticus. *Epilepsia* 1995; 36 (Suppl. 4): 90.

40 Kugler AR, Knapp LE, Eldon MA. Attainment of therapeutic phenytoin concentrations following administration of loading doses of fosphenytoin: A meta analysis. *Neurology* 1996; 46: A176.

41 Presutti M, Pollet L, Stordeur JM, Bruder N, Gouin F. Acute poisoning with phenytoin caused by an error in the administration of fosphenytoin. *Ann Franc Anesth Reanim* 2000; 19: 688–90.

42 DeToledo J, Lowe M, Rabinstein A, Villaviza N. Cardiac arrest after fast intravenous infusion of phenytoin mistaken for fosphenytoin. *Epilepsia* 2001; 42: 288.

43 Earnest MP, Marx JA, Drury LR. Complications of intraveneous phenytoin for acute treatment of seizures: Recommendations for usage. *J Royal Soc Med* 1983; 249: 762–5.

44 Katilavas JW. Soft tissue associated with intravenous phenytoin (reply). *N Engl J Med* 1984; 311: 1187.

45 Fierro L, Hudak J. Cost of fosphenytoin. *Ann Emerg Med* 1998; 31: 137–8.

46 Marchetti A, Magar R, Fischer J, Sloan E, Fischer P. A pharmacoeconomic evaluation of intravenous fosphenytoin (Cerebyx) versus intravenous phenytoin (Dilantin) in hospital emergency departments. *Clin Ther* 1996; 18: 953–66.

47 Armstrong EP, Sauer KA, Downey MJ. Phenytoin and fosphenytoin: A model of cost and clinical outcomes. *Pharmacotherapy* 1999; 19: 844–53.

35

Gabapentin

T.R. Browne

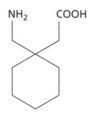

Primary indications	Adjunctive therapy or monotherapy in adults with partial or secondarily generalized epilepsy
Usual preparations	Capsules: 100, 300, 400 mg
Usual dosages	Initial: 300 mg/day. Maintenance: 900–3600 mg/day
Dosage intervals	2–3 times/day
Significant drug interactions	Felbamate clearance slowed
Serum level monitoring	Not useful
Target range	2–20 µg/mL
Common/important side-effects	Drowsiness, dizziness, seizure exacerbation, ataxia, headache, tremor, diplopia, nausea, vomiting, rhinitis, non-pitting leg oedema
Main advantages	Lack of side-effects (especially at low doses) and good pharmacokinetic profile
Main disadvantages	Lack of therapeutic effect in severe cases. Seizure exacerbation
Mechanisms of action	Not known. Possible action on calcium channels
Oral bioavailability	<65% (dose dependent)
Time to peak levels	2–3 h
Metabolism and excretion	Renal excretion without metabolism
Volume of distribution	0.65–1.04 L/kg
Elimination half-life	5–7 h
Plasma clearance	0.120–0.130 L/kg/h (varies with age)
Protein binding	None
Active metabolites	None
Comment	Novel anticonvulsant of uncertain relative efficacy, but easy to use and few side-effects

(*Note*: this summary table was formulated by the lead editor.)

Introduction and chemistry

Gabapentin is an antiepileptic drug related structurally to γ-aminobutyric acid (GABA), in which a GABA analogue portion is incorporated into a cyclohexane ring to allow it to be easily transported across the blood–brain barrier [1]. Although designed to act as a GABA agonist, experimental and clinical evidence shows that the drug has no action at the GABA receptor.

It was first studied as an antispastic agent. However, early trials showed its clinical antispastic action to be disappointing. Attention then turned to its antiepileptic action, and it is for this indication that the drug is currently licensed in the UK, US and other countries as adjunctive therapy for treatment of refractory partial seizures with or without secondary generalization in adults and as adjunctive therapy for refractory partial seizures in children over 3 years of age. It is also approved in 30 countries outside the US for monotherapy treatment of refractory partial seizures.

In addition, gabapentin has been approved in many countries for the treatment of neuropathic pain, including painful diabetic peripheral neuropathy and post-herpetic neuralgia (PHN). Recently, gabapentin was approved for treatment of PHN in adults in the US.

Gabapentin (1-[aminomethyl] cyclohexaneacetic acid, $C_9 H_{17} NO_2$) is an amorphous crystalline substance with a molecular mass of 171.24. The drug has pK_a of 3.68 and 10.70 at physiological temperatures and is freely soluble in water. Gabapentin is a zwitterion at physiological pH [2].

Analytical methods exist for measurement of gabapentin utilizing the following techniques: high-performance liquid chromatography with ultraviolet detection [3], high-performance liquid chromatography with electrospray tandem mass spectrometry detection [4], high-performance liquid chromatography with fluorometric detection [5,6], solid phase extraction with gas chromatography–mass spectrometry detection [7], solid phase extraction with gas–liquid and spectrofluorometry chromatography [8].

Mechanisms of action

Gabapentin has the same amino acid backbone as GABA with an additional cyclohexyl ring incorporated. Despite this close structural similarity to GABA, the drug does not act at either $GABA_A$ or $GABA_B$ receptors, is not converted into GABA and does not augment GABA-activated chloride current [9]. It does not bind to benzodiazepine, acetylcholine, opioid or glutaminergic receptor sites [10], nor does it have action on most central nervous system (CNS) enzymes [11].

In later work gabapentin has been reported to have multiple actions in relevant animal and cell models (Table 35.1). Indeed, the difficulty in defining the mechanism(s) of action of gabapentin lies in deciding which one of the relevant actions of gabapentin actually contribute to antiepileptic activity in man.

The multiple actions of gabapentin have been reviewed in detail elsewhere [12]. These actions are summarized in Table 35.1.

In animal models, gabapentin was most effective against maximal electroshock-induced seizures [3,12]. The drug was also effective against pentylenetetraole-induced seizures [3,12]. Gabapentin was not effective against animal models of absence seizures [12]. These and other preclinical results suggest gabapentin should have a spectrum of antiepileptic activity similar to that of phenytoin, and show efficacy against partial and tonic-clonic seizures but not against absence or myoclonic seizures.

Gabapentin increases GABA synthesis and inhibits GABA metabolism by inhibiting GABA transaminanase [3]. Gabapentin also inhibits the reuptake of GABA from the synaptic cleft [3,13]. The net effect of these actions is to increase brain GABA levels as demonstrated in both *in vitro* and *in vivo* studies [14].

Gabapentin binds to the α_2-δ subunit of the L-type voltage-regulated calcium channel [15,16]. The effect of this binding on inward calcium current is controversial [3].

Carbamazepine, phenytoin and other antiepileptic drugs inhibit high-frequency, repetitive firing of action potentials by blocking inward sodium current. Gabapentin also inhibits high-frequency,

Table 35.1 The effects of gabapentin on animal models of epilepsy and on biochemical and physiological mechanisms

Effects on animal models	
Maximal electroshock test	Potency equivalent to phenytoin
Pentylenetetrazole test	Effective in preventing pentylenetetrazole-induced seizures
Kindled rats	Effective against fully kindled seizures
GAERs	Not effective
Isoniazid-, semicarbazide- and bicuculline-induced seizures	Effective in inhibiting seizures induced by these drugs which inhibit or antagonize GABAergic action
Biochemical and physiological mechanisms	
Brain GABA levels	Increased by 50%. Gabapentin increases GABA synthesis and inhibits GABA metabolism by GABA transaminase
GABA release and reuptake	Gabapentin inhibits the reuptake of GABA from the synaptic cleft. It increases GABA release in an activity-dependent manner
Voltage-sensitive L-type calcium channel	Gabapentin binds to the α_2-delta subunit. The effects on conductance are controversial
Voltage-sensitive sodium channel	Gabapentin has no effect on the voltage clamped inward sodium current. However, it does inhibit high-frequency repetitive action potential firing
Glutamate receptors	No significant effect at therapeutic concentrations
Brain glutamate levels	Decreased by gabapentin. A possible effect on the glutamate transporter, which may be neuroprotective
Plasma serotonin levels	Increased by gabapentin which may indirectly increase GABAergic inhibition

repetitive firing of action potentials but does not block inward sodium current [3].

Gabapentin reduces brain content of glutamine and glutamate and reduces glutamate release [3,17,18]. These could result in decreased brain excitation and/or neuroprotection.

Pharmacokinetics

Absorption

Gabapentin is absorbed via the L-amino acid transport system located in the small intestine [19]. The time to maximum plasma concentration after oral administration is 2–3 h [3]. Bioavailability of gabapentin is dose dependent, presumably due to saturable absorption of the L-amino acid transport system. The bioavailability is 65% for doses <1800 mg/day and 35% or less for doses >3600 mg/day [3,20] given on a t.i.d. schedule. Food does not decrease the absorption of gabapentin [3]. Food rich in neutral amino acids or monosaccharides may enhance gabapentin absorption [3]. Absorption of gabapentin does not change in the elderly [21].

Distribution

Gabapentin minimally binds to plasma proteins (<3%). The volume of distribution of the drug is 0.65–1.04 L/kg [3].

Gabapentin readily crosses the blood–brain barrier and concentrates in the brain via the L-amino acid transport system [22]. In animals this system is saturable, and the plasma/brain extracellular concentration ratio decreases with increasing plasma concentration [23]. Two clearance mechanisms, active transport and passive diffusion, limit accumulation [24].

Gabapentin binds to a unique binding site in the brain with the highest binding in the outer layers of the cortex, hippocampus and cerebellum [3]. This site was later found to be the α_2-δ subunit of the L-type voltage-regulated calcium channel [25].

Metabolism

Gabapentin does not undergo metabolism in man [26].

Elimination

Gabapentin is eliminated unchanged entirely by renal excretion [27] with an elimination half-life of 5–7 h [3]. Clearance of gabapentin is linearly correlated with creatinine clearance and glomerular filtration rate [3]. Gabapentin clearance varies with age-related changes in creatinine clearance and glomecular filtration rate. Clearance is highest in young children [28]. Children 1 month to 5 years of age require approximately 30% higher dosing rates to achieve a given plasma concentration than children 5–12 years of age [28]. Between ages 20 and 78 there is a significant linear decrease in clearance [21]. Gabapentin clearance is not affected by gender [21].

Age- and disease-related decreases in renal function significantly reduce gabapentin clearance [3,21]. Guidelines have been published for adjusting gabapentin dosing rate in patients with reduced renal function [29].

Drug interactions

Gabapentin does not induce hepatic enzymes involved in drug metabolism [3]. Gabapentin does not alter the plasma concentration of the following antiepileptic drugs: carbamazepine and carbamazepine epoxide [29], phenobarbital [30], phenytoin [31,32] and valproate [29,33]; neither do these drugs affect the pharmacokinetics of gabapentin. Gabapentin significantly slows the elimination of felbamate, presumably by a renal interaction [3]. Cimetidine reduces gabapentin renal clearance, resulting in a small increase in gabapentin plasma concentration. Gabapentin does not alter the pharmacokinetics of the acetate/ethinyl/oestradiol combination oral contraceptive [34]. Aluminium hydroxide and magnesium hydroxide (Maalox TC) antacids reduce gabapentin absorption by 10–20% [3]

There is a growing appreciation of the 'antiepileptic drug burden' concept. This concept is that the larger the number of antiepileptic drugs a person is taking, the greater the probability that the next drug added will cause neurotoxicity. This pharmacodynamic interaction appears to apply to gabapentin.

Therapeutic plasma concentration

Plasma concentrations of 2 µg/mL or greater were necessary for good seizure control in double-blind studies [3]. Plasma concentrations of 20 µg/mL are obtained and well tolerated in patients taking 4800 mg/day of gabapentin [3]. Thus, the therapeutic range is often stated to be 2–20 µg/mL. Higher plasma concentrations have been well tolerated in some patients.

Animal toxicology

During the phase of animal experimentation of gabapentin, the only unfavourable toxicological finding was the induction of pancreatic acinar cell tumours [35,36]. These were only observed in male Wistar rats given very high doses of the drug (2 g/kg/day) for 2 years. No such effect was recorded in female rats, and no drug-induced pancreatic changes have been found to date in other species or in humans. The concentrations of gabapentin in rat pancreas are apparently much higher than occur in human subjects at normal dose ranges. These differences suggest that the rat is a poor model for human pancreatic cancer, and so the carcinogenic potential of gabapentin in humans is probably low. Male rat specific α_2-δ globulin is associated with many xenobiotics including gabapentin [3]. This species- and gender-specific effect has no clear relationship to human carcinogenic potential [3].

Teratogenicity

Animal studies demonstrate the following effects in fetal rats whose mothers were administered high doses of gabapentin: fetotoxicity, delayed ossification (long bones, skull and vertebrae), hydroureter and hydronephrosis [3]. Other malformations were not increased in frequency in mice, rats or rabbits administered doses between four and eight times the recommended daily human dose on a milligram per square metre basis. Gabapentin was not mutagenic in standard *in vitro* and *in vivo* tests [3]. There is little data on the risk of teratogenicity in humans. Gabapentin has been assigned a Category C rating for exposure during pregnancy by the US Food and Drug Administration.

Clinical efficacy

Early studies

Beginning in 1986, a series of open-label pilot studies showed efficacy (30–45% reduction in seizure frequency) against partial and secondarily generalized tonic-clonic seizures [11]. This led to a series of randomized, double-blind clinical trials to establish this effect in man.

Randomized controlled clinical trials

A large multicentre study was carried out by the UK Gabapentin Study Group [37] in patients with resistant partial seizures, using a double-blind, parallel group design. Patients were randomized, after a 3-month baseline period to establish baseline seizure frequency, to add-on therapy with either gabapentin (1200 mg) or placebo. The period of blinded observation was 3 months. Sixty-one patients were randomized to gabapentin and 66 to placebo. Fourteen patients dropped out during the baseline observation period (because of withdrawal of consent or the occurrence of insufficient seizures in the baseline period) and 127 patients entered the evaluation phase (61 on placebo and 53 on gabapentin). Of the gabapentin-treated patients, 25% showed a 50% or more reduction in partial seizures compared with 9.8% of those on placebo. The effectiveness of the drug was also assessed using the response ratio, defined as $t - b/t + b$, where t is the monthly seizure frequency on treatment and b the monthly seizure frequency in the baseline period. A response ratio of –1 indicated complete seizure control, and +1 indicated infinite worsening of seizures. A response ratio of –0.33 indicates a mean 50% improvement in seizures on treatment. The mean adjusted response ratio for gabapentin was –0.192, or a mean 26% decrement in seizures in patients randomized to gabapentin.

Sivenius *et al.* [38] have reported results from a smaller double-blind parallel group study of 43 patients with drug-resistant partial epilepsy, of whom 25 received gabapentin. Treatment at 900 mg/day was not statistically significant in this small group of patients, but at 1200 mg/day there was a significant mean decrease in seizure frequency of 57%.

The US Gabapentin Study Group [39] have reported results from a similar multicentre double-blind, placebo-controlled parallel group study in 306 patients with refractory partial epilepsy. Participants in this study had had at least six seizures during a 12-week baseline period, and were randomized to treatment with placebo or gabapentin treatment at 600, 1200 or 1800 mg/day. Eighteen patients were excluded who had inadequate numbers of seizures during the baseline period or who stopped treatment prior to randomization. The response ratio was –0.151 at 600 mg/day, –0.117 at 1200 mg/day and –0.233 at 1800 mg/day. The percentage of patients who experienced a 50% or more reduction in seizures ranged from 18 to 26% of patients treated with gabapentin and 8% on placebo. An increase in seizures was experienced by 19–26% of patients. These findings were very similar to those reported by the UK Gabapentin Study Group.

Open-label studies

Two large, prospective open-label, office-based studies of gabapentin for partial seizures have been performed: the Study of Titration to Effect Profile of Safety (STEPS) [40] and the Neurontin Evaluation of Outcomes in Neurology Practice (NEON) [41]. There were two principle findings in these studies. First, the CNS side-effects from gabapentin occurred early during therapy whilst on low doses of the drug, and if a patient tolerated low doses, increasing the dose to above 1800 mg was usually possible without the development of side-effects. Having said this, it is a common clinical observation that the higher doses (3000 mg/day or above) often result in CNS adverse effects. Second, the percentage of patients achieving complete seizure control was greater in open-label studies than in double-blind studies.

A large number of retrospective studies of gabapentin for partial seizures have been published [3]. In general, they report findings similar to the STEPS and NEON studies.

Long-term efficacy and safety studies

Long-term follow-up of up to 4.5 years is available from several single-blind and double-blind studies [3]. These studies show sustained benefit and did not show emergence of new toxicity. A multicentre retrospective study of 361 patients taking gabapentin found that less than 40% of patients taking gabapentin remained on the drug for 6 years and fewer than 4% became seizure free [42].

Monotherapy

Gabapentin is currently approved for monotherapy treatment of epilepsy in 30 countries outside the US, but not in the US.

Recently, a randomized, double-blind study was undertaken in 309 patients with newly diagnosed partial seizures with or without secondary generalization, or primary generalized seizures comparing gabapentin (1200–3600 mg/day) vs. lamotrigine (100–300 mg/day). Gabapentin demonstrated similar efficacy and adverse event profile to lamotrigine [57]. A randomized trial of newly diagnosed patients treated with gabapentin (300, 900 or 1800 mg/day) or carbamazepine (600 mg/day) found similar efficacy for gabapentin 900 mg/day, gabapentin 1800 mg/day and carbamazepine 600 mg/day [43]. Gabapentin had fewer side-effects than carbamazepine. A study of patients with refractory partial or tonic-clonic seizures evaluated response after attempting to limit treatment to gabapentin monotherapy at doses of of 600, 1200 or 2400 mg/day [44]. Reduction to gabapentin monotherapy was achieved in 15–26% of patients. Patients withdrawing from carbamazepine in combined carbamazepine/gabapentin therapy had more seizures and a smaller probability of achieving gabapentin monotherapy than with other drug combinations [3].

The use of gabapentin monotherapy is also supported by a study of hospitalized patients whose other antiepileptic drugs had been withdrawn for the purpose of provoking seizures for video/EEG monitoring [45].

Efficacy in childhood partial seizures

Four open-label trials of gabapentin for refractory partial seizures in children have been performed [3,46]. These studies report reductions in seizure frequency of complex partial and secondarily generalized tonic-clonic seizure similar to those reported in adults. Behavioural side-effects and increased seizure frequency occurred in some children, both with and without pre-existing behavioural problems and mental retardation [3].

Other seizure types

A double-blind trial of gabapentin for benign rolandic epilepsy (with centrotemporal spikes) demonstrated statistically significant superiority of gabapentin over placebo [47]. Gabapentin is not likely to be effective in primary generalized seizures, and studies have not shown efficacy (or exacebation) or absence seizures [3] nor efficacy in primary generalized tonic-clonic seizures [48]. Gabapentin has not proven superior to placebo for primarily generalized tonic-clonic seizures [48].

Side-effects

Safety

Gabapentin has been given to over 10 million patients, and remarkably few serious side-effects have been recorded. Amongst these serious adverse events have been a rash [49] in a patient who was allergic to phenytoin and carbamazepine. Ragucci and Cohen [50] reported a patient who developed altered mental status, fever, diffuse macular rash and an enlarged spleen 9 days after starting gabapentin. These signs rapidly resolved when gabapentin was stopped. Common less serious side-effects are listed below. Three cases of massive gabapentin overdose have been reported [3,51]. None resulted in serious sequelae. The abrupt withdrawal of gabapentin has been associated with a range of symptoms, many related to sympathetic overactivity [52].

Common side-effects

In the definitive double-blind studies from the UK and US Gabapentin Study Groups, similar levels of side-effects were recorded [37,39]. In the UK study, at 1200 mg/day, somnolence occurred in 15% of gabapentin-treated patients, fatigue in 13%, dizziness in 7% and weight increase in 5%. In the US study, at 1200 and 1800 mg/day, somnolence was recorded in 36% and 20%, dizziness at 24% and 18%, ataxia in 26% and 18%, nystagmus in 17% and 17%, headache in 9% and 20%, tremor in 15% and 13%, fatigue in 11% and 13%, diplopia in 11% and 4%, rhinitis in 11% and 4%, and nausea or vomitting in 6% and 9%, respectively. Most of the adverse effects were mild and only seven of the 61 and five of the 208 treated patients in the UK and US studies, respectively, withdrew medication because of adverse events.

In Table 35.2, a summary of the side-effects reported by 485 and 307 patients treated with gabapentin in controlled studies is shown [35]. Overall, only 7.4% of 1748 patients who received gabapentin in any clinical study have been withdrawn from the study due to adverse events. Nevertheless, there is a small number of individuals who develop severe CNS adverse effects, even with small doses of gabapentin.

Table 35.2 The 10 most common side-effects from gabapentin reported in the placebo-controlled trials

	Controlled studies		All studies
	Placebo $n = 307$	Gabapentin $n = 485$	Gabapentin $n = 1160$
Number (%) of patients with adverse effects	174 (56.7)	369 (76.1)	944 (81.4)
Adverse events			
Somnolence	30 (9.8)	98 (20.2)	283 (24.4)
Dizziness	24 (7.8)	87 (17.9)	235 (20.3)
Ataxia	16 (5.2)	64 (13.2)	202 (17.4)
Fatigue	15 (4.9)	54 (11.1)	171 (14.7)
Nyastagmus	15 (4.9)	45 (9.3)	174 (15.0)
Headache	28 (9.1)	42 (8.7)	176 (15.2)
Tremor	12 (3.9)	35 (7.2)	174 (15.0)
Diplopia	6 (2.0)	31 (6.4)	124 (10.7)
Nausea and/ or vomiting	23 (7.5)	29 (6.0)	108 (9.3)
Rhinitis	12 (3.0)	22 (4.5)	101 (8.7)

From [58].

Worsening of seizures

Not mentioned in the lists of adverse events in the trial was worsening of seizures, but this is a particularly marked phenomenon in a minority of patients treated with gabapentin. In the US study, 19% of patients treated with 1800 mg of gabapentin experienced a worsening of seizure frequency and 20% in the UK study of 1200 mg/day. In addition to worsening of partial seizures, gabapentin can ('has been reported to'?) worsen myoclonus [11].

Mood and behaviour

Gabapentin's effect on patient mood is unclear. It has been variously reported to improve, have no effect upon and adversely affect mood [13,53–55]. In mentally retarded individuals gabapentin has been associated with aggressive behaviour, increased seizure frequency, ataxia, lethargy, hyperactivity and irritability [3].

Cognitive effects

Martin *et al.* [55] found no adverse effects of gabapentin in tests of attention, psychomotor speed, language and speech in healthy volunteers. Dodrill *et al.* [53] found no cognitive changes in complex partial seizure patients treated with gabapentin (600, 1200 or 2400 mg/day). Meador *et al.* [56] compared cognitive toxicity in healthy volunteers given gabapentin (2400 mg/day) and carbamazepine (plasma concentration 8.3 μg/mL). Thirty-one variables were reviewed. Gabapentin showed statistical improvement on eight variables.

Place of gabapentin in the therapy of epilepsy

Gabapentin has been approved by the US Food and Drug Administration as adjunctive therapy in the treatment of partial seizures with and without secondary generalization in patients over 12 years of age with epilepsy and as adjunctive therapy in the treatment of partial seizures in paediatric patients aged 3–12 years. In addition, over 30 countries have approved gabapentin as monotherapy for the treatment of partial seizures.

The usual criteria for selecting among antiepileptic drugs are: efficacy (usually measured as responder rate), safety, tolerability, drug interactions and convenience (frequency of doses).

The principal advantages of gabapentin are safety, tolerability, and lack of drug interactions. Serious idiosyncratic reactions are very rare with the drug. CNS side-effects of gabapentin are uncommon and usually mild, but they can be severe in a small percentage of patients.

The efficacy of gabapentin reported in double-blind controlled studies was generally less than for other new antiepileptic drugs. However, the dosage of gabapentin used in these trials was less than that used now. Later single-blind studies using higher dosing rates showed better responder rates, but are subject to patient and observer bias. Worsening of seizures sometimes happens with gabapentin. Finally, the drug is more expensive than older drugs.

There are a number of groups for which gabapentin can be a particularly good therapeutic choice because of safety considerations. These include patients with allergy to older antiepileptic drugs, significant hepatic dysfunction, porphyria or patients receiving concomitant treatment with coumadin or oral contraceptive pills [3].

Administration and dosage

The starting dose recommended in the package insert is 300 mg TID. In refractory patients on multiple drugs, tolerance is improved with slower administration (e.g. 300 mg at bedtime × 1 week, than 300 mg BID × 1 week, then 300 mg TID). In emergency situations, the drug can be started very quickly. The author has started gabapentin at 1200 mg TID in patients with drug allergy requiring sudden cessation of old therapy and immediate coverage with new therapy. This was well tolerated.

The US package insert states that the recommended daily dose of gabapentin is 900–1800 mg/day based upon double-blind studies. In other countries, the recommended daily dose of gabapentin is 900–3600 mg/day. There is now evidence that doses of 1800–3600 mg/day produce better anticonvulsive effects in some persons and these doses are generally well tolerated. Many experts now routinely raise the dose to 3600 mg/day if needed for seizure control. There are reports that doses of 4800 mg/day produce higher plasma concentration and better seizure control in some patients, but these high doses are often limited by side-effects. Doses of 4800 mg/day should be divided into 4 daily doses because of the saturable absorption of gabapentin.

Because of the wide range of possible effective doses in individual patients receiving gabapentin, it may be necessary to escalate dosing. The author usually raises doses by 900–1200 mg/day and then allows 1 month or more to observe the efficacy and tolerability of the higher dose. More rapid escalation can be safely done. The dose should be increased until seizures are controlled or there are intolerable side-effects. Although not usually necessary during gabapentin therapy, plasma concentration determinations may be helpful to ascertain whether therapeutic failure is due to low plasma concentra-

tion (below 2 μg/mL). The package insert contains dosing directions for persons with renal insufficiency.

Gabapentin is available in 100-, 300- and 400-mg capsules, and in 600- and 800-mg tablets.

References

1 Satzinger G. Antiepileptics from gamma-aminobutyric acid. *Arzneim Forsch Drug Res* 1994; 44: 261–6.
2 Foot M, Wallace J. Gabapentin. *Epilepsy Res* 1991; 3 (Suppl.): 109–14.
3 McLean MJ. Gabapentin. In: Wyllie E, ed. *The Treatment of Epilepsy: Principles and Practice*, 3rd edn. Philadelphia: Lippincott Williams and Wilkins, 2001.
4 Ifa DR, Falci M, Moraes ME *et al.* Gabapentin quantification in human plasma by high-performance liquid chromatography coupled to electrospray tandem mass spectrometry. Application to bioequivalence study. *J Mass Spectrom* 2001; 36: 188–94.
5 Al-Zehouri J, al-Madi S, Belal F. Determination of the antiepileptics vigabatrin and gabapentin in dosage forms and biological fluids using Hantzsch reaction. *Arzneimittelforschung* 2001; 51: 97–103.
6 Jiang Q, Li S. Rapid high-performance liquid chromatographic determination of serum gabapentin. *J Chromatogr B Biomed Sci Appl* 1999; 30: 119–23.
7 Kushnir MM, Crossett J, Brown PL *et al.* Analysis of gabapentin in serum and plasma by solid-phase extraction and gas chromatography-mass spectrometry for therapeutic drug monitoring. *J Anal Toxicol* 1999; 23: 1–6.
8 Hassan EM, Belal F, Al-Deeb OA *et al.* Spectrofluorimetric determination of vigabatrin and gabapentin in dosage forms and spiked plasma samples through derivatization with 4-chloro-7-nitrobenzo-2-oxa-1,3-diazole. *J AOAC Int* 2001; 84: 1017–24.
9 Rock DM, Kelly KM, MacDonald RL. Gabapentin actions in ligand- and voltage-gated responses in cultured rodent neurons. *Epilepsy Res* 1993; 16: 89–98.
10 Rogowski MA, Porter RJ. Antiepileptic drugs: pharmacological mechanisms and clinical efficacy with consideration of promising developmental stage compounds. *Pharmacol Rev* 1990; 42: 223–86.
11 Shorvon SD. Gabapentin. In: Shorvon S, Dreifuss D, Fish D *et al.* eds. *The Treatment of Epilepsy.* Oxford: Blackwell Science, 1996.
12 Taylor CP, Gee NS, Su TZ *et al.* A summary of mechanistic hypotheses of gabapentin pharmacology. *Epilepsy Res* 1998; 29: 233–49.
13 Eckstein-Ludwig U, Fei J, Schwarz W. Inhibition of uptake, steady-state currents and transient charge movements generated by the neuronal GABA transporter by various anticonvulsant drugs. *Br J Pharmacol* 1999; 129: 92–102.
14 Petroff OA, Hyder F, Rothman DL *et al.* Effects of gabapentin on brain GABA, homocarnosine, and pyrroloidinone in epilepsy patients. *Biochem J* 1999; 342 (Pt 2): 313–20.
15 Marais E, Klugbauer N, Hofmann F. Calcium channel alpha(a)delta subunits—structure and gabapentin binding. *Mol Pharmacol* 2001; 59: 1243–8.
16 Wang M, Offord J, Oxender DL *et al.* Structural requirement of the calcium-channel subunit alpha2delta for gabapentin binding. *Biochem J* 1999; 342 (Pt 2): 313–20.
17 Meder WP, Dooley DJ. Modulation of K(+)-induced synaptosomal calcium influx by gabapentin. *Brain Res* 2000; 875: 157–9.
18 Dooley DJ, Donovan CM, Pugsley TA. Stimulus-dependent modulation of [(3)H] norepinephrine release from rat neocortical slices by gabapentin and pregabalin. *J Pharmacol Exp Ther* 2000; 295: 1086–93.
19 Maurer HH, Rump AFE. Intestinal absorption of gabapentin in rats. *Arzneimittelforschung* 1991; 41: 104–6.
20 Gidal BE, DeCerce J, Bockbrader HN *et al.* Gabapentin bioavailability: effect of dose and frequency of administration in adult patients with epilepsy. *Epilepsy Res* 1998; 31: 91–9.
21 Boyd RA, Turck D, Abel RB, Sedman AJ, Bockbrader HN. Effects of age and gender on single-dose pharmacokinetics of gabapentin. *Epilepsia* 1999; 40: 474–79.
22 Ben-Menachem E, Sodefelt B, Hamberger A *et al.* Seizure frequency and

CSF parameters in a double-blind placebo controlled trial of gabapentin in patients with intractable complex partial seizures. *Epilepsy Res* 1995; 21: 231–6.

23 Luer MS, Hamani C, Dujovny M *et al.* Saturable transport of gabapentin at the blood–brain barrier. *Neurol Res* 1999; 21: 559–62.

24 Wang Y, Welty DF. The simultaneous estimation of the influx and efflux blood–brain barrier permeabilities of gabapentin using a micro-dialysis-pharmacokinetic approach. *Pharm Res* 1996; 13: 398–403.

25 Gee NS, Brown JP, Dissamayake VUK *et al.* The novel anticonvulsant drug, gabapentin (Neurontin), binds to the subunit of a calcium channel. *J Biol Chem* 1996; 271: 5768–76.

26 Vollmer KO, von Hodenberg A, Kolle EU. Pharmacokinetics and metabolism of gabapentin in rat, dog and man. *Arzneimittelforschung* 1986; 36: 830–9.

27 Richens A. Clinical pharmacokinetics of gabapentin. In: Chadwick D, ed. *New Trends in Epilepsy Management: the Role of Gabapentin.* London: Royal Society of Medicine Services, 1993.

28 Haig GM, Bockbrader HN, Wesche DL *et al.* Single-dose gabapentin pharmacokinetics and safety in healthy infants and children. *Seizure* 2000; 9: 241–8.

29 Blum RA, Comstock TJ, Sica DA *et al.* Pharmacokinetics of gabapentin in subjects with various degrees of renal function. *Clin Pharmacol Ther* 1994; 56: 154–9.

30 Hooper WD, Kavanagh MC, Herkes GK *et al.* Lack of a pharmacokinetic interaction between phenobarbitone and gabapentin. *Br J Clin* 1990; 31: 171–4.

31 Anhut H, Leppik I, Schmidt B *et al.* Drug interaction study of the new anticonvulsant gabapentin with phenytoin in epileptic patients. *Naunyn Schmiedebergs Arch Pharmacol* 1988; 337 (Suppl.): R17.

32 Graves NM, Holmes GB, Leppik IE *et al.* Pharmacokinetics of gabapentin in patients treated with phenytoin. *Pharmacotherapy* 1989; 9: 196.

33 Uthman BM, Hammond EJ, Wilder BJ. Absence of gabapentin and valproate interaction: an evoked potential and pharmacokinetic study. *Epilepsia* 1990; 1: 645.

34 Eldon MA, Underwood BA, Randinitis EJ *et al.* Gabapentin does not interact with a contraceptive regimen of norethindrone acetate and ethinyl estradiol. *Neurology* 1998; 50: 1146–8.

35 Browne TR. Efficacy and safety of gabapentin. In: Chadwick D, ed. *New Trends in Epilepsy Management: the Role of Gabapentin.* London: Royal Society of Medicine Services, 1993.

36 Ramsey RE. Gabapentin. Toxicity. In: Levy RH, Mattson RH and Meldrum BS, eds. *Antiepileptic Drugs*, 4th edn. New York: Raven Press, 1995.

37 UK Gabapentin Study Group. Gabapentin in partial epilepsy. *Lancet* 1990; i: 1114–17.

38 Sivenius J, Kalviainen R, Ylinen A *et al.* Double-blind study on gabapentin in the treatment of partial seizures. *Epilepsia* 1991; 32: 539–42.

39 US Gabapentin Study Group. Gabapentin therapy in refractory epilepsy: a double-blind placebo-controlled parallel group study. *Neurology* 1993; 43: 2292–8.

40 Morrell MJ, McLean MJ, Willmore LJ *et al.* Efficacy of gabapentin as adjunctive therapy in a large multicenter study. The Steps Study Group. *Seizure* 2000; 9: 241–8.

41 Bruni J. Neurontin as first add-on therapy in epileptic patients with partial seizures: long term follow-up. *Can J Neurol Sci* 1998; 25: 134–40.

42 Wong IC, Chadwick DW, Fenwick PB *et al.* The long-term use of gabapentin, lamotrigine, and vigabatrin in patients with chronic epilepsy. *Epilepsia* 1999; 40: 1439–45.

43 Chadwick D, Anhut H. Murray GH *et al.* A double-blind trial of gabapentin monotherapy for newly diagnosed partial seizures. *Neurology* 1998; 51: 1282–8.

44 Beydoun A, Fakhoury T, Nasreddine W *et al.* Conversion to high-dose gabapentin monotherapy in patients with medically refractory partial epilepsy. *Epilepsia* 1998; 39: 188–93.

45 Bergey GK, Morris HH, Rosenfeld W *et al.* Gabapentin monotherapy, I: an 8-day, double-blind, dose-controlled, multicenter study in hospitalized patients with refractory complex partial or secondarily generalized seizures. The US Gabapentin Study Group 88/89. *Neurology* 1997; 49: 739–45.

46 Appleton R, Fichtner K, LaMoreaux L *et al.* Gabapentin as add-on therapy in children with refractory partial seizures: a 24-week, multicentre, open-label study. *Dev Med Child Neurol* 2001; 43: 269–73.

47 Bourgeois B, Brown LW, Pellock JM *et al.* Gabapentin (Neurontin) monotherapy in benign epileptiform centro-temporal spikes (BECTS): a 36-week, double-blind, placebo-controlled study. *Epilepsia* 1998; 39: 164 (abst.).

48 Chadwick D, Leiderman DB, Sauerman W *et al.* Gabapentin in generalized seizures. *Epilepsy Res* 1996; 25: 191–7.

49 DeToledo JC, Minagar A, Lowe MR *et al.* Skin eruption with gabapentin in a patient with repeated AED-induced Stevens–Johnson syndrome. *Ther Drug Monit* 1999; 21: 137–8.

50 Ragucci MV, Cohen JM. Gabapentin-induced hypersensitivity syndrome. *Clin Neuropharmacol* 2001; 24(2): 103–5.

51 Verma A, St Clair EW, Radtke RA. A case of sustained massive gabapentin overdose without serious side effects. *Ther Drug Monit* 1999; 21: 615–17.

52 Norton JW. Gabapentin withdrawal syndrome. *Clin Neuropharmacol* 2001; 24: 245–6.

53 Dodrill CB, Arnett JL, Hayes AG *et al.* Cognitive abilities and adjustment with gabapentin: results of a multisite study. *Epilepsy Res* 1999; 35: 109–21.

54 Harden CL, Lazar LM, Pick LH *et al.* A beneficial effect on mood in partial epilepsy patients treated with gabapentin. *Epilepsia* 1999; 40: 1129–34.

55 Martin R, Kuziecky R, Ho S *et al.* Cognitive effects of topirimate, gabapentin, and lamotrigine in healthy young adults. *Neurology* 1999; 52: 321–7.

56 Meador KJ, Loring DW, Ray PG *et al.* Differential cognitive effects of carbamazepine and gabapentin. *Epilepsia* 1999; 40: 1279–85.

57 Brodie *et al.* Gabapentin vs Lamotrigine monotherapy: a double blind comparison in newly diagnosed epilepsy. *Epilepsia* 2002; 45(9): 993–1000.

58 Chadwick D. Gabapentin. *Lancet* 1994; 343: 89–91.

36

Lamotrigine

F. Matsuo

Primary indications	Adjunctive or monotherapy in partial and generalized epilepsy. Also in Lennox–Gastaut syndrome and other childhood epilepsies
Usual preparations	Tablets: 25, 50, 100, 200 mg; chewtabs: 5, 25, 100 mg
Usual dosages	Initial: 12.5–25 mg/day. Maintenance: 200–600 mg (monotherapy); 100–200 mg (comedication with valproate); 200–700 mg (comedication with enzyme-inducing drugs)
Dosage intervals	2 times/day
Significant drug interactions	Autoinduction may occur. Lamotrigine levels are lowered by phenytoin, carbamazepine, methsuximide, phenobarbital and other enzyme-inducing drugs Lamotrigine levels increased by sodium valproate
Serum level monitoring	Value not established
Target range	1–15 mg/L
Common/important side-effects	Rash (sometimes severe), headache, blood dyscrasia, ataxia, asthenia, diplopia, nausea, vomiting, dizziness, somnolence, insomnia, depression, psychosis, tremor, hypersensitivity reactions
Main advantages	Effective and relatively well-tolerated
Main disadvantages	High instance of rash (occasionally severe) and other side-effects; complicated pharmacokinetics
Mechanisms of action	Blockage of voltage-dependent sodium conductance.
Oral bioavailability	<100%
Time to peak levels	1–3 h (1–6 h in children)
Metabolism and excretion	Hepatic glucuronidation (without phase I reaction)
Volume of distribution	0.9–1.3 L/kg
Elimination half-life	29 h (monotherapy approx.); 15 h (enzyme-inducing comedication); 60 h (valproate comedication). Auto-induction may occur
Plasma clearance	0.044–0.084 L/kg/h (but variable)
Protein binding	55%
Active metabolites	None
Comment	A useful medication in a wide variety of epilepsies both in monotherapy and in combination with other antiepileptic drugs

(*Note*: this summary table was formulated by the lead editor.)

Lamotrigine (LTG: 3.5-diamino-6-(2.3-dichlorophenyl)-1.2.4 triazine) was initially developed from a series of folate antagonists after the observation that patients with epilepsy treated with antiepileptic drugs (AED) had diminished levels of folic acid [1]. However, no correlation between antifolate activity and AED activity has ever been established. LTG is a weak folate antagonist and possesses a spectrum of activity in animal seizure models similar to those of phenytoin (PHT) and carbamazepine (CBZ) [2–4].

LTG was introduced for adjunctive treatment of partial seizures in the UK in 1991, in the US in 1994 and later worldwide, and its clinical use has since expanded [5]. Its extensive use has also highlighted some unique issues [6–8]. It is currently marketed in over 90 countries.

Mechanisms of action and experimental studies

LTG selectively increases the threshold for localized seizure activity, but the mechanisms of its antiepileptic action are not yet fully understood.

Mechanism of action

Although structurally unrelated to PHT and CBZ, LTG has been demonstrated to block sodium channels in a voltage-, use- and frequency-dependent manner, preventing propagation of action potentials [9–13] and the release of neurotransmitters, principally glutamate [14–17].

LTG inhibits voltage-sensitive sodium currents through a preferential interaction with the slow inactivated sodium channel [11], thereby suggesting that it may act selectively against high-frequency epileptiform discharges [9]. In keeping with its cellular actions, LTG suppresses burst firing in cultured rat cortical neurones and sustained repetitive firing in the mammalian spinal cord. LTG does not affect normal synaptic transmission in hippocampal slices, possibly due to preferential interaction with the slow-inactivation sodium channel [18]. Consistent with its effects on sodium channels, LTG also inhibits veratrine-induced γ-aminobutyric acid (GABA) release [19]. Furthermore, animal studies show that LTG is less active in inhibiting sodium-dependent glutamate release in vivo than in vitro [20].

Maximally effective anticonvulsant doses of LTG (15 mg/kg) produced no effect on veratridine-induced increases in extracellular glutamate levels in the rat striatum, whereas the sodium channel blocker tetrodotoxin showed potent inhibition. In addition, LTG showed less than 50% inhibition of veratridine-induced glutamate increases in the rat cortex, indicating that LTG has antiepileptic actions in vivo additional to its modulating effects on sodium-dependent glutamate release [20].

LTG has also been shown to modulate the calcium conductance involved in release of excitatory amino acid in the corticostriatal pathway [14,21–23]. At clinically relevant concentrations, LTG inhibits voltage-activated calcium currents in cortical and striatal neurones, an effect blocked by the N-type calcium channel blocker ω-conotoxin GVIA, but not nifedipine (a dihydropyridine calcium receptor blocker). This action could inhibit glutamate release presynaptically, as well as prevent calcium overload in neurones through postsynaptic antagonism of voltage-dependent calcium channels [24]. LTG potently inhibits glutamate and aspartate release (induced by the sodium channel opener veratrine) from rat cerebral cortical slices and displaces batrachotoxin from its sodium channel binding site [13,19]. LTG confers cerebral protection against local cerebral ischaemia and has reduced kainate-induced neurotoxicity in the rat, presumably by suppressing glutamate release [25–27].

Receptor binding assays show that LTG lacks any appreciable in vitro affinity for dopamine D_1 or D_2, adrenergic α- or β-, adenosine A1 or A2, muscarinic and γ-receptors, but has a weak inhibitory effect on serotonin 5-HT_3 receptors [9,28]. It has minimal effects on GABA-, glutamate-, N-methyl-D-aspartate (NMDA)- and kainate-activated ionic currents in rat cortical/hippocampal neuronal membranes [10,11]. LTG also appears to lack direct antagonistic activity at the glutamate receptor in vivo, being devoid of phencyclidine-like behavioural effects [28].

Current researches of LTG action are also directed to hippocampal neuronal networks potentially involved in its psychotropic action [29,30]. However, the full impact of data supporting the LTG inhibition of neurotransmitter release should be further examined.

Not readily understood is why LTG has a much broader spectrum of clinical activity than either PHT or CBZ [31]. This difference cannot be easily reconciled by citing the LTG blockade of glutamate neurotransmitter release because PHT and CBZ exhibit similar actions (again, under experimental conditions that may not be clinically relevant).

The broader spectrum of activity of LTG may be due to markedly preferential affinities to certain sodium channel–subunit combinations, exhibiting differential regional distributions in the brain [32]. Alternatively, there may be a yet unidentified mechanism of action for LTG that might shed light on this difference.

Effects in animal seizure models

In animal seizure models, LTG displays a broadly similar antiepileptic profile to PHT and CBZ [33,34]. A number of electrical, chemical and genetic models of epilepsy have indicated the therapeutic potential of LTG in the treatment of partial, generalized tonic-clonic and absence seizures [35]. LTG was more potent than both PHT and CBZ in these models and in suppressing sound-induced clonic seizures in the genetically epilepsy-prone rat [36]. Compared with other newer AED, LTG (intraperitoneal administration) was the only drug which antagonized tonic convulsions in the maximal electroshock (MES) test (gabapentin, tiagabine and vigabatrin had no effect) and was ranked above these agents (in terms of therapeutic index) in the inhibition of sound-induced seizures in DBA/2 mice [37]. LTG differs from CBZ and PHT in its effects in some models of absence epilepsy.

In contrast with these agents, oral LTG inhibited visually evoked after-discharge in the conscious rat [38]. In the lethargic model of human absence seizures, intraperitoneal LTG was shown to reduce seizure frequency by 65% compared with vehicle whereas vigabatrin and tiagabine significantly increased seizure frequency and gabapentin and topiramate had no effect [39]. However, in the classic absence model (ability to inhibit PTZ-induced clonus) LTG, like PHT and CBZ, failed to show any effect [34,37].

LTG showed a dose-dependent suppression of secondary generalized seizures and after-discharge duration in amygdaloid and hippocampal kindled seizures in rats (model of complex partial seizures), with the effect lasting as long as 24h in some cases [37,40]. This effect was also observed in kindled rats which had previously showed no response to PHT treatment. LTG is thought to produce this effect by increasing after-discharge threshold, i.e. by suppression of seizure initiation, not propagation. In another study of partial seizures, intravenous LTG showed a dose-dependent reduction or abolition of electrically evoked after-discharge duration in rat, dog and marmoset models [35].

EEG effects in patients with epilepsy

The EEG background was not modified by the addition of LTG [41]. In epileptic patients, single-dose LTG (120–240 mg) produced prolonged reduction in spontaneous interictal spike activity and photosensitivity [42]. In another trial in patients with refractory epilepsy, adjunctive LTG therapy (for 4 months) significantly reduced the total number of interictal spikes, and also decreased the frequency (but not significantly) as well as the duration of EEG ictal abnormalities in patients with focal and generalized epilepsies [43].

In a retrospective review of children younger than16 years with refractory epilepsy, the effect of adjunctive LTG therapy on EEG seizure activity closely correlated with clinical reductions in seizure frequency [44]. A total of 63 patients with partial epilepsy (65% of those studied), and 30 patients with primary generalized epilepsy (83%) showed a significant improvement in seizure frequency (generalized vs. focal) compared with baseline, following LTG therapy (mean 5.3 mg/kg/day) for an average of 2.3 years. Correspondingly, a greater than 50% reduction in EEG discharges was seen in 45 patients with focal epilepsy (47%) and in 25 patients with generalized epilepsy (70%).

Reduction in paroxysmal spike-wave activity is a valuable tool for assessing clinical response in patients with absence epilepsy [45]. Eight of 17 paediatric patients with refractory and frequent absence seizures had an approximately 80% reduction from baseline in spike-wave discharges when treated with LTG for 12–48 weeks [46]. A coincident reduction in overt seizures was seen in some but not all patients, and cognition was improved (subjective reporting only). In a study in children with absence seizures, 24-h ambulatory EEG was performed at the end of a double-blind dose escalation phase [47]. Of a total of 38 evaluable patients, 27 (71%) were free of electrographic seizure discharges.

A preliminary report showed a reduction in slow spike-wave discharges in patients with Lennox–Gastaut syndrome treated with LTG [48]. In 17 patients (aged 8–29 years) the mean overall percentage reduction from baseline in atypical seizures and drop attacks was 76.4% and 69.5%, respectively, after 12 months of LTG treatment. EEG abnormalities improved during treatment: the mean total number of slow spike-wave discharges decreased from 483 at baseline to 274 at 4 months and 207 at 12 months, with the mean total duration reduced by half. The finding is supported by findings from another study in patients with severe epileptic encephalopathies [49].

Cognitive and psychomotor effects

Studies in volunteers and patients with epilepsy show that LTG causes fewer adverse psychomotor and cognitive effects than traditional agents, as well as some of the newer agents; it is claimed by some also to produce positive cognitive effects.

In contrast with diazepam (10 mg), CBZ (400–600 mg) and PHT (1000 mg), LTG (120–300 mg) did not accentuate body sway and did not impair adaptive tracking (a measure of hand-to-eye coordination), smooth visual pursuit (a measure of cortical and cerebellar function) or saccadic eye movement (a measure of parapontine reticular formation function) after oral administration to healthy volunteers [50,51]. Moreover, single doses of LTG (240 mg), unlike diazepam (10 mg), produced no sedative effects in healthy adult volunteers and produced less sleepiness than CBZ in adult patients with newly diagnosed epilepsy [52]. Repeated doses of LTG (mean 7.1 mg/kg/day for 4 weeks) did not affect psychomotor speed, sustained attention, verbal memory, language and mood measures in 17 healthy volunteers; in contrast, topiramate (5.7 mg/kg/day) significantly impaired attention and word fluency [53–55].

In a smaller 4-week study, LTG (200 mg/day) was associated with improvements in memory (immediate and delayed visual memory and delayed logical memory) in five young healthy volunteers (mean age 19 years) but had no effect on mental attention; psychomotor function (finger tapping test) was, however, impaired [56]. In adult patients with refractory epilepsy, adjunctive LTG therapy (100–400 mg/day) produced no deleterious effect on attention, mental concentration or psychomotor response compared with placebo [57].

Pharmacokinetics

The pharmacokinetic profile of LTG in adult patients has previously been extensively reviewed [58–65] (Table 36.1), but data in children are less comprehensive [66] (Table 36.2).

The pharmacokinetic profile of LTG has been studied in the absence and presence of other antiepileptic agents in single [67–70] and multiple [71–73] dose studies in paediatric as well as adult patients.

Absorption and distribution

LTG is well absorbed following oral administration, displaying an absolute bioavailability of 98% in healthy adult volunteers: no first-pass effect is noted [74].

LTG pharmacokinetics are linear: a mean maximal plasma concentration (C_{max}) and area under the plasma concentration–time curve (AUC) values are directly proportional to LTG dose in the 30–450 mg range in both children and adults with epilepsy [59,60,75]. C_{max} occurs at approximately 1–3 h after oral administration in adults [58,59,76], and 1–6 h in children [69,70]. A second peak or plateau may occur at 4–6 h postdose, which is possibly due to gastric recycling of the drug [75]. The mean C_{max} was 1.6 mg/L after a single oral dose of 120 mg in adults, while after a single oral dose of 2 mg/kg, a mean C_{max} of 1.48 mg/L was attained in 12 children aged between 6 months and 12 years. These data indicate that the pharmacokinetics of LTG is not saturated at doses given clinically.

LTG absorption is not appreciably altered by the presence of food. LTG is approximately 55% bound to plasma protein *in vitro* and binding is constant over the plasma concentration range of

Table 36.1 Mean[a] pharmacokinetic parameters in adult patients with epilepsy or healthy volunteers (GlaxoSmithKline, product information, 2001)

Adult study population	No. subjects	t_{max}: time of maximum plasma concentration (h)	Elimination half-life (h)	Cl/F: apparent plasma clearance (mL/min/kg)
Patients taking EIAEDs[b]				
Single-dose LTG	24	2.3 (0.5–5.0)	14.4 (6.4–30.4)	1.10 (0.51–2.22)
Multiple-dose LTG	17	2.0 (0.75–5.93)	12.6 (7.5–23.1)	1.21 (0.66–1.82)
Patients taking EIAEDs + VPA				
Single-dose LTG	25	3.8 (1.0–10.0)	27.2 (11.2–51.6)	0.53 (0.27–1.04)
Patients taking VPA only				
Single-dose LTG	4	4.8 (1.8–8.4)	58.8 (30.5–88.8)	0.28 (0.16–0.40)
Healthy volunteers taking VPA				
Single-dose LTG	6	1.8 (1.0–4.0)	48.3 (31.5–88.6)	0.30 (0.14–0.42)
Multiple-dose LTG	18	1.9 (0.5–3.5)	70.3 (41.9–113.5)	0.18 (0.12–0.33)
Healthy volunteers taking no other medications				
Single-dose LTG	179	2.2 (0.25–12.0)	32.8 (14.0–103.0)	0.44 (0.12–1.10)
Multiple-dose LTG	36	1.7 (0.5–4.0)	25.4 (11.6–61.6)	0.58 (0.24–1.15)

EIAED, enzyme-inducing antiepileptic drug; LTG, lamotrigine; VPA, valproic acid.

[a] The majority of parameter means determined in each study had coefficients of variation between 20% and 40% for half-life and Cl/F and between 30% and 70% for t_{max}. The overall mean values were calculated from individual study means that were weighted based on the number of volunteers/patients in each study. The numbers in parentheses below each parameter mean represent the range of individual volunteer/patient values across studies.

[b] Examples of EIAEDs are carbamazepine, phenobarbital, phenytoin and primidone.

1–4 mg/L [33]. Plasma binding is unaffected by therapeutic concentrations of PHT, phenobarbital and valproic acid (valproate or divalproex sodium) [59]. The volume of distribution was 1.2 L/kg in healthy adult volunteers (range 0.87–1.2 L/kg) [58], and 1.5 L/kg in 12 children with epilepsy receiving single doses of LTG (2 mg/kg) in the absence of other AEDs [69,77].

Studies in animals show that LTG is widely distributed in all tissues and organs, but little is known of its differential tissue distribution in humans. In 11 adults undergoing neurosurgical intervention, LTG showed good penetration into the brain, with a brain/plasma LTG concentration ratio of 2.8 [78,79]. In another study, a 10-year-old patient with epilepsy was reported to have a brain tissue concentration of LTG 1.6 times higher than unbound plasma concentrations 4 h postdose [80]. Studies of cerebrospinal fluid (CSF) in children and young adults showed a CSF/plasma ratio of 43% [68].

Metabolism and elimination

LTG is extensively metabolized by the liver, predominantly via *N*-glucuronidation, which appears to be the rate-limiting step in LTG elimination [58,81]. Approximately 70% of a single oral dose of

LTG is recovered in the urine during the first 6 days, of which 80–90% is in the form of the 2-*N*-glucuronide metabolite, and the remainder in the form of the 5-*N*-glucuronide and parent drug [82,83]. About 2% of an oral dose is excreted in the faeces [60]. None of the metabolites are thought to be pharmacologically active [61].

Plasma clearance of LTG shows great interindividual variation and is significantly influenced by concomitant medication and age. Plasma clearance in children aged under 5 years is 2–3 times higher than that of adults [61]. In comparative studies of LTG monotherapy, plasma clearance and volume of distribution values were higher in children (0.038 L/h/kg and 1.5 L/kg) [69] than adults (0.021–0.035 L/h/kg and 0.9–1.3 L/kg, respectively) [7]; elimination half-lives were broadly similar in children and in adults (32.3 h in children vs. 23–37 h in adults). In the study in children, weight-normalized clearance appeared to be higher in children younger than 6 years (0.05 L/h/kg) than children aged 6–11 years (0.033 L/h/kg) [69]. The observed age-related differences in LTG clearance could be attributed to a relative reduction in liver size and hepatic blood flow in adolescents compared with young children [73] and diminished glucuronidation at older ages [8].

There is conflicting evidence about whether LTG induces its own

Table 36.2 Mean pharmacokinetic parameters in paediatric patients with epilepsy (GlaxoSmithKline, product information, 2001)

Paediatric study population	No. subjects	t_{max} (h)	Half-life (h)	Cl/F (mL/min/kg)
Ages 10 months–5.3 years				
Patients taking EIAEDs	10	3.0 (1.0–5.9)	7.7 (5.7–11.4)	3.62 (2.44–5.28)
Patients taking AEDs with no known effect on drug-metabolizing enzymes	7	5.2 (2.9–6.1)	19.0 (12.9–27.1)	1.2 (0.75–2.42)
Patients taking VPA only	8	2.9 (1.0–6.0)	44.9 (29.5–52.5)	0.47 (0.23–0.77)
Ages 5–11 years				
Patients taking EIAEDs	7	1.6 (1.0–3.0)	7.0 (3.8–9.8)	2.54 (1.35–5.58)
Patients taking EIAEDs plus VPA	8	3.3 (1.0–6.4)	19.1 (7.0–31.2)	0.89 (0.39–1.93)
Patients taking VPA only[a]	3	4.5 (3.0–6.0)	65.8 (50.7–73.7)	0.24 (0.21–0.26)
Ages 13–18 years				
Patients taking EIAEDs	11			1.3
Patients taking EIAEDs plus VPA	8			0.5
Patients taking VPA only	4			0.3

AED, antiepileptic drug; EIAED, enzyme-inducing antiepileptic drug; VPA, valproic acid.
[a]Two subjects were included in the calculation for mean t_{max}. Parameter not estimated.

metabolism. In adults, the pharmacokinetics of LTG after multiple dose administration conforms to those predicted from single dose studies [58], indicating that clinically significant autoinduction does not occur [60]. In keeping with this, LTG does not induce hepatic cytochrome P450 enzyme activity after repeated administration [84]. Autoinduction was demonstrated by Richens who showed a significant increase in clearance early after drug initiation, and in another pharmacokinetic analysis which demonstrated a 17% increase in oral clearance over 48 weeks of treatment [85]. There are no relevant steady-state pharmacokinetic data available to assess the autoinduction of LTG in children.

Diminished glucuronidation of LTG may account for an age-related decline in the plasma clearance of the drug. A comparison of the pharmacokinetics of LTG (150 mg oral dose) in healthy young (26–38 years) and elderly (65–76 years) volunteers revealed a 37% lower clearance in the elderly, associated with 27% higher C_{max} and 55% higher AUC values [86]. Plasma clearance of LTG has been reported to increase toward the end of pregnancy, but limited information is available concerning the pharmacokinetics of LTG [87,88].

LTG is excreted in considerable amounts in breast milk, which in combination with slow elimination in the infants, may result in LTG plasma concentrations comparable to active LTG therapy [71]. A group of nine mothers (10 infants) were investigated, as they delivered and breast-fed their infants for 2–3 weeks [87]. At delivery, maternal plasma LTG concentration was similar to the umbilical cord, indicating extensive placental transfer. There was slow decline in plasma levels in the newborn. At 72 h postpartum, median LTG plasma levels in the infants were 75% of the cord plasma level (range 50–100%). The median milk–maternal plasma concentra-

tion ratio was 0.61 (range 0.47–0.77) 2–3 weeks after delivery, and the nursed infant maintained LTG plasma concentrations of approximately 30% (median, range 23–50%) of the mother's plasma concentration. Maternal plasma concentrations increased during the first 2 weeks, the median increase in plasma concentration/dose ratio being 170%. No adverse effects were observed in the infants.

The pharmacokinetics of LTG is not significantly affected by renal impairment [89]. Gilbert's syndrome, a disorder of conjugation characterized by disturbances in bilirubin metabolism and uridine diphosphate glucuronyl transferase (UDGT) activity, is associated with impaired LTG clearance and prolongation (approximately 35%) of half-life, although this value remains within normal range [90].

Concentration vs. effect

A clear relationship between plasma LTG concentrations and clinical response has not been established in clinical trials [91]. A target range of between 1 and 4 mg/L was initially suggested [50,92–94] but children and adults with refractory epilepsy frequently require plasma concentrations in excess of 4 mg/L to gain optimum seizure control [95,96] and the more generally accepted concentration range is much wider, typically between 1 and 15 mg/L [97]. Although dose-related improvements in seizure control have been observed in children over the plasma concentration range of 4–21 mg/L [96], most investigators have not found this [72,98–101].

Likewise, there is also no clear relationship between plasma concentration and incidence of adverse events [72,99,102,103]. No toxic plasma LTG concentration has been established but one retrospective study demonstrated a significant relationship between plasma LTG concentrations above 15 mg/L and unsteadiness with or without vomiting in 176 patients aged 5–22 years [104]. Similarly, in a paediatric study of high-dose LTG therapy, increases in plasma LTG concentrations above 21 mg/L were prevented because of the development of unacceptable levels of nausea that did not resolve with reduction of concomitant medications [96].

The wide range of optimal plasma LTG concentrations (1–15 mg/L) implies that routine therapeutic drug monitoring is unwarranted with LTG [102,105,106]; dosage should be adjusted according to individual clinical response and tolerability [107,108].

Drug interactions

In current clinical practice, LTG is most often used in combination with other AEDs, so a clear understanding of possible drug interactions between LTG and coadministered drugs is important [109–111]. Although LTG has little influence on the pharmacokinetics of other AEDs, the pharmacokinetics of LTG can be influenced by concomitant medications via a number of pharmacokinetic and pharmacodynamic drug interactions. Investigators have shown that the presence of concomitant medication has little influence on the absorption or plasma binding of LTG [7,8,112], but drugs that affect the metabolism of LTG can increase or decrease its clearance.

Effects of coadministered drugs on LTG pharmacokinetics

Coadministration of valproate, an inhibitor of glucuronidation, markedly reduces the rate of LTG elimination [113] (Tables 36.1, 36.2). As shown in studies in children and adults, the half-life of LTG is approximately doubled (to approximately 45–65 h) in patients receiving concomitant valproate compared with values in those receiving LTG monotherapy. This pharmacokinetic interaction may be the cause of the increased incidence of rash seen in patients receiving combined LTG and valproate therapy. In contrast, coadministration of drugs that induce hepatic enzymes, such as phenytoin (PHT), carbamazepine (CBZ) and phenobarbital, increases the rate of elimination of LTG, more than halving the half-life of LTG (to approximately 7–14 h) in some clinical trials compared with LTG alone.

PHT appears to have a slightly greater effect on plasma LTG concentrations (decreases by 45–54%) than CBZ, phenobarbital or primidone (decreases by approximately 40%).

The effect of enzyme-inducing antiepileptic drugs (EIAED) on LTG appears to be more pronounced in children than in adults. This increased clearance, especially in children aged under 6 years, is likely to result in pronounced peak–trough fluctuations in plasma LTG concentrations [59].

LTG half-life is about 4- to 10-fold longer in patients given concomitant valproate than in those receiving EIAEDs (Table 36.2). Steady-state dose-normalized plasma concentrations are also increased or decreased, respectively, by this amount [71,73,114]. LTG dosage must therefore be adjusted according to the type of concomitant medication used. A recent population pharmacokinetic model for children has confirmed the effects of these other drugs on LTG clearance and has been used to develop new escalation schedules for concomitant therapy (GlaxoSmithKline, product information, 2001 and [115]). These new guidelines include lower initiation

dosages and a slower escalation rate designed to generate average plasma concentrations in children close to and not higher than those in adults under the current dosage guidelines [77].

The addition of methsuximide to an LTG regimen (which also included other AED therapies) significantly decreased LTG serum concentrations by a mean of 53% in 16 patients (mean age 15.5 years) with epilepsy. The effects of the newer AEDs have not been comprehensively investigated. Ethosuximide, vigabatrin, gabapentin, and possibly zonisamide and tiagabine, have no significant effect on hepatic metabolism and are therefore not expected to have an effect on LTG pharmacokinetics [111]. Gidal *et al.* reported no differences in LTG clearance between patients receiving it alone or in combination with felbamate [116]. Topiramate has either decreased or had no effect on LTG plasma concentrations in preliminary reports [117]. Although slight reductions in LTG AUC and plasma half-life values were noted on coadministration of paracetamol (acetaminophen) (900 mg 3 times daily) with LTG (300 mg) in healthy adult volunteers: this effect is unlikely to be of clinical importance [118].

Effects of LTG on the pharmacokinetics of coadministered drugs

In contrast with many other AEDs, LTG does not inhibit or induce hepatic cytochrome P450 drug-metabolizing enzymes [84] or displace other AEDs from plasma proteins [58]. Therefore, the pharmacokinetic profiles of PHT, CBZ, phenobarbital, primidone, methsuximide and ethosuximide are not markedly altered, when LTG is added to the regimen [67,92,119–122].

Valproate, like LTG, is extensively metabolized via the glucuronidation pathway; competition between these two agents for hepatic glucuronidation sites is thought to result in the observed inhibitory effect of valproate on LTG metabolism [113]. In one study, the addition of LTG to steady-state valproate treatment in adult volunteers resulted in a 25% reduction in valproate plasma concentrations; oral clearance of valproate was significantly increased over 3 weeks of concomitant LTG treatment [123]. However, LTG was shown to have no significant effect on valproate plasma concentrations in either adult [85] or paediatric patients in controlled trials [95,124].

Pharmacodynamic interactions

In addition to pharmacokinetic interactions, pharmacodynamic interactions between LTG and valproate, and LTG and CBZ, have been reported. Synergistic therapeutic effects, as well as some toxic effects have been observed [72,125–128] when combining LTG and valproate; this combination is thought to facilitate the development of tremor in some patients.

A toxic pharmacodynamic interaction between LTG and CBZ has also been observed: diplopia, dizziness, nausea, ataxia and nystagmus, classic signs of CBZ toxicity, have been reported when LTG has been added to CBZ therapy in adults and children [51,112,129]. This was originally thought to be attributable to increases in the plasma concentrations of the active metabolite, CBZ-10,11-epoxide. However, the effects of LTG on the plasma concentration of CBZ-epoxide are inconsistent. In adults, the addition of LTG to existing CBZ therapy has variously been reported to increase plasma CBZ-epoxide concentrations by 10–45% [112,129] or leave them unaltered [130,131]. In children, the mean plasma concentration of CBZ-epoxide decreased significantly when LTG was added to CBZ therapy in one study [132].

Oral contraceptives

A non-blind study in 12 healthy female volunteers demonstrated no effect of LTG on contraceptive steroids [133]. Women enrolled, serving as their own controls, received an ethinyloestradiol 30 µg/levonorgesterol 150 µg oral contraceptive preparation for three consecutive cycles. Menstrual progesterone levels indicated that no ovulation occurred. Likewise, no changes in menstrual pattern were reported in any women. LTG therefore is not expected to compromise oral contraceptive efficacy. The oral contraceptives may increase LTG clearance [134].

Clinical efficacy

Pivotal randomized clinical trials of the antiepileptic efficacy of LTG involved adult patients with refractory partial epilepsies, but an increasing number of postmarketing clinical trials have been directed to paediatric patients and patients with generalized epilepsies.

Medically refractory partial epilepsy

Various short-term randomized double-blind placebo-controlled studies, many in cross-over design, have confirmed the efficacy of LTG, when used as add-on therapy in patients with refractory partial epilepsy [57,92,94,135–141] (Table 36.3). One of the studies has been published in the abstract form only [141]. The result of meta-analysis, incorporating some unpublished data, is also available [119].

Addition of LTG 50–500 mg/day resulted in a 13–59% reduction in total seizure frequency, with 7–67% of patients experiencing seizure reduction of greater than 50%. In the largest of these studies, a multicentre parallel-group trial of 24 weeks' duration [136],

LTG 500 mg/day proved more effective than LTG 300 mg/day or placebo as add-on therapy, reducing total seizure frequency by 36% and producing a greater than 50% reduction in seizure frequency in 34% of patients. Analysis of the effects of LTG on specific seizure types indicated that both simple and complex partial seizures and secondarily generalized tonic-clonic seizures were significantly reduced, with secondarily generalized seizures tending to be more responsive. LTG-induced reductions in seizure frequency have been accompanied by significant and apparently independent improvements in patients' ratings of seizure severity and psychological well-being.

The results of a large double-blind paediatric US multicentre study were also published recently [140]. A total of 199 patients were randomized to LTG (n=98) and placebo (n=101), and the 6-week schedule of dose escalation was designed according to the patient's age and body weight. A total of 84 LTG-treated and 83 placebo-treated patients completed a 12-week maintenance phase. Over the entire study duration of 18 weeks, a greater than 50% reduction of partial seizures, compared with the baseline frequency, was seen in 42% of LTG-treated patient and 16% of placebo-treated patients. When partial seizures with secondary generalization were compared, a greater than 50% reduction was seen in 53% of LTG-treated patients, and 26% of placebo-treated patients. When analysis is restricted to the maintenance phase, difference remained significant, but somewhat less impressive.

Active control study

A double-blind, active-control study in adolescent and adult patients with refractory partial epilepsy further confirmed the efficacy of LTG in partial epilepsy [142]. A total of 156 patients on monotherapy of CBZ or PHT were assigned to LTG or valproate. While maintaining the concomitant drug at a steady dose level during baseline, the LTG group underwent dose escalation to the target dose of 500 mg daily (n=50), while the valproate group, to 1000 mg daily (a minimally effective dose) (n=64). When the concomitant drug was then gradually removed, monotherapy conversion was more often successful in the LTG group (56% vs. 20%). The medi-

Table 36.3 Double-blind, placebo-controlled efficacy trials of LTG as add-on therapy in partial epilepsy

Reference	No. patients randomized	Baseline seizure frequency (/month)	Dosage in mg (no. of patients in group)	Median seizure reduction (%)	50% or better seizure control (%)
[135]	30	4 or more	75–200 (30)	17	7
[92]	21	16	75–400 (21)	59	67
[120]	23	4 or more	75–300 (23)	23	30
[136]	191	4 or more	300 (65)	20	20
			500 (59)	36	34
[137]	88	3 or more	100–400 (88)	25	20
[121]	18	4 or more	100–300 (18)	18	11
[138]	41	17 (median)	150–400 (41)	24	22
[141]	21		Up to 300 (21)	21.9	29
[57]	62		100–400 (62)	30	18
[94]	20	3 or more	50–200 (20)	37	45
[139]	56	4 or more	100–400 (56)	30	24
[140]	199	4 or more	Age-weight adjusted	36.1	42

an time to escape was significantly shorter for the valproate group (57 days vs. 168 days).

Newly diagnosed patients

As monotherapy, LTG is as effective as CBZ and PHT against partial onset seizures and idiopathic generalized tonic-clonic seizures (Table 36.4).

Among adults with newly diagnosed epilepsy randomized to LTG 100–300 mg/day or CBZ 300–1400 mg/day for 48 weeks, the percentages of patients who remained seizure free over the final 24 weeks of treatment were similar, in terms of overall seizures (39 vs. 38%), partial seizures (35 vs. 37%) and idiopathic generalized seizures (both 47%) [52]. The likelihood of continuing treatment was, however, greater with LTG than with CBZ, primarily because LTG was the better tolerated drug.

In adolescent and adult patients with newly diagnosed or recurrent epilepsy, monotherapy with LTG 100 mg/day, LTG 200 mg/day or CBZ 600 mg/day for 30 weeks was equally effective in terms of seizure control and treatment compliance [143]. The proportion of patients remaining seizure free during maintenance treatment with LTG 100 mg/day (51%), LTG 200 mg/day (60%) and CBZ 600 mg/day (55%) were comparable.

Another multicentre double-blind study compared the efficacy of LTG and CBZ in elderly patients with newly diagnosed epilepsy [144]. A total of 150 patients participated and were randomized in a 2 : 1 ratio to treatment with LTG and CBZ for 24 weeks after a short titration period. The main difference was the rate of dropout due to adverse events (LTG 18% vs. CBZ 42%).

Although there was no difference between the drugs in time to the first seizure, a greater percentage of LTG-treated patients remained seizure free during the last 16 weeks of treatment (LTG 12% vs. CBZ 29%). In this study, the LTG group had a lower incidence of skin rash (LTG 3% vs. CBZ 19%).

In an European multicentre study, a total of 417 patients were randomized to treatment with LTG, while 201 patients to CBZ [145]. More patients receiving LTG completed the study (81%), compared with CBZ (77%), primarily related to adverse events. Small subsets of the patients were elderly (aged 65 years or older) and children (aged 2–12 years).

In a double-blind 48-week study comparing LTG and PHT, a total of 181 patients with newly diagnosed partial seizures were randomized to two treatment groups [146]. One group received LTG at modal dose of 150 mg/day, while the second received PHT at 300 mg/day. LTG and PHT were similarly effective, when compared as time to the first seizure and time to discontinuation. Adverse events led to discontinuation of 13 patients (15%) from LTG and 18 (19%) from PHT. Discontinuation from LTG was due to skin rash in 10 patients (12%) compared with five (5%) from PHT.

Use of LTG with valproate

In a complex non-randomized multicentre study, four groups of patients with monotherapy of valproate ($n=117$), CBZ ($n=129$), PHT ($n=92$) and phenobarbital ($n=9$) were recruited [147]. LTG was added to the concomitant drug to the target daily dose of 100 mg for the valproate group and 400 mg for others. The concomitant drug was then withdrawn and LTG monotherapy was attained. The LTG dose was adjusted in the valproate group, as valproate was withdrawn. The LTG plasma level in other groups rose, as the concomitant drug was withdrawn.

Seizure reduction of 50% or higher was seen in 47% (64%, valproate; 41%, CBZ; 38%, PHT) during the add-on phase, and the responder rate was higher in patients idiopathic tonic-clonic seizures (61%) than in those with partial seizures (43%). There were more responders in the valproate group, but statistical significance was reached in the partial seizure group only. The valproate group experienced better seizure control, after LTG was added ($n=$

Table 36.4 Comparative trials of LTG in newly diagnosed patient with epilepsy

Reference	No. patients on entry	Dosage (mg/day)	Study duration	Patients seizure free during final 24 weeks of treatment (%)	Patients completing study (%)
Versus CBZ					
[52]	131	LTG 100–300 (median 150)	48	39	65
	129	CBZ 300–1400 (median 600)		38	51
[143]	115	LTG 100	30	51	62
	111	LTG 200		60	69
	117	CBZ 600			65
[144]	102	LTG 75–300 (median 100)	24	38[a]	71
	48	CBZ 200–800 (median 400)		44[a]	42
[145]	417	LTG 50–300 (median 100)	24	65[b]	81
	201	CBZ 100–1500 (median 400)		73[b]	77
Versus PHT					
[146]	86	LTG 100 or more (mode 150)	48	43	48
	95	PHT 200 or more (mode 300)		36	47

CBZ, carbamazepine; LTG, lamotrigine; PHT, phenytoin.
[a] Data were collected for 16 weeks.
[b] For patients older than 13 years only.

81), than groups on other concomitant drug, and the benefit persisted, as the concomitant drug was withdrawn ($n=39$ remaining), while the LTG serum level was lower. The result was interpreted to reveal synergism between LTG and valproate. The results were supported by a larger study with a similar design [148].

Lennox–Gastaut syndrome

Efficacy of LTG in management of Lennox–Gastaut syndrome was shown in a pivotal double-blind, placebo-controlled study [95]. A total of 169 patients were randomized to 16 weeks of LTG ($n=79$) or placebo ($n=90$). The median frequency of all major seizures decreased in the LTG group (from 16.4 to 9.9 vs. 13.5–14.2, placebo). Seizure reduction of greater than 50% was seen significantly more often in the LTG group (33% vs. 16%).

Efficacy of LTG in Lennox–Gastaut syndrome was also confirmed in a single-centre study employing an innovative cross-over design [124]. After an 8-week baseline period, a total of 30 consecutive paediatric and adolescent patients with refractory generalized epilepsy were initiated on LTG in addition to concomitant drugs. LTG dose was titrated to the maximally tolerated, effective dose for each patient, and the seizure frequency was compared with the baseline. Seventeen patients (57%) experienced seizure reduction of greater than 50%. Fifteen of the responders were double-blindly assigned to LTG or placebo after a washout period. The two double-blind phases consisted of 12-week periods separated by 3-week cross-over. With the exception of a single patient, the seizure count was lower during the LTG phase.

Generalized epilepsy

In a multicentre study, a total of 26 patients with generalized epilepsies, including absence, were randomized to LTG at either 75 or 150 mg daily: a total of 22 patients completed the study [149]. There was significant reduction in frequency of both tonic-clonic and absence seizures with LTG. A greater than 50% reduction in tonic-clonic seizures occurred in 50%, and in absence seizures in 33%. In the continuation phase, five (25%) remained seizure free.

Absence seizures

The efficacy of LTG monotherapy in patients with newly diagnosed childhood typical absence epilepsy was demonstrated in a placebo-controlled trial [47]. During a non-blind dose escalation phase, 30 of 42 patients (71%) aged 2–16 years became seizure free at a median dose of 5 mg/kg/day. In the double-blind, placebo-controlled phase, significantly more patients remained seizure free with LTG treatment ($n=15$) compared with those receiving placebo ($n=14$): 62 vs. 21%. In an uncontrolled study of 15 patients of mixed ages [150], when LTG (1.6–3.0 mg/kg/day for children and 25–50 mg/day for adults) was added to valproate and continued for 3 months or longer, a total or near total control of absence was seen in 63% ($n=9$).

Non-controlled studies in paediatric mixed seizure types

In non-controlled studies, LTG (up to 15 mg/kg/day, 400 mg/day) has shown efficacy as add-on therapy in children and adolescents with refractory multiple seizure types (including those with accompanying neurological or developmental abnormalities), with approximately 40% of patients showing a reduction of 50% or higher in seizure frequency and approximately 10% achieving total control of seizures after 3 months' treatment [96,99,151–155].

Generalized seizures, including atypical and typical absence seizures, atonic and tonic seizures, and Lennox–Gastaut syndrome, were more responsive [63,98,100,156–159]. A retrospective analysis of 285 children with refractory epilepsy (frequently accompanied by neurological impairment) who responded to short to medium term (up to 12 months) adjunctive LTG therapy indicated that efficacy was maintained on long term (1–4.2 years) follow-up [100].

Special groups

Successful applications of LTG in refractory epilepsy have included conditions associated with underlying progressive neurological conditions, including neonatal seizures [160], infantile spasms [161], Rett's syndrome [162] and juvenile neuronal lipofuscinosis [163].

Myoclonus and myoclonic syndromes

As the scope of clinical uses of LTG has widened, including both partial and generalized epilepsies, it became known that LTG can aggravate myoclonus [164,165], while improved control has also been reported [100]. Exacerbation of myoclonus has been reported both in epilepsy syndromes including myoclonus and also in the myoclonic epilepsy syndrome [126,166,167]. The mechanisms involved in differential exacerbation of myoclonus are unknown.

Quality of life

A double-blind study compared LTG and CBZ in newly diagnosed epilepsy with health-related quality of life as an outcome measure [168]. The study population was identical to a report already reviewed [52] and the modified Side Effect and Life Satisfaction (SEALAS) inventory was applied at weeks 4, 12, 24 and 48. Analysis of SEALAS data by subscale showed that the CBZ group experienced more cognitive side-effects in general and more general changes in energy levels and affect during the first 4 weeks of treatment. These changes may help explain the difference in the study completion rate (LTG 65% vs. CBZ 51%).

LTG use in mood disorders

Soon after clinical trials of LTG as an antiepileptic were initiated, there were reports of a mood-elevating effect [46,169]. This lead to the investigation of LTG as a treatment of affective disorders [170,171]. A few double-blind studies as well as multiple open-label studies have demonstrated efficacy of LTG in a range of bipolar affective disorders [172,173]. LTG has also been shown to be effective in treatment of neuropathic pain, supported by one double-blind as well as open studies [174–176].

Table 36.5 Adverse experiences often reported by newly diagnosed patients on LTG monotherapy and active control groups

Study:	[52]	[143]	[143]	[146]	LTG total [52,143,146]	CBZ total [52,143]	PHT [146]
n	131	115	111	86	443	246	95
Median-modal dose	150 mg	100 mg	200 mg	150 mg	–	600	300 mg
Headache	39 (30%)	21 (18%)	20 (18%)	9 (10%)	89 (20%)	43 (17%)	18 (19%)
Asthenia	28 (21)	14 (12)	14 (13)	14 (16)	70 (16)	60 (24)	28 (29)
Rash	25 (19)	6 (5)	9 (8)	12 (14)	52 (12)	35 (14)	9 (9)
Nausea	23 (15)	7 (6)	7 (6)	7 (8)	44 (10)	25 (10)	4 (4)
Sleepiness	16 (12)	7 (6)	7 (6)	6 (7)	36 (8)	49 (20)	27 (29)
Dizziness	16 (12)	7 (6)	5 (5)	8 (9)	36 (8)	34 (14)	11 (12)

Side-effects

Assessment of the tolerability profile of LTG has been complicated by its frequent use in combination with other AEDs [177,178]. Information concerning the tolerability of LTG alone can be derived from controlled studies of LTG monotherapy. Pooled data from 443 patients with newly diagnosed recurrent epilepsy treated with LTG monotherapy identified headache (20%), asthenia (16%), rash (12%), nausea (10%), dizziness (8%) and somnolence (8%) as the most frequent adverse events [52,143,146] (Table 36.5).

When used as monotherapy, LTG compares favourably with other AEDs, particularly with respect to its lesser sedative effect. A comparison of LTG (100–300 mg/day) and CBZ (300–1400 mg/day) monotherapies in patients with newly diagnosed epilepsy noted similar incidences of adverse events with two drugs, apart from significantly higher incidence of drowsiness with CBZ (20% vs. 8%) [52,143]. A comparison of LTG and PHT (300–600 mg/day) as monotherapy reveals a greater frequency of reports of drowsiness with PHT (29% vs. 8%) [146]. A similar trend is noted for asthenia with PHT (29% vs. 16%). Weight gain (more than 10% increase in body weight) was a less common occurrence during medium term (30–48 weeks) monotherapy with LTG (1.8%) than with CBZ (6.5%) [52]. Analysis of the pooled clinical trial data indicated that adverse events necessitated withdrawal of adjunctive LTG therapy in 10.2% of patients (n=3501) [179]. Of these, skin rash was most frequently cited, responsible for discontinuation in 3.8% of patients. In a clinical trial of antiepileptic monotherapy in patients with newly diagnosed or recurrent epilepsy, withdrawal rates due to adverse events were lower with LTG (4–15%) than with CBZ (10–27%) [52]. Monotherapy data also indicated a lower rate of treatment withdrawal due to central nervous system (CNS)-related adverse effects (asthenia, dizziness, somnolence, insomnia) with LTG (2.5%) that with CBZ (7.7%). Although rash was equally prevalent with LTG (12%) and CBZ (14%), it necessitated treatment discontinuation in fewer LTG recipients (6.1%) than CBZ recipients (8.9%).

As noted with monotherapy, the most common adverse events associated with adjunctive LTG use are primarily neurological, gastrointestinal and dermatological. In a placebo-controlled study of the tolerability of add-on LTG (up to 500 mg/day) therapy in 334 adults patients with partial epilepsy, adverse events occurring significantly more often with LTG than with placebo included dizziness (50%), diplopia (33%), ataxia (24%), blurred vision (23%)

Table 36.6 Adverse experiences reported by 10% or more LTG patients in a double-blind, US tolerability study [180]

	LTG	Placebo
n	334	112
Dizziness	166 (50%)[a]	20 (18)
Headache	125 (37)	40 (36)
Diplopia	109 (33)[a]	12 (11)
Ataxia	80 (24)[a]	5 (5)
Blurred vision	77 (23)[a]	10 (9)
Nausea	73 (22)	17 (15)
Rhinitis	58 (17)	21 (19)
Somnolence	46 (14)[a]	8 (7)
Pharyngitis	42 (13)	13 (12)
Coordination abnormality	39 (12)	7 (6)
Flu syndrome	38 (11)	10 (9)
Cough	35 (10)	9 (8)
Rash	34 (10)	6 (5)
Dyspepsia	32 (10)	6 (5)
Vomiting	32 (10)	10 (9)

[a] Statistically significant against placebo.

and somnolence (14%) [180] (Table 36.6). Headache (37%), nausea (22%), abnormal coordination (12%) and skin rash (10%) were not more statistically significant than placebo. Available evidence suggests that LTG is well tolerated at higher maintenance doses (up to 700 mg/day) [181] and during long-term therapy [182,183] (Table 36.6).

Idiosyncratic effects

Of all adverse effects, skin rash has become most significant. Many AEDs cause allergic skin rash, and LTG is not unique in this regard [184]. LTG skin rash has typical characteristics of allergic drug rash, and its incidence is higher, when the patient has the history of allergic skin rash to some other AED with benzene ring [185,186]. While there has been a report of non-maculopapular rash [187], LTG-associated skin rash is typically maculopapular or erythematous, associated with pruritis, and displays the characteristics of a delayed hypersensitivity reaction, appearing within the first 4 weeks of initiating treatment and resolving rapidly on treatment withdrawal [188]. Occasionally the rash may be more severe (erythema multiforme) or progress to desquamation with involvement of the mucous membrane (Stevens–Johnson syndrome) and possibly to toxic epidermal necrolysis (TEN) [189–192].

The pathophysiology of Stevens–Johnson syndrome and TEN is different from common allergic skin rash, but a complete understanding of the mechanisms resulting in drug-related serious skin rashes is lacking. Therefore, the utility of lymphocyte toxicity assays to assess LTG hypersensitivity [193,194] is yet to be determined. In some patients, rash is accompanied by a flu-like syndrome of fever, malaise, myalgia, lymphadenopathy or eosinophilia, suggesting an immunological mechanism. No consensus exists as to which early dermatological features allow the clinician to differentiate potentially life-threatening from self-limited skin rash [195–198].

As LTG use increased among paediatric patient populations, multiple clinical studies suggested that the incidence of LTG-associated skin rash is higher in children than in adult patients [199–202]. On the other hand, the LTG group did not differ significantly from placebo (9% vs. 7%) in the incidence of skin rash, when elaborate dose escalation schedules were employed in a multicentre study of children with Lennox–Gastaut syndrome [95].

In view of a number of postmarketing clinical reports of serious skin rash, the manufacturer revised product information in 1997 (GlaxoSmithKline, product information, 2001 and [115]), warning the medical practitioner that the incidence of severe, potentially life-threatening rash in paediatric patients is very much higher than that reported in adults using LTG; specifically, reports from clinical trials suggested as many as 1 in 50 to 1 in 100 paediatric patients developed a potentially life-threatening rash [201,203]. The warning has been modified now to a 1% incidence of 'serious rash'.

Such experiential data highlighted issues related with LTG initiation in small children. There has been increasing recognition that the risk of skin rash is significantly increased when LTG therapy is initiated in patients already receiving valproate [192,204]. The risk, however, can be reduced by slow escalation from a low starting dose [177,188,205] (Table 36.7). In a multicentre, non-randomized study [138], multiple dose escalation schedules included valproate initial doses at 100, 25 and 12.5 mg/day, and initial doses of CBZ and PHT at 200 and 50 mg/day. When withdrawal due to skin rash was compared, the effect of lowering initial dose and slower escalation was statistically significant only for the valproate group (38%, 11% vs. 8% for respective initial doses).

Subsequent epidemiological data suggested that recommendation of lower starting doses and slow titration schedules was indeed followed by demonstrable reduction of the incidence of serious skin rash [206]. More recent epidemiological data further suggested that reduction in the incidence of serious skin rash associated with dosing adjustment of LTG introduction occurred, while the incidence of milder skin rash did not change [199] (Table 36.7). It is relevant that the most recent large US double-blind placebo-controlled study in children with refractory partial epilepsy [140] was carefully designed as to the dose escalation schedule, and skin rash was a reason for withdrawal. No statistically significant difference in the incidence of skin rash emerged between the LTG and placebo groups. Isolated cases of more severe skin rash, however, occurred in the LTG group.

It has been reported that LTG withdrawal was not necessary in all the patients who experienced skin rash in clinical trials [150]. Some patients experiencing skin rash at the initial exposure have been rechallenged later without recurrence of skin rash [207–209]. These rechallenges have not included patients with Stevens–Johnson syndrome or TEN.

Table 36.7 Paediatric and adult rash rates with different concomitant antiepileptic drugs [177]

AED therapy	Total no. patients	All rash (%)	DC rash (%)[a]	Hosp/SJS rash (%)[b]
Paediatric (younger than 16 years)				
LTG+EIAED	394	9.6	4.1	0.8
LTG+VPA+EIAED	155	4.5	0	0
LTG+VPA only	145	20.0	9.0	1.4
LTG+VPA+NEIAED	145	21.4	10.3	1.4
LTG+other	60	11.7	3.3	0
LTG monotherapy	192	13.5	3.1	1.6
Adult (older than 16 years)				
LTG+EIAED	2240	6.7	2.0	0.1
LTG+VPA+EIAED	303	7.6	3.3	0.7
LTG+VPA only	205	19.5	12.2	2.0
LTG+VPA+NEIAED	10	20.0	10.0	0
LTG+other	195	10.3	5.1	0.5
LTG monotherapy	420	14.5	6.0	0

EIAED, enzyme-inducing antiepileptic drugs; LTG, lamotrigine; NEIAED, non-enzyme-inducing antiepileptic drugs; VPA, valproic acid.
[a] Rash leading to treatment discontinuation (DC).
[b] Rash leading to hospitalization or Stevens–Johnson syndrome (SJS).

Multiorgan failure

Sporadic cases of multiorgan failure associated with disseminated intravascular coagulation have been reported. Multiorgan failure was initially attributed to status epilepticus [210] and/or concurrent serious systemic ilnesses [179], but cases of multiorgan failure attributable to LTG [211–213] have also been reported. More recent systematic analysis has suggested an overlap between multiorgan failure and a severe hypersensitivity syndrome associated with serious rash and fever [214].

Miscellaneous adverse experiences

There is a report of two children treated for diabetes insipidus who experienced an increase in desmopressin requirement, when LTG was added to treatment for their epilepsy [215]. There exist isolated reports of occurrences of pseudolymphoma [216], agranulocytosis [217] and hepatotoxicity [218]. LTG has not been associated with carcinogenesis (GlaxoSmithKline, product information, 2001).

A nationwide survey in UK patients evaluated association between AED use and acute psychological disorders [169]. In 19 incidences (30% of the total reported), the AED was judged responsible. LTG was implicated in three, and all three experienced interictal events, consisting of delirium in two and mood disorder in one.

British postmarketing surveillance of adverse events associated with LTG included rare single occurrences of hepatic failure, a severe flare-up of ulcerative colitis, disseminated intravascular coagulation and acute renal failure [219]. Additional neurobehavioural adverse experiences include aggression [220] and insomnia [221].

Sudden unexplained death in epilepsy (SUDEP)

Retrospective analysis of the LTG database indicates that the risk of sudden death in LTG-treated patients is no greater than that reported for other epileptic populations (GlaxoSmithKline, product information, 2001 and [222]). In a British postmarketing study, standardized mortality ratio was slightly higher than reported in the literature [219]; the result was interpreted to reflect severity of epilepsy in the study population.

Teratogenicity

LTG did not reveal significant teratogenic potential in preclinical animal testing (GlaxoSmithKline, product information, 2001 and [115]). Soon after introduction for clinical use under regulatory classification as a potential teratogen [223], the manufacturer established a pregnancy registry and empirical data have been collected on human teratogenicity of LTG [224,225].

As of March 2002, a total of 695 pregnancies had been prospectively registered with the pregnancy outcome pending in 102 [226]. Of the remaining 593, outcomes are known for 442 pregnancies (77.1%). Exposure to LTG occurred in the first trimester in 426 pregnancies with 430 outcomes (including four sets of twins). There were 16 live born infants with major defects and two pregnancy terminations involving major defects, following earliest exposure to LTG in the first trimester. One infant had a chromosome abnormality, not counted as a major defect, following exposure to LTG and CBZ during the entire pregnancy.

While the sample size is still considered insufficient to reach definitive conclusions about the teratogenic risk of LTG, a higher frequency of major malformations was seen within the group exposed to combinations including LTG and valproate compared with other polytherapies or compared with LTG monotherapy. It was not conclusive, however, that the published observations on valproate exposure explain the higher frequency of all major defects in the valproate groups.

Child development

The effects of LTG on children's physical maturation were evaluated in a group of 103 children over periods of 6–71 months [227]. The mean age at LTG introduction was 6.7 years (1.6–16.4), and the mean of daily LTG dose was 7.4 mg/kg body weight (3.5–14.2). Long-term LTG monotherapy was associated with normal body growth.

LTG overdose

Sporadic cases of accidental or deliberate overdose of LTG, involving quantities up to 15 g, have been reported, and some have been fatal (GlaxoSmithKline, product information, 2001). Observations from several cases of attempted suicide through LTG ingestion from 1350 to 4500 mg suggest that the drug does not cause respiratory depression [228–230]. Recorded peak plasma concentration varied from 18 to 53 mg/L. The main symptoms of LTG overdose included transient stupor [231], dizziness, nystagmus, ataxia, loss of reflexes, xerostomia and mild hyperkalaemia. Recovery occurred in 24–48 h. Activated charcoal [229,230] and paracetamol [232] can be used in treatment of acute LTG overdose.

Clinical therapeutics

Because of well-established difference in the pharmacokinetic characteristics, the method of LTG initiation is determined by whether the patient is currently treated with valproate or EIAEDs (GlaxoSmithKline, product information, 2001 and [115,117]). It has been shown that the risk of serious skin rash increases, when the recommended initial dose and/or rate of dose escalation of LTG is exceeded (GlaxoSmithKline, product information, 2001 and [115]). The flexibility of paediatric initiation and dosing has been appreciably improved by introduction of LTG in tablet sizes of 5 and 2 mg, and may help lower the incidence of skin rash further (GlaxoSmithKline, product information, 2001; Glaxo Wellcome Group, patient information leaflet, 2001). The manufacturer recommends the administration of whole tablets only. The dosing interval can be either once or twice daily.

Adjunctive LTG therapy with valproate

Patients over 12 years of age

- Weeks 1 and 2: 25 mg every other day.
- Weeks 3 and 4: 25 mg every day.
- Usual maintenance dose: 100–400 mg/day (1 or 2 divided doses).

- To achieve maintenance, doses may be increased by 25–50 mg/day every 1–2 weeks.
- Usual maintenance dose, when adding LTG to valproate alone, ranges from 100 to 200 mg/day.

Patients 2–12 years of age

- Weeks 1 and 2: 0.15 mg/kg/day in 1 or 2 divided doses, rounded down to the nearest whole tablet.
- Weeks 3 and 4: 0.3 mg/kg/day in 1 or 2 divided doses, rounded down to the nearest whole tablet.
- Weight-based dosing can be achieved by using the following guide: give this daily dose, using the most appropriate combination of LTG 2-mg and 5-mg tablets.

Patient's weight	6.7–14 kg (14.7–30.8 lb)	1.41–27 kg (31–59.4 lb)	2.71–34 kg (59.6–74.8 lb)	34.1–40 kg (75.0–88 lb)
Weeks 1 and 2	2 mg every other day	2 mg every day	4 mg every day	5 mg every day
Weeks 3 and 4	2 mg every day	4 mg every day	8 mg every day	10 mg every day

- Usual maintenance dose: 1–5 mg/kg/day in 1 or 2 divided doses (maximum 200 mg/day).
- To achieve the usual maintenance dose, subsequent doses should be increased every 1–2 weeks (calculate 0.3 mg/kg/day, round this amount down to the nearest whole tablet, and add this amount to the previously administered daily dose).

Adjunctive LTG therapy with EIAEDs

Patients over 12 years of age

- Weeks 1 and 2: 50 mg/day.
- Weeks 3 and 4: 100 mg/day in 2 divided doses.
- Usual maintenance dose: 300–500 mg/day in 2 divided doses.
- To achieve maintenance, doses may be increased by 100 mg/day every 1–2 weeks.

Patients 2–12 years of age

- Weeks 1 and 2: 0.6 mg/kg/day in 2 divided doses, rounded down to the nearest whole tablet.
- Weeks 3 and 4: 1.2 mg/kg/day in 2 divided doses, rounded down to the nearest whole tablet.
- Usual maintenance dose: 5–15 mg/kg/day in 2 divided doses (maximum 400 mg/day).
- To achieve the usual maintenance dose, subsequent doses should be increased every 1–2 weeks (calculate 1.2 mg/kg/day, round this amount down to the nearest whole tablet, and add this amount to the previously administered daily dose).

LTG monotherapy

Initial monotherapy with LTG is currently accepted in the UK [115] for patients older than 12 years only. In the US, conversion to LTG monotherapy only is accepted (GlaxoSmithKline, product information, 2001).

- Weeks 1 and 2: 25 mg/day.

- Weeks 3 and 4: 50 mg/day.
- Usual maintenance dose: 100–200 mg/day (up to 500 mg/day).
- To achieve maintenance doses may be increased 50–100 mg every 7–14 days.

Because of the faster rate of metabolism in children, those aged between 2 and 6 years may require a maintenance dose at the higher end of the recommended range, especially those receiving concomitant EIAEDs. The safety and effectiveness of LTG under 2 years of age has not been established and no dosage guidelines are available, but LTG dosing interval longer than 24 h has been employed [5]. There are published antiepileptic treatment recommendations for a range of paediatric epilepsy syndromes [97,233,234].

The highest maintenance dose reported is 1900 mg/day [103], and LTG plasma levels above 25 mg/L may be tolerated by some patients regularly receiving LTG for epilepsy treatment [235]. Some have been able to demonstrate benefit at small doses [236].

The use of LTG in the management of generalized adult epilepsy syndromes may have increased, partially because there has been increasing concern over possible long-term complications of valproate in women of reproductive age [237–239]. Weight gain is uncommonly associated with long-term LTG use, and its value as replacement for valproate has increased in popularity.

Laboratory monitoring guidelines

The value of monitoring plasma concentrations of LTG has not been established. Neither does the magnitude of adverse symptoms correlate with LTG plasma concentrations [102]. Because of possible pharmacokinetic interactions between LTG and other AEDs being taken concomitantly, monitoring of plasma levels of LTG and concomitant drugs may be indicated during dose adjustments. While no other laboratory monitoring is recommended during LTG treatment, clinical monitoring for adverse symptoms is important in view of rare reports of systemic complications attributed to LTG.

Long-term therapy

In the medical management of epilepsy, the clinician endeavours to develop the simplest, most effective AED regimen without adverse consequences often for lifetime use in a given patient [240–244]. There are a number of studies to determine how long a given agent is retained for chronic use, even when it may not be reasonably assumed that the last agent is the most effective, derived following serial replacement based on clinical assessment. In one study of longer than 3 years' duration, LTG was maintained in 29%, while 30% for topiramate and 10% for gabapentin [219]. Another multicentre study of 6 years' duration demonstrated the retention rate of somewhat less than 40% [183]. The same study demonstrated that fewer than 4% of the patients remained free of seizure recurrences. There is emerging literature of concurrent use of LTG and other newly introduced AEDs [245]. The use of LTG in the elderly has not been extensively studied, but the existing data suggest that it is a highly acceptable therapy [246]. There has been a recommendation to consider the use of LTG in patients who may represent a suicide risk, because overdose seems relatively easy to reverse and cumulating evidence has suggested positive psychotropic effect of LTG [230].

References

1 Hommes OR, Obbens EAMT. The epileptogenic action of Na-folate in the rat. *J Neurol Sci* 1972; 16: 271–81.
2 White HS. Comparative anticonvulsant and mechanistic profile of the established and newer antiepileptic drugs. *Epilepsia* 1999; 40 (Suppl. 5): S2–10.
3 Catterall WA. Molecular properties of brain sodium channels: an important target for anticonvulsant drugs. *Adv Neurol* 1999; 79: 441–56.
4 Kuo CC. A common anticonvulsant binding site for phenytoin, carbamazepine, and lamotrigine in neuronal Na+ channels. *Mol Pharmacol* 1998; 54: 712–21.
5 Matsuo F. Lamotrigine. *Epilepsia* 1999; 40 (Suppl 5): S30–6.
6 Culy CR, Goa KL. Lamotrigine. A review of its use in childhood epilepsy. *Paediatr Drugs* 2000; 2: 299–330.
7 Goa KL, Ross SR, Chrisp P. Lamotrigine. *Drugs* 1993; 46: 152–76.
8 Fitton A, Goa KL. Lamotrigine. *Drugs* 1995; 50: 691–713.
9 Cheung H, Kamp D, Harris E. An *in vitro* investigation of the action of lamotrigine on neuronal voltage-activated sodium channels. *Epilepsy Res* 1992: 13: 107–12.
10 Lang DG, Wang CM, Cooper BP. Lamotrigine, phenytoin and carbamazepine interactions on the sodium current present in N4TG I mouse neuroblastoma cells. *J Pharmacol Exp Ther* 1993: 266: 829–35.
11 Lees G, Leach MJ. Studies on the mechanism of action of the novel anticonvulsant lamotrigine (Lamnictal) using primary neuroglial cultures from rat cortex. *Brain Res* 1993: 612: 190–9.
12 Mutoh K, Dichter MA. Lamotrigine blocks voltage-dependent Na currents in a voltage-dependent manner with a small use-dependent component (abstract). *Epilepsia* 1993: 34 (Suppl. 6): 87.
13 Waldmeier PC, Baumann PA, Wicki P, Feldtrauer JJ, Stierlin C, Schmutz M. Similar potency of carbamazepine, oxcarbazepine, and lamotrigine in inhibiting the release of glutamate and other neurotransmitters. *Neurology* 1995; 45: 1907–13.
14 Wang S-J, Huang C-C, Hsu K-S, Tsai JJ, Gean PW. Inhibition of *N*-type calcium currcnts by lamotrigine in rat amygdalar neurones. *Neuroreport* 1996; 7: 3037–40.
15 Cunningham MO, Jones RS. The anticonvulsant, lamotrigine decreases spontaneous glutamate release but increases spontaneous GABA release in the rat entorhinal cortex *in vitro*. *Neuropharmacology* 2000; 39: 2139–46.
16 Meldrum BS, Excitatory amino acids in epilepsy and potential novel therapies. *Epilepsy Res* 1992; 12: 189–96.
17 Meldrum BS, Leach M. The mechanism of action of lamotrigine. *Rev Contemp Pharmacother* 1994: 5: 107–14.
18 Xie X, Lancaster B, Peakman T, Garthwaite J. Interaction of the antiepileptic drug lamotrigine with recombinant rat brain type IIA Na channels and with native Na channels in rat hipoccampal neurones. *Pflugers Arch* 1995; 430: 437–46.
19 Leach MJ, Marden CM, Miller AA. Pharmacological studies on lamotrigine, a novel potential antiepileptic drug: II. Neurochemical studies on the mechanism of action. *Epilepsia* 1986; 27: 490–7.
20 Waldemeier PC, Martin P, Stocklin K, Portet C, Schmutz M. Effects of carbamazepine, oxcarbazepine and lamotrigine on the increase in extracellular glutamate elicited by veratridine in rat cortex and striatum. *Naunyn Schmiedebergs Arch Pharmacol* 1996; 354: 164–72.
21 Stefani A, Hainsworth AH, Spadoni F, Bernardi G. On the inhibition of voltage activated calcium currents in rat cortical neurones by the neuroprotective agent 619C89. *Br J Pharmacol* 1998; 125: 1058–64.
22 Stefani A, Spadoni F, Sinicalchi A, Bernardi G. Lamotrigine inhibits Ca currents in cortical neurons: functional implication. *Eur J Pharmacol* 1996; 307: 113–16.
23 Grunze H, von Wegerer J, Greene RW, Walden J. Modulation of calcium and potassium currents by lamotrigine. *Neuropsychobiology* 1998; 38: 131–8.
24 Wang SJ, Sihra TS, Gean PW. Lamotrigine inhibition of glutamate release from isolated cerebrocortical nerve terminals (synaptosomes) by suppression of voltage-activated calcium channel activity. *Neuroreport* 2001; 12: 2255–8.
25 Smith SE, Meldrum BS. Cerebroprotective effect of lamotrigine afer focal ischemia in rats. *Stroke* 1995; 26: 117–22.
26 Meldrum BS. The role of glutamate in epilepsy and other CNS disorders. *Neurology* 1994; 44 (Suppl. 8): S14–23.
27 Halonen T, Nissinen J, Pitkanen A. Effect of lamotrigine treatment on status epilepticus-induced neuronal damage and memory impairment in rat. *Epilepsy Res* 2001; 46: 205–23.
28 Leach MJ, Baxiter MG, Critchley MAE. Neurochemical and behavioral aspects of lamotrigine. *Epilepsia* 1991; 32 (Suppl. 2): 4–8.
29 Langosch JM, Zhou XY, Frick A, Grunze H, Walden J. Effects of lamotrigine on field potentials and long-term potentiation in guinea pig hippocampal slices. *Epilepsia* 2000; 41: 1102–6.
30 Langosch JM, Zhou XY, Grunze H, Walden J. New insights into the mechanisms and sites of action of lamotrigine. *Neuropsychobiology* 2000; 42 (Suppl. 1): 26–7.
31 Coulter D. Antiepileptic drug cellular mechanisms of action: where does lamotrigine fit in? *J Child Neurol* 1997; 12 (Suppl. 1): S2–9.
32 Poolos NP, Miglore M, Johnston D. Pharmacologic upregulation of h-channels reduces the excitability of pyramidal neurone dendrites. *Nature Neurosci* 2002; 5: 767–74.
33 Miller AA, Sawyer DA, Ruth B *et al.* Lamotrigine. In: Meldrum BS, Porter RJ, eds. *New Anticonvulsant Drugs*. London: John Libbey, 1986: 165–77.
34 Miller AA, Wheatley P, Sawyer DA, Baxter MG, Roth B. Pharmacological studies on lamotrigine: a novel potential antiepileptic drug: I. Anticonvulsant profile in mice and rats. *Epilepsia* 1986; 27: 483–9.
35 Wheatley PL, Miller AA. Effects of lamotrigine on electrically induced afterdischarge duration in anaesthetised rat, dog, and marmoset. *Epilepsia* 1989; 30: 34–40.
36 Smith SE, Al-Zubaidy ZA, Chapman AG *et al.* Excitatory amino acid antagonists lamotrigine and BW 1003C87 as anticonvulsants in the genetically epilepsy-prone rat. *Epilepsy Res* 1993; 15: 101–11.
37 Dalby NO, Nielsen EB. Comparison of the preclinical anticonvulsant profiles of tiagabine, lamotriginc, gabapentin and vigabatrin. *Epilepsy Res* 1997: 28: 63–72.
38 Lamb RJ, Miller AA. Effect of lamotrigine and some known anticonvulsant drugs on visually-evoked after-discharge in the conscious rat (abstract). *Br J Pharmacol* 1985: 86: 765P.
39 Hosford DA, Wang Y. Utility of the lethargic (*lh/lh*) mouse model of absence seizures in predicting the effects of lamotrigine, vigabatrin, tiagabine, gabapentin, and topiramate against human absence seizures. *Epilepsia* 1997; 38: 408–14.
40 Otsuki K, Morimoto K, Sato K, Yamada N, Kuroda S. Effects of lamotrigine and conventional antiepileptic drugs on amygdala- and hippocampal-kindled seizures in rats. *Epilepsy Res* 1998: 31: 101–12.
41 Marciani MG, Stanzione P, Mattia D *et al.* Lamotrigine add-on therapy in focal epilepsy: electroencephalographic and neuropsychological evaluation. *Clin Neuropharmacol* 1998; 21: 41–7.
42 Binnie CD, Kasteleijn-Nolst Trenite TGA, de Korte RA. Photosensitivity as a model for acute anti-epileptic drug studies. *Electroencephalogr Clin Neurophysiol* 1985; 63: 35–41.
43 Marciani MG, Spanedda F, Bassetti MA *et al.* Effect of lamotrigine on EEC paroxysmal abnormalities and background activity: a computerized analysis. *Br J Clin Pharmacol* 1996; 42: 621–7.
44 Uberall MA, Wenzel D. Safety and efficacy of lamotrigine in pediatric epilepsy [abstract]. *Epilepsia* 1999; 40 (Suppl. 2): 167.
45 Milligan N, Richens A. Methods of assessment of antiepileptic drugs. *Br J Clin Pharmacol* 1981; 11: 35–41.
46 Besag F. The effect of lamotrigine on cognitive function in children. In: Loiseau P, edr. *Lamotrigine: a Brighter Future*. International Congress and Symposium Series no. 124. London: Royal Society of Medicine Press Limited, 1996: 81–7.
47 Frank LM, Enlow T, Holmes GL *et al.* Lamictal (lamotrigine) monotherapy for typical absence seizures in children. *Epilepsia* 1999; 40: 973–9.
48 Grinspan A, Chevalier Y, Hirsch E, Bidaut-Mazel C, Marescaux C. Efficacy and tolerability of adjunctive lamotrigine for the treatment of the Lennox–Gastaut syndrome: final results of an video/EEG open study [abstract]. *Epilepsia* 1997; 38 (Suppl. 8): 100.
49 Foletti C, Volanschi D. Influence of lamotrigine addition on computerized background EEG parameters in severe epileptogenic encephalopathies. *Eur Neurol* 1994: 34: (Suppl.) 1: 87–9.

50 Cohen AF, Ashby L, Crowley D, Peck AW, Miller AA. Lamotrigine (BW430C), a potential anticonvulsant: effects on the central nervous system in comparison with phenytoin and diazepam. *Br J Clin Pharmacol* 1985; 20: 619–29.

51 Hamilton MJ, Cohen AF, Yuen AWC, Land G, Weatherley BC, Peck AW. Carbamazepine and lamotrigine in healthy volunteers: relevance to early tolerance and clinical trial dosage. *Epilpsia* 1993; 34: 166–73.

52 Brodie MJ, Richens A, Yuen AWC. Double-blind comparison of lamotrigine and carbamazepine in newly diagnosed epilepsy. *Lancet* 1995; 345: 476–9.

53 Martin R, Kuzniecky R, Ho S *et al.* Cognitive effects of topiramate, gabapentin, and lamotrigine in healthy young adults. *Neurology* 1999; 52: 321–7.

54 Aldenkamp AP, Baker G. A systematic review of the effects of lamotrigine on cognitive function and quality of life. *Epilepsy Behav* 2001; 2: 85–91.

55 Meador KJ, Loring DW, Ray PG *et al.* Differential cognitive effects of carbamazepine and lamotrigine. *Neurology* 2002; 56: 1177–82.

56 Mervaala E, Koivisto K, Hanninen T *et al.* Electrophysiological and neuropsychological profiles of lamotrigine in young and age-associated memory impairment (AAMI) subjects. *Neurology* 1995; 45 (Suppl. 4): A259.

57 Smith D, Baker G, Davies G. Outcomes of add-on treatment with lamotrigine in partial epilepsy. *Epilepsia* 1993; 34: 312–22.

58 Cohen AF, Land GS, Breimer DD, Yuen WC, Winton C, Peck AW. Lamotrigine. A new anticonvulsant: pharmacokinetics in normal humans. *Clin Pharmacol Ther* 1987; 42: 535–41.

59 Rambeck B, Wolf P. Lamotrigine clinical pharmacokinctics. *Clin Pharmacokinet* 1993; 25: 433–43.

60 Peck AW. Clinical pharmacology of lamotrigine. *Epilepsia* 1991: 32 (Suppl. 2): S9–12.

61 Elwes RDC, Binnie CD. Clinical pharmacokinetics of newer antiepileptic drugs: lamotriginc, vigabatrin, gabapentin and oxcarbazepine. *Clin Pharmacokinet* 1996; 30: 403–15.

62 Dickins M, Sawyer DA, Morley TJ, Parsons DN. Lamotrigine: chemistry and biotransformation. In: Levy RH, Mattson RH, Meldrum BS, eds. *Antiepileptic Drugs*, 4th edn. New York: Raven Press, 1995: 871–5.

63 Parmeggiani L, Belmonte A, Ferrari AR, Perucca E, Guerrini R. Add-on lamotrigine treatment in children and young adults with severe partial epilepsy: an open, prospective, long-term study. *J Child Neurol* 2000; 15: 671–4.

64 Bialer M. Comparative pharmacokinetics of the newer antiepileptic drugs. *Clin Pharmacokinet* 1993; 24: 441–52.

65 Ramsay RE, Pellock IM, Garnett WR *et al.* Pharmacokinetics and safety of lamotrigine (Lamictal) in patients with epilepsy. *Epilepsy Res* 1991; 10: 191–200.

66 Garnett WR. Lamotrigine: pharmacokinetics. *J Child Neurol* 1997; 12 (Suppl. 1): S10–15.

67 Jawad S, Yuen WC, Peck AW *et al.* Lamotrigine: single-dose pharmacokinetics and initial 1 week experience in refractory epilepsy. *Epilepsy Res* 1987: 1: 194–201.

68 Eriksson A-S, Hoppu K, Nergardh A, Boreus L. Pharmacokinetic interactions between lamotrigine and other antiepileptic drugs in children with intractable epilepsy. *Epilepsia* 1996; 37: 769–73.

69 Chen C, Casale EJ, Duncan B, Culverhouse EH, Gilman J. Pharmacokinetics of lamotrigine in children in the absence of other antiepileptic drugs. *Pharmacotherapy* 1999; 19: 437–41.

70 Vauzelle-Kervroëdan F, Rey E, Cieuta C *et al.* Influence of concurrent antiepileptic medication on the pharmacokinetics of lamotrigine as add-on therapy in epileptic children. *Br J Clin Pharmacol* 1996; 41: 325–30.

71 Bar-Oz B, Nulman I, Koren G, Ito S. Anticonvulsants and breast feeding: a critical review. *Paediatr Drugs* 2000; 2: 113–26.

72 Battino D, Croci D, Granata T, Estienne M, Pisani F, Avanzini G. Lamotrigine plasma concentrations in children and adults: influence of age and associated therapy. *Ther Drug Monit* 1997 19: 620–7.

73 Armijo J, Bravo J, Cuadrado A, Herranz JL. Lamotrigine serum concentration-to-dose ratio: influence of age and concomitant antiepileptic drugs and dosage implications. *Ther Drug Monit* 1999; 21: 182–90.

74 Yuen AWC, Peck AW. Lamotrigine pharmacokinetics: oral and i.v. infusion in man. *Br J Clin Pharmacol* 1988; 26: 242P.

75 Mikati MA, Schachter SC, Schomer DL *et al.* Long-term tolerability, pharmacokinetic and preliminary efficacy study of lamotrigine in patients with resistant partial seizures. *Clin Neuropharmacol* 1989; 12: 312–21.

76 Yau MK, Garnett WR, Wargin WA, Pellock JM. A single dose, dose proportionality, and bioequivalence study of lamotrigine in normal volunteers [abstract]. *Epilepsia* 1991; 32 (Suppl.): 3–8.

77 Chen C. Validation of a population pharmacokinetic model for adjunctive lamotrigine therapy in children. *Br J Clin Pharmacol* 2000; 50: 135–45.

78 Meyer FP, Banditt P, Schubert A, Schoche J. Lamotrigine concentrations in human serum, brain tissue, and tumor tissue. *Epilepsia* 1999; 40: 68–73.

79 Levine B, Jufer RA, Smialek JE. Lamotrigine distribution in two postmortem cases. *J Anat Toxicol* 2000; 24: 635–7.

80 Remmel RP, Sinz MW, Graves NM *et al.* Lamotrigine and lamotrigine-N-glucuronide concentrations in human blood and brain tissue. *Seizure* 1992; 1 (Suppl. A): P7/34.

81 Parsons DN, Dickins M, Morley TJ. Lamotrigine: absorption, distribution and excretion. In: Levy RH, Mattson RH, Meldrum OS *et al.* eds. *Antiepileptic Drugs*, 4th edn. New York: Raven Press, 1995: 877–81.

82 Sinz MW, Remmel RP. Isolation and characterization of a novel quaternary ammonium-linked glucuronide of lamotrigine. *Drug Metab Dispos* 1991; 19: 149–53.

83 Doig MV, Clare RA. Use of thermospray liquid chromatography mass spectrometry to aid in the identification of urinary metabolites of a novel antiepileptic drug, lamotrigine. *J Chromatogr* 1999; 554: 181–9.

84 Posner J, Webster H, Yuen WC. Investigation of the ability of lamotrigine, a novel antiepileptic drug, to induce mixed function oxygenase enzymes [abstract]. *Br J Clin Pharmac* 1991; 32: 658P.

85 Richens A, ed. *Clinical Update on Lamotrigine: a novel antiepileptic agent*. Royal Tunbridge Wells: Wells Medical Limited, 1992.

86 Posner J, Holdich T, Crome P. Comparison of lamotrigine pharmacokinetics in young and elderly healthy volunteers. *Pharm Med* 1991; 1: 121–8.

87 Ohman I, Vitols S, Tomson T. Lamotrigine in pregnancy: pharmacokinetics during delivery, in the neonate, and during lactation. *Epilepsia* 2000; 41: 709–13.

88 Tran TA, Leppik IE, Blesi K, Sathanandan ST, Remmel R. Lamotrigine clearance during pregnancy. *Neurology* 2002; 59: 251–5.

89 Fillastre JP, Taburet AM, Fialaire A, Etienne I, Bidault R, Singlas E. Pharmacokinetics of lamotrigine in patients with renal impairment: influence of haemodialysis. *Drugs Exp Clin Res* 1993: 19: 25–32.

90 Posner J, Cohen AF, Land G, Winton C, Peck AW. The pharmacokinetics of lamotrigine (BW43OC) in healthy subjects with unconjugated hyperbilirubinaemia (Gilbert's syndrome). *Br J Clin Pharmacol* 1989; 28: 117–20.

91 Mahmood I, Tammara VK, Baweja RK. Dose percent reduction in seizure frequency correlate with plasma concentration of anticonvulsant drugs? *Clin Pharmacol Ther* 1998; 64: 547–52.

92 Jawad S, Richens A, Goodwin G, Yuen AWC. Controlled trial of lamotrigine (Lamictal) for refractory partial seizures. *Epilepsia* 1989; 30: 356–63.

93 Pisani F, Russo M, Trio R *et al.* Lamotrigine in refractory epilepsy: a long-term open study. *Epilepsy Res* 1991; 3 (Suppl.): 187–91.

94 Stolarek I, Blacklaw J, Forrest G, Thompson GG, Brodie MJ. Vigabatrin and lamotrigine in refractory epilepsy. *J Neurol Neurosurg Psychiatr* 1994; 57: 921–4.

95 Motte J, Trevathan E, Arvidsson JFV, Barrera MN, Mullens LL, Manasco P. The Lamictal Lennox-Gastaut Study Group. Lamotrigine for generalized seizures associated with the Lennox–Gastaut syndrome. *N Engl J Med* 1997; 337: 1807–12. (Erratum: *N Engl J Med* 1998; 339: 851–2.)

96 Mims J, Panovich P, Ritter F, Frost MD. Treatment with high doses of lamotrigine in children and adolescents with refractory seizures. *J Child Neurol* 1997; 12: 64–7.

97 Pellock JM. Managing pediatric epilepsy syndromes with new antiepileptic drugs. *Pediatrics* 1999; 104 (Pt 1): 1106–16.

98 Battino D, Buti D, Croci D *et al.* Lamotrigine in resistant childhood epilepsy. *Neuropediatrics* 1993; 24: 332–6.

99 Schumberger E, Chavez F, Palacios L, Rey E, Pajot N, Dulac O. Lamotrigine in treatment of 120 children with epilepsy. *Epilepsia* 1994; 35: 359–67.

100 Besag FMC, Wallace SJ, Dulac O, Aving J, Spencer SC, Hosking G. Lamotrigine for the treatment of epilepsy in childhood. *J Pediatr* 1995; 127: 991–7.

101 Bartoli A, Guerrini R, Belmonte A, Alessandri MG, Gatti G, Perucca E. The influence of dosage, age, and comedication on steady state plasma lamotrigine concentrations in epileptic children: a prospective study with preliminary assessment of correlations with clinical response. *Ther Drug Monit* 1997; 19: 252–60.

102 Kilpatrick ES, Forrest G, Brodie MJ. Concentration-effect and concentration-toxicity relations with lamotrigine: a prospective study. *Epilepsia* 1996; 37: 534–8.

103 Kanner AM, Chkenkely I, Frey M. Is there a relationship between the occurrence of adverse events from lamotrigine and its serum concentrations? *Epilepsia* 1998; 39 (Suppl. 6]: S72–3.

104 Betts T, Goodwin G, Withers RM. Human safety of lamotrigine. *Epilepsia* 1991: 32 (Suppl. 2): 17–21.

105 Hussein Z, Posner J. Population pharmacokinetics of lamotrigine monotherapy in patients with epilepsy: retrospective analysis of routine monitoring data. *Br J Clin Pharmacol* 1997; 43: 457–65.

106 Grasela TH, Fiedler-Kelly J, Cox E, Womble GP, Risner ME, Chen C. Population pharmacokinetics of lamotrigine adjunctive therapy in adults with epilepsy. *J Clin Pharmacol* 1999; 39: 373–84.

107 Perucca E. Is there a role for therapeutic drug monitoring of new anticonvulsants? *Clin Pharmacokinet* 2000; 38: 191–204.

108 Tomson T, Johannessen SI. Therapeutic monitoring of the new antiepileptic drugs. *Eur J Clin Pharmacol* 2000; 55: 697–705.

109 Anderson GD. A mechanistic approach to antiepileptic drug interactions. *Ann Pharmacother* 1998; 32: 554–63.

110 Sabers A; Gram L. Newer anticonvulsants: comparative review of drug interactions and adverse effects. *Drugs* 2000; 60: 23–33.

111 Riva R, Albani F, Contin M, Baruzzi A. Pharmacokinetic interactions between antiepileptic drugs: clinical considerations. *Clin Pharmacokinet* 1996; 31: 470–93.

112 Wolf P. Lamotrigine: preliminary clinical observations on pharmacokinetics and interactions with traditional antiepileptic drugs. *J Epilepsy* 1992; 5: 73–9.

113 Yuen AWC, Land G, Wheatherley BC, Peck AW. Sodium valproate acutely inhibits lamotrigine metabolism. *Br Clin Pharmacol* 1992; 33: 511–13.

114 Herranz JL, Arteaga R, Armijo JA. Three-year efficacy and tolerability of add-on lamotrigine in treatment-resistant epileptic children. *Clin Drug Invest* 1996: 11: 214–23.

115 Royal Pharmaceutical Society of Great Britain. Lamotrigine. *BNF* 2001; 42: 229.

116 Gidal BE, Kanner A, Maly M, Rutecki P, Lensmeyer GL. Lamotrigine pharmacokinetics in patients receiving felbamate. *Epilepsy Res* 1997; 27: 1–5.

117 Berry DJ, Besag FMC, Pool F, Natarajan J, Doose D. Does topiramate change lamotrigine serum concentrations when added to treatment? An audit of a dose-escalation study (abstract). *Epilepsia* 1998: 39 (Suppl. 6): 56–7.

118 Depot M, Powell JR, Messenheinier JJA, Clotier G, Dalton MJ. Kinetic effects of multiple oral doses of acetaminophen on a single oral dose of lamotrigine. *Clin Pharmacol Ther* 1990; 48: 346–55.

119 Ramaratnam S, Marson AG, Baker GA. Lamotrigine add-on for drug-resistant partial epilepsy. *Cochrane Database Syst Rev* 2000: CD001909.

120 Loiseau P, Yuen AWC, Duche B, Menager T, Arne-Bes MC. A randomized double-blind crossover add-on trial of lamotrigine in patients with treatment-resistant partial seizures. *Epilepsy Res* 1990; 7: 136–45.

121 Sander JWAS, Patsalos PN, Oxley JR, Hamilton MJ, Yuen WC. A randomized double-blind placebo-controlled add-on trial of lamotrigine in patients with severe epilepsy. *Epilepsy Res* 1990; 6: 221–6.

122 Matsuo F, Risner M, Valakas A, Womble GK, Yau M. Placebo-controlled evaluation of carbamazepine and phenytoin plasma concentraions during administration of add-on Lamictal (lamotrigine) in outpatients with partial seizures. *Epilepsia* 1994; 35 (Suppl. 8): 163.

123 Anderson GD, Yau MK, Gidal BE et al. Bidirectional interaction of valproate and lamotrigine in healthy subjects. *Clin Pharmacol Ther* 1996: 60: 145–56.

124 Eriksson A-S, Nergardh A, Hoppu K. The efficacy of lamotrigine in children and adolescents with refractory generalized epilepsy: a randomized, double-blind, crossover study. *Epilepsia* 1998; 39: 495–501.

125 Panayiotopoulos CP, Ferrie CD, Knott C, Robinson RO. Interaction of lamotrigine with sodium valproate (letter). *Lancet* 1993; 13; 341: 445.

126 Ferrie CD, Panayiotopoulos CP. Therapeutic interaction of lamotrigine and sodium valproate in intractable myoclonic epilepsy. *Seizure* 1994; 3: 157–9.

127 Pisani F, Di Perri P, Perucca E, Richens A. Interaction of lamotrigine with sodium valproate (letter). *Lancet* 1993: 341: 1224.

128 Pisani F, Oteri G, Russo MF, Di Perri R, Perucca E, Richens A. The efficacy of valproate-lamotrigine comedication in refractory complex partial seizures: evidence for a pharmacodynamic interaction. *Epilepsia* 1999; 40(8): 1141–6.

129 Warner T, Patsalos PN, Prevett M. Lamotrigine-induced carbamazepine toxicity: an interaction with carbamazepine-10,11-epoxide. *Epilepsy Res* 1992; 11: 147–50.

130 Besag FM, Berry DJ, Pool F, Newbery JE, Subel B. Carbamazepine toxicity with lamotrigine: pharmacokinetic or pharmacodynamic interaction? *Epilepsia* 1998; 39: 183–7.

131 Pisani F, Xiao B, Fazio A, Spina E, Perucca E, Tomson T. Single dose pharmacokinetics of carbamazepine-10, 11-epoxide in patients on lamotrigine monotherapy. *Epilepsy Res* 1994; 19: 245–8.

132 Eriksson A-S, Boreus LO. No increase in carbamazepine-10, 11-epoxide during addition of lamotrigine treatment in children. *Ther Drug Monit* 1997; 19: 499–501.

133 Wilbur K, Ensom MH. Pharmacokinetic drug interactions between oral contraceptives and second-generation anticonvulsants. *Clin Pharmacokinet* 2000; 38: 355–65.

134 Sabers A, Buchholt JM, Uldall P, Hansen EL. Lamotrigine plasma levels reduced by oral contraceptives. *Epilepsy Res* 2001; 47: 151–4.

135 Binnie CD, Debets RMC, Engelsman M et al. Double-blind crossover trial of lamotrigine (Lamictal) as add-on therapy in intractable epilepsy. *Epilepsy Res* 1989; 4: 222–9.

136 Matsuo F, Bergen D, Faught E et al. Placebo-controlled study of the efficacy and safety of lamotrigine in patients with partial seizures. *Neurology* 1993; 43: 2284–91.

137 Messenheimer J, Ramsey RE, Willmore LJ et al. Lamotrigine therapy for partial seizures: a multicenter, placebo-controlled, double-blind, crossover trial. *Epilepsia* 1994; 35: 113–21.

138 Schapel GJ, Beran RG, Vajda FJE et al. Double-blind, placebo-controlled, crossover study of lamotrigine in treatment resistant partial seizures. *J Neurol Neurosurg Psychiatr* 1993; 56: 448–53.

139 Boas J, Dam M, Friis ML, Kristensen O, Pedersen B, Gallagher J. Controlled trial of lamotrigine (Lamictal^R) for treatment-resistant partial seizures. *Acta Neurol Scand* 1996; 94: 247–52.

140 Duchowny M, Pellock JM, Graf WD et al. A placebo-controlled trial of lamotrigine add-on therapy for partial seizures in children. Lamictal Pediatric Partial Seizure Study Group. *Neurology* 1999; 53: 1724–31.

141 Schmidt D, Reid S, Rapp P. Add-on treatment with lamotrigine for intractable partial epilepsy: a placebo-controlled crossover trial (abstract). *Epilepsia* 1993; 34 (Suppl. 2): 66.

142 Gilliam F, Vazquez B, Sackellares JC et al. An active-control trial of lamotrigine monotherapy for partial seizures. *Neurology* 1998; 51: 1018–25.

143 Reunanen OM, Dam M, Yuen AWC. A randomized open multicenter comparative trial of lamotrigine and carbamazepine as monotherapy in patients with newly diagnosed or recurrent epilepsy. *Epilepsy Res* 1996; 23: 149–55.

144 Brodie MJ, Overstall PW, Giorgi L. Multicentre, double-blind, randomised comparison between lamotrigine and carbamazepine in elderly patients with newly diagnosed epilepsy. The UK Lamotrigine Elderly Study Group. *Epilepsy Res* 1999; 37: 81–7.

145 Nieto-Barrera M, Brozmanova M, Capovilla G et al. A comparison of monotherapy with lamotrigine or carbamazepine in patients with newly diagnosed partial epilepsy. *Epilepsy Res* 2001; 46: 145–55.

146 Steiner TJ, Dellaportas CI, Findley LJ et al. Lamotrigine monotherapy in newly diagnosed untreated epilepsy: a double-blind comparison with phenytoin. *Epilepsia* 1999; 40: 601–7.

147 Brodie MJ, Yuen AW. Lamotrigine substitution study: evidence for synergism with sodium valproate. *Epilepsy Res* 1997; 26: 423–32.

148 Jozwiak S, Terczynski A. Open study evaluating lamotrigine efficacy and safety in add-on treatment and consecutive monotherapy in patients with carbamazepine- or valproate-resistant epilepsy. *Seizure* 2000; 9: 486–92.

149 Beran RG, Berkovic SF, Dunagan FM *et al*. Double-blind, placebo-controlled, crossover study of lamotrigine in treatment-resistant generalised epilepsy. *Epilepsia* 1998; 39: 1329–33.

150 Ferrie CD, Robinson RO, Knott C, Panayiotopoulos PC. Lamotrigine as add-on drug in typical absence seizures. *Acta Neurol Scand* 1995; 91: 200–2.

151 Timmings PL, Richens A. Lamotrigine as an add-on drug in the management of Lennox–Gastaut syndrome. *Eur Neurol* 1992; 32: 305–7.

152 Buchanan N. The efficacy of lamotrigine on seizure control in 34 children, adolescents and young adults with intellectual and physical disability. *Seizure* 1995; 4: 233–6.

153 Buchanan N. Lamotrigine: clinical experience in 93 patients with epilepsy. *Acta Neurol Scand* 1995; 92: 28–32.

154 Farrell K, Connolly MB, Munn R, Peng S, MacWilliam LM. Prospective, open-label, add-on study of lamotrigine in 56 children with intractable generalized epilepsy. *Pediatr Neurol* 1997; 16: 201–5.

155 Donaldson JA, Glauser TA, Olberding LS. Lamotrigine adjunctive therapy in childhood epileptic encephalopathy (the Lennox–Gastaut syndrome). *Epilepsia* 1997; 38: 68–73.

156 Dulac O, Kaminska A. Use of lamotrigine in Lennox-Gastaut and related epilepsy syndromes. *J Child Neurol* 1997; 12 (Suppl. 1): S23–8.

157 Pimentel J, Guimaraes ML, Lima L, Leitao O, Sampaio MJ. Lamotrigine as add-on therapy in treatment-resistant epilepsy. Portuguese Lamotrigine as Add-on Therapy in Treatment-resistant Epilepsy Study Group. *J Int Med Res* 1999; 27: 148–57.

158 Coppola G, Pascotto A. Lamotrigine as add-on drug in children and adolescents with refractory epilepsy and mental delay: an open trial. *Brain Dev* 1997; 19: 398–402.

159 Uvebrant P, Bauzienè R. Intractable epilepsy in children: the efficacy of lamotrigine treatment, including non-seizure-related benefits. *Neuropediatrics* 1994; 25: 284–9.

160 Barr PA, Buettiker VE, Antony JH. Efficacy of lamotrigine in refractory neonatal seizures. *Pediatr Neurol* 1999; 20: 161–3.

161 Veggiotti P, Cieuta C, Rey E, Dulac O. Lamotrigine (Lamictal) in infantile spasms. *Lancet* 1994; 344: 1375–6.

162 Stenbom Y, Tonnby B, Hagberg B. Lamotrigine in Rett syndrome: treatment experience from a pilot study. *Eur Child Adolesc Psychiatr* 1998; 7: 49–52.

163 Aberg L, Kirveskari E, Santavuori P. Lamotrigine therapy in juvenile neuronal ceroid lipofuscinosis. *Epilepsia* 1999; 40: 796–9.

164 Perucca E, Gram L, Avanzini G, Dulac O. Antiepileptic drugs as a cause of worsening seizures. *Epilepsia* 1998; 39: 5–17.

165 Genton P. When antiepileptic drugs aggravate epilepsy. *Brain Dev* 2000; 22: 75–80.

166 Guerrini R, Belmonte A, Parmeggiani L, Perucca E. Myoclonic status epilepticus following high-dosage lamotrigine therapy. *Brain Dev* 1999; 21: 420–4.

167 Guerrini R, Dravet C, Genton P, Belmonte A, Kaminska A, Dulac O. Lamotrigine and seizure aggravation in severe myoclonic epilepsy. *Epilepsia* 1998; 39: 508–12.

168 Gillham R, Kane K, Bryant-Comstock L, Brodie MJ. A double-blind comparison of lamotrigine and carbamazepine in newly diagnosed epilepsy with health-related quality of life as an outcome measure. *Seizure* 2000; 9: 375–9.

169 Cockerell OC, Moriarty J, Trimble M, Sander JWAS, Shorvon SD. Acute psychological disorders in patients with epilepsy: a nation-wide study. *Epilepsy Res* 1996; 25: 119–31.

170 Post RM, Denicoff KD, Frye MA, Dunn RT, Leverich GS, Osuch E, Speer A. A history of the use of anticonvulsants as mood stabilizers in the last two decades of the 20th century. *Neuropsychobiology* 1998; 38: 152–66.

171 Xie X, Hagan RM. Cellular and molecular actions of lamotrigine: Possible mechanisms of efficacy in bipolar disorder. *Neuropsychobiology* 1998; 38: 119–30.

172 Zerjav-Lacombe S, Tabarsi E. Lamotrigine: a review of clinical studies in bipolar disorders. *Can J Psychiatr* 2001; 46: 328–33.

173 Calabrese JR, Suppes T, Bowden CL *et al*. A double-blind, placebo-controlled prophylaxis study of lamotrigine in rapid-cycling bipolar disorder. Lamictal 614 Study Group. *J Clin Psychiatr* 2000; 61: 841–50.

174 McCleane G. 200 mg daily of lamotrigine has no analgesic effect in neuropathic pain: a randomized, double-blind, placebo controlled trial. *Pain* 1999; 83: 105–7.

175 McCleane GJ. Lamotrigine in the management of neuropathic pain: a review of the literature. *Clin J Pain* 2000; 16: 321–6.

176 Devulder J, De Laat M. Lamotrigine in the treatment of chronic refractory neuropathic pain. *J Pain Symptom Manag* 2000; 19: 398–403.

177 Messenheimer JA, Giorgi L, Risner ME. The tolerability of lamotrigine in children. *Drug Saf* 2000; 22: 303–12.

178 Messenheimer J, Mullens EL, Giorgi L, Young F. Safety review of adult clinical trial experience with lamotrigine. *Drug Saf* 1998; 18: 281–96.

179 Richens A. Safety of lamotrigine. *Epilepsia* 1995; 35: S37–S40.

180 Schacter S, Leppik I, Matsuo F, Messenheimer JA, Faught E, Risner ME. Lamotrigine: six-month, placebo-controlled safety and tolerance study. *J Epilepsy* 1995; 8: 201–10.

181 Matsuo F, Gay P, Madsen J, Tolman KG, Rollins DE, Risner M, Lai AA. Lamotrigine high-dose tolerability and safety in patients with epilepsy: a double-blind, placebo-controlled, eleven-week study. *Epilepsia* 1996; 37: 857–62.

182 Mackay FJ, Wilton LV, Pearce GL, Freemantle SN, Mann RD. Safety of long-term lamotrigine in epilepsy. *Epilepsia* 1997; 38: 881–6.

183 Lhatoo SD, Wong IC, Polizzi G, Sander JW. Long-term retention rates of lamotrigine, gabapentin, and topiramate in chronic epilepsy. *Epilepsia* 2000; 41: 1592–6.

184 Ruble J, Matsuo F. Anticonvulsant-induced cutaneous reactions. *CNS Drugs* 1999; 12: 215–36.

185 Dooley J, Camfield P, Gordon K, Camfield C, Wirrell E, Smith E. Lamotrigine-induced rash in children. *Neurology* 1996; 46: 240–2.

186 Iametti P, Raucci U, Zuccaro P, Pacifici P. Lamotrigine hypersensitivity in chidhood epilepsy. *Epilepsia* 1998; 39: 502–7.

187 Hsiao CJ, Lee JY, Wong TW, Sheu HM. Extensive fixed drug eruption due to lamotrigine. *Br J Dermatol* 2001; 144: 1289–91.

188 Messenheimer JA. Rash in adult and pediatric patients treated with lamotrigine. *Can J Neurol Sci* 1998; 25: S14–18.

189 Elston DM. Photo quiz. *Cutis* 1999; 64: 202.

190 Dunn N, Wilton L, Shakir S. Stevens–Johnson syndrome and antiepileptics. *Lancet* 1999; 354: 1033–4.

191 Besag FM, Dulac O, Alving J, Mullens EL. Long-term safety and efficacy of lamotrigine (Lamictal) in paediatric patients with epilepsy. *Seizure* 1997; 6: 51–6.

192 Yalcin B, Karaduman A. Stevens–Johnson syndrome associated with concomitant use of lamotrigine and valproic acid. *J Am Acad Dermatol* 2000; 43 (Pt 2): 898–9.

193 Neuman MG, Malkiewicz IM, Shear NH. A novel lymphocyte toxicity assay to assess drug hypersensitivity syndromes. *Clin Biochem* 2000; 33: 517–24.

194 Schaub N, Bircher AJ. Severe hypersensitivity syndrome to lamotrigine confirmed by lymphocyte stimulation *in vitro*. *Allergy* 2000; 55: 191–3.

195 Bastuji-Garin S, Rzany B, Stern RS, Shear NH, Naldi L, Roujeau J-C. Clinical classification of cases of toxic epidermal necrolysis, Stevens–Johnson syndrome, and erythema multiforme. *Arch Dermatol* 1993; 129: 92–6.

196 Roujeau JC, Stern RS. Severe adverse cutaneous reactions to drugs. *N Engl J Med* 1994; 331: 1272–85.

197 Tennis P, Stern R. Risk of serious cutaneous disorders after initiation of phenytoin, carbamazepine, or sodium valproate: a record linkage study. *Neurology* 1997; 49: 542–6.

198 Rzany B, Correia O, Kelly JP, Naldi L, Auquier A, Stern R. Risk of Stevens–Johnson syndrome and toxic epidermal necrolysis during first weeks of antiepileptic therapy: a case-control study. Study Group of the International Case Control Study on Severe Cutaneous Adverse Reactions. *Lancet* 1999; 353: 2190–4.

199 Wong IC, Mawer GE, Sander JW. Factors influencing the incidence of lamotrigine-related skin rash. *Ann Pharmacother* 1999; 33: 1037–42.

200 Faught E, Morris G, Jacobson M *et al*. Adding lamotrigine to valproate: incidence of rash and other adverse effects. Postmarketing Antiepileptic Drug Survey (PADS) Group. *Epilepsia* 1999; 40: 1135–40.

201 Guberman AH, Besag FM, Brodie MJ et al. Lamotrigine-associated rash: risk/benefit considerations in adults and children. Epilepsia 1999; 40: 985–91.

202 Brown TS, Appel JE, Kasteler JS, Callen JP. Hypersensitivity reaction in a child due to lamotrigine. Pediatr Dermatol 1999; 16: 46–9.

203 Knowles SR, Shapiro LE, Shear NH. Anticonvulsant hypersensitivity syndrome: incidence, prevention and management. Drug Saf 1999; 21: 489–501.

204 Besag F, McShane T, Neville B, Robinson R. Factors associated with serious skin reactions in children aged 12 years and under taking lamotrigine. Dev Med Child Neurol 1999; 41: 68–9.

205 Messenheimer JA, Guberman AH. Rash with lamotrigine: dosing guidelines. Epilepsia 2000; 41: 488.

206 Schingmann J, Mockenhaup M, Schroeder W, Schlingmann E. Severe cutaneous reactions (SCAR) after the use of anticonvulsants. Pharmacoepidemiol Drug Saf 2000; 9: S85.

207 Tavenor SJ, Wong ICK, Newton R, Brown SW. Rechallenge with lamotrigine after initial rash. Seizure 1995; 4: 67–71.

208 Sorri A, Keranen T, Moilanen E et al. The effect of oral activated charcoal on the absorption and elimination of lamotrigine (abstract). Epilepsia 1998; 39 (Suppl. 6): 53.

209 Besag F, Ng GYT, Pool F. Successful reintroduction of lamotrigine after initial rash with lamotrigine. Seizure 2000; 9: 375–9.

210 Yuen AWC, Bihari DJ. Multiorgan failure and disseminated intravascular coagulation in severe convulsive seizures. Lancet 1992; 340: 618.

211 Schaub JE, Williamson PJ, Barnes EW, Trewby PN. Multisystem adverse reaction to lamotrigine. Lancet 1994; 344: 481.

212 Chattergoon D, McGuigan M, Koren M, Hwang P, Ito S. Multiorgan dysfunction and disseminated intravascular coagulation in children receiving lamotrigine and valproic acid. Neurology 1997; 49: 1142–4.

213 Makin AJ, Fitt S, Williams R, Duncan JS. Fulminant hepatic failure induced by lamotrigine. BMJ 1995; 311: 292.

214 Schlienger RG, Knowles SR, Shear NH. Lamotrigine–associated anticonvulsant hypersensitivity syndrome. Neurology 1998; 51: 1172–5.

215 Mewasingh L, Aylett S, Kirkham F, Stanhope R. Hyponatremia associated with lamotrigine in cranial diabetes insipidus. Lancet 2000; 356: 656.

216 Pathak P, McLachlan RS. Drug-induced pseudolymphoma secondary to lamotrigine. Neurology 1998; 50: 1509–10.

217 de Camargo OA, Bode H. Agranulocytosis associated with lamotrigine. Br Med J 1999; 318: 1179.

218 Fayad M, Choueiri R, Mikati M. Potential hepatotoxicity of lamotrigine. Pediatr Neurol 2000; 22: 49–52.

219 Wong IC, Chadwick DW, Fenwick PB, Mawer GE, Sander JW. The long-term use of gabapentin, lamotrigine, and vigabatrin in patients with chronic epilepsy. Epilepsia 1999; 40: 1439–45.

220 Beran RG, Gibson RJ. Aggressive behaviour in intellectually challenged patients with epilepsy treated with lamotrigine. Epilepsia 1998; 39: 280–2.

221 Sadler M. Lamotrigine associated with insomnia. Epilepsia 1999; 40: 322–5.

222 Leestma JE, Annegers JF, Brodie MJ et al. Incidence of sudden unexplained death in the Lamictal (lamotrigine) clinical development program. Epilepsia 1994; 35 (Suppl. 8): 12.

223 Arpino C, Brescianini S, Robert E et al. Teratogenic effects of antiepileptic drugs: use of an International Database on Malformations and Drug Exposure (MADRE). Epilepsia 2000; 41: 1436–43.

224 Reiff-Eldridge R, Heffner CR, Ephross SA, Tennis PS, White AD, Andrews EB. Monitoring pregnancy outcomes after prenatal drug exposure through prospective pregnancy registries: a pharmaceutical company commitment. Am J Obstet Gynecol 2000; 182 (Pt 1): 159–63.

225 White AD, Andrews EB. The Pregnancy Registry program at Glaxo Wellcome Company. J Allergy Clin Immunol 1999; 103 (Pt 2): S362–3.

226 GlaxoSmithKline. Lamotrigine Pregnancy Registry. Interim Report September 1, 1992 through March 31, 2002. London: GlaxoSmithKline, 2002: p.39.

227 Uberall MA. Normal growth during lamotrigine monotherapy in pediatric epilepsy patients—a prospective evaluation of 103 children and adolescents. Epilepsy Res 2001; 46: 63–7.

228 O'Donnell J, Bateman DN. Lamotrigine overdose in an adult. J Clin Toxicol 2000; 38: 659–60.

229 Briassoulis G, Kalabalikis D, Tamiolaki M, Hatzis T. Lamotrigine in childhood overdose. Pediatr Neurol 1998; 19: 239–42.

230 Buckley NA, Whyte IM, Dawson AH. Self-poisoning with lamotrigine (letter). Lancet 1993; 342: 1552–3.

231 Sbei M, Campellone JV. Stupor from lamotrigine toxicity. Epilepsia 2001; 1082–3.

232 Harchelroad F, Lang D, Valeriano J. Lamotrigine overdose. Vet Hum Toxicol 1994; 36: 372.

233 Delanty N, French J. Treatment of Lennox–Gastaut syndrome: current recommendations. CNS Drugs 1998; 10: 181–8.

234 Buoni S, Grosso S, Fois A. Lamotrigine treatment in childhood drug resistant epilepsy. J Child Neurol 1998; 13: 163–7.

235 Sander JWAS, Trevisol-Bittencourt PC, Hart YM, Patsalos PN, Shorvon SD. The efficacy and long-term tolerability of lamotrigine in the treatment of severe epilepsy. Epilepsy Res 1990; 7: 226–9.

236 Panayiotopoulos CP. Beneficial effect of relatively small doses of lamotrigine. Epilepsia 1999; 40: 1171–2.

237 Isojarvi JI, Rattya J, Myllyla VV et al. Valproate, lamotrigine, and insulin-mediated risks in women with epilepsy. Ann Neurol 1998; 43: 446–51.

238 Guo C-Y, Ronen GM, Atkinson SA. Long-term valproate and lamotrigine treatment may be a marker for reduced growth and bone mass in children with epilepsy. Epilepsia 2001; 42: 1141–7.

239 Stephen LJ, Kwan P, Shapiro D, Dominiczak M, Brodie MJ. Hormone profiles in young adults with epilepsy treated with sodium valproate or lamotrigine monotherapy. Epilepsia 2001; 42: 1002–6.

240 Cramer JA, Fisher R, Ben-Menachem E, French J, Mattson RH. New antiepileptic drugs: comparison of key clinical trials. Epilepsia 1999; 40: 590–600.

241 Leppik IE. The role of lamotrigine in the treatment of epilepsy. Neurology 1998; 51: 940–2.

242 Wallace SJ. Newer antiepileptic drugs: advantages and disadvantages. Brain Dev 2001; 23: 277–83.

243 Brodie MJ. Monostars: an aid to choosing an antiepileptic drug as monotherapy. Epilepsia 1999; 40 (Suppl. 6): S17–22 (discussion S73–4).

244 Wong IC, Lhatoo SD. Adverse reactions to new anticonvulsant drugs. Drug Saf 2000; 23: 35–56.

245 Stephen LJ, Sills GJ, Brodie MJ. Lamotrigine and topiramate may be a useful combination (letter). Lancet 1998; 351: 958–9.

246 Bourdet SV, Gidal BE, Alldredge BK. Pharmacologic management of epilepsy in the elderly. J Am Pharm Assoc 2001; 41: 421–36.

37   Levetiracetam

A. Sadek and J.A. French

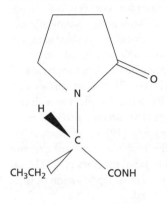

Primary indications	Adjunctive therapy in partial seizures with or without secondarily generalized seizures
Usual preparations	Tablets: 250, 500, 750, 1000 mg
Usual dosages	Initial: 1000 mg/day. Maintenance: 1000–3000 mg/day
Dosage intervals	2 times/day
Significant drug interactions	None
Serum level monitoring	Value not established
Target range	–
Common/important side-effects	Somnolence, asthenia, infection, dizziness, headache
Main advantages	A recently licensed drug which, on the basis of clinical trial evidence, is well-tolerated and highly effective
Main disadvantages	Limited experience in routine clinical practice, as it is recently licensed
Mechanism of action	Not known
Oral bioavailability	<100%
Time to peak levels	0.6–1.3 h
Metabolism and excretion	Partially hydrolysed in the blood to inactive compound
Volume of distribution	0.5–0.7 L/kg
Elimination half-life	6–8 h (lower in children; higher in the elderly and in renal impairment)
Plasma clearance	0.6 mL/min/kg
Protein binding	None
Active metabolites	None
Comment	A novel antiepileptic drug with promise in the therapy of partial onset seizures (with or without secondarily generalization)

(*Note*: this summary table was formulated by the lead editor.)

The antiepileptic drug (AED) levetiracetam [(*S*)-α-ethyl-2-oxo-1-pyrrolidine-acetamide] is a pyrrolidine derivative with a chemical structure that differs from all other AEDs, and reveals unique pharmacological properties [1,2]. Levetiracetam was approved in the USA in 1999, and subsequently has gained approval in Europe in 2000. This chapter will review preclinical data, efficacy, safety and clinical use of this unique compound.

Chemical properties

Levetiracetam is a white powder which is wholly soluble in water. It is a racemically pure S-enantiomer [3]. The R-enantiomer has been shown to be essentially devoid of anticonvulsant properties in animal models of epilepsy [4].

Preclinical data

Unlike other recently approved AEDs, levetiracetam is not active in the standard animal screening models used for determination of AED efficacy against acute seizures, namely the maximal electroshock (MES) and pentylenetetrazol (PTZ) seizure tests [5]. Levetiracetam also appears to lack anticonvulsant activity in other acute seizure tests utilizing chemoconvulsant agents, such as intracerebroventricular infusion of excitatory amino acids—N-methyl-D-aspartate (NMDA), kainate and α-amino-3-hydroxy-5-methyl-4-isoxazole propionic acid (AMPA)—as well as doses of chemoconvulsants inducing clonic convulsions in 97% of the animals tested, CD_{97} (bicuculline, picrotoxin, 3-mercaptoproprionic acid and caffeine) [5,6]. On the other hand, with agents such as pilocarpine (i.p.) and kainate (s.c.) that induce secondarily generalized seizures in rats (producing relatively drug-resistant seizures), levetiracetam provided potent seizure protection.

Despite its non-conventional and largely inactive profile against acute seizures, levetiracetam does possess activity in a variety of animal models which are thought to model chronic epilepsy, such as kindled and genetic animals with spontaneous, recurrent seizures or seizures that resemble human epileptic seizures [6]. Levetiracetam reduces seizure severity, duration of motor seizures as well as afterdischarge duration in fully amygdala-kindled rats [5]. Levetiracetam is also effective in preventing the acquisition of amygdala kindling (in rats) [5] and PTZ kindling in mice [7]. These results suggest that levetiracetam may possess antiepileptogenic properties (Silver et al. 1991). Phenytoin and carbamazepine do not prevent acquisition of kindling, although valproate and phenobarbital do. Recently, Löscher et al. [8] demonstrated that levetiracetam appears to be the only AED that is more effective in a subset of amygdala-kindled rats who were resistant to phenytoin, as compared to kindled rats sensitive to phenytoin. This indicates that levetiracetam might also be useful in patients who had been treatment resistant in the past. Some experiments indicate the potential for the development of tolerance in the amygdala-kindled rat model, but no tolerance was observed in a chronic mouse model of epilepsy and a bicuculline rat model [6,9,10]. The significance of these disparate findings in humans remains to be determined.

Levetiracetam was also shown to be effective in genetic animal models of epilepsy, such as the genetic absence epilepsy rat from Strasbourg (GAERS) (resembling human spike-wave conditions) and the audiogenic-seizure prone rat [11]. The seizures these animals display are thought to be primary generalized seizures as opposed to those in the kindling models which are thought to be representative of partial seizures. Thus, while levetiracetam is devoid of anticonvulsant activity in traditional seizure models, it does appear to possess a potent, broad spectrum of activity in animal models reflective of both partial and generalized epilepsy.

The preclinical safety profile of levetiracetam appears favourable. There is no evidence of carcinogenic or mutagenic potential. Levetiracetam did not produce motor impairment in the rotarod test in rats and mice except at doses markedly higher than protective doses nor did it cause obvious sedation in the open field test [5,6]. In

both the kindling model and the GAERS model, there was a wide safety margin between the effective dose (ED_{50}; dose protecting 50% of animals from seizures) and the dose impairing rotarod performance (TD_{50}; dose causing 50% of animals to lose equilibrium on the rotarod). As noted above, levetiracetam, in contrast to other AEDs, did not promote an increase in side-effects when used in kindled animals (which are more sensitive to central nervous system (CNS) adverse events) as compared to control animals [5,6] Additionally, levetiracetam did not produce cognitive impairment in the Morris water maze test in rats, in contrast to carbamazepine, valproate and clonazepam, when examined in both normal and amygdala-kindled rats [12].

The mechanism of action of levetiracetam appears to differ from those of other AEDs. Levetiracetam does not induce a conventional modulation of any of the three main mechanisms involved in the action of classical AEDs, i.e. inhibition of sodium [13] and T-type calcium channels [14] and direct enhancement of γ-aminobutyric acid (GABA)-ergic neurotransmission [15,16,17]. Recent studies suggest that levetiracetam moderately inhibits a specific high-voltage-activated calcium channel, the N-type [18] and may also inhibit the release of calcium from intracellular stores [19]. Levetiracetam has also been demonstrated to oppose the inhibitory action of zinc and β-carbolines on $GABA_A$- and glycine-gated currents [15]. The involvement of these mechanisms in the antiepileptic action of levetiracetam remains to be further elucidated.

Levetiracetam inhibits burst firing without affecting normal neuronal excitability [20,21]. This appears to relate to a novel ability to inhibit hypersynchronization of epileptiform activity, which distinguishes levetiracetam from other AEDs [22]. There does appear to be a stereoselective, saturable and reversible binding site specific for levetiracetam in the CNS, and there was a correlation between the degree of binding and the antiepileptic effect for a series of levetiracetam analogues, implying that this binding site appears to have a functional relevance [23]. Extensive in vitro binding experiments have not revealed any significant displacement of ligands specific for over 55 different binding sites, including various receptor systems, reuptake sites, second messenger systems and channel proteins. However, the involvement of this apparently novel binding site with the above-described mechanisms has yet to be determined.

Pharmacokinetics

The pharmacokinetics of levetiracetam have been studied in healthy adults, adults and children with epilepsy, the elderly and subjects with renal and hepatic impairment.

To date, there is only an oral form of levetiracetam available, although an intravenous form may become available in the future. Levetiracetam is a very water-soluble compound, which is rapidly and almost completely absorbed after oral administration. Administration of levetiracetam with food does not reduce the extent, but may slow the rate of absorption [24]. Bioavailability approaches 100% [24]. Peak plasma concentrations are reached in 1–2 h. The pharmacokinetics are linear, and unlike other recently approved AEDs, there is low intra- and intersubject variability. This means that the serum level can be estimated if weight and creatinine clearance are known. The extent of bioavailability of levetiracetam is not affected by food, although the absorption is slowed [24]. The volume of distribution is similar to intracellular and extracellular water, at 0.5–0.7 L/kg [24]. Despite its water-soluble nature, levetiracetam readily and freely crosses the blood–brain barrier [25]. Levetiracetam crosses the placenta, and fetal levels approximate maternal levels. Levetiracetam is <10% protein bound. Sixty-six per cent of the dose is excreted unchanged in the urine. Twenty-seven per cent of the dose is metabolized by an enzymatic hydrolysis of the acetamide group, mainly to L057 [26]. This process occurs diffusely in the body, and is not hepatically mediated. A study of levetiracetam using human liver microsomal enzymes revealed no inhibition of drug-metabolizing enzymes including CYP3A4, CYP1A2, CYP2C19, CYP2C9, CYP2E1, CYP2D6, epoxide hydrolase and various uridine glucuronyltransferases [27].

The metabolites of levetiracetam have no known pharmacological activity and are also renally excreted. Because there is no hepatic metabolism, and because levetiracetam does not induce or inhibit hepatic enzymes, it does not interfere with the metabolism of other AEDs, nor do other AEDs interact with its metabolism or elimination. However, because unpredictable interactions may occur, specific interaction studies were performed with commonly used agents, like oral contraceptives, digoxin and warfarin. No evidence of any specific interaction between levetiracetam and these products could be demonstrated [27]. Studies have also been done in patients receiving monotherapy phenytoin ($n=6$), carbamazepine ($n=4$), valproic acid ($n=6$) or combination carbamazepine/valproic acid ($n=2$). Up to 200 mg of levetiracetam was added without changes in plasma levels of the background drugs [28]. Another small study of 17 refractory epilepsy patients found no effect of levetiracetam on levels of carbamazepine, phenobarbital, valproic acid, primidone and clobezam [29]. In this study, there was a variable change in phenytoin levels when levetiracetam was added. This interaction was specifically investigated in a subsequent study. Tracer doses of deuterium-labelled (D_{10}) phenytoin were given intravenously 12 weeks before and after adding levetiracetam to the regimen of patients taking phenytoin as monotherapy. Phenytoin pharmacokinetic parameters (C_{max}, C_{min}, C_{ave}, AUC, CL, half-life, V_d) did not change after adding levetiracetam. The authors concluded that levetiracetam did not affect phenytoin disposition [30]. Drug interactions were also assessed during randomized controlled trials. Plasma levels of concomitant AEDs were not significantly altered in any of the placebo-controlled adjunctive trials of levetiracetam [31–33].

As might be expected in a drug which is not hepatically metabolized, other AEDs have no effect on the metabolism of levetiracetam [27]. Probenecid increases plasma levels of the levetiracetam metabolite L057 2.5-fold, by a reduction in renal clearance [24].

Plasma half-life of levetiracetam across studies is approximately 6–8 h. However, since the mechanism of action is unknown, this may not represent the functional half-life, and indeed there is evidence from studies of the effect on the photoparoxysmal response that the functional half-life may be much longer. After a single dose of levetiracetam, the photoparoxysmal response was suppressed for up to 30 h [34]. It was on this basis that a BID regimen was selected for clinical trials.

The half-life of levetiracetam in children, as for most drugs, is shorter than adults. After a single oral dose of 20 mg/kg, values for C_{max} and AUC equated for a 1-mg/kg dose were ~30–40% lower

than adults, whereas renal clearance was higher. The half-life was ~6 h [35].

Elderly individuals may have many reasons for altered drug metabolism, including gastric mucosal atrophy and decreased gastric motility leading to altered absorption, change in hepatic and renal function, and altered albumin levels. Studies of levetiracetam in 16 hospitalized patients demonstrated a prolonged half-life, which could be explained entirely by reduced creatinine clearance [36]. The elimination half-life is approximately 10–11 h, compared to 7.7 h in younger normal subjects [24]. Adjustments in dosage should be made based on estimated creatinine clearance, taking body mass into account.

Studies of levetiracetam disposition have been done in individuals with hepatic impairment. Mild to moderate (Child–Pugh class A or B) hepatic impairment do not alter the clearance of levetiracetam, and no dosage adjustments are required. However, in severe hepatic failure (Child–Pugh class C) there is a reduced clearance, most likely due to concomitant renal insufficiency [37]. Adjustments in dose should therefore be made based on renal rather than hepatic function.

As might be expected, renal impairment reduces clearance of levetiracetam and its metabolites. As a result, C_{max} and AUC are increased, and serum levels rise in proportion to creatinine clearance. Dose reductions are recommended, as outlined in Table 37.1. For patients with renal failure on dialysis, a dose of 500–1000 mg once daily is recommended, with a supplemental dose of 250–500 mg after dialysis treatment [36].

Serum levels

Serum levels can be measured using gas chromatography with nitrogen phosphorus detection after methanol extraction or by high-performance liquid chromatography (HPLC) with UV detection [38]. Levetiracetam exhibits little person-to-person variability in pharmacokinetics, as compared to other AEDs, and has no known drug–drug interactions. This reduces the need for frequent blood level monitoring. To date, the clinical utility of serum level monitoring has not been established. However, serum level monitoring would be appropriate for assessment of compliance, and in patients with renal failure.

Efficacy

Refractory partial seizures

Levetiracetam has been demonstrated to be very effective in reducing partial seizures in patients with treatment-resistant partial epilepsy, in three randomized well-controlled studies [2]. Charac-

Table 37.1 Levetiracetam dosing in patients with renal impairment [36]

Renal function	Creatinine clearance (ml/min/1.73 m²)	Dosage administered BID
Normal	>80	500–1500
Mild	50–80	500–1000
Moderate	30–50	250–750
Severe	<30	250–500

Table 37. 2 Randomized placebo-controlled trials of levetiracetam

Study	n	Design	Population	Doses	Evaluation period	% Responders (50% reduction)	% Seizure free
[33]	324	Double-blind randomized parallel	Refractory partial seizures; 4 szs/4 weeks; 1–2 AEDs	Placebo 1000 mg 2000 mg	12 weeks	Placebo: 10.4% 1000 mg: 22.8% 2000 mg: 31.6%	Placebo: .9% 1000 mg: 5% 2000 mg: 2%
[41]	286	Double-blind randomized parallel group followed by responder-selected withdrawal to monotherapy	Partial seizures; 2 complex partial seizures/4 weeks; one AED	Placebo 3000 mg	12 week (add-on phase only)	Placebo: 16.7% 3000 mg: 42.1%	Placebo: 1.0% 3000 mg: 8.2%
[32]	294	Double-blind randomized parallel	Refractory partial seizures; 12 szs/12 weeks; 1–2 AEDs	Placebo 1000 mg 3000 mg	14 weeks	Placebo: 10.8% 1000 mg: 33.0% 3000 mg: 39.8%	Placebo: 0.0% All Lev: 5.5%
[31]	119	Double-blind randomized parallel	Refractory partial, 1° or 2° GTCC; 1–3 AEDs; 4 szs/24 weeks	Placebo 2000 mg 4000 mg[a]	24 weeks	Placebo: 16.1% 2000 mg: 48.1% 4000 mg: 28.6%	Placebo: 2.5% 2000 mg: 9.5% 4000 mg: 5.2%

[a] No titration was used in this study.
GTCC, generalized tonic-clonic seizures.

teristics of these studies and an additional randomized study in both partial and generalized seizures can be found in Table 37.2. A total of 904 subjects were randomized to placebo, levetiracetam 1000 mg/day, 2000 mg/day or 3000 mg/day. Results from these studies have shown that levetiracetam-treated patients have significantly fewer seizures than placebo-treated patients, as measured by the responder rate (>50% reduction in weekly seizure frequency from baseline). Responder rates range from 23–33% (levetiracetam 1000 mg/day) to 42% (levetiracetam 3000 mg/day) compared to 10–17% on placebo. Up to 8% of patients were seizure free with 3000 mg/day [32,33,39]; 50%, 75% and 90% seizure-free rates for the various studies are indicated in Table 37.3. In the fourth study, patients with less refractory partial and generalized seizures were randomized to placebo, 2000 and 4000 mg of levetiracetam. Forty-eight per cent of patients had a 50% seizure reduction in the 2000 mg dose group [31]. This excellent response may be due to the less severe nature of the epilepsy studied. Some studies seem to indicate a dose–response relationship, while this is less clear in other cases [40]. For example, in the study by Betts *et al.* [31] of 2000 vs. 4000 mg of levetiracetam, patients randomized to 2000 mg were increased to 4000 mg in a non-blinded extension phase. No additional efficacy was gained (48.1% responder rate at 2000 mg vs. 46.2% at 4000 mg).

One study evaluated levetiracetam as monotherapy in refractory patients [41]. After the randomized placebo-controlled parallel study was completed, patients who had a 50% or greater reduction in seizures (whether on placebo or levetiracetam) underwent a 12-week gradual tapering of their background AED after which they entered a 12-week monotherapy phase. Patients exited this phase if they had worsening of seizures, as measured by pre-established criteria. By the end of the study, 19.9% of patients randomized to levetiracetam were able to complete the study, as compared to only

Table 37.3 Seizure reduction in clinical trials with levetiracetam (rate minus placebo)

Study/dose	>50% seizure reduction	>75% seizure reduction	>90% seizure reduction	Seizure free
[32]				
1000 mg	29.7	12.3	8.3	4.1
3000 mg	32.2	18.7	10.9	5.9
[33]				
1000 mg	14.5	6.7	3.8	1.0
2000 mg	28.9	14.4	5.8	2.0
[41]				
3000 mg	25.0	19.1	12.2	6.7

9.5% of placebo patients. Nine of the 49 patients who were successfully down-titrated to levetiracetam monotherapy were seizure free. This initial data suggests a role for levetiracetam as monotherapy. Further studies will be needed to confirm this.

The most important outcome of epilepsy therapy may arguably be an improvement in overall quality of life. Quality of life is a combined measure of seizure control and other factors, such as drug tolerability, and improvement in cognitive domains. Quality of life was measured in one double-blind placebo-controlled efficacy study of levetiracetam, using the QOLIE-31, a validated measure. Levetiracetam produced a dose-related improvement in several domains of quality of life when added to standard therapy [42]. There was a statistically significant improvement on total score and on seizure worry, overall quality of life and cognitive functioning subscales in patients taking levetiracetam. Responders (patients with

>50% seizure reduction) had improvement in all subscales, and did better than the placebo responder group.

Efficacy in other epilepsy syndromes

Levetiracetam has been approved by the American Food and Drug Administration as adjunctive therapy for partial onset seizures in adults since 1999 [43]. Several recent preliminary reports indicate that levetiracetam is also effective against other types of epilepsy. The efficacy of levetiracetam in treatment of primary generalized epilepsy including tonic-clonic, absence and myoclonic epilepsy was reported in a recent small case series. Among 36 patients with primary generalized epilepsy who failed other AEDs and were treated with levetiracetam for 8 months, 42% became seizure free and 75% were considered seizure responders with more than 50% reduction [44]. Another recent report further indicates that levetiracetam is effective in juvenile myoclonic epilepsy (JME). Among 30 patients with resistant JME who received levetiracetam, 62% became seizure free [45]. Other reports suggest that levetiracetam is potentially efficacious in photosensitive epilepsy. In 12 subjects with photosensitive epilepsy who received levetiracetam, the photoepileptiform response was abolished on EEG in 50%, and reduced in a further 25%, in a dose-dependent manner. Improvement lasted for up to 30h [34]. Since levetiracetam is an analogue of piracetam, a drug which has been used in the progressive myoclonic epilepsies, there has been enthusiasm for testing in this disorder. In early case series, patients with progressive myoclonic epilepsy have experienced dramatic improvements with the addition of levetiracetam to their regimen [46,47]. The use of levetiracetam in non-epileptic postanoxic myoclonus was also advocated recently by some reports [48,49]. Furthermore, there are some early indications that levetiracetam may also be useful in the treatment of other epilepsies including atypical absence and atonic seizures [50]. However the limited power of the above studies makes it very difficult to draw any meaningful conclusions, and larger placebo-controlled studies are needed to unequivocally test the efficacy of levetiracetam in different types of primary generalized epilepsies and progressive myoclonic epilepsies. Clinical research is currently being conducted in a number of areas within and outside of epilepsy treatment to further investigate the broad range of potential effectiveness of levetiracetam.

Side-effects

The side-effect profile of levetiracetam has been well characterized during phase II and III clinical trials. Collective safety data from 3347 patients receiving levetiracetam during trials including 1422 adult epilepsy patients indicates that levetiracetam is very well tolerated [2,51,52]. Furthermore, pooled safety data from several double-blinded studies suggests that the overall incidence of adverse events reported with levetiracetam 1000 mg/day (70.8 and 88.8%), 2000 mg/day (75 and 83.3%) and 3000 mg/day (55 and 89.1%) were similar to that observed with placebo (53–88.4%) [52].

Common side-effects

The most commonly reported side-effects of levetiracetam in the adult population were somnolence and asthenia. In a pooled analysis, somnolence was seen in 14.8% of epilepsy patients treated with levetiracetam vs. 8.4% of placebo patients [51]. The effect was not clearly dose related. For example, in one study somnolence was seen in 20.4% of patients on 1000 mg of levetiracetam vs. 18.8% on 3000 mg, as compared to 13.7% of placebo patients [32]. Asthenia had an overall incidence of 14.7% vs. 9.1% of placebo patients, and again was not dose related. Other adverse effects include nausea, dizziness and headache. Adverse effects from placebo-controlled trials are listed in Table 37.4. In a study where no titration was used, the incidence of somnolence, nausea and dizziness were most pronounced during the initiation (without up-titration) of the medication and at higher doses [31]. On the other hand, such clear dose-related effects for asthenia and headache were not established.

Infections including upper respiratory tract (rhinitis and pharyngitis) and urinary tract infections were reported to be increased in the levetiracetam group compared to placebo group in some of the controlled trials. The clinical relevance of this finding is still unclear especially since it was not associated with increase in the white blood cell count, and none of these symptoms led to discontinuation of levetiracetam. Increased infection rate was seen in some studies and not others, and may have been related to an artefact of which terms were used to report side-effects [53].

Premarketing studies indicate that behavioural symptoms including agitation, hostility, anxiety, apathy, emotional lability, depersonalization and depression were reported in 13.3% of levetiracetam patients compared to 6.2% in placebo group. Furthermore, 0.7% of levetiracetam patients reported psychotic symptoms compared to 0.2% placebo, and suicidal behaviour was reported in 0.5% vs. none for placebo group. Behavioural problems occurred at a lower rate in other populations treated with levetiracetam in early placebo-controlled trials, including patients with anxiety and cognitive disturbance [52]. This implies that either the epileptic condition or concomitant AED use may increase the potential for behavioural problems with levetiracetam use. Behavioural problems appear to remit when levetiracetam is discontinued. Premarketing studies may not be ideal for determination of behavioural side-effects, as patients on antidepressants and psychoactive medications are often excluded from trials. As postmarketing experience mounts, a better assessment of behavioural problems with levetiracetam will be possible. In a pooled analysis, >25% worsening of seizures occurred more frequently during add-on trials in the placebo group (26%) than in the levetiracetam-treated group (14%) [52]. A recent case series suggested that possible exacerbation of seizure could occur in a small number of patients with high doses of levetiracetam, especially in those with generalized abnormalities on the EEG [54]. Primary generalized epileptiform abnormalities on EEG may predict exacerbation.

Others have reported that patients may worsen at higher doses of levetiracetam, and in these cases a dose reduction may lead to improvement [55].

Hypersensitivity and skin rash appear to be uncommon adverse effects of levetiracetam. In placebo-controlled epilepsy trials, hypersensitivity led to dose reduction or discontinuation in one patient in the levetiracetam group, and six in the placebo group. There were no reports of Stevens–Johnson syndrome with levetiracetam. No clinically significant adverse effects were observed with any dosage of levetiracetam on physical or neurological examination,

Table 37.4 Overview of adverse events reported commonly with levetiracetam (LEV; different dosages) administered as adjunctive therapy than with placebo in the pivotal placebo-controlled trials in adult patients predominantly with refractory partial seizures with or without secondary generalization

Adverse events	Incidence (% of patients)				
	Placebo	LEV 1000 mg/day	LEV 2000 mg/day	LEV 3000 mg/day	LEV 4000 mg/day
[31]					
Somnolence	25.6		26.2		44.7
Dizziness	0		4.8		10.5
Asthenia	15.4		31		13.2
Infection	7.7		2.4		15.8
[32]					
Somnolence	13.7	20.4		18.8	
Dizziness	7.4	17.3		19.8	
Asthenia	11.6	16.3		12.9	
Headache	20	21.4		20.8	
Infection	12.6	27.6		26.7	
Rhinitis	8.4	13.3		6.9	
[33]					
Somnolence	4.5	9.4	11.3		
Dizziness	3.6	4.7	6.6		
Asthenia	8	7.5	13.2		
Headache	8.9	13.2	16		
Infection	6.3	9.4	6.6		
[41]					
Somnolence	3.8			6.1	
Asthenia	6.7			13.8	
Headache	10.5			3.3	
Infection	3.8			7.2	

blood or chemistry indices, ECG assessments or vital signs. Accidental injuries were reduced in patients receiving levetiracetam compared to placebo, perhaps due to improved seizure control [52].

Idiosyncratic adverse effects

Idiosyncratic reactions may be an uncommon occurrence. No reports of idiosyncratic adverse effects of levetiracetam are forthcoming to date. Only 3347 patients were included in the levetiracetam safety database [52], but as of 2002, 150 000 patients years of treatment have been recorded with levetiracetam (UCB, personal communication). Longer experience with levetiracetam is needed to draw any conclusions about its potential for idiosyncratic adverse effects, but the absence of problems to date is reassuring.

Teratogenicity

There are no well-controlled studies of levetiracetam in pregnancy. Currently levetiracetam is categorized in the US as a pregnancy category C drug (demonstrated teratogenicity in animals, human risk not known). Few pregnancies have been reported to the manufacturer in women who were treated with levetiracetam and the data are too limited to draw a conclusion about the effect of levetiracetam in human pregnancy. Of the pregnancies ending in live births during the clinical trials, one child was born with syndactyly and one with Fallot's tetralogy, but both patients were on AED polytherapy. Additional outcome data must be collected by pregnancy registry [51].

Adverse effects of levetiracetam in paediatric patients

Although a large multicentre-controlled adjunctive trial has been performed in paediatric patients with partial epilepsy, the results are not yet available. One open-label trial has been published, suggesting that levetiracetam as add-on therapy is effective, safe and well tolerated in children aged 6–12 years with treatment-resistant partial onset seizures [56]. Other data available on adverse effects of levetiracetam in paediatric epilepsy are derived from relatively smaller case series [50,57–60]. Adverse events occurred in between 24 and 44% of children who received levetiracetam. Most were mild and overall levetiracetam was well tolerated.

Behavioural problems were the most commonly reported adverse effect caused by levetiracetam in children, and occurred especially in those with a history of pre-existing behavioural disorder. Behavioural adverse effects from four open studies are shown in Table 37.5.

Table 37.5 Summary of published adverse effects of levetiracetam in paediatric patient population, in four open-label studies

Adverse effects	No. of patients (%)	Reference
Behavioural	10 (15.4)	[50] $n-70$
Lethargy	4 (6.2)	
Cognitive slowing	1 (1.5)	
Increased appetite/weight gain	1 (1.5)	
Dystonia	1 (1.5)	
Behavioural changes	2 (21.1)	[60] $n=19$
Ataxia	3 (6.7)	[57] $n=21$
Dizziness	3 (6.7)	
Lethargy	3 (6.7)	
Forced normalization	1 (2.2)	
Behavioural problems	6 (22.2)	[59] $n=27$
Drowsiness	2 (7.4)	
Decreased appetite	1 (3.7)	
Tremor	1 (3.7)	
Hypotonia	1 (3.7)	

Overdosage

The highest known dose of levetiracetam received in clinical development was 6000 mg/day. Reported overdosages caused only somnolence [51].

Tolerance

There has been interest in the question of whether levetiracetam produces tolerance over time, due to a report of this phenomenon in an animal model [9]. An analysis of patients continuing levetiracetam after the completion of controlled trials indicated that many patients maintained benefits of levetiracetam therapy for up to 5 years [61]. Thirteen per cent of treated patients were seizure free for at least 6 months.

Clinical therapeutics

Levetiracetam has a unique position among AEDs because of its pharmacokinetic and therapeutic properties. To summarize, it is highly water soluble, whereas almost all of the other AEDs are either only partially soluble or totally insoluble. Levetiracetam is not metabolized by the liver. It is free of non-linear metabolic kinetics, autoinduction and drug–drug interactions inherent to most AEDs. Furthermore, it lacks protein binding (<10%), which avoids the problem of displacement of highly protein-bound drugs. Its experimental antiepileptic profile differs from other drugs as does its mode of action. Its clinical efficiency is good, it has potentially broad-spectrum effects and a low rate of side-effects (at least, as reported to date). These unique properties permit easy addition of levetiracetam to other drug therapies without major concerns about drug–drug interactions.

The starting dose of levetiracetam is typically 500 mg BID, which is a therapeutic dose. Lately, there has been some enthusiasm for starting some or all patients on 250 mg BID to reduce the likelihood

of fatigue and irritability. Further clinical experience will determine whether this practice is beneficial. The dose can be titrated by 500–1000 mg every 1–2 weeks until maximum benefit has been obtained. A randomized controlled study was performed in which patients were initiated on up to 4000 mg of levetiracetam without titration. This dose was associated with higher rates of somnolence, dizziness and nausea. Dropout rates were no higher than initiation at 2000 mg, but responder rates also did not differ between the two doses, indicating that, while safe, starting at higher doses is probably not beneficial [31]. As noted above, very high doses of levetiracetam have not been proven effective, and there is preliminary evidence that such doses may exacerbate seizures in some patients [55]. The effects of levetiracetam are seen relatively quickly after initiation. In a pooled analysis of clinical trial data, seizure-free days were significantly increased even after the first day of levetiracetam therapy [62].

Children metabolize levetiracetam faster, and therefore might be expected to require higher doses per body weight. Clinical trials of children aged 6–12 years used mean doses of 40 mg/kg/day (according to the levetiracetam package insert). Initial doses used in children are typically 10–20 mg/kg/day [57,58]. The unique characteristics of levetiracetam and its lack of drug interactions make it potentially ideal for treating elderly epilepsy patients, particularly those patients who have other illnesses and are on several other medications.

In summary, levetiracetam has been established as an effective, safe and easy-to-use AED, with a novel mechanism. As experience with levetiracetam grows, it is likely to establish a prominent place in the therapeutic regimen, both for adjunctive and monotherapy use, in children, adults and the elderly, and in a broad spectrum of epilepsy syndromes.

References

1 Shorvon SD. New drug classes: Pyrrolidone derivatives. *Lancet* 2001; 200: 1885–92.
2 Shorvon SD, van Rijckevorsel K. A new antiepileptic drug. *J Neurol Neurosurg Psychiatr* 2002; 72: 426–9.
3 Genton P, Van Vleymen B. Piracetam and levetiracetam: close structural similarities but different pharmacological and clinical profiles. *Epileptic Disord* 2000; 2(2): 99–105.
4 Gower AJ *et al.* Ucb L059, a novel anti-convulsant drug: pharmacological profile in animals. *Eur J Pharmacol* 1992; 222(2–3): 193–203.
5 Löscher W, Honack D. Profile of ucb L059, a novel anticonvulsant drug, in models of partial and generalized epilepsy in mice and rats. *Eur J Pharmacol* 1993; 232(2–3): 147–58.
6 Klitgaard H *et al.* Evidence for a unique profile of levetiracetam in rodent models of seizures and epilepsy. *Eur J Pharmacol* 1998; 353(2–3): 191–206.
7 Löscher WD, Honack H, Rundfeldt C. Antiepileptogenic effects of the novel anticonvulsant levetiracetam (ucb L059) in the kindling model of temporal lobe epilepsy. *J Pharmacol Exp Ther* 1998; 284(2): 474–9.
8 Löscher W, Reissmuller E, Ebert U. Anticonvulsant efficacy of gabapentin and levetiracetam in phenytoin-resistant kindled rats. *Epilepsy Res* 2000; 40(1): 63–77.
9 Löscher W, Honack D. Development of tolerance during chronic treatment of kindled rats with the novel antiepileptic drug levetiracetam. *Epilepsia* 2000; 41(12): 1499–506.
10 Gower A *et al.* Anticonvulsant effects of UCB-L059 in rats: absence of tolerance or discontinuation after chronic administration. *Epilepsia* 1993; 34 (Suppl. 2): 50.
11 Gower AJ *et al.* Effects of levetiracetam, a novel antiepileptic drug, on con-

vulsant activity in two genetic rat models of epilepsy. *Epilepsy Res* 1995; 22(3): 207–13.

12 Lamberty Y, Klitgard M, Henrik G. Absence of negative impact of levetiracetam on cognitive function and memory in normal and amygdala-kindled rats. *Epilepsy Behav* 2000; 1: 333–42.

13 Zona C, Niespodziany I, Marchetti C, Klitgaard H, Bernardi G, Margineanu DG. Levetiracetam does not modulate neuronal voltage-gated Na⁺ and T-type Ca²⁺ currents. *Seizure* 2001; 10(4): 279–86.

14 Niespodziany I, Klitgaard H, Margineanu DG. Levetiracetam inhibits the high-voltage-activated Ca(2+) current in pyramidal neurones of rat hippocampal slices. *Neurosci Lett* 2001; 306(1–2): 5–8.

15 Rigo JM, Hans G, Nguyen L et al. The anti-epileptic drug levetiracetam reverses the inhibition by negative allosteric modulators of neuronal GABA- and glycine-gated currents. *Br J Pharmacol* 2002; 136(5): 659–72.

16 Sills GJ, Leach JP, Fraser CM et al. Neurochemical studies with the novel anticonvulsant levetiracetam in mouse brain. *Eur J Pharmacol* 1997; 325(1): 35–40.

17 Tong X, Patsalos PN. A microdialysis study of the novel antiepileptic drug levetiracetam: extracellular pharmacokinetics and effect on taurine in rat brain. *Br J Pharmacol* 2001; 133(6): 867–74.

18 Lukyanetz EA, Shkryl VM, Kostyuk PG. Selective blockade of N-type calcium channels by levetiracetam. *Epilepsia* 2002; 43(1): 9–18.

19 Angehagen M, Margineanu DG, Ben-Menachem E et al. Levetiracetam reduces caffeine-induced Ca²⁺ transients and epileptiform potentials in hippocampal neurons. *Neuroreport* 2003; 14(3): 471–5.

20 Margineanu DG, Wulfert E. Ucb L059, a novel anticonvulsant, reduces bicuculline-induced hyperexcitability in rat hippocampal CA3 in vivo. *Eur J Pharmacol* 1995; 286(3): 321–5.

21 Birnstiel S, Wulfert E, Beck SG. Levetiracetam (ucb LO59) affects in vitro models of epilepsy in CA3 pyramidal neurons without altering normal synaptic transmission. *Naunyn Schmiedebergs Arch Pharmacol* 1997; 356(5): 611–18.

22 Margineanu GD, Klitgaard H. Inhibition of neuronal hypersynchrony in vitro differentiates levetiracetam from classical antiepileptic drugs. *Pharmacol Res* 2000; 42(4): 281–5.

23 Noyer M et al. The novel antiepileptic drug levetiracetam (ucb L059) appears to act via a specific binding site in CNS membranes. *Eur J Pharmacol* 1995; 286(2): 137–46.

24 Patsalos PN. Pharmacokinetic profile of levetiracetam: toward ideal characteristics. *Pharmacol Ther* 2000; 85(2): 77–85.

25 Doheny HC et al. Blood and cerebrospinal fluid pharmacokinetics of the novel anticonvulsant levetiracetam (ucb L059) in the rat. *Epilepsy Res* 1999; 34(2–3): 161–8.

26 Perucca E, Bialer M. The clinical pharmacokinetics of the newer antiepileptic drugs. Focus on topiramate, zonisamide and tiagabine. *Clin Pharmacokinet* 1996; 31(1): 29–46.

27 Benedetti MS. Enzyme induction and inhibition by new antiepileptic drugs: a review of human studies. *Fund Clin Pharmacol* 2000; 14(4): 301–19.

28 DeDeyn P et al. Assessment of the safety of orally administered ucb L059 as add-on therapy in patients treated with antiepileptic drugs. *Seizure* 1992; 1 (Abstract): P7/15.

29 Sharief M et al. Efficacy and tolerability study of ucb L059 in patients with refractory epilepsy. *J Epilepsy* 1996; 9: 106–12.

30 Browne TR et al. Absence of pharmacokinetic drug interaction of levetiracetam with phenytoin in patients with epilepsy determined by new technique. *J Clin Pharmacol* 2000; 40(6): 590–5.

31 Betts T, Waegemans T, Crawford P. A multicentre, double-blind, randomized, parallel group study to evaluate the tolerability and efficacy of two oral doses of levetiracetam, 2000 mg daily and 4000 mg daily, without titration in patients with refractory epilepsy. *Seizure* 2000; 9(2): 80–7.

32 Cereghino JJ et al. Levetiracetam for partial seizures: results of a double-blind, randomized clinical trial. *Neurology* 2000; 55(2): 236–42.

33 Shorvon SD et al. Multicenter double-blind, randomized, placebo-controlled trial of levetiracetam as add-on therapy in patients with refractory partial seizures. European Levetiracetam Study Group. *Epilepsia* 2000; 41(9): 1179–86.

34 Kasteleijn-Nolst Trenite DG et al. Photosensitive epilepsy: a model to study the effects of antiepileptic drugs. Evaluation of the piracetam analogue, levetiracetam. *Epilepsy Res* 1996; 25(3): 225–30.

35 Pellock J et al. Single dose pharmacokinetics of levetiracetam in pediatric patients partial epilepsy. *Epilepsia* 1999; 40 (Suppl. 2): 238–9.

36 French J. Use of levetiracetam in special populations. *Epilepsia* 2001; 42 (Suppl. 4): 40–3.

37 Thomson T et al. No effect of liver impairment on the pharmacokinetics of levetiracetam. *Eur J Clin Pharmacol* 1999; 55: A25.

38 Ratnaraj N, Doheny HC, Patsalos PN. A micromethod for the determination of the new antiepileptic drug levetiracetam (ucb LO59) in serum or plasma by high performance liquid chromatography. *Ther Drug Monit* 1996; 18(2): 154–7.

39 Ben-Menachem E. New antiepileptic drugs and non-pharmacological treatments. *Curr Opin Neurol* 2000; 13(2): 165–70.

40 Boon P, Chauvel P, Pohlmann-Eden B, Otoul C, Wroe S. Dose-response effect of levetiracetam 1000 and 2000 mg/day in partial epilepsy. *Epilepsy Res* 2002; 48(1–2): 77–89.

41 Ben-Menachem E, Falter U. Efficacy and tolerability of levetiracetam 3000 mg/d in patients with refractory partial seizures: a multicenter, double-blind, responder-selected study evaluating monotherapy. European Levetiracetam Study Group. *Epilepsia* 2000; 41 (10): 1276–83.

42 Cramer JA et al. Effect of levetiracetam on epilepsy-related quality of life. N132 Study Group. *Epilepsia* 2000; 41(7): 868–74.

43 Leppik IE. The place of levetiracetam in the treatment of epilepsy. *Epilepsia* 2001; 42 (Suppl. 4): 44–5.

44 Krauss G et al. Efficacy of levetiracetam for treatment of drug-resistant generalized epilepsy. *Epilepsia* 2001; 42 (Suppl. 7): 179 (abstract).

45 Greenhill L, Betts T, Smith K. Effect of levetiracetam on resistant juvenile myoclonic epilepsy. *Epilepsia* 2001; 42 (Suppl. 7): 179 (abstract).

46 Kinirons P et al. Dramatic response to levetiracetam in progressive myoclonic epilepsy. *Epilepsia* 2001; 42 (Suppl. 7): 178 (abstract).

47 Genton P, Gelisse P. Antimyoclonic effect of levetiracetam. *Epileptic Disord* 2000; 2(4): 209–12.

48 Genton P, Gelisse P. Suppression of post-hypoxic and post-encephalitic myoclonus with levetiracetam. *Neurology* 2001; 57(6): 1144–5.

49 Krauss GL et al. Suppression of post-hypoxic and post-encephalitic myoclonus with levetiracetam. *Neurology* 2001; 56(3): 411–12.

50 Bourgeois B et al. Open-label assessment of levetiracetam efficacy and adverse effects in pediatric population. *Epilepsia* 2001; 42 (Suppl. 7): 53–4 (abstract).

51 Harden C. Safety profile of levetiracetam. *Epilepsia* 2001; 42 (Suppl. 4): 36–9.

52 French J, Edrich P, Cramer J.A. A systematic review of the safety profile of levetiracetam: a new antiepileptic drug. *Epilepsy Res* 2001; 47 (1–2): 77–90.

53 Ting T, French J, Cramer J. Infection rates among patients participating in clinical trials. *Epilepsia* 2000; 41 (Suppl. 7): 253 (abstract).

54 Goldstein JL. Levetiracetam: exacerbation of epilepsy. *Epilepsia* 2001; 42 (Suppl. 7): 254.

55 Montouris GD, Lippmann SM, Rosenfeld WE. Exacerbation of seizures: Any relationship to dose escalation of levetiracetam (Keppra)? *Epilepsia* 2001; 42(Suppl. 7): 184.

56 Glauser TA, Pellock JM, Bebin EM et al. Efficacy and safety of levetiracetam in children with partial seizures: an open-label trial. *Epilepsia* 2002; 43(5): 518–24.

57 Wannag E, Eriksson A, Brockmeier K. Tolerability of levetiracetam in children with refractory epilepsy. *Epilepsia* 2001; 42 (Suppl. 7): 57 (abstract).

58 Ng Y, Wheless J. Levetiracetam: Pediatric experience. *Epilepsia* 2001; 42 (Suppl. 7): 55 (abstract).

59 Faircloth VC et al. Levetiracetam adjunctive therapy for refractory pediatric focal-onset epilepsy. *Epilepsia* 2001; 42 (Suppl. 7): 54 (abstract).

60 Strunc M, Levisohn P. Tolerability and efficacy of levetiracetam in children. *Epilepsia* 2001; 42 (Suppl. 7): 92 (abstract).

61 Krakow K et al. Long-term continuation of levetiracetam in patients with refractory epilepsy. *Neurology* 2001; 56 (12): 1772–4.

62 French J et al. Rapid onset of action of levetiracetam in refractory epileptic patients. *Neurology* 2000; 7: A83 (abstract).

38

Oxcarbazepine

E. Faught and N. Limdi

Primary indications	Adjunctive or monotherapy in partial and secondarily generalized seizures
Usual preparations	Tablets: 150, 300, 600 mg
Usual dosages	Initial starting dose: 600 mg/day. Titration rate of 600 mg/week. The usual maintenance dose is 900–2400 mg/day
Dosage intervals	2 times/day
Significant drug interactions	Fewer than with carbamazepine
Serum level monitoring	Value not established
Target range	10–35 mg/L
Common/important side-effects	Somnolence, headache, dizziness, diplopia, ataxia, rash, hyponatraemia, weight gain, alopecia, nausea, gastrointestinal disturbance
Main advantages	Better tolerated and fewer interactions than with carbamazepine
Main disadvantages	25% cross-sensitivity with carbamazepine. Higher incidence of hyponatraemia than with carbamazepine
Mechanisms of action	Sodium-channel blockade. Also affects potassium conductance and modulates high-voltage activated calcium-channel activity
Oral bioavailability	>95%
Time to peak levels	4–6 h (MHD)
Metabolism and excretion	Hydroxylation then conjugation
Volume of distribution	0.3–0.8 L/kg
Elimination half-life	8–10 h (MHD)
Plasma clearance	–
Protein binding	38% (MHD)
Active metabolites	MHD
Comment	Close structural similarity to carbamazepine but better tolerated and with fewer drug interactions. Licensed in some countries only, and for use for partial and secondarily generalized seizures

(*Note*: this summary table was formulated by the lead editor.)

Carbamazepine (CBZ) and oxcarbazepine (OXC) were synthesized at the J.R. Giegy AG Laboratories in Basel, Switzerland, in 1963. CBZ was synthesized based on its structural similarity to chlorpromazine and imipramine. It was found to have anticonvulsant activ-

ity. Clinical trials of OXC as an antiepileptic agent did not begin until 1977.

Introduced in Denmark in 1990, OXC is now registered in 60 countries. It has been available in the EU since 1999 and in the USA since 2000. It is approved for use as monotherapy or add-on treatment of partial seizures with or without secondary generalization in most countries for adults and for children aged 4 years and above. Worldwide patient exposure to date is estimated at more than 600 000 patient-years based on a daily dose of 1200 mg.

Chemistry

OXC (10,11-dihydro-10-oxo-^{5}H-dibenz[b,f]azepine-5-carboxamide) is a 10-keto analogue of CBZ [1]. It is a highly lipophilic compound with very low water solubility. OXC is rapidly reduced to MHD (10,11-dihydro-10-hydroxy-^{5}H-dibenz[b,f]azepine-5-carboxamide) resulting in the formation of R-[–]-MHD [20%] and S-[+]-MHD [80%] enantiomers [4]. Both OXC and MHD are pharmacologically active [2–5], however, in humans OXC is almost completely metabolized to MHD, which is therefore primarily responsible for the pharmacological effect. MHD has greater water solubility, and an aqueous parenteral preparation was in development but is not currently available.

Mechanism of action and experimental studies

Preclinical *in vitro* studies

OXC and MHD modulate sodium, calcium and potassium channels [4–7]. Blockade of voltage-dependent sodium channels is implied by the decreased frequency of firing of sodium-dependent action potentials in central neurones in cell culture. MHD has been shown to produce a dose-dependent decrease in high-voltage activated calcium currents in isolated cortical pyramidal cells. In addition both MHD and OXC increase potassium conductance [1,4–7]. OXC may have other unidentified mechanisms of action [5].

Preclinical *in vivo* studies

CBZ, OXC and MHD exhibit similar activity in standard seizure models. In the maximal electroshock test, which identifies agents that prevent the spread of seizures, CBZ, phenytoin, OXC and MHD exhibited equal potency. This test predicts efficacy against partial onset and generalized tonic-clonic seizures [6]. CBZ, OXC and MHD lacked efficacy in seizure models used to identify agents that raise seizure threshold (strychnine, pentylenetetrazole and picrotoxin). These models predict efficacy against absence seizures [2,5].

Toxicology

The administration of OXC in intermediate and high doses to pregnant rats resulted in increased incidence of craniofacial, skeletal and cardiovascular malformations, decreased fetal body weights and fetal demise. In pregnant rabbits high doses of MHD increased the incidence of fetal mortality [1].

The increased incidence of structural and developmental toxicity observed in the offspring of animals treated with OXC and MHD, the lack of adequate well-controlled clinical studies of OXC in pregnant women and the structural similarity with CBZ suggest the teratogenic potential of OXC. OXC should be used during pregnancy only if the benefits outweigh the risk to the fetus (US Food and Drug Administration pregnancy category C) [1,8]. Additional data on the safety of OXC during pregnancy, as well as that of other new antiepileptic agents, are needed.

In some rodent species, increased incidences of hepatic and reproductive system tumours were observed among groups of animals given high doses of OXC for 2 years [1]. No carcinogenicity has been observed in humans.

Pharmacokinetics

Absorption

OXC is rapidly and completely absorbed (>95%) achieving peak concentrations within 1 h. It is rapidly reduced to MHD which reaches peak concentrations in 4–6 h [3–9]. The absorption of OXC from some older tablet formulations was slightly increased on administration with food (the C_{max} and AUC were increased by 23% and 16%, respectively, in older formulations) but this is not likely to be of clinical significance [10]. Therefore OXC can be administered with or without food [1].

Distribution

The volume of distribution for OXC is 0.3 L/kg and that of MHD is 0.7–0.8 L/kg, indicating distribution in total body water [2]. As a lipophilic substance, MHD is widely distributed in the body and has good blood–brain barrier permeability. Both OXC and MHD exhibit low protein binding (33–38% for MHD and 60–67% for OXC) [11]. There is no difference in binding between males and females and binding is independent of concentration within the therapeutically relevant range [2,11].

Therefore, OXC is unlikely to produce clinically significant protein binding interactions with other highly protein-bound drugs such as phenytoin and valproate.

Metabolism

OXC is rapidly eliminated from plasma, and therefore its half-life (1–2.5 h) is of no practical significance. The half-life of MHD is 9.3 ± 1.8 h. The elimination is monoexponential and follows linear kinetics in epileptic patients on OXC monotherapy or polytherapy. No autoinduction or accumulation occurred with OXC in healthy volunteers [12]. In contrast to CBZ, increases in OXC dosage during the first several weeks of therapy do not need to account for an autoinduction effect.

Although chemically similar, the metabolism of CBZ and OXC differs significantly (Fig. 38.1). CBZ is metabolized by cytochrome P450 oxidases with an epoxide intermediate [12]. OXC is rapidly and extensively metabolized by cytosolic (aldoketoreductases) enzymes in the liver to the active metabolite MHD (96%). A small fraction (4%) is oxidized to an inactive dihydroxy derivative. Aldoketoreductases are practically non-inducible enzymes. MHD is glucuronidated by microsomal uridine diphosphoglucuronyltransferases (UGTs). Mild to moderate hepatic dysfunction did not alter the pharmacokinetics of OXC or MHD. The pharmacokinetics of MHD have not been evaluated in severe hepatic dysfunction [9,12].

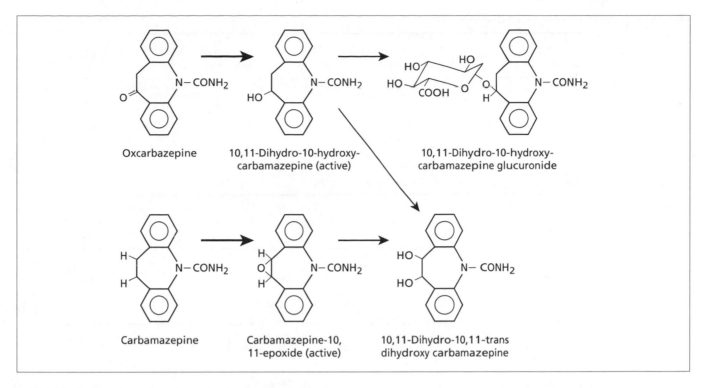

Fig. 38.1 Metabolism of oxcarbazepine and carbamazepine [9,12].

Elimination

The major route for OXC elimination is renal with most of the dose accounted for by MHD-glucuronide (51%) and unchanged MHD (28%). The dihydroxy derivative accounts for 13% of the dose excreted in the urine, with <1% of the drug excreted as minor conjugates of OXC and MHD [9].

The elimination of MHD is not significantly affected in patients with mild to moderate renal dysfunction. However patients with creatinine clearances of < 30 mL/min/1.73 m^2 exhibit a two-fold increase in the AUC, significant increases in elimination half-life and plasma concentrations of MHD [13,14].

Plasma concentrations

Due to rapid metabolic reduction, concentrations of OXC are negligible. Steady-state concentrations of MHD are reached in 2–3 days of twice daily dosing. At steady state, concentrations of MHD are about nine-fold higher than plasma concentrations of OXC. The dose–concentration relationship is linear across a wide dose range (300–2400 mg/day). The following relationship between MHD concentration and dose of OXC has been described, over the range 300–2700 mg/day [15]:

MHD mg/L $= 0.93 \times$ OXC dose mg/kg

Steady-state concentrations, adjusted for body weight, in children and adolescents were comparable to those in adults. However AUCs for MHD were 30% lower in children under 8 years of age. Higher doses may be required in children under the age of 8 years [1]. AUC values for MHD were significantly higher in elderly pa-

tients (> 60 years of age). This is probably explained by age-related decreases in creatinine clearance [13,16].

Drug interactions

In vitro studies indicate that both OXC and MHD are competitive inhibitors of cytochrome P450 (CYP) 2C19. High doses of OXC may produce clinically significant inhibition of CYP2C19, with consequent elevations of serum concentrations of substrates such as phenobarbital and phenytoin [1,17].

Interactions that occurred in controlled clinical trials are listed in Table 38.1. The addition of OXC to existing antiepileptic drug (AED) regimens produced increases in phenytoin, phenobarbital and CBZ-epoxide concentrations and a decrease in CBZ concentrations. When enzyme-inducing AEDs were added to OXC, plasma MHD concentrations decreased by 29–40%, an effect which may require an increase in OXC dose. Valproic acid has no significant interactions with OXC [18].

OXC induces CYP3A4 and 3A5 [19]. Breakthrough bleeding and loss of contraceptive efficacy was seen when OXC was added to a stable regimen of oral contraceptives due to increased metabolism of ethinyloestradiol [19]. Coadministration of OXC with felodipine resulted in a 28% decrease in systemic bioavailability of felodipine [20]. The interaction between verapamil and OXC is clinically insignificant [21]. OXC does not appear to have clinically significant interactions with warfarin [22], cimetidine [23] or erythromycin [24].

Because of their differing effects on the cytochrome P450 enzyme systems, substitution of OXC for CBZ may result in an increase in concentration of some concurrent drugs with subsequent dose-

Table 38.1 Summary of AED drug interactions with OXC

Drug	Influence of OXC on AED concentration	Influence of AEDs on MHD concentration
Phenytoin	0–40% increase	29–35% decrease
Phenobarbital	14–15% increase	30–31% decrease
Valproic acid	No influence	0–18% decrease
Carbamazepine	0–22% decrease	40% decrease
Carbamazepine-epoxide	30% increase	Not studied
Clobazam	Not studied	No influence
Felbamate	Not studied	No influence

Table 38.2 Randomized clinical trials comparing OXC to CBZ

Reference	No./type patients and study type	Mean dose per day OXC	Mean dose per day CBZ	Efficacy result OXC	Efficacy result CBZ	% dropouts, adverse events OXC	% dropouts, adverse events CBZ
[25] (adults)	48 inpatients on CBZ plus 1–3 drugs, crossover	2628 mg	1302 mg	OXC ↓ seizures 9% (NS)		None	None
[26] (adults)	40, unsatisfactory phenytoin treatment, conversion to OXC or CBZ, parallel	13.1 mg/kg	8.3 mg/kg	No difference		None	None
[27] (adults)	194 newly diagnosed PS or GTC, parallel (P=0.04)	1040 mg	684 mg	52% vs. 60% seizure-free (NS)		14%	25%

GTC, generalized tonic-clonic (seizures); NS, not significant; PS, partial onset seizures.

related toxicity. Therefore such a switch should be carefully monitored [17].

Efficacy

The efficacy of OXC has been evaluated in 12 randomized, controlled clinical trials as well as in several large open-label surveys. In contrast to most new AEDs, monotherapy trials of OXC preceded adjunctive therapy trials. From the eight controlled trials of monotherapy, we have available more data on OXC efficacy as a single agent than on any of the other new AEDs.

Six randomized controlled trials directly compared OXC to CBZ [25–27], phenytoin [28,29] and valproate [30]. Four other randomized monotherapy trials utilized non-equivalent controls: placebo in two [31,32] and low-dose OXC in two [33,34]. Three randomized controlled trials in which OXC was added to existing therapy in refractory patients included one enrolling patients aged 15–65 years [35] and one enrolling children aged 3–17 years [36].

All of these trials were designed to evaluate patients with partial onset seizures with or without secondary generalization, and some included patients with primary generalized onset tonic-clonic seizures. OXC is not indicated for absence, myoclonic and other types of generalized seizures other than tonic-clonic seizures. It may exacerbate the non-convulsive generalized seizure types, as one might expect from its similarity to CBZ [37].

Efficacy in comparison to CBZ

Three controlled trials compared OXC to CBZ (Table 38.2). In a randomized, double-blind cross-over study, 48 patients taking CBZ along with other drugs had their CBZ replaced by OXC [25]. Patients took OXC and CBZ for 12 weeks each. There was a significant reduction of tonic-clonic and tonic seizures on OXC compared to CBZ; there was no difference in other seizure types including complex partial seizures. However, interpretation of this study is complicated by the increases in serum concentrations of concomitant AEDs during the OXC intervals, due to changes in hepatic enzyme induction, which could have produced a more favourable result for OXC. Patients taking phenytoin monotherapy were converted to either OXC or CBZ in another double-blind trial; no efficacy differences were discovered [26]. The most convincing evidence for equipotency comes from a large trial enrolling 194 patients with newly diagnosed epilepsy [27]. Patients with previously untreated primary generalized tonic-clonic seizures or partial seizures with or without secondary generalization were enrolled and begun on either OXC 300 mg/day or CBZ 200 mg/day with dosages adjusted during a 4- to 8-week titration period. At the end of the 12-week maintenance phase, CBZ patients were taking a mean dose of 685 mg/day and OXC patients 1040 mg/day. Fifty-two per cent of OXC patients and 60% of CBZ patients were seizure free during this year-long study, not a significant difference.

In addition to these direct comparative trials, OXC was substituted for CBZ in some of the monotherapy trials as well as in reported open-label clinical experience. Data from these trials are not as compelling for demonstrating equal or superior efficacy for OXC because they involved sequential rather than parallel observations. Nevertheless, a substantial number of patients had fewer seizures when converted from CBZ to OXC. Although not the primary end point of one monotherapy trial [33], a 50% reduction in seizures occurred in 42% of patients randomized to 2400 mg/day of OXC, and 54% of these patients had been taking CBZ as one of their baseline drugs. This study did not report a comparison of OXC efficacy between those switched from CBZ-containing regimens and those switched from non-CBZ regimens. In another monotherapy trial, OXC 2400 mg/day was successfully substituted for CBZ in many patients [34]. Among 89 patients treated on a named-patient basis in the Netherlands [38] in whom CBZ was converted to OXC because of lack of efficacy, 50% were judged to be improved in terms of seizure control. It should be pointed out that there are no reports of the results of converting patients from OXC to CBZ.

In summary, the evidence suggests that OXC is approximately equally effective to CBZ in head-to-head comparisons. It appears to be more effective in certain patients, but the converse may or may not be true.

Efficacy in comparison to other drugs

In patients with newly diagnosed epilepsy, the efficacy of OXC is equivalent to that of phenytoin and valproate (Table 38.3). Fifty-nine per cent of patients with a new diagnosis of partial seizures with or without secondarily generalized seizures, or generalized tonic-clonic seizures without partial onset, were seizure free while taking OXC during a 48-month maintenance treatment period, compared to 58% receiving phenytoin [28]. The mean daily dose at the start of the maintenance period was 1028 mg for OXC and 313 mg for phenytoin (PHT). A similar result emerged from a study of 193 children aged 5–18 years, who were randomized to OXC or PHT after a new diagnosis of epilepsy [29]. Sixty per cent of each group was seizure free during the maintenance period. A single study comparing OXC to VPA enrolled 249 patients between the

ages of 15 and 65 years, with the same duration and similar procedures as the phenytoin comparisons [30]. The seizure-free rates were 57% for OXC and 54% for valproate, not significantly different. The median daily maintenance dose was 900 mg for each drug.

Monotherapy in refractory patients

The studies demonstrating monotherapy efficacy in newly diagnosed patients [27–30] led to the design of studies to evaluate monotherapy efficacy in patients with refractory partial onset seizures. These studies also served the purpose of registration for monotherapy use in the USA, where non-equivalent controls are required in order to eliminate the logical possibility that both comparative treatments are equally ineffective, rather than equally effective, in a particular study population.

The first of these was an inpatient trial [31] in which patients who had been completely removed from therapy for presurgical EEG and video monitoring were randomized to resume therapy with either OXC 2400 mg/day or placebo while remaining under close observation in the hospital. Patients exited the trial after completing 10 days of treatment, or after experiencing four partial seizures, two new onset secondarily generalized seizures, serial seizures or status epilepticus or if seizure severity or frequency became unsafe in the judgment of the investigator. Fifty-one patients were randomized to each arm, of whom 47% in the OXC arm and 84% in the placebo arm met one of the exit criteria. This study demonstrated that OXC has monotherapy efficacy in patients with frequent partial onset seizures. It also showed that, when necessary, OXC can be started quickly—1500 mg on the first day, 2400 mg on subsequent days—safely, and with acceptable tolerability. This study was not designed to compare OXC efficacy to the patient's previous treatment, but it is notable that one-third of the OXC patients were seizure free during the treatment period.

Rapid inpatient conversion of therapy is a relatively uncommon event in clinical practice; much more common is gradual outpatient conversion. Two studies have used this procedure to assess OXC monotherapy for refractory partial onset seizures [33,34]. Outpatients aged 12 years or older were enrolled in the first study [33] and converted from one or two baseline AEDs over a titration period of 14 days to either monotherapy with OXC 300 mg/day or 2400

Table 38.3 Randomized clinical trials comparing OXC to phenytoin or valproate

Reference	No./type patients and study type	Mean dose (mg)		Efficacy result (seizure-free %)		% dropouts, adverse events	
[28] (adults)	287 newly diagnosed PS or GTC, parallel	1028 OXC	313 Phenytoin	59 OXC	58 Phenytoin (NS)	3 OXC	11 Phenytoin (P=0.002)
[29] (children)	193 children 5–18 y newly diagnosed PS or GTC, parallel	672 (18.8 mg/kg) OXC	226 (5.8 mg/kg) Phenytoin	61 OXC	60 Phenytoin (NS)	2.5 OXC	18 Phenytoin (P=0.002)
[30] (adults)	249 newly diagnosed PS or GTC, parallel	1053 OXC	1146 Valproate	57 OXC	54 Phenytoin (NS)	12 OXC	8 Valproate (NS)

GTC, generalized tonic-clonic (seizures); NS, not significant; PS, partial onset seizures.

mg/day. Patients exited if there was a two-fold increase in partial seizure frequency over baseline during any 2-day or 28-day period, if a single tonic-clonic seizure occurred if none had occurred in the previous 6 months, or, in the judgment of the investigator, if there was a prolongation or worsening of generalized seizures necessitating a change in treatment. During the 112-day maintenance period, 41% of the high-dose group met one of the exit criteria compared to 93% of the low-dose group. It is interesting to note that most of the patients who did not get worse (that is, who did not meet one of the exit criteria) got better. Forty-two per cent of the 2400 mg/day patients had at least a 50% reduction in seizures compared to their previous baseline on other drugs. The second study used a very similar design, but all patients were initially on CBZ monotherapy before conversion to OXC 300 or 2400 mg/day as monotherapy [34]. Fifty-nine per cent of the OXC 2400 mg/day group and 89% of the OXC 300 mg/day group met one of the exit criteria. These studies conclusively demonstrate that OXC reduces the frequency of partial onset seizures as monotherapy. They do not, however, provide much confidence that it was superior in these groups of patients to previously used therapies, especially CBZ.

A true placebo control was used in another study of untreated patients with recent onset seizures, who received a placebo or 1200 mg OXC per day during the 90-day double-blind treatment phase [32]. The primary end point was the median time to the first seizure, which was 11.7 days in the OXC group and 3.2 days in the placebo group. Unlike many studies of new onset patients, this study incorporated a sufficiently long baseline phase—56 days—to derive some data on the absolute reduction produced by therapy. There was an 89% reduction in seizure frequency for each 28 days on OXC and a 37% reduction for placebo. The placebo reduction probably represents a combination of regression to the mean and intangibles related to medical care and close attention. Results of this study support the conclusions of the earlier studies in which OXC was directly compared with an active control drug in new onset patients because they provide natural history data on the course of newly diagnosed but untreated epilepsy.

Adjunctive therapy

There are two randomized controlled trials in which OXC or placebo was added to existing therapy for patients with inadequately controlled partial onset seizures (Table 38.4). A dose-ranging trial enrolled 694 patients aged 15–65 years in a parallel comparison of placebo and three doses of OXC [35]. An impressive dose–response association was generated, with reductions of 8%, 26%, 40% and 50% for placebo, 600, 1200 and 2400/day OXC, respectively. Among the 75% of patients who were taking CBZ as one of their baseline drugs, the percentage reductions in seizure frequency when OXC was added were virtually identical to the entire study group. Although this result does not answer the question of whether the addition of OXC to CBZ produces a qualitatively different effect on seizure frequency or merely an additive one—that is, whether the same effect could have been achieved by simply adding more CBZ—it does suggest that even patients on CBZ may derive some benefit from the addition of OXC. The 22% seizure-free rate among patients in the 2400 mg/day OXC group is quite high for studies of adjunctive therapy in refractory patients, but this may be partly because the duration of treatment with 2400 mg was relatively short for some patients who dropped out early due to adverse effects.

Children aged 3–17 years with inadequately controlled partial onset seizures taking one or two baseline drugs were enrolled in a study in which they were assigned to OXC 30–46 mg/kg/day or to placebo for a 112-day double-blind treatment phase, after a 56-day baseline [36]. The primary end point was percentage change in seizure frequency from baseline for 28 days, which was 35% for OXC and 9% for placebo, a highly significant difference. Baseline therapies included CBZ in about half of the patients.

In an open-label study, 53 children under the age of 7 years were treated with OXC [37]. Forty-three had failed other drugs, including 30 who had failed CBZ. Twenty-seven per cent became seizure-free and an additional 36% had at least a 50% reduction in seizure frequency. Side-effects led to discontinuation in 17%.

Open-label efficacy and tolerance

Of 260 patients treated at a single epilepsy centre on a named-patient basis, 161 remained on treatment with OXC for at least 3 months and for a mean of 43 months [38]. Seventy-three patients did not benefit sufficiently in terms of seizure control to continue OXC. Among 947 patients treated in Denmark between 1981 and 1990, 32–48% were judged to have had a decrease in seizure frequency after being changed to OXC treatment, with 1–10% having an increase in seizure frequency [39]. It is difficult to measure development of tolerance to antiepileptic therapy, but these large experiences suggest that tolerance to OXC efficacy is not a greater problem than with other standard drugs.

Table 38.4 Randomized clinical trials of OXC adjunctive therapy

Reference	No./type patients and study type	% Reduction in seizure frequency				% dropouts, adverse effects			
[35] (adults)	694, refractory partial onset, parallel	Placebo 8	600 mg 26	1200 mg 40	2400 mg 50	Placebo 9	600 mg 12	1200 mg 36	2400 mg 67
		($P=0.001$, all doses vs. placebo)							
[36] (children)	267 children, 3–17 y, refractory partial onset, parallel	Placebo 9	OXC 30–46 mg/kg/day 35 ($P=0.0001$)			Placebo 3	OXC 10		
		(median % change in seizure frequency)							

Side-effects

Central nervous system effects

The most common side-effects seen early in treatment and those which most often lead to OXC discontinuation affect the central nervous system (Table 38.5). Side-effect rates are best assessed in comparison to placebo in monotherapy studies. In these studies, the most common central nervous system effects were headache, somnolence and dizziness [1]. Ataxia and diplopia were remarkably uncommon with OXC monotherapy, though present significantly more often than placebo in adjunctive therapy trials, as was fatigue. These adverse effects closely resemble those of CBZ. Although diplopia was not commonly seen in OXC monotherapy trials, dosages were relatively low in these studies and clinical experience indicates that diplopia and ataxia can occur with OXC as dose-limiting side-effects at higher dosages.

In the OXC monotherapy trials, adverse effects judged as 'severe' by the investigators did not differ in incidence between placebo, valproate, phenytoin and OXC, ranging from 5.8% to 8.2% [27–30]. In these direct comparative trials, discontinuation rates were significantly lower for OXC in comparison to CBZ (14% vs. 26%) and in comparison to PHT. These conclusions do not change when all discontinuations for whatever reason are evaluated between OXC and the other drugs. Discontinuation rates are, as expected, higher in adjunctive therapy trials. They are also proportional to the dose of OXC added. Among adults, 9% of patients taking placebo and concomitant medications stopped treatment because of adverse effects, in comparison to 12%, 36% and 67% for patients taking OXC 600, 1200 and 1800–2400 mg/day, respectively [35]. Since patients in that study reached the target dosages within 2 weeks, it may be expected that slower titration would reduce these dropout rates substantially. However, a similar 14-day dose titration period in the study of OXC adjunctive therapy in children [36] resulted in only a 10% dropout rate in the OXC treatment group and 3% in the placebo group.

Gastrointestinal effects

Nausea occurred in 13% of patients taking OXC in monotherapy comparison trials, but this did not differ from the 12% rate for placebo. A substantial number of patients taking adjunctive thera-py, however, complained of nausea, 22.5% for all OXC doses compared to 8.1% for placebo [35]. Abdominal pain occurred in 10% taking OXC in this study, 4.6% taking placebo. Nausea was the most common reason for dropouts among children in the adjunctive therapy study [36].

Rash

OXC is less likely to cause skin rash than CBZ. 'Allergy' resulted in withdrawal of medication in 10% of OXC-treated and 16% of CBZ-treated patients in a comparative study [27]. Data from all clinical trials suggest that there is a 3% incidence of rash with OXC compared to 7% with CBZ [1]. Cross-reactivity with CBZ occurs: 25.5% of patients who had a history of skin rashes on CBZ also developed a rash when they were converted to OXC in one study [40]. To date, OXC has not been implicated in any case of Stevens–Johnson syndrome or toxic epidermal necrolysis.

Hyponatraemia

The only side-effect of OXC which is clearly more common than with CBZ is hyponatraemia. Although almost always asymptomatic, it could theoretically produce an increase in seizures and other clinical effects with levels below 125 mmol/L. Sachdeo et al. [41] reviewed the Novartis clinical safety database of 2026 OXC patients and found an incidence of serum sodiums <135 mmol/L of 24.5% and <125 mmol/L of 3%. There was a definite increase in this effect with age: 0.2% in children, 3.6% in adults aged 17–64 years and 7.3% in those 65 years or older. This analysis did not reveal a dose relationship, however, patients with pre-existing renal conditions associated with low sodium and patients treated concomitantly with sodium-lowering drugs (e.g. diuretics) may have a higher risk of developing hyponatraemia. The decrease in sodium occurred in nearly all patients by 3 months after initiation of therapy. The pathogenesis of the hyponatraemia for either CBZ or OXC is unclear, but some patients may be susceptible to its development because of their inability to generate an appropriate aldosterone response [42]. It was recently shown that the hyponatraemia due to OXC was not related to altered antidiuretic hormone (ADH) levels but might be caused by an increased sensitivity to ADH [43].

Other systems

No significant adverse effects on the liver, kidneys, blood, pancreas or other organs have been detected thus far [18]. Since most dangerous adverse effects of drugs occur early in treatment, the total number of patients exposed to a drug is more relevant than patient-years of exposure. For OXC, this figure is well over the 100 000 patient exposures usually considered a benchmark for the detection of dangerous and fatal effects on most organs.

Overdose

Six unsuccessful suicide attempts have occurred with OXC [1], with the maximum dose taken being 24 000 mg [43]. Symptoms with overdose are an exaggeration of the common central nervous system and gastrointestinal side-effects.

Table 38.5 Percentage of patients experiencing the five most common OXC central nervous system side-effects

Side-effect	Initial monotherapy trials		Adjunctive trials[a]	
	OXC ($n=440$)	Placebo ($n=66$)	OXC ($n=705$)	Placebo ($n=302$)
Headache	37	12	26	21
Somnolence	22	6	26	12
Dizziness	20	4	30	11
Ataxia	2	0	17	5
Diplopia	0.5	0	24	3

[a] Combined paediatric [36] and adults [35] data

Cognitive effects

Except for early, dose-initiation central nervous system side-effects such as somnolence, it is not clear that OXC has any significant effects on cognition. Small studies have reported no difference in cognitive function tests between OXC and phenytoin [44], and before and 4 months after initiation of OXC [45]. Further comparative studies with placebo, CBZ—especially timed-release formulations—and other drugs are needed.

Special populations

No unexpected side-effects or markedly different rates of side-effects occurred in the studies involving children [18,29] and in one study of patients with intellectual disability [46]. Few data are available on the elderly, except for the observation that hyponatraemia is more common [41].

Clinical therapeutics

OXC is an effective drug for the treatment of partial onset seizures and for primary or secondarily generalized tonic-clonic seizures when used as either monotherapy or adjunctive therapy. Its efficacy in the monotherapy of newly diagnosed patients is comparable to that of CBZ, phenytoin and valproate, but it is better tolerated than CBZ and phenytoin. Timed-release formulations of CBZ (extended-release CBZ) result in better tolerability than the immediate-release formulations, but there are no studies comparing OXC and timed-release CBZ. Its efficacy as adjunctive therapy for refractory partial onset seizures appears to be comparable to that of the more potent of the new AEDs tested in this fashion, although comparisons between different clinical trials cannot be considered scientifically sound (see Chapter 26). OXC tolerability as an adjunctive drug is good for children treated with 30–46 mg/day [36] and is good for adults treated with 600 mg/day, but tolerability diminishes for adults treated with 1200–2400 mg/day [35]. Since CBZ and OXC side-effects are often additive, the tolerability of OXC as an adjunct to CBZ is likely to be much better in clinical practice if concomitant CBZ dosage is reduced as OXC is added. Additional studies exploring the tolerability of OXC as adjunctive therapy with slower initial titration rates would be useful.

Dose initiation

The manufacturer recommends beginning OXC at 600 mg/day in two divided doses with weekly increases of 600 mg/day at weekly intervals to a recommended daily dose of 1200 mg [1]. Clinical experience suggests, however, that for most outpatients a slower titration schedule is better tolerated. An advisory board of UK physicians has recommended OXC monotherapy initiation at 300 mg/day, beginning with 150 mg at bedtime on the first day and then 150 mg twice daily thereafter [47]. Other authorities also suggest beginning with lower doses, such as 300 mg/day in two divided doses [18] or even 150 mg/day with increases of 150 mg/day every 2 days [48].

A simple schedule which can be used for most adults for monotherapy initiation, adjunctive therapy or substitution for CBZ is initiation of OXC 300 mg at bedtime for 1 week, with weekly increases of 300 mg/day, adhering to a twice-daily schedule.

It appears that the tolerability of rapid initiation of OXC is better than rapid initiation of CBZ. Attempts to orally load CBZ usually fail because of unacceptable initial side-effects. There were surprisingly few dropouts because of intolerance in the monotherapy conversion studies of OXC in which the dose reached 2400 mg in 2 weeks in outpatients [32–34], and in the inpatient trial in which 2400 mg was reached on the second day of treatment [31]. In the inpatient trial, only three of 51 OXC patients stopped treatment. Although 75% had a variety of central nervous system and gastrointestinal side-effects, 91% of these were rated as mild to moderate. Outpatients needing rapid attainment of an effective dose can be started at 600 mg/day in two divided doses, and inpatients 900–1200 mg/day in two or three divided doses.

Conversion from CBZ

Appropriate patients for conversion from CBZ to OXC therapy include those who have dose-limiting side-effects on CBZ or problems with CBZ-induced drug interactions. A good example is the patient taking CBZ and valproate, in whom adequate valproate levels cannot be achieved. Overnight conversion is not usually a problem for patients taking CBZ doses of 800 mg/day or less [47], but a more gradual conversion causes fewer problems for patients on higher doses of CBZ. Although the literature suggests a conversion ratio of 1:1.5 between CBZ and OXC, this dose of OXC often produces dose-related adverse effects. A lower ratio, especially if the conversion is from the timed-release preparations of CBZ, of 1:1 or 1:1.25, is commonly better tolerated. As with any conversion between AEDs, the clinician will need to decide whether the possibility of increased side-effects or the possibility of increased seizures is more to be avoided in a particular patient.

For children aged 4–16 years, the recommended starting dose is 8–10 mg/kg/day [1], but 4–5 mg/kg/day, not over 300 mg/day, is better tolerated [18]. Weekly increases of about 5 mg/kg/day are appropriate.

In patients with CBZ allergic reactions, rapid conversion to another drug is desirable as seizures are likely to occur as CBZ is removed. However, with the many choices now available, conversion to OXC may not be the best course of action because of the 25–30% cross-reactivity rate [1]. Patients being started on OXC should be questioned about any prior reactions to CBZ.

Maintenance treatment and serum levels

For adults with new onset epilepsy, OXC daily dosages of 900–1200 mg/day have been shown to be effective and well tolerated [27,28,30]. A reasonable target dose for children based on the childhood new onset monotherapy study [29] is 20 mg/kg/day. If no significant clinical response has been achieved, even without clinical toxicity, at 2400 mg/day in adults and 45 mg/kg/day in children, then further increases are unlikely to be productive. Measurement of the major metabolite of OXC (MHD) may be useful in determining compliance and in assessing the effects of concomitant medications which may lower serum levels. In a group of 214 patients treated to a clinically determined dose, the mean plasma level of

MHD was 15.3 µg/mL, but with a wide individual variation between patients [49]. Routine monitoring of serum levels is therefore not recommended.

Monitoring of serum sodium

Serum sodium concentrations of patients susceptible to hyponatraemia should be measured at baseline and a few times early in therapy, perhaps after 1, 2 and 6 months. These patients include the elderly, those with baseline sodium levels below 135 mmol/L, and those taking medications such as diuretics or non-steroidal anti-inflammatory drugs, which can lower serum sodium. Patients taking OXC who are started on one of these drugs, who experience prolonged vomiting or diarrhoea, or who have excessive free water intake for any reason, should also be monitored. There is no consensus about the need for monitoring other patients. The manufacturer states that measurement of serum sodium levels should be considered, particularly for patients taking medications known to decrease sodium levels (e.g. drugs associated with inappropriate ADH secretion) or symptoms possibly indicating hyponatraemia develop, such as nausea, malaise, headache, lethargy, confusion or obtundation [1]. It is not unreasonable to obtain a baseline serum sodium and another after 1–2 months of therapy in all patients.

Dosing interval

Although the elimination half-life of OXC and its monohydroxy metabolite (MHD) would suggest that three times daily dosing would be optimal, most of the clinical trials utilized twice daily dosing. No difference in efficacy was found in a study comparing twice daily with three times daily dosing [50]. Even though there was no difference in adverse event percentages by dosing interval in this study, an occasional patient may tolerate three daily doses better than two because of peak-dose central nervous system side-effects.

Conclusions

OXC is a good choice for initial monotherapy of partial onset seizures in adults and in children. It has efficacy equivalent to other first-line AEDs and tolerability is as good or better than older drugs. Some patients who do not tolerate maximal doses of CBZ will tolerate OXC. However, in many countries it is much more expensive than CBZ and superior efficacy to CBZ has not been demonstrated. Furthermore, as timed-release CBZ is better tolerated than the immediate-release (conventional) formulations, comparative tolerability studies of OXC and timed-release CBZ would be of interest.

OXC has clear advantages over CBZ in polytherapy situations involving valproate, phenytoin, phenobarbital, felbamate and other drugs affecting or affected by CBZ. If no reasonable alternative exists, OXC can be substituted in patients developing CBZ rashes, with the understanding that 25–30% of these patients may also develop a rash with OXC and in this situation less allergenic drugs may be preferred.

Adverse effects are similar to those of most other AEDs with the exception of an increased incidence of hyponatraemia, usually of no clinical significance. Serious adverse effects, especially those affecting the blood, liver or skin, so far have been encouragingly absent from OXC therapy. A reduced incidence of adverse effects as well as fewer drug interactions, in comparison to CBZ, may be related to the absence of the CBZ epoxide metabolite in the OXC metabolic pathway. Although this advantage may extend to reduced teratogenicity, this has not yet been demonstrated and thus it is not known whether OXC is safer for pregnancy than older drugs.

References

1 Novartis Pharmaceuticals Corporation. *Trileptal (oxcarbazepine) package insert.* East Hanover, NJ: 2000. Novartis Pharma AG (oxcarbazepine) Summary of Product characteristics (SPC). Basel: Novartis Pharmaceuticals Corporation, 30 November 1999.

2 Dam M, Ostergaard LH. Other antiepileptic drugs: oxcarbazepine. In: Levy RH, Matson RH, Meldrum BS, eds. *Antiepileptic Drugs*, 4th edn. New York: Raven Press, 1995: 987–95.

3 Faigle JW, Menge GP. Pharmacokinetics and metabolic features of oxcarbazepine and their clinical significance: comparison with carbamazepine. *Int Clin Psychopharmacol* 1990; 5 (Suppl. 1): 73–82.

4 Wamil AW, Portet C, Jensen PK *et al.* Oxcarbazepine and its mono-hydroxy derivative limit action potential firing by mouse central neurons in cell culture. *Epilepsia* 1991; 32 (Suppl. 3): S60–S65.

5 McLean MJ, Schmutz M, Wamil AW *et al.* Oxcarbazepine: mechanisms of action. *Epilepsia* 1994; 35 (Suppl. 3): S5–S9.

6 Schmutz M, Brugger F, Gentsch C *et al.* Oxcarbazepine: preclinical anticonvulsant profile and putative mechanisms of action. *Epilepsia* 1993; 35 (Suppl. 3): S47–S50.

7 Stefani A, Pisani A, Demurtas M *et al.* Action of GP 47779, the active metabolite of oxcarbazepine, on the corticostriatal system. II. Modulation of high voltage activated calcium currents. *Epilepsia* 1995; 36: 997–1002.

8 Schachter SC. Oxcarbazepine: current status and clinical applications. *Expert Opin Investig Drugs* 1999; 8: 1–10.

9 Schutz H, Feldmann KF, Faigle JW. The metabolism of oxcarbazepine in man. *Xenobiotica* 1986; 16(8): 769–78.

10 Degen PH, Flesch G, Cardot JM *et al.* The influence of food on the disposition of the antiepileptic oxcarbazepine and its major metabolites in healthy volunteers. *Biopharm Drug Dispos* 1994; 15: 519–26.

11 Pastalos PN, Elyas AA, Zakrzewska JM. Protein binding of oxcarbazepine and its primary active metabolite, 10-hydroxy carbazepine in patients with trigeminal neuralgia. *Eur J Clin Pharmacol* 1990; 39: 413–15.

12 Dickinson RG, Hooper WD, Dunstan PR *et al.* First dose and steady-state pharmacokinetics of oxcarbazepine and its 10-hydroxy metabolite. *Eur J Clin Pharmacol* 1989; 37: 69–74.

13 Augusteijn R, van Parys JAP. Oxcarbazepine (Trileptal, OXC) drug concentration relationship in patients with epilepsy. *Acta Neurol Scand* 1990; 82 (Suppl. 133): 37.

14 Battino D, Estienne M, Avanzini G. Clinical pharmacokinetics of antiepileptic drugs in pediatric patients. II. Phenytoin, carbamazepine, sulthiame, lamotrigine, vigabatrin, oxcarbazepine, felbamate. *Clin Pharmacokinet* 1995; 29: 341–69.

15 Van Heiningen P, Malcolm D, Oosterhuis B *et al.* The influence of age on the pharmacokinetics of the antiepileptic agent oxcarbazepine. *Clin Pharmacol Ther* 1991; 50: 410–19.

16 Rouan MC, Lecaillon JB, Godbillon J *et al.* The effect of renal impairment on the pharmacokinetics of oxcarbazepine and its metabolites. *Eur J Clin Pharmacol* 1994; 47: 161–7.

17 Cloyd JC, Remmel RP. Antiepileptic drug pharmacokinetics and interactions: impact on the treatment of epilepsy. *Pharmacotherapy* 2000; 20 (8 pt 2): S139–S151.

18 Glauser TA. Oxcarbazepine in the treatment of epilepsy. *Pharmacotherapy* 2001; 21: 904–19.

19 Sonnen AE. Oxcarbazepine in the treatment of epilepsy. *Pharmacotherapy* 1990; 82 (Suppl. 133): S34–S37.

20 Zaccara G, Gangemi PF, Bendoni L *et al.* Influence of single and repeated doses of oxcarbazepine on the pharmacokinetic profile of felodipine. *Ther Drug Monit* 1993; 15: 39–42.

21 Kramer G, Tettenborn B, Closterskov JP *et al.* Oxcarbazepine–verapamil

drug interaction in healthy volunteers. *Epilepsia* 1991; 30 (Suppl. 1): S70–S71.

22 Kramer G, Tettenborn P, Menge GP *et al*. Oxcarbazepine does not affect the anticoagulant activity of warfarin. *Epilepsia* 1992; 33(6): 1145–8.

23 Keranen T, Jolkkonen J, Klosterskov JP *et al*. Oxcarbazepine does not interact with cimetidine in healthy volunteers. *Acta Neurol Scand* 1992; 85: 239–42.

24 Keranen T, Jolkkonen J, Jensen PK *et al*. Absence of interaction between oxcarbazepine and erythromycin. *Acta Neurol Scand* 1992; 86: 120–3.

25 Houtkooper MA, Lammertsma A, Meyer JW *et al*. Oxcarbazepine (GP 47.680): a possible alternative to carbamazepine? *Epilepsia* 1987; 28: 693–8.

26 Reinikainen KJ, Keranen T, Halonen T *et al*. Comparison of oxcarbazepine and carbamazepine: a double-blind study. *Epilepsy Res* 1987; 1: 284–9.

27 Dam M, Ekberg R, Loyning Y, Waltimo O, Jacobsen K. A double-blind study comparing oxcarbazepine and carbamazepine in patients with newly diagnosed, previously untreated epilepsy. *Epilepsy Res* 1989; 3: 70–6.

28 Bill PA, Vigonius U, Pohlmann H *et al*. A double-blind controlled clinical trial of oxcarbazepine versus phenytoin in adults with previously untreated epilepsy. *Epilepsy Res* 1997; 27: 195–204.

29 Guerreiro MM, Vigonius U, Pohlmann H *et al*. A double-blind controlled clinical trial of oxcarbazepine versus phenytoin in children and adolescents with epilepsy. *Epilepsy Res* 1997; 27: 205–13.

30 Christe W, Kramer G, Vigonius U *et al*. A double-blind controlled clinical trial: oxcarbazepine versus sodium valproate in adults with newly diagnosed epilepsy. *Epilepsy Res* 1997; 26: 451–60.

31 Schachter SC, Vazquez B, Fisher RS *et al*. Oxcarbazepine: double-blind randomized, placebo-controlled, monotherapy trial for partial seizures. *Neurology* 1999; 52: 732–7.

32 Sachdeo R, Edwards K, Hasegawa H *et al*. Safety and efficacy of 1200 mg/day of oxcarbazepine monotherapy versus placebo in untreated patients with partial-onset seizures (abstr). *Epilepsia* 2000; 41: 113.

33 Beydoun A, Sachdeo RC, Rosenfeld WE *et al*. Oxcarbazepine monotherapy for partial onset seizures: a multicenter, double-blind, clinical trial. *Neurology* 2000; 54: 2245–51.

34 Sachdeo RC, Beydoun A, Schachter SC *et al*. Oxcarbazepine (Trileptal) as monotherapy in patients with partial seizures. *Neurology* 2001; 57: 864–70.

35 Barcs G, Walker EB, Elger CE *et al*. Oxcarbazepine placebo-controlled, dose-ranging trial in refractory partial epilepsy. *Epilepsia* 2000; 41: 1597–607.

36 Glauser TA, Nigro M, Sachdeo R *et al*. Adjunctive therapy with oxcarbazepine in children with partial seizures. *Neurology* 2000; 54: 2237–44.

37 Gaily E, Granstrom M-J, Liukkonen E. Oxcarbazepine in the treatment of early childhood epilepsy. *J Child Neurol* 1997; 12: 496–8.

38 Van Parys JAP, Meinardi H. Survey of 260 epileptic patients treated with oxcarbazepine (Trileptal) on named-patient basis. *Epilepsy Res* 1994; 19: 79–85.

39 Friis ML, Kristensen O, Boas J *et al*. Therapeutic experiences with 947 epileptic out-patients in oxcarbazepine treatment. *Acta Neurol Scand* 1993; 87: 224–7.

40 Dam M, Jacobsen K. Oxcarbazepine in patients hypersensitive to carbamazepine. *Acta Neurol Scand* 1984; 70: 223.

41 Sachdeo R, Wasserstein A, D'Souza J. Oxcarbazepine (Trileptal): effect on serum sodium (abstr). *Epilepsia* 1999; 40 (Suppl. 7): 103.

42 Isojarvi JIT, Huuskonen VEJ, Pakarinen AJ *et al*. The regulation of serum sodium after replacing carbamazepine with oxcarbazepine. *Epilepsia* 2001; 42: 741–5.

43 Sachdeo RC, Wasserstein A, Mesenbrink PJ, D'Souza J. Effects of oxcarbazepine on sodium concentration and water handling. *Ann Neurol* 2002; 51: 613–20.

44 Aikia M, Kalviainen R, Sivenius J *et al*. Cognitive effects of oxcarbazepine and phenytoin monotherapy in newly diagnosed epilepsy: one year followup. *Epilepsy Res* 1992; 11: 199–203.

45 Saber A, Moller A, Dam M. Cognitive function and anticonvulsant therapy: effect of monotherapy in epilepsy. *Acta Neurol Scand* 1995; 92: 19–27.

46 Gaily E, Granstrom M-J, Liukkonen E. Oxcarbazepine in the treatment of epilepsy in children and adolescents with intellectual disability. *J Int Dis Res* 1998; 42 (Suppl. 1): 41–5.

47 Smith PEM, for the UK Oxcarbazepine Advisory Board. Clinical recommendations for oxcarbazepine. *Seizure* 2001; 10: 87–91.

48 Schmidt D, Sachdeo R. Oxcarbazepine for treatment of partial epilepsy: a review and recommendations for clinical use. *Epilepsy Behav* 2000; 1: 396–405.

49 Gonzalez-Esquivel DF, Ortego-Gavilan M, Alcantara-Lopez G, Jung-Cook H. Plasma level monitoring of oxcarbazepine in epileptic patients. *Arch Med Res* 2000; 31: 202–5.

50 Kramer G, Canger R, Deisenhammer E *et al*. Double-blind, multicenter, non-comparative assessment of the retention rate of b.i.d. administration of oxcarbazepine 900–2700 mg/day as monotherapy for epilepsy in adults (abstr). *Epilepsia* 2000; 41.

39 Phenobarbital, Primidone and Other Barbiturates

R. Michelucci and C.A. Tassinari

Primary indications	Adjunctive or first-line therapy for partial or generalized seizures (including absence and myoclonus). Also for status epilepticus, Lennox–Gastaut syndrome, childhood epilepsy syndromes, febrile convulsions and neonatal seizures
Usual preparations	Tablets: 15, 30, 50, 60, 100 mg; elixir: 15 mg/5 mL; injection: 200 mg/mL
Usual dosages	Initial: 30 mg/day. Maintenance: 30–180 mg/day (adults); 3–8 mg/day (children); 3–4 mg/day (neonates)
Dosage intervals	1–2 times/day
Significant drug interactions	Phenobarbital has a number of interactions with antiepileptic and other drugs
Serum level monitoring	Useful
Target range	15–40 mg/L
Common/important side-effects	Sedation, ataxia, dizziness, insomnia, hyperkinesis (children), mood changes (especially depression), aggressiveness, cognitive dysfunction, impotence, reduced libido, folate deficiency, vitamin K and vitamin D deficiency, osteomalacia, Dupuytren's contracture, frozen shoulder, connective tissue abnormalities, rash
Main advantages	Highly effective and cheap antiepileptic drug
Main disadvantages	CNS side-effects
Mechanisms of action	Enhances activity of $GABA_A$ receptor, depresses glutamate excitability, affects sodium, potassium and calcium conductance
Oral bioavailability	80–100%
Time to peak levels	1–3 h (but variable)
Metabolism and excretion	Hepatic oxidation, glucosidation and hydroxylation, then conjugation
Volume of distribution	0.42–0.75 L/kg
Elimination half-life	75–120 h (in adults; varies with age in children)
Plasma clearance	0.006–0.009 L/kg/h (in adults; varies with age in children)
Protein binding	45–60%
Active metabolites	None
Comment	Highly effective antiepileptic, now not used as first-line therapy because of potential CNS toxicity, especially in children

(*Note*: this summary table was formulated by the lead editor.)

461

Barbiturates are a group of derivatives of barbituric acid, which was synthesized from condensation of malonic acid and urea in 1864. Initially believed to have only sedative properties, they have been recognized as antiepileptic agents since 1912, when Hauptmann described dramatic reduction in seizure frequency in patients with bromide-resistant epilepsy treated with phenobarbital (PB) [1]. PB (also called phenobarbitone) is the oldest antiepileptic drug still in use. However, because of its efficacy and low cost, it still has a role as a major antiepileptic drug, and indeed is the most commonly prescribed antiepileptic drug in the world. Over the years, attempts have been made to modify PB molecular structure in order to achieve agents with greater efficacy and lesser toxicity. Primidone (PRM) was introduced into clinical practice in 1952 and is still widely used. However, its effect can be attributed largely to the derived PB. Additionally, two N-methylderivates of barbituric acid, methylphenobarbital (or mephobarbital) (MPB) and metharbital, possess antiepileptic properties and were introduced into therapeutics in 1932 and 1948, respectively; neither drug, however, has achieved any widespread use. Barbexaclone (BBC), the propylhexedrine salt of PB, was marketed with the aim to decrease the sedation associated with PB use.

In this chapter, the comprehensive features of PB, PRM and other barbiturates will be outlined. A number of excellent reviews devoted to this subject matter are already available [2–14].

Phenobarbital

Chemistry

PB (5-ethyl-5-phenylbarbituric acid) is a substituted barbituric acid, with more potent anticonvulsant than sedative properties. Indeed, the presence of a phenyl group at the C5 position confers selective antiepileptic activity (Fig. 39.1). PB has a molecular weight of 232.23; the free acid of PB is a white crystalline substance, soluble in non-polar solvents (such as chloroform, ethyl ether, ethanol and propylene glycol) but relatively insoluble in water. In contrast, the sodium salt is freely soluble in water. PB is a weak acid with a pK_a of 7.3, similar to the normal PH of plasma. Changes in PH, which

are common in active epilepsy, can alter the ratio of ionized to non-ionized PB, resulting in significant modifications of both the distribution and excretion of the drug [4].

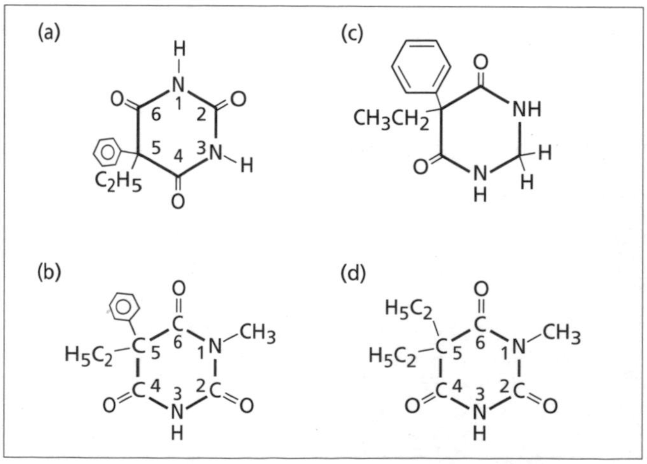

Mechanism of action and experimental studies

In experimental models of epilepsy, PB seems to act in a relatively non-selective manner. It protects against maximal electroshock (MES) convulsions, subcutaneous pentylenetetrazol (PTZ)-induced clonic seizures and electrically kindled seizures [5]. It also appears to prevent seizures induced by a variety of chemicals (such as strychnine, thiosemicarbazide, bicuculline) and photic seizures in the baboon [15]. In contrast, PB worsens spike-wave (SW) discharges in animal models of absence seizures, such as the γ-butyrolactone-induced SW seizures and the lethargic (lh/lh) mutant mouse [16]. This pattern of efficacy in multiple anticonvulsant tests and particularly its ability to limit the spread of seizure activity and also to elevate seizure threshold suggests utility in generalized tonic-clonic seizures and partial seizures in humans. This is bourne out in clinical practice, and PB has proven value in controlling generalized tonic-clonic seizures, partial seizures but not absence seizures.

The possible mechanisms of action of PB are still not completely elucidated. Different effects are noted at different serum concentrations [2]. At high concentrations—as those achieved in patients during treatment of status epilepticus—PB limits high-frequency repetitive firing of action potentials, presumably by interacting with Na and K transmembrane transport and conductance. PB also reduces the Ca influx in the presynaptic endings, which could result in a decreased release of excitatory neurotransmitters, such as glutamate and aspartate. However, these effects on ion transport appear more related to its sedative and/or anaesthetic properties than to its anticonvulsant action. At 'therapeutic' concentrations, PB produces modest changes in membrane conductance but exerts its anticonvulsant action mainly by increasing postsynaptic γ-aminobutyric acid (GABA)-ergic inhibition [5].

PB interacts with the GABA-A receptor, which is a macromolecular protein containing binding sites at least for GABA, picrotoxin, neurosteroids, barbiturates and benzodiazepines (BZDs) and a chloride ion selective channel [17]. GABA binds to GABA-A receptors to regulate gating (opening and closing) of the chloride ion channel [17]. Studies indicate that PB acts mainly by increasing the mean channel open duration without affecting channel conductances or opening frequency [18]; in contrast, the binding of a BZD to its allosterically coupled GABA-A binding site increases opening frequency without affecting open or burst duration [18]. A molecular basis for differential regulation of GABA receptor current by barbiturates and BZDs has been established by studying the more recently discovered GABA-A receptor subunits [19]. In particular, it has been observed that GABA-A receptors formed from α_1–β_1 subunits are sensitive to barbiturates but insensitive to BZDs, whereas the transient coexpression of the γ_2, α_1 and β_1 subunits results in both BZD and PB sensitivity [19]. This differential expression and assembly of various subunit subtypes in various cerebral regions—which is genetically determined [20]—could explain differences in the clinical profile between barbiturates and BZDs.

Fig. 39.1 Structural formula of PB (a), methylphenobarbital (b), primidone (c) and metharbital (d).

Pharmacokinetics

Absorption

PB can be administered by the i.v., i.m. and oral routes. Due to poor water solubility of free acid PB, formulations for i.v. and i.m. administration are prepared from the sodium salt in slightly alkaline solutions.

PB is readily absorbed after oral or i.m. administration (Fig. 39.2) and peak plasma levels are linearly related to dose within a wide range of doses [6,21]. Time to peak plasma concentrations usually occurs 1–3 h after oral dosing and within 4 h after i.m. injection [6,21–23]. As a whole, the differences between oral and i.m. absorption are not statistically significant. In newborns (<6 weeks old) and premature babies, however, the absorption of orally administered PB is delayed and incomplete when compared to i.m. route. Jalling [24] found that 90% of the peak plasma concentration of PB was achieved within 4 h in eight of 10 neonates following i.m. injection but only in three of six newborns after oral administration.

The rate and extent of gastrointestinal absorption after oral dosing may also be influenced by other factors [6]. In the acid environment of the stomach, PB is largely non-ionized and diffusible. The bulk of orally administered PB, however, is absorbed in the small intestine, where the non-ionized fraction is smaller but intraluminal dwell time is longer. Characteristics of the preparation administered (e.g. free acid or salt, crystal size), gastric blood flow, gastric emptying time, gastric acidity, presence of food and neutralizing agents, and small intestine pathologies may all alter PB absorption. PB has a nearly complete bioavailability in humans, ranging from 80 to 100%, whether administered by the oral or i.m. route [6,22,23].

Distribution

PB disseminates rapidly to all body tissues. The distribution of PB (whose pK$_a$ is similar to the normal PH of plasma) is very sensitive

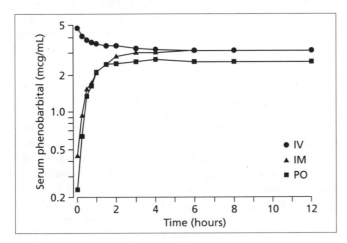

Fig. 39.2 Mean serum PB levels in six normal volunteers after single i.v. and i.m. injections of PB sodium 130 mg and single oral doses of PB acid 100 mg. Doses were given at least 1 month apart. From [23] with permission.

to variations in the plasma PH. Acidosis results in a higher percentage of non-ionized PB, enhancing its diffusion from plasma to tissues. On the other hand, alkalosis causes an increased transfer of PB from tissues to plasma.

In infants, children and adults PB is 45–60% protein bound [25]. Binding in newborns is even lower (36–43%) [24]. Therefore, changes in the extent of PB binding by hypoalbuminaemia or displacement by other agents have little effect on the unbound PB levels. Concentrations of PB in cerebrospinal fluid are 43–60% (in adults) and 48–83% (in infants) of plasma concentrations and correlate well with the unbound PB plasma levels [6]. They also provide a reliable index of PB concentration in brain. The brain to plasma concentration ratios in human epileptic brain specimens vary widely, ranging from 0.35 to 1.13 [6]. PB concentrations are higher in cerebrospinal fluid than in saliva and saliva to total serum concentration ratios in infants range from 0.21 to 0.52 [6].

PB rapidly crosses the placenta, so that maternally derived PB serum concentrations in neonates are similar to those in the mother. PB is also secreted in breast milk, where its concentrations are about 40% of those in the serum [6,26].

After i.v. administration, PB distribution into body organs is diphasic. In a first phase, PB distributes rapidly to the high blood flow organs including liver, kidney and heart, but not into the brain. During the second phase, PB achieves a fairly uniform distribution throughout the body except the fat tissue. This pattern of relatively slow entry into brain (12–60 min) and late exclusion from fat is related to PB's low lipid solubility; however, in status epilepticus, because of focal acidosis and increased blood flow, the transfer of PB to brain is much faster [6].

In adults, the relative volume of distribution for PB ranges from 0.36 to 0.67 L/kg after i.m. administration and from 0.42 to 0.73 L/kg after oral dosing [6]. The volume of distribution is larger in newborns, where it ranges from 0.39 to 2.25 L/kg after i.v. or i.m. injection [27].

Metabolism

PB is eliminated partly unchanged and is partly metabolized to inactive compounds.

There is considerable intersubject and intrasubject variability in the amount of PB excreted unchanged; however single dose and steady-state studies in volunteers and patients have shown that the fraction of the dose excreted unchanged accounts for approximately 20–25% of the total clearance (range: 7–55%) [4].

The majority of a PB dose appears to be eliminated by hepatic metabolism. The most common route of biotransformation is hydroxylation of the phenyl ring (aromatic hydroxylation) by the mixed function oxidase system to produce *p*-hydroxyphenobarbital (PBOH). This metabolite is excreted in urine partly in free form and partly conjugated with glucuronic acid to form PBOH glucuronide. The sum of the free and conjugated metabolite accounts for a range of 8–34% of the administered dose, with high intersubject variability. *N*-glucosidation is a more recently identified metabolic pathway, leading to the formation of a PB *N*-glucoside (PNG) metabolite. The *N*-glucosidation pathway is not active at birth but becomes effective only after 2 weeks of life. This may be the main reason for the long PB half-life observed in newborns. PNG accounts for a range of 6–30% of the dose of the parent drug. It has been suggested that the PNG undergoes significant breakdown to as yet unidentified derivatives while still present in the blood and tissues of the body, due to its high liability to PH variations and relatively short half-life. Therefore, N-glucosidation could be a more important metabolic pathway than originally thought [4].

Other less important routes of biotransformation are epoxidation with subsequent formation of PBOH or the dihydrodiol, aliphatic hydroxylation and hydrolysis [4].

Enterohepatic circulation and faecal excretion probably are not important contributors to PB distribution under usual circumstances.

Although PB is a well-known inducer of hepatic metabolism, it does not induce its own metabolism in humans. In animals, however, considerable autoinduction has been observed.

Elimination

Elimination of PB by all routes is slow and the average elimination half-life after single doses is between 75 and 126 h, the longest amongst the frequently used antiepileptic drugs [6,23]. Total renal clearance of PB ranges from 0.6 to 8.8 mL/kg/h in adults [22,23].

PB elimination follows first-order kinetics and thus is independent of concentration [28]. Several factors, however, contribute to variation in the rate of elimination of PB, including urinary PH and flow, age, nutritional states, drug interactions and liver or renal pathologies [6].

Urinary PH influences the passive reabsorption of PB from the distal tubule, whose membranes favour the transport of non-ionized compounds. Alkalinization of urine converts more drug to the ionized, non-diffusible form, thereby resulting in increased PB excretion. The opposite occurs with acidification of urine. Raising urinary PH to 8.0, with a corresponding plasma PH of 7.55, increases the fraction of ionized PB in renal tubular fluid from 69 to 86%. Renal clearance of PB is also enhanced by diuresis, either induced by water administration or dopamine and acetazolamide intake. These findings are the basis for the use of forced diuresis and urine alkalinization in overdose patients.

PB half-life also varies with age. Whereas premature and full-term newborns have the longest PB half-lives (ranging from 59 to 400 h), infants (aged 6 weeks to 12 months) have the shortest. Pitlick et al. [27] observed that the half-life diminishes from an average of 115 to 67 h between birth and the first month of life. Half-lives of 37–133 h were found in 33 infants older than 6 months after single doses in one study [29] and even shorter values (21–75 h) were reported in other studies [6,30].

PB clearance is also increased in children with protein–energy malnutrition [6]. Oral administration of activated charcoal increases intestinal elimination of PB [31].

Drug interactions

There is no clear proof of any significant pharmacodynamic interaction between PB and other drugs (except perhaps with the BZDs). However, there are many pharmacokinetic interactions [7].

PB is a potent inducer of the hepatic mixed-function oxidase system, which mediates the biotransformation of numerous drugs and endogeneous substances. This system includes cytochrome P450 (which exists in many subforms) and nicotinamide adenine dinu-cleotide phosphate (NADPH)–cytochrome c reductase. It seems likely that all the interactions of PB with other substances are due to this induction, which has been demonstrated in animals and humans [7]. Induction of the mixed-function oxidase system by PB is influenced to some extent by environmental factors (e.g. tobacco smoking, alcohol), age and genetic factors. Studies in identical and fraternal twins have shown that the extent of induction in each of the monozygotic twins within a pair was nearly identical despite different living habits. In contrast, in dizygotic twins, the intrapair differences in inducibility ranged from 8% to 31% [32]. Because of this strong genetic influence, the effects of induction by PB on other drugs in individual patients are largely unpredictable.

Effects of PB on the kinetics of other agents

PB induces the metabolism of numerous drugs, including a number of analgesics and antipyretics (antipyrine, amidopyrine, acetaminophen, meperidine and methadone), antiasthma agents (theophylline), antibiotics (chloramphenicol, doxicycline, griseofulvin), anticoagulants (bishydroxycoumarin and warfarin), antiulcer agents (cimetidine), immunosuppressants (ciclosporin), psychotropic drugs (chlorpromazine, haloperidol, desipramine, nortriptyline, BZDs), oral steroid contraceptives and antiepileptic agents. PB induces the metabolism of valproate (VPA) and decreases its plasma concentrations [33]. It has also been suggested that induction of VPA metabolism by PB may contribute to VPA hepatotoxicity, by stimulating the production of several VPA metabolites [34]. PB may cause a decline of plasma carbamazepine (CBZ) levels in some patients [35], but the effect is often negligible. The effect on phenytoin (PHT) is complex and not predictable in any individual: the interaction includes an inducing effect on PHT metabolism and a competitive inhibition with PHT as substrate, since both drugs undergo para-hydroxylation and glucuronidation [7].

Interestingly, the induction of drug metabolism by PB does not always results in a reduction of the effects of other drugs. There are instances in which the induction of metabolism causes an increased production of a toxic metabolite of the concomitant drug, leading to increased toxicity. This is the case of acetophenitidin, whose induction by PB may be responsible for methaemoglobin formation by increasing the production of a toxic intermediary metabolite (2-hydroxyphenetidin), particularly in patients with genetically determined deficient metabolic pathways [36].

Effects of other agents on the kinetics of PB

PHT, VPA, felbamate, clobazam and dextropropoxyphene may inhibit PB metabolism leading to elevation of PB levels. Accumulation of PB caused by VPA is the most constant, predictable and clinically important interaction in this group. The clinical manifestations include increasing somnolence, sometimes resulting in coma, within days or weeks after the initiation of VPA administration. Although the rate and magnitude of PB accumulation vary among individuals, PB dosage reductions are necessary in up to 80% of patients. The mechanism of this interaction is probably multifactorial but it mainly involves inhibition of PB metabolism [37]. Furthermore toxic signs might occur because of blood ammonia levels higher than those of patients taking only VPA. In man, the use of vigabatrin in combination with PB has been associated with small but significant decreases in serum PB concentrations. The mechanism of this interaction is unknown [7].

Clinical efficacy

As is the case with other drugs marketed so long ago, the assessment of PB efficacy is mainly based upon open studies and clinical anecdote rather than on information from controlled studies. There is however a large volume of uncontrolled data clearly demonstrating the value of PB in the treatment of both adult and childhood epilepsy. Neonatal seizures and status epilepticus are two other well-established indications for the use of PB.

PB use in adults and children

Controlled data concern the use of PB in previously untreated epileptic patients. The most authorative work in this field is the Veterans Administration (VA) Cooperative double-blind study conducted by Mattson et al. [38]. In this study the efficacy and tolerability of four drugs (PB, PRM, CBZ and PHT) were assessed in 622 adults with previously untreated or undertreated partial and secondarily generalized tonic-clonic seizures. PB, PRM, CBZ and PHT produced similar rates of overall seizure control (with percentages of 36, 35, 47 and 38%, respectively). While the prognosis for complete control of tonic-clonic seizures with the four drugs was also similar, CBZ provided significantly better total control of partial seizures (43%) than PB (16%) or PRM (15%), whereas PHT provided intermediate control (26%). These data were confirmed at every 6-month point during the 36 months of follow-up. In keeping with the data from this study, other open studies have also shown PB to be as successful as CBZ and PHT in the treatment of predominantly tonic-clonic seizures but with a higher failure rate in the management of partial seizures [39,40].

A large long-term prospective randomized pragmatic trial of the comparative efficacy and toxicity of PB, PHT, CBZ and VPA for newly diagnosed epileptic subjects has been performed in adults and children. Patients entered the trial with a minimum of two previously untreated tonic-clonic seizures or partial epilepsy with or without secondary generalization. Heller et al. [41] reported the findings in 243 adults. The overall outcome with all four drugs was good with 27% remaining seizure free and 75% entering 1 year of remission by 3 years of follow-up. There was no significant difference in efficacy between the four randomized major AEDs, in either time to first seizure recurrence or time to achieve 1 year of remission from all seizures. The same results were reported by de Silva et al.

[42] in the children of the trial. Of the 167 children (aged 3–16 years) who entered the study, 20% remained seizure free and 73% achieved 1-year remission by 3 years of follow-up. Again there was no difference in efficacy between the drugs for either measure of efficacy at 1, 2 or 3 years of follow-up. The divergence of findings in the VA trial, the study of Heller et al. [41] and that of de Silva et al. [42] in terms of relative efficacy in patients with partial seizures, was due probably to differences in study populations, with a larger proportion of tonic-clonic seizures (also of generalized origin) in the latter two studies. There have been a handful of other open studies confirming the equivalence of effect of PB, CBZ and VPA, both in adults [8] and children [43].

In drug-resistant patients, a few small trials are available showing that PB is equal in efficacy to established drugs [8]. However, large randomized controlled studies are lacking.

The above studies show that PB is useful in the treatment of partial and secondarily generalized seizures. The effects of PB in idiopathic generalized epilepsies have been also investigated. PB has been shown to be effective in the treatment of generalized tonic-clonic seizures [8,39,40] and could be used as an alternative drug for this seizure type if VPA is ineffective or not tolerated because of adverse effects. The drug is also effective against other generalized seizure types, including myoclonic, atonic and tonic seizures, although clinical trial evidence of its value in these attacks is largely lacking.

Neonatal seizures

PB is traditionally considered the drug of choice for the treatment of neonatal seizures. This extensive use is primarily due to years of familiarity and experience with PB in older children and adults. However, controlled evidence of its efficacy or superiority above other drugs is scanty. Moreover, neonatal seizures are a rather heterogeneous group of paroxysmal events and EEG confirmation of the diagnosis is remarkably absent in most studies.

Three series show very close agreement regarding the efficacy of PB as the initial agent in the treatment of neonatal seizures. In these open trials, involving a total of 197 neonates and utilizing loading doses of 15–20 mg/kg, seizure control was obtained in 32–36% of cases [44–46]. Gal et al. [47], however, reported efficacy in 85% of 71 neonates in whom PB was used as monotherapy, at doses as high as 40 mg/kg to achieve or surpass plasma concentrations of 40 μg/mL (Table 39.1). The lack of specific seizure definition, electrically or clinically, in all of these series makes the interpretation of the differences in data difficult.

Painter et al. [48] performed a randomized trial to assess the rela-

Table 39.1 Phenobarbital efficacy in neonatal seizures

Reference	Patients (no.)	Response rate (%)	Loading doses (mg/kg)
Lockman et al. [44]	39	32	15–20
Painter et al. [46]	77	36	15–20
VanOrman & Darrvish [45]	81	33	15–20
Gal et al. [47]	71	85	Up to 40

Modified from Painter and Gaus [8].

tive efficacy of PB and PHT in the treatment of seizures in neonates, using EEG criteria for diagnosis and to determine efficacy. Fifty-nine neonates with EEG-confirmed seizures mostly caused by asphyxia, haemorrhage or infarction of the brain, were randomly assigned to receive either PB or PHT i.v.; the doses were sufficient to achieve free plasma concentrations of 25 µg/mL for PB and 3 µg/mL for PHT. Seizures were controlled in 43% of neonates assigned to receive PB and in 45% of neonates treated with PHT. In refractory cases, the combined treatment with PB and PHT allowed interruption of seizures in 32% of cases. Interestingly, the severity of seizures was a stronger predictor of the success of treatment than the assigned treatment.

Status epilepticus

PB is a drug of choice in established status, both of tonic-clonic or partial type; it is given as i.v. infusion at 10 mg/kg at a rate of 100 mg/min.

PB achieves a maximum brain to plasma ratio more slowly than diazepam (DZ), and the response time in the treatment of status epilepticus might be expected to be slower. However, with a single dose of 250 mg of PB administered over 150 s, all patients in one study ceased convulsing within a few minutes [49]. In a randomized, non-blinded clinical trial, 36 consecutive patients with convulsive status epilepticus were treated with either a combination of DZ and PHT or with PB [50]. PB was administered i.v. at a rate of 100 mg/min until a dose of 10 mg/kg was achieved. DZ was infused at 2 mg/min i.v and PHT was administered simultaneously at a rate of 40 mg/min until a loading dose of 18 mg/kg was achieved. There were 18 episodes of status epilepticus in each group. Eleven of 18 patients in the PB group responded to PB monotherapy, a figure that compares favourably with that of alternative treatment. However, the cumulative convulsive time and the response latency was shorter for the PB group. The median response time was 5.5 min with PB. Effective brain concentrations of PB are achieved within 3 min [51]. Therefore PB has a rapid onset and long-lasting action, and can be administered much faster than PHT. Other advantages include its safety at high doses and its subsequent use as oral long-term therapy.

Special indications

PB has been extensively used as an anticonvulsant for the prophylaxis of febrile seizures. Although prophylaxis is now currently considered in only a minority of cases (showing prolonged or focal seizures, associated with transient or permanent neurological deficits), PB has been proven effective in preventing febrile seizures, whereas PHT has not [2]. If PB is chosen for prophylaxis, it should not be utilized intermittently, but must be administered daily. Faero et al. [52] compared 59 patients, all younger than 3 years, with 72 untreated children, and found that the febrile convulsion recurrence rate was 13% in the PB-treated group compared to 20% in the control group. However the risk decreased to 4% in those children whose PB plasma levels were maintained between 16 and 30 µg/mL.

PB has also been used in the treatment of seizures complicating cerebral malaria. In a randomized study performed in Kenya, 170 children were assigned to receive a single i.m. dose of PB (20 mg/kg) and 170 children identical placebo [53]. Seizure frequency was significantly lower in the PB group than in the placebo group (11% vs. 27%) but mortality was doubled (18% vs. 8% deaths). Mortality, due to respiratory arrest, however, was greatly increased in children who received PB plus three or more doses of DZ. The conclusion raised by the authors that 20 mg PB single i.m. dose should not be recommended in this special population because of an unacceptable risk of mortality has not been shared by other investigators [54].

Side-effects

After almost a century of worldwide use, PB has enjoyed a reputation of safety as it causes very few systemic or idiosyncratic side-effects. However, its sedative properties represent a common problem in daily practice. Overdose is also a specific issue of PB.

Neurotoxicity

Sedation is the most common side-effect associated with PB, particularly at the onset of treatment. In the VA Cooperative Study, however, acute sedation was not more frequent with PB than with other drugs (i.e. PRM, CBZ or PHT), probably because of cautious dose increases (32 mg as starting dose) [38]. In the study of Heller et al. [41] comparing the effects of four drugs (PB, CBZ, PHT and VPA) as monotherapies in adult newly diagnosed epileptic patients, PB was more likely to be withdrawn because of side-effects. Drowsiness and lethargy were the main reasons for early withdrawal, but the initial dosing was higher (60 mg/day) than in the VA Study [38].

Some tolerance to sedation may develop, particularly if the drug is introduced into therapy gradually and progressively. A subgroup of 58 patients taking PB in the VA Cooperative Study was examined at every visit for the first 3 months (1, 2, 4, 8, 12 weeks) to assess the incidence of acute adverse effects and development of tolerance. Of the subgroup studied for tolerance, 33% of patients started on PB reported initial sedation, declining significantly to 24% by 12 weeks ($P < 0.04$). Evidence of tolerance was taken to be decreasing symptoms despite increasing PB concentrations from a mean of 18 µg/mL at 2 weeks to 24 µg/mL at 12 weeks [38].

Instead of sedation, which is common in adults, insomnia and hyperkinetic activity may occur in children and the elderly subjects, as a paradoxical effect of the drug. In a study by Wolf and Forsythe [55], of 109 children treated daily with PB following their first febrile seizure, 42% developed behavioural disorders, primarily hyperactivity. The disturbance was not correlated with plasma PB concentrations. Hyperactivity improved in all children when PB was discontinued and disappeared entirely in 73%. Behavioural disturbances associated with PB were also more likely to occur in the presence of organic brain disease or deficits [9,56]. When compared to other first-line agents (PHT, CBZ and VPA) in newly diagnosed epileptic children, PB was associated with the highest chance of withdrawal, behavioural problems being the main cause of drop-out [42]. Problems with memory or compromised work and school performance can develop even in the absence of sedation and hyperkinetic activity, although these factors may play a contributory role. Changes in cognitive function have been measured by various standardized neuropsychological tests. A decrease in verbal and performance IQ scores, has been observed in children treated with PB compared to normal controls [9,56] or patients receiving VPA [57] or CBZ [9]. Memory and concentration scores, visuomotor performance and spatial memory, and short-term memory can also be significantly impaired in PB-treated subjects, especially children. Performance on vigilance tests requiring sustained effort may also be impaired, even after tolerance has developed [9].

Alteration of affect, particularly depression, has been associated with the use of PB in children [9]. A complex picture including depression, apathy, impotence, decreased libido and sluggishness is sometimes observed in adults [2]. In the VA Cooperative Study, decreased libido and/or potency was found to be more common in patients treated with PB or PRM than in those receiving CBZ or PHT [38].

During chronic therapy, dysarthria, incoordination, ataxia, dizziness and nystagmus may appear if serum levels exceed 40 µg/mL. Dyskinesia and peripheral neuropathy are very rare effects induced by PB [2].

Dependence and withdrawal

Prolonged use of PB produces physical dependence, with the appearance of abstinence symptoms following abrupt discontinuation. Special care should be taken during the neonatal period of children born to mothers who received PB. The neonatal withdrawal syndrome includes hyperexcitability, tremor, irritability and gastrointestinal upset and this can last for days or even months. An increase in seizure frequency or a relapse in controlled patients has often been noted during or after PB discontinuation. There is some evidence that this exacerbation of seizures is not only due to the underlying epilepsy but also to an additional barbiturate withdrawal mechanism [9]. In these cases, generalized tonic-clonic seizures are the rule, even when the patient habitually experiences partial seizures. Therefore, if a decision is made to stop PB therapy, the drug should be tapered very slowly to avoid these convulsive withdrawal seizures.

Overdose

A significant number of deaths have been associated with poisoning by barbiturates. In 27 such cases, observed in Ontario from 1955 to 1964, PB levels detected in postmortem blood ranged between 2.3 and 18.9 mg/100 mL [58]. Clinically, excessive high doses of PB first produce ataxia, dysarthria, nystagmus, incoordination and uncontrollable sleepiness. As the serum levels rise, these effects progress to stupor and coma. Death is due to depression of cardiorespiratory function. Drug-naive patients are more sensitive to the effects of PB but concentrations above 70 µg/mL cause coma in almost all individuals, including those on long-term therapy (Fig. 39.3). A level of 80 µg/mL is potentially lethal. The EEG features of PB overdose reflect the clinical severity, with pictures evolving from burst-suppression (Fig. 39.3) to electrical silence in fatal cases. In overdose patients, therapy includes maintenance of vital functions with assisted ventilation, as well as the need to accelerate PB elimination by alkalinization and forced diuresis. Charcoal and ion exchange resins have also been used [9].

Haematological toxicity

Folate deficiency is common in polymedicated patients, and PB monotherapy can also cause decreased folate levels and macrocytosis. Megaloblastic anaemia is rare, however, and the significance of folate deficiency is uncertain. A severe coagulation defect has been reported in neonates born to epileptic mothers taking PB [59]. The coagulation defect is similar to that observed in vitamin K deficiency. Supplementation of vitamin K administered to mothers prepartum will prevent this complication [59].

Metabolic bone disorders

PB can affect calcium and vitamin D metabolism, by inducing hydroxylation of vitamin D. This results in a high incidence of low calcium levels but overt rickets or osteomalacia are only occasionally observed.

Disorders of connective tissue

PB produces an increased tendency to fibrosis, including a higher incidence of Dupuytren's contractures with palmar nodules, frozen shoulder, plantar fibromatosis, Peyronie's disease, heel and knuckle pads and generalized joint pain. The incidence of barbiturate-related connective tissue disorders ranges from 5% to 38% depending on the population studied. A shoulder–hand syndrome was observed in 28% of 126 neurosurgical patients treated with barbiturates but in none of 108 control patients receiving CBZ or PHT [60].

Hypersensitivity reactions

Mild skin reactions, usually maculopapular, morbilliform or scarlatiniform rashes, occur in 1–3% of all patients receiving PB. Serious skin reactions, such as exfoliative dermatitis, erythema multiforme, Stevens–Johnson syndrome or toxic epidermal necrolysis are remarkably rare.

A barbiturate hypersensitivity syndrome, characterized by rash, eosinophilia and fever, is infrequent. Signs of hepatic injury (eosinophilic or granulomatous inflammation) may coexist. Systemic lupus erythematosus and acute intermittent porphyria may be unmasked or precipitated by PB.

Teratogenicity

Unfortunately, most studies of teratogenicity do not clarify the relative role of drugs, epilepsy, genetic and environmental factors. Overall, available studies seem to indicate that maternal intake of PB, as of any other AED, during pregnancy increases the risk of malformation in the offspring. This risk is enhanced if PB is used during pregnancy in combination with other drugs, particularly phenytoin [9].

Data from large-scale Japanese studies, however, suggest that PB is the least teratogenic of the AEDs in common use [61]. PB is also

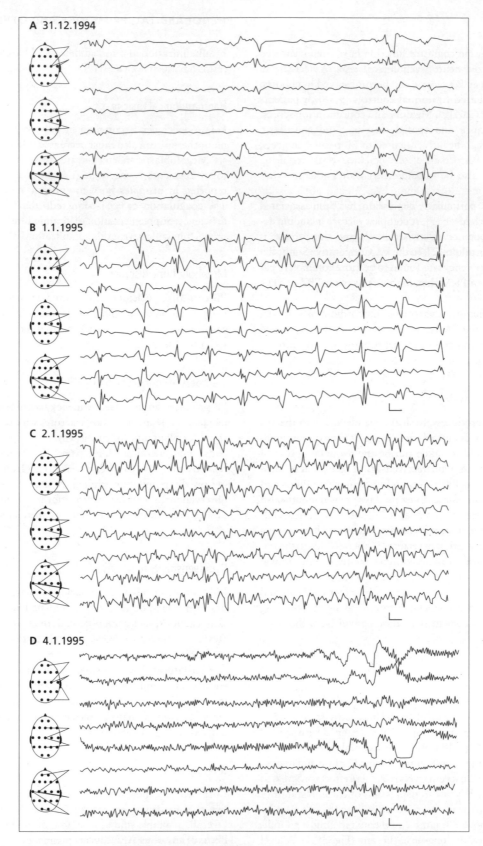

Fig. 39.3 PB overdose in a 47-year-old woman with a 34-year history of focal motor and secondarily generalized seizures, on chronic treatment with PB 100 mg daily. There was no apparent aetiology for epilepsy. The patient was found comatose in her bed; on admission to the hospital, the patient was in deep coma and required assisted ventilation; the EEG showed a burst-suppression pattern (A). The plasma levels of PB were 82 µg/mL. On the subsequent day, there was some improvement of the EEG, with shortening of the 'inter-bursts' flattenings (B). The corresponding plasma levels were 60 µg/mL. Progressive improvement of the EEG (C), with a normal tracing on the fifth day (D) after overdose. When awake, the patient admitted to have taken 'many' pills to attempt suicide (R. Michelucci, personal observation).

recommended by the American College of Obstetrics and Gynecology for pregnant women with epilepsy, probably because gross malformations appear to be less common with PB use. Forthcoming large prospective studies on pregnancies of epileptic women will hopefully clarify this issue in a near future [62].

Clinical therapeutics

PB has been marketed either as the acid or the sodium salt in 15-, 30-, 50-, 60- and 100-mg tablets, although not all sizes are available in all countries. Oral solutions (elixirs) are also available, as well as parenteral solutions of the drug, usually containing 100 or 200 mg sodium salt.

Introduction in therapy of PB should be gradual, with a starting dose in adults of 30 or 50 mg/day. The dose can be titrated with 5 or 30 mg increments every 1 or 2 weeks, accordingly to tolerability issues. The maintenance dose ranges between 60 and 240 mg/day, but in most adult patients it is restricted within 90 and 120 mg/day. A dosage interval of once a day is recommended.

In children, the starting dose is 3 mg/kg/day and the dose is titrated up to a maintenance dose of 3–8 mg/kg/day. Sometimes a twice daily dosing may be necessary due to the shorter half-life in children. PB dosages in status epilepticus and neonatal seizures are described in their specific sections.

Serum level measurements of PB are widely used. A therapeutic level for PB was first suggested by Buchthal et al. [63] who reported on the findings in 11 untreated patients with frequent seizures. PB was administered in small doses that were gradually increased. The average level at which the EEG and clinical response occurred was 10 µg/mL. By pooling the data from four studies (three retrospective and one prospective) Booker [10] commented on the results of a sample of 568 patients. On the whole, 84% of all subjects who were controlled had plasma levels between 10 and 40 µg/mL (Table 39.2). Some patients, however, may experience good seizure control above or below this limit. As the plama level increases above 40 µg/mL, the potential benefit must be weighed against the potential for side-effects.

The optimal PB plasma concentration might vary with the type of seizure. In a study of 78 patients with various seizure types, Schmidt et al. [40] observed that complete control of simple or complex partial seizures required significantly higher plasma concentrations of PB (38 ± 6 µg/mL) compared to concentrations required for complete control of tonic-clonic seizures alone (18 ± 10 µg/mL).

Though usually considered an old-fashioned drug, PB has a significant role in everyday therapeutic practice. Clear advantages are the low cost, the ease of use, the once daily dosing, lack of idiosyncratic reactions, safety in pregnancy and robust efficacy data. These characteristics render PB an important drug, particularly suitable for extensive use in the developing world. The main disadvantage consists in the perceived potential to cause central nervous system related side-effects, particularly sedation in adults and behavioural changes in children. While the sedative properties may be minimized by slow titration and development of tolerance, behavioural changes need close monitoring. When compared with other AEDs, PB shows the same efficacy in the control of tonic-clonic seizures, either primarily or secondarily generalized. PB is also effective against focal seizures, but probably to a lesser extent than CBZ. Neonatal seizures and status epilepticus are two other valuable indications.

Primidone

Chemistry

PRM (5-ethyldihydro-5-phenyl-4,6-$(1^H,5^H)$-pyrimidine-dione) is deoxyphenobarbital and differs from PB by the lack of the carbonyl group in position 2 of the pyrimidine ring (Fig. 39.1). PRM has a molecular weight of 218.25; it is an odourless crystalline white powder with a slightly bitter taste and a melting point of 218–282°C. It is almost insoluble in water and organic solvents, but is somewhat soluble in ethanol.

Mechanism of action and experimental studies

PRM itself is not easily studied for mechanism of action because of its rapid conversion to PB. Moreover, a second active metabolite of PRM, phenylethylmalonamide (PEMA), might also contribute to the overall pharmacodynamic effect of PRM. A number of experiments in animals suggest, however, that PRM has independent anticonvulsant activity. Indeed, a single dose of PRM was shown to protect rats against induced seizures before active metabolites were detectable [64]. Similar protection was achieved in mice when the biotransformation of PRM was delayed by the preadministration of a metabolic blocker [65]. PRM was effective in preventing MES seizures, but had virtually no effect against seizures induced chemically by PTZ or bicuculline [65]. In these models, PRM showed activity more characteristic of CBZ and PHT than PB, which is active in both MES- and PTZ-induced seizures [65]. PRM and PB differ pharmacodynamically not only on the basis of their anticonvulsant spectrum, but also on the basis of their protective or therapeutic index. In terms of brain concentrations in mice, PRM was found to be 2.5 times less neurotoxic than PB, with a correspondingly higher therapeutic index [65]. Coadministration of single doses of PB and PRM in mice resulted in a potentiation of their anticonvulsant activity without increase of side-effects.

In cultured mouse neurones, PRM had no effect on GABA and glutamate responses at concentrations up to 50 µg/mL but showed a synergistic action with PB to reduce sustained, high-frequency, repetitive firing [66].

Table 39.2 Plasma phenobarbital levels and seizure control

Plasma phenobarbital level (µg/mL)	Total number of subjects	Number of subjects controlled	Cumulative % of controlled subjects
<10	50	14	6.5
10–14	92	23	17.2
15–19	115	50	40.6
20–24	93	50	64.0
25–29	87	29	77.6
30–34	43	12	83.2
35–39	35	16	90.7
≥40	53	20	100.0

From Booker [10].

Pharmacokinetics

Absorption

Only oral preparations of PRM are available since the drug has an extremely low solubility which prevents parenteral administration. Time to peak plasma concentrations of PRM after oral ingestion of tablets ranged between 2.7 and 3.2 h in epileptic adults [11,67] and 4 and 6 h in children [11]. Oral bioavailability of PRM seems to be quite complete since approximately 92% of the daily dose was recovered in the urine as unchanged PRM or as metabolites in children.

Distribution

PRM distributes throughout body tissues and fluids in a similar pattern and at the same extent as PB. In humans, variable brain to blood concentration ratios of PRM have been reported, ranging from 40% to 87% [11]; these discrepancies may be due to the timing of specimen collections. PRM does not bind significantly to plasma proteins, the PRM bound fraction ranging from 0 to 20% [11]. Mean PRM volume of distribution was found to be between 0.64 and 0.72 L/kg in adult patients with epilepsy [11].

Metabolism

Although the majority of the dose is excreted in the urine unchanged, PRM does undergo some biotransformation. The primary and most relevant metabolic pathways of PRM biotransformation involve: (a) the formation of PEMA by cleavage of the pyrimidine ring; and (b) the formation of PB by oxidation of the methylene group. PB in turn is further oxidized to PBOH. Other metabolites of PRM have been identified (i.e. α-phenylbutyramide, p-hydroxyprimidone, and α-phenyl-p-butyrolactone) but they have no practical significance because of their low concentrations and lack of pharmacological activity. The time course of appearance in plasma of the metabolites is different for PEMA and PB; after a first dose of PRM, PEMA was detected in the blood within a few hours, whereas PB was often not measurable during the first 24 h [67]. Numerous clinical studies have addressed the quantitative aspects of the biotransformation of PRM to PB and PEMA. By comparing the level to dose ratios for PB and PRM in patients who had taken either drug for at least 6 months, Olesen and Dam [68] found that, on average, 24.5% of PRM administered was converted to PB. This finding was in keeping with the observation that, in order to achieve the same blood PB levels, the PRM dose (in mg/kg) has to be about five times higher than the corresponding dose of PB. The extent of the biotransformation of PRM is largely influenced by other antiepileptic drugs with enzyme-inducing action such as PHT, which may increase the conversion to PB.

Elimination

PRM and its metabolites are primarily eliminated by renal excretion. PRM elimination half-life is variable and is reported to range from 3.3 to 22.4 h, with factors such as age and concomitant therapy accounting for much of the variability [11]. The ability of newborns to metabolize PRM to PB appears to be very limited and in neonates the half-life of PRM was 23 h, on average, with a range of 8–30 h [11].

In adults taking other AEDs in addition to PRM, values for the half-life are reduced, ranging from 3.3 to 11 h [11,67]. Moreover, accumulation of PB during long-term PRM therapy could decrease PRM half-life as a result of microsomal enzyme induction [11].

Drug interactions

PRM is the cause as well as the object of numerous pharmacokinetic interactions. In principle, the conversion of PRM to PB and PEMA may be both markedly induced and inhibited by other drugs.

The most pronounced acceleration of the enzymatic biotransformation of PRM appears to be caused by PHT, which is a potent enzymatic inducer [69]. CBZ also accelerates biotransformation of PRM, but to a lesser extent, and may sometimes have an inhibitory effect.

Bourgeois [12] summarized the effects of comedication with PHT, CBZ or both on the concentration to dose ratio and on the ratios between the concentrations of PRM, PB and PEMA (Table 39.3). Compared with PRM monotherapy, the morning trough levels of PRM were reduced by about 50% and, conversely, PB levels were raised by a factor of 1.6 during comedication. Thus, when patients are taking PHT or CBZ the average PRM dose needed to maintain a given PB level is 1.6 times lower than that for PRM monotherapy. In addition, the morning trough serum concentration ratio of PB to PRM is more than three times higher during comedication. This implies that the serum levels of PB may increase

Table 39.3 Ratios of serum levels of PRM, PB and PEMA to PRM dose, and ratios of serum levels of PRM, PB and PEMA at steady state[a]

	n	Ratios of serum levels to PRM dose[b]			Ratios of serum levels[b]	
		PRM	PB	PEMA	PB : PRM	PEMA : PRM
Monotherapy	10	0.78 ± 0.25	1.47 ± 0.53	0.64 ± 0.39	1.65 ± 0.74	0.70 ± 0.36
Comedication[c]	53	0.40 ± 0.15	2.40 ± 0.98	0.75 ± 0.42	5.83 ± 2.62	1.71 ± 0.75

From Bourgeois *et al.* [12].

PB, phenobarbital; PEMA, phenylethylmalonamide; PRM, primidone.

[a] All blood samples were drawn before the first morning dose in hospitalized patients.

[b] Mean ± SD; PRM dose in mg/kg/day, serum levels in mg/L.

[c] Comedication consisted of phenytoin, carbamazepine or both.

from 'therapeutic' to 'toxic' levels if PHT or CBZ is added to pre-existing PRM therapy.

VPA does not induce significant modification of PB or PRM levels or may cause transitory elevations of PRM levels. Isoniazid and nicotinamide have been shown to inhibit the conversion of PRM to PB, causing high levels of PRM. PRM can also influence the levels of other drugs. Because of the derived PB, the effects of PRM are similar to those described in relation to PB treatment.

Clinical efficacy

Because PRM is metabolized to PB during long-term therapy, there has long been a controversy as to whether PRM is simply a prodrug of PB or whether it conveys added advantages. PRM generally has the same indications as PB. A number of comparative open clinical studies of PRM and other AEDs (usually PB, PHT and CBZ) have been performed in patients with partial and secondarily generalized seizures, mostly showing no significant difference in efficacy [12]. In one crossover study the efficacies of PRM and PB were compared sequentially in the same patients, 21 epileptic patients residing at the Chalfont Centre [70]. Similar PB levels were maintained during both therapies and PRM treatment was found to be slightly more effective against generalized tonic-clonic seizures than PB treatment [70]. In the authoritative VA Cooperative double-blind comparative study of the use of PRM, PB, CBZ and PHT in previously untreated or undertreated adult patients with partial and secondarily generalized tonic-clonic seizure, PRM produced an overall seizure control similar to that obtained with PB, PHT and CBZ but caused a significantly lower reduction (15%) of partial seizures than CBZ (43%) [38].

PRM was used as a drug of choice in the treatment of juvenile myoclonic epilepsy but has been largely replaced by VPA for this indication.

Toxicity

As with the antiepileptic effect, it is difficult to separate long-term side-effects of PRM therapy from those of PB therapy. It is usually stated that PRM shares all the side-effects of PB, both in adults and in children [13]. The same also applies to idiosyncratic side-effects and potential teratogenicity. Birth defects described in the offspring of women who took PRM during pregnancy are not specific and include ventriculoseptal defects, microcephaly and poor somatic development [71].

What clearly distinguishes PRM from PB is the occurrence of acute initial toxicity. Marked side-effects, including drowsiness, dizziness, ataxia, nausea and vomiting, can occur in some individuals even after a single low initial dose of PRM and may cause early interruption of treatment. These early adverse events were responsible for the higher rate of failures reported with PRM as compared with PB, PHT and CBZ in the VA Study [38]. Since acute toxicity has been shown to occur before PB and PEMA are detected in blood, it must therefore be caused by PRM itself. Tolerance to the side-effects of PRM develops rapidly, however, in a matter of hours to days. There is also some evidence that PB produces a cross-tolerance to acute PRM toxicity, as patients on long-term PB therapy are less prone to experience the same degree of toxicity when first exposed to PRM [13].

Overdose

PRM overdose causes signs of central nervous system depression, hypotonia, reduced deep tendon reflexes and marked crystalluria. Symptoms of central nervous system depression seem to correlate better with PRM plasma and cerebrospinal fluid levels than with PB or PEMA levels. Overdose should be treated with gastric lavage and supportive measures.

Clinical therapeutics

PRM is available only as oral formulation, i.e. 250-mg tablets. Because of the potential for acute adverse reactions occurring early in the treatment, it is important to begin with a small amount of the drug and to adopt a slow titration schedule. An average starting dose for an adult would be 125 mg at night, with increments every 3 days (or more) up to a final daily maintenance dose of 10–20 mg/kg. Because of the relatively short half-life of PRM, it is usually recommended to divide the daily dose into three doses, although the necessity to do so has never been documented.

There is a poor correlation between the oral dose of PRM and plasma levels of PRM or its derived PB. The VA Cooperative Study [38] suggests that the optimal mean plasma PRM level is 12 µg/mL with an associated PB level of 15 µg/mL, resulting in a PRM to PB ratio of 0.8. However, large variability occurs between patients and comedication with enzyme-inducing agents invariably lowers the PRM to PB ratio. Therefore although a therapeutic range of about 3–12 µg/mL has been suggested for PRM, monitoring PRM levels has very limited clinical value whereas monitoring the derived PB level is more useful in guiding therapy.

In summary, PRM is an intriguing drug because of its peculiar metabolic aspects. It is an antiepileptic drug in its own right, and also a PB prodrug. Most people believe, as does the author, that the main antiepileptic action of PRM is due to the derived PB; the contributory role of PRM itself or PEMA to the antiepileptic effects is controversial but is likely to be minor. The efficacy and tolerability profile of PRM does not differ significantly from that of PB and there is little reason to prescribe PRM instead of PB. When used, PRM has the same indications as PB, and since enzyme-inducing agents lower the PRM to PB ratio, it makes little sense to prescribe PRM in combination with such drugs.

Other barbiturates

Metharbital

Chemically, it is a 5,5-diethyl-1-methylbarbituric acid (Fig. 39.1). It is less polar than PB and more lipid soluble. There has been little interest in the drug for many years. There are no consistent published data on kinetics, clinical use and toxicity. Whether it has a role as an antiepileptic drug in contemporary practice is debatable.

Methylphenobarbital (or mephobarbital)

Chemistry

It is 5-ethyl-1-methyl-5-phenylbarbituric acid and is the N-methylated analogue of PB (Fig. 39.1). As usually supplied MPB is a racemic mixture (i.e. equal parts of the R(–) and S(+) enantiomers), with somewhat more lipophilic properties than PB, and has a pK$_a$ value of 7.8.

Kinetics and interactions

MPB is well absorbed but it undergoes appreciable presystemic metabolism; therefore oral bioavailability is about 75% [72]. MPB has a mean apparent volume of distribution of 132 L in adults, which is higher than that of PB; this correlates with the greater lipophilicity of the drug which tends to achieve higher concentrations in tissues than in plasma [3,14].

In human plasma, ~67% of the R enantiomer and ~59% of the S enantiomer were protein bound. In adults not being treated with other drugs, the mean half-life of the racemic MPB after the first oral dose is 49 ± 18.8 h, but it tends to be significantly shorter (19.6 ± 5 h) in comedicated patients with enzyme-inducing agents [3,14]. Moreover, continued MPB intake leads to the formation of considerable amounts of PB, which may cause significant induction of the body's capacity to biotransform this drug. The two enantiomers have different half-lives: 7.50 ± 1.7 h for the R enantiomer and 69.8 ± 14.8 h for the S enantiomer after a single oral dose. These differences reflect different clearance values, about 0.4 ± 0.18 L/kg/h for the R enantiomer and 0.017 ± 0.001 L/kg/h for the S enantiomer.

MPB is cleared from the human body almost entirely by means of biotransformation, since only 1.5–3% of the total amount of the drug administered orally is found unchanged in the urine [14]. The biotransformation of the drug is relatively stereoselective. The R enantiomer of MPB is metabolized mainly by aromatic hydroxylation (this being the pathway that is coregulated with mephenytoin hydroxylation) leading to the formation of phenolic, diol and O-methylcatechol derivatives; it may be also demethylated to PB. On the other hand, the S enantiomer is mainly oxidatively dealkylated to PB, though a small amount of hydroxylation occurs. From the standpoint of pharmacological activity, PB appears to be the significant biotransformation product. Therefore it is likely that any interaction that has been described for PB may also occur when MPB is the source of PB.

Clinical efficacy

MPB has the same indications as PB and, in nearly all clinical situations, PB and MPB may be considered interchangeable.

Toxicity

The tolerability profile of MPB is indistinguishable from that of PB. There seems to be no reason why any of the toxic manifestations of PB should not occur in patients taking MPB.

Clinical therapeutics

MPB has been marketed as 30-, 60- and 200-mg tablets. Considerations concerning dose titration, daily dosing and plasma serum concentrations are the same as PB. In general, there is only the need to use 1.7–2.0 mg of MPB for each milligram of PB to compensate the rapid elimination of the R enantiomer of MPB.

Although PB and MPB are virtually interchangeable, there is an argument for preferring MPB to PB. Within the range of plasma concentrations of PB usually encountered therapeutically, the relationship between steady-state plasma concentrations of PB and MPB dose is linear [73]. On the contrary, if PB itself is prescribed, the relationship in the individual between steady-state PB level and PB dose appears curvilinear [73]. Therefore, plasma concentrations of PB may be adjusted with a more predictable outcome when the drug is supplied as MPB than as PB itself. This may be part of the reason for the view that MPB is less likely than PB to produce unexpected side-effects and sedation.

Barbexaclone

BBC is the salt of the base propylhexedrine (indirect sympathomimetic) and PB. These two ingredients are contained in the proportions of 60% and 40%, respectively.

The kinetics of PB was compared after oral administration of equivalent doses of the drug as the acid or as the propylhexedrine salt (BBC) to seven normal volunteers. The absorption and elimination parameters were very similar and it was concluded that propylhexedrine did not affect the serum kinetics of PB given as BBC [74]. There has been a considerable interest in the use of BBC, mostly in the Italian and Spanish literature; several papers, mainly dealing with small series of patients openly receiving BBC as add-on or first-line agent or after switching from PB therapy, have claimed that this drug is at least as effective as PB but better tolerated, showing less sedative properties and improved compliance, both in adults and children. The favourable tolerability profile of BBC was attributed to the psychostimulant effect of propylhexedrine. These promising results, however, mostly published between 1977 and 1988, still await confirmation in controlled trials.

BBC is available as 25- and 100-mg tablets. Considerations concerning dose titration, daily dosing and plasma serum concentrations are the same as PB. When prescribing the drug, however, it should be remembered that 100 mg of BBC are equivalent to 60 mg of PB.

References

1 Hauptmann A. Luminal bei epilepsie. *Münch Med Wochenschr* 1912; 59: 1907–9.

2 Loiseau P, Duché B. Phenobarbital. In: Dam M, Gram L, eds. *Comprehensive Epileptology*. New York: Raven Press, 1990: 579–91.

3 Eadie MJ. Phenobarbital and other barbiturates. In: Engel J, Pedley TA, eds. *Epilepsy: a Comprehensive Textbook*. Philadelphia: Lippincott-Raven Publishers, 1997: 1547–55.

4 Anderson GD, Levy RH. Phenobarbital. Chemistry and biotransformation. In: Levy RH, Mattson RH, Meldrum BS, eds. *Antiepileptic Drugs*, 4th edn. New York: Raven Press, 1995: 371–7.

5 Prichard JW, Ranson BR. Phenobarbital. Mechanisms of action. In: Levy RH, Mattson RH, Meldrum BS, eds. *Antiepileptic Drugs*, 4th edn. New York: Raven Press, 1995: 359–69.

6 Dodson WE, Rust RS. Phenobarbital. Absorption, distribution, and excretion. In: Levy RH, Mattson RH, Meldrum BS, eds. *Antiepileptic Drugs*, 4th edn. New York: Raven Press, 1995: 379–87.

7 Kutt H. Phenobarbital. Interactions with other drugs. In: Levy RH, Mattson RH, Meldrum BS, eds. *Antiepileptic Drugs*, 4th edn. New York: Raven Press, 1995: 389–99.

8 Painter MJ, Gaus LM. Phenobarbital. Clinical use. In: Levy RH, Mattson RH, Meldrum BS, eds. *Antiepileptic Drugs*, 4th edn. New York: Raven Press, 1995: 401–7.

9 Cramer JA, Mattson RH. Phenobarbital. Toxicity. In: Levy RH, Mattson RH, Meldrum BS, eds. *Antiepileptic Drugs*, 4th edn. New York: Raven Press, 1995: 409–20.

10 Booker HE. Phenobarbital. Relation of plasma concentration to seizure control. In: Woodbury DM, Penry JK, Pippenger DE, eds. *Antiepileptic Drugs*. New York: Raven Press, 1982: 341–50.

11 Cloyd JC, Leppik IE, Primidone. Absorption, distribution and excretion. In: Levy RH, Mattson RH, Meldrum BS, eds. *Antiepileptic Drugs*, 4th edn. New York: Raven Press, 1995: 459–66.

12 Bourgeois BFD. Primidone. In: Resor SR, Kutt H, eds. *The Medical Treatment of Epilepsy*. New York: Marcel Dekker, 1992: 371–8.

13 Leppik IE, Cloyd JC. Primidone. Toxicity. In: Levy RH, Mattson RH, Meldrum BS, eds. *Antiepileptic Drugs*, 4th edn. New York: Raven Press, 1995: 487–90.

14 Eadie MJ, Hooper WD. Other barbiturates. Methylphenobarbital and metharbital. In: Levy RH, Mattson RH, Meldrum BS, eds. *Antiepileptic Drugs*, 4th edn. New York: Raven Press, 1995: 421–37.

15 Stark LG, Killam KF, Killam EK. The anticonvulsant effects of phenobarbital, diphenylhydantoin and two benzodiazepines in the baboon, *Papio papio*. *J Pharmacol Exp Therap* 1970; 173: 125–32.

16 Snead OC. Pharmacological models of generalised absence seizures in rodents. *J Neural Transm* 1992; 35: 7–19.

17 Delorey TM, Olsen RW. γ-Aminobutyric acid_A receptor structure and function. *J Biol Chem* 1992; 267: 6747–50.

18 Twyman RE, Rogers CJ, Macdonald RL. Differential regulation of γ-aminobutyric acid receptor channels by diazepam and phenobarbital. *Ann Neurol* 1989; 25: 213–20.

19 Pritchett DB, Sontheimer H, Shivers BD *et al*. Importance of a novel GABA_A receptor subunit for benzodiazepine pharmacology. *Nature* 1989; 338: 582–4.

20 Rabow LE, Russek SJ, Farb DH. From ion currents to genomic analysis: recent advances in GABA_A receptor research. *Synapse* 1995; 21: 189–274.

21 Viswanathan CT, Booker HE, Welling PG. Bioavailability of oral and intramuscular phenobarbital. *J Clin Pharmacol* 1978; 18: 100–5.

22 Nelson E, Powell JR, Conrad K *et al*. Phenobarbital pharmacokinetics and bioavailability in adults. *J Clin Pharmacol* 1982; 22: 141–8.

23 Wilensky AJ, Friel PN, Levy RH, Comfort CP, Kaluzny SP. Kinetics of phenobarbital in normal subjects and epileptic patients. *Eur J Clin Pharmacol* 1982; 23: 87–92.

24 Jalling B. Plasma concentrations of phenobarbital in the treatment of seizures in the newborn. *Acta Paediatr Scand* 1975; 64: 514–24.

25 Johannessen SI, Strandjord RE. Absorption and protein binding in serum of several antiepileptic drugs. In: Schneider H, Janz D, Gardner-Thorpe C, Meinardi M, Sherwin AL, eds. *Clinical Pharmacology of Antiepileptic Drugs*. Berlin: Springer, 1975: 262–73.

26 Nau H, Rating D, Hauser I, Jager E, Kock S, Helge H. Placental transfer and pharmacokinetics of primidone and its metabolites, phenobarbital, PEMA, and hydroxyphenobarbital in neonates and infants of epileptic mothers. *Eur J Clin Pharmacol* 1980; 18: 31–42.

27 Pitlick W, Painter M, Pippenger C. Phenobarbital pharmacokinetics in neonates. *Clin Pharmacol Ther* 1978; 23: 346–50.

28 Svensmark O, Buchtal F. Accumulation of phenobarbital in man. *Epilepsia* 1963; 4: 199–206.

29 Jalling P. Plasma and cerebrospinal fluid concentrations of PB in infants given single doses. *Dev Med Child Neurol* 1974; 11: 781–93.

30 Neimann G, Gladtke E. Pharmacokinetics of phenobarbital in childhood. *Eur J Clin Pharmacol* 1977; 12: 305.

31 Berg JM, Berlinger WG, Goldberg MJ, Spector R, Johnson GF. Acceleration of the body clearance of phenobarbital by oral activated charcoal. *N Engl J Med* 1982; 307: 642–4.

32 Vesell ES, Page JG. Genetic control of the phenobarbital-induced shortening of plasma antipyrine half-lives in man. *J Clin Invest* 1969; 48: 2202–9.

33 Perucca E, Gatti G, Frigo GM, Crema A, Calzetti S, Visintini D. Disposition of sodium valproate in epileptic patients. *Br J Clin Pharmcol* 1978; 5: 495–9.

34 Rettie AE, Rettenmeier AW, Howald WN, Baillie TA. Cytochrome P-450-catalyzed formation of delta-four VPA, a toxic metabolite of valproic acid. *Science* 1987; 235: 890–3.

35 Liu H, Delgado MR. Interactions of phenobarbital and phenytoin with carbamazepine and its metabolites' concentrations, concentration ratios, and level/dose ratios in epileptic children. *Epilepsia* 1995; 36: 249–54.

36 Shahidi NT. Acetophenetiden-induced methemoglobinemia. *Ann NY Acad Sci* 1968; 151: 822–31.

37 Kapetanovic IM, Kupferberg HJ, Porter RJ, Theodore W, Schulman E, Penry JK. Mechanism of valproate–phenobarbital interaction in epileptic patients. *Clin Pharmacol Ther* 1981; 29: 480–6.

38 Mattson RH, Cramer JA, Collins JF *et al*. Comparison of carbamazepine, phenobarbital, phenytoin, and primidone in partial and secondarily generalised tonic-clonic seizures. *N Engl J Med* 1985; 313: 145–51.

39 Feely M, O'Callaghan M, Duggan G, Callaghan N. Phenobarbitone in previously untreated epilepsy. *J Neurol Neurosurg Psychiatr* 1980; 43: 365–8.

40 Schmidt D, Einicke I, Haenel F. The influence of seizure type on the efficacy of plasma concentrations of phenytoin, phenobarbital and carbamazepine. *Arch Neurol* 1986; 43: 263–5.

41 Heller AJ, Chesterman P, Elwes RDC *et al*. Phenobarbitone, phenytoin, carbamazepine, or sodium valproate for newly diagnosed adult epilepsy: a randomised comparative monotherapy trial. *J Neurol Neurosurg Psychiatr* 1995; 58: 44–50.

42 deSilva M, MacArdle B, McGowan M *et al*. Randomised comparative monotherapy trial of phenobarbitone, phenytoin, carbamazepine, or sodium valproate for newly diagnosed childhood epilepsy. *Lancet* 1996; 347: 709–13.

43 Mitchell W, Chavez J. Carbamazepine versus phenobarbital for partial onset seizures in children. *Epilepsia* 1987; 28: 56–60.

44 Lockman LA, Kriel R, Zaske D. Phenobarbital dosage for control of neonatal seizures. *Neurology* 1979; 29: 1445–9.

45 VanOrman CB, Darrvish HZ. Efficacy of phenobarbital in neonatal seizures. *Can J Neurol Sci* 1985; 12: 95–9.

46 Painter MJ, Pippenger CE, Wasterlain C *et al*. Phenobarbital and phenytoin in neonatal seizures: metabolism and tissue distribution. *Neurology* 1981; 31: 1107–12.

47 Gal P, Tobock J, Boer H, Erkan N, Wells T. Efficacy of phenobarbital monotherapy in treatment of neonatal seizures – relationship to blood levels. *Neurology* 1982; 32: 1401–4.

48 Painter MJ, Scher MS, Stein AD *et al*. Phenobarbital compared with phenytoin for the treatment of neonatal seizures. *N Engl J Med* 1999; 341: 485–9.

49 Goldberg MA, McIntyre HB. Barbiturates in the treatment of status epilepticus. In: Delgado-Escueta AV, Wasterlain CG, Treiman DM, Porter RJ, eds. *Advances in Neurology: Status Epilepticus*, Vol. 34. New York: Raven Press, 1983: 499–503.

50 Shaner MD, McCurdy S, Herring M, Gabor A. Treatment of status epilepticus: a prospective comparison of diazepam and phenytoin versus phenobarbital and optional phenytoin. *Neurology* 1988; 38: 202–7.

51 Leppik IE, Sherwin AL. Intravenous phenytoin and phenobarbital: anticonvulsant action, brain content, and plasma binding in the rat. *Epilepsia* 1979; 20: 201–7.

52 Faero O, Kastrup KW, Nielsen E, Melchior JC, Thorn I. Successful prophylaxis of febrile convulsions with phenobarbital. *Epilepsia* 1972; 13: 279–85.

53 Crawley J, Waruiru C, Mithwani S *et al*. Effect of phenobarbital on seizure frequency and mortality in childhood cerebral malaria: a randomised, controlled intervention study. *Lancet* 2000; 355: 701–6.

54 Verhoef H, West CE, Kok FJ. Phenobarbital for children with cerebral malaria. *Lancet* 2000; 356: 256.

55 Wolf SM, Forsythe A. Psychology, pharmacotherapy and new diagnostic approaches. In: Meinardi H, Rowan AJ, eds. *Advances in Epileptology*. Amsterdam: Swets & Zeitlinger, 1977: 124–7.

56 Farwell JR, Lee YJ, Hirtz DG, Sulzbacher SI, Ellenberg JH, Nelson KB. Phenobarbital for febrile seizures – effects on intelligence and on seizure recurrence. *N Engl J Med* 1990; 322: 364–9.

57 Vining EPG, Mellits ED, Dorsen MM *et al*. Psychologic and behavioural effects of antiepileptic drugs in children: a double-blind comparison between phenobarbitone and valproic acid. *Pediatrics* 1987; 80: 165–74.

58 Gupta RC, Kofoed J. Toxicological statistics for barbiturates, other sedatives, and tranquillizers in Ontario: a 10-year survey. *Can Med Ass J* 1966; 94: 863–5.

59 Mountain KR, Hirsch J, Gallus AS. Neonatal coagulation defect due to anticonvulsant drug treatment in pregnancy. *Lancet* 1970; 1: 265–8.

60 De Santis A, Ceccarelli G, Cesana BM, Bello L, Spagnoli D, Villani RM.

Shoulder–hand syndrome in neurosurgical patients treated with barbiturates. A long term evaluation. *J Neurosurg Sci* 2000; 44: 69–75.

61 Kaneko S, Kondo Y. Antiepileptic agents and birth defects: incidence, mechanism and prevention. *CNS Drugs* 1995: 3641–55.

62 Holmes LB, Harvey EA, Coull BA *et al.* The teratogenicity of anticonvulsant drugs. *N Engl J Med* 2001; 344: 1132–8.

63 Buchthal F, Svensmark O, Simonsen H. Relation of EEG and seizures to phenobarbital in serum. *Arch Neurol* 1968; 19: 567–72.

64 Baumel IP, Gallagher BB, Di Micco D, Goico H. Metabolism and anticonvulsant properties of primidone in the rat. *J Pharmacol Exp Ther* 1973; 186: 305–14.

65 Bourgeois BFD, Dodson WE, Ferrendelli JA. Primidone, phenobarbital and PEMA. I. Seizure protection, neurotoxicity and therapeutic index of individual compounds in mice. *Neurology* 1983; 33: 283–90.

66 Macdonald RL, McLean MJ. Anticonvulsant drugs. mechanisms of action. In: Delgado-Escueta AV, Ward AA, Woodbury DM, Porter RJ, eds. *Basic Mechanisms of the Epilepsies: Molecular and Cellular Approaches.* New York: Raven Press, 1986: 713–36.

67 Gallagher BB, Baumel IP, Mattson RH. Metabolic disposition of primidone and its metabolites in epileptic subjects after single and repeated administration. *Neurology* 1972; 22: 1186–92.

68 Oleson OV, Dam M. The metabolic conversion of primidone to phenobarbitone in patients under long-term treatment. *Acta Neurol Scand* 1967; 43: 348–56.

69 Battino D, Avanzini G, Bossi L *et al.* Plasma levels of primidone and its metabolite phenobarbital: effect of age and associated therapy. *Ther Drug Monit* 1983; 5: 73–9.

70 Oxley J, Hebdige S, Laidlaw J, Wadsworth J, Richens A. A comparative study of phenobarbitone and primidone in the treatment of epilepsy. In: Johannessen SI, Morselli PL, Pippenger CE, Richens A, Schmidt D, Meinardi H, eds. *Antiepileptic Therapy. Advances in Drug Monitoring.* New York: Raven Press, 1980: 237–45.

71 Rating D, Nau H, Jäger-Roman E *et al.* Teratogenic and pharmacokinetic studies of primidone during pregnancy and in the offspring of epileptic women. *Acta Paediatr Scand* 1982; 71: 301–11.

72 Hooper WD, Kunze HE, Eadie MJ. Pharmacokinetics and bioavailability of methylphenobarbital in man. *Ther Drug Monit* 1981; 3: 39–44.

73 Eadie MJ, Lander CM, Hooper WD, Tyrer JH. Factors influencing plasma phenobarbitone levels in epileptic patients. *Br J Clin Pharmacol* 1977; 4: 541–7.

74 Perucca E, Grimaldi R, Ruberto G, Gelmi C, Trimarchi F, Crema A. Comparative kinetics of phenobarbital after administration of the acid and the propylhexedrine salt (barbexaclone). *Eur J Clin Pharmacol* 1986; 29: 729–30.

40 Phenytoin

M.J. Eadie

Primary indications	First-line or adjunctive therapy for partial and generalized seizures (excluding myoclonus and absence). Also for status epilepticus
Usual preparations	Capsules: 25, 30, 50, 100, 200 mg; chewtabs: 50 mg; liquid suspension: 30 mg/5 mL, 125 mg/50 mL; injection: 250 mg/5 mL
Usual dosages	Orally: 5 mg/kg/day (adults), 10 mg/kg/day (children); higher maintenance doses can be used guided by serum level monitoring and clinical response
Dosage intervals	1–2 times/day
Significant drug interactions	Phenytoin has a large number of interactions with antiepileptic and other drugs
Serum level monitoring	Useful
Target range	10–20 mg/L (40–80 μmol/L)
Common/important side-effects	Ataxia, dizziness, lethargy, sedation, headaches, dyskinesia, acute encephalopathy, hypersensitivity, rash, fever, blood dyscrasia, gingival hyperplasia, folate deficiency, megaloblastic anaemia, vitamin K deficiency, thyroid dysfunction, decreased immunoglobulins, mood changes, depression, coarsened facies, hirsutism, peripheral neuropathy, osteomalacia, hypocalcaemia, hormonal dysfunction, loss of libido, connective tissue alterations, pseudolymphoma, hepatitis, vasculitis, myopathy, coagulation defects, bone marrow hypoplasia
Main advantages	Highly effective and cheap antiepileptic drug
Main disadvantages	CNS and systemic side-effects; non-linear elimination kinetics
Mechanisms of action	Blockade of voltage-dependent sodium channels
Oral bioavailability	95%
Time to peak levels	4–12 h
Metabolism and excretion	Hepatic oxidation and hydroxylation, then conjugation
Volume of distribution	0.5–0.8 L/kg
Elimination half-life	7–42 h (mean, 20 h: dependent on plasma level)
Plasma clearance	0.003–0.02 L/kg/h in adults (dependent on plasma level)
Protein binding	85–95%
Active metabolites	None
Comment	Well-established first-line therapy. The side-effects profile and elimination kinetics may make it less desirable than carbamazepine in some patients

(*Note*: this summary table was formulated by the lead editor.)

Phenytoin was the first effective antiepileptic substance developed as the outcome of a systematic scientifically based screening process rather than chance discovery. The phenytoin molecule had been synthesized early in the 20th century, but was not initially considered as a possible antiepileptic agent. This was in part because at the time it was thought antiepileptic drugs must also have sedative properties as was the case for the bromides and phenobarbital. Phenytoin was a relatively mild sedative. The discovery of its antiepileptic potential was made by Putnam and Merritt, who in the late 1930s, sought from various chemical suppliers substances containing phenyl substituents and with a molecular structural resemblance to phenobarbital. This was in the belief that an aromatic ring substituent in members of a family of molecules probably enhanced any antiepileptic properties that were present in that family, as was the case for the barbiturates [1]. The substances were tested in an animal model of convulsive epileptic seizures, and phenytoin proved to combine antiseizure efficacy with a relative lack of sedation. The drug remains in quite extensive use worldwide more than 60 years after its introduction into therapeutics, and has served as the paradigm for the development of most of the subsequent antiepileptic substances which have been marketed. A number of accounts of the discovery of the drug are available, for example those of Glazko [1] and Friedlander [2].

Chemistry

Phenytoin (5,5′-diphenylhydantoin) for therapeutic use is usually provided as the free acid (molecular weight 252.3), or, more commonly, as the sodium salt (molecular weight 274.3). The molecular structure of phenytoin is shown in Fig. 40.1. It is a white crystalline, relatively poorly water-soluble acidic substance ($pK_a \sim 8.4$). The sodium salt is the more water soluble of the two, and is generally supplied in capsules or as a parenteral injection (pH about 12). The corresponding acid is available in tablets or in an oral suspension.

On a milligram-for-milligram basis, preparations of the drug in the form of the sodium salt contain about 8% less active substance than preparations containing the drug as the free acid.

Many methods have been described for measuring phenytoin at the concentrations at which it is present in the human body after therapeutic dosage. The early methods were chemical or spectrophotometric, but the drug at the present time is usually measured by one of a variety of immunoassays or, to measure other antiepileptic drugs simultaneously, by chromatographic methods, mainly high-performance liquid chromatography.

Pharmacodynamics

Molecular mechanisms

The antiepileptic effect of phenytoin is thought to depend on the drug's capacity to bind to, and prolong the inactivation of mammalian, including human [3], voltage-dependent Na^+ channels in neuronal cell membranes [4]. This effect is greater when the cell membrane is depolarized than when it is hyperpolarized. With repeated depolarizations the ion channel block becomes use dependent. Phenytoin binds to the same site on the outer surface of the cell membrane Na^+ channel as that to which carbamazepine and lamotrigine bind [5]. However phenytoin and carbamazepine have different binding affinities to this site [6] and quantitatively, though not qualitatively, possess somewhat different actions [4]. Inactivation of voltage- and frequency-dependent Na^+ channels makes partly depolarized axons less capable of transmitting rapid trains of action potentials (such as occur in epileptic discharges). However, there is less interference with action potential traffic which passes along axons at lower impulse frequencies.

Phenytoin at high concentration may also inhibit axonal and nerve terminal Ca^{2+} channels and this action might stabilize axonal cell membranes and diminish neurotransmitter release at axon ter-

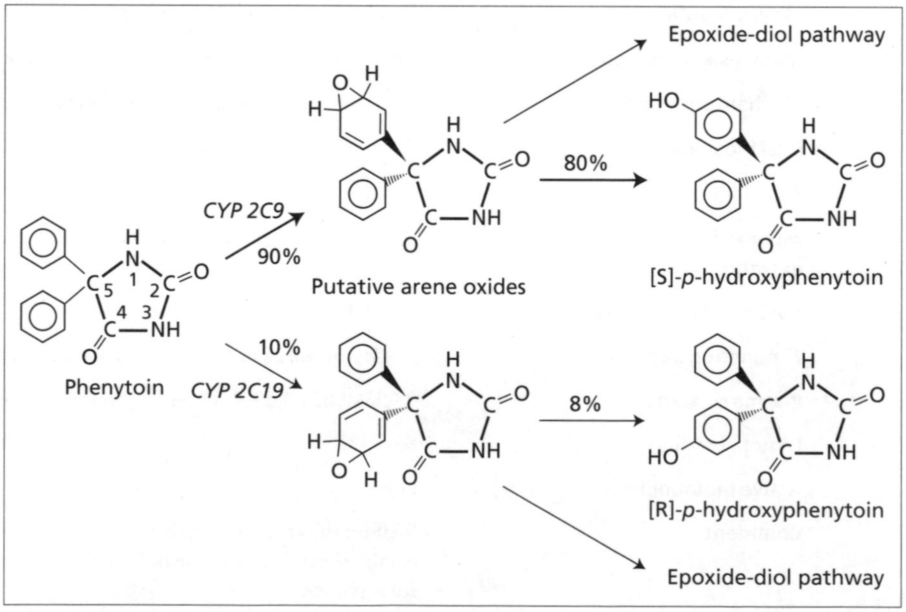

Fig. 40.1 Formulae for phenytoin and its known and putative stereoisomeric metabolites along the drug's major biotransformation pathway to p-hydroxyphenytoin.

minals in response to action potentials. However, the drug has no effect on the function of the T-type Ca^{2+} channels in the thalamus, which are important in the genesis of absence seizures [4]. Phenytoin at high concentrations inhibits Ca^{2+} calmodulin-mediated protein phosporylations [7]. The drug binds to the peripheral type of benzodiazepine receptor in brain membranes [8], but it is not clear whether this action leads to any antiepileptic effect. Phenytoin also has mild dopamine antagonist effects.

Electrophysiological effects

Phenytoin's inhibitory action on fast action potential traffic along axons results in various well-documented electrophysiological effects, for instance its ability in experimental preparations to prevent post-tetanic potentiation of synaptic transmission [9], and the fact that it tends not so much to suppress spike formation at experimental epileptic foci, as to prevent spike discharges spreading from such foci.

Effects in animal models of epileptic seizures

In various animal models of convulsive epileptic seizures (notably the maximal electroshock model) phenytoin has been shown effective in preventing or reducing the severity of induced seizures. The drug has also proved effective in models of partial (localization-related) epileptic seizures, for instance electrically or chemically kindled focal seizures in rats [10]. The drug is relatively ineffective against generalized seizures provoked by systemically administered chemical convulsants. Phenytoin also proved ineffective in what in the past were taken as animal models of absence seizures, but which are probably now better regarded as models of myoclonic seizures for instance pentylenetetrazole seizures. Phenytoin has also proved ineffective in preventing the attacks in the more recently developed and more realistic animal models of absence seizure, for instance the lethargic mouse and the rat with generalized absence epilepsy [10].

Pharmacokinetics

Absorption

The absorption rate of the drug from different oral preparations may vary. The importance of formulation was demonstrated 30 years ago when the oral bioavailability of phenytoin in the market leader's capsule formulation of the drug in Australasia changed due to an interaction between the drug in the capsule and the excipient calcium sulphate [11]. Since that time the usual branded preparation has a lactose excipient and in this formulation, phenytoin has a consistent and complete, or nearly complete (~95%) oral bioavailability. However reports continue to be published of generic phenytoin tablets whose oral bioavailabilities appear incomplete and to an extent inconsistent. The storage of phenytoin capsules under conditions of high temperature and humidity may also reduce the oral bioavailability of the drug [12]. Earlier reports suggested that the bioavailability of orally administered phenytoin was impaired during pregancy [13], but subsequent studies have shown that the drug has a reasonably complete oral bioavailability in this situation [14]. The topic of the bioavailability of phenytoin is reviewed by Neurvonen [15]. Variations in bioavailability should be unimpor-

tant clinically provided the same preparation of the drug is used in any individual patient.

Phenytoin is absorbed very slowly and inconsistently from intramuscular injection sites, making this route of administration unsatisfactory in clinical practice. Intravenous phenytoin is fully bioavailable, but the highly alkaline pH of the solution, and the presence of polyethylene glycol in it, make its very slow administration prudent to minimize unwanted effects. The drug may crystallize out if injected into any intravenous fluid reservoir containing a solution at a more physiological pH. The introduction of the phenytoin prodrug, fosphenytoin (see Chapter 34), is an attempt to overcome these practical issues.

The rectal bioavailability of phenytoin is low, around $24\pm3\%$ [16].

Distribution

After absorption, phenytoin is distributed throughout total body water, with relatively little selective regional concentration. Published values for the drug's apparent volume of distribution in humans have usually been in the range 0.5–0.8 L/kg. In the brain the drug comes to achieve a slightly higher concentration than in plasma. At steady state, it is present at a higher concentration in white than in grey matter, though soon after administration its concentrations are temporarily higher in grey matter [17]. Phenytoin is transported out of the brain by P-glycoprotein activity [18].

In whole blood the phenytoin concentration in red cells is lower than in plasma, so that whole blood phenytoin concentrations are lower than the simultaneous whole plasma (or serum) concentrations of the drug [19]. Some 90% of the phenytoin in plasma is bound to plasma proteins, mainly albumin [20]. The unbound fraction of the drug in plasma is higher in the neonate than the adult [21], and increases a little with advanced age [20], in later pregnancy [22], and in the presence of hypoalbuminaemia, as occurs in malnutrition, liver disease, nephrotic or uraemic states, AIDS, and with high levels of glycated albumin, as occur in diabetics [23]. Phenytoin concentrations in cerebrospinal fluid [24], routinely collected saliva [25], tears and sweat are very similar to simultaneous concentrations of the drug in plasma water. However, the saliva phenytoin concentration does vary with saliva flow rate and in the presence of gum disease [26]. Concentrations of the drug in maternal milk are lower (~19%) [27] than those simultaneously present in whole plasma, and to an extent vary with the fat and protein content of the milk. It is very unlikely that a breastfed infant would receive enough phenytoin from breast milk to produce any adverse effects, unless the mother was very substantially overdosed with the drug.

A number of acidic drugs, e.g. salicylates, valproate and certain endogenous substances (fatty acids, bilirubin), appear capable of displacing phenytoin from its plasma protein binding sites. In practice, such displacement is rarely of importance clinically.

Elimination

Very little phenytoin is excreted in urine as unchanged substance (Fu (∞) < 0.05). The great majority of a phenytoin dose is eliminated by hepatic metabolism. The main known metabolic pathways for the drug are indicated in Figs 40.1 and 40.2. Nearly all of the

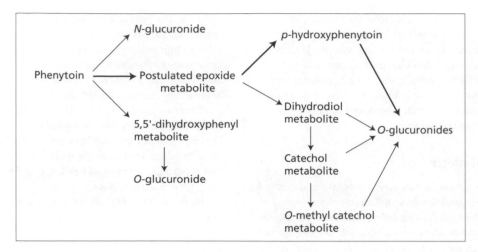

Fig. 40.2 Known metabolic pathways for phenytoin.

body's metabolism of the drug appears to occur in the liver, though some conversion of phenytoin to its major metabolite *p*-hydroxyphenytoin occurs in the gums and perhaps in other peripheral tissues, e.g. neutrophil leucocytes [28]. The major metabolite of phenytoin found in urine, *p*-hydroxyphenytoin (HPPH: 5-phenyl,5′-*p*-hydroxyphenylhydantoin), mainly in the form of its *O*-glucuronide conjugate, accounts for the elimination of some 60–80% of usual doses of the drug. This particular oxidative metabolite is formed via a postulated short-lived arene oxide intermediate in a reaction catalysed by the CYP450 isoforms 2C9 and 2C19 (Fig. 40.1). CYP2C9 activity accounts for some 90% of the metabolism of the drug in humans, at conventional dosage. *p*-Hydroxyphenytoin exists in the body in two stereoisomeric forms, the [S]-isomer being formed preferentially via CYP2C9 activity and the [R]-isomer via activity of 2C19 [29]. The glucuronide conjugate of the [S]-isomer of *p*-hydroxyphenytoin is the predominant one in human urine [29], accounting for 75–95% of the total phenytoin metabolite present. Neither *p*-hydroxyphenytoin isomer possesses any known biological activity [30], nor is either likely to achieve a high enough concentration in the plasma of patients with intact renal function to exercise any feedback inhibition on the biotransformation of phenytoin [31]. There is tentative evidence that the postulated arene oxide intermediate and also the postulated epoxide products of the drug's metabolism may interact with various tissue proteins and that the reaction products formed may be responsible for some unwanted effects of the drug. Poor metabolizers of mephenytoin (methoin) form relatively little of the [R]-isomer of *p*-hydroxyphenytoin [32]. About one per 500 of the Japanese population is a slow hydroxylator of phenytoin [33], and hereditary poor metabolizers of the drug have been encountered in other populations [34]. Mutations of the *CYP2C9* gene appear to be responsible for the slow metabolism.

Dickinson *et al.* [35] showed that, early in the course of its administration, phenytoin is capable of a degree of autoinduction of its own metabolism, via the *p*-hydroxy phenytoin pathway. The autoinduction process appears to involve CYP2C19 more than CYP2C9 [29]. The magnitude of the autoinduction is relatively small and the process is self-limiting.

Various minor metabolites of phenytoin have been described

(Fig. 40.2), mostly additional derivatives of the arene oxide pathway, e.g. *m*-hydroxyphenytoin (possibly an analytical artefact), dihydrodiol, catechol, *O*-methyl catechol derivatives, and a molecule *para*-hydroxylated on each aromatic ring. A possible hydantoin ring-opened product and a *N*-glucuronide conjugate of the drug have also been described [36].

Unlike most drugs, phenytoin does not exhibit linear kinetics at clinical dosages. The Michaelis constant of phenytoin is around 6 mg/L (24 μmol), lower than the usual plasma concentration in clinical practice. It is possible to calculate the half-life and clearance values for phenytoin, and this has often been done in the literature. However, these values are not constant for the individual. They vary depending on the concentration range of the drug over which they have been measured, the half-life being longer, and the clearance lower, at higher plasma phenytoin concentrations than at lower. Typical dose–concentration curves are shown in Fig. 40.3. A representative published value for the half-life of phenytoin over the concentration range likely to be encountered in treatment in humans would be the 22±9 h determined by Arnold and Gerber [37], with a clearance value for adults of 0.02 L/kg/h, and for children below 5 years of age of 0.06 L/kg/h. Numerous measurements of the Michaelis–Menten parameters of the drug both in individuals and in treated populations, have now been published. Most values of the K_m have been in the range 3–30 mg/L, with the mean around 6 mg/L (24 μmol). The maximum velocity of phenytoin elimination (V_{max}) has been in the range 6–16 mg/kg/day. The V_{max} is higher in young children than in adults [38].

The pharmacokinetic parameters are summarized in Table 40.1.

Clinical pharmacokinetics

Increasing phenytoin doses and the consequent increases in plasma phenytoin concentrations correlate with increasing degrees of seizure control in types of epilepsy responsive to the drug. Since the publications of Kutt *et al.* in 1964 [39] it has become widely accepted that plasma phenytoin concentrations in the range 10–20 mg/L (40–80 μmol) are usually associated with the best chance of achieving seizure control without producing manifestations of overdosage from the drug. This concentration range has come to be

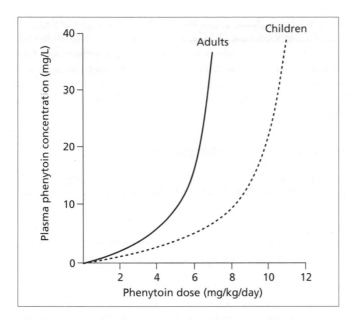

Fig. 40.3 Plot of mean steady-state plasma phenytoin concentration against drug dose in adults ($n=21$) and in children younger than 15 years ($n=15$), generated from the data of Eadie *et al.* [115] (mean K_m for adults 5.8 mg/L and for children 5.3 mg/L; mean V_{max} for adults 8.1 mg/kg/day, and for children 12.5 mg/kg/day).

Table 40.1 Phenytoin pharmacokinetic parameters

Absorption
Bioavailability (oral): ~ 0.95

Distribution
Apparent volume of distribution: 0.5–0.8 L/kg
Per cent protein bound: ~ 90%
Plasma water = CSF = saliva concentrations

Elimination
Per cent excreted in urine unmetabolized: < 5%
Half-life: 22 ± 9 h at 10–20 mg/L (40–80 μmol), but the value is
  concentration dependent
Clearance: adults 0.02 mL/kg/h; children 0.06 mL/kg/h, but the value is
  concentration dependent
Michaelis constant (K_m): ~ 6 mg/L (24 μmol)
Maximum velocity of elimination (V_{max}): adults 6–16 mg/kg/day;
  children higher
Time to steady state: ~ 1 week

Therapeutic range
Plasma: 10–20 mg/L or 7–25 mg/L (40–80 μmol or 28–100 μmol)
Plasma water: 1–2 mg/L (4–8 μmol)

accepted as the 'therapeutic' or 'target' range for the drug. However, certain authors, e.g. Loiseau [40], have set the lower limit of the range at around 7 mg/L (28 μmol), and the upper limit at 25 mg/L (100 μmol) [41]. Everyday clinical experience suggests that these wider limits are valid. There is evidence [42] that generalized tonic-clonic seizures may be fully controlled once plasma phenytoin levels are above 6–8 mg/L, but much higher levels may be needed before

partial seizures are controlled. Schmidt *et al.* [43] found a mean plasma phenytoin concentration of 14 mg/L (56 μmol) was associated with control of generalized tonic-clonic seizures, but a mean drug concentration of 23 mg/L (92 μmol) was needed before partial seizures were controlled. The therapeutic range values for the drug in plasma, water or saliva, are approximately one-tenth of those in whole plasma. In theory, it would be better always to measure the drug's concentration in plasma water, as this would obviate the effects of variation in the plasma protein binding of the drug in disease and in certain physiological states. In practice, the unbound (free) drug measurements are more expensive, and less accurate. They are rarely needed unless there is good reason to suspect altered plasma protein binding of the drug. The topic of the therapeutic range of plasma phenytoin concentrations is reviewed by Levine and Chang [44].

In practice, when plasma phenytoin concentrations are in the so-called 'therapeutic' or 'target' range of 10–20 mg/L (40–80 μmol), new steady-state conditions should apply some 4–8 days after a change in phenytoin dosage [24]. The delay will tend to be shorter at lower than higher plasma phenytoin concentrations. Under steady-state conditions in this drug concentration range the peak-to-trough fluctuation in plasma phenytoin concentration is likely to be of the order of ±10% over a 12-h dosage interval [45]. At lower phenytoin concentrations, under steady-state conditions, the inter-dosage fluctuations are likely to be wider.

There are wide interindividual variations in steady-state plasma phenytoin concentrations at conventional doses of the drug (300 or 400 mg/day) and an appreciable proportion of the values fall outside the therapeutic range. The correlation between dose and level is better if phenytoin dosage is expressed relative to body weight. As already mentioned, the maximum velocity of phenytoin biotransformation (or the clearance value) is higher in children than in adults [46]. A daily phenytoin dose of 5 mg/kg will yield a mean mid-therapeutic range steady-state plasma phenytoin concentration of 15 mg/L (60 μmol) in adults. However prepubertal children will need a mean daily phenytoin dose of 11 mg/kg to achieve a similar mean plasma drug concentration. The dose required is lower in neonates and in children in the first few months of life. It tends to be slightly lower in the elderly than in younger adults.

The pregnant woman's capacity to eliminate phenytoin begins to increase progressively after the first few weeks of pregnancy and plasma phenytoin concentrations, relative to drug dose, then begin to fall [47,48]. The drug concentration rises again to pre-pregnancy values over a few weeks after childbirth, if the drug dosage remains unchanged. This sequence of changes needs to be kept in mind if it is considered desirable to maintain plasma phenytoin concentrations at their pre-pregnancy values throughout the course of pregnancy, and afterwards. However, if this is done the reduced plasma protein binding of the drug in the third trimester of pregnancy needs to be taken into consideration. The altered disposition of the drug during pregnancy appears to be a consequence of increased drug metabolism. When Michaelis–Menten parameters of phenytoin during pregnancy were determined after intravenous administration of the stable isotope-labelled drug, and compared with those determined after parturition in the same women, Dickinson *et al.* [49] found the mean V_{max} had fallen from 1170 ± 600 mg/day to 780 ± 470 mg/day, and the K_m from 18.2 ± 8.4 to 10.2 ± 7.4 mg/L in whole plasma, and from 2.50 ± 0.85 mg/L to 1.16 ± 0.65 mg/L in plasma water. The latter change, and the change in the mean V_{max}, were statistically significant.

There may also be a premenstrual and menstrual fall in plasma (and saliva) phenytoin concentrations in some women, and this may correlate with the occurrence of breakthrough seizures, i.e. catamenial epilepsy [50].

In clinical practice, there will often be a need to adjust a patient's initial phenytoin dosage to achieve steady-state plasma phenytoin concentrations within a particular range of values or to adjust the continuing phenytoin dosage to maintain values in this range. Because of the Michaelis–Menten elimination kinetics of the drug, the steady-state plasma phenytoin concentrations will increase out of proportion to the relative size of an increase in phenytoin dosage [51] (Fig. 40.3). Failure to realize this, leading to prescribing phenytoin dosage increments in the expectation that the drug's plasma concentrations and effects will increase in proportion to the dosage increase, frequently results in the development of phenytoin intoxication. This phenomenon makes phenytoin dosage adjustment difficult in the hands of the uninformed.

In severe liver and renal disease the reduced plasma protein binding capacity for phenytoin needs to be taken into consideration when interpreting phenytoin concentrations in whole plasma. In such circumstances, measurement of plasma water, or salivary, phenytoin concentrations is likely to provide more reliable information.

Drug interactions

Phenytoin undergoes numerous reported interactions with endogenous biological substances and coadministered drugs [52–55]. A few of these interactions are pharmacodynamic in nature, and then mainly involve the occurrence of additional sedative effects when other drugs with sedative properties are taken. The great majority of interactions are pharmacokinetic in nature, and nearly all involve altered rates of metabolism of one or both drugs (see Tables 40.2–40.4). The individual interactions that have been described are now so numerous that limitations of space preclude their detailed discussion. The outcomes of many of them are listed in Tables 40.3–40.5. Their possible mechanisms are discussed below, but it should be pointed out that some of the recorded interactions

Table 40.2 Interactions which alter phenytoin absorption

Substances which may decrease the oral bioavailability of phenytoin
Antacids, calcium sulfate (within phenytoin capsules), charcoal (activated), protein hydrolysates for enteric feeding, sucralfate, theophylline

Table 40.3 Interactions which alter phenytoin distribution

Substances causing phenytoin displacement from plasma protein binding sites
Acetazolamide, ceftriaxone, diazoxide, heparin, ibuprofen, nafacillin, oxacillin, primidone, salicylates, sulphamethoxazole, tolbutamide, valproate

have unknown or uncertain mechanisms. Some interactions occur inconsistently, possibly because they involve more multiple mechanisms which can be mutually antagonistic. Therefore the final outcome of a given interaction can be the sum of two opposing processes, each of which may vary from person to person, and also in extent depending on the concentrations of the interacting substances.

Interactions affecting phenytoin absorption

Examples include the interaction between phenytoin and the calcium sulphate excipient which led to a local outbreak of phenytoin

Table 40.4 Metabolic interactions involving phenytoin

Interacting substances causing raised phenytoin concentrations
Allopurinol, amiodarone,[a] amphotericin, azapropazone,[a] carbamazepine, chloramphenicol, chlordiazepoxide, chlorpromazine, cimetidine,[b] clobazam, clofibrate, co-trimozazole,[a] dexamethasone, dextropropoxyphene,[a] diazepam,[b] dicoumarol, diltiazem, disulfiram, erythromycin, ethanol (acute intake), ethosuximide, famotidine, felbamate,[b] fluconazole,[a] fluctyosine, fluvoxamine,[a, b] fluoxetine,[b] halothane, imipramine,[b] isoniazid,[a] itraconazole, ketoconazole,[b] losarten,[a] methsuximide, methoin,[b] methylphenidate, methylphenobarbital,[b] metronidazole,[a] miconazole,[a] namifidone, nifedipine, nor-diazepam,[b] omeprazole,[b] paroxetine,[a] phenylacetylurea, pheneturide, phenylbutazone,[a] phenyramidol, pindolol, prochlorperazine, progabide, proguanyl,[b] propranolol,[b] ranitidine, remacemide, sertraline,[a] stiripentol,[a] sulfaphenazole,[a] sulthiame, thioridazine, ticlopidine,[a,b] tolbutamide,[a] topiramate,[b] torsemide,[a] trazoclone, trimethoprim,[a] troxidone, valproate, verapamil, viloxazine, [S]-warfarin[a]

Interacting substances causing lowered phenytoin concentrations
Aciclovir, aspirin, carbamazepine,[d] ciprofloxacin, cisplatin, dexamethasone, diazepam, diazoxide, dichloralphenazone, doxycycline, ethanol (chronic intake), folate, methotrexate, nitrofurantoin, oxacillin, phenobarbital, pyridoxine, reserpine, rifampicin,[c,d] salicylates, theophylline, tolbutamide, vigabatrin, vinblastine.

Phenytoin causing raised concentrations of interacting substances
Chloramphenicol, phenobarbital, tirilazad, warfarin

Phenytoin causing lowered concentrations of interacting substances
Antipyrine, atorvastatin, bromphenac, carbamazepine, chloramphenicol, clobazam, clonazepam, clozapine, ciclosporin, dexamethasone, dicoumarol, digoxin, disopyramide, doxycycline, felbamate, flunarizine, haloperidol, itraconazole, lamotrigine, lidocaine, methadone, metyrapone, mexilitine, midazolam, misonidazole, nisoldapine, nortriptyline, oral contraceptives, oxazepam, paracetamol, pethidine, phenazone, phenobarbital, prednisolone, primidone, praziquantel, quinidine, all *trans*- and β-*cis*-retinoic acid, simvastatin, theophylline, topiramate, tricyclic antidepressants, valproate, warfarin, zonisamide

Data from [52–55].
[a] Known substrate and/or inhibitor of CYP2C9.
[b] Known inhibitor and/or substrate of CYP2C19.
[c] Known inducer of CYP2C9.
[d] Known inducer of CYP2C19.

Table 40.5 More common and/or more serious adverse effects of phenytoin

Nervous system	Nystagmus, gait ataxia, diplopia, dyskinesias, mood and cognitive changes, depressed consciousness
Skin	Morbilliform rash in 5–10%, systemic lupus erythematosus, Stevens–Johnson syndrome, exfoliative dermatitis, epidermal necrolysis
Hypersensitivity	Aromatic anticonvulsant hypersensitivity syndrome
Gums	Hypertrophy
Bone	Osteomalacia
Reticuloendothelial	Lymphadenopathy (pseudolymphoma), megaloblastic anaemia, suppression of individual blood cell lines
Cardiovascular (intravenous therapy)	Cardiac conduction defects, arrhythmias, hypotension, cardiac depression
Biochemical alterations	*Increased*: γ-glutamyl transpeptidase, alkaline phosphatase, sex hormone binding globulin
	Reduced: folate, thyroid hormones, sex hormones
Teratogenesis	Various malformations—the risk is little raised in monotherapy but is higher if other antiepileptic drugs are used simultaneously, ?fetal hydantoin syndrome

intoxication when that excipient was replaced by lactose [11]. When phenytoin is given in solution via a gastrointestinal feeding tube at more or less the same time as certain protein hydrolysates used to provide enteral nutrition, the drug seems to fail to be fully absorbed [56]. Studies in volunteers have sometimes failed to reproduce this effect, and have also failed to elucidate its chemical mechanism [57]. It has been found that the problem can be avoided by administering the drug to patients several hours before, or after, the protein hydrolysate. Certain antacids, e.g. aluminium hydroxide, sucralfate and also activated charcoal, have been reported to interfere with the absorption of orally administered phenytoin.

Interactions affecting phenytoin distribution

In vitro, certain endogenous substances and various acidic drugs (e.g. salicylates, valproate, acetazolamide, heparin) displace phenytoin from its plasma protein binding sites. However, *in vivo*, these potential interactions are of small magnitude and are unlikely to be of clinical importance in most instances.

Interactions altering phenytoin metabolism

Phenytoin is eliminated from the body mainly by virtue of CYP2C9- and CYP2C19-catalysed oxidations to *p*-hydroxyphenytoin. As Levy [58] pointed out, coadministered drugs which induce the activity of either or both of these CYP isoenzymes are likely to cause increased phenytoin elimination, and hence lowered plasma concentrations of the drug. Coadministered drugs which competitively inhibit either or both of these CYP isoforms will tend to raise plasma phenytoin concentrations. Such inhibition occurs with the CYP2C9 substrates/inhibitors sulphaphenazole, phenylbutazole, fluconazole, azapropazone, disulfiram, metronidazole and stiripentol, and with the CYP2C19 substrates/inhibitors felbamate, omeprazole, cimetidine, fluoxetine, imipramine and diazepam. Because of the Michaelis–Menten elimination kinetics of phenytoin, a small degree of inhibition of the drug's metabolism can produce a disproportionately great increase in plasma phenytoin concentrations and therefore signs of drug toxicity. Interactions involving induction of the drug's metabolism, which reduce its plasma concentrations, are more likely to go unnoticed, unless plasma phenytoin concentrations are monitored, or seizure control deteriorates.

Despite the above explanation of interaction mechanisms, the metabolic basis of many of the interactions involving altered phenytoin concentrations remains unknown.

Phenytoin affecting other substances

Phenytoin is capable of altering the body's elimination of other substances by (a) inducing the synthesis of the CYP isoenzymes responsible for their metabolism, not only CYP2C isoforms, but also CYP3A4 [59] (which catalyses the oxidation of many drugs), and also by inducing the synthesis of certain glucuronyl transferases, important in drug conjugation; or (b) serving as a competitive inhibitor of the metabolism of other CYP2C9 or CYP2C19 eliminated drugs. It is not yet known to what extent other mechanisms are also important. As mentioned above, both induction and inhibition can occur simultaneously and the resultant clinical effect is difficult to predict.

Interactions between phenytoin and other antiepileptic drugs

Plasma phenytoin levels usually fall if primidone, clonazepam, vigabatrin, valproate, carbamazepine or phenobarbital are added as comedication, though sometimes contrary effects occur with carbamazepine and phenobarbital. Ethosuximide, felbamate or sulthiame comedication increase plasma phenytoin levels. Concentrations of carbamazepine, clobazam, clonazepam, felbamate, lamotrigine, primidone, topiramate, valproate and zonisamide can fall when phenytoin is added as comedication. The effect of phenytoin on phenobarbital concentrations are variable, and levels may rise or fall.

Side-effects

Phenytoin has been widely used for over 60 years, and numerous toxic effects of the drug are known (Table 40.5). Some of the unwanted effects of the drug are clearly related to the drug's concentration in the body, and many of these represent what would be regarded as drug overdosage effects. Some unwanted effects are hypersensitivity reactions, possibly related to immune-mediated attacks on chemical adducts formed between various tissue proteins, for instance liver microsomal membrane protein [60,61], and the arene-oxide intermediate derivative of phenytoin hydroxylation, or the drug's catechol metabolite. Adduct formation itself may also alter the composition of various body tissue elements and produce structural change in tissues. However, the mechanisms of some unwanted effects of the drug are currently unexplained. The common or important reported adverse effects of phenytoin are listed in Table 40.5.

Effects on the nervous system

In overdosage, phenytoin tends to produce vestibulocerebellar disturbance. The earliest manifestation is horizontal nystagmus which typically occurs at plasma concentrations above 20 mg/L (80 μmol). At concentrations above 30 mg/L (120 μmol) ataxia of gait and double vision occur, and at concentrations above 40 mg/L (160 μmol) drowsiness, sometimes with nausea and vomiting [39]. Coma will develop if the drug concentration is allowed to become high enough. However, there are large individual differences, and in some patients, effects are seen at serum levels above or below the usual optimal range. Conversely, absence of adverse effects can be seen at levels above 30 mg/L (120 μmol). Occasional patients may experience mood disorder, mainly depression, as the dose of the drug is increased. There have been reports that phenytoin, at therapeutic concentrations, may decrease performance in various tests of cognitive function [62]. However, this has been only inconsistently demonstrated, and may be partly an artefact of the drug's interference with motor coordination [63]. Despite the earlier suggestion that carbamazepine caused less interference with cognitive function than phenytoin, the literature reviews of Aldenkamp et al. [64] and Kalvainen et al. [65] suggested that, at therapeutic range concentrations, there was little real difference between the two drugs in this regard. Seizure control may worsen in some patients as plasma levels of phenytoin become 'supratherapeutic' [66].

Occasionally phenytoin overdosage results in dyskinetic and dystonic involuntary movements [67], or ophthalmoplegia. There are also reports of the drug causing subclinical and occasionally overt peripheral neuropathy [68]. Shorvon and Reynolds [69] found mild abnormalities of peripheral nerve conduction in 18% of a series of phenytoin-treated patients (with non-toxic levels) who had no clinically detectable evidence of peripheral neuropathy. At toxic levels, a more severe reversible demyelinating neuropathy may occur. Recently, phenytoin overdosage has been shown to cause decreased colour vision discrimination [70]. Cerebellar atrophy has been reported in persons with long-standing phenytoin overdosage [71], though whether there is a cause–effect relationship between the two has been argued. In one individual, cerebellar atrophy was reported to have followed a severe acute phenytoin overdose.

Effects on the skin

Some 5–10% of patients given phenytoin develop a measles-like rash which first appears on the trunk, usually in the second week of drug intake. If treatment with the drug is not ceased at that stage, more extensive skin and internal organ involvement can develop. Other cutaneous reactions, for example Stevens–Johnson syndromes, systemic lupus erythematosus, exfoliative dermatitis and toxic epidermal necrolysis are less common [72]. The incidence of

phenytoin-related rashes appears to be higher (22%) in patients taking the drug and receiving radiotherapy for intracranial tumours than in other patients taking the drug [73]. Phenytoin should be discontinued when a rash appears. Phenytoin may cause an overgrowth of body hair, particularly in dark-haired females. This can be cosmetically important.

Intravenous administration of phenytoin may lead to a 'purple glove' syndrome in the hand and forearm distal to the administration site, with local progressive skin discoloration, oedema and pain. The phenomenon occurred in 5.9% of one series of 152 patients given the drug intravenously [74], although clinical experience suggests a much lower rate. Thrombophlebitis may develop in the vein into which the drug has been administered.

The aromatic anticonvulsant hypersensitivity syndrome

The typical acute phenytoin toxic morbiliform rash described above may merge into the various expressions of the aromatic anticonvulsant hypersensitivity syndrome. In this condition the rash becomes more extensive whilst remaining erythematous, mucosal involvement with ulceration may develop, skin exfoliation may occur and eosinophilia, hepatitis and other evidence of systemic organ involvement may appear [75]. Cross sensitivity with other drugs is common, and 60% of affected persons experience similar reactions if subsequently exposed to carbamazepine or phenobarbital. The mechanism of the syndrome is thought to depend on an autoimmune response to adducts formed between phenytoin metabolites and various tissue protein components, e.g. microsomal proteins [61].

Effects on the gums

Since the drug was first introduced into clinical practice, the occurrence of gum hyperplasia has been recognized. The subject has been reviewed on a number of occasions e.g. [76]. Estimates of frequency have varied between 13 and 40% [77,78]. Most authors have noted a correlation between the degree of gum hyperplasia and serum level. Poor dental hygiene makes the hypertrophy more noticeable.

The causal mechanisms are unclear. Reduced immunoglobulin A (IgA) concentrations in saliva were thought originally to be of relevance [79]. More recently, the recognition that phenytoin is metabolized in gum tissue to p-hydroxyphenytoin [80] has led to the hypothesis that the resulting arene-oxide metabolic intermediate forms adducts with various tissue proteins in the gums leading to gum overgrowth. However, the degree of gum hypertrophy seemed unrelated to the salivary p-hydroxyphenytoin concentration [80]. The serum concentrations of basic fibroblast growth factor increase in the presence of phenytoin intake, and these concentrations seem to correlate with the degree of gum hyperplasia [81].

Effects on bone

Patients receiving long-term phenytoin therapy, with or without other of the older antiepileptic agents, can develop osteomalacia. Serum calcium levels may fall and alkaline phosphatase levels rise. Plasma 25-hydroxycholecalciferol concentrations are reduced. The risk of osteomalacia is highest in regions where diet is poor and there is little exposure to sunlight. Osteomalacia is likely to be due to the induction of vitamin D metabolism and possibly impaired intestinal absorption of dietary calcium.

Effects on lymphoid tissue

Rarely, continuing phenytoin intake has been associated with the development of widespread lymphadenopathy which disappears again when intake of the drug is ceased. The histological appearance of the affected lymph glands is reminiscent of that of Hodgkin's disease. The entity is referred to as a pseudolymphoma syndrome [82]. Even more uncommonly, instances of true lymphoma have been reported in association with phenytoin intake [83].

Effects on folates

Phenytoin intake causes a reduction in serum and red blood cell folate. The mechanisms of this effect have not been fully elucidated. The extent of the reduction is proportional to the phenytoin concentration [84]. There have been suggestions that this fall in folate concentration plays a role in the slowing in intellectual performance. Folate deficiency occasionally results in megaloblastic anaemia in patients receiving long-term phenytoin therapy.

Other effects

Phenytoin intake can precipitate attacks of porphyria in those who suffer from the disorder. Phenytoin can diminish insulin secretion from the pancreas, resulting in a tendency to hyperglycaemia. If the nature of paroxysmal hypoglycaemic symptoms is unrecognized and they are considered epileptic in nature, use of the drug can delay the diagnosis of an insulinoma. Rarely, the drug has caused hepatitis, vasculitis, interstitial lung infiltration, interstitial nephritis, myopathy, thyroiditis, arthritis and the suppression of the formation of particular lines of blood cell. The effects of phenytoin on cardiovascular function are considered in the section on intravenous administration.

Cardiovascular effects

Oral phenytoin therapy in usual dosages does not commonly cause cardiovascular disturbance. However, intravenous administration of phenytoin is potentially hazardous, especially if the rate of administration exceeds 50 mg/min in adults or 1–3 mg/min/kg in children or if the dose exceeds recommended levels. Effects can include hypotension, cardiovascular collapse and central nervous system depression. Severe cardiotoxic reactions and fatalities have been reported with atrial and ventricular conduction depression and ventricular fibrillation. Hypotension usually occurs when the drugs are administered rapidly by the intravenous route. Severe complications are most commonly encountered in elderly or gravely ill patients. Even at slower infusion rates, however, occasional problems arise.

Other biochemical effects

Phenytoin intake can result in a range of biochemical effects, which are often asymptomatic. These include raised serum or plasma levels of α-glutamyl transpeptidase, alkaline phosphatase, high-density lipoprotein (HDL) cholesterol, caeruloplasmin, copper, prolactin and sex hormone binding globulin. It has also been associated with reduced concentrations of folate (discussed above), IgA, IgG, IgE, IgM, fibrinogen, thyroxine, tri-iodothyronine, protein bound iodine, vitamin K, vitamin E, vitamin D metabolites (mentioned above), cortisol, oestrogens, progesterone, free testosterone, pyridoxal phosphate, tryptophan and thiamine. Neonatal blood coagulation defects, probably due to a relative deficiency of vitamin K-catalysed clotting factors in the neonate exposed to phenytoin during pregnancy, may cause bleeding on the fifth neonatal day unless the mother receives vitamin K before delivery and the baby receives prophylactic vitamin K immediately after birth. Presumably phenytoin induces the metabolism of the vitamin to inactive derivatives.

Teratogenicity

For more than 30 years, since the publications of Meadow [85] and Spiedel and Meadow [86] it has been known that in pregnant women the intake of antiepileptic drugs, including phenytoin, is associated with an approximate doubling or trebling in the rate of malformed infants being born to these women. The role of phenytoin is difficult to interpret, partly because there has been a tendency to treat the teratogenicity of antiepileptic drugs as a class effect. The literature has also sometimes not distinguished between the situation of the offspring of women who took phenytoin as monotherapy during pregnancy or in combination therapy. This is important because fetal malformation risk is increased if multiple antiepileptic drugs are taken [87,88].

In their literature review, Albengres and Tillement [89] noted a higher incidence of malformations in the offspring of phenytoin-treated as compared with normal pregnant women in three of four published series, and Dravet et al. [88] demonstrated a statistically significant association between use of the drug in pregnancy and fetal malformation. In contrast, Nakane et al. [90] failed to find any statistically significant excess of malformations in the offspring of pregnancies in which phenytoin was taken. There is only limited data for phenytoin taken in monotherapy. In 1988 Kaneko et al. [87] reported a 14.6% malformation rate in phenytoin-exposed neonates (with an average malformation rate of 14% in the offspring of all antiepileptic drug treated women), but in a subsequent series (1992) they found a rate of only 4.6%, compared with a rate of 5.7% in untreated control pregnancies [91]. The decrease in malformation rates between the two series was attributed to a reduction in antiepileptic drug dosage during pregnancy following the appearance of the 1988 paper. Samren et al. [92] carried out an analysis of five prospective European studies of malformation rates following fetal exposure to antiepileptic drugs during pregnancy. The malformation rate for phenytoin monotherapy was 6%, lower than for other established antiepileptic drugs; the relative risk for phenytoin being associated with malformations, compared with the background risk, was 2.2 (95% CI=0.7 – 6.7). Thus in that study phenytoin, used alone, appeared from the point of view of teratogenesis the safest of the established major antiepileptic drugs. In fact there was no statistically significant evidence that it was a teratogen.

A range of different malformations have been reported. The most severe include facial clefts, diaphragmatic hernias, hip dysplasias and congenital heart abnormalities. A 'fetal hydantoin' syndrome has been described [93]. This syndrome involves the presence of what is claimed to be a characteristic facies with wide-spaced eyes, together with deformities of the fingernails and slender and shortened terminal phalanges, mild mental retardation and poor infantile growth and development. Many of these minor abnormalities become unrecognizable within the first few years of life [88]. Partial rather than full syndromes are more commonly encountered. There is some controversy in the literature as to whether or not the fetal hydantoin syndrome is a genuine entity [94,95] and, if it is, whether or not it is specific to fetal exposure to phenytoin in pregnancy, or can occur associated with exposure to other antiepileptic drugs. A curious and potentially significant case was reported by Phelan *et al.* [96] of an epileptic woman treated with phenytoin who gave birth to a white and a black twin after a pregnancy which followed intercourse with a white man and an Afro-American during the same day. Only the black twin had features diagnosed as those of the fetal hydantoin syndrome, yet each twin must have been exposed to the same phenytoin concentrations in the same womb throughout pregnancy.

In summary, it seems likely that phenytoin has potential to cause fetal malformations. However, the risk is not high and may be less than that of alternative drugs, if phenytoin is taken as monotherapy. Phenytoin is less likely to cause serious spinal malformations than carbamazepine or valproate. The risk of malformation seems to an extent to be related to phenytoin dosage. The latter often bears some relationship to the severity of maternal epilepsy, and there is a possibility that the epilepsy itself may make some contribution to the risk of malformation occurring.

A good deal of experimental embryological work has been undertaken to explore the mechanisms of the phenytoin-associated malformations. It is possible that fetal maldevelopment results from reactive metabolic intermediates, e.g. arene-oxide derivatives which form adducts with fetal tissue proteins. Free radical intermediates produced by the activity of tissue peroxidases which metabolize phenytoin to hydroxyl radicals may also play a part if they are not inactivated by glutathione, and then oxidize various fetal macromolecules [28]. The arene-oxide adducts would be more likely to be present at higher concentrations if the activity of the enzyme epoxide hydrolase (which catalyses the further metabolism of arene oxides and epoxides) was deficient. Finnell *et al.* [60] found evidence that low levels of the enzyme epoxide hydrolase in amniocytes and fetal fibroblasts was associated with the occurrence of the fetal hydantoin syndrome.

Clinical effectiveness

The original studies of Merritt and Putnam in 1938 [97] demonstrated the efficacy of phenytoin against major seizures in the more common epileptic syndromes. They gave the drug for 2–11 months to 142 patients whose seizure disorders had failed to be controlled by phenobarbital and the bromides. Bromides were withdrawn but the phenobarbital was continued after phenytoin was commenced. 'Complete relief' was obtained in 58% of the 118 patients with frequent 'grand mal' seizures, and there was a 'marked decrease' in seizures in another 32%. The corresponding figures for the 74 patients with 'petit mal' (probably some cases would now be classified

as having complex partial seizures) were 35% and 49% respectively, and for the six with 'psychomotor seizures' 67% and 33%. By modern standards, the study design would not have been considered sufficient. The follow-up was short, the background therapy varied in different patients, there was no placebo-treated control group, and classification of cases was, to modern criteria, uncertain. Nonetheless, the study findings were confirmed in routine practice and in later investigations. For instance, Shorvon *et al.* [98] showed that phenytoin, given as monotherapy to newly diagnosed cases of generalized convulsive or partial epilepsy, yielded 78% full seizure control at 2 years from the inception of therapy.

Experience has also established that phenytoin is ineffective for treating myoclonic seizures (irrespective of their age of onset), and also the absence and atonic seizures of primary generalized epilepsy, infantile spasms and the seizures of the Lennox–Gastaut syndrome. The drug has also proved ineffective in treating two reasonably common varieties of situation-related human epilepsy, namely febrile convulsions of infancy [99], and the eclamptic seizures of pregnancy toxaemia [100]. Intravenous phenytoin has been used successfully in treating neonatal seizures.

North *et al.* [101] showed in a double-blind, placebo-controlled study, that phenytoin, commenced at the time of neurosurgery, substantially reduced (7.9% vs. 16.7%) the risk of epileptic seizures in the first few postoperative months. This was particularly the case if the plasma phenytoin concentration was kept in the therapeutic range throughout the study period. However, the use of prophylactic phenytoin after head injury does not seem to reduce the incidence of later onset post-traumatic epilepsy [102].

As new antiepileptic drugs have been marketed in more recent years, there have also been comparative studies with phenytoin, reviewed by Mitaki and Browne [103] and Marson and Chadwick [104]. The sizes, quality and adequacy of the various comparative studies have varied, and different criteria have been used to assess the antiepileptic efficacies of the agents concerned.

Phenytoin vs. carbamazepine, phenobarbital and primidone

Probably the methodologically most satisfactory comparison of the efficacy of the old antiepileptic drugs (phenytoin, carbamazepine, phenobarbital and primidone) was that of Mattson *et al.* [105], carried out in 622 patients in various veterans hospitals in the USA. The criterion of success of therapy was retention of patients in the study after 3 years, whilst still taking the drug to which the patient had originally been randomized. This criterion would more or less equate to satisfactory seizure control and lack of troublesome adverse effects of therapy. The retention rates were close to 60% for phenytoin and carbamazepine, and to 40% for phenobarbital and primidone. After the first year, complete control of generalized tonic-clonic seizures had been achieved in 48% of those taking carbamazepine, 43% taking phenytoin and phenobarbital and 45% taking primidone. For partial seizures the corresponding figures were 43%, 26%, 16% and 15%. Statistically, there were no differences at the $P < 0.05$ level between phenytoin and carbamazepine. In the study, phenytoin was not superior to phenobarbital in its capacity to control seizures, but was less likely to lead to adverse effects which caused therapy with the drug to be abandoned.

Phenytoin vs. valproate

Phenytoin has been compared with valproate in at least three trials [106–108]. The Shakir *et al.* [106] trial was a comparatively small study on a mixture of newly diagnosed and treatment-resistant cases of epilepsy, and was interpreted as showing that phenytoin and valproate had reasonably similar efficacies.

The study of Turnbull *et al.* [107] was larger (88 patients with generalized tonic-clonic or partial seizures and a follow-up period of at least 1 year, with drug dosage adjustments as indicated clinically). For 51 persons with generalized tonic-clonic seizures, 83% became fit free for at least a year if treated with valproate, and 71% if treated with phenytoin. For 37 patients with partial seizures, the corresponding figures were 30% for valproate, and 35% for phenytoin. In these studies, therefore, the two drugs had roughly similar efficacies.

Wilder *et al.* [108] compared phenytoin and valproate in 87 patients with partial, secondarily generalized or primary generalized tonic-clonic seizures, and considered the two agents equivalent, in terms of efficacy and toxicity.

Phenytoin vs. carbamazepine and valproate

Callaghan *et al.* [109] studied 181 previously untreated epileptic patients randomized to one or other of phenytoin, valproate and carbamazepine. For those with generalized tonic-clonic seizures, 73% who received phenytoin, 59% who received valproate and 39% who received carbamazepine became seizure free (a statistically significant difference between phenytoin and carbamazepine), whilst for those with partial seizures the corresponding figures were 57.1%, 44.4% and 33.5%. However, the proportions with poor responses (less than a 50% reduction in seizures) were similar for all three drugs. Probably largely on the basis of the latter finding, Callaghan *et al.* took the view that the three drugs compared were generally equal in efficacy, and were more effective for generalized tonic-clonic than for partial seizures.

Heller *et al.* [110] used time to the occurrence of the first seizure after initiating therapy, and time to 12 months duration of seizure remission as the criteria of therapeutic success in 234 patients with newly diagnosed epilepsy. Phenytoin, phenobarbital, carbamazepine and valproate proved of generally similar efficacy.

De Silva *et al.* [111] took a very similar approach and employed a similar set of efficacy criteria in 167 children with newly recognized generalized tonic-clonic or partial seizures (the latter with or without the attacks becoming secondarily generalized). They found the four agents equivalent in efficacy, though early in the course of their study, phenobarbital recruitment was stopped because of an excess of adverse effects. Phenytoin was withdrawn more often than the other two agents remaining in the comparison.

Phenytoin vs. lamotrigine

Steiner *et al.* [112] reported a comparative study of phenytoin and lamotrigine in 181 newly recognized cases of generalized tonic-clonic or partial epilepsies, with drug doses titrated to obtain optimal clinical responses. At 24 weeks of therapy, 48% of those with partial seizures who were taking phenytoin, and 41% of those who were taking lamotrigine, were seizure free. For secondarily general-ized partial seizures the corresponding figures were 50% and 50%, and for primary generalized tonic-clonic seizures 34% and 44%. At 40 weeks, the corresponding figures were: for partial seizures 22% and 16%, for secondarily generalized seizures 31% and 33%, and for primary generalized tonic-clonic seizures 32% and 30%.

Phenytoin vs. clobazam

The Canadian Study Group [113] compared phenytoin and clobazam as antiepileptic therapies in 76 children with treatment-resistant partial seizures or generalized tonic-clonic seizures. Seizures were reasonably fully controlled or controlled for 6 months in 40% of those taking phenytoin and 49% taking clobazam, a difference that was not statistically significant.

Clinical therapeutics

These various studies provide consistent evidence that phenytoin is as effective in suppressing seizures as other widely used established antiepileptic drugs in the common varieties of epilepsy. Its adverse effect profile, and its ease of use, may differ in some ways from the other agents with similar antiepileptic efficacies. A consensus appears to have emerged, at least in Europe, that carbamazepine is to be preferred to phenytoin in managing epilepsies with generalized tonic-clonic seizures, or with simple or complex partial seizures, a preference based on the better adverse effect profile of carbamazepine and greater ease of use (the latter probably in non-expert hands). Brodie and Kwan [114] have attempted to put the comparison of antiepileptic drugs onto a quantitative basis by developing a simple scoring system involving a number of criteria (a 'star' system) for grading the available antiepileptic agents. Phenytoin scores less well than other drugs, but there is little scientific basis for this scheme. Nonetheless, phenytoin still remains a satisfactory agent for treating many of the common epileptic syndromes. This is particularly the case if the drug is used by those familiar with its pharmacokinetics and adverse effect profile. It has the advantage also of very low cost and availability in parenteral formulations.

Phenytoin has also had some use in tic douloureux, certain cardiac arrhythmias, various neurogenic pain syndromes, as a prophylactic in occasional varieties of migraine, and in paroxysmal choreoathetosis and myotonia, though other agents are probably more efficient for many of these disorders.

Dosage in oral administration

An initial daily drug dose is 5 mg/kg in adults, and 10 mg/kg in prepubertal children. This will offer a good chance of obtaining a steady-state plasma phenytoin concentration in the range 10–20 mg/L (40–80 µmol) within 1 week, and is unlikely to cause the side-effects of overdosage. The full anticipated daily dose can be used from the commencement of therapy. Pharmacokinetic considerations suggest that once daily dosage should be satisfactory, and it often proves so in practice. However, twice daily intake does not appear to increase compliance problems, and allows greater security against the consequences of missed doses.

Once there is time for steady-state conditions to apply, the plasma phenytoin concentration should be measured. If in the light of the measurement, it appears clinically desirable to adjust the drug dose, this can be done but the non-linear relationship between steady-state plasma phenytoin concentrations and drug dosage should be kept in mind. Nomograms have been devised in an attempt to achieve quite precise phenytoin dosage adjustments to yield particular plasma phenytoin concentrations. However in practice the size of the available dosage units (generally 30, 50 and 100 mg) tends to determine the dosage adjustment that will be made. In most adults, a dose increment of 100 mg is unlikely to lead to overdosage manifestations if the patient's steady-state plasma phenytoin concentration is below 10 mg/L (40 µmol), and a dose increment of 30 or 50 mg is likely to be tolerated if the plasma phenytoin level is between 10 and 15 mg/L (40 and 60 µmol). In children, smaller sized increments are necessary.

The therapeutic range of plasma phenytoin concentrations is usually considered to be 10–20 mg/L (40–80 µmol). However, as mentioned earlier, some patients achieve seizure control at plasma phenytoin concentrations as low as 7 mg/L (28 µmol), whilst others require, and tolerate, levels of 25 mg/L (100 µmol) or higher before seizures cease. The latter is particularly the case in attempting to control partial seizures, whilst in the same patient lower concentrations of the drug may be associated with control of tonic-clonic convulsive seizures [43]. In varieties of epilepsy where the natural history of the disorder is not known, or when it is expected that seizures will recur only at long intervals, it is reasonable to try to achieve a steady-state plasma phenytoin concentration in the range 7–20 mg/L (28–80 µmol). Thereafter further dosage adjustment depends on the clinical response. In varieties of epilepsy in which seizures occur frequently, from the outset the clinical response provides the better guide to phenytoin dosage. Achieving therapeutic range plasma phenytoin concentrations guarantees neither obtaining the optimal possible control of seizures in the patient, nor the absence of adverse effects of therapy. Once a satisfactory phenytoin dosage regimen has been achieved in a particular patient, it will rarely be necessary to alter that regimen over many years, unless non-compliance occurs, the epilepsy is associated with progressive brain disease, late stage adverse effects of prolonged phenytoin intake occur, or another drug is prescribed which interacts with the phenytoin. Phenytoin dosage may need to be reduced in the presence of severe liver disease, though often not in the presence of renal failure. However, the reduced plasma albumin concentrations in patients with severe liver or renal disease may confound the interpretation of plasma phenytoin concentrations, and make measurement of the drug's concentration in plasma water, or saliva, desirable as a guide to therapy.

Intravenous administration

Intravenous phenytoin often provides effective therapy for convulsive status epilepticus. However, intravenous therapy carries a risk of cardiovascular complications (see p. 501). This can be minimized by ensuring that the rate of administration does not exceed 50 mg/min in adults and 1–3 mg/min/kg in neonates or children. Even in patients previously not receiving phenytoin, a total loading dose of 20 mg/kg should not be exceeded. Continuous monitoring of the ECG and blood pressure is strongly recommended. The parenteral formulation of phenytoin should be injected slowly into a large vein, through a large-gauge needle or intravenous catheter. An injection of intravenous phenytoin should be followed by a 'flushing' injection of sterile saline through the same needle or catheter to avoid local venous irritation. Prolonged infusions of phenytoin should not be given. Intravenous phenytoin therapy requires close medical supervision. The treatment of status epilepticus and acute seizures is dealt with in more detail in Chapter 18.

References

1 Glazko AJ. The discovery of phenytoin. *Ther Drug Monit* 1986; 8: 490–7.
2 Friedlander WJ. Putnam, Merritt, and the discovery of Dilantin. *Epilepsia* 1986; 27 (Suppl. 3): S1–S21.
3 Tomaselli G, Marban E, Yellen G. Sodium channels from human brain RNA expressed in *Xenopus* oocytes: basic electrophysiologic characteristics and their modification by diphenylhydantoin. *J Clin Invest* 1989; 83: 1724–32.
4 Macdonald RL. Cellular actions of antiepileptic drugs. In: Eadie MJ, Vajda FJE, eds. *Antiepileptic Drugs: pharmacology and therapeutics*. Berlin: Springer, 1999: 123–50.
5 Kuo CC. A common anticonvulsant binding site for phenytoin, carbamazepine, and lamotrigine in neuronal Na+ channels. *Mol Pharmacol* 1998; 54: 712–21.
6 Kuo CC, Chen RS, Lu L, Chen RC. Carbamazepine inhibition of neuronal Na+ currents: quantitative distinction from phenytoin and possible therapeutic implications. *Mol Pharmacol* 1997; 51: 1077–83.
7 DeLorenzo RJ. Phenytoin: mechanisms of action. In: Levy RH, Mattson RH, Meldrum BS, eds. *Antiepileptic drugs*, 4th edn. New York: Raven Press, 1995: 271–82.
8 Francis J, Eubanks JH, McIntyre-Burnham W. Diazepam-potentiated [3H]phenytoin binding is associated with peripheral-type benzodiazepine receptors and not with voltage-dependent sodium channels. *Brain Res* 2000; 876: 131–40.
9 Esplin DW. Effect of diphenylhydantoin on synaptic transmission in cat spinal cord and stellate ganglion. *J Pharmacol Exp Ther* 1957; 120: 301–23.
10 Loscher W. Animal models of epilepsy and epileptic seizures. In: Eadie MJ, Vajda FJE, eds. *Antiepileptic Drugs: pharmacology and therapeutics*. Berlin: Springer, 1999: 19–62.
11 Bochner F, Hooper WD, Tyrer JH, Eadie MJ. Factors involved in an outbreak of phenytoin intoxication. *J Neurol Sci* 1972; 16: 481–7.
12 Cloyd JC, Gumnit JR, Lesar TS. Reduced seizure control due to spoiled phenytoin capsules. *Ann Neurol* 1980; 7: 191–3.
13 Ramsay RE, Strauss RG, Wilder BJ, Willmore LJ. Status epilepticus in pregnancy: effect of phenytoin malabsorption on seizure control. *Neurology* 1978; 28: 85–9.
14 Lander CM, Smith MT, Chalk JB *et al.* Bioavailability and pharmacokinetics of phenytoin during pregnancy. *Eur J Clin Pharmacol* 1984; 27: 105–10.
15 Neurvonen PJ. Bioavailability of phenytoin: clinical pharmacokinetic and therapeutic implications. *Clin Pharmacokinet* 1979; 4: 91–103.
16 Chang SW, da Silva JH, Kuhl DR. Absorption of rectally administered phenytoin: a pilot study. *Ann Pharmacother* 1999; 33: 781–6.
17 Geary WA II, Wooten GF, Perlin JB, Lothman EW. In vitro and in vivo distribution and binding of phenytoin to rat brain. *J Pharmacol Exp Ther* 1987; 241: 704–13.
18 Tishler DM, Weinberg KI, Hinton DR, Barbaro N, Annett GM, Raffel C. MDR1 gene expression in brain of patients with medically intractable epilepsy. *Epilepsia* 1995; 36: 1–6.
19 Kurata D, Wilkinson GR. Erythrocyte uptake and plasma protein binding of diphenylhydantoin. *Clin Pharmacol Ther* 1974; 16: 355–62.
20 Hooper WD, Sutherland JM, Bochner F, Tyrer JH, Eadie MJ. The effect of certain drugs on the plasma protein binding of diphenylhydantoin. *Austral N Zeal J Med* 1973; 3: 377–81.
21 Bossi L. Neonatal period including drug disposition in newborns: review of the literature. In: Janz D, Bossi L, Dam M, Helge H, Richens A, Schmidt D, eds. *Epilepsy, Pregnancy, and the Child*. New York: Raven Press, 1982: 327–41.

22 Perucca E, Ruprah M, Richens A. Altered drug binding to serum proteins in pregnant women: therapeutic relevance. *J Roy Soc Med* 1981; 74: 422–6.

23 Kearns GL, Kemp SF, Turley CP, Nelson DL. Protein binding of phenytoin and lidocaine in pediatric patients with type I diabetes mellitus. *Dev Pharmacol Ther* 1988; 11: 14–23.

24 Triedman HM, Fishman RA, Yahr MD. Determination of plasma and cerebrospinal fluid levels of Dilantin in the human. *Trans Am Neurol Assoc* 1960; 85: 166–70.

25 Bochner F, Hooper WD, Sutherland JM, Eadie MJ, Tyrer JH. Diphenyl-hydantoin concentrations in saliva. *Arch Neurol* 1974; 31: 57–9.

26 Kamali F, Thomas SH. Effect of saliva flow rate on phenytoin concentrations: implications for therapeutic monitoring. *Eur J Clin Pharmacol* 1994; 46: 565–7.

27 Kaneko S, Fukushima Y, Sato T, Ogaea Y, Nomura Y, Shinagawa S. Breast feeding in epileptic mothers. In: Sato T, Shinagawa S, eds. *Antiepileptic Drugs and Pregnancy*. Amsterdam: Excerpta Medica, 1984: 38–45.

28 Mays DC, Pawluk LJ, Apseloff G *et al*. Metabolism of phenytoin and co-valent binding of reactive intermediates in activated human neutrophils. *Biochem Pharmacol* 1995; 50: 367–80.

29 Fritz S, Lindner W, Roots I, Frey BM, Kupfer A. Stereochemistry of aromatic phenytoin hydroxylation in various drug hydroxylation phenotypes in humans. *J Pharmacol Exp Ther* 1987; 241: 615–22.

30 Razman I. Pharmacodynamics of phenytoin-induced ataxia in rats. *Epilepsy Res* 1990; 5: 80–3.

31 Albert KS, Hallmark KR, Sakmar E, Weidler DJ, Wagner JG. Plasma concentrations of diphenylhydantoin, its para-hydroxylated metabolite, and corresponding glucuronide in man. *Res Comm Chem Pathol Pharmacol* 1974; 9: 463–9.

32 Ieiri I, Goto W, Hirata K *et al*. The effect of 5-(p-hydroxyphenyl)-5-phenylhydantoin (p-HPPH) enantiomers, major metabolites of phenytoin, on the occurrence of chronic-gingival hyperplasia: in vivo and in vitro study. *Eur J Clin Pharmacol* 1995; 49: 51–6.

33 Inaba T. Phenytoin: pharmacogenetic polymorphism of 4'-hydroxylation. *Pharmacol Ther* 1990; 464: 341–7.

34 Vermeij P, Ferrari MD, Buruma OJ, Veenema K, de Wolff FA. Inheritance of poor phenytoin parahydroxylation capacity in a Dutch family. *Clin Pharmacol Ther* 1988; 44: 588–93.

35 Dickinson RG, Hooper WD, Patterson M, Eadie MJ, Maguire B. Extent of urinary excretion of p-hydroxyphenytoin in healthy subjects given phenytoin. *Ther Drug Monit* 1985; 7: 283–9.

36 Browne TR, LeDue B. Phenytoin: chemistry and biotransformation. In: Levy RH, Mattson RH, Meldrum BS, eds. *Antiepileptic Drugs*, 4th edn. New York: Raven Press, 1995: 283–300.

37 Arnold K, Gerber N. The rate of decline of diphenylhydantoin in human plasma. *Clin Pharmacol Ther* 1970; 11: 121–34.

38 Bauer LA, Blouin RA. Phenytoin Michaelis-Menten pharmacokinetics in Caucasian pediatric patients. *Clin Pharmacokinet* 1983; 8: 545–9.

39 Kutt H, Winters W, Kokenge R, McDowell F. Diphenylhydantoin metabolism, blood levels, and toxicity. *Arch Neurol* 1964; 11: 642–8.

40 Loiseau P, Brachet Liermain A, Legroux M, Jogeix M. Intérêt du dosage des anticonvulsivants dans le traitement des épilepsies. *Nouv Presse Med* 1977; 16: 813–17.

41 Norrell E, Lilenberg G, Gamstorp I. Systematic determination of the serum phenytoin level as an aid in the management of children with epilepsy. *Eur Neurol* 1975; 13: 232–44.

42 Turnbull DM, Rawlings MD, Weightman D, Chadwick DW. 'Therapeutic' serum concentrations of phenytoin: the influence of seizure type. *J Neurol Neurosurg Psychiatr* 1984; 47: 231–4.

43 Schmidt D, Einicke I, Haenel F. The influence of seizure type on the efficacy of plasma concentrations of phenytoin, phenobarbital, and carbamazepine. *Arch Neurol* 1986; 43: 263–5.

44 Levine M, Chang T. Therapeutic drug monitoring of phenytoin. Rationale and current status. *Clin Pharmacokinet* 1990; 19: 341–58.

45 Svensmark O, Schiller PJ, Buchthal F. 5,5'-diphenylhydantoin (Dilantin) blood levels after oral or intravenous dosage in man. *Acta Pharmacol Toxicol* 1960; 16: 331–46.

46 Battino D, Estienne M, Avanzini G. Clinical pharmacokinetics of antiepileptic drugs in paediatric patients. Part II. Phenytoin, carba-mazepine, sulthiame, lamotrigine, vigabatrin, oxcarbazepine and felba-mate. *Clin Pharmacokinet* 1995; 29: 341–69.

47 Dam M, Mygind KI, Christiansen J. Antiepileptic drugs: plasma clearance during pregnancy. In: Janz D, ed. *Epileptology*. Stuttgart: Thieme, 1976: 179–83.

48 Lander CM, Edwards VE, Eadie MJ, Tyrer JH. Plasma anticonvulsant concentrations during pregnancy. *Neurology* 1977; 27: 128–31.

49 Dickinson RG, Hooper WD, Wood B, Lander CM, Eadie MJ. The effect of pregnancy on the pharmacokinetics of stable isotope labelled phenytoin. *Br J Clin Pharmacol* 1989; 28: 17–27.

50 Herkes GK, Eadie MJ. Possible roles for frequent salivary antiepileptic drug monitoring in the management of epilepsy. *Epilepsy Res* 1990; 6: 146–54.

51 Bochner F, Hooper WD, Tyrer JH, Eadie MJ. The effect of dosage increments on blood phenytoin concentrations. *J Neurol Neurosurg Psychiatr* 1972; 35: 873–6.

52 Eadie MJ, Tyrer JH. *Anticonvulsant Therapy: pharmacological basis and practice*, 3rd edn. Edinburgh: Churchill-Livingstone, 1989.

53 Nation RL, Evans AM, Milne RW. Pharmacokinetic drug interactions with phenytoin. *Clin Pharmacokinet* 1990; 18: 37–60, 131–50.

54 Kutt H, Harden CL. Phenytoin and congeners. In: Eadie MJ, Vajda FJE, eds. *Antiepileptic Drugs: pharmacology and therapeutics*. Berlin: Springer, 1999: 229–65.

55 Anderson GD, Graves NM. Drug interactions with antiepileptic agents. Prevention and management. *CNS Drugs* 1994; 2: 268–79.

56 Bauer LA. Interference of oral phenytoin absorption by continuous naso-gastric feedings. *Neurology* 1982; 32: 570–2.

57 Kreuger KA, Garnett WR, Comstock CJ, Fitxsimmons WE, Karnes HT, Pellock JM. Effect of two administration schedules of an enteral nutrient formula on phenytoin bioavailability. *Epilepsia* 1987; 28: 706–12.

58 Levy RH. Cytochrome P450 isoenzymes and antiepileptic drug interactions. *Epilepsia* 1995; 35 (Suppl. 5): S8–S13.

59 Brackett CC, Bloch JD. Phenytoin as a possible cause of acetaminophen hepatotoxicity: case report and review of the literature. *Pharmacotherapy* 2000; 20: 229–33.

60 Finnell RH, Buehler BA, Kerr BM, Ager PL, Levy RH. Clinical and experimental studies linking oxidative metabolism to phenytoin-induced teratogenesis. *Neurology* 1992; 42 (Suppl. 5): 25–31.

61 Leeder JS. Mechanism of idiosyncratic hypersensitivity reactions to antiepileptic drugs. *Epilepsia* 1998; 39 (Suppl. 7): S8–S16.

62 Trimble MR. Anticonvulsant drugs and cognitive function: a review of the literature. *Epilepsia* 1987; 28 (Suppl. 3): S37–S45.

63 Dodrill CB, Temkin NR. Motor speed is a contaminating factor in evaluating the 'cognitive' effect of phenytoin. *Epilepsia* 1989; 30: 453–7.

64 Aldenkamp AP, Alpherts WC, Diepman L, van 't Slot B, Overweg J, Vermuelen J. Cognitive side-effects of phenytoin compared with carbamazepine in patients with localization-related epilepsy. *Epilepsy Res* 1994; 19: 37–43.

65 Kalviainen R, Aikia M, Riekkinen PJS. Cognitive adverse effects of antiepileptic drugs: incidence, mechanisms and therapeutic implications. *CNS Drugs* 1996; 5: 358–68.

66 Chua HC, Venketasubramanian N, Tan CB, Tjia H. Paradoxical seizures in phenytoin toxicity. *Singapore Med J* 1999; 40: 276–7.

67 McLellan DL, Swash M. Choreo-athetosis and encephalopathy induced by phenytoin. *Br Med J* 1974; 2: 204–5.

68 Yoshikawa H, Abe T, Oda Y. Extremely acute phenytoin-induced peripheral neuropathy. *Epilepsia* 1999; 40: 528–9.

69 Shorvon S, Reynolds EH. Anticonvulsant peripheral neuropathy. A clinical and electrophysiological study of patients on single drug treatment with phenytoin, carbamazepine or barbiturates. *J Neurol Neurosurg Psychiatr* 1982; 47: 621–6.

70 Bayer AU, Thiel HJ, Zrenner E *et al*. Color vision tests for early detection of antiepileptic drug toxicity. *Neurology* 1997; 48: 1394–7.

71 Luef G, Chemelli A, Birbamer G, Aichner F, Bauer G. Phenytoin over-dosage and cerebellar atrophy in epileptic patients: clinical and MRI findings. *Eur Neurol* 1994; 34 (Suppl. 1): 79–81.

72 Leong KP, Chng HH. Allergic reaction to phenytoin in a general hospital in Singapore. *Asian Pacific J Allergy Immunol* 1996; 14: 65–8.

73 Mamon HJ, Wen PY, Burns AC, Loeffler JS. Allergic skin reactions to an-

ticonvulsant medications in patients receiving cranial radiation therapy. *Epilepsia* 1999; 40: 341–4.

74 O'Brien TJ, Cascino GD, So EL, Hanna DR. Incidence and clinical consequences of the purple glove syndrome in patients receiving intravenous phenytoin. *Neurology* 1998; 51: 1034–9.

75 Schjlienger RG, Shear NH. Antiepileptic drug hypersensitivity syndrome. *Epilepsia* 1998; 39 (Suppl. 7): S3–S7.

76 Meraw SJ, Sheridan PL. Medically induced gingival hyperplasia. *Mayo Clin Proc* 1998; 73: 1196–9.

77 Thomason JM, Seymour RA, Rawlins MD. Incidence and severity of phenytoin-induced gingival overgrowth in epileptic patients in general medical practice. *Commun Dentr Oral Epidemiol* 1992; 20: 288–91.

78 Casetta I, Granieri E, Desidera M *et al.* Phenytoin-induced gingival overgrowth: a community-based cross-sectional study in Ferrara, Italy. *Neuroepidemiology* 1997; 16: 296–303.

79 Aarli JA, Tonder O. Effect of antiepileptic drugs on serum and salivary IgA. *Scand J Immunol* 1975; 4: 391–6.

80 Zhou LX, Pihlstrom B, Hardwick JP, Park SS, Wrighton SA, Holzman JL. Metabolism of phenytoin by the gingiva of normal humans: the possible role of reactive metabolites of phenytoin in the initiation of gingival hyperplasia. *Clin Pharmacol Ther* 1996; 60: 191–8.

81 Sasaki T, Maita E. Increased bFGF level in the serum of patients with phenytoin-induced gingival overgrowth. *J Clin Periodontol* 1998; 25: 42–7.

82 Salzstein SL, Ackermann LV. Lymphadenopathy induced by anticonvulsant drugs and mimicking clinically and pathologically malignant lymphoma. *Cancer* 1959; 12: 164–82.

83 Olsen JH, Schulgen G, Boice JDJ *et al.* Antiepileptic treatment and risk for hepatobiliary cancer and malignant lymphoma. *Cancer Res* 1995; 55: 294–7.

84 Berg MJ, Fincham RW, Ebert BE, Schottelius DD. Decrease of serum folates in healthy male volunteers taking phenytoin. *Epilepsia* 1988; 29: 67–73.

85 Meadow SR. Congenital abnormalities and anticonvulsant drugs. *Proc Roy Soc Med* 1970; 63: 48–9.

86 Speidel BD, Meadow SR. Maternal epilepsy and abnormalities of the fetus and newborn. *Lancet* 1972; 2: 839–43.

87 Kaneko S, Otani K, Fukushima Y *et al.* Teratogenicity of antiepileptic drugs: analysis of possible risk factors. *Epilepsia* 1988; 29: 459–67.

88 Dravet C, Julian C, Magaudda A *et al.* Epilepsy, antiepileptic drugs, and malformations in children of women with epilepsy: a French prospective study. *Neurology* 1992; 42 (Suppl. 5): 75–82.

89 Albengres E, Tillement JP. Phenytoin in pregnancy: a review of the reported risks. *Biol Res Pregnancy* 1983; 4: 71–4.

90 Nakane Y, Okuma T, Takahashi R *et al.* Multi-institutional study on the teratogencicty and fetal toxicity of antiepileptic drugs: a report of a collaborative study group in Japan. *Epilepsia* 1980; 21: 663–80.

91 Kaneko S, Otani K, Kondo T *et al.* Malformations in infants of mothers with epilepsy receiving antiepileptic drugs. *Neurology* 1992; 42 (Suppl. 5): 68–74.

92 Samren EB, van Duijn CM, Koch S *et al.* Maternal use of antiepileptic drugs and the risk of major congenital malformations: a joint European prospective study of human teratogenesis associated with maternal epilepsy. *Epilepsia* 1997; 38: 981–90.

93 Hanson JW, Smith DW. The fetal hydantoin syndrome. *J Pediatr* 1975; 87: 285–90.

94 Janz D. On major malformations and minor abnormalities in the offspring of parents with epilepsy: review of the literature. In: Janz D, Bossi L, Helge H, Richens A, Schmidt D, eds. *Epilepsy, Pregnancy, and the Child*. New York: Raven Press, 1982: 211–22.

95 Gaily E, Granstrom ML, Hiilesmaa V, Bardy A. Minor abnormalities in offspring of epileptic mothers. *J Pediatr* 1988; 112: 520–9.

96 Phelan MC, Pellock JM, Nance WE. Discordant expression of fetal hydantoin syndrome in heteropaternal dizygotic twins. *N Engl J Med* 1982; 307: 99–101.

97 Merritt HH, Putnam TJ. Sodium diphenyl hydantoinate in the treatment of convulsive disorders. *J Am Med Assoc* 1938; 111: 1068–73.

98 Shorvon SD, Chadwick D, Galbraith AW, Reynolds EH. One drug for epilepsy. *Br Med J* 1978; 1: 474–6.

99 Bacon CJ, Hierons AM, Mucklow JC, Webb JKG, Rawlins MD, Weightman D. Placebo-controlled study of phenobarbitone and phenytoin in the prophylaxis of febrile convulsions. *Lancet* 1981; 2: 600–4.

100 Naidu S, Moodley J, Botha J, McFadyen L. The efficacy of phenytoin in relation to serum levels in severe pre-eclampsia and eclampsia. *Br J Obstet Gynaecol* 1992; 99: 881–6.

101 North JB, Hanieh A, Challen R, Penhall RK, Hann CS, Frewin DB. Postoperative epilepsy: a double-blind trial of phenytoin after craniotomy. *Lancet* 1980; 1: 384–6.

102 Salazar AM, Jabbari B, Vance SC, Grafman J, Amin D, Dillon JD. Epilepsy after penetrating head injury. I. Clinical correlates: a report of the Vietnam head injury study. *Neurology* 1985; 35: 1406–14.

103 Mitaki MA, Browne TR. Comparative efficacy of antiepileptic drugs. *Clin Neuropharmacol* 1988; 11: 130–40.

104 Marson AG, Chadwick D. Comparing antiepileptic drugs. *Curr Opin Neurol* 1996; 9: 103–6.

105 Mattson RH, Cramer JA, Collins JF *et al.* Comparison of carbamazepine, phenobarbital, phenytoin, and primidone in partial and secondarily generalized tonic-clonic seizures. *N Engl J Med* 1985; 313: 145–51.

106 Shakir RA, Johnson RH, Lambie DG, Melville ID, Nanda RN. Comparison of sodium valproate and phenytoin as single drug treatment in epilepsy. *Epilepsia* 1981; 22: 27–33.

107 Turnbull DM, Rawlings MD, Weightman D, Chadwick DW. A comparison of phenytoin and valproate in previously untreated adult epileptic patients. *J Neurol Neurosurg Psychiatr* 1982; 45: 55–9.

108 Wilder BJ, Ramsay RE, Murphy JV, Karas BJ, Marquardt K, Hammond EJ. Comparison of valproic acid and phenytoin in newly diagnosed tonic-clonic seizures. *Neurology* 1983; 33: 1474–6.

109 Callaghan N, Kenny RA, O'Neill B, Crowley M, Goggin T. A prospective study between carbamazepine, phenytoin and sodium valproate as monotherapy in previously untreated and recently diagnosed patients with epilepsy. *J Neurol Neurosurg Psychiatr* 1985; 48: 639–44.

110 Heller AJ, Chesterman P, Elwes RD *et al.* Phenobarbitone, phenytoin, carbamazepine, or sodium valproate for newly diagnosed adult epilepsy: a randomised comparative monotherapy trial. *J Neurol Neurosurg Psychiatr* 1995; 58: 44–50.

111 de Silva M, MacArdle B, McGowan M *et al.* Randomized comparative monotherapy trial of phenobarbitone, phenytoin, carbamazepine, or sodium valproate for newly diagnosed childhood epilepsy. *Lancet* 1996; 347: 709–13.

112 Steiner TJ, Dellaportas CI, Findley LJ *et al.* Lamotrigine monotherapy in newly diagnosed untreated epilepsy: a double-blind comparison with phenytoin. *Epilepsia* 1999; 40: 601–7.

113 Canadian Study Group for Childhood Epilepsy. Clobazam has equivalent efficacy to carbamazepine and phenytoin as monotherapy for childhood epilepsy. *Epilepsia* 1998; 39: 952–9.

114 Brodie MJ, Kwan P. The star system. Overview and use in determining antiepileptic drug choice. *CNS Drugs* 2001; 15: 1–12.

115 Eadie MJ, Tyrer JH, Bochner F, Hooper WD. The elimination of phenytoin in man. *Clin Exp Pharmacol Physiol* 1976; 3: 217–24.

41 Piracetam

S.D. Shorvon

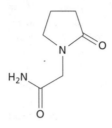

Primary indications	Adjunctive therapy for myoclonus
Usual preparations	Tablets or capsules: 400, 800, 1200 mg; solution: 20, 33%
Usual dosages	Initial: 7.2 g/day. Maintenance: up to 24 g/day
Dosage intervals	2–3 times/day
Significant drug interactions	None
Serum level monitoring	Not useful
Target range	–
Common/important side-effects	Dizziness, insomnia, nausea, gastrointestinal discomfort, hyperkinesis, weight gain, tremulousness, agitation, drowsiness, rash
Main advantages	Well-tolerated and very effective in some resistant cases
Main disadvantages	Not effective in many cases
Mechanisms of action	Unclear
Oral bioavailability	<100%
Time to peak levels	30–40 min
Metabolism and excretion	Renal excretion without metabolism
Volume of distribution	0.6 L/kg
Elimination half-life	5–6 h
Plasma clearance	–
Protein binding	None
Active metabolites	None
Comment	Useful drug for some patients with refractory myoclonus

(*Note*: this summary table was formulated by the lead editor.)

The pyrrolidone (2-oxo-pyrrolidine) derivatives form a family of compounds which have unique properties in a variety of neurological settings. Over 1600 compounds in this chemical group have been synthesized in the past three decades, and over 300 compounds seriously studied by at least 10 different pharmaceutical companies. Experimental and clinical work was focused initially on the so-called nootropic effect [1–3], and then more recently on the possibilities for neuroprotection after stroke and as an antiepileptic.

Piracetam was the first drug of the class to be developed, following pioneering research by Giurgea and Salama [2], working in the laboratories of UCB. It was Giurgea who also coined the term nootropic for this drug class to mean (a) enhancement of learning and memory; (b) facilitation of cross-hemispheric information flow; (c) neuroprotection; and (d) lack of other psychopharmacological actions (e.g. sedation, analgesia, or motor or behavioural changes) which distinguishes this class from other psychoactive drugs. The clinical value of piracetam in this role is contentious, and the findings are not, for instance, considered strong enough currently to allow licensing for this indication in the USA or the UK. However, piracetam is widely used in many other countries, particularly in the developing world, and the manufacturers report that over 1 000 000 people worldwide are currently receiving the drug largely for nootropic indications. It is also worth commenting on the geographical aspects of the interest in this drug class. There are expanding programmes of clinical studies in Japan and in Asia, and whilst the geographical differences are likely to be due to cultural regulatory factors, it remains at least possible that there are racial differences in drug response.

The major impact of piracetam in the field of epilepsy is its antimyoclonic effect and this is the main concern of this chapter. The drug is currently also being investigated for a beneficial effect in mild cognitive impairment (MCI) and to aid functional recovery after stroke, and in various countries is licensed for other indications (Table 41.1). The remarkable antimyoclonic effect of piracetam was first reported in 1978 in a case of postanoxic myoclonus after cardiac arrest [4], and in the past decade the effectiveness of this drug in cortical myoclonus of various aetiologies has been confirmed. Its use in epilepsy is confined to this indication.

A striking feature of the entire drug class is its stereospecificity [5,6] (Fig. 41.1). Minor changes in structure result in remarkable differences in pharmaceutical action. The l-isomer of piracetam, for instance, levetiracetam exhibits quite different cerebral binding and very strong broad-spectrum antiepileptic properties as well as effects in myoclonus (see Chapter 37). Other drugs in this class also have antimyoclonic and antiepileptic properties, including some in the early experimental phase and others in late phase trials (e.g. nefiracetam).

Another notable aspect of the whole class is their lack of side-effects or of central nervous system toxicity, and this distinguishes the group from other psychotropic drug classes (for example, the N-methyl-D-aspartate (NMDA) antagonists) which have been investigated in the same general therapeutic areas. This lack of toxicity has been an important impetus to further studies, and remains one of the primary attractions of this drug class.

Mechanism of action

The antimyoclonic action of the drug is unexplained, as indeed are its other putative effects. Piracetam has been shown to enhance oxidative glycolysis, to have anticholinergic effects, positive effects of the cerebral microcirculation under certain conditions and increases in cerebral blood flow, effects on membrane physics and also rheological properties including reduction of platelet aggregation and improvement in erythrocyte function [3,7–10]. How any of these properties might contribute to the suppression of myoclonus is quite unclear. Although disturbances of serotonergic and γ-aminobutyric acid (GABA)-ergic function are implicated in cortical myoclonus, piracetam does not seem to modify GABAergic activity, or affect cerebral serotonin or dopamine levels.

Pharmacology and pharmacokinetics

Piracetam, 2-oxo-1-pyrrolidine acetamide, is a white, almost odourless crystalline powder. The pharmacokinetics of the drug have been widely studied in humans and animals. The human and animal pharmacology are very similar. The drug has favourable properties for both acute and chronic oral use [11,12]. Studies in healthy volunteers have shown rapid and complete absorption after

Table 41.1 Licensed indication of piracetam in Europe and the USA

	Myoclonus	Cognitive impairment[a]	Post-stroke	Other
Austria	–	+	+	Alcohol withdrawal, alcoholism, head injury (sequelae)
Belgium	+	+	–	Alcohol withdrawal, learning disorder, vertigo, dyslexia
France	+	+	–	Dyslexia, vertigo
Germany	+	+	+	Head injury (sequelae), dyslexia, learning disorder
Italy	–	+	+[b]	Dyslexia, learning disorder, alcohol withdrawal
Netherlands	–	–	–	Vertigo
Norway	+	–	–	None
Portugal	+	+	+	Learning disorder, dyslexia, head injury (sequelae), post-traumatic vertigo and coma, sickle-cell anaemia, alcoholism, epilepsy, alcohol withdrawal, Raynaud's disease, Parkinson's disease
Spain	+	+	+	None
Sweden	+	–	–	None
Switzerland	+	+	–	Dyslexia
UK	+	–	–	None
USA	–	–	–	None

From [3].

[a] Cognitive impairment is variously defined in different countries as chronic organic brain disorders, Alzheimer's disease, senile dementia of the Alzheimer's type, multi-infarct dementia.

[b] Mental symptoms caused by cerebral insufficiency.

In the developing world and in Asia, piracetem is widely used with varying indications.

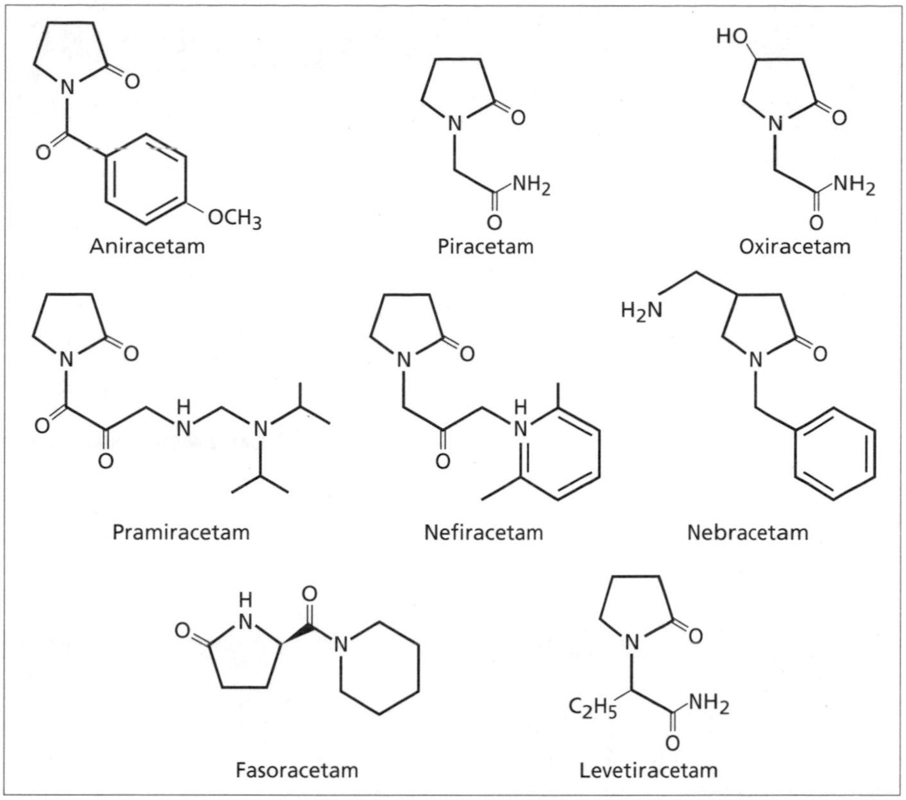

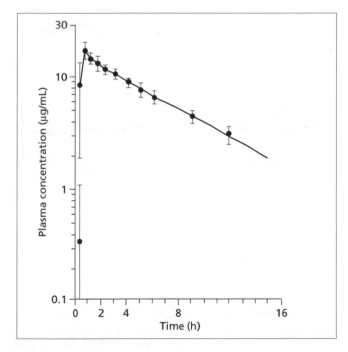

Fig. 41.1 Structure of piracetam and seven other pyrrolidone drugs which are licensed or in clinical trials.

oral administration, with peak concentrations reached between 30 and 50 min. The C_{max} values are 15–37 mg/L after a single dose of 800 mg, and 30–54 mg/L after a dose of 1600 mg. The volume of distribution of piracetam is 0.5–0.75 L/kg, and there is no significant protein binding. Piracetam crosses the blood–brain barrier with a delayed peak, and the mean half-life in cerebrospinal fluid is 7.7 h after IV injection in healthy volunteers. The dose–serum level ratio is linear (Fig. 41.2). The drug does not undergo metabolism, and is excreted unchanged through the kidneys, with renal excretion accounting for 85–100% of the dose in various studies; figures which are similar in acute or chronic administration (Fig. 41.3). After oral administration of single doses between 800 and 1200 mg, an elimination half-life of 4–5 h is found, and similar findings have been reported in the elderly. The drug crosses the placental barrier freely. The distribution of the molecule has been investigated in the rat with radioactive labelled drug, with some evidence of preferential concentration in brain. Limited experience in humans also shows the drug to be somewhat more slowly eliminated from cerebrospinal fluid (half-life, 7.4 h) than from blood. No drug interactions have been recorded, and none indeed would be expected in view of the lack of metabolism or protein binding and its mode of elimination. Over the years, the studies of potential interaction have included comedication with antibiotics, antiepileptic drugs, muscle relaxants, corticosteroids, antifibrinolytic drugs, antidepressants, antihypertensive drugs and hormone replacement therapy.

Clinical effectiveness

The first case report demonstrating an antimyoclonic effect was by

Fig. 41.2 Plasma concentrations following oral administration of 800-mg tablets. From manufacturer's literature.

Terwinghe *et al.* [4], in which a dramatic acute effect on postanoxic myoclonus was recorded. Subsequent uncontrolled reports in small numbers of patients confirmed this action [13–20]. Following the early anecdotal reports, Obeso and colleagues then published a

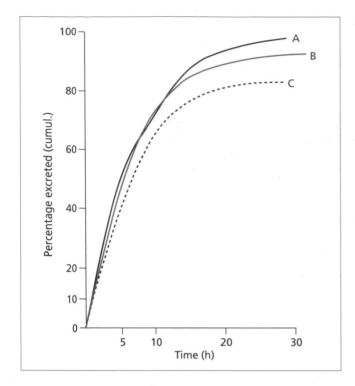

Fig. 41.3 Urinary excretion of labelled piracetam in three subjects following a single oral dose of 2 g. From manufacturer's literature.

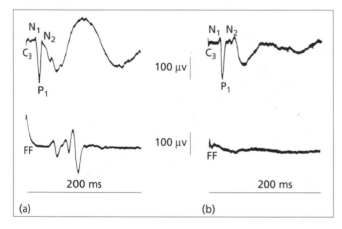

Fig. 41.4 Giant cortical somatosensory evoked potential to electrical stimulation of the forefinger and the reflex EMG discharge recorded from the finger flexor (FF) muscles of the right arm. (a) Prior to treatment with piracetam, and (b) following treatment, showing the abolition of the reflex myoclonus after treatment with oral piracetam. From [24].

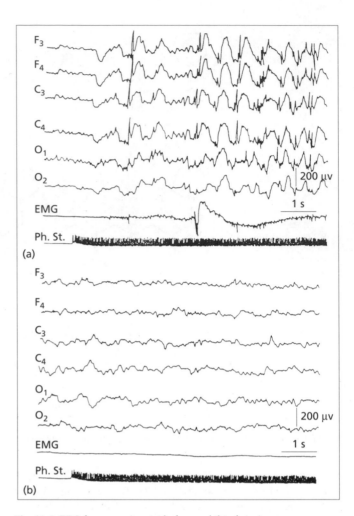

Fig. 41.5 EEG from a patient (a) before and (b) after piracetam treatment. The pretreatment EEG shows spike-and-wave activity associated with generalized muscle jerks, induced by photic stimulation at 18 flashes/s. The post-treatment EEG shows a complete suppression of the spike-wave bursts and also the reflex myoclonic jerking after oral treatment with piracetam on 9 g/day for 7 days. From [24].

series of papers [21–26], exploring the effects of piracetam in myoclonus more systematically (e.g. in a patient with myoclonic encephalopathy of uncertain aetiology; Figs 41.4, 41.5). These studies included a series of 40 patients with myoclonus, with differing clinical and electrophysiological features [25], and subsequently a further report of 10 patients extensively studied and treated with up to 18 g/day of piracetam [26]. In 1993, a placebo-controlled double-blind crossover trial was reported confirming the undoubted effectiveness of the drug in myoclonus [27]; the drug was then licensed for use in myoclonus in the UK and elsewhere.

The 40 patients reported by Obeso *et al.* [25] were heterogeneous. The myoclonus was secondary to anoxia in 12 cases, associated with the Ramsey–Hunt syndrome in five cases, multisystem atrophy in four, torsion dystonia in seven, birth anoxia in three, Creutzfeldt–Jakob disease in two, and occurred in single cases of Alzheimer's disease, herpes encephalitis, Lafora body disease and essential myoclonus. In three cases, the cause was unknown. Piracetam was given as short-term monotherapy to six patients. Two with cortical myoclonus showed electrophysiological improvement, but none of the four with electrophysiological evidence of subcortical myoclonus improved. Nine patients with cortical and subcortical myoclonus showed no clinical improvement on monotherapy. Twenty-eight patients had piracetam added to existing antimyoclonic therapy, and in 16 there was improvement. A dramatic response was seen in one case on clonazepam, who was bedbound with severe postanoxic action myoclonus. When piracetam was added she could walk, dress and feed herself; within 2 days of withdrawal of piracetam she was again bedbound. Five out of eight other patients with postanoxic myoclonus also improved, but less dramatically. All of the 16 patients who showed improvement had cortical myoclonus, and the aetiology underlying the cases was varied. Five other patients with cortical myoclonus did not improve, nor did any of the seven patients with subcortical myoclonus.

The study of Brown et al. [27] was a well-conducted double-blind placebo-controlled crossover trial in 21 patients. All patients had cortical myoclonus and received piracetam or placebo for 14-day trial periods, in addition to their routine antimyoclonic therapy. Patients were rated on scales of stimulus sensitivity, motor, writing, functional disability, and also were scored on global assessments and visual analogue scales. Ten of the 21 patients failed to complete the placebo phase due to a severe exacerbation of their myoclonus, and none from the piracetam phase. Significant improvements were noted in all the scales on piracetam, and there was a median 22% improvement on piracetam on the global rating scale. There were also more seizures of other types in the placebo than piracetam phase. These results are impressive and confirm that piracetam can have a marked effect on cortical myoclonus. The study also showed that abrupt withdrawal of piracetam may lead to a marked exacerbation of myoclonus and withdrawal seizures. Longer term follow-up of some of the patients in these trials has confirmed the effect of piracetam, and in at least one of the cases (treated by the author), the effect was profound and has been maintained without evidence of tolerance. This patient, with myoclonus and epilepsy of unknown aetiology, was bedbound and dependent prior to piracetam therapy. There was an immediate response to piracetam, and immediate relapse on the three occasions that the drug has been withdrawn. After 6 years of therapy (at a daily dose of 21 g piracetam), she is still almost entirely free of myoclonus, has completed a university education and lives a normal life. Peuvot [28] reported the effect of piracetam in 13 patients (12 with postanoxic myoclonus), of whom five were 'cured' and all except one improved. It was also noted that temporary withdrawal of piracetam led to a 'spectacular reappearance of myoclonus'.

Other reports of effectiveness against myoclonus, often dramatic, have been published: Paulus et al. [29] in three patients with progressive myoclonic epilepsy; Kim et al. [30] in myoclonus due to carbon monoxide poisoning; Straub [31] in two sisters with myoclonus due to sialidosis type 1; Akpinar et al. [32] in six cases of dyssinergia cerebellis myoclonica; Karacostas et al. [33] in postelectrocution myoclonus; and Thompson et al. [34] in three patients with Huntington's disease and myoclonus.

Cortical myoclonus, with or without additional epilepsy, can result in profound disability. The jerks are often exacerbated by action, and the patients may be bedbound and immobile, unable to move without severe myoclonic jerking disrupting all motor responses. In some cases, piracetam can have a truly remarkable effect, suppressing the myoclonus, and reversing completely even severe disability. In such patients, the drug is nearer to a 'magic bullet' than any other I have experience of. There does not appear to be tolerance to the antimyoclonic effect, but withdrawal of medication will often return the patient to the pretreatment state within a few days [35]. Whether or not the effects are confined to cortical myoclonus is uncertain, and I have personal cases with myoclonus, controlled by piracetam, which was more likely to be subcortical in origin. Not all patients with cortical myoclonus respond to the

drug, and what differentiates these cases from others is quite unclear. It is the only drug that improves the myoclonus in some patients with progressive myoclonic epilepsy syndromes. There are no systematic studies of the myoclonus of idiopathic generalized epilepsy (e.g. in juvenile myoclonic epilepsy), although these would be of great interest. The effect of piracetam on other types of seizures has not been studied in a controlled fashion, although anecdotal experience is disappointing.

Long-term efficacy is maintained, and there is no evidence of habituation or tolerance. It has been said that the drug works best in combination, for example with clonazepam, although personal and anecdotal experience shows that piracetam monotherapy can be highly efficacious. It is usual to reserve piracetam therapy as a second line for patients resistant to treatment with valproate or benzodiazepine drugs. Its effectiveness in some patients combined with its almost complete lack of side-effects give the drug a special place in the therapy of myoclonus. The dosing in myoclonus has to be extremely high. The initial dose is 4.8 g/day and this may be rapidly increased (in 1600-mg incremental steps weekly) to 18–32 g/day in two or three divided doses. The major drawback at these higher doses is the number of tablets taken and their bulk, although occasionally drowsiness is dose limiting in this high range. Serum level monitoring is not available.

As mentioned earlier, piracetam has been widely used clinically for other indications. Its cognitive enhancing properties have been the subject of numerous open studies but most were uncontrolled and do not meet modern assessment standards. About 50 controlled studies exist, with some showing modest benefits, but others are negative. The picture is very mixed, and a Cochrane meta-analysis was carried out in 1998 which concluded that evidence of effects on cognition and other measures were inconclusive [36]. There are also on-going studies of the effect of piracetam on the syndrome of mild cognitive impairment. A distinctive and convincing neuroprotective function, separate from cognitive enhancement, has been demonstrated experimentally. Both properties clearly carry promise for use after stroke, both to limit functional impairment and for rehabilitation [37–39]. Initial uncontrolled clinical evidence in acute stroke had been encouraging, but the major randomized control trial, of 927 patients randomized to placebo or piracetam (12 g IV, followed by 12 g daily for 4 weeks and 4.8 g daily for 8 weeks), showed no difference in the primary or secondary endpoints (the neurological outcome after 4 weeks or functional outcome after 12 weeks) [37,38]. It is possible that earlier treatment confers more benefit, and also that those with more severe symptoms following stroke do better than those with mild symptoms, and also those with aphasia [39,40].

Side-effects

In animal experimentation, few adverse effects have been reported, and acute toxicological studies showed the drug to be lethal only at very high doses (in mice at 18.2 g/kg, in rats at 21 g/kg and in dogs at 10 g/kg).

Because of its extensive use as a cognitive-enhancing drug, there is considerable experience of adverse events in clinical use, at least at low dosage. The drug seems well tolerated, and there is a very low incidence of reported side-effects. Even in the placebo-controlled trials, side-effects were often reported at a significantly greater frequency in placebo than with the active drug. In these studies, the side-effects include dizziness, insomnia, nausea, gastrointestinal discomfort, hyperkinesis, weight gain and agitation (all reported at a frequency of less than 10%). Rash occurs in less than 1% of patients, and there have been no serious idiosyncratic reactions. In the placebo-controlled double-blind crossover study of Brown et al. [27], the only adverse events were a sore throat and headache in one patient, and single seizures in two; these side-effects may well not have been treatment related. In routine clinical treatment of myoclonus, it is not uncommon to use daily doses of up to 24 g or more, and the adverse event profile at these doses is much less well studied. Anecdotal clinical evidence suggests, however, that most patients tolerate even these high doses well, and that side-effects are rarely a serious problem. In the controlled trials, there have been no significant effects on haematological or biochemical parameters.

Administration and dosage

Piracetam is available in 800 and 1200 mg white tablets or as a solution of 333.3 mg/mL. In myoclonus, early experience and the first clinical series used doses of piracetam which were high by previous standards, but modest by current standards: Terwinghe et al. [4] used 4.8 g/day in the first reported case; 6.4 g/day [41]; 8–9 g/day [16,21,24]; and 10 g/day [13,29,32,35]. More recently, higher doses have been used—up to 16.8 g/day [27]; up to 18 g/day [26]; and in my personal clinical practice doses of up to 24 g/day or even higher are commonly used. The optimal dosage is therefore unclear, and it would seem sensible advice to recommend initial therapy of between 4.8 and 8.0 g/day, and to progressively increase this to up to 24 g/day, guided by clinical response and limited by side-effects. The drug can be given in two or three divided doses; its major drawback at higher doses being the number of tablets taken and their bulk. For other indications, lower doses are used.

There is little experience of the drug in pregnancy, but as the drug readily crosses the placenta and into breast milk, it should be avoided in pregnancy and lactation. As the drug is almost exclusively excreted by the kidneys, the dose should be lowered in patients with renal impairment. Recommended adjustments are 50% reduction in dose at creatinine clearances of 40–60 mL/min (serum creatinine of 112–153 μmol/L) and 75% reduction at creatinine clearances of 20–40 mL/min (serum creatinine of 153–270 μmol/L). The drug is contraindicated in patients with creatinine clearances below 20 mL/min, and in those with severe hepatic impairment. There is no published experience of the drug in children.

References

1 Gouliaev AH, Senning A. Piracetam and other structurally related nootropics. Brain Res Rev 1994; 19: 180–2.
2 Giurgea C, Salama M. Nootropic drugs. Prog Neuropsychopharmacol Biol Psychiatr 1997; 1: 235–47.
3 Shorvon S. Pyrrolidone derivatives. Lancet 2001; 358: 1885–92.
4 Terwinghe G, Daumerie J, Nicaise CL, Rosillon O. Therapeutic effect of piracetam in a case of postanoxic action myoclonus. Acta Neurol Belg 1978; 78: 30–6.
5 Noyer M, Gillard M, Matagne A, Hénichart J-P, Wülfert E. The novel antiepileptic drug levetiracetam (ucb L059) appears to act via a specific binding site in CNS membranes. Eur J Pharmacol 1995; 286: 137–46.
6 Genton P, Van Vleymen B. Piracetam and levetiracetam: close structural
7 Peuvot J, Schanck A, Deleers M, Brasseur R. Piracetam-induced changes to membrane physical properties: a combined approach by 31P nuclear magnetic resonance and conformational analysis. Biochem Pharmacol 1995; 50: 1129–34.
8 Müller W, Koch S, Scheuer, Rostock A, Bartsch R. Effects of piracetam on membrane fluidity in the aged mouse, rat and human brain. Biochem Pharmacol 1997; 53: 135–40.
9 Verloes R, Scotto AM, Gobert J, Wülfert E. Effects of nootropic drugs in scopolamine-induced amnesia model in mice. Psychopharmacology 1988; 95: 226–30.
10 Sara SJ, Lefevre D. Hypoxia induced amnesia in one trial learning and pharmacological protection by piracetam. Psychopharmacologia (Berlin) 1972; 25: 32–40.
11 Hitzenberger G, Rameis H, Manigley C. Pharmacological properties of piracetam: rationale for use in stroke patients. CNS Drugs 1998; 9 (Suppl. 1): 19–27.
12 Parnetti L. Clinical pharmacokinetics of drugs for Alzheimer's disease. Clin Pharmacokinet 1995; 29: 110–29.
13 Cremieux C, Serratrice G. Post-anoxic intention myoclonus. Amelioration with piracetam. Nouv Presse Med 1979; 8 (412): 3357–8.
14 Petit HA, Destee J-L, Salomez J-L, Gomel JJ. Syndromes Myocloniques et Dystoniques. Action du piracetam. Proceedings of Le Congrès de Psychiatrie et de Neurologie de Langue Française, 1981.
15 Bourrin JC, Chopard JL, Lassauge F, Boillot A, Dintroz M, Rousselot JP. Lance and Adams syndrome. Report of an observation. Favorable evolution under treatment. Lyon Med 1982; 247: 39–43.
16 Fahn S. Newer drugs for posthypoxic action myoclonus: observation from a well-studied case. Adv Neurol 1986; 43: 197–9.
17 Barreiro Tella P, Diez-Tejedor E, Frank Garcia A, Vinals Torras M. Therapeutic effect of piracetam in action myoclonus and the Ramsay–Hunt syndrome. Neurologia 1986; 1 (Suppl. 1): 5.
18 Van Vleymen B, Van Zandijcke M. Piracetam in the treatment of myoclonus; an overview. Acta Neurol Belg 1996; 96: 270–80.
19 Koskiniemi M, Van Vleymen B, Hakamies L, Lamusuo S, Taalas J. Piracetam relieves symptoms in progressive myoclonus epilepsy: a multicentre, randomised, double blind, crossover study comparing the efficacy and safety of three dosages of oral piracetam with placebo. J Neurol Neurosurg Psychiatr 1998; 64: 344–8.
20 Genton P, Guerrini R, Remy P. Piracetam in the treatment of cortical myoclonus. Pharmacopsychiatry 1999; 32 (Suppl.): 49–53.
21 Martinez-Lage JM, Obseo JA, Artieda J et al. Treatment of myoclonus with piracetam. J Neurol 1985; 232 (Suppl. 1): 112.
22 Artieda J, Obseo JA, Luquin MR, Vaamonde J, Martinez-Lage JM. Piracetam in the treatment of myoclonus of various origin. Neurology 1986; 36/4 (Suppl. 1): 1.
23 Artieda J, Obeso JA, Luquin MR, Vaamonde J, Martinez-Lage JM. Photosensitive myoclonus: physiologic and pharmacologic study. Neurology 1987; 37: 263.
24 Obeso JA, Artieda J, Luquin MR, Vaamonde J, Martinez-Lage JM. Antimyoclonic action of piracetam. Clin Neuropharmacol 1986; 9: 58–64.
25 Obeso JA, Artieda J, Quinn M et al. Piracetam in the treatment of different types of myoclonus. Clin Neuropharmacol 1988; 11: 529–36.
26 Obeso JA, Artieda J, Rothwell JC, Day B, Thompson P, Marsden CD. The treatment of severe action myoclonus. Brain 1989; 112: 756–77.
27 Brown P, Steiger MJ, Thompson PD et al. Effectiveness of piracetam in cortical myoclonus. Mov Disord 1993; 8(1): 63–8.
28 Peuvot J. Piracetam. 5 year progress in pharmacology. Athens Fund Crenc Med 1990; 22: 101–7.
29 Paulus W, Ried S, Stodieck SRG, Schmidt D. Abolition of photoparoxysmal response in progressive myoclonus epilepsy. Eur Neurol 1991; 31: 388–90.
30 Kim JS, Lee SA, Kim JS. Myoclonus delayed sequelae of carbon monoxide poisoning, piracetam trial. Yonsei Med J 1987; 28(3): 231–4.
31 Straub H-B. Treatment of myoclonus in sialidosis type 1 with piracetam. Neurology 1993; 43: 4.
32 Akpinar S, Yardium M, Vural O, Tanndag O, Alver T, Gunduz D. Action of myoclonus treatment with high dose piracetam. Psychopharmacology 1988; 96: 366.

similarities but different pharmacological and clinical profiles. Epileptic Dis 2000; 2: 99–105.

33 Karacostas D, Giannopoulos S, Artemis N, Milonas I. Effect of piracetam on myoclonus secondary to electrocution. A case report. *Acta Ther* 1993; 19: 401–4.

34 Thompson PD, Bhatia KP, Brown P *et al*. Cortical myoclonus in Huntingdon's disease. *Mov Disord* 1994; 9(6): 633–41.

35 Papyrakis JC. Management of a case of myoclonia. *Acta Ther* 1987; 13/1: 109–14.

36 Flicker L, Grimley Evans J. Piracetam for dementia or cognitive impairment. *The Cochrane Library* 1999; 1: 1–43.

37 Herrschaft H, ed. Advances in the management of stroke: the role of piracetam. *CNS Drugs* 1998; 9 (Suppl. 1): 1–59.

38 Orgogozo J-M. Piracetam in the treatment of acute stroke. *CNS Drugs* 1998; 9 (Suppl. 1); 41–9.

39 Enderby P, Broeck J, Hospers W *et al*. Effect of piracetam on recovery and rehabilitation after stroke: a double blind placebo controlled study. *Clin Neuropharmacol* 1994; 17: 320–31.

40 Huber W, Willmes K, Poeck R *et al*. Piracetam in aphasia: a double blind study. *Arch Phys Med Rehab* 1997; 72: 245–50.

41 Fernandez Ortega JD, Arnal Garcia C, Togores Veguero JM. Piracetam in myoclonus of the trunk. *Revista Españ Neurol* 1987; 2/5: 282.

Pregabalin

E. Ben-Menachem and A.R. Kugler

Primary indication	Adjunctive therapy in the treatment of partial seizures with or without secondary generalization in adults
Usual preparation	Capsules: 25 mg, 50 mg, 75 mg, 150 mg, 300 mg
Usual dosage	Initial: 75 mg 2 times/day (150 mg/day). Maintenance: 150–600 mg/day
Dosage intervals	2 times/day
Significant drug interactions	Nil
Serum level monitoring	Not required
Target range	–
Common/important side-effects	Somnolence, dizziness, ataxia
Main advantages	On the basis of clinical trial experience, is effective and well tolerated
Main disadvantages	Limited clinical practice experience
Mechanism of action	Binds to alpha$_2$-delta subunits of voltage-gated calcium channels
Oral bioavailability	90%
Time to peak levels	1 h
Metabolism and excretion	No metabolism. Excreted via the kidney
Volume of distribution	42 L following oral administration
Elimination half-life	6.3 h
Plasma clearance	83 mL/min following oral administration
Protein binding	Nil
Active metabolites	Nil
Comment	Antiepileptic; under regulatory review, for adjunctive therapy in partial seizures with or without secondary generalization, and for treatment of neuropathic pain in adults

(*Note*: this summary table was formulated by the lead editor.)

Pregabalin is a new antiepileptic drug (AED) that is currently in Phase III clinical trials. Registration activities and submissions to regulatory bodies are underway at the time of manuscript preparation. The drug is being developed for epilepsy, neuropathic pain and generalized anxiety disorder [1–3].

Pharmacology

The compound itself is a structural analogue of γ-aminobutyric acid (GABA) and is also known as S-(+)-3-isobutyl GABA. It is a white solid and is stable for > 18 months at 25°C. Although pregabalin has structural similarities to gabapentin, the potency in animal models of epilepsy, pain and anxiety is significantly greater. Effective doses of pregabalin are lower than for gabapentin and the clinical effect longer per dose. The R-isomer of S-pregabalin, R-isobutyl GABA, appears to be 10-fold less potent in animal models of epilepsy and pain than the isomer being developed [4].

The mechanism of action of pregabalin is not fully understood. Pregabalin is an α_2-δ ligand that has analgesic, anxiolytic, and anticonvulsant activity. α_2-δ is an auxiliary protein associated with voltage-gated calcium channels. Pregabalin binds potently to the α_2-δ subunit [5]. Potent binding at this site reduces calcium influx at nerve terminals and therefore reduces the release of several neurotransmitters, including glutamate, noradrenaline and substance P [6–9]. These activities and effects result in the analgesic, anxiolytic and anticonvulsant activity exhibited by pregabalin. Pregabalin is inactive at GABA-A and GABA-B receptors, it is not converted metabolically into GABA or a GABA antagonist, and it does not alter GABA uptake or degradation [1,10].

Animal models of epilepsy

In animal models of epilepsy, pregabalin has a similar profile in all animal models tested to gabapentin but pregabalin was consistently three- to six-fold more potent on a milligram per kilogram dose basis compared with gabapentin [11].

In the maximal electric shock (MES) model, which is an indicator of efficacy in generalized tonic-clonic seizures, pregabalin prevented tonic extensor seizures in mice at doses similar for both p.o. and i.v. delivery suggesting high bioavailability (ED_{50} 20 mg/kg p.o.), and in rats (ED_{50} 1.5 mg/kg p.o.) with maximal effect 2–4 h after dosing.

The pentylenetetrazrol test is an indicator for effect in primary generalized seizures. Pregabalin had less effect in this model than for the MES, preventing threshold clonic seizures at ED_{50} 97 mg/kg p.o. in mice and >125 mg/kg p.o. in rats. Pregabalin only partially blocked the response in the bicucullin, picrotoxin and strychnine models, which are indicative of effect on the central nervous GABAergic system.

In the hippocampal kindling rat model, pregabalin at doses of 9.5 mg/kg reduced behavioural seizures while higher doses prevented both behavioural seizures and afterdischarges, suggesting that pregabalin might be effective for the treatment of focal seizures [12].

There was no effect of pregabalin on audiogenic seizures neither in the DBA/2 mice nor in the genetically susceptible rats with spontaneous absence seizures (genetic absence epilepsy in rats from Strasbourg (GAERS)). High doses (>200 mg/kg i.p.) increased the amount of absence seizures in GAERS. That dose is 20-fold higher than the highest recommended dose in humans of 600 mg/day [4].

Pharmacokinetics

Pregabalin exhibits predictable linear pharmacokinetics [13]. In the studies elucidating the pharmacokinetics in healthy normal human volunteers, single rising doses of 1–300 mg and multiple rising doses of 25–300 mg given every 8 h and 300 mg given every 12 h for 14 days were used. Pregabalin was found to be rapidly absorbed with a bioavailability of > 90%. T_{max} was 1 h with both C_{max} and overall exposure (AUC, area under the plasma pregabalin concentration–time curve) proportional to dose and similar following both single and multiple doses. The plasma pregabalin half-life was approximately 6 h, independent of dose and repeated administration. Plasma pregabalin concentration–time profiles were similar following twice or three times daily dosing [13].

Pregabalin is not metabolized to any extent in man nor does it bind to plasma proteins. It does not affect the cytochrome P450 system in humans at therapeutic doses. Approximately 98% of the drug can be recovered unchanged in the urine. The per cent excreted is independent of dose and is not significantly different whether given as single or repeated administrations (82–108%). There have been no reports of drug interactions.

Pregnancy

No information is yet available on the effect of pregabalin on pregnancy since the drug is still undergoing clinical trials. Female patients in these studies are instructed not to become pregnant. However, pregabalin is not teratogenic in mice or rabbits, but teratogenicity was observed in rats at very high doses of 1250–2500 mg/kg. That dose range is > 100-fold higher than the upper end of the human recommended dose range of 600 mg/day, representing a body weight normalized dose of < 10 mg/kg (data on file; Pfizer, Ann Arbor, Michigan, USA).

Clinical efficacy

Randomized control trials (RCT)

As of 14 February 2003, more than 9400 subjects have received oral pregabalin including over 1600 epilepsy patients, 2500 neuropathic pain patients and 1900 patients with generalized anxiety disorder (data on file; Pfizer, Ann Arbor, Michigan, USA).

One pilot, inpatient, double-blind, monotherapy study in refractory partial epilepsy has been reported (Study 1008-007; [14]). Patients were in the monitoring unit for epilepsy surgical evaluation. During this period patients had their concomitant AEDs down titrated and then randomized to either 600 mg/day pregabalin (n = 42) or 300 mg/day gabapentin (n=51) daily for 8 days. Pregabalin 600 mg/day exhibited anticonvulsant activity in patients with refractory epilepsy as demonstrated by a longer time to exit and by a greater proportion of patients completing the study with pregabalin compared to gabapentin 300 mg/day. Pregabalin 600 mg/day was well tolerated

The results of three major outpatient, multicentre, double-blind, placebo-controlled, parallel-group, randomized trials of pregabalin as add-on therapy in patients with refractory partial epilepsy have been presented and reported in abstract form, with full publication underway. Seizure counts were collected based on entries in daily seizure diaries, made by patients or their guardian. Seizure frequencies were assessed during 8-week baseline periods, in which patients were required to experience at least six partial seizures with no 4-week seizure-free period. Treatment periods were 12 weeks with drug titrated over 1 week or initiated without titration. The patients enrolled were highly refractory with a mean epilepsy duration of approximately 25 years and a mean 28-day seizure rate in baseline of approximately 22. Patients could be taking one to three concomitant AEDs, which were not changed during the entire study period. Approximately one-quarter of patients were taking one, half taking two and one-quarter taking three concomitant AEDs. After the double-blind phases, patients were allowed to continue pregabalin therapy in optional, long-term, open-label extension studies. Overall, pregabalin was well tolerated as 83% of pregabalin-treated patients enrolled in the open-label extensions. The primary efficacy measure was reduction in all partial seizure frequency during treatment compared with baseline. Efficacy was also assessed on the basis of responder rate, defined as the percentage of patients with a 50% or greater reduction in seizure frequency during treatment compared with baseline, and seizure freedom assessed over the last 28 days of treatment. Individual results for the three adjunctive double-blind trials are given below.

The first RCT enrolled 453 patients at 76 centres in the USA and Canada (Study 1008-034; [15]). Patients were randomized to one of five treatment groups: placebo, 50, 150, 300 or 600 mg/day pregabalin given b.i.d., with no titration phase. There was a percentage reduction in seizure frequency between baseline and treatment periods of 7, 12, 34, 44 and 54 for the placebo (n=100) and the pregabalin 50 (n=88), 150 (n=86), 300 (n=90) and 600 (n=89) mg/day groups, respectively. Seizure reduction for all partial seizures was statistically significantly lower in the pregabalin 150, 300 and 600 mg/day groups compared with the placebo group ($P \leq 0.0001$). Responder rates were 14, 15, 31, 40 and 51%, respectively, and was significantly greater than placebo in the pregabalin 150 (P=0.006), 300 ($P \leq 0.001$) and 600 ($P \leq 0.001$) mg/day groups. The analysis of seizure reduction ($P \leq 0.0001$) and responder rate ($P \leq 0.001$) also indicated a significant pregabalin dose–response. Seizure-free rates were 8, 5, 6, 11 and 17%, respectively. Adverse events resulted in the discontinuation of 5, 7, 1, 14 and 24% patients, respectively. Common adverse events were dizziness and somnolence and both appeared to be dose related. Most adverse events were transient and mild to moderate in intensity.

The second study enrolled 287 patients at 45 international centres in Europe, South Africa and Australia (Study 1008-011; [16]). Patients were treated with placebo, 150 or 600 mg/day pregabalin given t.i.d., with up to 1 week of titration. There was a percentage reduction in seizure frequency between baseline and treatment periods of –2 (slight worsening in placebo), 21 and 48 for the placebo (n=96), pregabalin 150 (n=99) and pregabalin 600 (n=92) mg/day groups, respectively. Seizure reduction for all partial seizures was statistically significantly lower in the pregabalin 150 (P=0.0007) and 600 ($P \leq 0.0001$) mg/day groups compared with the placebo group. Responder rates were 6, 14 and 44%, respectively. The analysis of seizure reduction ($P \leq 0.0001$) and responder rate ($P \leq 0.001$) also indicated a significant pregabalin dose–response. Seizure-free rates were 1, 7 and 12%, respectively. Adverse events resulted in the discontinuation of 6, 10 and 19% patients, respectively. The adverse events most frequently experienced by patients in the active treatment groups were somnolence, dizziness, ataxia and asthenia. Most adverse events were transient and mild to moderate in intensity.

The third study enrolled 312 patients at 43 centres in the USA and Canada (Study 1008-009; [17]). Patients were given placebo, 600 mg/day pregabalin in three divided doses (t.i.d.), or 600 mg/day pregabalin in two divided doses (b.i.d.), with up to 1 week of titration. There was a percentage reduction in seizure frequency between baseline and treatment periods of –1, 53 and 44 for the placebo (n=98), pregabalin 600 mg/day t.i.d. (n=111, $P \leq 0.0001$) and pregabalin 600 mg/day b.i.d. (n=103, $P \leq 0.0001$) groups, respectively. The percentage reduction in seizure rate for the pregabalin b.i.d. and t.i.d. groups were similar and not statistically significantly different ($P \leq 0.1092$). Responder rates were 9%, 49% ($P \leq 0.001$) and 43% ($P \leq 0.001$), respectively. The responder rates for the pregabalin b.i.d. and t.i.d. groups were similar and not sta-

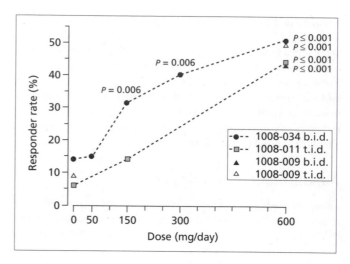

Fig. 42.1 Responder rate ($\geq 50\%$ seizure frequency reduction from baseline) by study, regimen and daily dose for all partial seizures. The dotted lines connect data from the two dose–response studies. On the x axis, 0 = placebo. Only significant P-values are shown.

tistically significantly different (P=0.430). Seizure-free rates were 3, 14 and 3%, respectively. Adverse events resulted in the discontinuation of 7, 19 and 26% patients, respectively. Adverse events most often reported were dizziness, somnolence and ataxia. Most adverse events were transient and mild to moderate in intensity.

The responder rates for pregabalin compare favourably with those seen for other AEDs tested as adjunctive therapy in similar patient populations. Figure 42.1 shows the dose response (linear for both dose response; Studies 1008-011 and 1008-034 at $P \leq 0.001$) and overall consistency in efficacy results across all three adjunctive therapy studies for the secondary efficacy measure responder rate.

Side-effects reported from other studies

In normal volunteers given doses up to 900 mg/day, the main side-effects seen were headache, dizziness and somnolence, which were judged to be mild or moderate in intensity. No major serious adverse events due to pregabalin treatment were reported. Mild transient increases in hepatic enzymes in the multiple dose study at 900 mg/day were observed [13]. Therefore, the highest recommended dose in clinical trials is 600 mg/day.

Two epilepsy investigators published papers concerning their single-site observations of myoclonus. One [18] reported myoclonus in 21% (four out of 19 pregabalin-treated patients), and another [19] reported myoclonus in 33% (two out of six pregabalin-treated patients). However, myoclonus has only been reported in 1.2% (60 of 5026 patients) of all patients treated with pregabalin in all 29 controlled and uncontrolled epilepsy and analgesic studies. It has led to withdrawal in 0.12% (six of 5026 patients (data on file; Pfizer, Ann Arbor, Michigan, USA). Of the 60 cases, 56 had epilepsy and were receiving one to three other AEDs. The overall incidence of myoclonus in the controlled epilepsy trials was 3.5% (56 of 1160 patients). EEGs were obtained in six of the cases and none showed visible correlates, suggesting that the myoclonus may not be of cortical origin.

Clinical therapeutics

Place of the drug in therapy

At the time of writing, one peer-reviewed publication concerning the RCTs with pregabalin is in print and the others are still in review. However, pregabalin appears to be an AED that is effective, well tolerated and with excellent overall ease of use (lack of drug–drug interactions, linear pharmacokinetics, b.i.d. dosing, etc.). There was a favourable and statistically significant increase in efficacy with dose in the two dose–response studies of pregabalin as adjunctive therapy in patients with partial seizures. The potential clinical use of pregabalin for patients with other seizure types, in special populations, and as monotherapy needs to be explored.

Dose and titration rates

From information taken from the RCTs, the starting dose of pregabalin currently recommended is 150 mg/day given in two divided doses. Titration should then be made depending on individual tolerability and response to the drug. In the clinical studies titration was either over 1 week or done without titration up to 600 mg/day. Two placebo-controlled studies demonstrated a significant dose–response relationship up to the maximum dosages tested of 600 mg/day.

Conclusions

Current efficacy and safety data indicate pregabalin, combined with a linear pharmacokinetic profile and the potential for b.i.d. or t.i.d. dosing, suggest that pregabalin is a promising new AED for the treatment of partial seizures (all partial seizures with and without secondary generalization). However, additional data will be needed to define further the safety, efficacy and clinical utility of pregabalin.

References

1 Bialer M, Johannessen SI, Kupferberg HJ, Levy RH, Loiseau P, Perucca E. Progress report on new antiepileptic drugs: a summary of the fourth Eilat conference (EILAT IV). *Epilepsy Res* 1999; 34: 1–41.
2 Bialer M, Johannessen SI, Kupferberg HJ, Levy RH, Loiseau P, Perucca E. Progress report on new antiepileptic drugs: a summary of the Fifth Eilat Conference (EILAT V). *Epilepsy Res* 2001; 43: 11–58.
3 Ben-Menachem E, Kugler AR. Pregabalin. In: Levy RH, Mattson RH, Meldrum BS, Perucca E eds. *Antiepileptic Drugs*, 5th edn. Philadelphia: Lippincott Williams & Wilkins, 2002: 901–5.
4 Bryans JS, Wustrow DJ. 3-substituted GABA analog with central nervous system activity: A review. *Med Res Rev* 1999; 19: 149–77.
5 Gee NS, Brown JP, Dissanayake VU, Offord J, Thurlow R, Woodruff GN. The novel anticonvulsant drug, gabapentin (Neurontin), binds to the $\alpha_2\delta$ subunit of a calcium channel. *J Biol Chem* 1996; 271(10): 5768–76.
6 Fink K, Dooley DJ, Meder WP, Suman-Chauhan N, Duffy S, Clusmann H, Gothert M. Inhibition of neuronal Ca^{2+} influx by gabapentin and pregabalin in the human neocortex. *Neuropharmacology* 2002; 42(2): 229–36.
7 Dooley DJ, Mieske CA, Borosky SA. Inhibition of K^+-evoked glutamate release from rat neocortical and hippocampal slices by gabapentin. *Neurosci Lett* 2000; 280: 107–10.
8 Dooley DJ, Donovan CM, Pugsley TA. Stimulus-dependent nodulation of [3H]norepinephrine release from rat neocortical slices by gabapentin and pregabalin. *J Pharmacol Exp Ther* 2000; 295: 1086–93.
9 Maneuf YP, Hughes J, McKnight AT. Gabapentin inhibits the substance P-facilitated K^+-evoked release of [3H]glutamate from rat caudal trigeminal nucleus slices. *Pain* 2001; 93: 191–6.
10 Welty D, Wang Y, Busch JA, Taylor CP, Vartanian MG, Radulovic LL. Pharmacokinetics (PK) and pharmacodynamics (PD) of CI-1008 (pregabalin) and gabapentin in rats with maximal electroshock. *Epilepsia* 1997; 38 (Suppl. 8): 35.
11 Taylor CP, Vartanian MG. Profile of the anticonvulsant activity of CI-1008 (pregabalin) in animal models. *Epilepsia* 1997; 38 (Suppl. 8): 8.
12 Williamson J, Lothman CTE, Bertran E. Comparison of S(+)-3 Isobutyl GABA and gabapentin against kindled hippocampal seizures. *Epilepsia* 1997; 38 (Suppl. 8): 29.
13 Bockbrader HN, Hunt T, Strand J, Posvar E, Sedman A. Pregabalin pharmacokinetics and safety in healthy volunteers: results from two phase 1 studies. *Neurology* 2000; 54 (Suppl. 3): A421.
14 Abou-Khalil BW, Vazquez BR, Beydoun AA *et al.* Pregabalin 7/8 Study Group. Pregabalin in-patient monotherapy trial-study results and impact of seizure frequency on efficacy evaluations. *Epilepsia* 1999; 40 (Suppl. 7): 109.
15 French JA, Kugler AR, Robbins JL, Knapp LE, Garofalo EA. Dose–response trial of pregabalin adjunctive therapy in patients with partial seizures. *Neurology* 2003; 60: 1631–7.
16 Arroyo S, Anhut H, Messmer S, Mathe H. Pregabalin double-blind add-on study in patients with partial seizures. *Epilepsia* 2001; 42 (Suppl. 7): 83.
17 Beydoun AA, Uthman BM, Ramsay RE *et al.* and The Pregabalin 1008–009/010 Study Group. Pregabalin add-on trial: double-blind, multicenter study in patients with partial epilepsy. *Epilepsia* 2000; 41 (Suppl. 7): 253–4.
18 Huppertz H-J, Feuerstein TJ, Schulze-Bonhage A. Myoclonus in epilepsy patients with anticonvulsive add-on therapy with pregabalin. Brief communication. *Epilepsia* 2001; 42: 790–2.
19 Asconape JJ, Hartman LM, Salanova V. Pregabalin-associated myoclonus. *Epilepsia* 1999; 40 (Suppl. 7): 143.

43 Rufinamide

V. Biton

Primary indications	Evaluated for treatment in focal and primary generalized epilepsy
Usual preparation	Tablets: 100, 200, 400 mg
Usual dosages	In clinical trials, up to 3200 mg/day
Dosage intervals	2 times/day
Significant drug interactions	Rufinamide levels are elevated by phenobarbital, phenytoin and primidone. Rufinamide levels are lowered by valproate
Serum level monitoring	Unknown
Common/important side-effects	Dizziness, headache, nausea, somnolence, diplopia, fatigue and ataxia
Main advantages	Well-tolerated, broad spectrum of activity
Main disadvantages	Moderate potency
Mechanisms of action	Limits excessive firing of Na+ dependent action potentials
Oral bioavailability	60–85% (affected by food)
Time to peak levels	5–6 h
Metabolism and excretion	Extensively metabolized, excretion is primarily renal
Volume of distribution	–
Elimination half-life	8.5–12 h
Plasma clearance	–
Protein binding	34%
Active metabolites	Nil
Comment	Novel antiepileptic drug emerging from clinical trials

(*Note*: this summary table was formulated by the lead editor.)

Rufinamide (Ruf 331, CGP 33101), a triazole derivative structurally unrelated to any currently marketed antiepileptic drug (AED), was discovered by Novartis Pharma AG (Switzerland) and was evaluated within the National Institutes of Health (NIH)-sponsored anticonvulsant drug-screening programme [1]. Development of this compound was started by Novartis AG in Switzerland in the 1980s. Based on the broad-spectrum preclinical profile, favourable clinical pharmacological characteristics, and safety and efficacy results from early clinical trials, Phase III development is ongoing [2,3]. Development for other potential uses such as neuro-

pathic pain started in mid 1999 [4]. The drug received a proprietary name of Xilep in the USA.

Chemical characteristics

Rufinamide, 1-(2,6-difluoro-benzyl)-^{1}H-1,2,3-triazole-4-carboxide, is a white crystalline substance, which is odourless and slightly bitter. Rufinamide has a low solubility in water and limited solubility in 0.1 N-HCl (63 mg/L) and simulated intestinal fluid (59 mg/L). Rufinamide has the molecular formula of $C_{10}H_8F_2N_4O$ with the molecular weight of 238.20. The drug is available as 100, 200 and 400 mg film-coated tablets. The drug does not show any hygroscopicity, and no water was absorbed by the drug when placed in an environment of up to 100% relative humidity [1,5].

Mechanism of action

Seizure suppression by most conventional AEDs is achieved by their interaction with neurotransmitter receptors or ion channels [6,7], but the mechanism of action of rufinamide is not clearly established. However, voltage-dependent sodium channels may mediate in part the anticonvulsant properties of this drug; rufinamide limits the frequency of excessive firing of sodium-dependent action potentials in neurones. This effect could contribute to blocking the spread of seizure activity from an epileptogenic focus [8,9]. In radioligand binding studies, rufinamide did not significantly interact with various neurotransmitter systems, including adenosine, γ-aminobutyric acid (GABA), N-methyl-D-asparate (NMDA), monoaminergic and cholinergic binding sites and other excitatory amino acid binding sites.

Rufinamide was evaluated within the framework of the NIH-sponsored anticonvulsant drug screening programme. Studies conducted within that programme show that rufinamide is effective in blocking both the tonic and clonic phases in a number of electrical and chemical animal seizure models [8].

Maximimal electroshock (MES) test

The MES test is known to identify AEDs with the potential to suppress generalized tonic-clnic seizures and, in part, partial seizures [7,9–12].

In rodent models of epilepsy, rufinamide is particularly effective at inhibiting MES-induced tonic-clonic seizures. The oral effective dose in 50% of the animals or ED_{50} was 5–17 mg/kg. The anticonvulsant effect was maintained for at least 4 h in mice and 8 h in rats [8]. There was no evidence of tolerance development in the rodent model.

Pentylenetetrazole (PTZ) test

The PTZ test is widely used to evaluate the ability of a potential AED to prevent clonic seizures. It may also correlate with drug activity against absence seizures [7,10–13]. PTZ given subcutaneously or intraperitoneally to mice typically generates a seizure pattern expressed by short periods of generalized clonic hind limb movements. Compared to the MES test, the efficacy of rufinamide against PTZ-induced seizures was lower, $ED_{50} = 300$ mg/kg.

Bicuculline and picrotoxin

Bicuculline-induced and picrotoxin-induced seizures are thought to be due to antagonism of the inhibitory neurotransmitter GABA. Compared to the MES test, the potency of rufinamide in blocking bicuculline-induced seizures and picrotoxin-induced seizures was lower, the $ED_{50} = 50.5$ mg/kg and 76.3 mg/kg, respectively [3,8].

Kindling

Once-daily threshold electrical stimulation of the amygdala in animals induces epileptic EEG after-discharges and results in a kindling phenomenon [10,11]. Rufinamide (oral doses 100–300 mg/kg) has been found to be effective in delaying the development of kindling and suppressing after-discharges in amygdala-kindled cats with generalized tonic-clonic convulsions. It has shown effectiveness in reducing seizure frequency in rhesus monkeys with chronic alumina foci in the motor cortex. Hippocampal and cortical after-discharges induced by electrical stimulation in non-kindled cats are also inhibited by rufinamide. A drug's therapeutic potential can be quantified by calculating its protective index that is defined as the ratio of median toxic dose to median effective dose; the protective index of rufinamide is generally higher than that of most common AEDs [3,8].

The profile of rufinamide in animals would predict effectiveness against partial and generalized (including absence) seizures in humans.

Effects on learning and memory

Evaluation of rufinamide for its potential effects on learning and memory in mice revealed that this compound effectively improved learning performance in the step-down passive avoidance paradigm and partially counteracted electroshock-induced amnesia [8]. The enhanced cognitive functions were observed at doses of rufinamide at and below effective anticonvulsant doses. Such a cognition-promoting effect could offer an important advantage over current AED treatments for which negative effects on cognitive functions have been described in clinics [14].

Pharmacokinetics

Absorption and bioavailability

The oral absorption of ^{14}C-labelled rufinamide was investigated in various animals including mice, rats, cats, dogs, baboons and rhesus monkeys.

The peak plasma concentration of rufinamide is typically reached within 5–6 h of oral administration independent of dose. The mean plasma elimination half-lives of rufinamide ranged from 8 to 12 h, with an overall mean of 9.5 h. An important indicator of potential interactions due to drug displacement is the percentage of protein binding; rufinamide is only about 34% bounded to protein, predominantly albumin (27%). The drug is evenly distributed between erythrocytes and plasma.

In a study designed to evaluate the metabolism and disposition of rufinamide in humans, adult healthy male volunteers received single oral doses of 600 mg of ^{14}C-labelled microcrystalline rufinamide in gelatin capsules with food. Concentrations of radioactivity, rufinamide and its metabolites were measured in blood, plasma, urine and faeces. The absorption was demonstrated to be at least 85%. The main radioactive compound in plasma was rufinamide. Excretion was largely renal (85%) and was complete (98%) within 7 days. Rufinamide was extensively metabolized with only 4% recovered unchanged in urine (2%) and in faeces (2%) [15]. The most prominent metabolite was the carboxylic acid derivative CGP 47292, which was inactive [15,16]. A few minor metabolites were detected in the urine that appear to be acyl-glucuronides of CGP 47292. Otherwise, no relevant metabolites were detected in the urine and faeces. Results show that rufinamide exhibits a simple disposition in man. Biotransformation by hydrolysis appears to be the essential clearance mechanism. It did not appear that oxidative metabolic processes by cytochrome P450 enzymes were involved. Rufinamide demonstrated little or no significant activity of the P450 enzymes [3,17]. For that reason, it was postulated that rufinamide is not expected to inhibit the kinetics or biotransformation of coadministered drugs metabolized by the P450 enzyme system [15].

The overall variability in pharmacokinetic parameters of rufinamide were assessed after oral administration of two 200-mg tablets of rufinamide relative to that of 400-mg powder suspended in 100 mL water (suspension). Using a replicate designed trial, 16 healthy male volunteers were randomly assigned to four different treatment groups to receive tablets or suspension twice in four different dosing sequences. The peak concentration (C_{max}), time at which C_{max} was reached (t_{max}), and the extent of absorption or AUC were calculated. Results showed that rufinamide, despite its low solubility in aqueous solution, had small variabilities in its absorption kinetics with AUC (0–48) and C_{max} less than 26% for both tablets and suspension. Intrasubject variability was also small, around 20%, between the two formulations. The tablet formulation was bioequivalent to the suspension in terms of rate and extent of absorption based on 90% conventional confidence intervals [1,18].

The effect of food on the pharmacokinetics of rufinamide has been investigated in healthy volunteers. When rufinamide was administered with food, the average AUC increased by ~40% compared to those after administration without food. The C_{max} values after administration without food were twice as high as without, and the t_{max} was shorter (8 h under fasting conditions and 6 h under fed conditions). The terminal half-life decreased by only 3% (from 9.4 to 9.1 h) on average [1,5,19].

The drug appeared more rapidly in the systemic circulation with food as confirmed by the absorption kinetics (Fig. 43.1) and the shorter t_{max} associated with the higher C_{max}. The half-life from plasma was not significantly influenced by the concomitant intake of food, indicating unchanged elimination kinetics [5].

In a study designed to evaluate the pharmacokinetics of rufinamide in elderly, healthy subjects as compared to younger healthy subjects was conducted by Chang et al. [20]. This was an oral single-dose (400 mg) and multiple-dose (400 mg given twice daily for nine doses), open-label, parallel study. Pharmacokinetic evaluation included seven elderly subjects (age range 66–77 years) and seven gender-matched younger subjects (age range 18–40 years) under both single-dose and multiple-dose treatments. Rufinamide plasma levels were determined using a validated HPLC (high-performance liquid chromatography) method. Steady-state conditions under multiple-dose treatment were confirmed by the subjects' trough levels. The extent of absorption (AUC 0–infinity) and the absorption rates (C_{max}) were similar between the elderly and the younger volunteers under both single-dose (mean ratio of elderly/younger: AUC 0–infinity, 1.04; C_{max} 1.08) and multiple-dose (mean ratio of elderly/younger: AUC 0–infinity, 0.89; C_{max}, 1.01) treatments.

Elimination half-life values were also similar in the elderly subjects (single-dose 8.6 ± 1.3 h; multiple-dose 8.3 ± 1.1 h) and younger subjects (single-dose 10.8 ± 3.2 h; multiple-dose 10.2 ± 2.4 h) and were not altered after multiple-dose treatment [21]. Rufinamide (<2% of dose) and its major metabolite (CGP 47292; 60% of dose) were recovered in urine after single-dose treatment and between dosing intervals at steady state. Linear kinetics were observed in multiple-dose treatment for both the elderly subjects and the younger subjects, as shown by comparable AUC 0–12 at steady-state conditions and AUC 0–infinity under single-dose treatment. No significant differences were shown in these comparisons. The results showed no significant differences found in the plasma and urine pharmacokinetic parameters between elderly subjects and younger subjects with either single-dose treatment or multiple-dose treatment [20].

Sachdeo et al. [22] conducted a clinical study to obtain rufinamide safety and pharmacokinetic data in paediatric patients with epilepsy. The pharmacokinetic profile of rufinamide was evaluated in a 2-week, open-label, ascending-dose study stratified by age (2–6, 7–12 and 13–17 years of age). Rufinamide was administered orally in equally divided twice-daily doses of 10 mg/kg/day (week 1) and 30 mg/kg/day (week 2) to 16 paediatric patients. At the end of each week, plasma samples were taken for pharmacokinetic profiling.

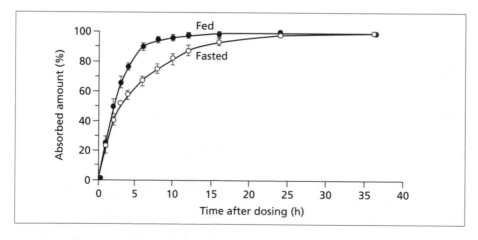

Fig. 43.1 Mean absorption profile of rufinamide (+SEM) in healthy volunteers treated with a single oral dose of 600 mg without (○) and with (●) food.

Table 43.1 Pharmacokinetic parameters at two dose levels in paediatric patients [22]

Dose (mg/kg/day)	AUC (h × µg/mL)	C_{max} (µg/mL)	C_{min} (µg/mL)	t_{max} (h)
10	37.8 (47)	4.01 (44)	2.28 (59)	4
30	89.3 (58)	8.68 (52)	5.37 (75)	4

The pharmacokinetic parameters AUC (0–12 h), C_{max}, C_{min} (minimum plasma concentration), and t_{max} were calculated. The pharmacokinetic parameters at the two dose levels in those patients are summarized in Table 43.1. The data showed a less than dose proportional increase in AUC, C_{max} and C_{min} when the dose was increased from 10 mg/kg/day to 30 mg/kg/day, similar to the data obtained from studies in the adult population. No significant differences in pharmacokinetic parameters as a function of age were noted.

All 16 patients completed the core study with good tolerability. The most frequently reported adverse experiences were mild in severity and related to the central nervous and gastrointestinal systems. There was no evidence that any of the adverse experiences were dose related; no patients discontinued the study medication prematurely due to an adverse experience [22].

Toxicology

Rufinamide has demonstrated an excellent safety profile in toxicology studies, and showed no evidence of mutagenicity or teratogenicity in preclinical studies [3].

Drug interactions

A pharmacokinetic evaluation involving 471 patients has revealed that the relative extent of absorption was lower at 1600 mg/day compared with doses of 200, 400 and 800 mg/day administered twice daily. This study showed that valproate decreased the plasma clearance of rufinamide by approximately 22% (compared with patients not receiving valproate), while any combination of phenobarbital, phenytoin and primidone increased the plasma clearance of rufinamide by approximately 25% (compared with patients not receiving these AEDs). The mechanism of these interactions has not yet been clarified. The same study showed that the plasma pharmacokinetics of rufinamide oral clearance was found not to be affected by comedication of carbamazepine, vigabatrin, oxcarbazepine and clobazam. Additionally, rufinamide had no effect on the trough concentrations of the eight commonly used concomitant AEDs in this study (carbamazepine, phenytoin, clobazam, phenobarbital, primidone, oxcarbazepine, clonazepam and valproate [3,18,19]).

An in vitro evaluation of potential drug interactions was performed by Kapeghian et al. [17]. Rufinamide was incubated at concentrations up to 300 µM, with various substrates, in human liver microsomal fractions to evaluate any potential inhibitory effect on the activities of various human P450 isoenzymes that are known to be responsible for the metabolism of several clinically important anticonvulsant agents, as well as other drugs that may be used in combination or supportive therapy. Rufinamide did not demonstrate

any inhibition on the activities of these human P450 isoenzymes: CYP1A2, CYP2A6, CYP269, CYP2619, CYP2D6, CYP2E1, CYP3A4/5 and CYP4A9/11. This suggested that clinically important drug interactions are unlikely with this drug for those medications metabolized through the cytochrome P450 [17].

An interaction study was conducted to determine the effect of rufinamide on coadministered low-dose oral contraceptives. In this single-centre, open-label, multiple-dose study, 18 healthy female volunteers were maintained on Ortho-Novum 1/35 for at least two cycles before randomization and throughout days 1–56 of the study. Rufinamide 800 mg was administered twice daily on days 22–35. The results demonstrated that coadministration of rufinamide and Ortho-Novum 1/35 produced a statistically significant decrease in the systemic concentrations of both norethindrone and ethinyl oestradiol. Because markers of ovulation were not measured, the clinical significance of this decrease is unknown [23]. However, it is clear that rufinamide has the potential to reduce the efficacy of oral contraceptives.

Rufinamide level determination

Preclinical data has suggested that rufinamide (CGP 33101) would be a well-tolerated, effective drug with a long duration of action in the treatment of partial and generalized tonic-clonic seizures. Plans for large-scale clinical trials have necessitated development of a method to analyse concentrations of rufinamide. Therefore, an automated analytical method utilizing laboratory robotics has been developed and validated for quantifying the concentrations of rufinamide in human plasma samples over the concentration range of 50–4000 ng/mL [2]. The further development of an analytical method for determination of rufinamide (CGP 33101) plasma and its main metabolite, CGP 47292, in urine were required for pharmacokinetic investigations. Subsequently, a method was developed (involving high-performance liquid chromatography and liquid–solid extraction) for the simultaneous determination of the level of rufinamide (CGP 33101) and its main carboxylic metabolite, CGP 47292, in urine [24]. The recovery and reproducibility assessments indicated a good level of accuracy with an overall mean relative recovery of 102.7% and precision for rufinamide over the concentration range of 50–4000 ng/mL. The limit of quantification was reported to be 50 ng/mL.

Multiple dose studies

In multiple dose studies, the rufinamide disposition was linear. Repeated administration of rufinamide at weekly increment doses of 300, 600, 900 and 1200 mg/day given as b.i.d. regimen were not significantly different.

The pharmacokinetic profile of rufinamide has been evaluated in a study conducted on 12 fasting patients with epilepsy. The drug was given at 400, 800 and 1200 mg/day as an adjunctive therapy. The C_{max} and AUC showed a dose proportional increase between the 400 mg/day and the 800 mg/day dose. The value was reduced for the 1200 mg/day dose.

The pharmacokinetic profile was also evaluated in normal volunteers as well as epileptic patients who received multiple doses of rufinamide with weekly rising doses of 1200, 1600, 2000 and 2400 mg given on a b.i.d. regimen. Again, the pharmacokinetic characteristics of rufinamide did not change. There was no indication of autoinduction. The plasma half-life before and after multiple dosing did not change [10,11].

Efficacy and safety data

The efficacy of rufinamide has been demonstrated in two adjunctive therapy, double-blind, placebo-controlled studies, AE/PT2 and AE/ET1.

Study AE/PT2 was designed to assess the pharmacokinetic and safety profile in patients with refractory epilepsy. Fifty patients (34 males, age range 20–60, median age of 34 years) with partial seizures or primary generalized tonic-clonic seizures who were receiving up to two concomitant AEDs were randomized to rufinamide or placebo according to a parallel-group design [25]. Weekly ascending doses of 400, 800, 1200 and 1600 mg/day or matching placebo were administered in a twice-daily dosing regimen over the duration of the 4-week study. Efficacy endpoints were the seizure frequency ratio (primary efficacy variable) defined as the seizure frequency per 28 days in the double-blind treatment phase divided by that in the baseline phase and the 25 and 50% responder rates (secondary efficacy variables) [16,25]. The median seizure frequency was reduced by 42% in the rufinamide group as compared to an increase of 52% in the placebo-treated patients ($P=0.00397$). The 25% responder rate was significantly higher in the patients treated with rufinamide than in patients treated with placebo (52% vs. 15%; $P=0.014$). The 50% responder rate also showed a trend toward significance in the rufinamide-treated group relative to the placebo-treated group (39% vs. 16%; $P=0.096$). Despite the small sample size, the efficacy results indicated that rufinamide reduced the number of seizures in patients with epilepsy.

During the course of clinical study AE/PT2, no fatal or life-threatening events occurred. Two patients discontinued the study prematurely after experiencing adverse events. One patient reported symptoms of vertigo, fatigue, headache and diplopia, and the other patient reported symptoms of fatigue, dizziness and tremor. Both patients had reported similar adverse events with other AEDs. The most commonly reported adverse events were headache (20% in the placebo group, 12% in the rufinamide group), tiredness/fatigue/lethargy (20% rufinamide, 4% placebo), tremor (12% rufinamide, 0% placebo) and gait disturbance/balance difficulty (8% rufinamide, 4% placebo). These findings are summarized in Table 43.2. There were no clinically significant changes in vital signs, EEG, ECG or sleep. There was no evidence of any clinically significant change in laboratory parameters with the study treatment [25].

Study AE/ET1 was designed to assess the efficacy and tolerability of rufinamide (400–1600 mg/day) as adjunctive therapy in patients with partial or generalized seizures. In study AET/ET1, 647 patients with refractory epilepsy receiving one to three concomitant AEDs were randomized to one of four rufinamide-treatment groups (200, 400, 800 or 1600 mg/day administered twice daily) or placebo in a double-blind, add-on, five-arm parallel-group design. The primary efficacy variable, seizure frequency per 28 days, was improved significantly by rufinamide ($P=0.003$, multiple linear regression model assuming normal-error, logarithmic transformation) using a linear trend of dose–response. A secondary efficacy variable, seizure frequency ratio, demonstrated statistical significance of the individ-

Table 43.2 Study AE/PT2: adverse events reported by at least 5% of patients in either treatment group [25]

IMN preferred term	Rufinamide n (%) (n=25)	Placebo n (%) (n=25)
Tiredness/fatigue/lethargy	5 (20%)	1 (4%)
Headache	3 (12%)	5 (20%)
Tremor	3 (12%)	0 (0%)
Balance difficulty/gait disturbance	2 (8%)	1 (4%)
Dizziness	2 (8%)	0 (0%)

IMN, International Medical Nomenclature.

ual rufinamide dose 400, 800 and 1600 mg/day relative to placebo (all $P<0.027$) based on pair-wise Wilcoxon rank-sum tests [3,4,16,18]. An additional secondary variable, the 50% responder rate, was analysed using the linear dose–response trend ($P=0.0319$) [3].

During the course of clinical study AET/ET1, no fatal or life-threatening adverse events occurred. The most frequently reported adverse events were central nervous system-related. In general, reports of adverse events were more common in patients who received rufinamide (~53%) than in patients who received placebo (46%). There was no evidence of a dose–response relationship for any of the adverse events. The percentage of patients who discontinued the study prematurely due to adverse events was similar between treatments (10% rufinamide, ~7% placebo). Rufinamide was found to have no clinically significant adverse effects on pulse rate or blood pressure and there were no clinically significant abnormal findings in any of the laboratory parameters assessed [3,16].

Litzinger et al. [26] reported the preliminary safety and efficacy data of adjunctive therapy rufinamide in a small cohort of paediatric patients in the open-label extension of an ongoing double-blind, placebo-controlled study of rufinamide in the treatment of partial seizures. Nine paediatric patients (age range 4–16 years old; two males and seven females; minimum of three seizures per month in the double-blind baseline, and receiving up to two concomitant AEDs) entered the open-label extension study. Rufinamide was titrated over 1 week to a target dose of 45 mg/kg while the concomitant AEDs were maintained at the same doses. Seizure frequency during the 14-day baseline (prior to double-blind randomization) was compared to the seizure frequency in the first 14 days of the extension study after 1 week of rufinamide titration. Four of the nine patients (45%) had a 50% reduction in their complex partial seizure frequency as compared to baseline. No adverse events were reported and there were no reported changes in haematological, hepatic or urinary parameters [26].

One thousand and fifty-four patients with epilepsy participated in five completed clinical studies (AE/ET1, AE/PT2, AE/PT3, 3310101027 and RUF3310021A) of rufinamide. Seven hundred and sixty of those patients received rufinamide. The most frequently reported adverse events were central nervous system related. Overall, they were more common in the rufinamide-treated than in the placebo-treated patients. Adverse events reported by at least 10% of the patients included in declining frequency, dizziness, headaches, nausea, somnolence, diplopia, fatigue, ataxia, vomiting, abnormal vision and infection. The last one occurred more in the placebo group.

Two hundred and ninety-five volunteers participated in open-label and double-blind studies. Adverse events reported by 5% or more of the patients were headaches, tiredness, drowsiness, concentration difficulties and nausea. Most adverse experiences were reported soon after the initiation of treatment and were mild to moderate in severity. Moreover, the adverse experiences reported were transient and generally did not lead to premature discontinuation of the study medication. Three other controlled clinical trials are currently underway which will further define the efficacious dose range and safety profile of rufinamide as monotherapy and adjunctive therapy. The first, which was recently completed, is a multicentre, double-blind, placebo-controlled study designed to assess the safety and efficacy of rufinamide as adjunctive therapy in children and adults with primary generalized tonic-clonic seizures. The second is a study designed to determine the safety and efficacy of high-dose versus low-dose rufinamide monotherapy in patients with inadequately controlled partial seizures. The third is a multicentre, double-blind, placebo-controlled study designed to evaluate the safety and efficacy of rufinamide as monotherapy in patients with refractory partial seizures who have completed an inpatient evaluation for epilepsy surgery.

Non-epileptic use

Various AEDs, including carbamazepine, phenytoin and lamotrigine, are known to be clinically effective in neuropathic pain [27–29]. Although structurally different, these AEDs share two common actions; they suppress MES-induced generalized tonic-clonic seizures in rodents [7,9,12,30–32) and they stabilize neuronal membranes by inhibiting sustained repetitive firing of sodium-dependent action potentials [6,7,9,33–35]. Rufinamide exhibits both of these properties; it inhibits sustained repetitive firing of sodium-dependent action potentials and suppresses MES-induced seizures. Therefore, rufinamide may be effective in treating neuropathic pain.

Conclusions

Rufinamide is a novel AED with a molecular structure unlike any of the other available AEDs. Animal studies in various models of epilepsy suggest potential efficacy in focal as well as generalized epilepsy. In clinical trials, the drug was well tolerated by normal volunteers as well as patients with epilepsy. Safety data from clinical studies indicate adverse events to be similar in type and occurred with a frequency less than that reported in most other clinical AED studies utilizing similar design and patient populations [36–38]. Various phase III studies were recently completed, including an outpatient monotherapy study, an inpatient monotherapy study on patients being evaluated for epilepsy surgery, a study on patients with primary generalized epilepsy and a paediatric study. The outcome of these studies will have a major impact on further development of this drug.

References

1 Cheung WK, Kianifard F, Wong A et al. Intra- and inter-subject variabilities of CGP 33101 after replicate single oral doses of two 200-mg tablets and 400-mg suspension. Pharm Res 1995; 12(12): 1878–82.

2 Brunner LA, Powell ML. An automated method for the determination of a new potential antiepileptic agent (CGP 33101) in human plasma using high performance liquid chromatography. Biomed Chromatogr 1992; 6(6): 278–82.

3 Bialer M, Johannessen SI, Kupferberg HJ, Levy RH, Loiseau P, Perucca E. Progress report on new antiepileptic drugs: a summary of the Fifth Eilat Conference (EILAT V). Epilepsy Res 2001; 43 (1): 11–58.

4 Jain KK. An assessment of rufinamide as an anti-epileptic in comparison with other drugs in clinical development. Expert Opin Invest Drugs 2000; 9(4): 829–40.

5 Cardot JM, Lecaillon JB, Czendlik C, Godbillon J. The influence of food on the disposition of the antiepileptic rufinamide in healthy volunteers. Biopharm Drug Dispos 1998; 19(4): 259–62.

6 Macdonald RL. Cellular effects of antiepileptic drugs. In: Engel J, Pedley TA, eds. Epilepsy: A Comprehensive Textbook. New York: Lippincott-Raven Publishers, 1997: 1383–91.

7 Rogawski MA, Porter RJ. Antiepileptic drugs: pharmacological mechanisms and clinical efficacy with consideration of promising development stage compounds. Pharmacol Rev 1990; 42 (3): 223–86.

8 Schmutz M, Allgeier H, Jeker A, Klebs K, McLean MJ, Mondadori C. Anticonvulsant profile of CGP 33101 in animals. Epilepsia 1993; 34(2): 122.

9 Wamil AW, Schmutz M, Portet CH, Feldmann KF, McLean MJ. Effects of oxcarbazepine and 10-hydroxycarbamazepine on action potential firing and generalized seizures. Eur J Pharmacol 1994; 271: 301–8.

10 Kupferberg HJ, Schmutz M. Screening of new compounds and the role of the pharmaceutical industry. In: Engel J, Pedley TA, eds. Epilepsy: A Comprehensive Textbook. Philadelphia: Lippincott-Raven Publishers, 1997: 1417–34.

11 Löscher W, Schmidt D. Which animal models should be used in the search for new antiepileptic drugs? A proposal based on experimental and clinical considerations. Epilepsy Res 1988; 2: 145–81.

12 Schmutz M, Bernasconi R, Portet CH, Baltzer V. Effects of antiepileptic drugs in tests related to GABA. In: Manelis J, Bental E, Loeber J, Dreifuss FE, eds. Advances in Epileptology. XVIIth Epilepsy International Symposium. New York: Raven Press, 1989: 229–32.

13 Swinyard EA, Woodhead JH, White HS, Franklin MR. Experimental selection, quantification and evaluation of anticonvulsants. In: Levy R, Mattson R, Meldrum B, Penry JK, Dreifuss FE, eds. Antiepileptic Drugs. New York: Raven Press, 1989: 85–102.

14 Trimble MR. Neuropsychiatric consequences of pharmacotherapy. In: Engel J, Pedley TA, eds. Epilepsy: A Comprehensive Textbook. Philadelphia: Lippincott-Raven Publishers, 1997: 2161–70.

15 Waldmeier F, Gschwind HP, Rouan MC, Sioufi A, Czendlik C. Metabolism of the new anticonvulsive trial drug rufinamide (CGP 33101) in healthy male volunteers. Epilepsia 1996; 37 (Suppl. 5): 167.

16 Bialer M, Johannessen SI, Kupferberg HJ, Levy RH, Loiseau P, Perucca E. Progress report on new antiepileptic drugs: a summary of the fourth Eilat conference (EILAT IV). Epilepsy Res 1999; 34(1): 1–41.

17 Kapeghian JC, Madan A, Parkinson A, Tripp SL, Probst A. Evaluation of rufinamide (CGP 33101), a novel anticonvulsant, for potential drug interactions in vitro. Epilepsia 1996; 37 (Suppl. 5): 26.

18 Willmore LJ. Clinical pharmacology of new antiepileptic drugs. Neurology 2000; 55(11 Suppl. 3): S17–24.

19 Perucca E, Bialer M. The clinical pharmacokinetics of the newer antiepileptic drugs. Focus on topiramate, zonisamide and tiagabine. Clin Pharmacokinet 1996; 31(1): 29–46.

20 Chang SW, Choi L, Karolchyk MA. A pharmacokinetic evaluation of rufinamide in elderly and younger subjects. Epilepsia 1998; 39 (Suppl. 6): 59.

21 Chang SW, Yeh CM, Van Logtenberg M, Sêdek G, Karolchyk MA. A geriatric pharmacokinetic evaluation of rufinamide. Clin Pharmacol Ther 2000; 67(2): 154.

22 Sachdeo RC, Rosenfeld WE, Choi L, Yeh CM, Cooper AN, Karolchyk MA. Pharmacokinetics and safety of adjunctive rufinamide therapy in pediatric patients with epilepsy. Epilepsia 1998; 39 (Suppl. 6): 166–7.

23 Svendsen K, Choi L, Chen BL, Karolchyk MA. Single-center, open-label, multiple-dose pharmacokinetic trial investigating the effect of rufinamide

administration on ortho-novum 1/35 in healthy women. *Epilepsia* 1998; 39 (Suppl. 6): 59.

24 Rouan MC, Souppart C, Alif L, Moes D, Lecaillon JB, Godbillon J. Automated analysis of a novel anti-epileptic compound, CGP 33,101, and its metabolite, CGP 47,292, in body fluids by high-performance liquid chromatography and liquid-solid extraction. *J Chromatogr B Biomed Appl* 1995; 667(2): 307–13.

25 Palhagen S, Canger R, Henriksen O, Van Parys JA, Karolchyk MA. Efficacy and safety of rufinamide in patients with refractory epilepsy. *Epilepsia* 1997; 38 (Suppl. 8): 207–8.

26 Litzinger MJ, Annajill H. Safety and efficacy of open-label rufinamide as adjunctive therapy in pediatric patients with partial seizures. *Epilepsia* 1999; 40 (Suppl. 7): 114.

27 Lunardi G, Leandri M, Albano C *et al.* Clinical effectiveness of lamotrigine and plasma levels in essential and symptomatic trigeminal neuralgia. *Neurology* 1997; 48: 1714–17.

28 McQuay H, Carroll D, Jadad AR, Wiffen P, Moore A. Anticonvulsant drugs for management of pain: a systematic review. *Brit Med J* 1995; 311: 1047–52.

29 Tremont-Lukats IW, Megeff C, Backonja MM. Anticonvulsants for neuropathic pain syndromes: mechanisms of action and place in therapy. *Drugs* 2000; 60(5): 1029–52.

30 Krall RL, Penry JK, White BG, Kuperferberg HJ, Swinyard EA. Antiepileptic drug development: II. Anticonvulsant drug screening. *Epilepsia* 1978; 19: 409–28.

31 Miller AA, Wheatley P, Sawyer DA, Baxter MG, Roth B. Pharmacological studies on lamotrigine, a novel potential antiepileptic drug: I. Anticonvulsant profile in mice and rats. *Epilepsia* 1986; 27: 483–9.

32 Schmutz M, Brugger F, Gentsch C, McLean MJ, Olpe HR. Oxcarbazepine: preclinical anticonvulsant profile and putative mechanisms of action. *Epilepsia* 1994; 35 (Suppl. 5): 47–50.

33 Cheung H, Kamp D, Harris E. An in vitro investigation of the action of lamotrigine on neuronal voltage activated sodium channels. *Epilepsy Res* 1992; 13: 107–12.

34 Macdonald RL. Anticonvulsant drug actions on neurons in cell culture. *J Neural Transm* 1988; 72: 173–83.

35 Macdonald RL, Kelly KM. Mechanisms of action of currently prescribed and newly developed antiepileptic drugs. *Epilepsia* 1994; 35 (Suppl. 4): 41–50.

36 Leppik IE, Dreifeuss FE, Pledger GW *et al.* Felbamate for partial seizures: results of a controlled clinical trial. *Neurology* 1991; 41: 1785–9.

37 Matsuo F, Bergen D, Faught E *et al.* Placebo-controlled study of the efficacy and safety of lamotrigine in patients with partial seizures. *Neurology* 1993; 43: 2284–91.

38 US Gabapentin Study Group No. 5. Gabapentin as add-on therapy in refractory partial epilepsy: a double-blind, placebo-controlled, parallel-group study. *Neurology* 1993; 43: 2292–8.

44

Tiagabine

R. Kälviäinen

Primary indications	Adjunctive therapy or monotherapy in partial and secondarily generalized seizures
Usual preparations	Tablets: 5, 10, 15 mg
Usual dosages	Initial: 15 mg/day. Maintenance: 30–45 mg/day (combination with enzyme-inducing drugs), 15–30 mg/day (comedication with non-enzyme-inducing drugs)
Dosage intervals	2–3 times/day
Significant drug interactions	Tiagabine levels are lowered by comedication with hepatic enzyme-inducing drugs
Serum level monitoring	Not useful
Target range	0.001–0.234 mg/L
Common/important side-effects	Dizziness, tiredness, nervousness, tremor, diarrhoea, headache, confusion psychosis, flu-like symptoms, ataxia, depression, word-finding difficulties
Main advantages	Clinical experience is too limited to define the place of tiagabine in clinical practice, but initial experience is favourable
Main disadvantages	CNS side effects
Mechanisms of action	Inhibits GABA reuptake
Oral bioavailability	96%
Time to peak levels	30–90 min (slowed by food)
Metabolism and excretion	Hepatic oxidation then conjugation
Volume of distribution	1.0 L/kg
Elimination half-life	5–9 h (reduced to 2–3 h in patients taking enzyme-inducing comedication)
Plasma clearance	12.8 L/kg/h
Protein binding	96%
Active metabolites	None
Comment	Newly licensed antiepileptic drug with promise for use in therapy of refractory partial seizures

(*Note*: this summary table was formulated by the lead editor.)

Tiagabine is a γ-aminobutyric acid (GABA) uptake inhibitor which is structurally related to nipecotic acid but has an improved ability to cross the blood–brain barrier. Tiagabine has proven effective as add-on therapy in patients with refractory partial seizures with or without secondary generalization.

Mechanism of action and experimental studies

Potentiation of GABA is regarded as one of the most important mechanisms of action for novel antiepileptic agents. GABA uptake inhibitors represent a new class of antiepileptic drugs (AEDs), of which tiagabine was the first to be introduced into clinical practice. This approach is thought to offer two potential advantages over direct GABA-A receptor agonists and benzodiazepine-receptor agonists [1]. Firstly, unlike direct agonists, which produce a continuous or perhaps non-physiological pattern of receptor stimulation, the inhibition of GABA uptake enhances only the effect of endogenously released GABA, thus retaining physiological specificity. Secondly, the extent of enhancement of GABA-A receptor-mediated function by a GABA uptake inhibitor will be limited by the amount of GABA released, which is under constant physiological control, thus potentially limiting the side-effect liability of a GABA uptake inhibitor.

Tiagabine prevents GABA uptake by inhibiting selectively the GAT-1 GABA transporter with little or no activity on GAT-2, GAT-3 or BGT-1 which are the GABA transporters responsible for the uptake of the neurotransmitter into neurones and glial cells after synaptic release [1,2]. Tiagabine's affinity for inhibiting glial GABA uptake is 2.5-fold greater than that for neuronal uptake [3]. Tiagabine is not a substrate for the GABA uptake carrier and is therefore unlikely to act as a false transmitter at GABAergic neurones [3]. Blockade of GABA uptake temporarily sustains levels of endogenously released GABA in the synapse [1]. This is the only known mechanism of tiagabine action.

Although both tiagabine and vigabatrin act by enhancing GABA neurotransmission in the central nervous system (CNS), preclinical data show that vigabatrin and tiagabine have different pharmacological profiles and different mechanisms of action at the cellular level [4]. Tiagabine prolongs the duration, but not the magnitude, of the peak inhibitory postsynaptic current, consistent with temporarily sustained levels of endogenously released GABA in the synapse [5]. By contrast, vigabatrin inhibits presynaptic GABA degradation by selective, enzyme-activated irreversible blockade of the mitochondrial enzyme GABA transaminase, and thus induces a persistent five-fold increase in whole brain GABA concentration, and also high concentrations in the retina [6]. Tiagabine does not induce the widespread increase in total brain GABA concentrations that accompanies GABA-T inhibition. Moreover, vigabatrin seems to accumulate in the retina, whereas tiagabine does not [6].

The anticonvulsant action of tiagabine has been studied in animal models of epilepsy induced by electrical, chemical and sensory stimuli and in genetic models of epilepsy. When administered intraperitoneally to amygdala-kindled rats, tiagabine attenuates the expression of secondarily generalized seizures and completely blocks the expression of partial seizures [7]. Tiagabine also suppresses amygdala kindling-induced epileptogenesis in a dose-dependent manner in the rat [8].

Intraperitoneal tiagabine was shown to be an active anticonvulsant in experimental studies by protecting against audiogenic and methyl-6,7-dimethoxy-4-ethyl-α-carboline-3-carboxylate- and pentylenetetrazol (PTZ)-induced tonic or clonic seizures in mice and PTZ-induced tonic or clonic seizures in rats [9]. However, tiagabine did not protect against maximal electroshock-induced tonic seizures in mice or rats [7,9]. Tiagabine did not prevent tonic or clonic seizures induced by the potassium channel antagonists dendrotoxin or 4-aminopyridine in mice [10,11].

In common with GABA agonists, tiagabine may enhance the occurrence of spike-wave discharges in animal models of non-convulsive epilepsy. In WAG/Rij rats, a genetic model of generalized non-convulsive absence epilepsy, spike-and-wave discharges were increased by tiagabine 3 and 10 mg/kg administered intraperitoneally, but not by a 1-mg/kg dose [12]. Walton et al. [13] reported that tiagabine was effective in treating status epilepticus in cobalt-lesioned rats. At doses ≥ 5 mg/kg intraperitoneally, it was also associated with rhythmic high-voltage discharges. At even higher doses, a similar pattern could be produced in normal rats as well. Exacerbation of absence seizures has been found also in rats with genetic absence epilepsy (GAERS) and in the lethargic mouse model [14,15].

Tiagabine reduced both seizure-induced damage to pyramidal cells in the hippocampus and impairment of spatial memory associated with hippocampal damage in the perforant pathway stimulation model of status epilepticus in the rat [16]. Neuronal cell death was also reduced by tiagabine in the hippocampus of gerbils subjected to cerebral ischaemia [17] and in the rat cerebral ischaemia model of delayed pyramidal cell death [18].

Pharmacokinetics

Tiagabine is rapidly and nearly completely absorbed after oral administration with peak concentrations seen within 30–90 min of dosing [19]. Food delays the time to peak concentration from a mean of 0.9 to a mean of 2.6 h but does not change the total quantity absorbed. Because tiagabine has a short elimination half-life, the smoother absorption produced by concomitant intake of food helps in reducing excessive fluctuations in plasma drug levels during the dosing interval, and for this reason it is recommended that the drug be taken at meal times, preferably at the end of the meal.

Protein binding is high at 96%, but tiagabine does not displace highly protein-bound drugs such as phenytoin and valproic acid from their binding sites. The volume of distribution is approximately 1 L/kg. Tiagabine is widely metabolized in humans, mainly by isoform CYP3A4 of the cytochrome P450 family. Less than 1% is excreted unchanged in the urine, and no active metabolites have been identified [20].

Tiagabine pharmacokinetics are linear at doses up to 80 mg/day [21]. There is no evidence that tiagabine either causes induction or inhibition of cytochrome P450 enzymes [19]. Consequently, tiagabine has shown no action on hepatic metabolism which would be expected to alter the pharmacokinetics of cimetidine, carbamazepine, digoxin, erythromycin, oral contraceptives, phenytoin, theophylline, valproate and warfarin [22]. However, enzyme-inducing AEDs such as carbamazepine, phenytoin, phenobarbital or primidone increase the hepatic clearance of tiagabine when given in combination [23]. The plasma half-life which is normally 5–9 h

[19], is reduced to 2–3 h in combination with enzyme-inducing drugs.

Clinical efficacy

Evidence from randomized controlled trials

Tiagabine has proven effective as add-on therapy in patients with refractory partial seizures with or without secondary generalization. The primary clinical evidence for this efficacy is based on five controlled add-on trials in adults with epilepsy unsatisfactorily controlled with current AEDs (Table 44.1).

The first phase II multicentre trials were two small placebo-controlled cross-over studies. In an initial titration period lasting up to 8 weeks, patients started with a tiagabine dose of 8 mg/day, and the dose was titrated either to reduce seizures sufficiently or to produce unacceptable adverse events. Patients then entered a 4-week fixed-dose period on the dose attained in titration. The maximal dose allowed in the first study was 52 mg/day [24]. Patients were eligible to enter the double-blind cross-over phase if their seizure frequency had been reduced by at least 25% during the fixed-dose period. In this two-period cross-over study, patients were randomized to placebo/tiagabine or their previously determined dose of tiagabine/placebo, remaining on each of these two regimens for 7 weeks. The 7-week treatment periods were separated by a 3-week washout period. The median daily dose of tiagabine in the double-blind phase was 32 mg/day. Of the total of 42 patients who contributed data for both periods of the cross-over phase, 26% of those with complex partial seizures and 63% with secondarily generalized tonic-clonic seizures ($n=27$) experienced a reduction of at least 50% in seizure frequency during the tiagabine period compared to the placebo period. The median seizure rate during the tiagabine treatment period was significantly lower than during the placebo treatment period for complex partial seizures ($P=0.05$) and secondarily generalized tonic-clonic seizures ($P=0.009$).

The second phase II study used the same design but allowed a maximal dose of 64 mg/day [25]. The intent-to-treat group comprised 36 patients who received a mean total daily dose of 46 mg in the tiagabine treatment periods. Tiagabine was significantly better than placebo in reducing all partial seizures ($P=0.002$), complex partial seizures ($P<0.001$) and partial seizures with secondary generalization ($P=0.030$). A total of 46% of patients with complex partial seizures had at least a 50% reduction in weekly seizure rates.

Altogether 769 patients took part into the three multicentre, parallel-group, double-blind add-on studies in which tiagabine was compared with placebo—a dose–response study, a dose–frequency study and a thrice-a-day (t.i.d) dosing study [26–28]. The dose-ranging multicentre study in the USA had a fixed-dose, placebo-controlled parallel-group design ($n=297$) [28]. During a 4-week period, tiagabine-treated patients were given increasing doses until the dose level to which they had been randomized was reached (16, 32 or 56 mg/day divided in four equal doses). The patients then remained on a fixed dose for 12 weeks of double-blind treatment. Median decreases in 4-week complex partial seizure frequency for 32 mg (–2.2) and 56 mg (–2.8) tiagabine groups were significantly greater than for placebo (–0.7) group ($P=0.03$ and $P<0.03$, respectively); 20% and 29% of patients in the 32- and 56-mg groups had a 50% or greater reduction in the frequency of complex partial seizures compared with 4% in the placebo group ($P=0.002$ and $P<0.001$, respectively).

The dose–frequency study was also a randomized, double-blind, placebo controlled USA multicentre study with a parallel-group, add-on design ($n=318$) [26]. The study lasted for 24 weeks and consisted of an 8-week baseline, a 12-week double-blind treatment phase and a 4-week termination period. During the first month of treatment, doses were increased weekly to 32 mg/day. The treatment groups were placebo, 16 mg tiagabine twice a day (b.i.d.) and 8 mg tiagabine four times a day (q.i.d.). The median changes in 4-week complex partial seizure rates were –1.6 ($P=0.055$) for the 16

Table 44.1 Data from five double-blind placebo-controlled trials and from an integrated analysis of these studies showing the efficacy of tiagabine as add-on therapy in partial epilepsy

Reference	Number of patients	Daily dose	Responder rate (>50% seizure reduction) for all partial seizures mg/day	
			Tiagabine (%)	Placebo (%)
[24]	42	33	52	24[b]
[25]	36	46	40	14[a]
[28]	297	16	10	4
		32	20	4[b]
		56	31	4[c]
[26]	318	32 (16 mg b.i.d.)	28	8[c]
		32 (8 mg q.i.d.)	23	8[b]
[27]	154	30	10	5
[32]	951	16–56	23	9

[a] $P<0.05$.
[b] $P<0.01$.
[c] $P<0.001$.

mg b.i.d. group and −1.2 (P < 0.05) for the 8 mg q.i.d. group, versus −0.2 for placebo. Statistically significant differences between placebo and two tiagabine groups occurred in the proportion of patients experiencing > 50% rate reduction for complex partial, simple partial and all partial seizure rates.

The t.i.d. dosing study was a Northern-European multicentre parallel-group study which compared a dose of 30 mg/day tiagabine with placebo as add-on therapy (n = 154) [27]. The study included 12-week baseline, an 18-week double-blind treatment phase, and a 4-week termination period. The median change from baseline in complex partial seizure rates was −1.3 for patients on tiagabine, while placebo patients had a median increase of 0.1 in complex partial seizure rates (P < 0.05). Tiagabine was significantly more effective than placebo in patients with simple partial seizures with respect to the proportion of patients achieving a seizure reduction of at least 50% (21% vs. 6%; P < 0.05).

The meta-analysis across all these three trials for 50% responders showed an odds ratio of 3.03 (95% CI 2.01–4.58) in favour of tiagabine [29]. The summary odds ratios for each dose indicate increasing efficacy with increasing doses, with no suggestion that the effect of the drug had reached a plateau at the doses examined in these studies. A 16-mg dose has a fairly small effect of 2.40 (95% CI 0.65–8.87). There is a substantial increase with doses of 30 or 32 mg to odds ratio of 3.17 (95% CI 2.03–4.96) and a smaller additional gain for a dose level 56 mg, odds ratio 7.95 (95% CI 3.09–20.49).

A multicentre, open-label, randomized, parallel-group study compared the efficacy, tolerability and safety of t.i.d. and b.i.d. dosing of tiagabine as an adjunctive therapy for the treatment of refractory patients with partial seizures [30]. A total of 347 patients were randomized and treated (175 t.i.d. and 172 b.i.d.). Each group was administered the same daily dose of tiagabine incremented stepwise during a 12-week fixed-schedule titration period to a target 40 mg/day. The patients were followed for a further 12-week flexible continuation phase. A significantly greater number of patients in the t.i.d. group completed the fixed schedule titration period (81.4% vs. 73.1%; 95% CI = 0.331, 0.970; P = 0.038). The proportion of responders (patients showing at least 50% decrease in all-seizure frequency from baseline) was similar for both groups (44% for b.i.d. and 48% for t.i.d.) during the last 8 weeks of treatment and seven (4%) patients in the b.i.d. group were seizure free compared to 14 (8%) patients in the t.i.d. group.

A multicentre trial has also been performed to determine whether the combination of AEDs with different mechanisms of action may be superior to the combination of AEDs with similar mechanisms of action. In this study patients on carbamazepine or phenytoin monotherapy with inadequately controlled complex partial seizures were randomized to add-on tiagabine or phenytoin (if previously on carbamazepine) or add-on tiagabine or carbamazepine (if previously on phenytoin) and titrated to an optimal dose in a double-blind trial [31]. In this trial tiagabine (n = 170) showed similar efficacy to traditional AEDs (carbamazepine or phenytoin) (n = 175) adjunctive therapy for complex partial seizures at low average doses of 24–28 mg/day. The study also suggested that tiagabine may be better tolerated when added to phenytoin or carbamazepine than when carbamazepine or phenytoin are added to each other.

Evidence from other studies

There are data from six long-term open-label trials. More than half of the 2248 patients have been treated with tiagabine for more than 1 year. For each type of partial seizure, 30–40% of the patients obtained considerable treatment effect, which was maintained after 12 months of treatment [32]. Daily dosages in the long-term studies were between 24 and 60 mg in the majority of patients and mean and median doses were 45 mg/day for most studies. However, up to 15% of patients received a dose of between 80 and 120 mg/day after their first year of treatment [33].

Pragmatic trials use larger patient numbers and a longer follow-up than the trials required for drug registration and more closely mimic routine clinical practice. Three such pragmatic studies — in Germany, Poland and Spain — have been conducted with add-on tiagabine in patients with refractory partial epilepsy [34–36]. All have a longer follow-up than that of the pivotal studies, and together have included considerably more patients than the studies submitted in the registration dossier. These trials used the newly recommended titration schedule in a total of 1151 patients, aged 3–93 years, who were followed for up to 6 months. Tiagabine was given thrice daily, at an initial dose of 5 mg/day and following the titration schedule, with increases of 5 mg/week. The maintenance dose was titrated individually according to the labelling. The average dose was 30 (range 5–90) mg/day. Rates for 50% responder varied from 41 to 61%, and 8–22% of patients became seizure free.

Efficacy as monotherapy

The efficacy of tiagabine during monotherapy in patients with chronic partial epilepsy not satisfactorily controlled by other drugs has been studied in a double-blind parallel-group study in 198 patients with refractory epilepsy comparing 6 mg/day tiagabine with 36 mg/day after gradual withdrawal of other AEDs over 29 weeks [37]. Altogether 33% of the patients on the low dose completed the study compared with 47% taking the higher dose. For both dose groups the median complex partial seizure rates decreased significantly during treatment compared with baseline (P < 0.05). However a higher proportion of patients in the 36 mg/day group experienced a reduction in complex partial seizures of at least 50% compared with the 6 mg/day group (31% vs. 18%, P < 0.05). In addition to showing a dose–response relationship, this study suggested that even as low a dose as 6 mg/day of tiagabine may be effective when used as monotherapy or with non-inducing AEDs.

The second study was a double-blind, randomized comparison of a slow and fast switch to tiagabine monotherapy from another monotherapy, followed by an open-label evaluation of the safety and efficacy of tiagabine as monotherapy for chronic partial epilepsy [38]. If the patients did not tolerate the double-blind titration scheme for tiagabine even slower open-label up-titration of tiagabine could be used. Thirty-four (85%) out of the 40 patients were successfully switched to tiagabine monotherapy in either the double-blind or open-label drug switching schemes. According to this trial it seems that the open label up-titration with 5 mg/day with weekly increments of 5 mg/day should be recommended in clinical practice. The retention rate in the study for 12 weeks on tiagabine monotherapy was 63% (25/40) and 48% for 48 weeks (19/40). The initial target dose of tiagabine monotherapy was 10 mg b.i.d. but in the open-label phase tiagabine could be adjusted up or down in individual patients according to the clinical judgment of the investigator up to a maximum daily dose of 70 mg. The median dose was 20 mg/day and the range was from 7.5 mg/day to 42.5 mg/day during the first 48 weeks.

Monotherapy in newly diagnosed partial epilepsy has been studied comparing the efficacy and safety of tiagabine versus carbamazepine as monotherapy in a double-blind, randomized, parallel group trial ($n=290$) [39]. During the 6-week titration period patients were titrated from tiagabine 5 mg/day or carbamazepine 200 mg/day to tiagabine 10 or 15 mg/day or carbamazepine 400 or 600 mg/day in a step-wise fashion. During the 44-week assessment period the dose could be adjusted within the ranges tiagabine 10–20 mg/day or carbamazepine 400–800 mg/day. All doses were administered b.i.d. The study has so far only been published in abstract form, showing a significant difference between the study groups with regard to the endpoint 'time to meeting the exit criterion' ($P<0.05$). An exit criterion was either status epilepticus or the occurrence of the second seizure at maximum tolerated or maximum allowed dose level. In the tiagabine group 41% (77/144) and in the carbamazepine group 53% (77/144) completed the assessment period either seizure free or with a single seizure ($P<0.05$). It has been suggested that failure of tiagabine monotherapy to show efficacy comparable to carbamazepine in this trial might have been related to the relatively low maximum dose of tiagabine that was used.

Efficacy in paediatric patients

Use of tiagabine in children has been studied as adjunctive therapy in over 200 paediatric patients. A European study was carried out at two centres in Denmark and one centre in France [40]. This 4-month, single-blind study evaluated the tolerability, safety and preliminary efficacy of ascending doses (0.25–1.5 mg/kg/day) of tiagabine add-on therapy in 52 children over 2 years with different syndromes of refractory epilepsy. Tiagabine appeared to reduce seizures more in localization-related epilepsy syndromes than generalized epilepsy syndromes. Seventeen of the 23 patients with localization-related epilepsy syndromes entered the fourth dosing period. The 17 patients had a median reduction of seizure rate in the fourth month of treatment of 33% compared with baseline. In comparison 13, of 22 children with seven different generalized epilepsy syndromes entered the fourth dosing period with a median change of seizure rate of 0%. Among generalized seizures, tonic seizures and atypical absences responded best, with median percentage reductions in the weekly seizure rate of 77% and 63%. The overall maximum daily tiagabine dose level received and tolerated (mean ± SD) was 0.65 ± 0.37 mg/kg.

In the USA the long-term use of tiagabine has been studied also in an open-label extension study in 152 children aged 2–11 years from antecedent double-blind studies [41]. Of the 140 evaluatable patients 10 patients were seizure free with tiagabine add-on therapy and 13 patients achieved seizure freedom with tiagabine monotherapy for periods ranging from 9 to 109 weeks. The shortest seizure-free or monotherapy durations represented patients with recent enrolment dates at the time of report. Dose range was from 4 to 66

mg/day and average dose 23.5 mg/day. In a recent preliminary open trial in infantile spasms, six of 12 infants had at least 50% seizure reduction at dosages of 0.5–3.1 mg/kg/day [42].

Clinical safety

At the time of writing, exposure to tiagabine amounted to about 50 000 patient-years. From short-term trials compared with placebo, it was clear that some CNS-related adverse effects are particularly common with tiagabine treatment (Table 44.2). Dizziness is most frequent. This is a feeling of light-headedness or unsteadiness, and develops usually within 1–2 h of taking a tiagabine dose. It is associated with the peak concentration of the drug. Also more common with tiagabine than with placebo were: asthenia (lack of energy), nervousness, tremor, concentration difficulties, depressive mood and language problems (difficulty in finding words or initiation of speech). The increased risk of CNS-related adverse events compared to placebo was in the titration period only. There was no difference in side-effects during the fixed-dose period [33]. This experience suggests that tiagabine should be titrated slowly. The CNS-related adverse effects are also shown to be clearly dose related in the US monotherapy study in which low-dose (6 mg/day) and high-dose (36 mg/day) monotherapy were compared [37]. It is recommended, on the bases of these studies, that initial dosages of tiagabine can be given twice a day, but a change to thrice daily dosing is recommended with dosages above 30 mg/day. Tiagabine should always be taken with food to avoid rapid rises in plasma concentrations. Individually four times daily dosing may also be helpful at least with higher doses. Somnolence or drowsiness were not seen more frequently in tiagabine patients than in patients receiving placebo.

No idiosyncratic reactions have as yet been linked to the use of tiagabine [43]. No systematic abnormalities have been noted in haematology values or common chemistry values and therefore there are no specific guidelines for routine monitoring of laboratory values during tiagabine treatment [33]. The relationship of adverse events has correlated more strongly with dose than with the plasma

Table 44.2 Significantly higher treatment emergent CNS-related adverse events reported by ≥ 1% of tiagabine-treated patients during the experiment period in the three placebo-controlled, parallel-group, add-on epilepsy studies [33]

Adverse event	Placebo ($n=275$), n (%)	Tiagabine ($n=494$), n (%)
Dizziness	41 (15)	131 (27)[b]
Asthenia	39 (14)	99 (20)[a]
Nervousness	8 (3)	50 (10)[b]
Tremor	9 (3)	46 (9)[a]
Difficulty with concentration/attention	6 (2)	30 (6)[a]
Depression	2 (<1)	17 (3)[a]
Language problems	0 (0)	8 (2)[a]

[a] $P<0.05$.
[b] $P<0.01$.

concentration of tiagabine [33]. Therefore it is most important to up-titrate the dosage according to the tolerability of the individual patient and there is no need to follow-up routinely the plasma concentration.

Because of its action on GABAergic mechanisms, the question has been raised as to whether tiagabine, like vigabatrin, can result in visual field abnormalities. To date, however, there is no evidence that the increased risk of concentric visual field defects is a class effect of GABAergic drugs. The first ophthalmological study of 15 patients using tiagabine as monotherapy (mean daily dosage 21 mg, range 5–60 mg; mean duration of therapy 38 months, range 23–55 months) did not show any evidence of a relationship between visual field constriction and tiagabine treatment [44]. A larger cross-sectional study was set up in newly diagnosed patients with partial epilepsy, receiving tiagabine, carbamazepine or lamotrigine as initial monotherapies [45]. Neurological and ophthalmological tests including Goldmann and Humphrey perimetries were performed. A neuro-ophthalmological expert blindly reviewed all visual charts. Seventy-three patients were included and completed the study. The population eligible for analysis included 68 patients, of whom 32 were treated with tiagabine (median duration, 25 months), 24 with carbamazepine (21 months) and 12 with lamotrigine (15 months). No patient treated with tiagabine showed a concentric visual field defect on Goldmann perimetry testing. No clinically relevant abnormalities in visual fields resembling those known with vigabatrin were detected, particularly in patients treated initially with tiagabine monotherapy. These findings support the evidence that tiagabine is not associated with retinal toxicity.

There has also been concern that tiagabine may be associated with an increased incidence of psychosis, particularly with rapid titration. Evaluation of psychosis-related adverse effects showed there was no excess risk of this disorder attributable to tiagabine beyond what would be expected from the population with difficult to control partial seizures. The incidence of psychosis was 0.8% in the tiagabine-treated patients and 0.4% in the placebo-treated patients in the three parallel group add-on trials [33]. However, the addition of tiagabine in clinical trials was associated significantly more often with depression than the use of placebo (5 vs. 2%) [33]. Because of this concern, if there is a history of behavioural problems or depression, treatment with tiagabine should be initiated at a low initial dose under close supervision as there may be an increased risk of recurrence of these symptoms during treatment with tiagabine.

No adverse effect on cognitive abilities has been demonstrated, and the neuropsychological effects of tiagabine add-on therapy and monotherapy have been widely evaluated. In the largest short-term double-blind study 162 adults completed a multicentre, dose–response study with random assignment to placebo or 16, 32 or 56 mg/day tiagabine [46]. Results on 19 measures of cognitive abilities and 18 measures of adjustment and mood showed only findings attributable to chance. Long-term cognitive results have been presented in a double-blind, placebo-controlled, parallel-group add-on study with an open-label extension study with 18–24 months follow-up [47]. The neuropsychological and EEG evaluation did not indicate any adverse effects of tiagabine during the double-blind phase at low doses or long-term open phase at higher doses up to 80 mg/day. The daily dosages in the long-term follow-up of this study were higher than in the previous reports. Dose-related im-

pacts of tiagabine on cognition and mood were studied in a conversion-to-monotherapy study comparing doses of 6 mg/day and 36 mg/day of tiagabine as monotherapy in previously uncontrolled epilepsy patients [48]. The study showed modest improvements in cognitive abilities and adjustment compared to the more traditional AEDs given at baseline. Tiagabine dose was related to the type of improvement, with the low dose more likely to be associated with improvement in adjustment and mood and the high dose more likely to be associated with improvement in cognitive abilities. In the other study, doses were individually titrated between 7.5 and 35 mg/day and also in this conversion to tiagabine monotherapy study tiagabine did not produce cognitive or behavioural adverse effects as compared to the previous treatment with standard AEDs [49]. However, successful tiagabine monotherapy seemed to be associated with improvement in simple psychomotor speed and to cause less fatigue compared with standard AEDs.

Teratogenic effects were seen in the offspring of rats exposed to maternally toxic doses of tiagabine, but not in animals receiving non-toxic dosages. Only limited pregnancy data involving tiagabine, which show no clear teratogenicity, are available [50]. Therefore tiagabine cannot be recommended for women who are pregnant or at risk of becoming pregnant, and should be used only if the potential benefit justifies the potential risk to the fetus.

Several cases of non-convulsive status epilepticus have been reported, with disappearance of the status after withdrawal of the drug or reduction in dosage. In double-blind, placebo-controlled trials on patients with partial epilepsy, however, the incidence of spike-wave status or any kind of status epilepticus was 3% (8/275 patients) on placebo and 4% (22/494 patients) on tiagabine, the difference being not statistically significant [51]. Further study of individual cases suggested that most of the subjects with apparently tiagabine-associated non-convulsive status had pre-existing spike/wave patterns and, that, in some cases, the condition was related to drug-induced encephalopathy rather than status epilepticus. However, it might be wise not to use tiagabine in patients with unclassified epilepsy or patients with generalized epilepsy, especially those with a history of absence or myoclonic seizures, with a history of spike-and-wave discharges on EEG or non-convulsive status epilepticus [52]. Tiagabine has not yet been shown to be effective in these patients, and there is other evidence that AEDs increasing GABAergic transmission may exacerbate or induce absences or myoclonus [53]. In patients with a history of spike-and-wave discharges, cognitive or neuropsychiatric disturbances can be associated with exacerbation of the EEG abnormalities. However, in the documented cases of spike-and-wave discharges on EEG with cognitive/neuropsychiatric events, some patients with partial epilepsies have been able to continue tiagabine, but required dosage adjustment [33].

Clinical therapeutics

Tiagabine is recommended as add-on treatment of adults and children over 12 years with partial seizures with or without secondary generalization which cannot be satisfactorily controlled with other AEDs. In the preclinical and clinical studies, the tiagabine dose was expressed in terms of milligrams of hydrochloride. A conversion factor of 0.91 has been used to calculate the dose as tiagabine free base, which is available as 2.5-, 5-, 10- and 15-mg tablets, except in the USA, Canada and Mexico where 2-, 4-, 12-, 16- and 20-mg tablets of tiagabine hydrochloride are used.

The current labelling with tiagabine free base states that the initial dosage is 7.5–15 mg/day, followed by weekly increments of 5–15 mg/day. In the USA, Canada and Mexico, labelling was already modified towards lower initial dose of 4 mg/day tiagabine hydrochloride, followed by weekly increments of 4–8 mg/day.

Phase IV trial and clinical experience to date would suggest starting tiagabine with 4 or 5 mg/day and gradually increasing the dosage by weekly increments of 4 or 5 mg/day, in order to minimize CNS-related side-effects. Initial dosages can be given twice a day, but a change to thrice-daily dosing is recommended with dosages above 30–32 mg/day. Tiagabine should always be taken with food, and preferably at the end of meals, to avoid rapid rises in plasma concentrations. Individual dosing four times daily may also be helpful, at least with higher doses.

Population pharmacokinetic analyses indicate that tiagabine clearance is 60% greater in patients taking enzyme-inducing AEDs. The usual initial target maintenance dosage in patients taking enzyme-inducing drugs is 30–32 mg/day and in patients not taking enzyme-inducing drugs 15–16 mg/day [52]. The usually recommended range of maintenance dosage in patients taking enzyme-inducing drugs is up to 50–56 mg/day and in patients not taking enzyme-inducing drugs up to 30–32 mg/day. However, high daily doses of at least 70–80 mg are well tolerated for some individual patients. Patients taking a combination of inducing and non-inducing drugs (e.g. carbamazepine and valproate) should be considered to be enzyme induced. No AED should be suddenly withdrawn, and although there are no clinical data, it seems sensible to withdraw tiagabine gradually over at least 2–3 weeks [52].

The pharmacokinetics of tiagabine in elderly patients are similar to those observed in younger patients, hence there should be no need for dosage modification [54]. The pharmacokinetics of tiagabine have not been investigated in adequate and well-controlled clinical trials in patients below the age of 12 years. The apparent clearance and volume of distribution of tiagabine per unit body surface area or per kilogram of body weight were fairly similar in 25 children (age: 3–10 years) and in adults taking enzyme-inducing AEDs. In children who were taking a non-inducing AED, the clearance of tiagabine based upon body weight and body surface area was 2 and 1.5-fold higher, respectively, than in non-induced adults with epilepsy suggesting that dosage requirements (on a milligram per kilogram basis) may be higher in children [55]. In the paediatric study the maximal tolerated doses for children over 2 years old on inducing AEDS were only slightly higher than in children on non-inducing AEDs, but the difference was not significant (0.73 ± 0.44 mg/kg vs. 0.61 ± 0.32 mg/kg) [40].

The pharmacokinetics of tiagabine is unaffected in patients with renal impairment or in subjects with renal failure requiring haemodialysis [56]. Patients with mild or moderate liver function impairment have been shown to have higher and more prolonged plasma concentrations of both total and unbound tiagabine after administration compared with normal subjects. The patients with hepatic impairment also had more neurological side-effects. Tiagabine should therefore be given with caution to patients with epilepsy who have impaired hepatic function. Patients with impaired liver function may require reduced initial and maintenance doses of tiagabine and/or longer dosing intervals compared to

patients with normal hepatic function. The patients should be monitored closely because of the potential for increased incidence of neurological side-effects [57]. Tiagabine should not be used in patients with severely impaired liver function.

Role of tiagabine in epilepsy treatment

Tiagabine, a selective GABA-uptake inhibitor, is effective against all partial seizures and has a relatively favourable safety profile. The frequency of idiosyncratic drug-related reactions, including cutaneous reactions, is low with tiagabine. Moreover, tiagabine has a favourable cognitive profile. The characteristic concentric visual field defect seen with vigabatrin treatment has not been observed in two tiagabine monotherapy trials. Thus, tiagabine is recommended for use as an add-on treatment in partial epilepsy, for example after failure with the first-line sodium-channel blocking AED or if the first-line AED has caused idiosyncratic reactions. Tiagabine is suitable also for patients for whom it is particularly important that the AED does not cause any deterioration in cognitive performance. If there is a history of behavioural problems or depression, treatment with tiagabine should be initiated at a low initial dose under close supervision as there may be an increased risk of recurrence of these symptoms during treatment with tiagabine. Tiagabine should not be used in patients with unclassified epilepsy or patients with generalized epilepsy, especially those with a history of absence or myoclonic seizures, with a history of spike-and-wave discharges on the EEG or non-convulsive status epilepticus.

References

1 Suzdak PD, Jansen JA. A review of the preclinical pharmacology of tiagabine: a potent and selective anticonvulsant GABA uptake inhibitor. *Epilepsia* 1995; 36: 612–26.
2 Borden LA, Murali Dhar TG, Smith KE *et al*. Tiagabine, SKF 89976-A, CI-966 and NNC-711 are selective for the cloned GABA transporter GAT-1. *Eur J Pharmacol* 1994; 269: 219–24.
3 Braestrup C, Nielsen EB, Sonnewald U *et al*. (R)-N-[4,4-bis(3-methyl-2-thienyl)but-3-en-1-yl]nipecotic acid binds with high affinity to the brain γ-aminobutyric acid uptake carrier. *J Neurochem* 1990; 54: 639–47.
4 Sills G, Butler E, Thompson G, Brodie M. Vigabatrin and tiagabine are pharmacologically different drugs. A preclinical study. *Seizure* 1999; 8: 404–11.
5 Roepstorff A, Lampert JD. Comparison of the effect of the GABA uptake blockers, tiagabine and nipecotic acid, on inhibitory synaptic efficacy in hippocampal CA1 neurones. *Neurosci Lett* 1992; 146: 131–4.
6 Sills G, Patsalos P, Butler E, Forrest G, Ratnaraj N, Brodie M. Visual field constriction: accumulation of vigabatrin but not tiagabine in the retina. *Neurology* 2001; 57(2): 196–200.
7 Dalby NO, Nielsen EB. Comparison of the preclinical anticonvulsant profiles of tiagabine, lamotrigine, gabapentin and vigabatrin. *Epilepsy Res* 1997; 28: 63–72.
8 Dalby NO, Nielsen EB. Tiagabine exerts an antiepileptogenic effect in amygdala kindling epileptigenesis in the rat. *Neurosci Lett* 1997; 229: 135–7.
9 Nielsen EB, Suzdak PD, Andersen KE *et al*. Characterization of tiagabine (No-328), a new potent and selective GABA uptake inhibitor. *Eur J Pharmacol* 1991; 196: 257–66.
10 Coleman MH, Yamaguchi S, Rogawski MA. Protection against dendrotoxin-induced clonic-seizures in mice by anticonvulsant drugs. *Brain Res* 1992; 575: 138–42.
11 Yamaguchi S, Rogawski MA. Effects of anticonvulsant drugs on 4-aminopyridine-induced clonic seizures in mice. *Epilepsy Res* 1992; 11: 9–16.

12 Coenen AML, Blezer EHM, van Luijtelaar ELJM. Effects of the GABA uptake inhibitor tiagabine on electroencephalogram, spike-wave discharges and behaviour of rats. *Epilepsy Res* 1995; 21: 89–94.

13 Walton NY, Gunawan S, Treiman DM. Treatment of experimental status epilepticus with the GABA uptake inhibitor, tiagabine. *Epilepsy Res* 1994; 19: 237–44.

14 Marescaux C. *Effects of tiagabine in rats with genetic absence epilepsy (GAERS)*. Unpublished report, data on file Novo Nordisk.

15 Hosford DA, Wang Y. Utility of the lethargic (lh/lh) mouse model of absence seizures in predicting the effects of lamotrigine, vigabatrin, tiagabine, gabapentin, and topiramate against human absence seizures. *Epilepsia* 1997; 38: 408–14.

16 Halonen T, Nissinen J, Jansen JA *et al*. Tiagabine prevents seizures, neuronal damage and memory impairment in experimental status epilepticus. *Eur J Pharmacol* 1996; 299: 69–81.

17 Inglefield JR, Perry JM, Schwartz RD. Postischemic inhibition of GABA reuptake by tiagabine slows neuronal death in the gerbil hippocampus. *Hippocampus* 1995; 5(5): 460–8.

18 Johansen FF, Diener NH. Enhancement of GABA neurotransmission after cerebral ischaemia in the rat reduces loss of hippocampal CA1 pyramidal cells. *Acta Neurol Scand* 1991; 84: 1–6.

19 Gustavsson LE, Mengel HB. Pharmacokinetics of tiagabine, a gamma-aminobutyric acid-uptake inhibitor, in healthy subjects after single and multiple doses. *Epilepsia* 1995; 36: 605–11.

20 Mengel HB. Tiagabine. *Epilepsia* 1994; 35 (Suppl. 5): 81–4.

21 So EL, Wolff D, Graves NM *et al*. Pharmacokinetics of tiagabine as add-on therapy in patients taking enzyme-inducing antiepilepsy drugs. *Epilepsy Res* 1995; 22: 221–6.

22 Brodie MJ. Tiagabine pharmacology in profile. *Epilepsia* 1995; 36 (Suppl. 6): 7–9.

23 Krämer G. Pharmacokinetic interactions of new antiepileptic drugs. In: Stefan H, Krämer G, Mamoli B, eds. *Challenge in Epilepsy—New Antiepileptic Drugs*. Berlin: Blackwell Science Publications, 1998: 87–103.

24 Richens A, Chadwick DW, Duncan JS *et al*. Adjunctive treatment of partial seizures with tiagabine: a placebo-controlled trial. *Epilepsy Res* 1995; 21: 37–42.

25 Crawford PM, Engelsman M, Brown SW. Tiagabine: phase II study of efficacy and safety in adjunctive treatment of partial seizures. *Epilepsia* 1993; 34 (Suppl. 2): S182.

26 Sachdeo RC, Leroy R, Krauss G *et al*. Tiagabine therapy for complex partial seizures. A dose-frequency study. *Arch Neurol* 1997; 54: 595–601.

27 Kälviäinen R, Brodie MJ, Chadwick D *et al*. A double-blind, placebo-controlled trial of tiagabine given three-times daily as add-on therapy for refractory partial seizures. *Epilepsy Res* 1998; 30: 31–40.

28 Uthman B, Rowan J, Ahman PA *et al*. Tiagabine for complex partial seizures: a randomised, add-on, dose–response trial. *Arch Neurol* 1998; 55: 56–62.

29 Marson AG, Kadir ZA, Hutton JL *et al*. The new antiepileptic drugs: a systematic review of their efficacy and tolerability. *Epilepsia* 1997; 38(8): 859–80.

30 Biraben A, Beaussart M, Josien E *et al*. Comparison of twice- and three times daily tiagabine for the adjunctive treatment of partial seizures in refractory patients with epilepsy: an open label, randomized, parallel-group study. *Epileptic Disord* 2001; 3(2): 91–100.

31 Biton V, Vasquez KB, Sachdeo RC *et al*. Adjunctive tiagabine compared with phenytoin and carbamazepine in the multicenter, double-blind trial of complex partial seizures. *Epilepsia* 1998; 39 (Suppl. 6): 125–6.

32 Ben-Menachem E. International experience with tiagabine add-on therapy. *Epilepsia* 1995; 36: 14–21.

33 Leppik IE, Gram L, Deaton R. Safety of tiagabine: summary of 53 trials. *Epilepsy Res* 1999; 33: 235–46.

34 Bergmann A, Bauer J, Stodieck S. Treatment of epilepsy with tiagabine as add-on antiepileptic drug in patients with refractory seizures: Experiences in 574 patients. *Epilepsia* 2000; 41 (Suppl. Florence): 40.

35 Czapinski P, Jedrzejczak J, Kozik A *et al*. Open multicentre study of tiagabine as add on treatment in patients with partial seizures. *Epilepsia* 2000; 41 (Suppl. Florence): 40.

36 Salas-Puig J, Arroyo and the Epilepsy Observational Investigation Group of Spain. Tiagabine adjunctive therapy: An observational study. *Epilepsia* 2000; 41 (Suppl. Florence): 40.

37 Schachter S. Tiagabine monotherapy in the treatment of partial epilepsy. *Epilepsia* 1995; 36 (Suppl. 6): S2–S6.

38 Kälviäinen R, Salmenperä T, Jutila L *et al*. Slow versus fast drug switch from established AED to tiagabine monotherapy. *Epilepsia* 1998; 39: 66.

39 Brodie MJ, Bomhof MAM, Kälviäinen R *et al*. Double-blind comparison of tiagabine and carbamazepine monotherapy in newly diagnosed epilepsy: preliminary results. *Epilepsia* 1997; 38 (Suppl. 3): S66–S67.

40 Uldall P, Bulteau C, Pedersen SA *et al*. Tiagabine adjunctive therapy in children with refractory epilepsy: a single-blind dose escalating study. *Epilepsy Res* 2000; 42: 159–68.

41 Collins SD, Fugate J, Sommerville KW. Long-term use of Gabitril (tiagabine HCl) monotherapy in pediatric patients. *Neurology* 1999; 52 (Suppl. 2): A392.

42 Kugler SL, Mandelbaum DE, Patel R *et al*. Efficacy and tolerability of tiagabine in infantile spasms. *Epilepsia* 1999; 40 (Suppl. 7): 127.

43 Leach JP, Brodie MJ. Tiagabine. *Lancet* 1998; 351: 203–7.

44 Nousiainen I, Mäntyjärvi M, Kälviäinen R. Visual function in patients treated with the GABAergic anticonvulsant drug tiagabine. *Clin Drug Invest* 2000; 20(6): 393–400.

45 Kälviäinen R, Hache J-C, Renault-Djouadi J. A study of visual fields in patients receiving tiagabine as monotherapy versus carbamazepine or lamotrigine monotherapy. *Epilepsia* 2001; 42 (Suppl. 7): 256.

46 Dodrill CB, Arnett JL, Sommerville KW, Shu V. Cognitive and quality of life effects of differing doses of tiagabine in epilepsy. *Neurology* 1997; 48: 1025–31.

47 Kälviäinen R, Äikiä M, Mervaala E *et al*. Long-term cognitive and EEG effects of tiagabine in drug-resistant partial epilepsy. *Epilepsy Res* 1996; 25: 291–7.

48 Dodrill CB, Arnett JL, Shu V *et al*. Effects of tiagabine monotherapy on abilities, adjustment and mood. *Epilepsia* 1998; 39: 33–42.

49 Äikiä M, Kälviäinen R, Salmenperä T, Riekkinen PJ. Cognitive effects of tiagabine monotherapy. *Epilepsia* 1997; 38: 107.

50 Collins S, Donnelly J, Krups D, Sommerville KW. Pregnancy and tiagabine exposure. *Neurology* 1997: 48 (Suppl. 2): abstract P01.039.

51 Shinnar S, Berg A, Treiman D *et al*. Status epilepticus and tiagabine therapy: Review of safety data and epidemiologic comparisons. *Epilepsia* 2001; 42(3): 372–9.

52 Schmidt D, Gram L, Brodie M *et al*. Tiagabine in the treatment of epilepsy – a clinical review with a guide for prescribing physician. *Epilepsy Res* 2000; 41: 245–51.

53 Loiseau P. Review of controlled trials of tiagabine; a clinician's viewpoint. *Epilepsia* 1999; 40 (Suppl. 9): 145.

54 Snel S, Jansen JA, Mengel HB *et al*. The pharmacokinetics of tiagabine in healthy elderly volunteers and elderly patients with epilepsy. *J Clin Pharmacol* 1997; 37: 1015–20.

55 Gustavson LE, Boellner SW, Grannemann GR *et al*. A single-dose study to define tiagabine pharmacokinetics in pediatric patients with complex partial seizures. *Neurology* 1998; 48: 1032–7.

56 Cato A.III, Gustavson LE, Qian J *et al*. Effects of renal impairment on the pharmacokinetics and tolerability of tiagabine. *Epilepsia* 1998; 39: 43–7.

57 Lau AH, Gustavson LE, Sperelakis R *et al*. Pharmacokinetics and safety of tiagabine in subjects with various degrees of hepatic function. *Epilepsia* 1997; 38(4): 445–51.

45 Topiramate

J.H. Cross

Primary indications	Adjunctive therapy or monotherapy in partial and secondarily generalized seizures. Also for Lennox–Gastaut syndrome and primary generalized tonic–clonic seizures
Usual preparations	Tablets: 25, 50, 100, 200 mg; sprinkle: 15, 25 mg
Usual dosages	Initial: 25–50 mg/day (adults), 0.5–1 mg/kg/day (children). Maintenance: 100–500 mg/day (adults), 5–9 mg/kg/day (children)
Dosage intervals	2 times/day
Significant drug interactions	Topiramate levels are lowered by carbamazepine, phenobarbital and phenytoin
Serum level monitoring	Not generally useful
Target range	9–12 mg/L
Common/important side effects	Dizziness, ataxia, headache, paresthesia, tremor, somnolence, cognitive dysfunction, confusion, agitation, amnesia, depression, emotional lability, nausea, diarrhoea, diplopia, weight loss
Main advantages	Highly effective, recently introduced antiepileptic drug
Main disadvantages	CNS side effects
Mechanisms of action	Blockade of sodium channels; potentiation of GABA-mediated inhibition at the GABAA receptor; reduction of excitatory actions of glutatmate via the AMPA receptor; inhibtion of high voltage calcium channels
Oral bioavailability	<100%
Time to peak levels	2–4 h
Metabolism and excretion	Mainly renal excretion without metabolism
Volume of distribution	0.6–1.0 L/kg
Elimination half-life	19–25 h (but varies with comedication)
Plasma clearance	0.022–0.036 L/kg/h
Protein binding	13–17%
Active metabolites	None
Comment	Highly effective recently introduced antiepileptic drug

(*Note*: This summary table was formulated by the lead editor)

Over the past 10 years more anticonvulsant medications have emerged than in the previous 30. Of all the medication now available, topiramate remains one of the most potent. Animal model studies have suggested the drug to have a broad spectrum of action,

corroborated in clinical practice by randomized controlled clinical trials and subsequent open-label studies.

Topiramate, 2,3:4,5-*bis-O*-(1-methylethylidene)-α-D-fructo-pyranose sulphamate is a sulphamate substituted monosaccharide,

Table 45.1 Proposed mechanisms of action of topiramate

Site	Action
Voltage-activated Na$^+$ channels	Limits sustained repetitive firing via state-dependent blockade of Na$^+$ channels
GABA-A receptor	Potentiates GABA-mediated neuroinhibition at GABA-A site not modulated by benzodiazepines or barbiturates
Glutamate receptor subtype (kainate/AMPA)	Blocks glutamate-mediated neuroexcitation with no apparent effect on NMDA receptor activity
Ca^{2+} channel subtypes	Mild reduction of high voltage-activated Ca^{2+} current amplitude
Carbonic anhydrase	Antagonizes type II and IV CA

derived from D fructose. Its empirical formula is $Cl_2H_{21}NO_8S$ and its molecular weight 339.36. Neurochemical and neurophysiological studies as well as findings in predictive animal models of epilepsy have suggested that it may have up to five different modes of action which may account for why it has a relatively broad spectrum of activity (Table 45.1). The relative contribution of each mechanism determined is not known, and may of course differ in individuals and types of epilepsy.

Mechanisms of action and experimental studies

In cultured rat pyramidal neurones and slices, which displayed spontaneous epileptiform discharges, topiramate dose-dependently reduced the duration and frequency of action potentials associated with repetitive firing [1,2]. These actions are consistent with an effect of topiramate involving modulation of sodium and/or calcium channel conductance. Topiramate was subsequently shown to reduce subicular cell excitability in a dose-dependent manner and depress their bursting ability and repetitive firing properties [3]. Whole cell patch recordings of cerebellar granule cells [4], slice preparations of entorhinal cortex [2] and whole cell patch-clamp recordings in dissociated neocortical neurones and intracellular recordings in neocortical sites [5] further support an effect of topiramate on voltage-gated sodium conductance. Recent studies with cultured mouse spinal neurones have extended this [6]. In this model topiramate caused a voltage-sensitive limitation of spontaneous repetitive firing. However, even at high concentrations this effect of topiramate was not as rapid and complete as that of phenytoin and lamotrigine suggesting that sodium channel blockade may not be the primary mechanism of the anticonvulsant action of topiramate.

A separate potential mechanism is enhancement of γ-aminobutyric acid (GABA) activity at some types of receptors. Topiramate potentiates GABA-evoked opening of chloride channels in mouse cortical neurones not blocked by flumazenil (and therefore independent of benzodiazepines), enhances the rate of GABA-mediated chloride flux into chloride-depleted cerebellar granule cells and potentiates GABA-evoked chloride currents in cortical neurones in a rapid and reversible manner [7,8]. It has also been shown to block the kainate-elicited excitatory response in studies of cultured rat

hippocampal pyramidal neurones, possibly by exerting an effect at the aminohydroxymethylisozole propionic acid (AMPA) glutamate receptor subtype site. It had no effect on the N-methyl-D-aspartate (NMDA) receptors [1,9]. In spontaneously epileptic rats, topiramate reduced the abnormally high levels of glutamate and aspartate by about 45%, the decrease corresponding with a decrease in tonic seizures [10,11]. Further evidence arises from the effect of the drug on the excitability of CA3 neurones of spontaneously epileptic rats that topiramate inhibits the release of glutamate and therefore inhibition of excitatory neurotransmission may contribute to the mechanism of action of the drug. Topiramate has also been shown selectively to inhibit L-type high-voltage activated calcium channels in whole cell patch clamp recordings from dentate granule cells of rats [12].

Topiramate structurally resembles acetazolamide, and similarly inhibits carbonic anhydrase. However, this is not thought to be a major contributor to the action of the drug as it only weakly inhibits the enzyme compared to acetazolamide, which is 10–100 times more potent. The inhibitory effect has been shown to be selective, affecting mostly two of the six carbonic anhydrase isoenzymes (CAII and CAIV) [13]. This action may however be responsible for some of the side-effects of the medication (for example, the increased incidence of renal stones and paraesthesia).

Topiramate exerts a relatively broad spectrum of activity in animal seizure models. This includes the maximal electroshock (MES) test in mice and rats, the genetically seizure-prone DBA/2 mouse and the spontaneously epileptic rat and the amygdala kindled rat. Topiramate blocked tonic-clonic seizures in the DBA/2 mouse, and such seizures and absence seizures in the spontaneously epileptic rat. However, it is virtually ineffective in preventing pentylenetetrazol-induced seizures or seizures induced by bicuculline or picrotoxin [14,15], although it has been shown to elevate seizure threshold using the pentylenetetrazol threshold test. The drug is also ineffective in the genetic lethargic (lh/lh) mouse model, known to be predictive of efficacy against absence seizures in humans [16].

Pharmacokinetics

Topiramate is rapidly and well absorbed with peak plasma concentrations occurring approximately 2–4 h after administration [17] with oral bioavailability of at least 81% [18]. Although ingestion with food delays topiramate absorption by about 2 h, there is no alteration to the extent of absorption with no effect on the maximal plasma concentrations for a given dose [19,20]. This is independent of whether the sprinkle or tablet formulation is used [21]; topiramate can therefore be given without regard to mealtimes. Topiramate has a long elimination half-life of 19–25 h [20]. It distributes into all tissues including the brain. At a steady state achieved after multiple dose administration the elimination of topiramate was indistinguishable from that observed in single dose administration in healthy volunteers [22]. Plasma protein binding is minimal (13–17%) [23] and it is minimally metabolized. Serum concentrations are linear and dose related and there is not much intersubject variability. The trace metabolites that have been identified have little or no anticonvulsant activity and are not thought to have significant clinical activity.

Topiramate is excreted primarily unchanged through the kidneys, probably through tubular reabsorption. Approximately 40%

of a single 100-mg dose of [^{14}C]topiramate administered to six healthy volunteers was excreted unchanged over a 48-h period with 80% radioactivity recovered in the urine [24].

Overall, in most patients, topiramate has no significant effects on plasma concentrations of concomitant antiepileptic drugs. Topiramate in theory may inhibit phenytoin metabolism; it inhibits cytochrome P450 isoenzyme CYP2C19. This isoenzyme is responsible for only 20% of phenytoin metabolism so one would expect only a slight effect. However, although in a study of 12 patients, six had no change in phenytoin level, in six this was increased by a mean 25%. They were increased primarily in patients receiving twice daily administration [25]. The phenytoin metabolism may have been nearer saturation in these patients, so the small change in inhibition may have been sufficient to lead to the increase in plasma concentration, and in some be clinically significant. No change from baseline has been seen in the steady-state plasma concentrations of carbamazepine or the metabolite carbamazepine-10,11-epoxide from monotherapy suggesting there is no effect of topiramate on their metabolism [26]. When topiramate has been added to sodium valproate, an increase in clearance of valproate was noted with a small but significant decrease in plasma concentration. However, these changes do not appear to be clinically significant [27]. In addition, topiramate may displace valproate from its plasma binding sites, but again the clinical significance of this is uncertain. In children with partial onset seizures, changes in lamotrigine levels were significantly different in the topiramate and placebo groups ($P = 0.017$) with a 20% increase in the placebo group and a 10% decrease in the topiramate group [28]. Possible synergistic action has been reported in animals and humans between lamotrigine and topiramate [29].

Hepatic enzyme-inducing antiepileptic drugs such as phenytoin, phenobarbital and carbamazepine induce the metabolism of topiramate. Concomitant carbamazepine therapy lowered the topiramate concentration by 40% when compared to topiramate monotherapy [26]. Topiramate may compromise the effectiveness of certain oral contraceptives, and this appears to be related to the oestrogenic component [30]. It has also been suggested that digoxin clearance may be increased although the clinical significance of this is uncertain [31]

Children

In children renal clearance between the ages of 4 and 7 years has been found to be 40% higher than children over 8 years; for the entire group of children 4–17 years old the average topiramate clearance has been found to be twice that of those taking enzyme-inducing antiepileptic drugs with a correspondingly shorter half-life [32]. When compared with adults, the topiramate clearance in this group of children was 50% higher both among enzyme-induced and non-induced individuals. The elimination half-lives are correspondingly reduced. The effect of concomitant therapy with enzyme inducers is the same in children as in adults, with topiramate clearance being increased and its half-life reduced (from 15.4 h without enzyme inducers to 7.5 h with). In infants topiramate half-life is shorter and clearance values higher than in older children, the latter more than two times that in adults, suggesting that for the steady-state level the topiramate dose in milligrams per kilogram per day would be two times that for infants than in adults

[33]. Concurrent treatment with enzyme inducers increased clearance by 50–100% reducing half-life to 6.4 h.

Elderly

No change in clearance or elimination half-life of topiramate has been seen amongst adults up to 67 years of age [34]. However, normal ageing may be associated with a decline in renal function and this may need to be taken into consideration as this may affect drug clearance as outlined below.

Impaired renal function

Topiramate clearance is reduced in patients with impaired renal function. This has been studied by giving a single 100-mg dose to patients with moderate creatinine clearance (CL_{cr} 30–69 mL/min) or severe ($CL_{cr} < 30$ mL/min) renal impairment and matched volunteers with normal renal function ($CL_{cr} < 70$ mL/min) [35]. Topiramate clearance was reduced 42% in patients with moderate renal impairment and 54% in patients with severe renal impairment. As a consequence, topiramate doses should be reduced in such patients. Concentrations are however significantly affected by haemodialysis. The mean haemodialysis plasma clearance of topiramate in patients with end-stage renal disease is 4–6 times higher than that for an individual with normal renal function [25]. This can remove a significant amount of drug from the system and therefore a supplemental dose may be required in patients undergoing haemodialysis.

Impaired hepatic function

Compared with healthy matched controls, mean oral plasma clearance decreased by 26% and topiramate plasma concentrations were increased by 29% in five patients with moderate to severe liver impairment [36]. These changes were not considered clinically significant.

Clinical efficacy

Topiramate has been evaluated in placebo-controlled trials as adjunctive therapy in adults and children with refractory partial onset seizures, primary generalized tonic-clonic seizures and Lennox–Gastaut syndrome. Three randomized controlled trials have been conducted with topiramate as monotherapy in newly and recently diagnosed epilepsy, including a trial comparing topiramate with valproate and carbamazepine. A number of prospective, inpractice open-label studies have further characterized the broad-spectrum profile of topiramate and its effectiveness during long-term treatment.

Randomized controlled trials

Topiramate as adjunctive therapy in refractory epilepsy

The design of the topiramate adjunctive therapy trials included a prospective baseline phase and a double-blind, parallel-arm treatment phase. During the baseline phase, seizure frequency data were collected while patients received stabilized dosages of at least one

AED (usually an enzyme-inducing AED). Following randomization to add-on therapy with topiramate or placebo, the study drug was titrated to preassigned target dosages, which were then maintained until completion of double-blind treatment; dosages of concomitant AEDs remained fixed. The primary efficacy analysis in most studies was median per cent reduction from baseline in average monthly (28-day) seizure frequency. Secondary analyses included proportion of patients who were treatment responders with ≥ 50%, ≥75% and 100% seizure reduction, as well as global evaluation by investigators and parents/guardians in the case of children and patients with Lennox–Gastaut syndrome. Analyses were reported for intent-to-treat populations, with the last observation carried forward.

Double-blind placebo-controlled trials in adults with refractory partial onset seizures

The initial double-blind, placebo-controlled trials in adults with refractory partial onset seizures included two dose-ranging trials (200, 400 and 600 mg/day; and 600, 800 and 1000 mg/day) [37,38] and four single-dose trials (400, 600, 800 and 1000 mg/day) [39–42]. Data from animal and human volunteer studies had suggested that a dosage of 600–800 mg/day topiramate would provide a clear therapeutic effect. Consequently, most patients (79%, n = 395) in the early Phase II studies were randomized to 600–1000 mg/day topiramate; only 9% (n=45) of patients were randomized to 200 mg/day; and 13% (n=68) to 400 mg/day topiramate.

The similarity of study design and patient populations among the six trials allowed data to be pooled [43]. Among 527 patients randomized to topiramate and 216 patients randomized to placebo, the median baseline seizure frequency was three seizures/week, and the median duration of epilepsy was 22 years. There was a rapid dose escalation schedule used in the initial trials (starting dose 100 mg/day topiramate, increased weekly in 100–200 mg/day increments), and although 98% and 92% of patients achieved the 200 and 400 mg/day target doses, respectively, only 57% of patients were able to reach 1000 mg/day.

A pooled analysis showed that median per cent reduction in topiramate-treated patients was 44% compared with 2% in placebo-treated patients (P≤0.001). Overall, more topiramate-treated patients achieved ≥ 50% (43% vs. 12%, P≤0.001), ≥75% (21% vs. 3%, P≤0.001) and 100% (5% vs. 0%, P<0.001) seizure reduction. Topiramate was similarly effective against simple partial, complex partial and secondarily generalized tonic-clonic seizures. The therapeutic effect of topiramate was consistent regardless of age, gender, baseline seizure rate or concomitant AED therapy.

Seizure reduction was greater in topiramate-treated patients at each dosage studied. The difference in median per cent seizure reduction between topiramate and placebo achieved statistical significance at dosages ≥ 400 mg/day. The difference at 200 mg/day was not statistically significant but sample size was small. Population response seemed to plateau at ≥ 600 mg/day, which suggested that these early studies evaluated the upper end of the therapeutic dose range. As a conclusion to this study, suggested optimal dose ranges were put forward as 400–600 mg. On review of the graph (Fig. 45.1) it could be concluded that the curve seen was the upper end of

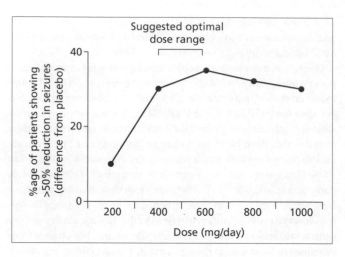

Fig. 45.1 Results of two dose ranging placebo-controlled double-blind studies of topiramate, suggesting maximal efficacy at 400–600 mg/day, from which the conclusion was made that this should be the target dose range.

the dose–response curve expected and a lower optimal dose range should be considered.

Subsequent double-blind, placebo-controlled studies explored what initially appear to be the lower limits of the dosing range, i.e. 200 and 300 mg/day, in adults with refractory partial onset seizures [44,45]. In a study of 300 mg/day topiramate [44], patients were titrated to the target dose over 6 weeks, which was maintained for an additional 8 weeks. Overall, 48% of patients receiving 300 mg/day topiramate (n=23) achieved ≥ 50% seizure reduction compared to 13% of placebo-treated patients (n=23; P = 0.01). Topiramate-treated patients also had significantly better investigator (P=0.014) and patient (P=0.0005) global evaluation scores (using a non-standardized questionnaire) than patients in the placebo group. Two patients (9%) in each treatment group discontinued treatment due to adverse events. In a study using 200 mg/day [45], patients receiving stabilized dosages of carbamazepine were randomized to placebo (n=92), to 200 mg/day topiramate escalated in 4 weeks (50 mg starting dose increased 50 mg weekly; n=86), or to 200 mg/day topiramate escalated in 8 weeks (25 mg starting dose, increased 25 mg weekly; n=85). After 12 weeks treatment, median per cent reduction was 44% in topiramate-treated patients vs. 20% with placebo (P≤0.05). The proportion of topiramate-treated patients who achieved ≥ 50% seizure reduction was 45% compared with 24% in placebo-treated patients (P=0.001). Notably, after 2 weeks' treatment at a topiramate dose of 100 mg/day, median per cent seizure reduction was 60% vs. 17% with placebo (P<0.001); 48% of topiramate-treated patients compared with 30% in the placebo group had ≥ 50% seizure reduction (P=0.01). Discontinuations due to adverse events occurred in 8% of topiramate-treated patients and 2% of patients receiving placebo. Thus, topiramate dosages of 100–200 mg/day appear to be appropriate target dosages to initially evaluate therapeutic response in adults receiving enzyme-inducing AEDs. Topiramate plasma concentrations are reduced about 50% by enzyme induction [46], and therefore lower topiramate dosages (e.g. 70–130 mg/day) may be appropriate initial target dosages in the absence of enzyme induction.

Double-blind placebo-controlled trial in children with refractory partial onset seizures

Once apparent efficacy in adults with partial onset seizures was established, topiramate was evaluated in children with partial onset seizures during a 16-week randomized, double-blind, placebo-controlled trial [28] and long-term, open-label extension phase [47]. During an 8-week baseline period, children (1–16 years of age) had to have at least six partial onset seizures, with or without secondary generalization, while being treated with one or two standard AEDs at optimal dosages. Children were then randomized to placebo or topiramate, which was titrated over 8 weeks to a maximum of 400 mg/day (mean, 6 mg/kg/day), and maintained an additional 8 weeks. As outlined above, topiramate clearance is higher in children than in adults so the 400 mg/day dose was equivalent to an adult dose of approximately 270 mg/day.

Median per cent seizure reduction was 33% in topiramate-treated compared with 11% in placebo-treated children ($P=0.03$) [28]. The proportion of topiramate-treated children achieving ≥ 50% seizure reduction was higher than in the placebo group (39% vs. 20%, $P = 0.08$). With a baseline seizure rate of 20 seizures/month, 5% of children receiving topiramate were seizure free during the 16-week study; no placebo-treated children were seizure free. No children discontinued topiramate treatment because of adverse events.

Double-blind placebo-controlled trials in adults and children with primary generalized tonic-clonic seizures

Topiramate was evaluated in a double-blind, placebo-controlled trial in which patient enrollment was limited to patients with primary generalized tonic-clonic seizures (PGTCS), with or without other generalized seizure types. Two 20-week trials with identical protocols and similar patient populations were conducted in patients ≥ 4 years of age [48,49]. Patients had to have at least three PGTCS a month during an 8-week baseline and an EEG consistent with a diagnosis of generalized epilepsy. Patients with Lennox–Gastaut syndrome or partial onset seizures were excluded.

Topiramate was introduced more gradually than in the earlier trials in adults with refractory partial onset seizures. In this study, 50 mg/day topiramate was maintained for 4 weeks, then increased over 8 weeks to weight-based target dosages of 5–9 mg/kg/day (maximum, ~400 mg/day in adults). Stabilized dosages were maintained for an additional 12 weeks.

For the primary endpoint (median per cent reduction in PGTCS), the difference between treatment groups was statistically significant ($P=0.02$) in favour of topiramate in one trial [48]; the treatment difference did not reach statistical significance in the second trial [49]. When data from both studies were pooled [50], median per cent reduction in PGTCS was 57% in topiramate-treated patients and 27% in the placebo group ($P=0.003$). More than half (55%) of topiramate-treated patients had ≥ 50% seizure reduction compared to 28% in the placebo group ($P=0.001$). Topiramate was equally effective in children (≤ 16 years of age) and adults (> 16 years of age). Adverse events led to discontinuation of therapy in 10% of topiramate-treated patients and 8% in the placebo group.

Juvenile myoclonic epilepsy (JME) was the most frequently reported generalized epilepsy syndrome ($n=22$) in these trials [51]. In addition to reducing the frequency of PGTCS in the subset of patients with JME, topiramate had a greater effect on myoclonus-free weeks than placebo (topiramate, 171% reduction; placebo, 130% reduction). The number of absence-free weeks in topiramate-treated patients increased 15% while the number of absence-free weeks decreased 7% in the placebo group. Clinical experience also supports the effectiveness of topiramate in patients with JME, including reports of seizure freedom and monotherapy use [29,52–55].

Double-blind placebo-controlled trial in Lennox–Gastaut syndrome

Patients with Lennox–Gastaut syndrome experience multiple seizure types that are difficult to control. Given its broad spectrum of anticonvulsant activity, topiramate was evaluated in an 11-week double-blind, placebo-controlled trial [56], which was followed by a long-term, open-label extension [57]. Patients (1–30 years of age) receiving at least one standard AED had to have a confirmed EEG showing a slow spike-and-wave pattern with multiple seizure types including drop attacks (i.e. tonic or atonic seizures) and a history of atypical absence (≥ 60 seizures in the month preceding baseline). Following randomization, topiramate was started at 1 mg/kg/day and increased at weekly intervals to 3 mg/kg/day and then 6 mg/kg/day. Stabilized dosages were maintained for an additional 8 weeks.

In patients receiving topiramate ($n=46$), the median per cent reduction in drop attacks was 15% compared to a 5% increase in drop attacks in patients receiving placebo ($n=49$; $P=0.04$). The median per cent reduction in major motor seizures (drop attacks and tonic-clonic seizures combined) was 26% with topiramate treatment compared to a 5% increase in major motor seizures with placebo ($P<0.02$). The proportion of patients achieving ≥ 50% reduction in drop attacks was higher in the topiramate group than in placebo-treated patients (28% vs. 14%, $P = 0.07$). With 33% of topiramate-treated patients and 8% of placebo-treated patients achieving ≥ 50% reduction in major motor seizures ($P=0.002$), the effectiveness of topiramate against major motor seizures was comparable to that reported with lamotrigine [58].

Topiramate as monotherapy in newly and recently diagnosed epilepsy

Topiramate was evaluated as monotherapy in three double-blind dose-comparison studies to document its efficacy as monotherapy, two of which were in newly/recently diagnosed epilepsy [59–61]. Topiramate has also been compared with traditional first-line agents in a randomized double-blind trial to evaluate its relative role as single-agent therapy in newly diagnosed epilepsy [62].

A conversion-to-monotherapy trial in adults with refractory partial onset seizures receiving one or more traditional AEDs served as a 'proof of principle' study [59]. Patients were randomized to one of two topiramate dosages, 100 mg/day ($n=24$) or 1000 mg/day ($n=24$) topiramate. The baseline AED was gradually withdrawn as the topiramate dose was increased. With the higher topiramate dose, fewer patients exited the study due to seizure-related exit criteria (P

=0.002). In some patients converted to topiramate monotherapy, seizure control actually improved.

A subsequent dose–comparison study evaluated the effectiveness of topiramate as initial/early therapy in patients with less severe epilepsy [60]. In this study, 252 patients (≥3 years of age) with an epilepsy diagnosis within 3 years before study entry and one to six partial onset seizures during a 3-month retrospective baseline were randomized to double-blind treatment with 50 mg/day (n = 125) or 500 mg/day (n = 127). Patients weighing ≤ 50 kg were randomized to 25 or 200 mg/day, respectively. The primary efficacy analysis was time-to-exit, which was time-to-second seizure in 98% of patients. Although time-to-exit was longer in the 200/500 mg/day group (422 days vs. 293 days with 25/50 mg/day topiramate), the difference was not statistically significant. However, a *post-hoc* analysis of time-to-exit using time-to-first seizure as a dependent variable did show a statistically significant difference (P = 0.01) between treatment groups in favour of patients receiving 200/500 mg/day topiramate. Moreover, during double-blind treatment, 54% of patients receiving 200/500 mg/day topiramate were seizure free compared with 39% of patients receiving 25/50 mg/day topiramate (P = 0.02). Treatment differences favoured the higher dose group in two other seizure-related outcome variables (time-to-first seizure and treatment effect vs. plasma concentration). However it is notable that efficacy was seen in the lower dose group.

In a double-blind study limited to patients with newly diagnosed epilepsy (i.e. diagnosis within 3 months of study entry; partial onset and/or PGTCS at baseline), a strongly significant dose–response effect was observed with topiramate monotherapy [61]. In this study, the difference in time-to-first seizure was statistically significant (P = 0.0002) in favour of 400 mg/day topiramate (n = 236) vs. 50 mg/day (n = 234) topiramate. Statistically significant differences in favour of 400 mg/day were also observed in 6-month (83% vs. 71% with 50 mg/day, P = 0.005) and 1-year (76% vs. 59% with 50 mg/day, P = 0.001) seizure-free rates. During double-blind treatment, 6% of patients receiving 50 mg/day and 17% of patients receiving 400 mg/day discontinued therapy due to adverse events. The seizure-free rates with 400 mg/day topiramate exceed those reported with other AEDs (6 months, 35–48% [63,64]; 1-year, 54–61% [65–67]) during double-blind trials in patients with newly diagnosed epilepsy.

A randomized controlled trial was designed to evaluate initial target dosages in patients with newly diagnosed epilepsy. Topiramate monotherapy (100 and 200 mg/day) was compared with carbamazepine (600 mg/day) and valproate (1250 mg/day). Results from this study showed that topiramate was as effective as carbamazepine and valproate in a broad spectrum of patients with newly diagnosed epilepsy. The 6-month seizure-free rate with 100 mg/day topiramate was 49%; with 200 mg/day topiramate, carbamazepine and valproate, the 6-month seizure-free rate was 44% in each group. With treatment duration up to 2 years, discontinuation rates due to adverse events for 100 mg/day topiramate, 200 mg/day topiramate, carbamazepine, and valproate were 19%, 28%, 25% and 23%, respectively. Although 100 mg/day and 200 mg/day dosages of topiramate were similarly effective, 100 mg/day was better tolerated, with fewer discontinuations due to adverse effects [62].

Based on this series of monotherapy studies in newly/recently diagnosed epilepsy, 50 mg/day topiramate provides a modest degree of seizure control with 100 mg/day being the recommended initial target dose. The topiramate dose can be individualized as needed to provide effective seizure control, with 400–500 mg/day shown to be safe and effective.

Open-label experience

Adults with partial onset or generalized seizures

Controlled clinical studies are generally of short duration and can give relatively limited data on longer-term efficacy. In addition, they give little information on the optimal use of a drug, in particular target and maintenance doses. Prospective open-label studies in which dosages are adjusted according to clinical need can provide valuable information regarding long-term clinical performance, tolerability and safety.

Patients with generalized epilepsy who completed double-blind treatment in the placebo-controlled trials could enter a long-term, open-label extension phase during which dosages of topiramate and concomitant AEDs could be individually adjusted. During long-term treatment, 16% of patients (n = 96) receiving topiramate ≥ 6 months had no GTCS for at least 6 months (mean topiramate dose, 500 mg/day or 7 mg/kg/day for children). In patients treated up to 2.5 years (n = 131), 5% discontinued due to inadequate seizure control and 8% discontinued due to adverse events [56].

Among patients who entered the long-term, open-label extension of the Lennox–Gastaut study [68] during which dosages of topiramate and concomitant AEDs could be adjusted according to patient response, drop attacks were reduced ≥ 50% in 55% of patients receiving topiramate (mean dose, 10 mg/kg/day) for at least 6 months (n = 82). Despite having an average of 90 drop attacks per day, 15% of patients had no drop attacks for at least 6 months. Substantial reductions were also observed in atypical absence, myoclonic, and tonic-clonic seizures. During treatment up to 3.4 years (n = 97), 12% of patients discontinued treatment due to inadequate seizure control and 10% discontinued due to adverse events.

From the controlled trial of the use of topiramate in children with partial onset seizures, 83 continued and doses adjusted according to clinical response (mean 9 mg/kg/day). A total of 14% had been seizure free for at least 6 months since the last visit; seizure frequency over the last 3 months of therapy was reduced in 57% of children. During treatment periods up to 2.5 years 6% of children discontinued treatment in view of adverse events and 13% because of inadequate seizure control [47].

To supplement information from initial randomized controlled trials with topiramate, a large, pragmatic trial was conducted to explore dosing needs for patients typically found in clinical practice [69]. In this 20-week, open-label, multicentre study in 901 adults with partial onset seizures, topiramate was initiated at 50 mg/day with weekly dosage increases of 25–50 mg/day according to patient response. With a mean topiramate dosage of 323 mg/day, median seizure reduction was 73%, with 68% of patients achieving ≥ 50% seizure reduction. In patients with less than four baseline seizures per month, the mean topiramate dosage was 303 mg/day compared with 341 mg/day in patients with four or more baseline seizures per month, a difference that was statistically significant (P = 0.005). Topiramate tolerability was improved, with fewer discontinuations due to adverse effects, when dosages of concomitant AEDs were reduced.

In a prospective observational study in adults with refractory localization-related ($n=134$) or idiopathic generalized epilepsy ($n=36$), topiramate dosages substantially lower than those used in randomized controlled trials provided effective seizure control. With a mean dose of 250 mg/day, 23% of patients became seizure free. Twenty-nine of 119 patients (24%) who achieved ≥ 50 seizure reduction, including 13 of 31 patients (42%) who became seizure free, were receiving ≤ 100 mg/day topiramate [70].

Patient retention rates also provide a measure of long-term effectiveness. In a retrospective review of patients with refractory partial and/or generalized epilepsy in an adult tertiary referral centre [71,72] 1-year retention rates were 52% for topiramate ($n=393$), 46% for lamotrigine ($n=424$), and 23% for gabapentin ($n=158$); 3-year retention rates were 30%, 29% and 10%, respectively. Estimated retention rates at 5 years were 28% (topiramate), 12% (lamotrigine) and 2% (gabapentin). Perceived lack of efficacy resulted in treatment withdrawal in 19% of topiramate-treated patients compared with 39% of those receiving lamotrigine and 34% of those treated with gabapentin. Factors associated with long-term retention in topiramate-treated patients included higher maximal daily doses and younger age of epilepsy onset; patients with prior exposure to fewer than two new AEDs and those receiving no more than one concurrent AED were more likely to continue topiramate treatment [72].

A similar 1-year retention rate (55%) was reported for 174 patients receiving topiramate in a specialist regional epilepsy clinic [53]. When topiramate was substituted for another drug, the retention rate was 56% compared with 41% when topiramate was added to existing therapy ($P<0.05$). Adverse events were more frequent in add-on patients than in substitution patients, which may reflect pharmacodynamic interactions. Overall, nine (5%) patients became seizure free, including eight patients with partial epilepsy and one patient with JME.

Children with refractory epilepsy

During the long-term, open-label extension of children with refractory partial epilepsy [47], dosages of topiramate and concomitant AEDs could be adjusted according to patient response. Increasing the topiramate dose to a mean of 9 mg/kg/day (compared to 6 mg/kg/day during double-blind treatment) was associated with greater seizure control; 14% of children receiving topiramate were seizure free at least 6 months. With topiramate treatment up to 2.5 years ($n=83$), 13% of children discontinued due to inadequate seizure control and 6% due to adverse events.

West's syndrome (infantile spasms)

The effectiveness of topiramate in children with West's syndrome, characterized by infantile spasms, mental retardation and hysarrhythmia, was evaluated in a pilot study ($n=11$) [73] with a long-term follow-up [74]. Topiramate was started at 25 mg/day and then increased 25 mg every 2–3 days until spasms were controlled, the maximally tolerated topiramate dose was reached, or a maximal topiramate dose of 24 mg/kg/day was achieved. Spasm frequency was reduced from a baseline mean of 26 per day to six per day ($P<0.003$). Spasms were reduced ≥ 50% in nine patients (82%), and five patients (45%) became spasm free (EEG documentation).

Seven patients were successfully converted to topiramate monotherapy [73]. During long-term treatment, four of the five spasm-free children remained spasm free for an average of 18 months (mean topiramate dose, 29 mg/kg/day) [74].

Childhood absence epilepsy

During a pilot study, children with typical absence seizures (documented as 3 Hz spike-wave on EEG) who were untreated or taking only one AED received topiramate at a starting dose of 1 mg/kg/day titrated twice weekly in 1 mg/kg/day increments to 12 mg/kg/day or maximally tolerated dose. Among five children (6–11.5 years of age) completing the 6-week study, one previously untreated child became seizure free (5 mg/kg/day) with no residual spike-wave activity. In two children, absence seizures were reduced early but then increased with higher topiramate dosages. With topiramate dose reduction to 6 mg/kg/day, seizure control improved (one seizure free; one with > 50% seizure reduction) with substantial reduction in spike-wave activity over a 24-h period. Seizure counts and EEG were not improved in two patients [75].

Other patient populations with seizures

Clinical reports suggest that topiramate is effective in other seizure disorders, including tuberous sclerosis ($n=14$) [76], and patients with learning difficulties [77,78]. Among 64 patients with refractory epilepsy who were learning disabled, 70% achieved ≥ 50% seizure reduction with topiramate adjunctive therapy. Sixteen (25%) patients became seizure free, including 10 patients who were receiving topiramate doses ≤ 200 mg/day [77]. In 20 patients with intractable epilepsy (mixed seizures), mental retardation and developmental disabilities who were treated with topiramate adjunctive therapy, 69% of patients had ≥ 50% seizure reduction and two patients (13%) were seizure free [78].

The use of topiramate has also been reported in children with severe myoclonic epilepsy of infancy [79]. This is a syndrome first described by Dravet, where children initially present with prolonged, often lateralized seizures, and later in the second year go on to develop myoclonus and developmental arrest. It can be very resistant to treatment. Nineto-Barrera *et al.* [79] report 18 children with this diagnosis who had been treated with a mean of 6.7 drugs at the time of study. Topiramate was added to current therapy, at a starting dose of 1 mg/kg/day and titrated to a maximum 6–8 mg/kg/day, with a mean observation time of 10.5 months (6–18 months). At the end of the study 72% of patients had reached a > 50% reduction in seizure rate, 50% >75% reduction and 16.6% were seizure free.

Five children with Angelman's syndrome have also been reported to show a good response. After a mean 8.8 months on the medication four children were on monotherapy with topiramate, two of whom were seizure free, and one had discontinued the drug [80]. The mean dosage was 12 mg/kg/day. Studies have also shown that topiramate is effective in patients with neuropsychiatric disorders that can occur in patients with epilepsy [81–85].

Adverse events

Obviously the efficacy of any anticonvulsant drug has to be balanced with the possible adverse event profile. Early evidence of side-

Table 45.2 Percentage of patients in placebo-controlled trials experiencing side-effects

| | Percentage of patients in each target mg/kg dosage group | | | | | |
Adverse event	Placebo (n=174)	200 (n=45)	400 (n=68)	600 (n=124)	800 (n=76)	1000 (n=47)
Ataxia	7	20	22	17	16	21
Concentration impaired	1	11	9	12	15	21
Confusion	5	9	15	18	14	28
Dizziness	13	36	22	31	32	40
Fatigue	16	13	18	31	49	32
Somnolence	10	27	26	17	20	28
Abnormal thinking	2	20	12	29	28	26
Anorexia	3	4	4	8	9	21
Paraesthesia	3	18	20	13	18	13

Adapted from [86].

effects has to be gleaned from randomized controlled trials, although these may be misleading. The medication is introduced over a predefined period of time, and to a set target dose. No data is available from these trials on events seen long term. In addition, such trials are performed on small selected populations. Open-label extensions and observational studies therefore contribute further information on the side-effect profile as they do with efficacy.

Data from the five early randomized controlled trials suggested central nervous system (CNS) effects to be the most troublesome. In these trials six patients (3%) receiving placebo and 51 patients (14%) receiving topiramate withdrew prematurely because of an adverse event. The most common reasons were CNS-related events, and such events increased in occurrence as the dose of topiramate increased [86](Table 45.2). Most were classified as mild to moderate in severity. On further examination of trial data, it has become apparent that such adverse events are also more commonly seen with a faster rate of titration, and concomitant use of other AEDs. In all these studies, topiramate was used as add-on therapy; titration was over a 4–6-week period with an 8–12 week stabilization period. Of the discontinuations from the trial 70% were due to adverse events during the titration period. These effects appeared far more prevalent in the early trials where higher doses were titrated over a relatively shorter period of time, and those more recently where a faster rate of titration were seen (e.g. Lennox–Gastaut 3 weeks vs. generalized seizures 6 weeks, Table 45.3) as well as in add-on trials compared to the monotherapy trials (Table 45.4). A multicentre randomized parallel double-blind trial evaluated two rates at which topiramate was titrated to a maximum dosage of 400 mg/day, with increments either by 50 mg or 100 mg/day. The 50-mg titration was better tolerated, with 11% discontinuing or interrupting treatment compared to 22% in the 100/200 group [87]. Other side-effects reaching greater than 10% incidence in trials included anorexia, weight loss and paraesthesia.

Cognitive effects

In view of the concern expressed about cognitive effects of topiramate, investigators have attempted to evaluate such effects in more detail. Martin et al. set out to evaluate the acute and steady-state

Table 45.3 Side-effect profile of topiramate in generalized tonic-clonic seizure placebo-controlled trial and the Lennox–Gastaut trial (%)

| | GTCS[a] | | LGS[b] | |
	Placebo	TPM	Placebo	TPM
Somnolence	16	24	22	42
Anorexia	6	16	20	40
Nervousness	1	15	10	21
Fatigue	12	19	4	19
Weight loss	4	14	0	10

[a]Titration over 6 weeks.
[b]Titration over 3 weeks.

Table 45.4 Side-effect profile of topiramate in children in add-on and monotherapy trials (%)

| | Add-on | | |
Adverse event	Placebo + AEDs (n=101)	TPM + AEDs (n=98)	Monotherapy[a] (n=114)
Somnolence	16	26	10
Anorexia	15	24	13
Fatigue	5	16	19
Nervousness	7	14	4
Concentration/ attention difficulty	2	10	8
Aggressiveness	4	9	4
Weight loss	1	9	5
Memory difficulty	0	5	5

Events with ≥ 5% difference in incidence vs. placebo: 6 mg/kg/day topiramate.
[a]25–500 mg/day topiramate.

cognitive effects of three anticonvulsant drugs, gabapentin, topiramate and lamotrigine [88]. Seventeen healthy young adults were evaluated; six received topiramate, five lamotrigine and six gabapentin as a single oral dose. Three hours after this single dose the individuals underwent a series of neuropsychological tests. They then received no further anticonvulsant medication for 72 h. After this period, if well and free of side-effects, a regular dose of the relevant anticonvulsant medication was initiated (topiramate 25 mg/day, lamotrigine 50 mg/day or gabapentin 300 mg/day) and titrated to a therapeutic dose (topiramate 5.7 mg/kg/day, lamotrigine 7.1 mg/kg and gabapentin 35 mg/kg) by day 30. For each of the groups, the neurobehavioural performances were compared at baseline, week 2 and week 4. The verbal fluency rate of the topiramate group dropped an average of 50% per subject compared with a negligible change for the other two groups, and a three-fold error occurred for the visual attention task. The other two AED groups had no performance changes. At the 2- and 4-week test periods only the topiramate subjects continued to display neurocognitive effects from drug administration. Although marked changes were seen, this study reflects changes at a very rapid rate of dose escalation and subjects were tested before individuals could have become habituated to the effects of topiramate therapy [89]. Aldenkamp et al. [90] have subsequently reported on a study comparing the cognitive effects of topiramate compared to those of valproate. This was a multicentre randomized, observer-blinded, parallel group clinical trial with sodium valproate or topiramate given as first-line add-on therapy to steady-state treatment with carbamazepine, with medication increased in stages to 200–400 mg/day for topiramate (with weekly increments of 25 mg) and 1800 mg/day for valproate. The study evaluated changes in cognitive function from baseline (performed up to 2 weeks before start of medication) to endpoint (after 20 weeks treatment) and during titration (after 8 weeks of treatment). Of 10 baseline to endpoint comparisons, one test measuring short-term verbal memory (the Rey Auditory Verbal Learning Test) yielded a statistically significant difference between the treatments with worsening for topiramate and improvement for valproate. The 10 baseline to titration comparisons showed a similar difference. None of the mood tests or tests for subjective complaints showed statistically significant differences between the treatments, although more were in the negative direction for topiramate during titration.

These results suggest that the cognitive effects seen with topiramate may be related to rapid dose escalation, particularly with titration to higher doses. However, the studies also illustrate that physicians need to be vigilant in monitoring for cognitive effects, especially during titration. In a further study, Thompson et al. compared neuropsychological test scores of 18 patients obtained before and after the introduction of topiramate (median dose 300 mg) with changes in test performance of 18 patients who had undergone repeat neuropsychological assessments at the same time intervals [91]. The results showed an overall decline in performance on testing after a period of topiramate treatment and when compared to those not treated. The most significant differences in change of score between the groups were recorded for word fluency, list learning and verbal IQ ($P < 0.001$) with the topiramate group showing a decline in performance and comparison group an improvement from the first to the second session. Patients who underwent topiramate withdrawal or reduction all produced better scores after the drug change on all tests administered. The median dose was relatively high which may account for some differences compared to some of the trials. However as these are retrospective studies they are likely to be subject in part to selection bias.

In most individuals it appears that such side-effects can be avoided by a slow cautious introduction of the medication whilst minimizing polytherapy. However, there appears to be a small proportion of patients who are extremely sensitive to this medication and are unable to tolerate topiramate regardless how cautious the introduction. Further work is required to evaluate risk factors for this.

Weight loss

In early trials weight reductions appeared to be dose related, with mean decreases ranging from 1.1 kg in patients receiving 200 mg/day to 5.9 kg in patients receiving ≥ 800 mg/day [86]. These decreases tended to plateau during long-term therapy. Weight loss also appears to be greatest in heavier patients; 8% weight loss was seen in topiramate patients who had baseline weight of more than 100 kg compared to 3% in those who initially weighed less than 60 kg [92]. Anorexia appeared to be a common complaint amongst patients taking topiramate in clinical trials but rarely led to discontinuation.

Other effects

The paraesthesia is almost certainly related to carbonic anhydrase inhibition and the extent dose related. In addition renal calculi are estimated to occur in 1–2% of patients taking topiramate. Stone formation is believed to be related to an increase in urinary pH and reduced excretion of citrate associated with the drugs' carbonic anhydrase inhibiting activity [93]. Stones are passed spontaneously in two-thirds of those effected and in one study most patients elected to continue topiramate despite their occurrence [94]. These adverse events were seldom therapy limiting. Fulminant hepatic failure has been reported in one case thought to be linked to topiramate therapy; a 39-year-old woman with complex partial seizures on polytherapy with carbamazepine as well as paracetamol developed fulminant hepatic failure requiring transplant after reaching 300 mg/day [95]. Rare cases of hyperammonaemia in patients on combination therapy with valproate and topiramate have been reported [96,97]. Cases are emerging of acute myopia associated with increased intraocular pressure, presenting with an acute red eye (or eyes) that resolves with discontinuation of treatment [98]. There have been no reports of haematological toxicity with topiramate.

Pregnancy

Topiramate has been found to be teratogenic in animals but its possible effects on the human fetus is unknown. With the advent of pregnancy registers, data are accumulating with regard to safety in monotherapy but relative or exact risk is unknown. There have been some reports of hypospadias but in these cases topiramate has been used in combination with carbamazepine and/or lamotrigine.

Children

Adverse events seen in trials in children have been similar to those seen in the adults with CNS effects and weight loss being the most notable. Paraesthesia appear to be less prevalent but of course may be underreported. It has been considered to be the cause of agitation in some learning disabled children. Cognitive slowing and weight loss have been two key side-effects about which concern has been demonstrated; cognitive slowing in view of any possible subtlety as well as the confounding factors of an underlying encephalopathy, as well as weight loss in view of the possible influence on growth. The most common adverse events seen in children in randomized trials are seen in Table 45.4. Somnolence, anorexia, fatigue, agitation and concentration difficulties were the most common side-effects seen. Again these effects were more prevalent in the polytherapy rather than monotherapy, and with a more rapid titration of the dose.

The possible long-term implications of weight loss in children are uncertain and further studies with regard to this are planned. This is particularly difficult, as the exact mechanisms responsible for the weight loss are unclear. It does not appear to be directly related to anorexia. Further evaluation has shown the drug rarely to be discontinued as the result of weight loss and it appears unlikely to be a long-term problem. In addition, few children show > 10% weight change; in fact most stabilize and regain after a period of time. Renal stones appear to be rare in children (one in 313 reported by Shields and Wu [99]). A decrease in serum bicarbonate has been documented, particularly in children [100], although clinical acidosis is rare. This may only be of importance to susceptible individuals such as those on the ketogenic diet or the very young.

Neuroprotection

Anticonvulsants to date have only acted to *prevent* seizure occurence. None have been definitively shown either to ameliorate the disease or prevent epilepsy in those who are susceptible due to genetics, injury or other neuronal insults. In certain epilepsy syndromes in the very young, the reasons why the advent of unrelenting seizures herald developmental arrest and compromise are likely to be multifactorial, but as yet unknown. The debate about the possibility of preventing hippocampal sclerosis in susceptible individuals also continues. Many anticonvulsants have been assessed in animal models as to whether they inhibit either epileptogenesis as defined by kindling acquisition or the development of chronic epilepsy as defined by kindled seizures. A number of AEDs have also been evaluated in status epilepticus (SE) although few have been evaluated in models designed to separate antiepileptogenic effects from their ability to suppress seizures. In experimental SE, recurrent spontaneous seizures often develop weeks or months after an episode. Alterations in GABA receptors precede or coincide with the development of spontaneous seizures. This suggests that such changes may be epileptogenic and not just a response to seizures. In a rat model where SE was interrupted on discontinuation of the stimulus, topiramate was given immediately after experimentally induced SE had ended [101]. A significant reduction in hippocampal neuronal degeneration was observed, not seen with lorazepam, valproate, fosphenytoin, pentobarbitol, dextromorphan or ketamine; as electroclinical activity ceased prior to administration of topiramate this suggests this reduction to be caused by the drug and not cessation of seizure activity. However further studies are required to determine whether the prevention of neuronal injury in this model can decrease subsequent seizure susceptibility.

Few anticonvulsants have been studied for their antiepileptogenic effects in preclinical models of important and prevalent childhood syndromes. Topiramate has been tested for potential protective/preventative effects in models of febrile seizures, neonatal hypoxia and neonatal seizures. Prolonged hyperthermic seizures in immature rats do not cause spontaneous seizures but increase susceptibility to seizures later in life following a 'second hit' such as low-dose kainate. In addition they produce transient but widespread structural changes in the hippocampus and amygdala, and long-lasting molecular [102] and functional changes in hippocampal excitability [103–106]. Baram and colleagues used this model to address whether there was any evidence that topiramate prevented these proepileptogenic functional changes. Because administration of topiramate before the seizures may attenuate them, these authors initiated subchronic administration of the drug in very high doses (90 mg/kg, six times) immediately following experimental prolonged febrile seizures. Using the established alterations in hippocampal GABAergic inhibition, typifying the proepileptogenic state created by these seizures as a surrogate marker, the authors found no epileptogenic effect of topiramate (T.Z. Baram, personal communication).

Rats exposed to a perinatal hypoxic insult have both acute seizures as well as subsequent seizure susceptibility and induced neuronal injury [107]. Changes were seen to be age specific, with hypoxic seizures induced in rats on postnatal day 10 increasing seizure susceptibility to a chemical convulsant but not with oxygen deprivation on day 5 or 60. When topiramate was administered to P10 rats prior to hypoxia, acute seizures were not observed. In addition, subsequent challenge with kainate 4 days and 20 days later showed reduced tendency to seizures and neuronal injury [108]. A study to evaluate long-term treatment with topiramate after recurrent neonatal seizures and SE in immature rats demonstrated a trend toward improved function in the animals with recurrent neonatal seizures and modest beneficial effects on cognitive function following SE. Furthermore, chronic administration of topiramate in the normal developing rat brain did not alter subsequent cognitive function [109]. These data suggest some degree of neuroprotective effect but further evaluation is required, particularly in transfer to clinical practice.

Clinical therapeutics

Topiramate has proved to be an effective broad-spectrum agent in the treatment of epilepsy. Efficacy has been demonstrated against all seizure types in placebo-controlled and open-label trials, with little evidence of aggravation of seizures. However, it is likely that lower doses are more effective than initially predicted from trial data. It has a particular place in the treatment of apparently resistant focal seizures, and symptomatic generalized epilepsies where certain anticonvulsants have been shown to be ineffective or contraindicated. Side-effects may also be minimized or avoided by reducing concomitant medication rather than topiramate itself. Because of the risk of side-effects, topiramate should be introduced at a low dose (0.5 mg/kg or 25 mg/day), and titration upwards should be slow and cautious (no more than 0.5 mg/kg or 25 mg/day per week). Efficacy should be reviewed at 50 mg or 2 mg/kg/day, although much higher doses can sometimes be required and tolerated. There remains, however, a small group who are unable to tolerate the medication, regardless of the dose or rate of titration used. Good tolerance and efficacy has been demonstrated in monotherapy and newly diagnosed trials, in which the side-effect profile appears to have been minimized.

In current clinical practice, topiramate may be used as first or second line for focal and generalized epilepsies. In children with symptomatic generalized epilepsies, particularly those including myoclonus, the medication should be considered earlier rather than later in view of the efficacy relative to other existing anticonvulsant agents.

References

1 Coulter D, Sombati S, Delorenzo R. Topiramate effects on excitatory amino acid-mediated responses in cultured hippocampal neurons: selective blockade of kainate currents. *Epilepsia* 1995; 36: S40.

2 Avoli M, Lopantsev V. Topiramate blocks ictal like discharges in the entorhinal cortex. *Epilepsia* 1997; 37: 44.

3 Kawasaki H, Tancredi V, D'Arcangelo G, Avoli M. Multiple actions of the novel anticonvulsant drug Topiramate in the rat subiculum *in vitro*. *Brain Res* 1998; 807: 125–34.

4 Zona C, Ciotti M, Avoli M. Topiramate attenuates voltage gated sodium currents in rat cerebellar granule cells. *Neurosci Lett* 1997; 231: 123–6.

5 Taverna S, Sancini G, Mantegazza M, Franceschetti S, Avanzini G. Inhibition of transient and persistent Na^+ current fractions by the new anticonvulsant topiramate. *J Pharmacol Exp Ther* 1999; 288: 960–8.

6 McLean MJ, Bukhari AA, Wamil AW. Effects of Topiramate on sodium-dependent action-potential firing by mouse spinal cord neurons in cell culture. *Epilepsia* 2000; 41 (Suppl. 1): s21–s24.

7 White H, Brown S, Skeen G, Wolf H, Twymann R. The anticonvulsant Topiramate displays a unique ability to potentiate GABA-evoked chloride currents. *Epilepsia* 1995; 36: s39–s40.

8 White H, Brown S, Woodhead J, Skeen G, Wolf H. Topiramate enhances GABA mediated chloride flux and GABA evoked chloride currents in murine brain neurons and increase seizure threshold. *Epilepsy Res* 1997; 28: 167–79.

9 Coulter D, Sombati S, Delorenzo R. Selective effects of topiramate on sustained repetitive firing and spontaneous bursting in cultured hippocampal neurones. *Epilepsia* 1993; 34: s123.

10 Kanda T, Nakamura J, Kurokawa M *et al.* Inhibition of excessive releases of excitatory amino acids in hippocampus of spontaneously epileptic rat (SER) by topiramate (KW-6485). *Jpn J Pharmacol* 1992; 58: 92P.

11 Kanda T, Kurokawa M, Tamura S *et al.* Topiramate reduces abnormally high extracellular levels of glutamate and aspartate in the hippocampus of spontaneous epileptic rats (SER). *Life Sci* 1996; 59: 1607–16.

12 Zhang XL, Velumian A, Jones O, Carlen PL. Modulation of high voltage-activated calcium channels in dentate granule cells by topiramate. *Epilepsia* 2000; 41 (Suppl. 1): 52–60.

13 Dodgson S, Shank R, Maryanoff B. Topiramate as an inhibitor of carbonic anhydrase isoenzymes. *Epilepsia* 2000; 41: s35–s39.

14 Shank R, Gardocki J, Vaught J. Topiramate: preclinical evaluation of a structurally novel anticonvulsant. *Epilepsia* 1994; 35: 450–60.

15 Kimishima K, Wang Y, Tanabe T *et al.* Anticonvulsant activities and properties of topiramate. *Jpn J Pharmacol* 1992; 58: 211P.

16 Hosford D, Wang Y. Utility of lethargic (*lh/lh*) mouse model of absence seizures in predicting the effects of lamotrigine, vigabatrin, tiagabine, gabapentin, and topiramate against human absence seizures. *Epilepsia* 1997; 38: 408–14.

17 Easterling D, Zakszewski T, Moyer M, Margul B, Marriott T, Nayak R. Plasma pharmacokinetics of topiramate, a new anticonvulsant in humans. *Epilepsia* 1988; 29: 662.

18 Nayak R, Gisclon L, Curtin C, Benet L. Estimation of the absolute bioavailability of topiramate in humans without intravenous data. *J Clin Pharmacol* 1994; 34: 1029.

19 Doose, DR, Gisclon, LG, Stellar SM, Riffets JM, Hills JF. The effect of food on the bioavailability of topiramate from 100- and 400-mg tablets in healthy male subjects. *Epilepsia* 1992; 33 (Suppl. 3): 105.

20 Doose D, Walker SA, Gisclon L, Nayak R. Single dose pharmacokinetics and effect of food on the bioavailability of topiramate, a novel antiepileptic drug. *J Clin Pharmacol* 1996; 36: 884–91.

21 Doose DR, Walker SA, Scott VV *et al.* The comparative bioavailability of topiramate from two investigational pediatric sprinkle formulations relative to a tablet formulation. *Epilepsia* 1996; 37 (Suppl. 5): 112.

22 Doose DR, Scott VV, Margul BL, Marriott TB, Nayak RK. Multiple dose pharmacokinetics of topiramate in helathy male subjects. *Epilepsia* 1988; 29 (Suppl. 6): 131.

23 Ben-Menachem E. Potential antiepileptic drugs: topiramate. In: Levy RH, Mattson RH, Meldrum BS, eds. *Antiepileptic Drugs*. New York: Raven Press, 1995: 1063–70.

24 Wu W, Heebner J, Streeter A *et al.* Evaluation of the absorption, excretion, pharmacokinetics and metabolism of the anticonvulsant, topiramate in healthy men. *Pharm Res* 1994; 11 (Suppl.): s336.

25 Gisclon L, Curtin C. The pharmacokinetics (PK) of topiramate (T) in subjects with end stage renal disease undergoing haemodialysis. *Clin Pharmacol Ther* 1994; 55: 196.

26 Sachdeo R, Sachdeo S, Walker S, Kramer L, Nayak R, Doose D. Steady state pharmacokinetics of topiramate and carbamazepine in patients with epilepsy during monotherapy and concomitant therapy. *Epilepsia* 1996; 37: 774–80.

27 Rosenfield W, Liao S, Kramer L *et al.* Comparison of the steady state pharmacokinetics of topiramate and valproate in patients with epilepsy during monotherapy and concomitant therapy. *Epilepsia* 1997; 38: 324–33.

28 Elterman RD, Glauser TA, Wyllie E, Reife R, Wu S-C, Pledger GW, and the Topiramate YP Study Group. A double blind, randomized trial of Topiramate for partial-onset seizures in children. *Neurology* 1999; 52: 1338–44.

29 Stephen LJ, Sills GJ, Brodie MJ. Lamotrigine and topiramate may be a useful combination. *Lancet* 1998; 351: 958–9.

30 Rosenfeld WE, Doose D, Walker SA, Nayak R. Effect of topiramate on the pharmacokinetics of an oral contraceptive containing norethindrone and ethinyl estradiol in patients with epilepsy. *Epilepsia* 1997; 38: 317–23.

31 Liao S, Palmer, M. Digoxin and topiramate drug interaction study in male volunteers. *Pharm Res* 1993; 10 (Suppl.): S405.

32 Rosenfield W, Doose D, Walker S, Baldessarre J, Reiffe R. A study of topiramate pharmacokinetics and tolerability in children with epilepsy. *Pediatr Neurol* 1999; 20: 339–44.

33 Glauser T, Miles M, Tang P *et al.* Topiramate pharmacokinetics in infants. *Epilepsia* 1999; 40: 788–91.

34 Privitera M. Topiramate: a new antiepileptic drug. *Ann Pharmacother* 1997; 31: 1164–73.

35 Gisclon L, Curtin C. The pharmacokinetics (PK) of topiramate (T) in subjects with renal impairment (RI) as compared to matched subjects with normal renal function (NRF). *Pharm Res* 1993; 10: s397.

36 Doose DR, Walker SA, Venkataramanan R, Rabinovitz M. Topiramate pharmacokinetics in subjects with liver impairment. *Pharm Res* 1994; 11: s446.

37 Faught E, Wilder BJ, Ramsey RE *et al.* Topiramate placebo controlled dose-ranging trial in refractory partial epilepsy using 200-, 400-, and 600-mg daily dosages. *Neurology* 1996; 46: 1684–90.

38 Privitera M, Fincham R, Penry J, Reife R, Kramer L, Pledger G. Topiramate placebo-controlled dose-ranging trial in refractory partial epilepsy using 600-, 800-, and 1000-mg daily dosages. *Neurology* 1996; 46: 1678–83.

39 Sharief M, Viteri C, Ben-Menachem E, Weber M, Reife R. Double blind placebo-controlled study of topiramate in patients with refractory epilepsy. *Epilepsy Res* 1996; 25: 217–24.

40 Tassinari CA, Michelucci R, Chauvel P *et al.* Double blind, placebo-controlled trial of topiramate (600 mg daily) for the treatment of refractory partial epilepsy. *Epilepsia* 1996; 37: 763–8.

41 Ben-Menachem E, Henriksen O, Dam M *et al.* Double blind, placebo-controlled trial of topiramate as add-on therapy in patients with refractory partial seizures. *Epilepsia* 1996; 37: 539–43.

42 Rosenfeld W, Abou-Khalil B, Reife R, Hegadus R, Pledger G, and Topiramate YF/YG study group. Placebo-controlled trial of topiramate as adjunctive therapy to carbamazepine or phenytoin for partial onset epilepsy. *Epilepsia* 1996; 37 (Suppl. 5): s153.

43 Reife R, Pledger G, Wu S-C. Topiramate as add-on therapy: pooled analy-

sis of randomised controlled trials in adults. *Epilepsia* 2000; 41 (Suppl. 1): s66–s71.

44 Yen D-J, Yu H-Y, Guo Y-C *et al*. A double-blind, placebo-controlled study of topiramate in adult patients with refractory partial epilepsy. *Epilepsia* 2000; 41: 1162–6.

45 Guberman A, Neto W, Gassmann-Mayer C. Efficacy of 200 mg/day topiramate in treatment-resistant partial seizures when added to an enzyme-inducing antiepileptic drug (AED). *Epilepsia* 2001; 42 (Suppl. 7): 179–80.

46 Garnett WR. Clinical pharmacology of topiramate: a review. *Epilepsia* 2000; 41: s61–s65.

47 Ritter F, Glauser TA, Elterman RD, Wyllie E, Topiramate YP study group. Effectiveness, tolerability, and safety of topiramate in children with partial onset seizures. *Epilepsia* 2000; 41: s82–s85.

48 Biton V, Montouris GD, Ritter F *et al*. A randomised, placebo-controlled study of topiramate in primary generalised tonic-clonic seizures. *Neurology* 1999; 52: 1330–7.

49 Ben-Menachem E and Topiramate YTC-E study group. A double blind trial of topiramate in patients with generalised tonic-clonic seizures of non-focal origin. *Epilepsia* 1997; 38: s60.

50 Chadwick D, Reife R, Hughson C. Topiramate in generalised seizures without focal onset. *Eur J Paediatr Neurol* 1997; 1: A10.

51 Biton V, Rosenfeld WE, Twyman R, Lim P. Topiramate (TPM) in juvenile myoclonic epilepsy (JME): observations from randomised controlled trials in primary generalised tonic-clonic seizures (PGTCS). *Epilepsia* 1999; 40: 218.

52 Harden CL, Martin SM, Liporace J, Labar DR, French JA. Comparison of patients who became seizure free taking lamotrigine, Topamax or tiagabine: data from the PADS study group. *Epilepsia* 1998; 39: 147.

53 Kellett MW, Smith DF, Stockton PA, Chadwick D. Topiramate in clinical practice: a first years postlicensing experience in a specialist epilepsy clinic. *J Neurol Neurosurg Psychiatry* 1999; 66: 759–63.

54 Kugler SL, Mandelbaum DE, Traeger EC *et al*. Broad-spectrum efficacy of topiramate in children. *Epilepsia* 1998; 39: 164.

55 Rosenfeld WE, Schaefer PA, Lippmann SM. Topiramate in patients with juvenile myoclonic epilepsy. *Epilepsia* 1998; 39: 139.

56 Montouris GD, Biton V, Rosenfeld WE, Topiramate YTC/YTCE study group. Nonfocal generalised tonic-clonic seizures: response during long term topiramate treatment. *Epilepsia* 2000; 41: s77–s81.

57 Glauser TA, Levisohn PM, Ritter F, Sachdeo RC, Topiramate YL study group. Topiramate in Lennox–Gastaut syndrome: open label treatment of patients completing a randomised controlled trial. *Epilepsia* 2000; 41: s86–s90.

58 Motte J, Trevathan E, Arvidson JFV *et al*. Lamotrigine for generalized seizures associated with the Lennox–Gastaut syndrome. *N Engl J Med* 1997; 337: 1807–12.

59 Sachdeo R, Reife R, Lim P, Pledger G. Topiramate monotherapy for partial onset seizures. *Epilepsia* 1997; 38: 294–300.

60 Gilliam FG, Veloso F, Bomhof MAM *et al*. and the Topiramate EPMN 104 Study Group. A dose comparison trial of topiramate as monotherapy in recently diagnosed partial epilepsy. *Neurology* 2003; 60: 196–202.

61 Arroyo S, Squires L, Twyman R. Topiramate (TPM) monotherapy in newly diagnosed epilepsy: effectiveness in dose–response study. *Epilepsia* 2002; 43: 47–8.

62 Privitera M, Brodie MJ, Neto W, Wang S. Topiramate, carbamazepine and valproate in the spectrum of newly diagnosed epilepsy. *Neurology* 2001; 56: A332.

63 Brodie MJ, Richens A, Yuen AWC, for UK Lamotrigine/Carbamazepine Monotherapy Trial Group. Double-blind comparison of lamotrigine and carbamazepine in newly diagnosed epilepsy. *Lancet* 1995; 345: 476–9.

64 Steiner TJ, Dellaportas CI, Findley LJ *et al*. Lamotrigine monotherapy in newly diagnosed untreated epilepsy: A double blind comparison with phenytoin. *Epilepsia* 1999; 40: 601–7.

65 Christe W, Kramer G, Vigonius U *et al*. A double-blind controlled clinical trial: oxcarbazepine versus sodium valproate in adults with newly diagnosed epilepsy. *Epilepsy Res* 1997; 26: 451–60.

66 Bill PA, Vigonius U, Pohlmann H *et al*. A double-blind controlled clinical trial of oxcarbazepine versus phenytoin in adults with previously untreated epilepsy. *Epilepsy Res* 1997; 27: 195–204.

67 Guerriero MM, Vigonius U, Pohlmann H *et al*. A double-blind controlled

68 Sachdeo RC, Glauser TA, Ritter F *et al*. A double-blind randomised trial of topiramate in Lennox–Gastaut syndrome. *Neurology* 1999; 52: 1882–7.

69 Dodson WE, Kamin M, Kraut L, Olson WH, Wu S-C. Individualized topiramate therapy in an open lable, in-practice study of 800+ patients. *Ann Pharmacother* 2003; 37: 615–20.

70 Stephen LJ, Sills GJ, Brodie MJ. Topiramate in refractory epilepsy: a prospective observational study. *Epilepsia* 2000; 41: 977–80.

71 Lhatoo SD, Wong ICK, Polizzi G, Sander JWAS. Long term retention rates of lamotrigine, gabapentin and topiramate in chronic epilepsy. *Epilepsia* 2000; 41: 1592–6.

72 Lhatoo SD, Wong ICK, Sander JWAS. Prognostic factors affecting long-term retention of topiramate in patients with chronic epilepsy. *Epilepsia* 2000; 41: 338–41.

73 Glauser TA, Clark PO, Strawsburg R. A pilot study of topiramate in the treatment of infantile spasms. *Epilepsia* 1998; 39: 1324–8.

74 Glauser TA, Clark PO, McGee K. Long term response to topiramate in the treatment of infantile spasms. *Epilepsia* 2000; 41: S91–S94.

75 Cross JH. Topiramate monotherapy for childhood absence seizures: results from an open lable pilot study. *Seizure* 2002; 11: 406–10.

76 Franz DN, Tudor C, Leonard J. Topiramate as therapy for tuberous sclerosis complex-associated seizures. *Epilepsia* 2000; 41: 87.

77 Kelly K, Stephen LJ, Sills GJ, Brodie MJ. Topiramate in patients with learning disability and refractory epilepsy. *Epilepsia* 2002; 43: 399–402.

78 Singh BK, White-Scott S. Role of topiramate in adults with intractable epilepsy, mental retardation, and developmental disabilities. *Seizure* 2002; 11: 47–50.

79 Nieto Barrera M, Candau R, Nieto-Jimenez M, Correa A, Ruiz Del Portal L. Topiramate in the treatment of severe myoclonic epilepsy of infancy. *Seizure* 2000; 9: 590–4.

80 Franz DN, Glauser TA, Tudor C, Williams S. Topiramate therapy of epilepsy associated with Angelman's syndrome. *Neurology* 2000; 54: 1185–8.

81 Chengappa KNR, Gershon S, Levine J. The evolving role of topiramate among other mood stabilizers in the management of bipolar disorders. *Bipolar Disord* 2001; 3: 215–32.

82 Chengappa KNR, Levine J, Rathore D, Parepally H, Atzert R. Long-term effects of topiramate on bipolar mood instability, weight change and glycemic control: a case series. *Eur Psychiatr* 2001; 16: 186–90.

83 Letmaier M, Schreinzer D, Wolf R, Kasper S. Topiramate as a mood stabilizer. *Int Clin Psychoparmacol* 2001; 16: 295–8.

84 Marcotte D. Use of topiramate, a new anti-epileptic as a mood stabilizer. *J Affective Disord* 1998; 50: 245–51.

85 McElroy SL, Suppes T, Keck PE *et al*. Open-label adjunctive topiramate in the treatment of bipolar disorders. *Biol Psychiatry* 2000; 47: 1025–33.

86 Shorvon, S. D. Safety of Topiramate: adverse events and relationships to dosing. *Epilepsia* 1996; 37: S18–S22.

87 Biton V, Edwards KR, Montouris GD *et al*. Topiramate titration and tolerability. *Ann Pharmacother* 2001; 35: 173–9.

88 Martin R, Kuzniecky R, Ho S *et al*. Cognitive effects of topiramate, gabapentin, and lamotrigine in healthy young adults. *Neurology* 1999; 52: 321–7.

89 Aldenkamp AP. Cognitive effects of topiramate, gabapentin, and lamotrigine in healthy young adults [letter; comment]. *Neurology* 2002; 54: 271–2.

90 Aldenkamp AP, Baker G, Mulder OG *et al*. A multicenter, randomized clinical study to evaluate the effect on cognitive function of Topiramate compared to valproate as add-on therapy to carbamazepine in patients with partial onset seizures. *Epilepsia* 2000; 41: 1167–78.

91 Thompson PJ, Baxendale SA, Duncan JS, Sander JW. Effects of topiramate on cognitive function. *J Neurol Neurosurg Psychiatry* 2000; 69: 636–41.

92 Lhatoo SD, Walker MC. The safety and adverse event profile of topiramate. *Rev Contemp Pharmacother* 1999; 10: 185–91.

93 Wasserstein A, Reife R, Rak I. Mechanistic basis for topiramate associated nephrolithiasis. *Epilepsia* 1995; 36: S153.

94 Wasserstein A, Reife R, Rak I. Topiramate and nephrolithiasis. *Epilepsia* 1995; 36: S153.

95 Bjoro K, Gjerstad L, Bentdal O, Osnes S, Schrumpf E. Topiramate and fulminant hepatic failure. *Lancet* 1998; 352: 1119.

96 Hamer HM, Knake S, Schomburg U, Rosenow F. Valproate-induced hyperammonemic encephalopathy in the presence of topiramate. *Neurology* 2000; 54: 230–2.

97 Longin E, Teich M, Koelfen W, Konig S. Topiramate enhances the risk of valproate-associated side effects in three children. *Epilepsia* 2002; 43: 451–4.

98 Banta JT, Hoffman K, Budenz DL, Ceballos E, Greenfield DS. Presumed topiramate-induced bilateral acute angle-closure glaucoma. *Am J Ophthalmol* 2001; 132: 112–14.

99 Shields D, Wu S-C. Safety of Topiramate (TPM) in children with epilepsy. *Epilepsia* 1999; 40: 126.

100 Takeoka M, Holmes GL. Topiramate and metabolic acidosis in pediatric epilepsy. *Epilepsia* 1999; 40: 127.

101 Niebauer M, Gruenthal M. Topiramate reduces neuronal injury after experimental status epilepticus. *Brain Res* 1999; 837: 263–9.

102 Brewster A, Bender RA, Chen Y, Eghbal-Ahmadi M, Dube C, Baram TZ. Developmental febrile seizures modulate hippocampal gene expression of hyperpolarization-activated channels in an isoform and cell-specific manner. *J Neurosci* 2002; 22: 4591–9.

103 Toth Z, Yan XX, Heftoglu S, Ribak CE, Baram TZ. Seizure induced neuronal injury: vulnerability to febrile seizures in an immature rat model. *J Neurosci* 1998; 18: 4285–94.

104 Chen K, Baram TZ, Soltesz I. Seizures in the immature brain result in persistent modification of neuronal excitability in limbic circuits. *Nature Med* 1999; 5: 888–94.

105 Dube C, Chen K, Eghbal-Ahmadi M, Brunson K, Soltesz I, Baram TZ. Prolonged febrile seizures in the immature rat model enhance hippocampal excitability long-term. *Ann Neurol* 2000; 47: 336–44.

106 Dube C. Do prolonged febrile seizures in an immature rat model cause epilepsy? In: Baram TZ, Shinnar S, eds. *Febrile Seizures*. London: Academic Press, 2002: 215–29.

107 Jensen FE, Holmes GL, Lombroso CT *et al*. Age-dependent changes in long-term seizure susceptibility and behavior after hypoxia in rats. *Epilepsia* 1992; 33: 971–80.

108 Koh S, Jensen FE. Topiramate blocks acute and chronic epileptogenesis in a rat model of perinatal hypoxic encephalopathy. *Epilepsia* 1999; 40: 5–6.

109 Cha BH, Silveira DC, Liu X, Hu Y, Holmes GL. Effect of topiramate following recurrent and prolonged seizures during early development. *Epilepsy Res* 2002; 51: 217–32.

46

Valproate

S. Arroyo

COOH

Primary indications	First-line or adjunctive therapy in generalized seizures (including myoclonus and absence) and also partial seizures, Lennox–Gastaut syndrome and drug of first choice in the syndrome of primary generalized epilepsy. Also for childhood epilepsy syndromes and febrile convulsions
Usual preparations	Enteric-coated tablets: 200, 500 mg; crushable tablets: 100 mg; capsules: 150, 300, 500 mg; syrup: 200 mg/5 mL; liquid: 200 mg/5 mL; slow-release tablets; 200, 300, 500 mg; Divalproex tablets: 125, 300, 500 mg; sprinkle
Usual dosages	Parenteral formulation. Initial: 400–500 mg/day (adults); 20 mg/kg/day (children under 20 kg); 40 mg/kg/day (children over 20 kg). Maintenance: 500–2500 mg/day (adults); 20–40 mg/kg/day (children under 20 kg); 20–30 mg/kg/day (children over 20 kg) (slow-release formulation not suitable for children)
Dosage intervals	2–3 times per day
Significant drug interactions	Valproate has a number of complex interactions with antiepileptic and other drugs
Serum level monitoring	Not generally useful
Target range	300–700 μmol/L
Common/important side effects	Nausea, vomiting, hyperammonaemia and other metabolic effects, endocrine effects, severe hepatic toxicity, pancreatitis, drowsiness, cognitive disturbance, aggressiveness, tremor, weakness, encephalopathy, thrombocytopenia, neutropenia, aplastic anemia, hair thinning and hair loss, weight gain, polycystic ovarian syndrome
Main advantages	Drug of choice in primary generalized epilepsy and a wide spectrum of activity
Main disadvantages	Cognitive effects, weight gain, tremor and hair loss Potential for severe hepatic and pancreatic disturbance in children
Mechanism of action	Uncertain but may affect GABA glutaminergic activity, calcium (T) conductance and potassium conductance
Oral bioavailability	<100%
Time to peak levels	1–10 h (dependent on formulation)
Metabolism and excretion	Hepatic glucuronidation and oxidation and then conjugation
Volume of distribution	0.1–0.4 L/kg
Elimination half-life	12–15 h (adults); 14–17 h (elderly); 30–60 h (neonates)
Plasma clearance	0.010–0.115 L/kg/h
Protein binding	85–95%
Active metabolites	None
Comment	Drug of choice in primary generalized epilepsy and useful in a wide spectrum of other epilepsies

(*Note*: this summary table was formulated by the lead editor.)

Valproic acid (VPA) is a simple branched-chained carboxylic acid and differs structurally from other antiepileptic drugs (AEDs). VPA was discovered by chance when it was used as an organic solvent for testing potential epileptic compounds. It was marketed in Europe in the 1960s and in the USA in 1978.

There are several marketed forms of the drug: the parent compound (VPA), its sodium salt (sodium valproate), its amide derivative (depamide) and an oligomeric combination of the parent compound and its sodium salt (divalproex sodium). None of these derivatives have shown obvious advantages among themselves. In this chapter the term VPA will be used for all forms, except when otherwise stated. VPA is available in capsule, tablet, sprinkle, liquid, enteric-coated tablet, controlled-release tablet (chrono formulation using a mixture of sodium valproate and VPA) and in an intravenous formulation.

Mechanisms of action and experimental studies

Until now the mechanism of action of VPA has not been fully elucidated. However, most animal studies have emphasized the effect of VPA on the γ-aminobutyric acid (GABA) system. VPA increases synaptosomal GABA concentrations through the activation of the GABA-synthesizing enzyme glutamic acid decarboxylase. In addition, VPA inhibits GABA catabolism through inhibition of GABA transaminase and succinic semialdehyde dehydrogenase. VPA also inhibits the excitatory neurotransmission mediated by aspartic acid, glutamic acid and γ-hydroxybutyric acid. Furthermore, VPA reduces cellular excitability through modulation of voltage-dependent sodium currents [1].

VPA has shown efficacy in animal models of absence, partial and generalized seizures induced by chemical (bicuculline, pentylenetetrazol, picrotoxin, strychnine, quinolinic acid), electrical (maximal electroshock) or sensory stimuli (photic). VPA prevents the development of kindled seizures (thus, has an antiepileptogenic effect) [2].

VPA is highly effective in reducing spike-wave EEG discharges in humans with idiopathic generalized epilepsy (childhood absences, for example) [3] and in photosensitive patients [4].

Pharmacokinetics (Table 46.1)

Absorption and distribution

The mean bioavailability of oral formulations of VPA approaches 100% [5]. Peak plasma concentrations (C_{max}) increase proportionally with dose following oral administration. The mean time to reach C_{max} depends on the presentation: 1–3 h for capsules, uncoated tablets or oral solution, 3–5 h for enteric-coated tablets. Total and free C_{max} are lower by approximately 25% with controlled-release tablets but with a relatively stable plateau from 4 to 14 h [6]. Administration with food delays the rate but not the extent of absorption. There is a significant diurnal variation in VPA absorption. The apparent volume of distribution ranges from 0.1 to 0.4 L/kg, suggesting confinement principally to the circulation and extracellular fluid. VPA is highly protein bound (85–95%), but the unbound fraction increases in a non-linear fashion with total plasma VPA concentrations above 80–85 mg/L. A diurnal variation

Table 46.1 Valproate pharmacokinetic properties

Oral bioavailability (%)	96–100
t_{max} (h)	
tablets	1.5
enteric-coated tablets	3–5
slow release	5–10
V_d (L/kg)	0.1–0.4
Protein binding (%)	85–95
CSF and brain concentration (%)	7–28% of the plasma concentration
% in milk	1–3
Plasma clearance	0.01–0.1 L/kg/h
Metabolism	Glucuronidation and oxidation
Major metabolites	2-en-VPA and 4-en-VPA
Urinary excretion (%)	3–7
Half-life	
adults	12–15 h (~9 h in polytherapy)
elderly	14–17 h
neonates	30–60 h

in VPA's plasma protein binding has also been observed, possibly due to fluctuations in the levels of free fatty acids that displace the drug from its binding sites.

Metabolism and elimination

VPA metabolism is complex and undergoes biotransformation through glucuronidation and oxidation [5]. Only 1–3% of the dose is excreted unchanged in the urine, while most of the parent drug and metabolites undergo conjugation with glucuronic acid. Approximately 14% of the total plasma VPA concentration is in the form of metabolites: 2-En-VPA (with anticonvulsant effect) and 4-En-VPA (probably responsible for hepatotoxicity and teratogenicity) [7]. Plasma clearance ranges from 0.4 to 0.6 L/h. Increased clearance is seen in patients receiving enzyme-inducing AEDs. Plasma elimination half-life ranges from 8 to 16 h. VPA has linear pharmacokinetics at usual therapeutic doses. However at high doses, as drug binding to plasma proteins is saturated, the pharmacokinetics become non-linear due to an increased clearance [8].

Age effects

In neonates the percentage of unbound VPA is higher than in children. Mean half-life in untreated neonates born to epileptic mothers is from 30 to 60 h, and from 17 to 40 h in neonates treated with VPA [5]. In children (2–10 years) a higher plasma clearance and lower half-life values are observed than in adults. Children over 10 years have pharmacokinetic parameters similar to adults. In elderly patients unbound plasma concentrations are about 67% higher due to a reduction in clearance and drug binding to plasma proteins. Thus, a slight dose reduction is recommended in the elderly.

Hepatic disease

VPA is contraindicated in patients with acute liver disease or patients with close family history of drug-induced hepatitis due to its increased risk of hepatotoxicity (see below). In patients with alcoholic cirrhosis there is a decreased binding to plasma protein and a decrease in clearance of the unbound drug [9].

Renal disease

VPA's half-life is not altered by renal impairment. However, plasma protein binding of VPA may be reduced. Thus, dosage adjustments should be considered.

Diabetes mellitus

Patients with uncompensated diabetes mellitus and high free fatty acid levels may have an increased unbound VPA plasma level giving rise to adverse effects [10]. Nevertheless, in patients with well-controlled diabetes, this alteration in VPA plasma protein binding is unlikely to be of any clinical significance [5].

Pregnancy

VPA's plasma protein binding decreases during pregnancy. Total plasma VPA concentration is also reduced due to an increased volume of distribution and clearance. Free drug fraction concentration is double from the first to the third trimester. In addition, the free fraction at birth is 50% higher in mothers treated with oxytocin. Concentrations of VPA in the breast milk range from 1 to 3% of those in maternal plasma. In animal models of teratogenicity, high peak plasma levels of VPA (but not the doses) are correlated with the incidence of neural tube defects. In these models, teratogenicity has been greatly reduced or abolished by avoiding peak plasma levels. Thus, slow-release VPA formulations are preferred for women.

Pharmacodynamic effects

Several studies (human and animal) have shown that it often takes days or weeks of VPA treatment before maximum antiepileptic efficacy is obtained despite having previously reached therapeutic plasma levels [11]. In addition, in the photosensitive model of epilepsy, the antiepileptic effect remains for a few days after discontinuing the drug [12]. The cause of this increased and long-lasting anticonvulsant effect is unknown, but does not appear to be due to slow VPA accumulation in the brain or the action of VPA metabolites [11].

VPA drug interactions with AEDs (Table 46.2)

VPA can affect the plasma concentration of other drugs by displacement from plasma proteins and inhibition of hepatic metabolism. VPA can produce clinically significant increases in plasma concentrations of phenobarbital (PB) reaching up to 30–40% in adults and 52–68% in children. VPA displaces phenytoin (PHT) from its albumin binding sites increasing PHT free fraction. This increases PHT clearance resulting in a reduction in total plasma PHT concentration. In addition, VPA-induced hepatic inhibition leads to an increase in total and unbound PHT concentration. Thus, VPA effect can result in PHT total plasma concentrations within the therapeutic range but an increased unbound free fraction, giving rise to toxicity. Thus, it is necessary to follow closely unbound PHT plasma concentrations after adding VPA.

Carbamazepine (CBZ) epoxide increases when VPA is added (from 25 to 100%). This effect is more pronounced with valpromide (concentration increases by 330%). This interaction is, however, of variable magnitude and is probably only relevant at high doses.

VPA increases plasma ethosuximide (ESM) concentrations up to 53% by reducing its metabolism. Similarly, VPA can increase the plasma concentration of benzodiazepines through metabolic inhibition and displacement from protein binding sites.

The addition of VPA to a lamotrigine (LTG) treatment reduces the clearance of LTG, leading to large LTG serum concentration increases (up to 164%). Interestingly, the degree of inhibition of

Table 46.2 Valproate's pharmacological interactions

Drug	VPA effect on the drug	Effect of the drug on VPA
Phenytoin (PHT)	Increase PHT unbound fraction	Reduced VPA serum concentrations (30–40%)
Carbamazepine (CBZ)	Increase CBZ epoxide (25–100%)	Reduced VPA serum concentrations (30–40%)
Phenobarbital (PB)	Increase PB concentration (30–40%)	Reduced VPA serum concentrations (30–40%)
Primidone (PRM)	Increase PB concentration (30–40%)	Reduced VPA serum concentrations (30–40%)
Ethosuximide (ESM)	Increase ESM concentration (50%)	No effect
Benzodiazepines	Increase plasma benzodiazepine concentration	No significant effect (clobazam may increase VPA plasma concentration)
Felbamate (FLM)	Increase FLM concentration	Increase VPA plasma concentration
Vigabatrin (VGB)	No effect	No effect
Lamotrigine (LTG)	Increase LTG concentration (up to 164%)	No effect
Gabapentin (GBP)	No effect	No effect
Topiramate (TPM)	No effect	No effect
Tiagabine (TGB)	No effect	No effect
Oxcarbazepine (OXC)	No effect	No effect
Zonisamide (ZNS)	No effect	No effect
Levetiracetam (LEV)	No effect	No effect

LTG clearance is independent of the dose of VPA [13]. This pharmacokinetic interaction appears to be only in part responsible for the synergism observed between these two drugs, and the increase in efficacy of LTG–VPA combination is claimed by some to be independent of LTG serum concentrations [14].

The addition of felbamate (FLM) to a patient treated with VPA, induces a reduction of VPA clearance between 28 and 54% depending on the FLM dose, increasing the steady-state plasma concentrations. Thus, on starting FLM, a reduction of the dose of VPA is suggested.

AEDs with hepatic enzyme induction properties (PHT, CBZ, PB or primidone) can reduce plasma VPA concentrations by increasing the intrinsic clearance and decreasing the plasma half-life of VPA (reduced to 9 h) [5]. Plasma VPA concentrations are usually reduced from 30 to 40% in adults and up to 50% in children. Thus, VPA doses should be increased when used with enzyme-inducing drugs and conversely its dose should be reduced if an enzyme-inducing drug is discontinued.

No clinically significant VPA interactions have been observed with tiagabine (TGB), vigabatrin (VGB), gabapentin (GBP), topiramate (TPM), levetiracetam (LEV) and oxcarbazepine (OXC).

VPA drug interactions with other medications

Salicylates increase plasma concentrations of VPA by decreasing its metabolism and by displacing it from plasma albumin binding sites. Although the clinical relevance is probably minimal, it is sometimes recommended that alternative analgesics/anti-inflammatories be used in patients taking VPA. Acetaminophen and non-steroidal anti-inflammatory drugs do not appear to provoke interactions. VPA displaces warfarin from its albumin binding sites increasing the active unbound drug. VPA may increase serum concentrations of amitriptyline, nortryptilin, zidovudine, cimetidin, chlorpromazine, erythromycin, nimodipine through metabolic inhibition. Certain cytotoxics (cisplatin) and cholestyramine may reduce the absorption of VPA. Plasma VPA concentration might vary (increase or decrease) with fluoxetine or fluvoxamine. Rifampin may produce a 40% increase in the oral clearance of VPA.

VPA has no interaction with oral contraceptives, lithium and clozapine.

Clinical efficacy

VPA has a wide spectrum of action and is widely used in monotherapy or add-on for generalized and partial seizures both in children and adults.

Localization-related epilepsies

The efficacy of VPA on partial seizures has been demonstrated in multiple trials in adults comparing the efficacy of VPA to other AEDs [15–24]. However, in this review only randomized double-blind trials (RDBT) will be discussed.

Add-on VPA for partial seizures

Two RDBT have been conducted using VPA as add-on in partial onset seizures. Richens et al. carried out a cross-over RDBT comparing VPA to placebo as add-on in 20 patients with 'chronic uncontrolled epilepsy'. VPA 1200 mg/day significantly reduced the frequency of both tonic-clonic and 'minor seizures' in these patients [25]. In another RDBT, Willmore et al. compared VPA versus placebo as adjunctive therapy in 137 patients with uncontrolled complex partial seizures concomitantly treated with CBZ or PHT [26]. VPA-treated patients experienced a significant seizure reduction compared to placebo. Responder rate (percentage of patients with more than 50% seizure reduction) was 38% compared with 19% in those receiving placebo. Six VPA and one placebo-treated patient became seizure free.

VPA in monotherapy for partial seizures

Mattson et al. conducted a large RDBT comparing VPA with CBZ in monotherapy in 480 adults with partial or secondarily generalized seizures previously untreated or undertreated [27]. The dosages in this study were flexible in order to achieve VPA concentrations of 80–100 µg/mL and CBZ concentrations of 7–8 µg/mL. If seizures were not controlled with these serum concentrations, further increments were administered until either seizures stopped or unacceptable adverse events appeared. Mean doses and serum concentrations attained were 2099 mg/day and 89.6 µg/mL of VPA and 722 mg/day and 7.8 µg/mL for CBZ. The study showed that both VPA and CBZ were similarly effective in the main outcome of the trial (the proportion of patients remaining treated during the first 12 months). Analysis of the results by seizure types showed that VPA and CBZ were similarly efficacious in controlling secondarily generalized seizures, but a significantly greater percentage of patients with partial seizures remained seizure free on CBZ than on VPA. However, full 12-month data were available for only 150 of the total 480 patients.

Brodie et al. conducted a multicentre RDBT randomizing the substitution of CBZ monotherapy with VPA or VGB in patients with uncontrolled partial seizures [28]. A total of 215 patients (107 VPA, 108 VGB) entered the study. No significant differences in efficacy were seen between the two groups: 51% of the patients on VPA and 53% of those in VGB group were responders (achieved a monthly reduction in seizures greater than 50%); 31% and 27% maintained alternative monotherapy, respectively. Of the VPA-treated patients 19% and of the VGB-treated patients 17% remained seizure free during the final 3-month treatment period. The percentage of patients who were discontinued due to adverse events was also similar (11% on VPA versus 13% on VGB).

A double-blind, concentration–response design clinical trial analysed the safety and efficacy of VPA (divalproex sodium) in monotherapy in patients with uncontrolled partial epilepsy [29]. The study included 143 patients that were randomly assigned to high (80–150 µg/mL) or low (25–50 µg/mL) plasma VPA concentrations. Initially, VPA was introduced and its dose was adjusted while the baseline AEDs were tapered and discontinued. There was a statistically significant reduction from baseline in the 8-week frequency of complex partial and secondarily generalized tonic-clonic seizures for patients in the high compared with the low plasma VPA group. Compared to baseline, there was a 30% median reduction in complex partial seizures for patients in the high group and a 19% increase for those in the low group. The median reduction for secondarily generalized tonic-clonic seizures was 70% for patients in the high group compared with a 22% increase in the low group. Adverse events occurred significantly more frequently in the high group, the three most frequent being tremor in 64%, thrombocytopenia in 31% and alopecia in 28%.

VPA in monotherapy for new onset epilepsy (partial and generalized seizures)

Christe *et al.* conducted a RDBT comparing VPA with OXC in 249 adults with new onset epilepsy (partial and generalized seizures) with a 1-year follow-up [30]. Both drugs showed similar efficacy: 53.8% of the VPA-treated patients were seizure free during maintenance treatment compared with 56.6% in the OXC group. Tolerability was not significantly different: 41 patients in the VPA group discontinued treatment prematurely (10 due to tolerability reasons) and 52 patients discontinued in the OXC group (15 because of tolerability reasons).

A recent comparative RDBT between VPA and LTG in monotherapy in patients with partial or generalized seizures showed that the proportions of seizure-free patients during the 8-month study were no different: 26% on VPA and 29% on LTG [31]. However, the study was powered to analyse weight gain and safety, not efficacy.

VPA in children with partial or generalized seizures

No RDBT on paediatric localization-related epilepsy has been published. Verity *et al.* conducted an open-label randomized study comparing VPA to CBZ [32]. The trial included 260 children with new onset epilepsy, of whom 133 had 'primary generalized seizures'. Remission rates were similar for both drugs at 6, 12 and 24 months. Mean dosage of VPA was relatively low (17 mg/kg/day). There were no significant differences in withdrawal from the trial due to adverse events. However, adverse event profile was different: there were significantly more children with somnolence and dizziness on the CBZ arm and a greater number with appetite increase and weight gain in the VPA arm.

Reynolds *et al.* undertook an open-label study of 410 children and adults with new onset epilepsy comparing PB, PHT, CBZ and VPA [33]. There were no significant differences in the proportion of patients achieving 1-year remission, the time to first seizure or the number of patients withdrawing because of adverse events.

Another open-label study compared VPA, PB and PHT in 167 children (3–16 years) with newly diagnosed partial or generalized seizures [34]. No differences in efficacy were seen, but PB was more frequently withdrawn due to adverse events.

Generalized epilepsies

VPA is considered the drug of choice for generalized epilepsies and has shown efficacy for a wide range of generalized epileptic disorders: childhood and juvenile absences, juvenile myoclonic epilepsy, photosensitive epilepsies, Lennox–Gastaut syndrome, West's syndrome and myoclonic epilepsies. However, most of the information on the efficacy of VPA in these indications is based on open-label or retrospective studies.

Two RDBT have compared VPA to ESM in children with absence epilepsy [3,35]. Both of them had a cross-over design. VPA was as effective as ESM in reducing absences and spike-wave discharges and had similar adverse event frequency. However, the superior efficacy of VPA for convulsive seizures and the knowledge of the rarity of severe VPA-associated hepatotoxicity in children over 2 years of age (see below), has made VPA the drug of choice for this type of epilepsy.

Despite VPA being considered as the AED of first choice for Lennox–Gastaut syndrome [36], only one small RDBT has been conducted on this indication. Vassella *et al.* in a cross-over RDBT compared PB to VPA on 17 children with Lennox–Gastaut syndrome [37]. The study concluded that VPA plus PB was more effective than PB monotherapy.

VPA's efficacy in West's syndrome has been assessed in several controlled studies. Dyken *et al.* conducted a cross-over RDBT in children with infantile spasms who had not responded to ACTH and corticosteroid therapy [38]. Twenty-one patients were randomly assigned to either the baseline–VPA–placebo treatment or the baseline–placebo–VPA treatment groups. The VPA group had lower total mean spasm frequency than the placebo group. However, this difference was not apparent after the cross-over. In any case, VPA treatment had significant lower mean spasm index scores than the baseline treatments. Other open-label studies have shown VPA efficacy in infantile spasms [39,40]. VPA dosages used for this indication have generally been high (100–300 mg/kg/day) [39]. In one study 16/22 children were free of spasms after 3 months of therapy (14 of them in monotherapy) [40]. After 6 months of therapy, total seizure control was achieved in 20 of 22 patients (16 children VPA monotherapy). No direct comparative trial has been conducted between VPA and VGB for this indication.

Retrospective studies have acknowledged the high efficacy of VPA in patients with juvenile myoclonic epilepsy [41,42]. In most of them, around 85% of the patients became seizure free. There is only one small RDBT that, curiously enough, gave very different results. Sundqvist *et al.* conducted a cross-over RDBT of 16 patients with juvenile myoclonic epilepsy comparing 1000 and 2000 mg VPA daily during a 6-month observation period on each dose [43]. There was no significant difference in seizure frequency between the two doses. Only 25% of the patients were seizure free throughout the study. During the higher dose, 37.5% of the patients had an improved seizure control, but 25% of the patients had an increase in seizure frequency compared to the lower dose. Their results dramatically contrast with common clinical experience and retrospective data. Inadequate patient selection (classification) might account for them.

Jeavons *et al.* followed 142 patients (84% aged less than 20 years) with various forms of generalized epilepsies treated with VPA (monotherapy or add-on) [44]. Half of the patient population had daily seizures. Dosage varied from 23 to 54 mg/kg/day. Seizures were controlled in 63% of all cases and a further 18% showed improvement greater than 50%. Of the 69 patients with 3 Hz spike-wave discharges, 81% became seizure free, as did 77% of those with myoclonic jerks. VPA also controlled the seizures in 8/32 patients with myoclonic-astatic epilepsy and 8/32 were improved greater than 50%. In this study, only 21 patients received VPA monotherapy from the start of treatment and all other drugs were withdrawn in another 38.

Dulac *et al.* analysed 154 children (mean age of 6 years) who were followed on VPA monotherapy for a period ranging from 5 to 27 months (mean 22 months) [45]. In this open-label study all types of partial and generalized epilepsies were included. Children with generalized epilepsies (absence epilepsies, benign myoclonic epilepsies, epilepsies with tonic-clonic seizures on awakening) were the best controlled, followed by benign partial epilepsies and infantile spasms.

VPA is effective in controlling photosensitivity and abolishes it in more than half of the patients [46]. In patients with photosensitive seizures, total seizure control is attained in 84% of them [47].

VPA is considered the drug of first choice for patients with degenerative/metabolic myoclonic epilepsies (Lafora body, Univerricht–Lundborg, etc.), although this choice is based on anecdotal information [48].

Status epilepticus

Several reports have acknowledged the use of intravenous VPA in patients with convulsive or non-convulsive status epilepticus [49]. VPA is generally well tolerated and is not associated with adverse cardiovascular effects sometimes associated with the use of PHT [50]. However, due to the lack of controlled data, the role of VPA as a primary drug in the management of status epilepticus remains to be established. On the other hand, intravenous VPA appears to be a first choice for the treatment of absence status or myoclonic status.

Seizure-epilepsy prophylaxis

VPA has been successful in preventing febrile seizures [51]. However, continuous use of any AED is not warranted for this indication, due to poor benefit to risk ratio.

A RDBT has compared PHT and VPA as anticonvulsant prophylaxis after craniotomy [52]. Fifty patients in each group were included and were followed for a year after surgery. Patients were given 1500 mg/day of VPA and 300 mg/day of PHT. There were no significant differences in efficacy or tolerability between the drugs. Seven patients in each group experienced seizures and seizures were of similar severity.

Another RDBT has compared VPA with PHT for prevention of seizures following traumatic brain injury [53]. A total of 379 patients at high risk for seizures entered the study: 132 were assigned to receive a 1-week course of PHT, 120 a 1-month course of VPA and 127 a 6-month course of VPA. Patients were followed for up to 2 years. The rates of early seizures were similarly low using either VPA or PHT (1.5% in the PHT treatment group and 4.5% in the VPA arms of the study). The rates of late seizures did not differ among treatment groups (15% in patients receiving the 1-week course of PHT, 16% in patients receiving the 1-month course of VPA and 24% in those receiving the 6-month course of VPA). The rates of mortality were not significantly different between treatment groups, but there was a trend toward a higher mortality rate in patients treated with VPA (7.2% in patients on PHT and 13.4% on VPA). The incidence of serious adverse events, including coagulation problems and liver abnormalities, was similar in PHT- and VPA-treated patients. No significant adverse or beneficial neuropsychological effects of VPA were detected [54]. Thus, VPA showed no benefit over short-term PHT therapy for prevention of early seizures and neither treatment prevented late seizures. Current data on prophylaxis of epilepsy after traumatic injury or craniotomy does support short-term treatment (either with PHT or VPA) but not a long-term use [55].

Adverse events

Central nervous system adverse events

Somnolence, tremor and dizziness can occur in up to 25% of the patients treated with VPA, and most frequently are of mild severity. An intention–action tremor similar to essential tremor is the most characteristic adverse event, and it is usually dose dependent. Reducing the daily dosage of VPA or treatment with propanolol may be effective in controlling the tremor. Although VPA is not usually associated with drowsiness within the therapeutic range, some sedation may occur with serum levels above 100 µg/mL. There is, however, a wide variation in tolerance for VPA, and some patients complain of drowsiness at lower serum levels.

Cognition and psychomotor function

VPA has little effect on cognitive function and behaviour compared with other AEDs. In healthy volunteers VPA 800–1000 mg/day has minimal effects on psychomotor functions compared with placebo [56]. Cognitive functioning has also been assessed in adult patients with newly diagnosed partial epilepsy undergoing the Veteran Administration 264 study comparing VPA with CBZ [57]. This study showed no significant differences between VPA or CBZ on motor speed, coordination, memory, concentration and mental flexibility. There was no significant decline in neuropsychological performance from pretreatment baseline levels for either drug. In addition, there were no significant differences in performance between patients with low (mean, 52.8 µg/mL) and high (mean, 94.4 µg/mL) serum VPA levels. Thus, the impact on cognitive functioning of VPA monotherapy appears to be similar to CBZ and both drugs produce minimal negative effects.

Aldenkamp *et al.* compared the cognitive effects of VPA and TPM as adjunctive therapy to CBZ in a randomized observer-blinded clinical study [58]. Mean dose of VPA was 1384 mg/day and mean dose of TPM 251.1 mg/day. Patients on TPM had significantly worst short-term verbal memory and word recognition than those treated with VPA.

VPA effects on cognition have also been tested in children with new onset epilepsy. One study showed that VPA monotherapy can impair psychomotor performance at higher doses (27 vs. 16 mg/kg/day) [59]. However, the effect of VPA appears to be less than that of PB [60] or CBZ [61].

Encephalopathy

Occasional cases of encephalopathy have been reported in association to VPA, and some of these cases have led to coma [62]. Patients clinically present with asterixis, confusion, aggravation of pre-existing neurological deficits and increase in seizure frequency. Encephalopathy usually occurs in the first weeks of treatment but may appear months after the initiation of therapy. VPA serum concentrations are within normal limits. Ammonia is within normal limits, thus differentiating this event from hyperammonaemic encephalopathy (see below). EEG shows diffuse slowing and increase in the number of spike-wave discharges. This encephalopathy worsens if treated with benzodiazepines, and, in fact, an improvement with flumazenil (benzodiazepine receptor antagonist) has been reported.

Systemic adverse events

Most frequent adverse events with VPA are related to gastrointestinal tolerability (nausea, dyspepsia, diarrhoea, vomiting, anorexia, abdominal pain). Gastrointestinal complaints are especially frequent at treatment initiation (in up to 45% of the patients) and of variable severity. These adverse events are much less frequent using the enteric-coated formulation [63].

Alopecia

VPA can precipitate alopecia in up to 12% of patients in a dose-dependent manner. Alopecia appears to be dose dependent and at high VPA serum concentrations its incidence may reach 28% of the treated patients. In addition, VPA can change hair colour and structure. In general, discontinuation of the medication or dose reduction almost always leads to complete hair regrowth. The therapeutic value of mineral supplements is unclear [64].

Weight gain

Weight gain is relatively frequent in patients on VPA and appears in over half of those undergoing long-term treatment. A recent RDBT has compared weight gain in patients older than 12 years treated either with VPA or LTG [31]. Average VPA dose was 1822±633 mg/day (with an average plasma concentration of 90.2±45.4 μg/mL) and LTG dose of 254±69 mg/day (with an average plasma concentration of 4.1±2.9 μg/mL). Weight remained stable among LTG-treated patients, but a significant weight gain was observed among the VPA-treated patients within 10 weeks of treatment initiation. At 8 months mean weight gain among VPA-treated patients was 5.8±4.2 kg compared with 0.6±5.4 kg among those treated with LTG. Thirty eight per cent of the VPA-treated patients gained more than 10% of weight compared with 8% of the patients treated with LTG. Weight gain was observed in both men and women. It appears that weight gain is not correlated to plasma VPA concentration or dose. The cause of weight gain is not completely known and is probably multiple: increase in appetite and food intake, impaired β-oxidation of fatty acids with reduction of thermogenesis and, possibly, hyperinsulinaemia.

Hyperammonaemic encephalopathy

Asymptomatic elevation of ammonia is sometimes observed in patients treated with VPA and, when present, requires more frequent monitoring. Encephalopathy or coma has occasionally been observed in patients undergoing VPA treatment [65]. The disorder usually appears during the first weeks of therapy and is manifested by drowsiness, gastrointestinal symptoms and lethargy. Liver enzymes are normal or mildly elevated. A high degree of suspicion is necessary for diagnosing this entity and patients with excessive drowsiness should have an ammonia serum determination. VPA discontinuation and carnitine supplementation resolves the disorder [66].

Pancreatitis

Treatment with VPA may increase serum amylase concentration in up to 24% of the asymptomatic patients [67]. In these patients discontinuing VPA is not necessary provided that other pancreatic enzymes (elastase, lipase, trypsin) are within normal limits.

VPA has been rarely associated with fatal pancreatitis [67]. Pancreatitis usually presents with progressive epigastric pain, nausea and vomiting. Symptoms may occur for days, weeks or months. Asconape et al. [67] reviewed 39 patients with pancreatitis associated with VPA. Most cases (77%) occurred before the age of 20 years and a third of them in the first decade of life. Twenty-four per cent of these patients were treated with monotherapy. Approximately half of them had been exposed to VPA for less than 3 months and in two-thirds pancreatitis appeared during the first year of treatment. However, in six patients (18.8%) pancreatitis emerged after more than 2 years of treatment.

VPA pancreatitis appears to be an idiosyncratic reaction and is not dose or serum concentration related. In most of the cases the illness is mild to moderate and the patients recover promptly, although occasionally it has been fatal [67]. It is not appropriate to rechallenge patients with VPA after having suffered pancreatitis because all of them relapse [67].

Blood disorders

VPA has been associated with aplastic anaemia, thrombocytopenia, leucopenia, platelet dysfunction and low fibrinogen levels. Thrombocytopenia is relatively frequent occurring in up to 31% of patients with high serum VPA concentrations (80–150 μg/mL) [29]. VPA-related thrombocytopenia is usually dose related (appearing at high doses) and moderate [68]. There have been some case reports of haematoma and increased bleeding after surgery, possibly related to moderate thrombocytopenia and altered platelet function. However, a retrospective study on bleeding complications in a large sample (313 patients) of neurosurgical patients (111 receiving VPA) has shown no significant difference between patients treated with VPA and other patients in estimated blood loss during surgery or qualitative wound discharge postsurgery [69].

Hepatotoxicity

Dose-related elevation of liver enzymes has been detected in up to 44% of VPA-treated patients [70]. However, those elevations are usually not associated with clinical symptoms and resolve with drug reduction or withdrawal.

VPA has rarely been associated with severe liver damage and this adverse event has been extensively assessed by Dreifuss et al. in three consecutive epidemiological studies. They initially reviewed all cases of fatal hepatotoxicity coincident with VPA therapy that were reported in the USA between 1978 and 1984 [71]. They reported 37 hepatic fatalities coincident with the use of VPA. The highest risk of fatal hepatic dysfunction was found to be in children younger than 2 years old receiving VPA as polytherapy and with developmental delay (1/500). The risk declined with age and was low in patients receiving VPA as monotherapy (1/37 000). In a subsequent study, these authors continued the previous one analysing the period from 1985 to 1986 [72]. They observed a nearly fivefold decrease in the incidence of hepatic fatality during that period when the overall use of VPA had increased significantly. The incidence decreased from 1/10 000 in 1978–1984 to 0.2 per 10 000 in 1985–86. This reduction could be due to changes in the prescribing patterns of physicians in relation to the greater awareness of a higher risk in children and the use of monotherapy. A third subsequent study (1987–93) found 29 patients with fatal liver failure and confirmed the same risk factors for hepatotoxicity [73]. In these studies no hepatic fatalities associated with VPA monotherapy occurred in patients above the age of 10 years. However, cases of fatal liver toxicity have exceptionally been reported in adults [74]. Thus, high risk factors for VPA-related hepatotoxicity are: children aged less than 2 years, use in polytherapy, children with psychomotor retardation or certain metabolic disorders (organic acidaemias, mitochondrial disorders, etc.). As the pathology of the hepatic failure is similar to Reye's syndrome, avoidance of salicylates in patients treated with VPA is recommended.

Hepatotoxicity-associated VPA usually appears during the first 3 months of therapy [75]. Enzyme and bilirubin abnormalities are not a good predictor of serious hepatic involvement, but prolonged prothrombin time may provide a more accurate indicator [75]. The pathology is microvesicular steatosis with necrosis. Liver damage induced by VPA appears to be caused by an unsaturated metabolite of the drug (2-n-propyl-4-pentenoic acid) that is a potent inducer of microvesicular steatosis. However, routine measurement of metabolites has not been useful in predicting hepatic disease [76].

Therapy for VPA-related hepatotoxicity requires, in addition to the general supportive measures, infusion of intravenous L-carnitine (100 mg/kg/day, up to a maximum of 2 g/day) [77]. VPA induces serum and tissue depletion of carnitine through inhibition of cell membrane carnitine uptake. Oral L-carnitine has also been advocated for patients with symptomatic VPA-associated hyperammonaemia, patients with multiple risk factors for VPA hepatotoxicity, and infants and young children taking VPA [77].

Polycystic ovarian syndrome (PCOS)

There is evidence that PCOS (polycystic ovaries, hyperandrogenism, obesity, hirsutism, anovulatory cycles and menstrual disorders) occurs more frequently in women with epilepsy compared to the general female population (prevalence data of 13–25% versus 4–6%) [78]. PCOS was described in women with epilepsy treated with valproate, especially those who start treatment before 20 years of age [79,80]. In fact, VPA has been associated with alteration in the reproductive hormonal function beginning in the first month of treatment. Serum androgen concentrations increase in VPA-treated patients but with different profile of hormonal changes in women than in men. Animal studies have corroborated the adverse ovarian and endocrine changes of VPA [81].

The frequency of PCOS in VPA-treated women appears to be high: in a cross-sectional study on women on VPA monotherapy ($n=22$), 59% of the women on VPA were obese and 64% had poly-

cystic ovaries, hyperandrogenism or both [80]. Most of the abnormalities were reversed when VPA was discontinued [82].

Although the evidence of the association between PCOS and VPA treatment is solid, current published studies are limited due to the small sample size and the diverse definitions for PCOS. Thus, the true clinical relevance and frequency of the association needs further investigation by means of large multicentre prospective studies. Women undergoing treatment with VPA should be interrogated about menstrual disorders. The presence of a menstrual disorder, hirsutism or weight gain should trigger a thorough evaluation and if necessary VPA discontinuation.

Stimulation of the replication of human immunodeficiency virus (HIV)

It has been demonstrated that VPA may increase viral burden in infected individuals by potentiating replication of HIV. The clinical consequences of this effect for HIV-positive patients are unknown [83].

Bone resorption and low mineral bone density

A recent publication has reported a 14% reduction in bone mineral density during long-term treatment with VPA, both in men and women [84]. Its pathogenesis is unknown.

Parkinsonism

In some patients undergoing long-term treatment (more than 12 months) with VPA, varying degrees of parkinsonism and cognitive impairment have been observed. In one report, discontinuation of VPA in 32 affected patients led to subjective and objective improvement on follow-up testing [85].

Clinical therapeutics

Dosages (Table 46.3)

The recommended initial dose in adults is 500 mg daily, increasing at 2–3-day intervals by 250–500 mg. Maximum dosage is 2500 mg/day, although higher doses might be used in certain individuals. In children the starting dose is 20 mg/kg/day with increases of 10 mg/kg/day every 2–3 days to 40–60 mg/kg/day or even higher in certain situations (infantile spasms, for example). VPA is to be given twice a day, although three times a day is recommended for patients in polytherapy with enzyme-inducing AEDs. The sustained-release formulation allows once-a-day prescription. Gastrointestinal adverse events are minimized by administration with food, slow introduction and using the enteric-coated formulation.

Therapeutic plasma serum concentrations

The therapeutic range of VPA has been established to be between 40 and 100 mg/L (c. 300–700 μmol/L). However, the relationship between plasma concentration and clinical response is not well documented and has been largely based on poorly controlled studies of patients on polytherapy.

Table 46.3 Valproate dosing

	Adults	Children
Initiation of oral therapy	500 mg/day 10–15 mg/kg/day	20 mg/kg/day
Range of maintenance doses	500–2500 mg/day 20–30 mg/kg/day	20–60 mg/kg/day
Initiation of IV therapy	20 mg/kg in 5 min	20 mg/kg in 5 min
Maintenance of IV therapy	0.5 mg/kg/h, starting 30 min after loading dose (1 mg/kg/h if concomitant enzyme-inducing AED)	1 mg/kg/h, starting 30 min after loading dose (1.5 mg/kg/h if concomitant enzyme-inducing AED)

Two studies in patients on monotherapy have observed a significant linear correlation between VPA dose and serum concentration [86,87]. However, considerable interindividual variability in this ratio was demonstrated (coefficient of variation of 28.9%) and only 40% of the variance in plasma concentration could be attributed to dosage. This could be due to multiple factors: non-linear protein binding, large diurnal fluctuations of free fatty acids that displace VPA from proteins and the presence of active metabolites. However, even though patients receiving similar doses have large variations of serum concentrations, dose and plasma concentration are highly correlated in individual patients and thus clinically useful for monitoring compliance [87].

It is discussed if VPA plasma concentration is related to therapeutic effect [87,88]. A recent dose–response trial in a relatively large population has shown that there is a plasma concentration–response relationship in patients with refractory partial seizures [29]. Adverse effects were also more common in patients with higher dose/serum concentration. Low VPA serum concentrations (25–50 µg/mL) may, nevertheless be sufficient for adequate control of patients with less refractory epilepsy, as is frequently observed in patients with idiopathic generalized epilepsies or recent onset partial epilepsy [23,88]. Thus, the optimum dosage is to be determined by seizure control and the occurrence of adverse effects. VPA serum concentrations could be useful for testing compliance, evaluating adverse events and for dose adjustment in patients on polytherapy.

Contraindications and precautions

A whole blood count, liver enzymes and coagulation parameters should be available before initiating therapy with VPA. In patients using high VPA doses, periodic monitoring of platelets is suggested. In patients with persistent gastrointestinal upset, pancreatic enzymes (amylase, lipase, elastase) and serum ammonia concentration should be obtained.

VPA in contraindicated in patients with hepatic disease or with chronic pancreatitis. VPA in children younger than 2 years should be used with caution and close monitoring.

Pregnancy

Animal studies have demonstrated VPA-induced teratogenicity. The most common abnormalities observed have been malformations of the skeletal systems, although other systems can be affected. As with other AEDs, growth retardation and death in the offspring have also been observed. However, the role played by the AEDs and by the underlying disease *per se* have to be taken into account. Women treated with VPA have a 1–2% increased risk of spina bifida in the offspring. In addition, other congenital anomalies (cardiovascular malformations, craniofacial defects, etc.) have been reported [89]. Prospective studies have shown a significant relationship between the incidence of spina bifida and the maternal daily dosage or dose per administration of valproate and serum peak levels [90]. As a result of these findings, practical advice should be given to women with epilepsy treated with VPA and who are planning to conceive [91]: optimum seizure control should be reached with monotherapy by the lowest effective dose (dose under 1000 mg daily having shown to be associated with a lower incidence of spina bifida). Moreover, the required daily dose should be divided into three or more administrations per day to avoid high peak plasma levels of VPA and it is recommended that the controlled release formulation of VPA which reduces peak plasma concentrations should be used in women planning to become pregnant.

Fertile women should be advised that all classic AEDs have an increased potential for offspring malformation and on the use of systematic folate supplementation for reducing the risk of neural tube defects [92]. If this decision is made supplementation should be commenced 4 weeks prior to conception.

During pregnancy close monitoring with frequent serum concentrations and if possible free (unbound) VPA serum concentrations is suggested. Alpha-fetoprotein determination and high-resolution ultrasound may allow early diagnosis of malformations [92].

Role of VPA in antiepileptic therapy

VPA is considered a first-line agent for the treatment of generalized epilepsies (childhood and juvenile absence epilepsy, juvenile myoclonic epilepsy, benign myoclonic epilepsy in infants, myoclonic astatic epilepsy, epilepsy with myoclonic absences, eyelid myoclonia with absences), progressive myoclonus epilepsy and photosensitive epilepsy. LTG appears to have similar efficacy and has been proposed as an alternative to VPA in these disorders. In fact, LTG has demonstrated efficacy in childhood absence epilepsy (in a placebo-controlled double-blind trial [93]), juvenile myoclonic epilepsy (open studies [94]) and in the treatment-resistant generalized epilepsy (double-blind trial [95]). However, LTG can aggravate severe myoclonic epilepsy or progressive myoclonic epilepsies [96]. LTG may not be associated with the hormonal changes associated with VPA, but has a much higher risk of severe skin reaction, especially in children. Due to the absence of trials comparing VPA with LTG in the treatment of generalized epilepsies, the choice rests in the particular patient condition and in the experience of the physician.

VPA is considered a first-line agent for the treatment of localization-related epilepsies. In clinical trials VPA have been found as effective as PHT, PB, OXC, VGB and LTG. In one RDBT, CBZ was found to be as effective as VPA for secondarily generalized seizures but more effective for partial seizures. From this trial, many neurologists have been prescribing CBZ as the first agent for localization-related epilepsies. However, the methodological limitations of the trial do not support with certainty the superiority of CBZ over VPA. A recent meta-analysis of the randomized trials comparing CBZ with VPA in monotherapy has shown that there is no overall difference between both drugs. In any case, confidence intervals are too wide to confirm equivalence [97]. In fact, the choice of drug depends on a risk–benefit analysis for the particular patient.

VPA and VGB are first-line agents for West's syndrome [36]. No direct comparison has been conducted between both drugs in this indication. VPA is also considered the drug of first choice for Lennox–Gastaut syndrome. Although newer AEDs (TPM, LTG and FLM) have also demonstrated efficacy for this indication through RDBT, there are no comparative trials for this indication.

In conclusion, VPA is a first-line wide-spectrum AED. In recent years, and after decades of extensive use, high efficacy on the broadest spectrum of epilepsy and seizure types has been confirmed but new adverse events have also emerged with time (teratogenesis, liver failure in infants, pancreatitis, PCOS, etc.). In most cases, patients at risk for these adverse events, or methods to prevent or diagnose them early, have been described. Newer AEDs with wide-spectrum efficacy have a different safety profile without some of the adverse events associated with VPA. Nevertheless, other yet undisclosed adverse events might emerge with years of use in large populations. Thus the clinician is now challenged with the choice between a well-known safety profile drug versus a possibly safer new one with a complete safety profile yet to be discovered.

References

1 Vreugdenhil M, Wadman WJ. Modulation of sodium currents in rat CA1 neurons by carbamazepine and valproate after kindling epileptogenesis. *Epilepsia* 1999; 40: 1512–22.

2 Silver JM, Shin C, McNamara JO. Antiepileptogenic effects of conventional anticonvulsants in the kindling model of epilepsy. *Ann Neurol* 1991; 29(4): 356–63.

3 Sato S, White BG, Penry JK, Dreifuss FE, Sackellares JC, Kupferberg HJ. Valproic acid versus ethosuximide in the treatment of absence seizures. *Neurology* 1982; 32: 157–63.

4 Jeavons PM, Bishop A, Harding GF. The prognosis of photosensitivity. *Epilepsia* 1986; 27(5): 569–75.

5 Davis R, Peters DH, McTavish D. Valproic acid. A reappraisal of its pharmacological properties and clinical efficacy in epilepsy. *Drugs* 1994; 47: 332–72.

6 Hussein Z, Mukherjee D, Lamm J, Cavanaugh JH, Granneman GR. Pharmacokinetics of valproate after multiple-dose oral and intravenous infusion administration: gastrointestinal-related diurnal variation. *J Clin Pharmacol* 1994; 34(7): 754–9.

7 Sokolova S, Schmitz D, Zhang CL, Loscher W, Heinemann U. Comparison of effects of valproate and trans-2-en-valproate on different forms of epileptiform activity in rat hippocampal and temporal cortex slices. *Epilepsia* 1998; 39: 251–8.

8 Bowdle AT, Patel IH, Levy RH, Wilensky AJ. Valproic acid dosage and plasma protein binding and clearance. *Clin Pharmacol Ther* 1980; 28(4): 486–92.

9 Klotz U, Rapp T, Muller WA. Disposition of valproic acid in patients with liver disease. *Eur J Clin Pharmacol* 1978; 13(1): 55–60.

10 Bowdle TA, Patel IH, Levy RH, Wilensky AJ. The influence of free fatty acids on valproic acid plasma protein binding during fasting in normal humans. *Eur J Clin Pharmacol* 1982; 23(4): 343–7.

11 Loscher W, Fisher JE, Nau H, Honack D. Valproic acid in amygdala-kindled rats: alterations in anticonvulsant efficacy, adverse effects and drug and metabolite levels in various brain regions during chronic treatment. *J Pharmacol Exp Ther* 1989; 250(3): 1067–78.

12 Rowan AJ, Binnie CD, Warfield CA, Meinardi H, Meijer JW. The delayed effect of sodium valproate on the photoconvulsive response in man. *Epilepsia* 1979; 20(1): 61–8.

13 Kanner AM, Frey M. Adding valproate to lamotrigine: a study of their pharmacokinetic interaction. *Neurology* 2000; 55: 588–91.

14 Brodie MJ, Yuen AW. Lamotrigine substitution study: evidence for synergism with sodium valproate? 105 Study Group. *Epilepsy Res* 1997; 26: 423–32.

15 Wilder BJ, Ramsay RE, Murphy JV, Karas BJ, Marquardt K, Hammond EJ. Comparison of valproic acid and phenytoin in newly diagnosed tonic-clonic seizures. *Neurology* 1983; 33: 1474–6.

16 Crawford P, Chadwick D. A comparative study of progabide, valproate, and placebo as add-on therapy in patients with refractory epilepsy. *J Neurol Neurosurg Psychiatr* 1986; 49: 1251–7.

17 Turnbull DM, Howel D, Rawlins MD, Chadwick DW. Which drug for the adult epileptic patient: phenytoin or valproate? *Br Med J (Clin Res Ed)* 1985; 290: 815–19.

18 Loiseau P, Cohadon S, Jogeix M, Legroux M, Dartigues JF. Efficacité du valproate de sodium dans les épilepsies partielles. *Rev Neurol (Paris)* 1984; 140: 434–7.

19 Callaghan N, Kenny RA, O'Neill B, Crowley M, Goggin T. A prospective study between carbamazepine, phenytoin and sodium valproate as monotherapy in previously untreated and recently diagnosed patients with epilepsy. *J Neurol Neurosurg Psychiatr* 1985; 48: 639–44.

20 Turnbull DM, Rawlins MD, Weightman D, Chadwick DW. A comparison of phenytoin and valproate in previously untreated adult epileptic patients. *J Neurol Neurosurg Psychiatr* 1982; 45: 55–9.

21 Livanainen M, Waltimo O, Tokola O et al. A controlled study with taltrimide and sodium valproate: valproate effective in partial epilepsy. *Acta Neurol Scand* 1990; 82: 121–5.

22 Richens A, Davidson DL, Cartlidge NE, Easter DJ. A multicentre comparative trial of sodium valproate and carbamazepine in adult onset epilepsy. Adult EPITEG Collaborative Group. *J Neurol Neurosurg Psychiatr* 1994; 57: 682–7.

23 Heller AJ, Chesterman P, Elwes RDC et al. Phenobarbitone, phenytoin, carbamazepine, or sodium valproate for newly diagnosed adult epilepsy: a randomised comparative monotherapy trial. *J Neurol Neurosurg Psychiatr* 1995; 58: 44–50.

24 Gram L, Wulff K, Rasmussen KE et al. Valproate sodium: a controlled clinical trial including monitoring of drug levels. *Epilepsia* 1977; 18(2): 141–8.

25 Richens A, Ahmad S. Controlled trial of sodium valproate in severe epilepsy. *Br Med J* 1975; 4: 255–6.

26 Willmore LJ, Shu V, Wallin B. Efficacy and safety of add-on divalproex sodium in the treatment of complex partial seizures. The M88-194 Study Group [see comments]. *Neurology* 1996; 46: 49–53.

27 Mattson RH, Cramer JA, Collins JF. A comparison of valproate with carbamazepine for the treatment of complex partial seizures and secondarily generalized tonic-clonic seizures in adults. The Department of Veterans Affairs Epilepsy Cooperative Study No. 264 Group. *N Engl J Med* 1992; 327: 765–71.

28 Brodie MJ, Mumford JP. Double-blind substitution of vigabatrin and valproate in carbamazepine-resistant partial epilepsy. 012 Study group. *Epilepsy Res* 1999; 34: 199–205.

29 Beydoun A, Sackellares JC, Shu V. Safety and efficacy of divalproex sodium monotherapy in partial epilepsy: a double-blind, concentration-response design clinical trial. Depakote Monotherapy for Partial Seizures Study Group. *Neurology* 1997; 48: 182–8.

30 Christe W, Kramer G, Vigonius U et al. A double-blind controlled clinical trial: oxcarbazepine versus sodium valproate in adults with newly diagnosed epilepsy. *Epilepsy Res* 1997; 26: 451–60.

31 Biton V, Mirza W, Montouris G, Vuong A, Hammer AE, Barrett PS. Weight

change associated with valproate and lamotrigine monotherapy in patients with epilepsy. *Neurology* 2001; 56(2): 172–7.

32 Verity CM, Hosking G, Easter DJ. A multicentre comparative trial of sodium valproate and carbamazepine in paediatric epilepsy. The Paediatric EPITEG Collaborative Group. *Dev Med Child Neurol* 1995; 37: 97–108.

33 Reynolds EH, Heller AJ, Chadwick D. Valproate versus carbamazepine for seizures. *N Engl J Med* 1993; 328(3): 207–8.

34 de Silva M, MacArdle B, McGowan M *et al*. Randomised comparative monotherapy trial of phenobarbitone, phenytoin, carbamazepine, or sodium valproate for newly diagnosed childhood epilepsy. *Lancet* 1996; 347: 709–13.

35 Callaghan N, O'Hare J, O'Driscoll D, O'Neill B, Daly M. Comparative study of ethosuximide and sodium valproate in the treatment of typical absence seizures (petit mal). *Dev Med Child Neurol* 1982; 24(6): 830–6.

36 Schmidt D, Bourgeois B. A risk-benefit assessment of therapies for Lennox–Gastaut syndrome. *Drug Saf* 2000; 22(6): 467–77.

37 Vassella F, Rudeberg A, Da SV, Pavlincova E. [Double-blind study on the anti-convulsive effect of phenobarbital and valproate in the Lennox syndrome]. *Schweiz Med Wochenschr* 1978; 108(19): 713–16.

38 Dyken PR, DuRant RH, Minden DB, King DW. Short term effects of valproate on infantile spasms. *Pediatr Neurol* 1985; 1: 34–7.

39 Prats JM, Garaizar C, Rua MJ, Garcia-Nieto ML, Madoz P. Infantile spasms treated with high doses of sodium valproate: initial response and follow-up. *Dev Med Child Neurol* 1991; 33(7): 617–25.

40 Siemes H, Spohr HL, Michael T, Nau H. Therapy of infantile spasms with valproate: results of a prospective study. *Epilepsia* 1988; 29(5): 553–60.

41 Salas PJ, Tunon A, Vidal JA, Mateos V, Guisasola LM, Lahoz CH. Janz's juvenile myoclonic epilepsy: a little-known frequent syndrome. A study of 85 patients. *Med Clin (Barc)* 1994; 103: 684–9.

42 Penry JK, Dean JC, Riela AR. Juvenile myoclonic epilepsy: long-term response to therapy. *Epilepsia* 1989; 30 (Suppl. 4): S19–23; discussion S24–7, S19–S23.

43 Sundqvist A, Tomson T, Lundkvist B. Valproate as monotherapy for juvenile myoclonic epilepsy: dose-effect study. *Ther Drug Monit* 1998; 20: 149–57.

44 Jeavons PM, Clark JE, Maheshwari MC. Treatment of generalized epilepsies of childhood and adolescence with sodium valproate ('epilim'). *Dev Med Child Neurol* 1977; 19: 9–25.

45 Dulac O, Steru D, Rey E, Perret A, Arthuis M. Sodium valproate monotherapy in childhood epilepsy. *Brain Dev* 1986; 8: 47–52.

46 Harding GF, Herrick CE, Jeavons PM. A controlled study of the effect of sodium valproate on photosensitive epilepsy and its prognosis. *Epilepsia* 1978; 19(6): 555–65.

47 Harding GF, Edson A, Jeavons PM. Persistence of photosensitivity. *Epilepsia* 1997; 38(6): 663–9.

48 Wallace SJ. Myoclonus and epilepsy in childhood: a review of treatment with valproate, ethosuximide, lamotrigine and zonisamide. *Epilepsy Res* 1998; 29: 147–54.

49 Chez MG, Hammer MS, Loeffel M, Nowinski C, Bagan BT. Clinical experience of three pediatric and one adult case of spike-and-wave status epilepticus treated with injectable valproic acid. *J Child Neurol* 1999; 14: 239–42.

50 Sinha S, Naritoku DK. Intravenous valproate is well tolerated in unstable patients with status epilepticus. *Neurology* 2000; 55: 722–4.

51 Mamelle N, Mamelle JC, Plasse JC, Revol M, Gilly R. Prevention of recurrent febrile convulsions—a randomized therapeutic assay: sodium valproate, phenobarbital and placebo. *Neuropediatrics* 1984; 15(1): 37–42.

52 Beenen LF, Lindeboom J, Trenit DG *et al*. Comparative double blind clinical trial of phenytoin and sodium valproate as anticonvulsant prophylaxis after craniotomy: efficacy, tolerability, and cognitive effects. *J Neurol Neurosurg Psychiatr* 1999; 67: 474–80.

53 Temkin NR, Dikmen SS, Anderson GD *et al*. Valproate therapy for prevention of posttraumatic seizures: a randomized trial. *J Neurosurg* 1999; 91: 593–600.

54 Dikmen SS, Machamer JE, Winn HR, Anderson GD, Temkin NR. Neuropsychological effects of valproate in traumatic brain injury: a randomized trial. *Neurology* 2000; 54: 895–902.

55 Temkin NR. Antiepileptogenesis and seizure prevention trials with antiepileptic drugs: meta-analysis of controlled trials. *Epilepsia* 2001; 42(4): 515–24.

56 Thompson PJ, Trimble MR. Sodium valproate and cognitive functioning in normal volunteers. *Br J Clin Pharmacol* 1981; 12(6): 819–24.

57 *Prevey ML, Delaney RC, Cramer JA, Cattanach L, Collins JF, Mattson RH. Effect of valproate on cognitive functioning. Comparison with carbamazepine. The Department of Veterans Affairs Epilepsy Cooperative Study 264 Group. *Arch Neurol* 1996; 53: 1008–16.

58 Aldenkamp AP, Baker G, Mulder OG *et al*. A multicenter, randomized clinical study to evaluate the effect on cognitive function of topiramate compared with valproate as add-on therapy to carbamazepine in patients with partial-onset seizures. *Epilepsia* 2000; 41(9): 1167–78.

59 Aman MG, Werry JS, Paxton JW, Turbott SH. Effect of sodium valproate on psychomotor performance in children as a function of dose, fluctuations in concentration, and diagnosis. *Epilepsia* 1987; 28(2): 115–24.

60 Vining EPG, Mellits ED, Dorsen MM *et al*. Psychologic and behavioral effects of antiepileptic drugs in children: A double-blind comparison between phenobarbital and valproic acid. *Pediatrics* 1987; 80: 165–74.

61 Forsythe I, Butler R, Berg I, McGuire R. Cognitive impairment in new cases of epilepsy randomly assigned to carbamazepine, phenytoin and sodium valproate. *Dev Med Child Neurol* 1991; 33: 524–34.

62 Marescaux C, Warter JM, Micheletti G, Rumbach L, Coquillat G, Kurtz D. Stuporous episodes during treatment with sodium valproate: report of seven cases. *Epilepsia* 1982; 23(3): 297–305.

63 Wilder BJ, Karas BJ, Penry JK, Asconape J. Gastrointestinal tolerance of divalproex sodium. *Neurology* 1983; 33: 808–11.

64 Mercke Y, Sheng H, Khan T, Lippmann S. Hair loss in psychopharmacology. *Ann Clin Psychiatr* 2000; 12(1): 35–42.

65 Duarte J, Macias S, Coria F, Fernandez E, Claveria LE. Valproate-induced coma: case report and literature review. *Ann Pharmacother* 1993; 27: 582–3.

66 De VD, Bohan TP, Coulter DL *et al*. L-carnitine supplementation in childhood epilepsy: current perspectives. *Epilepsia* 1998; 39: 1216–25.

67 Asconape JJ, Penry JK, Dreifuss FE, Riela A, Mirza W. Valproate-associated pancreatitis. *Epilepsia* 1993; 34: 177–83.

68 Delgado MR, Riela AR, Mills J, Browne R, Roach ES. Thrombocytopenia secondary to high valproate levels in children with epilepsy. *J Child Neurol* 1994; 9: 311–14.

69 Anderson GD, Lin YX, Berge C, Ojemann GA. Absence of bleeding complications in patients undergoing cortical surgery while receiving valproate treatment. *J Neurosurg* 1997; 87: 252–6.

70 Sussman NM, McLain LW. A direct hepatotoxic effect of valproic acid. *JAMA* 1979; 242: 1173–4.

71 Dreifuss FE, Santilli N, Langer DH, Sweeney KP, Moline KA, Menander KB. Valproic acid hepatic fatalities: a retrospective review. *Neurology* 1987; 37(3): 379–85.

72 Dreifuss FE, Langer DH, Moline KA, Maxwell JE. Valproic acid hepatic fatalities. II. US experience since 1984. *Neurology* 1989; 39(2 Pt 1): 201–7.

73 Bryant AE, Dreifuss FE. Valproic acid hepatic fatalities. III. US experience since 1986. *Neurology* 1996; 46: 465–9.

74 Konig SA, Schenk M, Sick C *et al*. Fatal liver failure associated with valproate therapy in a patient with Friedreich's disease: review of valproate hepatotoxicity in adults. *Epilepsia* 1999; 40: 1036–40.

75 Dreifuss FE, Langer DH. Hepatic considerations in the use of antiepileptic drugs. *Epilepsia* 1987; 28 (Suppl. 2): S23–9.

76 Tennison MB, Miles MV, Pollack GM, Thorn MD, Dupuis RE. Valproate metabolites and hepatotoxicity in an epileptic population. *Epilepsia* 1988; 29(5): 543–7.

77 De Vivo DC, Bohan TP, Coulter DL *et al*. L-Carnitine supplementation in childhood epilepsy: currrent perspectives. *Epilepsia* 1998; 39: 1216–25.

78 Herzog AG, Schachter SC. Valproate and the polycystic ovarian syndrome: final thoughts. *Epilepsia* 2001; 42(3): 311–15.

79 Isojarvi JI, Laatikainen TJ, Pakarinen AJ, Juntunen KT, Myllyla VV. Polycystic ovaries and hyperandrogenism in women taking valproate for epilepsy. *N Engl J Med* 1993; 329(19): 1383–8.

80 Isojarvi JI, Laatikainen TJ, Knip M, Pakarinen AJ, Juntunen KT, Myllyla VV. Obesity and endocrine disorders in women taking valproate for epilepsy. *Ann Neurol* 1996; 39: 579–84.

81 Roste LS, Tauboll E, Berner A, Isojarvi JI, Gjerstad L. Valproate, but not lamotrigine, induces ovarian morphological changes in Wistar rats. *Exp Toxicol Pathol* 2001; 52(6): 545–52.

82 Isojarvi JI, Rattya J, Myllyla VV *et al*. Valproate, lamotrigine, and insulin-mediated risks in women with epilepsy. *Ann Neurol* 1998; 43: 446–51.

83 Jennings HR, Romanelli F. The use of valproic acid in HIV-positive patients. *Ann Pharmacother* 1999; 33: 1113–16.

84 Sato Y, Kondo I, Ishida S *et al*. Decreased bone mass and increased bone turnover with valproate therapy in adults with epilepsy. *Neurology* 2001; 57: 445–9.

85 Armon C, Shin C, Miller P *et al*. Reversible parkinsonism and cognitive impairment with chronic valproate use. *Neurology* 1996; 47: 626–35.

86 Tisdale JE, Tsuyuki RT, Oles KS, Penry JK. Relationship between serum concentration and dose of valproic acid during monotherapy in adult outpatients. *Ther Drug Monit* 1992; 14(5): 416–23.

87 Turnbull DM, Rawlins MD, Weightman D, Chadwick DW. Plasma concentrations of sodium valproate: their clinical value. *Ann Neurol* 1983; 14(1): 38–42.

88 Gram L, Flachs H, Wurtz-Jorgensen A, Parnas J, Andersen B. Sodium valproate, serum level and clinical effect in epilepsy: a controlled study. *Epilepsia* 1979; 20(3): 303–11.

89 Lindhout D, Meinardi H, Meijer JW, Nau H. Antiepileptic drugs and teratogenesis in two consecutive cohorts: changes in prescription policy paralleled by changes in pattern of malformations. *Neurology* 1992; 42: 94–110.

90 Lindhout D, Omtzigt JGC. Pregnancy and the risk of teratogenicity. *Epilepsia* 1992; 33 (Suppl. 33): S41–S48.

91 American Academy of Neurology. Practice Parameter: management issues for women with epilepsy (summary statement). Report of the Quality Standards Subcommittee of the American Academy of Neurology. *Neurology* 1998; 51: 944–8.

92 Zahn CA, Morrell MJ, Collins SD, Labiner DM, Yerby MS. Management issues for women with epilepsy: a review of the literature. *Neurology* 1998; 51: 949–56.

93 Frank LM, Enlow T, Holmes GL *et al*. Lamictal (lamotrigine) monotherapy for typical absence seizures in children. *Epilepsia* 1999; 40: 973–9.

94 Buchanan N. The use of lamotrigine in juvenile myoclonic epilepsy. *Seizure* 1996; 5: 149–51.

95 Beran RG, Berkovic SF, Dunagan FM *et al*. Double-blind, placebo-controlled, crossover study of lamotrigine in treatment-resistant generalised epilepsy. *Epilepsia* 1998; 39: 1329–33.

96 Guerrini R, Dravet C, Genton P, Belmonte A, Kaminska A, Dulac O. Lamotrigine and seizure aggravation in severe myoclonic epilepsy. *Epilepsia* 1998; 39: 508–12.

97 Marson AG, Williamson PR, Hutton JL, Clough HE, Chadwick DW. Carbamazepine versus valproate monotherapy for epilepsy. In: *The Cochrane Library*, 1. 2001. Oxford: Update Software.

47 Vigabatrin

G. Krämer

Primary indications	Adjunctive therapy in partial and secondarily generalized epilepsy. Also for infantile spasm and Lennox–Gastaut syndrome
Usual preparations	Tablets: 500 mg; powder sachet: 500 mg
Usual dosages	Initial: 1000 mg/day (adults). Maintenance: 1000–3000 mg/day (adults); 40 mg/kg/day (children) or 500–1000 mg/day (body weight 10–15 kg), 1000–1500 mg (body weight 15–30 kg), 1500–3000 mg (body weight over 30 kg)
Dosage intervals	2 times/day
Significant drug interactions	Vigabatrin may lower phenytoin levels
Serum level monitoring	Not useful
Target range	–
Common/important side-effects	Sedation, dizziness, headache, ataxia, paraesthesia, agitation, amnesia, mood change, depression, psychosis, aggression, confusion, weight gain, insomnia, changes in muscle tone in children, tremor, diplopia, severe visual field constriction
Main advantages	Highly effective recently introduced antiepileptic drug
Main disadvantages	CNS side-effects and visual field constriction
Mechanisms of action	Inhibition of GABA transaminase activity
Oral bioavailability	<100%
Time to peak levels	0.5–2 h
Metabolism and excretion	Renal excretion without metabolism
Volume of distribution	0.8 L/kg
Elimination half-life	4–7 h
Plasma clearance	0.102–0.114 L/kg/h
Protein binding	None
Active metabolites	None
Comment	Highly effective antiepileptic drug whose usage is limited by potential for neuropsychiatric side-effects and effects on visual field

(*Note*: this summary table was formulated by the lead editor.)

γ-Aminobutyric acid (GABA) is the major inhibitory neurotransmitter in the mammalian brain. Vigabatrin (γ-vinyl-GABA, 4-amino-5-hexenoic acid; VGB) was synthesized in 1974 as a structural GABA analogue with a vinyl appendage. The aim was to achieve enzyme-activated inhibition of GABA catabolism. It has been regarded as a prime example of a drug developed on a rational scientific basis for treatment of a disease. VGB was first marketed for adults in the UK in 1989 and thereafter in most European countries. The application was extended in 1990 to the use of VGB in children suffering from refractory epilepsy, and later to its use as monotherapy for infantile spasms. Although VGB has been approved in over 65 countries worldwide, its usage has currently declined dramatically because of the detection of persistent peripheral visual field defects (VFD) in up to 40% of the patients.

Pharmacology and mechanism of action

Pharmacology

VGB is a white to off-white crystalline amino acid which is highly water soluble and only slightly soluble in ethanol and methanol. The molecular weight is 129.16, and the conversion factor is 7.75 (mg/L × 7.75 = μmol/L). VGB exists as a racemic mixture of S(+) and R(−)-enantiomers in equal proportions. The S(+)-enantiomer is responsible for the pharmacological and toxic effects and the R(−)-enantiomer is entirely inactive [1]. The only available forms of VGB are oral formulations (tablets and sachets, containing 500 mg).

Mechanism of action

VGB acts by replacing GABA as a substrate of GABA-transaminase (GABA-T). However, because VGB possesses an inert appendage it prevents the transamination of GABA to form succinic acid semialdehyde by irreversible and covalent binding to GABA-T, causing its permanent inactivation [2]. This results in prolonged elevation of brain GABA levels without any major influence on other enzymes involved in GABA synthesis and metabolism. The effect is maximal 3–4 h after administration and maintained for at least 24 h. Because GABA-T has a much longer half-life, the major pharmacological effects of VGB are determined not by the half-life of the drug itself but by that of GABA-T. Restoration of normal enzyme activity by resynthesis after withdrawal of VGB takes several days [3]. In addition, VGB significantly reduces the activity of the plasma alanine aminotransferase (ALAT) between 20 and 100% [4].

In patients with epilepsy, a dose-related (up to 3 g/day) elevation of free GABA, total GABA and homocarnosine (a dipeptide of GABA) in cerebrospinal fluid (CSF) levels could be demonstrated [5]. ^{1}H-MR spectroscopy has shown that the brain GABA content in the occipital region of patients with epilepsy increased two- to three-fold [6,7]. Increasing VGB dosage from 3 to 6 g/day did not result in a further increase in brain GABA concentrations, most probably because of a feedback inhibition of glutamic acid decarboxylase (GAD), the GABA-synthesizing enzyme, at high GABA concentrations.

Pharmacokinetics and drug interactions

Pharmacokinetics

Infants and children

Following single oral doses of 125 mg VGB racemate in six neonates, the mean values of C_{max} and AUC were significantly lower for the active S(+)-enantiomer whereas no difference was found for the time to reach peak plasma concentrations (t_{max}). Repeated administration of 125 mg twice daily over 4 days was without evidence of accumulation of either enantiomer [8]. A pharmacokinetic study after a single 50 mg/kg VGB dose in six infants (5–24 months old) and six children (4–14 years old) with intractable epilepsy showed comparable results as in adults, mainly with regard to the elimination of the active S(+)-enantiomer which seem to be age independent. In contrast to adults, in whom t_{max} of the inactive R(−)-enantiomer is about twice that of the active S(+)-enantiomer, no differences were found for t_{max} of the two allosteric forms in children. However, the mean AUC of the R(−)-enantiomer was also significantly greater. In addition, the AUC values for both isomers were significantly lower in infants than in children, which in turn were lower than in adults. Despite lower AUC values in children, pharmacokinetics of VGB appeared to be little influenced by age, and VGB accumulation during multiple dose administration (5 days) did not occur [9].

Adults

VGB is rapidly and almost completely absorbed from the gastrointestinal tract. Food does not influence absorption [10], and peak C_{max} are reached within 0.5–2 h after single doses [11]. AUC as well as C_{max} indicate linear pharmacokinetics over the dose range of 0.5–4 g. VGB is widely distributed in the body with a volume of distribution of 0.8 L/kg; levels in the CSF are approximately 10% of those in the blood [12]. It is neither bound to proteins nor does it influence the protein binding of other drugs or cytochrome P450-dependent enzymes. Elimination is primarily renal with a renal clearance of unchanged drug accounting for 60–70% of the total clearance, which indicates an oral bioavailability of at least that magnitude. The elimination half-life is between 5 and 7 h but, in patients taking hepatic enzyme-inducing drugs, slightly shorter half-life values of 4–6 h have been observed [13]. Because about 60% of the drug is removed from the blood during haemodialysis, VGB should be administered thereafter [14]. The passage of both enantiomers of VGB across the human placenta is slow, and the concentration ratio in breast milk compared to plasma for the active S(+)-enantiomer is below 0.5 [15].

Drug interactions

VGB has no effect on the plasma concentrations of valproate (VPA) [16], and felbamate (FBM) [17]. Usually there is also no effect on carbamazepine levels. After a latency of some weeks VGB reduces phenytoin (PHT) levels about 25% without altered absorption [18] or plasma protein binding [19]. In children with epilepsy, the drop of PHT levels can be even more pronounced [20]. Serum levels of phenobarbital and primidone can also be slightly reduced by VGB

[13]. VPA has no effect on VGB plasma levels [16] and, generally, nor do other established AEDs [21], although a shorter half-life of VGB in patients on enyzme-inducing drugs has been observed [13]. FBM leads to a slight increase of the active S(+)-enantiomer [17]. VGB has no effect on oral steroid contraceptives [22].

Drug monitoring

VGB concentrations can be determined in biological fluids by high-performance liquid chromatographic (HPLC) and gas chromatography–mass spectroscopy [23]. A sensitive HPLC method for the simultaneous determination of VGB and gabapentin in serum and urine has been described [24]. Plasma level does not correlate with clinical efficacy. In 16 children with refractory epilepsy there was no strong correlation between VGB dosages, plasma concentrations and clinical efficacy [25]; given its mode of action none would be expected.

Animal studies

The anticonvulsant effect of VGB has been studied in numerous animal models. It is inactive in models such as maximal electroshock or pentylenetetrazol, it protects against bicuculline-induced myoclonic activity, strychnine-induced tonic seizures, isoniazid-induced generalized seizures, audiogenic seizures in mice, light-induced seizures in the baboon and amygdala-kindled seizures in the rat [26].

The usual animal preclinical safety studies carried out in rats, mice, dogs and monkeys demonstrated no significant adverse effects on the liver, kidney, lung, heart or gastrointestinal tract. Studies revealed no evidence of mutagenic or carcinogenic effects. However, in the brain, microvacuolation has been observed in white matter tracts of rats, mice and dogs at doses of 30–50 mg/kg/day. In the monkey, these lesions were minimal or equivocal. This effect is caused by a separation of the outer lamellar sheath of myelinated fibres, a change characteristic of intramyelinic oedema. In both rats and dogs the intramyelinic oedema was reversible upon discontinuation of VGB, and even with continued treatment histological regression was observed. In rodents, minor residual changes consisting of swollen axons and mineralized microbodies have been observed [27,28].

VGB-associated retinotoxicity has been observed in albino rats, but not in pigmented rats, dogs or monkeys. The retinal changes in albino rats were characterized as focal or multifocal disorganization of the outer nuclear layer with displacement of nuclei into the rod and cone area. The other layers of the retina were not affected. Although the histological appearance of these lesions was similar to that found in albino rats following excessive exposure to light, the retinal changes may also represent a direct drug-induced effect [27].

Although there is no evidence of intramyelinic oedema in humans, the American Food and Drug Administration halted clinical studies with VGB because of these findings for 5 years between 1983 and 1988. Tests done to confirm lack of significant adverse effect on neurological function include evoked potentials, CT and MRI scans, and CSF analyses. Neuropathological studies have been carried out on patients who have died or who had epilepsy surgery during VGB treatment. Sixty case reports have been published comprising 10 postmortem and 50 surgical samples. Treatment periods were up to 108 months. None of the material examined has shown vacuolation [28,29].

Further animal experiments have shown that VGB has no negative influence on fertility or pup development. No teratogenicity was seen in rats at doses up to 150 mg/kg (3 times the human dose) or in rabbits in doses up to 100 mg/kg. However, in rabbits, a slight increase in the incidence of cleft palate at doses of 150–200 mg/kg was seen. Therefore, the usage of VGB is presently not recommended for women with childbearing potential [30].

Clinical studies

Infants and children

The approval of VGB in childhood refractory epilepsies in several countries has been granted on the basis of several open studies and compassionate experience [31]. Since the efficacy of VGB had been demonstrated in adults and the safety profile was reassuring in adults, it was not deemed necessary to repeat those studies in children. Nevertheless, the paediatric file was supplemented with two single-blind, placebo run-in dose-ranging studies [32,33] and one additional open dose-ranging study [34]. These studies also allowed for a better definition of the profile of activity of VGB in different types of resistant epilepsies, including the epileptic syndromes specific to childhood and for the assessment of the tolerability of VGB in children.

The two dose–response studies performed in a total of 86 children with refractory epilepsy [32,33] demonstrated an optimal efficacy at the first dose step (40–80 mg/kg/day, mean: 60 mg/kg/day), which is higher than in adults (35–65 mg/kg/day). Further dose increases in non-responders, although well tolerated, did not result in a higher number of patients being controlled.

On the basis of pharmacokinetic and dose–response studies, the following dosage regimen for children was recommended and approved: starting dose: 40 mg/kg/day, increasing to 80–100 mg/kg/day, depending on response. Children with partial seizures seemed to show similar benefits to those seen in adults with difficult-to-control partial epilepsy. Greater than 50% seizure suppression was seen in 38–54% of patients in three studies [31,34–36] but in more than 80% of the patients in the study of Herranz et al. [32]. VGB was effective against both simple and complex partial seizures and secondary generalization. Among different epilepsies, best efficacy was seen in localization-related epilepsies with symptomatic or cryptogenic aetiology. Anecdotal case reports described favourable effects in neonatal seizures due to Ohtahara syndrome [37] or Sturge–Weber syndrome [38].

Two double-blind, placebo-controlled, parallel design efficacy/safety studies in paediatric patients with treatment-resistant complex partial seizures with or without secondary generalization were recently completed in the US. There were four arms in protocol 118, placebo and three fixed-dose VGB groups, at 20, 60 and 100 mg/kg/day, respectively. All patients had uncontrolled seizures, VGB (or placebo) was administered as add-on treatment. VGB exhibited a linear dose–response trend in reducing mean seizures frequency ($P=0.057$). Although reductions in mean seizure frequency occurred in all VGB treatment groups, only the 100 mg/kg/day dose was statistically significantly more effective than placebo (median change in mean seizures frequency −5.00 vs. −2.75 for placebo; $P < 0.05$). In the 100 mg/kg/day group, therapeutic success rate was 56% versus 31% for placebo ($P < 0.05$), and both caregiver and investigator evaluations showed more improvement in VGB patients than placebo patients ($P < 0.05$). Adverse events occurred somewhat more frequently in the 100 mg/kg/day VGB group than placebo, but were mostly mild or moderate in severity and did not cause patient withdrawal from the study (Aventis, formerly Hoechst Marion Roussel, data on file, 1999).

The second study was a two-arm parallel trial with placebo and VGB administration in variable doses between 1.5 and 4.0 g/day, primarily dependent on body weight. The therapeutic success rate (defined as percentage of responders) was 50% with VGB and 27% with placebo ($P < 0.01$). Change in seizure-free days (number/28 days) was greater with VGB than placebo ($P < 0.01$), and caregiver evaluations showed improvement in significantly more patients receiving VGB than receiving placebo ($P < 0.05$) (Aventis, formerly Hoechst Marion Roussel, data on file, 1999).

There are several further add-on open-label studies of VGB in the treatment of uncontrolled epilepsies in children, which have been mostly published as abstracts. A single-blind, dose-increasing study in 46 children with refractory partial seizures demonstrated a decrease of the average monthly seizure rate from 97 during placebo add-on to 21, 12 and 9 after 2, 4 and 6 months of VGB treatment, respectively [20]. The study of Chiron et al. [39] was a randomized withdrawal study of placebo vs. VGB in children who had responded earlier to VGB. In these studies, over 50% decreases in seizure frequency were observed in 40–64% of the children. There were no differences in efficacy between children with simple or complex partial seizures and children with secondarily generalized seizures. Of the children 10–40% became seizure free.

Long-term efficacy data of VGB treatment in children who have been followed up to 6 years have been published. The findings in one of these studies (follow-up 1.5–5.5 years) of a cohort of 196 children with drug-resistant epilepsy and VGB as add-on therapy were as follows [40].

1 Increase of seizure frequency occurred in only 10% of patients, with half occurring during the first month of treatment. Patients with atypical absences had the highest incidence of increase in seizure frequency (38%) compared with less than 8% of those with partial seizures. Non-progressive myoclonic epilepsy and Lennox–Gastaut syndrome showed the greatest increase in seizure frequency, 38% and 29%, respectively.

2 Loss of efficacy was reported in 12% of children who were on VGB (25–50% of responders, some of them had been seizure free). Three-quarters of these patients had never had their seizures controlled prior to the introduction of VGB. Loss of efficacy was not connected to any specific seizure type except atypical absences and clonic seizures. The average time to reported loss of efficacy was 7 months. In 38%, the loss of efficacy was consecutive to an attempt to decrease concomitant antiepileptic medication.

3 Eleven per cent of the children developed new seizure types, mainly myoclonus and new partial seizures, after a quite variable time lag. Partial seizures were better tolerated than the initial seizure type and had little impact on the patient's overall clinical development.

The satisfactory results obtained with VGB in children with drug-resistant epilepsy have prompted some investigators to use it as first-line treatment in partial epilepsy. Preliminary uncontrolled data showed trends in favour of a disappearance of seizures in around 50% of patients with similar reported side-effects as in add-on therapy. However, no controlled study has been implemented so far to confirm these data. In addition, uncontrolled trials of VGB monotherapy after successful add-on effect have usually been disappointing (e.g. [36,41]).

Infantile spasms (West's syndrome)

There are three controlled studies on VGB in infantile spasms. Only one study was blinded, the other two studies were open label. All studies used cessation of infantile spasms by caregiver observation as the primary efficacy endpoint. Initial doses of VGB varied between 50 and 150 mg/kg/day, but in all studies dose was titrated up to 150 mg/kg/day.

In the blinded study in 40 children with newly diagnosed infantile spasms comparing VGB and placebo over 5 days [42], VGB showed only a slight and not statistically significant advantage over placebo using a 2-h intensive monitoring period. However, using a 24-h window based on observation of nursing staff or parents, VGB showed a large significant difference in seizure reduction. This difference was also supported by the investigator's overall assessment, which noted a marked or moderate improvement in 80% of VGB patients compared to 15% of placebo patients. Other efficacy measures (complete cessation of infantile spasms on the final treatment day and disappearance of hypsarrhythmia on the EEG) showed a trend toward advantage of VGB, but did not reach statistical significance [42].

The second randomized, prospective study compared VGB (100–150 mg/kg/day) with adrenocorticotrophic hormone (ACTH; 10 IU/day) as first-line therapy in 42 infants with infantile spasms [43]. In non-responders (within 20 days) or in cases of intolerance to the initial therapy, the alternative drug was administered. Contrary to the other two studies, only four out of 42 patients had symptomatic infantile spasms due to tuberous sclerosis, where VGB has its best efficacy [44]. Cessation of infantile spasms was observed in 48% (11/23) under VGB and 74% (14/19) under ACTH. The response to VGB was seen within 14 days. Follow-up data for up to 44 months showed only one relapse. In the ACTH group, when treatment was stopped after 40–45 days and replaced with a benzodiazepine, six patients had a relapse.

The third prospective randomized multicentre monotherapy study in 22 newly diagnosed patients [39] with an optional cross-over for non-responders showed a highly significant difference between oral hydrocortisone (15 mg/kg/day) and VGB (150 mg/kg/day) both before and after cross-over, with 100% (11/11) of patients on VGB but less than half (5/11) on hydrocortisone responding. All seven patients crossed from hydrocortisone to VGB (six for inefficacy, one for adverse events) and also became totally controlled. In addition, there was a statistically significant difference for the mean time to disappearance of infantile spasms favouring VGB (3.5 days vs. 13 days), and side-effects were less common.

In addition to these controlled studies, there have been many reports on VGB treatment in newly diagnosed or refractory infantile spasms. Most of the reports have been published either as an abstract or letter to editor and they included different patient groups regarding symptomatic or cryptogenic aetiology. In the fully published reports, the percentage of complete control of infantile spasms without relapse seemed to be comparable for newly diagnosed patients ([45]: 43%; [46]: 45%) and refractory patients ([47]: 43%; [48]: 48%).

Retrospective survey analyses were conducted of the safety and efficacy data from infantile spasm patients treated initially with VGB monotherapy at 59 European centres [49]. The dose of VGB in the efficacy evaluable patients ranged from 20 to 400 mg/kg/day (mean dose, 99 mg/kg/day) and the duration of therapy ranged from 0.2 to 28.6 months. Complete disappearance of infantile spasms was reported in 131/192 (68%) patients. Treatment with VGB did not result in any improvement in 24 (12.5%) patients and one patient deteriorated. Of the subgroups of infantile spasm, patients with tuberous sclerosis had the highest response rate (27/28 = 97%) and VGB was least effective in patients with dysplasia (45%). Of the 131 patients who demonstrated a complete initial response to VGB, 28 (21.3%) relapsed.

A prospective US study of VGB as initial therapy in newly diagnosed infantile spasms was designed as a randomized, open-label comparison of low-dose (18–36 mg/kg/day) and high-dose (up to 150 mg/kg/day) VGB. Preliminary efficacy data are available before a cut-off date of 30 June 1997 for 62 patients, 29 in the high-dose group and 33 in the low-dose group. In the first 2-week period of the study, 13/62 were free from infantile spasms by caregiver observation and EEG criteria. Five out of 33 (15%) low-dose patients and 8/29 (28%) of high-dose patients responded. The 62 patients were then also evaluated by caregiver report only (not to include EEG criteria). The total number of patients who were infantile spasm free, including both new responders and continuing responders, was 5/61 (8%) at 2 weeks, 19/58 (33%) at 1 month, 20/47 (43%) at 2 months and 26/43 (61%) at 3 months (Aventis, formerly Hoechst Marion Roussel, data on file, 1999).

In an open-label, prospective add-on study in 45 infants with refractory infantile spasms (2 months to 13 years of age, most < 2 years) VGB was titrated up to 105 mg/kg/day and treatment duration was up to 23 months. Two patients discontinued the study prematurely due to adverse events and were not included in the efficacy evaluation. At the end of the initial evaluation phase (mean duration of therapy, 3.8 months), 20/43 (47%) patients included in the efficacy analysis were seizure free. Of the eight patients with tuberous sclerosis, six (75%) were seizure free. Out of the 33 patients with adequate response to VGB who were entered into a long-term phase, decreased frequency of infantile spasms was maintained in 22 patients (Aventis, formerly Hoechst Marion Roussel, data on file, 1999).

The efficacy of a protocol using VGB as the first and ACTH or VPA as the second drug was studied in the patients with newly diagnosed infantile spasms in a population-based design. Only total disappearance of infantile spasms for a minimum duration of 1 month was accepted as treatment success, and the response was confirmed by video-EEG study. Altogether 42 infants, 10 with cryptogenic and 32 with symptomatic aetiology were treated. Eleven (26%) responded to VGB, five (50%) with cryptogenic and six (19%) with symptomatic aetiology. Ninety-one per cent of infants responded to doses of 50–100 mg/kg/day and 82% of them within 1 week. ACTH was given in combination with VGB to 22 and VPA to four infants who failed VGB. Eleven responded to ACTH and one to VPA. In total, 26 (62%) infants responded to the treatment protocol; all

(100%) with cryptogenic aetiology and 16 (50%) with symptomatic aetiology. ACTH treatment was associated with more severe side-effects than VGB or VPA. Only one infant relapsed after a spasm-free period on VGB of more than 4 months but none after ACTH was combined to VGB [50].

Lennox–Gastaut syndrome

In the treatment of children with Lennox–Gastaut syndrome, results have been controversial. In a first European add-on clinical study, 26 children with Lennox–Gastaut syndrome were included. Good seizure response was observed in less than 30% of them [31]. Only a small number of children with Lennox–Gastaut syndrome has been included in other studies, and most of them have not been regarded as treatment successes. A good response rate to VGB was observed in only one open study [51]. Twenty children aged 2–20 years with refractory Lennox–Gastaut syndrome were first treated with high-level VPA monotherapy, and after that for 12 months with add-on VGB. Eighty-five per cent experienced more than 50% seizure reduction and 40% became seizure free. A decrease by at least 50% was observed in all seizure types (tonic, atonic, atypical absences, tonic-clonic and complex partial seizures), except myoclonic seizures which increased by 5%. VGB may therefore play a limited role as add-on treatment in the management of Lennox–Gastaut syndrome but not in case of myoclonic seizures as the main seizure type.

The precipitation or exacerbation of myoclonic seizures, absence seizures and non-convulsive status epilepticus have also been reported [52,53]. Therefore, the prescription of VGB in idiopathic generalized epilepsies is not recommended and has been mentioned as a contraindication in some countries.

Adults

Clinical studies with VGB have included over 2000 patients. After initial open and single-blind dose finding studies, several randomized, double-blind, placebo-controlled crossover studies in adult patients with refractory partial epilepsies and add-on therapy with VGB were conducted.

An Australian study in 97 patients with uncontrolled partial seizures comparing 2 and 3 g/day showed a similar efficacy with 42% of the patients experiencing a 50% or greater reduction of their seizure frequency in comparison to placebo. In addition, the number of seizure-free days and longest seizure-free period were significantly longer during VGB and more patients had less severe and shorter seizures [54].

In addition to the crossover studies, several double-blind, placebo-controlled parallel group studies were carried out. The therapeutic efficacy of VGB add-on in treatment-resistant epilepsy, as assessed by the percentage of patients having at least a 50% reduction in seizure frequency, was quite similar across the studies with about 40% of patients being responders (for review of the earlier studies see [44,55,56]). In the first of more recent studies from the US 92 patients received VGB 3 g/day add-on and were compared to 90 patients in the placebo group [57]. Significantly more patients under VGB were responders with 50–99% reduction of seizure frequency (37% vs. 18%) or seizure freedom (6% vs. 1%). The second study examined three different VGB daily doses (1, 3 or 6 g) in a total of 174 patients [58]. Whereas only 7% in the placebo group were responders, the corresponding figures for the VGB groups were 24, 51 and 54%.

A double-blind, double-dummy substitution trial comparing add-on VGB (2–4 g daily) and VPA (1–2 g daily) in CBZ-resistant partial epilepsy allowing withdrawal of CBZ in responders showed similar percentages of responders (53% vs. 51%) and maintanance of alternative monotherapy (27% vs. 31%) [59].

Two open, single-centre randomized monotherapy studies using CBZ as comparator included 100 [60] and 51 patients [61], respectively. Both studies failed to show differences in efficacy, but demonstrated a more favourable side-effect profile of VGB (prior to the knowledge of VFDs related to VGB). In addition, several open, long-term studies on the add-on use of VGB in adult patients with treatment-resistant partial epilepsy have been reported. The length of the follow-up varied between 9 and 78 weeks. Most of the patients included had a favourable initial response to VGB, which was maintained in 22–75% of the patients.

More recently, two larger randomized, double-blind, parallel-group studies have been carried out to compare the efficacy of VGB as monotherapy with CBZ and VPA in newly diagnosed epilepsy. In the VGB/CBZ study, 53% of the 229 patients on 2 g VGB daily and 57% of the 230 patients on 600 mg CBZ daily achieved a 6-month period of remission. However, significantly more patients on VGB withdrew due to lack of efficacy than with CBZ and time to first seizure after the first 6 weeks from randomization also showed CBZ to be more effective. It was concluded that VGB cannot be recommended as a first-line drug for monotherapy of newly diagnosed partial epilepsies [62].

In the VGB/VPA study in a total of 215 patients (age range 12–76 years), an initial open monotherapy with CBZ was followed by a blinded add-on of VGB (1–4 g/day) or VPA (0.5–2 g/day) and polytherapy in those patients resistant to optimal CBZ monotherapy before CBZ was withdrawn and monotherapy with VGB or VPA was maintained in the final study phase. The therapeutic efficacy was similar for the two study drugs (Aventis, formerly Hoechst Marion Roussel, data on file, 1999).

In most double-blind trials in adults, the daily dose of VGB was 2–3 g. Initial studies suggested that 1 g might also have some therapeutic efficacy, and there are patients who benefit from doses of 4 g or more. In the US study comparing daily doses of 1, 3 and 6 g, no improvement in efficacy was observed in patients given 6 g vs. 3 g, but side-effects increased substantially [58]. Although VGB is usually administered twice daily, a double-blind pilot study in 50 patients comparing once-daily versus twice-daily add-on administration demonstrated no statistical difference [63].

Long-term efficacy

Several studies of long-term efficacy have been performed. One indicator is the proportion of patients remaining on treatment over time. Presumably, patients for whom the treatment loses efficacy will stop treatment. In several long-term studies, from 39 to 72% of patients remained on VGB for more than 3 years. Among the patients electing to continue treatment, the majority had maintained their initial positive response, and in this particular subset, there was no evidence of tachyphylaxis [64,65].

Adverse events

Side-effects during VGB treatment are usually mild and well tolerated even with high doses. In adults and older children fatigue, drowsiness, dizziness, nystagmus, agitation, amnesia, abnormal vision, ataxia, weight increase, confusion, depression and diarrhoea were most often reported [58]. In children and infants receiving VGB, drowsiness, insomnia, hyperactivity, agitation, hypotension, weight gain, and hypertonia or hypotonia were the most frequently reported adverse events [29,35,66]. A VGB-induced encephalopathy with stupor, confusion and EEG slowing has been described [67,68]. A fatal hepatoxicity in a child treated with VGB [69] was later attributed most likely to an undetected metabolic disorder (Kellermann 1999, personal communication). Most side-effects are dose related and can be reversed when the drug is stopped or the dose reduced.

An adverse event possibly related to the GABAergic mechanism of action is an increased incidence of psychosis [70], sometimes as forced normalization. A retrospective survey of behaviour disorders in 81 patients described 50 cases meeting the criteria for either psychosis ($n=28$) or depression ($n=22$). A comparison with psychotic events in epilepsy patients never treated with VGB described an increased risk for more severe epilepsies, right-sided EEG focus and suppression of seizures. Depression as a treatment-emergent effect of VGB is associated with a past history of depressive illness [71]. A formal testing of mood disturbances in 73 adult patients with refractory epilepsy before and under treatment with VGB revealed that mood problems were the main reason for discontinuation [72]. Repeated testing with a series of eight cognitive measures in a double-blind, placebo-controlled, parallel group dose–response study in patients with difficult-to-control focal seizures detected a decreased performance in only one cognitive test (digit cancellation test) [73].

A recent review of US and non-US double-blind, placebo-controlled trials of VGB as add-on therapy for refractory partial epilepsy in a total of 717 patients revealed a significantly higher incidence of depression (12.1% vs. 3.5%, $P < 0.001$) and psychosis (2.5% vs. 0.3%, $P = 0.028$). There was no significant differences between treatment groups for aggressive reactions, manic symptoms, agitation, emotional liability, anxiety or suicide attempt [74]. Depression and psychosis were usually observed during the first 3 months. Depression was usually mild, and psychosis was reported to respond to reduction or discontinuation of VGB or to treatment with neuroleptics.

As a secondary effect of treatment with VGB a significant increase of α-aminoadipic acid in plasma and urine occurs which may mimic α-aminoadipic aciduria, a known rare metabolic disease. Therefore, when a genetic metabolic disease is suspected, amino acid chromatography should be performed before initiation of VGB treatment [75]. In addition, VGB can interfere with urinary amino acid analysis due to inhibition of catabolism of β-alanine [76].

In 1997, three cases of severe symptomatic and persistent visual field constriction associated with VGB treatment were described [77]. During 1997–98, similar concentric visual field constrictions were described in patients with drug-resistant epilepsy who were receiving VGB concurrently with other AEDs [78,79]. However, a study of patients treated with VGB monotherapy alone showed that there was a causal relationship between VGB treatment and the specific bilateral concentric visual field constriction. The Marketing Authorisation Holders survey (involving 335 VGB recipients aged >14 years) indicated that 31% of patients (95% CI 26–36%) had a VFD attributable to VGB, compared with a 0% incidence of VFDs (upper 95% CI 3%) in an unexposed control group. Other studies in adults have given similar overall prevalences, with a total of 169 of 528 patients diagnosed with VGB-associated field defects (32%, 95% CI 28–36%). Male gender seems to be associated with an increase in the relative risk of visual field loss of approximately two-fold. The pattern of defect is typically a bilateral, absolute concentric constriction of the visual field, the severity of which varies from mild to severe [80]. Data gathered so far suggest that the cumulative incidence increases rapidly during the first 2 years of treatment and within the first 2 kg of VGB intake, stabilizing at 3 years and after a total VGB dose of 3 kg. The prevalence of VGB-associated field defects seems to be lower in children, but there are also methodological problems and greater variability in the assessment of visual fields in children.

In addition to the persistent VFDs, discrete non-haemorrhagic focal lesions in the splenium of the corpus callosum have been described in six patients with epilepsy and treatment with VGB and/or PHT. In two of the patients, the lesions disappeared on follow-up MRI after withdrawal of VGB and/or PHT [81].

VGB should currently be used only in combination with other AEDs for patients with resistant partial epilepsy when all other appropriate drug combinations have proved inadequate or have not been tolerated. Regular visual field testing should be performed before the start of treatment and at regular intervals during treatment. Patients with pre-existent VFDs due to other causes should not be treated with VGB.

References

1 Ben-Menachem E. Vigabatrin. Chemistry, absorption, distribution, and elimination. In: Levy RH, Mattson RH, Meldrum BS, eds. *Antiepileptic Drugs*, 4th edn. New York: Lippincott-Raven, 1995: 915–23.

2 Patsalos PN, Duncan JS. The pharmacology and pharmacokinetics of vigabatrin. *Rev Contemp Pharmacother* 1995; 6: 447–56.

3 Jung MJ, Palfreyman MG. Vigabatrin. Mechanisms of action. In Levy RH, Mattson RH, Meldrum BS, eds. *Antiepileptic Drugs*, 4th edn. New York: Raven Press, 1995: 903–13.

4 Richens A, McEwan JR, Deybach JC, Mumford JP. Evidence for both in vivo and in vitro interaction between vigabatrin and alanine transaminase. *Br J Clin Pharmacol* 1997; 43: 163–8.

5 Schechter PJ, Hanke, NFJ, Grove J, Huebert N, Sjoerdsma A. Biochemical and clinical effects of γ-vinyl GABA in patients with epilepsy. *Neurology* 1984; 34: 182–6.

6 Petroff OAC, Rothman DL, Behar RL, Mattson RH. Human brain GABA levels rise after initiation of vigabatrin therapy but fail to rise further with increasing dose. *Neurology* 1996; 46: 1459–63.

7 Petroff OAC, Hyder F, Collins T, Mattson RH, Rothman DL. Acute effects of vigabatrin on brain GABA and homocarnosine in patients with complex partial seizures. *Epilepsia* 1999; 40: 958–64.

8 Vauzelle-Kervroëdan F, Rey E, Pons G et al. Pharmacokinetics of the individual enantiomers of vigabatrin in neonates with uncontrolled seizures. *Br J Clin Pharmacol* 1996; 42: 779–81.

9 Rey E, Pons G, Richard MO et al. Pharmacokinetics of the individual enantiomers of vigabatrin (gamma-vinyl-GABA) in epileptic children. *Br J Clin Pharmacol* 1990; 30: 253–7.

10 Frisk-Holmberg M, Kerth P, Meyer P. Effect of food on the absorption of vigabatrin. *Br J Clin Pharmacol* 1889; 27 (Suppl.): 23S–25S.

11 Haegele KD, Schechter PJ. Kinetics of the enantiomers of vigabatrin after an oral dose of the racemate or the inactive S-enantiomer. *Clin Pharmacol Ther* 1986; 40: 581–6.

12 Ben-Menachem E, Persson LI, Schechter PJ et al. Effects of single doses of vigabatrin on CSF concentrations of GABA, homocarnosine, homovanillic acid and 5-hydroxyindoleacetic acid in patients with complex partial epilepsy. *Epilepsy Res* 1988; 2: 96–101.

13 Browne TR, Mattson TH, Penry JK et al. Vigabatrin for refractory complex partial seizures: multicenter single-blind study with long-term follow-up. *Neurology* 1987; 37: 184–9.

14 Bachmann D, Ritz R, Wad N, Haefeli E. Vigabatrin dosing during haemodialysis. *Seizure* 1996; 5: 239–42.

15 Tran A, O'Mahoney T, Rey E, Mai J, Mumford JP, Olive G. Vigabatrin: placental transfer in vivo and excretion into breast milk of the enantiomers. *Br J Clin Pharmacol* 1998; 45: 409–11.

16 Armijo JA, Arteaga R, Valdizán EM, Herranz JL. Coadministration of vigabatrin and valproate in children with refractory epilepsy. *Clin Neuropharmacol* 1992; 15: 459–69.

17 Reidenberg P, Glue P, Banfield CR et al. Pharmacokinetic interaction studies between felbamate and vigabatrin. *Br J Clin Pharmacol* 1995; 40: 157–60.

18 Gatti G, Bartoli A, Marchiselli R. Vigabatrin-induced decrease in phenytoin concentration does not involve a change in phenytoin bioavailability. *Br J Clin Pharmacol* 1993; 36: 603–6.

19 Rimmer EM, Richens A. Interaction between vigabatrin and phenytoin. *Br J Clin Pharmacol* 1989; 27: 27S–33S.

20 Dalla Bernadina B, Fontana E, Vigevano F et al. Efficacy and tolerability of vigabatrin in children with refractory partial seizures: a single-blind dose-increasing study. *Epilepsia* 1995; 36: 687–91.

21 Szylleyko OJ, Hoke JF, Eller MG, Weir SJ, Zobrist RH, Sussman NM. A definitive study evaluating the pharmacokinetics of vigabatrin in patients with epilepsy. *Epilepsia* 1993; 34 (Suppl. 6): 41–2.

22 Bartoli A, Gatti G, Cipolla G et al. A double-blind, placebo-controlled study on the effect of vigabatrin on in vivo parameters of hepatic microsomal enzyme induction and on the kinetics of steroid oral contraceptives in healthy female volunteers. *Epilepsia* 1997; 38: 702–7.

23 Rey E, Pons G, Olive G. Vigabatrin. Clinical pharmacokinetics. *Clin Pharmacokinet* 1992; 23: 267–78.

24 Wad N, Krämer G. Sensitive high-performance liquid chromatographic method with fluorometric detection for the simultaneous determination of gabapentin and vigabatrin in serum and urine. *J Chromatography B* 1998; 705: 154–8.

25 Arteaga R, Herranz JL, Valdizan, EM, Armilo JA. Gamma-vinyl-GABA (vigabatrin): relationship between dosage, plasma concentrations, platelet GABA-transaminase inhibition, and seizure reduction in children. *Epilepsia* 1992; 33: 923–31.

26 Ben-Menachem E, French J. Vigabatrin. In: Engel J Jr, Pedley TA, eds. *Epilepsy. A comprehensive textbook*. Philadelphia: Lippincott-Raven, 1997: 1609–18.

27 Butler WH. The neuropathology of vigabatrin. *Epilepsia* 1989; 30 (Suppl. 3): S15–S17.

28 Cannon DJ, Buttler WH, Mumford JP, Lewis PJ. Neuropathologic findings in patients receiving long-term vigabatrin therapy for chronic intractable epilepsy. *J Child Neurol* 1991; 6 (Suppl. 2): 2S17–2S24.

29 Fisher RS, Kerrigan JF III. Vigabatrin. Toxicity. In: Levy RH, Mattson RH, Meldrum BS, eds. *Antiepileptic Drugs*, 4th edn. New York: Raven Press, 1995: 931–9.

30 Morrell MJ. The new antiepileptic drugs and women: efficacy, reproductive health, pregnancy, and fetal outcome. *Epilepsia* 1996; 37 (Suppl. 6): S34–S44.

31 Livingston JH, Beaumont D, Arzimanoglou A, Aicardi J. Vigabatrin in the treatment of epilepsy in children. *Br J Clin Pharmacol* 1989; 27 (Suppl. 1): 109–12.

32 Herranz JL, Arteaga R, Farr IN et al. Dose–response study of vigabatrin in children with refractory epilepsy. *J Child Neurol* 1991; 6 (Suppl. 2): 2S45–2S51.

33 Luna D, Dulac O, Pajot N, Beaumont D. Vigabatrin in the treatment of childhood epilepsies: a single-blind placebo-controlled study. *Epilepsia* 1989; 30: 430–7.

34 Uldall P, Alving J, Gram L, Beck S. Vigabatrin in pediatric epilepsy—an open study. *J Child Neurol* 1991; 6 (Suppl. 2): 2S38–2S44.

35 Dulac O, Chiron C, Luna C *et al*. Vigabatrin in childhood epilepsy. *J Child Neurol* 1991; 6 (Suppl. 2): 2S38–2S44.

36 Uldall P, Alving J, Gram L, Høgenhaven H. Vigabatrin in childhood epilepsy: a 5-year follow-up study. *Neuropediatrics* 1995; 26: 253–6.

37 Baxter PS, Gardner-Medwin D, Barwick DD, Ince P, Livingston J, Murdoch-Eaton D. Vigabatrin monotherapy in resistant neonatal seizures. *Seizure* 1995; 4: 57–9.

38 Buchanan N, Kearney B. Vigabatrin in Sturge–Weber syndrome. *Med J Aust* 1993; 158: 652.

39 Chiron C, Dumas C, Jambaqué I, Mumford J, Dulac O. Randomized trial comparing vigabatrin and hydrocortisone in infantile spasms due to tuberous sclerosis. *Epilepsy Res* 1997; 26: 389–95.

40 Lortie A, Chiron C, Dumas C, Mumford JP, Dulac O. Optimizing the indication of vigabatrin in children with refractory epilepsy. *J Child Neurol* 1997; 12: 253–9.

41 Nabbout RC, Chiron C, Mumford J, Dumas C, Dulac O. Vigabatrin in partial seizures in children. *J Child Neurol* 1997; 12: 172–7.

42 Appleton RE, Peters ACB, Mumford JP, Shaw DE. Randomised, placebo-controlled study of vigabatrin as first-line treatment of infantile spasms. *Epilepsia* 1999; 40: 1627–33.

43 Vigevano F, Cilio MR. Vigabatrin versus ACTH as first-line treatment for infantile spasms: a randomized, prospective study. *Epilepsia* 1997; 38: 1270–74.

44 Ferrie CD, Robinson RO. The clinical efficacy of vigabatrin in children. *Rev Contemp Pharmacother* 1995; 6: 469–76.

45 Wohlrab G, Boltshauser E, Schmitt B. Vigabatrin as a first-line drug in West syndrome: clinical and electroencephalographic outcome. *Neuropediatrics* 1998; 29: 133–6.

46 Covanis A, Theodorou V, Lada C, Skiadas K, Loli N. The first-line use of vigabatrin to achieve complete control of seizures. *J Epilepsy* 1998; 11: 265–9.

47 Chiron C, Dulac O, Beaumont D, Palacios L, Pajot N, Mumford J. Therapeutic trial of vigabatrin in refractory infantile spasms. *J Child Neurol* 1991; 6 (Suppl. 2): 2S52–2S59.

48 Siemes H, Brandl U, Spohr HL, Völger S, Weschke B. Long-term follow-up study of vigabatrin in pretreated children with West syndrome. *Seizure* 1998; 7: 293–7.

49 Aicardi J, Sabril IS investigator and peer review groups, Mumford J, Dumas C, Wood S. Vigabatrin as initial therapy for infantile spasms: a European retrospective survey. *Epilepsia* 1996; 37: 638–42.

50 Granström ML, Gaily E, Liukkonen E. Treatment of infantile spasms: results of a population-based study with vigabatrin as the first drug for spasms. *Epilepsia* 1999; 40: 950–7.

51 Feucht M, Brantner-Inthaler S. γ-vinyl-GABA (vigabatrin) in the therapy of Lennox–Gastaut syndrome: an open study. *Epilepsia* 1994; 35: 993–8.

52 Appleton RE. Vigabatrin in the management of generalized seizures in children. *Seizure* 1995; 4: 45–8.

53 Vogt H, Krämer G. Vigabatrin und Lamotrigin. Erfahrungen mit zwei neuen Antiepileptika an der Schweizerischen Epilepsie-Klinik. *Schweiz Med Wochenschr* 1995; 125: 125–32.

54 Beran RG, Berkovic SF, Buchanan N *et al*. A double-blind, placebo-controlled crossover study of vigabatrin 2 g/day and 3 g/day in uncontrolled partial seizures. *Seizure* 1996; 5: 259–65.

55 Grant SM, Heel RC. Vigabatrin. A review of its pharmacodynamic and pharmacokientic properties, and therapeutic potential in epilepsy. *Drugs* 1991; 41: 889–926.

56 Ferrie CD, Panayiotopoulos CP. The clinical efficacy of vigabatrin in adults. *Rev Contemp Pharmacother* 1995; 6: 457–68.

57 French JA, Mosier M, Walker S, Sommerville K, Sussmann N, and the Vigabatrin Protocol 024 Investigative Cohort. A double-blind, placebo-controlled study of vigabatrin 3 g/day in patients with uncontrolled complex partial seizures. *Neurology* 1996; 46: 54–61.

58 Dean C, Mosier M, Penry K. Dose–response study of vigabatrin as add-on therapy in patients with uncontrolled complex partial seizures. *Epilepsia* 1999; 40: 74–82.

59 Brodie MJ, Mumford JP, 012 study group. Double-blind substitution of vigabatrin and valproate in carbamazepine-resistant partial epilepsy. *Epilepsy Res* 1999; 34: 199–205.

60 Kälviäinen R, Äikiä M, Saukkonen AM, Mervaala E, Riekkinen PJ Sr. Vigabatrin vs carbamazepine monotherapy in patients with newly diagnosed epilepsy. A randomized, controlled study. *Arch Neurol* 1995; 52: 989–96.

61 Tanganelli P, Regesta G. Vigabatrin vs. carbamazepine monotherapy in newly diagnosed focal epilepsy: a randomized response conditional cross-over study. *Epilepsy Res* 1996; 25: 257–62.

62 Chadwick D, for the Vigabatrin European Monotherapy Study Group. Safety and efficacy of vigabatrin and carbamazepine in newly diagnosed epilepsy: a multicentre randomised double-blind study. *Lancet* 1999; 354: 13–19.

63 Zahner B, Stefan H, Blankenhorn V *et al*. Once-daily versus twice-daily vigabatrin: Is there a difference? The results of a double-blind pilot study. *Epilepsia* 1999; 40: 311–15.

64 Browne TR, Mattson RH, Penry JK *et al*. Multicenter long-term safety and efficacy study of vigabatrin for refractory complex partial seizures; an update. *Neurology* 1991; 41: 363–4.

65 Michelucci, R, Veri L, Passarelli D *et al*. Long-term follow-up study of vigabatrin in the treatment of refractory epilepsy. *J Epilepsy* 1994; 7: 88–93.

66 Gherpelli JLD, Guerreiro MM, da Costa JC *et al*. Vigabatrin in refractory childhood epilepsy. The Brazilian multicenter study. *Epilepsy Res* 1997; 29: 1–6.

67 Sälke-Kellermann A, Baier H, Rambeck B, Boenigk HE, Wolf P. Acute encephalopathy with vigabatrin. *Lancet* 1993; 342: 185.

68 Sharif MK, Sander JWA, Shorvon SD. Acute encephalopathy with vigabatrin. *Lancet* 1993; 342: 619.

69 Kellermann K, Soditt V, Rambeck B, Klinge O. Fatal hepatotoxicity in a child treated with vigabatrin. *Acta Neurol Scand* 1996; 93: 380–1.

70 Sander JWAS, Hart YM, Trimble MR, Shorvon SD. Vigabatrin and psychosis. *J Neurol Neurosurg Psychiatr* 1991; 54: 435–9.

71 Thomas L, Trimble M, Schmitz B, Ring H. Vigabatrin and behaviour disorders: a retrospective survey. *Epilepsy Res* 1996; 25: 21–7.

72 Aldenkamp AP, Vermeulen J, Mulder OG *et al*. γ-vinyl GABA (vigabatrin) and mood disturbances. *Epilepsia* 1994; 35: 999–1004.

73 Dodrill CB, Arnett JL, Sommerville KW, Sussman NM. Effects of differing dosages of vigabatrin (Sabril) on cognitive abilities and quality of life in epilepsy. *Epilepsia* 1995; 36: 164–73.

74 Levinson DF, Devinsky O. Psychiatric adverse events during vigabatrin therapy. *Neurology* 1999; 53: 1503–11.

75 Vallat C, Rivier F, Bellet H *et al*. Treatment with vigabatrin may mimic γ-aminoadipic aciduria. *Epilepsia* 1996; 37: 803–5.

76 Preece MA, Sewell IJ, Taylor JA, Green A. Vigabatrin—interference with urinary amino acid analysis. *Clin Chimica Acta* 1993; 218: 113–16.

77 Eke T, Talbot JF, Lawdon MC. Severe persistent visual field constriction associated with vigabatrin. *Br Med J* 1997; 314: 180–1.

78 Krauss GL, Johnson MA, Miller NR. Vigabatrin-associated retinal cone system dysfunction. Electroretinogram and ophthalmologic findings. *Neurology* 1998; 50: 614–18.

79 Kälviäinen R, Nousiainen I, Mäntyjärvi M *et al*. Vigabatrin, a gabaergic antiepileptic drug, causes concentric visual field defects. *Neurology* 1999; 53: 922–6.

80 Kalviainen R, Nousiainen I. Visual field defects with vigabatrin: epidemiology and therapeutic implications. *CNS Drugs* 2001; 15: 217–30.

81 Kim SS, Chang K-H, Kim ST *et al*. Focal lesion of the splenium of the corpus callosum in epileptic patients: antiepileptic drug toxicity? *Am J Neuroradiol* 1999; 20: 125–9.

48

Zonisamide

M. Seino and B. Fujitani

Primary indication	Adjunctive therapy in refractory partial epilepsy. Also in generalized epilepsy (all types). Also in Lennox–Gastaut syndrome, Infantile spasm and progressive myoclonic epilepsy of Univerricht–Lundborg type
Usual preparation	Capsules: 100 mg (USA) Tablets: 100 mg (Japan, Korea) Powder: 20% (Japan, Korea)
Usual dosage	Initial: 100–200 mg (adults); 2–4 mg/kg/day (children). Maintenance: 200–600 mg/day (adults); 4–8 mg/kg/day (children)
Dosage intervals	1–2 times/day
Significant drug interactions	Zonisamide can reduce the carbamazepine : epoxide ratio on comedication with carbamazepine. Enzyme-inducing drugs reduce zonisamide plasma concentrations. Lamotrigine increases zonisamide plasma concentrations
Serum level monitoring	Useful
Target range	20–30 µg/ml
Common/important side-effects	Somnolence, ataxia, dizziness, fatigue, nausea, vomiting, irritability, anorexia, impaired concentration, mental slowing, itching, diplopia, insomnia, abdominal pain, depression, skin rashes. Significant risk of renal calculi (in US and European studies, but not in Japanese studies). Oligohidrosis and risk of heat stroke
Main advantages	Effective in broad spectrum of epilepsies. Also, a particular place in Lennox–Gastaut syndrome, infantile spasm and PME
Main disadvantages	Side-effect profile, including the risk of renal stones (in US and European populations)
Mechanism of action	Not known
Oral bioavailability	<100%
Time to peak levels	2–4 h
Metabolism and excretion	Hepatic acetylation iisoxazole ring cleavage and then glucuronidation
Volume of distribution	–
Elimination half-life	49–69 h (monotherapy); 27–38 h (comedication with enzyme-inducing drugs); 46 h (comedication with valproate)
Plasma clearance	–
Protein binding	30–60%
Active metabolites	–
Comment	Licensed only for adjunctive therapy of refractory partial epilepsy in USA. Wider licensing indications in Japan and Korea

(*Note*: this summary table was formulated by the lead editor.)

Novel classes of antiepileptic drugs (AEDs) had been required because a substantial population of patients with epilepsy suffer from refractory seizures with administration of conventional AEDs. Zonisamide (ZNS) is a sulfonamide derivative chemically distinct from any of the previously established AEDs, and was discovered by serendipity in 1974 in Dainippon Pharmaceutical Co., Ltd [1]. ZNS showed anticonvulsant activity in various models and it did not show any neurotoxic action at anticonvulsant doses in experimental animals [2].

The pharmacokinetic profile of ZNS is favourable for clinical use, as it has rapid and virtually complete absorption, a relatively long half-life and low protein binding in humans [3,4]. ZNS is partially metabolized in the liver and unchanged compound and metabolites are mostly excreted in urine. Metabolism of ZNS is accelerated under presence of some other AEDs [5], but its effect on metabolism of other AEDs is rather small [6–8].

Before approval for manufacture in Japan in 1989, the clinical efficacy of ZNS had been extensively studied [9]. ZNS was shown to be particularly beneficial in the treatment of partial epileptic seizures, such as simple and/or complex partial seizures, or secondarily generalized seizures, and it was also effective in the treatment of generalized seizures and combined seizures, although to a more variable extent. Two double-blind studies conducted in Japan using adults and children demonstrated that the efficacy of ZNS was at least comparable to that of carbamazepine (CBZ) in partial seizures, or valproate (VPA) in generalized seizures [10,11]. Furthermore, three double-blind placebo-controlled studies for the treatment of refractory partial seizures conducted in the US and Europe demonstrated a comparable clinical effect to the studies performed in Japan [12–14].

Chemistry

ZNS, 1,2-benzisoxazole-3-methanesulfonamide, is a non-hygroscopic white to pale yellow crystal or a crystalline powder with a slightly bitter taste. Its molecular formula is $C_8H_8N_2O_3S$ with molecular weight of 212. Since the pK_a of ZNS is 9.66, it is only slightly soluble in acidic and neutral aqueous solutions, but the solubility markedly increases as pH increases into the alkaline range. ZNS was proven to be highly stable in acidic, neutral and alkaline solutions and in the solid state even when exposed to heat and light [15].

Pharmacology

Anticonvulsant properties

ZNS protects animals from seizures in various models of epilepsy. Orally administered ZNS prevents tonic extensor components of seizures caused by maximum electroshock (MES) in rats, rabbits, dogs and monkeys [2]. In comparison with other AEDs, ZNS is as potent as CBZ and phenobarbital (PB), and more potent than phenytoin (PHT) in preventing convulsions in the same species. The plasma concentrations of ZNS that exhibited anti-MES effects were approximately 10 mg/L and those that caused acute neurological side-effects were over 70 mg/L in the same species, demonstrating a wider therapeutic range of plasma concentrations than the other AEDs. In a rat MES model, the anticonvulsant effect of ZNS, as well

as that of PHT and PB, peaks 2 h after administration and lasts for at least 10 h after oral administration, but with the administration of CBZ the effect disappeared earlier. In the same model, Masuda et al. [16] also examined the anticonvulsant effect of these AEDs after repeated dosing once a day for a week. The strength and duration of the anticonvulsant effect of ZNS was unaffected by repeated dosing, but the anticonvulsant effect of other AEDs waned, suggesting development of drug tolerance.

ZNS, like PHT or CBZ, protects mice from a maximal seizure induced by either electroshock or pentylenetetrazole but it does not prevent the development of a minimum seizure induced by pentylenetetrazole, suggesting that ZNS exerts anticonvulsant effects by inhibiting the spread or propagation of seizures in these models [2,17]. The above theory is supported by EEG studies in feline models, in which ZNS restricted the spread of focal seizures induced by electrical stimulation of the visual cortex [18], and prevented the propagation of seizures induced by focal cortical freezing from the cortex to the subcortical structures [19]. ZNS also suppresses focal seizure activity in the cortex induced by electrical stimulation in a visual cortex-kindled model in cats [20], and prevents the spread of seizures induced by intra-amygdaloid application of kainic acid from the amygdala to the hippocampus and cortex in rats [21].

Other EEG studies suggest that ZNS also suppresses focal epileptogenic activity. ZNS, like VPA, decreased the amplitude and frequency of spikes induced by cortical freezing in cats [18], and stopped interictal spikes induced by cortical application of tungstic acid gel or conjugated oestrogen in rats [19], whereas PHT, CBZ and PB did not. However, ZNS was almost without effect against thalamic after-discharges induced by electrical stimulation of the nucleus centralis in cats and the reticularis thalami in rats, while some standard AEDs were effective against these after-discharges [18]. ZNS failed to suppress focal epileptogenic activity while blocking seizure propagation from the amygdala to the hippocampus and cortex in the aforementioned kainate-induced model [21]. These results suggest that ZNS had suppressing activity on focal epileptogenic activity only within the cortical foci but not in the subcortical regions.

In the kindled model, ZNS was usually found to suppress convulsive seizures and after-discharges in cortex- and hippocampus-kindled rats [22], amygdala-kindled rats [23] and amygdala-kindled cats [24], although one study failed to show the effect in amygdala-kindled rats [22]. ZNS also suppressed photically induced seizures [25]. The effect was also reported in some kinds of hereditary epileptic models [26–29].

In summary, ZNS has been demonstrated to suppress seizures in a wide range of models of epilepsy, suggesting its wide-spectral nature of antiepileptic activity. It may exert antiepileptic action mainly by suppressing propagation of seizures. It may also suppress focal cortical epileptogenic activity.

Mechanism of anticonvulsant action

The exact mechanism(s) of action remains unknown, although several possible conduit mechanisms have been identified. An electrophysiological study demonstrated that ZNS, like PHT, blocked the sustained repetitive firing of the intracellular action potential at clinically relevant concentrations in cultured human spinal cord neurones [30]. Since ZNS selectively blocked only the latter phase of action potentials, it seems likely that repetitive firing is inhibited by an effect on the Na^+ current inactivation kinetics. In accordance with this, Shauf reported that ZNS caused a hyperpolarizing shift in the steady-state fast inactivation curve and retarded recovery from fast and slow inactivation [31].

ZNS also reduces T-type Ca^{2+} current in the cultured neurones of rat cerebral cortex without affecting the L-type Ca^{2+} current, within the therapeutic plasma concentration range [32]. Reduction of T-type Ca^{2+} current was attributable to a shift of the channel population toward the inactivation state, thereby allowing fewer channels to open during membrane depolarization [33].

Both voltage-dependent Na^+ and Ca^{2+} channels have a pivotal role in membrane excitability [34]. Blockade of Na^+ channels suppresses Na^+-dependent action potentials, and suppression of T-type Ca^{2+} channels prevents sharp depolarization of the membrane potential supporting Na^+ action potentials. The effect of ZNS on these ion channels could be sufficient to disrupt synchronized neuronal firing and epileptic activity, thereby limiting the spread or propagation of seizures [32].

The suppressive effect of ZNS on focal epileptogenic activity, may be activated by the binding of ZNS to the benzodiazepine/ γ-aminobutyric acid (GABA) receptor. ZNS inhibited [3H]-flunazepam or [3H]-mucimol binding to crude membranes of rat brain [35]. [3H]-ZNS bound to rat brain membranes with a low kDa value of 90 nmol/l in a saturable manner, and the ligand was partially displaced by clonazepam [36]. Indeed, studies on excitatory and inhibitory mechanisms in the feline spinal trigeminal nucleus demonstrated that ZNS had a VPA-like profile of activity, which could support a GABAergic mechanism of action [37]. However, ZNS did not alter responses to GABA in cultured spinal cord neurones [30]. Thus, further study is required to clarify the involvement of this mechanism in the suppression of epileptogenic activity of ZNS.

Other mechanisms have been suggested for the anticonvulsant effect of ZNS, such as inhibition of excitatory glutaminergic transmission [38], increased release and metabolism of acetylcholine [39] and inhibition of dopamine turnover [40]. However, relevance of these actions to the anticonvulsant action of ZNS still remains to be clarified.

As ZNS, like acetazolamide, possesses a sulfamoyl moiety in the molecule, the antiepileptic action could be considered to be due to the inhibition of carbonic anhydrase in the brain. In fact, ZNS was reported to inhibit the enzyme *in vitro* and *ex vivo*. The effect is, however, considerably less than that of acetazolamide [41,42]. The 7-methylated analogue of ZNS, which had the same potency as the parent compound in inhibiting carbonic anhydrase, did not exert any anticonvulsant effect in experimental animals [43]. Support for the view that the mechanism of antiepileptic action of ZNS is not related to its carbonic anhydrase activities are studies which have demonstrated contrasting central nervous system (CNS) effects of ZNS and acetazolamide. Acetazolamide decreased cerebral pH and increased cerebral blood flow in rats but ZNS did not [44]. ZNS reduced the turnover rate of monoamines, such as noradrenaline and dopamine, in the rat brain, but acetazolamide enhanced it [40,44]. Taking these results into consideration, it is unlikely that ZNS exerts its anticonvulsant action through the inhibition of carbonic anhydrase.

Free radical scavenging and neuroprotective effects

Head trauma, hyperoxygenation and hypoxia, which often lead to seizure development and neurodegeneration, are associated with a massive generation of free radicals [45]. Topical application of free radical generating systems, such as an alumina gel [46] or an iron salt [47], into brain tissue induced seizures in experimental animals. Recent studies demonstrated the production of free radicals during seizures in an *in vitro* model of epilepsy [48] and amygdala-kindled rats [49]. These observations suggested the implication of free radicals and a subsequent neurodegeneration in seizure development and epileptogenic focus formation.

ZNS has unique and interesting properties in relation to free radicals. ZNS scavenged the 1,1-diphenyl-2-picryl-hydroxyl (DPPH) radical, a lypophilic free radical, at millimolar concentrations *in vitro*, but PHT, PB, VPA and CBZ did not [50,51]. ZNS scavenged the hydroxyl radical in a concentration-dependent manner with an IC_{50} value of about 0.9 mmol/l and the effect was observed even at the lowest concentration of 0.078 mmol/l [52]. It also scavenged nitric oxide with the IC_{50} value of 6.8 mmol/l and carbon-centred radicals generated by ferric chloride and ascorbic acid at concentrations over 0.005 mmol/l, but it did not scavenge superoxide anion [51,53].

Several studies have demonstrated the antioxidant effect of ZNS *in vivo*. Tokumaru *et al.* perfused synthetic nitroxide radicals into the hippocampal tissue of rats, and examined the effect of ZNS on the elimination rate of nitric oxide by using a microdialysis–electronic spin resonance method [54]. ZNS (40 mg/kg) administered intraperitoneally shortened the half-life of nitric oxide in the tissue, suggesting that ZNS exerted free radical scavenging action within the neuronal cells. Oral administration of ZNS prevented the increase of lipid peroxides in rat cerebral cortex induced by topical application of ferric chloride [51]. ZNS also prevented the accumulation of 8-hydroxy-2′-deoxyguanosine, an indicator of oxidative stress to DNA, in rat cerebral cortex using the same model [55]. Mean plasma concentrations of ZNS in these studies were within or slightly higher than its therapeutic plasma concentrations in humans.

Several study experiments have also shown the preventative neuroprotective effect of ZNS. A brief period of global cerebral ischaemia produces substantial damage in the CA1 region of the hippocampus 2–3 days after insult in gerbils [56], which is thought to result from excitotoxic amino acid accumulation [57]. ZNS pretreatment prevented neuronal death, occurrence of abnormal behaviours and memory impairment in this model [58–60]. It also prevented the increase in excitatory amino acids in the hippocampus of this model [60].

ZNS prevented neuronal damage induced by a unilateral carotid artery ligation followed by hypoxia, without suppression of seizures during hypoxia, in neonatal rats [61], and by the middle cerebral artery occlusion-reperfusion in rats at clinically relevant plasma concentrations [62]. CBZ and PB did not have the protective effect in a latter study.

Free radical scavenging and neuroprotection may contribute to the efficacy of ZNS in patients with progressive myoclonus epilepsy (PME) [63] or postsurgical epileptic seizures [64]. Free radical formation and the neurodegenerative process are thought to have a prominent contribution in the genesis of these types of epilepsies [65,66].

Preclinical toxicology

Acute toxicity

The acute toxicity of ZNS has been studied in mice and rats by oral, i.v. and s.c. routes, and in dogs and monkeys by the oral route [67]. The results are summarized in Table 48.1.

Multiple-dose toxicity

One-month and 9-month multiple-dose toxicity studies were carried out in rats. In the 9-month study, rats were administered ZNS at 10, 30, 100 and 300 mg/kg/day [68], and the outcome of the study was as follows:
1 Decreased locomotor activity and abdominal myotonus, and ataxia (300 mg/kg).
2 Suppression of body weight gain and food consumption (≥ 100 mg/kg).
3 Renal effect: increased urinary Na, Na/K ratio (≥ 30 mg/kg), increased urine volume and plasma urea nitrogen levels and increased relative kidney weight (≥ 100 mg/kg).
4 Hepatic effect: increased plasma total bilirubin levels, total cholesterol levels and relative liver weight (≥ 100 mg/kg).
5 Slight decrease of haematocrit, haemoglobin contents or erythrocyte numbers (≥ 100 mg/kg).
6 The maximum non-toxic dose was estimated to be 10 mg/kg in males and 30 mg/kg in females; all toxic signs mentioned above disappeared during the recovery phase.

Toxic signs observed in the 1-month study, in which ZNS was administered at 20, 60, 200 and 600 mg/kg p.o. were essentially the same as those observed in the 9-month study, although toxic signs appeared at somewhat higher doses in the 1-month study than in the 9-month study [69].

Reproductive studies

No adverse effects on fertility were observed in a fertility study in which rats were orally administered ZNS at 20, 60 and 200 mg/kg/day [70].

Teratology studies

Teratogenic effects of ZNS were observed in rats (200 mg/kg/day), mice (500 mg/kg/day) and dogs (30 and 60 mg/kg/day), but no teratogenic effects were observed in monkeys administered up to 20 mg/kg [71,72]. Observed teratogenic abnormalities were an increased incidence of persistent cords of thymic tissue, ventricular septal defect, abnormal lumber vertebrae, cleft palate, open eye, dilatation of the cerebral ventricles and dilatation of the renal pelvis. Various kinds of visceral abnormalities, mainly cardiovascular anomalies, and fusion and deformity of caudate vertebrae were also noted.

In humans, of all the known 25 births or pregnancies during the ZNS pre- and postmarketing periods, two had malformations, including one child with anencephaly who was born to a woman treated with ZNS and PHT. The other child was born with septal defect of the atria to a women treated with a combination therapy that included PB and VPA [73].

Pharmacokinetics

Preclinical studies

ZNS is rapidly and fully absorbed, and its elimination half-life was long, after oral administration to rats, dogs and monkeys. [^{14}C] ZNS was absorbed with bioavailability of more than 83% and its plasma concentration reached the maximum level within 3 h. It was then eliminated from plasma with the half-life of 8–24 h [4]. The time course of plasma concentration after repeated administration of ZNS was essentially similar to that of the single oral administration in rats [74].

The protein binding of ZNS is 30–60% in the plasma or the serum [4,75,76]. The distribution profile of ZNS was studied after a single dose or consecutive doses of [^{14}C] ZNS in rats. The radioactivity in most tissues was similar to that in the plasma, but the radioactivity in erythrocytes, liver, kidney and adrenal gland was twice that of the plasma [4]. ZNS was distributed at a higher concentration in the cerebral cortex than in the midbrain [77]. The level of ZNS in the fetus was similar to that in the plasma of maternal rats suggesting its transport across the placenta. The concentration in milk was also similar to that in the plasma of lactating rats [4].

Table 48.1 Acute toxicity of zonisamide in mice, rats, dogs and monkeys

Species and sex		Lethal dose (LD_{50}, mg/kg)			Behavioural abnormality at sublethal doses
		p.o.	s.c.	i.v.	
Mouse	Male	1917	1195	854	Marked sedation such as decreased
	Female	2134	1009	816	locomotor activity and ataxia
Rat	Male	1992	1128	816	
	Female	2049	925	672	
Dog		3/6 dogs died at 1000 mg/kg, p.o.			Decreased locomotor activity, vomiting and ataxia
Monkey		No deaths were observed at 1000 mg/kg, p.o.			

Clinical studies

Human studies have also demonstrated the rapid and full absorption of ZNS from gastrointestinal tract. In healthy volunteers who were orally administered ZNS at 200, 400 and 800 mg/kg in a crossover manner, ZNS was absorbed with the mean t_{max} between 2.4 and 3.6 h and the bioavailability was approximately 100% [78]. ZNS was eliminated from plasma in an apparently first-order fashion and the half-life of ZNS ranged between 49.7 and 62.5 h for the above 3 doses. Similar pharmacokinetic properties were demonstrated after single administration of ZNS in two Japanese studies [3,4].

From the results of a single dose study, plasma ZNS concentration was predicted to reach its steady state 10 days after administration of ZNS at 200 mg [3]. In fact, steady-state serum concentrations were achieved within 7 days after administering 100 mg ZNS [79] or about 15 days after the last dose adjustment [80]. The half-life of ZNS in steady state (63–69 h) was consistent with that in single dose studies. Diurnal fluctuation of steady-state serum concentrations (C_{ss}) of ZNS was very small—peak-through difference in C_{ss} with q.i.d. or b.i.d. dosing was 27% and 14%, respectively [80].

Dose-proportional serum concentration during the steady state was demonstrated in a repeated dosing study in which 22 paediatric patients with epilepsy were administered ZNS up to the maximum of 800 mg/day [81]. Another study with adult patients also demonstrated a linear relationship between the dosage of ZNS and its serum concentration over the dose range of 1.3 mg/kg to 18.6 mg/kg [79]. In contrast to these findings, the plasma clearance value of ZNS after multiple dosing was 46% smaller than that after single administration indicating, non-linear pharmacokinetics [82].

In humans, ZNS is mainly excreted in urine. Analysis of urine samples in healthy human volunteers who were orally administered ZNS revealed that the parent compound was metabolized by acetylation, and cleavage of the isoxazole ring followed by conjugation with glucuronic acid [3,4]. The major enzyme involved in its cleavage is reported to be CYP3A species [83].

In patients treated with ZNS, adjunctive administration of AEDs that induce hepatic drug-metabolizing enzymes shortened the half-life of ZNS; the half-life was reduced from 52 to 66 h when administered alone to < 27 h with PHT, 38 h with CBZ and 38 h with PB [5]. Concomitant administration of VPA was also reported to shorten the half-life of ZNS to 46 h [5]. Concomitant administration of PB, PHT or CBZ with ZNS significantly decreased the ratio of steady-state plasma concentration to dosage of ZNS, whereas clonazepam

or VPA did not [8]. Although extensive drug interaction studies of ZNS with newer AEDs have not been completed, a case report suggested that lamotrigine may inhibit the clearance of ZNS [84]. These results suggest that doses of ZNS may need to be modified on the basis of concomitant AED therapy.

Reports concerning the effect of ZNS on the metabolism of other AEDs are a little confusing. In a US controlled study, ZNS was reported to raise plasma concentrations of most other concomitant drugs, particularly CBZ [85]. It also resulted in a small but significant increase in the serum concentration of PHT [6]. The ratio of the plasma concentration of CBZ-10,11-epoxide to that of CBZ was significantly decreased by concomitant administration of ZNS [8]. However, it has been reported that concomitant administration of ZNS does not alter the plasma or serum concentration of CBZ or PHT [86], CBZ [6], and PHT or VPA [7].

Efficacy

Randomized controlled clinical trials and placebo-controlled studies

Five randomized controlled trials on ZNS have been performed: three placebo-controlled studies and two comparative studies with active reference drugs, either CBZ or VPA. All of the three placebo-controlled studies were an evaluation of ZNS for add-on treatment for patients with refractory partial or generalized epileptic seizures. The designs and the results of these placebo-controlled studies are summarized in Table 48.2.

Schmidt et al. reported a European multicentre placebo-controlled study of ZNS in adult patients who had four or more partial or secondarily generalized tonic-clonic seizures per month and were refractory to other existing AEDs, either in monotherapy or in bitherapy [12]. One hundred and thirty-nine patients were randomly allocated to the ZNS group ($n = 71$) or the placebo (PLC) group ($n = 68$). ZNS was administered once a day for 12 weeks in an add-on manner at an average maintenance dose of 430 mg/day after a 1-month baseline period. Although the study involved patients either with partial or with secondarily generalized tonic-clonic seizures, the majority of the patients were having complex partial seizures. In patients with complex partial seizures, the median seizure frequency decreased by 27.7% in the ZNS group and increased by 3.9% in the PLC group from baseline ($P < 0.05$). Responder rates—defined as the percentage of patients whose seizure frequency decreased by 50% or more—were 30.3% in the ZNS group and 12.7% in the PLC group ($P < 0.05$). The median daily doses and plasma concen-

Table 48.2 Summary of placebo-controlled studies of zonisamide in patients with refractory partial seizures (adjunctive therapy)

Reference	No. of patients	Duration (months)	Dose (mg/day)	Responder rate (%)	Median reduction of seizure frequency (%)
Schmidt et al. [12]	66 (63)	5–12	100–600	30.3 (12.7)	27.7 (−3.9)
Sackellares et al. [13]	69 (72)	5–12	100–600	26.1 (16.7)	29.5 (−1.8)
Faught et al. [14]	98 (72)	8–12	400	41.8 (22.2)	40.5 (9.0)

Data were analysed for all types of partial seizures.

Figures in parentheses are patient numbers, responder rate and median reduction of seizure frequency in placebo control group, respectively.

trations of ZNS did not differ between responders and non-responders—7.8 and 6.8 mg/kg/day, and 17.0 and 15.2 µg/mL, respectively.

A multicentre double-blind placebo-controlled study was conducted by Sackellares et al. [13] in the US under a similar protocol to the study by Schmidt et al. [12]. One hundred and fifty-two patients (ZNS group, 78; PLC group, 74) with refractory partial seizures were enrolled in the study, and the efficacy was evaluated in 141 patients (ZNS group, 69; PLC group, 72). After a 2–3-month baseline period, ZNS was administered twice a day for 12 weeks in an add-on manner with an average maintenance dose of 530 mg/day. The median seizure frequency decreased by 29.5% in the ZNS group (n=69) and increased by 0.8% in the PLC group (n=72). The difference was statistically significant with $P < 0.05$. Responder rates were 26.1% in the ZNS group and 16.7% in the PLC group ($P < 0.05$). The final median plasma concentrations of ZNS were 16.9 µg/mL responders and 13.0 µg/mL in non-responders.

The third placebo-controlled ZNS study, a randomized, double-blind, placebo-controlled study, was conducted to assess the efficacy and dose–response of ZNS as an adjunctive therapy for refractory partial seizures [14]. After a 4-week baseline period, the 203 patients enrolled were randomly allocated to group A (n=85), group B1 (n=60) and group B2 (n=58). Group A patients received placebo, along with their concomitant AEDs, for 12 weeks. At week 13, they were then crossed over to ZNS treatment, starting at 100 mg/day and the dose was incremented weekly by 100 mg/day up to 400 mg/day for the final 5 weeks (weeks 16–20). Group B1 patients received 100 mg/day of ZNS for weeks 1–5, 200 mg/day during week 6, 300 mg/day during week 7, and 400 mg/day for weeks 8–20. Group B2 patients received 100 mg/day of ZNS for week 1, 200 mg/day for weeks 2–6, 300 mg/day during week 7, and 400 mg/day for weeks 8–20. This unique study protocol allowed parallel comparisons with placebo for three fixed doses and a final crossover to 400 mg/day for all patients. During weeks 8–12, median seizure frequency in patients treated with ZNS at 400 mg (n=98) decreased 40.5% from baseline, compared with 9.0% decrease in the PLC group (n=72) ($P < 0.01$). During these weeks, the responder rate of all seizures was 41.8% in patients treated with 400 mg/day of ZNS, compared with 22.2% in the PLC group ($P < 0.05$). As for the dose–efficacy relationship to ZNS, the median reduction of seizure frequency in patients treated with ZNS at 100 mg/day for weeks 1–5 was 24.7%, compared with 8.3% in the PLC group during the same period ($P < 0.05$). Median reduction in patients administered 200 mg/day of ZNS for weeks 2–6 was 20.4% compared with 4.0% in the PLC group ($P < 0.05$), and that in patients administered 400 mg/day of ZNS (weeks 8–12) was 40.5% compared with 9.0% in the PLC group ($P < 0.01$). The significant reduction of seizure frequency by administration of ZNS was consistent between the doses of 100, 200 and 400 mg/day.

Controlled comparative study with active reference drugs

The design and results of two controlled comparative studies with active reference drugs were summarized in Table 48.3. Seino et al. compared the efficacy of ZNS with that of CBZ in their double-blind controlled study [10]. One hundred and twenty-three patients with partial seizures, two seizures a month or more, who had been untreated with other AEDs, or were refractory to one to three other AEDs, were assigned to the ZNS group (n=59) or the CBZ group (n=64). Based on a preclinical study [24] and a preliminary clinical study [87], 100 mg ZNS was equated with 200 mg CBZ. The patients were administered either ZNS (mean dose 330 mg/day) or CBZ (mean dose 600 mg/day) for 16 weeks. After the 16-week treatment period, the average frequency of simple and/or complex partial seizures were reduced by 68.4% in the ZNS group and 46.6% in the CBZ group compared with baseline. The average frequency of secondarily generalized tonic-clonic seizures was also markedly reduced in the ZNS group (69.7%), and in the CBZ group (70.2%). There were no statistical differences in the reduction of seizure frequency between the two groups. Responder rates were 81.8% in the ZNS group and 70.7% in the CBZ group (NS). Overall improvement rates in terms of seizure frequency and interseizure condition were also similar for the ZNS group (66.1%) and for the CBZ group (65.4%).

A controlled study in paediatric patients with generalized seizures was carried out in which efficacy of ZNS was compared with that of VPA [11]. Thirty-four patients with convulsive and/or non-convulsive generalized seizures, four seizures or more per month, who were refractory to between one and three other AEDs were allocated to the ZNS group (n=18) or the VPA group (n=16). The patients were on medication for 8 weeks with ZNS or VPA at the mean daily dose of 7.3 mg/kg/day or 27.6 mg/kg/day, respectively. Overall improvements rates based on the assessment of seizure frequency, EEG findings and interseizure condition were 50.0% in the ZNS group and 43.8% in the VPA group. It was concluded that the efficacy of ZNS was at least comparable to that of VPA for children with convulsive or non-convulsive generalized seizures.

Table 48.3 Summary of controlled comparative studies of zonisamide with active reference drugs

Reference	Subjects	Test drug	No. of patients	Duration (weeks)	Dose	Overall improvement (%)
Seino et al. [10]	Adults with partial seizures	Zonisamide	59	16	330 mg/day	66.1
		Carbamazepine	64	16	600 mg/day	65.4
Oguni et al. [11]	Children with generalized seizures	Zonisamide	18	8	2–8 mg/kg/day	50.0
		Valproate	16	8	400–1200 mg/day	43.8

Overall improvement rate was assessed by seizure frequency, EEG findings and interseizure condition.

Other clinical studies

Non-comparative multicentre study

Leppik *et al.* studied the efficacy of ZNS in a non-comparative multicentre study in the US [88]. The study enrolled 167 patients with simple and/or complex partial seizures including secondarily generalized tonic-clonic seizures. The study patients were refractory to one or two other AEDs and had four or more seizures per month. After a 12-week baseline period, patients were administered ZNS, 50–1100 mg/day, for 16 weeks in an add-on manner. Treatment of patients with ZNS resulted in a significant reduction in seizure frequency per month from 11.5 during baseline to 5.5 (a 51.8% reduction) during the final month of administration. At least 50% reduction of seizure frequency was noted in 41% of all patients, 43.2% of those with complex partial seizures and 67.5% of those with secondarily generalized tonic-clonic seizures.

Ono *et al.* conducted a multicentre non-comparative clinical study in 538 adult patients with partial seizures (*n*=433) or secondarily generalized tonic-clonic seizures (*n*=105) [79]. ZNS was administered in an add-on manner with a daily dose of 6.08± 2.89 mg/kg for at least 3 months. The mean duration of administration was 273 days. At the completion of the trial, at least 50% reduction of seizure frequency was obtained in 254 out of 506 patients (50.2%). Overall improvement rates based on an assessment of severity and duration of seizures, interseizure condition and EEG findings were 41.4% (213/514) in all patients, 48.1% (13/27) in those with simple partial seizures, 38.3% (23/60) in those with simple followed by complex partial seizures, 41.2% (98/238) in those with complex partial seizures and 50% (45/90) in those with secondarily generalized tonic-clonic seizures. There were no statistically significant differences in the overall improvement rates between patients with these seizure types.

Oguni *et al.* carried out an open-label trial in 393 patients with partial or generalized epilepsies [11]. Patients, either adults or children that were refractory to previous AEDs—in whom the average number of AEDs concomitantly used was 2.8—were administered ZNS at a dose of 2–8 mg/kg/day, with an average final dose of 7.3 mg/kg/day. The overall responder rate was 44.4%. The overall improvement rate based on an assessment of severity and duration of seizures, interseizure condition and EEG findings was 51.0% in all patients. According to seizure types, the overall improvement rates were 50–70% in patients with simple and/or complex partial seizures or secondarily generalized tonic-clonic seizures. Improvement rates in patients with generalized seizures were lower than in those with partial seizures—47% in patients with generalized tonic-clonic seizures, 31.3% in those with generalized tonic seizures and 20.0% in those with myoclonic seizures.

Yagi and Seino [9] analysed the clinical efficacy of ZNS in a total of 1008 adult and paediatric patients with various epilepsies (605 adults and 403 children), who were enrolled in the controlled studies and non-comparative multicentre studies cited previously in this chapter [10,11,79]. Mean daily doses of ZNS ranged between 5.9 and 8.8 mg/kg, and their mean serum concentrations ranged between 19.6 and 20.7 µg/mL at steady state. The efficacy was assessed by responder rate, i.e. the percentage of patients whose seizure frequency decreased by 50% or more from the baseline. ZNS showed efficacy in 50% or more of patients with simple and/or complex seizures, and secondarily generalized tonic-clonic seizures. It was also beneficial for the treatment of convulsive and non-convulsive generalized seizures and combined seizures, although efficacy rates varied between 26% and 100% by the seizure type (Table 48.4). The responder rate of ZNS was also analysed according to epileptic syndromes in this study (Table 48.5). ZNS showed efficacy in more than 50% of patients with symptomatic partial epilepsies: including temporal lobe epilepsy, extratemporal lobe epilepsy and unclassifiable symptomatic partial epilepsies. As for generalized epilepsies, responder rates to ZNS were 66% in patients with idiopathic generalized epilepsy, 32% in those with Lennox–Gastaut syndrome, 22% in those with West's syndrome and 47% in those with other symptomatic generalized epilepsies. This study suggested that ZNS had a wide spectrum of efficacy for the treatment of patients with various seizure types and syndromes. Supporting this analysis, more than 20 open-label studies have demonstrated the efficacy of ZNS in the treatment of adults and children with partial, generalized or combined seizures in the late 1980s and early 1990s in Japan [89].

Table 48.4 Clinical efficacy of zonisamide by seizure types with 1008 patients in controlled and open-label studies in Japan

Seizure type	No. of patients	Responder rate (%)
Partial		
Simple partial	63	57
Simple partial followed by complex partial	82	50
Complex partial	362	50
Partial-onset generalized tonic-clonic	168	60
Generalized		
Generalized tonic-clonic	46	59
Generalized tonic	74	26
Atypical absences	9	67
Typical absences	4	50
Atonic	10	50
Myoclonic	7	43
Clonic	1	100
Combination	129	41

Table 48.5 Clinical efficacy of zonisamide by epilepsy classification with 1008 patients in controlled and open-label studies

Epilepsies	No. of patients	Responder rate (%)
Partial		
Temporal lobe	428	54
Extratemporal lobe	224	51
Unclassifiable	21	57
Generalized		
Idiopathic generalized	41	66
West's syndrome	9	22
Lennox–Gastaut syndrome	132	32
Other symptomatic generalized	100	47

Long-term efficacy

Yagi and Seino also analysed the efficacy of ZNS in 155 patients who were treated for at least 1 year with ZNS in controlled comparative studies and non-comparative studies conducted in Japan [9]. The responder rates were 75% in patients with simple partial seizures ($n=4$), 65% in those with simple partial followed by complex partial seizures ($n=26$), 64% in those with complex partial seizures ($n=47$), 61% in those with secondarily generalized tonic-clonic seizures ($n=28$), 67% in those with generalized tonic-clonic seizures ($n=6$), 40% in those with tonic seizures ($n=20$) and 50% in those with combined seizures ($n=24$). This analysis demonstrated the long-term efficacy of ZNS.

Three open-label trials were completed to assess the long-term efficacy of ZNS in the US. One of these trials, a multicentre study, enrolled 103 patients who were refractory to other AEDs [90]. Patients were administered ZNS (generally 400–600 mg/day) for up to 24 months. The median reduction of seizure frequency and responder rates were 37.6% and 36.4% (35/96) after 5–16-week treatment and those after 5–24-month treatment were 45.5% and 42.3% (33/78), respectively.

In the second trial, long-term efficacy was investigated in 137 patients with partial seizures who were refractory to other existing AEDs [91]. ZNS was administered for at least 5 months in an add-on fashion, and the dose did not exceed the smaller of 20 mg/kg/day or the amount producing a plasma concentration of 40 µg/mL. Forty patients were treated with ZNS for longer than 16 months. Overall median seizure frequency was reduced by 64.9% ($n=129$). Responder rates were constantly higher than 40% throughout the study period: the responder rates were 44% (53/120), 46% (44/95), 51% (38/74) and 49% (31/63) during the 5–7, 8–10, 11–13 and 14–16 month periods, respectively, and 40% (16/40) for more than 16 months.

The third trial was an extension of a US placebo-controlled study [92]. A total of 123 patients having documented refractory partial seizures, with or without secondary generalization, received open-label ZNS therapy (median dose 450 mg/day). Of the 123 patients who began open-label therapy, 47 patients received ZNS for at least 12 months, and 40 patients received ZNS for 15 months or more before the study terminated. The median per cent reduction in seizure frequency from the baseline was 50.1% for patients with any kind of partial seizures and 50.8% for those with complex partial seizures only. The responder rate ranged from 42.1% to 55.0% depending on the treatment period. Ota *et al.*, Kohsaka *et al.*, Nishiura and Oiwa, Kanazawa *et al.*, Wilder *et al.*, Shimizu *et al.* and Sugihara *et al.* also showed the long-term efficacy of ZNS [93–99].

ZNS monotherapy

Analysis of 1008 epileptic patients recruited in controlled studies and multicentre open-label studies in Japan included 55 patients who were treated with ZNS alone [9]. The percentage of patients who showed at least a 50% reduction of seizure frequency was 72% of these 55 patients. Kumagai *et al.* investigated the efficacy and safety of ZNS monotherapy in 44 paediatric patients [100]. ZNS was administered for between 4 months and 4.5 years (mean treatment period 1.1 years). The starting doses were 2–4 mg/kg/day and increased to 12 mg/kg/day, unless a satisfactory response

was obtained at a previous dose. The seizures completely disappeared in 30 out of 38 patients (78.9%) whose efficacy could be evaluated (5/5 in patients with idiopathic generalized epilepsy, 7/8 in those with symptomatic generalized epilepsy, 1/1 in those with idiopathic partial epilepsy and 17/24 in those with symptomatic partial epilepsy). Hosoda *et al.* also investigated the efficacy of ZNS monotherapy in 72 paediatric patients with cryptogenic localization-related epilepsies. ZNS was administered once daily at 2–8 mg/kg/day for 6–43 months [101]. During this period, complete seizure control was achieved in 57 out of 72 patients (79%), including eight patients whose dosage was increased at an early stage of the treatment because of seizure recurrence with the initial maintenance dose. Suzuki *et al.* reported the efficacy of ZNS monotherapy for infantile spasms [102]. Eleven newly diagnosed children with infantile spasms who failed to respond to vitamin B_6 were treated with ZNS at 3–10 mg/kg/day. Four of the 11 infants had cessation of spasms and disappearance of hypsarrhythmia within a few days after starting treatment, although two of them relapsed into spasms several weeks after cessation of seizures. Two other patients showed a reduction of seizure frequency, but seizure frequency did not change in the remaining five patients.

ZNS therapy for specific syndromes

Progressive myoclonus epilepsy (PME)

PME is a group of syndromes mainly consisting of generalized convulsive seizures, fragmentary myoclonus, status epilepticus, ataxia and progressive dementia. Henry *et al.* first reported in 1988 dramatic improvement of seizures after treatment with ZNS at separate doses of 8.8 and 10.5 mg/kg/day in two patients with PME of Unverricht–Lundborg type [103]. Later, Kyllerman and Ben-Menachem treated seven cases of PME with ZNS at 100–600 mg/day [63]. They demonstrated that it dramatically reduced the number of myoclonus and generalized convulsive seizures in six out of seven cases, although the initial effect on myoclonus wore off after 2–4 years of the treatment in three of them. Yagi and Seino also reported that ZNS monotherapy resulted in the complete disappearance of seizures in one patient having mitochondrial encephalopathy with ragged-red fibres, and a significant improvement in two paediatric patients with other PMEs [9].

ZNS has been thought to exert its antiepileptic effect through the blockade of the sodium channel [31] and the T-type calcium channel [32]. Since other sodium channel blocking agents, such as PHT or CBZ, do not improve seizures of PMEs, ZNS seems to exhibit its improving effect on PMEs through its blockade on the T-type calcium channel and/or some unknown mechanisms. In relation to the therapeutic effect of ZNS on PME, it should be noted that ZNS has free radical scavenging action, because treatment with N-acetylcysteine, an antioxidant, markedly decreased frequency of seizures and normalized somatosensory evoked potential in patients with PME of Unverricht–Lundborg type [104]. As described elsewhere in this chapter, ZNS has free radical scavenging and antioxidant actions *in vitro* and *in vivo*. It also exerts neuroprotective action at an anticonvulsive dose. Considering these findings, ZNS may, at least partly, exert therapeutic effects on PMEs and other symptomatic generalized epilepsies through its free radical scavenging action in addition to its blocking action on the T-type calcium channel.

Prevention of postsurgical seizures

After demonstrating the cerebral protective effect of ZNS in animal models of cerebral ischaemia or traumatic head injury, Fukuda and Masuda first tried to treat six craniotomy patients with ZNS and showed its efficacy in five of these six patients [105]. Later, Nakamura *et al.* conducted a randomized controlled study of ZNS in postoperative seizures using PB as an active placebo [64]. High-risk patients ($n=278$) for seizures who had craniotomy for their brain tumours, cerebrovascular diseases or head injuries were recruited into this study and were randomly assigned to the ZNS group ($n= 141$) or the PB group ($n=137$). ZNS (100–400 mg/day) or PB (40–160 mg/day) was administered from 1 week before to 1 year after the surgery, thereafter the patients were followed-up for 3 years. An occurrence of seizures was recorded in 255 patients (ZNS group, 129; PB group, 126) during the treatment period and in 219 patients (ZNS group, 112; PB group, 107) during the follow-up period. The development of epileptic seizures during medication were 5.4% (7/129) and 6.3% (8/126) in the ZNS group and the PB group, respectively (NS), and those during the follow-up period were 7.1% (8/112) and 12.1% (13/107), respectively (NS). While six patients (5.6%) in the PB group experienced partial seizures during follow-up period, none in the ZNS group experienced such seizures (Fisher test; $P = 0.013$). In addition to the antiepileptic action, free radical scavenging action of ZNS may, at least in part, contribute to its preventive effect on postsurgical seizures.

Safety

In the pooled data of three double-blind placebo-controlled studies conducted in the US and Europe, the incidence of adverse drug reactions (ADRs) was 78.1% in the ZNS group and 61.3% in the PLC group [106]. Somnolence, ataxia, anorexia, dizziness, fatigue, nausea and vomiting and irritability were the most common ADRs (Table 48.6). ADRs observed more than twice in the ZNS group were ataxia, anorexia, irritability, diplopia, impaired concentration, insomnia, abnormal pain and discomfort, and depression. Thirty-one out of 269 patients (11.5%) in the ZNS group, and 15 out of 230 patients (6.5%) in the PLC group discontinued treatment due to ADRs. Frequently reported ADRs in dropped-out patients in the ZNS group were psychiatric or behavioural symptoms (28.6%), cognitive impairment (10.7%), fatiguability (10.7%) and anorexia. Skin rash and asymptomatic renal calculi were reported in one patient each.

In pooled data of preapproval clinical studies in Japan, ADRs were reported in 517 out of 1008 patients (51%), and 185 patients (18%) discontinued ZNS treatment due to ADRs [107]. The most common ADRs reported were drowsiness (24.3%), followed by ataxia (12.7%), anorexia (11%), gastrointestinal discomfort (6.2%), decreased spontaneity (5.5%) and mental slowing (5.3%). Skin rash/itching occurred in 6% of patients.

The most striking difference between the Japanese studies and the US and European studies is the occurrence of urinary lithiasis. In preapproval studies in Japan, only two out of 1008 patients (0.2%) developed urinary stones. In early studies in the US and Europe, however, 13 out of 505 patients (2.6%) developed urinary stones

Table 48.6 Treatment emergent adverse events of zonisamide (%) in double-blind placebo-controlled studies (pooled data: events occurred in more than 5% of patients)

Adverse event	Placebo ($n=230$)	Zonisamide (mg/day)				
		Total ($n=269$)	<200 ($n=249$)	200–399 ($n=258$)	400–599 ($n=256$)	≥600 ($n=92$)
All events	*61.3*	*78.1*	*33.3*	*47.3*	*51.2*	*29.3*
Somnolence	12.2	19.3	7.6	8.9	8.2	2.2
Ataxia	5.7	16.7	4.4	6.6	9.8	7.6
Anorexia	6.1	15.6	2.8	5.0	7.0	1.1
Dizziness	10.9	15.6	3.6	5.0	5.9	7.6
Fatigue	10.4	14.1	2.0	4.7	7.4	5.4
Nausea and or vomiting	11.7	11.5	2.4	4.7	4.7	6.5
Irritability	5.2	11.5	2.0	4.3	5.9	2.2
Diplopia	4.3	8.9	2.0	4.3	5.5	2.2
Headache	8.3	8.6	2.4	4.3	2.0	1.1
Decreased concentration	0.9	8.2	0.4	2.3	5.9	7.6
Insomnia	3.5	7.8	2.8	1.9	1.2	1.1
Abdominal pain/discomfort	1.7	7.4	0.8	3.5	3.1	2.2
Depression	3.0	7.4	0.8	1.9	4.7	1.1
Forgetfulness	2.2	7.1	0.8	2.3	3.1	5.4
Rhinitis	6.1	6.7	2.8	3.1	1.2	0
Confusion	1.3	5.6	0.8	1.9	2.7	2.2
Anxiety	2.6	5.6	0.4	2.3	2.3	0
Nystagmus	2.6	5.2	0.8	0.8	3.1	2.2

[88]. Another US study examined the occurrence of renal stones by means of a renal ultrasound technique in 514 epileptic patients; 429 patients treated with ZNS and 85 patients with placebo (later 72 patients in the placebo group were crossed over to ZNS group) were examined prior to entry and then at yearly intervals. Renal ultrasound technique demonstrated calculi in two out of 85 patients (2.4%) during the placebo-treated period and in 17 out of 501 patients (3.4%) treated with ZNS. Among these 17 patients, four (0.8%) showed symptomatic lithiasis, but calculi disappeared while receiving ZNS in three other patients [108]. The reason for this differentiation in the US/European and Japanese studies is not known.

Oligohidrosis seems to be another characteristic ADR associated with ZNS. During Japanese development, only one case (0.1%) developed oligohidrosis among 1008 patients treated with ZNS [107] and there were no cases in the US and European development. However, oligohidrosis was reported in 12 (17.1%) of 70 children with epilepsy [109], and in 38 (24.8%) of 153 children [110]. ZNS suppressed sweating response to acetylcholine loading in humans [109]. Decrease in sweating may predispose to heat stroke in infants and severely handicapped children taking ZNS, especially in summer.

Clinical therapeutics

ZNS is a chemically distinct AED with several potential mechanisms underlying its antiepileptic activity. Preclinical pharmacological studies have shown potent antiepileptic activity in various models of epilepsy. Furthermore ZNS has free radical scavenging and neuroprotective action. The ZNS is rapidly and entirely absorbed and has a long half-life. ZNS does not have an overt effect on the metabolism of other AEDs. It has proven efficacy in adults and children for a wide variety of partial and generalized seizures and has been launched in Japan since 1989. Many studies demonstrated the efficacy of ZNS in the treatment of simple and complex partial seizures, and secondarily generalized tonic-clonic seizures. For generalized seizures, the efficacy was demonstrated in patients with generalized tonic-clonic seizure, atypical absence, tonic, atonic, myoclonic or clonic seizures. It is also effective to some extent in the treatment of West's syndrome, and tonic and atypical absence seizures in Lennox–Gastaut syndrome. Some investigators have reported a dramatic improvement of seizures in patients with PME. Although the indications of ZNS is limited to adjunctive therapy for adult patients with refractory partial epilepsy in the US, studies on its monotherapy, or paediatric use is currently ongoing. The most common ADRs associated with ZNS are CNS related and psychiatric ones. Hence ZNS is an important addition to the ranks of available AEDs.

References

1 Uno H, Kurokawa M, Masuda Y et al. Studies on 3-substituted 1,2-benz-isoxazole derivatives. Syntheses of 3-(sulfamoylmethyl)-1,2-benzisoxazole derivatives and their anticonvulsant activities. J Med Chem 1979; 22: 180–3.
2 Masuda Y, Karasawa T, Shiraishi Y et al. 3-Sulfamoylmethyl-1, 2- benzisoxazole, a new drug. Pharmacological profile. Arzneim-Forsch/Drug Res 1980; 30: 477–83.
3 Ito T, Yamaguchi T, Miyazaki H et al. Pharmacokinetic studies of AD-810, a new antiepileptic compound, Phase I trials. Arzneim-Forsch/Drug Res 1982; 32: 1581–6.
4 Matsumoto K, Miyazaki H, Fujii T et al. Absorption, distribution and excretion of 3-(sulfamoyl[^{14}C]methyl)-1,2-benzisoxazole (AD-810) in rats, dogs and monkeys and of AD-810 in man. Arzneim-Forsch/Drug Res 1983; 33: 961–8.
5 Buchanan RA, French JA, Leppik IE, Padgett CS. Zonisamide drug interactions. Epilepsia 1997; 38 (Suppl. 8): 107.
6 Kaneko S, Hayashimoto A, Niwayama H et al. Effects of zonisamide on serum levels of phenytoin and carbamazepine. Jpn J Epilepsy Soc 1993; 11: 31–5.
7 Tasaki K, Minami T, Ieiri I et al. Drug interactions of zonisamide with phenytoin and sodium valproate: serum concentrations and protein binding. Brain Dev 1995; 17: 182–5.
8 Shinoda M, Akita M, Hasegawa M et al. The necessity of adjusting the dosage of zonisamide when coadministered with other anti-epileptic drugs. Biol Pharmacol Bull 1996; 19: 1090–2.
9 Yagi K, Seino M. Methodological requirements for clinical trials in refractory epilepsies – our experience with zonisamide. Prog Neuro-Psychopharmacol Biol- Psychiatr 1992; 16: 79–85.
10 Seino M, Ohkuma T, Miyasaka M et al. Efficacy evaluation of AD-810 (zonisamide) – results of a double blind comparison with carbamazepine [in Japanese]. Igaku no Ayumi 1988; 144: 275–91.
11 Oguni H, Hayashi K, Fukuyama Y et al. Phase III clinical study of the new antiepileptic drug, AD-810 [zonisamide (ZNS)], in patients with childhood epilepsy [in Japanese]. Shonika Rinsyo 1989; 41 (Suppl.): 439–50.
12 Schmidt D, Jacob R, Loiseau P et al. Zonisamide for add-on treatment of refractory partial epilepsy: a European double-blind trials. Epilepsy Res 1993; 15: 67–73.
13 Sackellares CJ, Ramsay RE, Wilder BJ et al. Controlled clinical trial of zonisamide: an effective adjunctive treatment for refractory partial seizures. Osaka, Japan: Files of Dainippon Pharm. Co., Ltd. (#912 US).
14 Faught E, Ayala R, Montouris GG et al. Randomized controlled trial of zonisamide for the treatment of refractory partial onset seizures. Neurology 2001; 57: 1774–9.
15 Seino M, Naruto S, Ito T et al. Other antiepileptic drugs: Zonisamide. In: Levy RH, Mattson RH, Meldrum BS, eds. Antiepileptic Drugs, 4th edn. New York: Raven Press, 1995: 1011–23.
16 Masuda Y, Utsui Y, Shiraishi Y et al. Relationship between plasma concentration of diphenylhydantoin, phenobarbital, carbamazepine, and 3-sulfamoyl-methyl-1,2-benzisoxazole (AD-810), a new anticonvulsant agent, and their anticonvulsant or neurotoxic effects in experimental animals. Epilepsia 1979; 20: 623–33.
17 Ibba M, Vanasia A, Testa R. Differential antagonism of denzimol to various components of metrazole-induced seizures in rats and mice. Pharmacol Res Commun 1985; 17: 1169–80.
18 Ito T, Hori M, Masuda Y et al. 3-Sulfamoylmethyl-1,2-benzisoxazole, a new type of anticonvulsant drug. Electroencephalographic profile. Arzneim-Forsch/Drug Res 1980; 30: 603–9.
19 Ito T, Hori M, Kadokawa T. Effects of zonisamide (AD-810) on tungstic acid gel-induced thalamic generalized seizures and conjugated estrogen-induced cortical spike wave discharge in cats. Epilepsia 1986; 27: 367–74.
20 Wada Y, Hasegawa H, Yamaguchi N. Anticonvulsant effects of zonisamide and phenytoin on seizure activity of the feline visual cortex. Brain Dev 1990; 12: 206–10.
21 Takano K, Tanaka T, Fujita T et al. Electrophysological and metabolic changes in kainic acid-induced limbic seizure in rats. Epilepsia 1995; 36: 644–8.
22 Kamei C, Oka M, Masuda Y et al. Effects of 3-sulfamoylmethyl-1,2-benzisoxazole (AD-810) and some antiepileptics on the kindled seizures in neocortex, hippocampus and amygdala in rats. Arch Int Pharmacodyn 1981; 249: 164–76.
23 Hamada K, Ishida S, Yagi K, Seino M. Anticonvulsant effects of zonisamide on amygdala kindling in rats. Neurosciences 1990; 16: 407–12.
24 Kakegawa N. An experimental study on the modes of appearance and disappearance of suppressive effect of antiepileptic drugs on kindled seizures. Psychiatr Neurol Jpn 1986; 88: 81–98.

25 Wada Y, Hasegawa H, Yamaguchi N. Effect of novel anticonvulsant, zonisamide (AD-810, CI-912), in an experimental model of photosensitive epilepsy. *Epilepsy Res* 1990; 7: 117–20.

26 Bartoszyk GD, Hamer M. The genetic animal model of reflex epilepsy in Mongolian gerbil: differential efficacy of new anticonvulsive drugs and prototype antiepileptics. *Pharmacol Res Commun* 1986; 19: 429–41.

27 Sasa M, Hanaya R, Iida K *et al*. Novel hereditary epileptic model (NER) [in Japanese]. *Nippon Shinkei seishin Yakurigaku Zasshi* 1997; 17: 35–8.

28 Hashiguchi S. Studies on the hippocampal neuronal activity and deep EEG in EL mice: Effect of phenytoin, zonisamide and muscimol. *Kyusyu Seishin Igaku* 1993; 39: 157–70.

29 Miura Y, Kitahara H, Amono S *et al*. Effect of antiepileptics on two different types of seizures in novel epileptic mutant rats (IGER). *Jpn J Pharmacol* 1999; (Suppl. 1): 228.

30 Rock DM, McDonald RL, Taylor CP. Blockade of sustained repetitive action potentials in cultured spinal cord neurons by zonisamide (AD-810, CI 912), a novel anticonvulsant. *Epilepsy Res* 1989; 3: 138–43.

31 Schauf CL. Zonisamide enhances slow inactivation in *Myxicola*. *Brain Res* 1987; 413: 185–8.

32 Suzuki S, Kawakami K, Nishimura S *et al*. Zonisamide blocks T-type calcium channel in cultured neurons of rat cerebral cortex. *Epilepsy Res* 1992; 12: 21–7.

33 Kito M, Maehara M, Watanabe K. Mechanism of T-type calcium channel blockade by zonisamide. *Seizure* 1996; 5: 115–19.

34 Adams PR, Galvin M. Voltage-dependent current of vertebrate neurons and their role in membrane excitability. In: Delgado-Escueta *et al*., eds. *Basic Mechanism of the Epileptics, Advances in Neurology*, Vol. 44. New York: Raven Press, 1986: 137–70.

35 Mimaki T, Suzuki Y, Tagawa T *et al*. [³H] Zonisamide binding in rat brain. *Med J Osaka Univ* 1990; 39: 19–22.

36 Mimaki T, Suzuki Y, Tagawa T *et al*. Interaction of zonisamide with benzodiazepine and GABA receptors in rat brain. *Med J Osaka Univ* 1990; 39: 13–17.

37 Fromm GH, Shibuya T, Terrence CF. Effect of zonisamide (CI-912) on a synaptic system model. *Epilepsia* 1987; 28: 673–9.

38 Okada M, Kawata Y, Mizuno K *et al*. Interaction between Ca⁺⁺, K⁺, carbamazepine and zonisamide on hippocampal extracellular glutamate monitored with microdialysis electrode. *Br J Pharmacol* 1998; 124: 1277–85.

39 Mizuno K. Effect of carbamazepine and zonisamide on acetylcholine levels in rat striatum. *Jpn J Psychopharmacol* 1997; 17: 17–23.

40 Okada M, Kaneko S, Hirano T *et al*. Effect of zonisamide on dopaminergic system. *Epilepsy Res* 1995; 22: 193–205.

41 Hammond EJ, Perchelski RJ, Wilder BJ *et al*. Neuropharmacology of zonisamide, a new antiepileptic drug. *General Pharmacol* 1987; 18: 303–7.

42 Masuda Y, Karasawa T. Inhibitory effect of zonisamide on human carbonic anhydrase *in vitro*. *Arzneim-Forsch/Drug Res* 1993; 43: 416–17.

43 Masuda Y, Noguchi H, Karasawa T. Evidence against a significant implication of carbonic anhydrase inhibitory activity of zonisamide in its anticonvulsant effects. *Azneim-Forsch/Drug Res* 1994; 44: 267–9.

44 Hori M, Ito T, Oka M *et al*. General pharmacology of the novel antiepileptic compound zonisamide – 1st communication: effect on the central nervous system. *Arzneim-Forsch/Drug Res* 1987; 37: 1124–30.

45 Frantseva MV, Velazquez JLP, Carlen AP. Changes in membrane and synaptic properties of thalamocortical circuitory caused by hydrogen peroxide. *J Neurophysiol* 1998; 80: 1317–26.

46 Kusske JA, Wyler AR, Ward AA Jr. Tungstic acid gel as a focal epileptogenic agent. *Exp Neurol* 1974; 42: 587–92.

47 Willmore LJ, Rubin JJ. Antiperoxidant pretreatment and iron-induced epileptiform discharge in the rat: EEG and histopathologic studies. *Neurology* 1981; 31: 63–9.

48 Frantseva MV, Verazquez JLP, Hwang PA, Carlen PL. Free radical production correlates with cell death in an in vitro model of epilepsy. *Eur J Neurosci* 2000; 12: 1431–9.

49 Frantseva MV, Velazquez JLP, Tsorakilidis G *et al*. Oxidative stress is involved in seizure-induced neurodegeneration in the kindling model of epilepsy. *Neuroscience* 2000; 97: 431–5.

50 Komatsu M, Hiramatsu M, Okamura Y. Free radical scavenging activity of zonisamide and its inhibitory effect on lipid peroxidation. *Neuroscience* 1995; 21: 21–9.

51 Hiramatsu M, Komatsu M, Shi H. Free radical scavenging activity of anticonvulsants on in vivo study of iron-induced epileptogenic foci of rats [in Japanese]. *Ann Rep Jpn Epi Res Found* 1997; 9: 91–6.

52 Mori A, Noda Y, Kaneyasu T, Packer L. Antiepileptic mechanism of zonisamide involves its antioxidant effect in the brain. In Nesaretnam K, Packer L, eds. *Micronutrient and Health: Molecular Biological Mechanisms*. Illinois: AOCS Press, 2001: 236–46.

53 Mori A, Noda Y, Packer L. The anticonvulsant zonisamide scavenges free radicals. *Epilepsy Res* 1998; 30: 153–8.

54 Tokumaru J, Ueda Y, Yokoyama H *et al*. In vivo evaluation of hippocampal anti-oxidant ability of zonisamide in rats. *Neurochem Res* 2000; 25: 1107–11.

55 Komatsu M, Hiramatsu M, Willmore LJ. Zonisamide reduces the increase in 8-hydroxy-2′-deoxyguanosine levels formed during iron-induced epileptogenesis in the brain of rats. *Epilepsia* 2000; 41: 1091–4.

56 Kirino T. Delayed neuronal death in the gerbil hippocampus following ischemia. *Brain Res* 1981; 239: 57–69.

57 Benveniste H, Drejer J, Schousboe A, Diemer N. Elevation of the extracellular concentrations of glutamate and aspartate in rat hippocampus during transient cerebral ischemia monitored by intracerebral microdialysis. *J Neurochem* 1984; 43: 1369–74.

58 Fukuda M, Masuda Y. Effect of anticonvulsant on delayed neuronal death in hippocampus of gerbils [in Japanese]. *Med Biol* 1991; 122: 175–8.

59 Fukuda A, Aoki M, Masuda Y. Abnormal behaviors and histological changes induced by ligation of the unilateral common carotid artery in gerbils [in Japanese]. *Med Biol* 1991; 122: 201–3.

60 Owen AJ, Ijas S, Miyashita H *et al*. Zonisamide as a neuroprotective agent in an adult gerbil model of global ischemia: histological, in vitro microdialysis and behavioral study. *Brain Res* 1997; 770: 115–22.

61 Hayakawa T, Higuchi Y, Nigami H *et al*. Zonisamide reduces hypoxic-ischemic brain damage in neonatal rats irrespective of its anticonvulsant effect. *Eur J Clin Pharmacol* 1994; 257: 131–6.

62 Minato H, Kikuta C, Fujitani B *et al*. Protective effect of zonisamide, an antiepileptic drug, against transient focal cerebral ischemia with middle cerebral artery occlusion-reperfusion in rats. *Epilepsia* 1997; 38: 975–80.

63 Kyllerman M, Ben-Menachem E. Zonisamide for progressive myoclonus epilepsy: long term observation in seven patients. *Epilepsy Res* 1998; 29: 109–14.

64 Nakamura N, Ishijima B, Mayanagi Y, Manaka S. A randomized controlled trial of zonisamide in postoperative epilepsy: a report of the cooperative group study [in Japanese]. *Jpn J Neurosurg* 1999; 8: 647–56.

65 Ben-Menachem E, Kyllerman M, Marklund S. Superoxide dismutase and glutathion peroxidase function in progressive myoclonus epilepsies. *Epilepsy Res* 2000; 40: 33–9.

66 Willmore LJ. Post-traumatic seizures. *Neurol Clin* 1993; 11: 823–34.

67 Takemoto Y, Senda H, Yamazoe H *et al*. Toxicity studies of zonisamide (AD-810), a new antiepileptic drug: (1) Acute toxicity study in mice, rats, dogs, monkeys and juvenile rats [in Japanese]. *Jpn Pharmacol Ther* 1993; 15: 4337–46.

68 Takemoto Y, Senda H, Sato Y *et al*. Toxicity studies of zonisamide (AD-810), a new antiepileptic drug: (3) Nine-month chronic toxicity study in rats [in Japanese]. *Jpn Pharmacol Ther* 1987; 15: 4361–86.

69 Takemoto Y, Senda H, Matsuoka N *et al*. Toxicity studies of zonisamide (AD-810), a new antiepileptic drug: (2) One-month subacute toxicity study in rats [in Japanese]. *Jpn Pharmacol Ther* 1987; 15: 4347–60.

70 Terada Y, Ichikawa H, Nishimura K *et al*. Reproduction studies of zonisamide (1) Fertility study in rats [in Japanese]. *Jpn Pharmacol Ther* 1987; 15: 4387–98.

71 Terada Y, Satoh K, Funabashi H *et al*. Reproduction studies of zonisamide (2) Teratogenicity study in rats (Cesarean section and natural delivery studies) [in Japanese]. *Jpn Pharmacol Ther* 1987; 15: 4399–416.

72 Terada Y, Fukagawa S, Shigematsu K *et al*. Reproduction studies of zonisamide (3) Teratogenicity study in mice, dogs, and monkeys [in Japanese]. *Jpn Pharmacol Ther* 1987; 15: 4435–53.

73 Kondo K, Kaneko S, Amano Y *et al*. Preliminary report on teratogenic effect of zonisamide in the offspring of treated women with epilepsy. *Epilepsia* 1996; 37: 1242–4.

74 Masuda Y, Utsui Y, Shiraishi Y *et al*. Pharmacokinetic and pharmacodynamic tolerance of a new anticonvulsant agent (3-sulfamoylmethyl-1,2-

benz-isoxazole) compared to phenobarbital, diphenylhydantoin, and carbamazepine in rats. *Arch Int Pharmacodyn* 1979; 240: 79–89.

75 Kimura M, Tanaka N, Kimura Y *et al*. Pharmacokinetic interaction of zonisamide in rats; effect of other antiepileptics on zonisamide. *J Pharmacobio Dyn* 1992; 15: 631–9.

76 Nishiguchi K, Ohnishi N, Iwakawa S *et al*. Pharmacokinetics of zonisamide: saturable distribution into human and rat erythrocytes and into rat brain. *J Pharmacobio Dyn* 1992; 15: 409–15.

77 Mimaki T, Tonoue H, Matsunaga Y *et al*. Regional distribution of [^{14}C] zonisamide in rat brain. *Epilepsy Res* 1994; 17: 223–6.

78 Taylor CP, Mclean JR, Rockbrader HN *et al*. Zonisamide (AD-810, CI-912). In Meldrum BS, Poret RJ, eds. *New Anticonvulsant Drugs*. London: Libbeya & Co. Ltd., 1986: 277–94.

79 Ono T, Yagi K, Seino M. Clinical efficacy and safety of a new antiepileptic drug, zonisamide: a multi-institutional phase III study [in Japanese]. *Clin Psychiatr* 1988; 30: 471–82.

80 Kochak GM, Page JG, Buchanan RA *et al*. Steady-state Pharmacokinetics of zonisamide, an antiepileptic agent for treatment of refractory complex partial seizures. *J Clin Pharmacol* 1998; 38: 166–71.

81 Yagi K, Seino M, Mihara T *et al*. Open clinical trial of a new antiepileptic drug, zonisamide (ZNA) on 49 patients with refractory epileptic seizures [in Japanese]. *Seishin Igaku* 1987; 29: 111–19.

82 Wagner JG, Sackellares JG, Donofrio PD *et al*. Non-linear pharmacokinetics of CI-912 in adult epileptic patients. *Ther Drug Monitor* 1984; 6: 277–83.

83 Nakasa H, Komiya M, Ohmori S *et al*. Characterization of human liver microsomal cytochrome p450 involved in the reductive metabolism of zonisamide. *Mol Pharmacol* 1993; 44: 216–21.

84 McJilton J, De Tolendo J, De Cerce J *et al*. Cotherapy of lamotrigine/zonisamide results in significant elevation of zonisamide levels [Abstract]. *Epilepsia* 1996; 37 (Suppl. 5): 172.

85 Sackellares JC, Donofrio PD, Wagner JG *et al*. (1985) Pilot study of zonisamide (1,2-benzisoxazole-3-methansulfonamide) in patients with refractory partial seizures. *Epilepsia* 1985; 26: 206–11.

86 Browne TR, Szabo GK, Kres J *et al*. Drug interactions of zonisamide (CI-912) with phenytoin and carbamazepine [Abstract]. *J Clin Pharmacol* 1986; 26: 555.

87 Wilensky AJ, Friel PN, Ojemann LM *et al*. Zonisamide in epilepsy: a pilot study. *Epilepsia* 1985; 26: 212–20.

88 Leppik IE, Willmore LJ, Homan RW *et al*. Efficacy and safety of zonisamide: results of multicenter study. *Epilepsy Res* 1993; 14: 165–73.

89 Peters DH, Sorkin EM. Zonisamide, a review of its pharmacodynamic and pharmacokinetic properties, and therapeutic potential in epilepsy. *Drugs* 1993; 45: 760–87.

90 Baseline controlled safety and efficacy evaluation of zonisamide in the treatment of seizure in medically refractory patients. Files on Dainippon Pharmaceutical Co., Ltd, Osaka, Japan. #810-920.

91 Efficacy and safety report of the extended phase of a baseline-controlled 16 week multicenter study of the efficacy and safety of zonisamide (CI-912) in refractory patients with seizure, USA. Files on Dainippon Pharmaceutical Co., Ltd, Osaka, Japan. #Baseline-contr. Ext.

92 Overall report of the extended phase of the multicenter placebo-controlled double-blind study of the efficacy and safety of zonisamide (CI-912) in the treatment of complex partial seizures in medially refractory patients (USA). Files on Dainippon Pharmaceutical Co., Ltd, Osaka, Japan. #912-US-Ext.

93 Ota Y, Nakane Y, Hironaka I *et al*. Therapeutic effect of zonisamide (AD-810, ZNS) on refractory partial epilepsy [in Japanese]. *J Clin Ther Med* 1987; 3 (Suppl.): 1079–87.

94 Kohsaka M, Sumi T, Hiba T *et al*. The long term treatment of zonisamide for epileptic patients with intractable epilepsy [in Japanese] *J Clin Ther Med* 1987; 3 (Suppl.): 1343–52.

95 Nishiura N, Oiwa N. Clinical study of a new antiepileptic drug, AD-810 (zonisamide): long-term use in intractable patients [in Japanese]. *Jpn Pharmacol Ther* 1987; 15: 4217–23.

96 Kanazawa O, Sengoku A, Kawai I. Experiences of zonisamide treatment on adults and children with refractory epilepsy: follow up for more than 1 year. *J Jpn Epileptic Soc* 1990; 8: 29–38.

97 Wilder BJ, Sackellares JC, Wilensky AJ *et al*. Zonisamide as long-term treatment for refractory partial and generalized tonic-clonic seizures. *Neurology* 1987; 37 (Suppl. 1): 351–2.

98 Shimizu A, Ikoma R, Shimizu T. Effects and side effects of zonisamide during long-term medication. *Curr Ther Res Clin Exp* 1990; 47: 696–706.

99 Sugihara H, Yoneyama K, Kamo C *et al*. Long-term clinical efficacy of zonisamide in patients with symptomatic epilepsies [in Japanese]. *Jpn Pharmacol Ther* 1992; 20: 4657–61.

100 Kumagai N, Seki T, Yamawaki H *et al*. Monotherapy for childhood epilepsies with zonisamide. *Jpn J Psychiatr Neurol* 1991; 45: 357–9.

101 Hosoda N, Miura H, Takahashi S *et al*. Once-daily dose of zonisamide monotherapy in the control of partial seizures in children with cryptogenic localization-related epilepsies: clinical efficacy and their pharmacokinetic basis. *Jpn J Psychiatr Neurol* 1994; 48: 335–7.

102 Suzuki Y, Nagai T, Ono J *et al*. Zonisamide monotherapy in newly diagnosed infantile spasms. *Epilepsia* 1997; 38: 1035–8.

103 Henry TR, Leppik IE, Robert J *et al*. Progressive myoclonus epilepsy treated with zonisamide. *Neurology* 1988; 38: 928–31.

104 Hurd RW, Wilder GJ, Wendell R *et al*. Treatment of four siblings with progressive myoclonus epilepsy of the Unverricht-Lundborg type with N-acetylcysteine. *Neurology* 1996; 47: 1264–8.

105 Fukuda M, Masuda Y. Cerebral protective effect of zonisamide and its clinical experience on post operative seizures [in Japanese]. *Jpn Pharmacol Ther* 1991; 19: 2011–18.

106 Integrated summary of safety in NDA of zonisamide in the US. Files on Dainippon Pharmaceutical Co., Ltd, Osaka, Japan. Zonisamide capsules 100 mg: 8h-A.9. Number of patients reporting TEAEs in placebo-controlled studies.

107 Seino M, Ito T. Zonisamide. In: Engel J Jr, Pedlley TA, eds. *Epilepsy: A comprehensive textbook*. Philadelphia: Lippincott-Raven, 1997: 1619–26.

108 Padgett CS, Bergen DC, French JA *et al*. Renal calculi associated with zonisamide. *Epilepsia* 1996; 37 (Suppl. 5): 173.

109 Okumura A, Hayakawa F, Kuno K *et al*. Oligohidrosis caused by zonisamide [in Japanese]. *No to Hattatsu* 1996; 28: 44–7.

110 Hosoda N, Miura H, Shirai H *et al*. Clinical study on oligohidrosis in patients treated with zonisamide [in Japanese]. *Shonika Rinsyo* 1996; 49: 2445–9.

Other Drugs More Rarely Used in the Treatment of Epilepsy

H. Meierkord

Adrenocorticotropic hormone (ACTH)

ACTH is an endogenous hormone released by the anterior pituitary gland that regulates secretion of glucocorticoids and sex hormones. Since the 1950s ACTH has been used to treat a variety of seizure types and epileptic syndromes.

Chemistry

ACTH is a peptide consisting of 39 amino acids.

Mechanisms of action

The anticonvulsant mechanisms of action of ACTH is unclear. It differs from other anticonvulsants, in that its effect in stopping seizures and normalizing the EEG in infantile spasms is frequently an all or none phenomenon. Furthermore, the seizure-free state, when achieved, is frequently long lasting even when the drug is withdrawn. These clinical observations indicate that ACTH is able to improve deranged homeostatic mechanisms in the brain during a discrete period of postnatal development [1]. Huttenlocher [2] has suggested that ACTH might accelerate the retarded brain development in patients with infantile spasms. Croiset and de Wied [3] investigated the anticonvulsant effect of various ACTH fragments on pilocarpine-induced epilepsy. Pilocarpine is a cholinergic muscarine agonist, which induces epileptic seizures. These attacks show a characteristic sequential development of behavioural features and EEG activity [4]. Only the sequences 4–7 and 7–16 of the ACTH molecule, but not the other longer fragments, were found to reduce epileptiform activity in this model. The effective fragments do not possess a peripheral endocrine activity suggesting an independent anticonvulsant activity of ACTH. The precise mechanism is not yet known, but ACTH may act on the cholinergic system.

Recently, Brunson *et al.* [5] published experimental data supporting direct central nervous system actions of ACTH. The substance given either systemically or directly into the cerebral ventricles influences gene expression in specific brain regions.

Pharmacokinetics

Since ACTH is inactivated in the gastrointestinal tract, it must be administered parenterally. ACTH is rapidly metabolized and has a short half-life of only 15 min.

Biotransformation

Although the precise metabolic fate of ACTH is not known, circulating ACTH is probably enzymatically cleaved at the 16–17 lysine–arginine bond by the plasmin–plasminogen system.

Drug interaction

Drugs that induce hepatic enzymes, such as phenobarbital or phenytoin, may increase the clearance of corticosteroids. Therefore, increases in corticoid dose may be required to achieve the desired response.

Clinical efficacy

Infantile spasms

ACTH is used for the treatment of infantile spasms or West's syndrome, a condition consisting of infantile spasms, disturbed psychomotor development and the characteristic EEG pattern of hypsarrhythmia. There has been some discussion as to whether corticosteroids are more effective compared to ACTH. Although Hrachovy *et al.* [6] in a double-blind, placebo-controlled, crossover study did not find any difference in the effectiveness of ACTH or prednisone, the majority of physicians prefer ACTH [7–11]. Snead recommends the following dosage: $150\,U/m^2$/day in two divided doses for 1 week, followed by $75\,U/m^2$/day in a single dose for another week and then this same dose only on alternate days for 2 weeks. Four weeks after starting treatment the alternate-day dose of ACTH is gradually reduced over 8 or 9 weeks, until discontinued.

ACTH has an all or nothing effect in infantile spasms [6]; monitoring is therefore relatively straightforward. In about 70–75% of children, ACTH is effective in stopping the seizures and valproate, gabapentin and benzodiazepines may also be effective. Pietz *et al.* [12] reported encouraging results using high-dosage vitamin B_6 in the treatment of infantile spasms. Such a regimen has the advantage of avoiding the toxicity of ACTH therapy.

Lennox–Gastaut syndrome (LGS)

ACTH has been reported to be effective in patients with LGS [13,14]. Although response rates of 40–60% have been reported, it is not clear which seizures types are most responsive. The marked variability in seizure frequency over time and the lack of objective criteria for evaluating response to treatment makes it difficult to determine anticonvulsant efficacy in such patients. At present, there is no controlled evidence that ACTH therapy significantly alters the course of these patients.

Rasmussen's syndrome

Hart *et al.* [15] reported that 10 of 17 patients with Rasmussen's syndrome who were treated with steroids (ACTH or prednisone) showed some reduction (25–73%) in seizure frequency. However, only two patients showed prolonged benefit after steroid withdrawal.

Further studies are needed before specific recommendations can be made.

Side-effects

Treatment with ACTH may have a number of severe side-effects.

Hypertension develops in 4–33% of patients with infantile spasms who are treated with ACTH or corticosteroids [16]. A variety of infections have also been reported in patients treated with ACTH and corticosteroids, including pneumonia, septicaemia, urinary tract infections, gastroenteritis, ear infection, candidiasis and encephalitis [16]. Pneumonia is one of the most commonly occurring infections and may result in death. Hypokalaemia may occur rarely in patients receiving higher doses and longer durations of hormonal therapy [16]. Myocardial hypertrophy develops in 72–90% of patients with infantile spasms who are treated with ACTH. These ECG changes are reversible within months after discontinuation of ACTH therapy [17]. Transient brain shrinkage may occur in 63% of patients with infantile spasm with ACTH [18]. This phenomenon reverses on discontinuance of therapy. Finally, most children will develop cushingoid features and exhibit irritability.

Clinical therapeutics

With the exception of infantile spasms the therapeutic benefit of the substance remains to be demonstrated.

Allopurinol

Developing antiepileptic agents that are specifically tailored to a patient's individual biochemistry has long been a goal of neurology.

Allopurinol was introduced initially by Coleman *et al.* [19] for the treatment of epilepsy in patients with additional hyperuricaemia. Subsequently, DeMarco and Zagnoni [20] reported that the drug was also effective in patients with epilepsy without hyperuricosuria.

Chemistry

Allopurinol (4-hydroxypyrazolo-3,4-D-dipyramidine) is a structural analogue of hypoxanthine with a molecular weight of 136.1.

Mechanisms of action

Allopurinol inhibits the enzyme xanthine oxidase with subsequent reduction of uric acid in the blood, but the mechanism of antiepileptic action is unclear. It is also unknown if the anticonvulsant effect is based on allopurinol only, or on oxypurinol, the main and active metabolite or on both.

Experimental studies have shown that allopurinol suppresses epileptiform activity induced by penicillin in the rat hippocampus [21]. Hoppe *et al.* [22] on the other hand, did not find anticonvulsant effects on a model of oxygen-induced seizures in mice. The effect of allopurinol on hippocampal-kindled seizures has been investigated by Wada *et al.* [23], employing two different doses (5 and 50 mg/kg). It was found that the high dose had a significant effect on the behavioural seizures, but the duration of after-discharges was not affected by either dose. Thus, allopurinol is an effective anticonvulsant in some models. The underlying mechanisms of action may be due to the effect on excitotoxicity. Allopurinol inhibits tryptophan-2,3-dioxygenase which causes a reduction in quinolinic acid, an endogenous glutamate analogue with strong antiepileptic action. It has been postulated that this is the underlying mechanism of at least part of its antiepileptic mechanisms [24]. In addition, the substance appears to suppress free radical generation [25].

Pharmacokinetics

The drug is quickly absorbed in the gastrointestinal tract, the bioavailability is > 80%. After oral intake peak levels of allopurinol are reached within 30–120 min The peak levels of oxypurinol, which is the active metabolite of allopurinol, is found after 2–5 h after both, oral and intravenous application [26].

Biotransformation

Twenty per cent of allopurinol is excreted in faeces within 48–72 h after oral intake. The main active metabolite oxypurinol is completely excreted in urine without further metabolism [27].

Drug interactions

Various reports [20,28,29] suggest that plasma concentrations of most anticonvulsant drugs are not affected by the additional administration of allopurinol. There is, however, one report of allopurinol-induced elevation of carbamazepine levels [30].

Clinical efficacy

The effectiveness of allopurinol in epilepsy is controversial. Sander and Patsolos [31] did not find the drug effective in intractable epilepsy, nor did So and Ptacek [32]. Other clinical trials suggest that allopurinol is most effective in patients with focal epilepsy and secondary generalized seizures. DeMarco and Zagnoni [20,28] found it effective in generalized tonic-clonic seizures. Tada *et al.* [29] reported the anticonvulsant efficacy of allopurinol in generalized tonic-clonic seizures and focal epilepsy, but found it ineffective in LGS. Conversely, Marrosu *et al.* [33] found it effective in particular in LGS, but not in other forms of epilepsy. Zagnoni *et al.* [34] assessed the anticonvulsant effect of allopurinol in a double-blind, randomized, placebo-controlled, crossover trial in 84 patients with epileptic seizures refractory to standard anticonvulsant drugs. Allopurinol significantly reduced total seizures ($P=0.005$), and secondarily generalized seizures ($P=0.0015$). Median seizure reduction for total seizures was 10.5 and 27.9% for secondarily generalized seizures. Another double-blind, placebo-controlled crossover trial with allopurinol as add-on therapy in childhood refractory epilepsy had less favourable results [35]. Seventeen patients received allopurinol and matched placebo for 12 weeks in two doses (10 mg/kg/day during the first week and 15 mg/kg/day thereafter with a washout period of 2 weeks between treatment phases). The total number of seizures was reduced by 50–98% in four patients (23.5%) and by 25–49% in another four (23.5%). However, the number of seizures remained unchanged in five patients (29.4%) and worsened in four (23.5%). A mean follow-up of 10 months of the responders did not show any relevant efficacy of allopurinol as an adjuvant therapy for refractory epilepsy, even at high doses. Thus, further studies are needed to determine the exact place for allopurinol as an anticonvulsant.

Allopurinol is used as an add-on therapy with dosages of up to 15 mg/kg/day twice or three times a day.

Side-effects

Side-effects, in general, are mild and may occur in up to 25% of patients including headache, diarrhoea and malaise [31], decreased appetite, drowsiness and abdominal pain [29]. It is unclear if the side-effects are dose dependent.

Adverse side-effects (17.6%) were generally mild and transient, suggesting that allopurinol is well tolerated.

Clinical therapeutics

Allopurinol may play a minor role as an adjuvant therapy for refractory epilepsy.

Bromide

Bromides were the first effective anticonvulsants [36] but their use in the treatment of epilepsy dropped dramatically after the introduction of phenobarbital and phenytoin [37]. Since then the drug gained a reputation of having a very narrow target range and being less effective than other anticonvulsant drugs [38]. However, there are also studies which have shown that bromides are more effective than other drugs in the treatment of special syndromes such as refractory tonic-clonic seizures of childhood [39–41], of severe myoclonic epilepsy in infants [42], and of malignant migrating partial seizures in infancy [43].

Chemistry

Bromide is formulated in various salts. In clinical practice the salts most commonly used are sodium bromide, calcium bromide and ammonium bromide. Bromine itself is a non-metallic element which does not occur in pure form in nature because of its high reactivity.

Mechanisms of action

The mechanisms by which bromide produces anticonvulsant effects are still not entirely clear. According to Balcar et al. [44] bromide does not affect the γ-aminobutyric acid (GABA)-ergic inhibitory system. This was indicated by a lack of changes in the metabolism or transport of GABA and also by unchanged characteristics of the receptor-associated GABA binding sites under acute or chronic bro-

mide exposure. In contrast, Suzuki et al. [45] have shown that bromide potentiates GABA-activated currents in cultured cerebral neurones. To clarify such contradictory results we have recently tested the effect of the substance on GABAergic inhibition in a paired-pulse protocol and on inhibitory postsynaptic currents [46]. A significant increase in paired-pulse inhibition was seen in a paired-pulse stimulation protocol used to monitor the efficacy of GABAergic inhibition at concentrations of 5 mmol sodium bromide (NaBr). This finding was confirmed in whole cell patch clamp recordings from cultured hippocampal neurones showing an increase in inhibitory postsynaptic current amplitude.

It has also been suggested that bromide may interact with the enzyme CA resulting in extracellular acidosis and consequent inhibition of epileptiform activity [47]. This prompted us to compare the effect of both the CA blocker AZM and NaBr on extracellular pH changes at rest and following electrical stimulation [46]. Using pH-sensitive microelectrodes different effects of NaBr compared to those of AZM on extracellular pH under control conditions and after stimulation were seen. AZM at 1 mmol caused a reversible acidification of ΔpH: 0.2 ± 0.14 at rest whereas no change on extracellular pH was seen with 5 mmol NaBr. AZM increased the transient alkalosis induced by repetitive stimulation of the stratum radiatum in area CA1 and reduced the subsequent acidosis. NaBr also increased the alkalosis but had no effect on the subsequent acidosis. The results indicate that the anticonvulsant properties of bromide are unlikely to be caused by its effect on extracellular pH. In preclinical studies Grewal et al. [48] demonstrated the anticonvulsant potency of NaBr using six different procedures, four electrical and two chemical. The electrical procedures included the maximal electroshock seizure pattern test, the minimal electroshock seizure pattern test, the minimal electroshock seizure pattern in hyponatraemic (low-threshold) mice test and a test in which unidirectional currents of four times threshold intensity are delivered. The chemical procedures were based on pentylenetetrazole injections. It could be demonstrated that NaBr is effective by all tests employed and modifies seizure pattern as well as elevates seizure threshold.

Using combined rat hippocampus–entorhinal cortex slices Meierkord et al. [46] analysed the effects of NaBr on four types of epileptiform discharges in two different models of epilepsy, the low Ca^{2+} and the low Mg^{2+} model.

NaBr concentration-dependently reduced the frequency and finally blocked the low Ca^{2+}-induced discharges. Low Mg^{2+}-induced short recurrent discharges were also reduced in a concentration-dependent manner. In the entorhinal cortex the frequency of seizure-like events was reduced by 3 and 5 mmol and the discharges were blocked by 7 mmol NaBr. Also, the late recurrent discharges in the entorhinal cortex which do not respond to most clinically employed anticonvulsants were reduced by concentrations of 10 and 15 mmol and completely blocked by 30 mmol NaBr (Fig. 49.1).

Pharmacokinetics

Bromide is completely resorbed from the gastrointestinal tract and distributed throughout the body in an almost identical fashion to chloride [49]. It replaces chloride in extracellular fluids and the equivalent amount of chloride is excreted. Intracellularly, bromide is found largely in red blood cells. The rate of distribution to the cerebrospinal fluid, gastrointestinal tract and muscle is slower. The

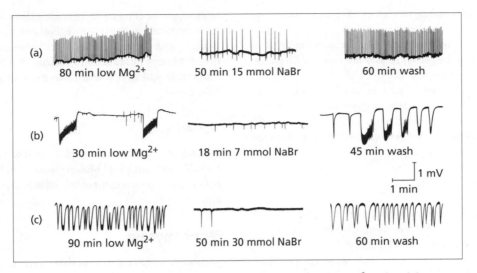

Fig. 49.1 Effects of NaBr on different types of spontaneous epileptiform activities. (a) Effects on low Mg^{2+}-induced short recurrent discharges. Low Mg^{2+}-induced activity in hippocampal area CA1 is characterized by short recurrent discharges associated with positive field potentials superimposed by repetitively bursting spikes following 80 min of washout of Mg^{2+}. SRDs in hippocampal region CAI are reduced under 15 mmol NaBr in frequency but not in amplitude while under 20 mmol the short recurrent discharges were completely blocked (not shown). Reversibility of the anticonvulsant effects. (b) Low Mg^{2+}-induced seizure-like events. Seizure-like events characterized by tonic- and clonic-like electrographic activity superimposed on slow negative field potentials appear in the entorhinal cortex but not in hippocampus proper after 30 min of washout of Mg^{2+}. NaBr in concentrations of 7 mmol blocked these discharges reversibly. (c) Effects on low Mg^{2+}-induced late recurrent discharges. Following prolonged washout of Mg^{2+} (90 min) the seizure-like events in the entorhinal cortex change to late recurrent discharges. NaBr in concentrations of 30 mmol blocked such activity reversibly.

ion easily crosses the placenta and with the breast milk it can cause fetal hypotonia and irritability when used during pregnancy or nursing [50,51]. Bromide is excreted unchanged by the kidneys. In the distal tubule there is a competitive reabsorption of chloride and bromide, a fact that can be exploited in cases of bromide intoxication since administration of chloride will speed up bromide excretion. The elimination half-life ranges between 10.5 and 14 days [50], so the steady-state concentration is not reached for 40–50 days [52].

Biotransformation

There is no biotransformation and bromide is excreted unchanged.

Drug interactions

Bromide does not bind to plasma proteins and there is no evidence that it induces or inhibits hepatic enzymes responsible for the metabolism of other anticonvulsants. For these reasons, no metabolic drug interactions are expected. However, bromide may enhance the depressant effect of other AEDs. It should also be kept in mind that there is a drug–food interaction with the chloride ion. When NaCl is ingested in the form of table salt, the chloride ion in NaCl displaces the bromide ion so that the bromide does not accumulate as expected. Therefore, it is recommended that the ingestion of NaCl is held fairly constant during administration of bromides.

Clinical efficacy

There are no randomized, placebo-controlled trials with bromides to determine their efficacy. Much of the available literature is in the form of single case reports and anecdotal information. Most therapeutic efforts and recent reports focus on the treatment of infants, children and adolescents.

Livingston and Pearson [53] reported the effects of triple bromide elixir (ammonium bromide, potassium bromide and sodium bromide) in 196 children with epilepsy. Sixty-one patients had complete seizure control, 39 were markedly improved (75% reduction in number of seizures), 15 had less than a 50% improvement and 81 did not improve. Of the various seizure types, bromides appeared most effective against generalized tonic-clonic, partial, myoclonic and akinetic seizures. There was no beneficial effect on absence seizures. Dreifuss and Bertram [52] reported six patients treated with bromides. Two patients with complex partial seizures and two patients with generalized tonic-clonic seizures became seizure free. Two patients with absence seizures did not show an improvement. Boenick et al. [39] reported the effects in 68 children and adults. Thirty-three per cent of patients with tonic-clonic seizures of early childhood became seizure free. No improvement in patients with LGS was seen.

Woody et al. [50] carried out a study in children with different types of epilepsy including photosensitive epilepsy, acquired epileptic aphasia, LGS and focal seizures. Six of 11 patients had at least a 75% improvement in seizure control. Three patients had transient improvement, and two had no reduction in seizure frequency. Steinhoff and Kruse [41] reported the results of bromide in 60 cases with generalized tonic-clonic seizures resistant to treatment with standard medication. There was a 50% reduction in seizure frequency in 58% of patients.

Oguni et al. [42], in a study on 22 infants with severe epilepsy and various seizure types, saw KBr reduce the frequency of tonic-clonic seizures in 17 of 22 patients. In addition, focal seizures were reduced in all seven patients and myoclonic or absence seizures were also reduced in four patients.

Okuda *et al.* [43] reported complete seizure control in one and 95% reduction in seizure frequency in another infant with malignant migrating partial seizures in infancy.

The usual dosage in children under 6 years of age ranges from 300 mg twice a day to 600 mg three times a day; over 6 years of age, a dose of 300 mg to 1 g is given three times a day. The therapeutic blood bromide concentration has been reported to range between 10 and 20 mmol/L [50,52].

Side-effects

Apart from bromide exanthema, side-effects are generally dose dependent and these may be divided into those affecting the gastrointestinal tract, the skin and the nervous system.

Effects on the gastrointestinal tract include anorexia, constipation and weight loss [47]. Pancreatitis as a side-effect of potassium bromide therapy has also been described [54].

In cases of bromism the tongue may feel coated and sore. When large quantities of bromide salts are ingested, nausea and vomiting may occur [55].

The three main dermatological manifestations are bromide exanthema, acneiform eruptions and bromoderma tuberosum [56]. Acneiform rashes usually occur on the face but may also spread over the neck, chest and arms [52]. If a rash develops the medication should be discontinued. The bromoderma tuberosum is in most cases fully reversible after cessation of the medication. The mechanisms by which the lesions and the associated intraepidermal abscesses are formed is unknown.

Neuropsychiatric side-effects (bromism) are sedation, action myoclonus, cerebellar signs such as ataxia and dysarthria, decreased libido, dysphagia, decreased tendon jerks, somnolence, tremor and hallucinations [47]. Severe bromism is associated with bromide concentrations above 200 mg/100 mL and manifest as restlessness, headache, delirium and dementia. Other features consist of diminished deep tendon reflexes, loss of pupil reflexes, papilloedema, increased cerebrospinal fluid pressure, slowing on EEG and loss of gag reflex [57].

Clinical therapeutics

Bromides are no longer a mainstay of treatment for epilepsy. However, given the fact that bromides are cheap and widely available anticonvulsants with powerful anticonvulsant properties their use should be considered more frequently in severe forms of childhood epilepsy.

Ethotoin

Ethotoin is a phenyl derivative with a structure and mechanism of action similar to phenytoin. Today, it is rarely used in clinical practice.

Therapeutic use

The drug has a lower anticonvulsant potency than phenytoin and has hypnotic properties; both factors limit its clinical use. It is at-

tractive, on the other hand, because it lacks the side-effects of gingival hyperplasia and hirsutism. Ethotoin is mostly used as an adjunct in cases with generalized tonic-clonic seizures. Carter *et al.* [58] found it useful in reduction of seizure frequency in children with intractable epilepsy. Ethotoin is given in divided doses of 20–40 mg/kg/day.

Side-effects

Side-effects include ataxia, visual disturbances, rash and gastrointestinal problems [59]. Malformations such as cleft lip and cleft palate have been reported in infants born to mothers taking ethotoin [60].

Mephenytoin

Mephenytoin has a structure that clearly resembles phenytoin and ethotoin.

Mechanisms of action

The mechanisms of action are presumed to be similar to phenytoin, but its effectiveness against pentylenetetrazole-induced seizures is greater. It inhibits post-tetanic potentiation and prevents the tonic phase in tonic-clonic seizures. It is also effective against seizures induced by bicucculline and picrotoxin [59].

Therapeutic use

Mephenytoin has the same spectrum of indications as phenytoin, but because of its common side-effects its use should be limited to those cases unable to tolerate other drugs. It is effective in complex partial seizures and tonic-clonic attacks, but it may exacerbate absence seizures [59]. The usual daily dose is 300–600 mg in adults, given in divided doses.

Side-effects

Side-effects include skin rashes, hepatotoxicity, periarteritis nodosa and lupus erythematosus. Other adverse effects are psychotic reactions and behavioural disturbances.

Paraldehyde

Paraldehyde is a hypnotic drug that has been used primarily for the treatment of withdrawal seizures and status epilepticus.

Mechanisms of action

The mechanisms of this drugs anticonvulsant actions are unclear.

Pharmacokinetics and clinical efficacy

The drug is rapidly and completely absorbed and reaches a peak concentration in the plasma within 30–60 min after oral, rectal or intramuscular administration. About 30% is eliminated via the lungs and the remainder is metabolized in the liver. The half-life can be greatly increased in hepatic disease. Today, the sole indication for paraldehyde is in the treatment of acute seizures or status epilepticus. The literature concerning efficacy comprises case reports and small case series, and there are no modern assessments or controlled studies. It is apparent that paraldehyde is highly effective in stopping seizures, and although there are no controlled comparisons, paraldehyde probably has similar efficacy in acute epilepsy as the benzodiazepines, barbiturates or phenytoin.

Side-effects

The main toxicity results from the use of inappropriately diluted or decomposed paraldehyde. Paraldehyde has a short shelf life, and to prevent decomposition, the drug should be freshly made and not be unduly exposed to light. The decomposed compound can result in precipitation, microembolism, thrombosis or cardiovascular collapse. The drug also reacts with rubber and plastic, therefore IV infusions must be given via glass giving sets and syringes. Paraldehyde has the advantage that hypotension and respiratory arrest are less common than with the benzodiazepines, phenytoin or phenobarbital. Direct injury from arterial injection leading to both arterial and venous thrombosis has been reported [61]. It can also result in lactic acidosis. The intramuscular injection is extremely painful and can result in a sterile abscess and inflammatory response. Sciatic nerve damage is a risk if the injection is too close to the nerve.

Clinical therapeutics

Paraldehyde has a small but useful place in contemporary therapy. It is mainly used as an alternative or sequel to the administration of diazepam in acute seizures or the stage of early status epilepticus [62,63]. It has the great advantage of little sedation or cardiorespiratory risk, and so can be given rectally in situations where there are no facilities for resuscitation (e.g. at home or in residential institutions). The drug can be administered intravenously, intramuscularly or rectally. The drug should never be administered intra-arterially. The usual rectal or IM dosage is 5–10 mL diluted with the same volume of water (adults) or 0.07–0.34 mL/kg (children). The dose can be repeated after 15–30 min. For intravenous use, according to Lockman [64], the drug is diluted with saline to a concentration of 10% which is slowly infused in a dose of 0.3 mL/kg. In contemporary clinical practice, the intramuscular and the intravenous route are now rarely used as safer alternatives are available.

Phenacemide

Phenacemide was introduced by Gibb *et al.* [65] for patients with intractable complex partial seizures.

Mechanisms of action

Phenacemide prevents maximal electroshock-induced seizures and elevates seizure threshold to pentylenetetrazol [66,67].

Therapeutic use

Because of its serious side-effects, the drug is rarely used, although efficacy may be greater and toxicity less than previously thought [68]. It is only indicated in intractable complex partial seizures when other drugs have failed. The total daily dose ranges from 20 to 40 mg/kg.

Side-effects

The major problem with this drug is its tendency to induce personality changes, aggression and acute psychosis [69]. Other side-effects include sedation, insomnia, vertigo, headache and drowsiness.

Trimethadione

Trimethadione was the first drug of choice for absence seizures until the introduction of ethosuximide and valproic acid. It was one of the first drugs that was shown to act selectively on specific epileptic symptoms [70]. The production of trimethadione had stopped in most countries by the end of 1994.

Absorption, distribution and excretion

The drug is rapidly absorbed after oral administration and reaches a peak plasma concentration in 0.5–2 h. The half-life is 240 h and trimethadione is eliminated to 95% by the liver.

Mechanisms of action

The compound is more effective against pentylenetetrazol-induced seizures than against electrically induced seizures. Several mechanisms of action have been suggested, including augmentation of GABA [71], blocking of extracellular potassium accumulation [72] and induction of extracellular acidosis [73].

Therapeutic use

The main indication for trimethadione is absence seizures in patients who are not adequately controlled by other anticonvulsants, or who do not tolerate these. It is not effective in focal seizures or generalized tonic-clonic attacks. The usual daily dose is 20–40 mg/kg/day. The therapeutic plasma concentration ranges between 500 and 1200 µg/mL.

Side-effects

The drug is intensely teratogenic and must not be given to women of childbearing age [74]. Side-effects are dose related and include sedation and blurred vision [75]. Other adverse effects are skin reactions such as rash and erythema multiforme. Pancytopenia has been reported and a myasthenic syndrome may also occur [76].

References

1 Snead OC. How does ACTH work against infantile spasms? Bedside to bench. *Ann Neurol* 2001; 49: 288–9.
2 Huttenlocher PR. Dendritic development in neocortex of children with mental defect and infantile spasms. *Neurology* 1974; 24: 203–10.
3 Croiset G, de Wied D. ACTH: a structure-activity study on pilocarpine-induced epilepsy. *Eur J Parmacol* 1992; 229: 211–16.

4 Turski L, Ikonomidou C, Turski W, Bortolotto ZA, Cavalheiro EA. Review: cholinergic mechanisms and epileptogenesis. The seizures induced by pilocarpine: a novel experimental model of intractable epilepsy. *Synapse* 1989; 3: 154–71.

5 Brunson KL, Khan N, Eghbal-Ahmadi M, Baram TZ. Corticotropin (ACTH) acts directly on amygdala neurons to down-regulate corticotropin-releasing hormone gene expression. *Ann Neurol* 2001; 49: 304–12.

6 Hrachovy RA, Frost JD, Kellaway P, Zion TE. Double-blind study of ACTH vs. Prednisone therapy in infantile spasms. *J Pediatr* 1983; 103: 641–5.

7 Hrachovy RA, Frost JD, Kellaway P, Zion TE. A controlled study of prednisone therapy in infantile spasms. *Epilepsia* 1979; 20: 403–7.

8 Hrachovy RA, Frost JD, Kellaway P, Zion TE. A controlled study of ACTH therapy in infantile spasms. *Epilepsia* 1980; 21: 631–6.

9 Snead OC. Adrenocorticotropic hormone (ACTH). In: Levy R *et al.*, eds. *Antiepileptic Drugs*, 3rd edn. New York: Raven Press, 1989.

10 Snead OC. Treatment of infantile spasms with highdose ACTH: efficacy and plasma levels of ACTH and cortisol. *Neurology* 1989; 39: 1027–31.

11 Holmes GL. Effect of non-sex hormones on neuronal excitability, seizures, and the electroencephalogram. *Epilepsia* 1991; 32 (Suppl. 6): S11–S18.

12 Pietz J, Benninger H, Sontheimer D, Mittermaier G, Rating D. Treatment of infantile spasms with high-dosage vitamin B_6. *Epilepsia* 1993; 34: 757–63.

13 Yamatogi Y, Ohtsuka Y, Ishida T *et al.* Treatment of the Lennox syndrome with ACTH: a clinical and electroencephalographic study. *Brain Dev* 1979; 1: 267–76.

14 Kurokawa T, Goya N, Fukuyama Y *et al.* West syndrome and Lennox–Gastaut syndrome: a survey of natural history. *Pediatrics* 1980; 65: 81–8.

15 Hart YM, Cortez M, Andermann F *et al.* Medical treatment of Rasmussen's syndrome (chronic encephalitis and epilepsy): effect of high-dose steroids or immunoglobulins in 19 patients. *Neurology* 1994; 44: 1030–6.

16 Hrachovy RA, Frost JD Jr, Glaze DG. High-dose, long-duration versus low-dose, short-duration corticotropin therapy for infantile spasms. *J Pediatr* 1994; 124: 803–6.

17 Bobele GB, Ward KE, Bodensteiner JB. Hypertrophic cardiomyopathy during corticotropin therapy for infantile spasms. A clinical and echocardiographic study. *Am J Dis Child* 1993; 147: 223–5.

18 Glaze DG, Hrachovy RA, Frost JD Jr, Zion TE, Bryan RN. Computed tomography in infantile spasms: effects of hormonal therapy. *Pediatr Neurol* 1986; 2: 23–7.

19 Coleman M, Landgrebe M, Landgrebe A. Progressive seizures with hyperuricosuria reversed by allopurinol. *Arch Neurol* 1974; 31: 238–42.

20 DeMarco P, Zagoni P. Allopurinol and severe epilepsy. *Neurology* 1986; 37: 1691–2.

21 Makhailov IB, Gusel WA. Pharmaco-dynamic mechanisms for reducing the activity of an epileptogenic focus with allopurinol. *Neuropatol Psikiatr* 1983; 83: 870–3.

22 Hoppe, SA, Terrell DJ, Gottlieb SF. The effect of allopurinol on oxygen-induced seizures in mice. *Aviat Space Environ Med* 1984; 55: 927–30.

23 Wada Y, Hasegawa H, Nakamura M, Yamaguchi N. Anticonvulsant effects of allopurinol on hippocampal-kindled seizures. *Pharmacol Biochem Behav* 1992; 42: 899–901.

24 Stober T, Jacobi P. Allopurinol and epilepsy. *Neurology* 1987; 37: 1691.

25 Murashima YL, Kasamo K, Suzuki J. Antiepileptic effects of allopurinol on EL mice are associated with changes in SOD isoenzyme activities. *Epilepsy Res* 1998; 32: 254–65.

26 Breithaupt B, Tittel M. Kinetics of allopurinol after single intravenous and oral doses. Noninteraction with benzobromarone and hydrochlorothiazide. *Eur J Clin Pharmacol* 1982; 22: 77–84.

27 Turnheim K, Krivanek P, Oberbauer R. Pharmacokinetics and pharmacodynamics of allopurinol in elderly and young subjects. *Br J Clin Pharmacol* 1999; 48: 501–9.

28 DeMarco P, Zagoni P. Allopurinol and severe epilepsy. A preliminary report. *Neuropsychobiology* 1988; 19: 51–3.

29 Tada H, Morooka K, Arimoto K, Matsuo T. Clinical effects of intractable epilepsy. *Epilepsia* 1991; 32: 279–83.

30 Mikati M, Erba G, Skouteli H, Gadia C. Allopurinol–carbamazepine drug interactions in resistant epilepsy. *Neurology* 1990; 40 (Suppl. 1): 139.

31 Sander JW, Patsolos PN. Allopurinol as an add-on drug in the management of intractable epilepsy. *Epilepsy Res* 1988; 2: 323–5.

32 So EL, Ptacek L. Failure of allopurinol as an adjunct therapy in intractable epilepsy. *Epilepsia* 1988; 29: 671.

33 Marrosu F, Marrosu G, Rachele MG, Masala C, Giagheddu M. Allopurinol add-on treatment in intractable seizures. *Acta Neurol Napoli* 1990; 12: 207–13.

34 Zagnoni PG, Bianchi A, Zolo P *et al.* Allopurinol as add-on therapy in refractory epilepsy: a double-blind placebo-controlled randomized study. *Epilepsia* 1994; 35: 107–12.

35 Coppola G, Pascotto A. Double-blind, placebo-controlled, cross-over trial of allopurinol as add-on therapy in childhood refractory epilepsy. *Brain Dev* 1996; 18: 50–2.

36 Locock C. Discussion of paper by EH Sieveking: analysis of 52 cases of epilepsy observed by author. *Lancet* 1857; 1: 527.

37 Friedlander WJ. The rise and fall of bromide therapy in epilepsy. *Arch Neurol* 2000; 57: 1782–5.

38 Joynt RJ. The use of bromides for epilepsy. *Am J Dis Child* 1974; 128: 362–3.

39 Boenick HE, Lorenz JH, Jürgens U. Bromide heute als antiepileptische Substanzen noch nützlich? *Nervenarzt* 1985; 10: 579–82.

40 Ernst JP, Doose H, Baier WK. Bromides were effective in intractable epilepsy with generalized tonic-clonic seizures and onset in early childhood. *Brain Dev* 1988; 10: 385–8.

41 Steinhoff BJ, Kruse R. Bromide treatment of pharmaco-resistent epilepsies with generalized tonic-clonic seizures: a clinical study. *Brain Dev* 1992; 14: 144–9.

42 Oguni H, Hayashi K, Oguni M *et al.* Treatment of severe myoclonic epilepsy in infants with bromide and its borderline variant. *Epilepsia* 1994; 35: 1140–5

43 Okuda K, Yasuhara A, Kamei A, Araki A, Kitamura N, Kobayashi Y. Successful control with bromide of two patients with malignant migrating partial seizures in infancy. *Brain Dev* 2000; 22: 56–9.

44 Balcar VJ, Erdo SL, Joo F, Kasa P, Wolff JR. Neurochemistry of GABAergic system in cerebral cortex chronically exposed to bromide in vivo. *J Neurochem* 1987; 48: 167–9.

45 Suzuki S, Kawakami K, Nakamura F, Nishimura S, Yagi K, Seino M. Bromide, in the therapeutic concentration, enhances GABA-activated currents in cultured neurons of rat cerebral cortex. *Epilepsy Res* 1994; 19: 89–97.

46 Meierkord H, Grunig F, Gutschmidt U *et al.* Sodium bromide: effects on different patterns of epileptiform activity, extracellular pH changes and GABAergic inhibition. *Naunyn Schmiedebergs Arch Pharmacol* 2000; 361: 25–32.

47 Woodbury DM, Pippenger CE. Bromides. In: Woodbury DM, Penry JK, Pippenger CE, eds. *Antiepileptic Drugs*, 2nd edn. New York: Raven Press, 1982: 791–801.

48 Grewal MS, Swinyard EA, Jensen HV, Goodman LS. Correlation between anticonvulsant activity and plasma concentration of bromide. *J Pharmacol* 1956; 112: 109–15.

49 Vaiseman N, Koren G, Pencharz P. Pharmacokinetics of oral and intravenous bromide in normal volunteers. *Clin Toxicol* 1986; 23: 403–13.

50 Woody RC, Steele RW, Knapple WL, Pilkington NS. Impaired neutrophic function in children with seizures treated with ketogenic diet. *J Pediatr* 1989; 115: 427–30.

51 Rossiter EJ, Rendle-Short TJ. Congenital effects of bromism? *Lancet* 1979; 30: 705.

52 Dreifuss FE, Bertram EH. Bromide therapy for intractable seizures. *Epilepsia* 1986; 27: 593.

53 Livingston S, Pearson PH. Bromides in the treatment of epilepsy in children. *Am J Dis Child* 1953; 86: 717–20.

54 Diener W, Kruse R, Berg P. Halogenpannikulitis auf Kaliumbronid. *Monatsschr Kinderheilkd* 1993; 141: 705–7.

55 Goodman LS, Gilman A. Hypnotics and sedatives. In: Goodman LS, Gilman, eds. *The Pharmacological Basis of Therapeutics*, 2nd edn. New York: Macmillan Company, 1955: 156–63.

56 Pfeifle J, Grieben U, Bork K. Bromoderma tuberosum durch antikonvulsive Behandlung mit Kaliumbromid. *Hautarzt* 1992; 43: 792–4.

57 Steinhoff B. Zur antiepileptischen Therapie mit Bromiden. MD thesis, Heidelberg, 1988.

58 Carter CA, Helms RA, Boehm R. Ethotoin in seizures of childhood and adolescence. *Neurology* 1984; 34: 483–4.

59 Kupferberg HJ. Other hydantoins: mephenytoin and ethotoin. In: Levy R, Mattson R, Meldrum B, Penry JK, Dreifuss FE, eds. *Antiepileptic Drugs*, 3rd edn. New York: Raven Press, 1989: 257–66.

60 Zablen M, Brand N. Cleft lip and palate with the anticonvulsant ethotoin. *N Engl J Med* 1977; 297: 855–76.

61 Gooch WM III, Kennedy J, Banner W Jr, McGuire HJ. Generalized arterial and venous thrombosis following intra-arterial paraldehyde. *Clin Toxicol* 1979; 15: 39–44.

62 Shorvon S. Tonic clonic status epilepticus. *J Neurol Neurosurg Psychiatr* 1993; 56: 125–34.

63 Shorvon S. *Status Epilepticus: Clinical Features and Treatment in Children and Adults*. Cambridge: Cambridge University Press, 1994.

64 Lockman LA. Paraldehyde. In: Levy R, Mattson R, Meldrum B, Penry JK, Dreifuss FE, eds. *Antiepileptic Drugs*, 3rd edn. New York: Raven Press, 1989; 881–6.

65 Gibb FA, Everett GM, Richards RK. Phenurone in epilepsy. *Dis Nerv Syst* 1949; 10: 47–9.

66 Everett GM. Pharmacological studies of phenacetylurea (Phenurone), an anticonvulsant drug. *Fed Proc* 1949; 8: 289.

67 Swinyard EA. Laboratory assay of clinically effective antepileptic drugs. *J Am Pharm Assoc Sci Ed* 1949; 38: 201–4.

68 Coker SB, Holmes EW, Egel RT. Phenacemide therapy of complex partial epilepsy in children: determination of plasma drug concentrations. *Neurology* 1987; 37: 1861–6.

69 Tyler MW, King EQ. Phenacemide in treatment of epilepsy. *J Am Med Assoc* 1951; 147: 17–21.

70 Everett GM, Richards RK. Comparative anticonvulsant action 3,5,5,-trimethyloxazolidine-2-4-dione (tridone), dilantin and phenobarbital. *J Pharmacol Exp Ther* 1944; 1: 402–7.

71 Pellmar TC, Wilson WA. Synaptic mechanism of pentylenetetrazol: selectivity for chloride conductance. *Science* 1977; 179: 912–14.

72 Woodbury DM. Convulsant drugs: mechanisms of action. In: Glaser GH, Penry JK, Woodbury DM, eds. *Antiepileptic Drugs: Mechanisms of Action, Advances in Neurology*, Vol. 27. New York: Raven Press, 1980: 249–304.

73 Butler TC, Kuroiwa Y, Waddell WJ, Poole DT. Effects of 5-,5-dimethyl 2.4-oxazolidinedione (DMO) on acid-base and electrolyte equilibria. *J Pharmacol Exp Ther* 1966; 152: 62–6.

74 Futagi Y, Otani K, Abe J. Growth suppression in children receiving acetazolamide with antiepileptic drugs. *Pediatr Neurol* 1996; 15: 323–6.

75 Sloan LL, Golger AP. Visual effects of triadione. *Am J Ophthalmol* 1947; 30: 1387–405.

76 Booker HE, Chun R, Sanguino M. Myasthenia gravis syndrome associated with trimethadione. *J Am Med Assoc* 1970; 212: 2262–3.

Despite the introduction into clinical practice of 10 new antiepileptic drugs (AEDs) during the past 15 years these drugs have had no significant impact on the prognosis of intractable epilepsy. Thus, the treatment of patients with intractable epilepsy still relies on the development of new AEDs and the need for new AEDs is undiminished. There is a substantial market for drugs with novel therapeutic targets that are more efficacious, that have improved side-effect profiles and better pharmacokinetic characteristics.

The current emphasis of AED development is to develop novel drugs that achieve and maintain seizure freedom, with no side-effects, and to enable the patient to lead as normal a lifestyle as possible. AEDs that improve the prognosis of epilepsy, that prevent epileptogenesis and the secondary cerebral damage which occurs in epilepsy, and that prevent mortality in those patients at increased risk of premature death, particularly sudden unexplained death, are needed. Drugs that prevent the development of epilepsy following head injury, neurosurgery and in particular stroke are very much needed.

There are currently more than 50 molecules that have been granted a patent for possible development as AEDs, with varying biological targets and proposed mechanisms of action. There are also endogenous substances with multiple actions in addition to potential antiepileptic effects. It should also not be forgotten that drug effects may differ in patients with epilepsy compared to unaffected persons. Indeed some potential drug targets are present only during the actual depolarization or repetitive firing of neurones during a seizure. Targeting use-dependent mechanisms represents an important strategy in our quest for novel AEDs.

In this chapter, the 11 novel AEDs that are presently undergoing clinical development are summarized in terms of their mechanism of action, pharmacokinetic and interaction profiles, efficacy and adverse effect characteristics. The putative targets for AED development are listed in Table 50.1. The drugs are reviewed in alphabetical order in Table 50.2.

AWD 131–138

Mechanism of action

AWD 131–138, 1-[4-chlorophenyl]-4-morpholino-imidazolin-2-one, exerts anticonvulsant effects in a broad spectrum of animal seizure models including maximal electroshock, pentylenetetrazole, bicuculline and audiogenic models. Additionally, AWD 131–138 shows high activity in the amygdala kindling model in rats, which is predictive of efficacy against complex partial seizures [1]. The oral ED_{50} for neurotoxicity in the rotarod test was 105 mg/kg and 998 mg/kg in mice and rats, respectively, so that overall it possesses a high therapeutic index. It acts as a partial agonist of the benzodiazepine receptor, however its low affinity and low intrinsic activity suggest that its primary action is via some other mechanism [2]. AWD 131–138 exhibits a dose-dependent block of voltage gated Ca^{2+} channels, although as yet it is unclear which channel subtype is affected.

Pharmacokinetics

To date the pharmacokinetics of AWD 131–138 has not been reported in detail. After oral ingestion AWD 131–138 is rapidly and extensively absorbed.

Drug interactions

The drug interaction profile AWD 131–138 is at present unknown.

Efficacy and side-effects

The efficacy and side-effect profiles of AWD 131–138 are at present unknown.

Carabersat (SB-204269)

Mechanism of action

Carabersat, *trans*-(+)-6-acetyl-4*S*-(4-fluoro-benzoyl amino)-3,4-dihydro-2,2-dimrethyl-^{2}H-benzo(b)pyran-3*R*-ol hemihydrate, is a compound that is structurally unrelated to other AEDs. Carabersat is effective in numerous seizure models (maximal electroshock, pentylenetetrazole), with virtually no neurotoxicity so that its therapeutic index is very high [3]. It may act by preventing seizure spread by a stereoselective interaction with a novel but as yet uncharacterized binding site in the brain [4]. The mechanism of action of carabersat is unknown, although it does not appear to act via γ-aminobutyric acid (GABA) inhibition of excitatory amino acid receptors or to act via voltage-gated ion channels [5].

Pharmacokinetics

No data are currently available on the pharmacokinetics of carabersat in man.

Drug interactions

The drug interaction profile carabersat is at present unknown.

Table 50.1 Putative targets for AED development

Target	Comment
Ion channels	To date, voltage-dependent Na$^+$ channels have been the most important target. However, vital targets for novel AEDs are Ca^{2+} and K$^+$ channels
Carbonic anhydrase inhibition	The possible mechanism whereby carbonic anhydrase inhibition modifies GABA-mediated inhibitory potentials and may therefore produce an antiepileptic effect has recently been described
GABA-mediated inhibition	Uptake of synaptic GABA is mediated by specific carriers, of which there are four. Tiagabine, increases the extracellular concentration of GABA and therefore prolongs the inhibitory effects of synaptically released GABA, is specific for GAT-1. Other GAT transporters may represent a target for novel AEDs
Glutamate/NMDA antagonists	The competitive NMDA antagonist, D-CPPene, and the non-competitive antagonists, dizocilpine and dextromethorphan, have proved disappointing. However, there remains scope for development for a low affinity, non-competitive antagonist or a glycine site antagonist. Other allosteric sites on the NMDA receptor (e.g. the redox site) are potential sites for AED development
Glutamate transporters	Multiple glutamate transporter subtypes exist. The neuronal transporter EAAC-1 appears most important in epilepsy, but the glial transporter GLAST may also contribute to seizure susceptibility. The potential exists for the development of AEDs that might augment excitatory amino acid transporter function and reduce excitability
Metabotropic glutamate receptors	Metabotropic glutamate receptors (mGluR) are G-protein-coupled and respond to their ligands by generating second messengers and produce transient or sustained changes in neuronal excitability. There are at least three subclasses and eight subtypes of mGluR. One of the more interesting features of these receptors is that the group I subclass is proconvulsive and the group II and III subclasses are anticonvulsive
AMPA receptors	AMPA receptors are another glutamate receptor subclass. AMPA/kainate receptors, which participate in a broad range of pathological processes, include GluR1–4 (AMPA), GluR5–7 (kainate) and KA1–2 (kainate). Development of selective AMPA/kainate receptor antagonists or even against specific subunits could result in innovative AEDs
Neuromodulators	Adenosine is released during seizure activity and has been proposed as an endogenous anticonvulsant
Protein kinase activity	There are several thousand protein kinases expressed in the brain, they affect the excitability and function of neurones and glia and may play a crucial role in epileptogenesis. Pharmacological or genetic manipulation of these kinases may prove useful in blocking or reversing epileptogenesis
Neurotrophin receptors	Neurotrophins increase synaptic efficacy and are thought to play a role in epileptogenesis. Compounds acting on neurotrophin receptors may also affect epilepsy or seizure expression
Serotonin	Since the characterization of serotonin receptors, there has been an increased interest in the potential role of serotonin in epilepsy
Drug resistance proteins	It is known that drug resistance proteins are responsible for the efflux of some AEDs. The proteins (MDR1, MDR and PgP), which are overexpressed in epileptic tissues, may provide novel targets for AED development
Gene expression	Neuronal activity, growth factors and cytokines (plus other factors) modify gene expression. In the future, a major approach to suppressing or reversing epileptogenesis is manipulation of gene expression

Efficacy and side-effects

The efficacy and side-effect profiles of carabersat are at present unknown. Phase II clinical trials with carabarat, as add-on therapy in patients with refractory epilepsy are currently in progress.

CGX-1007 (conantokin-G)

Mechanism of action

CGX-1007 is a synthetic 17 amino acid derivative of a version of conopeptide that is derived from cone snail venom (*Conus geographus*). It is effective in numerous seizure models (threshold and maximal electroshock, pentylenetetrazole, bicuculline and picrotoxin and in rat kindling models) and has a highly favourable therapeutic index [6]. CGX-1007 specifically acts as an *N*-methyl-D-aspartate (NMDA) antagonist and appears not to act on other receptor types [7,8].

Pharmacokinetics

No data are currently available on the pharmacokinetics of CGX-1007 in man. As it is proposed that CGX-1007 be administered intrathecally to patients with epilepsy, its pharmacokinetic characterization can be expected to be somewhat different to that commonly undertaken for AEDs [6]. Furthermore, since the pump and

Table 50.2 Antiepileptic drugs in development

AWD 131–138	1-(4-chlorophenyl)-4-morpholino-imidazolin-2-one	Drug is in phase I development
Carabersat	*Trans*-(+)-6-acetyl-4*S*-(4-fluoro-benzoyl amino)-3,4-dihydro-2, 2-dimrethyl-^{2}H-benzo(b)pyran-3*R*-ol hemihydrate	Drug is in phase II development
CGX-1007	A synthetic 17 amino acid	Drug is in phase I development
Ganaxolone	3α-hydroxy-3β-methyl-5α-pregnan-20-one	Drug is in phase III development
Harkoseride	*R*-2-acetamido-*N*-benzyl-3-methoxypropionamide	Drug is in phase II development
NPS 1776	3-methylbutanamide	Drug is in phase I development
Retigabine	*N*-(2-amino-4-(4-fluorobenzylamino)-phenyl) carbamic acid ethyl ester	Drug is in phase III development
Safinamide	(*S*)-(+)-2-(4-(3-fluorobenzyloxy) benzylamino) propanamide methansulfonate	Drug is in phase I development
SPD421	Phospholipid prodrug of valproic acid	Drug is in phase II development
Talampanel	(*R*)-7-acetyl-5-(4-aminophenyl)-8,9-dihydro-8-methyl-^{7}H-1,3-dioxolo-(4,5-h) (2,3) benzodiazepine	Drug is in phase II development
Valrocemide	*N*-valproyl-glycinamide	Drug is in phase II development

drug reservoir will be implanted into the abdomen and the catheter placed intrathecally, the digestive tract and the blood–brain barrier will be bypassed.

Drug interactions

The drug interaction profile CGX-1007 is at present unknown.

Efficacy and side-effects

The efficacy and side-effect profiles of CGX-1007 are at present unknown. Phase II clinical trials with CGX-1007, as add-on therapy in patients with refractory epilepsy, are planned.

Ganaxolone

Mechanism of action

Ganaxolone, 3α-hydroxy-3β-methyl-5α-pregnan-20-one, is chemically related to progesterone but seems to be devoid of any hormonal activity. It is a member of a novel class of neuroactive steroids, called epalons, which allosterically modulate the GABA-A receptor complex via a unique recognition site [9]. It exhibits potent activity against seizures induced by pentylenetetrazole, bicuculline, aminophylline and corneal kindling, whilst it is less potent against maximal electroshock-induced seizures. Ganaxolone appears to have a pharmacological action similar to that seen with ethosuximide and valproate suggesting that the drug could have efficacy in humans against primary generalized seizures of the absence type [9]. However, a study using two specific animal models of absence seizures suggests that ganaxolone has the potential to exacerbate absence seizures [10].

Pharmacokinetics

In healthy volunteers (87 adult males) ganaxolone was rapidly absorbed, after oral ingestion and after a high-fat meal, with peak plasma ganaxolone concentrations achieved within 1–3 h [11]. Plasma concentrations increased essentially dose dependently and subsequently declined bioexponentially with a terminal half-life of 37–70 h. Plasma concentration versus time profiles after multiple doses of ganaxolone did not suggest any significant accumulation. There is no gender difference in respect to its pharmacokinetic characteristics, however fasting significantly reduces the absorption of ganaxolone [11]. It is highly bound (>99%) to plasma proteins. Ganaxolone is metabolized to yet unknown metabolites which are eliminated from plasma at a rate 3–6 times the terminal half-life of ganaxolone [11].

Drug interactions

Preliminary trials have not identified any potential significant drug interactions with concomitant AEDs [12,13].

Efficacy and side-effects

Side-effects seen in healthy volunteers include sedation, dizziness, headache, gastrointestinal disturbances and fatigue. Interestingly, these side-effects were twice as common in females as in males, even though plasma ganaxolone concentrations were indistinguishable in the two genders [14]. A double-blind, randomized, placebo-controlled clinical trial to examine the safety, tolerability and antiepileptic activity of ganaxolone in patients after withdrawal from other AEDs as part of a presurgical evaluation has been published [15]. This 'proof of concept' study comprising 52 patients (24 on ganaxolone, 28 on placebo) showed that ganaxolone monotherapy was well tolerated and that ganaxolone does have antiepileptic activity in patients with intractable complex partial seizures (with or without secondary generalization). Adverse events comprised of a variety of central nervous system-related events, primarily dizziness, and were very similar in the two treatment groups.

Ganaxolone is effective in children with infantile spasms, which is particularly refractory to currently available AEDs [13]. Of a total of 20 children with refractory infantile spasms, 16 subjects completed the open-label study. Spasm frequency was reduced by at least 50% in 33% of subjects, with an additional 33% experiencing a 25–50% reduction in spasm frequency. The most frequent (>10%) drug-related adverse events were somnolence, diarrhoea, nervousness and vomiting.

Harkoseride (SPM 927; ADD 234037)

Mechanism of action

Harkoseride, R-2-acetamido-N-benzyl-3-methoxypropionamide, exhibits potent anticonvulsant activity in several seizure models, including maximal electroshock seizures in rats and mice, the hippocampal kindling model and it protects against sound-induced seizures in the Frings mouse. Harkoseride is also effective in two models of status epilepticus [16]. The mechanism of action of harkoseride is considered to be via an action on the glycine strychnine-insensitive recognition site of the NMDA–receptor complex.

Pharmacokinetics

In healthy male volunteers, harkoseride was rapidly and completely absorbed after oral ingestion with peak concentrations achieved 1–5 h later. Its bioavailability is 100% and plasma protein binding is about 15%. Harkoseride is metabolized in the liver to as yet unknown metabolites and elimination is primarily by renal excretion. The elimination half-life of harkoseride is approximately 12 h. In patients with epilepsy receiving concomitant AED treatment, serum harkoseride concentrations were dose dependent and comparable to those seen in healthy volunteers.

Drug interactions

Preliminary data suggest that harkoseride does not interact with carbamazepine, phenytoin or valproic acid.

Efficacy and side-effects

A multicentre, open-label study of harkoseride as add-on therapy in 13 patients with refractory partial seizures, has been very encouraging [17]. Harkoseride dose was escalated weekly for 3 weeks and then tapered down during the fourth week. After 3 weeks of treatment, nine of the 13 patients experienced a significant reduction in seizures with two patients becoming seizure free. Side-effects comprised dizziness, headache and ataxia and were mild in intensity for most patients. For three patients, the side-effects were intolerable and required a reduction in harkoseride dosage.

NPS 1776

Mechanism of action

NPS 1776, 3-methylbutanamide, possesses a broad spectrum of activity in that it is effective against maximal electroshock, pentylenetetrazole, picrotoxin and bicuculline-induced seizure. It is also effective against audiogenic seizures in the Frings mouse model and kindled seizures in the amygdala-kindled rat [18]. The mechanism of action of NPS 1776 is unknown but does not involve a direct action on receptor-mediated events associated with classical neurotransmitter systems.

Pharmacokinetics

In healthy volunteers NPS 1776 (ingested as a solution) is rapidly absorbed with maximum concentration achieved within 30–45 min [19]. Binding to plasma proteins is not significant and concentrations increase linearly and dose dependently. The elimination half-life of NPS 1776 is approximately 2–3 h in males whilst in females, at the higher dose, it is a little longer. Renal excretion represents a minor route of elimination, with approximately 2–4% of an administered dose excreted unchanged within 24 h.

Drug interactions

In vitro studies using a variety of cytochrome P450 (CYP) isoenzymes associated with the metabolism of commonly used AEDs suggest that NPS 1776 has no inhibitory action.

Efficacy and side-effects

In healthy volunteers NPS 1776 is well tolerated with no serious side-effects observed during two studies; a double-blind, placebo-controlled, ascending single-dose study in 18 healthy male volunteers, and a multiple-dose study where NPS 1776 was administered for 10 days to 36 healthy male and female volunteers [19].

Retigabine (D-23129)

Mechanism of action

Retigabine, N-(2-amino-4-(4-fluorobenzyl-amino)-phenyl) carbamic acid ethyl ester, exhibits anticonvulsant activity in a broad range of seizure models including maximal electroshock, pentylenetetrazole, picrotoxin and kainate [20]. In particular, it possesses remarkable potency in delaying epileptogenesis and in protecting against amygdala-kindled seizures [21]. Its action is not receptor specific, with action on various ion channels (K^+, Na^+ and Ca^{2+}) and it prevents the synthesis of glutamate and aspartate via allosteric modulation of the GABA-B receptor. Retigabine has been reported to stimulate the de novo synthesis of GABA and to amplify GABA-induced currents in the isolated rat hippocampus [22,23]. However, more recent in vivo mouse whole brain evidence would suggest that retigabine blocks GABA metabolism rather than enhancing GABA synthesis [24]. Retigabine also exhibits antiepileptic activity in a variety of slice preparations including human neocortical slices [25–27].

Pharmacokinetics

In healthy volunteers, retigabine peak plasma concentrations occur within 2 h after oral ingestion and its pharmacokinetics are linear after both single (50, 100, 200 and 600 mg) and repeat administration (50, 100 and 200 mg b.i.d.) [28]. Food co-ingestion does not affect the absorption of retigabine and its elimination half-life is about 9 h. In the elderly the elimination half-life of retigabine is approximately 12 h and there appears to be some gender differences. Retigabine undergoes metabolic biotrasformation primarily by N-glucuronidation and acetylation. The primary metabolite of retigabine, AWD21-360, is rapidly formed after retigabine ingestion and its pharmacokinetics follow that of the parent compound [29,30].

Drug interactions

In patients with epilepsy whilst the pharmacokinetics of retigabine are unaffected by valproate or topiramate, its clearance is significantly enhanced by phenytoin and carbamazepine [30]. Retigabine does not affect the pharmacokinetics of valproic acid, topiramate, phenytoin or carbamazepine [30]. In healthy volunteers, neither phenobarbital nor lamotrigine affect the pharmacokinetics of retigabine and indeed phenobarbital and lamotrigine are not affected by retigabine [31,32]. Retigabine does not appear to affect the metabolism of a low-dose oral contraceptive pill (0.03 mg ethinyl oestradiol, 0.3 mg norgestrel) and thus retigabine can be used by women taking oral contraceptives without the need for back-up contraception [33].

Efficacy and side-effects

A study designed to determine the maximum tolerated dose of retigabine in healthy volunteers reported mild to moderate adverse effects which were generally central nervous system related and disappeared after the first day [34]. Also the tolerability of retigabine has been investigated in two open-label studies in patients with refractory partial seizures. Of the 46 patients enrolled, 11 were withdrawn due to non-compliance ($n=8$), seizure exacerbation ($n=2$) and adverse events ($n=1$). Overall, retigabine was well tolerated with somnolence, vertigo, blurred vision and ataxia being dose limiting. A total of 12 patients out of 35 patients showed a > 50% reduction in seizure frequency and preliminary data of the 18 patients that proceeded to enter a long-term extension study suggest that the therapeutic dose of retigabine will be 600–1200 mg/day.

Safinamide (NW-1015; PNU-151774E)

Mechanism of action

Safinamide, (S)-(+)-2-(4-(3-fluorobenzyloxy) benzylamino) propanamide, methansulfonate, is effective in a variety of seizure models (bicuculline, picrotoxin, 3-methyl-aspartate, strychnine, NMDA and electrically induced seizures) where it acts by preventing seizure spread [35,36]. In these models, safinamide is associated with a very high therapeutic index, suggesting minimal toxicity. In the kainic acid model, safinamide protects against both the seizures and the ensuing neuronal damage [37]. Safinamide acts via an action on site 2 of the Na^+ channel [38]. It also modulates Ca^{2+} currents (inhibits aspartate and glutamate release) and inhibits monoamine oxidase B (MAOB) activity [39].

Pharmacokinetics

In healthy volunteers, safinamide is rapidly absorbed after oral ingestion with peak concentrations occurring within 2 h. Plasma safinamide concentrations increase linearly and dose dependently and the elimination half-life of safinamide is 21–23 h.

Drug interactions

In vitro studies suggest that safinamide has no inducing or inhibiting activity on the different CYP isoenzymes that are known to be involved in the metabolism of other AEDs. Although no formal in vivo drug interaction studies have yet been undertaken, it is considered unlikely that safinamide will be associated with pharmacokinetic interactions at the metabolic level.

Efficacy and side-effects

Formal efficacy studies in patients with epilepsy are in progress. In healthy volunteer studies, headache, somnolence and light headedness were reported as side-effects by a few subjects at the highest safinamide dose.

SPD421 (DP16; DP-VPA)

Mechanism of action

SPD421 is a novel AED intended to provide a targeted delivery of valproate (valproic acid) within the neurone at the time of epileptiform discharge. It comprises valproate covalently bound to a lysolecithin moiety. The lipophilicity of SPD421 enables penetration into the central nervous system where it is believed that increased phospholipase A_2 activity within affected cells cleaves the molecule to provide intracellular valproic acid. This targeted delivery should produce effective control of seizures but reduce the systemic exposure of valproic acid and thereby reduce the risk of side-effects.

SPD421 suppresses seizures associated with pentylenetetrazole administration and is also effective in suppressing audiogenic seizures in Frings mice. ED_{50} values for SPD421 in these models are substantially smaller than that for valproic acid. Although it is without effect in the genetic absence epilepsy in rats from Strasbourg (GAERS) model of absence seizures, absence seizures are inhibitory in origin so increased phospholipase A2 activity would not be expected to occur [19].

Pharmacokinetics

In 29 healthy male volunteers (aged 18–37 years), SPD421 was administered at five single doses (0.31, 0.62, 1.25, 2.5 and 5.00 g) using a double-blind, randomized study design. After oral ingestion of a liquid formulation, SPD421 was rapidly absorbed, with peak plasma concentrations (t_{max}) achieved within 9–11 h. Maximum plasma concentrations (C_{max}) increased dose dependently and essentially linearly. The elimination half-life of SPD421 was 5.1–12.1 h. The concurrent valproic acid pharmacokinetic parameters were as follows: t_{max} range 9–24 h; elimination half-life range 15.1–21.1 h. Valproic acid C_{max} values also increased with increasing dose. Preliminary results from a further study indicated that administration of SPD421 after food increased systemic exposure of SPD421 approximately four-fold without increasing exposure of valproic acid [19].

Drug interactions

Preliminary data from animals suggest that SPD421 is not metabolized by cytochrome P450. Therefore the propensity for any significant pharmacokinetic interactions with SPD421 can be expected to be negligible. Of course any valproic acid in the circulation that may arise from SPD421 might be expected to have an interaction profile typically associated with valproic acid administration. *In vitro* protein binding studies using human plasma suggest that SPD421, at concentrations significantly greater than those likely to be encountered clinically, is unlikely to interfere with the binding of phenytoin, carbamazepine and valproic acid [19].

Efficacy and side-effects

Clinical trials are presently ongoing to ascertain the efficacy of SPD421 in patients with epilepsy.

Tolerability has been assessed in a total of 39 healthy volunteers who have received repeat daily doses of 314.5–2400 mg SPD421 for 7–14 days and was compared with placebo groups. SPD421 has been generally well tolerated with principal adverse events reported being of gastrointestinal or central nervous system origin [19].

Talampanel (LY300164; GIKY 53773)

Mechanism of action

Talampanel, (R)-7-acetyl-5-(4-aminophenyl)-8,9-dihydro-8-methyl-7H-1,3-dioxolo-(4,5-h) (2,3) benzodiazepine, is a noncompetitive antagonist at the AMPA (a receptor subtype of glutamate) receptor site with very weak affinity for benzodiazepine receptors. It has a broad spectrum of anticonvulsant activity in animal seizure models including maximal electroshock and pentylenetetrazole-induced seizures in mice, chemically and electrically kindled seizures in mice and is effective in a mouse model of phenytoin-resistant status epilepticus. Interestingly, talampanel enhances the efficacy of conventional AEDs (phenytoin, phenobarbital, valproate and clonazepam) when administered in combination [40].

Pharmacokinetics

After oral ingestion, talampanel is rapidly absorbed with peak plasma concentrations occurring within 2.5 h. Binding to plasma proteins is of the order of 75% (range 67–88%).

The elimination of talampanel is probably via a combination of first-order and capacity-limited processes. Its elimination half-life in healthy volunteers is 6–8 h. Although its metabolic pathways have not been completely characterized in man, acetylation appears to be an important route. Thus, acetylation status is likely to impact on the metabolism of talampanel and potentially a two-fold difference in talampanel concentrations can be expected. In addition, concomitant AEDs are likely to impact on the metabolism of talampanel.

Drug interactions

Talampanel has been shown in an *in vitro* setting to be an irreversible inhibitor of the cytochrome P450 isoenzyme CYPA3 and consequently it would be anticipated that talampanel may inhibit the metabolism of CYP3A substrates such as carbamazepine. Indeed carbamazepine plasma concentrations are elevated during carbamazepine and talampanel coadministration. In patients with epilepsy the clearance of talampanel is enhanced by hepatic enzyme-inducing AEDs (carbamazepine and phenytoin) whilst it is decreased by valproate [41].

Efficacy and side-effects

In a series of 24 healthy male volunteers, who received a single dose (100 mg) of talampanel, and a second series of 16 healthy male volunteers, who received multiple doses (20–50 mg t.i.d.) of talampanel, the drug was well tolerated. Adverse effects included mild drowsiness, dizziness, ataxia and paraesthesia and occurred at doses above 50 mg [42].

A double-blind cross-over study evaluated talampanel in 49 patients with intractable partial seizures. Concomitant AED concentrations were kept within 30% of baseline levels, necessitating a carbamazepine dose reduction in six patients. Compared to placebo, talampanel was associated with a 21% reduction in median seizure frequency. The only significant adverse effects were dizziness (52%) and ataxia (26%).

Valrocemide (TV 1901)

Mechanism of action

Valrocemide, N-valproyl-glycinamide, exhibits a broad-spectrum anticonvulsant activity in numerous seizure models including maximal electroshock, pentylenetetrazole, picrotoxin and bicuculline-induced seizures as well as sound-induced seizures in Frings mice. Valrocemide is also effective against hippocampal-kindled seizures and focal seizures from corneally kindled rats [43]. The metabolic profile of valrocemide does not suggest that it is a valproic acid prodrug (indeed valrocemide exhibits a better therapeutic index than that of valproic acid) and therefore the observed anticonvulsant action can be considered to be that of valrocemide *per se*. However, the mechanism of action of valrocemide is unknown; an effect on GABA or glutamate-sensitive ion channels has been ruled out.

Pharmacokinetics

In healthy volunteers, valrocemide is rapidly absorbed and its elimination half-life is 6.4–9.4 h after single dose administration and 7.2–8.5 h after multiple dose administration. Approximately 20% of the administered dose is excreted unchanged, 40% is in the form of valproyl glycine and 4–6% is valproic acid. Protein binding of valrocemide is < 25% [19].

Drug interactions

In vitro studies using CYP isoenzymes suggest that significant drug interactions with other AEDs should not be anticipated. Nevertheless, in a series of 22 patients with epilepsy receiving concomitant AEDs, higher valrocemide clearance and shorter valrocemide half-life values were observed in those patients on enzyme-inducing AEDs whilst values were indistinguishable from those of healthy volunteers in those patients not on enzyme-inducing AEDs (phenytoin and carbamazepine) [19].

Efficacy and side-effects

The efficacy of valrocemide has been investigated in a series of 22 patients with epilepsy using an open-study design during a 13-week period. Valrocemide was observed to be very efficacious in 15 patients, two of which become seizure free. No serious side-effects were observed; most were mild to moderate and were central nervous system or gastrointestinal tract related [19].

Conclusions

Seizure freedom with no side-effects for all patients is the treatment aim in epilepsy. This utopian ideal has not been realized by the new AEDs licensed around the world since 1989.

Therefore, there is still a need for new AEDs that are effective in patients with refractory epilepsy, that improve the prognosis of epilepsy, that prevent epileptogenesis and the secondary cerebral damage caused by epilepsy, and that prevent mortality in those patients at increased risk of premature death. Most drugs are being screened using a standard range of animal seizure models, and it is self-evident that this approach may identify mainly those drugs that act on the same molecular targets as the established AEDs. New paradigms are required to identify new drugs. Drug development is now increasingly targeted at differing pathophysiological and chemical mechanisms. Some of the AEDs reviewed in this chapter act by novel targets by hitherto unique mechanisms. These drugs will hopefully particularly enhance the prognosis of patients with intractable epilepsy.

References

1 Tober C, Stark B, Bartsch R, Kronbach T. Effect of AWD 131–138 in a model of focal epilepsy, the amygdal kindling in rats. *Epilepsia* 2000; 41 (Suppl. 7): 53.

2 Sigel E, Baur R, Netzer R, Rundfeldt C. The antiepileptic drug AWD 131–138 stimulates different recombinant isoforms of the rat GABA(A) receptor through the benzodiazepine binding site. *Neurosci Lett* 1998; 3: 85–8.

3 Upton N, Blackburn TP, Cooper D et al. Profile of SB-2-4-4269, a novel anticonvulsant drug, in rat models of focal and generalized epileptic seizures. *Br J Pharmacol* 1997; 121: 1679–86.

4 Herdon HJ, Jerman JC, Stean TO et al. Characterization of the binding of (^{3}H)-SB-204269, a radioactive form of the new anticonvulsant SB-204269, to a novel binding site in rat brain membranes. *Br J Pharmacol* 1997; 121: 1687–91.

5 Ceaser M, Evans ML, Benham CD. Lack of effect of the novel anticonvulsant SB-204269 on voltage-dependent currents in neurones cultured from rat hippocampus. *Neurosci Lett* 1999; 271: 57–60.

6 Bialer M, Johannessen SI, Kupferberg HJ, Levy RH, Loiseau P, Perucca E. Progress report on new antiepileptic drugs: a summary of the sixth Eilat conference (Eilat VI). *Epilepsy Res* 2002; 51: 31–71.

7 Donevan SD, McCabe RT. Conantokin G is an NR2B selective competitive antagonist of NMDA receptors. *Mol Pharmacol* 2000; 58: 614–23.

8 Jimenez EC, Donevan SD, Walker C et al. Conantokin-L a new NMDA receptor antagonist: determinants for anticonvulsant potency. *Epilepsy Res* 2002; 51: 73–80.

9 Carter RB, Wood PL, Wieland S et al. Characterization of the anticonvulsant properties of ganaxolone (CCD 1042; 3alpha-hydroxy-3beta-methyl-5alpha-pregnan-20-one), a selective, high affinity, steroid modulator of the gamma-aminobutyric acid(A) receptor. *J Pharmacol Exp Ther* 1997; 280: 1284–95.

10 Snead OC. Ganaxolone, a selective, high-affinity steroid modulator of the γ-aminobutyric acid-A receptor, exacerbates seizures in animal models of absence. *Ann Neurol* 1998; 44: 688–91.

11 Monaghan EP, Navalta LA, Shum L, Ashbrook DW, Lee DA. Initial human experience with ganaxolone, a neuroactive steroid with antiepileptic activity. *Epilepsia* 1997; 38: 1026–31.

12 Lechtenberg R, Villeneuve N, Monaghan EP, Densel MB, Rey E, Dulac O. An open-label dose-escalation study to evaluate the safety and tolerability of ganaxolone in the treatment of refractory epilepsy in pediatric patients. *Epilepsia* 1996; 37 (Suppl. 5): 204.

13 Kerrigan JF, Shields WD, Nelson TY et al. Ganaxolone for treating intractable infantile spasms: a multicenter, open-label, add-on trial. *Epilepsy Res* 2000; 42: 133–9.

14 Monaghan EP, Densel MB, Lechtenberg R. Gender differences in sensitivity to ganaxolone, a neuroactive steroid under investigation as an antiepileptic drug. *Epilepsia* 1996; 37 (Suppl. 5): 171.

15 Laxer K, Blum D, Abou-Khalil BW et al. Assessment of ganaxolone's anticonvulsant activity using a randomized, double-blind, presurgical trial design. *Epilepsia* 2000; 41: 1187–94.

16 Walton NY. Harkoseride, a novel anticonvulsant: efficacy in treatment of experimental status epilepticus, plasma protein binding, plasma and brain pharmacokinetics. *Epilepsia* 1999; 40 (Suppl. 7): 24–6.

17 Fountain NB, French JA, Privitera MD. Harkoseride: safety and tolerability of a new antiepileptic drug (AED) in patients with refractory partial epilepsy. *Epilepsia* 2000; 41 (Suppl. 7): 169.

18 White HS. Anticonvulsant profile of NPS 1776: a broad-spectrum antiepileptic drug. *Epilepsia* 1999; 40 (Suppl. 7): 28.

19 Bialer M, Johannessen SI, Kupferberg HJ, Levy RH, Loiseau P, Perucca E. Progress report on new antiepileptic drugs: a summary of the fifth Eilat Conference (EILAT V). *Epilepsy Res* 2001; 42: 11–58.

20 Rostock A, Tober G, Rundfeldt C et al. D-23129: a new anticonvulsant with a broad spectrum of activity in animal models of epileptic seizures. *Epilepsy Res* 1996; 23: 211–23.

21 Tober C, Rostock A, Rundfeldt C, Bartsch R. D-23129: a potent anticonvulsant in the amygdala kindling model of complex partial seizures. *Eur J Pharmacol* 1996; 303: 163–9.

22 Kapetanovic IM, Yonekawa WD, Kupferburgh HJ. The effects of D-23129, a new experimental anticonvulsant drug, on neurotransmitter amino acids in the rat hippocampus in vitro. *Epilepsy Res* 1995; 22: 167–73.

23 Rundfeldt C. Characterization of the K$^+$ channel opening effect of the anticonvulsant retigabine in PC12 cells. *Epilepsy Res* 1999; 35: 99–107.

24 Sills GJ, Rundfeldt C, Butler E, Forrest G, Thompson GG, Brodie MJ. A neurochemical study of the novel antiepileptic drug retigabine in mouse brain. *Pharmacol Res* 2000; 42: 553–7.

25 Armand V, Rundfeldt C, Heinemann U. Effects of retigabine (D-23129) on different patterns of epileptiform activity induced by low magnesium in rat entorhinal cortex hippocampal slices. *Epilepsia* 2000; 41: 28–33.

26 Dost R, Rundfeldt C. The anticonvulsant retigabine potently suppresses epileptiform discharges in the low Ca^{++} and low Mg^{++} model in the hippocampal slice preparation. *Epilepsy Res* 2000; 38: 53–6.

27 Straub H, Kohling R, Hohling JM et al. Effects of retigabine on rhythmic synchronous activity of human neocortical slices. *Epilepsy Res* 2001; 44: 155–65.

28 Troy SM, Paul J, Knebel N, Richards LS, Getsy JA, Ferron GM. Linear dose-proportional pharmacokinetics of single and multiple twice-a-day dosing. *Epilepsia* 2000; 41 (Suppl.): 149.

29 Herman R, Knebel N, Troy SM, Russ P. Effects of age and gender on the pharmacokinetics of retigabine. *Epilepsia* 2000; 41 (Suppl.): 176.

30 Sachdeo RC, Ferron GM, Partiot AM et al. An early determination of drug–drug interaction between valproic acid, phenytoin, carbamazepine, or topiramate and retigabine in epileptic patients. *Epilepsia* 2001; 42 (Suppl. 7): 298–9.

31 Ferron GM, Paul J, Richards LS, Knebel N, Getsy JA, Troy SM. Lack of

pharmacokinetic interaction between retigabine and lamotrigine. *Epilepsia* 2000; 41 (Suppl. 7): 111.

32 Ferron GM, Patat A, Parks V, Rolan P, Troy SM. Lack of pharmacokinetic interactions between retigabine and phenobarbital at steady state in healthy subjects. *Epilepsia* 2001; 42: (Suppl. 7): 89.

33 Paul J, Ferron GM, Richards LS, Getsy JA, Troy SM. Retigabine does not alter the pharmacokinetics of a low-dose oral contraceptive in women. *Epilepsia* 2001; 42 (Suppl. 7): 259.

34 Paul J, Feron GM, Troy SM, Richards LS, Francillo RJ, Getsy JA. Establishment of retigabine safety and tolerability: An ascending, multiple dose study in healthy volunteers. *Epilepsia* 2000; 41 (Suppl. 7): 221.

35 Fariello RG, McArthur RA, Bonsignori A *et al.* Preclinical evaluation of PNU-151774E as a novel anticonvulsant. *J Pharmacol Exp Ther* 1998: 397–403.

36 Fariello RG, Maj R, Marrari P, Beard D, Algate C, Salvati P. Acute behavioral and EEG effects of NW-1015 on electrically-induced afterdischarge in conscious monkeys. *Epilepsy Res* 2000; 39: 37–47.

37 Maj R, Fariello RG, Ukmar G *et al.* PNU-151774E protects against kainate-induced status epilepticus and hippocampal lesions in the rat. *Eur J Pharmacol* 1998; 359: 27–32.

38 Salvati P, Maj R, Caccia C *et al.* Biochemistry and electrophysiology of PNU-151774E, a novel and broad spectrum anticonvulsant. *J Pharmacol Exp Ther* 1999; 288: 1151–9.

39 Strolin Benedetti M, Marrari P, Colombo M *et al.* The anticonvulsant FCE 26743 is a selective and short-acting MAO-B inhibitor devoid of inducing properties towards cytochrome P450-dependent testosterone hydroxylation in mice and rats. *J Pharm Pharmacol* 1994; 46: 814–19.

40 Czuczwar SJ, Swiader M, Kuzniar H, Gasior M, Kleinrok Z. LY 300164, a novel antagonist of AMPA/kainate receptors, potentiates the anticonvulsant activity of antiepileptic drugs. *Eur J Pharmacol* 1998; 359: 103–9.

41 Lanyan Y, Lucas R, Jewell H *et al.* Talampanel, a new antiepileptic drug: single- and multiple-dose pharmacokinetics and initial 1-week experience in patients with chronic intractable epilepsy. *Epilepsia* 2003; 44: 46–53.

42 Meng CQ. Talampanel. *Curr Opin CPNS Invest Drugs* 1999; 1: 637–43.

43 Isoherranen N, Woodhead JH, White HS, Bialer M. Anticonvulsant profile of valrocemide (TV1901): a new antiepileptic drug. *Epilepsia* 2001; 42: 832–6.

Section Four
Presurgical Evaluation of Epilepsy and Epilepsy Surgery

51 Introduction to Epilepsy Surgery and its Presurgical Assessment

S.D. Shorvon

The treatment of epilepsy by surgical means has a long history. Archaeological evidence shows trephination and trepanation to have been practised in many ancient civilizations, a logical approach given the beliefs, widely held over many centuries, that epilepsy is due to possession by evil spirits, or occupation of the body by noxious substances or humours. It follows that the removal or release of these influences might effect a cure, and indeed this is echoed in contemporary surgical philosophy which aims to remove 'epileptogenic (bad) tissue' from the brain.

The modern history of epilepsy surgery is usually dated from the operation on 26 May 1886 carried out by Sir Victor Horsley, at the National Hospital, Queen Square in London. Horsley was a remarkable man and a first-rate scientific investigator (Fig. 51.1 [1,2]). His major theoretical contribution was the recognition that some forms of epilepsy were due to focal lesions and that the location in the brain of these lesions could be deduced by analysis of the clinical symptomatology (clinical localization). He carried out a series of definitive studies using electrical stimulation and ablation in over 100 monkeys to identify the function of brain areas and tracts. He produced detailed maps of motor and sensory function, and produced a prototype homunculus. These experimental studies are a masterpiece of functional anatomy, and pre-date Penfield's similar work by over half a century. He also made contributions to operative technique and these included impeccable antisepsis, the introduction of the long semi-lunar incision, the importance of clean removal of bone, the use of bone wax and the clear appreciation of the scope and limitations of anaesthesia. Horsley's first patient was a Scotsman who had sustained a depressed fracture and developed epilepsy. He had 2870 seizures in the first 13 days of hospitalization. Using the newly discovered principles of cerebral localization by clinical symptomatology, Horsley predicted a scar in the 'hinder part of the left superior frontal sulcus'. He operated, found the scar and resected it. By the end of 1886, he had carried out 10 operations, of which nine were judged successful [3]. The techniques were widely copied and Andriezen [4] reported that in the next 10 years, about 400 operations carried out for Jacksonian epilepsy were known to the medical literature. Another landmark in epilepsy surgery was the use by Krause in 1893 of electrical stimulation peroperatively in man, based on the method that Horsley had used years earlier in monkeys, and the publication of the first map of the human motor cortex [2]. This first wave of enthusiasm for surgery, which was largely concerned with the resection of neocortical lesions (trauma, tumours, postinfective scarring), waned in the early part of the 20th century. Presumably this was in part due to the injudicious widening of indications and the failure to adopt strict criteria for cerebral localization. As Turner noted in 1901, operations had been carried out 'in cases of genuine idiopathic epilepsy' to no avail and Turner considered that generally epilepsy surgery 'had not fulfilled the favourable anticipations formed during the early years of surgical treatment' [5]. Horsley's approach established the principle, still adhered to, that focal epilepsy arises in discrete identifiable areas in the brain and that the presurgical assessment should be directed at localizing these areas. To what extent epilepsy is in reality physiologically localized is arguable, but this principle still underpins all resective surgery today, and has been shown pragmatically to be efficacious, at least in some patients and some types of epilepsy syndrome.

The next major development in epilepsy surgery was the discovery, by Wilder Penfield in Montreal, that resection of the temporal lobe could have dramatic results in epilepsy [6,7]. Penfield was trained by Foerster in the cerebral localization techniques pioneered by Horsley. His first patient had developed severe epilepsy, with up to 20 seizures a day, following a subdural haematoma. This young man was operated upon on three occasions by Penfield. At the first operation, the motor strip was defined by stimulation and a small cortical excision made. There was no improvement. In the second, the contralateral frontal lobe was exposed but no abnormalities found and no resection made. In the third operation, 3 years later in 1931, a scar was found in the temporal cortex and a wide excision of the temporal cortex (but not hippocampus) was made (Penfield referred to this case as his first temporal lobectomy). The patient made a dramatic recovery, with four seizures only in the next 14 years.

A striking feature of the evolution of epilepsy surgery has been its reliance on technological advance, and epilepsy surgery is above all the triumph of applied technology. Advances in anaesthesia, antisepsis, neurophysiology, neuroimaging and surgical instrumentation have all shaped surgical practice more than basic theory. A major technological stimulus was the introduction of EEG into clinical practice in 1937. This was rapidly exploited to enhance the potential for localization of epileptogenic tissue. In 1939 Penfield and his colleagues adopted EEG in a series of pioneering operations, combining an anatomical and electroencephalographic approach to resective surgery with great effect. Over the next 15 years, the recognition that scalp EEG could localize epileptic discharges arising in the temporal lobe led to the rapid adoption of temporal lobectomy as a standard operation for epilepsy. The operation has become the dominant form of epilepsy surgery and is now performed in many centres throughout the world. Although Penfield's technique has been modified over the years by successive surgeons, his basic approach remains to this day.

More and more sophisticated EEG techniques were developed in the subsequent 30 years. Intracranial recording was first carried out in Oxford in 1944 [8]. The technique was refined by Tailarach and

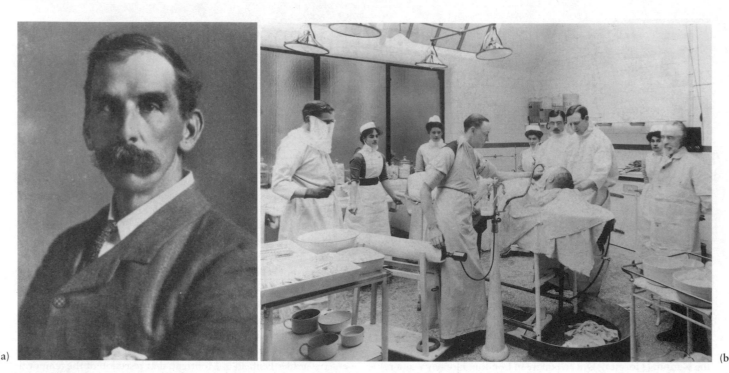

Fig. 51.1 (a) Sir Victor Horsley. (b) The operating theatre at the National Hospital, Queen Square, London, at the end of the 19th century. Horsley is the figure on the left, gowned and masked.

Bancaud who introduced depth recording into routine practice using stereotactic methods, and depth EEG has subsequently developed in enormous complexity, especially in continental Europe and the US. At the Sainte-Anne Hospital in Paris for instance, by 1990, 11 intracranial electrodes with 15 contacts each were routinely implanted as part of the SEEG work-up [9–11]. In parallel to these developments has been the evolution of techniques for long-term monitoring of EEG, with the primary aim of providing recordings of ictal rather than interictal events. The longest recording-paper length available to Berger (who originated EEG) was 7.5 m which allowed recording for only 4 min at normal paper speeds. Continuous paper recording was introduced in the late 1930s and became rather widely used in sleep research in the 1960s. Even then, a typical night recording would require over a kilometre of paper, and the review of such recordings was clearly impractical in an epilepsy setting [12].

The development of computerized data reduction techniques, computerized data storage, the transmission of EEG via radio or cable telemetry and the miniaturization of recording equipment during and after the 1960s has revolutionized this situation. Chronic recording using simultaneous EEG and video telemetry was introduced in the mid 1960s, and since then ictal recordings using video EEG telemetry, with both scalp and depth electrodes, have become a routine part of presurgical evaluation worldwide.

The increasingly sophisticated nature of EEG investigation has refined electrical localization to what is now probably the limits of its potential, and it is difficult to escape the feeling that many complex SEEG examinations have exceeded the bounds of clinical utility. At the root of the problem is the fact that the concept of an 'epileptic focus' is an oversimplification in many situations (it remains perhaps most valid in relation to the epilepsy caused by small discrete neocortical lesions). In many instances, the epileptic seizure is the result of simultaneous or near-simultaneous involvement and activation of large-scale and widespread neuronal networks and circuits. This is true for instance of mesial temporal lobe epilepsy, and although temporal lobectomy may cure the seizures, it probably does not do so by simply 'removing the focus'. The persistence of auras after surgery and the findings from preoperative intracranial stimulation experiments [13] are evidence of this, as for instance is the lack of correlation between surgical outcome and the presence of spiking cortex in residual tissue in peroperative EcoG recordings. The non-focal nature of such 'partial' epilepsies limits the value of efforts to exquisitely localize epilepsy by functional investigations.

In the past 30 years, other methods for functional localization have also been developed, notably PET scanning, first used in epilepsy in the late 1970s, and MEG introduced in the mid 1980s. Neither has achieved widespread acceptance in spite of long years of experimentation, although both can be useful in individual cases. SPECT scanning was introduced into clinical epilepsy practice in the early 1980s and ictal SPECT particularly has proved more useful generally than PET. However, PET and SPECT provide poor temporal resolution and furthermore rely on blood flow changes which have generally a greater anatomical extent than the electrographic activity. Many centres in the world carry out epilepsy surgery without the routine use of any of these technologies, without any obvious detriment to quality or outcome.

The second approach to localization, again driven largely by technological development, is to detect structural (anatomical) rather than functional abnormalities underpinning epilepsy. The importance of structural change was well recognized by Horsley who had no imaging technologies available, and who relied on per-

Table 51.1 The impact of CT on epilepsy practice: the percentage of CT abnormalities found in five series of patients with epilepsy published between 1977 and 1982

CT findings	Unselected cases ($n = 367$)	Consecutive cases ($n = 150$)	New adult referrals ($n = 237$)	Consecutive children ($n = 256$)	Unselected focal epilepsy ($n = 50$)
Normal	47%	60%	65%	68%	65%
Diffuse atrophy	18%	13%	28%	12%	10%
Focal atrophy	4%	9%	12%	8%	4%
Porencephaly	0%	3%	1%	1%	12%
Hydrocephalus	3%	3%	0%	1%	2%
Hemiatrophy	0%	0%	0%	2%	0%
AVM/aneurysm	2%	4%	1%	0%	0%
Infarction	5%	4%	0%	0%	0%
Neoplasm	14%	4%	4%	2%	4%
Calcification	5%	0%	0%	3%	0%
Other (misc.)	1%	0%	0%	5%	2%

Adapted from [14].

AVM, arteriovenous malformation.

operative inspection of the brain. He noticed that the absence of a visible pathological abnormality reduced the likelihood that surgery would succeed in relieving the seizures. This principle has been reiterated by Penfield in the 1940s and many others since. In Penfield's time, anatomical imaging was confined to ventriculography, pneumoencephalography and angiography. These techniques relied on mass effect to deform the normal patterns of the ventricles or blood vessels—and none were sensitive nor specific. The neuroimaging revolution in the last 30 years has had a profound effect on presurgical studies in epilepsy, by the increasingly sensitive rendition of the visible anatomical lesions underpinning the epileptic seizures. The first CT scan in a patient was carried out in London in 1971, and the first major report of CT in epilepsy was made in 1975 at the 21st European Congress of Electroencephalography and Epilepsy. Table 51.1 is taken from a review of CT in epilepsy in 1987 [14], and provides a snapshot of the impact of CT on epilepsy practice at that time. An interesting comparison can be made with a similar survey of MRI two decades later (Table 51.2) [15]. As was the case with EEG, this technology produced a sense of intense excitement and new frontiers for surgical therapy seemed in prospect. CT remains to this day a highly sensitive and specific method of diagnosing many lesions underlying epilepsy, but its principal clinical role was, however, quickly overtaken. In 1980, the first images of the human brain using MRI were made in Nottingham, UK, and the first clinical image in the brain of a patient with epilepsy was published in 1982 [16]. Although initially thought to be not superior to CT [17], the potential of MRI and its superiority in defining more subtle lesions of the brain was well recognized by the late 1980s. As written in the proceedings of the NATO Advanced Scientific Workshop on MRI and Epilepsy held in London in 1992, 'A true revolution in medicine has ensued [since the first publication of clinical scans]; in only a few years of development, the esoteric physics of nuclear spin, angular momentum and magnetic vector precession were harnessed to provide exquisite images of living anatomy: modern science has no greater tribute' [16]. MRI has a number of advantages over CT. It provides better grey–white matter contrast, there is no artefact due to bone and resolution is better than in CT.

Table 51.2 The impact of MRI on epilepsy practice: the percentage of MRI abnormalities found in a consecutive series of patients with chronic epilepsy

Abnormality detected	n	%
None	87	26
Hippocampal atrophy	109	32
Cortical dysgenesis	43	13
Tumour	40	12
Vascular malformation	28	8
Infarct / contusion	20	6
Other abnormalities*	38	11

Note: 24 (7%) patients had two abnormalities detected.

*Abnormalities mostly thought to be non-contributory to the epilepsy. The results of MRI scanning in a series of 341 consecutive patients, from the tertiary epilepsy clinics at the National Hospital for Neurology and Neurosurgery, London. A highly selected group with severe epilepsy. Prior CT showed a causal lesion in only about 5%. This population is typical of the patient group referred for pre-surgical assessment. From [15].

Image contrast can be altered by varying sequences, and thus examination can be tailored to an individual problem. The data collection allows postprocessing, reformatting and detailed measurement. MRI carries no risk of radiation, and thus long or repeated studies are possible. MRI has the ability to detect and visualize hippocampal sclerosis and cortical dysplasia and, as a result, interest in both pathologies, and in their surgical treatment, has greatly intensified. MRI also has promoted the development of microsurgery and stereotactic approaches to surgery.

Advances in operative technology have also driven the development of epilepsy surgery. As mentioned above, Horsley's work was possible at least in part due to advances in antisepsis and anaesthesia. In the first half of the 20th century, neurosurgical instrumentation greatly improved, and this had a great impact, for instance, on

Penfield's work. The stereotactic atlas, published by Tailarach and co-workers in 1957, was the basis for the subsequent development of stereotactic surgery [9]. By 1973, the results of over 400 instances of SEEG in over 300 patients in a 14-year period were published by Tailarach and colleagues [10]. Stereotaxy was improved by computerized surgical navigation systems and the use of the relocatable frame (for instance the CRW frame introduced in the 1980s). Frameless stereotaxy was made possible by the computerized coregistration of neuroimaging modalities. The operating microscope was another landmark in the development of neurosurgical technique, although introduced into neurosurgical practice, remarkably, only after several decades of routine use in other specialities (e.g. otological surgery). The microscope has allowed increasingly selective resective surgery and the development of a range of microsurgical techniques. Gazi Yasargil, a Turkish neurosurgeon in Zurich, was an early pioneer, using the operative microscope in epilepsy from the late 1960s. He developed new surgical procedures using subarachnoid approaches to lesions throughout the brain, and in epilepsy, particularly, the trans-sylvian selective amygdalohippocampectomy from 1973 [18]. The introduction of focused beam radiotherapy has also stimulated interest in the potential for radiation-induced lesioning in temporal lobe epilepsy. Irradiation has in fact been occasionally used to control seizures since the 1930s, but the potential for highly focused radiation has been possible only with the development of gamma knife and other technology. Similarly, stereotactic lesioning and stimulation of many midline structures (notably the thalamic nuclei and fields of Forel) were popularized in the 1940s and 1950s, but the advent of advanced technology allowing increasing accuracy and selectivity has resulted in a resurgence of interest.

Indeed, most contemporary surgical approaches are modifications of procedures used for at least 50 years. Modern temporal lobectomy is a case in point. Although Penfield initially carried out wide cortical excision only, he soon recognized the importance of removing mesial structures. Since then, various methods for mesial resection have been devised, and these developments are essentially variations on the same theme. Murray Falconer and others proposed the standard *en bloc* operation. Amygdalohippocampectomy with limited cortical resection was then introduced using the trans-sylvian approach of Yasargil, the transcortical transventricular approach of Niemeyer [19], an approach through the middle temporal gyrus by Thomas [20] or the occipital lobe by Kelly [21], and via a resection of the cortical pole [22,23]. Similar variations in techniques occurred with corpus callosectomy and hemispherectomy. The former has an interesting history. In 1931, Dandy resected a sectum pellucidal cyst in a 4 year old, via a callosal approach, and in doing so sectioned the corpus callosum. This operation was noticed to terminate the child's seizures and this chance observation led Van Wagenen to carry out the first corpus callosum section for epilepsy on 6 February 1939 [24]. Since then the extent of the recommended extension has varied—anterior, posterior, complete, one stage, two stage—but the essential concept is unchanged. Dandy was also the first to carry out hemispherectomy, although for an infiltrating glioma not for epilepsy. Krynauw was the first to propose this for intractable epilepsy [25]. He reported 12 cases in 1950, and the operation was then rapidly adopted for specific types of infantile epilepsies. By 1961 over 250 cases had been reported in the medical literature [26]. Since then operative techniques have evolved to

Table 51.3 A lesson from history—some of the largely spurious surgical procedures carried out for epilepsy during the first part of the 20th century

Trephination
Trepanation
Carotid occlusion
Bilateral vertebral artery ligation
Cervical sympathectomy
Castration
Circumcision
Hysterectomy or oophorectomy
Colectomy and other large bowel resections
Adrenalectomy
Dural splitting
Arterialization of the internal jugular vein

avoid late complications and have included the creation of a subdural space to replace the subpial cavity by Adams [27], the functional hemispherectomy by Rasmussen [28], the hemispherotomy by Delalande and colleagues [29], hemidecortication by Hoffman and colleagues [30], peri-insular hemispherotomy by Villemure and Mascott [31].

Finally, a note of caution. Even in fairly recent times, largely spurious surgical procedures continued to be carried out. In the first part of the 20th century, operative approaches included an intimidating list of ineffective procedures (Table 51.3), some carried out in the best institutions and on a large scale. Trephination is a case in point, persisting as it did from antiquity until the mid 20th century. It was, in the 19th century, a common procedure. Billings [32] mentions that a single surgeon in St Louis had carried out over 100 cases, and Gowers [33] cites its widespread use in the US and by Kocher in Berne. It was still a recommended operation in Kinnear Wilson's standard neurology textbook of 1940 [34]. New but equally inappropriate therapies were introduced in the 20th century, for instance the use of cerebellar stimulation in the 1970s, or of bilateral temporal lobectomy which persisted throughout the 1950s in some centres in spite of its great morbidity. The impressive advances of modern science and technology should not induce complacency. Our contemporary practice, embedded as it is in largely pragmatic observation and the opportunistic application of new technology to older procedures, may prove ridiculous to future generations. Fallibility is a major lesson of history, and critical appraisal should temper the exuberance and exaggerated claims which seem inevitably to flow from all new ideas in technology or surgical theory. The chapters which follow in this section aim to provide such a critical view.

The need for epilepsy surgery

Various epidemiological studies have been carried out to determine the number of patients who might be suitable for epilepsy surgery. This is not the place to review these in detail, but a few words on potential surgical volume are appropriate. The crude incidence of epilepsy in most countries is between 50 and 100/100 000 persons/year, and the crude prevalence of active epilepsy is 5–8/1000 cases. An estimate based on prospective follow-up of a cohort of

564 patients followed from the time of diagnosis for 10 years or more has suggested that up to 3% of new cases of epilepsy may prove to be suitable candidates for epilepsy surgery [35]. A suitable candidate was defined, in this survey, as one who fulfilled the following criteria: (a) had partial onset seizures; (b) had seizures occurring at an average frequency of more than one a week; (c) was under the age of 60 years; (d) had no epilepsy aetiology which was a contraindication to surgery; and (e) had no other known contraindication to surgery. These figures approximate to at least 10 new cases per million persons in the population per year. The underlying assumptions are obviously broad generalizations; some patients in these categories would not wish to be considered for surgery and conversely others who do not fulfil all these criteria might well benefit from surgery. Nevertheless, the figures provide the basis for rough estimation.

A landmark in epilepsy surgery was the workshop, held on 20–24 February 1986 in Palm Desert Springs [36]. This brought together many of the world figures in epilepsy surgery, and was instrumental in both stimulating interest and activity in epilepsy surgery and also in providing figures about numbers of operated cases worldwide. At this conference, it was estimated that in the US (with its population of about 250 000 000) there were about 25 000 persons who might be considered to be candidates for epilepsy surgery, and yet only about 300 operations were being performed annually. Exactly how the figure of 25 000 was calculated is not made clear, and probably overestimates the true potential number; nevertheless, the workshop left no doubt that a substantial treatment gap existed. A second conference was convened in 1992, and by then the number of operated cases had increased sizeably [37]. A survey of surgical activity in 100 centres then suggested that over 8000 cases had been operated worldwide in the 5 years between 1986 and 1990 (Table 51.4). These data were based largely on uncorroborated retrospective estimations, and reflect in some cases good intentions rather than solid achievement. Nevertheless, the figures demonstrated that there was an undoubted increase in surgical numbers during the period since the first conference and this expansion is continuing to this day.

One prospective national study has been carried out. This was of all neurosurgeons in the UK, who were surveyed monthly over a 6-month period [35]. Each surgeon was asked to list the number and type of epilepsy surgeries performed in the previous month. An annualized figure of 512 operated cases was ascertained (in a population of approximately 50 million persons; see Table 51.5). Thus, the

number of surgeries was thought to be approximately equal to the new cases added to the pool of potential cases annually, but was inadequate to dent the residual backlog of existing patients. It is likely that a similar gap exists in many other countries, although figures are not widely available.

Types of epilepsy surgery

Epilepsy surgery is defined as surgery carried out specifically to control epileptic seizures. This will include operations on tumours and vascular lesions where epilepsy is the primary indication for surgery. There is clearly an overlap with lesional surgery carried out for other primary reasons, if the lesion is causing epilepsy and even if the operation influences the epilepsy. Such operations are not generally classified as epilepsy surgery, but this is clearly a grey area. There are many such cases in whom the control of epilepsy is an important consideration in the decision to undertake surgery. Epilepsy surgery also implies a particular approach to presurgical assessment which is discussed further below.

There are various types of operation possible, and the main categories are shown in Table 51.6. Each is described in detail in the Chapters that follow.

The results of the survey in 2001 (Table 51.5) show the range of current practice in the UK. Practice has changed substantially since the introduction of MRI, with a trend towards lesional surgery and away from non-lesional resections guided by EEG. Notable also is the rapid and some would say unjustifiable increase in the number of cases of vagal nerve stimulation, in spite of the modest results in most instances from this operation.

The process of presurgical assessment– selection of patients for epilepsy surgery

As a general rule, surgical treatment should at least be considered in any patient with partial seizures that are intractable to medical therapy. When surgery is to be contemplated, the patient should be referred to an experienced epilepsy surgery team for presurgical evaluation. The evaluation will depend on the type of surgery being proposed, but in general terms should have the following aims.
1 To confirm that the patient has medically intractable epilepsy.
2 To define the outcome goals of the chosen surgical procedure (e.g.

Table 51.4 Number of surgical procedures performed worldwide between 1986 and 1990

Anterior temporal lobectomy	4862 (59%)
Amygdalohippocampectomy	568 (7%)
Extratemporal resection	1073 (13%)
Lesionectomy	440 (5%)
Hemispherectomy and large lobar resections	448 (5%)
Corpus callosectomy	843 (10%)
Total	*8234*

These figures are estimates only and derive from a retrospective survey of interested centres. It is likely that the proportion of lesionectomies is underestimated and of non-lesional extratemporal lobe resections overestimated. From [44].

Table 51.5 A survey of the numbers of epilepsy surgical procedures performed in the UK over a 12-month period

Type of surgical procedure	Annual no.	%
Temporal lobe resection for mesial temporal sclerosis	208	41
Lesion surgery for epilepsy	114	22
Non-lesional resective surgery	6	1
Hemispherectomy	14	3
Functional surgery		
corpus callosotomy	14	3
vagal nerve stimulation	156	30

From [35].

Table 51.6 The major categories of epilepsy surgery in contemporary practice

Resection of hippocampal sclerosis—which includes the standard temporal lobectomy, selective operations and other variants

Resections of overt lesions (lesionectomy)—for instance, for tumours, post-trauma lesions, postinfective lesions and cortical dysplasia. These include lesions in temporal and non-temporal areas

Non-lesional focal resections—for cases in which no structural lesion can be demonstrated preoperatively, and in whom the evidence for localization is based entirely on functional investigation (e.g. EEG, PET, MEG, SPECT)

Large resections—for instance of whole lobes or of a cerebral hemisphere (multilobar resection, frontal lobectomy, hemispherectomy). These are carried out for large, widely distributed or multifocal lesions

Functional surgery—these are non-resective procedures in which the purpose of surgery is to interrupt pathways or inhibit seizure production in other ways. Examples are multiple subpial transection, corpus callosectomy, stereotactic lesioning or stimulation, vagal nerve stimulation

seizure freedom (usually), 50% reduction in seizures etc.) and estimate the chances of attaining this successful outcome.

3 To define the likely gains in terms of quality of life if surgery is carried out.

4 To determine the risks of carrying out the surgical procedure—for instance in terms of mortality, neurological morbidity, psychological and social effects; also the risks of not operating.

5 To determine that the person is medically fit for surgery.

6 To counsel the patient appropriately about the outcome and risks.

The process of presurgical evaluation is usually emotionally demanding and time-consuming. The patient should be made aware of this at the outset. Not infrequently, surgery will prove not to be possible, and this rejection can be devastating for a person who has made a considerable emotional investment in the process. The decision to proceed with surgery is in view of its risks and uncertainties often difficult, and the balance of risks and benefits seldom clearcut. The decision must always be an individual one, and one made by the patient; the doctor's role is to provide information and to advise. The decision should be a considered choice on the basis of the information provided. The patient must feel confident that sufficient information has been given, and that this information is accurate and unbiased. Surgery should not be performed if the patient is reluctant or undecided.

The specific investigations and operations are covered in detail in subsequent chapters of this section. However, a few general points can be made here.

The approach to the selection of patients for epilepsy surgery

Intractable epilepsy

Strictly speaking, epilepsy can be defined as intractable only in retrospect. However, for pragmatic reasons, in the author's usual practice, epilepsy is regarded as sufficiently intractable to contemplate surgery if it has been continuously active for 5 years (or less in severe epilepsy) in spite of adequate therapy with three or more mainline antiepileptic drugs, and if seizures are frequent (more than one a month). The chances of further medical therapy controlling seizures after 5 years of intractability thus defined are slight (probably less than 5–10% with currently available drugs). There has been a recent trend to define intractability earlier (after 2 or 3 years of failure to respond to medical therapy) based on studies which show that an early failure of treatment is predictive of a continuing poor response

to medical therapy [38–40]. However, some patients do respond later and 2–3 years seems, to this author at least, generally too short a time to make appropriate judgements about surgery. These are guidelines only, and there will be patients in whom epilepsy surgery is appropriate, and yet who do not fulfil these criteria. The merits of each case should be considered individually, and this requires skill and experience.

Estimation of seizure outcome and risk of surgery

The outcome of surgery will depend on the type and severity of the epilepsy and its underlying anatomical and physiological bases. Accurate prediction can only be made after the presurgical evaluation is completed. However, a patient should be given estimates from the outset, so that he/she can decide whether or not to proceed with investigation. Estimates are usually given in percentage terms; a common example might be, for instance, the 60% chance of seizure freedom following anterior temporal lobectomy in an uncomplicated case of mesial temporal epilepsy (and see Chapter 60). The estimate should be based both on the literature and the audited record of the surgical unit. The estimation of surgical risk will also depend on the nature of the surgery being offered, and the extent and location of brain resection. Again, accurate prediction is only possible after the presurgical evaluation is completed. At the end of the assessment period, the estimations of risk and of outcome should be given in writing to the patient who must be given time for careful consideration and who should also be offered the opportunity for discussion and counselling.

Quality of life gain

The prediction of the extent of the expected quality of life gain due to surgery is a key part of the presurgical assessment. Surgery should be offered only to those whose quality of life is seriously compromised by the occurrence of seizures and in whom the expected outcome of surgery (usually seizure freedom) is likely to result in major quality of life improvement. This may seem obvious, but it is in fact often difficult to decide. There are many patients who have had surgery which successfully controls seizures but who regret having had the operation, and whose life has shown little improvement. Frequent seizures are not necessarily disabling—for instance mild seizures, simple partial seizures or seizures occurring only at night. In some situations, even severe seizures are not the key determinant of quality of life, for instance in patients with multiple disabling features. Emotional factors are important, and surgery which is successful in controlling seizures will not automatically alleviate other negative lifestyle aspects, even if these had been moulded by the epilepsy. Social structures and interpersonal relationships may be predicated on a lifetime of seizures, and their sudden cure by surgery may result in change, not necessarily for the best. Skilful counselling is vital in this area.

Non-epileptic seizures

It is not uncommon for a patient to be referred for surgery who on investigation turns out to have non-epileptic seizures, either alone or in combination with genuine epileptic attacks. Generally speaking, the occurrence of non-epileptic attacks—even in combination with genuine attacks—is a contraindication for surgery. Therapy should be directed at the physical causes or the psychological pressures which underpin these attacks. If surgery is carried out in patients with a combination of genuine and psychogenic attacks, the psychogenic attacks frequently worsen even if the genuine attacks are relieved. Decisions about treatment in this area should be made only in a specialist setting.

Learning disability, behavioural disorder and psychosis

Learning disability in some cases implies widespread cerebral dysfunction and, because of this, resective surgery is less likely to control seizures. However, many patients with learning disability are severely handicapped by severe epilepsy, and such people have great potential benefit from surgery. Expert evaluation is needed in such cases, and the risk–benefit equation needs careful formulation and discussion with the patient and carers. Ethical issues of informed consent are important and can be difficult. Surgery is generally also contraindicated in individuals who show severely dysfunctional behaviour. Such patients generally cannot tolerate the intensive or prolonged hospitalizations required for epilepsy surgery, nor make informed and considered judgements about the potential risks and benefits of epilepsy surgery. The presence of a chronic psychosis is also generally a contraindication to surgery, as the psychosis can worsen dramatically after surgery. Again, individual decisions in this situation require a detailed and experienced assessment.

Medical fitness and age

Some patients have added risks due to general medical problems, for instance cervical spinal or vascular disease. Surgery should only be contemplated in those who can withstand prolonged anaesthesia. In general terms, surgery is usually restricted to those under the age of 50 years. Above this age, lifestyle is often adapted well to the epilepsy and may be difficult to change. The risks of surgery may be greater, and in the ageing brain the adverse consequences can be more severe. Age though is not an absolute criteria, and the key assessments are the estimation of risks and of the potential for quality of life gain, whatever the patient's age.

The timing of epilepsy surgery

In recent years, there has been a vogue for recommending surgery at an early stage in the epilepsy. This is to minimize the impact of the seizure disorder on education and social development, to minimize the potential for morbidity or death due to epileptic seizures, to prevent the possibility of secondary epileptogenesis (either through injury or 'kindling') and the possibility of progressive intellectual or behavioural decline and to minimize the psychological impact of epilepsy. The recommendation for early surgery applies particularly in children and for the surgically remediable childhood epilepsy syndromes. Seizures may pose additional risks to the developing brain of infants and young children. Uncontrolled seizures also jeopardize the chances for an independent lifestyle, and children with intractable epilepsy are likely to be excluded from normal schools and from social and vocational opportunities. Also, the potential for functional recovery from cerebral resection is greatest when surgery is performed in childhood.

The approach to investigation in presurgical assessment

The approach to resective surgery for epilepsy can, since the time of Horsley, be summarized as follows. In many cases of epilepsy, the seizures originate in a small area of brain (the epileptic focus). Surgery aims to resect this epileptogenic tissue, sufficient in extent to lead to the resolution of the seizures.

The epileptogenic, irritative and ictal onset zones

The aim of resecting brain tissue sufficient to abolish the epileptic seizures rests philosophically on the presumption that there is an 'epileptic focus' underpinning the epilepsy. This is undoubtedly true of some cases, especially in acquired neocortical epilepsy. However, in many cases seizures are in fact underpinned by widespread and complex neuronal networks and circuits. In such cases, the concept of a discrete focus is both naïve and untenable (see for instance [41]). Because of this, the concept of the 'epileptogenic zone' has gained currency. This term is defined as the anatomical area necessary and sufficient for initiating seizures and whose removal or disconnection is necessary for abolition of seizures. It has arisen in recognition of the fact that the epilepsy may arise in distributed areas that are wider, for instance, than simply that of the overt electrographic or structural abnormalities. The presurgical evaluation of a patient therefore, it is argued, aims to define the anatomical boundaries of the epileptogenic zone, and having done so, the feasibility of resection and its potential risks can then be estimated.

Unfortunately, there are no preoperative clinical or laboratory tests which can define the area in any individual patient. It is only possible to ascertain whether an 'epileptogenic zone' was successfully resected after years of postoperative seizure freedom—and even then without knowing how much unnecessary resection of additional brain tissue was carried out. This is unsatisfactory and the concept of the epileptogenic zone, in the author's opinion, adds little to that of the epileptic focus. The concept however has one virtue—it emphasizes what has been known for more than half a century, that the amount of brain resection necessary often extends beyond the lesion visualized on neuroimaging or the cortical area which generates interictal spikes. This latter area is often known as the irritative zone. The irritative zone can extend beyond the epileptogenic zone, and it is common, for instance, for residual tissue left after surgery to exhibit active spiking on ECoG. Furthermore, the apparent extent of the irritative zone will vary with differing types of EEG investigation. If ictal rather than interictal EEG recording is carried out, the electrographic onset of a seizure can sometimes be defined—sometimes known as the ictal onset zone. This area provides a rough indication of where to target surgery, but again its value depends on the extent to which the epileptic network is localized, and is also dependent on the method of investigation employed.

It has been shown pragmatically that the resection of structurally abnormal areas of brain tissue will sometimes result in seizure control. In other words, in such cases, the epileptogenic zone is often included in the areas of structural abnormality. Complete excision is generally better than partial excision, but even complete excision of structurally abnormal tissue does not always result in seizure control. The success depends on the aetiology of the lesion—the resection of areas of cortical dysplasia, for instance, has a low success rate, whereas the resection of mesial temporal sclerosis has a higher rate. The reasons are complex. The presence of subtle anatomical changes beyond the resolution of neuroimaging may be part of the reasons for surgical failure, but it is more likely that the complex neuronal networks spread well beyond the primary anatomical defects.

The complexity of seizure generation can be well demonstrated in mesial temporal lobe epilepsy. Here there is good experimental and clinical evidence that the seizures are underpinned by a network which extends well beyond the mesial temporal lobe, yet resection of the hippocampus which will remove only part of this network is often successful in controlling seizures. Conversely, resection of large areas of frontal cortex in apparently well-localized frontal lesional epilepsy will stop seizures in a relatively small proportion of patients.

The principle of concordance of investigations

An observation fundamental to presurgical assessment is that resective surgery is more likely to be successful if the findings from the different modalities of presurgical investigations are concordant—i.e. if each points to a similar localization of seizure onset. Conversely, if results are discordant, resective surgery is likely to be less successful. It follows that all patients require multimodal investigation aimed at defining the seizure localization. There are four main components of investigation—radiological, neurophysiological, psychological and clinical. Different centres use different methods of investigation in these four areas (see below) but all four modalities should be carried out in the majority of patients being worked up for surgery. It follows also that incomplete or unfocused investigation is fraught with danger. It is for this reason that presurgical evaluation is best carried out in a designated centre with multidisciplinary experience.

The importance of aetiology and syndrome

Key determinants of successful surgery are the underlying aetiology and epilepsy syndrome. It is because of the importance of demonstrating aetiology that MRI has had such a great impact on presurgical evaluation. Indeed, MRI should be the starting point of all investigation. Resective surgery is best for those with well-localized lesions shown on MRI, especially those with unilateral mesial temporal lobe atrophy, small focal neocortical or temporal cavernomas

or benign or low-grade tumours, or other small and entirely discrete lesions. The demonstration of aetiology is also of prognostic importance in other types of surgery, for instance hemispherectomy, frontal lobe and other large resections, and also for corpus callosectomy. The different surgical approaches to these are outlined in subsequent chapters.

MRI as a screening test, and MRI-negative cases

Prior to MRI many cases of epilepsy (including virtually all cases of hippocampal sclerosis) were 'non-lesional', in the sense that no lesion could be detected preoperatively. The nature and extent of the surgery in these cases depended heavily on scalp and invasive EEG. It was realized even then that if no pathology was found in the pathological examination of the operated specimen, the prognosis for seizure control was likely to be poor.

The advent of MRI has radically altered the clinical situation, as preoperative MRI can identify many of these previously occult lesions. The dependency on EEG for localization has been lost, and the requirement for invasive EEG has been greatly reduced. It has been shown that if MRI shows no lesion preoperatively, a so-called MRI-negative epilepsy, the chances of successful surgery are greatly diminished, even after intensive work-up using other modalities. In routine practice, therefore, MRI has become in effect a screening test for further surgical evaluation and has now displaced EEG in this role.

In one study of 40 MRI-negative patients investigated with a view to surgery, only five such cases were found to have a well-localized electrographic focus concordant with other (non-MRI) investigations: operation proved possible in only three, and only one had a successful surgical outcome. Other groups have found better results (see [42]). It is clear however that MRI-negative cases should be offered surgery only after careful assessment by an experienced unit, that surgery will not prove possible in many patients investigated and that extensive and costly investigations will usually be needed. This is not surgery for the faint-hearted.

It is important to stress that a patient should not be considered MRI-negative unless a detailed MRI examination has been made, applying the correct sequences and techniques (see Chapter 55). A critical approach is needed. Many patients have apparently normal MRI scans using inappropriate examinations, who show clear lesions when scanned using the epilepsy-orientated MRI protocols—this is especially true of patients harbouring such lesions as hippocampal atrophy, small vascular lesions or tumours or cortical dysplasia. These pseudo-MRI-negative cases emphasize the importance of a tailored MRI approach.

The selection of patients for temporal lobe surgery

The most common indication for epilepsy surgery is temporal lobe epilepsy, and this subject deserves special mention.

The epilepsy is usually divided into two categories, mesial temporal epilepsy and lateral temporal neocortical epilepsy, although there is a marked overlap in causative aetiologies, symptomatology and treatment. Temporal lobe epilepsy has been the subject of a number of extensive reviews (see [41]).

Causative aetiologies and pathologies in temporal lobe epilepsy

Many different temporal lobe abnormalities can result in temporal lobe epilepsy. The commonest pathology underlying mesial temporal lobe epilepsy is mesial temporal sclerosis (sometimes known as hippocampal sclerosis). The principal abnormality is hippocampal neuronal cell loss. The cell loss has a characteristic distribution, with maximum loss in the CA1 and CA4 regions and in the dentate gyrus, and relative sparing of the CA2 region. There is a dense fibrous gliosis associated with the cellular loss. The cell loss and gliosis result in atrophy, and on hippocampus is shrunken and hardened. Another common abnormality is an alteration in the laminar arrangement of the dentate gyrus. The cells are frequently more dispersed than is normal, and there is sometimes duplication of the laminar structure. The dispersed granule cells expand into the molecular layer to a variable degree, and the boundaries of the layer can be indistinct. Another typical feature is extensive aberrant mossy fibre innervation of the dentate gyrus (mossy fibre sprouting). The mossy fibres form excitatory synapses on the dendrites of the neurones of the inner molecular layer and elsewhere. A large number of neurochemical changes have been documented in the sclerotic hippocampus, although the extent to which these are primary changes or simply consequential to the hippocampal injury is often unclear. There are also pathological changes outside the hippocampus, for instance widespread subpial fibrillary gliosis (Chaslin's gliosis) and nerve cell loss in the neocortex. Cerebellar atrophy and widespread cerebral atrophy are also not uncommon. In some series, over 70% of patients with hippocampal sclerosis also show some evidence of microdysgenesis. The commonest pattern of microdysgenesis is the clustering of abnormal neurones, abnormal in structure and abnormally positioned, in the temporal lobe white matter, although changes in widely dispersed parts of the brain are not infrequently encountered. MRI morphometry has also recently shown, in cases of unilateral hippocampal sclerosis, a mean 15% reduction of the volume of the rest of the temporal lobe, reductions of similar magnitude in the parahippocampal gyrus and middle and inferior temporal gyri, and a 25% reduction in mean size of the superior temporal gyrus [43]. Volumetric analysis of grey and white matter ratios and volumes has also demonstrated changes well away from the hippocampus, both in and outside the temporal lobe. It is possible that extrahippocampal abnormalities define the widely distributed neuronal aggregate which underpins the hippocampal seizure.

Mesial temporal lobe epilepsy can also be caused by other pathologies. These include tumours (in about 10–15% of all cases of surgically treated mesial temporal lobe epilepsy). The most common are low-grade gliomas, oligodendroglioma and other astrocytic or glial tumours. Developmental abnormalities of various types account for a further 15–25% of cases, and these are sometimes associated with mesial temporal sclerosis. These include neuronal migrational disorders, heterotopia, focal dysplasia and developmental tumours. Trauma, cavernous haemangioma (cavernoma) and other vascular disease, and cerebral infections (meningitis or encephalitis) can also result in temporal lobe epilepsy. The latter two categories carry a generally poorer surgical prognosis. Sometimes acquired or congenital pathologies, both within and without the temporal lobe, are associated with mesial temporal lobe sclerosis. Surgery in such patients with 'dual pathology' is generally less successful.

Lateral temporal lobe epilepsy can similarly be caused by tumours, trauma, cavernoma and other vascular disorders, abnormalities of development and cerebral infection.

Symptomatology of mesial temporal lobe epilepsy

The clinical seizures in patients with mesial temporal lobe epilepsy are rather distinctive. The seizures take the form of simple or complex partial seizures. The complex partial seizure typically has a relatively gradual evolution (compared to extratemporal seizures), develops over 1–2 min, has an indistinct onset with partial awareness at the onset and lasts longer than most extratemporal complex partial seizures (2–10 min). The typical complex partial seizure of temporal lobe origin has three components: aura, absence and automatism.

The aura can occur in isolation as a simple partial seizure or the initial manifestation of a complex partial seizure. It typically comprises visceral, cephalic, gustatory, dysmnesic or affective symptoms. A rising epigastric sensation is the commonest. Autonomic symptoms include changes in skin colour, blood pressure, heart rate, pupil size and piloerection. Speech usually ceases or is severely reduced if the seizure is in the dominant temporal lobe. In the nondominant lobe, speech may be retained throughout the seizure or meaningless repetitive vocalizations may occur. Simple auditory phenomena such as humming, buzzing, hissing and roaring may occur if the discharges occur in the superior temporal gyrus; and olfactory sensations, which are usually unpleasant and difficult to define, occur in seizures in the sylvian region. More complex hallucinatory or illusionary states are produced with seizure discharges in association areas (e.g. structured visual hallucinations, complex visual patterns, musical sounds and speech). A cephalic aura can also occur in focal temporal lobe seizures, although this is more typical of a frontal lobe focus.

The absence takes the form of a motor arrest or absence (the so-called 'motionless stare'). This is prominent especially in the early stages of seizures arising in mesial temporal structures, and probably more so than in extratemporal lobe epilepsy. During the seizure, there is often spasm or dystonic posturing of the arm contralateral to the side of the seizure discharge; this can be a very useful localizing sign.

The automatisms of mesial temporal lobe epilepsy are typically oroalimentary (lip smacking, chewing, swallowing), or gestural (e.g. fumbling, fidgeting, repetitive motor actions, undressing, sexually directed actions, walking, running) and sometimes prolonged. They are usually less violent than in frontal lobe seizures.

Postictal confusion and headache are common after a temporal lobe complex partial seizure, and if dysphasia occurs this is a useful lateralizing sign indicating seizure origin in the dominant temporal lobe. Amnesia for the events of the absence and the automatism is the rule—and if awareness of these events is retained it is likely that the seizure is not of temporal lobe origin.

Secondary generalization can occur, but usually infrequently. Rather typically, the secondary generalized seizures occur only in patients who are not taking antiepileptic drugs. Psychiatric or behavioural disturbances often accompany the epilepsy.

The clinical syndrome of mesial temporal sclerosis is highly characteristic, and it is often possible to predict the presence of this lesion from the clinical history. Typically, seizures of the mesial temporal type (see above) develop in mid to late childhood. There is often also a history of febrile seizures (single or recurrent) between the ages of 2 and 5 years, and some years before the onset of the habitual seizures. The more characteristic the history, the more successful surgery is likely to be. A history of frequent secondary generalized seizures is predictive of a poorer outcome, as is the absence of a history of febrile seizures in patients with mesial temporal sclerosis. The frequency of attacks does not seem to influence surgical outcome.

Symptomatology of lateral temporal lobe epilepsy

There is considerable overlap between the clinical and EEG features of mesial and lateral temporal lobe epilepsy. However, differences in degree exist. The typical aura includes hallucinations which are often structured and of visual, auditory, gustatory or olfactory forms, and which can be crude or elaborate, or illusions of size (macropsia, micropsia), shape, weight, distance or sound. An auditory aura is characteristic of one form of inherited lateral temporal lobe epilepsy. Affective, visceral or psychic auras are less common than in mesial temporal lobe epilepsy. Consciousness may be preserved for longer than in a typical mesial temporal seizure. The automatisms can be unilateral and have more prominent motor manifestations than in mesial temporal lobe epilepsy. Postictal phenomena, amnesia for the attack and the psychiatric accompaniments are indistinguishable from the mesial temporal form.

There is usually a detectable underlying structural pathology, the commonest being a glioma, angioma, hamartoma, dysembryoplastic neuroepithelial tumour, other benign tumour, neuronal migration defect and post-traumatic change. There is no association with a history of febrile convulsions.

A protocol for presurgical assessment

A range of tests should be undertaken as part of the presurgical evaluation. Different centres use different testing protocols and there is a striking lack of consensus internationally or indeed within the same country. This is unsatisfactory, and reflects both the rapid development of technologies and also a failure to undertake objective and evidence-based evaluations of technologies. Some of the tests pose little or no risk, but others are invasive and have the potential for discomfort and injury and some incur great cost without clear evidence of benefit. The local availability of often expensive tests also influences their usage. The multiplicity of approaches is well demonstrated in the published appendices of presurgical evaluation protocols in standard textbooks (e.g. [37,42]).

Some investigations are of marginal proven value. The use of evidence-based protocols and guidelines would be a great improvement on the current, rather chaotic situation where investigatory approaches vary considerably without any striking differences in outcome. An objective evaluation of the contribution to patient selection and outcome is clearly needed for many of the tests

currently in common usage. It is only in this way that cost effectiveness and clinical value can be ultimately assessed.

The range of tests applied depends on the type of surgery being offered. The various investigations are discussed in more detail in the chapters which follow in this section. Here a summary outline of each investigatory modality is presented, and a protocol which reflects the personal bias of the author and the approach to presurgical assessment taken at the author's institution (the National Hospital for Neurology and Neurosurgery in London; see Table 51.7).

Medical history and examination

A detailed neurological history is taken in all patients, at the onset of the presurgical assessment programme. The following aspects are carefully documented: the observable features of the seizures, the aura and seizure manifestations as experienced by the patient, postictal features, seizure precipitants, the onset and temporal evolution of the seizures, their pattern over time, seizure frequency and timing, family history and response to therapy. The aetiology of the epilepsy can often be ascertained from the history and enquiry should be directed towards this. The clinical history will often provide clues to the localization and discordance between the clinical and investigatory localization should warn against surgery. The clinical examination should be meticulously recorded to document the epilepsy history and the preoperative deficit and as a baseline for comparison with postoperative findings.

Psychiatric assessment

A detailed neuropsychiatric evaluation is routinely carried out in the early stages of a presurgical assessment. The evaluation has three purposes.

1 To establish the risk of psychosis or affective disorder postoperatively.
2 To estimate the ability of the person to withstand the long process of surgical evaluation and any adverse consequences of surgery.
3 To estimate the potential for psychological and psychiatric quality of life gains postoperatively, if seizure control is achieved.

Details of the psychiatric assessment are given in Chapter 59. One should recognize however that psychiatry is not an exact science, and the predictive value of premorbid psychiatric features is not fully understood. In broad terms, a history of psychosis is a contraindication to surgery, unless the psychosis was entirely confined to a postictal period. Similarly, psychopathy or personality disorder is a relative contraindication as is significant depression. The patient and the family should be counselled about the possible psychological and psychiatric consequences of surgery, so that any postoperative psychiatric problems can be swiftly identified. Both temporal and frontal lobe surgery carry specific risks—in temporal lobe surgery, for instance, the risk of postoperative psychosis and depression. For this reason, patients undergoing temporal or frontal resections require specific psychiatric counselling.

Scalp EEG

The work-up of all patients includes a routine review 24-channel scalp EEG and a review of previous EEGs.

Most patients with mesial temporal sclerosis have anterior tem-

Table 51.7 The approach to presurgical investigation taken at the National Hospital for Neurology and Neurosurgery, London

Medical history and examination	All patients
Psychiatric assessment	All patients
24-channel scalp EEG (and review of previous EEG)	All patients
Seizure recordings using video-EEG telemetry	>95% of patients
MRI imaging using 1.5 T scanner—T1-weighted thin slice volumetric, T2 and FLAIR acquisitions	All patients
Regional measurement of hippocampal volume and of T2 signal intensity	All patients undergoing investigation with a view to hippocampal surgery >50% of patients with extrahippocampal lesions to determine outcome and guide surgical planning
Other MRI techniques are used, selected from the following: MR angiography, diffusion imaging, perfusion imaging, MR spectroscopy, fMRI, 3D reconstruction and rendering of the cortical surface, surface area/volume measurements. Coregistration with EEG, angiographic, SPECT or PET	All patients with normal MRI ('MRI-negative cases') being investigated with a view to resective surgery In selected patients, techniques are selected to answer specific questions. MRS used mainly in hippocampal epilepsy, and other tests in extrahippocampal epilepsy Usage of diffusion scanning, perfusion scanning, surface area/volume measurements fMRI and fMRI-EEG is still confined largely for research
Other neuroimaging techniques (CT, plain skull radiography, angiography)	In a few selected patients
Neuropsychological assessment of general intellectual ability, language and memory	All patients
Other neuropsychological tests	Selected patients to address specific questions. Used mainly in extrahippocampal epilepsy
Sodium amytal test	Selected patients undergoing hippocampal surgery (about 30% of the total)
Intracranial EEG	5–10% of patients (see text for indications)
Functional imaging using HMPAO-SPECT or FDG PET	5–10% of patients (see text for indications)
Other functional imaging investigations (ligand or receptor PET, MEG, SISCOM), TMS	Usage still confined largely for research
Individual counselling	All patients

poral spiking interictally, and the presence of persisting unilateral focal interictal spikes is taken as a generally reliable guide to lateralization. However, in some series false localization is recorded in over 10% of cases [44]. The spiking is often bilateral—although usually with a predominance over the affected temporal lobe. This is not in itself a contraindication to surgery, and unilateral temporal lobe resection results in the cessation of seizures in many patients with bilateral and independent spikes. However, the presence of frequent independent bilateral spiking interictally is a warning that hippocampal pathologies may be bilateral. However, the presence of wide field abnormalities in an apparently focal epilepsy disorder raises the possibility of more widespread disturbance, a potential contraindication to surgical therapy.

In extratemporal epilepsy, the interictal spatial distribution of the scalp EEG focus is often distant from the site of the lesion, and the interictal scalp EEG is an unreliable guide to precise localization. In many cases of focal temporal and extratemporal epilepsy, the interictal EEG cannot clearly localize the epileptic focus, and non-specific changes are not taken to exclude a surgically remediable focal disorder.

Ictal recordings on scalp video-EEG telemetry

The recording of seizures on video-EEG telemetry is seen as an absolute requirement in almost all patients undergoing an epilepsy surgical work-up. Exceptions are those whose interictal EEG abnormalities are very clear-cut and concordant with other findings (for a further elaboration of this point, see Chapter 52). Patients are usually booked in for telemetry for a week (or less if seizures are very frequent) although the sessions are terminated early if sufficient seizures are recorded. The recording is needed for the following reasons:

1 To document that the attacks are epileptic in nature. A small but important proportion of patients in all presurgical programmes, often in spite of extensive prior neurological attention, are found unexpectedly to have non-epileptic seizures of psychogenic origin. Clearly resective surgery in these cases would be disastrous.

2 To identify the seizure type and syndrome. The observed seizure semiology is often rather different from that obtained from witnessed accounts. Seizure classification and clinical localization can only reliably be obtained by a careful review of the telemetry records. The number of seizures required to be recorded varies in different centres, but decisions are best tailored to the patient's clinical presentation. In complex cases, for instance where multiple seizure types occur, it is necessary to record many attacks, whilst in uncomplicated patients, a single attack can be sufficient.

3 To provide information about the localization of seizure onset. The ictal EEG is often more informative than the interictal record in providing good functional evidence of localization and lateralization.

In temporal lobe epilepsy, unilateral temporal rhythmic theta activity within 30 s of the clinical onset of the seizure is usually a reliable lateralizing sign, and occurs during telemetry in about one-half to two-thirds of cases of temporal lobe epilepsy (Fig. 51.2). However, scalp ictal recordings can be morphologically variable and the ictal EEG is not always helpful in localization. Not uncommonly, the ictal EEG will show widespread changes even in focal lesions (Fig. 51.3), and the absence of focal features during the ictal discharge is not in itself a contraindication to surgery, although clearly such patients need a particularly careful assessment. A normal EEG during a seizure raises the strong possibility but not certainty that the seizure was non-epileptic (usually a pseudoseizure). Routine 24-channel EEG is often supplemented with superficial sphenoidal electrodes in temporal lobe epilepsy. Occasionally, the ictal EEG is falsely localizing, and this is discussed further in Chapter 52.

In extratemporal epilepsy, the scalp ictal EEG is often non-localizing (Fig. 51.4) and indeed can be highly misleading. The use of closely spaced electrodes crowded around a potential focus are sometimes used to add information. The use of EEG in presurgical evaluation is considered in more detail in Chapters 52 and 53.

MRI

MRI is undertaken in all patients undergoing evaluation for epilepsy surgery. Indeed, it is now the primary screening test for entry into the process of presurgical evaluation. The use of MRI in presurgical assessment is the subject of Chapter 55. For presurgical assessment in my unit, the minimum MRI dataset applied, using high-quality 1.5 tesla scanning, is as follows.

1 A volume acquisition T1-weighted coronal dataset that covers the whole brain in slices of 1 or 1.5 mm thickness. This sequence provides approximately cubic voxels which can be used for reformatting in any orientation, quantitation of hippocampal volume and other morphological measures, three-dimensional reconstruction and surface rendering.

2 An oblique inversion recovery sequence, heavily T1 weighted, and oriented perpendicularly to the long axis of the hippocampus.

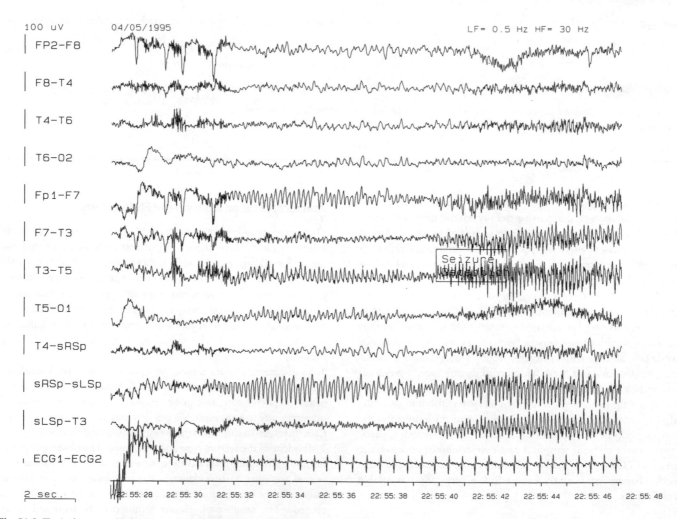

Fig. 51.2 Typical temporal lobe seizure with rhythmic lateralized theta activity.

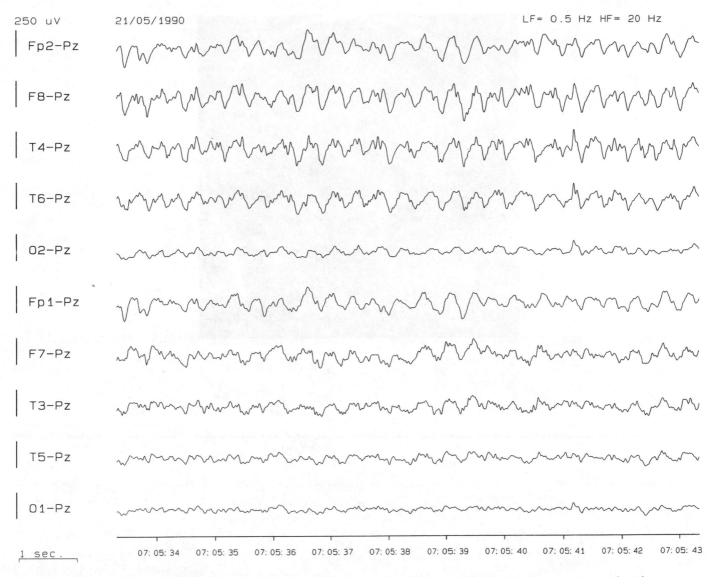

250 uV   21/05/1990   LF= 0.5 Hz HF= 20 Hz

Fp2–Pz

F8–Pz

T4–Pz

T6–Pz

O2–Pz

Fp1–Pz

F7–Pz

T3–Pz

T5–Pz

O1–Pz

1 sec.   07:05:34   07:05:35   07:05:36   07:05:37   07:05:38   07:05:39   07:05:40   07:05:41   07:05:42   07:05:43

Fig. 51.3 Ictal EEG findings from a patient with a large left temporal lobe tumour. The EEG shows widespread rhythmic activity over the right hemisphere and irregular slowing over the left temporal region (the site of the lesion).

This sequence provides good hippocampal anatomical definition and contrast.

3 An oblique T2-weighted sequence orientated perpendicularly to the long axis of the hippocampus. This sequence provides the basis for regional hippocampal T2 intensity measurement.

4 FLAIR sequence, which increases the perspicacity of some of the lesions, including hippocampal sclerosis, which commonly underpin focal epilepsy.

This MRI approach can demonstrate hippocampal sclerosis with high specificity and sensitivity. However, care must be taken not to misinterpret the MRI signs. Occasionally, for instance, hippocampal atrophy is the result not the cause of epilepsy (e.g. after status or in lesional cortical epilepsies) or a consequence of trauma or previous hippocampal surgery. A swollen hippocampus on one side due to tumour can lead to the mistaken diagnosis of an atrophic contralateral hippocampus. Increased hippocampal T2 signal is also relatively non-specific and occurs in patients with hippocampal tumour, vascular or developmental abnormalities. Also, in a sizeable

proportion of patients with epilepsy, this MRI approach will demonstrate more than one potentially causative lesion (so-called 'dual pathology'); for example, about 15% of patients with hippocampal sclerosis exhibit other extrahippocampal dysgenetic lesions (Table 51.8, Fig. 51.5). It is imperative to identify those that are epileptogenic, for clearly hippocampal resection in such cases will not be successful.

Quantitative volumetric analysis (Fig. 51.6) and T2 measurement of the hippocampus are also routinely undertaken in patients being assessed for hippocampal surgery. These provide objective information about the severity of the hippocampal sclerosis and also allow the detection of bilateral damage. Volumetry is also used in many patients with extrahippocampal lesions, as coexisting hippocampal atrophy worsens prognosis in extrahippocampal lesional epilepsy and assists in the decision to include hippocampal resection during extrahippocampal surgery.

In extrahippocampal epilepsy, a similar MRI approach is taken and range of sequences applied. Particular attention is taken to re-

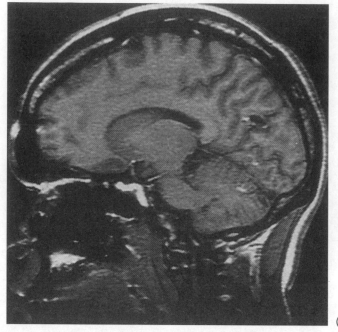

(a)

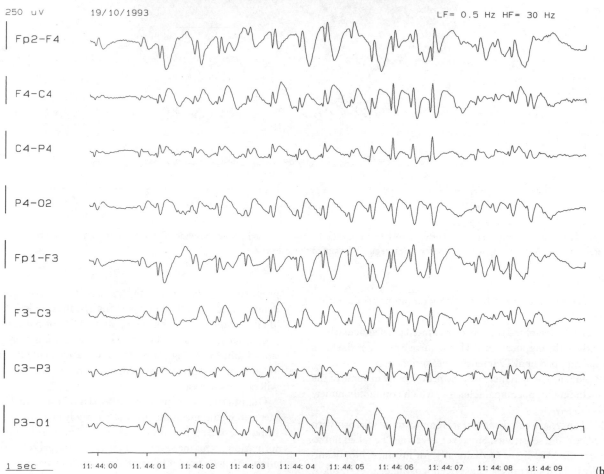

Fig. 51.4 Findings from a patient with a parasagittal pareito-occipital oligodendroglioma (biopsy proven) and brief complex partial seizures comprising eyelid blinking and motor arrest. (a) MRI showing lesion; and (b) EEG showing widespread bilateral slow spike-and-wave discharges.

Table 51.8 Dual pathology: the findings in 100 consecutive patients with MRI-defined hippocampal sclerosis

Coexistent cortical dysgenesis in	15 (15%)
subependymal heterotopia	6
tuberose sclerosis	2
focal macrogyria	2
focal cortical dysplasia	1
band heterotopia	1
schizencephaly	1
other gyral abnormalities	2

Dysgenesis often mild: two of the 15 had a history of childhood febrile convulsions.
Adapted from [45].

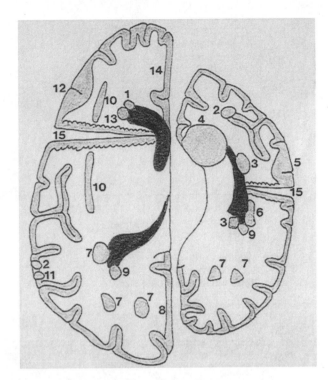

Fig. 51.5 Location of areas of cortical dysgenesis in 15 patients with dual pathology from a series of 100 patients with hippocampal sclerosis (from [45]).

formatting the T1-weighted sequences to provide better lesional definition. This is discussed further in Chapter 55.

A range of other techniques is also used in selected cases, including MR angiography, diffusion imaging, perfusion imaging, MR spectroscopy, fMRI and three-dimensional reconstruction and rendering of the cortical surface, surface area and volume measurements. Each technique assists in addressing specific issues and the interpretation of the tests requires a good understanding of the clinical context. The importance of tailoring the MRI examination to address specific questions cannot be overemphasized, and in this sense MRI differs from CT. Coregistration of MRI and other investigatory modalities (such as EEG, angiography, fMRI, SPECT or PET) is used in complex cases to add localization of abnormal findings and to aid surgical planning.

Other imaging modalities

CT has a limited role in detecting small calcified lesions (for instance in cysticercosis, small low-grade tumours) which are overlooked on MRI, and where MRI is contraindicated (e.g. patients with pacemakers, intracranial metal, etc.). CT cannot detect hippocampal atrophy nor many cases of cortical dysgenesis. Plain skull radiography is now largely redundant. Angiography is used mainly to determine the anatomical features of blood supply to vascular malformations and also prior to depth electrode placement, where angiographic findings can be coregistered with other neuroimaging techniques to guide electrode positioning. MRI angiography is likely to replace invasive angiography in these roles over the next few years.

Neuropsychological assessment

Psychometric assessment is mandatory in all patients being investigated with a view to temporal lobe surgery. The assessment should include tests of general intellectual ability, language and memory. These are vital components of the presurgical work-up for several reasons.

1 To identify dysfunctioning cortex. In temporal lobe epilepsy, if the findings are discordant from those of imaging and neurophysiology, the epileptogenic zone is likely to extend beyond the damaged hippocampus and the outcome of surgery will be generally unfavourable. The verbal and non-verbal memory tests have proved to be reliable lateralizing signs. A discrepancy between verbal and performance IQ indicates lateralized dysfunction and this should be concordant with the side of the hippocampal sclerosis. Verbal memory deficits indicate dominant temporal lobe dysfunction and non-verbal deficits non-dominant dysfunction. Discordant findings on memory tests suggest either that other tests are falsely lateralized or that there is bilateral hippocampal disease. Also, in general an overall IQ below 70 usually indicates widespread cerebral dysfunction and is a relative contraindication to surgery.

2 To assess the risk of amnesia as a consequence of temporal lobe resection. The better the preoperative verbal memory, the worse will be the memory outcome following dominant temporal lobectomy. Conversely, a poor verbal memory seldom is significantly worse after surgery, as it implies that hippocampal memory function is already damaged by the hippocampal sclerosis. A similar, but less striking, pattern is encountered in regard to non-verbal memory and the non-dominant temporal lobe. Generally, non-verbal memory deficits are less troublesome and disabling than verbal memory deficits. Bilateral hippocampal dysfunction should be suspected if both verbal and non-verbal memory tests are affected. If temporal lobectomy is planned in the presence of contralateral hippocampal memory dysfunction, the risk of severe postoperative memory disturbance is greatly increased.

3 To determine which hemisphere is dominant, where this is in doubt. In a proportion of patients with epilepsy, dominance is bilateral.

In focal extratemporal epilepsy, the neuropsychological assessment needs to be tailored according to the brain region under consideration for resection. Speech, visual and higher cognitive

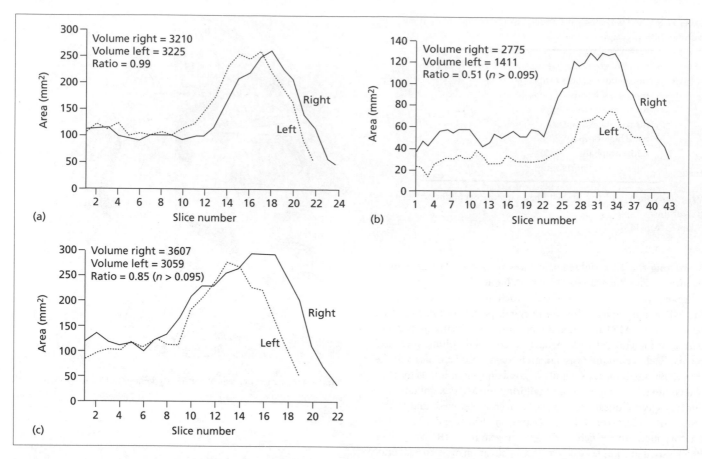

Fig. 51.6 Three graphs showing regional hippocampal volume. In the graphs, the cross-sectional areas of the hippocampus are measured from successive slices of volumetric T1-weighted coronal MRI images of the hippocampus covering the whole anterior to posterior extent of the hippocampus and amygdala. The MRI slices are spaced 1.5 mm apart. (a) Normal hippocampus. (b) Gross generalized hippocampal atrophy. (c) Focal anterior hippocampal atrophy.

functions will need to be documented and mapped to resection in eloquent cortex, and the patient counselled about the risks of surgery to cortical function. Details of the psychometric tools used in presurgical assessment are given in Chapter 58.

Sodium amytal test (Wada test)

This is required if dominance is uncertain or if there appears on routine psychological testing to be an unexpected or significant risk to memory, either because the hippocampal disease is bilateral or wrongly lateralized. About 30% of cases of temporal lobe epilepsy passing through the epilepsy surgical programme at the National Hospital, for instance, require a Wada test. The sodium amytal test though is not infallible and a favourable amytal test is not an absolute guarantee of postoperative freedom from memory impairment.

Intracranial EEG

In some centres, intracranial EEG recordings are frequently used to identify the epileptic focus (see Chapter 53). Various techniques are used, most commonly intracerebral multicontact depth electrodes and subdural grid and strip electrodes. With the advent of MRI,

however, this practice seems now obsolete for the majority of patients. At the National Hospital, for instance, chronic intracranial monitoring is used in only about 5–10% of all cases proceeding to epilepsy surgery. Depth EEG records from otherwise functionally inaccessible cortex, but it should not be forgotten that the EEG data comes from only small areas of brain (a < 1 cm core), and unless the electrodes are placed logically to address specific questions, negative results can be misleading. Grid and strip electrodes cover larger areas than depth electrodes but localization is less precise.

In the National Hospital protocols, invasive intracranial EEG is used to answer the following questions in the work-up for hippocampal surgery:
1 To determine from which temporal lobe seizures are arising in patients with MRI, neuropsychological or other evidence of bilateral hippocampal sclerosis.
2 To determine whether or not seizures are arising from the temporal lobe in patients in whom imaging shows dual pathology and the scalp EEG is indeterminate.
3 To localize the seizure discharge in patients with discordant MRI and functional data.

Electrodes are usually placed bitemporally and in other sites as determined by the questions being addressed. There is a 1–2% risk of haemorrhage or infection from each electrode placement, and the overall risk of the procedure increases with the number of electrodes inserted. There is no place for insertion of multiple electrodes without a prior idea about the most likely sites of seizure onset.

In most patients with neocortical extratemporal focal lesions detected by MRI, the additional information gathered by ictal scalp EEG and video recording will be sufficient to allow a decision about surgery to be made without the need for invasive monitoring. However, in a minority of cases of extratemporal epilepsies, invasive EEG using either subdural strips or grids or depth electrodes is needed to address the following questions:

1 To define the position and extent of the irritative cortex (cortex with spike discharges) in relation to an identified causative lesion.

2 To localize epileptic disturbances in patients who have a normal MRI despite the application of advanced MRI methods, and who have evidence of focal disturbance from clinical, prior electrographic or functional imaging investigation.

3 To localize epileptic disturbances in patients with discordant data from other test modalities. In this sense, the intracranial EEG is intended to provide gold standard information, but nevertheless prognosis is generally less good than in concordant cases even if the depth EEG identifies well-defined focal epileptic discharges.

4 To define the boundaries of the epileptogenic zone in relation to eloquent cortex.

Chronic recording using intracranial electrodes is always carried out in conjunction with video telemetry, typically for 1–2 weeks, to ensure that a good number of seizures are recorded. Brain stimulation is also occasionally undertaken during chronic depth recording.

Peroperative ECoG can assist the surgeon in deciding the extent of the resection, although the relative value of all these techniques is controversial. For instance, while the complete resection of all spiking areas identified at corticography does not always succeed in stopping seizures, nor does incomplete resection always fail.

Cortical mapping has an essential role in resections in eloquent areas of the brain, to assess the surgical risks to normal cortical function and thus to plan the extent of the surgical resection. The lesions which cause epilepsy often distort normal cerebral functional anatomy, which only careful mapping can demonstrate. Mapping is usually carried out preoperatively using chronically implanted subdural grids, or acutely at operation in an awake patient, using cortical stimulation or by recording evoked potentials. Preoperative functional mapping by fMRI is in a stage of rapid development and has replaced invasive mapping in some situations.

Foramen ovale electrode placement, in which the electrode tip is inserted through the foramen ovale to lie medial to the hippocampus, is a form of extracerebral intracranial electrode placement. It is a straightforward technique and does not require a craniotomy or stereotactic equipment, but has a significant complication rate, including facial pain, meningitis and vascular damage to the brainstem. It is not used at the National Hospital, and there is a diminishing place for this technique in modern practice.

Functional imaging (PET, SPECT or fMRI)

The usage of HMPAO-SPECT and FDG-PET varies greatly in different centres. Financial and logistical considerations seem influential in determining local patterns, and no consensus about their role has yet been reached. In the author's view, there is little convincing evidence to support their routine use in straightforward cases.

Both techniques have a more important role in extratemporal epilepsy (lesional or not) than in temporal lobe epilepsy. Their use is mainly in demonstrating large areas of dysfunction thus excluding surgery rather than assisting in precise surgical planning. The techniques are relatively crude as tools for localization, and usually detailed EEG or MRI are needed to provide more definitive data. In some centres, SPECT is also commonly used as a method of lateralizing seizure foci in temporal lobe epilepsy. The interictal SPECT shows a decreased tracer uptake in the relevant temporal lobe and the ictal SPECT an increased tracer uptake. However, usually both MRI and EEG provide similar information (and are more specific and sensitive). Little new information is gained and the number of cases who require this test as part of a surgical work-up at the National Hospital is small.

Other functional imaging techniques are currently in research development, and include MR spectroscopy, ligand- or receptor-based PET, optical imaging and coregistered fMRI and EEG (physiological imaging). Exactly what their role will prove to be in routine practice is uncertain, although PET scanning with flumazenil has recently been shown to be useful in identifying electrographic foci in MRI-negative cases. SPECT can be coregistered with MRI (e.g. in the SISCOM system) and the combined images are routinely used in some centres. MEG is another modality of investigation, currently in the experimental phase, which provides data for electrographic localization that is potentially superior to that from EEG, especially for deeply placed foci. The various functional techniques are described in Chapters 54, 56 and 57.

Counselling

During presurgical assessment, all patients are counselled in detail about the medical and psychosocial aspects of epilepsy and epilepsy surgery. The patients are encouraged to discuss all their concerns, and not uncommonly counselling will reveal issues which have a major impact on surgical decision making. Counselling also identifies issues for postoperative rehabilitation. At the end of the presurgical assessment, patients are also counselled in detail about the perceived risks and benefits of the surgical options.

Organizational aspects of an epilepsy surgery programme

The surgical planning meeting

It will be clear from the above that presurgical assessment involves input from diverse disciplines and sources. Effective coordination is key, and at the National Hospital, as at all other major epilepsy surgery centres, weekly epilepsy surgery planning meetings are held. At these meetings, the investigations of all patients undergoing presurgical assessment during the current week are reviewed. The meetings are attended by the neurologists, neurosurgeons, neurophysiologists, neuroradiologists, neuropsychiatrists, neuropsychologists, EEG technicians, epilepsy nurses and counsellors. The patient's history is outlined. The results of investigations are given, and the seizure recordings on video-EEG telemetry and MRI scans displayed. An ensuing discussion is then held and decisions made about further investigation or surgical approach. Estimates (in percentage terms) are made about the potential risks of surgery and the seizure outcome. Special risks, for instance in terms of psychological or psychiatric disability, are identified. The salient points from the meetings are recorded and minuted and these minutes form the basis of a letter that is written by the supervising consultant to the referring doctor summarizing the findings. The conclusions reached are then discussed in a subsequent meeting between the supervising neurologist and the patient. The categories included in a typical written summary are shown in Table 51.9.

There are a number of important benefits to regular meetings. The quality of patient care is greatly enhanced. Every patient presents specific problems and the multidisciplinary approach ensures that therapy is tailored to individual needs. The standard format ensures efficiency, thoroughness and avoids errors of omission. The multidisciplinary input allows discussion of points which might not be covered in written reports. The meetings provide an efficient forum for gathering opinions from colleagues. The meetings also have a significant team-building function and improve communcation between team members. They are the focus for education and training activities in epilepsy (for both medical and allied health professionals). Regular timetabling is a good way to ensure adequate attendance. A typical case will require 15 min of discussion, and complex cases will often be discussed repeatedly over a period of weeks or months as investigations progress.

Such meetings should be at the core of all epilepsy programmes, and are an integral part of the presurgical assessment process.

Epilepsy surgery centres

It has been proposed that there should be two levels of epilepsy surgery centre: basic epilepsy surgery centres (level 1) and reference epilepsy surgery centres (level 2). Both should be sited within a comprehensive neuroscience centre with access to all the specialties listed above. The basic centre should have a throughput of at least 25 operated cases/year, a bed occupancy of at least 700 patient-days and facilities should include advanced MRI, amytal testing and video-EEG telemetry. The reference epilepsy surgery centres should have a throughput of 50–100 operated cases and bed occupancy potential of between 30 and 70 days per patient, and ancillary operative facilities including electrocorticography, cerebral functional mapping and evoked potential studies. An illustrative example of the differentiation of facilities is shown in Table 51.10. In the age of clinical governance and audit, it is inevitable as well as desirable that epilepsy surgery services are organized in a formal and regulated fashion. However, the demarcation which is made will differ from country to country and from centre to centre, and depends as much on the enthusiasms of individuals as on the health-care systems within which they work. The level 1 centres should be able to provide surgical therapy for at least two-thirds of the patients referred—and carry out standard lesional resective operations (including anterior temporal lobectomy). Each level 2 centre should have formal links to several level 1 centres for on-ward referral of complex cases. The range of facilities required in level 2 centres will be greater, especially in relation to functional and invasive investigation. As emphasized above, there is wide regional variation in the testing facilities utilized and the investigatory protocols followed; this is unsatisfactory, and level 2 centres should be in a position to provide both health technology assessment and health service research evidence to support their higher level provision.

Postoperative care

Postoperative counselling and rehabilitation

Prior to surgery, detailed counselling on the risks of surgery as well as its potential benefits is mandatory. After successful surgery, most patients experience the need for a major readjustment to a life without epilepsy. This can be difficult and painful, as is the realization that the problems in life are not automatically resolved. There is

Table 51.9 Categories covered in a typical written summary of an epilepsy surgery management meeting

Demographic data (age, gender, identifiers, contact details)
Handedness
Epilepsy history (observable seizure phenomena, aura, seizure manifestations experienced by the patient, seizure precipitants, temporal evolution of the seizures, postictal features, epilepsy onset and pattern over time, response to therapy, aetiology, seizure frequency and timing, family history, previous investigations and results)
Examination—summary findings (including preoperative neurological deficit and visual fields)
MRI—summary findings (including quantitative hippocampal volumetric and T2 signal intensity readings)
Interictal scalp EEG—summary findings (current and past) and frequency and focal distribution of spike discharges
Ictal clinical phenomenology and EEG—summary findings from video telemetry
Neuropsychological test—summary findings (full-scale IQ, VIQ, PIQ)
Sodium amytal test—summary findings
Specialized MRI and other neuroimaging—summary findings
Invasive EEG—summary findings
Functional imaging (PET, SPECT)—summary findings
Neuropsychiatric assessment—summary findings
Psychosocial and counselling—summary findings
Summary—seizure classification, epilepsy classification, aetiology, other medical or psychosocial issues
Conclusions—surgical options, estimate of percentage chance of seizure freedom (or in selected cases percentage chance of improvement), estimate of percentage chance of adverse outcomes (specified), other issues of importance for postoperative rehabilitation
Actions re: place on surgical waiting list and schedule, patient follow-up and counselling, further investigation

Table 51.10 The characteristics of level 1 and level 2 epilepsy centres

	Level 1 centre	Level 2 centre
Patients	Adults (and children in centres with paediatric facilities)	Adults, children and infants (in centres with paediatric facilities).
Types of surgery	Anterior temporal lobectomy, lesionectomy	All types of temporal lobe surgery, all types of lesional resections, hemispherectomy, callosotomy, non-lesional surgery, functional surgery, awake craniotomy
General facilities	Full range of general neurological and neurosurgical inpatient and outpatient facilities, and neurosurgical ITU	As for level 1 centre
MRI facilities	1.5 Tesla MRI with facilities for thin slice volumetric imaging	As for level 1 centres with additional facilities for a range of techniques which could include: MRS, volume quantitation, T2 relaxometry, 3D reconstruction, co-registration, fMRI and fMRI-EEG
Other neuroimaging facilities	CT	CT Also a range of other functional imaging facilities which could include: FDG PET, PET with other ligands, SPECT, SISCOM, or MEG
Neuropsychological facilities	Routine neuropsychology Facility for Wada testing	As for level 1 centre with additional facilities which could include fMRI
EEG facilities	Routine scalp EEG Scalp video telemetry	Routine scalp EEG, scalp video telemetry, and a range of invasive EEG facilities which might include: depth, subdural strips and grids, extradural EEG, foramen ovale recordings, chronic recording with intracranial stimulation
Intraoperative EEG	Corticography	Corticography and preoperative stimulation
Other investigations	Angiography	Angiography TMS
Staffing (with specialized training and experience in epilepsy; and also paediatrical training for those treating childhood epilepsy)	Neurologist, neurosurgeon, clinical neurophysiologist, neuroradiologist, neuropsychiatrist, neuropsychologist, intensive nurse specialists, counsellors, EEG technicians	As for a level 1 centre, but staff require more specialized experience in the greater range of presurgical assessment tools and surgical procedures
Audit	A full audit of surgical volume and results should be available	As for level 1 centres, with evaluative data on additional facilities

Table 51.11 Follow-up protocol for patients without complications after successful temporal lobe epilepsy surgery

Neurosurgical follow-up	6 weeks, 1 year and then annually
Neurological follow-up	3, 6, 9, 12 months then annually
Psychiatry	1 month, 6 months, 12 months and then annually
Psychology	3, 12 months
Field testing	6 months
MRI	3 months
Counsellor	3, 12 months

This is based on the protocol used at the National Hospital for Neurology and Neurosurgery, London. Adapted from [46].

often a sense of anticlimax, at least in the first 12 months following the operation. Furthermore, if the operation fails, disappointment and depression are almost inevitable. Seizure freedom will not immediately reverse years of social isolation, a lack of self confidence or a strong sense of identity, missed educational or career opportunities. Becoming seizure free can alter interpersonal relationships, which might have been based on dependency or a sickness role. Appropriate preoperative counselling can help prepare people, and in some instances a structured postoperative rehabilitation programme can be helpful.

Postoperative follow-up

A minimum follow-up protocol is needed for all patients who have undergone epilepsy surgery. This should be orchestrated by the supervising consultant neurologist, and the typical protocol adopted at the National Hospital for patients rendered seizure free is as shown in Table 51.11. Of course, additional follow-up is needed for patients in whom surgery was not successful or those in whom complications have arisen.

References

1 Shorvon SD, Sander JWAS. The treatment of epilepsy at the National Hospital Queen Square, 1857–1939: a mirror of the first phase of the modern history of medical and surgical therapy. In: Shorvon SD, Dreifuss F, Fish D, Thomas D, eds. *The Treatment of Epilepsy*. Oxford: Blackwell Science, 1996: xvii–xliv.

2 Paget S. *Sir Victor Horsley*. London: Baillière, Tindall and Cox, 1919.

3 Horsley V. Brain surgery. *Br Med J* 1886; 2: 670–5.

4 Andriezen WL. On some of the newer aspects of the pathology of insanity. *Brain* 1894; 18: 548–692.

5 Turner WA. *Epilepsy – a Study of the Idiopathic Disease*. London: Macmillan, 1907.

6 Penfield W, Flanigin H. Surgical therapy of temporal lobe seizures. *Arch Neurol Psychiatr* 1950; 4: 491–500.

7 Feindel W. Towards a surgical cure for epilepsy. The work of Wilder Penfield and his school at the Montreal Neurological Institute. In: Engel J, ed. *Surgical Treatment of the Epilepsies*, 2nd edn. New York: Raven Press, 1993: 1–9.

8 Engel J. Principles of epilepsy surgery. In: Shorvon SD, Dreifuss F, Fish D, Thomas D, eds. *The Treatment of Epilepsy*. Oxford: Blackwell Science, 1996: 519–29.

9 Tailarach J, David M, Tournoux P *et al. Atlas d'Anatomie Stéréotaxique des Noyaux Gris Centraux*. Paris: Masson & Cie, 1957.

10 Bancaud J, Talairach J, Bonis A *et al. La Stéréoélectroencéphalographie dans l'Epilepsie: informations neurophysiopathologiques apportées par l'investigation fonctionnelle stéréotaxique*. Paris: Masson & Cie, 1965.

11 Chauvel P. Contributions of Jean Talairach and Jean Bancaud to epilepsy surgery. In: Luders H, Comair Y, eds. *Epilepsy Surgery*, 2nd edn. Philadelphia: Lippincott, Williams and Wilkins, 2001: 35–41.

12 Gloor P. General introduction. In: Gotman J, Ives JR, Gloor P, eds. *Long-term Monitoring in Epilepsy. Electroenceph Clin Neurophysiol* 1985 (Suppl. 37): xiii–xx.

13 Fish DR, Gloor P, Quesney LF, Olivier A. Clinical responses to electrical brain stimulation of the temporal and frontal lobes in patients with epilepsy: pathophysiological implications. *Brain* 1993; 116: 397–414.

14 Shorvon SD. Imaging in the investigation of epilepsy. In: Hopkins A, ed. *Epilepsy*. London: Chapman and Hall, 1987: 201–28.

15 Li LM, Fish DR, Sisodiya SM, Shorvon SD, Alsanjari N, Stevens JM. High resolution magnetic resonance imaging scanning in adults with partial or secondarily generalised epilepsy attending a tertiary referral unit *J Neurol Neurosurg Psychiat* 1995; 59: 384–7.

16 Shorvon SD, Fish DR, Andermann F, Bydder GM, Stefan H. *Magnetic Resonance Scanning and Epilepsy*. Nato ASI Series A. *Life Sciences*, Vol. 264. New York: Plenum Press, 1994.

17 Sperling M, Wilson C, Engel J. Magnetic resonance imaging in intractable partial epilepsy: correlative studies. *Ann Neurol* 1986; 20: 57–62.

18 Fandino J, Wieser H-G. Contributions of Hugo Kravenbuhl and M. Gazi Yasargil to epilepsy surgery. In: Luders H, Comair Y, eds. *Epilepsy Surgery*, 2nd edn. Philadelphia: Lippincott, Williams and Wilkins, 2001: 43–53.

19 Niemeyer P. The transventricular amygdalohippocampectomy in temporal lobe epilepsy. In: Baldwin M, Bailey P, eds. *Temporal Lobe Epilepsy*. Springfield: CC Thomas, 1958: 461–82.

20 Kratimenos GP, Pell MF, Thomas DGT, Shorvon SD, Fish DR, Smith SJN. Open selective amygdalohippocampectomy for drug resistant epilepsy. *Acta Neurochir* 1992; 116: 150–4.

21 Kelly PJ, Sharbrough FW, Kall BA *et al.* Magnetic resonance imaging-based computer-assisted stereotactic resection of the hippocampus and amygdala in patients with temporal lobe epilepsy. *Mayo Clin Proc* 1987; 62: 103–8.

22 Spencer DD, Spencer SS, Mattson RH, Williamson PD, Novelly RA. Access to the posterior medial structures in the surgical treatment of temporal lobe epilepsy. *Neurosurgery* 1984; 15: 667–71.

23 Olivier A. Surgery of mesial temporal epilepsy. In: Shorvon SD, Dreifuss F, Fish D, Thomas D, eds. *The Treatment of Epilepsy*. Oxford: Blackwell Science, 1996: 689–98.

24 Van Wagenen WP, Herren RY. Surgical division of the commissural pathways in the corpus callosum: relation to spread of an epileptic attack. *Arch Neurol Psychiatr* 1940; 44: 740–59.

25 Krynauw RA. Infantile hemiplegia treated by removing one cerebral hemisphere. *J Neurol Neurosurg Psychiatr* 1950; 13: 243–67.

26 White HH. Cerebral hemispherectomy in the treatment of infantile hemiplegia: Review of the literature and report of two cases. *Confin Neurol* 1961; 21: 1–50.

27 Adams CBT. Hemispherectomy: a modification. *J Neurol Neurosurg Psychiatr* 1983; 46: 617–19.

28 Rasmussen T. Hemispherectomy for seizures revisited. *Can J Neurol Sci* 1983; 10: 7.

29 Delalande O, Pinard JM, Basdevant C, Gauthe M, Plouin P, Dulac O. Hemispherotomy: a new procedure for central disconnection. *Epilepsia* 1992; 33 (Suppl. 3): 99–100.

30 Hoffman HJ, Hendrick EB, Dennis M, Armstrong D. Hemispherectomy for Sturge–Weber syndrome. *Childs Brain* 1979; 5: 233–48.

31 Villemure JG, Mascott CR. Peri-insular hemispherotomy: surgical principles and anatomy. *Neurosurgery* 1995; 37: 975–81.

32 Billings JF. The surgical treatment of epilepsy. *Qincinnati Lancet Observer* 1861; 4: 334–41.

33 Gowers WA. *Epilepsy and Other Chronic Convulsive Disorders: Their Causes, Symptoms and Treatment*, 2nd edn. London: Churchill, 1901.

34 Wilson SA. *Neurology*, Vol. 1. London: Edward Arnold, 1940.

35 Lhatoo SD, Solomon JK, McEvoy A, Kitchen ND, Shorvon SD, Sander JW. A prospective study of the requirement for and the provision of epilepsy surgery in the United Kingdom. *Epilepsia* 2003; 44: 673–6.

36 Engel J, ed. *Surgical Treatment of the Epilepsies*. New York: Raven Press, 1987.

37 Engel J, ed. *Surgical Treatment of the Epilepsies*, 2nd edn. New York: Raven Press, 1993.

38 Shorvon SD. The temporal aspects of prognosis in epilepsy. *J Neurol Neurosurg Psychiatr* 1984; 47: 1157–65.

39 Cockerell OC, Johnson AL, Sander JWAS, Shorvon SD. Prognosis of epilepsy: further analysis of the first nine years of the British National General Practice Study of Epilepsy, a prospective population based study. *Epilepsia* 1997; 38: 31–46.

40 Lhatoo SD, Sander JW, Shorvon SD. The dynamics of drug treatment in epilepsy: an observational study in an unselected population based cohort with newly diagnosed epilepsy followed up prospectively over 11–14 years. *J Neurol Neurosurg Psychiatr* 2001; 71: 632–7.

41 Gloor P. *The Temporal Lobe and Limbic System*. Oxford: Oxford University Press, 1997.

42 Luders H, Comair Y, eds. *Epilepsy Surgery*, 2nd edn. Philadelphia: Lippincott, Williams and Wilkins, 2001.

43 Moran NF, Lemieux L, Kitchen ND, Fish DR, Shorvon SD. Extrahippocampal temporal lobe atrophy in temporal lobe epilepsy and mesial temporal sclerosis. *Brain* 2001; 124: 167–75.

44 Engel J Jr, Shewmon DA. Overview: who should be considered a surgical candidate? In: Engel J Jr, ed. *Surgical Treatment of the Epilepsies*, 2nd edn. New York: Raven Press, 1993: 23–4.

45 Raymond AA, Fish DR, Sisodiya S, Alsanjari M, Stevens J, Shorvon SD. Association of hippocampal sclerosis with cortical dysgenesis in patients with epilepsy. *Neurology* 1994; 44: 1841–4.

46 Duncan J, Fish DR, Shorvon SD. *Clinical Epilepsy*. Edinburgh: Churchill Livingstone, 1995.

52 The Scalp EEG in Presurgical Evaluation of Epilepsy

D.R. Fish

Since its development in the late 1920s, the EEG has become established as a robust clinical test in epilepsy. It is one of the few medical investigations which has remained useful over many decades, providing unique evidence of epileptogenicity that cannot be matched by structural or other currently available functional imaging techniques. As such, it has a central role in the presurgical evaluation of patients with medically intractable epilepsy. However, its contemporary role must be continually revised in view of the evolution of alternative investigative modalities. Until the early 1990s, the lack of preoperative information concerning the underlying structural basis for the individual patient's seizure disorder forced the clinician to work backwards on the basis of the clinical history, neurological and psychological features and EEG parameters in order to try and predict this substrate prior to surgery [1]. The advent of high-resolution MRI, which provided clinicians with the ability to detect the underlying structural abnormality in most patients prior to surgery (see Chapter 55), redefined this paradigm. Far from removing the need for the EEG, this structural information has allowed the clinician to utilize the EEG in a more productive manner, appropriate to the information that it can best provide. In this setting the EEG can confirm the clinical diagnosis of epilepsy, and syndromic classification, and may demonstrate that an identified lesion is associated with an area of epileptogenesis rather than being a coincidental finding. In consequence of this major shift during the early 1990s, earlier studies on scalp EEG patterns in patients being evaluated for epilepsy surgery (e.g. [2–13]) provided useful background information, but do not define optimum current usage. High-resolution MRI studies may divide patients presurgically into the following categories: hippocampal sclerosis, focal structural lesions (e.g. indolent glioma, cavernoma), multiple pathology (e.g. concurrent hippocampal sclerosis and malformations of cortical development, multiple angiomas), specific structural pathologies that are often more diffuse or multifocal, including malformations of cortical development or post-traumatic changes, and MRI-negative cases (Fig. 52.1). Some of these categories may be amenable to further subdivision, particularly hippocampal sclerosis which may be unilateral or bilateral and diffuse or focal, and may occur either in isolation or in association with other cerebral abnormalities. Also, there are many subtypes of cortical maldevelopment. It is increasingly evident that information from MR is a major predictor of postoperative outcome [14,15].

Over the last decade there has been increasing sophistication of structural MRI techniques as well as enhanced application of functional imaging techniques to the problems of presurgical evaluation. The latter include PET (metabolism, blood flow and ligand studies), interictal and ictal SPECT and fMRI. This changing and evolving context reduces the possibility of large multivariate prospective studies to determine a set of optimum or most efficient pathways for individual patient presurgical assessments but there is increasing interest in specific issues relating to scalp interictal/ictal EEG recordings (e.g. [15–24]).

The use of the EEG in individual cases must also take account of the likely surgical options. For example, in a patient with isolated unilateral hippocampal sclerosis on structural imaging, different electrographic information may be required, depending on whether the patient is being evaluated for an amygdalohippocampectomy or a standard *en bloc* temporal lobectomy. The role of the EEG in different pathologies will also be influenced by the site of the abnormality (e.g. temporal, frontal, central, parietal occipital) and its relationship to eloquent structures that may influence the surgical technique.

Technical considerations—scalp electrodes

The standard 10–20 electrode system of scalp electrode placement unfortunately does not cover the anterior temporal region. In consequence, several investigators developed recording techniques using indwelling electrodes, introduced through the cheek, with the recording tip lying in the region superficial to the foramen ovale (sphenoidal electrodes) (e.g. [25–28]) or, subsequently, minisphenoidals inserted to a shorter distance [29]. The use of sphenoidal electrodes has become standard practice at most epilepsy surgery centres. However, little work has been done on their evaluation and comparisons were often made with the standard 10–20 electrode positions rather than other more useful extracranial sites. Subsequently, several authors have shown that indwelling sphenoidal electrodes offer little if any benefit over suitably placed skin electrodes covering the same region, i.e. placed over the anterior temporal region (e.g. [30,31]). Binnie *et al.* [32] studied 111 patients with epilepsy evaluated with sphenoidal EEG recordings, using additional anterior temporal superficial electrodes. In 17 patients a superficial electrode recorded all discharges seen at the sphenoidal and, out of 165 epileptic foci, in only two instances were less than 90% of sphenoidal discharges recognized at the surface. Goodin *et al.* [33] confirmed the very low rate of additional pick-up of interictal spikes using sphenoidal electrodes. In their study, 70% of spikes were detected using an anterior temporal electrode (T1 or T2) placed 1 cm above and one-third the distance along the line from the external auditory meatus to the external canthus of the eye. In the study of Binnie *et al.* [32], a multipolar sphenoidal electrode was used in six patients and this showed a shallow potential gradient between the standard sphenoidal site and the surface; in other words, while spike amplitudes may appear larger with indwelling sphenoidal electrodes, the spikes usually remain of sufficient amplitude

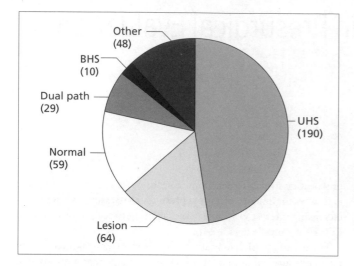

Fig. 52.1 Relative frequency of different structural abnormalities identified by high-resolution MRI in 400 consecutive patients referred for presurgical video-EEG scalp telemetry at a specialist epilepsy centre [24]. BHS, bilateral hippocampal sclerosis; UHS, unilateral hippocampal sclerosis.

to be seen at the surface. Few data are available on the potential benefit of indwelling sphenoidal or minisphenoidal electrodes during ictal recordings. Wilkus *et al.* [34] were able to demonstrate slightly earlier detection of the seizure onset using sphenoidal electrodes as opposed to surface electrodes, but this remains of questionable clinical significance in scalp recordings of temporal lobe seizures as the localized changes, such as rhythmic temporal theta, usually take more than 10 s to become apparent. There is always the possibility that occasional patients may have brief but low-amplitude ictal electrographic activity of a sufficiently small potential to be detected with an indwelling sphenoidal electrode but missed at the surface. Such cases would appear to be extremely rare. Given the discomfort of indwelling sphenoidal electrodes and their potential, albeit small, for complications and for degradation during the course of studies due to repetitive movement, there are insufficient data to support their routine use in presurgical evaluation. Similar considerations have led to the (earlier) widespread discontinuation of nasopharyngeal or other such electrodes [35–37].

The use of additional scalp electrodes interspaced between the 10–20 electrode system of contacts over the scalp convexity may refine the description of specific EEG potentials [8]. However, physical constraints limit the number of additional electrodes that can be applied. The additional information derived may be of research interest regarding the generators of cortical potentials but is unlikely to reveal new information concerning deeply placed epileptogenic foci, because the EEG recorded using scalp electrodes reflects electrical changes in the superficial neocortex. There is only a minimal contribution from deep generators. Alarcon *et al.* [38] studied 12 patients with simultaneous mesial temporal recordings and surface electrodes. The ratio of deep to surface activity during interictal epileptiform spikes was of the order of 1:2000. The authors concluded that most of the electrical activity recorded on the scalp does not represent volume conduction from deep structures but rather propagation of activity with activation of relatively large areas of

neocortex. This finding is of importance because it demonstrates the physiological inappropriateness of attempts to derive deep-seated dipole analogues to scalp EEG recorded potentials.

Types of scalp EEG recording

Routine scalp interictal records during wakefulness reveal interictal epileptiform discharges in approximately 40–50% of patients with epilepsy. This figure rises to approximately 70–80% if daytime sleep is induced [39–41], although care is needed to exclude non-specific EEG patterns mimicking epileptic activity [42]. However, reliability of interictal EEG localization may be affected by the sleep state. Sammaritano *et al.* [43] demonstrated that interictal spikes recorded during wakefulness and REM sleep showed a significantly better concordance with the eventual electroclinical localization than spikes recorded during non-REM sleep; in other words, the additional pick-up rate of spiking during non-REM sleep may be at the expense of reduced specificity. The potential for interictal spiking to be bilateral and independent or multifocal, even in cases in whom there is a surgically resectable discrete pathology (hippocampal sclerosis or foreign-tissue lesion), makes it essential that such findings are not used to preclude a patient with medically intractable epilepsy from undergoing high-resolution MRI as part of the presurgical evaluation. Notwithstanding these concerns, well-localized stereotyped interictal spikes have been shown repeatedly to be a strong predictor of a good outcome from epilepsy surgery (e.g. [19,44–46]).

Most epilepsy surgery centres include dedicated video-EEG monitoring services, providing simultaneous recording of the EEG and clinical behaviour during seizures as part of their routine assessment to help localize the epileptogenic zone, assess the possibility of additional non-epileptic attacks and/or facilitate peri-ictal SPECT recordings [47]. Various commercial and inhouse developed systems are available, with processing techniques to reduce the volume of data for visual analysis by the electroencephalographer [48,49]. The use of digital recording techniques offers a significant advantage by allowing remontaging and refiltering to be performed on the EEG previously acquired during seizures, thereby reducing the number of ictal electrographic events that may need to be recorded. The possibility that scalp EEG may predict seizure occurrence by many minutes also raises the possibility of using this test to identify crucial periods for other studies [50]. Ambulatory cassette recordings have been used to a lesser extent in presurgical assessment due to the limited number of recording channels and the usual lack of video but may be effective for a subset of patients who can be evaluated on an outpatient basis [51]. The advent of 16 (or more) channel recorders may overcome some of these problems and allow their use in patients with well-established clinical seizure patterns in whom other data are strongly concordant, particularly when combined with handheld or other mobile ictal video recordings. In selected patients with frequent seizures, in whom antiepileptic drug reduction is not necessary and who have ready outpatient access, it may be worthwhile using repeated periods of outpatient recordings rather than inpatient facilities [52].

It is also important to consider whether these interictal studies can effectively 'screen out' patients unlikely to benefit from expensive inpatient video EEG telemetry (which may also reduce false raising of hopes or delays in exploring other non-surgical therapies). DellaBadia *et al.* [53] studied the predictive value of interictal sleep-deprived EEG, MRI and PET, prior to comprehensive evaluation, in a total of 69 patients, 35 of whom eventually were accepted for epilepsy surgery. When all three tests were 'negative' only one of 13 patients (7.7%) eventually proceeded to surgery. Any two positive tests together had a high predictive value of proceeding to surgery (77–83%). Detailed analysis of the cost–benefit ratio indicated that the most financially efficient predictive pair of tests was sleep-deprived EEG and MRI.

Postoperative EEG has been seen as of less important long-term predictive value, possibly because of the confounding effects of the craniotomy [54]. However, Patrick *et al.* [55] have reported that persistent abnormalities at 1 year are associated with a less favourable long-term prognosis.

Seizure activation and drug withdrawal

The use of chemically induced seizures has been discontinued in presurgical assessment because of potential unreliability, i.e. the induction of non-habitual seizure types [56]. In contrast, anticonvulsant drug withdrawal is routinely utilized to facilitate seizure recordings. Several authors have demonstrated that seizure activation is more likely to occur once the anticonvulsant levels become subtherapeutic rather than during the period when the levels are falling [57,58] although drug changes have little direct effect on interictal spike frequency [59,60]. For the most part, it would appear that seizures recorded during acute anticonvulsant withdrawal have a similar clinical symptomatology and electrographic onset to those occurring habitually [57,58]. Occasional patients have been reported in whom it was thought that new foci were revealed by antiepileptic withdrawal (e.g. [61–64]), but the significance of these isolated case reports is uncertain. In practice, concern about ictal electrographic localization in the setting of anticonvulsant withdrawal is largely restricted to seizures which differ clinically from the habitual semiology. There are clear clinical, and medicolegal advantages to the use of standard protocols for antiepileptic drug reduction and restitution during video-EEG monitoring [65], given the risks of injury during seizures, postictal psychosis or sudden unexpected death in epilepsy. Haut *et al.* [66] studied seizure clustering during video-EEG monitoring. Of 91 patients 56 exhibited three or more seizures during monitoring. Particular risk factors in that study were a history of seizure clustering at home, MRI evidence of mesial temporal sclerosis and multiple seizure types. Surprisingly, antiepileptic drug withdrawal was not identified as a risk factor and the seizures recorded during clusters appeared to be as useful in localizing the epileptogenic zone as those that occurred in isolation.

Scalp ictal EEG changes

Ictal scalp EEG changes during partial seizures have been well described (e.g. [2,3,5,6,9,22,67,68]). Simple partial seizures often fail to show any scalp EEG correlates [69,70], presumably because of lack of synchronous involvement of a sufficient area of superficial cortex. In temporal lobe complex partial seizures, there is often widespread attenuation followed by sustained rhythmic activity (Fig. 52.2). Areas of seizure onset that are deeply placed, involve small or convoluted areas of neocortex or are associated with rapid

seizure spread reduce the proportion of extratemporal cases with localized/lateralized scalp ictal EEG changes [6,10,71,72] (see below). Postictal slowing or attenuation of normal rhythms (Fig. 52.3) are usually lateralized to the side of seizure onset. Kaibara and Blume [73] reported concordance in 35/35 patients. Jan *et al.* [74] studied postictal scalp EEG changes in 80 seizures from 29 patients with temporal lobe epilepsy. Lateralized postictal changes were present in 64% of recordings and concordant with the side of eventual surgery in 96%. Occasional patients will, however, have false lateralizing postictal changes, presumably due to shifting side emphasis during the ictus.

Scalp EEG in patients with mesial temporal lobe epilepsy

Hippocampal sclerosis is the commonest pathology in patients undergoing epilepsy surgery. It may be subdivided, on the basis of neuroimaging, into focal or diffuse [75] and unilateral or bilateral [76,77], as well as being isolated or being associated with another pathology, such as cortical maldevelopment, a porencephalic cyst, reactive gliosis or a foreign tissue lesion [78]. There are only limited EEG studies currently available in these MRI defined categories. However, previous studies of scalp and sphenoidal ictal EEG have demonstrated good reliability and accuracy of positive interictal and ictal findings.

Interictal spikes may be unilateral (Fig. 52.2), but bilateral independent spikes are common in temporal lobe epilepsy, even with well-lateralized pathology, in both children and adults [2,79–81]. The degree to which this is observed may depend upon the patient population, aetiological factors, duration of recording and sleep states examined. Although previous studies have considered spike frequency, relative morphology and distribution may influence their significance; further studies are required, especially in light of the potential for neuroimaging to better define the range of patients who can proceed to surgery without ictal recordings (see below).

Risinger *et al.* [9] analysed 706 ictal records from 110 patients who subsequently underwent intracerebral evaluation. They specifically defined the ictal scalp electrographic onset into morphological categories. The presence of a unilateral temporal/sphenoidal rhythmic discharge of 5 Hz or faster within the first 30 s of the ictal recording occurred in 57 patients, and correctly predicted an ipsilateral temporal depth onset in 82% of cases. Other scalp lateralizing features were seen in 27 patients but showed a lower predictive value, while 26 patients showed no lateralizing or localizing features in the scalp ictal recordings. Furthermore, the predictive accuracy of a localized scalp ictal EEG onset at 5 Hz or faster within the first 30 s was increased to 94% when only cases showing this pattern consistently were included.

Walczak *et al.* [82] studied the reliability of ictal scalp and sphenoidal EEG in 138 complex partial seizures (119 temporal and 18 extratemporal) recorded in 35 patients who had subsequently undergone epilepsy surgery and had been seizure free for 2 or more years. Of all temporal lobe seizures, 76–83% were correctly lateralized. However, when seizures showing generalized features or those obscured by artefact were excluded, this figure rose to 93–99%, with excellent interobserver reliability.

Murro *et al.* [83], who studied 50 patients who became seizure free or who had rare seizures following temporal lobectomy,

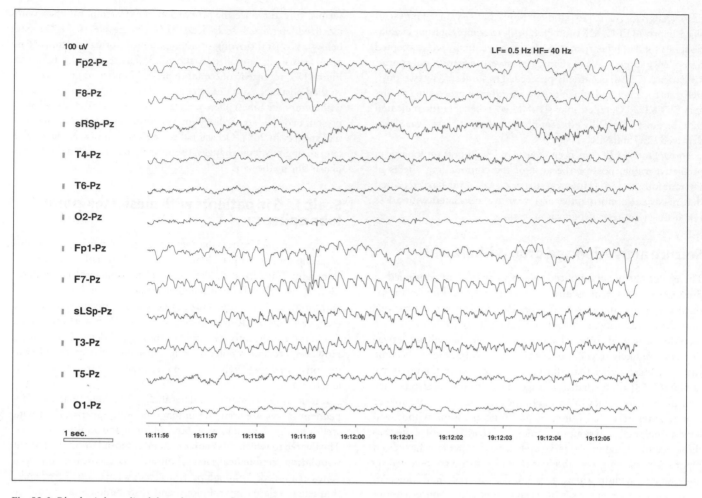

Fig. 52.2 Rhythmic lateralized theta during a temporal lobe seizure in a patient with underlying hippocampal sclerosis.

reported similar findings. Localization from scalp EEG disagreed with the side of eventual surgery in only 2% of cases. While such retrospective studies necessarily suffer from the problems of case selection, they cast doubts on the significance of the previously reported high incidence of false lateralization of ictal scalp EEG [7], possibly because of the recording paradigms or case mix used in the latter study.

Lateralization of scalp ictal video-EEG recordings may be further refined by a study of the clinical seizure semiology: dystonic posturing is usually contralateral, while unilateral automatisms are mainly ipsilateral to the site of onset [84].

Occasional patients (approximately 5%) with temporal lobe epilepsy show additional generalized spike-and-slow-wave discharges. There have only been small surgical case series including such patients. Although some authors have suggested that this may be associated with a less favourable outcome [85–87], this has not been a uniform experience [88–90]. In any case, the presence of such additional neurophysiological abnormalities must necessitate comprehensive ictal EEG assessment prior to surgery and careful exclusion of clinical phenomenology suggestive of an additional primary generalized epilepsy.

Isolated hippocampal sclerosis

In 50 patients with a clinical history of temporal lobe epilepsy and MRI evidence of isolated hippocampal sclerosis studied with EEG telemetry at the National Hospital for Neurology and Neurosurgery, London, the ictal EEG was concordant (33/50), non-lateralized (12/50), obscured (3/50) or showed bilateral and independent onset (2/50), but in none of these 50 cases was it discordant (only changes seen within 30 s of seizure onset were included). Furthermore, the two cases with bilateral independent ictal onsets both showed a majority of seizures arising from the side of the presumed hippocampal sclerosis. Subsequent confirmation of the scalp EEG findings with intracranial EEG was possible in one of these subjects [91]. However, Spencer [92], reviewing previous series, suggested a higher degree of discordance between the neuroimaging and EEG findings. Similarly, the Yale group reported a higher degree of discordance between the EEG findings and patients with hippocampal pathology defined only by quantitative MRI without recourse to additional neuroimaging features, such as T2 signal change and loss of internal structure, in a series of 101 patients. The interictal EEG in 98 patients was unlocalized in 48%, localized to the atrophic temporal

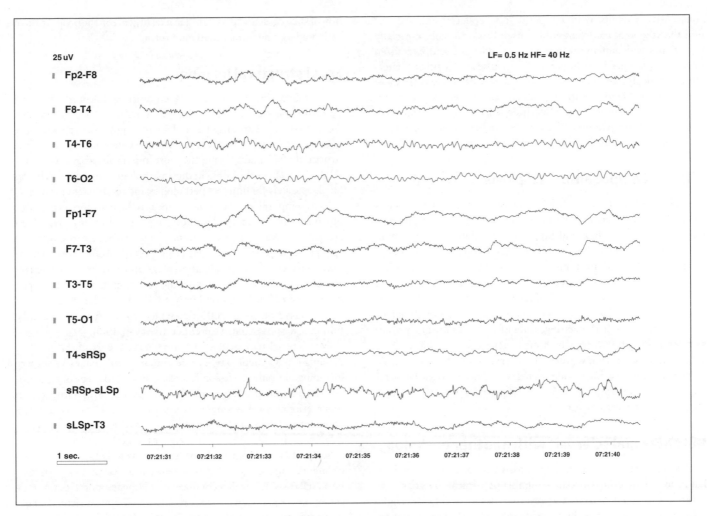

Fig. 52.3 Asymmetrical postictal scalp EEG changes, with well formed alpha on the right and lack of alpha on the left posteriorly.

lobe in 40% and localized elsewhere in 12%. The ictal scalp EEG in 99 patients was unlocalized in 53%, localized to the atrophic temporal lobe in 38% and localized elsewhere in 9% [93]. It is the author's current view that whilst ictal scale EEG recordings may be beneficial in some patients with MRI evidence of isolated hippocampal sclerosis, in order to confirm the clinical seizure type and/or exclude pseudoseizures, it is becoming apparent that some of these patients can proceed to epilepsy surgery without any ictal EEG recordings based on other information [94]. Once the predictive value of other tests is sufficiently secure, the benefit from scalp ictal EEG monitoring within this category that might accrue to the relatively infrequent discordant cases could be outweighed by false-positive results, hazards of subsequent invasive studies or delay in treatment [93]. In this regard, it is noteworthy that a retrospective analysis of operated cases failed to reveal specific EEG characteristics that independently predicted outcome in patients undergoing temporal lobe surgery in whom the pathology subsequently showed hippocampal sclerosis [95]. Of course, it must be recognized that, in assessing the literature, historical cases are likely to have included concordant EEG in the criteria for surgery, thereby reducing the potential of this variable to be identified as an independent predictor of outcome.

Scalp ictal EEG recordings are likely to have a small but definite false lateralizing rate in patients with mesial temporal lobe epilepsy, due to rapid (undetected) contralateral propagation. Alarcon *et al.* [96] studied 314 seizures in 110 patients with temporal lobe epilepsy who underwent simultaneous scalp and foramen ovale ictal recordings. Approximately three-quarters of seizures showed lateralized scalp onset, with largest amplitude at T1/T2 or T3/T4. While 65% of such scalp recordings were indeed associated with a mesial temporal onset on the foramen ovale recordings, 10.9% of the scalp EEG recordings were falsely lateralized, i.e. the true seizure onset was contralateral. Scott [24] studied 400 patients evaluated with scalp video-EEG telemetry, undergoing presurgical evaluation. Of these, 154 had unilateral hippocampal sclerosis on MRI and ictal scalp EEG recordings. Ictal scalp EEGs lateralized to the contralateral side in 10/152 (6.6%). The 10 patients subsequently underwent intracerebral recordings. In all cases the intracerebral recordings lateralized to the side of the hippocampal sclerosis. Nine of these patients proceeded to ·surgery (the other died in a seizure). Six had an excellent outcome (Engel class I/II), two had less favourable and one was lost to follow-up. This rate of false lateralization is less than reported for occipital (28%) or parietal (16%) epilepsy using scalp ictal EEG [97,98].

Cendes *et al.* [98] have revisited the question whether or not ictal recording is mandatory in temporal lobe epilepsy. They studied 184 consecutive patients with temporal lobe epilepsy and did not find that the ictal recording added useful information, especially in patients with unilateral hippocampal sclerosis and lateralized interictal spiking. Given the possibility of false ictal scalp EEG lateralization, delays and expense of scalp video EEG telemetry there seems reasonable justification (both clinical and economic) to bypass this test if all other data is clearly concordant with the unilaterial hippocampal sclerosis, there is a reliable history of seizure semiology and no suspicion of non-epileptic attacks.

Bilateral hippocampal sclerosis

The advent of quantitative MRI using volumetric or T2 measures offers the opportunity to identify patients with bilateral hippocampal pathology [76]. Bilateral hippocampal sclerosis is seen more often in patients with a history of previous encephalitis or meningitis than in those with prolonged febrile seizures in childhood [76]. Given the pathological and aetiological basis of these epilepsies, it is unlikely that scalp EEG will be sufficiently well lateralized in an individual patient to allow confident selection for surgery without invasive monitoring. In this setting, scalp EEG studies are likely to act as a screening procedure, which may exclude some patients from surgical assessment, but will otherwise serve as a prelude to invasive studies. It is notable that Cendes *et al.* [98] reported discordant ictal scalp EEG lateralization in 6/33 (18%) patients with asymmetric, bilateral hippocampal sclerosis.

Hippocampal sclerosis with another pathology

The occurrence of hippocampal sclerosis with a second pathology has been well described in a small number of surgical cases based on histological findings from the resected tissue (see [99]). High-resolution MRI with the ability to identify subtle lesions in non-resected tissue has demonstrated a higher incidence of such dual pathology than was previously recognized. Raymond *et al.* [100] identified areas of cortical dysgenesis separate from the mesial temporal structures in 15 patients out of 100 with hippocampal sclerosis. In a further study of 167 patients with lesional epilepsy, Cendes *et al.* [78] reported the frequent occurrence of hippocampal sclerosis in association with porencephalic cysts (30%), reactive gliosis (25%) and cortical dysgenesis (20%), but a lower incidence in association with vascular abnormalities (9%) or tumours (2%).

Surgical strategies in this increasingly recognized subgroup of hippocampal sclerosis and a second lesion remain poorly defined [78,99,100]. Resection of the mesial temporal structures alone appears to be associated with an unfavourable outcome [99,100]. An alternative approach, based on lesion resection in a first operation, followed, if necessary, by removal of the mesial temporal structures in those in whom seizures are not controlled, may be considered in some patients with discrete second pathologies, but is unlikely to be a realistic option in many patients with cortical dysgenesis, given its diffuse nature. Li *et al.* [101] reported the results of surgical intervention in 38 patients with dual pathology. Lesionectomy plus mesial temporal resection was associated with an excellent outcome in 11/15 (73%) compared to only 2/10 patients with mesial resection or 2/16 with lesionectomy alone. The spatial resolution of scalp EEG is unlikely to provide sufficient discrimination. Further advances in neuroimaging are likely to identify an increasing population of such cases and may result in a resurgence in the proportion of cases undergoing intracranial monitoring.

Focal structural lesions

Small indolent lesions, such as cavernomas, indolent gliomas and dysembryoplastic neuroepithelial tumours (DNET), are readily recognized on neuroimaging and increasingly such patients are undergoing limited lesional resections, the extent of removal of the structural abnormality being the most important prognostic factor [102–104]. The role of EEG in these pathologies may need to be defined separately for different pathologies and for different locations.

Extratemporal lesionectomies appear to have a more favourable outcome than temporal lesionectomies, possibly because of increased involvement of the mesial temporal structures with the epileptogenic process in the latter group [105,106]. However, the optimum methods for localization of the epileptogenic zone remain uncertain even in patients with discrete tumours. For example, Zaatreh *et al.* [107] reported only 13/37 (35%) class 1 and 12/37 (32%) class 2 outcomes following epilepsy surgery for frontal lobe tumours, despite extensive preoperative evaluation.

With regard to vascular abnormalities, Yeh *et al.* [108] have demonstrated a highly favourable outcome with extensive surgery including not only the lesion but also associated areas of epileptogenicity identified using neurophysiological criteria. However, in other lesional epilepsy surgery series, the role of EEG has been less apparent and there are few data to indicate which neurophysiological factors should influence the extent of resection [102,104].

Scalp EEG may sometimes provide apparently falsely localizing or lateralizing changes in lesional epilepsy as well as in mesial temporal sclerosis. It is well recognized that large temporal lesions may sometimes be associated with scalp EEG interictal and ictal changes that predominate over the contralateral side [43]. Williamson *et al.* [72] reported scalp EEG findings in 11 patients with parietal lesions. Of these, nine showed interictal spikes but only one had spikes restricted to the parietal region. Three others had spiking in parietal and other regions, while in five of the 11 spiking was outside the parietal region, being either frontal or temporal. Only one of the 11 showed a focal EEG onset concordant with the parietal lesion. Three of the 11 showed a lateralized onset appropriate to the lesion but eight showed no focal changes at ictal onset. Despite this poor correlation with the EEG, 10 of the patients underwent lesional surgery, all with an excellent outcome. Similarly, occipital lobe lesions may be associated with more anterior scalp EEG changes. Williamson *et al.* [71] reported 25 patients undergoing occipital lobe surgery. Only two of the 25 had interictal spikes restricted to the appropriate occipital lobe, although four had occipital and other appropriately lateralized interictal spikes. Most (22/25) showed temporal spikes, especially over the posterior temporal region. While this study demonstrates the need to scrutinize carefully the occipital cortex in patients thought to have temporal lobe epilepsy in whom the interictal spikes are more posterior than usual, the excellent outcome from occipital surgery seen in this group also demonstrates the need to interpret with caution the scalp EEG findings in the presence of an occipital lesion. The relative distribution of such abnormalities does not appear to be of prognostic significance. Similar problems may be seen with lesions occupying the frontal lobes, in that the scalp EEG often shows an absence of interictal spiking or apparently widespread or bilateral epileptiform discharges, in part due to the relative inaccessibility of much of the frontal lobe to study with scalp EEG recordings and the rapid propagation of epileptiform activity within the frontal lobes [80]. It remains to be established in which pathological substrates/ anatomical localizations additional neurophysiological investigations (scalp or intracranial) will add predictive data. Worrell *et al.* [109] studied the predictive value of ictal onset focal β activity in 54 patients with lesional and non-lesional frontal lobe epilepsy, 52% of whom subsequently became seizure free following surgery. Interestingly, in both groups the presence of this activity on the scalp EEG was strongly associated with a good outcome with 90% of such patients being seizure free. This was independent of lesion resection—and interestingly neither lateralized ictal onset or postresection ECoG were helpful. The potential for misleading or multifocal scalp EEG changes in patients with surgically resectable focal structural lesions is important in planning investigative strategies: a patient with medically intractable epilepsies should not be excluded from high-resolution neuroimaging merely because of such electrographic findings. However, the failure of a significant number of lesionectomy cases to become and remain seizure free clearly identifies this as an important area of study [93].

Malformations of cortical development, hemispherectomy and other diffuse pathologies

The role of scalp EEG in patients with diffuse pathologies, including cortical dysgenesis, will be dependent upon the surgical options. In patients with severe unilateral hemisphere disease, consideration may be given to functional or anatomical hemispherectomy. Initial series [110–112] suggested that scalp EEG findings were of limited value in the assessment of such patients for surgery. Subsequently, Smith *et al.* [113] suggested that independent interictal spiking over the good hemisphere may be a poor prognostic factor in that three of five such patients continued to have seizures postoperatively. Carmant *et al.* [114] reported the neurophysiological prognostic factors in 12 children undergoing hemispherectomy. Although many of their cases had bilateral independent spikes, they were able to combine different EEG factors to produce a prognostic guide. The single most important predictive factor appeared to be depression of the EEG over the damaged hemisphere. Generalized epileptiform discharges, bilateral independent spikes or contralateral slowing also appeared to be unfavourable factors. Ictal scalp EEG recordings were largely unhelpful, with only two of the 12 patients showing definite lateralization, probably due to rapid interhemispheric propagation, and this is also the author's experience.

Criteria for the preoperative evaluation of patients with malformation of cortical development remain poorly defined. Preliminary observations suggest that the most important predictive outcome may be the extent of the removal of the visually identified abnormal areas based on neuroimaging [115]. However, the range of scalp EEG features seen in patients with cortical dysgenesis shows a wide spectrum. In lissencephaly, there may be high-amplitude rhythmic activity or abnormal fast rhythms [116]. In more localized forms of cortical dysgenesis, background rhythms are often preserved, localized areas of slow activity may be seen in relation to the visually identified areas of structural abnormality and epileptiform discharges are often coexistent but more extensive than the identified structural abnormalities [106,117]. Somewhat characteristically, the interictal spiking is often continuous or near-continuous (6/22 patients) or occurs, in repetitive bursts (6/22 patients) [117]. Interestingly, there appears to be a significant association between areas of relatively localized cortical dysgenesis apparent on neuroimaging and generalized 3/s spike and waves [117]. Further studies will be needed to determine whether or not these changes represent secondary bilateral synchrony [118] or, more probably, a generalized epileptogenic process and therefore, presumably, of poor prognostic significance for resective surgery.

MRI-negative cases

The proportion of truly MRI-negative cases undergoing epilepsy surgery continues to fall. With the various combined MRI techniques for the assessment of the mesial temporal lobe structures, hippocampal sclerosis can be detected preoperatively with a very high degree of sensitivity and specificity. The most likely pathologies to be undetected by high-resolution MRI are areas of localized cortical dysgenesis, focal atrophy and gliosis. Truly MRI-negative cases may be considered for epilepsy surgery on the basis of medically intractable partial seizures with well-defined ictal semiology and localized scalp interictal and ictal EEG changes. It is unlikely that these will be sufficiently clear to allow surgery to proceed on the basis of non-invasive studies alone. For example, Scott *et al.* [119] reported only 3/40 non-lesional patients proceeded eventually to epilepsy surgery compared with over half who had MRI abnormalities. However, such scalp EEG studies are essential for the planning of invasive strategies. It is likely that these will only be contemplated in patients with relatively discrete localizing data from the other investigative modalities, supported by the scalp EEG findings. Hong *et al.* [120] reported ictal scalp EEG, interictal FDG PET and ictal SPECT in 41 non-lesional patients with neocortical epilepsy. Thirty-nine per cent were reported to be seizure free at 1 year and 81% to be seizure free or at least 90% improved. While all three tests were of similar lateralizing value, apparently ictal EEG showed the highest localizing value (70% vs. 43% and 33%, respectively) amongst those with a good outcome. Clearly more sophisticated (and probably multicentre) large-scale studies are needed to define optimum protocols to select and evaluate non-lesional cases.

EEG in patients being evaluated for corpus callosal section

Corpus callosal section may be undertaken in patients with medically intractable drop attacks without an identified surgically resectable focal abnormality responsible for their seizure disorder. Such patients are normally evaluated on the basis of the clinical history, neuroimaging and non-invasive EEG. Earlier studies suggested that a more favourable outcome is seen when there is evidence of predominantly lateralized disease, but this has not been a consistent finding [121] and ictal scalp EEGs were usually performed to ensure that there is evidence of bilateral seizure spread in association with the drop attacks. Hanson *et al.* [122] studied the ictal scalp EEG pattern in 41 patients who subsequently had undergone corpus callosal section for drop attacks. There was a significant association between a favourable outcome on ictal EEG recordings showing generalized slow spike-wave, electrodecremental non-evolving fast activity rather than other EEG ictal onset patterns.

Conclusions

Scalp EEG remains one of the fundamental tests in the presurgical evaluation of patients with epilepsy. It is a reliable, robust technique and has dominated this clinical field for several decades. The advent of modern high-resolution MRI, with the ability to identify the underlying anatomical/pathological substrate in most patients being evaluated for surgery, is now allowing a more appropriate use of EEG techniques. The relative importance of the role of EEG in individual patients being assessed for epilepsy surgery will vary according to the MRI-defined category. In a small but increasing number of patients with discrete isolated MRI abnormalities, it is possible to define criteria that allow surgery to proceed based on a well-established history, concordance of other data and interictal scalp EEG alone. The majority of patients, however, continue to require ictal scalp EEG recording to confirm the diagnosis and classification of the epilepsy, as well as to demonstrate the epileptogenicity of identified structural abnormalities. An important group has emerged with dual pathologies, in whom scalp EEG may need to be seen as a prelude to move invasive studies in order to identify the optimum surgical strategy. While truly MRI-negative cases are unlikely to be able to proceed to epilepsy surgery without invasive monitoring, scalp interictal and ictal EEG recordings remain of much importance to determine whether or not there are possible invasive strategies which could be employed in order to plan future resections.

References

1 Fish DR. The anatomical bases of epilepsy. In: Shorvon SD, Fish DR, Andermann F, Stefan H, Bydder G, eds. *MR and Epilepsy.* New York: Plenum Press, 1994: 15–20.

2 King DW, Ajmone-Marsan C. Clinical features and ictal patterns in epileptic patients with EEG temporal lobe foci. *Ann Neurol* 1977; 2: 138–47.

3 Geiger LR, Harrier RN. EEG patterns at the time of focal seizure onset. *Arch Neurol* 1978; 35: 276–86.

4 Escueta AV, Bacsal FE, Treiman DM. Complex partial seizures on closed-circuit television and EEG: a study of 691 attacks in 79 patients. *Ann Neurol* 1982; 11(3): 292–300.

5 Blume WT, Young GB, Lemieux JF. EEG morphology of partial epileptic seizures. *Electroencephalogr Clin Neurophysiol* 1984; 57: 295–302.

6 Quesney LF, Gloor P. Localization of epileptic foci. In: Gotman J, Ives JR, Gloor P, eds. *Long Term Monitoring in Epilepsy. Electroencephalogr Clin Neurophysiol* 1985; 37(Suppl.): 165–200.

7 Spencer SS, Williamson PD, Bridges SL, Mattson RH, Cicchetti DV, Spencer DD. Reliability and accuracy of localization by scalp ictal EEG. *Neurology* 1985; 35: 1567–75.

8 Morris HH III, Luders H, Lesser RP, Dinner DS, Klem GH. The value of closely spaced scalp electrodes in the localization of epileptiform foci: a study of 26 patients with complex partial seizures. *Electroencephalogr Clin Neurophysiol* 1986; 63: 107–11.

9 Risinger NW, Engel J Jr, Van Ness PC, Henry TR, Crandall PH. Ictal localization of temporal lobe seizures with scalp/sphenoidal recordings. *Neurology* 1989; 39: 1288–93.

10 Quesney LF, Constain M, Fish DR, Rasmussen T. Frontal lobe epilepsy: a field of recent emphasis. *Am J EEG Technol* 1990; 30: 177–93.

11 Quesney LF, Risinger MW, Shewmon DA. Extracranial EEG evaluation. In: Engel J Jr, ed. *Surgical Treatment of the Epilepsies.* New York: Raven Press, 1993: 173–96.

12 Swartz BE, Walsh GO, Delgado-Escueta AV, Zolo P. Surface ictal electroencephalographic patterns in frontal vs. temporal lobe epilepsy. *Can J Neurol Sci* 1991; 18: 549–53.

13 Walczak TS, Lewis DV, Radtke R. Scalp EEG differs in temporal and extratemporal complex partial seizures. *J Epilepsy* 1991; 4: 25–8.

14 Antel SB, Li LM, Cendes F *et al.* Predicting surgical outcome in temporal lobe epilepsy patients using MRI and MRSI. *Neurology* 2002; 28: 1505–12.

15 Engel J Jr. When is imaging enough? *Epileptic Disord* 1999; 1: 249–53.

16 Cendes F, Li LM, Watson C, Andermann F, Dubeau F, Arnold DL. Is ictal recording mandatory in temporal lobe epilepsy? Not when the interictal electroencephalogram and hippocampal atrophy coincide. *Arch Neurol* 2000; 57: 497–500.

17 Gilliam F, Bowlings S, Bilir E *et al.* Association of combined MRI, interictal EEG, and ictal EEG results with outcome and pathology after temporal lobectomy. *Epilepsia* 1997; 38(12): 1315–20.

18 Gilliam F, Faught E, Martin R *et al.* Predictive value of MRI-identified mesial temporal sclerosis surgical outcome in temporal lobe epilepsy: an intent-to-treat analysis. *Epilepsia* 2000; 41(8): 963–6.

19 McIntosh AM, Wilson SJ, Berkovic DF. Seizure outcome after temporal lobectomy: current research practice and findings. *Epilepsia* 2001; 42: 1288–307.

20 Pataraia E, Lurger S, Serles W *et al.* Ictal scalp EEG in unilateral mesial temporal lobe epilepsy. *Epilepsia* 1998; 39(6): 608–14.

21 Rosenow F, Luders H. Presurgical evaluation of epilepsy. *Brain* 2001; 124: 1683–700.

22 Schulz R, Luders HO, Hoppe M *et al.* Interictal EEG and ictal EEG propagation are highly predictive of surgical outcome in mesial temporal lobe epilepsy. *Epilepsia* 2000; 41(5): 564–70.

23 Sadler M, Desbiens R. Scalp EEG in temporal lobe epilepsy surgery. *Can J Neurol Sci* 2000; 27 (Suppl. 1): S22–8.

24 Scott CA. Current role of scalp ictal EEG in evaluation for epilepsy surgery. M Phil degree, London University, 2002.

25 Jones DP. Recording of the basal electroencephalogram with sphenoidal needle electrodes. *Electroencephalogr Clin Neurophysiol* 1952; 3: 100.

26 Pampiglione G, Kerridge J. EEG abnormalities from the temporal lobe studied with sphenoidal electrodes. *J Neurol Neurosurg Psychiatr* 1956; 19: 117.

27 Christodoulou G. Sphenoidal electrodes. *Acta Neurol Scand* 1967; 43: 587–93.

28 Kristensen O, Sindrup EH. Sphenoidal electrodes, their use in the electroencephalographic investigation of complex partial epilepsy. *Acta Neurol Scand* 1978; 58: 157–66.

29 Laxer KD. Mini-sphenoidal electrodes in the investigation of seizures. *Electroencephalogr Clin Neurophysiol* 1984; 58: 127–9.

30 Silverman D. The anterior temporal electrode and the ten-twenty system. *Electroencephalogr Clin Neurophysiol* 1960; 12: 735–7.

31 Howman RW, Jones MC, Rawat S. Anterior temporal electrodes in complex partial seizures. *Electroenceph Clin Neurophysiol* 1998; 70: 105–9.

32 Binnie CD, Marston D, Polkey CE, Amin D. Distribution of temporal spikes in relation to the sphenoidal electrode. *Electroencephalogr Clin Neurophysiol* 1989; 73: 403–9.

33 Goodin DS, Aminoff MJ, Laxer KD. Detection of epileptiform activity by different noninvasive EEG methods in complex partial epilepsy. *Ann Neurol* 1990; 27: 330–4.

34 Wilkus RJ, Vossler DG, Thompson PM. Comparison of EEG derived from sphenoidal, infrazygomatic, anterior temporal and midtemporal electrodes during complex partial seizures. *J Epilepsy* 1993; 6: 152–61.

35 Gastaut H. Presentation d'une électrode pharyngée bipolaire. *Rev Neurol* 1948; 80: 623–4.

36 Roubicek J, Hill D. Electroencephalography with pharyngeal electrodes. *Brain* 1948; 71: 77–87.

37 Lehtinen LOJ, Bergstrom L. Naso-ethmoidal electrode for recording the electrical activity of the inferior surface of the frontal lobe. *Electroencephalogr Clin Neurophysiol* 1970; 29: 303–5.

38 Alarcon G, Guy CN, Binnie CD, Walker SR, Elwes RD, Polkey CE. Intracerebral propagation of interictal activity in partial epilepsy: implications for source localization. *J Neurol Neurosurg Psychiatr* 1994; 57 (4): 435–49.

39 Ellingson RJ, Wilken K, Bennett DR. Efficacy of sleep deprivation as an activation procedure in epilepsy patients. *J Clin Neurophysiol* 1985; 1: 83–101.

40 Gastaut H, Gomez-Almanzar M, Taury M. The enforced nap: a simple method of inducing sleep activation in epileptics. *Epilepsy Res* 1991; S2: 31–6.

41 Fish DR. Electroencephalography. In: Hopkins J, Cascino G, Shorvon SD, eds. *Clinical Epilepsy*. London: Churchill, 1995.

42 Klass DW, Westmoreland BF. Non-epileptic epileptiform electroencephalographic activity. *Ann Neurol* 1985; 18: 627–35.

43 Sammaritano M, Gigli GL, Gotman J. Interictal spiking during wakefulness and sleep and localization of foci in temporal lobe epilepsy. *Neurology* 1991; 41: 290–7.

44 Holmes MD, Kutsy RL, Ojemann GA, Wilensky AJ, Ojemann LM. Interictal, unifocal spikes in refractory extratemporal epilepsy predict ictal origin and postsurgical outcome. *Clin Neurophysiol* 2000; 111: 1802–8.

45 Hennessy MJ, Elwes RD, Rabe-Hesketh S, Binnie CD, Polkey CE. Prognostic factors in the surgical treatment of medically intractable epilepsy associated with mesial temporal sclerosis. *Acta Neurol Scand* 2001;103: 344–50.

46 Hennessy MJ, Elwes RD, Honavar M, Rabe-Hesketh S, Binnie CD, Polkey CE. Predictors of outcome and pathological considerations in the surgical treatment of intractable epilepsy associated with temporal lobe lesions. *Neurol Neurosurg Psychiatr* 2001; 70: 450–8.

47 Cascino GD. Video-EEG Monitoring in adults. *Epilepsia* 2002; 43: 80–93.

48 Gotman J, Gloor P. Automatic recognition and quantification of interictal epilepsy activity in the human scalp EEG. *Electroencephalogr Clin Neurophysiol* 1976; 41: 513–29.

49 Gotman J. Automatic recognition of epileptic seizures in the EEG. *Electroencephalogr Clin Neurophysiol* 1982; 54: 530–40.

50 Litt B, Lehnertz K. Seizure prediction and the preseizure period. *Curr Opin Neurol* 2002; 15: 173–7.

51 Chang BS, Ives JR, Schomer DL, Drislane FW. Outpatient EEG monitoring in the presurgical evaluation of patients with refractory temporal lobe epilepsy. *Clin Neurophysiol* 2002; 19: 152–6.

52 Guerreiro CA, Montenegro MA, Kobayashi E, Noronha AL, Guerreiro MM, Cendes F. Daytime outpatient versus inpatient video-EEG monitoring for presurgical evaluation in temporal lobe epilepsy. *Clin Neurophysiol* 2002; 19: 204–8.

53 DellaBadia J Jr, Bell WL, Keyes JW Jr, Mathews VP, Glazier SS. Assessment and cost comparison of sleep-deprived EEG, MRI and PET in the prediction of surgical treatment for epilepsy. *Seizure* 2002; 11: 303–9.

54 Cobb WA, Guiloff RJ, Cast J. Breach rhythm: the EEG related to skull defects. *Electroencephalogr Clin Neurophysiol* 1979; 47: 251–71.

55 Patrick S, Berg A, Spencer SS. EEG and seizure outcome after epilepsy surgery. *Epilepsia* 1995; 36 (3): 236–40.

56 Wieser HG, Bancaud J, Talairach G. Comparative value of spontaneous and chemically and electrically induced seizures in establishing the lateralization of temporal lobe seizures. *Epilepsia* 1979; 20: 47–59.

57 So N, Gotman J. Changes in seizure activity following anticonvulsant drug withdrawal. *Neurology* 1990; 40: 407–13.

58 Marks DA, Katz A, Scheyer R, Spencer SS. Clinical and electrographic effects of acute anticonvulsant withdrawal in epileptic patients. *Neurology* 1991; 41: 508–12.

59 Gotman J. Electroencephalographic spiking activity, drug levels and seizure occurrence in epileptic patients. *Ann Neurol* 1985; 17: 597–603.

60 Gotman J, Koffler DJ. Interictal spiking increases after seizures but does not after decrease in medication. *Electroencephalogr Clin Neurophysiol* 1989; 72: 7–15.

61 Spencer SS, Spencer DD, Williamson PD, Mattson RH. Ictal effects of anticonvulsant medication withdrawal in epileptic patients. *Epilepsia* 1981; 22: 297–307.

62 Engel J Jr, Crandall PH. Falsely localizing ictal onset with depth EEG telemetry during anticonvulsant withdrawal. *Epilepsia* 1983; 24: 344–55.

63 Marciana MG, Gotman J, Andermann F, Olivier A. Patterns of seizure activation after withdrawal of antiepileptic medication. *Neurology* 1985; 35: 1537–43.

64 Marciani MG, Gotman J. Effects of drug withdrawal on location of seizure onset. *Epilepsia* 1986; 27: 423–31.

65 Scott CA, Fish TR, Allen PJ. Design of an intensive epilepsy monitoring unit. *Epilepsia* 2000; 41: 83–8.

66 Haut SR, Swick C, Freeman K, Spencer S. Seizure clustering during epilepsy monitoring. *Epilepsia* 2002; 43: 711–15.

67 Walczak TS. Neocortical temporal lobe epilepsy: characterizing the syndrome. *Epilepsia* 1995; 36(7): 633–5.

68 Walczak TS, Radtke RA, McNamara JO et al. Anterior temporal lobectomy for complex partial seizures: evaluation, results, and long-term follow-up in 100 cases. *Neurology* 1990; 40(3): 413–18.

69 Lieb JP, Walsh GO, Babb TL, Walter RD, Crandall PH. A comparison of EEG seizure patterns recorded with surface and depth electrodes in patients with temporal lobe epilepsy. *Epilepsia* 1976; 17: 137–60.

70 Devinsky O, Kelly K, Porter R, Theodore WH. Clinical and electrographic features of simple partial seizures. *Neurology* 1988; 38: 1347–52.

71 Williamson PD, Thadani VM, Darcey TM, Spencer DD, Spencer SS, Mattson RH. Occipital lobe epilepsy: clinical characteristics, seizure spread patterns and results of surgery. *Ann Neurol* 1992; 31: 3–13.

72 Williamson PD, Boon PA, Thadani VM et al. Parietal lobe epilepsy: diagnostic considerations and results of surgery. *Ann Neurol* 1992; 31: 193–201.

73 Kaibara M, Blume WT. The postictal electroencephalogram. *Electroencephalogr Clin Neurophysiol* 1988; 70: 99–104.

74 Jan MM, Sadler M, Rahey SR. Lateralized postictal EEG delta predicts the side of seizure surgery in temporal lobe epilepsy. *Epilepsia* 2001; 42: 402–5.

75 Cook MJ, Fish DR, Shorvon SD, Straughan K, Stevens JM. Hippocampal volumetric and morphometric studies in frontal and temporal lobe epilepsy. *Brain* 1992; 115: 1001–15.

76 Free SL, Bergin PS, Fish DR et al. Methods for normalization of hippocampal volumes measured with MR. *Am J Neuroradiol* 1995: 16(4): 637–43.

77 Jack CR Jr, Trenerry MR, Cascino GD et al. Bilaterally symmetric hippocampi and surgical outcome. *Neurology* 1995; 45(7): 1353–8.

78 Cendes F, Cook MJ, Watson C et al. Frequency and characteristics of dual pathology in patients with lesional epilepsy. *Neurology* 1995; 45(11): 2058–64.

79 So N, Gloor P, Quesney LF, Jones-Gotman M, Olivier A, Andermann F. Depth electrode investigations in patients with bitemporal epileptiform abnormalities. *Ann Neurol* 1989; 25: 423–31.

80 Quesney LF, Fish DR, Rasmussen T. Extracranial EEG and electrocorticography in children with medically refractory partial seizures. *J Epilepsy* 19906; 3 (Suppl.): 55–67.

81 Chung MY, Walczak TS, Lewis DV et al. Temporallobectomy and independent bitemporal interictal activity: what degree of lateralization is sufficient? *Epilepsia* 1991; 32: 195–201.

82 Walczak TS, Radtke RA, Lewis DV. Accuracy and interobserver reliability of scalp ictal EEG. *Neurology* 1992; 42: 2279–85.

83 Murro AM, Park YD, King DW, Gallagher BB, Smith JR, Littleton W. Use of scalp-sphenoidal EEG for seizure localization in temporal lobe of epilepsy. *J Clin Neurophysiol* 1994; 11 (2): 216–19.

84 Kotagal P, Luders H, Morris HH et al. Dystonic posturing in complex partial seizures of emporal lobe onset: a new lateralizing sign. *Neurology* 1989; 39(9): 196–201.

85 Jasper H, Pertuisset B, Flanigin H. EEG and cortical electrograms in patients with temporal lobe seizures. *Arch Neurol Psychiatr* 1951; 65: 272–90.

86 Engel J, Drive MV, Falconer MA. Electrophysiological correlates of pathology and surgical results in temporal lobe epilepsy. *Brain* 1975; 98: 129–56.

87 Delgado-Escueta AV, Walsh GO. The selection process for surgery of intractable complex partial seizures: surface EEG and depth electrocorticography. In: Ward AA, Penry JK, Purpura D, eds. *Epilepsy*. New York: Raven Press, 1983: 295–326.

88 Bergen D, Morrel F, Bleck TP, Whisler WW. Predictors of success in surgical treatment of intractable epilepsy. *Epilepsia* 1984; 25: 656.

89 Dodrill CB, Wilkus RJ, Ojemann GA et al. Multidisciplinary prediction of seizure relief from cortical resection surgery. *Ann Neurol* 1986; 20: 2–12.

90 Sadler RM, Blume W. Significance of bisynchronous spike-waves in patients with temporal lobe spikes. *Epilepsia* 1989; 30: 143–6.

91 Scott C, Quirk J, Fish DR. Correlation of ictal electrographic activity and MRI. In: *Proceedings of the Fifth International Cleveland Clinic/Bethel.* Epilepsy Symposium, 1994: 80.

92 Spencer SS. The relative contributions of MRI, SPECT and PET imaging in epilepsy. *Epilepsia* 1994; 35 (Suppl. 6): S72–S89.

93 Fish DR, Spencer SS. Clinical correlations: MRI and EEG. *Magnetic Res Imag* 1995; 13: 1113–17.

94 Antel SB, Li LM, Cendes F *et al.* Predicting surgical outcome in temporal lobe epilepsy patients using MRI and MRSI. *Neurology* 2002; 58(10): 1505–12.

95 Williamson PD, French JA, Thadani VM *et al.* Characteristics of medial temporal lobe epilepsy: interictal and ictal scalp electroencephalography, neuropsychological testing, neuroimaging, surgical results and pathology. *Ann Neurol* 1993; 34: 781–7.

96 Alarcon G, Kissani N, Dad M *et al.* Lateralizing and localizing values of ictal onset recorded on the scalp: evidence from simultaneous recordings with intracranial foramen ovale electrodes. *Epilepsia* 2001; 42: 1426–37.

97 Foldvary N, Klem G, Hammel J, Bingaman W, Najm I, Luders H. The localizing value of ictal EEG in focal epilepsy. *Neurology* 2001; 11: 2022–8.

98 Foldvary N, Bingaman WE, Wyllie E. Surgical treatment of epilepsy. *Neurol Clin* 2001; 19: 491–515.

99 Fish DR, Andermann F, Olivier A. Complex partial seizures and posterior temporal or extratemporal lesions: surgical strategies. *Neurology* 1991; 41: 1781–4.

100 Raymond AA, Fish DR, Stevens JM, Sisodiya SM, Shorvon SD. Association of hippocampal sclerosis with cortical dysgenesis in patients with epilepsy. *Neurology* 1994; 44: 1841–4.

101 Li LM, Cendes F, Andermann F *et al.* Surgical outcome in patients with epilepsy and dual pathology. *Brain* 1999; 122(5): 799–805.

102 Boon PA, Williamson PD, Fried I *et al.* Intracranial, intraaxial, space-occupying lesions in patients with intractable partial seizures: an anatomical, clinical, neuropsyiological and surgical correlation. *Epilepsia* 1991; 32: 467–76.

103 Boon P, Calliauw L, De Renck J *et al.* Clinical and neurophysiological correlations in patients with refractory partial epilepsy and intracranial structural lesions. *Acta Neurochir (Wien)* 1994; 128: 68–83.

104 Cascino G, Boon P, Fish DR. Surgically remedial lesional syndromes. In: Engel J, ed. *Surgical Treatment of the Epilepsies*, 2nd edn. New York: Raven Press, 1993: 77–85.

105 Cascino GD, Kelly PJ, Hirschorn KA, Marsh WR, Sharborough FW. Stereotactic lesion resection in partial epilepsy. *Mayo Clin Proc* 1990; 65: 1053–60.

106 Raymond AA, Fish DR, Sisodiya S, Alsanjari M, Stevens J, Shorvon SD. Abnormalities of gyration, heterotopias, tuberous sclerosis, focal cortical dysplasia, microdysgenesis, dysembryoplastic neuroepithelial tumour and dysgenesis of the archicortex in epilepsy. Clinical, EEG and neuroimaging features in 100 adult patients. *Brain* 1995; 118: 629–60.

107 Zaatreh MM, Spencer DD, Thopson JL *et al.* Frontal lobe tumoral epilepsy: clinical, neurophysiologic features and predictors of surgical outcome. *Epilepsia* 2002; 43: 727–33.

108 Yeh H, Kashiwagi S, Tew JM, Berger TS. Surgical management of epilepsy associated with cerebral arteriovenous malformations. *J Neurosurg* 1990; 72: 216–23.

109 Worrell GA, So EL, Kazemi J *et al.* Focal ictal beta discharge on scalp EEG predicts excellent outcome of frontal lobe epilepsy surgery. *Epilepsia* 2002; 43: 277–82.

110 David M, Oradat P, Mikol F, Miribel J. Valeurs des différents critères dans les indications de l'hémisphérectomie. *Neurochirugie* 1967; 3: 339–411.

111 Wilson PJE. Cerebral hemispherectomy for infantile hemiplegia: a report of 50 cases. *Brain* 1970; 93: 147–80.

112 Lindsay J, Ounstead C, Richards P. Hemispherectomy for childhood epilepsy: a 36 year study. *Den Med Child Neurol* 1987; 29: 592–600.

113 Smith SJM, Andermann F, Villemure JG *et al.* Functional hemispherectomy: EEG findings, spiking from isolated brain postoperatively and prediction of outcome. *Neurology* 1991; 41: 1790–4.

114 Carmant L, Kramer U, Riviello JJ *et al.* EEG prior to hemispherectomy: correlation with outcome and pathology. *Electroencephalogr Clin Neurophysiol* 1995; 94: 265–70.

115 Palmini A, Andermann F, Olivier A, Tampieri D, Robitaille Y. Focal neuronal migration disorders: results of surgical treatment. *Ann Neurol* 1991; 30: 750–7.

116 Quirk JA, Kendall B, Kingsley DPE, Boyd SG, Pitt MC. EEG features of cortical dysplasia in children. *Neuropaediatrics* 1993; 24: 193–9.

117 Raymond AA, Fish DR, Boyd SG, Smith SJM, Pitt MC, Kendall B. Cortical dysgenesis: serial EEG findings in children and adults. *Electroencephalogr Clin Neurophysiol* 1995; 94: 389–97.

118 Tukel K, Japser H. The electroencephalogram in parasagittal lesions. *Electroencephalogr Clin Neurophysiol* 1952; 4: 481–94.

119 Scott CA, Fish DR, Smith SJ *et al.* Presurgical evaluation of patients with epilepsy and normal MRI: role of scalp video-EEG telemetry. *J Neurol Neurosurg Psychiatry* 1999; 66(1): 69–71.

120 Hong KS, Lee SK, Kim JY, Lee DS, Chung CK. Pre-surgical evaluation and surgical outcome of 41 patients with non-lesional neocortical epilepsy. *Seizure* 2002; 11: 184–92.

121 Gates JR, Wada JA, Reeves AG *et al.* Reevaluation of corpus callosal section. In: Engel J Jr, ed. *Surgical Treatment of the Eptlepsies.* New York: Raven Press, 1993: 637–48.

122 Hanson RR, Risinger M, Maxwell R. The ictal EEG as a predictive factor for outcome following corpus callosum section in adults. *Epilepsy Res* 2002; 49: 89–97.

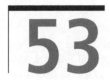

53 Invasive EEG in Presurgical Evaluation of Epilepsy

D.K. Nguyen and S.S. Spencer

Contemporary indications for intracranial monitoring

General considerations

Intracranial electrodes are indicated when it is reasonable to assume that all or most seizures originate from a single epileptogenic focus and that a surgical procedure can be performed to help the patient's intractable condition with some additional localizing information [1,2]. This assumption is based on the clinical history, surface EEG and tests of focal functional deficit and structural abnormalities, all part of a comprehensive presurgical work-up. In some patients, the non-invasive evaluation alone is conclusive enough to guide a clear decision whereas in others it is inconclusive, reveals discordant findings or requires additional cortical mapping before surgery can be done.

The spectrum of presurgical findings should allow a hypothesis about the region(s) to be further investigated. All intracranial electrodes will overcome the sensitivity limitations of extracranial electrodes because they are closer to generators of epileptiform activity. Whereas a large cortical surface (~6 cm^2) is required to generate a recordable signal by extracranial electrodes, intracranial electrodes can pick up potential changes occurring over only a few millimetres of cortex. However, because sampling is restricted by the number of electrodes that can safely be used, there is a risk that the intracranial study may fail to identify the epileptogenic zone if suspected areas are insufficiently covered. The key to a successful intracranial study is the strength of the hypothesis produced by the non-invasive evaluation [3].

Indications in mesial temporal lobe epilepsy (MTLE)

There appears to be general agreement that surgery can be offered without intracranial study to certain patients who exhibit all or some of the following congruent findings compatible with unilateral MTLE, as long as some structural and functional localization concordant with EEG is obtained, and no discordant localization is present [4]:

1 Seizure semiology is compatible with temporal lobe origin.
2 MRI reveals unilateral mesial temporal sclerosis (MTS).
3 Interictal activity consists of ipsilateral unilateral or predominantly (>75%) lateralized anterior temporal spikes.
4 Ictal surface recordings show ipsilateral lateralized rhythmic activity maximal over the anterior temporal/subtemporal/sphenoidal head regions.
5 Neuropsychological evaluation detects deficits compatible with ipsilateral temporal lobe dysfunction.

6 SPECT shows interictal hypoperfusion and ictal hyperperfusion over the epileptogenic temporal lobe.
7 PET reveals ipsilateral hypometabolism.

When these criteria are not satisfied, invasive EEG is recommended prior to anteromedial temporal resection.

Special issues in MTLE

Bitemporal epilepsy

Evidence from animal and human studies suggests that MTS is often a bilateral disease, albeit asymmetrical [5,6]: (a) bilateral hippocampal damage noted in 47–90% on autopsy studies; (b) observation of bilateral independent temporal epileptiform discharges and/or ictal onsets; and (c) bilateral MRI evidence of hippocampal damage. Despite these observations, patients with signs of bilateral epileptogenesis on non-invasive modalities should not necessarily be excluded from epilepsy surgery.

Independent bitemporal spikes

The presence of bilateral temporal spikes is not synonymous with bilateral epileptogenesis or poor surgical outcome [6–8]. So *et al.* [6] showed that 44% of patients who harboured bitemporal spikes on scalp EEG were found to have seizures originating from only one temporal lobe on depth electrode studies. Hirsch *et al.* [8] reported that 36/49 patients (71%) with bitemporal abnormalities on interictal scalp EEG were found to have unilateral seizure onset on ictal EEG. In most centres, patients with bitemporal independent spikes will have surgery without a precedent invasive study if all surface recorded seizures arise over one temporal lobe in concordance with MRI, neuropsychological and functional data.

Bitemporal independent seizure onsets

Bilateral independent scalp ictal onset is a strong indicator of bilateral temporal epileptogenesis. However, in about 7% of patients with unilateral MTLE, the ictal pattern is first noted on scalp EEG over the contralateral temporal lobe [9]. Even in those who have bilateral independent temporal lobe seizure onset documented by invasive recordings, many centres will consider temporal lobectomy if most of their seizures originate from one side [3,7,8]. What represents a reasonable cut-off to determine adequate predominance is, however, not clear. In a study by So *et al.* [7], patients with less than 80% of seizures originating from the resected temporal lobe fared significantly worse than those with ≥ 80% of seizures arising from the resected lobe. Hirsch *et al.* [10] suggested that even bitemporal patients who have as few as 55% of seizures from the resected temporal lobe can obtain excellent surgical results with temporal lobectomy when complementary tests strongly favour the resected side.

It is also important to recognize that apparent bitemporal epileptogenesis may be due to extratemporal seizure onset with bitemporal seizure spread [10]. This is not an uncommon finding in individuals with parietal or occipital seizure onset which may be difficult to identify on scalp EEG, and is an important reason to consider invasive EEG with posterior sampling, if other findings are compatible with such a scenario.

Non-lesional non-MTLE

Recent studies have defined a syndrome of neocortical temporal lobe epilepsy (NTLE) with characteristic clinical and electroencephalographic features [11,12]. These patients, who frequently have normal or non-localizing MRIs, always require invasive studies to better define the epileptogenic zone. Their surgical management is more challenging (especially when the epileptogenic region overlies the language area) and outcome is not as good as with MTLE patients [11,12].

Lesional epilepsy

Next to MTS, tumours, vascular malformations and cortical dysplasia are the most common aetiologies of uncontrolled epilepsy considered for surgery. Although interictal spikes can be widespread and even bilaterally independent, scalp ictal recordings should show that seizures arise in the vicinity of the lesion. PET studies should at least be lateralizing and preferably localizing. Because of the structural evidence, less precision is needed from EEG localization as long as it is consistent and regionally concordant. Indications for an intracranial study may include the following.
1 Non-localizing or discordant ictal scalp recordings suggesting the lesion might not be responsible for the seizures.
2 Determination of the necessity to remove the MTL also in patients with lesions adjacent to it who are at risk of memory decline following surgery.
3 Definition of the margins of the epileptogenic zone to guide the extent of resection (although other strategies such as ECoG, radiological or pathological evaluation of margins may be used) [13].
4 Cortical stimulation for brain mapping with lesions overlying or adjacent to eloquent cortex.
5 Cortical dysplasia: contrary to tumours and vascular malformations, limits of dysplastic lesions seen on MRI are poorly defined, often not reflecting the real extent of the epileptogenic zone [14].

Dual pathology

Dual pathology is defined as the coexistence of hippocampal atrophy and another lesion on MRI, either of which has the potential to be the source of the uncontrolled seizures. Dual pathology is not synonymous with dual epileptogenesis. When presurgical noninvasive modalities are unable to unequivocally distinguish if only one or both are responsible for the patient's seizure condition, intracranial recordings are necessary to resolve the matter.

Non-lesional extratemporal epilepsies

In non-lesional extratemporal epilepsies, intracranial recordings are necessary due to the limited value of interictal epileptic discharges and poorly localized (or even sometimes lack of) scalp ictal rhythms. Furthermore, cortical mapping may be necessary if the probable epileptogenic zone overlies eloquent areas.

Currently, invasive recordings are used in approximately 25–50% of adult patients at most tertiary care epilepsy surgery centres in North America [1,2]. Most patients suffer from extrahippocampal epilepsies, as 'pure' cases of MTLE no longer require invasive studies. The overall frequency of intracranial studies has fallen in recent years, and continues to do so at most institutions.

Specific intracranial electrode techniques

A wide array of intracranial electrodes is available [1–3]. The major goal for each intracranial study is to design it such that all suspected epileptogenic zones are sampled. Intracranial electrodes differ by the parts of the brain from which they can best record, method of insertion, accuracy, risks and limitations. In order to maximize the yield of the specific study, one must capitalize on the singular advantages of each technique.

Depth electrodes

Technical aspects

Depth electrodes are inserted into deep cerebral structures. Although they may be flexible or rigid, the former is now more commonly used because they have less potential for brain injury in the advent of movement [15]. The main disadvantage of flexible electrodes is the requirement of a rigid stylet for their insertion with the potential risk for a variable degree of withdrawal of the electrode as the stylet is removed, a problem which can be minimized with an electrode placement device. Depth electrodes can carry 4–18 contacts along their length, usually spaced 5–10 mm apart at constant intervals. Electrode contacts can be made of stainless steel, platinum or nichrome, all MRI compatible.

Depth electrodes are stereotactically inserted by way of burr holes under local or general anaesthesia (the latter method being preferred for longer procedures). While electrode introduction was traditionally done with the help of a stereotaxic frame, it can now be carried out with frameless MRI-guided stereotaxy [15]. The cortical surface is inspected through the burr holes to assure absence of superficial cortical vessels. After a hollow electrode introducer is passed to the target, a wire electrode is then inserted as far as the tip of the introducer, positioning the electrode at the exact target point. The introducer is then withdrawn while the wire electrode is gradually fed downward. A carrier electrode placement device may be used to help feed the wire downward through the introducer at the same rate as the introducer is withdrawn, preventing displacement of the electrode from the target. The cable is fixed to the skin at the outlet by sutures or a burr hole button may be used to secure the electrode cable following depth electrode placement. Postimplantation MRI are often used to verify the exact location of each electrode contact (although there are some issues to resolve concerning the possibility of induced current flow during imaging).

Use

Amongst the available intracranial electrodes, only depth electrodes penetrate brain tissue directly. They are hence the electrodes of choice when evaluating deep buried structures such as the amygdala or the hippocampus or the vicinity of deep brain lesions.

Medial temporal lobe epilepsy

Depth electrodes represent the method of choice for the study of MTLE since it is the only technique which can sample directly from the hippocampus, whether they are placed orthogonally or longitudinally. With the longitudinal method of placement, multicontact depth electrodes are inserted in an anteroposterior fashion, from the occipital lobe (through occipital burr holes) towards the ipsilateral hippocampus [15,16] (Fig. 53.1). This method allows sampling of electrical activity throughout the whole longitudinal axis of the hippocampus. With the orthogonal method, multiple bipolar or multicontact depth electrodes are inserted transversely from lateral to medial at various locations, usually through punctures in the middle or inferior temporal gyri into the amygdala and anterior and posterior hippocampus (Fig. 53.2). This method allows sampling of multiple hippocampal sites and also of the lateral temporal neocortex. However, the small contact strands have very limited spatial resolution, and in many situations additional cortical electrodes are required to afford adequate lateral coverage [16]. When necessary bilateral homotopic depth electrodes are inserted.

Neocortical temporal lobe epilepsy

NTLE cases will often require additional invasive intracranial recording, especially in the absence of a lesion, to delineate the epileptogenic zone. There are various ways to study NTLE [12].

Some centres will use multiple orthogonally placed depth electrodes to sample the lateral as well as the medial temporal lobe as discussed above. Unfortunately, these electrodes commonly pro-vide minimal or no coverage of basal, tip or inferolateral temporal neocortex from which NTLE seizures often arise. Others use subdural electrodes (without depth electrodes) for the diagnosis of mesial versus NTLE [15,16]. The use of a subdural grid over the lateral temporal region combined with multiple subdural strips may also allow adequate localization as well as language mapping by cortical stimulation in the dominant temporal lobe. Subdural strips passed beneath the temporal lobe provide excellent recording from the uncus, amygdala and hippocampus if their placement is medial enough. Claims that the electrical activity detected by depth electrodes is not always reflected by subdural electrodes may be a result of inadequate subdural placement [17,18]. Eisenschenk et al. [18] reported that seven seizures in three patients (out of 22) were falsely localized on subdural electrode analysis alone (compared with depth recordings) due to the suboptimal placement of subtemporal subdural electrodes.

Extratemporal epilepsy

Depth electrodes may also target deep structures such as the orbitofrontal region or the medial occipital region. Depth extratemporal electrodes may also be placed orthogonally or parasagittally. Bilateral symmetrical sampling is not as routine as in bitemporal epilepsy, but is used in cases of suspected medial occipital and frontal lobe epilepsy due to the rapid spread of the activity to contralateral homologous regions [15].

Advantages

Access

The main advantage of depth electrodes is the direct access to generators buried deep in the brain, allowing detection of the earliest electrographic changes in seizures arising from these regions. In some cases, especially auras and subclinical seizures, the ictal discharges may only be seen on depth electrode recordings [15,19,20].

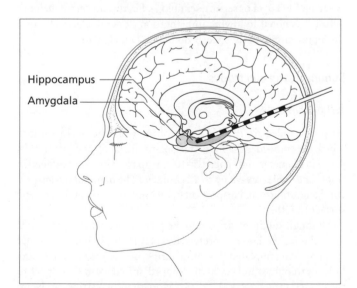

Fig. 53.1 Longitudinal depth electrode inserted in an anteroposterior fashion from the occipital lobe toward the ipsilateral hippocampus.

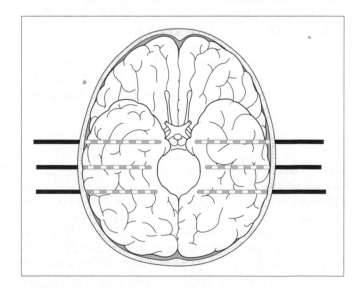

Fig. 53.2 Orthogonal depth electrodes inserted transversely from lateral to medial temporal lobe at various locations.

Accuracy of placement

Depth electrodes are also unique in the exquisite precision with which they can be placed using modern computer-assisted image-based stereotaxy [15].

Seizure cure

An infrequently mentioned 'advantage' is the (extremely rare) occurrence of seizure cure after depth electrode implantation without any resective procedure, tentatively explained by a well-placed injury in the epileptogenic zone by the depth electrodes [2,15].

Disadvantages

Restricted sampling

The major limitation of depth electrodes is limited spatial sampling. Depth electrode contacts reveal activity from a very focused region. One can never be certain that the earliest seizure activity truly comes from the area where it was first recorded [3].

Haemorrhage

Early studies reported a 1–4% risk of intracranial haemorrhage after depth electrode studies, accounting for more than half their major complications [21]. Reviewing the combined results of depth electrode studies in 14 institutions in the pre-MRI era, Van Buren [21] found an overall morbidity of 4% among 879 cases, with 12 infections, seven haemorrhages with permanent sequelae (0.8%), 17 haemorrhages without sequelae and two cases of Creutzfeldt–Jakob disease. Pilcher *et al.* [22] in a later literature review reported a 2.5% rate of haemorrhage in 1582 patients who were assessed with depth electrodes. However, with the subsequent use of digital subtraction angiography, MRI-guided depth electrode placement and direct cortical visualization through burr holes to avoid major vascular structures, the rate of haemorrhage has been reduced. In later series using modern techniques, the risk of intraparenchymal haemorrhage was <1% [6]. The use of postoperative MRI also confirmed a very low incidence of asymptomatic haemorrhage. A retrospective review of MR scans in 57 patients who underwent stereotactic implantation of 210 depth electrodes reported only one case of occipital lobe haematoma, and four tracks (2%) showing punctate signal voids consistent with microhaemorrhage [23].

Infection

Infection occurs in 1–5% of patients [21,22]. Meningitis is most common while intracerebral abscesses, scalp infections, cerebritis and subdural empyemas are less commonly observed. Creutzfeldt–Jakob disease transmission through re-used depth electrodes was reported in the literature, but not since the institution of disposable electrodes. Although infections may sometimes prompt the early removal of electrodes, they are easily treated. To minimize their occurrence, some epilepsy centres will instigate prophylactic antibiotic coverage from the time of depth electrode insertion until removal.

Damage to brain parenchyma

Since depth-electrode placement requires brain penetration, theoretical concerns were raised about damage to brain parenchyma. Pathological studies have shown gliosis, cystic degeneration and microbial abscesses [3,15]. Signal abnormalities were noted in 67% of patients, mostly consisting of punctate hyperintensities on long-repetition-time images, in 57 patients who underwent stereotaxic placement of 210 depth electrodes [23]. Despite these findings, no significant deficits have yet been observed in the absence of subsequent complications or resective surgery [24,25]. Novelly *et al.* [24] analysed the neuropsychological profiles before and after depth electrode implantation (but prior to any surgery) in 17 patients and reported no cognitive sequelae. More recently, Fernandez *et al.* [25] showed that intrahippocampal depth electrode implantation into an unaffected hippocampus of the speech-dominant hemisphere did not result in any verbal memory deficit.

Epileptogenesis

Animal studies have suggested that depth electrode implantation alone may cause epileptogenesis [26]. However, centres which use depth electrodes report similar short- and long-term success and relapse rates after resection as those not using them [15].

Fernandez *et al.* [25] systematically re-evaluated the safety of depth electrodes by retrospectively reviewing surgical complications, epileptogenesis and neuropsychological deficits in 115 patients undergoing bilateral longitudinal depth electrode implantation. Clinically significant complications occurred in 4.3% of patients but only one was specifically related to depth electrode implantation. Asymptomatic complications in 2.6% of patients detected by imaging studies consisted of a thin layer of blood on the trigonal ventricular plexus in two patients and a folded electrode in another. No differences of seizure outcome were noted between patients with and without intrahippocampal depth electrodes. Postoperatively, there was no evidence of bilateral epileptogenesis based on EEG data or seizure semiology. Finally, no verbal memory deficit was noted following implantation of depth electrodes into the hippocampus of the speech-dominant hemisphere.

Subdural strip electrodes

Technical aspects

Strip electrodes are flexible strips of inert Silastic or Teflon into which are embedded stainless steel, platinum or silver contact disks 4 mm in diameter and spaced 5–10 mm apart. They are designed in single or double rows of up to 12 contacts. The material is transparent, facilitating visual inspection upon implantation on the cortical surface [27,28].

Although subdural strips may be placed under local or general anaesthesia, the latter is preferred when multiple burr holes and strips are contemplated. Subdural strips are inserted through burr holes or trephines and manually 'slipped' into the subdural space to the desired target areas [2,27,28]. More than two strips can be inserted through each burr hole with different planned trajectories, and a wider burr hole could accommodate more strips if necessary.

In patients requiring a combined study with a subdural grid, multiple strips with different trajectories can be easily inserted through the craniotomy. Precise anatomic location of electrodes is documented after implantation with MRI. In order to limit risks of cerebrospinal fluid (CSF) leak and infection, the exit cables are passed through a separate stab wound away from the main incision. At the end of the monitoring session, the subdural strips can be removed under general anaesthesia or at the bedside with adequate sedation [2,28].

Use

Subdural electrodes are used to better localize the epileptogenic zone by recording directly over the brain. Subdural strips are used over any lateral neocortical surface location but also to cover the medial temporal structures as well as the interhemispheric fissure [1–3,27,28].

Temporal lobe epilepsy

If a temporal focus is strongly suspected, adequate coverage of medial and lateral surfaces can be achieved in experienced hands using several strips terminating in basal anterior/middle and posterior hippocampal/entorhinal cortex inserted through temporal burr holes (Fig. 53.3) [18–20]. Increasingly, multiple bilateral subdural strips are advocated to replace depth EEG because they can provide chronic intracranial recording without brain penetration. Prior studies have however demonstrated greater sensitivity of intrahippocampal depth electrodes over inferior temporal subdural electrodes for the detection of medial temporal seizures [19,20]: (a) some subclinical or simple partial seizures are only detected by the depth electrodes; (b) ictal rhythms never appear earlier in subdural strips and take an average latency of 36 s to spread from the depth

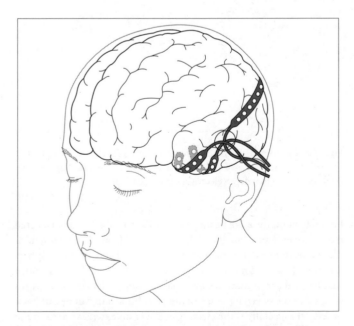

Fig. 53.3 Subdural strip electrodes inserted through a temporal burr hole to study lateral and medial temporal neocortex.

electrode to the subdural electrode; and (c) rare cases of false lateralization have been reported by Sperling and O'Connor [20] although Spencer et al. [19] reported that despite the decreased sensitivity, lateralization was always accurate in strips with adequate medial placement. Subdural electrodes offer the advantages of obviating brain penetration, and better and broader coverage of lateral and basal temporal neocortical structures. When MTLE is being studied only to differentiate the predominant epileptogenic medial temporal lobe, either type of electrode may be used. When it is still unclear whether seizures originate more from lateral than medial structures, a combined study is probably preferable. In either case, one must strive for extreme medial subdural electrode placement to maximize such studies.

Extratemporal epilepsy

If a combined study with a subdural grid is required, placement of subdural electrodes may take advantage of the craniotomy required for the implantation of the grid. Strips can be inserted through frontal burr holes into the interhemispheric fissure to record from the medial frontal lobe and cingulate gyrus or more laterally to record the orbital frontal and lateral frontal cortex. Similarly, medial or lateral occipital or parietal placement is used as needed.

Advantages

Subdural strip electrodes have the same increased sensitivity and lower signal to noise ratio as other intracranial electrodes. Since they do not penetrate the brain, subdural strip electrodes are associated with a lower morbidity rate than depth electrodes. Finally, although mainly performed with subdural grids, cortical mapping by stimulation can also be done with subdural strips when sufficiently represented in adequate locations.

Disadvantages

Restricted sampling

As for all intracranial electrodes, increased sensitivity is obtained at the expense of limited sampling [2,3].

Inaccurate placement

One of the main limitations of subdural strip electrodes is the relative inaccuracy of the placement method. Whereas depth electrodes are inserted with stereotactic guidance such that the trajectory and endpoint can be accurately predicted [15], subdural strip electrodes are 'slid' more or less 'blindly' to targeted areas with uncertainty about final location. Furthermore, placement may be impeded by surgical adhesions related to prior events, deviating the strip from the intended target. Ross et al. [29] reported on the morbidity and efficacy of placement of electrodes in 50 consecutive patients studied with a combination of subdural strip electrodes and depth electrodes. Despite adequate intraoperative fluoroscopic appearance, the subdural strips were found to have penetrated into the temporal white matter in two patients on postimplantation MRI, and two subdural electrodes were found to have entered sulci as well as the parenchyma. Eisenschenk et al. [18] recently reported seven seizures in three of 22 patients with false localization on subdural electrode analysis alone when compared with depth electrode recordings (and verified by postsurgical outcome). After careful retrospective review of the postimplantation MRIs for these three patients, the authors found suboptimal placement of subtemporal subdural electrodes with the most mesial electrode lateral to the collateral sulcus. Furthermore, four additional patients were found to have suboptimal placement of subtemporal subdural electrodes (without resulting in false localization however). Strict precision is not always required, however, and this disadvantage can be limited to some degree by the skill and experience of the surgeon. Furthermore, precise anatomical localization of the contacts obtained by postimplantation MRI allows insightful analysis of recordings.

Surgical complications

In experienced hands, the morbidity of strip electrodes is small (1%) and usually associated with no long-term sequelae [27,30]. Infection is the most common complication, which usually responds to antibiotics, and can be minimized by prophylactic antibiotics and by tunnelling the electrode wires to exit the skin several centimetres from the burr hole incision. Incorporating all wires into a mono-strand cable minimizes CSF leakage. Haemorrhagic complications are extremely rare but have been seen due to the tearing of bridging veins in medial temporal and interhemispheric regions. Cerebral oedema is unusual with strip electrodes. Epileptogenesis is not a concern since there is no brain penetration. Patients complain of some degree of headache, nausea and malaise related to meningeal irritation. Wyler *et al.* [30] reported a general morbidity rate of 0.85% associated with long-term ictal monitoring with subdural strip electrodes in 350 patients (half of whom received continuous antibiotic coverage and half of whom received only one dose of antibiotics on the morning of surgery). The only major complications were infections (two cases of meningitis and three superficial wound infections treated without sequelae, and one brain abscess with permanent left hemiplegia). Rosenbaum *et al.* [17] reported no morbidity or mortality in 50 patients studied with subdural electrodes.

Subdural grid electrodes

Technical aspects

Subdural grid electrodes are flexible sheets of Silastic or Teflon into which are embedded multiple stainless steel, platinum, silver or nichrome electrode contact disks 2–4 mm in diameter and usually spaced 10 mm apart arranged into multiple parallel rows of variable dimension. Grids are approximately 1.5 mm thick and are manufactured in different shapes and sizes. Commonly available designs include 8×8 cm, 8×6 cm and 4×5 and 4×4 cm (Fig. 53.4). Grids can also be trimmed to fit the desired cortical region [1,2,28].

Because of their size, placement of subdural grid electrodes requires a craniotomy. The scalp and bone flaps are tailored to allow grid coverage of all suspected zones of epileptogenicity as determined by non-invasive studies and nearby functional brain, to allow adequate access for surgical resection if such a decision is made, and to avoid cosmetic sequelae. After the dura is opened, the grid is placed under direct visual inspection. Additional strips may

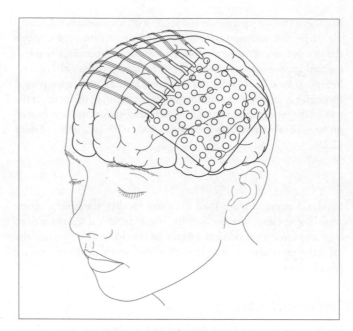

Fig. 53.4 Subdural grid electrode implanted for localization of the epileptogenic zone and functional topographic mapping.

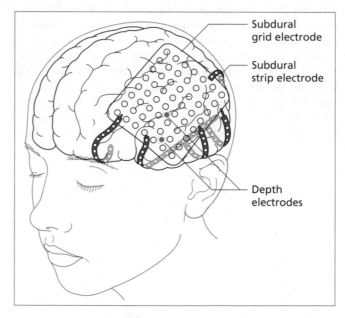

Fig. 53.5 Combined study including a subdural grid electrode implanted through a craniotomy, five additional strips 'slid' beyond the edges of the craniotomy and two depth electrodes inserted freehandedly.

be slid beyond the edge of the craniotomy to cover other suspected regions of epileptogenicity such as the basal frontal, anterior, middle and posterior temporal, temporal occipital and interhemispheric regions (Fig. 53.5). Although grid insertion is usually unilateral, a smaller grid can sometimes be inserted contralaterally. The grid is sutured to the overlying dura mater. The bone flap can be put back or left off especially if the electrodes cover an extensive area of the brain and cerebral oedema is a concern. If the bone flap is replaced, it should be turned in an osteoplastic fashion (i.e. attached to a vascularized muscle and periosteal pedicle) when possible to minimize risk of osteomyelitis from bacterial invasion along electrode cables or from aseptic necrosis. Exit cables are tunnelled under the galea out through a separate stab incision to prevent CSF leakage. The craniotomy site is then closed and the head is wrapped in a sterile bandage [1,2,28].

After implantation, precise localization of contacts with respect to anatomical landmarks as well as verification of grid placement with respect to the epileptogenic lesion is accomplished with MRI. After an adequate number of seizures are recorded and cortical stimulation accomplished (if necessary), the patient is returned to the operating room for the reopening of the craniotomy, removal of electrodes and often resection of the identified epileptogenic zone.

Use

Subdural grids are the intracranial electrodes of choice when the suspected epileptogenic zone overlies or is near functionally critical regions. Brain mapping by stimulation allows identification of crucial areas that should be spared during resection to avoid post-operative functional deficits. Grids are hence useful in many circumstances including (a) definition of a lateral frontal or parietal focus in relation to sensorimotor areas; (b) assessing the localization of a dominant lateral temporal focus with respect to Wernicke's language area; (c) localizing the primary leg motor cortex and the supplementary motor area when the epileptogenic zone lies in the interhemispheric region (mesial frontal or mesial parietal); (d) evaluating the reorganization of functional areas in patients with an epileptogenic cortical developmental malformation; (e) defining the boundaries of the epileptogenic zone in epileptogenic tumours or vascular malformations in relation to underlying functional areas; and (f) mapping of residual epileptogenicity in failed temporal lobectomies using a subdural grid wrapped on the stump to localize the remaining epileptogenic zone and define adjacent speech areas [28].

Advantages

Subdural grids have the distinct advantage of allowing cortical mapping of eloquent cortex. Multiple subdural strips cannot be placed with the same precision to achieve the desired spatial array for ideal mapping [1–3]. Accuracy of placement is not a problem with grids as it is for subdural strip electrodes since insertion is done under direct visual control.

Disadvantages

Restricted sampling

Although the extensive array of electrodes is ideal for mapping, coverage of other regions must be restricted (especially the contralateral region due to technical considerations) so as to limit complications of cerebral oedema.

Surgical complications

Surgical implantation of subdural grid electrodes is associated with a morbidity rate of approximately 4%, weighed towards infection

and cerebral oedema [1–3]. In 1987, van Buren reported on the morbidity of subdural or epidural grids in nine epilepsy centres which had responded to a questionnaire [21]. Out of 228 cases, 10 patients (4.4%) suffered complications including three cases of infection, one case of aseptic bone flap necrosis, four cases of transient rise in intracranial pressure, one case of haemorrhage and one case of increased hemiparesis. Uematsu *et al.* [31] reported two cases of grid-related infections in 28 patients and no other major persistent complications. More recently, Silberbusch *et al.* [32] reviewed the medical records and imaging studies of 51 consecutive patients undergoing 54 craniotomies for subdural grid implantation between 1988 and 1993. Sixteen complications were detected by imaging in 14 patients. Only two patients had clinically apparent manifestations: one patient with tension pneumocephalus and the other with transtentorial herniation and hyponatraemia due to salt wasting. Two patients, although asymptomatic, required treatment for abscess and cerebritis. One patient required premature removal of the grid for aphasia with resolution after removal.

Infection

Infection is the most common surgical complication. Earlier studies have reported incidence rates of 5–14% [3,22]. With additional precautions, this rate has decreased: the bone flap is attached to vascularized muscle flaps, the dura is closed in a watertight fashion, antibiotic ointment is applied, the head bandage is changed daily and prophylactic intravenous antibiotic coverage is implemented perioperatively.

Haemorrhage

Subdural or epidural haemorrhage occur in approximately 2% of patients [3]. Behrens *et al.* [33], however, reported a higher rate of subdural haematoma. Out of 25 patients with grid electrodes (in combination with other types of electrodes), two (8%) had an asymptomatic subdural haematoma and another two (8%) had a symptomatic subdural haematoma with transient hemiparesis. Removal of electrodes and haemorrhage evacuation may be necessary at times.

Cerebral oedema

Occurrence of oedema is directly proportional to the size of the grid and the number of additional electrodes inserted [1–3]. Although the oedema may prompt removal of electrodes, patients rarely sustain permanent deficits.

Neurological deficits

In the absence of obvious cerebral oedema or brain infarction, neurological signs may occur in rare instances. Jobst *et al.* [34] reported a patient who developed right hemiplegia and aphasia 2 days after grid implantation and another patient who returned obtunded following implantation of interhemispheric and right convexity grids. Despite the removal of subdural electrodes in both patients, the former remained dysphasic and hemiplegic for 5 weeks and the latter remained comatose with bilateral intermittent decerebrate posturing. Because both patients had received prior cranial radiotherapy and chemotherapy, authors suggested that the subdural grids had exacerbated some inapparent underlying cerebral tissue damage caused by prior irradiation and chemotherapy. Behrens *et al.* [33] mentioned complications of permanent dysphasia (which later improved partially) following implantation of a subdural grid over the speech area of two patients who had previously undergone surgery of their dominant temporal or frontal lobe.

Impact on recorded signals

The 'blanketing' of cortex by grids may possibly have physiological repercussions on the quality or character of recorded signals. The Yale group have noted delayed electrical seizure onset, an unreasonable incidence of initial electrical charge at the edge of the grid and occasional difficulty in recording spontaneous ictal events at all [1,2].

Combined studies

Technical aspects

Method of insertion will depend on which types of electrodes are used. One will usually take advantage of the craniotomy opening if a subdural grid is necessary to insert the other electrodes. Depth electrodes may need to be inserted freehand with less precision than usual since the craniotomy limits the use of the stereotactic apparel or frameless stereotactic insertion [2].

Use

Over the last decade, combination studies have become the standard for intracranial studies (Fig. 53.5).

Temporal lobe epilepsy

Studies have shown increased sensitivity of depth electrodes over subdural strips for seizures originating from MTL structures, although multiple subdural strips inserted medially enough can obviate the need for depth electrodes. The extent of coverage and the type of electrodes needed over the temporal lobe depends on the situation at hand. Patients with bilateral MTLE who require lateralization more than localization can be studied with intrahippocampal depth electrodes or subdural strip electrodes. In patients where doubt exists about the lateral or medial or anterior or posterior origin of seizures, more widespread coverage of both mesial and lateral structures is necessary. For this, a combination of different types of intracranial electrode is best, such as multiple strips in addition to depth electrodes or a subdural grid with strips and depth electrodes. If there is a concern that the seizures may originate from the frontal region although most non-invasive findings suggest a temporal onset of seizures, one might be inclined to include subdural strips and/or depth electrodes over the ipsilateral frontal region in addition to the electrodes chosen to cover the temporal lobe [2,15].

Extratemporal lobe epilepsy

The same logic applies to extratemporal lobe epilepsies. When it is

unclear if seizures originate from deep or neocortical structures, a combination of depth and subdural electrodes is required. If the epileptogenic zone lies near eloquent cortex, the combination should include a subdural grid.

Advantages

The main advantage of combined studies is more thorough sampling [2]. The advantages of each different type of electrode are synergistically combined.

Disadvantages

Studies combining depth and subdural strip electrodes have not shown a significant difference in morbidity or mortality compared to either alone. (a) Out of 70 patients, van Veelen and Debets [35] reported only one patient (1.4%) with possibly permanent neurological deficit related to an intracerebral haemorrhage and 4.2% transient complications. (b) Out of 50 patients, Ross *et al.* [29] reported one extra-axial haematoma and another asymptomatic temporal pole haematoma. (c) Out of 141 patients, van Roost *et al.* [16] reported 0.7% of permanent neurological deficits and an overall morbidity rate of 5.7% with three cases of meningitis, one occipital brain prolapse through the burr hole, three subcortical haemorrhages not requiring intervention but leading to persisting enlargement of a pre-existing visual field deficit in one and resulting in slowly reversible amnesia in another.

Morbidity may be higher when the combination study includes a subdural grid. Luders *et al.* [36] reported one symptomatic subdural haematoma and one case of CSF pleocytosis out of 26 patients studied with subdural grid and strip electrodes. Spencer *et al.* [19] reported only one serious complication—diffuse cerebral oedema—in 47 patients studied with a combination of depth, subdural strip or grid electrodes. Behrens *et al.* [33] reported 0.7% of permanent neurological complications and 2.9% of transient surgical complications out of 279 invasive diagnostic procedures using various combinations of strip, grid and depth electrodes: four meningitis, four subacute subdural haemorrhages related to grids associated with transient hemiparesis in two, and two cases of permanent dysphasia (which later partially improved) when the subdural grid was placed over the speech area of patients who had already undergone previous surgery of their dominant temporal or frontal lobe. Out of 38 patients studied with various combinations of grid, strip and depth electrodes, Wiggins *et al.* [37] reported no permanent morbidity, individual cases of atrial fibrillation, pulmonary oedema, epidural haematoma and transient fever with negative cultures. The authors also found positive cultures in five patients (13.2%), three of which were symptomatic (7.9%). Of note, all positive cultures were found in intracranial studies done prior to 1997 when their institution had not yet started using antibiotics for the whole duration of implantation. Positive cultures correlated with the number of electrode contacts (>100), number of cables (>10), number of scalp cable exit sites and number of days implanted (>14).

Epidural electrodes

Technical aspects

Intracranial recordings with depth, subdural strip or grid electrodes provide a higher signal-to-noise ratio than extracranial electrodes at the expense of potential risks such as haemorrhage or infection. Epidural electrodes are an attractive alternative because placement in the epidural space is associated with fewer complications [38].

Epidural electrodes come in various forms including ball electrodes, bolts, strips, grids, pegs and screws. Epidural strip or grid electrodes are simply strip or grid electrodes which are laid in the epidural space instead of the subdural space. Technical aspects of electrode insertion and management are similar to those of subdural electrodes [1,2,27,38]. Epidural peg electrodes are flexible mushroom-shaped epidural electrodes (Fig. 53.6). After small twist-drilled skull holes are made under local or general anaesthesia, the pegs are inserted through the scalp incision and skull holes until they reach a final epidural position to record from the underlying dura. Pegs can be inserted over any area of the cortical convexity, even over the midline vertex to record from the interhemispheric fissure. If pegs are used over a limited region, the pegs can be inserted under a scalp flap instead of using separate scalp incisions. When used over dural venous sinuses, pegs are inserted into a partial thickness of the skull with a rim of cortical bone preserved. Epidural screw electrodes are 5 mm in diameter, made of titanium and are available in different lengths (18, 22 and 24 mm) (Fig. 53.6). The tip is a blunt disc electrode insulated from the shaft by a 3-mm Silastic sleeve. The electrode may be placed under local or general anaesthesia through a stab incision and a twist-drill hole. The screw is first hand-tightened and then securely anchored with a wrench. When recording is completed, the epidural screw electrodes are removed at the bedside with a wrench.

Use

The main use of epidural strip or grid electrodes has been to allow better definition of the epileptogenic zone in patients who have had prior brain surgeries and in whom subdural adhesions are likely to be found. Once the epileptogenic region is delineated, risky lysis of dense subdural adhesions is only done over that area, leaving uninvolved areas undisturbed. Subdural electrodes or depth electrodes are preferable for mesial structures such as the mesial temporal, mesial frontoparietal or orbitofrontal regions [3].

Epidural peg electrodes were initially designed to determine surgical suitability in patients in whom the exact placement of a subdural grid was uncertain based on non-invasive presurgical studies [27]. Because of limited information, many centres have abandoned this technique [3]. Pegs have also been used as 'sentinel' electrodes to provide negative information, i.e. confirming that seizures do not arise from a certain region. They have also been used in combination with extracranial electrodes or semi-invasive electrodes to provide additional data used to determine if more invasive recordings could be helpful [1].

Epidural screw electrodes have been used to monitor seizures in patients with severe muscle artefacts consistently obscuring the ictal onsets during scalp EEG monitoring.

Advantages

Because they lie in the epidural space and because the dura is not opened, there are fewer risks of serious haemorrhage or infection. Wyllie and Awad reported only one case of asymptomatic brain contusion in 500 consecutive placements of pegs. The risk of bacterial colonization was 22% but with no clinical infection [1,39].

Occasional damage to the underlying dura has been observed but can be minimized by the use of drill guards and careful technique.

Disadvantages

Epidural strips and grids are only useful in sampling the lateral hemispheric convexities and are not suited for patients with suspected epileptogenic areas over basal temporal, orbitofrontal or interhemispheric regions. Furthermore, accuracy of electrode placement is limited by the fact that epidural grids are not as easily slid beyond the edges of a burr hole or craniotomy and that direct visualization of cortical surface is not possible. Cortical stimulation cannot be performed with epidural grids since leaving the dura intact causes tremendous pain from concomitant stimulation of meningeal nociceptive fibres. The exposed dura may be denervated to allow painless cortical stimulation. Goldring and Gregorie [38] noted minimal complications with epidural electrodes but the electrodes were in place for 3 or fewer days. Wennberg et al. [40] reported a case of small intraparenchymal haemorrhage following epidural electrode implantation, resulting in mild aphasia, right hemiparesis and inducing a transient epileptic foci distinct from the region responsible for the patient's stereotypical seizures.

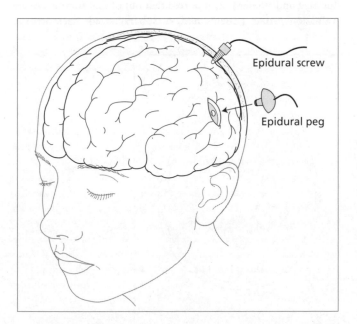

Epidural screw

Epidural peg

Fig. 53.6 A percutaneous epidural screw tightened into a twist drill hole through the cranium and an epidural peg electrode placed in another twist drill hole.

Foramen ovale electrodes

Technical aspects

Foramen ovale electrodes were developed in Zurich in the 1980s [41]. Monopolar electrodes were subsequently modified into multipolar/multicontact electrodes. Several types are available commercially containing from four up to 12 contacts.

These thin electrodes are inserted under local or general anaesthesia. A special cannula is inserted through the cheek and is directed percutaneously under fluoroscopic guidance 5–10 mm below the sella turcica within or near the foramen ovale with the needle tip resting within Meckel's cave cistern [3]. Through the cannula, a thin silver wire multicontact electrode is inserted freehand into Meckel's cave and gently advanced into the ambient or perimesencephalic cistern next to the MTL to allow recording from the anterior and posterior hippocampus, with the proximal contact located in the foramen ovale. The cannula is withdrawn and the electrode is fixed to the cheek by adhesive tape or sutures [3,42]. An electrode is usually also implanted on the other side. This procedure usually takes 30 min to 1 h. A lateral X-ray is used to confirm the subtemporal location of the electrodes and an anteroposterior view to confirm their positions above the incisura trigemini. A CT scan can also be used to verify the location of the electrodes alongside the brainstem [42] (Fig. 53.7).

Use

Because of their site of placement, which allows them to record from the medial aspect of the temporal lobe, foramen ovale electrodes are mainly indicated in patients with temporal lobe epilepsy. Some authors have recommended the use of foramen ovale electrodes in patients with good evidence of bilateral temporal but clearly mesial lobe epilepsy to establish the side of seizure onset mainly because of the relative greater risk of depth electrodes [41]. Foramen ovale electrodes are frequently used in Europe for patients with MTLE and have obviated the use of more invasive intracranial studies in some cases.

Foramen ovale electrodes have been used in combination with subdural strip and/or grid electrodes for better delineation of the epileptogenic zone, or with epidural peg electrodes to determine whether seizures begin from an extratemporal or temporal location on one side, or for patients with vascular malformations near the epileptogenic zone [41,42]. Foramen ovale electrodes have also been used during selective temporal lobe amobarbital memory procedures to assess reliably the amobarbital-induced brain dysfunction. This allows better analysis of data obtained during the selective Wada procedure knowing the time course of inactivation and reactivation of temporal lobe functions following the injection of amobarbital into the bloodstream [42].

Advantages

Foramen ovale electrodes are semi-invasive so they provide a definite advantage over extracranial electrodes and sphenoidal electrodes for the detection of epileptiform activity over MTL structures [41]. Compared to intrahippocampal depth electrodes, the method of insertion is easier and morbidity is lower due to the lack of brain penetration [3]. In patients without clear localization of ictal onset after scalp recordings but clinical and electroencephalographic evidence of MTLE involvement, foramen ovale electrodes can 'streamline' evaluation by confirming and lateralizing their medial temporal origin [41,42].

Disadvantages

Foramen ovale electrodes are less sensitive than depth electrodes for early seizure discharges with significant delay before detection [2]. False lateralization of seizure onset has also been reported [2,43].

Foramen ovale electrodes are not devoid of complications. Zumsteg and Wieser [42] reported that out of 224 foramen ovale evaluations, one patient had a subarachnoid haemorrhage

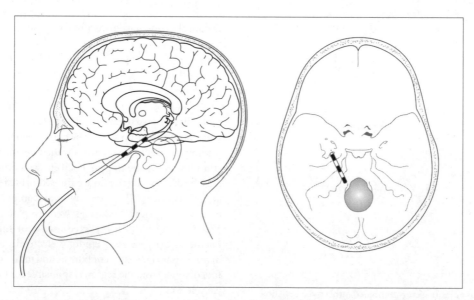

Fig. 53.7 Foramen ovale electrode inserted through the cheek and then the foramen ovale into the ambient or perimesencephalic cistern to lie next to the mesial temporal lobe.

associated with a transient upper pontine syndrome, two had small subarachnoid haemorrhages without neurological deficits and one had brainstem penetration resulting in a transient brainstem syndrome. Awad et al. [44] reported a 2% rate of infection [3]. Other complications include facial bruising and facial pain, which are not uncommon and can be troublesome. Death following electrode insertion has also been recorded.

Foramen ovale electrodes produce facial discomfort in the majority of patients due to irritation of the trigeminal nerve [42,45]. Wieser et al. [41] reported hypaesthesia or dysaesthesia of one corner of the mouth in 9% of patients at their centre. Steude et al. [45] reported a case of transient hypaesthesia which lasted 3 months. From the same series of 39 patients studied with bilateral foramen ovale electrodes, one case of subarachnoid haemorrhage after electrode withdrawal and seven cases of transient herpes simplex on the lips were noted.

Morbidity may be higher in patients evaluated a second time with foramen ovale electrodes. Schuler et al. [46] reported that out of the four patients who failed to be controlled after the first surgery and who underwent a foramen ovale electrode investigation, two suffered a brainstem lesion compared to none of the 55 patients who had the same procedure only once over 3 years at their centre. Although both improved, recovery was incomplete. MRI revealed pontine lesions in both, probably related to misdirected electrodes due to subdural adhesions (as supported by X-ray documentation in one patient).

Cortical stimulation

General comments

Eloquent cortices are areas of the brain which cannot be surgically removed because they subserve important functions. To define these areas, cortical stimulation is often used [47]. It is possible that in the future, fMRI will replace cortical stimulation; available studies already show good concordance. Cortical stimulation involves the passage of a small electrical current through pairs of adjacent contacts, with close observation for symptoms (positive phenomena) or inhibition of, or interference with, cortical function (negative phenomena). Correlation with intraoperative photographs of grids and postimplantation MRI allows the production of a functional map with regards to each electrode position to guide safe resections.

Technical aspects

Electrical stimulation can be performed either intraoperatively or extraoperatively using chronically implanted electrodes.

For extraoperative mapping, stimulation is done by generating trains of electrical pulses at selected pairs of adjacent contacts in an incremental fashion. Stimulation at each site usually consists in 100–300 μs monophasic square wave pulses delivered at 50 Hz at a constant current for a duration of 5 s. A low intensity current (around 0.5–1 mA) is commonly used at first with subsequent increments of 0.5–1 mA until a functional change, after-discharges, clinical seizure or a maximum current of 10 mA is reached (whichever occurs first). Because large currents can evoke local after-discharges, which sometimes propagate, care is taken to detect these after-discharges by monitoring the patient's EEG. Most centres premedicate patients with a small dose of a benzodiazepine prior to cortical mapping to prevent the advent of a clinical seizure which would temporarily end the stimulation session. For the same reason, stimulation is often begun at sites distant from or surrounding the epileptogenic zone when possible to avoid the occurrence of a seizure until the majority of contact pairs has been assessed.

Intraoperative stimulation is usually performed using a handheld device at the end of which are two stimulating electrodes. Because of time restraints, the neurosurgeon will often select a single intensity of stimulation for a particular region and then use the same intensity throughout this region. Although this approach is not optimal, it is usually successful, probably because of greater current densities [47].

Use

Cortical stimulation is used to allow identification of eloquent cortices that need to be preserved during resective epilepsy surgery to avoid postoperative functional deficits. The areas of greatest concern are those subserving hand motor, sensory or language function over the motor and sensory strip and superior temporal language regions. When extensive temporal resections are planned, cortical stimulation to map language areas is required. The use of stimulation techniques when a standard temporal resection is contemplated is more controversial. Although it has been maintained that resection of only the anterior 4–5 cm of temporal tip, sparing the superior temporal gyrus, avoids risk to language, rare aphasias have been reported, albeit transient, and sites identified as essential to language have been reported to be present in that area. This controversy is not so relevant with the recent tendency to perform selective amygdalohippocampectomy with resection of only the anterior 3 cm of temporal tip.

Electrical stimulation can be used to confirm the location of the epileptogenic zone, seeking an area of lower after-discharge threshold and trying to reproduce a seizure. Almost all centres have relinquished this technique as inaccurate compared to spontaneous seizures [48,49]. Although we no longer try to obtain electrically induced seizures voluntarily for localization purposes, one should not simply discard seizures unintentionally obtained during mapping but rather benefit from their analysis. Bernier et al. [49] sought to determine the concordance between the epileptogenic zone as determined by three spontaneous seizures and that determined by electrically induced seizures (auras, seizures and after-discharges) recorded during stimulation of 126 patients with refractory epilepsy. Concordance between spontaneous and induced auras or seizures was >90% with single unilateral foci and less with multiple foci. Stimulation findings reliably predicted the resection area in temporal lobe epilepsies but not in extratemporal epilepsies. A prior study showed a concordance rate of 77% between spontaneous and electrically induced seizures [50].

Advantages and disadvantages

Extraoperative mapping allows testing to be done in greater detail and over a longer period of time using the same subdural electrodes inserted for localization of the epileptogenic zone. Intraoperative mapping is still preferred by some centres because of its flexibility.

Intraoperative stimulation electrodes can be positioned precisely where one wishes. Because the electrodes are small in diameter (1–2 mm), a smaller area of the brain will receive maximal stimulation and thus allows better resolution. Once language mapping is completed, resection can be done while the patient is awake, allowing continuous monitoring.

A global assessment of the patient's condition is required to decide whether intra- or extraoperative cortical stimulation should be used. If long-term monitoring is necessary to delineate the epileptogenic area, if one feels the patient will not tolerate an awake craniotomy, if more time-consuming mapping of language is required, then extraoperative cortical stimulation is preferred. If the epileptogenic zone has already been defined by other criteria such as in patients with tumours or arteriovenous malformations, or in dealing with infants and young children, intraoperative stimulation may be preferred. In infants and young children, cortical stimulation studies are more challenging because of the lack of cooperation and the poor tolerance threshold.

Electrocorticography

Technical aspects

ECoG refers to the intraoperative acute recording of electrical activity directly from the cortical surface. Temporal lobe ECoG can be performed in many different ways using commercial or custom-made electrodes arranged in various montages. The actual method of electrode placement varies widely between institutions. At Yale, we employ an L-shaped 37 contact Silastic grid and two 1×8 contact subdural strips. The grid is placed over the anterior, inferior and lateral temporal neocortex. The first strip is positioned over the middle temporal gyrus and is wrapped around the temporal pole. The second strip is placed over the posterior inferior temporal region [51]. Some use an ECoG headset which consists of a rigid frame anchored at the craniotomy site to allow the surgeon to place individual electrodes according to the anatomy using various reusable cortical contacts attached by springs to pivoting metal arms. Others include acute depth electrodes to sample the amygdala and hippocampus. Others insert a strip in the opened temporal horn after partial resection to sample the hippocampal surface [52]. Extratemporal ECoG is usually performed with an 8×8 subdural Silastic grid placed directly over the epileptogenic lesion or region [53].

The recording equipment is the same as for scalp EEG, preferably using a large number of channels for simultaneously recording from as many contacts as possible (or else adequate sampling requires montage adjustments with prolongation of the recording time). Filters are set at 0.3–70 Hz avoiding 60 Hz notch filters, and sensitivity at 50–75 µV/mm, otherwise clipping of spikes (often 1–3 mV) and excessive amplification of other activity impairs discrimination. Reasonable pre- and postexcision sampling requires up to 20 min each, depending on spike frequency.

Intraoperative ECoG can be performed under local anaesthesia with the patient fully awake or under general anaesthesia [55]. Some authors prefer recordings obtained in awake patients because general anaesthesia can affect the quality of the ECoG survey. General anaesthesia using drugs such as barbiturates, benzodiazepines and inhalational agents (halothane, high-dose isoflurane and nitrous oxide) can suppress epileptiform activity. Propofol can also attenuate or suppress epileptiform activity at sedative doses although some have also reported activation. Local anaesthesia avoids these problems but is technically more difficult and arduous for children.

Many centres are moving towards the use of 'light' anaesthesia. Pain control is achieved through local anaesthesia and narcotics, which have little influence on spike activity. Sedation can be achieved with benzodiazepines, barbiturates or propofol early in the procedure, but these short-acting anaesthetics are discontinued many minutes before and withheld during recording with ECoG to minimize their detrimental effect on interictal activity. A majority of epilepsy centres employ low-dose isoflurane for its lack of proconvulsant activity and absence of deleterious effect on interictal activity at very low concentrations. No premedication is given prior to induction with thiopental and fentanyl. Nitrous oxide, which potentiates the anaesthetic effect of isoflurane, is not used. If used, it should be discontinued 30–50 min prior to ECoG [54].

Following resection, a postexcision ECoG survey can be carried out with attention to cortical areas surrounding the excised region in extratemporal epileptogenic processes and cortices of the three temporal gyri posteriorly beyond the confines of the lobectomy, the stump of the hippocampus, the parahippocampal gyrus and the insular cortex in temporal lobe epileptogenic processes [1,2].

Use

Because seizures are rarely obtained during ECoG, on-line interpretation relies on interictal activity. However, spikes might be rare or absent, widespread and multifocal, be only a partial representation of the epileptic activity, consist of propagated spikes, 'injury spikes' due to surgical manipulation or postexcisional activation spikes. Despite these interpretative limitations, ECoG is used by many centres to guide the extent of resection. It is theoretically assumed that the irritative zone delineated by interictal activity from all recorded sites will contain within its limits the epileptogenic zone. The irritative zone, while probably (but not always) containing the epileptogenic zone, may be much more widespread, even bilateral or multifocal, limiting the usefulness of ECoG [52,53]. Removal of a large irritative zone extending well beyond the confines of a lesion or the suspected area of epileptogenesis may not be feasible or may result in unnecessarily large resections.

Temporal lobe epilepsy

Controversy exists regarding the need for intraoperative ECoG in guiding temporal lobe resections. Several studies suggested that postresection ECoG findings correlated with outcome [55,56] while other reports failed to reproduce these findings [51,53,57]. Moreover, some contend that only certain postresection ECoG spikes should be analysed by specific regions: (a) anterior hippocampal spikes and not neocortical spikes in MTLE [58]; (b) persisting spikes far from the resection margins and not 'injury' spikes at the resection margins [53,55]; and (c) independent spikes and not synchronous spikes [52].

Frontal lobe epilepsy

The significance of residual ECoG spikes after frontal lobe surgery is uncertain. One study suggested that surgical failure was more likely in the presence of large epileptogenic zones and postexcisional residual spiking [59]. However, a recent study [60] specified that only persistence of seizure patterns (and not sporadic ECoG spikes) was associated with poor surgical outcome. Not surprisingly, these seizure patterns were found mainly in patients with cortical dysplasia, reproducing findings by Palmini et al. [14].

Structural lesions

The value of intraoperative ECoG in planning resection of structural lesions such as tumours and arteriovenous malformations is also controversial. In a comprehensive review of 100 brain tumour patients with epilepsy at the Montreal Neurological Institute from 1945 to 1960, Gonzalez and Eldridge [61] found that resection including surrounding epileptogenic foci on ECoG was necessary to offer patients complete cure of their seizures. More recent studies have promoted wide resections to include spikes in the surrounding tissue as well as the lesion [13]. Other studies found that lesionectomies were sufficient. Goldring et al. [62] reported 80% seizure freedom with this technique. Cascino [63] reported 80% improvement in seizure control in 86% of patients undergoing stereotactic lesionectomy. Tran et al. [53] showed that spikes occurring in tissues surrounding a tumour are common and do not affect the seizure outcome.

Clearly a diversity of opinion exists regarding the usefulness of ECoG and there are no conclusive data to resolve these controversies.

Procedural issues and interpretation of invasive EEG recordings

Recording sessions

Sixty-four or more channels of simultaneous EEG recording are required for adequate display and interpretation of the information. In combined studies or studies involving more than 10 subdural strips, 128 channels are preferred. The simultaneous recording of behaviour and EEG using digital recording equipment allows considerable flexibility for EEG interpretation since reformatting and display of recordings can be made in referential or bipolar montages, with any desired electrode combinations, and at different filter settings. Review of synchronized clinical and electrophysiological data is critical for interpretation since one suspects electrodes might be recording spreading epileptic activity instead of actual onset of epileptic activity when clinical symptoms precede the first ictal rhythms on available recordings [1,2,15].

In order to record an adequate number of seizures in a limited time frame, several activation procedures may be used such as sleep deprivation, physical exertion and medication withdrawal. Studies assessing the reliability of antiepileptic withdrawal seizures have suggested that carbamazepine, phenytoin and valproate withdrawal seizures are equally localizing as spontaneous seizures, but that barbiturate and benzodiazepine withdrawal seizures have the potential to be falsely localized [64]. The newer antiepileptic drugs have not been assessed in this regard.

Although there are no strict rules, most centres agree that at least three seizures are required to be reasonably assured of the repro-

ducibility and exclusivity of an epileptogenic zone. It is unknown whether auras, simple partial, complex partial or subclinical seizures are sufficient for localization. In Sperling and O'Connor's series [65] of 40 patients implanted with bilateral temporal depth electrodes and subdural grids, 58% of patients had 352 subclinical seizures and 50% had 117 auras/simple partial seizures. All subclinical seizures arose from the temporal lobe (345 in the hippocampus and seven in the temporal neocortex) usually having the same origin as complex partial seizures (14 of 16 patients with complex partial seizures in the temporal lobe had subclinical and complex partial seizures arising from the same region) but not always. Interestingly, of the patients whose seizures were localized to a temporal lobe, those with subclinical seizures were more likely to be free of complex partial seizures after temporal lobectomy than those who did not have subclinical seizures. The localizing implications of subclinical seizures in extratemporal epilepsy have not been established. Seizures that occur earlier or later during the recording session have the same level of accuracy for localization purposes. Recording sessions may last from 3 days to 4 weeks but most longterm intracranial monitoring sessions average 2 weeks. Long-term monitoring sessions with subdural grids tend to be lengthier than those with other intracranial electrodes.

General comments

Considering that intracranial studies have been around since the 1960s, it is remarkable that so little has been written on their proper interpretation. Few systematic studies of morphology, frequency, extent, spread and termination of intracranial epileptic activity in different cerebral locations have been published. We still rely on old-fashioned 'pattern recognition'. Correlation of signal characteristics with surgical outcome is biased by variable selection criteria. Over the last quarter of century, a set of rules for the interpretation of intracranial recordings has partly been achieved for medial temporal lobe epilepsies, whereas interpretation of extrahippocampal epilepsies remains rudimentary [1,2,15].

Background

Background activity recorded by intracranial electrodes conforms to rhythms detected by extracranial electrodes. Commonly encountered normal patterns include occipital alpha rhythm, central mu rhythm, frontal beta predominance, lambda waves and sleep spindles. Because of the loss of frequency filtering from scalp and skull and because recordings are made from a small volume of tissue, the waveforms appear sharper and higher frequencies are found, at times mistaken for epileptiform activity by inexperienced readers [2,15]. For instance, mu rhythm can take a particularly sharp high-amplitude appearance which may be erroneously interpreted as epileptiform activity although its regularity, lack of propagation, lack of clinical ictal activity, response to sleep and activity and typical central location should serve to define its nature accurately.

Other rhythms, albeit only seen on intracranial recordings, are also probably normal. Hippocampal spindles detected by depth electrodes and an alpha-like pattern recorded over temporal neocortex called the 'third rhythm' are two such examples [66]. The latter is seen in the awake state, in drowsiness and occasionally in light sleep, and does not show a blocking response. Recognition of these rhythms unique to intracranial studies minimizes localization errors.

Non-epileptiform findings

Apart from bitemporal depth or strip electrode studies, asymmetry can rarely be assessed in tailored intracranial studies. If asymmetrical activity is defined, it has the same implications as extracranial studies. Slow-wave foci are commonly found over previously identified structural lesions. *De novo* or progressive or unexpected asymmetrical or localized flattening or focal slowing may suggest progressive haemorrhage, fluid collection or infection [1,2,15]. Haemorrhage following electrode insertion has been noted to induce not only focal slowing but also focal periodic epileptiform discharges and even transient epileptogenic foci [40].

With hippocampal depth electrodes, disturbances of background activity may at times occur in the absence of any structural lesion, manifested by a mild transient increase in slow activity, rarely localized, gradually dissipating over the first or second day of implantation and tentatively explained by electrode insertion injury or anaesthetic effects [15]. The independent localizing significance of intracranial background abnormalities has not been studied rigorously.

Interictal EEG

Intracranially recorded interictal activity may differ from extracranially recorded activity in many aspects. The morphology of interictal spikes differs in regard to its higher amplitude, steeper slope and briefer duration [1,2]. When spikes share time, phase and morphology along an electrode, it is reasonable to assess the spike generator by looking for phase reversals on bipolar montages or the spike of highest amplitude on referential montages. However, interictal activity is much more widespread in intracranial EEG [2,15]. Spikes from multiple locations with various morphologies and polarities are often observed in individual patients. The presence of multiple phase reversals along an electrode makes it difficult to know whether one or multiple foci exist. Distinction between propagated spikes and focal spikes is difficult when spikes appear diffusely. The occurrence of multiple divergent spike populations in patients despite a single epileptogenic zone as proven by seizure freedom following surgical resection has led to the minimization of their use for localization purposes and it is generally believed that localization of the epileptogenic region on intracranial EEG should rely on ictal studies far more than interictal spike analyses. Reports vary on the concordance of the predominant spike focus with the ictal onset focus.

Possibly related to anaesthetic effects, interictal epileptic discharges appear to be less frequent immediately postoperatively [15,67]. Interictal epileptic activity also varies with different physiological states [67]. Many patients have maximal spike frequency during slow-wave sleep and decreased spike activity in REM sleep. Variability seems to be greater with frontal lobe interictal activity and less within the epileptogenic region. Absence or paucity of interictal spiking is not known to be a negative prognostic factor for ictal onset localization [2].

Medial temporal lobe epilepsy

Interictally, intracranial recordings reveal medial temporal spikes in >95% of patients. Supporting the concept that hippocampal sclerosis is a bilateral disorder, up to 80% of patients will have bilateral independent interictal discharges [6–8]. Even in patients who will subsequently be found to have unilateral onset of seizures, at least 50% will show bilateral spike distribution [6,7].

There is some indication that a more quantitative rather than qualitative approach to interictal spike analysis (allowed by the advent of computerized spike detection) may provide additional localizing information. Most studies of spike frequency have noted an increase in the postictal period possibly more in the specific area of ictal onset [67,68]. Two types of hippocampal spikes have been isolated in simultaneous scalp, depth, subdural and sphenoidal electrode studies: one detected by surface or sphenoidal electrodes which is associated with an inferior temporal or vertical dipole with positive polarity in the hippocampus and negative polarity over the inferior temporal neocortex; the other more spatially restricted, associated with negative polarity in the hippocampus [68]. Electropositive hippocampal spikes seem to increase preictally, while electronegative hippocampal spikes seem to increase postictally. Recently, Hufnagel *et al.* [69] gave further evidence of the usefulness of intracranial interictal spike quantification by reviewing electrocorticograms of 32 patients studied with depth and subdural electrodes. The authors found that the location of the earliest spike of one cluster of interictal discharges was exactly at the electrode of seizure onset or ≤2 cm away in 84% of patients and that the higher averaged amplitude of all clusters was located at the site of seizure onset or ≤2 cm away in 75% of patients. The authors also confirmed some prior notions: (a) the predominant spike focus is not always the ictal focus since the highest spike frequency was congruent with the site of seizure onset (or ≤2 cm away) in only 53%; and (b) removal of all brain areas showing spike clusters is unnecessary since there was no evidence for decreased surgical outcome in patients with several multilobar or bihemispheric spike clusters.

Extrahippocampal epilepsies

A variety of intracranial interictal epileptic discharges may be found, some focal, others widespread. Their significance remains unclear. Some value this information to determine the extent of surgical resection and are strong proponents of intraoperative ECoG. These proponents cite studies showing that persistence of epileptiform discharges seen after resection is associated with poor outcome [14,70]. Others cite studies denying an association with the ictal onset zone [53,57]. Part of the reason for the conflicting results on the value of interictal activity may be related to the limited amount of time and sampling available. Whether interictal activity as assessed during long-term monitoring can be useful has been assessed by Bautista *et al.* [71] who reviewed intracranial recordings of patients undergoing extrahippocampal resection. Their study showed that the spatial extent of extrahippocampal interictal epileptiform discharges is important. Patients with widespread discharges extending beyond the limits of the resection continued to do poorly after surgery, even if the region of ictal onset was resected. Conversely, patients with focal discharges included in the surgical field of resection did well following surgery. Accumulating evidence indicates that interictal extrahippocampal epileptiform discharges are important because they provide insight into the extent of pathological abnormalities. Patients with extrahippocampal epilepsy due to structural lesions tend to have more focal interictal discharges (and a better outcome) whereas those with less restricted lesions such as cortical dysplasia or encephalomalacia tend to have more variability in the extent of spiking and poorer surgical outcome. In the latter group, interictal discharges are not necessarily contiguous to the lesions as seen on structural imaging studies. Interictal epileptiform discharges may be a more accurate estimate of the extent of these pathologies than current structural imaging studies.

Ictal EEG

Identification of the earliest EEG change during the seizure is the most crucial step for localization. This is more easily said than done. First, one must assume that the intracranial electrodes implanted cover the area where seizures originate. It is not yet possible to determine with certainty if the first recorded signal represents the seizure origin or ictal activity that has propagated to the recording electrode unless clinical manifestations precede first electrographic changes. Second, there is no consensus on what constitutes an appropriate definition of seizure onset: (a) Five seconds of high-amplitude spikes? (b) Paroxysmal rhythmic sustained activity? (c) Significant change of electrical activity with spike attenuation or rhythmic change? Confusion worsens with recent evidence suggesting that epileptic seizures may begin hours in advance of clinical onset [72]. Although mechanisms underlying seizure generation are traditionally thought to occur over seconds to minutes before clinical seizure onset, quantitative EEG changes occurring up to 7 h before seizures have been reported.

We currently consider a pattern to be ictal based on traditional terms. Clues include: (a) a sudden change in baseline activity; (b) rhythmicity; (c) focality; (d) higher frequency at onset; (e) sustained presence (tens of seconds); (f) evolution of frequency, amplitude and spatial distribution; and (g) presence of ictal behaviour. An exception to these rules includes the electrodecremental pattern with loss or flattening of background activity. A variety of EEG patterns occurs at the onset of seizures whether they are recorded from deeper structures or cortical surfaces, with variable morphology, frequency and even location.

Medial temporal lobe epilepsy

Preictal stage A preictal stage, characteristic of hippocampal epileptogenesis, has been found in > 70% of patients with MTLE and MTS studied with depth electrodes [73]. This preictal stage consists of periodic sharp waves or spikes occurring in a rhythmic fashion with a frequency of < 2 Hz lasting from 5 to over 100 s confined to the hippocampus, and transitioning into an ictal pattern characterized by the superimposition of a 10–15 Hz activity over the same electrode contacts. This periodic spiking was found to be directly correlated with reduced neuronal counts in the CA1 subfield, inversely with glial density in CA2/CA3 and absence of synaptically evoked inhibition in hippocampal slice preparations [5,74].

Onset Hippocampal seizure onset usually presents with one of two patterns. The first pattern consists of a high-voltage 10–16 Hz paroxysmal rhythm which is superimposed over the characteristic preictal slow 1–2 Hz periodic spike activity described above [73] (Fig. 53.8). This hippocampal preictal spiking and the initial ictal discharge as demonstrated on intrahippocampal depth electrodes can often be minimally reflected in basal and lateral subdural strip electrode contacts [75]. The second pattern begins as a low-voltage, high-frequency discharge, without the preictal spiking [73] (Fig. 53.9). This pattern is commonly seen in both hippocampal depth electrode contacts and basomedial subdural strip electrodes recording from the entorhinal cortex. Furthermore, propagation is faster to adjacent temporal cortex than with the first pattern [73,76].

1 Morphology: these two ictal onset morphologies can vary in the same patient even when the location of discharge at seizure onset is consistent [77]. Patients may exhibit one or both types of patterns, occurring in combination or following one another [2].

2 Frequency: analyses of frequency with respect to neuropathological findings have yielded conflicting results with some [78] showing that frequencies >13 Hz were correlated with MTS whereas slower frequencies were correlated with normal tissue, while others did not [79]. Comparative analyses of frequency have revealed that (a) temporal neocortical seizure onsets have significantly faster frequencies (usually >35 Hz) than hippocampal ictal onsets (usually 10–15 Hz); (b) seizures of hippocampal onset which later appear over the temporal neocortex have lower onset frequencies than seizures of simultaneous medial and lateral onsets (12 Hz vs. 23 Hz); (c) the onset frequency of hippocampal seizures is always higher than the frequency of hippocampal seizures resulting from their contralateral spread (11 Hz vs. 15 Hz) [80,81]; and (d) the onset frequency and maximal frequency (at any time during a seizure) is higher when amygdala and hippocampal structures are part of a small epileptogenic zone than when they are part of a large zone [82].

3 Location: there is variability in the exact medial temporal location of onset, ranging from variations in one to two adjacent depth electrode contacts to a widespread regional pattern involving mesial and lateral temporal regions, as well as the length of the hippocampus. Between 20 and 50% of seizures in patients with MTLE arise focally from the hippocampus, 6–20% from posterior hippocampus, 5–10% from the amygdala and 2–5% from lateral neocortex [73].

This variability in morphology, frequency and location suggests that seizures might begin in different parts of a medial temporal lobe circuit or loop between entorhinal cortex and hippocampus [77].

Propagation Most hippocampal-onset seizures (60%) propagate initially to ipsilateral temporal neocortical areas, with variable subsequent involvement of contralateral temporal and frontal lobe regions [73,83]. As adjacent entorhinal and temporal neocortex are recruited, a synchronous and regular 5–9 Hz ictal rhythm evolves that is readily seen in subtemporal and anterior temporal scalp EEG electrodes [84]. About 25–30% of hippocampal-onset seizures will spread first to the contralateral hippocampus and the remaining 10% of seizures involve the contralateral hippocampus and ipsilateral temporal neocortex simultaneously [83]. Long propagation time from one hippocampus to the other (>8–50 s) correlates with excellent outcome after MTL resection [76,85]. Spencer *et al.* [76] reported an inverse correlation between interhippocampal seizure

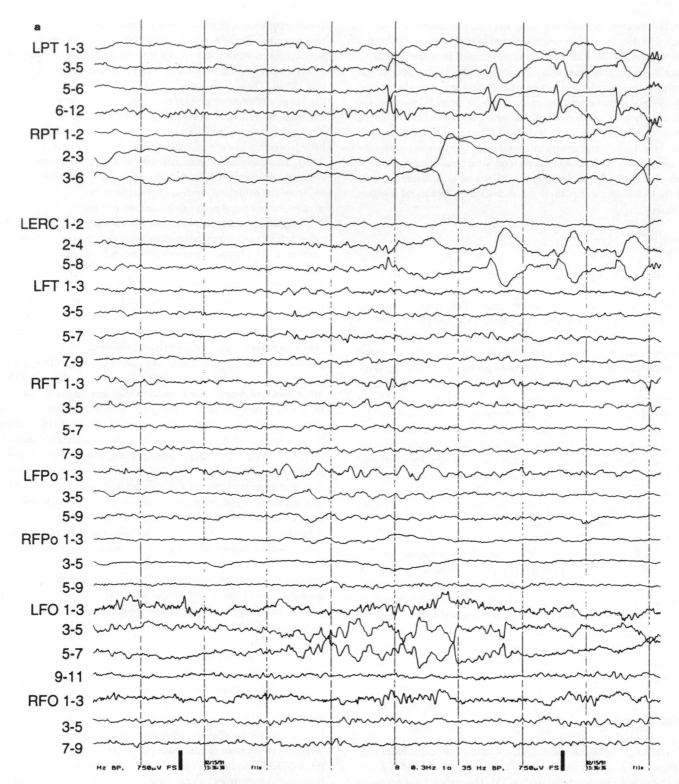

Fig. 53.8 Continuous depth and subdural EEG recording of a spontaneous seizure with a typical medial temporal lobe onset morphology characterized by periodic high-amplitude sharp waves preceding lower-voltage fast discharge. This is seen optimally in LPT 3–5, 5–6 (left hippocampal depth-electrode middle contacts) but also in left entorhinal cortex depth electrode (LERC 2–4, 5–8). LFT, RFT, LFPo, RFPo, LFO, RFO, left and right frontotemporal, frontopolar and fronto-occipital subdural strips placed from frontal burr holes and labelled distal (1) to proximal. Full-scale 750 μV; each division, 1 s. Reproduced with permission from [1].

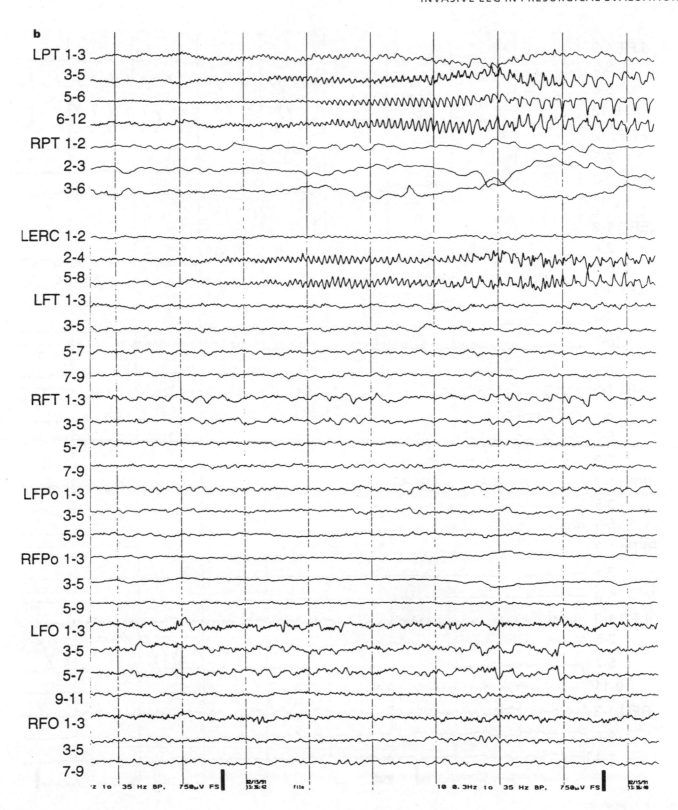

Fig. 53.8 *Continued.*

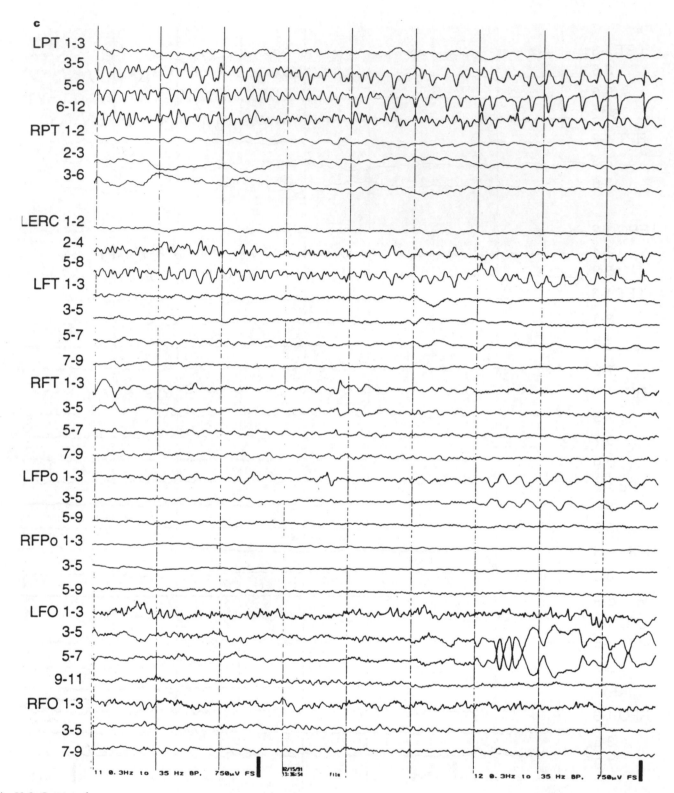

Fig. 53.8 *Continued.*

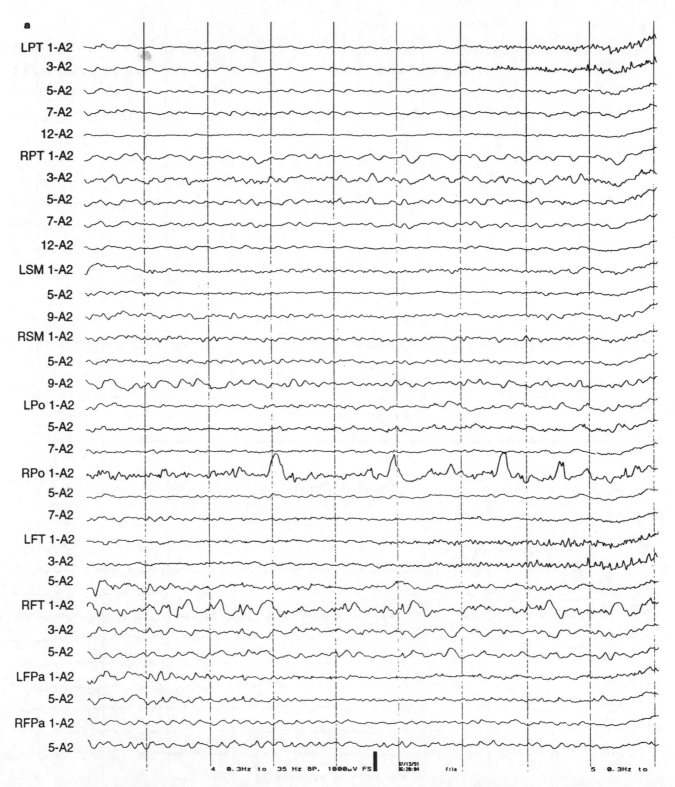

Fig. 53.9 Another typical medial temporal seizure onset pattern is seen in these continuous EEG segments as low-voltage fast discharge in LPT 1, 3 (left depth electrode contacts at tip). Simultaneous seizure onset of similar morphology is identified in distal contacts of left temporal subdural strip (LFT 1, 3) overlying entorhinal cortex. Electrode contacts are labelled from distal (1) to proximal. LPT, RPT, left and right hippocampal depth electrodes; LSM, RSM, supplementary motor subdural strips; LPo, RPo, LFT, RFT, LFPa, RFPa, left and right frontopolar, frontotemporal and frontoparietal subdural strips. Full-scale 1000 μV; each division 1 s. Reproduced with permission from [1].

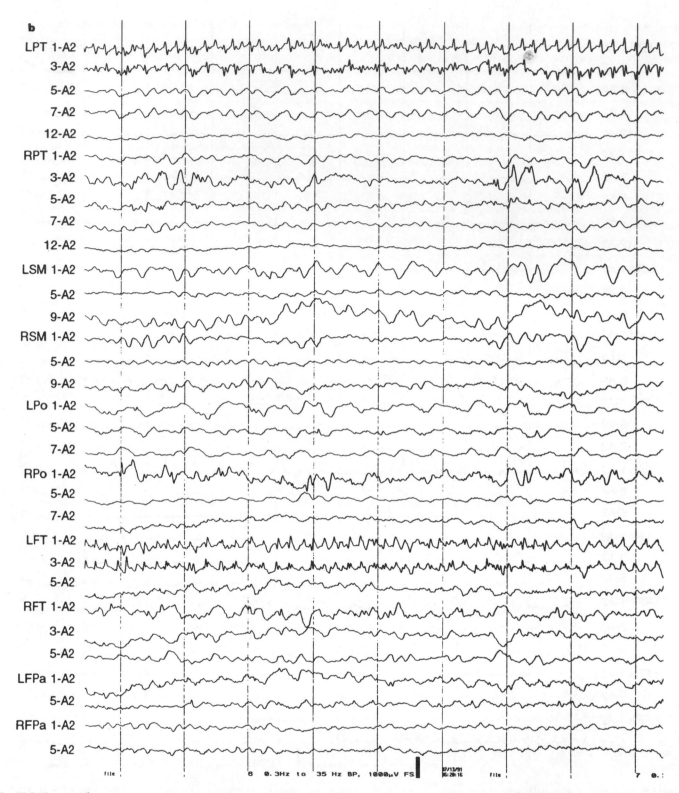

Fig. 53.9 *Continued.*

propagation time and cell counts in the CA4 region of the hippocampus, supporting the concept that longer interhippocampal propagation time is a characteristic of MTLE with MTS.

Termination There are three typical patterns of termination: sudden cessation of seizure activity diffusely or focally; gradual decrease in frequency and increase in amplitude, usually focally; and decreased frequency of a burst-suppression-like pattern, usually diffusely. Spencer and Spencer [86] reported on 50 patients with TLE operated on and monitored for >1 year. Patients who were seizure free after surgery had a significantly greater proportion of their recorded seizures terminating in the onset location (67%) than did patients with persistent seizures (36%, P <0.01). The seizure-free patients also had a significantly lower proportion of seizures with localized termination somewhere other than the onset site (13%) than did patients with persistent seizures (45%, P <0.005). In contrast, Brekelmans *et al.* [87] published a study of 44 surgically treated patients with refractory TLE in which intracranial seizure-offset patterns were unreliable in predicting seizure outcome.

The start–stop–start phenomenon Blume and Kaibara [88] first described this pattern of apparent abortive ictal signal in subdurally recorded seizures (Fig. 53.10). The start phase is defined as rhythmic waves, spikes and/or spike/waves compatible with a clinical or subclinical ictus lasting at least 1 s. The stop phase is defined as complete cessation of the ictal discharge or marked voltage attenuation. The restart phase consists of recurrent, sustained electrographic ictal activity usually with ensuing clinical ictal manifestations. The authors found this phenomenon in 23/98 patients (23%) studied with subdural electrodes and stressed the importance of recognizing this phenomenon since the initial start is more reliable in terms of localization due to the wider field of the restart activity or simply incorrect location. Failure to recognize the initial start phase may have mislocalized the actual origin of seizures in 22 of 52 seizures (35%) involving eight of 23 patients (35%) in their study. Proposed mechanisms for this phenomenon include actual brief stop of

seizure activity but restart due to the lack of adequate seizure-terminating factors, or migration of ictal activity to deeper structures or uncovered regions before re-emerging at the restart location. Atalla *et al.* [89] subsequently noted this phenomenon on scalp-sphenoidal recordings as well.

Neocortical temporal lobe epilepsy

Neocortical temporal lobe seizure onsets also vary in terms of onset morphology, discharge frequency, focality, spread pattern and anterior versus posterior location [12]. In some cases, seizure onsets may occur simultaneously in lateral and mesial temporal structures [11]. The most common ictal onset is characterized by a low-voltage high-frequency discharge often associated with a more widely distributed loss of background activity (electrodecremental pattern) and not apparent on simultaneous recorded scalp EEG [12] (Fig. 53.11). The first changes on scalp EEG occur after seizure build-up and manifest as background attenuation or lateralized, irregular, low-frequency (<5 Hz) activity [75,84].

Using high digital sampling and spectral analysis, one study of neocortical electrodecremental ictal discharge revealed significant power in the gamma frequency band (>40 Hz) localized to the region of the seizure focus [90]. Electrodecremental neocortical seizures have also been shown to have restricted areas of ictal DC shift even when the region of voltage attenuation is large [91]. It is unknown if resection of these restricted regions of ictal gamma activity or DC shifts is associated with better surgical outcome in NTLE patients.

Distinct from the highly localized hippocampal spiking in MTLE, neocortical temporal lobe seizure onsets may also be associated with more regional, repetitive, sometimes periodic sharp waves (<5 Hz). A more focal, low-voltage, high-frequency discharge may precede these repetitive potentials and probably represents the true seizure onset [92].

Jung *et al.* [12] analysed ictal intracranial EEG recordings in 31 patients with NTLE to identify features that predicted surgical

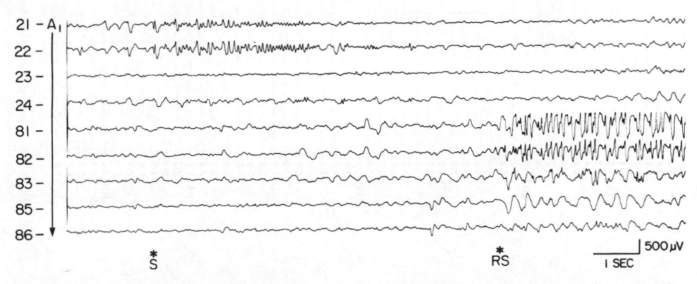

Fig. 53.10 The start–stop–start phenomenon. Sequential rhythmic waves with intermingled spikes occur at right inferior temporal region anteriorly (22,21). These stop completely for 2 s and restart as sequential spikes at right orbital-frontal region (92,81). Reproduced with permission from [88].

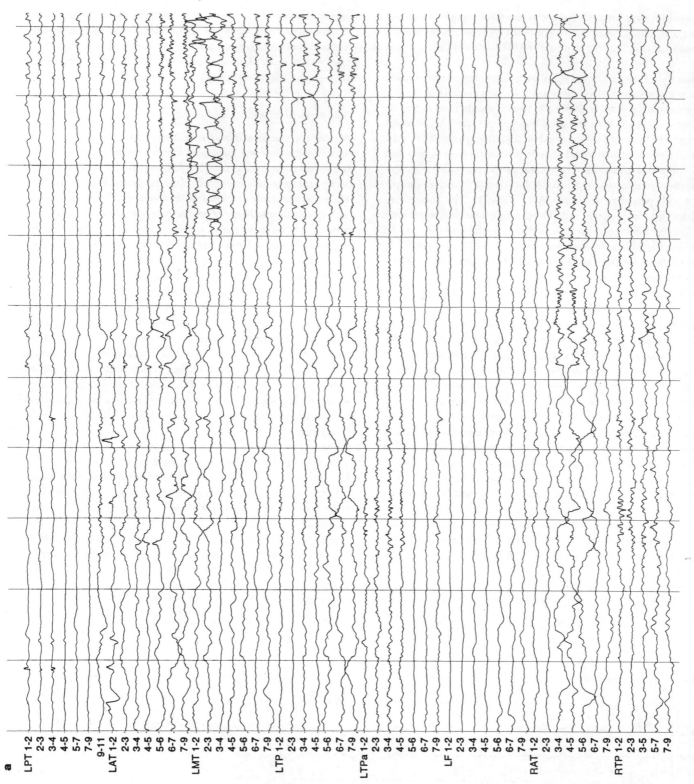

Fig. 53.11 Continuous segments of intracranial EEG during spontaneous seizure activity in lateral temporal lobe. Mixed slow (4 Hz) and low-voltage fast frequencies characterize neocortical seizure onset, seen at LMT 2–3, 3–4 (left mid-temporal subdural strip). LPT, left hippocampal depth electrode; LAT, LMT, LTP, left anterior, mid and posterior temporal subdural strips; LTPa, LF left temporoparietal and frontal strips; RAT, RTP, right anterior and posterior temporal strips. Reproduced with permission from [1].

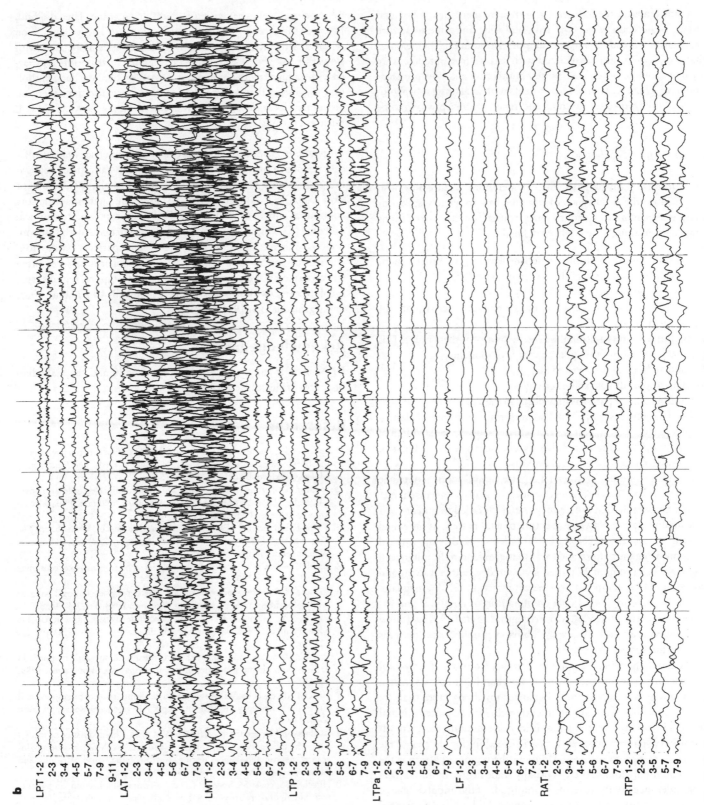

b

LPT 1-2
2-3
3-4
4-5
5-7
7-9
9-11
LAT 1-2
2-3
3-4
4-5
5-6
6-7
7-9
LMT 1-2
2-3
3-4
4-5
5-6
6-7
7-9
LTP 1-2
2-3
3-4
4-5
5-6
6-7
7-9
LTPa 1-2
2-3
3-4
4-5
5-6
6-7
7-9
LF 1-2
2-3
3-4
4-5
5-6
6-7
7-9
RAT 1-2
2-3
3-4
4-5
5-6
6-7
7-9
RTP 1-2
2-3
3-5
5-7
7-9

Fig. 53.11 *Continued.*

outcome amongst the following features: frequency, extent of ictal onset, localization within the temporal lobe and time to seizure propagation outside the temporal lobe. Intracranial EEG features that were significantly associated with seizure-free outcome were focal or sublobar onset, anterior temporal onset and slow propagation time. There was a trend for patients with ictal onset morphologies of slow ictal-onset rhythms and repetitive sharp waves to be seizure free.

Extratemporal epilepsy

Preictal stage Many patients with extratemporal seizure onset also demonstrate the occurrence of periodic low-frequency spikes or sharp waves in the 10s prior to seizure onset, but their correlations or specific meaning have not been defined.

Ictal onset Several patterns of neocortical seizure onset can be observed [93]. Earliest ictal changes may consist of:
1 Low-voltage fast activity, generally >13 Hz.
2 Rhythmic spike, spike-wave or sharp-wave activity in the alpha–theta range.
3 Rhythmic round sinusoidal waves, in the alpha–theta range. This pattern did not show any spike or sharp component.
4 Semirhythmic slow waves <5 Hz.
5 High-amplitude beta spike activity.

Multiple seizure patterns may occur in the same patient. In Lee's series of 53 patients [93], 70% had uniform appearance of electrographic seizures. Low-voltage fast activity was the most common pattern (56.6%), often preceded by one sharp wave, a burst of spikes or an electrodecremental response.

Correlation studies between ictal patterns and surgical outcome have been inconclusive. Wieser considered localized fast discharges to be a favourable sign [94]. Kutsy *et al.* [95] failed to find any significant correlation between structure of ictal pattern at onset and surgical outcome. Schiller *et al.* [96] failed to predict the surgical outcome using the pattern and local spatial extent of the initial ictal discharge in a group of 77 patients who underwent extratemporal resection (34%), temporal neocortical resection (3%), amygdalo-hippocampectomy (54%) or a combination of temporal and extratemporal resection (5%). More recently, Lee *et al.* [93] also failed to show correlation between the above-mentioned ictal patterns with overall surgical outcome.

The size of the epileptogenic zone can vary from (a) a strictly focal pattern (initial changes involving fewer than five to six contacts); (b) to a regional pattern (initial changes involving more than six contacts, usually > 20); (c) or an extremely diffuse pattern (initial changes involving essentially the entire grid simultaneously); or (d) a multifocal pattern at onset (for patients exhibiting shifting of the foci from seizure to seizure). Although the regional pattern is the most commonly found, there is usually some degree of initial focal preponderance usually in terms of amplitude of the initial discharge or small time differences. Against common thinking and findings in temporal lobe epilepsy, Kutsy *et al.* [95] found no statistically significant difference between the size of epileptogenic zone and surgical outcome in extratemporal epilepsies. In Schiller's group [96] of temporal and extratemporal patients, surgical outcome was similar whether patients had focal or widespread initial ictal discharges, with half of patients rendered seizure free. Lee *et al.* [93] also failed

to associate focal onset with a favourable outcome. They did find, however, that spatial distribution at seizure onset had a signification relation with onset frequency, with focal onset associated with slower (usually beta) frequency, and regional distribution associated with gamma frequency at onset, regardless of underlying pathology, suggesting that seizure characteristics are also dependent on anatomical location and network connections (as shown for MTLE seizures previously).

Propagation Propagation may occur by continuous spread to adjacent regions or by non-contiguous spread to distant sites. Propagation may further be subdivided into rapid (usually 50–200 ms) or slow (usually > 10s). Kutsy *et al.* [95] found that patients with slow continuous spread of ictal activity had significantly better surgical outcome (62.5% seizure free) compared to patients with fast continuous spread (23% seizure free) and patients with non-contiguous spread (0% seizure free). Neocortical seizures often spread to medial temporal regions. Whether temporal regions were involved early (within 1–2s) or late (usually 10–40s) had no effect on surgical outcome [95].

Acknowledgements

Dr Nguyen is supported by Epilepsy Canada and the Canadian Institutes of Health Research.

References

1 Spencer SS, Lamoureux DL. Invasive EEG evaluation for epilepsy surgery. In: Shorvon SD, Dreifuss FE, Fish DF, Thomas DGT, eds. *The Treatment of Epilepsy*. Oxford: Blackwell, 1994: 562–88.
2 Spencer SS, Sperling MR, Shewmon DA. Intracranial electrodes. In: Engel J Jr, Pedley TA, eds. *Epilepsy: a comprehensive textbook*. Philadelphia: Lippincott-Raven Publishers, 1997: 1719–47.
3 Wyllie E. Intracranial EEG and localization studies. In: Wyllie E, ed. *The Treatment of Epilepsy: Principles and Practice*, 2nd edn. Baltimore: Williams and Wilkins, 1996: 988–99.
4 Diehl B, Luders HO. Temporal lobe epilepsy: when are invasive recordings needed? *Epilepsia* 2000; 41 (Suppl. 3): 61–74.
5 Spencer SS. Substrates of localization-related epilepsies: biologic implications of localizing findings in humans. *Epilepsia* 1998; 39(2): 114–23.
6 So N, Gloor P, Quesney F *et al.* Depth electrode investigations in patients with bitemporal epileptiform abnormalities. *Ann Neurol* 1989; 25: 423–31.
7 So NK, Olivier A, Andermann F *et al.* Results of surgical treatment in patients with bitemporal epileptiform abnormalities. *Ann Neurol* 1989; 25: 432–9.
8 Hirsch LJ, Spencer SS, Williamson PD *et al.* Comparison of bitemporal and unitemporal epilepsy defined by depth electroencephalography. *Ann Neurol* 1991; 30: 340–6.
9 Williamson PD, French JA, Thadani VM *et al.* Characteristics of medial temporal lobe epilepsy: II. Interictal and ictal scalp electroencephalography, neuropsychological testing, neuroimaging, surgical results and pathology. *Ann Neurol* 1993; 34: 781–7.
10 Hirsch LJ, Spencer SS, Spencer DD *et al.* Temporal lobectomy in patients with bitemporal epilepsy defined by depth electroencephalography. *Ann Neurol* 1991; 30: 347–56.
11 Buergermann GJ, Sperling MR, French JA *et al.* Comparison of mesial versus neocortical onset temporal lobe seizures: neurodiagnostic findings and surgical outcome. *Epilepsia* 1995; 36: 662–70.
12 Jung WY, Pacia SV, Devinsky O. Neocortical temporal lobe epilepsy: intracranial EEG features and surgical outcome. *J Clin Neurophysiol* 1999; 16(5): 419–25.
13 Jooma R, Yeh HS, Privitera MD, Gartner M. Lesionectomy versus electro-

physiologically guided resection for temporal lobe tumors manifesting with complex partial seizures. *J Neurosurg* 1995; 83: 231–6.

14 Palmini A, Gambardella A, Andermann F *et al*. Intrinsic epileptogenicity of human dysplastic cortex as suggested by corticography and surgical results. *Ann Neurol* 1995; 37: 476–87.

15 Spencer SS, So NK, Engel J Jr *et al*. Depth electrodes. In: Engel J Jr, ed. *Surgical Treatment of the Epilepsies*, 2nd edn. New York: Raven Press, 1993: 359–76.

16 Van Roost DV, Solymosi L, Schramm J *et al*. Depth electrode implantation in the length axis of the hippocampus for the presurgical evaluation of medial temporal lobe epilepsy: a computed tomography-based stereotactic insertion technique and its accuracy. *Neurosurgery* 1998; 43: 819–27.

17 Rosenbaum TJ, Laxer KD, Vessely M *et al*. Subdural electrodes for seizure focus localization. *Neurosurgery* 1986; 19: 73–81.

18 Eisenschenk S, Gilmore RL, Cibula JE *et al*. Lateralization of temporal foci: depth versus subdural electrodes. *Clin Neurophysiol* 2001; 112: 836–44.

19 Spencer SS, Spencer DD, Williamson PD, Mattson R. Combined depth and subdural electrode investigation in uncontrolled epilepsy. *Neurology* 1990; 30: 74–9.

20 Sperling M, O'Connor M. Comparison of depth and subdural electrodes in recording temporal lobe seizures. *Neurology* 1989; 39: 1497–504.

21 Van Buren JM. Complications of surgical procedures in the diagnosis and treatment of epilepsy. In: Engel J Jr, ed. *Surgical Treatment of the Epilepsies*. New York: Raven Press, 1987: 465–75.

22 Pilcher WH, Roberts DW, Flanigan HF. Complications of epilepsy surgery. In: Engel Jr J, ed. *Surgical Treatment of the Epilepsies*. New York: Raven, 1993: 565–81.

23 Merriam MA, Bronen RA, Spencer DD *et al*. MR findings after depth electrode implantation for medically refractory epilepsy. *AJNR* 1993; 14: 1343–6.

24 Novelly RA, Augustine EA, Mattson RH *et al*. Selective memory improvement and impairment in temporal lobectomy for epilepsy. *Ann Neurol* 1984; 15: 64–7.

25 Fernandez G, Hufnagel A, van Roost D *et al*. Safety of intrahippocampal depth electrodes for presurgical evaluation of patients with intractable epilepsy. *Epilepsia* 1997; 38(3): 922–9.

26 Loscher W, Honack D, Gramer M. Effect of depth electrode implantation with or without subsequent kindling on GABA turnover in various rat brain regions. *Epilepsy Res* 1999; 37: 95–108.

27 Arroyo S, Lesser RP, Awad IA *et al*. Subdural and epidural grids and strips. In: Engel J Jr, ed. *Surgical Treatment of the Epilepsies*. New York: Raven Press, 1993: 377–86.

28 Luders H, Awad I, Burgess R *et al*. Subdural electrodes in the presurgical evaluation for surgery of epilepsy. In: Theodore WH, ed. *Surgical Treatment of Epilepsy*. Holland: Elsevier Science Publishers, 1992: 147–56.

29 Ross D, Brunberg J, Drury I *et al*. Intracranial depth electrode monitoring in partial epilepsy: the morbidity and efficacy of placement using magnetic resonance image-guided stereotactic surgery. *Neurosurgery* 1996; 39(2): 327–34.

30 Wyler AR, Walker G, Somes G. The morbidity of long-term seizure monitoring using subdural strip electrodes. *J Neurosurg* 1991; 74: 734–7.

31 Uematsu S, Lesser R, Fisher R *et al*. Resection of the epileptogenic area in critical cortex with the aid of a subdural electrode grid. *Stereotact Funct Neurosurg* 1990; 54: 34–45.

32 Silberbusch MA, Rothman MI, Bergey GK *et al*. Subdural grid implantation for intracranial EEG recording: CT and MR appearance. *AJNR* 1998; 19: 1089–93.

33 Behrens E, Schramm J, Zenter J *et al*. Surgical and neurological complications in a series of 708 epilepsy procedures. *Neurosurgery* 1997; 41: 1–10.

34 Jobst BC, Williamson PD, Coughlin CT *et al*. An unusual complication of intracranial electrodes. *Epilepsia* 2000; 41(7): 898–902.

35 Van Veelen CWM, Debets RMC. Functional neurosurgery evaluation and the contribution of subdural and stereotactically implanted depth electrodes in the Dutch Workgroup for Functional Surgery. *Acta Neurochir* 1993; 124: 7–10.

36 Luders H, Hanh JF, Lesser RP *et al*. Basal temporal subdural electrodes in the evaluation of patients with intractable epilepsy. *Epilepsia* 1989; 30: 131–42.

37 Wiggins GC, Elisevich K, Smith BJ. Morbidity and infection in combined subdural grid and strip electrode investigation for intractable epilepsy. *Epilepsy Res* 1999: 37: 73–80.

38 Goldring S, Gregorie EM. Surgical management using epidural recordings to localize the seizure focus: review of 100 cases. *Neurosurgery* 1984; 60: 457–66.

39 Wyllie E, Awad I. Intracranial EEG and localization studies. In: Wyllie E, ed. *The Treatment of Epilepsy: Principle and Practice*. Philadelphia: Lea and Febiger, 1993: 1023–38.

40 Wennberg R, Gross D, Quesney F *et al*. Transient epileptic foci associated with intracranial hemorrhage in patients with subdural and epidural electrode placement. *Clin Neurophysiol* 1999; 110: 419–23.

41 Wieser HG, Quesney LF, Morris HS. Foramen ovale and peg electrodes. In: Engel J Jr, ed. *Surgical Treatment of the Epilepsies*. New York: Raven Press, 1993: 331–9.

42 Zumsteg D, Wieser HG. Presurgical evaluation: current role of invasive EEG. *Epilepsia* 2000; 41 (Suppl. 3): 55–60.

43 Binnie CD, Elwes RDC, Polkey CE *et al*. Utility of stereoelectroencephalography in preoperative assessment of temporal lobe epilepsy. *J Neurol Neurosurg Psychiatr* 1994; 57: 58–65.

44 Awad I, Assirati JA, Brugess R *et al*. A new class of electrodes of 'intermediate invasiveness': preliminary experience with epidural pegs and foramen ovale electrodes in the mapping of seizure foci. *Neurol Res* 1991; 13: 177–83.

45 Steude U, Stodieck S, Schmiedek P. Multiple contact foramen ovale electrode in the presurgical evaluation of epileptic patients for selective amygdala-hippocampectomy. *Acta Neurochir* 1993; (Suppl.) 58: 193–4.

46 Schuler P, Neubauer U, Schulemann H *et al*. Brain-stem lesions in the course of a presurgical re-evaluation by foramen ovale electrodes in temporal lobe epilepsy. *Electroencephal Clin Neurophys* 1993; 86: 301–2.

47 Lesser RP, Arroyo S, Crone N *et al*. Motor and sensory mapping of the frontal and occipital lobes. *Epilepsia* 1998; 39 (Suppl. 4): 69–80.

48 Ojemann GA, Sutherling WW, Lesser RP *et al*. Cortical stimulation. In: Engel J Jr, ed. *Surgical Treatment of the Epilepsies*. New York: Raven Press, 1993: 399–414.

49 Bernier GP, Richer F, Giard N *et al*. Electrical stimulation of the human brain in epilepsy. *Epilepsia* 1990; 31(5): 513–20.

50 Wieser HG, Bancaud J, Talairach J *et al*. Comparative value of spontaneous and electrically induced seizures in establishing the lateralization of temporal seizures. *Epilepsia* 1979; 20: 47–59.

51 Tran TA, Spencer SS, Marks D *et al*. Significance of spikes recorded on electrocorticography in nonlesional medial temporal lobe epilepsy. *Ann Neurol* 1995; 38: 763–70.

52 MacDonald DB, Pillay N. Intraoperative electrocorticography in temporal lobe epilepsy surgery. *Can J Neurol Sci* 2000; 277 (Suppl. 1): 85–91.

53 Tran TA, Spencer SS, Javidan M *et al*. Significance of spikes recorded on intraoperative electrocorticography in patients with brain tumor and epilepsy. *Epilepsia* 1997; 38(10): 1132–9.

54 Kraemer DL, Spencer DD. Anesthesia in epilepsy surgery. In: Engel J, ed. *Surgical Treatment of the Epilepsies*, 2nd edn. New York; Raven, 1993: 527–38.

55 Wennberg RA, Quesney LF *et al*. Increased neocortical spiking and surgical outcome after selective amygdalohippocampectomy. *Electroencephalogr Clin Neurophysiol* 1998; 48 (Suppl.): 105–11.

56 Kanner AM, Kaydanova Y, de Toledo-Morrell L *et al*. Tailored anterior temporal lobectomy. Relation between extent of resection of mesial structures and postsurgical seizure outcome. *Arch Neurol* 1995; 52: 173–8.

57 Schwartz TH, Bazil CW, Walczak TS *et al*. The predictive value of intraoperative electrocorticography in resections for limbic epilepsy associated with mesial temporal sclerosis. *Neurosurgery* 1997; 40: 302–11.

58 McKhann GM, Schoenfeld-McNeill J, Born DE *et al*. Intraoperative hippocampal electrocorticography to predict the extent of hippocampal resection in temporal lobe epilepsy surgery. *J Neurosurg* 2000; 93: 44–52.

59 Salanova V, Morris HH, van Ness PC *et al*. Comparison of scalp electroencephalograph with subdural electrocorticogram recordings and functional mapping in frontal lobe epilepsy. *Arch Neurol* 1993; 50: 294–9.

60 Ferrier CH, Alarcon G, Engelsman J *et al*. Relevance of residual histologic and electrocorticographic abnormalities for surgical outcome in frontal lobe epilepsy. *Epilepsia* 2001; 42(3): 363–71.

61 Gonzalez D, Eldridge AR. On the occurrence of epilepsy caused by astrocytoma of the cerebral hemispheres. *J Neurosurg* 1962: 19: 470–82.

62 Goldring S, Rich K, Picker S. Experience with gliomas in patients presenting with a chronic seizure disorder. In: Little JR, ed. *Clinical Neurosurgery*, Vol. 33. Baltimore: William & Wilkins, 1986: 15–42.

63 Cascino GD. Epilepsy and brain tumors: implication for treatment. *Epilepsia* 1990; 31 (Suppl. 3): 537–44.

64 Marks DA, Katz A, Scheyer R *et al*. Clinical and electrographic effects of acute anticonvulsant withdrawal in epileptic patients. *Neurology* 1991; 41: 508–12.

65 Sperling MR, O'Connor MJ. Auras and subclinical seizures: characteristics and prognostic significance. *Ann Neurol* 1990; 28: 320–8.

66 Niedermeyer E. The 'third rhythm': further observations. *Clin Electroencephalogr* 1991; 22: 83–6.

67 Masuoka LK, Spencer SS. Clinical neurophysiology in epilepsy. *Curr Opin Neurol* 1994; 7: 148–52.

68 Katz A, Marks D, Spencer S *et al*. Human hippocampal spikes of reverse polarity respond differently to seizures and anticonvulsants and antiepileptic drugs. *Epilepsia* 1991; 32 (Suppl. 3): 45.

69 Hufnagel A, Dumpelmann M., Zentner J *et al*. Clinical relevance of quantified intracranial interictal spike activity in presurgical evaluation of epilepsy. *Epilepsia* 2000; 41(3): 467–78.

70 McBride MC, Binnie CD, Janota I *et al*. Predictive value of intraoperative electrocorticograms in resective epilepsy surgery. *Ann Neurol* 1991; 30: 526–32.

71 Bautista RED, Cobbs MA, Spencer DD *et al*. Prediction of surgical outcome by interictal epileptiform abnormalities during intracranial EEG monitoring in patients with extrahippocampal seizures. *Epilepsia* 1999; 40(7): 880–90.

72 Litt B, Esteller R, Echauz J *et al*. Epileptic seizures may begin hours in advance of clinical onset: a report of five patients. *Neuron* 2001; 30: 51–64.

73 King D, Spencer S. Invasive electroencephalography in mesial temporal lobe epilepsy. *J Clin Neurophysiol* 1995; 12(1): 32–45.

74 Williamson A, Spencer SS, Spencer DD. Depth electrode studies and intracellular dentate granule cell recordings in temporal lobe epilepsy. *Ann Neurol* 1995; 38: 778–87.

75 Pacia SV, Ebersole JS. Intracranial EEG in temporal lobe epilepsy. *J Clin Neurophysiol*. 1999; 16(5): 399–407.

76 Spencer SS, Marks D, Katz A *et al*. Anatomic correlates of interhippocampal seizure propagation time. *Epilepsia* 1992; 33(5): 862–73.

77 Spencer SS, Spencer DD. Entorhinal–hippocampal interactions in medial temporal lobe epilepsy. *Epilepsia* 1994; 35(4): 721–7.

78 Spencer SS, Guimaraes P, Katz A *et al*. Morphological patterns of seizures recorded intracranially. *Epilepsia* 1992; 33: 537–45.

79 Lieb JP, Engel J Jr, Brown WJ *et al*. Neuropathological findings following temporal lobectomy related to surface and deep EEG patterns. *Epilepsia* 1981; 22: 539–49.

80 Javidan M, Katz A, Tran T *et al*. Frequency characteristics of neocortical and hippocampal onset seizures. *Epilepsia* 1992; 33 (Suppl. 3): 58.

81 Javidan M, Katz A, Pacia S *et al*. Onset and propagation frequencies in temporal lobe seizures. *Epilepsia* 1992; 33 (Suppl. 3): 59.

82 Gotman J, Levtova V, Olivier A. Frequency of the electroencephalographic discharge in seizures of focal and widespread onset in intracerebral recordings. *Epilepsia* 1995; 36(7): 697–703.

83 Spencer SS, Williamson PD, Spencer DD *et al*. Human hippocampal seizure spread studied by depth and subdural recording: the hippocampal commissure. *Epilepsia* 1987; 28(5): 479–89.

84 Pacia SV, Ebersole JS. Intracranial EEG substrates of scalp ictal patterns from temporal lobe foci. *Epilepsia* 1997; 38: 642–54.

85 Lieb JP, Engel J Jr, Babb TL. Interhemispheric propagation time of human hippocampal seizures. I. Relationship to surgical outcome. *Epilepsia* 1986; 27: 286–93.

86 Spencer SS, Spencer DD. Implications of seizure termination location in temporal lobe epilepsy. *Epilepsia* 1996; 37(5): 455–8.

87 Brekelmans GJF, Velis DN, van Veelen CWM *et al*. Intracranial EEG seizure-offset termination patterns: relation to outcome of epilepsy surgery in temporal lobe epilepsy. *Epilepsia* 1998; 39(3): 259–66.

88 Blume WT, Kaibara M. The start-stop-start phenomenon of subdurally recorded seizures. *Electroenceph Clin Neurophysiol* 1993; 86: 94–9.

89 Atalla N, Abou-Khalil B, Fakhoury T. The start-stop-start phenomenon in scalp-sphenoidal ictal recordings. *Electroencephalogr Clin Neurophysiol* 1996; 98: 9–13.

90 Fisher RS, Webber WR, Lesser RP *et al*. High-frequency EEG activity at the start of seizures. *J Clin Neurophysiol* 1992; 9: 441–8.

91 Ikeda A, Terada K, Mikuni N *et al*. Subdural recording of ictal DC shifts in neocortical seizures in humans. *Epilepsia* 1996; 37: 662–74.

92 Ebersole JS, Pacia SV. Localization of temporal lobe foci by ictal EEG patterns. *Epilepsia* 1996; 37: 386–99.

93 Lee SA, Spencer DD, Spencer SS. Intracranial EEG seizure-onset patterns in neocortical epilepsy. *Epilepsia* 2000; 41(3): 297–307.

94 Wieser HG. Data analysis. In: Engel J Jr, ed. *Surgical Treatment of Epilepsies*. New York: Raven Press, 1987: 335–60.

95 Kutsy RL, Farrell DF, Ojemann GA. Ictal patterns of neocortical seizures monitored with intracranial electrodes: correlation with surgical outcome. *Epilepsia* 1999; 40(3): 257–66.

96 Schiller Y, Cascino GD, Busacker NE *et al*. Characterization and comparison of local onset and remote propagated electrographic seizures recorded with intracranial electrodes. *Epilepsia* 1998; 39: 380–8.

54 MEG in Presurgical Evaluation of Epilepsy

H. Stefan, C. Hummel and R. Hopfengärtner

Epilepsy surgery primarily aims to control seizures in pharmaco-resistant epilepsies; in addition, neurological or neuropsychological deficits should be avoided and social integration improved. Before imaging techniques became increasingly important, EEG had been the only functional investigation technique for presurgical evaluation for a long time. The individual determination of the localization and extent of interictal (irritative) and ictal epileptic (seizure onset) brain region is the main task during presurgical evaluation of partial epilepsies. Another important issue concerns the delineation of functionally important areas (e.g. motor, somatosensory, language). Therefore, functionally important areas have to be correlated with the localization of the epileptogenic area.

Since neurosurgical approaches have become routine procedures in the treatment of pharmacoresistant focal epilepsies, the diagnostic challenge culminates in determining the site and extent of epileptogenic tissue to be removed without risk of functional deficits. To this purpose, the combined findings of diagnostic methods may contribute anatomical (CT, MRI), blood flow (SPECT), metabolism-related (PET) and electrophysiological information, the latter comprising long-established non-invasive surface EEG and invasive EEG recordings, and, as a comparatively new method, MEG (magneto-encephalography). MEG being a non-invasive method with high temporal and potentially high spatial resolution, and offering data on electrophysiological phenomena from a point of view somewhat different to the EEG, has been found a potentially useful addition to the pool of techniques applied in preoperative focus localization of pharmacologically intractable epilepsies. As the standard procedure for MEG processing includes corecording with MRI, centres of activity localized from MEG data are usually displayed in the corresponding anatomical images. This particularly advantageous combined technique [1,2] has been labelled 'magnetic source imaging' (MSI).

Focal epileptic activity can be generated both in superficial cortex and in deeper brain regions. The feasibility of localization has to be considered for any given type of focal epilepsy (neocortical or limbic). Basically, a certain amount of cortex has to be involved by epileptic discharges to be accessible non-invasively [3,4]. Therefore, presurgical evaluation requires extensive experience in deciding whether non-invasive interictal or ictal recordings are sufficient for the localization of focal epileptic activity in any individual case, or if invasive recordings have to be carried out in order to improve the accuracy of preliminary non-invasive results.

If the generator is, for instance, located in the hippocampus, non-invasive detection of focal epileptic activity may be difficult or impossible. The distribution of interictal spikes in deep hippocampal electrodes and surface electrodes was analysed by Alarcon *et al.* [3]. The results of this study indicate that single hippocampal dis-charges could not always be detected by scalp EEG, but excision of 'leading regions of spike activity' in the temporal lobe yielded good surgical outcome [5].

According to our experience with simultaneous invasive recordings from hippocampus, temporal basal, mesial temporal and temporal neocortical areas in many patients with cryptogenic temporal lobe epilepsies, hippocampal and parahippocampal or basal areas or inferior temporal gyrus are involved in the epileptic aggregate. Rather frequently we observed spike onset in the entorhinal, parahippocampal cortex and sometimes in the lateral neocortex. Invasive ictal recordings revealed that the entorhinal cortex of the basal temporal cortex itself can be the region of ictal onset [6]. Thus, it may happen that the hippocampus is only secondarily involved in the epileptic excitation process. The epileptic network in such an instant involves temporomesiobasal areas as well as the hippocampus.

As only discharges involving several thousand neurones are assessable non-invasively, only approximated localizations within the neuronal network of the brain are possible. The question arises if magnetoelectroencephalography is able to define 'critical hot spots' in the neuronal network which are necessary and sufficient for seizure generation and control. In the following chapter procedures and applications of MSI in epileptic patients for the detection of focal epileptic interictal and ictal activity and functionally important areas are discussed.

Method

It is well known that activated groups of neurones in the human brain produce electrical potentials which can be recorded with scalp EEG. At the same time, the neuronal activity also produces very small magnetic fields outside the head in the range of 50–1000 fT, which can be detected by MEG. Essential for the assessment of these small magnetic fields are special sensors (superconducting quantum interferometer devices or SQUIDs). In addition, MEG recording is usually performed in a specific shielding chamber to attenuate the influence of external magnetic noise. For technical details about registration and instrumentation of MEG, see [7,8].

MEG is a non-invasive method requiring neither referencing nor direct contact between the recording equipment and the patient's head. Its high temporal resolution in the milliseconds range is comparable to that of the EEG. Due to the use of multichannel systems, and particularly the so-called whole head systems with up to more than 200 sensors, good spatial resolution has also been achieved.

The so-called neuromagnetic 'inverse problem'—the tracing of an unknown source in the brain from magnetic field data recorded outside the head—is approached using special model assumptions concerning the type of underlying source which produces the magnetic field and the shape of the volume conductor. For the determination of the location, orientation and strength of focal activity in the brain, the model of a single equivalent current dipole is often used (with a specific physical feature of magnetic field recording being its 'blindness' to radial portions of the dipoles). However, when sources overlap both spatially and temporally (i.e. in the case of multifocal sources) the approach of a multidipole model might be more appropriate [9–11]. Furthermore, different current density reconstruction approaches (e.g. minimum norm, weighted minimum norm and LORETA) [12,13] are also used for the localization of more extended generators.

As to the volume conductor, besides the most frequently used spherical model, more realistically shaped models are also available (e.g. boundary element method or BEM). In this case, the volume conductor model consists of the three different compartments—brain, skull and skin—assuming that each compartment has homogeneous and isotropic conductivity [14]. The BEM is based upon segmentation of MRI data sets, thus accounting for the individual patient's anatomy.

Clinical aspects of MEG methodology are presented in Stefan and Hummel [15].

Applications of MSI in epileptic patients

Evoked activity

In cases where neurosurgery remains the only therapeutic hope for epileptic patients, it is essential that not only the site of the epileptogenic region be known (see below), but also to determine whether removal of the tissue in question may cause functional deficits.

Recently, functional validation of MSI has been obtained with various sensory modalities, source localization being based upon evoked magnetic responses to repeated stimulation, in accordance with the well-established technique for evoked potentials, averaged over a number of stimulus-related EEG epochs [16].

Evoked magnetic responses to acoustic (AEF) [17,18], visual (VEF) [19,20] somatosensory (SEF) [21] and olfactory (OEF) [22] stimulation can be obtained. Magnetic fields representing motor activity (motor evoked fields, MEF) generated by voluntary finger and limb movements have long been assessed [23,24]. Thus, localization of cortical generators calculated from magnetic evoked activity could become an established tool to provide information about functionally significant areas, and particularly so, if MSI and neurosurgery have access to compatible systems of space coordinates ('neuronavigation' systems are already being established in operation theatres—see Plate 54.1, shown in colour facing p. 670). Using a variety of stimulating sites, SEF localizations illustrate the 'homuncular' organization and its variations of the somatosensory cortex [15,25,26]. It is also possible to localize functional regions for language [27].

Spontaneous activity

An increasing number of publications are dealing with the application of MEG in presurgical evaluation, giving evidence of its capability to localize spontaneous epileptic activity.

Validation of source localizations with respect to the 'true' source is necessary. MEG findings on epileptogenic foci need to be compared with the results of other diagnostic techniques considered as most reliably detecting the epileptogenic brain tissue. Whether ictal video EEG, which is generally regarded as 'gold standard' [28], invasive EEG monitoring or intraoperative ECoG are wanted to check the accuracy of MEG focus localization has to be decided upon in each individual case, depending on other clinical findings. Initial results indicate that MEG indeed yields fairly good accuracy, even though the activity investigated is mostly interictal [29–33].

Eliashiv et al. [34] reported congruency of MEG localizations with other findings of presurgical evaluation in 70–80%. We found a similar percentage (72%) of patients after successful temporal lobe epilepsy surgery with good spatial correlation between predominant focal epileptic activity in MEG and other localization results from presurgical evaluation and intraoperative ECoG [35]. In another study, a comparison of MEG localizations with MRI and various video EEG findings in 58 patients with pharmacologically intractable epilepsy showed that in patients who, after surgery, were seizure free (class 1, according to Engel's classification) or had only rare seizures, MEG was inferior only to subdural video EEG recordings in predicting the epileptogenic zone. MEG was superior to MRI, interictal and ictal non-invasive video EEG and interictal invasive subdural EEG [36]. The data suggest that in temporal and extratemporal lobe epilepsies MEG is at least as effective as the established methods for localizing the epileptogenic region. In a study comparing MEG with PET and SEEG, MEG localizations agreed with PET and SEEG results in seven out of nine patients. If PET and MEG findings agreed, the outcome after surgery was favourable [37].

King et al. [38] reported outcome data (according to Engel's classification) in 19 patients after resection of the primary MEG spike region: 14 patients were grouped in class 1, four in class 2, one was in class 3 and none in class 4. On the other hand, out of 17 patients after resection of tissue with marginal or no relationship to MEG spike localization, only three were in each of the best and second best outcome category, whereas in four cases the outcome ranked in class 3 and a major portion of seven cases were graded in the worst outcome class.

These results indicate that resection of the primary MEG spike focus correlates strongly with excellent outcome. In this context, it seems important to note that MSI dipole localizations are considered neither to represent point-shaped sources with millimetre accuracy nor to yield an outline of the epileptogenic tissue, but rather to indicate centres of epileptic activity, revealing compartmental information on a sublobar level. In many patients with pharmacoresistant focal epilepsies, circumscribed clusters of localizations indicating centres of predominant focal epileptic activity can be found [39]. If MEG localizations in temporal lobe epilepsy showed more than one distinct cluster in different regions, this was interpreted as a hint towards multifocal temporal lobe epilepsy.

Although, in many cases, cerebral MRI of epileptic patients shows abnormal morphology, varying from subtle alterations to extensive mass lesions, abnormal MRI findings are not necessarily epileptogenic, and even if so, it may be important to clarify the relation between anatomical and functional pathology in detail. Furthermore, if there is more than one lesion, those crucial to epileptogenicity must be determined. In a considerable number of patients with neocortical temporal or extratemporal epilepsies, MSI yielded localizations of epileptiform activity in proximity to an epileptogenic structural lesion [31,40].

On the other hand, there is sometimes, prior to surgery, no evidence of morphological pathology associated with epilepsy [41,42]. Although with the availability of new powerful imaging systems, and more sophisticated software to identify discrete alterations, the number of patients with 'cryptogenic' aetiology is decreasing, it is not yet possible to identify a structural abnormality to account for any epileptic focus. The lack of morphological clues renders the functional diagnostic methods more significant. MSI has been found to offer useful source locations of cryptogenic epileptic activity in accordance with other non-invasive results, thus facilitating the detailed planning of invasive procedures and neurosurgical regimen. In a study by Knowlton et al. [40] 11 out of 12 patients without focal abnormality on MRI, MEG discharges were localized to the epileptogenic zone as determined by standard preoperative evaluation.

A recent review about numerous studies showing that MEG can detect interictal epileptiform discharges in patients with intractable epilepsies was done by King et al. [38].

There are, however, cases where MEG spike localization does not result in focal source findings.

A major problem in using MEG for focus localization arises from the fact that sources of spontaneous epileptic activity are often located less superficially than, for example, the comparatively easily accessible cortical generators of evoked responses. As, with increasing depth of the source, the signals recorded at the surface decline drastically, deep sources are more difficult to locate than superficial ones. A crucial question in the management of drug-resistant epilepsy is the capacity of magnetic field recordings of spontaneous brain activity to assess deep sources in the mesial structures of the temporal lobe. Initial attempts have been made to approach this issue. In an unpublished study where experimental dipoles were established at the tips of foramen ovale electrodes, we found that the dipoles were localized in deeper parts of temporal brain regions, with the distance between estimated source and experimental dipole ranging from 8 to 22 mm. This result gives some encouragement to the use of MSI localizations for presumed deep epileptic foci. However, the circular arrangement of cell layers, e.g. in the amygdala, may cause cancellation of magnetic fields, thus jeopardizing detection of the signals. In addition, an unfavourable sensor configuration may also impair sensitivity. The possibility to record from deeper sources depends on sensor configuration. Comparing MEG localization with 'standard localizations' (based upon MRI, non-invasive and invasive EEG) an agreement was found by Smith et al. [43] in about two-thirds, with spontaneous spikes available in approximately half the mesial temporal lobe epilepsy (MTLE) cases. Knowlton et al. confirmed that the yield of MEG is higher in patients with neocortical epilepsies than in those with MTLE [40].

A frequently used measure to increase the signal-to-noise ratio when dealing with small amplitudes of epileptic discharges in patients with foci in deeper brain regions is averaging of similar specific patterns. The resulting signals, subjected to spatiotemporal analysis, are more likely to produce a reliable estimate of focal epileptic activity than the unaveraged data [44,45].

Based primarily on dipole analyses of EEG spikes, Ebersole stressed the usefulness of interpreting dipole orientation in order to obtain additional information about sublobar attribution of localizations in the temporal lobe [29].

Owing to the distribution of focal origins of seizure disorders, early clinical MSI studies in epileptic patients were mostly restricted to temporal lobe cases [29,31,44–47]. Nevertheless, presurgical evaluation of patients with extratemporal epilepsies has also been reported sporadically to benefit from MSI [15,48,49]. In frontal and other extratemporal epilepsies, intralobar localizations (predominantly lateral and frontobasal) could be confirmed by invasive recordings, but until now the number of investigated patients is rather small. Plate 54.2 (shown in colour between pp 670 and 671) gives an example of localization results in a patient with frontal lobe epilepsy. A special challenge in frontal lobe cases is propagation analysis [50].

The newer generations of biomagnetic systems, allowing for simultaneous examination of large fields of interest, both hemispheres or the entire head, are particularly suited for the investigation of epileptic spikes [39,51], as they offer the opportunity to investigate temporal relationships of events with extended spatial distribution, for example mirror foci [49].

Due to relatively short MEG recording times (as compared with long-term EEG monitoring), spikes are not detected in all patients with focal epilepsy. The rate of MEG spike detection in focal epilepsies varies between 70 and 90% of spontaneous spikes. In order to induce more frequent spiking, activation using methohexital and/or clonidine can be used [52].

Furthermore, with limited recording duration, most MEG recordings miss ictal activity, even in inpatients whose antiepileptic medication is reduced for presurgical evaluation purposes. The restricted access to ictal recording presently remains one of the basic problems of MSI. Even if ictal activity is obtained, motor artefacts are likely to disturb the brain signals, as is known from EEG. Yet, MEG data recorded during auras or seizure onset [29,33,35,53,54] may yield dipole localizations reflecting focal activity (see Plate 54.3, shown in colour between pp. 670 and 671). According to investigations by Ebersole et al. [29] and Tilz et al. [55], ictal recordings permitted the detection of epileptiform signals in the MEG in 40–50%. Prolonged MEG recordings, split into repeated sessions and interspersed with breaks for the patient to have a stretch, might be a strategy to provide ictal data during spontaneous seizures. Another way to obtain seizure-related MEG measurements is to take advantage of procedures which provoke the attacks. For seizure precipitation, sleep deprivation and antiepileptic drug withdrawal can be used.

The correlation of ictal and interictal localizations is among the important issues that have to be assessed systematically in future research in different types of epilepsies.

In small children, limited cooperation and small head size may impose limitations on recording and analysis. Still, even under these conditions, MEG proved advantageous. In childhood epilepsy with Landau–Kleffner's syndrome, Paetau et al. [56], using a whole-head system, showed that in all investigated patients the earliest spike activity originated in the intrasylvian cortex. In one subject, activity spread to the contralateral sylvian cortex within 20 ms. Secondary spikes occurred within 10–60 ms in the ipsilateral perisylvian temporo-occipital and parietal-occipital areas. In these cases, MEG provided useful presurgical information regarding cortical spike dynamics.

Studies comprising MEG and EEG data recorded and analysed simultaneously [46,57] are of particular interest, enabling clinicians to take full advantage of the merits of both methods and to overcome their respective drawbacks.

In spite of the specific limitations of the MSI technique—MEG being apt to detect only tangential dipoles and the comparatively short recording periods rendering spontaneous ictal recordings unlikely—the advantages of MSI are undeniable. Its non-invasiveness, high spatial and temporal resolution, superior accuracy due to magnetic fields' independence of conductivities and its merging functional and anatomical information suggest that MSI plays a significant role among the diagnostic methods that contribute to finding epileptic foci. MSI being non-invasive, it is neither restricted to inpatients, nor to presurgical evaluation, but is also applicable to projects screening outpatients. It may be particularly useful in cases where, after an operation, seizures have decreased, but not altogether ceased, and where, due to asymmetrical conductivities, the defect of the cranial vault and the cavity resulting after resection impede EEG but not MEG analysis.

The applications of MSI in presurgical epilepsy evaluation can be summarized as follows.

1 Delineation of functionally significant areas (which must be spared in neurosurgery) by means of evoked activity.

2 Localization of focal epileptic activity to guide invasive procedures and thus reduce invasive regimens.

3 Localization of focal epileptic activity to guide detailed planning of neurosurgical procedures, e.g. with neuronavigation, aiming at the removal of as little tissue as possible.

4 Contribution to elucidating spatial relationships of epileptic spike generation and—even subtle—anatomical pathologies.

5 Postoperative follow-up and, in cases where the first neurosurgical treatment has failed to render the patient seizure free, facilitation of the decision concerning the possibility of a second operation.

Acknowledgement

The authors gratefully acknowledge the permission to reproduce Fig. 54.1 from Ganslandt *et al.* [58].

References

1 Gallen CC, Sobel DF, Iragui-Madoz V *et al.* Use of MEG focal slow wave localizations to identify epileptic regions: Comparisons with EEG monitoring. *Epilepsia* 1993; 34 (Suppl. 6): 84.

2 Stefan H, Bauer J, Neubauer PU, Feistel H, Schulemann H, Huk W. Vergleich von Untersuchungsbefunden der präoperativen Epilepsiediagnostik unter Einbezug eines Mehrkanal-MEG. In: *Deutsche EEG-Gesellschaft*, 33. Hamburg: Jahrestagung, 1988.

3 Alarcon G, Guy CN, Binnie CD, Walker SR, Elwes RD, Polkey CE. Intracerebral propagation of interictal activity in partial epilepsy: implications for source localisation. *J Neurol Neurosurg Psychiatr* 1994; 57(4): 435–49.

4 Sutherling WW, Crandall PH, Darcey TM, Becker DP, Levesque MF, Barth DS. The magnetic and electric fields agree with intracranial localizations of somatosensory cortex. *Neurology* 1988; 38(11): 1705–14.

5 Alarcon G, Garcia SJ, Binnie CD *et al.* Origin and propagation of interictal

6 Spencer SS, Spencer DD. Entorhinal–hippocampal interactions in medial temporal lobe epilepsy. *Epilepsia* 1994; 35(4): 721–7.

7 Baumgartner C, Deecke L, Stroink G, Williamson SJ, eds. *Biomagnetism: Fundamental Research and Clinical Applications*. Vienna: Elsevier, 1995.

8 Hämäläinen M, Hari R, Ilmoniemi LJ, Knuutila J, Lounasmaa OV. Magnetoencephalography – theory, instrumentation, and applications to noninvasive studies of the working human brain. *Rev Modern Phys* 1993; 65(2): 413–97.

9 Scherg M, Bast T, Berg P. Multiple source analysis of interictal spikes: goals, requirements, and clinical value. *J Clin Neurophysiol* 1999; 16(3): 214–24.

10 Hämäläinen MS. Magnetoencephalography: a tool for functional brain imaging. *Brain Topography* 1992; 5(2): 95–102.

11 Mosher JC, Lewis PS, Leahy RM. Multiple dipole modeling and localization from spatio-temporal MEG data. *IEEE Trans Biomed Engineering* 1992; 39(6): 541–57.

12 Ebersole JS. EEG source modeling. The last word [editorial]. *J Clin Neurophysiol* 1999; 16(3): 297–302.

13 Pascual Marqui RD, Michel CM, Lehmann D. Low resolution electromagnetic tomography: a new method for localizing electrical activity in the brain. *Int J Psychophysiol* 1994; 18(1): 49–65.

14 Fuchs M, Drenckhahn R, Wischmann HA, Wagner M. An improved boundary element method for realistic volume-conductor modeling. *IEEE Trans Biomed Engineering* 1998; 45(8): 980–97.

15 Stefan H, Hummel C. Magnetoencephalography. In: Meinardi A, ed. *Handbook of Clinical Neurology*. Amsterdam: Elsevier, 1999: 319–36.

16 Hari R, Hämäläinen H, Hämäläinen M, Kekoni J, Sams M, Tiihonen J. Separate finger representations at the human second somatosensory cortex. *Neuroscience* 1990; 37(1): 245–9.

17 Paetau R, Ahonen A, Salonen O, Sams M. Auditory evoked magnetic fields to tones and pseudowords in healthy children and adults. *J Clin Neurophysiol* 1995; 12(2): 177–85.

18 Hari R, Aittoniemi K, Jarvinen ML, Katila T, Varpula T. Auditory evoked transient and sustained magnetic fields of the human brain. Localization of neural generators. *Exp Brain Res* 1980; 40(2): 237–40.

19 Aine CJ, Supek S, George JS. Temporal dynamics of visual-evoked neuromagnetic sources: effects of stimulus parameters and selective attention. *Int J Neurosci* 1995; 80(1–4): 79–104.

20 Drasdo N, Thompson DA. An optical stimulator for studying the topography of electrical and magnetic visual evoked responses. *Doc Ophthalmol* 1992; 81(2): 219–25.

21 Baumgartner C. *Clinical Electrophysiology of the Somatosensory Cortex*. Wien: Springer Verlag, 1993.

22 Kettenmann B, Jousmäki V, Portin K, Salmelin R, Kobal G, Hari R. Odourants activate the human superior temporal sulcus. *Neurosci Lett* 1996; 203: 1–3.

23 Cheyne D, Kristeva R, Deecke L. Homuncular organization of human motor cortex as indicated by neuromagnetic recordings. *Neurosci Lett* 1991; 122(1): 17–20.

24 Deecke L, Kornhuber HH, Lang W, Lang M, Schreiber H. Timing function of the frontal cortex in sequential motor and learning tasks. *Hum Neurobiol* 1985; 4(3): 143–54.

25 Ganslandt O, Steinmeier R, Kober H *et al.* Magnetic source imaging combined with image-guided frameless stereotaxy: a new method in surgery around the motor strip. *Neurosurgery* 1997; 41(3): 621–8.

26 Yang TT, Gallen CC, Schwartz BJ, Bloom FE. Noninvasive somatosensory homunculus mapping in humans by using a large-array biomagnetometer. *Proc Natl Acad Sci USA* 1993; 90(7): 3098–102.

27 Papanicolaou AC, Breier JI, Gormley W *et al.* Comparison of language mapping using extra and intraoperative electrocortical stimulation and magnetoencephalography. *Epilepsia* 1998; 39(6): 107.

28 Engel J. *Surgical Treatment of the Epilepsies*. New York: Raven Press, 1993.

29 Ebersole JS, Squires KC, Eliashiv SD, Smith JR. Applications of magnetic source imaging in evaluation of candidates for epilepsy surgery. *Neuroimag Clin N Am* 1995; 5(2): 267–88.

30 Nakasato N, Levesque MF, Barth DS, Baumgartner C, Rogers RL,

discharges in the acute electrocorticogram. Implications for pathophysiology and surgical treatment of temporal lobe epilepsy. *Brain* 1997; 120(12): 2259–82.

Sutherling WW. Comparisons of MEG, EEG, and ECoG source localization in neocortical partial epilepsy in humans. *Electroencephalogr Clin Neurophysiol* 1994; 91(3): 171–8.

31 Stefan H, Schüler P, Abraham Fuchs K *et al*. Magnetic source localization and morphological changes in temporal lobe epilepsy: comparison of MEG/EEG, ECoG and volumetric MRI in presurgical evaluation of operated patients. *Acta Neurol Scand Suppl* 1994; 152: 83–8.

32 Smith JR, Gallen C, Orrison W *et al*. Role of multichannel magnetoencephalography in the evaluation of ablative seizure surgery candidates. *Stereotactic Functional Neurosurg* 1994; 62(1–4): 238–44.

33 Sutherling WW, Crandall PH, Engel J Jr, Darcey TM, Cahan LD, Barth DS. The magnetic field of complex partial seizures agrees with intracranial localizations. *Ann Neurol* 1987; 21(6): 548–58.

34 Eliashiv SD, Squires K, Fried I, Engel JJ. Magnetic source imaging as a localization tool in patients with surgically remediable epilepsies. *Epilepsia* 1998; 39 (Suppl. 6): 80–90.

35 Stefan H, Abraham Fuchs K, Schneider S, Schuler P, Huk WJ. Multichannel magneto-electroencephalography recordings of interictal and ictal activity. *Physiol Measure* 1993; 14 (Suppl. 4A): A109–11.

36 Wheless JW, Willmore LJ, Breier JI *et al*. A comparison of magnetoencephalography, MRI, and V-EEG in patients evaluated for epilepsy surgery. *Epilepsia* 1999; 40(7): 931–41.

37 Lamusuo S, Forss N, Ruottinen HM *et al*. [18F]FDG-PET and whole-scalp MEG localization of epileptogenic cortex. *Epilepsia* 1999; 40(7): 921–30.

38 King DW, Park YD, Smith JR, Wheless JW. Magnetoencephalography in neocortical epilepsy. *Adv Neurol* 2000; 84(415): 23.

39 Stefan H, Schneider S, Abraham Fuchs K *et al*. The neocortico to mesiobasal limbic propagation of focal epileptic activity during the spike-wave complex. *Electroencephalogr Clin Neurophysiol* 1991; 79(1): 1–10.

40 Knowlton RC, Laxer KD, Aminoff MJ, Roberts TP, Wong ST, Rowley HA. Magnetoencephalography in partial epilepsy: clinical yield and localization accuracy. *Ann Neurol* 1997; 42(4): 622–31.

41 Cascino GD, Jack CR Jr, Parisi JE. Magnetic resonance imaging in intractable frontal lobe epilepsy. Pathologic correlation and prognostic significance. *Epilepsy Res* 1992; 11(51): 171–8.

42 Swartz B, Halgren E, Delgado-Escuetta AV. Neuroimaging in patients with seizures of probable frontal lobe origin. *Epilepsia* 1989; 30(5): 547–58.

43 Smith JR, Schwartz BJ, Gallen C *et al*. Utilization of multichannel magnetoencephalography in the guidance of ablative seizure surgery. *J Epilepsy* 1995; 8: 119–30.

44 Stefan H, Schneider S, Abraham Fuchs K *et al*. Magnetic source localization in focal epilepsy. Multichannel magnetoencephalography correlated with magnetic resonance brain imaging. *Brain* 1990; 113(Pt 5): 1347–59.

45 Sutherling WW, Barth DS. Neocortical propagation in temporal lobe spike foci on magnetoencephalography and electroencephalography. *Ann Neurol* 1989; 25(4): 373–81.

46 Ebersole JS, Squires K, Gamelin J, Lewine J, Scherg M. Simultaneous MEG and EEG provide complementary dipole maps of temporal lobe spikes. *Epilepsia* 1993; 34 (Suppl. 6): 143.

47 Rose DF, Sato S, Smith PD *et al*. Localization of magnetic interictal discharges in temporal lobe epilepsy. *Ann Neurol* 1987; 22(3): 348–54.

48 Stefan H, Quesney LF, Feistel HK, Schüler P, Weis M, Hummel C, Pauli E. Presurgical evaluation in frontal lobe epilepsy. A multimethodological approach. *Adv Neurol* 1995; 66: 213–20.

49 Hari R, Ahonen A, Forss N *et al*. Parietal epileptic mirror focus detected with a whole-head neuromagnetometer. *Neuroreport* 1993; 5(1): 45–8.

50 Ossenblok P, Fuchs M, Velis DN, Veltman E, Pijn JP, da-Silva FH. Source analysis of lesional frontal-lobe epilepsy. *IEEE Eng Med Biol Mag* 1999; 18(3): 67–77.

51 Paetau R, Kajola M, Karhu J *et al*. Magnetoencephalographic localization of epileptic cortex – impact on surgical treatment. *Ann Neurol* 1992; 32(1): 106–9.

52 Kirchberger KG, Schmitt H, Hummel C, Peinemann A, Pauli E, Stefan H. Clonidine and Methohexital induced epileptic MEG discharges in patients with focal epilepsies. *Epilepsia* 1998; 39: 1104–12.

53 Watanabe Y, Fukao K, Watanabe M, Seino M. Epileptic events observed by multichannel MEG. *Electroencephalogr Clin Neurophysiol Suppl (Ireland)* 1996; 47: 383–91.

54 Stefan H, Schneider S, Feistel H *et al*. Ictal and interictal activity in partial epilepsy recorded with multichannel magnetoelectroencephalography: correlation of electroencephalography/electrocorticography, magnetic resonance imaging, single photon emission computed tomography, and positron emission tomography findings. *Epilepsia* 1992; 33(5): 874–87.

55 Tilz C, Hummel C, Hopfengärtner R, Kettenmann B, Stefan H. Ictal source localization from standard MEG recordings. 10th European Congress of Clinical Neurophysiology, oral presentation, 2000.

56 Paetau R, Granström M-L, Blomstedt G, Jousmäki V, Korkman M, Liukkonen E. Magnetoencephalography in presurgical evaluation of children with the Landau–Kleffner syndrome. *Epilepsia* 1999; 40(3): 326–35.

57 Stefan H, Hummel C, Hopfengärtner R *et al*. Magnetoencephalography in extratemporal epilepsy. *J Clin Neurophysiol* 2000; 17(2): 190–200.

58 Ganslandt O, Fahlbusch R, Nimsky C *et al*. Functional neuronavigation with magnetoencephalography: outcome in 50 patients with lesions around the motor cortex. *J Neurosurg* 1999; 91(1): 73–9.

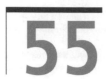

55 MRI in Presurgical Evaluation of Epilepsy

C.E. Elger and J. von Oertzen

The increased use of high-resolution MRI in recent years has changed the presurgical evaluation of patients with pharmacoresistant epilepsies. While in former times electrophysiological focus localization was the primary diagnostic tool, MRI is now becoming an increasingly important guide to focus localization, and is quite often the first step in presurgical evaluation [1,2]. This is based on the experience that epilepsy surgery is most successful if a lesion found on the MRI scan to be epileptogenic is removed completely [3]. This means that:

1 The MRI has to be of the highest possible quality to detect and identify a lesion or to rule out that a further lesion or lesions exist.

2 The MRI investigation should be based on a hypothesis regarding the probable localization of the focus since the temporal lobes should be investigated differently from extratemporal areas. Suitable specific examination protocols are discussed below.

3 MRI should be interpreted on the basis of an understanding of the pathophysiological process of epileptogenicity. Epileptogenic lesions are most often located (sub-)cortically. If they are found elsewhere, they usually contain neurones in atypical allocations.

4 Epileptologists and the neurophysiologists involved in presurgical evaluation should be able to interpret structural MRI of the brain since the radiological detection of a lesion, and interpretation of the neurophysiological tests, and semiology should ideally be a two-way interactive process.

In the authors' opinion, MRI has changed the presurgical work-up to the extent that the first question should be: 'Is there a lesion detectable on MRI?' If so, one should not ask whether this is the epileptic focus but rather if there is any reason to suspect that the epileptic focus is not closely related to the lesion. If no lesion is visible, the question is whether the quality of the MRI scan was sufficient. Otherwise the scan should be repeated according to a dedicated epilepsy MRI protocol. If this also fails to show a lesion, other methods such as ictal EEG recording, ictal SPECT and analysis of the semiology may generate a hypothesis on the basis of which the MRI scan is re-evaluated and repeated in some cases. If no lesion has been found at this stage one should discuss whether a sufficiently strong hypothesis exists to warrant the placement of intracranial electrodes (with attendant risks) or whether further evaluation should be postponed until a new generation of MRI is available which may detect a lesion.

Epilepsy surgery is not possible without structural MRI. Current studies on magnetic resonance spectroscopy and functional MRI show that these modes of investigation are also useful. However, it seems that these techniques might either still be used on a research basis, or provide redundant clinical data. Therefore these techniques will only be addressed briefly at the end of this chapter, especially as the reader may wish to refer to Chapter 57 for more details.

Structural imaging

It appears to be accepted worldwide that epilepsy surgery should only take place when drugs have failed and the patient has been proven to be suffering from so-called pharmacoresistant epilepsy. There is a lively discussion about what the term 'pharmacoresistant epilepsy' actually means. Definitions range from treatment failure with two to three or more antiepileptic drugs used in monotherapy to continuing seizures on antiepileptic drug combination therapy [4]. On the other hand, the increasing use of epilepsy surgery has shown that it is usually safe and very successful, especially considering the groups of patients operated on. Therefore, a modern concept defining the term 'pharmacoresistance' should take the probable chances of success with epilepsy surgery into account. The following example illustrates this concept.

A patient suffers from seizures of right temporal origin. Two first-line drugs in appropriate dosage have failed to control seizures. Hence, the chance of controlling seizures using additional drugs has to be assumed to be less than 10%. The standard MRI scan performed after his first seizure showed no obvious lesion. On the basis of this information, one might conclude that the patient would not be a good candidate for epilepsy surgery evaluation. However, reinvestigation with MRI shows Ammon's horn sclerosis (AHS) on the right side, thus identifying the patient as an ideal candidate for epilepsy surgery with a low risk of morbidity or mortality and an 80% chance of becoming seizure free postoperatively. This example demonstrates that only a correct characterization of lesional and non-lesional MRI makes it possible adequately to plan further treatment.

Based on these considerations, the different MRI protocols as shown in Fig. 55.1 should be applied. After the first seizure, an MRI examination according to the initial protocol should be performed in every patient to rule out abnormalities which have to be treated irrespective of epileptological considerations such as brain tumours, metastases, etc. Such an MRI may be repeated where appropriate to exclude progressive processes with certainty. However, this protocol is inadequate for the consideration of presurgical evaluation, and even more inadequate for use in a presurgical work-up. If the first and the second drug have failed, MRI re-examination should be performed following the protocol for difficult-to-treat patients with epilepsy. If this MRI shows a lesion, which appears to be concordant with other data such as EEG and seizure semiology, the chances of becoming seizure free by resection and the risk involved should be discussed with the patient. If the patient remains non-lesional after dedicated MRI scanning, the process of proving drug resistance should continue in the first instance. Should the epilepsy remain difficult to treat, the evaluation protocol for

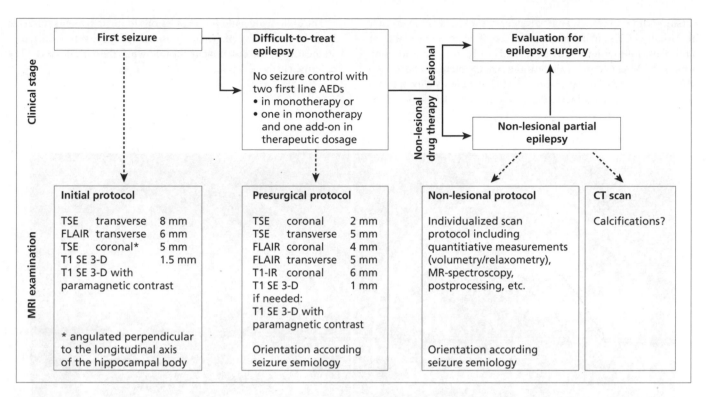

Fig. 55.1 Diagram of clinical stages and MRI examination protocols. MRI according to the dedicated 'difficult-to-treat epilepsy' protocol should be performed early to identify candidates with a good prospect of successful epilepsy surgery from the group of patients with pharmacoresistant epilepsy.

Table 55.1 Characteristic MRI signal abnormalities associated with the commonest epileptogenic lesions

Aetiology	Preferred MRI sequence	Signal changes	Other features
Hippocampal sclerosis	T2, FLAIR	T2↑, T1↔	Hippocampal atrophy
Focal cortical dysplasia	FLAIR, T2	T2↑↔, T1↔	Thickened cortex, blurred g/w junction
Nodular heterotopia	T1 IR, 3D-T1	T1↔, T2↔	Periventricular/subcortical cortex nodules
Polymicrogyria	3D-T1, T1 IR	T1↔, T2↔	Multiple small gyri
Pachygyria	3D-T1, T1 IR	T1↔, T2↔	Focally thickened gyri and cortex
Hemimegalencephaly	All	T1/T2↑↓↔	Unilateral volume↑, possibly other MCDs
Dysembryoplastic neuroepithelial tumour (DNT)	T1, T2	T1↓↔, T2↑↔	Often multicystic elements
Ganglioglioma	T1, T2	T1↓↔, T2↑↔	Often cystic parts, < 50% calcifications, < 50% CM enhancement
Cavernoma	T2*	T2↑↓↔	Haemosiderin ring
Arteriovenous malformation	T2, T2*	T2↑↓↔	Notch-like configuration, haemosiderin
Post-traumatic lesion	T2, T2*, FLAIR	T2↑↓↔	Contre coupe
Tuberous sclerosis	T2, FLAIR	T2↑	Tubers, calcifications
	T1, CM	T1↑↔	Subependymal nodules, CM enhancement: giant cell astrocytoma
Sturge–Weber syndrome	T2, FLAIR, T1, CM	T2↑↔	Calcifications, atrophy, angioma: CM enhancement
Hypothalamic hamartoma	(3D-)T1, T2	T1↑↔, T2↔	Gelastic seizures
Rasmussen's encephalitis	T2	T2↑↔	Initially focal swelling, signal intensities vary as condition progresses

3D-T1, three-dimensional T1-weighted images; CM, contrast medium; g/w, grey/white (matter); MCDs, malformations of cortical development; T1, T1-weighted images; T2, T2-weighted images, T2*, T2-weighted gradient echo images.

patients with non-lesional partial epilepsy should be initiated later on. Usually a CT scan has been performed. If this is not available, or if the quality is low, it should be repeated in all cases where no lesion is found by MRI to detect calcifications, which might not be seen on MRI scans. For the interpretation of MRI in patients with epilepsy by the consulting neurologist, the major characteristics of structural lesions are summarized in Table 55.1.

The underlying pathologies of lesions found in patients suffering from long-standing pharmacoresistant epilepsy were reported in studies of surgical outcome. In the following, the pathologies will be described in more detail.

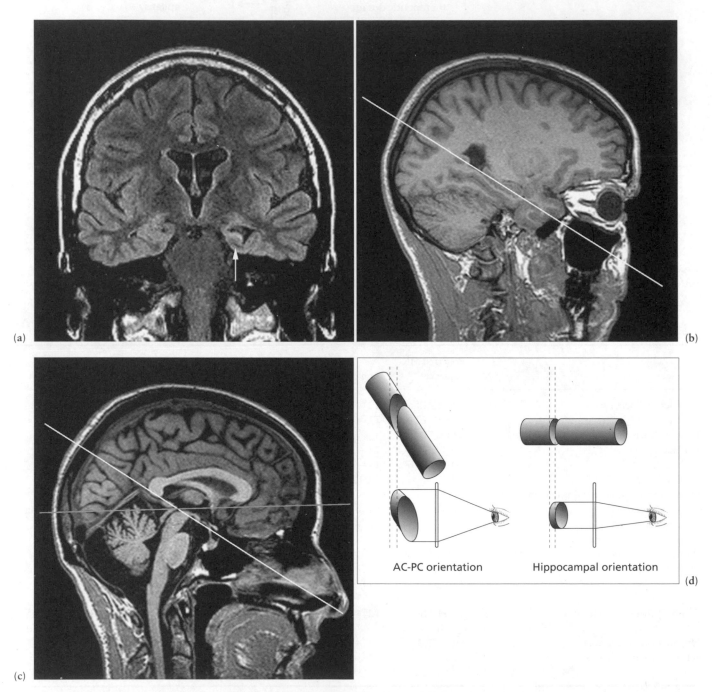

Fig. 55.2 (a–c) MRI in temporal lobe epilepsy. For detection of typical lesions like Ammon's horn sclerosis (a, FLAIR sequence, arrow) orientation should be parallel or orthogonal to the longitudinal axis of the hippocampus (b, T1 weighted). Difference between temporal orientation and orientation according to the AC–PC plain is demonstrated in (c) (T1 weighted, white line: hippocampal orientation white; grey line: AC–PC orientation). The scheme (d) clarifies the difference of AC–PC and hippocampal-orientated scans. As the former orientation slices the hippocampus (depicted as tube) in (a) non-orthogonal angle, the structure appears larger on the two-dimensional scan. Only in an orthogonal slice orientation (hippocampal orientation) the extent of the structure can be assessed accurately.

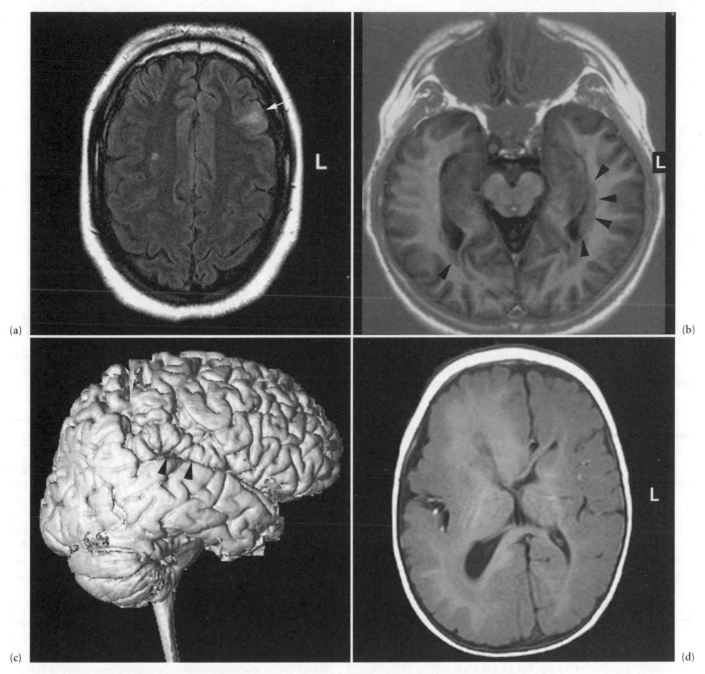

Fig. 55.3 (a–f) Malformations of cortical development (a–d): (a) axial FLAIR image: focal cortical dysplasia (arrow) presenting as increased subcortical signal intensity, often with radial striation towards the ventricle. (b) Axial IR image: nodular heterotopia adjacent to the lateral ventricle (arrowheads) and isointense with cortex. Images have to be surveyed carefully to detect or exclude bilateral changes. (c) Three-dimensional surface rendering of segmented brain viewed from the right (T1-weighted dataset): polymicrogyria in the centroparietal region (arrowheads). (d) Axial T1-weighted image of an 8-month-old girl: enlargement of the right hemisphere with ipsilateral ventriculomegaly representing hemimegalencephaly. The intrahemispheric cleft is shifted to the contralateral side. It can be difficult to decide if the right hemisphere is enlarged or the left hemisphere is atrophic.

Ammon's horn sclerosis (AHS)

AHS is the result of cell loss within the Ammon's horn formation together with an increase of axonal sprouting. Most often these structural changes are not only found in the hippocampus but also in the amygdala. The terms hippocampal sclerosis or mesial temporal sclerosis are often used synonymously. AHS and/or amygdala sclerosis are some of the main causes of pharmacoresistant temporal lobe epilepsy. Due to the anatomical location of the Ammon's horn and the temporal lobe, standard MRI protocols of the head often fail to detect temporal lesions [5,6]. This is due to partial volume effects caused by images slicing through the hippocampus in a non-orthogonal direction and by a relatively thick slice of (usually) 6 mm. This results in difficulties with visualizing the amygdala and

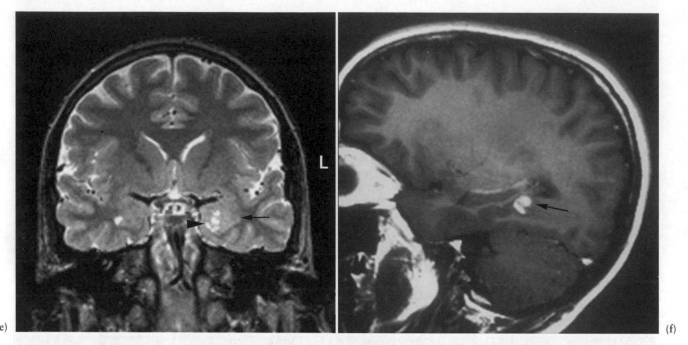

Fig. 55.3 *Continued.* (e) Coronal T2-weighted TSE image (temporal orientation): cortical lesion with solid and multicystic parts in the temporomesial region representing a dysembryoplastic neuroepithelial tumour. (f) Sagittal T1-weighted image with contrast medium: this temporobasal, cortical ganglioglioma presents as a cystic structure and showing enhancement of contrast medium (arrow).

hippocampus clearly, and with detecting alterations by comparing both sides (Fig. 55.2). The orientation of the scan should therefore be orthogonal or longitudinal to the axis of the hippocampus, thus providing a clear view of hippocampal volume and signal and minimizing partial volume effects.

On MR scans, typical signs of AHS are loss of volume, increased signal intensity in T2-weighted images, loss of internal structure and loss of digitations of the hippocampal head [7–12]. Secondary changes, seen inconsistently, are ipsilateral atrophy of the temporal lobe, the fornix, the mamillary body and the white matter between hippocampus and grey matter of the collateral sulcus as well as dilatation of the temporal horn [13]. Depending on the preference of the MRI unit, the assessment of these characteristics can be done on T1-weighted images, T1-weighted inversion recovery, T2-weighted images or FLAIR images. The authors prefer T2-weighted turbospin echo (2 mm slice thickness) and FLAIR images (Fig. 55.2a). In unclear cases, quantitative MRI is recommended (for details see below). It is important not to miss AHS or any other lesions. In some cases, particularly in patients with bilateral hippocampal atrophy, malformations of cortical development (MCDs) are found reflecting dual pathology [14]. In such cases in particular, the relevance of structural MRI for the detection of focal lesions becomes obvious: if unilateral AHS is found in a patient with temporal lobe epilepsy, the major concern is not the localization of the epileptic focus but whether there is a contraindication to its resection.

Limbic encephalitis

In some cases the pathology underlying the MRI changes of increased signal intensity and hippocampal atrophy is that of limbic encephalitis rather than AHS. Limbic encephalitis is most often

paraneoplastic but there are rare cases without any evidence of an underlying neoplasm [15–17]. In the early stages, swelling and oedema of temporomesial structures may be present producing increased signal intensity in T2-weighted images on MRI. In the later stages, sclerosis of temporomesial structures appears. The differentiation of the causes of sclerosis is very difficult by MRI scanning alone, even retrospectively when the postoperative histological diagnosis is known. Combined with the patient's history of a short duration of illness, a frequently high seizure frequency, dramatic memory impairment and sometimes psychiatric alterations (i.e. psychosis), the diagnosis of limbic encephalitis needs more consideration. The decision about further treatment depends on the results of an intensive tumour screen and the histological diagnosis, respectively (cytostatic/resective or immunosuppressive). If tumour screening was negative it should be repeated every 3–6 months for up to 2 years as paraneoplastic symptoms may present before a primary tumour is detectable.

Malformations of cortical development (MCDs)

MCD is a term used for a range of different abnormalities. There is additionally no generally accepted single classification. In 1996, a useful approach divided MCDs into malformations due to disturbance of (a) neuronal and glial proliferation; (b) neuronal migration; (c) cortical organization; or (d) malformations which do not fit into one of the other groups [18]. Currently, efforts are underway to develop a new classification of MCDs but work is still in progress [19]. For developmental reasons some types of MCD are frequently localized in the temporal lobe. The following paragraphs give an overview of the most common focal or multifocal MCDs (Fig. 55.3a–d).

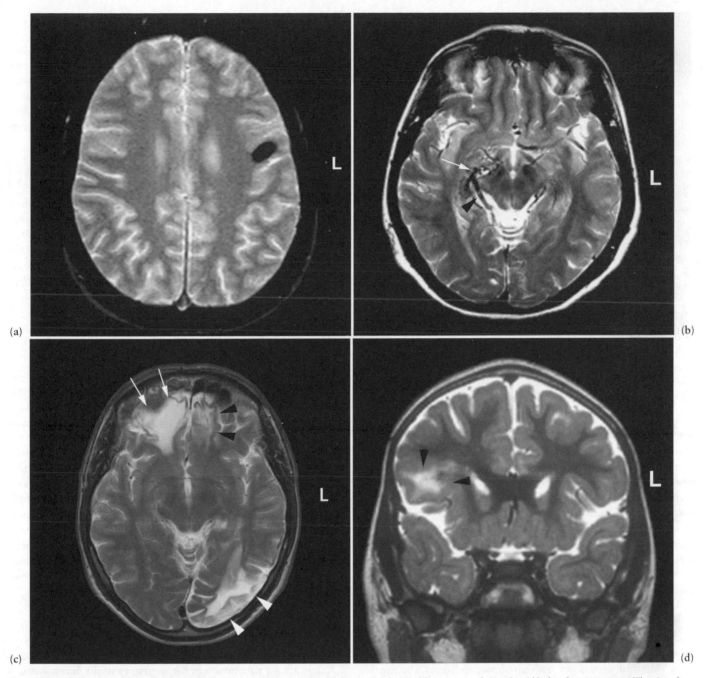

Fig. 55.4 (a–e) Vascular malformations (a and b): (a) axial T2-weighted GE image: left-sided frontocentral signal void halo of a cavernoma. The signal void is due to susceptibility artefacts of haemosiderin deposits best demonstrated on a gradient echo sequence. (b) Axial T2-weighted TSE image: irregular hyper- and hypointensities in the right-sided temporomesial structures (white arrow) with an enlarged communicating vessel (black arrowhead) representing an arteriovenous malformation. Hypointense areas represent changes caused by haemosiderin deposits or blood vessels, hyperintense areas reflect changes like gliosis and oedema due to thrombosed vessels. (c) Axial T2-weighted TSE image: postcontusional lesions after a right anterolateral head trauma. Right frontal defect with sclerotic edge (white arrows) and contralateral sclerosis (black arrowheads). Note the additional left parieto-occipital defect representing the contre coup (white arrowheads). Neurocutaneous syndromes (d and e): (d) coronal T2-weighted image: subcortical almost ring-shaped hyperintense tuber in a patient with tuberous sclerosis and epilepsy.

Focal cortical dysplasia (FCD)

With the improvement of MRI, FCDs are detected more frequently. In the classification mentioned above, two kinds of FCD are distinguished, histologically differentiated by the appearance of balloon cells (BC, without BC type IIa, with BC type IIb) [18–20]. Recently,

FCD-BCs have been linked to tuberous sclerosis (TS) [21]. The differentiation of these two types of FCD by MRI may be difficult. In general, the MRI signs of FCD include thickening of the cortex with blurring of the grey matter–white matter interface. Signal intensity in the adjacent white matter is increased or normal on T2-weighted images and especially FLAIR images (Fig. 55.3a) [22].

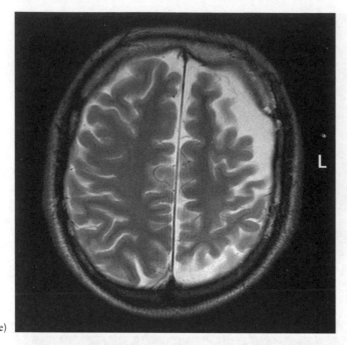

(e)

Fig. 55.4 *Continued.* (e) Axial T2-weighted TSE image: typical unilateral atrophy in Sturge–Weber syndrome. Leptomeningeal angiomatosis is best demonstrated by CT (calcifications) or by MRI with contrast enhancement.

MR postprocessing techniques can provide additional information. One of these is curvilinear reformatting of three-dimensional T1-weighted images, where the grey matter–white matter junction can be assessed by peeling away millimetre by millimetre the extracted brain surface [23,24]. Other techniques apply algorithms for voxel-based analysis to find disturbances of the grey matter–white matter junction [25,26]. The sensitivity of MRI for FCD is clearly improved by these techniques. In the presurgical evaluation of patients with MCD and in particular FCD, it remains unclear whether we are able to visualize most abnormalities or whether we visualize only the tip of the iceberg, but postoperative outcome in patients with FCD who have undergone extended lesionectomy appearing complete on MRI is often excellent [22]. The most substantial recent progress of MRI in epilepsy has been made with regard to the FCD. Postprocessing techniques now allow the prediction of 'good' surgical candidates with circumscribed focal abnormalities and 'bad' surgical candidates with widespread or multifocal abnormalities.

Nodular heterotopia

Nodular heterotopias are another kind of MCD which is of special interest in presurgical evaluation of patients with epilepsy. There are several issues to take into account. Nodular heterotopias are found subcortically, periventricularly or in both locations (Fig. 55.3b). MRIs have to be assessed carefully as 33% of heterotopias are bilateral [27,28]. T1-weighted inversion recovery images or three-dimensional T1-weighted images are best suited to assess heterotopias. Some radiologists also suggest inverted T2-weighted images but the authors prefer T1-weighted inversion recovery sequences which show the grey matter–white matter contrast best.

Focal polymicrogyria/pachygyria

Disturbances of gyration include focal polymicrogyria and pachygyria, the latter describing focally thickened gyri with a thickened layer of cortex. Again three-dimensional T1-weighted images and T1-weighted inversion recovery images are best suited to detect these abnormalities, and postprocessing of MRI data can help to identify abnormalities by curve linear reformatting or three-dimensional reconstruction of brain surface (Fig. 55.3c) [24].

Hemimegalencephaly

Seizures caused by hemimegalencephaly, a further MCD, can be treated successfully by epilepsy surgery. On MRI, hemimegalencephaly is characterized by a unilaterally increased brain volume, enlarged ventricles and a shift of the intrahemispheric fissure (Fig. 55.3d). These changes are frequently combined with other types of MCD in the same hemisphere. Hemispherectomy may be appropriate after careful evaluation [27,29–31].

Dysembryoplastic neuroepithelial tumour (DNT)/ganglioglioma

Some low-grade tumours include elements of dysplasia. DNTs contain neurones, cells of the oligodendrite line as well as undifferentiated cells. On MRI, they are hypointense on T1-weighted images, hyperintense on T2-weighted images and often include multicystic parts. They are located in the cortex and found most often in the temporal lobe (Fig. 55.3e). In about one-third of cases DNTs show enhancement with contrast. Rarely, they contain calcifications which may be demonstrable with CT. Gangliogliomas are very similar, containing neuronal cells, glial cells and astrocytes. Their MRI appearance is almost identical to that of DNTs although gangliogliomas only contain cystic but no multicystic parts. Contrast enhancement or calcification on CT scans are present in less than 50% (Fig. 55.3f). Usually, DNTs and gangliogliomas are low-grade tumours but rare anaplastic types have been described [32–35].

Vascular abnormalities

Cavernous haemangiomas or cavernomas of the central nervous system are the commonest of the angiographically occult vascular malformations. It is likely that two variants of cavernomas exist, a single sporadic form and a multiple familial form with an assumed dominant inheritance. If localized within the hemispheres, they may cause partial epilepsy. Susceptibility artefacts in gradient echo sequences are the most sensitive MRI indicator of haemosiderin deposits caused by (micro-)bleeds into the surrounding tissue (Fig. 55.4a). The annual risk of intracranial haemorrhage ranges from 1 to 3%, the risk being greater with deep localization and after a first haemorrhage. The neurosurgical resection of a cavernoma after a first intracranial haemorrhage is being discussed controversially [36]. In drug-resistant epilepsy, surgical intervention after presurgical evaluation reduces seizure frequency in most patients [37]. It remains unclear whether a lesionectomy suffices or whether the resection of surrounding tissue is required to achieve good postoperative seizure control.

After bleeding, seizures are the second most common mode of presentation of arteriovenous malformations. They are usually identified by angiography. On MRI, high flow in arteriovenous shunts causes a high signal intensity in T2-weighted images, usually with a notch-like configuration. This may be accompanied by areas with decreased signal intensity which represent residuals of intralesional bleeding (Fig. 55.4b). Surgery should not only be considered to reduce the risk of intracranial haemorrhage, but also to help control seizures if present. Given that seizures arise from neurones, adjacent tissue should probably be removed to improve postoperative outcome in terms of seizure control although no sufficient data exist to support such an approach.

Post-traumatic lesions

Hippocampal sclerosis as well as neocortical lesions may be caused by traumatic brain injury. Non-penetrating traumatic brain injuries have a predilection for the anterior frontal and frontobasal as well as anterior temporal, temporobasal and temporomesial regions. An additional area of brain injury may be located on the opposite side representing the contre coup (Fig. 55.4c). Gradient echo sequences may help to detect sites of former injuries using the susceptibility artefacts caused by haemosiderin. Post-traumatic epilepsies are often caused by bilateral or multifocal brain injury. Therefore epilepsy surgery should only be considered after careful evaluation [38,39].

Neurocutaneous syndromes

Neurocutaneous syndromes are malformations caused by disturbances in the germinal sheet. Only two of these conditions may cause epilepsy: tuberous sclerosis and Sturge–Weber syndrome.

Tuberous sclerosis (TS)

TS has many other clinical symptoms than the classical triad of seizures, mental retardation and facial angiofibroma. Sometimes the only manifestation affects the central nervous system (forme fruste). Neuroimaging may show the typical central nervous lesions of subependymal nodules and subcortical tubers. Subependymal nodules are located periventricularly, or flanking the ventricles. These small lesions are best detected by T1-weighted images appearing isointense to white matter and iso- to hyperintense to grey matter. Calcifications are common. Contrast enhancement is unusual except after transformation of lesions to giant cell astrocytomas. Because of the calcifications associated with TS lesions, CT scanning can be very helpful. Tubers are found subcortically or, less frequently, cortically and appear hyperintense on T2-weighted images, sometimes as a ring-shaped structure with irregular hyperintensities at the centre (Fig. 55.4d) [40,41]. Recent studies have shown that the cerebral manifestations of TS can be diagnosed antenatally [42]. If only one tuber is present or one tuber can be identified as the dominant epileptogenic zone, occasional patients can benefit from epilepsy surgery [43,44].

Sturge–Weber syndrome

This syndrome is characterized by a venous leptomeningeal angioma in the central nervous system causing chronic ischaemia in the underlying cortex. MRI or CT scanning can demonstrate calcifications associated with the venous angioma as well as atrophy or even hemiatrophy (Fig. 55.4e). Angiomatose changes are best demonstrated using intravascular contrast agents. The surgical options include lobectomy or hemispherectomy. They are associated with good seizure outcome and better cognitive outcome when surgery is undertaken early in life [45].

Hypothalamic hamartomas

Hypothalamic hamartomas frequently cause gelastic seizures, most often in children. The hypothalamic region has to be examined very carefully by MRI, as these hamartomas may be very small lesions within the tuber cinereum. Their signal is isointense to cortex in T1-weighted images and T2-weighted images, but the authors prefer T1-weighted images for optimal visualization. Surgical intervention may be difficult because of the high risk of complications. Treatment options include surgery, radiosurgery or thermocoagulation [46–48].

Rasmussen's encephalitis

It has recently been shown that the MRI changes associated with Rasmussen's encephalitis go through five distinct stages during the course of the disease. Initially, no abnormalities are detectable, then there is swelling and subcortical focal hyperintensities on T2-weighted images. The swelling disappears after some time and is replaced by focal atrophy, still combined with increased signal intensities. As atrophy progresses, the signal abnormalities return to normal resulting in hemiatrophy in the final stage [49]. In the earlier stages an extended lesionectomy can help to control seizures and/or to clarify the underlying diagnosis by providing a specimen for histopathological examination. In the final stage, when Rasmussen's encephalitis has caused hemiparesis, hemispherectomy may be indicated to help with seizure control.

MRI in children

As in adults, MRI is one of the most important diagnostic tools in children, especially as the localizing value of the seizure semiology in younger children is limited. Once again, MRI leads the way to the diagnosis of the underlying pathology, the definition of epilepsy syndrome and therapeutic strategy. MRI in children differs from that in adults in some aspects.

The scanning procedure itself is different as most young children may need to be examined under sedation or general anaesthesia. This requires special equipment and interdisciplinary cooperation. Thus, scanning has to be planned and supervised carefully to obtain as much MRI information as required during one examination.

Apart from this, images have to be interpreted in the light of different distribution of pathological entities during childhood, and some pathologies have to be considered which are much more likely to present in childhood. Probably the most common group of MRI lesions in children are MCDs. Most characteristics of these lesions are described above. MCDs presenting in childhood may be more severe, as lissencephaly and other major malformations manifest early. Moreover, neurocutaneous syndromes, hypothalamic hamartomas and Rasmussen's encephalitis are more frequent in children than adults. AHS remains common: it has been demonstrated in children with the minimum age of 9 months and seizures caused by AHS often start in early childhood [50]. It has recently been noted that AHS is underrepresented in MRI series of children with epilepsy [51]. With improving imaging techniques and more high-resolution imaging in children with partial epilepsy, this lesion should be found more often. The early detection of AHS is important as early surgical intervention may lead to better socioeconomic outcome [52].

Quantitative MRI

It has been shown that hippocampal volumetry (HCV) and hippocampal relaxometry identify hippocampal sclerosis with high specificity and sensitivity, and are superior to visual analysis in some cases. However, most studies of qualitative assessment of the Ammon's horn formation were undertaken by experienced epilepsy experts. These experts are able to diagnose AHS visually with a sensitivity of 90% or more. Assessment by epileptologically less experienced MRI readers has been shown to have a much lower sensitivity for the detection of AHS [5,6]. Therefore, apart from increasing sensitivity and specificity in the small number of cases who are visually difficult to assess (i.e. bilateral atrophy/AHS), quantitative MRI could increase sensitivity and specificity in the great number of cases examined by non-expert radiologists. But unfortunately, quantitative MRI techniques are quite time-consuming, and still not widely or routinely available.

Hippocampal volumetry (HCV)

HCV can be undertaken using standard three-dimensional T1-weighted images. If images are not obtained with a temporal orientation, they have to be resliced. In the coronal plain both hippocampi have to be outlined manually or semiautomatically on each slice. The first and last slice as well as the anatomical borders of hippocampus have to be defined in detail to ensure reproducible results. To determine the volume, cross-sectional areas are summed up and multiplied by the slice thickness (Cavalieri's principle). A trained investigator needs 30–45 min to complete the off-line analysis for a single patient [53].

Hippocampal relaxometry

For hippocampal relaxometry, an additional MRI relaxometry sequence has to be obtained. This sequences measure echos at two to 16 different times before the relaxation time of each pixel is calculated. A region of interest representing the hippocampus has to be placed on each slice of the calculated map (one to six, depending on the sequence). This technique requires 10–13 min additional scan time and a few minutes for off-line analysis [54–57]. Recently, a faster sequence with shorter scan time was described [58]. As with all quantitative studies there needs to be reliable scanner-specific baseline control data and good quality assurance.

MR spectroscopy

The measurement of tissue metabolites with proton magnetic reso-nance spectroscopic imaging (MRSI) has shown some use in addition to structural imaging in the presurgical evaluation of patients with epilepsy over the past 5 years. MRSI is able to lateralize TLE in 97–98% of cases [59,60]. In patients with bilateral hippocampal atrophy MRSI may predict good surgical outcome if changes of metabolites are present or more pronounced ipsilateral to the EEG focus [61]. Furthermore, MRSI also discriminates TLE and extratemporal lobe epilepsy (X-TLE) but it is less good at this than at lateralization. The reason for this may be that temporal damage also occurs in patients with X-TLE [60]. MRSI has been shown to detect abnormalities in patients with FCDs, but it has, so far, not proven useful for other MCDs [56,62]. Besides the localizing value of MRSI, the pathophysiology of MRSI changes remains unclear. Neuronal and glial cell counts have shown no significant correlation with metabolic abnormalities. MRSI after surgery only revealed normalization of metabolites in those patients who became seizure free [63]. Given the significant correlation of seizure frequency and metabolic abnormalities in MRSI, it is possible that some metabolic changes are generated by seizures themselves rather than by the underlying pathology.

Imaging of the epileptogenic area

For successful epilepsy surgery, both the epileptogenic lesion (the structural lesion) and the pacemaker zone have to be excised. However, information about other components of the epileptogenic area (the irritative and functional deficit zones) is also important as, for example, surgical intervention may cause dramatic memory impairment [64]. EEG is the most important investigation in the localization of irritative and pacemaker zones. Neuropsychological testing provides information about the functional deficit zone. It has been shown that MRI is able to contribute data about these zones but these techniques are currently still at a research level, or provide redundant clinical information. Hence, these techniques will only be addressed briefly below.

The irritative zone

The zone of interictal spiking, called the irritative zone, can be demonstrated by functional MRI (fMRI). fMRI requires scans with susceptibility sensitive sequences (e.g. echo planar imaging sequences) during at least two different conditions to detect changes in cerebral blood flow (CBF) and deoxygenation which develop 4–6 s after an event. Analysis is done by statistical parametrical mapping. In spike detection fMRI the two conditions are the appearance or absence of a spike. Image data are obtained by scanning immediately after an event (spike) and after periods without an event, or with continuous measurement and event-related off-line analysis. This technique makes it possible to localize the spike-generating zone [65,66]. The disadvantage of this method is that it can only be used in patients with periods of frequent spike activity but also periods of normal interictal EEG and that the technique is rather time-consuming. Hence, its use is limited to a small group of patients in whom continuous interictal spike activity allows the localization of the irritative zone by EEG anyway. The role of spike-triggered fMRI in routine clinical practice may therefore be limited. The possible use of continuous and simultaneous EEG fMRI is considered in Chapter 57.

Pacemaker zone

In the area where ictal activity is generated, the pacemaker zone, CBF increases as seizures begin. Blood flow changes can be detected by fMRI as described above. The problem is that most patients move during seizures and are therefore unsuitable for fMRI examination. CBF changes have been detected by fMRI prior to clinical manifestation of a seizure. Interestingly, apart from an initial increase in CBF, a decrease of CBF has also been detected although the relevance of this is still unclear [67]. As with spike detection fMRI the clinical application of this method is very limited, to patients with non-convulsive status epilepticus or non-convulsive seizures. Imaging of the pacemaker zone is more easily achieved by ictal SPECT and may be enhanced by subtraction of interictal SPECT and coregistration to structural MRI (SISCOM) [68].

Functional deficit zone

The functional deficit zone has traditionally been identified by neuropsychological testing [64]. In recent studies of patients with TLE, memory fMRI showed changes on the epileptogenic side. The contrast between complex visual scenes and visual noise produced almost symmetrical activations in normal controls whereas there was a significant ipsilateral diminution of activation in patients with TLE. In patients, the affected side showed decreased activation compared to normal controls as well as to the contralateral side [69–71]. However, as yet, determination of the extent of the functional deficit is not possible with fMRI. For the decision about surgery or the extent of surgical intervention, the significance of the exact extent of the functional deficit zone remains to be fully assessed.

Localization of eloquent areas

Like the localization of the epileptogenic area, the delineation of eloquent brain areas is very important. The latter has traditionally been determined by suppression, either using the intracarotid amytal test (Wada test) or cortical electrostimulation via sub-dural electrodes. By contrast, fMRI has begun to contribute information about localization of brain functions by demonstrating activation.

With respect to epilepsy surgery, the sensitivity and specificity of fMRI for lateralization of speech dominance is acceptable in clearly unilateral dominance. Using real-time fMRI this can be determined in 15 min [72]. Recent studies have shown that there is close correlation of speech areas mapped by fMRI and cortical electrostimulation but fMRI results depended on the paradigm and the way of presentation (i.e. visual, auditory) [73,74]. It seems necessary to combine different paradigms and presentations. The localization of the precentral region has been described but the precision of mapping is still under review. Furthermore, problems and artefacts inherent in the method have to be considered in the interpretation of results [75].

Future perspectives

In the last two decades the development of new MRI techniques has continuously enhanced the role of this diagnostic tool. The best way of translating this development into progress with the selection of patients for presurgical evaluation may be to improve the teaching of radiologists who are unfamiliar with high-resolution imaging in epilepsy. However, even when epileptologically experienced radiologists read high-resolution, dedicated MR images, 10–15% of patients with medically resistant epilepsy appear to have no abnormalities. There are also patients with clear, focal, unilateral lesions who, contrary to expectations, do not benefit from epilepsy surgery. The technical progress of structural MRI should help us to detect more lesions in normal and abnormal MRI scans so that the number of patients with cryptogenic epilepsy and the number of 'surgical failures' should decrease. Technical progress includes 3 tesla MRI scanners with new sequences as well as new postprocessing facilities. Furthermore, retest reliability studies of fMRI techniques as well as further comparison with 'traditionally' suppressive techniques like the Wada test or cortical electrostimulation have to define the accuracy of mapping of eloquent areas by this technique. Additionally, fMRI will provide us with further information about the cognitive status of patients with epilepsy. This may enable us better to predict the cognitive outcome after surgical intervention in the future. As MRS currently needs a clear localization hypothesis, this technique may prove more useful in basic neuroscience and in research than in the clinical setting. However, prediction is difficult; 20 years ago no one would have predicted the diagnostic possibilities offered by MRI as it is available today.

Acknowledgement

We wish to thank M. Reuber, MD, for helpful comments on the manuscript.

References

1 Duncan JS. Imaging and epilepsy. *Brain* 1997; 120: 339–77.
2 Rosenow F, Luders H. Presurgical evaluation of epilepsy. *Brain* 2001; 124: 1683–700.
3 Engel J Jr, ed. *Surgical Treatment of the Epilepsies*, 2nd edn. New York: Raven Press, 1993.
4 Hauser WA, Hesdorffer DC. Epidemiology of intractable epilepsy. In: Luders HO, Comair YG, eds. *Epilepsy Surgery*. Philadelphia: Lippincott Williams & Wilkins, 2001.
5 McBride MC, Bronstein KS, Bennett B, Erba G, Pilcher W, Berg MJ. Failure of standard magnetic resonance imaging in patients with refractory temporal lobe epilepsy. *Arch Neurol* 1998; 55: 346–8.
6 von Oertzen J, Urbach H, Jungbluth S, Reuber M, Fernández G, Elger CE. Standard magnetic resonance imaging is inadequate for patients with refractory focal epilepsy. *J Neurol Neurosurg Psychiatr* 2002; 73: 643–7.
7 Berkovic SF, Andermann F, Olivier A *et al*. Hippocampal sclerosis in temporal lobe epilepsy demonstrated by magnetic resonance imaging. *Ann Neurol* 1991; 29: 175–82.
8 Bronen RA, Cheung G, Charles JT *et al*. Imaging findings in hippocampal sclerosis: correlation with pathology. *Am J Neuroradiol* 1991; 12: 933–40.
9 Jackson GD, Berkovic SF, Tress BM, Kalnins RM, Fabinyi GC, Bladin PF. Hippocampal sclerosis can be reliably detected by magnetic resonance imaging. *Neurology* 1990; 40: 1869–75.
10 Jackson GD, Berkovic SF, Duncan JS, Connelly A. Optimizing the diagnosis of hippocampal sclerosis using MR imaging. *Am J Neuroradiol* 1993; 14: 753–62.

11 Oppenheim C, Dormont D, Biondi A *et al*. Loss of digitations of the hippocampal head on high-resolution fast spin-echo MR: a sign of mesial temporal sclerosis. *Am J Neuroradiol* 1998; 19: 457–63.

12 Wieshmann UC, Free SL, Everitt AD *et al*. Magnetic resonance imaging in epilepsy with a fast FLAIR sequence. *J Neurol Neurosurg Psychiatr* 1996; 61: 357–61.

13 Bronen R. MR of mesial temporal sclerosis: how much is enough? *Am J Neuroradiol* 1998; 19: 15–18.

14 Kuzniecky R, Ho SS, Martin R *et al*. Temporal lobe developmental malformations and hippocampal sclerosis: epilepsy surgical outcome. *Neurology* 1999; 52: 479–84.

15 Corsellis JA, Goldberg GJ, Norton AR. 'Limbic encephalitis' and its association with carcinoma. *Brain* 1968; 91: 481–96.

16 Dirr LY, Elster AD, Donofrio PD, Smith M. Evolution of brain MRI abnormalities in limbic encephalitis. *Neurology* 1990; 40: 1304–6.

17 Bien CG, Schulze-Bonhage A, Deckert M *et al*. Limbic encephalitis not associated with neoplasm as a cause of temporal lobe epilepsy. *Neurology* 2000; 55: 1823–8.

18 Barkovich AJ, Kuzniecky RI, Dobyns WB, Jackson GD, Becker LE, Evrard P. A classification scheme for malformations of cortical development. *Neuropediatrics* 1996; 27: 59–63.

19 Palmini A, Luders HO. Classification issues in malformations caused by abnormalities of cortical development. *Neurosurg Clin N Am* 2002; 13: 1–16.

20 Guerrini R, Andermann E, Avoli M, Dobyns WB. Cortical dysplasias, genetics, and epileptogenesis. *Adv Neurol* 1999; 79: 95–121.

21 Becker AJ, Urbach H, Scheffler B *et al*. Focal cortical dysplasia of Taylor's balloon cell type: mutational analysis of the TSC1 gene indicates a pathogenic relationship to tuberous sclerosis. *Ann Neurol* 2002; 52: 29–37.

22 Urbach H, Scheffler B, Heinrichsmeier T *et al*. Focal cortical dysplasia of Taylor's Balloon cell type: a clinicopathological entity with characteristic neuroimaging and histopathological features, and favorable postsurgical outcome. *Epilepsia* 2002; 43: 33–40.

23 Bastos AC, Comeau RM, Andermann F *et al*. Diagnosis of subtle focal dysplastic lesions: curvilinear reformatting from three-dimensional magnetic resonance imaging. *Ann Neurol* 1999; 46: 88–94.

24 Bastos AC, Korah IP, Cendes F *et al*. Curvilinear reconstruction of 3D magnetic resonance imaging in patients with partial epilepsy: a pilot study. *Magn Reson Imaging* 1995; 13: 1107–12.

25 Bernasconi A, Antel SB, Collins DL *et al*. Texture analysis and morphological processing of magnetic resonance imaging assist detection of focal cortical dysplasia in extra-temporal partial epilepsy. *Ann Neurol* 2001; 49: 770–5.

26 Woermann FG, Free SL, Koepp MJ, Ashburner J, Duncan JS. Voxel-by-voxel comparison of automatically segmented cerebral gray matter – a rater-independent comparison of structural MRI in patients with epilepsy. *Neuroimage* 1999; 10: 373–84.

27 Dubeau F, Tampieri D, Lee N *et al*. Periventricular and subcortical nodular heterotopia. A study of 33 patients. *Brain* 1995; 118: 1273–87.

28 Li LM, Dubeau F, Andermann F *et al*. Periventricular nodular heterotopia and intractable temporal lobe epilepsy: poor outcome after temporal lobe resection. *Ann Neurol* 1997; 41: 662–8.

29 Edwards JC, Wyllie E, Ruggeri PM *et al*. Seizure outcome after surgery for epilepsy due to malformation of cortical development. *Neurology* 2000; 55: 1110–14.

30 Battaglia D, Di Rocco C, Iuvone L *et al*. Neuro-cognitive development and epilepsy outcome in children with surgically treated hemimegalencephaly. *Neuropediatrics* 1999; 30: 307–13.

31 Palmini A, Gambardella A, Andermann F *et al*. Operative strategies for patients with cortical dysplastic lesions and intractable epilepsy. *Epilepsia* 1994; 35 (Suppl. 6): S57–S71.

32 Daumas-Duport C, Scheithauer BW, Chodkiewicz JP, Laws ER Jr, Vedrenne C. Dysembryoplastic neuroepithelial tumor: a surgically curable tumor of young patients with intractable partial seizures. Report of thirty-nine cases. *Neurosurgery* 1988; 23: 545–56.

33 Ostertun B, Wolf HK, Campos MG *et al*. Dysembryoplastic neuroepithelial tumors: MR and CT evaluation. *Am J Neuroradiol* 1996; 17: 419–30.

34 Zentner J, Wolf HK, Ostertun B *et al*. Gangliogliomas: clinical, radiologi-

cal, and histopathological findings in 51 patients. *J Neurol Neurosurg Psychiatr* 1994; 57: 1497–502.

35 Daumas-Duport C, Varlet P, Bacha S, Beuvon F, Cervera-Pierot P, Chodkiewicz JP. Dysembryoplastic neuroepithelial tumors: nonspecific histological forms – a study of 40 cases. *J Neurooncol* 1999; 41: 267–80.

36 Dorsch NWC, McMahon JHA. Intracranial cavernous malformations – natural history and management. *Crit Rev Neurosurg* 1998; 8: 154–68.

37 Casazza M, Broggi G, Franzini A *et al*. Supratentorial cavernous angiomas and epileptic seizures: preoperative course and postoperative outcome. *Neurosurgery* 1996; 39: 26–32.

38 Marks DA, Kim J, Spencer DD, Spencer SS. Seizure localization and pathology following head injury in patients with uncontrolled epilepsy. *Neurology* 1995; 45: 2051–7.

39 Diaz-Arrastia R, Agostini MA, Frol AB *et al*. Neurophysiologic and neuroradiologic features of intractable epilepsy after traumatic brain injury in adults. *Arch Neurol* 2000; 57: 1611–16.

40 McMurdo SK Jr, Moore SG, Brant-Zawadzki M *et al*. MR imaging of intracranial tuberous sclerosis. *Am J Roentgenol* 1987; 148: 791–6.

41 Roach ES, Williams DP, Laster DW. Magnetic resonance imaging in tuberous sclerosis. *Arch Neurol* 1987; 44: 301–3.

42 Levine D, Barnes P, Korf B, Edelman R. Tuberous sclerosis in the fetus: second-trimester diagnosis of subependymal tubers with ultrafast MR imaging. *Am J Roentgenol* 2000; 175: 1067–9.

43 Bebin EM, Kelly PJ, Gomez MR. Surgical treatment for epilepsy in cerebral tuberous sclerosis. *Epilepsia* 1993; 34: 651–7.

44 Koh S, Jayakar P, Dunoyer C *et al*. Epilepsy surgery in children with tuberous sclerosis complex: presurgical evaluation and outcome. *Epilepsia* 2000; 41: 1206–13.

45 Arzimanoglou AA, Andermann F, Aicardi J *et al*. Sturge–Weber syndrome: indications and results of surgery in 20 patients. *Neurology* 2000; 55: 1472–9.

46 Palmini A, Chandler C, Andermann F *et al*. Resection of the lesion in patients with hypothalamic hamartomas and catastrophic epilepsy. *Neurology* 2002; 58: 1338–47.

47 Dunoyer C, Ragheb J, Resnick T *et al*. The use of stereotactic radiosurgery to treat intractable childhood partial epilepsy. *Epilepsia* 2002; 43: 292–300.

48 Sisodiya SM, Free SL, Shorvon SD. Surgical treatment of hypothalamic hamartoma. *Ann Neurol* 1998; 43: 273–5.

49 Bien CG, Urbach H, Deckert M *et al*. Diagnosis and staging of Rasmussen's encephalitis by serial MRI and histopathology. *Neurology* 2002; 58: 250–7.

50 Risse JH, Menzel C, Grunwald F *et al*. Early childhood MRI findings in complex partial seizures and hippocampal sclerosis. *J Magn Reson Imaging* 1999; 10: 93–6.

51 Gaillard WD. Structural and functional imaging in children with partial epilepsy. *Ment Retard Dev Disabil Res Rev* 2000; 6: 220–6.

52 Lendt M, Helmstaedter C, Elger CE. Pre- and postoperative socioeconomic development of 151 patients with focal epilepsies. *Epilepsia* 1997; 38: 1330–7.

53 Cook MJ, Fish DR, Shorvon SD, Straughan K, Stevens JM. Hippocampal volumetric and morphometric studies in frontal and temporal lobe epilepsy. *Brain* 1992; 115: 1001–15.

54 Duncan JS, Bartlett P, Barker GJ. Technique for measuring hippocampal T2 relaxation time. *Am J Neuroradiol* 1996; 17: 1805–10.

55 Jackson GD, Connelly A, Duncan JS, Grunewald RA, Gadian DG. Detection of hippocampal pathology in intractable partial epilepsy: increased sensitivity with quantitative magnetic resonance T2 relaxometry. *Neurology* 1993; 43: 1793–9.

56 Kuzniecky RI, Bilir E, Gilliam F *et al*. Multimodality MRI in mesial temporal sclerosis: relative sensitivity and specificity. *Neurology* 1997; 49: 774–8.

57 Van Paesschen W, Sisodiya S, Connelly A *et al*. Quantitative hippocampal MRI and intractable temporal lobe epilepsy. *Neurology* 1995; 45: 2233–40.

58 von Oertzen J, Urbach H, Blümcke I *et al*. Time-efficient T2-relaxometry of the entire hippocampus is feasible in temporal lobe epilepsy. *Neurology* 2002; 58: 257–64.

59 Kuzniecky R, Hugg JW, Hetherington H *et al*. Relative utility of 1H

spectroscopic imaging and hippocampal volumetry in the lateralization of mesial temporal lobe epilepsy. *Neurology* 1998; 51: 66–71.

60 Li LM, Caramanos Z, Cendes F *et al*. Lateralization of temporal lobe epilepsy (TLE) and discrimination of TLE from extra-TLE using pattern analysis of magnetic resonance spectroscopic and volumetric data. *Epilepsia* 2000; 41: 832–42.

61 Li LM, Cendes F, Antel SB *et al*. Prognostic value of proton magnetic resonance spectroscopic imaging for surgical outcome in patients with intractable temporal lobe epilepsy and bilateral hippocampal atrophy. *Ann Neurol* 2000; 47: 195–200.

62 Stefan H, Feichtinger M, Pauli E *et al*. Magnetic resonance spectroscopy and histopathological findings in temporal lobe epilepsy. *Epilepsia* 2001; 42: 41–6.

63 Cendes F, Andermann F, Dubeau F, Matthews PM, Arnold DL. Normalization of neuronal metabolic dysfunction after surgery for temporal lobe epilepsy. Evidence from proton MR spectroscopic imaging. *Neurology* 1997; 49: 1525–33.

64 Luders HO, Awad IA. Conceptual considerations. In: Luders HO, ed. *Epilepsy Surgery*. New York: Raven Press, 1992.

65 Krakow K, Woermann FG, Symms MR *et al*. EEG-triggered functional MRI of interictal epileptiform activity in patients with partial seizures. *Brain* 1999; 122: 1679–88.

66 Krakow K, Messina D, Lemieux L, Duncan JS, Fish DR. Functional MRI activation of individual interictal epileptiform spikes. *Neuroimage* 2001; 13: 502–5.

67 Krings T, Topper R, Reinges MH *et al*. Hemodynamic changes in simple partial epilepsy: a functional MRI study. *Neurology* 2000; 54: 524–7.

68 O'Brien TJ, So EL, Mullan BP *et al*. Subtraction ictal SPECT co-registered to MRI improves clinical usefulness of SPECT in localizing the surgical seizure focus. *Neurology* 1998; 50: 445–54.

69 Billingsley RL, McAndrews MP, Crawley AP, Mikulis DJ. Functional MRI of phonological and semantic processing in temporal lobe epilepsy. *Brain* 2001; 124: 1218–27.

70 Detre JA, Maccotta L, King D *et al*. Functional MRI lateralization of memory in temporal lobe epilepsy. *Neurology* 1998; 50: 926–32.

71 Jokeit H, Okujava M, Woermann FG. Memory fMRI lateralizes temporal lobe epilepsy. *Neurology* 2001; 57: 1786–93.

72 Fernandez G, de Greiff A, von Oertzen J *et al*. Language mapping in less than 15 minutes: real-time functional MRI during routine clinical investigation. *Neuroimage* 2001; 14: 585–94.

73 Carpentier A, Pugh KR, Westerveld M *et al*. Functional MRI of language processing: dependence on input modality and temporal lobe epilepsy. *Epilepsia* 2001; 42: 1241–54.

74 FitzGerald DB, Cosgrove GR, Ronner S *et al*. Location of language in the cortex: a comparison between functional MR imaging and electrocortical stimulation. *Am J Neuroradiol* 1997; 18: 1529–39.

75 Krings T, Reinges MH, Erberich S *et al*. Functional MRI for presurgical planning: problems, artefacts, and solution strategies. *J Neurol Neurosurg Psychiatr* 2001; 70: 749–60.

56 PET and SPECT in Presurgical Evaluation of Epilepsy

B. Sadzot and W. van Paesschen

Epilepsy is first and foremost a disorder of brain function. EEG was the first tool for the non-invasive diagnostic investigation of seizure disorders. Fifty years later, EEG and related techniques remain essential for the diagnosis of epilepsy and the localization of the epileptic focus. They may however provide unclear or even misleading information due to the rapid propagation of epileptic discharges or to the occurence of interictal spikes in areas that do not generate seizures.

PET and SPECT are nuclear medicine techniques that have proved extremely useful for epileptologists in providing information on other aspects of brain function. They can be combined with electrophysiological and structural data to define non-invasively the cerebral area generating partial seizures, and permit non-invasive confirmation of functional disturbances. In consequence, a panel of experts has recognized the clinical usefulness of PET for the presurgical evaluation of patients with refractory seizure disorders [1].

Despite dramatic improvements in morphological imagery with MRI showing in many patients subtle or discrete brain lesions related to the epileptic focus, interictal PET and/or ictal SPECT have become commonly used at many centres for the presurgical evaluation of epileptic patients considered for surgery. They have a significant impact on diagnostic evaluation and surgical planning. They are particularly useful in patients with normal MRI, diffuse morphological abnormalities and discordant seizure semiology, electrophysiology and morphological data.

PET

Method

PET is based upon the detection of radioactive tracers and computerized tomographic reconstruction methods. It permits the non-invasive measurement of the regional biodistribution of trace amounts of radioligand in a slice of organ at any time after its administration and therefore the monitoring of its regional kinetics. The measured radioactive concentrations can be translated into colour-coded images and, with an appropriate calibration, it is also possible to quantify the true regional tracer concentration at any given time.

A major advantage of PET methodology is related to the large variety of radioactive tracers that are available. The measurements are highly specific to the biological system of interest. Though many biochemical and physiological brain parameters can be studied *in vivo* by PET, it has been used, in epilepsy, to study mostly glucose consumption and neuroreceptors (Table 56.1).

PET methods developed to image these parameters usually re-quire a steady state in the patient's condition. They are not designed to study short-term events like epileptic fits. Measurement of glucose consumption, for example, requires an incubation period (or steady state) of 30–45 min after tracer administration before scanning. During this time, ^{18}FDG is trapped and accumulates into cells as a function of hexokinase activity. The ^{18}FDG scan reflects cerebral glucose metabolism during the uptake, weighted towards the beginning of that period, primarily the first 10 min after injection. The method underestimates changes in metabolic rates associated with changes in cerebral function of short duration [2]. PET is designed for studying cooperative patients during the interictal state. Some ictal PET studies have been reported but they will not be discussed here [3–6], as technical constraints preclude their regular use in epilepsy surgery.

Another important limitation of PET is its spatial resolution. The first tomographs had an in-plane resolution of 15 mm. In using current technology, this has been reduced to 5 mm. One of the consequences of the limited spatial resolution is the so-called partial volume effect, which can be defined as an averaging of the signal between neighbouring areas. This effect concerns structures smaller than approximately twice the spatial resolution of the system [7]. It results in a blurring of boundaries between adjacent structures and therefore in poor definition of anatomical details, as well as in an underestimation of true isotope concentration for smaller structures.

Spatial resolution definitely affects the sensitivity of PET studies. With the old single slice ECAT scanner (in-plane resolution of 16 mm), Engel *et al.* [8] had a 52% yield of positive scans in their overall epileptic population, while it increased to 86% with their multislice CTI-831 (in plane resolution of 5 mm). With limited spatial resolution and the resulting partial volume effect, the apparent size of the hypometabolic zone is increased but the degree of hypometabolism is underestimated. Methods to correct for this variable have been designed and implemented [9–11]. Partial volume correction increased the sensitivity of detecting a lateralizing asymmetry of hippocampal metabolic activity by 15–20% over that without partial volume correction [12].

Coregistration of structural (MRI) and metabolic images (PET or SPECT) may further enhance the anatomical accuracy of functional data [13–16], but is seldom used in clinical routine.

To date, there is no consensus concerning the best method for PET data analysis. Interpretation of PET images may be achieved through visual inspection alone, which is often sufficient for clinical purposes, particularly when studying a focal pathology, such as partial epilepsy. Quantification of PET studies may be relative (raw counts) or absolute (after modelling, to obtain for example glucose metabolic rates, or receptor densities (B_{max})). Measurements are obtained in regions of interest (ROI) which are affected by several source of variations (size, shape, positioning) and biases (partial volume effect). These data are used for comparison with a control population or calculation of asymmetry indices, or normalized to global counts. Quantitative analysis can help validate or negate contradictory or questionable visual interpretation.

Automated, non-interactive, voxel-by-voxel based techniques of scan analysis such as statistical parametric mapping (Wellcome Department of Cognitive Neurology, Institute of Neurology, London, UK) offer more objective, extensive, rigorous and detailed analysis of brain metabolic activity [17,18]. Comparisons with a control group may be performed for groups of patients but also for each patient individually [19] (Plate 56.1; parts (c–e) also shown in colour between pp. 670 and 671). Use of SPM maps may facilitate comparisons and exchanges of standardized data between epilepsy centres. There has been little application of this method of analysis for PET in epileptic patients [11,19–21]. Using SPM analysis of quantitative (CMRGlu) and non-quantitative (radioactive counts) data, the same pattern of results was obtained, further suggesting that it no longer appears justified to perform invasive arterial catheterization and blood sampling for ^{18}FDG-PET scans in epileptic patients to obtain valuable and reliable functional information [22].

Glucose metabolism

Because of the above methodological and technical considerations, the vast majority of ^{18}FDG-PET studies have been carried out during the interictal state. There have been only a few reports of ictal ^{18}FDG-PET studies [3–6,23].

Kuhl et al. [2] were the first to demonstrate that interictal ^{18}FDG scans are characterized by a localized depression in cerebral glucose consumption that correlated anatomically with the EEG spike foci in patients with partial epilepsy. The metabolic defect on PET was larger than atrophic lesions found on CT scan and than the structural damage found at pathological examination. Interictal EEG electrical activity did not seem to influence glucose metabolism.

Table 56.1 Radiolabelled molecules for PET in epilepsy

Studied parameters	Radiolabelled molecule	Original publication
Blood flow	H$_2$^{15}O	[109]
Glucose metabolism	^{18}F-fluorodeoxyglucose	[2]
Central benzodiazepine receptors	^{11}C-flumazenil	[131]
Opiate receptors	^{11}C-carfentanil	[88]
	^{11}C-diprenorphine	[119]
	^{18}F-cyclofoxy	[54]
	^{11}C-methyl-naltrindole	[124]
MAO-B Enzymes	^{11}C-deprenyl	[194]
Serotonin synthesis	^{11}C-a-methyl-L-tryptophan	[195]
Peripheral benzodiazepine receptors	^{11}C-PK11195	[196]
Muscarinic receptors	^{11}C-methyl-4-piperidyl benzylate	[197]

These original findings were later expanded by Engel et al. [24–26] and largely confirmed by many others [23,27,29–35] (Fig. 56.1).

More than 70% of patients with partial epilepsy show a localized area of decreased brain glucose metabolism on ^{18}FDG-PET. PET however may be normal even in patients with well-defined EEG focus; and inversely, PET may show an area of decreased CMRGlu in patients with non-localizing EEG or IC-EEG [25]. The hypometabolism may be regional or lobar and usually has a progressive demarcation from the normal cortex; it may also be more widespread and multilobar; in this case, the most hypometabolic lobe is usually the lobe of seizure onset [32]. The hypometabolic region may include an area with more severe hypometabolism and a sharp demarcation from the adjacent cortex. This metabolic pattern often corresponds to a structural lesion. The site of ictal onset always lies within any demonstrated hypometabolic area.

The hypometabolism is thus always on the side of the brain with the epileptic focus and false lateralizations are exceptional [8,32,36,37]. False lateralizations may be due to postictal effects or to unrecognized, subclinical seizure activity during the uptake phase. EEG monitoring during the hours preceding the PET scan minimizes the risk of false lateralization (to exclude unreported seizures). Following complex partial seizures, the ipsilateral temporal metabolic rate is relatively increased for 48 h before falling significantly later [38]. Falsely localizing information obtained by ^{18}FDG-PET have been reported in patients with extratemporal epilepsies.

The sensitivity of PET is influenced by several factors, including location of seizure focus. Complex partial seizures may arise from many areas of the brain [39–42]. Patients with extratemporal epilepsy, however, are less likely to have an abnormal PET study than patients with a temporal epilepsy [35,43–45]. Based on a review of the literature, Spencer et al. [46] reported that overall sensitivity of interictal ^{18}FDG-PET to temporal lobe epilepsy as judged by EEG criteria was 84% with a specificity of 86%, while sensitivity for extratemporal epilepsy was 33% with 95% specificity. When a lesion is detected by CT or MRI, ^{18}FDG-PET is abnormal as well; the hypometabolic zone is larger and more extensive than the lesion itself [5,23,27,32,47]. This discrepancy between anatomical and functional imaging is explained by partial volume effect and biochemical factors (loss of neurones and their projections). The sensitivity of PET is lower when MRI is normal [48]. The relative sensitivity of PET and MRI will vary according to the case-mix and aetiologies. For example, small gliomas, hamartomas and arteriovenous malformations may not disturb glucose metabolism [47,49–51]. Such functional and anatomical tests should clearly be seen as complimentary rather than competitive.

Neuronal migration disorders (NMD) can present with either hypometabolism or displaced grey matter activity to a white matter area [52]. This latter metabolic pattern is a unique feature of NMD and it is highly suggestive of this pathology. It represents glucose metabolism of abnormally located grey matter rather than subclinical ictal phenomenon.

The pathophysiology underlying the regional changes in glucose consumption in the brain of epileptic patients remains speculative. If one considers the mesiotemporal epilepsy syndrome, which is a convenient model, it appears from the first studies that the size of the hypometabolic zone is larger than the epileptic focus defined as

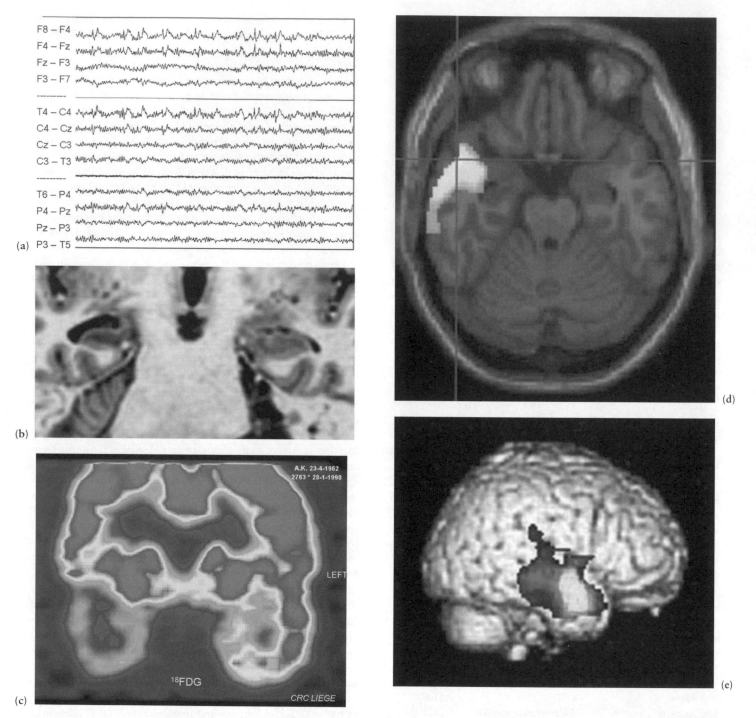

Fig. 56.1 Complex partial seizures in a 32-year-old man. (a) EEG showing very frequent spiking over the right temporal cortex. (b) MRI with right hippocampal atrophy on a coronal IR slice. (c) ^{18}FDG-PET with important glucose hypometabolism over the entire right temporal lobe. (d, e) SPM analysis of this PET study comparing the patient's PET to a group of 30 age-matched controls: pixels with a significant hypometabolism are projected over a transverse slice of a standard MRI in the Talairach's frame (d) or on a standard three-dimensional MRI (e). (Parts (c–e) also shown in colour between pp. 670 and 671.)

the site of seizure onset during intracranial EEG recordings [23,26,27,32,34,49,51,53]. The hypometabolism sometimes extends to homolateral frontal and parietal cortex, as well as to subcortical structures such as homolateral basal ganglia and thalamus, and contralateral cerebellar lobe [19,28,32,34,51,55–57].

Pathological studies have indicated that the majority of temporal

lobe epilepsies are characterized by neuronal loss and gliosis in the hippocampus [58,59]. There is however no relation between the degree of interictal PET hypometabolism and the amount of hippocampal gliosis or cell loss [47,60–63]. Furthermore, temporal lobe hypometabolism has been observed in the absence of hippocampal sclerosis or any other identifiable pathology [60,64].

Hippocampal glucose metabolism is not closely correlated to hippocampal volume [65–67], suggesting that hippocampal atrophy is not a major determinant of the hippocampal hypometabolism. Localized neuronal loss cannot therefore be held solely responsible for the interictal hypometabolism.

Attempts to correlate clinical data and both the extent and the degree of glucose hypometabolism have been deceptive. There is no correlation between the hypometabolism and the frequency of EEG spikes in the interictal state, the presence of EEG slow waves, seizure frequency, lifetime number of generalized tonic-clonic seizures, duration of the seizure disorder, type of partial seizure, presence of multiple seizure type or secondary generalized seizures, age, sex, age at seizure onset or a history of febrile convulsions [23,26–28,32,68]. Antiepileptic drugs (phenobarbital and to a lesser degree, phenytoin and carbamazepine) cause a uniform drug-induced depression of glucose metabolism without change in the degree of asymmetry between the hypometabolic region and the normal, contralateral cortex [69,70]. This is important since these patients are usually under one (or more) of these drugs at the time of their PET study.

Synapses are the major source of glucose utilization in the brain [71]. Any reduction in synaptic activity should lead to a remote reduction in metabolic activity: it is the deafferentation hypothesis. The hypometabolism may thus reflect decreased synaptic activity in the projection fields of inhibited, dysfunctioning or damaged neurones, or a loss of 'activating' influences [24,51,61,64]. Such a transsynaptic effect (the so-called 'diaschisis') explains the hypometabolism sometimes observed at sites distant from the temporal lobe such as the cerebellar lobe contralateral to the area of cortical hypometabolism, the homolateral thalamus and basal ganglia. In primates, the hippocampus and the amygdala have extensive connections with the striatum, thalamus and cerebral cortex [72–75]. Subcortical structures play an important role in controlling neuronal cortical excitability and seizure propagation [76,77].

There are also the strong anatomical and functional links between the temporal pole and the limbic structures. Animal studies have reported afferent projection from both the amygdala and the hippocampus to the temporopolar cortex [78], as well as efferent projections from temporal pole to orbitofrontal regions, temporal neocortex and anterior cingulate cortex [75,79]. Polar temporal lobe hypometabolism worsened in patients who underwent a selective hippocampoamygdalectomy [80].

The hypometabolism in the lateral temporal cortex is thus probably not directly related to a loss of neurones nor glial cells. The lobectomy specimens of many patients display normal cortical temporal neuronal density [24,62,81]. However, loss of dentritic spines (and therefore of synaptic density and connectivity) has been demonstrated in chronic human epileptogenic lesions but is not well appreciated on routine light microscopy and requires special Golgi and electronic preparations [82]. More recent pathological studies of anterior temporal lobectomy specimens have described widespread microdysgenesis in the temporal neocortex of many patients with hippocampal sclerosis [83,84], or subpial gliosis [36]. Careful examination of MRI sometimes reveals temporal neocortical structural changes like decreased volume of temporal lobe ipsilateral to the side of the seizure focus, or the loss of grey–white matter differentiation in the temporal lobe of patients with temporal lobe epilepsy [85–87]. Subtle structural or functional regional neocortical

abnormalities not associated with cell loss may thus play a role in this hypometabolism. Neocortical increase in mu opiate receptors may reflect altered synaptic activity in patients with temporal lobe epilepsy [88].

Alternatively, interictal inhibitory processes that promote or retard seizure discharges may cause widespread interictal hypometabolism [89]. In favour of this hypothesis is the observation of improvement of metabolic activity in the orbitofrontal cortex and in the contralateral medial temporal structures after surgery [80], and a trend towards normalization of regional glucose utilization in the ipsilateral temporal neocortex 1 year after surgery [90].

Glucose metabolism is, on average, significantly lower in all cortical regions on the side of the epileptic focus compared to the same regions on the non-focus side, with the exception of the sensorimotor cortex [19,32,34]. This suggests that the spatially limited epileptic focus may influence or disturb the function of a whole hemisphere. The clinical significance of extratemporal hypometabolism in temporal lobe epilepsy is unclear but it might explain the cognitive or affective disturbances often observed in these patients. Correlations with depressed glucose consumption in remote cortical areas and neuropsychological deficit suggests that impaired language function in patients with left temporal lobe epilepsy could result from functional changes beyond the temporal lobe [21].

Prediction of seizure outcome on the basis of PET data is an important issue in patients with uncontrolled partial seizures as PET results may influence patient selection for surgery.

In patients with temporal lobe epilepsy, temporal hypometabolism on ^{18}FDG-PET predicts successful temporal lobectomy even when surface EEG is non-localizing [36,60,91–93]. Both the degree and the extent of relative hypometabolism, or the metabolic pattern, in the temporal lobe predictive of outcome is still a matter of debate. For some, mesial hypometabolism is not a predictor of outcome [60,91,92], while for others it is associated with better outcome [55,93]; diffuse hypometabolism or lateral temporal hypometabolism may be a better indication of a good outcome [49,91].

Using multivariate analysis of metabolic data in three temporal ROI and one basofrontal region, Dupont et al. [94] showed that postoperative outcome is better predicted by describing metabolic abnormalities over a network of cortical regions rather than in a single, highly focused cortical area. The temporal pole played the most determining role, exhibiting the higher and the more discriminant coefficient. They could correctly predict the 2-year prognosis in 100% of the 30 patients who underwent anterior temporal lobectomy.

Multilobar hypometabolism [91], or extratemporal hypometabolism [36,92,95], is associated with a higher likelihood of postsurgical seizure activity. Interestingly, it has been found that patients with thalamic hypometabolism ipsilateral to the temporal lobe seizure focus were at higher risk of postoperative seizures than were patients with no thalamic asymmetry; furthermore, patients with relative contralateral thalamic hypometabolism were not seizure free postoperatively [55].

Normal scans are associated with suboptimal surgical outcome [92] and intracranial EEG studies may be less likely to disclose an epileptogenic region when ^{18}FDG-PET shows no hypometabolism [91]. Nevertheless, these patients without hypometabolism may benefit from surgery but may need further scrutiny [33].

Epileptic syndromes are proportionally more frequent and numerous in infants and children than in adults [96]. A description of the cerebral metabolic patterns is not yet available for each of these syndromes however. For some, functional imaging has changed the therapeutic approach or improved the understanding of their pathogenesis.

Cryptogenic partial epilepsy in infants and children is characterized during the interictal period by focal or regional decreases in glucose metabolism similar in nature and extent to those found in adults [97,98]. The location of the metabolic abnormality is also in good agreement with EEG findings and electrocorticographic recordings [99]. The presence of such hypometabolic areas should raise the possibility of a surgical cure of the epilepsy given the deleterious effects of repeated seizures in children. The extension of the metabolic abnormality may guide the surgical strategy: focal resection for limited hypometabolic foci, hemispherectomy when metabolic disturbances are widespread, if the other clinical and investigative findings are congruent.

Exceptionally, a paradoxical increase in glucose metabolism [100] or cerebral blood flow (CBF) [101] has been observed during the interictal period in children with partial epilepsy. This phenomenon is not well understood. This hypermetabolism might be specifically observed in highly spiking foci or might be a transitory stage of recent epileptic foci.

In patients with cryptogenic infantile spasms, the interictal metabolic pattern is also characterized by focal areas of decreased glucose metabolism, the topography of which usually corresponds to the lateralized EEG findings [102]. An increase in glucose metabolism was observed in the lenticular nuclei of all patients [103]. Given their extremely poor prognosis, some have proposed the resection of the cortex that looks abnormal on PET. The results are encouraging since amongst 30 operated infants, 75% were reported seizure free [104] with the remainder often showing improvement. In many cases, neuropathological examination of the resected tissue revealed a microscopic cortical dysplasia that had gone undetected by available MRI.

The Landau–Kleffner syndrome associates an acquired aphasia with spike-and-wave discharges that are activated by slow-wave sleep, behavioural disturbances and epileptic seizures. In most cases, PET studies revealed a focal increase in glucose metabolism during the active phase of the disease even during wakefulness when spike-and-wave discharges are sporadic. After recovery, a focal decrease in glucose metabolism was observed. The metabolic abnormalities essentially involved cortical associative areas and in all cases the temporal cortex [105].

In Lennox–Gastaut syndrome, the distribution of cerebral glucose metabolism is variable [106,107]. During the interictal state, hypometabolic areas of various extension are observed: focal, diffuse unilateral, diffuse bilateral or multifocal [108]. These localized metabolic defects are usually not suspected from clinical, EEG or MRI findings.

As with partial epilepsies, PET findings may help to influence the appropriate surgical strategy for these refractory epilepsies within the overall clinical and investigative context. A focal cortical resection may be considered when there is a focal hypometabolism, whereas hemispherectomy or corpus callosum section might be helpful in unilateral diffuse cases.

Cerebral blood flow

CBF has also been studied with PET in patients with complex partial epilepsy using $^{13}NH_3$ [2] and ^{15}O [5,109,110] in the early years of PET. These studies involving patients suspected of having complex partial epilepsy showed an interictal decrease in blood flow in the temporal lobe ipsilateral to the surface EEG focus. There was also a decrease in oxygen consumption. While blood flow and metabolism are normally tightly coupled, Bernardi et al. [109] found that the decrease in oxygen consumption ($CMRO_2$) was of a lesser magnitude than the decrease of CBF, and accordingly, oxygen extraction rate was increased in the area of low blood flow. To interpret these findings, it was argued that at the site of the focus the reserve of oxygen supply is diminished and the tissue metabolic requirements are high, even interictally, while for others [5,110], there was no significant change in the rate of oxygen extraction and the decreases in CBF and in $CMRO_2$ were coupled. More recently, Breier et al. [111] found in patients with complex partial seizure that the degree of interhemispheric asymmetry in the temporal lobe in both glucose and blood flow increased with duration of seizure disorder, but the rate of increase in asymmetry was significantly greater for glucose metabolism than for blood flow, suggesting a progressive uncoupling between these parameters. Gaillard et al. [112] also found that glucose metabolism was more decreased than blood flow in the temporal cortex ipsilateral to the EEG focus, suggesting that glucose metabolism and blood flow may be uncoupled in the epileptogenic cortex.

Oxygen-15 emits positrons that are more energetic than those from ^{18}F (1.72 vs. 0.64 MeV); hence the positron range is longer for ^{15}O than for ^{18}F (8.2 vs. 2.39 mm). Images obtained with ^{15}O-labelled molecules are more fuzzy, have a poorer resolution and a higher statistical noise than images obtained with ^{18}F-labelled compounds. This explains that the ^{15}O-radiolabelled molecules are no longer used for static imaging. Leiderman et al. [113] investigated 28 patients with medically intractable partial epilepsy undergoing presurgical evaluation with PET scanning using both ^{18}FDG and $H_2^{15}O$. Amongst the 15 patients who had surgery or subdural electrodes, three showed falsely lateralizing $H_2^{15}O$-PET and four were normal. False lateralizations with ^{15}O-water have been reported elsewhere [112]. Only one ^{18}FDG-PET was normal and there was no discordant lateralization. ^{18}FDG-PET is more sensitive and specific for the lateralization and the localization of the epileptogenic area than methods using ^{15}O.

$H_2^{15}O$ is currently used for activation studies to map specific brain functions. Non-invasive functional brain mapping with dynamic $H_2^{15}O$-PET for language localization may alleviate the need for Wada test or cortical stimulation [114,115], but fMRI may be superior to PET in this area.

Receptor studies

While ^{18}FDG-PET is a sensitive and reliable method of localization in partial epilepsies, it suffers from some drawbacks and limitations. The hypometabolism is often widespread and it extends beyond the epileptic focus. It therefore does not allow a precise localization of the seizure onset. The observed changes in glucose metabolism are not specific. In order to overcome these limitations, and in the hope of obtaining new insights into the pathophysiology of epilepsies and the biochemistry of the epileptic focus, radioligands have been developed to study specific neuroreceptor systems. While receptor studies have proved useful in some situations, [18]FDG-PET remains the PET method of preference.

Opiate receptors

A role for opioid peptides in seizure mechanisms (modulation of neuronal excitability or seizure threshold) has been documented extensively in experimental animal models. Morphine and the opioid peptides elicit proconvulsant or anticonvulsant effects depending on the dose, route and rate of administration, and the animal model used [116]. At low doses, they are predominantly anticonvulsant [116]. Induced generalized seizures are associated with the release of β-endorphine and a met-enkephalin precursor [117,118].

Using PET and the selective mu opiate ligand ^{11}C-carfentanil, an extremely potent fentanyl analogue and opiate agonist, Frost et al. [88] found a 9–15% increase in mu opiate receptor binding in the lateral temporal neocortex of 13 patients with epilepsy, on the side of electrical foci, during the interictal state. The cortical increase in ^{11}C-carfentanil correlated with the decrease in glucose metabolism and occurred distant to the amygdalohippocampal region, the presumed primary site of the epileptic focus. In the amygdala, ^{11}C-carfentanil binding was reduced, reflecting non-specific tissue damage or receptor downregulation in the region of the presumed epileptogenic focus [119].

Several interpretations can be proposed to explain the increased cortical binding: (a) an increase in the total number of opiate receptors; (b) a decrease in opiate receptor occupation by endogenous opioids; and (c) an increase in receptor affinity, or any combination of the above. Tracer kinetic modelling indicated that this increase in binding was not due to changes in blood flow or blood–brain barrier transport [88]. Carfentanil is such a potent agonist that side-effects, including respiratory depression, occur for doses greater than 0.05 µg/kg. Therefore, ^{11}C-carfentanil can only be administered at high specific activity, which means that it is mathematically not possible, in vivo, to estimate separately the affinity and the density of opiate receptors.

Mu, delta and kappa receptors may each play a role in anticonvulsant mechanisms. Anticonvulsant effects of D-ala-D-leu-enkephalin and dynorphin, acting respectively at delta and kappa receptors, have been demonstrated [120]. Satisfactory ligands for selectively labelling kappa opiate receptors in vivo do not exist. ^{11}C-diprenorphine, a weak partial opiate agonist, has a similar and high affinity for mu, delta and kappa receptors. Sequential PET studies in the same individuals with ^{11}C-carfentanil and ^{11}C-diprenorphine provide images with different patterns in accordance with the pharmacology of these tracers. By comparing the ^{11}C-carfentanil and ^{11}C-diprenorphine scans, the contribution of non-mu opiate receptors to ^{11}C-diprenorphine images can be evaluated [121]. Interictal paired PET measurements were made using ^{11}C-diprenorphine and ^{11}C-carfentanil in patients with unilateral complex partial seizures. ^{11}C-diprenorphine binding was not significantly altered between homologous regions of the focus and the non-focus side, even in the presence of an increase in mu opiate receptor binding and a decrease in glucose consumption [119]. Cyclofoxy (6-deoxy-6β-fluoronaltrexone) is a potent opiate antagonist which binds to both mu and kappa but not to delta receptors [122].

An acetylated analogue, 3-[^{18}F]acetyl cyclofoxy (^{18}F-ACF), has been developed for PET studies. It retains the original pharmacological properties of cyclofoxy [123]. ^{18}F-ACF scans showed regional radioactive concentrations in agreement with other studies of opiate receptors.

Theodore et al. [54] studied 14 patients with uncontrolled CPS, 11 of whom had clearly lateralized temporal epileptiform focus. No consistent patterns of ^{18}F-ACF activity attributable to the focus side could be detected.

The discrepancies between ^{11}C-carfentanil on the one hand and less specific ligands like ^{11}C-diprenorphine or ^{18}F-cyclofoxy on the other in epileptic patients could be explained by differential regulation of mu and kappa opiate receptor. Delta receptors which are in low concentration in the cortex are less likely to be involved. A decrease in kappa opiate receptor could 'cancel' the increase in mu opiate receptor, resulting in an apparent normal signal with ^{11}C-diprenorphine or ^{18}F-ACF. Thus using only these less specific ligands would have falsely led to the conclusion that no change in opiate receptor occurs in human epilepsy. This emphasizes the need for selective PET ligands. Imaging studies using a kappa selective ligand may help clarify the hypothesized decrease in this receptor subtype.

Binding of the selective delta antagonist ^{11}C-methyl-naltrindole was not changed in the amygdala, and increased in the temporal neocortex in patients with unilateral temporal lobe epilepsy [124]. Alterations in the delta opioid receptor subtype are greater and observed in more regions of the temporal cortex than the changes in mu opiate receptors as assessed by ^{11}C-carfentanil in the same subjects, suggesting distinctive roles of the two opioid receptor subtypes in cellular mechanisms associated with seizure phenomena.

These data strongly support the idea that the endogenous opioid system plays a role in human seizure disorders.

Benzodiazepine receptors

Epilepsy is often considered as the result of an imbalance between excitatory and inhibitory influences on populations of neurones. γ-aminobutyric acid (GABA) is the major inhibitory neurotransmitter in the central nervous system and could thus play an important role in seizure susceptibility. Reduced GABA-mediated inhibitory control may underlie paroxysmal and inappropriate neuronal discharges. Autoradiographic works have demonstrated a decrease in central benzodiazepine receptors in the hippocampus from patients with temporal lobe epilepsy and mesiotemporal sclerosis, without changes in the temporal neocortex [125–127]. The loss of central benzodiazepine receptors was particularly pronounced in the CA1 field. The decrease of central benzodiazepine receptors is of greater magnitude than the decrease in neuronal cell density, suggesting that there might be a decrease in central benzodiazepine receptors on the remaining neurones and therefore a reduced inhibitory tone in the epileptic focus [125,128].

No GABA agonist or antagonist labelled with a positron emitter is available for satisfactory in vivo imaging with PET. The GABA receptor is a macromolecular complex with binding sites for barbiturates and benzodiazepines. Imaging central benzodiazepine receptors is therefore an indirect but accepted way of assessing GABA receptors. ^{11}C-flumazenil (^{11}C-Ro 15–1788) is a benzodiazepine antagonist highly suitable for mapping central benzodiazepine receptors with PET in humans [129,130].

In 10 patients with simple or complex partial seizures and a normal MRI scan, a 15–35% decrease in ^{11}C-flumazenil concentration (central benzodiazepine receptors density (B_{max})) was found in limited brain regions corresponding to the EEG localization, without change in receptor affinity [131].

Numerous PET studies have further confirmed the existence of a focal reduction in ^{11}C-flumazenil binding in the hippocampus of patients with temporal lobe epilepsy [11,15,132–138]. As with opiate receptors, several interpretations are theoretically possible: (a) increased release of an endogenous ligand competing with ^{11}C-flumazenil for binding to central benzodiazepine receptors that are normal in density and affinity; (b) downregulation of benzodiazepine receptors (in response to an increased release of endogenous ligands); (c) change in receptor characteristics, affecting (lowering) affinity; or (d) a loss of neurones and synapsis expressing benzodiazepine–GABA receptors, and (e) any combination of the above.

In patients with refractory mesiotemporal epilepsy and an MRI diagnosis of hippocampal sclerosis, no correlation was found between reduction in central benzodiazepine receptor binding and reduced hippocampal volume, implying that atrophy with neuronal loss is not the sole determinant of reduced central benzodiazepine receptor binding [11,138].

In some of these patients with temporal lobe epilepsy, the hippocampus on the focus side is atrophic on MRI scans and the apparent decrease in ^{11}C-flumazenil binding could simply be the result of partial volume averaging and not from a true decrease in binding per unit of volume. The use of partial-volume correction is laborious and complicated, and its clinical utility has not been determined [137]. Further, it has been suggested that ^{11}C-flumazenil PET without correcting for partial volume effect underestimates rather than overestimates its ability to localize the epileptogenic area [138]. ^{11}C-flumazenil binding was abnormal even in patients with normal or mildly damaged hippocampus on quantitative MRI which suggests a greater sensitivity of ^{11}C-flumazenil PET over MRI [138]. After application of an MRI-based method for partial-volume effect correction, all 17 patients reported by Koepp *et al.* [11] showed significant unilateral reduction of ^{11}C-flumazenil binding; using the same methodology, more confusing results were obtained by the same group in 10 patients with temporal lobe epilepsy and a normal MRI; ^{11}C-flumazenil PET showed focal increases as well as decreases of ^{11}C-flumazenil binding in 80% and was not therefore consistently helpful in localizing the epileptic foci [139]. *In vivo* ^{11}C-flumazenil PET measurement of hippocampal central benzodiazepine receptor binding when corrected for partial volume effects were highly correlated with *ex vivo* ^{3}H-flumazenil autoradiographic findings in patients with mesiotemporal epilepsy and histologically verified hippocampal sclerosis [140].

Because of the fast clearance of ^{11}C-flumazenil from the brain and the rapid radioactive decay of ^{11}C, it is possible to carry out sequential PET studies with ^{11}C-flumazenil followed approximately 75 min later by ^{18}FDG, in the same patient in one session, allowing a direct comparison between the regional changes in benzodiazepine receptor binding and those in glucose consumption, the 'reference method'. Patients with temporal lobe epilepsy are characterized on the epileptogenic side by a reduction in ^{11}C-flumazenil binding limited to the mesial temporal region with little change in the lateral

temporal cortex, while glucose metabolism is reduced in the mesial and the lateral temporal cortex, and sometimes in extratemporal areas [15,132–134] (Plates 56.2 and 56.3, shown in colour between pp. 670 and 671).

In frontal lobe epilepsy, the cortical focus of decreased ^{11}C-flumazenil binding corresponded with the location of seizure onset determined with subdural electrodes, whereas the hypometabolic zone shown on ^{18}FDG-PET appeared larger than the ^{11}C-flumazenil focus [141]. In two patients with frontal lobe epilepsy caused by focal dysplasia documented by histology, a regional reduction of central benzodiazepine receptor ^{11}C-flumazenil binding was found and correlated well with the site of seizure onset documented by invasive EEG recordings. In contrast, the hypometabolic region documented by ^{18}FDG-PET was more widespread and extended beyond the seizure onset zone and the dysplastic cortex [142]. In 10 children with extratemporal lobe epilepsy, ^{11}C-flumazenil PET detected at least part of the seizure onset zone identified by subdural EEG in all subjects, whereas ^{18}FDG-PET failed to detect the seizure onset in two [143]. Furthermore, in young patients with both nonlesional and extratemporal epilepsies, large preoperative ^{11}C-flumazenil PET abnormalities were associated with poor outcome and patients who became seizure free after surgery had smaller nonresected cortex with ^{11}C-flumazenil abnormalities than those who continued to have seizures. By contrast, the size of non-resected ^{18}FDG-PET abnormalities which were considerably larger than corresponding ^{11}C-flumazenil abnormalities was not a predictor of outcome after neocortical epilepsy surgery. ^{11}C-flumazenil PET could therefore be an effective tool for guiding subdural electrode placement to ensure coverage of the epileptogenic zone in patients with extratemporal lobe epilepsy [143].

In patients with partial seizures caused by various malformations of cortical development (MCD), abnormalities of central benzodiazepine receptors were usually more extensive than MRI-defined abnormalities, were often multiple and were sometimes seen at distant sites where the neocortex had a normal MRI appearance. Both increases and decreases in receptor availability were found [144]. It remains to be determined whether these areas correspond to occult dysgenesis.

Falsely lateralizing and sometimes transient ^{11}C-flumazenil PET asymmetries have been reported on several occasions [11,15,136,145]. The potentially lower clinical reliability of this technique must be kept in mind.

These changes in ^{11}C-flumazenil binding may sometimes reflect more dynamic and more functional changes in central benzodiazepine receptors. Indeed, in patients with frequent seizures, decreases in central benzodiazepine receptor density were observed in projection areas from the epileptogenic zone [146]. Furthermore, central benzodiazepine receptor density normalized in several (but not all) of the affected projection areas 1 year after surgery in four patients with temporal lobe epilepsy [147].

Both ^{11}C-flumazenil and ^{18}FDG-PET appear extremely sensitive in temporal lobe epilepsy. The area of decreased ^{11}C-flumazenil binding is spatially more limited and could therefore have a closer relationship with the epileptic focus than the area of glucose hypometabolism. These new data are extremely relevant for the non-invasive evaluation of patients with refractory temporal lobe epilepsy. Further experience will define the respective indications, advantages and limitations of ^{11}C-flumazenil and ^{18}FDG scans.

SPECT

SPECT studies in partial epilepsy have been carried out with blood flow tracers. Iodinated tracers were first used (^{123}I-isopropyl-iodo-amphetamine, IMP; trimethyl-(hydroxy-methyl-^{123}I-iodobenzyl)-propanediamine, HIDPM) [148–150], but these cyclotron-produced ^{123}I-labelled radioisotopes were poorly available and often contained high-energy contaminants that degraded image quality and restricted patient dosage. More recent studies have used ^{99m}Tc-labelled compounds, such as ^{99m}Tc hexamethyl-propyleneamine oxime (^{99m}Tc-HMPAO) or ^{99m}Tc ethyl cysteinate dimer (^{99m}Tc-ECD). These lipophilic amines rapidly cross the blood–brain barrier (around 85% of brain uptake on the first pass). Once inside the brain, they form a hydrophilic compound that is trapped within cells, which prevents washout. Cerebral uptake is complete within 2 min and less than 5% is redistributed later. The activity in the brain remains essentially constant and proportional to regional perfusion at the time of administration. Its distribution is not affected by subsequent changes in CBF or pharmacological intervention. These radiopharmaceuticals are therefore more precise than [18]FDG-PET in terms of temporal resolution, and allow imaging of transient changes in CBF. Given the long half-life of these radiopharmaceuticals, static SPECT scans can be acquired up to 180 min after their intravenous administration. Radiopharmaceuticals can be prepared any time, without the requirement of running a complex cyclotron. These technological particuliarities allow for injecting the patient at distance from the SPECT camera, for example in the epilepsy monitoring unit, during or just after a seizure, which is a major advantage. Scanning is then carried out when the patient has recovered full consciousness and is able to collaborate. During the initial ictal studies in epilepsy, ^{99m}Tc-HMPAO had to be reconstituted rapidly at the bedside during a seizure [151], which made the implementation of ictal injections of ^{99m}Tc-HMPAO more difficult compared with ^{99m}Tc-ECD, which is a stable ligand, and which allowed for earlier ictal injections [152]. A stabilized form of ^{99m}Tc-HMPAO is now available [153]. ^{99m}Tc-ECD is cleared from the body more rapidly than ^{99m}Tc-HMPAO, giving a higher brain/background ratio of activity and a superior SPECT image quality [154].

With the availability of more stable radiopharmaceuticals, ictal SPECT can be a safe, non-invasive procedure completed on a routine basis in the epilepsy monitoring unit, provided appropriately trained support staff are utilized as part of a structured multidisciplinary programme [155,156]. Several methods for a rapid and safe ictal injection have been described [157–159].

SPECT is now often used in the presurgical evaluation of patients with intractable partial epilepsy. The localizing value of SPECT performed with cerebral perfusion imaging agents in patients with partial epilepsy is based on cerebral metabolic and perfusion coupling, i.e. an increase in neuronal metabolic activity is associated with an increase in CBF, and a decrease in neuronal metabolic activity with a decrease in CBF.

An interictal SPECT is obtained when the ligand is injected between seizures. Interictal SPECTs in partial epilepsy have shown areas of low perfusion in a proportion of patients, mainly with temporal lobe epilepsy. The usefulness of interictal SPECT for preoperative seizure focus localization, however, is limited by a low sensitivity of around 44% and a false positive rate of around 7%

[160–164]. It is now recommended that an interictal SPECT is obtained to compare the ictal SPECT, and to obtain subtraction ictal SPECT coregistered to MRI (SISCOM), i.e. an analysis technique comparing ictal and interictal studies and coregistering to MRI [165,166].

Ictal SPECT is obtained by injecting the ligand during a seizure, and a postictal SPECT by postictal injection. A time delay, however, of around 30 s should be taken into account between the injection of the ligand into an arm vein and first pass through the brain for a correct interpretation of the SPECT study. Ictal injection should be performed as soon as possible after seizure onset, since seizure activity may propagate. If ictal SPECT injection is late during the seizure, the hyperperfusion may reflect the propagated activity [157,159,167,168], and not the ictal onset zone, which may be hypoperfused [169,170]. The sequence of perfusion changes in temporal lobe complex partial seizures has been well documented. During the ictus, there is hyperperfusion of the whole temporal lobe. Up to 2 min postictally, there is hyperperfusion of the mesial temporal structures with hypoperfusion of lateral temporal structures, and from 2 to 15 min postictally, there is hypoperfusion of the whole temporal lobe. A return to normal is seen in 10–30 min [161,171]. Sensitivity for ictal SPECT localization in patients with temporal lobe complex partial seizures relative to diagnostic evaluation is around 97%, and for postictal SPECT studies around 75% [46,160–163,172]. False lateralizations due to rapid seizure spread are uncommon [159,173]. The sensitivity of ictal SPECT localization during simple partial seizures has been less well studied and is probably much lower [159,174]. Ictal SPECT studies of complex partial seizures of extratemporal lobe origin also have an excellent localizing value, but may be more difficult to obtain when the seizures are brief in duration [161,175,176]. The sensitivity of ictal SPECT in extratemporal seizures has been reported to be around 90%, but for postictal studies only around 46%, probably due to a fast switch from hyper- to hypoperfusion in the postictal period [161,175]. Two cases of preictal SPECT in temporal lobe epilepsy showed an increased regional CBF prior to EEG seizure onset [177]. The study of the preictal state may be feasible using SPECT if the preictal state can be determined more reliably [178,179].

Difference images calculated from ictal and interictal ^{99m}Tc-HMPAO or ^{99m}Tc-ECD SPECT scans and coregistered with MRI [165] or subtraction ictal SPECT coregistered to MRI (SISCOM) [166] has been shown to be more sensitive and specific in localizing the seizure focus in the presurgical evaluation (Plate 56.4, shown in colour between pp. 670 and 671). SPECT perfusion difference analysis has been shown to localize epileptogenic regions with accuracy comparable with that of intracranial EEG [180,181]. Ictal SPECT, and in particular SISCOM images, are predictive of postsurgical outcome [166,171,182] independently of MRI or scalp ictal EEG findings [183]. The extent of resection of the cortical region of the SISCOM focus was significantly associated with the rate of excellent outcome [183].

[18]FDG-PET has been compared with SPECT imaging in epilepsy. Interictal [18]FDG-PET is more sensitive than interictal SPECT [184,185]. The area of interictal hypoperfusion tends to be concordant with but smaller than the areas of hypometabolism. This discordance of perfusion and metabolic abnormalities represents an uncoupling of perfusion and metabolism in the epileptogenic zones,

and could explain the lower diagnostic accuracy of interictal perfusion imaging in partial epilepsy [186]. Interictal ^{18}FDG-PET and ictal SPECT are both sensitive techniques for the detection of the epileptic focus. Interictal ^{18}FDG-PET provides a broad approximate nature of the epileptogenic zone, which may not be adequate for precise surgical localization of the epileptogenic zone [187]. Ictal SPECT may be more easy to interpret and more sensitive and specific than interictal ^{18}FDG-PET [173,180]. Both techniques are considered complementary when localization is difficult [46,173,181,187,188].

Cerebral perfusion changes in partial seizures other than the ictal hyperperfusion and postictal hypoperfusion of the epileptic focus have received little attention. Ictal frontal hypoperfusion during temporal lobe complex partial seizures has been described, and it has been postulated that this may represent frontal cortical inhibition and be responsible for the loss of consciousness [189]. Cerebellar hyperperfusion has been reported in 48–75% of patients with refractory partial epilepsy, mainly when unilateral clonic motor activity was present [190] or frontal hyperperfusion [191], and in frontal lobe seizures [192], and is probably mediated via the corticopontocerebellar pathway. Ipsilateral thalamic hypoperfusion on interictal SPECT was noted in 26% of patients with temporal lobe epilepsy [193]. Further studies of the perfusion changes associated with partial seizures may provide new insights into the pathophysiology of epileptic seizures.

References

1 American Academy of Neurology Expert Technology Assessment Panel. Positron emission tomography. *Neurology* 1991; 41: 163–7.

2 Kuhl DE, Engel J Jr, Phelps ME, Selin C. Epileptic patterns of local cerebral metabolism and perfusion in humans determined by emission computed tomography of 18FDG and 13NH3. *Ann Neurol* 1980; 8: 348–60.

3 Barrington SF, Koutroumanidis M, Agathonikou A *et al.* Clinical value of 'ictal' FDG-positron emission tomography and the routine use of simultaneous scalp EEG studies in patients with intractable partial epilepsies. *Epilepsia* 1998; 39: 753–66.

4 Engel J Jr, Kuhl DE, Phelps ME, Rausch R, Nuwer M. Local cerebral metabolism during partial seizures. *Neurology* 1983; 33: 400–13.

5 Franck G, Sadzot B, Salmon E *et al.* Regional blood flow and metabolic rates in human focal epilepsy and status epilepticus. In: Delgado-Escueta AV, Ward AA Jr, Woodbury DM, Porter RJ. *Advances in Neurology: Basic Mechanisms of the Epilepsies*, Vol. 44. New York: Raven Press, 1986: 935–48.

6 Meltzer CC, Adelson PD, Brenner RP *et al.* Planned ictal FDG PET imaging for localization of extratemporal epileptic foci. *Epilepsia* 2000; 41: 193–200.

7 Hoffman EJ, Huang SC, Phelps ME. Quantitation in positron emission computed tomography. 1. Effect of object size. *J Comput Assist Tomogr* 1979; 3: 299–308.

8 Engel J Jr, Henry TR, Risinger MW *et al.* Presurgical evaluation for partial epilepsy: relative contribution of chronic depth-electrode recordings versus FDG-PET and scalp-sphenoidal ictal EEG. *Neurology* 1990; 40: 1670–7.

9 Meltzer CC, Zubieta JK, Brandt J, Tune LE, Mayberg HS, Frost JJ. Regional hypometabolism in Alzheimer's disease as measured by positron emission tomography after correction for effects of partial volume averaging. *Neurology* 1996; 47: 454–61.

10 Meltzer CC, Zubieta JK, Links JM, Brakeman P, Stumpf Frost JJ. MR-based correction for brain PET measurements for heterogenous grey matter radioactivity distribution. *J Cereb Blood Flow Metab* 1996; 16: 650–8.

11 Koepp MJ, Richardson MP, Labbé C *et al.* 11C-Flumazenil PET, volumet-

12 Knowlton RC, Laxer KD, Klein G *et al.* In vivo hippocampal glucose metabolism in mesial temporal lobe epilepsy. *Neurology* 2001; 57: 1184–90.

13 Parker F, Levesque MF. Presurgical contribution of quantitative stereotactic positron emission tomography in temporo limbic epilepsy. *Surg Neurol* 1999; 51: 202–10.

14 Heinz R, Ferris N, Lee EK *et al.* MR and positron emission tomography in the diagnosis of surgically correctable temporal lobe epilepsy. *Am J Neuroradiol* 1994; 15: 1341–8.

15 Szelies B, Weber-Luxenburger G, Pawlik G *et al.* MRI-guided flumazenil- and FDG-PET in temporal lobe epilepsy. *Neuroimage* 1996; 3: 109–18.

16 Valk PE, Laxer KD, Barbaro NM, Knezevic S, Dillon WP, Budinger TF. High resolution (2.6-mm) PET in partial epilepsy associated with mesial temporal sclerosis. *Radiology* 1993; 186: 55–8.

17 Friston KJ, Ashburner J, Poline JB, Frith CD, Heather JD, Frackowiak RSJ. Spatial registration and normalization of images. *Hum Brain Map* 1995; 2: 165–8.

18 Friston KJ, Holmes AP, Worsley KJ *et al.* Statistical parametric maps in functional imaging: a general linear approach. *Hum Brain Map* 1995; 2: 189–210.

19 Van Bogaert P, Massager N, Tugendhaft P *et al.* Statistical parametric mapping of regional glucose metabolism in mesial temporal lobe epilepsy. *Neuroimage* 2000; 12: 129–38.

20 Swartz BE, Thomas K, Simpkins F, Kovalik E, Mandelkern MM. Rapid quantitative analysis of individual ^{18}FDG-PET scans. *Clin Pos Imag* 1999; 2: 47–56.

21 Arnold S, Schlaug G, Niemann H *et al.* Topography of interictal glucose hypometabolism in unilateral mesiotemporal epilepsy. *Neurology* 1996; 46: 1422–30.

22 Signorini M, Paulesu E, Friston L *et al.* Rapid assessment of regional cerebral metabolic abnormalities in single subjects with quantitative and nonquantitative [^{18}F]FDG PET: A clinical validation of statistical parametric mapping. *Neuroimage* 1999; 9: 63–80.

23 Theodore WH, Newmark ME, Sato S *et al.* [^{18}F]fluorodeoxyglucose positron emission tomography in refractory complex partial seizures. *Ann Neurol* 1983; 14: 429–37.

24 Engel J Jr, Brown WJ, Kuhl DE *et al.* Pathological findings underlying focal temporal lobe hypometabolism in partial epilepsy. *Ann Neurol* 1982; 12: 518–28.

25 Engel J Jr, Kuhl DE, Phelps ME, Crandall PH. Comparative localization of epileptic foci in partial epilepsy by PCT and EEG. *Ann Neurol* 1982; 12: 529–37.

26 Engel J Jr, Kuhl DE, Phelps ME, Mazziotta JC. Interictal cerebral glucose metabolism in partial epilepsy and its relation to EEG changes. *Ann Neurol* 1982; 12: 510–17.

27 Abou-Khalil BW, Siegel GJ, Sackellares *et al.* Positron emission tomography studies of cerebral glucose metabolism in chronic partial epilepsy. *Ann Neurol* 1987; 22: 480–6.

28 Theodore WH, Fishbein D, Dubinsky R. Patterns of cerebral glucose metabolism in patients with partial seizures. *Neurology* 1988; 38: 1201–6.

29 Holmes MD, Kelly K, Theodore WH. Complex partial seizures. Correlation of clinical and metabolic features. *Arch Neurol* 1988; 45: 1191–3.

30 Stefan H, Pawlik G, Böcher-Schwarz HG *et al.* Functional and morphological abnormalities in temporal lobe epilepsy: a comparison of interictal and ictal EEG, CT, MRI, SPECT and PET. *J Neurol* 1987; 234: 377–84.

31 Hajek M, Antonini A, Leenders KL, Wieser HG. Mesiobasal versus lateral temporal lobe epilepsy: metabolic differences in the temporal lobe shown by interictal 18F-FDG positron emission tomography. *Neurology* 1993; 43: 79–86.

32 Sadzot B, Debets RM, Maquet P *et al.* Regional brain glucose metabolism in patients with complex partial seizures investigated by intracranial EEG. *Epilepsy Res* 1992; 12: 121–9.

33 Chee MW, Morris HH III, Antar MA *et al.* Presurgical evaluation of temporal lobe epilepsy using interictal temporal spikes and positron emission tomography. *Arch Neurol* 1993; 50: 45–8.

34 Henry TR, Mazziotta JC, Engel J Jr *et al.* Quantifying interictal metabolic activity in human temporal lobe epilepsy. *J Cereb Blood Flow Metab* 1990; 10: 748–57.

35 Radtke RA, Hanson MW, Hoffman JM *et al*. Positron emission tomography: Comparison of clinical utility in temporal lobe and extratemporal epilepsy. *J Epilepsy* 1994; 7: 27–33.

36 Swartz BE, Tomiyasu U, Delgado-Escueta AV, Mandelkern M, Khonsari A. Neuroimaging in temporal lobe epilepsy: test sensitivity and relationships to pathology and post-operative outcome. *Epilepsia* 1992; 33: 624–34.

37 Sperling MR, Alavi A, Reivich M, French JA, O'Connor MJ. False lateralization of temporal lobe epilepsy with FDG positron emission tomography. *Epilepsia* 1995; 36: 722–7.

38 Leiderman DB, Albert P, Balish M, Bromfield E, Theodore WH. The dynamics of metabolic change following seizures as measured by positron emission tomography with fludeoxyglucose F 18. *Arch Neurol* 1994; 51: 932–6.

39 Williamson PD, Spencer DD, Spencer SS, Novelly RA, Mattson RH. Complex partial seizures of frontal lobe origin. *Ann Neurol* 1985; 18: 497–504.

40 Williamson PD, Boon PA, Thanadi VM *et al*. Parietal lobe epilepsy: diagnostic considerations, and results of surgery. *Ann Neurol* 1992; 31: 193–201.

41 Williamson PD, Thanadi VM, Darcey TM *et al*. Occipital lobe epilepsy: clinical characteristics, seizure spread patterns, and results of surgery. *Ann Neurol* 1992; 31: 3–13.

42 Wieser HG. *Electroclinical Features of the Psychomotor Seizure. A stereoelectroencephalographic study of ictal symptoms, and chronotopographical seizure patterns including clinical effects of intracranial stimulation.* Stuttgart: Fisher, Butterworth.

43 Henry TR, Sutherling WW, Engel J Jr *et al*. Interictal cerebral metabolism in partial epilepsies of neocortical origin. *Epilepsy Res* 1991; 10: 174–82.

44 Swartz BE, Halgren E, Delgado-Escueta AV *et al*. Neuroimaging in patients with seizures of probable frontal lobe origin. *Epilepsia* 1989; 30: 547–58.

45 Swartz BE, Mandelkern M, Delgado-Escueta AV *et al*. 18FDG-PET scans in parietal lobe epilepsy. *J Nucl Med* 1992; 39: 1017.

46 Spencer SS. The relative contributions of MRI, SPECT, and PET imaging in epilepsy. *Epilepsia* 1994; 35 (Suppl. 6): S72–89.

47 Theodore WH, Katz D, Kufta C *et al*. Pathology of temporal lobe foci: Correlation with CT, MRI and PET. *Neurology* 1990; 40: 797–803.

48 Ryvlin P, Cinotti L, Froment JC *et al*. Metabolic patterns associated with non-specific magnetic resonance imaging abnormalities in temporal lobe epilepsy. *Brain* 1991; 114: 2363–83.

49 Theodore WH, Sato S, Kufta C *et al*. Temporal lobectomy for uncontrolled seizures: the role of positron emission tomography. *Ann Neurol* 1992; 32: 789–94.

50 Henry TR, Engel J Jr, Sutherling WW, Risinger MR, Phelps ME. Correlation of structural and metabolic imaging with electrographic localization and histopathology in refractory complex partial epilepsy. *Epilepsia* 1987; 28: 601.

51 Sperling MR, Gur RC, Alavi A *et al*. Subcortical metabolic alterations in partial epilepsy. *Epilepsia* 1990; 31: 145–55.

52 Lee N, Radtke RA, Gray L *et al*. Neuronal migration disorders: positron emission tomography correlations. *Ann Neurol* 1994; 35: 290–7.

53 Theodore WH, Brooks R, Sato S *et al*. The role of positron emission tomography in the evaluation of seizure disorders. *Ann Neurol* 1984; 15: S176–S179.

54 Theodore WH, Carson RE, Andreasen P *et al*. PET imaging of opiate receptor binding in human epilepsy using [18F]cyclofoxy. *Epilepsy Res* 1992; 13: 129–39.

55 Newberg AB, Alavi A, Berlin J *et al*. Ipsilateral and contralateral thalamic hypometabolism as a predictor of outcome after temporal lobectomy for seizures. *J Nucl Med* 2000; 41: 1964–8.

56 Rubin E, Dhawan V, Moeller JR *et al*. Cerebral metabolic topography in unilateral temporal lobe epilepsy. *Neurology* 1995; 45: 2212–23.

57 Juhàsz C, Nagy F, Watson C *et al*. Glucose and [11C]flumazenil positron emission tomography abnormalities of thalamic nuclei in temporal lobe epilepsy. *Neurology* 1999; 53: 2037–45.

58 Margerison JH, Corsellis JAN. Epilepsy and the temporal lobes. A clinical, electroencephalographic and neuropathological study of the brain in epilepsy, with particular reference to the temporal lobes. *Brain* 1966; 89: 499–530.

59 Bruton CJ. The neuropathology of temporal lobe epilepsy. In: *Maudsley Monographs*, Number 31. Oxford: Oxford University Press, 1988.

60 Radtke RA, Hanson MW, Hoffman JM *et al*. Temporal lobe hypometabolism on PET. *Neurology* 1993; 43: 1088–92.

61 Henry TR, Babb TL, Engel J, Jr *et al*. Hippocampal neuronal loss and regional hypometabolism in temporal lobe epilepsy. *Ann Neurol* 1994; 36: 925–7.

62 Sackellares JC, Siegel GJ, Abou-Khalil BW *et al*. Differences between lateral and mesial temporal metabolism interictally in epilepsy of mesial temporal origin. *Neurology* 1990; 40: 1420–6.

63 Foldvary N, Lee N, Hanson MW *et al*. Correlation of hippocampal neuronal density and FDG-PET in mesial temporal lobe epilepsy. *Epilepsia* 1999; 40: 26–9.

64 Gaillard WD, Bhatia S, Bookheimer SY, Fazilat S, Sato S, Theodore WH. FDG-PET and volumetric MRI in the evaluation of patients with partial epilepsy. *Neurology* 1995; 45: 123–6.

65 Theodore WH, Gaillard WD, DeCarli C, Bhatia S, Hatta J. Hippocampal volume and glucose metabolism in temporal lobe epileptic foci. *Epilepsia* 2001; 42: 130–2.

66 O'Brien TJ, Newton MR, Cook MJ *et al*. Hippocampal atrophy is not a major determinant of regional hypometabolism in temporal lobe epilepsy. *Epilepsia* 1997; 38: 74–80.

67 Semah F, Baulac M, Hasboun D *et al*. Is interictal temporal hypometabolism related to mesial temporal sclerosis? A positron emission tomography/magnetic resonance imaging confrontation. *Epilepsia* 1995; 36: 447–56.

68 Spanaki MV, Kopylev L, Liow K *et al*. Relationship of seizure frequency to hippocampus volume and metabolism in temporal lobe epilepsy. *Epilepsia* 2000; 41: 1227–9.

69 Theodore WH. Antiepileptic drugs and cerebral glucose metabolism. *Epilepsia* 1988; 29 (Suppl. 2): S48–S55.

70 Theodore WH, Di Chiro G, Margolin R *et al*. Barbiturates reduce human cerebral glucose metabolism. *Neurology* 1986; 36: 60–4.

71 Schwartz WJ, Smith CB, Davidsen L *et al*. Metabolic mapping of functional activity in the hypothalamo-neurohypophysial system of the rat. *Science* 1979; 205: 723–5.

72 Nauta WJH. Circuitous connections liking cerebral cortex, limbic system and corpus striatum. In: Doane BK, Livingston KE, eds. *The Limbic System: Functional Organization and Clinical Disorders*. New York: Raven Press, 1986: 43–54.

73 Van Hoesen GW. The parahippocampal gyrus: new observations regarding its cortical connections in the monkey. *Trends Neurosci* 1982; 5: 345–50.

74 Van Hoesen GW, Rosene DC, Mesulam MM. Subicular input from temporal cortex in the rhesus monkey. *Science* 1979; 205: 608–10.

75 Van Hoesen GW, Pandya DN. Some connections of the entorhinal (area 28) and perirhinal (area 35) cortices of the rhesus monkey III: efferent connections. *Brain Res* 1975; 95: 39–59.

76 La Grutta V, Sabatino M, Ferraro G *et al*. Hippocampal seizures and striatal regulation: a possible functional pathway. *Neurosci Lett* 1986; 72: 277–82.

77 Mirski MA, Ferrendelli JA. Interruption of the mamillothalamic tracts prevents seizures in guinea pigs. *Science* 1984; 226: 72–4.

78 Moran MA, Mufson EJ, Mesulam MM. Neural inputs into the temporopolar cortex of the rhesus monkey. *J Comp Neurol* 1987; 256: 88–103.

79 Van Hoesen GW, Mesulam MM, Haaxma R. Temporal cortical projection to the olfactory tubercle in the rhesus monkey. *Brain Res* 1976; 109: 375–81.

80 Dupont S, Croizé AC, Semah F *et al*. Is amygdalohippocampectomy really selective in medial temporal lobe epilepsy? A study using positron emission tomography with 18fluorodeoxyglucose. *Epilepsia* 2001; 42: 731–40.

81 Babb TL, Brown WJ. Pathological findings in epilepsy. In: Engel J Jr, ed. *Surgical Treatment of the Epilepsies*. New York: Raven Press, 1987: 511–40.

82 Scheibel ME, Crandall PH, Scheibel AB. The hippocampal-dentate complex in temporal lobe epilepsy: a Golgi study. *Epilepsia* 1974; 15: 55–80.

83 Armstrong DD. The neuropathology of temporal lobe epilepsy. *J Neuropathol Exp Neurol* 1993; 52: 433–42.

84 Cook MJ, Gonzalez MF, Kilpatrick CE, Kaye A. Hippocampal sclerosis and cortical dysplasia: an association suggesting a prenatal aetiology. *Epilepsia* 1995; 36 (Suppl. 3): S54.

85 Raymond AA, Fish DR, Stevens JM, Cook JM, Sisodiya SM, Shorvon SD. Association of hippocampal sclerosis with cortical dysgenesis in patients with epilepsy. *Neurology* 1994; 44: 1841–5.

86 Mitchell LA, Jackson GD, Kalnins RM *et al.* Anterior temporal abnormality in temporal lobe epilepsy: a quantitative MRI and histopathologic study. *Neurology* 1999; 52: 327–36.

87 Lencz T, McCarthy G, Bronen R *et al.* Quantitative magnetic resonance imaging in temporal lobe epilepsy: relationship to neuropathology and neuropsychological function. *Ann Neurol* 1992; 31: 629–37.

88 Frost JJ, Mayberg HS, Fisher RS *et al.* Mu-opiate receptors measured by positron emission tomography are increased in temporal lobe epilepsy. *Ann Neurol* 1988; 23: 231–7.

89 Henry TR. Functional neuroimaging with positron emission tomography. *Epilepsia* 1996; 37: 1141–54.

90 Hajek M, Wieser HG, Khan N *et al.* Preoperative and postoperative glucose consumption in mesiobasal and lateral temporal lobe epilepsy. *Neurology* 1994; 44: 2125–32.

91 Theodore WH, Sato S, Kufta CV, Gaillard WD, Kelley K. FDG-positron emission tomography and invasive EEG: seizure focus detection and surgical outcome. *Epilepsia* 1997; 38: 81–6.

92 Manno EM, Sperling MR, Ding X *et al.* Predictors of outcome after anterior temporal lobectomy: positron emission tomography. *Neurology* 1994; 44: 2331–6.

93 Delbeke D, Lawrence SK, Abou-Khalil BW, Blumenkopf B, Kessler RM. Postsurgical outcome of patients with uncontrolled complex partial seizures and temporal lobe hypometabolism on 18FDG-positron emission tomography. *Invest Radiol* 1996; 31: 261–6.

94 Dupont S, Semah F, Clemenceau S, Adam C, Baulac M, Samson Y. Accurate prediction of post-operative outcome in mesial temporal lobe epilepsy. *Arch Neurol* 2000; 57: 1331–6.

95 Blum DE, Ehsan T, Dungan D, Karis JP, Fisher RS. Bilateral temporal hypometabolism in epilepsy. *Epilepsia* 1998; 39: 651–9.

96 Roger J, Bureau M, Dravet C, Dreifuss FE, Perret A, Wolf P. In: *Epileptic Syndromes in Infancy, Childhood and Adolescence*, 2nd edn. London: John Libbey, 1992.

97 Gaillard WD, White S, Malow B *et al.* FDG-PET in children and adolescents with partial seizures: role in epilepsy surgery evaluation. *Epilepsy Res* 1995; 20: 77–84.

98 Chugani HT, Shewmon DA, Peacock WJ *et al.* Surgical treatment of intractable neonatal-onset seizures: the role of positron emission tomography. *Neurology* 1988; 38: 1178–88.

99 Olson DM, Chugani HT, Shewmon DA, Phelps ME, Peacock WJ. Electrocorticographic confirmation of focal positron emission tomographic abnormalities in children with intractable epilepsy. *Epilepsia* 1990; 31: 731–9.

100 Chugani HT, Shewmon DA, Khanna S, Phelps ME. Interictal and postictal focal hypermetabolism on positron emission tomography. *Pediatr Neurol* 1993; 9: 10–15.

101 Chiron C, Raynaud C, Tzourio N *et al.* Regional cerebral blood flow by SPECT imaging in Sturge-Weber disease: an aid for diagnosis. *J Neurol Neurosurg Psychiatry* 1989; 52: 1402–9.

102 Chugani HT, Shields WD, Shewmon DA *et al.* Infantile spasms: I. PET identifies focal cortical dysgenesis in cryptogenic cases for surgical treatment. *Ann Neurol* 1990; 27: 406–13.

103 Chugani HT, Shewmon DA, Sankar R, Chen BC, Phelps ME. Infantile spasms: II. Lenticular nuclei and brainstem activation on positron emission tomography. *Ann Neurol* 1992; 31: 212–19.

104 Chugani HT. Functional brain imaging in pediatrics. *Pediatr Neurol* 1992; 39: 777–99.

105 Maquet P, Hirsch E, Dive D *et al.* Cerebral glucose utilization during sleep in Landau–Kleffner syndrome: a PET study. *Epilepsia* 1990; 31: 778–83.

106 Theodore WH, Rose D, Sat S *et al.* Cerebral glucose metabolism in the Lennox–Gastaut syndrome. *Ann Neurol* 1987; 21: 14–21.

107 Ferrie CD, Maisey M, Cox T, Polkey C, Barrington SF, Panayiotopoulos CP, Robinson RO. Focal abnormalities detected by 18FDG-PET in epileptic encephalopathies. *Arch Dis Child* 1996; 75: 102–7.

108 Chugani HT, Mazziotta JC, Engel J, Phelps ME. The Lennox–Gastaut syndrome: metabolic subtypes determined by 2-deoxy-2[18F]fluoro-D-glucose positron emission tomography. *Ann Neurol* 1987; 21: 4–13.

109 Bernardi S, Trimble MR, Frackowiak RSJ, Wise RJS, Jones T. An interictal study of partial epilepsy using positron emission tomography and the oxygen-15 inhalation technique. *J Neurol Neurosurg Psychiatr* 1983; 46: 473–7.

110 Yamamoto YL, Ochs R, Gloor P *et al.* Patterns of rCBF and focal energy metabolic changes in relation to electroencephalographic abnormality in the interictal phase of partial epilepsy. In: Baldy-Moulinier M, Ingvar DH, Meldrum BS. *Current Problems in Epilepsy*, Vol 1. *Cerebral Blood Flow, Metabolism and Epilepsy*. London: John Libbey, 1983: 51–62.

111 Breier JI, Mullani NA, Thomas AB *et al.* Effects of duration of epilepsy on the uncoupling of metabolism and blood flow in complex partial seizures. *Neurology* 1997; 48: 1047–53.

112 Gaillard WD, Fazilat S, White S *et al.* Interictal metabolism and blood flow are uncoupled in temporal lobe cortex of patients with complex partial epilepsy. *Neurology* 1995; 45: 1841–7.

113 Leiderman DB, Balish M, Sato S *et al.* Comparison of PET measurements of cerebral blood flow and glucose metabolism for the localization of human epileptic foci. *Epilepsy Res* 1992; 13: 153–7.

114 Bookheimer SY, Zeffiro TA, Blaxton T *et al.* A direct comparison of PET activation and electrocortical stimulation mapping for language localization. *Neurology* 1997; 48: 1056–65.

115 Pardo JV, Fox PT. Preoperative assessment of the cerebral hemispheric dominance for language with CBF PET. *Hum Brain Map* 1993; 1: 57–68.

116 Frenk H. Pro- and anticonvulsant actions of morphine and the endogenous opioids: involvement and interactions of multiple opiate and non-opiate systems. *Brain Res Rev* 1983; 6: 197–210.

117 Tortella FC, Long JB. Characterization of opioid peptide-like anticonvulsant activity in rat cerebrospinal fluid. *Brain Res* 1988; 456: 139–46.

118 Tortella FC, Long JB. Endogenous anticonvulsant substance in rat cerebral spinal fluid following a generalized seizure. *Science* 1985; 228: 1106–7.

119 Mayberg HS, Sadzot B, Meltzer CC *et al.* Quantification of mu and non-mu opiate receptors in temporal lobe epilepsy using positron emission tomography. *Ann Neurol* 1991; 30: 3–11.

120 Nataka Y, Chang KJ, Mitchell CL, Hon JS. Repeated electroconvulsive shock downregulates the opioid receptors in rat brain. *Brain Res* 1985; 346: 160–3.

121 Frost JJ, Mayberg HS, Sadzot B *et al.* Comparison of 11C-diprenorphine and 11C-carfentanil binding to opiate receptors in man by positron emission tomography. *J Cereb Blood Flow Metabol* 1990; 10: 484–92.

122 Rothman RB, McLean S. An examination of the opiate receptor subtypes labeled by [3H]CycloFOXY: an opiate antagonist suitable for positron emission tomography. *Biol Psychiatr* 1988; 23: 435–58.

123 Pert CB, Danks JA, Channing MA *et al.* 3-[18F]acetylcyclofoxy: a useful probe for the visualization of opiate receptors in living animals. *FEBS* 1984; 177: 281–6.

124 Madar I, Lesser RP, Krauss G *et al.* Imaging of delta- and mu-opioid receptors in temporal lobe epilepsy by positron emission tomography. *Ann Neurol* 1997; 41: 358–67.

125 Johnson EW, de Lanerolle NC, Kim JH *et al.* 'Central' and 'peripheral' benzodiazepine receptors: opposite changes in human epileptogenic tissue. *Neurology* 1992; 42: 811–15.

126 McDonald JW, Garofalo EA, Hood T *et al.* Altered excitatory and inhibitory amino acid receptor binding in hippocampus of patients with temporal lobe epilepsy. *Ann Neurol* 1991; 29: 529–41.

127 Olson RW, Bureau M, Houser CR *et al.* GABA/benzodiazepine receptors in human focal epilepsy. In: Avanzini G, Engel Jr J, Fariello R. *Neurotransmitters in Epilepsy*. Holland: Elsevier Science Publishers, 1992: 383–91.

128 Hand KS, Baird VH, Van Paesschen W *et al.* Central benzodiazepine receptor autoradiography in hippocampal sclerosis. *Br J Pharmacol* 1997; 122: 358–64.

129 Samson Y, Hantraye P, Baron JC. *et al.* Kinetics and displacement of [11C]Ro 15–1788, a benzodiazepine antagonist, studied in human brain in vivo by positron emission tomography. *Eur J Pharmacol* 1985; 110: 247–51.

130 Persson A, Ehrin E, Eriksson L *et al.* Imaging of [11C]-labelled Ro

15–1788 binding to benzodiazepine receptors in the human brain by positron emission tomography. *J Psychiatr Res* 1985; 19: 609–22.

131 Savic I, Persson A, Roland P, Pauli S, Sedvall G, Widen L. In vivo demonstration of reduced benzodiazepine receptor binding in human epileptic foci. *Lancet* 1988; 2: 863–6.

132 Henry TR, Frey KA, Sackellares JC *et al*. In vivo cerebral metabolism and central benzodiazepine-receptor binding in temporal lobe epilepsy. *Neurology* 1993; 43: 1998–2006.

133 Savic I, Ingvar M, Stone-Elander S. Comparison of [11C]flumazenil and [18F]FDG as PET markers of epileptic foci. *J Neurol Neurosurg Psychiatr* 1993; 56: 615–21.

134 Sadzot B, Debets RM, Delfiore G *et al*. Decrease of 11C-flumazenil binding is more localized than glucose hypometabolism in patients with TLE studied by PET. *Neurology* 1994; 44 (Suppl. 2): A351–A352.

135 Koepp MJ, Richardson MP, Brooks DJ *et al*. Cerebral benzodiazepine receptors in hippocampal sclerosis. An objective in vivo analysis. *Brain* 1996; 119: 1677–87.

136 Debets RMC, Sadzot B, van Isselt JW *et al*. Is 11C-flumazenil PET superior to 18FDG PET and 123I-iomazenil SPECT in presurgical evaluation of temporal epilepsy? *J Neurol Neurosurg Psychiatr* 1997; 62: 141–50.

137 Ryvlin P, Bouvard S, Le Bars D *et al*. Clinical utility of flumazenil-PET versus [18F]fluorodeoxyglucose-PET and MRI in refractory partial epilepsy. A prospective study in 100 patients. *Brain* 1998; 121: 2067–81.

138 Lamusuo S, Pitkanen A, Jutila L *et al*. [11 C]Flumazenil binding in the medial temporal lobe in patients with temporal lobe epilepsy: correlation with hippocampal MR volumetry, T2 relaxometry, and neuropathology. *Neurology* 2000; 54: 2252–60.

139 Koepp MJ, Hammers A, Labbe C *et al*. 11C-flumazenil PET in patients with refractory temporal lobe epilepsy and normal MRI. *Neurology* 2000; 54: 332–9.

140 Koepp MJ, Hand KS, Labbe C *et al*. In vivo [11C]flumazenil-PET correlates with ex vivo [3I I]flumazenil autoradiography in hippocampal sclerosis. *Ann Neurol* 1998; 43: 618–26.

141 Savic I, Thorell JO, Roland P. 11C-Flumazenil positron emission tomography visualises frontal epileptogenic regions. *Epilepsia* 1995; 36: 1225–332.

142 Arnold S, Berthele A, Drzezga A *et al*. Reduction of benzodiazepine receptor binding is related to the seizure onset zone in extratemporal focal cortical dysplasia. *Epilepsia* 2000; 41: 818–24.

143 Muzik O, da Silva EA, Juhasz C *et al*. Intracranial EEG versus flumazenil and glucose PET in children with extratemporal lobe epilepsy. *Neurology* 2000; 54: 171–9.

144 Richardson MP, Koepp MJ, Brooks DJ, Fish DR, Duncan JS. Benzodiazepine receptors in focal epilepsy with cortical dysgenesis: an 11C-flumazenil PET study. *Ann Neurol* 1996; 40: 188–98.

145 Ryvlin P, Bouvard S, Le Bars D, Mauguiere F. Transient and falsely lateralizing flumazenil-PET asymmetries in temporal lobe epilepsy. *Neurology* 1999; 53: 1882–5.

146 Savic I, Svanborg E, Thorell JO. Cortical benzodiazepine receptor changes are related to frequency of partial seizures: a positron emission tomography study. *Epilepsia* 1996; 37: 236–44.

147 Savic I, Blomqvist G, Halldin C, Litton JE, Gulyas B. Regional increases in [11C]flumazenil binding after epilepsy surgery. *Acta Neurol Scand* 1998; 97: 279–86.

148 Hill TC, Holman BL, Lovett R *et al*. Initial experience with SPECT (single-photon computerized tomography) of the brain using N-isopropyl I-123 p-iodoamphetamine: concise communication. *J Nucl Med* 1982; 23: 191–5.

149 LaManna MM, Sussman NM, Harner RN *et al*. Initial experience with SPECT imaging of the brain using I-123 p-iodoamphetamine in focal epilepsy. *Clin Nucl Med* 1989; 14: 428–30.

150 Brinkmann BH, O'Connor MK, O'Brien TJ, Mullan BP, So EL, Robb RA. Dual-isotope SPECT using simultaneous acquisition of ^{99m}Tc and ^{123}I radioisotopes: a double-injection technique for peri-ictal functional neuroimaging. *J Nucl Med* 1999; 40: 677–84.

151 Newton MR, Austin MC, Chan JG, McKay WJ, Rowe CC, Berkovic SF. Ictal SPECT using technetium-99m-HMPAO: methods for rapid preparation and optimal deployment of tracer during spontaneous seizures. *J Nucl Med* 1993; 34: 666–70.

152 O'Brien TJ, Brinkmann BH, Mullan BP *et al*. Comparative study of 99mTc-ECD and 99mTc-HMPAO for peri-ictal SPECT: qualitative and quantitative analysis. *J Neurol Neurosurg Psychiatr* 1999; 66: 331–9.

153 Koslowsky IL, Brake SE, Bitner SJ. Evaluation of the stability of (99m)Tc-ECD and stabilized (99m)Tc-HMPAO stored in syringes. *J Nucl Med Technol* 2001; 29: 197–200.

154 Leveille J, Demonceau G, Walovitch RC. Intrasubject comparison between technetium-99m-ECD and technetium-99m-HMPAO in healthy human subjects. *J Nucl Med* 1992; 33: 480–4.

155 Smith BJ, Karvelis KC, Cronan S *et al*. Developing an effective program to complete ictal SPECT in the epilepsy monitoring unit. *Epilepsy Res* 1999; 33: 189–97.

156 Huntington NA. The nurse's role in delivery of radioisotope for ictal SPECT scan. *J Neurosci Nurs* 1999; 31: 208–15.

157 Sepkuty JP, Lesser RP, Civelek CA, Cysyk B, Webber R, Shipley R. An automated injection system (with patient selection) for SPECT imaging in seizure localization. *Epilepsia* 1998; 39: 1350–6.

158 Herrendorf G, Steinhoff BJ, Bittermann HJ, Mursch K, Meller J, Becker W. An easy method to accelerate ictal SPECT. *J Neuroimaging* 1999; 9: 129–30.

159 Van Paesschen W, Dupont P, Van Heerden B *et al*. Self-injection ictal SPECT during partial seizures. *Neurology* 2000; 54: 1994–7.

160 Jack CR Jr, Mullan BP, Sharbrough FW *et al*. Intractable nonlesional epilepsy of temporal lobe origin: lateralization by interictal SPECT versus MRI. *Neurology* 1994; 44: 829–36.

161 Newton MR, Berkovic SF, Austin MC, Rowe CC, McKay WJ, Bladin PF. SPECT in the localisation of extratemporal and temporal seizure foci. *J Neurol Neurosurg Psychiatr* 1995; 59: 26–30.

162 Runge U, Kirsch G, Petersen B *et al*. Ictal and interictal ECD-SPECT for focus localization in epilepsy. *Acta Neurol Scand* 1997; 96: 271–6.

163 Devous MD Sr, Thisted RA, Morgan GF, Leroy RF, Rowe CC. SPECT brain imaging in epilepsy: a meta-analysis. *J Nucl Med* 1998; 39: 285–93.

164 Rowe CC, Berkovic SF, Austin MC *et al*. Visual and quantitative analysis of interictal SPECT with technetium-99m-HMPAO in temporal lobe epilepsy. *J Nucl Med* 1991; 32: 1688–94.

165 Zubal IG, Spencer SS, Imam K *et al*. Difference images calculated from ictal and interictal technetium-99m-HMPAO SPECT scans of epilepsy. *J Nucl Med* 1995; 36: 684–9.

166 O'Brien TJ, So EL, Mullan BP *et al*. Subtraction ictal SPECT co-registered to MRI improves clinical usefulness of SPECT in localizing the surgical seizure focus. *Neurology* 1998; 50: 445–54.

167 Laich E, Kuzniecky R, Mountz J *et al*. Supplementary sensorimotor area epilepsy. Seizure localization, cortical propagation and subcortical activation pathways using ictal SPECT. *Brain* 1997; 120: 855–64.

168 Wichert-Ana L, Velasco TR, Terra-Bustamante VC *et al*. Typical and atypical perfusion patterns in periictal SPECT of patients with unilateral temporal lobe epilepsy. *Epilepsia* 2001; 42: 660–6.

169 Lee HW, Hong SB, Tae WS. Opposite ictal perfusion patterns of subtracted SPECT. Hyperperfusion and hypoperfusion. *Brain* 2000; 123: 2150–9.

170 Avery RA, Zubal IG, Stokking R *et al*. Decreased cerebral blood flow during seizures with ictal SPECT injections. *Epilepsy Res* 2000; 40: 53–61.

171 Duncan R, Patterson J, Roberts R, Hadley DM, Bone I. Ictal/postictal SPECT in the pre-surgical localisation of complex partial seizures. *J Neurol Neurosurg Psychiatr* 1993; 56: 141–8.

172 Oliveira AJ, da Costa JC, Hilario LN, Anselmi OE, Palmini A. Localization of the epileptogenic zone by ictal and interictal SPECT with 99mTc-ethyl cysteinate dimer in patients with medically refractory epilepsy. *Epilepsia* 1999; 40: 693–702.

173 Ho SS, Berkovic SF, Berlangieri SU *et al*. Comparison of ictal SPECT and interictal PET in the presurgical evaluation of temporal lobe epilepsy. *Ann Neurol* 1995; 37: 738–45.

174 Sakai K, Hidari M, Fukai M, Okamura T, Asaba H, Sakai T. A chance SPECT study of ictal aphasia during simple partial seizures. *Epilepsia* 1997; 38: 374–6.

175 Harvey AS, Hopkins IJ, Bowe JM, Cook DJ, Shield LK, Berkovic SF. Frontal lobe epilepsy: clinical seizure characteristics and localization with ictal 99mTc-HMPAO SPECT. *Neurology* 1993; 43: 1966–80.

176 Weil S, Noachtar S, Arnold S, Yousry TA, Winkler PA, Tatsch K. Ictal ECD-SPECT differentiates between temporal and extratemporal epil-

epsy: confirmation by excellent postoperative seizure control. *Nucl Med Commun* 2001; 22: 233–7.

177 Baumgartner C, Serles W, Leutmezer F *et al.* Preictal SPECT in temporal lobe epilepsy: regional cerebral blood flow is increased prior to electroencephalography-seizure onset. *J Nucl Med* 1998; 39: 978–82.

178 Le Van Quyen M, Martinerie J, Navarro V *et al.* Anticipation of epileptic seizures from standard EEG recordings. *Lancet* 2001; 357: 183–8.

179 Elger CE, Lehnertz K. Seizure prediction by non-linear time series analysis of brain electrical activity. *Eur J Neurosci* 1998; 10: 786–9.

180 Spanaki MV, Spencer SS, Corsi M, MacMullan J, Seibyl J, Zubal IG. Sensitivity and specificity of quantitative difference SPECT analysis in seizure localization. *J Nucl Med* 1999; 40: 730–6.

181 Spanaki MV, Zubal IG, MacMullan J, Spencer SS. Periictal SPECT localization verified by simultaneous intracranial EEG. *Epilepsia* 1999; 40: 267–74.

182 Lynch BJ, O'Tuama LA, Treves ST, Mikati M, Holmes GL. Correlation of 99mTc-HMPAO SPECT with EEG monitoring: prognostic value for outcome of epilepsy surgery in children. *Brain Dev* 1995; 17: 409–17.

183 O'Brien TJ, So EL, Mullan BP *et al.* Subtraction peri-ictal SPECT is predictive of extratemporal epilepsy surgery outcome. *Neurology* 2000; 55: 1668–77.

184 Ryvlin P, Philippon B, Cinotti L, Froment JC, Le Bars D, Mauguiere F. Functional neuroimaging strategy in temporal lobe epilepsy: a comparative study of 18FDG-PET and 99mTc-HMPAO-SPECT. *Ann Neurol* 1992; 31: 650–6.

185 Nagata T, Tanaka F, Yonekura Y *et al.* Limited value of interictal brain perfusion SPECT for detection of epileptic foci: high resolution SPECT studies in comparison with FDG-PET. *Ann Nucl Med* 1995; 9: 59–63.

186 Lee DS, Lee JS, Kang KW *et al.* Disparity of perfusion and glucose metabolism of epileptogenic zones in temporal lobe epilepsy demonstrated by SPM/SPAM analysis of 15O water PET, [18F]FDG-PET, and [99mTC]-HMPAO SPECT. *Epilepsia* 2001; 42: 1515–22.

187 Won HJ, Chang KH, Cheon JE *et al.* Comparison of MR imaging with PET and ictal SPECT in 118 patients with intractable epilepsy. *Am J Neuroradiol* 1999; 20: 593–9.

188 Markand ON, Salanova V, Worth R, Park HM, Wellman HN. Comparative study of interictal PET and ictal SPECT in complex partial seizures. *Acta Neurol Scand* 1997; 95: 129–36.

189 Menzel C, Grunwald F, Klemm E, Ruhlmann J, Elger CE, Biersack HJ. Inhibitory effects of mesial temporal partial seizures onto frontal neocortical structures. *Acta Neurol Belg* 1998; 98: 327–31.

190 Bohnen NI, O'Brien TJ, Mullan BP, So EL. Cerebellar changes in partial seizures: clinical correlations of quantitative SPECT and MRI analysis. *Epilepsia* 1998; 39: 640–50.

191 Shin WC, Hong SB, Tae WS, Seo DW, Kim SE. Ictal hyperperfusion of cerebellum and basal ganglia in temporal lobe epilepsy: SPECT subtraction with MRI coregistration *J Nucl Med* 2001; 42: 853–8.

192 Seto H, Shimizu M, Watanabe N *et al.* Contralateral cerebellar activation in frontal lobe epilepsy detected by ictal Tc-99m HMPAO brain SPECT. *Clin Nucl Med* 1997; 22: 194–5.

193 Yune MJ, Lee JD, Ryu YH, Kim DI, Lee BI, Kim SJ. Ipsilateral thalamic hypoperfusion on interictal SPECT in temporal lobe epilepsy. *J Nucl Med* 1998; 39: 281–5.

194 Kumlien E, Bergstrom M, Lilja A *et al.* Positron emission tomography with [11C] deuterium-deprenyl in temporal lobe epilepsy. *Epilepsia* 1995; 36: 712–21.

195 Chugani DC, Chugani HT, Muzik O *et al.* Imaging epileptogenic tubers in children with tuberous sclerosis complex using alpha-[11C]methyl-L-tryptophan positron emission tomography. *Ann Neurol* 1998; 44: 858–66.

196 Goerres GW, Revesz T, Duncan J, Banati RB. Imaging cerebral vasculitis in refractory epilepsy using [(11)C](R)-PK11195 positron emission tomography. *Am J Roentgenol* 2001; 176: 1016–18.

197 Pennell PB, Henry TR, Koeppe RA, Kilbourn MR, Frey KA. PET imaging of benzodiazepine and muscarinic receptor losses in mesial temporal lobe epilepsy. *Epilepsia* 1995; 36: (Suppl. 4): 24.

New Physiological and Radiological Investigations in the Presurgical Evaluation of Epilepsy

A. Salek-Haddadi, I. Merlet, F. Mauguière, H. Meierkord, K. Buchheim, D.R. Fish, M.J. Koepp and E.L. So

There have been many advances in structural imaging over the last two decades which have greatly enhanced the processes of presurgical evaluation. We have already seen considerable advances in associated functional imaging techniques, such as PET, interictal and ictal SPECT and MEG described elsewhere. This chapter outlines the principles, and current or future potential applications, of five specific functional imaging techniques: EEG dipole source modelling, optical imaging, simultaneous EEG-correlated functional MRI (EEG/fMRI), functional MRI (fMRI) and subtraction ictal SPECT coregistered on MRI (SISCOM).

Dipole source modelling (Chapter 57a)

I. Merlet and F. Mauguière

Although qualitative information may be gained from the visual analysis of scalp potential fields, or from voltage maps [1–7], conventional scalp EEGs are inadequate in localizing the origins of epileptic paroxysms. More than 50 years ago, Marie Brazier proposed the application of physical and mathematical principles to the localization of EEG sources [8] based on the assumption that an active current source within a finite conductive medium will produce volume currents that lead to potential differences on the surface.

In this section, we will first review the methodological aspects of dipole modelling methods, then examine the results for interictal spikes, and their relation to other data such as MRI or PET, and invasive recordings. Finally, we will assess the peculiar difficulties encountered in modelling ictal discharges and examine the overall clinical relevance of dipole modelling results in the presurgical evaluation of epileptic patients.

The wording used in dipole modelling is sometimes confusing; in what follows the term 'generator' refers to the anatomical structure generating the events, while the words 'source' or 'dipolar source' refer to the dipole used to model the generator.

Methodological aspects

Principle

Dipole modelling of EEG and MEG is based on an iterative statistical estimation of the locations, orientations and amplitudes of the intracerebral generators from surface signals and this requires models for both generators and conductive media.

Modelling the sources

The easiest way to represent a current source is with a current dipole. If we consider an excitatory synapse on a dendrite of a pyramidal cell, synaptic activation (membrane depolarization) will induce a massive inflow of Na^+ ions (a current entrance or sink) and therefore a deficit in positive charge outside the membrane. This massive inflow is counterbalanced by an exiting current downstream along the postsynaptic membrane, resulting in a group of negative and a group of positive charges, separated by a small distance (i.e. a dipole).

Since pyramidal cells are organized in columns orientated perpendicular to the cortical surface, if a sufficient number of focal neurones are synchronously activated, currents may be obtained with sufficient amplitude to produce a measurable potential difference at the surface. The geometry of neuronal aggregates is of particular importance since 'closed field' configurations, i.e. groups of neurones with different or random orientations (as in amygdala or thalamus for example), will theoretically give rise to very small or nil equivalent dipoles with no recordable electrical potential outside. Conversely, if neurones are orientated in a parallel way ('open field', as is for most cortex), their activity can be modelled by an equivalent dipole, representing the vectorial sum of each of the unitary dipoles [9].

Modelling the conductive volume

Besides anatomical constraints, the potential differences recorded at the scalp also have physical constraints. In particular, these depend on the source intensity and the different conductivities of brain tissues. A model for the head therefore has to describe mathematically the physical properties of brain tissues and liquids, i.e. brain itself, cerebrospinal fluid (CSF), skull and scalp. In order to simplify this calculation, it is usually assumed that all these properties are purely resistive. The geometry of head models used for dipole modelling is either spherical or realistic. The human head can be modelled by spherical shells of different conductivity representing the scalp, skull, CSF and brain [10], and although this sphere is quite well adapted to the shape of the brain, particularly over central regions, the real shape of the head is clearly different from a sphere in occipital, frontal or basal regions, which could potentially give rise to localization errors [11]. In order to improve the localization of intracerebral sources, realistic models of the head have been proposed [12–15], based on the extraction of scalp, skull and brain surfaces from individual MRI data.

The forward and inverse problems

If, at a given time, the source distributions and configurations within the brain as well as the conductive properties of the tissues are known, the resulting potentials at the scalp surface can be calculated on the basis of physical principles. This is generally referred to as the 'forward problem' and has a unique solution. Inversely, dipole modelling methods search for the location of intracerebral generators whose activity might explain scalp potentials and this is referred to as the 'inverse problem'. Since each dipole is characterized by three spatial location parameters (Cartesian x, y, z or spherical r, theta, phi, coordinates), and three vector parameters (sense, direction and amplitude), the inverse problem is equivalent to an estimation of these parameters in a system involving $6 \times N$ unknowns for N generators.

As there are only a finite number of sites on the scalp where potentials are recorded, it is theoretically possible to obtain an infinite number of intracerebral source configurations for a given surface potential distribution. In practice, however, knowledge of the underlying pathology and physiology allows for the definition of some constraints which considerably help in reducing the number of solutions (for example, sources cannot be located in ventricles, white matter, eyes, etc.). Dipole inverse solutions are calculated by an iterative process in which the dipole location, orientation and amplitudes are changed step by step to obtain the best fit between the real scalp potential distribution and the theoretical distributions predicted (the solutions of the individual forward problems). The quality of the solution is evaluated by 'goodness of fit' or 'residual variance' parameters, respectively, reflecting the percentage of data variance explained or left unexplained by the model.

Preprocessing the data

Spike averaging

Interictal spikes usually occur over the background EEG or MEG which can act as a noise and potentially contaminate the real spike topography. In order to increase the signal-to-noise ratio, spikes can be averaged but, since spikes are often polyphasic, averaging has to be triggered from the same time reference so that phases from different polarities do not cancel. Although spike averaging is used often, this technique has been criticized for the risks of mixing spikes from different generators. The averaging of spikes from different foci gives a composite spike and can falsely suggest a spreading process by blurring the localization process [16,17]. In our experience, however, non-averaged (even filtered) spikes are difficult to model and in most cases, a dipole solution can obtain only around the maximal amplitude peak. Another advantage of averaging is that it may reveal small voltage deflections during the paroxysm otherwise indiscernible, but it remains a risky procedure and requires careful checks on the similarities of the spikes selected.

Averaged-spike topography

Averaged spikes are usually characterized by several phases with inverse polarity. The typical deflections observed are an early positive peak, a main negative peak and a late positive peak sometimes followed by a negative wave. Analysis of the temporal sequence of voltage maps during the interictal spike can help to understand better the spatiotemporal dynamics and to formulate hypotheses regarding the underlying generators. For an example a 'dipolar' distribution of voltage fields at the scalp surface, i.e. two maxima of inverse polarity, can be considered as due to a source tangential to the scalp surface, localized approximately under the zero potential line. In a similar way, a 'radial' topography, characterized by a single polarity maximum at the surface, may suggest a source orientated radially to the scalp, localized under the voltage maximum itself. In the example provided in Fig. 57.1, the topographies during the main and late phases of the spike are similar, suggesting that the

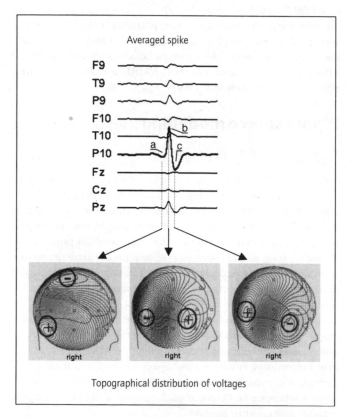

Fig. 57.1 Topographical analysis of an averaged interictal spike. Averaging is time-locked to the main negative peak of interictal spikes. The averaged spike is usually made of three to four phases with inverse polarity, i.e. (a) an early positive peak, (b) a high-amplitude negative peak, (c) a late positive peak, sometimes followed by a negative slow-wave. The scalp voltage distribution observed at these different peaks alludes to the number of underlying generators. In this example, voltage maps at the main and late peaks are almost identical, suggesting that the same source is activated during both phases. On the contrary, the early peak voltage map is clearly different, suggesting that another source might be active during this period.

same generator(s) might be active during both phases. Conversely, during the early peak, as the topography differs, different sources may be active. Spike topography is an important consideration in model selection.

Dipole modelling approaches

Instantaneous dipoles

The simplest of these approaches consists of estimating the instantaneous equivalent dipole which best fits the scalp voltage distribution at a single point: the single instantaneous fit (Plate 57.2a, shown in colour between pp. 670 and 671). This solution will have reasonable accuracy only if the actual generator is very focal and simple in space and over time, otherwise the solution will merely estimate the centre of mass for the activated area. The major limitations are (a) to assume that those equivalent sources are well separated, without time-overlapping; and (b) to choose the time points within the spike complex where the sources are to be calculated, ignoring other parts of the signal which might be of physiological interest.

Single equivalent dipole analysis can also be applied to time intervals, producing a pattern of multiple sequential sources (as many as the number of sampling points in the interval) which vary in location and orientation: the 'multiple instantaneous fit', or 'moving dipole' (Plate 57.2b, shown in colour between pp. 670 and 671). This pattern can be interpreted as reflecting the sequential activation of multiple brain regions, limited in space and time, but the question arises as to whether the whole sequence of dipoles is relevant or not with regard to the anatomical propagation of transients.

Multiple spatiotemporal dipoles

Rather than assuming discrete cerebral regions to be activated shortly and sequentially, it seems physiologically more reasonable to consider that larger cortical regions are activated for a longer period, with their activities overlapping in time. The 'spatiotemporal approach' takes into account the course of the signals as a whole instead of considering each time sample separately. This method, first described by Michael Scherg [18], is based on the assumptions of several 'static' dipolar sources, fixed in position and orientation, but varying in magnitude over the time interval of interest. A 'spatiotemporal dipole solution' thus characterizes the position and orientation of the sources, as well as their time of activation during the event (Plate 57.2c, shown in colour between pp. 670 and 671). The underlying concept is that the earliest part of the EEG or MEG spike is more likely to reflect the activity of a single source rather than the peaks for example. In some instances, the early source also explains the later segments and the generator is assumed to be very focal but, in other instances, additional sources are needed to explain the residual activity.

In practice, it is useful to combine dipole modelling approaches. The 'single moving dipole' approach provides a pattern of dipolar sources often grouped into 'clusters' for the time interval under consideration. This allows the estimation of both the number of active sources and the timings of their maximal activity. Next, in order to take into account the spatiotemporal evolution of the paroxysms,

static dipoles with fixed location and orientation but time varying activity are useful. In practice, a first source is fitted over the early phase of the spike, then a second to model the main peak and the residual signal unexplained by the first, and this procedure can be repeated at increasing intervals from spike onset until an acceptable fit is achieved (Plate 57.2c, shown in colour between pp. 670 and 671).

Projection of sources onto three-dimensional MRI

The frame of the dipole model is defined by orthogonal axes passing through vertex (Cz electrode, vertical z-axis), right ear (T4, lateral x-axis), and frontopolar (Fpz, anteroposterior y-axis) electrodes. Coregistration of dipole modelling and anatomical data implies that both are in the same frame which may be done by calculations using external landmarks, or by estimating the mean location of the model centre with respect to anatomy [19]. Most available software packages now allow for automatic registration of dipole modelling results onto individual or averaged MRI data.

Quality of solution and accuracy of localization

The quality of the solution is usually assessed in terms of 'residual variance' or 'goodness of fit' but these are difficult to interpret without a reliability threshold and it is important to use other criteria. For example, the stability of the solution should be systematically taken into account by checking that (a) for one given spike, dipole results are stable as the modelling process is replayed using different starting points prior to fit; and that (b) for a given patient, different spike averages with similar scalp distributions yield similar dipole configurations. The existence of interactions is another criterion which should be considered. Sources are interacting when they tend to converge on the same location and display a very similar activity waveform during the fitting process, in which case only one is sufficient to explain the data.

In addition to the quality, accuracy is a frequently raised issue. Error measurements would require reference information as to the actual source locations and this is seldom the case in relation to epileptic paroxysmal transients. In some cases, error may be calculated directly by modelling simulated data from known sources, or alternatively by creating current dipoles between two adjacent intracerebral electrodes *in vivo*. The results of such studies are summarized in Table 57.1. A mean localization error of around 10 mm may be accepted [20–23], but this can vary from a few millimetres to as much as a few centimetres.

Indeed it is generally well accepted that the localization error (a) is larger when the source is located deep [23–25]; (b) is smaller when realistic head models are used, as compared with spherical models [24–26]; (c) is smaller when the spatial sampling of EEG electrodes or MEG captors is increased [27–29]; and finally (d) increases with signal-to-noise ratio. Knowing this, it is reasonable to hold that superficial dipoles calculated from 32-channel data with a good signal-to-noise ratio, in a realistic head model, can be localized with an error of about 5 mm.

It is noteworthy that the above estimations derive from simulated data. For physiological signals such as epileptic spikes, the locations of dipole sources can be validated when scalp and intracerebral

Table 57.1 (a–d) Localization errors with dipole modelling

(a) Mean errors or range

Reference	Localization errors
Smith *et al.* 1985 [20]	<20 mm
Cohen *et al.* 1990 [21]	10 mm (max. 17 mm)
Cuffin *et al.* 1991 [22]	11 mm (max. 28 mm)
Mosher *et al.* 1999 [24]	25 mm
Cuffin 1996 [27]	2–17 mm
Yvert *et al.* 1997 [25]	5–6 mm
Cuffin 2001 *et al.* [23]	10.6 mm

(b) Mean errors according to mesiolateral localization of sources

| Reference | Error | |
	Superficial sources	Mesial sources
Mosher *et al.* 1999 [24]	20 mm	35 mm
Yvert *et al.* 1997 [25]	5–6 mm	15–25 mm
Cuffin *et al.* 2001 [23]	9 mm	13 mm

(c) Influence of electrode number

Reference	Number of electrodes	Error improvement
Mosher *et al.* 1999 [24]	37 vs. 21	10 mm
	127 vs. 37	5 mm
Yvert *et al.* 1997 [25]	32 vs. 19	3 mm
	63 vs. 32	1 mm
Krings *et al.* 1999 [26]	41 vs. 21	5 mm

(d) Improvement in localization error according to the type of head model used

Reference	Realistic vs. spherical: error improvement
Cuffin 1996 [27]	2.6 mm
Leahy *et al.* 1998 [28]	0.4 mm (phantom)
Crouzeix *et al.* 1999 [29]	2.5 mm (superficial sources)
	12 mm (deep sources)

signals are recorded simultaneously. Here, intracranial spikes can be used as triggers for averaging the corresponding scalp signal, which in turn can be modelled. Dipole localization can then be compared with intracranial electrodes where spikes are maximally recorded.

Using this technique, Lantz *et al.* could identify different intracranial distributions associated with temporal scalp EEG spikes [30]. Spikes with similar distributions were averaged together with the concomitant scalp EEG activity and the authors showed that the analysis of scalp-averaged activity allowed for the separation of different types of intracranial distributions, and the identification of the temporal regions involved during the paroxysm. Dipole loca-

tions, however, were difficult to assess because there was no projection onto MRI. This averaging technique was also used to analyse the scalp EEG signals associated with interictal mesiotemporal spikes recorded from foramen ovale (FO) electrodes [31]. Spikes detected visually on FO traces were used to trigger surface EEG averaging (Fig. 57.3) and although there was initially no paroxysmal activity detectable on surface EEG, a low-voltage EEG transient ($5–20\,\mu V$) was clearly seen to emerge from the noise post-averaging. Dipole modelling of this transient consistently permitted the identification of a source located in the mesial temporal structures (Plate 57.4, shown in colour between pp. 670 and 671), close to the FO electrode where the maximal spike had been recorded. These results show that dipole modelling methods can localize the mesiotemporal sources of interictal spikes with an acceptable spatial accuracy.

Such validation studies, however, focus on specific intracranial signals, while epileptologists would prefer to know whether dipole models of scalp data can localize the actual generators of interictal spikes. This question can be indirectly addressed by comparing spike modelling data with results from other modalities such as MRI, PET or invasive (stereo-EEG) recordings. In the following, we review data addressing these points.

Dipole modelling of the interictal spikes: interictal network

Dipole modelling of the interictal spikes: spikes as 'simple' or 'distributed' phenomena

When dipole modelling methods are applied to interictal spikes, several source distributions may be obtained. In rare instances interictal spikes can be adequately modelled by a single dipole. For example Fig. 57.5a shows that spikes from a patient with parieto-occipital epilepsy could be modelled by a single source within an occipital heterotopic lesion. In the majority of cases, however, several dipoles are required. These sources are usually located in distinct anatomical regions, are activated sequentially, but overlap in time as illustrated in Fig. 57.5b. Such patterns lead to the concept of 'spreading' activity and distributed sources during a single spike. It is historically noteworthy that all teams interested in spike dipole modelling have gradually been moving from 'unique source' [3,32,33] to 'multiple source' activation models of interictal paroxysms [4,34–36].

Temporal lobe epilepsy (TLE)

Modelling spikes in TLE is helpful to address whether mesial, lateral or both temporal cortices are involved in spike generation. In general, the majority of spikes culminating at temporal electrodes can be modelled by dipoles localized to the ipsilateral temporal lobe. However, within this group it is possible to distinguish between 'early mesial' and 'early neocortical' involvement depending on whether early sources localize to mesial or lateral temporal structures. Early mesial involvement seems to be more frequently observed, suggesting that mesiotemporal structures function as a trigger in the interictal network [36–41]. However, the opposite may also be observed and suggests that mesiotemporal structures can also work as a secondary relay [35,40,42] in this process.

Whatever the model of sequential activation, interictal spikes appear as distributed phenomena involving both mesial and neo-

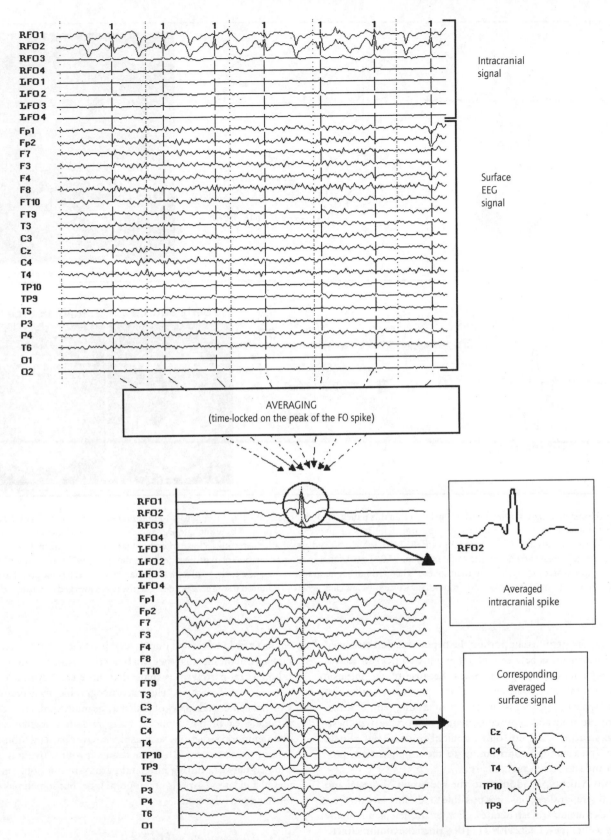

Fig. 57.3 Averaging of scalp EEG triggered by intracranial spikes recorded with foramen ovale (FO) electrodes. Non-averaged simultaneous FO and scalp EEG is illustrated at the top. Spikes are lateralized to one FO electrode and the concomitant raw EEG does not show a significant signal. The main peaks of the FO paroxysms are used to trigger scalp EEG averaging. Following this, synchronized low-amplitude EEG deflections are detectable and this signal is used for dipole modelling. R, right; L, left—these label the FO electrode (as in Plate 57.4, shown in colour between pp. 670 and 671). Scalp electrode sites are labelled according to the extended international 10/20 system [106].

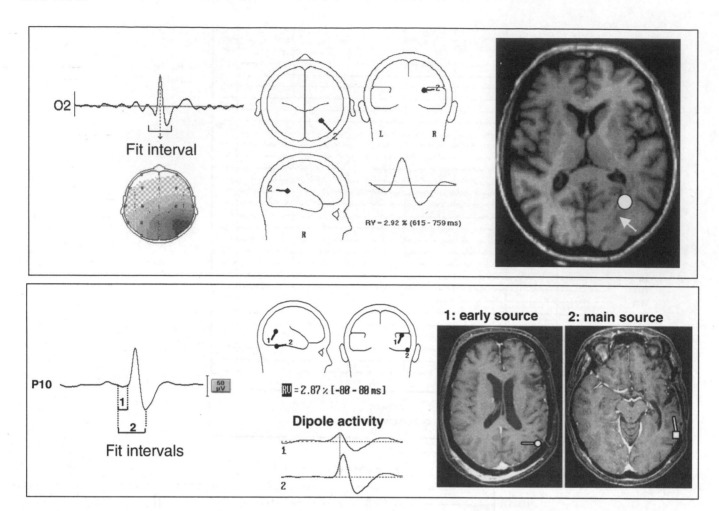

Fig. 57.5 (a) Simple vs. (b) complex interictal spikes. (a) In this patient with right parieto-occipital epilepsy, voltage maps at different peaks of the averaged interictal spike showed identical scalp distributions. This type of spike can be explained by a single source and adding others does not improve the residual variance. This source was concordant with the MRI, which showed grey matter heterotopia located in the right occipital white matter (arrow). (b) The complex case reported here is the same as in Fig. 57.2. Two distinct sources are necessary to properly explain the spikes in this patient with extensive frontotemporal atrophy of the right hemisphere. They activate sequentially, and suggest early involvement of the temporoparieto-occipital junction, followed by involvement of the posterior temporal neocortex. In this case, when an additional source was added, it always converged towards the main source.

cortical temporal regions supporting the hypothesis that sustained reciprocal interactions between mesial and neocortical structures exist during interictal temporal spikes. Because of the intrinsic properties of the mesiotemporal regions, particularly the hippocampus which appears essential to maintaining temporal discharges, results from spike source modelling support the hypothesis that these structures act not only as initial triggers, but also as secondary 'pacemakers' contributing to the amplification, prolongation and spread of ictal discharges.

In certain patients, in addition to the activation of mesial and neocortical temporal regions, it is possible to identify late involvement of extratemporal structures. For example, using dipole modelling techniques, Lantz *et al.* [17] described the combined activation of temporal and orbitofrontal regions during spikes culminating at the temporal scalp electrodes.

In our experience, the most frequently involved extratemporal regions are orbitofrontal, inferior parietal, insular and central oper-

cular. Their involvement during ictal propagation is not really surprising, but the fact that they can be recruited during a rapid temporal interictal paroxysm is somewhat more so. Nevertheless, such data are confirmed by electrocorticographic measurements in which the interictal spikes of TLE may be multifocal, often covering a large area of the temporal lobe, and may involve adjacent extratemporal structures such as the inferior parietal lobule or the orbitofrontal cortex [43]. These results favour activation of a distributed network during interictal paroxysms, not only involving mesial and lateral aspects of temporal lobe, but sometimes exceeding temporal lobe limits.

Frontal lobe epilepsy (FLE)

There have been few reports of dipole modelling results in FLE. In general, frontal spikes are recognized as more complex that temporal spikes. They are characterized by a more diverse range of

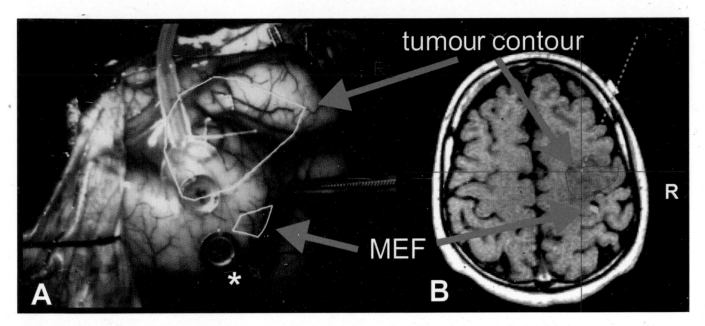

Plate 54.1 (a) Intraoperative view showing that in this patient the MEF dipole representing the motor cortex is displayed on the same gyrus as the tumour, which indicates that a resection is not possible. The white asterisk represents the SEF phase reversal and indicates the central sulcus. (b) Axial MRI showing the tumour contour and MEF dipole yellow triangle in the precentral gyrus, as displayed in the operating theatre for navigation purposes (with kind permission reproduced from Ganslandt et al. 1999).

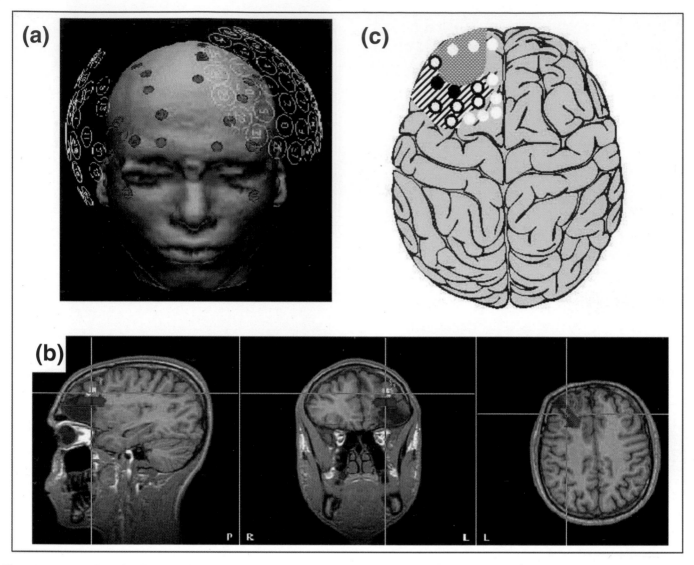

Plate 54.2 MEG and EEG localizations of interictal spikes in a patient with symptomatic frontal lobe epilepsy; with EEG spikes only identifiable after averaging according to MEG templates: (a) EEG electrode (magneta) and MEG sensor (cyan, yellow) locations. (b) Dipole sites, displayed in sagittal, coronal and axial MRI slices. Red: MEG results. Yellow: EEG results (showing higher variability). (c) Sketch of the intraoperative situation. Circles indicate ECoG contacts. Black: maximum spiking activity, in accordance with localization results in (b). White open: no spiking observed. Black-white: medium spiking activity. Shaded area: lesion. Hatched area: resection.

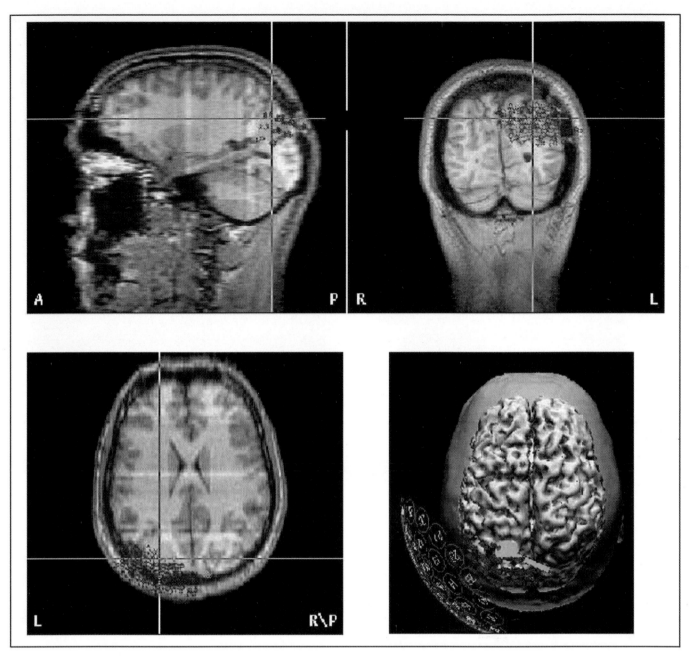

Plate 54.3 Ictal MSI localizations in a patient with symptomatic epilepsy of the left occipito-parietal region, displayed in sagittal, coronal and axial MRI slices (top and bottom left), and in a 3D reconstruction of the cortex and skin compartments (bottom right). Red: area resulting from current density reconstruction. Green: dipole site. Numbers in magenta circles indicate MEG sensor positions.

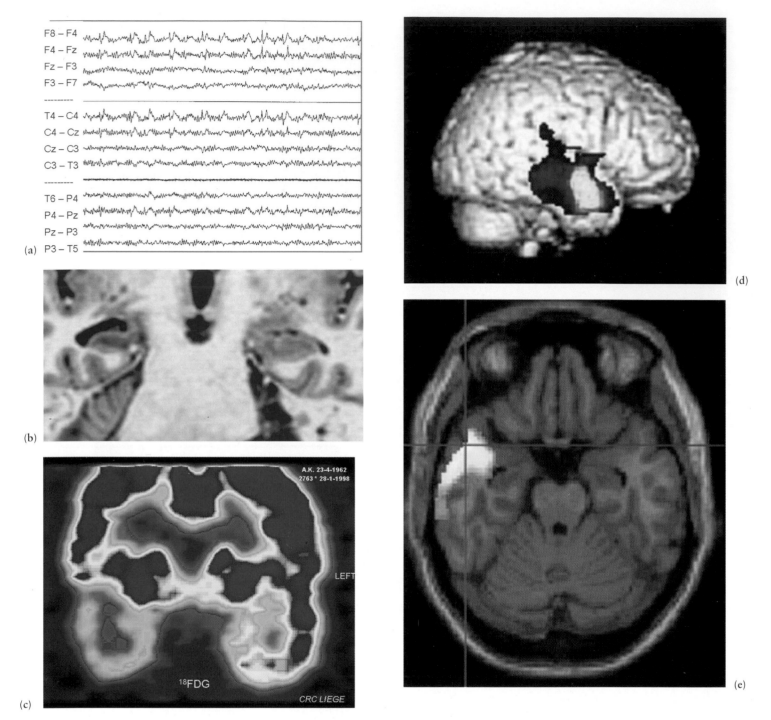

Plate 56.1 Complex partial seizures in a 32-year-old man. (a) EEG showing very frequent spiking over the right temporal cortex. (b) MRI with right hippocampal atrophy on a coronal IR slice. (c) ^{18}FDG-PET with important glucose hypometabolism over the entire right temporal lobe. (d, e) SPM analysis of this PET study comparing the patient's PET to a group of 30 age-matched controls: pixels with a significant hypometabolism are projected over a transverse slice of a standard MRI in the Talairach's frame (d) or on a standard three-dimensional MRI (e).

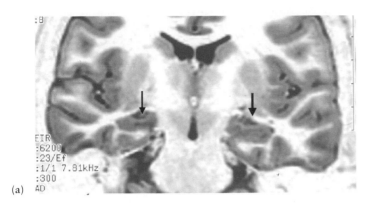

(a)

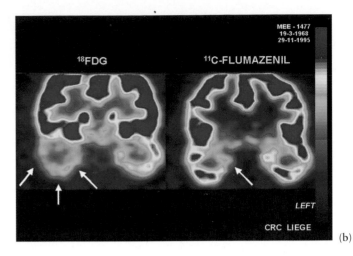

(b)

Plate 56.2 Combined ^{11}C-flumazenil and [18]FDG-PET in a case of temporal lobe epilepsy in a 26-year-old male with complex partial seizures resistant to drug treatment. Seizure semiology was suggestive of a temporal lobe epilepsy. (a) MRI showed a right hippocampal atrophy. (b) Representative PET images showing two adjacent coronal slices obtained with a 951 Siemens tomograph: glucose metabolism (left) and ^{11}C-flumazenil uptake (right). Glucose metabolism is decreased in the lateral, basal and mesial part of the right temporal lobe while ^{11}C-flumazenil binding is decreased only in the hippocampal region.

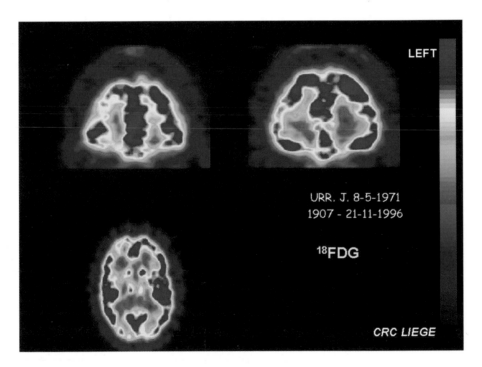

Plate 56.3 [18]FDG-PET of a 28-year-old male with a long history of typical frontal lobe seizures, non-contributive scalp EEG and normal MRI. IC-EEG indicated a right frontal lobe seizure focus and pathological examination of the resected cortex showed a focal Taylor's cortical dysplasia. [18]FDG-PET helped to focus IC-EEG recording by showing a right frontal lobe hypometabolism.

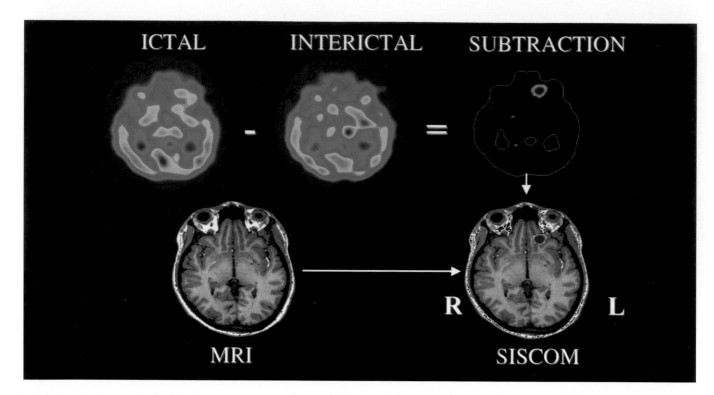

Plate 56.4 Ictal and interictal cerebral perfusion SPECT images were acquired after injection of ^{99m}Tc-ECD. The ictal scan was registered to the same patient's interictal scan. Normalization of the three-dimensional data was applied to account for global per cent brain uptake and total injected activity. After registration and normalization the ictal and interictal SPECT scans were subtracted. This subtraction or difference image gives a quantitative measure of perfusion alterations during ictus. The resulting difference images were also registered with the patient's MRI scan which permits localization of perfusion changes associated with ictal activity onto anatomical structures.

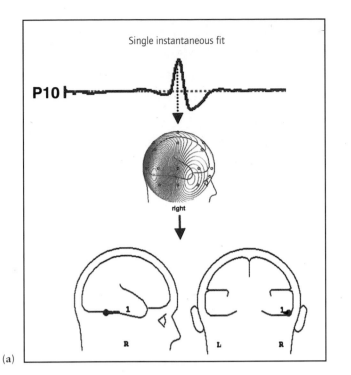

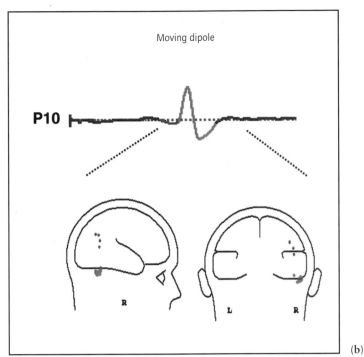

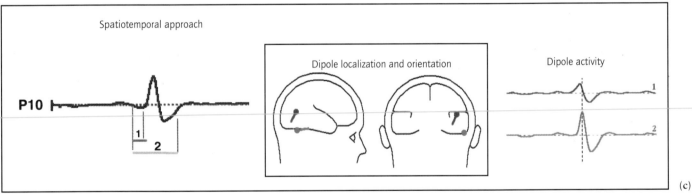

(a)

(b)

(c)

Plate 57.2 Dipole modelling approaches. (a) The 'single instantaneous fit' approach gives a dipole at one time point. (b) The 'moving dipole' approach (also called 'multiple instantaneous fit') gives one dipole for each sampling point over the entire spike interval. This approach helps in estimating the number of active sources during the spike as well as the time interval over which they are spatially stable. In this example, sources calculated over the early positive peak are grouped in the posterior parietotemporal regions, while sources calculated over the main and late peaks localize to the basal temporal regions. This suggests that two distinct sources might be active during the spike. (c) The spatiotemporal approach can be used to calculate the position and orientation of sources over the intervals previously defined by the moving dipole approach. In the same example as (b), a first dipole can be calculated over the early peak interval (early source); this source being fitted, another source can be calculated over the interval including the main (main source) and late (late source) peaks. Here, the same dipole explains both main and late peaks. This approach gives dipole location and orientation as well as activation sequence over time.

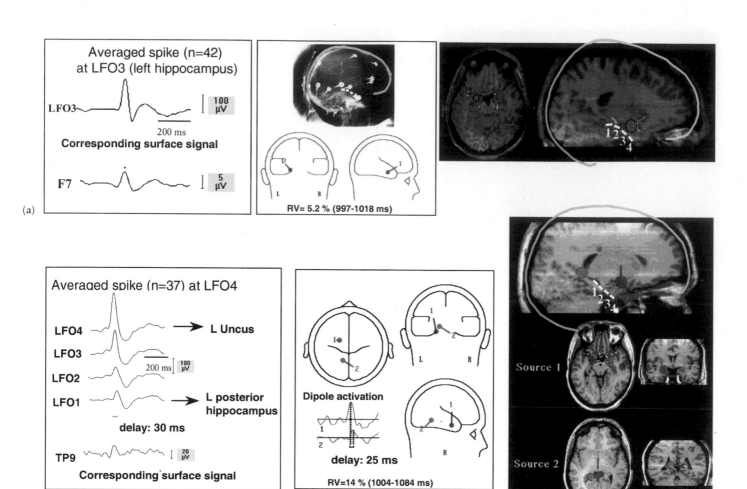

Plate 57.4 Reliability of mesiotemporal sources. Averaged scalp EEG and FO traces are illustrated on the left, and the results of dipole modelling, as well as the location of intracranial recording sites on MRI, are shown on the right (see [35] for methods). (a) In patient 1, paroxysms were culminating at the contact LFO3, facing the left uncus where the dipole explaining the surface EEG data was located. (b) In patient 2, FO spikes were first maximal at the fourth contact (facing the anterior hippocampus) and peaked 30 ms later at the LFO1 contact, facing the posterior hippocampus. Since this delay was reproducible across all spikes, it was possible to use the peaking time of the earlier LFO4 spike as a trigger for surface EEG averaging. The averaged signal was a biphasic wave of low amplitude, culminating at TP9 in synchrony with the early LFO4 intracranial spike. This signal could be modelled by two dipoles, showing sequential but overlapping activation first in the left amygdala and 25 ms later in the left posterior hippocampus.

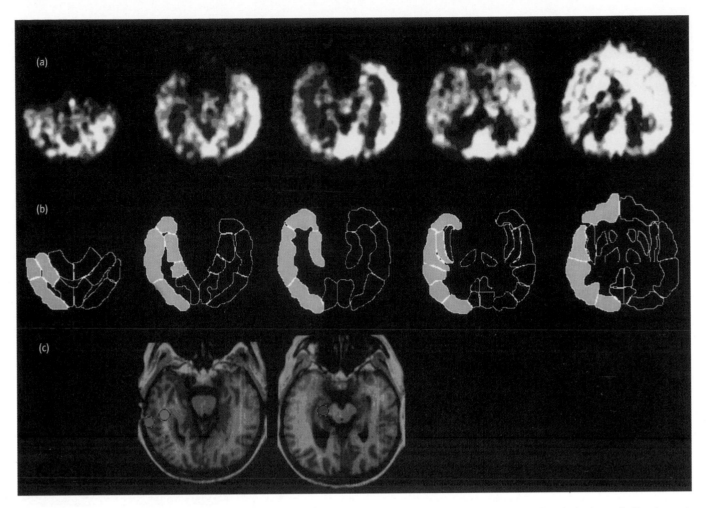

Plate 57.7 Glucose hypometabolism on PET and spikes dipoles. (a) [18]FDG-PET images showing regional glucose uptake. The hypometabolism is massive and involves the bulk of the left hemisphere. (b) ROI where significant hypometabolism was found. (c) Dipole localization in the same patient. All spike sources were localized to the left temporal lobe, within the significant hypometabolic region, where they delimit a smaller area.

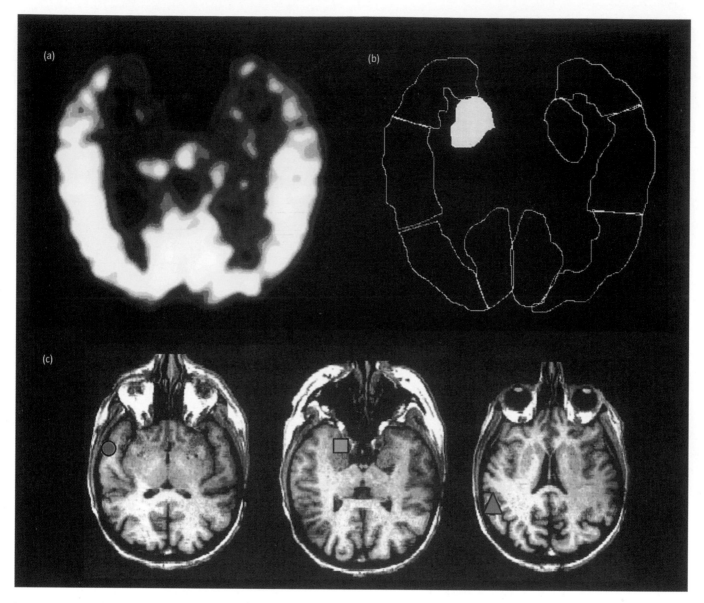

Plate 57.8 Late involvement of extratemporal regions and glucose hypometabolism. (a) ^{18}FDG-PET slice in the bihippocampal plane. (b) ROI for the corresponding slice. The filled area in the left anterior hippocampus showed a significant decrease in glucose uptake. (c) Spike dipole localization. Dipole modelling results suggest that spikes originate in the temporal lobe, and spread extratemporally. Only the main source was located within the focal hypometabolic area. Red circle, early source; green square, main source; blue triangle, late source.

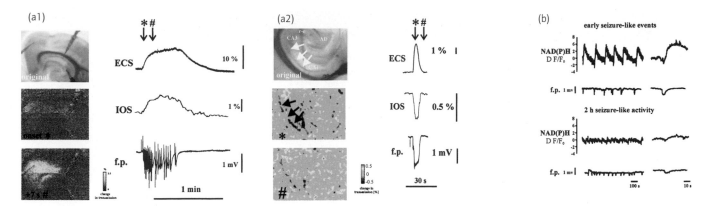

Plate 57.14 Different experimental applications of intrinsic optical signal (IOS) analysis. (a1) Low Mg^{2+}-induced seizure activity. Left: original image of the slice preparation. Illumination from below, through which myelin-rich regions such as the alveus appear dark and regions in which neurones are densely packed such as the cornu ammonis appear bright. The two pseudocoloured subtraction images indicate that the onset (*) of seizure activity is in the medial entorhinal cortex and in all other regions only noise is seen. Seven seconds later (#) the activity has spread along the lateral entorhinal cortex and into the subiculum. Right: traces of extracellular space volume (ECS) changes, IOS and extracellular field potentials (f.p.) during the seizure-like event. Shrinkage of the ECS volume is accompanied by an increase in light transmittance. The black arrows indicate the time points at which images were taken. (a2) Low Ca^{2+}-induced seizure activity: the original image is focused on the hippocampal formation. The arrows indicate the stratum pyramidale of CA1 were the seizure activity occurs. During seizure activity (*) a decrease in light transmittance took place, whereas the ECS volume shrunk. Outside seizure activity (#) only optical noise is seen. (b) Low magnesium-induced seizure activity. Left: time course of NAD(P)H autofluorescence in relation to extracellular f.p. during the first six subsequent seizure-like events and after 2 h of seizure-like activity. Note the decline of the NAD(P)H autofluorescence overshoot already appears within the first six seizure-like events. Right: expanded time scales for the first and the 40th seizure-like event.

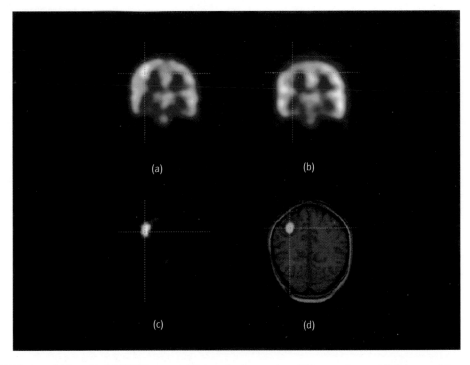

Plate 57.20 (a) Ictal SPECT image. (b) Interictal SPECT image. (c) Focus of subtracted, or difference, image. (d) Subtracted focus coregistered on MRI. With permission from [238].

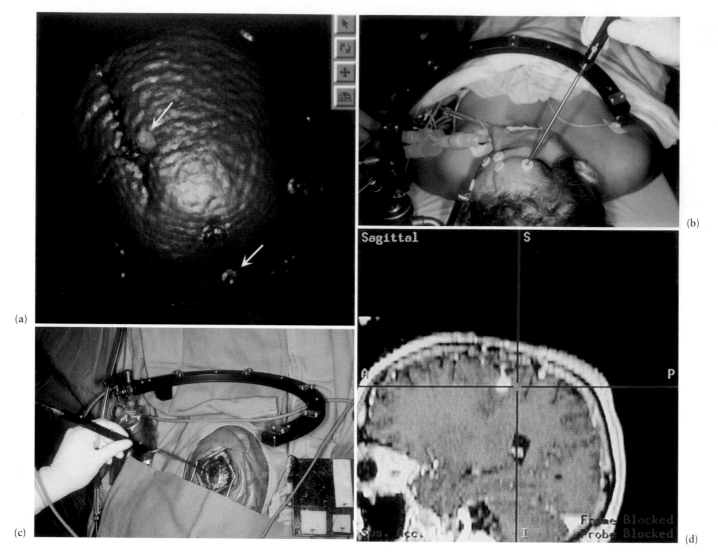

Plate 57.21 (a) Three-dimensional reconstruction of the patient's head from the frameless stereotactic MRI procedure, showing scalp markers (lower arrow) and the surface-rendered SISCOM focus (upper arrow). (b) The scalp markers are then registered into a computer to create a transformation matrix, so that the MRI image space can be related to the physical space of the patient's head. (c) During operation, the surgeon uses a wand to point at locations in the surgical field. (d) The surgeon views the computer monitor screen, where the crosshairs indicate how close the tip of the wand is to the SISCOM abnormality. This observation is used to guide the implantation of subdural electrodes and the resection of the SISCOM focus. With permission from [247].

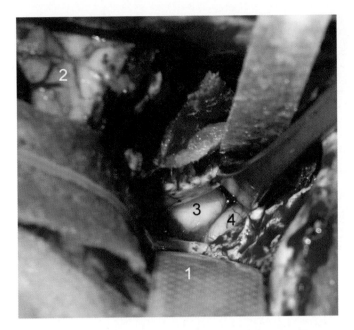

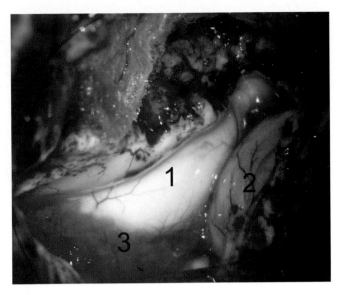

Plate 60.6 Operative photograph of a left temporal lobectomy. The lateral cortex has been resected, exposing the temporal horn. A retractor (1) elevates the roof of the ventricle. Residual lateral cortex is seen to the left (2). The surface of the anterior hippocampus (3) and lateral amygdala (4) are immediately visible upon entry into the ventricle.

Plate 60.7 The ventricle has been opened further. The anterior hippocampus (1) and amygdala (2) are visible. Posteriorly, the choroids plexus is found atop the medial border of the hippocampus (3).

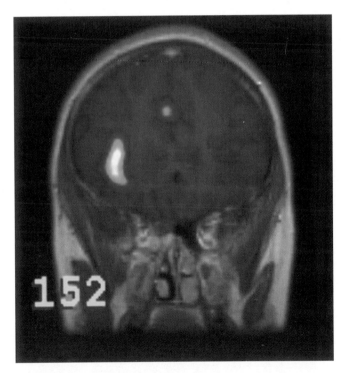

Plate 61.2 Subtraction ictal SPECT scan coregistered to a structural MRI (SISCOM) in a patient with a previously resected right insular glioma. There is a region of hypoperfusion that is intimately associated with the site of the previous tumour resection.

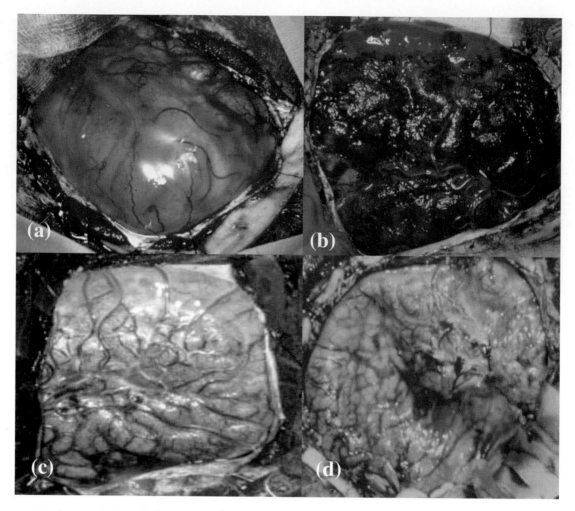

Plate 66.1 Preoperative photographs in hemispherectomies of: (a) right porencephaly (courtesy Dr J.P. Farmer); (b) left Sturge–Weber syndrome; (c) left Rasmussen's chronic encephalitis (early); and (d) right hemisphere atrophy (infantile hemiplegia).

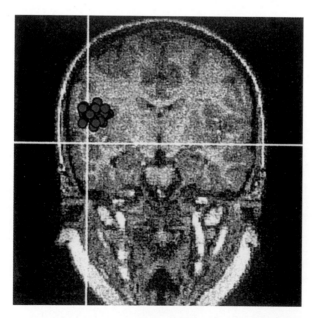

Plate 68.1 Magnetic source imaging in a case of Landau–Kleffner syndrome. Changes in magnetic field induced by paroxysmal cerebral activity are detected by an array of extracranial sensors. The position of the source of each episode is calculated and projected on an MRI scan of the patient's brain. Each of these dipoles appears deep in the right Sylvian fissure.

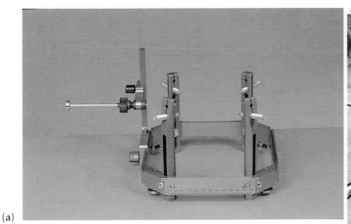

(a)

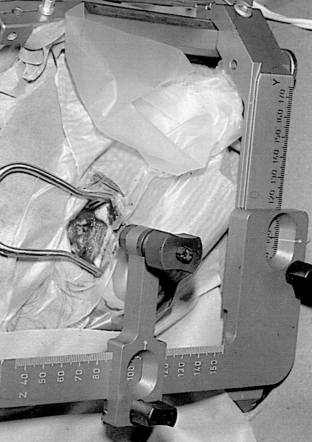

(b)

Plate 70.1 Following electrode placement confirmatory radiological imaging is used to show the final position achieved, since it is critical to know precisely where the EEG recordings are emanating from in order to obtain an accurate three-dimensional picture of seizure activity. Usually, disposable multiple contact platinum electrodes are used. (a) The Lexell stereotactic frame. (b) The Lexell frame being used intraoperatively for the insertion of depth electrodes. (c,d) Axial and coronal MRI showing depth electrodes bilaterally placed in the temporal lobes. (e) AP radiograph of the skull showing bilateral placement of subdural grid electrodes and right-sided frontal depth electrodes. (b) to (e) shown on p. 835.

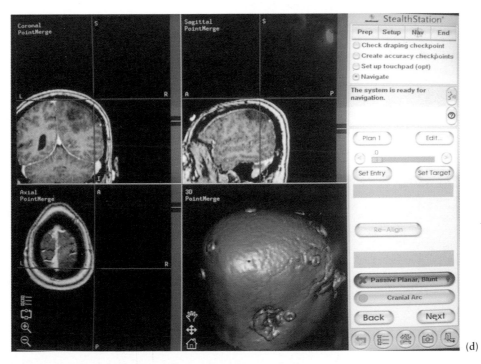

(d)

Plate 70.3 Modern frameless stereotaxy. The Stealth neuronavigation system in use for tumour resection. (a) The patient's head must be fixed in Mayfield pins throughout the procedure. There must be unrestricted lines of sight between the exploratory probe and the camera receiver. (b) The fiducial points are carefully loaded into the computer so that image space can be accurately mapped to patient space. (c) The system is then ready for neuronavigation with a light-emitting diode probe. (d) The position of the probe tip is demonstrated relative to multiplaner preoperative imaging enabling the margins of the lesion to be accurately delineated and an accurate trajectory taken. (a–c) appear in black and white on p. 835.

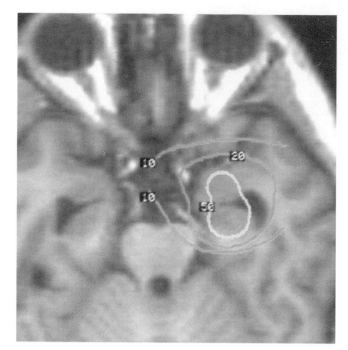

Plate 70.5 Planning scan using stereotactic radiosurgery in the form of the gamma knife in the treatment of medial temporal sclerosis.

Plate 73.4 PET studies in patients undergoing intermittent vagus nerve stimulation. Statistical mapping of regional blood flow increases (yellow) and decreases (blue) in the high and low stimulation groups (see text), with schemata for locations of predetermined structures of interest. The subjects' left is displayed on image right. The first two rows consist of axial images with ~1 cm spacing, arranged from interior (top left) to superior (bottom right) of the high stimulation group (see text for parameter settings). The middle two rows are similarly arranged data for the low stimulation group. The bottom two rows are axial brain schemata at the same levels as the other rows, with numbers inserted to indicate locations of structures. 1, Dorsal-rostral medulla; 2, 3, inferior cerebellar hemisphere; 4, cerebellar vermis; 5, hypothalamus; 6, 7, thalamus; 8, 9, hippocampus; 10, 11, amygdala; 12, 13, posterior cingulate gyrus; 14, 15, anterior insula; 16, 17, orbitofrontal cortex; 18, 19, inferior frontal gyrus; 20, 21, entorhinal cortex; 22, 23, temporal pole; 24, 25, inferior postcentral gyrus; 26, 27, inferior parietal lobule. Reproduced with permission from [48].

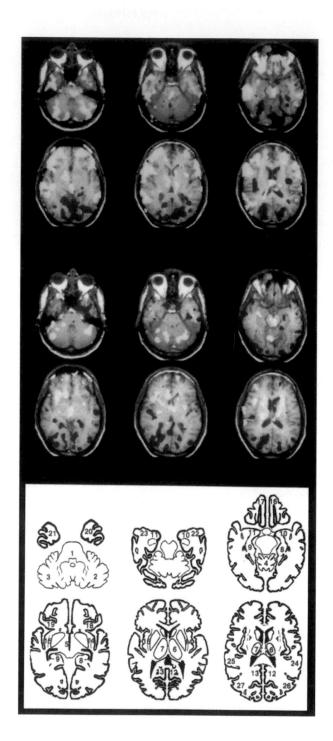

Table 57.2 Concordance between the location of spike sources and MRI lesions. For each type of lesion (columns), we summed the total number of patients and concordant cases according to the type of model used (spherical vs. realistic), and the signal recorded (EEG vs. MEG)

Study	Model and approach	Event	Data	Hippocampal atrophies	Tumours	Focal dysplasia or heterotopia	Other	Total
				Lesion/dipole concordance (<10 mm)				
Stefan et al. 1994 [42]	Spherical spatiotemporal	Spikes	MEG	5/5	6/8	—	2/3	81%
Nakasato et al. 1994 [99]	Spherical single dipole	Spikes	EEG	—	—	—	1/2	50%
			MEG	—	—	—	2/2	100%
Knowlton et al. 1997 [100]	Spherical single dipole	Spikes	MEG	2/3	2/2	—	1/1	83%
Merlet et al. 1997 [52]	Spherical spatiotemporal	Spikes	EEG	7/8	1/1	2/2	2/3	86%
Diekmann et al. 1998 [251]	Spherical moving dipole	Spikes	EEG	—	1/4	—	1/1	40%
			MEG	—	0/4	—	1/1	20%
Krings et al. 1998 [83]	Spherical single dipole	Spikes		2/2	1/1	1/1	4/4	100%
		Seizures	EEG	3/3	1/1	—	—	100%
Shindo et al. 1998 [49]	Realistic dipole unique	Spikes	EEG	2/2	—	0/1	3/4	71%
Ossenblok et al. 1999 [50]	Realistic spatiotemporal	Spikes	EEG	—	—	—	1/1	100%
Scherg et al. 1999 [51]	Spherical spatiotemporal	Spikes	EEG	—	—	1/1	—	100%
Morioka et al. 1999 [65]	Spherical single dipole	Spikes	MEG	—	—	3/3	—	100%
Baumgartner et al. 2000 [252]	Spherical single dipole	Spikes	MEG	—	—	—	8/8	100%
Huppertz et al. 2001 [7]	Realistic single dipole	Spikes	EEG	1/4	0/1	—	4/6	45%
		Delta		0/2	1/1	—	5/6	67%
Total	Spherical	Spikes	EEG	9/10	3/6	4/4	8/10	79.3%
			MEG	7/8	8/14	3/3	13/14	79.4%
	Realistic	Spikes	(EEG)	3/6	0/1	0/1	8/11	57.8%
				79%	52%	87%	83%	

topographies for a given patient (greater number of different types of spikes), requiring more sources to model, and wider spatial extents suggesting interlobar and interhemispheric propagation.

In a recent Japanese study correlating the locations of frontal spike dipole sources with ictal semiology, the author shows frequent orbitofrontal involvement, rapid bilateral involvement, and in some instances, propagation to extrafrontal regions [44]. Accordingly, studies using frequency analysis, in particular coherence and phase measurements [45,46] during bilaterally synchronous spike-wave activity, reported high coherence values between homologous EEG channels on both hemispheres which favour direct interfrontal connections potentially through the corpus callosum or anterior commissure.

Finally, using principal component analysis (PCA) in a group of 39 children, Rodin et al. showed a greater complexity of frontal interictal spikes, compared to temporal and occipital ones [47]. These results are in favour of a posteroanterior gradient of complexity reflecting recruitment within the interictal network of an increasing number of structures, as anterior regions are involved in the spiking process. In practice, the high complexity of frontal interictal spikes

together with the multifocal distributions of their dipolar sources, does cast some doubt on the reliability of such models, in the context of FLE [48].

Dipole sources and MRI lesions

Most studies exploring the relationships between MRI abnormalities and the generators of interictal paroxysms conclude fairly good spatial agreement (summarized in Table 57.2). Most have used spherical head models and single instantaneous dipole fits at the maximum of the interictal spike peak. These results come from series of various sizes (1–16 patients) including epilepsies of different types, and may therefore be contradictory. However, global analysis shows dipole sources to be located within lesions or close to (within 10 mm) in about 80% of cases, regardless of the techniques used to record the spikes (EEG or MEG). Thus, both techniques seem to provide a similar degree of accuracy.

Surprisingly, the concordance between dipole locations and MRI lesion was poorer in studies using realistic head models (58%) [7,49,50] than in studies using spherical head models (79%) but the former are far fewer. As far as the type of lesion is concerned, the best agreements between dipole results and lesions are found in focal dysplasia or heterotopia (86%), and next, hippocampal atrophies (79%), whereas a dipole is identified close to tumours in only 50%.

Some of these authors studied the spatiotemporal relationships between lesions and the activation sequence of spike sources. From a series of five hippocampal atrophies [42], one frontal gliotic lesion [50] and one frontal dysplasia [51], it has been suggested that sources calculated from the first part of the spike (early and main sources) are more concordant. Our own results, obtained from a series of 14 patients [52], are less affirmative. Although, in heterotopia or tumour cases, the best agreement is obtained for early and main sources (Fig. 57.6b,c), for hippocampal atrophies, dipole sources (indifferently early, main or late) may be located in the atrophic hippocampus, or outside the atrophic hippocampus, in the temporal and extratemporal neocortical areas (Fig. 57.6a). In some cases, sources may be located in the hippocampus, even in the absence of any atrophic lesion. Results from space-occupying lesions are very similar (Fig. 57.6b).

Considering these data, the spatial relationships between lesions and the localization of interictal spikes can vary and seem to depend on the lesion type. In the majority of cases, an overlap exists between the lesional zone and the network involved during interictal spikes, but when timing is considered, dipole results may suggest either origin or propagation within the lesion. Obviously the relationships are complex and echo the relations between electrophysiological and structural abnormalities. Indeed intracerebral spikes have been recorded inside the lesion, at the edge or further afield [53–55].

Dipole sources of interictal spikes and PET metabolic abnormalities

Most [18F] fluorodeoxyglucose PET studies show interictal hypometabolism in 60–80% of partial epilepsies (see [54,56,57]). However, these values vary according to whether a lesion was detected or not, and the type of epilepsy. In TLE both FDG-PET and flumazenil-PET [58] appear sensitive but abnormalities may be widespread [56]. The relation between epileptogenesis and FDG or flumazenil change is not straightforward and thus far no specific PET markers of epileptogenicity have been identified from interictal studies. For instance, it appears that the ability of perilesional cortex to generate seizures bears no relation to the presence of glucose hypometabolism in focal lesions such as cavernous angiomas (see [59]).

Whilst comparing, in the same group of TLE patients, the location of interictal spike sources with that of the FDG-PET hypometabolic zone [40], we found that when spikes are modelled by unilateral temporal sources, the latter were located within the hypometabolic zone. Conversely, glucose hypometabolism was not significantly more pronounced in regions where dipoles were localized. The example illustrated in Plate 57.7 (shown in colour between pp. 670 and 671) shows how the hypometabolic zone can be more widespread than networks involved in interictal spikes. Surprisingly, in a majority of patients in whom late extratemporal involvement was suggested by interictal spike modelling, hypometabolism was restricted to mesiotemporal areas (Plate 57.8, shown in colour between pp. 670 and 671).

In FLE, the spatial relationships between glucose hypometabolism and spike source can be extremely diverse. Dipole sources can be located either within the hypometabolic area where several lobes are involved, or outside the hypometabolic zone in cases where the metabolic abnormality is very focal.

The above findings are in agreement with those reported by Lantz et al. describing the relations between the focal interictal decreases in cerebral blood flow (CBF) on SPECT images, and the localization of spike sources [17]. These authors found a better concordance between the low CBF zone and sources of interictal spikes when dipoles were localized within one temporal lobe. These results have recently been corroborated by two similar studies showing a good concordance between 18FDG-PET abnormalities and dipole sources in both interictal MEG [60] and EEG [61] spikes, when these were unilateral temporal. As with our group of patients, these authors failed to find a correlation between the degree of decrease in glucose uptake and dipole location. They also found less agreement between PET and dipoles where extratemporal involvement was suggested by interictal spike modelling.

All together, the above studies converge on the conclusion that when spike sources are localized to one temporal lobe, FDG images tend to confirm the dipole locations and this could suggest some functional link between the metabolic dysfunction and the processes responsible for spikes. Conversely, when spikes are spread outside the temporal lobe or a frontal origin is suggested by dipole modelling, the metabolic and electrophysiological processes seem partly independent.

Dipole sources of interictal spikes and intracranial recordings

Since the non-invasive presurgical evaluation techniques reflect different pathophysiological aspects in epilepsy, they are not ideal for validating the localization of dipole sources in epileptic paroxysms. Such validation needs to rely upon more direct tools such as invasive or semi-invasive recordings but it is necessary to differentiate studies in which scalp and intracranial data were obtained simultaneously from otherwise. When ECoG or SEEG is not recorded during the scalp EEG session, dipoles are difficult to validate since the risk exists that the scalp and intracranial spikes might not share the same generator.

Several case reports have been published showing a perfect agreement between dipole location and ECoG spikes in lesional cases [62] or in complex cases where multiple foci are suspected [63,64]. Larger series generally show good concordance between dipole locations and intracranial interictal data. In a group of four patients with focal cortical dysplasia, the localization of MEG spike sources were consistent with interictal intracranial recordings in all cases [65] and Lantz et al. showed that when spike dipoles were spatially stable, their locations were concordant with ECoG recordings [17].

Some studies also demonstrate good concordance between spike dipoles and intracranial ictal onset in mesial TLE [41,66]. Although some found such concordance higher in TLE over FLE [49], spike sources and intracranial ictal data are also reported to have matched in 75% of adults [67] and 90% of children [68] presenting with extratemporal non-lesional epilepsies.

Studies in which simultaneous scalp and intracranial recording could be achieved are fewer. We recently addressed this issue [69] to answer the following questions: (a) when a spike is recorded at the

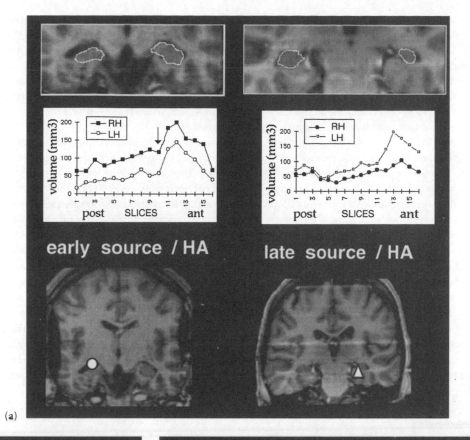

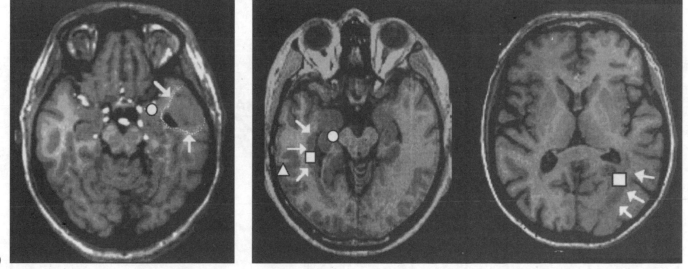

Fig. 57.6 Spike dipoles and MRI lesions. (a) Hippocampal atrophy. Two examples are given. The curves represent the volumes of the right (RH) and left (LH) hippocampi measured on coronal slices between the anterior (ant) and posterior (post) aspects of the hippocampus. The top of the figure illustrates diffuse LH atrophy (on the left), also atrophy of the anterior aspect of the hippocampus (on the right). In both cases at least one source was located in the atrophic hippocampus but this source was the early one in the first case (white circle), and the late one in the second case (white triangle). (b) Example of a tumour. In this patient, the early source of interictal spikes is located in the vicinity of a grade III xanthoastrocytoma (arrows and dotted line). (c) Concordance between heterotopia and spike sources in two patients (left: left temporal periventricular heterotopia; right: right occipital heterotopia). The main sources (white squares) of interictal spikes were localized to within the abnormal grey matter in both patients. In the patient with periventricular heterotopia (left), the dipole modelling results suggest that spikes originate from the hippocampus and spread within the lesion, whereas in the other patient (right), they originate from the lesion without involving other regions.

surface, what are the spatial characteristics of the underlying activated area? (b) Is the dipole that models a scalp spike located in the region of maximal electric field? (c) When dipole modelling suggests propagation between distinct areas, do intracerebral recordings show spike activity in each of these areas, and are there any intracerebral indices of propagation?

The current finding is that when a spike is recorded at the scalp surface, the intracerebral activity always involves several contacts suggesting the participation of a large cortical area (Fig. 57.9). Conversely, when intracerebral spikes are very focal, either in mesiotemporal structures or even in neocortical regions, no discernible scalp EEG signal is recorded. This result is now widely accepted and was suggested more than 30 years ago from simulated data using a polythene sheet connected to a low-frequency oscillator in an empty skull [70]. These findings have also more recently been confirmed in epileptic patients, in particular by Ebersole's team, using simultaneous EEG and ECoG or SEEG recordings [66,71,72] and it is held that a minimal cortical area of 6–8 cm^2 is necessary for a spike to be recorded on scalp EEG. The accuracy of such estimations are, however, limited by the low spatial resolution of intracranial recordings exploring a restricted number of regions.

A second interesting finding is that in some instances scalp interictal spikes are associated with 'simple' distributions of intracerebral fields (i.e. characterized by a maximum culminating at the time of the surface EEG spikes, and by synchronous activity gradually decreasing along the adjacent contacts; see Fig. 57.10a). This does not however, represent the majority, and in most instances asynchronous activities can be detected in addition to the maximal synchronous peak (Fig. 57.10b) [69]. This complex arrangement of intracerebral fields may be interpreted as reflecting spreading phenomena between regions where the asynchronous activities are recorded.

Interestingly, dipole modelling techniques might be able to predict reliably the type of field distribution since in almost all cases where intracerebral activity is simple, spikes can be modelled by one source. However, in cases where intracerebral activity is complex, several dipoles are needed and when a single model is used, dipoles are usually located at the centre of mass of the intracerebral area activated [73].

Simultaneously combining MEG and ECoG recordings in two patients, Mikuni et al. found good concordance when spikes were recorded from the lateral temporal cortex, whereas dipoles were ill-localized when spikes arose from mesiotemporal structures [74]. In our series, no such differences were observed. The main dipole source was located on average 11 mm from the SEEG contact showing the maximal intracerebral potential. In two-thirds of cases good concordance was obtained between (a) main dipole sources and maximal intracerebral fields; and (b) early or late sources and early

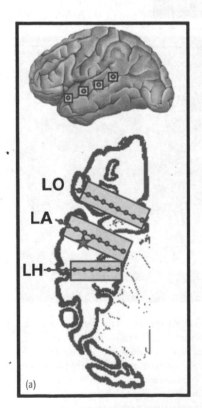
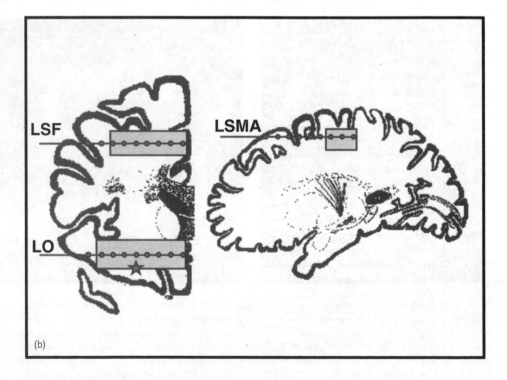

Fig. 57.9 Cortical area involved during scalp EEG spikes. In case (a) scalp spikes were located in the temporal area, in case (b) scalp spikes were right frontal. The figure illustrates the locations of the intracerebral electrode tracks and the position of epidural electrodes in case (a). Stars indicate intracerebral contacts where maximal activity was recorded. Grey rectangles represent the contacts that recorded the spike activity. For example, in (a), contacts 1–8 of the LO electrode, 1–8 of the LA electrode, 1–6 of the LH electrode, as well as the four subdural electrodes on the superior temporal gyrus, are active during the scalp EEG spike. This figure illustrates the fact that generators of a spike restricted to a focal scalp region can be distributed over a large cortical area. LO, left orbitofrontal; LA, left amygdala and anterior middle temporal; LH, left anterior hippocampus and middle temporal gyrus; LSF, left superior frontal; LSMA, left supplementary motor area.

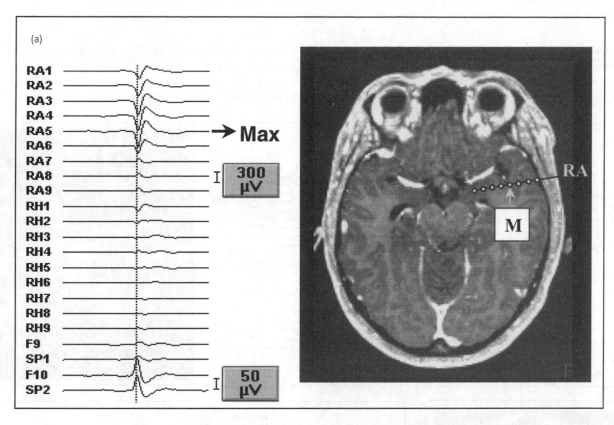

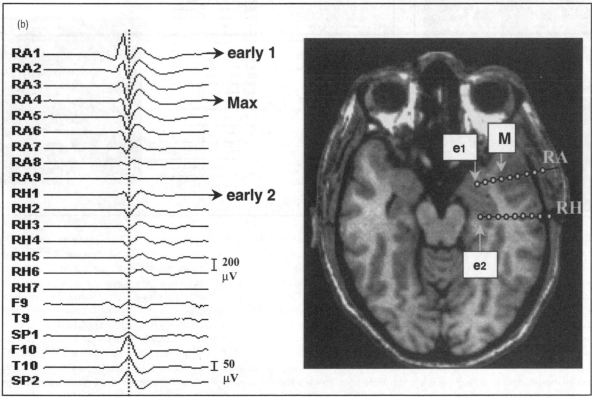

Fig. 57.10 Simple vs. complex intracerebral fields associated with surface EEG spikes. (a) Simple spikes. On scalp EEG recordings, the spike is maximal at F10 in the right anterior temporal region. Concomitantly, the maximal intracerebral field is recorded in the right temporal pole (RA5) and gradually decreases along the adjacent intracerebral contacts. No asynchronous activity is recorded elsewhere. (b) Complex spikes. Concomitant with the scalp EEG spike and culminating in the right anterior temporal region (electrode F10), the maximal intracerebral field occurs at RA4 (right temporal pole). Two earlier asynchronous activities can also be detected in the right amygdala (RA1) and hippocampus (RH1). Intracerebral electrodes: contacts 1 are the deepest, and contacts 9 are the most superficial; RA, right amygdala; RH, right anterior hippocampus; e1 and e2, early intracerebral field(s); M, maximal intracerebral field. Scalp electrodes: F9, F10 (anterior low temporal), T9, T10 (middle low temporal) and SP1, SP2 (zygomatic).

or late intracerebral fields; in general associated with good temporal concordance, i.e. the delay between the different intracerebral activities was perfectly congruent with the delay between dipole activation curves (Fig. 57.11a). Spatial discordance was found in 16% of cases (Fig. 57.11b), and in 10%, dipole locations could not be validated as they were situated in unexplored areas (Fig. 57.11c) [69].

These data confirm that surface EEG spikes are associated with intracerebral fields distributed over broad cortical areas and rarely

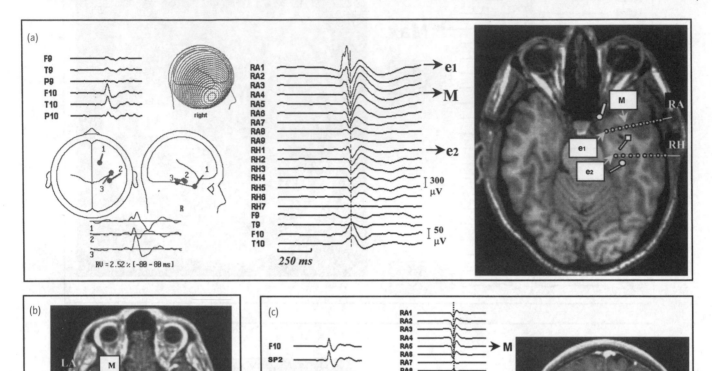

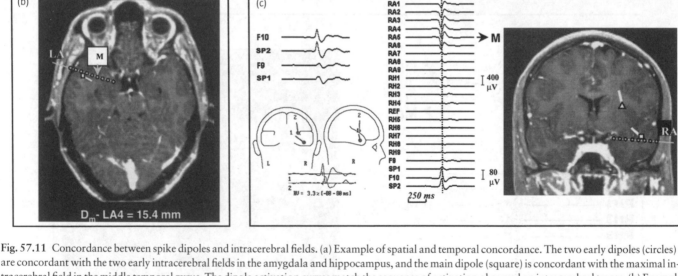

Fig. 57.11 Concordance between spike dipoles and intracerebral fields. (a) Example of spatial and temporal concordance. The two early dipoles (circles) are concordant with the two early intracerebral fields in the amygdala and hippocampus, and the main dipole (square) is concordant with the maximal intracerebral field in the middle temporal gyrus. The dipole activation curves match the sequence of activation observed on intracerebral traces. (b) Example of spatial discordance. The maximal intracerebral field is recorded at LA4 whereas the main source (square) is more lateral and closer to LA6. The distance between the main source and the maximal intracerebral field at LA4 (Dm-LA4) was 15.4 mm. (c) Example of non-validated source. The late source (triangle) is located in the right insula which was not explored with intracerebral electrodes. In this case the location of this source cannot be confirmed by intracerebral recordings. Intracerebral electrodes: contacts 1 are the deepest, and contacts 9 are the most superficial; RA, right amygdala; RH, right anterior hippocampus; LA, left amygdala; e1 and e2, early intracerebral fields; M, maximal intracerebral field; circle, early dipoles; square, main dipole; triangle, late dipole. Scalp electrodes: F9, F10 (anterior low temporal), T9, T10 (middle low temporal), P9, P10 (posterior low temporal) and SP1, SP2 (zygomatic).

Fig. 57.12 Dipole modelling of ictal discharges. The top of the figure (session 1) shows the scalp EEG recordings. At seizure onset, an initial period of ictal activity (pattern 1) can be identified, which consists of 11 Hz spiking culminating at AF8 (inferior frontal electrode). This period stops when the spike frequency shifts and becomes irregular. During this period, a trigger is placed at the negative maximum of each spike for averaging. The middle of the figure shows simultaneous scalp and intracerebral recordings. The same ictal pattern as for session 1 is identified on scalp electrodes of session 2 recordings. On the concomitant intracerebral signals, we identified the discharge onset (boxes) and the maximal intracerebral activity occurring at the time of scalp EEG change. In this case, the seizure starts synchronously in the amygdala (RA2-4), in the hippocampus (RH1-2), and in the lateral neocortex (RH5-7) with no detectable scalp activity. The first scalp EEG changes are detected 4 s later, when maximal intracerebral activity is recorded on orbitofrontal contacts. The main source, modelling the averaged ictal activity, is concordant with the maximal orbitofrontal fields. An additional source is necessary to explain the ictal EEG spikes but this source is contralateral, within an unexplored region. Intracerebral electrodes: contacts 1 are the deepest, and contacts 9 are the most superficial. RA, right amygdala; RH, right anterior hippocampus; RC, middle hippocampus; RO, right orbitofrontal cortex.

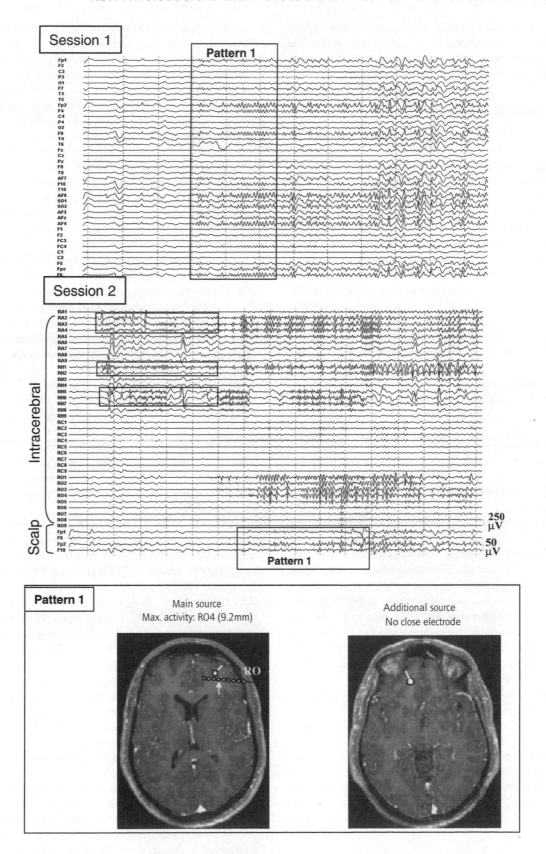

occur simultaneously with a focal activity, especially when it is limited to mesiotemporal structures. They imply that modelling the scalp spike by a *single* source located in the mesial aspect of the temporal lobe may be unreliable.

Dipole modelling of ictal discharges

Studies which assess the spatial relationship between interictal and ictal events give extremely variable results. The concordance between regions generating interictal and ictal paroxysms is generally good according to the type of epilepsy, the localizing method and its accuracy. In terms of hemispherical lateralization, excellent agreement between interictal and ictal events is observed in partial unifocal epilepsies, even perfect agreement in certain series [75]. In terms of lobar localization, concordance remains good, especially for TLEs [76,77] but in terms of sublobar localization, concordance drops [78]. Using combined scalp and invasive EEGs, Marks *et al.* showed that interictal spikes and ictal discharges originate from the same area in only 58% of TLEs [79]. By means of intracerebral recordings, Rougier estimated that the zones from which interictal spikes and seizures arose were similar in 55% of patients suffering from TLE, but in only 30% of patients suffering from frontal seizures [80]. .

Seizure modelling is more complex than interictal spike modelling owing to a low signal-to-noise ratio, the presence of artefacts and spread of activity which may be extensive and entail rapid changes in the complex source configurations over time. Some authors have demonstrated the feasibility of ictal dipole models [36,81] with good agreement sometimes in the locations of interictal and ictal events [17,41,82,83]. More recent studies indicate low yield (30–40% of patients) when dipole modelling is applied directly to ictal signals [84–86].

Interestingly, in cases where dipole models fail, the intracranial field correlates of the first scalp EEG change are bilateral and maximal in the mesiotemporal regions. This suggests that bilateral involvement at seizure onset may lead to dipoles located at the centre of the head or reaching different locations when initial conditions change. In case reports of one and two patients, respectively, good agreement was also found between the dipole sources of ictal events and ictal onsets as defined on non-simultaneous ECoG recordings [87,88]. During simultaneous recordings, ictal dipole sources are usually concordant with ictal onset, provided the latter does not occur in mesiotemporal regions [86].

When maximal activity was located within mesiotemporal structures, dipoles were usually displaced more laterally. Comparisons between ictal dipoles and ictal intracerebral fields were hampered when ictal onsets occurred very focally, so that no scalp EEG activity could be simultaneously detected (Fig. 57.12). Finally, additional sources were often found scattered in diverse cortical regions so that in a majority, their significance could not be established. It is possible for example, that apart from noise, these additional sources reflect spreading to regions beyond the primary epileptic zone.

Clinical relevance of dipole modelling results

Few studies have examined sensitivity for localizing the epileptogenic zone and most have compared the location of dipoles with resection margins in good outcome patients (Engel class I and II). When dipole modelling was performed in ictal systems, concordance rates between ictal sources and resection margins were very poor (only 10% of cases) [84], but concordance was higher for interictal spike sources. Comparing source models of interictal MEG spikes, MRI, interictal/ictal video-EEG and interictal/ictal intracerebral recordings, some found dipole modelling to be the second most sensitive method (57% concordance) for predicting the epileptogenic zone after ictal intracerebral recordings (62%) in TLE [89]. In extratemporal cases this dropped to 44% vs. 81% for ictal intracerebral recordings. In another recent study, sensitivity reached 94% [90]; however, this result is not very specific since good concordance between spike dipoles and resection localization was also found in 85% of patients with bad surgical outcome (Engel class III and IV).

In some instances, dipole distributions can help identify specific syndromes. For example, in benign rolandic epilepsy, dipole modelling of interictal spikes may differentiate an atypical group of children with intellectual deficits [91]. In adult TLE, interictal and ictal spike distributions allow distinction between mesial and lateral seizure onsets [4,46,92] which might be of particular interest in planning lobectomies without invasive recordings.

In other instances, the distribution of interictal spike dipoles might have lateralizing value. Indeed, in some cases of independent bilateral temporal spiking, early sources for both can be localized to the same side (Fig. 57.13). In our experience, this also corresponds to the side of most frequent spiking and this is clinically relevant since hemispheric predominance is observed in 80% of TLEs with bilaterally asynchronous spiking [93–96] and the laterality is (a) well correlated with the side from where seizures originate [75,96]; and (b) associated with better surgical outcome when operating on the same side [97].

Even though source accuracy has been assessed by means of simulated data (see above), the clinical relevance of spike modelling cannot be evaluated without examining concordance between source locations, and structural (MRI) or functional neuroimaging data. Stefan *et al.* [98], though reporting on three patients, observed surgical success when dipole sources of MEG spikes were spatially congruent with PET, SPECT and interictal ECoG results. Lamusuo *et al.* have also reported good outcome in cases where dipole modelling results agreed with PET data, whereas the others were not cured by surgery [60]. Good agreement between dipole locations and MRI lesions have likewise been widely reported to predict good surgical outcome [65,83,99,100]. Similarly, Smith *et al.* found concordance between ECoG results and the localization of MEG interictal spikes in 75%, amongst which surgical results were good in 61%, and surgery failed in all discordant cases [67].

No studies however, have addressed directly the question of whether the spatial extent of the spiking network (as defined by spike modelling) may help in delineating the epileptogenic zone and planning resection. The fact that a single spike may reflect the activation of several sources does not imply that all need be removed to control seizures and conversely, seizure spread may include areas uninvolved in interictal spiking. It is likely, for instance, that a number of TLEs remedied by mesial temporal surgery may actually have shown interictal spike sources in the lateral neocortex prior to surgery and this remains to be demonstrated through a dedicated prospective study.

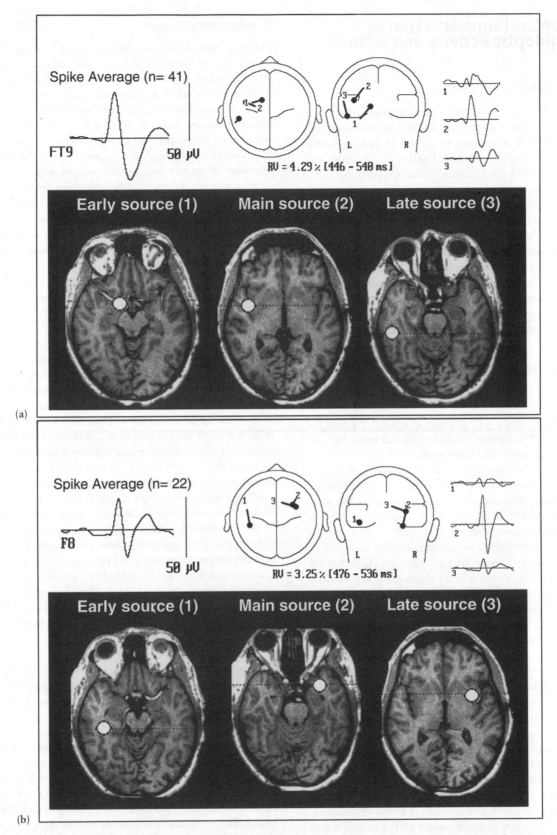

Fig. 57.13 Dipole modelling of bitemporal interictal spikes. In this example, independent bilateral temporal spikes could be averaged. (a) The left-sided (FT9) spikes are the most frequent and can be modelled by three left temporal dipoles, suggesting spread from mesial to lateral temporal regions. (b) The right-sided (F8) spikes are less frequent but have an early source still located in the left mesiotemporal region, as for FT9 spikes. Dipole modelling here suggests spreading from the left mesiotemporal region to the right temporal pole, and later the right insula. These data suggest predominance of the left temporal areas over the right side.

Intrinsic optical signals: a tool to analyse epileptic activity and seizures
(Chapter 57b)

H. Meierkord and K. Buchheim

To analyse epileptiform activity and the pathways through which it spreads, tools are required that provide both excellent temporal and spatial resolution. Optical imaging is capable of yielding pathophysiological information on this scale [101] and is therefore well suited to both experimental and clinical studies in epilepsy.

There are two main forms of optical imaging. 'Extrinsic' optical imaging relies on the use of indicators that change their optical properties (e.g. fluorescence or absorbance) with variations in cellular activity, i.e. membrane potential. With the use of voltage-sensitive dyes, temporal resolution is excellent (within milliseconds) but as dyes are toxic, this approach is used in experimental studies only [102]. In contrast, 'intrinsic' optical imaging is based on signal changes associated with tissue itself and is entirely non-invasive [103]. This section deals with intrinsic optical imaging and its relevance to the study of epileptic activity and seizures.

Basics of intrinsic optical imaging

Optical physics

The processes which occur when light interacts with living cells, tissues and organs, leading to loss of light intensity (attenuation), include scattering, absorption and fluorescence.

During scattering photons undergo elastic collisions, i.e. no energy is lost and the photon merely changes direction [104]. Light reflectance and transmittance are affected in opposite ways. The more a medium scatters, the more the light is reflected and the less it is transmitted. Higher frequency (shorter wavelength) light at the blue end of the visible spectrum is scattered considerably more in cells and tissues than lower frequency (longer wavelength) light. For this reason, near-infrared radiation is more effective for non-invasive optical detection through bone and tissue.

When light is absorbed by tissue, its energy is dissipated as either thermal energy or fluorescence (see below). There are many absorbing molecules in nervous tissue, and information can be obtained by measuring changes in absorption that are specific to a certain chromophore. An important example is the use of light in the near-infrared region (650–1000 nm) to study the absorption peaks for oxy-, deoxy- and total haemoglobin as is done by near-infrared spectroscopy (NIRS). It is thus possible to measure dynamic changes in blood flow and haemoglobin oxygenation during various forms of physiological and pathophysiological activation as seen during seizure activity.

Fluorescence occurs if the electromagnetic energy absorbed in the tissue is re-emitted. The emitted light can be detected by microfluorometric techniques and nicotinamide adenine dinucleotide (NAD(P)H) is an important example since it plays a central role in oxidative phosphorylation and is frequently investigated in studies of energy metabolism and epilepsy (see below).

Physiological processes

The physiological processes associated with brain activation and of interest in optical imaging, may be subdivided into those that occur at a cellular level and those that are mediated by the neurovascular coupling. There are important differences between these. Changes in the intrinsic optical signal (IOS) associated with changes on a cellular level are based mainly on scattering and are therefore wavelength independent. In contrast, signal changes mediated by the neurovascular coupling are based on absorption and are therefore dependent on specific wavelengths. Signal changes due to scattering are much smaller than those linked to neurovascular coupling. Finally, there is a latency of about 3 s from activating stimulus to vascular response but scattering occurs virtually without delay [105]. Scattering changes do occur together with absorption changes in vivo and it is still difficult to separate the two [106].

The physiological processes underlying the IOS change are still elusive but important published data and opinions with respect to the systems studied will be summarized next.

Processes in peripheral nerves and non-verterbrate neurones In their pioneering study, Hill and Keynes found optical changes in the nerve trunk of the walking leg of the shore crab (*Carcinus maenas*) to correlate with nerve activation [107]. The signal change consisted of an increase in light transmission in association with the period of electrical stimulation, followed by a prolonged decrease in transmission afterwards. Using optical and mechanoelectric movement detectors it can be demonstrated that rapid swelling in nerve fibres is responsible for IOS change, related directly to the mechanisms underlying the action potential. Cohen, after experiments with combined electrophysiological and optical methods in single giant axons of the squid, identified both fast and slow scattering changes [108]. The fast scattering changes were dependent on membrane voltage, the slow scattering change was caused by periaxonal volume changes. Stepnoski *et al.* [109] used single *Aplysia* neurones in culture and dark-field microscopy to identify an IOS change that was linearly proportional to the change in membrane potential. Since the static optical properties of the nerve were determined by the cytoplasm, the dynamic changes were attributed to conformational changes within the membrane.

Processes at the level of brain slices A system of considerably higher complexity is represented by the brain slice preparation, permitting the study of neuronal activation induced by electrical stimulation, and changes due to spontaneous neuronal activity under pathological conditions, across a fabric of cortical regions. In brain slice preparations, both transmitted and reflected light can be analysed. The first optical studies using this preparation were carried out by Lipton [110]. Since stimulation-induced IOSs could be abolished in the presence of Ca^{2+}-free artificial CSF (ACSF) or by addition of kynurenic acid in hippocampal slices, MacVicar and Hochman suggested that postsynaptic activation may be important for an IOS [111]. At odds with this however, Buchheim *et al.* have demonstrated that postsynaptic activation is not a prerequisite for an IOS to be evoked, since a reproducible IOS is associated with epileptiform discharges induced by low Ca^{2+} ACSF in which synaptic transmission is blocked [112].

A widely held hypothesis is that cell swelling or shrinkage of the extracellular space (ECS) linked to neuronal activation may be the most important factor in generating the IOSs. This assumption is based on the results of N-methyl-D-aspartate (NMDA) or kainate application [113] on simultaneous measurements of the ECS volume, the IOS [114,115] and the effects of pharmacological manipulation of the ECS [114,116,117].

Only recently it was suggested that IOS changes might reflect the extent of excitotoxic damage associated with excessive neuronal discharges [118–120]. This hypothesis was derived from experiments in which an irreversible signal was shown after the excessive application AMPA and NMDA receptor agonists with the histological demonstration of beading dendritic processes.

Thus, changes in plasma viscosity, cellular volume and membrane potential have all been suggested to underlie the IOS change and in slice preparations, postsynaptic activation and shrinkage of the ECS are assumed to be important.

Whole brain in vivo *(neurovascular coupling)* It has long been established that energy demand, oxygen consumption and CBF increase in response to neuronal activation. The increase in CBF exceeds the increase in oxygen consumption culminating in a local increase in oxygenation [105], i.e. an increase in oxyhaemoglobin concentration and a decrease in deoxyhaemoglobin [101]. Since oxy- and deoxyhaemoglobin have different light absorption patterns such changes may be measured using optical methods. A characteristic pattern of haemoglobin change has been demonstrated during physiological activation consisting of an increase in oxyhaemoglobin concentration of 1–2 μmol/L and a decrease in deoxyhaemoglobin concentration of 0.5–1 μmol/L [121]. As the absorption change is rather large, it is possible to measure this even through the intact skull but it is important to bear in mind that this is an indirect way of assessing brain function, one which also forms the basis of fMRI.

Epileptic activity and seizures

Different forms of epileptiform activity

Buchheim *et al.* compared the effects of three different forms of spontaneous epileptiform activity on IOS changes *in vitro* [112]. The seizure-like events (SLE) that were analysed in this study are based on different pathophysiological mechanisms. In the low Mg^{2+} model there is increased synaptic excitation which mainly results from unblocking the NMDA receptor [122]. Addition of 4-aminopyridine (4-AP) to ACSF also causes SLEs from the blockade of different K^+ channels [123]. In the low Ca^{2+} model, in contrast to other models, epileptiform discharges depend on non-synaptic mechanisms including excitability increases through field effects, electrical coupling by gap junctions and fluctuations in extracellular K^+ concentration [124,125]. On comparing the IOS changes associated with these three types of discharges, characteristic differences are seen. In the two models of enhanced synaptic transmission, spontaneous activity leads to an immediate increase in light transmission (Plate 57.14a1, shown in colour between pp. 670 and 671) but decreases in light transmission take place during low Ca^{2+}-induced discharges (Plate 57.14a2, shown in colour between pp. 670 and 671). Furthermore, the relative durations of IOS change as-

sociated with SLEs in the low Mg^{2+} model were significantly longer than those occurring in the 4-AP model, despite no significant difference in the duration of electrophysiological parameters such as field potentials between the two models. Thus, IOS change not only reflects tissue activation, but appears to be influenced by seizure generation mechanisms directly.

Origin and spread

Intrinsic optical imaging is advantageous in studying the spread of epileptiform activity since it allows for simultaneous monitoring of changes over an entire preparation. In the low Mg^{2+} model, it was demonstrated for example that discharges originated in the entorhinal cortex and spread to the temporal neocortex [126]. Buchheim *et al.* compared origin and spread patterns of discharges in both the low Mg^{2+} model, and in the 4-AP model [127]. While SLEs induced by low Mg^{2+} solutions occurred predominately in the entorhinal region, there was no consistent region of onset or spread in the 4-AP model. This was explained by the differing mechanisms of action: in the low Mg^{2+} model, epileptiform discharges result from unblocking the NMDA receptor which is more richly expressed in entorhinal cortices, whilst 4-AP is an antagonist of various K^+ channels found ubiquitously.

Age dependency

It is well known that infants and young children carry a higher risk of developing seizures and epilepsy than adults [128]. Experimental studies have suggested that this is due to discrete periods of altered seizure susceptibility and expression during development [129]. The effect that this increase in seizure susceptibility may have on regions of seizure onset, spread patterns and spread velocity during development is poorly understood.

Weissinger *et al.* combined extracellular microelectrode (ion-sensitive electrode) recordings with intrinsic optical imaging to study the spatiotemporal patterns of seizure onset and spread during development in rats [130]. Three age groups were analysed: 4–6 days (age group I), 10–14 days (group II) and 20–23 days (group III). Seizure susceptibility was highest in age groups II and III. In age group I SLEs originated mainly in the hippocampus proper. SLEs in age group II originated mainly in the entorhinal cortex and this tendency was even more pronounced in age group III. Invasion of the hippocampal formation via the perforant path–dentate gyrus and via the subiculum was seen in age groups I and II. By contrast, in age group III the hippocampus was invaded exclusively via the subicular pathway. The velocity of spread at which SLEs propagated within different regions of the slice increased with postnatal age. The characteristics of onset, spread patterns and propagation velocities as revealed by this study allow insight into the evolving properties of the developing brain.

The highest incidence of epileptic seizures has been reported to occur in the elderly [131]. It would therefore be of considerable interest and therapeutic relevance to determine the effects of old age on onset, spread patterns and propagation velocities in the absence of structural lesions.

Energy changes associated with seizure activity

Monitoring NAD(P)H autofluorescence can elucidate patterns of cellular metabolism during epileptiform activity. The NAD(P)H signal displays a characteristic time course during SLEs *in vitro*. A brief initial decrease, which occurs synchronously with the electrical onset, is followed by a long-lasting increase. Schuchmann *et al.* demonstrated this dynamic pattern for the first time using microfluometry [132]. The initial decrease reflects Ca^{2+}-induced depolarization of the mitochondrial membrane with increased activation of the mitochondrial chain and therefore energy consumption. From previous studies in which biochemical metabolites were calculated in frozen sections, a decrease in $NAD^+/NAD(P)H$ ratio has long been recognized to parallel the second phase of the signal time course [133–135]. This heralds the activation of Ca^{2+}-dependent citric acid cycle enzymes and therefore increased energy supply. There is, in fact, energy overproduction in response to the increased neuronal requirements during the early phase of repetitive seizure activity in the low Mg^{2+} model but, after subsequent SLEs, a gradual decline of the overshoot was demonstrated, disappearing after some 30–40 SLEs (Plate 57.14b, shown in colour between pp. 670 and 671). The transition of this model into late activity is well established and supports various hypotheses implicating energy failure as being responsible for the acute drug resistance encountered not only in this model, but also after prolonged status epilepticus in man [136].

Chen [137] applied IOS analysis to the *in vivo* study of penicillin-induced seizure activity in the rat. Reflection changes were monitored through the thinned skull illuminated with white light. Decreases in light reflection were seen ipsi- and contralaterally to the seizure induction site and surrounding areas of increased reflection were interpreted as areas of surround inhibition. This approach allowed monitoring of seizure spread, and occasionally optical changes even preceded EEG changes.

Schwartz and Bonhoeffer carried out *in vivo* optical mapping of interictal spikes, after-discharges, ictal events and secondary foci in the ferret cerebral cortex [138]. Interictal activity was induced by focal bicuculline application and each interictal spike was followed by a decrease in light reflection. The IOS changes correlated well in size and duration with the electrophysiological features of the spike and in the areas surrounding the spike, an inverse optical signal was recorded again reflecting surround inhibition. After-discharges were also associated with optical signals that were significantly larger than those recorded with interictal spikes. Surrounding non-propagating after-discharges were large areas of increased reflection possibly also indicating surround inhibition. Horizontally propagated SLEs induced by 4-AP had much smaller surrounding inhibitory signals. Clear IOS change was also seen over contralateral homotopic areas, though delayed and smaller. This report was the first to demonstrate the feasibility of intrinsic optical imaging of isolated interictal spikes without averaging.

Clinical studies

In the first study of its kind, Haglund *et al.* demonstrated that intrinsic optical imaging is possible intraoperatively in the human cerebral cortex [139]. The cortical surface was illuminated and changes in light reflection associated with various activations were analysed. Epileptiform after-discharges of varying intensity and duration, following electrical stimulation, were associated with IOS change that correlated with electrographic changes. In the surrounding areas an IOS change was seen in the opposite direction. Changes in the IOS were also seen within somatosensory cortex during tongue movement and in Broca's and Wernicke's areas during naming exercises.

Later studies have extended the work of Haglund *et al.* on the time course and morphology of IOSs, following peripheral median and ulnar nerve stimulation in patients undergoing brain surgery [140]. The spatial extent of the IOS correlated well with evoked potential maps collected during the same experiments. Peak signal was reached at 3s, and disappeared by 9s. Similar results were also demonstrated in human and rodent cortex [141].

Studies using NIRS

The technique of NIRS relies upon two important phenomena: (a) that, in tissue, there are compounds whose absorption of light is oxygenation status dependent; and (b) that biological tissue is relatively transparent to light in the near-infrared region of the spectrum. Indeed at near-infrared wavelengths (650–1000 nm), the attenuation of light is significantly lower, and with appropriate instrumentation it is possible to detect light that has traversed up to 8 cm of tissue [105,142].

The principles of transcranial NIRS have been described in detail [143]. Light from laser diodes (wavelengths 775, 825, 850 and 904 nm) is guided through a fibre optic bundle. The first 'optode' is placed over the region of interest (ROI) and the detecting optode (second optode), leading to a photomultiplier-based optical detection system, is placed at a distance of 4 cm in a horizontal line occipital to the first optode. The NIRS signals are deemed to stem from a banana-shaped volume between the two optodes, with a penetration depth of approximately 2–3 cm from the head surface. The analysis procedure converts the obtained optical densities (OD) to concentrations of oxy- and deoxyhaemoglobin, expressed in µmol/L using Beer–Lambert's law and an algorithm developed by Wyatt *et al.* [144].

Since its first description [145], the method has successfully been applied to the assessment of regional physiological stimulation [105], states of global cerebral hypoperfusion [146] and changes during epileptic seizures. During complex focal seizures, massive increases in blood flow, oxyhaemoglobin and decreases in deoxyhaemoglobin have been described [147–150].

Findings regarding interictal seizure activity are more controversial. Adelson *et al.* [147] described reduced oxyhaemoglobin concentrations but no changes were seen by Sokol *et al.* [148]. Comparing the effects of complex focal and rapidly generalized complex focal seizures, decreases in oxyhaemoglobin concentrations during the generalized seizures were demonstrated [148].

We have recently applied this method to the study of focal seizures and generalized absences and directly compared the oxygenation signals. There were marked differences in the NIRS signal as illustrated in Fig. 57.15. In absence seizures, ictal NIRS shows a homogeneous pattern of decrease in oxyhaemoglobin concentration, increase in deoxyhaemoglobin concentration and subsequent decrease in total haemoglobin concentration with a return to baseline values within a few seconds after the EEG seizure end (Fig. 57.15a1).

These data are in line with findings using transcranial doppler ultrasonography [151,152] and laser doppler flowmetry [153] that showed reduction in CBF during absence seizures in humans and animals. A slight increase in CBF velocity during the preictal and early ictal phases of childhood absence seizures, and an abrupt decrease during the final part outlasting the seizure for 15–20 s, was also demonstrated recently [154]. The decrease in deoxyhaemoglobin that we found may indicate an increase in oxygen consumption, probably reflecting elevated metabolic activity as seen in children [155,156], young adults [157] and a genetic rat model [158] during

ictal PET. However, as PET studies have poor temporal resolution, with 70–80% of cerebral uptake over 15 min following i.v. injection, there is an amalgam of ictal and interictal periods contributing to any one scan [57].

We did not see uniform changes in the NIRS parameters during focal seizures: although an increase in oxy- and total haemoglobin concentration occurred in all seizures, the changes in deoxyhaemoglobin concentration varied between patients. An increase in CBF velocity during focal seizures has been shown recently using doppler sonography [159] and this may correspond to the increase in oxy- and total haemoglobin concentration seen in our patients. A marked decrease in deoxyhaemoglobin in one, and small increases in the majority of patients, over the EEG-defined focus, were ac-

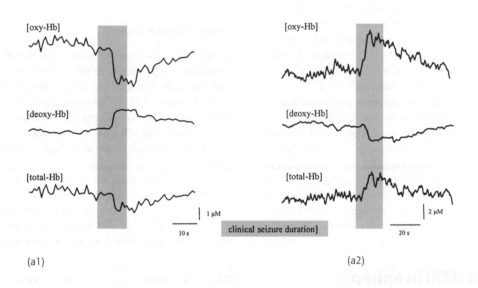

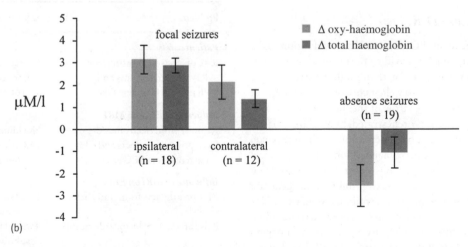

Fig. 57.15 Near-infrared (NIRS) signals during focal and absence seizures. (a1) Cerebral oxygenation changes during an absence seizure in a 21-year-old male patient with juvenile myoclonic epilepsy, who was non-compliant with treatment. Optodes were placed on the patient's forehead. (b) Summary of oxy- and total haemoglobin concentration changes across all patients and seizures. Total haemoglobin concentration changes differ significantly between ipsi- and contralateral recordings in focal seizures. (a2) NIRS findings during focal seizure of a 27-year-old female patient with simple focal epileptic seizures since adolescence. The seizure started in the left arm with muscle stiffness. The optodes were placed over the right (focus) and centroparietal regions. The grey bar indicates the phase of the clinical seizures assessed by simultaneously video-EEG monitoring which was applied throughout in all patients.

companied by marked increases in oxy- and total haemoglobin concentration. This indicated a focal hyperperfusion far exceeding oxygen demand and, similarly, focal hyperoxygenation has also been demonstrated during focal seizures by two groups monitoring oxy- and/or total haemoglobin concentration (but not deoxyhaemoglobin concentration) using NIRS [147,148]. This is in line with a recent study using subtraction SPECT describing focal hyperperfusion over an epileptic focus in the majority of the patients with temporal and extratemporal lobe epilepsies [160].

Summary and perspectives

Imaging IOS change allows the mapping of physiological and pathophysiological brain activation non-invasively and with high spatial and temporal resolution. In bloodless *in vitro* preparations, the IOS change is primarily based on light scattering. The physiological changes that give rise to scatter are largely elusive and represent challenges for future studies. Onset, spread patterns and propagation velocities can be analysed in detail and compared between different age groups using intrinsic optical imaging. In addition, employing NAD(P)H autofluorescence, the energy changes associated with epileptic activity can be analysed.

Intrinsic optical imaging can be used to study functional activation, epileptiform activity and seizures *in vivo*. In this case, signal changes are due both to scattering and absorption. The absorption changes that reflect concentration changes in oxy- and deoxyhaemoglobin are affected with a time delay of several seconds due to the inherent properties of the neurovascular coupling. Successful separation of scattering and absorption changes has already been achieved. Optical mapping in the clinical setting can be applied to the intraoperative determination of eloquent cortex and to the study of seizure spread.

EEG-correlated fMRI in epilepsy
(Chapter 57c)

A. Salek-Haddadi and D.R. Fish

Blood oxygen level dependent (BOLD) fMRI has revolutionized the field of human brain mapping by providing the means to study focal neuronal activity non-invasively and with submillimetre resolution.

Focal changes in neuronal activity elicit concomitant changes in blood flow and blood volume by virtue of the 'neurovascular coupling' [161,162]. This response is orchestrated, by and large, via the glia [163] and serves to induce subtle fluctuations in the intravoxel concentrations of paramagnetic deoxyhaemoglobin. In biophysical terms, this functions as an endogenous contrast agent to bring about focal changes in magnetic susceptibility and generate 'BOLD contrast' [164]. Whole-brain susceptibility-weighted (T2*-weighted) scans may be acquired successively in seconds (individual slices in just tens of milliseconds), using ultra-fast imaging sequences such as echo planar imaging, such that BOLD changes at each and every voxel may be monitored continuously during an experiment.

Virtually every aspect of normal brain activity has or is being investigated using fMRI and increasingly, attention is focusing on studies of abnormal activity such as following stroke and in epilepsy. The localization of seizure activity should present an obvious

application, given the enormous clinical interest in mapping the 'epileptogenic zone', even if invasively. Clinically, the potential exists for such findings to help guide invasive studies and help tailor surgical resections in focal epilepsy. Scientifically, the opportunity also exists to study the complex metabolic and neurovascular responses to epileptiform activity *in vivo*.

The use of fMRI for mapping eloquent cortex in the presurgical evaluation of epilepsy is covered elsewhere in this chapter. Conventional fMRI studies rely on specific experimental manipulations or paradigms to elicit optimally the relevant pattern of neuronal activity, and hence focal changes in BOLD, for subsequent detection and localization. In contrast, however, 'spontaneous' patterns of human EEG activity such as epileptiform activity, in general, cannot be replicated or manipulated. 'Paradigmless' EEG/fMRI studies therefore need to be performed within the same session and there are several difficulties.

Methodological aspects

The technical challenges of acquiring simultaneous EEG/fMRI are formidable, beginning with the earliest attempts in 1993 [165], with the recent release of several commercial solutions.

Simultaneous EEG/fMRI acquisition is essentially subject to three sets of problems: patient safety issues, the deleterious effects of EEG recording on MR imaging and vice versa. A referenced summary of the technical problems in EEG/fMRI is presented in Table 57.3.

The use of MR-compatible electrodes, pastes, safety resistors and fibre-optic isolation now provides excellent patient safety [166,167] and we are unaware of any adverse incidents having ever occurred anywhere in this regard. Together with appropriately shielded cables and hardware, the impact on image quality can also

Table 57.3 Summary of technical problems and solutions in simultaneous EEG/fMRI

Problem	Solutions
Patient safety	
Risk of electrode heating from RF-induced currents and changes in magnetic flux	Current limiting resistors, and fibre-optic isolation of patients [166, 167]
Influence of EEG on MRI	
RF noise from electronics/digitizer	Shielding, RF filters
Susceptibility artefacts and eddy currents from EEG electrodes	MR-compatible electrodes [166–170]
Influence of MRI on EEG	
Motion artefacts from static field	Head support, subject selection, cable arrangement
Pulse artefact (ballistocardiogram)	Twisted leads, pulse artefact subtraction algorithm [170, 171]
Imaging artefact	Bipolar recording. Interleaved acquisition or imaging artefact subtraction algorithm with hardware modifications [170, 173, 175, 176, 253]

be minimized [168,169]. Our own particular set-up is shown in Fig. 57.16.

The issues surrounding EEG quality are several. Scanner EEG is exquisitely prone to motion-related artefacts which arise by virtue of Faraday's law which states that for a closed circuit, the induced voltage is proportional to the rate of change in magnetic flux. Two specific artefacts are very well recognized in the scanner and occur in addition to the familiar sources of noise in EEG. Pulse artefact (also called 'cardiobalistogram') tends to present in the majority of subjects, arising principally from subtle head motion in relation to the cardiac cycle, and is observed throughout EEG recordings [170]. Imaging artefacts however, arise from the application of time-varying magnetic fields (gradients) during image acquisition only, but would ordinarily tend to obscure the EEG completely during this time.

Interleaved EEG/fMRI

Until relatively recently (see below), the interpretation of scanner EEG was strictly restricted to periods devoid of imaging artefact. Indeed the majority of EEG/fMRI studies to date have been performed using an interleaved acquisition. Interleaved acquisitions may be either periodic, with a sufficiently long duty cycle to allow for limited EEG interpretation in between bursts of imaging [170], or more commonly aperiodic (e.g. EEG-triggered fMRI) [173,174]. In spike-triggered fMRI, the haemodynamic delay is exploited by triggering single-volume acquisitions, either manually or automatically, following individual EEG events so as to selectively capture the peak BOLD response (Fig. 57.17). This is made possible by the application of unsupervised software algorithms for real-time pulse artefact removal to allow online EEG monitoring [171] during the interscan interval. Equivalent 'resting' time points are also acquired such that statistical parametric maps [172] may be created using voxel-wise *t*-tests or equivalents [173,174].

Simultaneous EEG/fMRI

More recently, advances in hardware and signal processing have allowed the removal of EEG imaging artefact, and therefore the continuous acquisition of uninterrupted high-quality EEG throughout fMRI (Fig. 57.18). For the purposes of detecting discrete events, this has been achieved both through the accurate subtraction of an adequately sampled channel-specific artefact waveform from an unsaturated EEG trace in combination with adaptive noise cancellation [175], and through removal of the dominant imaging artefact frequencies by way of band-stop filtering [176]. These methods may be used online, and in combination with pulse artefact removal, to provide diagnostic quality EEG throughout imaging experiments.

The theoretical advantages of continuous acquisition are that BOLD changes may be studied prior to, during and after a host of EEG phenomena within the same experimental session and signal dynamics may be fully explored. Therefore, a whole new 'physiological' dimension is added to the anatomical. At a practical level, experiments are also easier to perform as EEG analyses need no longer be done at the scanner console and in real time.

The analysis of continuous fMRI time series is, however, substantially more complex. A lot of this added complexity centres on the implementation of strategies for dealing with the complex spatiotemporal autocorrelation structure of the data so that significance testing may take place in an unbiased manner. There are several dynamic sources of noise that also need to be dealt with. These may be physical (hardware related), physiological (e.g. cardiac, respiratory, vasomotor, etc.) or neuronal (i.e. other unaccounted neuronal activity). Statistical modelling is also problematic. In contrast to studying state-related changes (e.g. finger tapping vs. no finger tapping), event-related signal changes are both more subtle (more difficult to detect above noise) and, within the context of spontaneous EEG events, more enigmatic. Indeed there are sever-

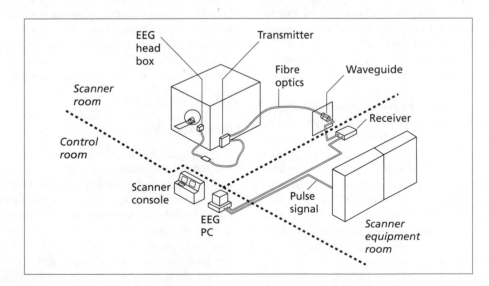

Fig. 57.16 Equipment schematic. Twelve gold electrodes fitted with 10K Ohm current-limiting safety resistors are applied using the 10/20 system. EEG (plus ECG) is sampled at 5000 Hz. Shielded fibre-optics carry the signal away from the room. A timing signal is sourced from the scanner and used to synchronize imaging artefact subtraction. The EEG is monitored online and throughout the experiment.

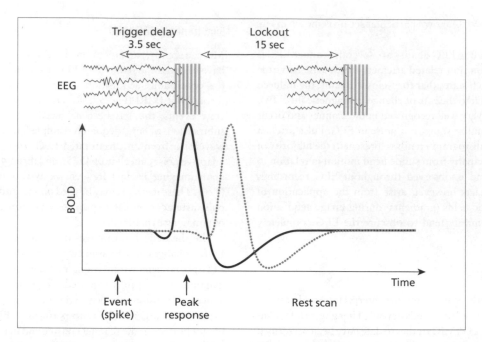

Fig. 57.17 EEG-triggered fMRI. A haemodynamic response function is shown, as arising from a single interictal epileptiform discharge (indicated). The haemodynamic latency allows for the delayed acquisition of a single scan capturing the peak signal change and by the same virtue, it is reasoned that epileptiform activity taking place during missing EEG segments will not be of consequence (dotted response). Resting scans are acquired at other time points free of activity for statistical comparison and a lockout is used to ensure equal T1 weighting throughout.

al unknowns regarding the precise manner in which the generators of EEG phenomena may engender changes in BOLD [250].

EEG/fMRI in epilepsy

Ictal EEG/fMRI

EEG/fMRI can resolve seizure activity *in vivo* but its use is largely prohibited by practical considerations. BOLD fMRI is not sensitive to detecting state-related (low-frequency) signal changes, due to noise, and this would tend to necessitate the capture of both seizure onset and termination within the same experimental session. As most seizures are generally unpredictable, infrequent and associated with a degree of movement, the practical difficulties are apparent.

Using fMRI alone, Jackson *et al.* first described concordant areas of activation, based on the visual inspection of subtraction images, in a child experiencing partial motor seizures [177]. Other reports [178–180] have since followed, describing concordant BOLD changes in relation to either assumed seizure activity or overt ictal symptomatology but with ever-present risks of motion-related artefact. Recently, using continuous EEG-correlated fMRI we were able to capture a focal subclinical electrographic seizure, for the first time, in its entirety. A cluster of activation was apparent and concordant with the EEG focus, and displaying a significant rise in BOLD, followed by a deep and prolonged undershoot in keeping with ictal physiology data from several other techniques [181].

Where obtainable, ictal fMRI activation would be expected to reflect both seizure generation and propagation sites (e.g. the symptomatogenic zone) but low temporal resolution together with in-

terregional variations in the haemodynamic response [182,183] have prevented more detailed studies of seizure spread and propagation using fMRI.

More recently, we have obtained EEG/fMRI recordings in a patient with intractable idiopathic generalized epilepsy experiencing frequent spontaneous absences [254]. A very different pattern of activation was demonstrated during generalized spike-and-wave activity, comprising thalamic activation but symmetrical and widespread cortical deactivation (i.e. a sustained decrease in BOLD and blood flow). This is generally consistent with findings from both animal and human studies [153], including optical imaging as presented elsewhere in this chapter. This does raise the interesting question of whether EEG/MRI in this setting may potentially serve to differentiate primary and secondary generalized activity, a subject of ongoing work.

Interictal EEG/fMRI

It is well established that brief bursts of focal neuronal activity give rise to characteristic changes in BOLD [184], the subsequent detection/localization of which is the basis of event-related fMRI [185]. The event-related fMRI of interictal epileptiform discharges (IEDs) presents an obvious alternative to mapping epileptogenic cortex as imaging the 'irritative zone' in preference to the 'ictal onset zone', is potentially safer, more practical, more applicable and more effective given the relative abundance of such activity.

Over the last few years, several spike-triggered studies from a number of centres have explored the feasibility of studying the fMRI correlates of IEDs using EEG-triggered fMRI and an outline of the main literature is presented in Table 57.4.

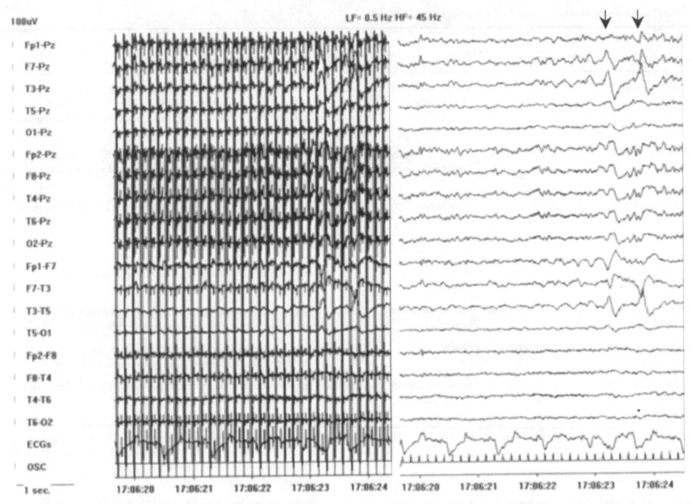

Fig. 57.18 Continuously acquired EEG. A segment of EEG is shown as obtained during image acquisition from the same experiment referred to in Fig. 57.19c. Two temporal chains are shown as referenced to Pz (top 10 channels), followed by a bipolar montage and the ECG. Slice-timing signals are shown at the bottom (OSC) as recorded from the scanner. The same segment is shown on the right-hand side, following imaging and pulse artefact removal. Two focal left temporal sharp waves are clearly visible (arrows).

Despite several shortcomings, plausible fMRI activations are reported overall in approximately half of all published cases, with evidence of reproducibility in addition. Where high-density EEG data and other corroborative investigations are available, results are also, on the whole, encouraging. The most impressive activations have generally tended to appear in relation to focal cortical dysplasias, within encephalitic cortex, and surrounding porencephalic cysts on MRI, as well as in relation to frequent stereotyped unifocal high-amplitude IEDs on EEG. An example from our own work, demonstrating concordant and reproducible BOLD activations in relation to focal IEDs, is provided in Fig. 57.19.

Unfortunately any meaningful meta-analysis of the EEG/fMRI literature is precluded by low numbers and major methodological differences. Some general criticisms include: lack of significance testing and motion correction in earlier studies, inadequate thresholding, selective reporting of results and ambiguities in the manner in which multifocal spikes and more complex EEGs were dealt with. Moreover, single experiments in unclear clinical syndromes often render face validation difficult and, where corroborative measures

of the irritative zone are available, the want of objective criteria for cross-validation is a prevailing theme.

Using continuous EEG-correlated fMRI, both ourselves [186] and other groups [187] have also begun a more detailed exploration of the event-related reponses to IEDs and their time courses (Fig. 57.19d). It is reassuring to note that whilst there appears to be significant variability, on the whole, this appears physiological. Addressing the sources of such variability and their relevance is the subject of ongoing efforts.

Limitations of EEG/fMRI

Whilst it is tempting to relate EEG/fMRI findings directly to electro-clinical data, there are several caveats and some important limitations deserve emphasis.

The control of type I error lies at the heart of statistical hypothesis testing, particularly where multiple comparisons are involved such as in the voxel-based analysis of neuroimaging data. In the present context, however, the identification of any false positives may prove

Table 57.4 Summary of published interictal EEG-triggered fMRI data

Reference	Fld	Motion correction	Analysis	n	I	Reported conclusions
Warach et al. 1996 [191]	1.5	None	Thresholded % change images	2	2	Bilateral activation where EEG suggested left temporal localization and anterior cingulate activation in relation to generalized epileptiform activity. '. . . we cannot make conclusions about the source of the discharge from the present data'
Seeck et al. 1998 [192]	1.5	Coregistration	Cross-correlation with Bonferroni correction	1	1	Multiple areas of signal enhancement on fMRI. Confirmed on 3D-EEG source localization with evidence of a focal onset. Focus later confirmed on subdural recordings
Patel et al. 1999 [193]	1.5	2 patients excluded	Largely based on comparison of individual spike images with rest	20	2	9/10 overall reported as showing 'activation corresponding to the EEG focus'
Symms et al. 1999 [194]	1.5	Coregistration	Pixel-by-pixel two-tailed t-test	1	1	Reproducible and concordant activation across 4 sessions
Krakow et al. 1999 [195]	1.5	Coregistration	Pixel-by-pixel two-tailed t-test	10	2	Reproducible activations (same lobe and overlapping) obtained in 6/10 patients in close spatial relation to EEG focus
Krakow et al. 1999 [196]	1.5	Coregistration	SPM96	1	1	Focal activation within a large malformation of cortical development in response to focal epileptiform discharges
Lazeyras et al. 2000 [197]	1.5	Coregistration	Cross-correlation with Bonferroni correction	11	4	Activation confirmed clinical diagnosis in 7/11. In 5/6 intracranial EEG confirmed result
Krakow et al. 2001 [190]	1.5	Coregistration	SPM96	1	1	Focal concordant activation within encephalitic cortex also obtained in relation to 15/43 individual spikes. 'Single event-related fMRI of interictal spikes is feasible in selected patients, giving complementary information . . .'
Baudewig et al. 2001 [198]	2.0	Scan removal	Cross-correlation with shifted boxcar	1	1	Unilateral insular activation shown in relation to generalized epileptiform discharges. '. . . strategy resulted in robust BOLD MRI responses to epileptic activity that resemble the same characteristics as are commonly observed for functional challenges'
Krakow et al. 2001 [195,199]	1.5	Coregistration	SPM99	24	0	12/24 patients showed activations concordant with EEG focus, 7/12 of which also had concordant structural lesions. 2/24 were discordant and 10/24 showed no significant activation. 64-channel EEG dipole solutions were later concordant in 6/6 [200]
Jager et al. 2002 [201]	1.5	Coregistration + exclusion	Cross-correlation	10	1	Focal activation in 5/5 patients, concordant with EEG amplitude mapping. Mean signal increase was 15±9%. Spike amplitude correlated with volume of activation

Fld, MRI field strength in tesla; I, number of fMRI results illustrated; n, total number of cases studied.

particularly problematic. Even where clear lesions exist, the range of anatomically plausible spike- or seizure-related activation patterns remains wide and the possibility of propagation is often raised. Distinction from 'genuine' effects is particularly troublesome where 'stimulus-correlated motion' is present, for example in cases where subtle epileptic myoclonus may coexist.

Conversely and as a general rule, lack of activation in fMRI is not informative. This stems directly from the crucial fact that type II error control (against false negatives) is not provided for in functional neuroimaging, as precise specification of the alternate hypothesis (i.e. the 'ordinary' behaviour of each and every voxel) is not possible. This notion is particularly important for surgery, where fMRI is used to map eloquent cortices, as lack of activation can never be used to infer lack of function confidently.

Together with signal-to-noise ratio considerations, these also dictate that thresholded activations will represent 'tips of the icebergs'

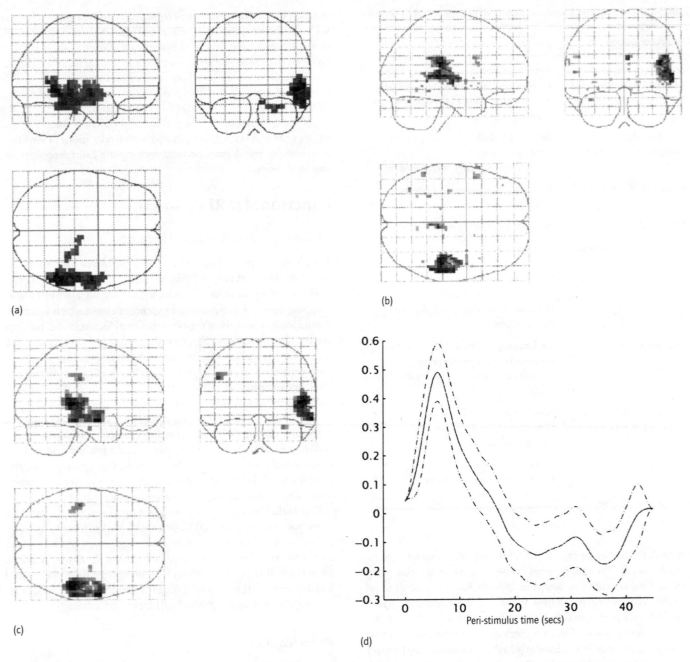

Fig. 57.19 Interictal EEG/fMRI. Three sets of EEG/fMRI results are shown from separate studies on the same patient, a 51-year-old lady with biopsy confirmed left temporal lobe encephalitis and refractory partial seizures, reported previously in [190]. These studies were performed approximately 1 year apart on two different scanners. The EEG-triggered fMRI result is shown in (a) [190]. Results from a continuous EEG/fMRI study at 2 T are shown in (b) [186] and results from a similar study at 1.5 T are shown in (c). All SPMs were thresholded at the $P < 0.05$ level following correction for multiple comparisons. The physiological time course shown in (d) was derived from the maximally activated voxel in (c), and was based on 233 focal discharges of the type shown in Fig. 57.18. The functional activations were reproducible, and anatomically concordant with the EEG focus, clinical picture and previous ECoG recordings.

and, given that the largest contributors to BOLD signal at low field strengths are veins, the so-called 'brain or vein' problem [188] imposes an important biophysical constraint on spatial resolution.

Both the chances of success in EEG/fMRI and results are profoundly influenced by a multitude of experimental and biological factors, presiding over the experimental variables of interest (e.g. patient characteristics or pathology). A list of these is provided in

Table 57.5, as reviewed elsewhere [250]. One theoretical dilemma is that statistical hypothesis testing in fMRI relies on the specification of appropriate models (null hypotheses) of expected signal change, but the precise manner in which EEG events translate into focal changes in BOLD remains unclear. This is partly because studies of BOLD signal dynamics, for this purpose and in general, need focus on specific regions of interest (ROIs). In studies of normal brain

Table 57.5 Essential conditions and assumptions in interictal EEG/fMRI

Condition/assumption	Confounds/issues
Focal changes in metabolic demand arise in relation to EEG events	Relative effects of excitation vs. inhibition Changes in synchrony vs. changes in firing Misclassification of EEG events/variable generators
Neurovascular transduction is intact	Effects of pathology Influence of drugs Consequences of epileptiform activity
Adequate EEG signal-to-noise ratio	Imaging, pulse and motion artefact Safety resistors
EEG is 'fMRI-efficient'	Non-optimal EEG event presentation
Adequate fMRI signal-to-noise ratio	Field strength Choice of head coil Choice of sequence Artefacts, e.g. susceptibility Influence of EEG setup, e.g. RF noise Head motion
No head motion	Lack of cooperation Involuntary movement/epilepsy Discomfort/noise/long experimental time Sleep
Adequate modelling of expected BOLD change	Non-canonical HRF Non-linear behaviour Unexpected interactions
Adequate control of type I error	Inappropriate statistical model Unaccounted spatiotemporal autocorrelations

function, ROIs may be prespecified, for example, in terms of functionally specific Broadman areas across a range of subjects using standardized coordinates, and their exact behaviour studied using optimal experimental paradigms. In focal epilepsy again, the equivalent ROIs are both variable across subjects, largely unknown (no 'gold standard') and studied using non-optimal experimental paradigms (spontaneous EEG). Similarly in this context, the assessment of validity can be problematic.

However, the possibility of optimizing EEG activity pharmacologically (e.g. drug reduction) or physiologically remains to be fully explored, as does the possibility of enhancing BOLD signal-to-noise ratio pharmacologically [189] or through advances in MRI (e.g. better sequences at higher field strengths). The advent of simultaneous intracranial EEG/fMRI, already on the horizon, should also ensure several breakthroughs on the above fronts.

Conclusions

Seizure- or spike-related BOLD activations may be envisaged to contribute both directly to the pool of presurgical investigations, or indirectly, for example, through the provision of more realistic (fMRI-derived) constraints for the purposes of EEG dipole modelling.

EEG-correlated fMRI may be regarded as a developing technique with significant scientific potential but also important theoretical, methodological and practical limitations. Future clinical roles in epilepsy, such as in seizure disorder classification (e.g. in conjunction with EEG) or the localization of epileptogenic cortex during presurgical evaluation, will depend on the accumulation of further EEG/fMRI data and, specifically, in combination with other markers of the epileptogenic zone and surgical outcome data. Clinical value needs ultimately to be dictated by considerations of sensitivity, specificity and diagnostic yield versus practicality, applicability and limitations.

Functional MRI (Chapter 57d)

M.J. Koepp and A. Salek-Haddadi

The identification of eloquent cortex is important for minimizing postoperative morbidity in epilepsy surgery. Since we cannot practically test all putative functions for a given region, eloquent cortex mapping relies on pre-existing hypotheses about which functions should localize to a given region (functional localization). Intraoperative electrocorticography, recording from and stimulation with invasive electrodes and the intracarotid amytal procedure (IAP) are frequently used for this purpose but all have limitations of risk and restricted sampling.

fMRI provides direct observation of brain activity during cognitive processes using BOLD contrast [164]. Various tasks may be performed during fMRI to target specific cortical networks but task-related BOLD changes are subtle; just a few per cent at 1.5 T [202]. Paradigms also need to be tailored so that patients can perform them. Studies with no or little activation suggest poor cooperation, sleep or an inability to perform the task.

fMRI relies heavily on the paradigms employed and the assumptions that underlie them [203,204]. fMRI studies identify areas involved in cognitive functions, but these areas may not be critical. Similarly, critical areas not identified by one task may be activated by another. If there is insufficient distinction between the control and experimental conditions during the paradigm [205], lack of activation may not necessarily indicate lack of a function.

Motor function

An early fMRI study showed that in simple tests of language and motor function the haemodynamic response function was very similar between epilepsy patients and normal controls, demonstrating the feasibility of the technique for patient studies [206]. Presurgical sensory motor mapping is a widely used clinical application of fMRI for patients with mass lesions in the vicinity of the central sulcus and has repeatedly been found to be in agreement with intraoperative cortical stimulation studies [207–209]. In patients without neurological deficits, tasks involving the hand and foot produce more reliable activations with a lesser degree of movement-related artefacts than tasks involving additional proximal muscles [210]. In patients with a paresis, different paradigms can be used to avoid artefacts while maintaining functional information including sensory stimulation, passive movements or motor imagery tasks.

Only a few studies have focused on the potential of fMRI to explore the participation of aberrant tissue in physiological functions in patients with malformation of cortical development (MCD). Functional overlap between MCD and normal brain tissue is well recognized as is wider functional reorganization within MCD brains [211,212]. Pinnard et al. [213] were able to demonstrate coactivation within the MCD itself in a child with subcortical laminar heterotopia during a finger-tapping task. Spreer et al. [214] reported on three similar patients showing coactivation of the outer part of the inner neuronal band during performance of a motor task. During visual stimulation in one patient, coactivation was also evident inwards along the route of embryonic neuronal migration from the occipital cortex towards the ventricular wall.

Language lateralization

The IAP remains the most widely used tool to assess language dominance, but does not provide detailed information on the localization of specific language skills, which may be widely distributed both within and between hemispheres. Naming and reading abilities are the language skills most at risk following dominant temporal lobe surgery and IAP determined language lateralization is generally too broad to allow an assessment of such risks for individual patients [215].

fMRI language paradigms readily and reliably identify the language dominant hemisphere [216–223]. All studies, apart from one [222], report impressive concordance rates between fMRI and IAP despite the use of different language tasks and IAP protocols [216,218,220,221,223]. fMRI language tasks are specifically designed to provide strong lateralizing data. Benson et al. [221] compared three language tasks including object naming, single word reading and verb generation; only the verb generation task was reliably lateralizing with laterality determined by IAP or electrocortical stimulation mapping. Using a semantic decision task relative to an auditory tone discrimination task Binder et al. [218] found an extremely strong correlation ($r = 0.96$, $P < 0.0001$) between a laterality index for the IAP and a laterality index from fMRI calculated as an asymmetry in the number of voxels activated in each hemisphere.

In a larger series using the same paradigm, Springer et al. [224] reported atypical or less strong language dominance in 11 out of 50 patients on both fMRI and IAP measures. Since these are the very patients who are at risk for postoperative deficits, the lack of a sufficient fMRI sample size in such patients is troubling and complicated further by performance factors: most patients with right hemisphere or mixed dominance have reorganized language because of a lesion, and patients with lesions in the left hemisphere may have deficits in language processing. How language deficits might influence the magnitude and perceived direction of laterality is not known.

Verbal fluency and semantic decision paradigms have proved to be robust activators of frontal cortex but not temporal language areas [225]. This is problematic as most epilepsy surgery is performed on the temporal lobe. Language paradigms that stress comprehension of a text rather than single words do identify temporal language areas in controls [226]. Contrary to expectations, patients with left TLE showed increased left frontal rather than altered temporal activity compared with controls during semantic processing suggestive of both inter- and intrahemispheric functional reorganization of language representation in left TLE [227].

One practical limitation is the age limit above which fMRI studies may be performed in children; 7 years is thought to be the lower limit for most cognitive studies, but studies can be performed in well-motivated children as young as 5 years [228]. There may also be a difference in the appropriate thresholds for children as opposed to adults which also may depend upon the imaging methods [216]. The haemodynamic response of the immature brain appears similar to adults [216,229]. Children have tended to activate more widely than adults in a test of verbal fluency [230] and this may reflect developmental plasticity for the ongoing organization of neural networks. Language networks appear to lateralize and localize by middle to late childhood [231].

Memory

The IAP is primarily used to ensure mnemic adequacy of the contralateral temporal lobe, but does not reliably indicate the risk of verbal memory impairment following surgery to the speech dominant temporal lobe [215]. fMRI can provide maps of temporal lobe activation potentially identifying functionally hypoactive memory areas which may have predictive value for postoperative memory deficits.

Bellgowan et al. [232] utilized a semantic encoding task that produced unilateral activations in normal controls and found increased fMRI activations in the left hippocampus and parahippocampal gyrus in right TLE patients, whereas the left TLE group showed little significant activation in these regions. Importantly neither group showed activation of any of these regions in the right hemisphere. Whilst these results demonstrate the feasibility of predicting the side of seizure focus in TLE patients, they are based on group data that need to be extended to individual patient studies.

Detre et al. [233] used a complex visual scene encoding task, which was partly chosen because it produced bilateral and broadly symmetrical anterior temporal lobe activations in normals, and so allowed calculation of an asymmetry index in patients, relatively insensitive to individual variability. In TLE patients the activation was asymmetrical and strongly correlated with IAP measures of memory. Interestingly, the significance of the task-correlated activity was greater in controls and in the patients with good performance, although successful lateralization was seen even in patients who complained that the task was too difficult or who performed poorly on the recognition task.

In a recent fMRI study [234], a mental navigation task reliably activated mesial temporal structures symmetrically in individual control subjects, but identified interhemispheric differences lateralized to the side of seizure onset in 90% of patients with symptomatic unilateral TLE including children, older subjects and patients with low IQ.

Dupont et al. [235] used a verbal memory encoding and retrieval paradigm to compare patients with left TLE against controls. Normals activated parahippocampal regions, right more than left, during retrieval. This pattern was less marked in patients, but in the patient group a left frontal region participated. The authors interpreted this as a dysfunctional response due to epilepsy and left hippocampal sclerosis, but overlooked the vast difference in performance, with patients recalling with far less accuracy than normals ($P < 0.007$).

Maguire et al. [236] reported the fMRI results of successful retrieval in a patient with bilateral hippocampal damage confirming the functionality of remaining tissue in the damaged hippocampi and this study underlines the value of scanning patients while they undertake tasks they can actually perform. The recruitment of bilateral regions during memory retrieval and altered pattern of effective connectivity between brain regions may be important indicators of a diseased memory.

Conclusions

fMRI is a powerful tool for investigating cognitive function in both normal and patient populations. Its main clinical application is in the non-invasive mapping of motor, language and memory functions, and in epilepsy surgery this information can be used to minimize the risks of postoperative neuropsychological deficit. fMRI mapping of sensory and motor function is fairly well established. Localization of the language dominant hemisphere has been well validated in normal volunteers and in left hemisphere dominant patients, but is less developed for patients with mixed or right hemisphere language dominance. Characteristic activations identified in normals are not always seen in patients and importantly these altered patterns appear to represent functional rearrangements rather than just the anatomical pathology. At present, fMRI memory paradigms do not confidently assess the risk of a postoperative amnesic syndrome. Further work is needed quantitatively to assess sensitivity, specificity and reliability prior to wider implementation within the clinical setting.

Subtraction ictal SPECT coregistered on MRI (SISCOM) (Chapter 57e)

E.L. So

Over the past two decades, SPECT has been widely used to help identify the epileptogenic zone for surgical resection in patients with intractable epilepsy. This diagnostic test is based on the phenomenon of increased blood flow associated with localized seizure activity, which is a reproducible phenomenon in animals and a frequent observation made in humans during brain surgery [237].

Until recently, the conventional method of interpreting ictal SPECT studies consisted of visual comparison of ictal (Plate 57.20a, shown in colour between pp. 670 and 671) and interictal SPECT images (Plate 57.20b, shown in colour between pp. 670 and 671). However, this method of detecting an increase in blood flow at the seizure focus has several drawbacks. The interictal and ictal images may vary in signal intensity, because of differences in the amount of radiotracer injected and the time between injection and image acquisition. The level of slices in acquired images often varies between the interictal and the ictal SPECT studies. Furthermore, an interictal focus that is hypoperfused may not stand out visually from the background on the ictal images despite an ictal increase in perfusion. Finally, both ictal and interictal SPECT images lack the anatomical landmarks of the brain that are needed for clinical correlation and surgical planning.

To overcome these drawbacks, the technique of SISCOM was developed [238].

Technique

The technique of SISCOM is based on concepts of subtracting the interictal from the ictal images [239], and on the concept of registering SPECT images onto MRI or CT [240]. The SISCOM technique begins with coregistering the interictal to the ictal SPECT study by a surface matching method [241], or by the voxel-based matching method, which is even more accurate [242].

As a means of accounting for global differences in image intensity between the interictal and ictal studies, the mean cerebral pixel intensities of each study are normalized to a mean intensity of 100. The normalized interictal data are then subtracted from the normalized ictal data to derive the difference or subtraction image. The difference image is then set at a threshold to display only pixels with intensities more than 2 standard deviations above zero (Plate 57.20c, shown in colour between pp. 670 and 671). Finally, the thresholded difference image is registered to the MRI (Plate 57.20d, shown in colour between pp. 670 and 671).

Clinical validation and application

The SISCOM method substantially improves interobserver agreement between blinded reviewers when compared with the conventional method of visual comparison of interictal and ictal studies [243]. The rates of interobserver agreement were 84% with SISCOM and 41% with conventional visual comparison. The sensitivity of detecting an abnormal focus was also much higher with SISCOM (88%) than with conventional visual comparison (39%), and these results were actually obtained from patients whose seizure foci could not be sufficiently localized by standard diagnostic tests such as MRI and EEG.

Thus, SISCOM has been shown to provide independently useful data for localization of the seizure focus and, in addition, SISCOM gives important prognostic information regarding seizure outcome following surgical resection. The probability of excellent seizure control after surgical resection of the focus is 62% when the SISCOM focus is resected and 20% when the SISCOM focus is either absent or not resected.

Non-lesional extratemporal epilepsies are notorious for being very difficult to localize for epilepsy surgery but SISCOM has also been proved to be useful in patients with this disorder. The chances of excellent postsurgical seizure control are 55% when a SISCOM focus is present and is surgically resected, and zero when a SISCOM focus is absent or not resected [244]. This result should be considered from the perspective that the chances of excellent outcome in this group of patients were only 25% prior to the use of SISCOM [245].

It is often difficult to inject the SPECT radiotracer before the seizure has ended, especially with short extratemporal seizures. Thus, the radiotracer is often injected after the seizure has terminated. The seizure focus becomes *hypo*perfused during the immediate postictal period and then eventually recovers its baseline degree of perfusion. Thus, detection of a *hyper*perfusion abnormality loses sensitivity when the SPECT injection is postictal in timing. However, the SISCOM technique can be used to display the postictal *hypo*perfusion. With the SISCOM technique, a postictal hypoperfusion focus can be demonstrated in about 75% of patients.

Nonetheless, both hypoperfusion and hyperperfusion subtraction images must be reviewed with each study, because the two in combination yield a better sensitivity for detecting the potential seizure focus than each reviewed alone [246,247].

SISCOM and computer image-guided epilepsy surgery evaluated with intracranial electrode implantation

This is best accomplished with computer-aided techniques, such as the Stealth image-guided system [248]. With this technique, a frameless stereotactic MRI is first performed with 10 external markers attached to the scalp (Plate 57.21a, shown in colour between pp. 670 and 671). The same markers are then manually registered into a computer to create a transformation matrix, so that the MRI image space can be related to the physical space of the patient's head (Plate 57.21b, shown in colour between pp. 670 and 671).

During operation, the surgeon uses a wand to point at areas in the surgical field (Plate 57.21c, shown in colour between pp. 670 and 671). In doing so, the surgeon is able to view the computer screen to observe how close the tip of the wand is to the SISCOM abnormality (Plate 57.21d, shown in colour between pp. 670 and 671). This observation is used to guide the placement of electrodes and subsequent surgical resection of the SISCOM focus.

The use of computer image-guided surgery is critical to the success of the evaluation and resection of the SISCOM focus, especially in patients with non-lesional epilepsy, in whom the gross anatomy is normal and therefore there is no obvious target in the surgical field for electrode implantation or surgical resection. The computer-aided surgical technique allows integration of the SISCOM focus with the surgical field, so that intracranial electrodes can be accurately implanted and the focus can be fully resected [249].

Acknowledgements

H. Meierkord and K. Buchheim were supported by a DFG Grant BV 1331–1.

References

1 Gregory DL, Wong PK. Topographical analysis of the centrotemporal discharges in benign rolandic epilepsy of childhood. *Epilepsia* 1984; 25: 705–11.

2 Wong PK, Bencivenga R, Gregory D. Statistical classification of spikes in benign rolandic epilepsy. *Brain Topogr* 1988; 1: 123–9.

3 Ebersole JS, Wade PB. Spike voltage topography and equivalent dipole localization in complex partial epilepsy. *Brain Topogr* 1990; 3: 21–34.

4 Ebersole JS. EEG dipole modeling in complex partial epilepsy. *Brain Topogr* 1991; 4: 113–23.

5 Do Marcolino C, Baulac M, Samson-Dollfus D. Topographic analysis of interictal spikes in the presurgical evaluation of severe partial epilepsy. *Neurophysiol Clin* 1994; 24: 20–34.

6 Koszer S, Moshe SL, Legatt AD, Shinnar S, Goldensohn ES. Surface mapping of spike potential fields: experienced EEGers vs. computerized analysis. *Electroencephalogr Clin Neurophysiol* 1996; 98: 199–205.

7 Huppertz HJ, Hof E, Klisch J, Wagner M, Lucking CH, Kristeva-Feige R. Localization of interictal delta and epileptiform EEG activity associated with focal epileptogenic brain lesions. *Neuroimage* 2001; 13: 15–28.

8 Brazier MA. A study of electrical fields at the surface of the head. *Electroencephal Clin Neurophysiol Suppl* 1949; 2: 38–52.

9 Lorente de No R. Analysis of the distribution of action currents of nerve. *Studies Rockefeller Inst Med Res* 1947; 132: 384–477.

10 Fender DH. Source localization of brain electric activity. In: Gevins, A Rémond, A, eds. *Methods of Analysis of Brain Electrical and Magnetic Signals.* Amsterdam: Elsevier, 1987: 355–403.

11 Roth BJ, Balish M, Gorbach A, Sato S. How well does a three-sphere model predict positions of dipoles in a realistically shaped head? *Electroencephalogr Clin Neurophysiol* 1993; 87: 175–84.

12 Hamalainen MS, Sarvas J. Realistic conductivity geometry model of the human head for interpretation of neuromagnetic data. *IEEE Trans Biomed Eng* 1989; 36: 165–71.

13 Cuffin BN. A method for localizing EEG sources in realistic head models. *IEEE Trans Biomed Eng* 1995; 42: 68–71.

14 Yvert B, Bertrand O, Echallier JF, Pernier J. Improved forward EEG calculations using local mesh refinement of realistic head geometries. *Electroencephalogr Clin Neurophysiol* 1995; 95: 381–92.

15 Yvert B, Bertrand O, Echallier JF, Pernier J. Improved dipole localization using local mesh refinement of realistic head geometries: an EEG simulation study. *Electroencephalogr Clin Neurophysiol* 1996; 99: 79–89.

16 Binnie CD, MacGillivray BB. Brain mapping – a useful tool or a dangerous toy? [editorial]. *J Neurol Neurosurg Psychiatr* 1992; 55: 527–9.

17 Lantz G, Ryding E, Rosen I. Three-dimentional localization of interictal epileptiform activity with dipole analysis: Comparison with intracranial recordings and SPECT findings. *J Epilepsy* 1994; 7: 117–29.

18 Scherg M. Fundamentals of dipole source potential analysis. In: Grandori, F Hoke, M Romani, GL, eds. *Auditory Evoked Electric and Magnetic Fields.* Basel: Karger, 1990: 40–69.

19 Merlet I, Garcia-Larrea L, Froment JC, Mauguiere F. Simplified projection of EEG dipole sources onto human brain anatomy. *Neurophysiol Clin* 1999; 29: 39–52.

20 Smith DB, Sidman RD, Flanigin H, Henke J, Labiner D. A reliable method for localizing deep intracranial sources of the EEG. *Neurology* 1985; 35: 1702–7.

21 Cohen D, Cuffin BN, Yunokuchi K et al. MEG versus EEG localization test using implanted sources in the human brain [see comments]. *Ann Neurol* 1990; 28: 811–17.

22 Cuffin BN, Cohen D, Yunokuchi K et al. Tests of EEG localization accuracy using implanted sources in the human brain. *Ann Neurol* 1991; 29: 132–8.

23 Cuffin BN, Schomer DL, Ives JR, Blume H. Experimental tests of EEG source localization accuracy in spherical head models. *Clin Neurophysiol* 2001; 112: 46–51.

24 Mosher JC, Baillet S, Leahy RM. EEG source localization and imaging using multiple signal classification approaches. *J Clin Neurophysiol* 1999; 16: 225–38.

25 Yvert B, Bertrand O, Thevenet M, Echallier JF, Pernier J. A systematic evaluation of the spherical model accuracy in EEG dipole localization. *Electroencephalogr Clin Neurophysiol* 1997; 102: 452–9.

26 Krings T, Chiappa KH, Cuffin BN, Cochius JI, Connolly S, Cosgrove GR. Accuracy of EEG dipole source localization using implanted sources in the human brain. *Clin Neurophysiol* 1999; 110: 106–14.

27 Cuffin BN. EEG localization accuracy improvements using realistically shaped head models. *IEEE Trans Biomed Eng* 1996; 43: 299–303.

28 Leahy RM, Mosher JC, Spencer ME, Huang MX, Lewine JD. A study of dipole localization accuracy for MEG and EEG using a human skull phantom. *Electroencephalogr Clin Neurophysiol* 1998; 107: 159–73.

29 Crouzeix A, Yvert B, Bertrand O, Pernier J. An evaluation of dipole reconstruction accuracy with spherical and realistic head models in MEG. *Clin Neurophysiol* 1999; 110: 2176–88.

30 Lantz G, Holub M, Ryding E, Rosen I. Simultaneous intracranial and extracranial recording of interictal epileptiform activity in patients with drug resistant partial epilepsy: patterns of conduction and results from dipole reconstructions. *Electroencephalogr Clin Neurophysiol* 1996; 99: 69–78.

31 Merlet I, Garcia-Larrea L, Ryvlin P, Isnard J, Sindou M, Mauguière F. Topographical reliability of mesio-temporal sources of interictal spikes in temporal lobe epilepsy. *Electroencephalogr Clin Neurophysiol* 1998; 107: 206–12.

32 Barth DS, Sutherling W, Engel J Jr, Beatty J. Neuromagnetic localization of epileptiform spike activity in the human brain. *Science* 1982; 218: 891–4.

33 Stefan H, Schneider S, Abraham-Fuchs K *et al*. Magnetic source localization in focal epilepsy. Multichannel magnetoencephalography correlated with magnetic resonance brain imaging. *Brain* 1990; 113 (5): 1347–59.

34 Barth DS, Sutherling W, Engle J Jr, Beatty J. Neuromagnetic evidence of spatially distributed sources underlying epileptiform spikes in the human brain. *Science* 1984; 223: 293–6.

35 Stefan H, Schneider S, Abraham-Fuchs K *et al*. The neocortico to mesiobasal limbic propagation of focal epileptic activity during the spike-wave complex. *Electroencephalogr Clin Neurophysiol* 1991; 79: 1–10.

36 Ebersole JS. Non-invasive localization of the epileptogenic focus by EEG dipole modeling. *Acta Neurol Scand Suppl* 1994; 152: 20–8.

37 Chauvel P, Buser P, Badier JM, Liegeois-Chauvel C, Marquis P, Bancaud J. The 'epileptogenic zone' in humans: representation of intercritical events by spatio-temporal maps. *Rev Neurol (Paris)* 1987; 143: 443–50.

38 Sutherling WW, Barth DS. Neocortical propagation in temporal lobe spike foci on magnetoencephalography and electroencephalography. *Ann Neurol* 1989; 25: 373–81.

39 Baumgartner C, Lindinger G, Ebner A *et al*. Propagation of interictal epileptic activity in temporal lobe epilepsy. *Neurology* 1995; 45: 118–22.

40 Merlet I, Garcia-Larrea L, Gregoire MC, Lavenne F, Mauguière F. Source propagation of interictal spikes in temporal lobe epilepsy. Correlations between spike dipole modelling and [18F]fluorodeoxyglucose PET data. *Brain* 1996; 119: 377–92.

41 Boon P, D'Have M, Vandekerckhove T *et al*. Dipole modelling and intracranial EEG recording: correlation between dipole and ictal onset zone. *Acta Neurochir (Wien)* 1997; 139: 643–52.

42 Stefan H, Schuler P, Abraham-Fuchs K *et al*. Magnetic source localization and morphological changes in temporal lobe epilepsy: comparison of MEG/EEG, ECoG and volumetric MRI in presurgical evaluation of operated patients. *Acta Neurol Scand Suppl* 1994; 152: 83–8.

43 Tsai ML, Chatrian GE, Pauri F *et al*. Electrocorticography in patients with medically intractable temporal lobe seizures. I. Quantification of epileptiform discharges prior to resective surgery. *Electroencephalogr Clin Neurophysiol* 1993; 87: 10–24.

44 Ito T, Shibata T, Koseki K, Iwasa H, Sato T, Nakajima Y. Estimation of electrical sources of interictal spikes in frontal lobe epilepsy with the dipole tracing of the scalp-skull-brain head model: comparison with temporal lobe epilepsy. *Epilepsia* 1996; 37 (Suppl. 3): 78–9.

45 Gotman J. Interhemispheric relations during bilateral spike-and-wave activity. *Epilepsia* 1981; 22: 453–66.

46 Gotman J. Interhemispheric interactions in seizures of focal onset: data from human intracranial recordings. *Electroencephalogr Clin Neurophysiol* 1987; 67: 120–33.

47 Rodin E, Litzinger M, Thompson J. Complexity of focal spikes suggests relative epileptogenicity. *Epilepsia* 1995; 36: 1078–83.

48 Yoshinaga H, Kobayashi K, Sato M, Mizukawa M, Ohtahara S. Clinical application of spike averaging to dipole tracing method. *Brain Topogr* 1993; 6: 131–5.

49 Shindo K, Ikeda A, Musha T *et al*. Clinical usefulness of the dipole tracing method for localizing interictal spikes in partial epilepsy. *Epilepsia* 1998; 39: 371–9.

50 Ossenblok P, Fuchs M, Velis DN, Veltman E, Pijn JP, da Silva FH. Source analysis of lesional frontal-lobe epilepsy. *IEEE Eng Med Biol Mag* 1999; 18: 67–77.

51 Scherg M, Bast T, Berg P. Multiple source analysis of interictal spikes: goals, requirements, and clinical value. *J Clin Neurophysiol* 1999; 16: 214–24.

52 Merlet I, Garcia-Larrea L, Isnard J, Ryvlin P, Froment JC, Mauguière F. The problem of spike focus versus MRI lesion incongruence as assessed by source modeling. *Epilepsia* 1997; 38 (Suppl. 8): 72.

53 Engel J Jr. Clinical neurophysiology, neuroimaging, and the surgical treatment of epilepsy. *Curr Opin Neurol Neurosurg* 1993; 6: 240–9.

54 Spencer SS. The relative contributions of MRI, SPECT, and PET imaging in epilepsy. *Epilepsia* 1994; 35 (Suppl. 6): S72–S89.

55 Cendes F, Dubeau F, Andermann F *et al*. Significance of mesial temporal atrophy in relation to intracranial ictal and interictal stereo EEG abnormalities. *Brain* 1996; 119 (4): 1317–26.

56 Mauguière F, Ryvlin P. Morphological and functional neuro-imaging of surgical partial epilepsies in adults. *Rev Neurol (Paris)* 1996; 152: 501–16.

57 Duncan JS. Imaging and epilepsy. *Brain* 1997; 120 (2): 339–77.

58 Ryvlin P, Bouvard S, Le Bars D *et al*. Clinical utility of flumazenil-PET versus [18F]fluorodeoxyglucose-PET and MRI in refractory partial epilepsy. A prospective study in 100 patients. *Brain* 1998; 121 (11): 2067–81.

59 Ryvlin P, Mauguière F, Sindou M, Froment JC, Cinotti L. Interictal cerebral metabolism and epilepsy in cavernous angiomas. *Brain* 1995; 118 (3): 677–87.

60 Lamusuo S, Forss N, Ruottinen HM *et al*. [18F]FDG-PET and whole-scalp MEG localization of epileptogenic cortex. *Epilepsia* 1999; 40: 921–30.

61 Pozo M, Pascau J, Rojo P *et al*. Correlation between FDG PET data and EEG dipole modeling. *Clin Positron Imaging* 2000; 3: 173.

62 Shibata N, Kubota F, Machiyama Y, Takahashi A, Miyamoto K. Mapping epileptic foci by the dipole tracing method in a brain tumor patient with olfactory seizures: comparison with intraoperative electrocorticograms. *Clin Electroencephalogr* 1998; 29: 91–5.

63 Otsubo H, Sharma R, Elliott I, Holowka S, Rutka JT, Snead OC III Confirmation of two magnetoencephalographic epileptic foci by invasive monitoring from subdural electrodes in an adolescent with right fronto-central epilepsy. *Epilepsia* 1999; 40: 608–13.

64 Yoshinaga H, Nakahori T, Hattori J *et al*. Dipole analysis in a case with tumor-related epilepsy. *Brain Dev* 1999; 21: 483–7.

65 Morioka T, Nishio S, Ishibashi H *et al*. Intrinsic epileptogenicity of focal cortical dysplasia as revealed by magnetoencephalography and electrocorticography. *Epilepsy Res* 1999; 33: 177–87.

66 Ebersole JS. Magnetoencephalography/magnetic source imaging in the assessment of patients with epilepsy. *Epilepsia* 1997; 38 (Suppl. 4): S1–S5.

67 Smith JR, Schwartz BJ, Gallen C *et al*. Multichannel magnetoencephalography in ablative seizure surgery outside the anteromesial temporal lobe. *Stereotact Funct Neurosurg* 1995; 65: 81–5.

68 Minassian BA, Otsubo H, Weiss S, Elliott I, Rutka JT, Snead OC III Magnetoencephalographic localization in pediatric epilepsy surgery: comparison with invasive intracranial electroencephalography. *Ann Neurol* 1999; 46: 627–33.

69 Merlet I, Gotman J. Reliability of dipole models of epileptic spikes. *Clin Neurophysiol* 1999; 110: 1013–28.

70 Cooper R, Winter AL, Crow HJ, Walter WG. Comparison of subcortical, cortical, and scalp activity using chronically indwelling electrodes in man. *Electroencephalogr Clin Neurophysiol* 1965; 18: 217–28.

71 Ebersole JS, Squires KC, Eliashiv SD, Smith JR. Applications of magnetic source imaging in evaluation of candidates for epilepsy surgery. *Neuroimaging Clin N Am* 1995; 5: 267–88.

72 Pacia SV, Ebersole JS. Intracranial EEG substrates of scalp ictal patterns from temporal lobe foci. *Epilepsia* 1997; 38: 642–54.

73 Rubboli G, Francione S, Parmeggiani L *et al*. Dipole source estimation of focal epileptic spikes: correlation with stereo-electroencephalographic findings. In: Angeleri F, Butler SR, Giaquinto S, Majkowski J, eds. *Analysis of the Electrical Activity of the Brain*. New York: John Wiley & Sons, 1997: 309–25.

74 Mikuni N, Nagamine T, Ikeda A *et al*. Simultaneous recording of epileptiform discharges by MEG and subdural electrodes in temporal lobe epilepsy. *Neuroimage* 1997; 5: 298–306.

75 Blume WT, Borghesi JL, Lemieux JF. Interictal indices of temporal seizure origin. *Ann Neurol* 1993; 34: 703–9.

76 King DW, Ajmone Marsan C. Clinical features and ictal patterns in epileptic patients with EEG temporal lobe foci. *Ann Neurol* 1977; 2: 138–47.

77 Sammaritano M, Gigli GL, Gotman J. Interictal spiking during wakefulness and sleep and the localization of foci in temporal lobe epilepsy. *Neurology* 1991; 41: 290–7.

78 Lieb JP, Engel J Jr, Gevins A, Crandal PH. Surface and deep EEG correlates of surgical outcome in temporal lobe epilepsy. *Epilepsia* 1981; 22: 515–38.

79 Marks DA, Katz A, Booke J, Spencer DD, Spencer SS. Comparison and correlation of surface and sphenoidal electrodes with simultaneous in-

tracranial recording: an interictal study. *Electroencephalogr Clin Neurophysiol* 1992; 82: 23–9.

80 Rougier A. Relation between inter-critical and critical stereoelectroencephalographic elements: consequences on the results of cortectomies. *Rev Neurol (Paris)* 1987; 143: 437–42.

81 Pacia SV, Ebersole JS. EEG dipole models of spikes versus seizures. *Electroencephalogr Clin Neurophysiol* 1993; 86: 57p.

82 Boon P, D'Have M. Interictal and ictal dipole modelling in patients with refractory partial epilepsy. *Acta Neurol Scand* 1995; 92: 7–18.

83 Krings T, Chiappa KH, Cuffin BN, Buchbinder BR, Cosgrove GR. Accuracy of electroencephalographic dipole localization of epileptiform activities associated with focal brain lesions. *Ann Neurol* 1998; 44: 76–86.

84 Wiederin TBJ, Chiappa KH, Krings T *et al.* The utility of dipole source analysis of seizure onsets in the localization of epileptogenic zones as assessed by postsurgical outcome. *J Contemp Neurol* 1999; 1: 1–10.

85 Boon P, D'Have M, Vanrumste B *et al.* Ictal source localization in presurgical patients with refractory epilepsy. *Clin Neurophysiol* 2000; 111 (Suppl. 1): S100.

86 Merlet I, Gotman J. Dipole modeling of scalp electroencephalogram epileptic discharges: correlation with intracerebral fields. *Clin Neurophysiol* 2001; 112: 414–30.

87 Mine S, Yamaura A, Iwasa H, Nakajima Y, Shibata T, Itoh T. Dipole source localization of ictal epileptiform activity. *Neuroreport* 1998; 9: 4007–13.

88 Ishibashi H, Morioka T, Shigeto H, Nishio S, Yamamoto T, Fukui M. Three-dimensional localization of subclinical ictal activity by magnetoencephalography: correlation with invasive monitoring. *Surg Neurol* 1998; 50: 157–63.

89 Wheless JW, Willmore LJ, Breier JI *et al.* A comparison of magnetoencephalography, MRI, and V-EEG in patients evaluated for epilepsy surgery. *Epilepsia* 1999; 40: 931–41.

90 Rojo P, Caicoya AG, Martin-Loeches M, Sola RG, Pozo MA. Localization of the epileptogenic zone by analysis of electroencephalographic dipole. *Rev Neurol* 2001; 32: 315–20.

91 Wong PK. The importance of source behavior in distinguishing populations of epileptic foci. *J Clin Neurophysiol* 1993; 10: 314–22.

92 Boon P, D'Have M, Adam C *et al.* Dipole modeling in epilepsy surgery candidates. *Epilepsia* 1997; 38: 208–18.

93 Theodore WH, Porter RJ, Penry JK. Complex partial seizures: clinical characteristics and differential diagnosis. *Neurology* 1983; 33: 1115–21.

94 Quesney LF. Extracranial EEG evaluation. In: Engel J Jr, ed. *Surgical Treatment of the Epilepsies.* New York: Raven Press, 1987: 129–66.

95 Quesney LF, Abou-Khalil B, Cole A, Olivier A. Pre-operative extracranial and intracranial EEG investigation in patients with temporal lobe epilepsy: trends, results and review of pathophysiologic mechanisms. *Acta Neurol Scand Suppl* 1988; 117: 52–60.

96 So N, Gloor P, Quesney LF, Jones-Gotman M, Olivier A, Andermann F. Depth electrode investigations in patients with bitemporal epileptiform abnormalities. *Ann Neurol* 1989; 25: 423–31.

97 So N, Olivier A, Andermann F, Gloor P, Quesney LF. Results of surgical treatment in patients with bitemporal epileptiform abnormalities. *Ann Neurol* 1989; 25: 432–9.

98 Stefan H, Schneider S, Feistel H *et al.* Ictal and interictal activity in partial epilepsy recorded with multichannel magnetoelectroencephalography: correlation of electroencephalography/electrocorticography, magnetic resonance imaging, single photon emission computed tomography, and positron emission tomography findings. *Epilepsia* 1992; 33: 874–87.

99 Nakasato N, Levesque MF, Barth DS, Baumgartner C, Rogers RL, Sutherling WW. Comparisons of MEG, EEG, and ECoG source localization in neocortical partial epilepsy in humans. *Electroencephalogr Clin Neurophysiol* 1994; 91: 171–8.

100 Knowlton RC, Laxer KD, Aminoff MJ, Roberts TP, Wong ST, Rowley HA. Magnetoencephalography in partial epilepsy: clinical yield and localization accuracy. *Ann Neurol* 1997; 42: 622–31.

101 Malonek D, Grinvald A. Interactions between electrical activity and cortical microcirculation revealed by imaging spectroscopy: implications for functional brain mapping. *Science* 1996; 272 (5261): 551–4.

102 Grinvald A, Frostig RD, Lieke E, Hildesheim R. Optical imaging of neuronal activity. *Physiol Rev* 1988; 68 (4): 1285–366.

103 Aitken PG, Fayuk D, Somjen GG, Turner DA. Use of intrinsic optical signals to monitor physiological changes in brain tissue slices. *Methods* 1999; 18 (2): 91–103.

104 Hochman DW. Intrinsic optical changes in neuronal tissue. Basic mechanisms. *Neurosurg Clin N Am* 1997; 8 (3): 393–412.

105 Villringer A, Chance B. Non-invasive optical spectroscopy and imaging of human brain function. *Trends Neurosci* 1997; 20 (10): 435–42.

106 Steinbrink J, Kohl M, Obrig H *et al.* Somatosensory evoked fast optical intensity changes detected non-invasively in the adult human head. *Neurosci Lett* 2000; 291 (2): 105–8.

107 Hill DK, Keynes RD. Opacity changes in stimulated nerve. *J Physiol* 1949; 108: 278–81.

108 Cohen LB. Changes in neuron structure during action potential propagation and synaptic transmission. *Physiol Rev* 1973; 53 (2): 373–418.

109 Stepnoski RA, LaPorta A, Raccuia BF, Blonder GE, Slusher RE, Kleinfeld D. Noninvasive detection of changes in membrane potential in cultured neurons by light scattering. *Proc Natl Acad Sci USA* 1991; 88 (21): 9382–6.

110 Lipton P. Effects of membrane depolarization on light scattering by cerebral cortical slices. *J Physiol Lond* 1973; 231 (2): 365–83.

111 MacVicar BA, Hochman D. Imaging of synaptically evoked intrinsic optical signals in hippocampal slices. *J Neurosci* 1991; 11 (5): 1458–69.

112 Buchheim K, Schuchmann S, Siegmund H, Gabriel HJ, Heinemann U, Meierkord H. Intrinsic optical signal measurements reveal characteristic features during different forms of spontaneous neuronal hyperactivity associated with ECS shrinkage in vitro. *Eur J Neurosci* 1999; 11 (6): 1877–82.

113 Andrew RD, Adams JR, Polischuk TM. Imaging NMDA- and kainate-induced intrinsic optical signals from the hippocampal slice. *J Neurophysiol* 1996; 76 (4): 2707–17.

114 Holthoff K, Witte OW. Intrinsic optical signals in rat neocortical slices measured with near-infrared dark-field microscopy reveal changes in extracellular space. *J Neurosci* 1996; 16 (8): 2740–9.

115 Holthoff K, Witte OW. Directed spatial potassium redistribution in rat neocortex. *Glia* 2000; 29 (3): 288–92.

116 Andrew RD, MacVicar BA. Imaging cell volume changes and neuronal excitation in the hippocampal slice. *Neuroscience* 1994; 62 (2): 371–83.

117 Hochman DW, Baraban SC, Owens JW, Schwartzkroin PA. Dissociation of synchronization and excitability in furosemide blockade of epileptiform activity. *Science* 1995; 270 (5233): 99–102.

118 Jarvis CR, Lilge L, Vipond GJ, Andrew RD. Interpretation of intrinsic optical signals and calcein fluorescence during acute excitotoxic insult in the hippocampal slice. *Neuroimage* 1999; 10 (4): 357–72.

119 Polischuk TM, Andrew RD. Real-time imaging of intrinsic optical signals during early excitotoxicity evoked by domoic acid in the rat hippocampal slice. *Can J Physiol Pharmacol* 1996; 74 (6): 712–22.

120 Polischuk TM, Jarvis CR, Andrew RD. Intrinsic optical signaling denoting neuronal damage in response to acute excitotoxic insult by domoic acid in the hippocampal slice. *Neurobiol Dis* 1998; 4 (6): 423–37.

121 Obrig H, Wenzel R, Kohl M *et al.* Near-infrared spectroscopy: does it function in functional activation studies of the adult brain? *Int J Psychophysiol* 2000; 35 (2–3): 125–42.

122 Mody I, Lambert JD, Heinemann U. Low extracellular magnesium induces epileptiform activity and spreading depression in rat hippocampal slices. *J Neurophysiol* 1987; 57 (3): 869–88.

123 Rutecki PA, Lebeda FJ, Johnston D. 4-Aminopyridine produces epileptiform activity in hippocampus and enhances synaptic excitation and inhibition. *J Neurophysiol* 1987; 57 (6): 1911–24.

124 Haas HL, Jefferys JG. Low-calcium field burst discharges of CA1 pyramidal neurones in rat hippocampal slices. *J Physiol (Lond)* 1984; 354: 185–201.

125 Jefferys JG. Nonsynaptic modulation of neuronal activity in the brain: electric currents and extracellular ions. *Physiol Rev* 1995; 75 (4): 689–723.

126 Meierkord H, Schuchmann S, Buchheim K, Heinemann U. Optical imaging of low Mg (2+)-induced spontaneous epileptiform activity in combined rat entorhinal cortex-hippocampal slices. *Neuroreport* 1997; 8 (8): 1857–61.

127 Buchheim K, Schuchmann S, Siegmund H, Weissinger F, Heinemann U, Meierkord H. Comparison of intrinsic optical signals associated with low

Mg^{2+}- and 4-aminopyridine-induced seizure-like events reveals characteristic features in adult rat limbic system. *Epilepsia* 2000; 41 (6): 635–41.

128 Hauser WA. Incidence and prevalence. In: Engel J, Pedley TA, eds. *Epilepsy: a Comprehensive Textbook.* New York: Demos Press, 1997: 47–57.

129 Holmes GL. Epilepsy in the developing brain: lessons from the laboratory and clinic. *Epilepsia* 1997; 38 (1): 12–30.

130 Weissinger F, Buchheim K, Siegmund H, Heinemann U, Meierkord H. Optical imaging reveals characteristic seizure onsets, spread patterns, and propagation velocities in hippocampal-entorhinal cortex slices of juvenile rats. *Neurobiol Dis* 2000; 7 (4): 286–98.

131 Stephen LJ, Brodie MJ. Epilepsy in elderly people. *Lancet* 2000; 355 (9213): 1441–6.

132 Schuchmann S, Buchheim K, Meierkord H, Heinemann U. A relative energy failure is associated with low-Mg^{2+} but not with 4-aminopyridine induced seizure-like events in entorhinal cortex. *J Neurophysiol* 1999; 81 (1): 399–403.

133 Folbergrová J, Ingvar M, Nevander G, Siesjö BK. Cerebral metabolic changes during and following fluorothyl-induced seizures in ventilated rats. *J Neurochem* 1985; 44: 1419–26.

134 Fujikawa DG, Vannucci RC, Dwyer BE, Wasterlain CG. Generalized seizures deplete brain energy reserves in normoxemic newborn monkeys. *Brain Res* 1988; 454: 51–9.

135 Merrill DK, Guynn RW. Electroconvulsive seizure: an investigation into the validity of calculating the cytoplasmic free [NAD+]/[NADH][H+] ratio from substrate concentrations of brain. *J Neurochem* 1976; 27: 459–64.

136 Walker MC. The epidemiology and management of status epilepticus. *Curr Opin Neurol* 1998; 11 (2): 149–54.

137 Chen JW. Optical intrinsic signal imaging in a rodent seizure model. *Neurology* 2000; 55 (2): 312–15.

138 Schwartz TH, Bonhoeffer T. In vivo optical mapping of epileptic foci and surround inhibition in ferret cerebral cortex. *Nat Med* 2001; 7 (9): 1063–7.

139 Haglund MM, Ojemann GA, Hochman DW. Optical imaging of epileptiform and functional activity in human cerebral cortex. *Nature* 1992; 358 (6388): 668–71.

140 Toga AW, Cannestra AF, Black KL. The temporal/spatial evolution of optical signals in human cortex. *Cereb Cortex* 1995; 5 (6): 561–5.

141 Cannestra AF, Blood AJ, Black KL, Toga AW. The evolution of optical signals in human and rodent cortex. *Neuroimage* 1996; 3 (3 Part 1): 202–8.

142 Svaasand LO. Properties of thermal waves in vascular media; application to blood flow measurements. *Med Phys* 1982; 9 (5): 711–14.

143 Cope M, Delpy DT. System for long-term measurement of cerebral blood and tissue oxygenation on newborn infants by near infra-red transillumination. *Med Biol Eng Comput* 1988; 26 (3): 289–94.

144 Wyatt JS, Cope M, Delpy DT *et al.* Quantitation of cerebral blood volume in human infants by near-infrared spectroscopy. *J Appl Physiol* 1990; 68 (3): 1086–91.

145 Jobsis FF. Noninvasive, infrared monitoring of cerebral and myocardial oxygen sufficiency and circulatory parameters. *Science* 1977; 198 (4323): 1264–7.

146 Kirkpatrick PJ, Smielewski P, Czosnyka M, Menon DK, Pickard JD. Near-infrared spectroscopy use in patients with head injury. *J Neurosurg* 1995; 83 (6): 963–70.

147 Adelson PD, Nemoto E, Scheuer M, Painter M, Morgan J, Yonas H. Noninvasive continuous monitoring of cerebral oxygenation periictally using near-infrared spectroscopy: a preliminary report. *Epilepsia* 1999; 40 (11): 1484–9.

148 Sokol DK, Markand ON, Daly EC, Luerssen TG, Malkoff MD. Near infrared spectroscopy (NIRS) distinguishes seizure types. *Seizure* 2000; 9 (5): 323–7.

149 Steinhoff BJ, Herrendorf G, Kurth C. Ictal near infrared spectroscopy in temporal lobe epilepsy: a pilot study. *Seizure* 1996; 5 (2): 97–101.

150 Villringer A, Planck J, Stodieck S, Botzel K, Schleinkofer L, Dirnagl U. Noninvasive assessment of cerebral hemodynamics and tissue oxygenation during activation of brain cell function in human adults using near infrared spectroscopy. *Adv Exp Med Biol* 1994; 345: 559–65.

151 Bode H. Intracranial blood flow velocities during seizures and generalized epileptic discharges. *Eur J Pediatr* 1992; 151 (9): 706–9.

152 Klingelhofer J, Bischoff C, Sander D, Wittich I, Conrad B. Do brief bursts of spike and wave activity cause a cerebral hyper- or hypoperfusion in man? *Neurosci Lett* 1991; 127 (1): 77–81.

153 Nehlig A, Vergnes M, Waydelich R *et al.* Absence seizures induce a decrease in cerebral blood flow: human and animal data. *J Cereb Blood Flow Metab* 1996; 16 (1): 147–55.

154 De Simone R, Silvestrini M, Marciani MG, Curatolo P. Changes in cerebral blood flow velocities during childhood absence seizures. *Pediatr Neurol* 1998; 18 (2): 132–5.

155 Engel J, Kuhl DE, Phelps ME. Patterns of human local cerebral glucose metabolism during epileptic seizures. *Science* 1982; 218 (4567): 64–6.

156 Engel J Jr, Lubens P, Kuhl DE, Phelps ME. Local cerebral metabolic rate for glucose during petit mal absences. *Ann Neurol* 1985; 17 (2): 121–8.

157 Theodore WH, Brooks R, Margolin R *et al.* Positron emission tomography in generalized seizures. *Neurology* 1985; 35 (5): 684–90.

158 Nehlig A, Vergnes M, Marescaux C, Boyet S, Lannes B. Local cerebral glucose utilization in rats with petit mal-like seizures. *Ann Neurol* 1991; 29 (1): 72–7.

159 Niehaus L, Wieshmann UC, Meyer B. Changes in cerebral hemodynamics during simple partial motor seizures. *Eur Neurol* 2000; 44 (1): 8–11.

160 Lee HW, Hong SB, Tae WS. Opposite ictal perfusion patterns of subtracted SPECT. Hyperperfusion and hypoperfusion. *Brain* 2000; 123 (Part 10): 9.

161 Buxton RB, Wong EC, Frank LR. Dynamics of blood flow and oxygenation changes during brain activation: the balloon model. *Magn Reson Med* 1998; 39 (6): 855–64.

162 Mandeville JB, Marota JJ, Ayata C *et al.* Evidence of a cerebrovascular postarteriole windkessel with delayed compliance. *J Cereb Blood Flow Metab* 1999; 19 (6): 679–89.

163 Magistretti PJ. Cellular bases of functional brain imaging: insights from neuron-glia metabolic coupling. *Brain Res* 2000; 886 (1–2): 108–12.

164 Ogawa S, Lee TM, Kay AR, Tank DW. Brain magnetic resonance imaging with contrast dependent on blood oxygenation. *Proc Natl Acad Sci USA* 1990; 87 (24): 9868–72.

165 Ives JR, Warach S, Schmitt F, Edelman RR, Schomer DL. Monitoring the patient's EEG during echo planar MRI. *Electroencephalogr Clin Neurophysiol* 1993; 87 (6): 417–20.

166 Lemieux L, Allen PJ, Franconi F, Symms MR, Fish DR. Recording of EEG during fMRI experiments: patient safety. *Magn Reson Med* 1997; 38 (6): 943–52.

167 Huang-Hellinger F, Hans C, McCormack G *et al.* Simultaneous functional magnetic resonance imaging and electrophysiological recording. *Hum Brain Mapping* 1995; 3: 13–23.

168 Krakow K, Allen PJ, Symms MR, Lemieux L, Josephs O, Fish DR. EEG recording during fMRI experiments: Image quality. *Hum Brain Mapping* 2000; 10: 10–15.

169 Bonmassar G, Hadjikhani N, Ives JR, Hinton D, Belliveau JW. Influence of EEG electrodes on the BOLD fMRI signal. *Hum Brain Mapping* 2001; 14 (2): 108–15.

170 Goldman RI, Stern JM, Engel J, Cohen MS. Acquiring simultaneous EEG and functional MRI. *Clin Neurophysiol* 2000; 111 (11): 1974–80.

171 Allen PJ, Polizzi G, Krakow K, Fish DR, Lemieux L. Identification of EEG events in the MR scanner: The problem of pulse artifact and a method for its subtraction. *Neuroimage* 1998; 8: 229–39.

172 Friston KJ, Holmes AP, Worsley KJ, Poline JB, Frith CD, Frackowiak RS. Statistical parametric maps in functional imaging: a general linear approach. *Hum Brain Mapping* 1995; 2: 189–210.

173 Krakow K, Allen PJ, Lemieux L, Symms MR, Fish DR. Methodology: EEG-correlated fMRI. *Adv Neurol* 2000; 83: 187–201.

174 Schomer DL, Bonmassar G, Lazeyras F *et al.* EEG-linked functional magnetic resonance imaging in epilepsy and cognitive neurophysiology. *J Clin Neurophysiol* 2000; 17 (1): 43–58.

175 Allen PJ, Josephs O, Turner R. A method for removing imaging artifact from continuous EEG recorded during functional MRI. *Neuroimage* 2000; 12 (2): 230–9.

176 Hoffmann A, Jager L, Werhahn KJ, Jaschke M, Noachtar S, Reiser M. Electroencephalography during functional echo-planar imaging: Detec-

tion of epileptic spikes using post-processing methods. *Magn Reson Med* 2000; 44 (5): 791–8.

177 Jackson GD, Connelly A, Cross JH, Gordon I, Gadian DG. Functional magnetic resonance imaging of focal seizures. *Neurology* 1994; 44 (5): 850–6.

178 Detre JA, Sirven JI, Alsop DC, O'Connor MJ, French JA. Localization of subclinical ictal activity by functional magnetic resonance imaging: correlation with invasive monitoring. *Ann Neurol* 1995; 38 (4): 618–24.

179 Detre JA, Alsop DC, Aguirre GK, Sperling MR. Coupling of cortical and thalamic ictal activity in human partial epilepsy: demonstration by functional magnetic resonance imaging. *Epilepsia* 1996; 37 (7): 657–61.

180 Krings T, Topper R, Reinges MH *et al.* Hemodynamic changes in simple partial epilepsy: a functional MRI study. *Neurology* 2000; 54 (2): 524–7.

181 Salek-Haddadi A, Merschhemke M, Lemieux L, Fish DR. Simultaneous EEG-correlated ictal fMRI. *Neuroimage* 2002; 16 (1): 32–40.

182 Lee AT, Glover GH, Meyer CH. Discrimination of large venous vessels in time-course spiral blood oxygen level dependent magnetic resonance functional neuroimaging. *Magn Reson Med* 1995; 33 (6): 745–54.

183 Miezin FM, Maccotta L, Ollinger JM, Petersen SE, Buckner RL. Characterizing the hemodynamic response: effects of presentation rate, sampling procedure, and the possibility of ordering brain activity based on relative timing. *Neuroimage* 2000; 11 (6 Part 1): 735–59.

184 Buckner RL, Bandettini PA, O'Craven KM *et al.* Detection of cortical activation during averaged single trials of a cognitive task using functional magnetic resonance imaging. *Proc Natl Acad Sci USA* 1996; 93 (25): 14878–83.

185 Josephs O, Henson RN. Event-related functional magnetic resonance imaging: modelling, inference and optimization. *Philos Trans R Soc Lond B Biol Sci* 1999; 354 (1387): 1215–28.

186 Lemieux L, Salek-Haddadi A, Josephs O *et al.* Event-related fMRI with simultaneous and continuous EEG: description method initial case report. *Neuroimage* 2001; 14 (3): 780–7.

187 *Benar CG, Gross DW, Wang Y *et al.* The BOLD response to interictal epileptiform discharges. *Neuroimage* 2002; 17 (3): 1182–92.

188 Frahm J, Merboldt KD, Hanicke W, Kleinschmidt A, Boecker H. Brain or vein – oxygenation or flow? On signal physiology in functional MRI of human brain activation. *NMR Biomed* 1994; 7 (1–2): 45–53.

189 Mulderink TA, Gitelman DR, Mesulam MM, Parrish TB. On the use of caffeine as a contrast booster for BOLD fMRI studies. *Neuroimage* 2002; 15 (1): 37–44.

190 Krakow K, Messina D, Lemieux L, Duncan JS, Fish DR. Functional MRI activation of individual interictal epileptiform spikes. *Neuroimage* 2001; 13 (3): 502–5.

191 Warach S, Ives JR, Schlaug G *et al.* EEG-triggered echo-planar functional MRI in epilepsy. *Neurology* 1996; 47 (1): 89–93.

192 Seeck M, Lazeyras F, Michel CM *et al.* Non-invasive epileptic focus localization using EEG-triggered functional MRI and electromagnetic tomography. *Electroencephalogr Clin Neurophysiol* 1998; 106 (6): 508–12.

193 Patel MR, Blum A, Pearlman JD *et al.* Echo-planar functional MR imaging of epilepsy with concurrent EEG monitoring. *Am J Neuroradiol* 1999; 20 (10): 1916–19.

194 Symms MR, Allen PJ, Woermann FG *et al.* Reproducible localization of interictal epileptiform discharges using EEG-triggered fMRI. *Phys Med Biol* 1999; 44 (7): 161–168.

195 Krakow K, Woermann FG, Symms MR *et al.* EEG-triggered functional MRI of interictal epileptiform activity in patients with partial seizures. *Brain* 1999; 122 (9): 1679–88.

196 Krakow K, Wieshmann UC, Woermann FG *et al.* Multimodal MR imaging: functional, diffusion tensor, and chemical shift imaging in a patient with localization-related epilepsy. *Epilepsia* 1999; 40 (10): 1459–62.

197 Lazeyras F, Blanke O, Perrig S *et al.* EEG-triggered functional MRI in patients with pharmacoresistant epilepsy. *J Magn Reson Imaging* 2000; 12 (1): 177–85.

198 Baudewig J, Bittermann HJ, Paulus W, Frahm J. Simultaneous EEG and functional MRI of epileptic activity: a case report. *Clin Neurophysiol* 2001; 112 (7): 1196–200.

199 Krakow K, Lemieux L, Messina D *et al.* Spatio-temporal imaging of focal interictal epileptiform activity using EEG-triggered functional MRI. *Epileptic Disord* 2001; 3 (2): 67–74.

200 Lemieux L, Krakow K, Fish DR. Comparison of spike-triggered functional MRI BOLD activation and EEG dipole model localization. *Neuroimage* 2001; 14 (5): 1097–104.

201 Jager L, Werhahn KJ, Hoffmann A *et al.* Focal epileptiform activity in the brain: detection with spike-related functional MR imaging preliminary results. *Radiology* 2002; 223 (3): 860–9.

202 Duyn JH, Yang Y, Frank JA *et al.* Functional magnetic resonance neuroimaging data acquisition techniques. *Neuroimage* 1996; 4: S76–83.

203 Gaillard WD, Bookheimer SY, Cohen M. The use of fMRI in neocortical epilepsy. *Adv Neurol* 2000; 84: 391–404.

204 Price CJ, Friston KJ. Scanning patients with tasks they can perform. *Human Brain Mapping* 1999; 8: 102–8.

205 Binder JR, Frost JA, Hammeke TA, Bellgowan PSF, Rao SM, Cox RW. Conceptual processing during the conscious resting state: a functional MRI study. *J Cogn Neurosci* 1999; 11: 80–93.

206 Morris GL, Mueller WM, Yetkin FZ. *et al.* Functional magnetic resonance imaging in partial epilepsy. *Epilepsia* 1994; 35: 1194–8.

207 Achten E, Jackson GD, Cameron JA *et al.* Presurgical evaluation of the motor hand area with functional MR imaging in patients with tumours and dysplastic lesions. *Radiology* 1999; 210: 529–38.

208 Jack CR Jr, Thompson RM, Butts RK *et al.* Sensory motor cortex: correlation of presurgical mapping with functional MR imaging and invasive cortical mapping. *Radiology* 1994; 190: 85–92.

209 Puce A, Constable RT, Luby ML *et al.* Functional magnetic resonance imaging of sensory and motor cortex: comparison with electrophysiological localization. *J Neurosurg* 1995; 83: 262–70.

210 Krings T, Reinges MHT, Erberich S *et al.* Functional MRI for presurgical planning: problems, artefacts, and solution strategies. *J Neurol Neurosurg Psychiatr* 2001; 70: 749–60.

211 Richardson MP, Koepp MJ, Brooks DJ *et al.* Cerebral activation in malformations of cortical development. *Brain* 1998; 121: 1295–304.

212 Sisodiya SM. Surgery for malformations of cortical development causing epilepsy. *Brain* 2000; 123: 1075–91.

213 Pinard J, Feydy A, Carlier R *et al.* Functional MRI in double cortex: functionality of heterotopia. *Neurology* 2000; 54: 1531–3.

214 Spreer J, Martin P, Greenlee MW *et al.* Functional MRI in patients with band heterotopia. *Neuroimage* 2001; 14: 357–65.

215 Baxendale SA. Carotid amytal testing and other amytal procedures. In: Oxbury JM, Polkey CE, Duchowny M, eds. *Intractable Focal Epilepsy: Medical and Surgical Treatment*. London: W.B. Saunders, 1999.

216 Hertz-Pannier L, Gaillard WD, Mott SH. Non-invasive assessment of language dominance in children and adolescents with functional MRI. *Neurology* 1997; 48: 1003–12.

217 Stapleton SR, Kiriakipoulos E, Mikulsi D *et al.* Combined utility of functional MRI, cortical mapping, and frameless stereotaxy in the resection of lesions in eloquent areas of brain in children. *Pediatr Neurosurg* 1997; 26: 68–82.

218 Binder JR, Swanson SJ, Hammeke TA. *et al.* Determination of language dominance using functional MRI. A comparison with the Wada test. *Neurology* 1996; 46: 978–84.

219 Fitzgerald DB, Cosgrove GR, Ronner S. *et al.* Location of language in the cortex: a comparison between functional MR imaging and electrocortical stimulation. *Am J Neuroradiol* 1997; 18: 1529–39.

220 Yetkin FZ, Swanson S, Fischer M *et al.* Functional MR of frontal lobe activation: comparison with Wada language results. *Am J Neuroradiol* 1998; 19: 1095–8.

221 Benson RR, FitzGerald DB, LeSueur LL *et al.* Language dominance determined by whole brain functional MRI in patients with brain lesions. *Neurology* 1999; 52: 798–809.

222 Worthington C, Vincent DJ, Bryant AE *et al.* Comparison of functional magnetic resonance imaging for language localization and intracarotid speech amytal testing in presurgical evaluation for intractable epilepsy. Preliminary results. *Stereotact Funct Neurosurg* 1997; 69: 197–201.

223 Benbadis SR, Binder JR, Swanson SJ *et al.* Is speech arrest during Wada testing a valid method for determining hemispheric representation of language? *Brain Lang* 1998; 65: 441–6.

224 Springer JA, Binder JR, Hammeke TA *et al.* Language dominance in neurologically normal and epilepsy subjects. A functional MRI study. *Brain* 1999; 122: 2033–45.

225 Bahn MM, Lin W, Silbergeld DL *et al.* Localization of language cortices by

functional MR imaging compared with intracarotid amobarbital hemispheric sedation. *Am J Radiol* 1997; 169: 575–9.

226 Lehericy S, Cohen L, Bahin B *et al*. Functional MR evaluation of temporal and frontal language dominance compared with the WADA test. *Neurology* 2000; 54: 1625–33.

227 Billingsley RL, McAndrews MP, Crawley AP, Mikulis DJ. Functional MRI of phonological and semantic processing in temporal lobe epilepsy. *Brain* 2001; 124: 1218–27.

228 Gaillard WD. Structural and functional imaging in children with partial epilepsy. *MRDD Res Rev* 2000; 6: 220–6.

229 Benson RR, Logan WJ, Cosgrove GR *et al*. Functional MRI localization of language in a 9-year-old child. *Can J Neurol Sci* 1996; 23: 213–19.

230 Gaillard WD, Hertz-Pannier L, Mott SH, Barnett AS, LeBihan D, Theodore WH. Functional anatomy of cognitive development. FMRI of verbal fluency in children and adults. *Neurology* 2000; 54: 180–5.

231 Gaillard WD, Pugliese M, Grandin CB *et al*. Cortical localisation of reading in normal children. An fMRI language study. *Neurology* 2001; 57: 47–54.

232 Bellgowan PS, Binder JR, Swanson SJ *et al*. Side of seizure focus predicts left medial temporal lobe activation during verbal encoding. *Neurology* 1998; 51: 479–84.

233 Detre JA, Maccotta BS, King MD *et al*. Functional MRI lateralization of memory in temporal lobe epilepsy. *Neurology* 1998; 50: 926–32.

234 Jokeit H, Okujava M, Woermann FG. Memory fMRI lateralizes temporal lobe epilepsy. *Neurology* 2001; 57: 1786–92.

235 Dupont S, Van de Moortele PF, Samson S *et al*. Episodic memory in left temporal lobe epilepsy: a functional MRI study. *Brain* 2000; 123: 1722–32.

236 Maguire EA, Vargha-Khadem F, Mishkin M. The effects of bilateral hippocampal damage on fMRI regional activations and interactions during memory retrieval. *Brain* 2001; 124: 1156–70.

237 Penfield W, von Santha K, Cipriani A. Cerebral blood flow during induced epileptiform seizures in animals and man. *J Neurophysiol* 1939; 2: 257–67.

238 O'Brien TJ, O'Connor MK, Mullan BP *et al*. Subtraction ictal SPECT co-registered to MRI in partial epilepsy: description and technical validation of the method with phantom and patient studies. *Nucl Med Comm* 1998; 19 (1): 31–45.

239 Zubal IG, Spencer SS, Imam K *et al*. Difference images calculated from ictal and interictal technetium-99m-HMPAO SPECT scans of epilepsy. *J Nucl Med* 1995; 36: 684–9.

240 Erickson BJ, Jack CR Jr. Correlation of single photon emission CT with MR image data using fiduciary markers. *Am J Neuroradiol* 1993; 14: 713–20.

241 Brinkmann BH, O'Brien TJ, Aharon S *et al*. Quantitative and clinical analysis of SPECT image registration for epilepsy studies. *J Nucl Med* 1999; 40: 1098–105.

242 Woods RP, Grafton ST, Watson JD, Sicotte NL, Mazziotta JC. Automated image registration. II. Intersubject validation of linear and nonlinear models. *J Comput Assist Tomogr* 1998; 22: 153–65.

243 O'Brien TJ, So EL, Mullan BP *et al*. Subtraction ictal SPECT co-registered to MRI improves clinical usefulness of SPECT in localizing the surgical seizure focus. *Neurology* 1998; 50: 445–54.

244 O'Brien TJ, So EL, Mullan BP *et al*. Subtraction peri-ictal SPECT is predictive of extratemporal epilepsy surgery outcome. *Neurology* 2000; 55: 1668–77.

245 Mosewich RK, So EL, O'Brien TJ *et al*. Factors predictive of the outcome of frontal lobe epilepsy surgery. *Epilepsia* 2000; 41: 843–9.

246 O'Brien TJ, So EL, Mullan BP *et al*. Subtraction SPECT co-registered to MRI improves postictal SPECT localization of seizure foci. *Neurology* 1999; 52: 137–46.

247 So EL. Integration of EEG, MRI, and SPECT in localizing the seizure focus for epilepsy surgery. *Epilepsia* 2000; 41 (Suppl. 3): S48–S54.

248 Smith KR, Frank KJ, Bucholz RD. The NeuroStation—a highly accurate, minimally invasive solution to frameless stereotactic neurosurgery. *Comput Med Imaging Graph* 1994; 18: 247–56.

249 So EL, O'Brien TJ, Brinkmann BH, Mullan BP. The EEG evaluation of single photon emission computed tomography abnormalities in epilepsy. *J Clin Neurophysiol* 2000; 17: 10–28.

250 Salek-Haddadi A, Friston KJ, Lemieux L, Fish DR. Studying spontaneous EEG activity with fMRI. *Brain Res Brain Res Rev* 2003; 43(1): 110–33.

251 Diekmann V, Becker W, Jurgens R *et al*. Localisation of epileptic foci with electric, magnetic and combined electromagnetic models. *Electroencephalogr Clin Neurophysiol* 1998; 106(4): 297–313.

252 Baumgartner C, Pataraia E, Lindinger G, Deecke L. Magnetoencephalography in focal epilepsy. *Epilepsia* 2000; 41 (Suppl. 3): S39–47.

253 Anami K, Mori T, Tanaka F *et al*. Stepping stone sampling for retrieving artifact-free electroencephalograms during functional magnetic resonance imaging. *Neuroimage* 2003; 19 (2 Pt 1): 281–95.

254 Salek-Haddadi A, Lemieux L, Merschhemke M *et al*. Functional magnetic resonance imaging of human absence seizures. *Ann Neurol* 2003; 53(5): 663–7.

58 Psychological Testing in Presurgical Evaluation of Epilepsy

J. Djordjevic and M. Jones-Gotman

Neuropsychological evaluation is an essential part of the comprehensive investigation of patients who are candidates for surgical treatment of epilepsy. The decision as to whether a patient is an appropriate surgical candidate is based upon data gathered by a team of professionals. Some of the necessary information is anatomical, derived from neuroimaging, some is physiological (EEG) and some is based on clinical history and seizure pattern. The contribution of neuropsychology is unique in providing data about function through evaluation of a patient's strengths and weaknesses on cognitive tests. In recent years there has been an increase in the use of functional neuroimaging to localize critical sites for different cognitive functions in individual patients; this is an important new aspect of neuropsychological evaluation, but is beyond the scope of this chapter.

The information obtained through traditional neuropsychological testing methods is used in several ways. Interpretation of the pattern of results on neuropsychological tests gives information about the site of epileptic focus, inferred from the pattern of cognitive dysfunction. Although the sophisticated imaging techniques that are now able to evaluate brain structure and function overlap partially with neuropsychological information, they do not supplant it. In terms of their usefulness in localizing dysfunction, neuropsychological findings can reinforce or, if the findings disagree, question data from other sources about the site of seizure focus. When disagreement with other data occurs, those discrepancies can provoke further investigation. An unsuspected atypical representation of language is sometimes exposed in this way, and discrepant or unexpected findings from memory assessment can have a strong and direct impact on surgical management, as will be discussed below.

Because neuropsychological results show the functional effect of a lesion or of abnormally discharging tissue, they allow evaluation of the impact of an individual's epilepsy on his/her life and provide a basis for offering guidance. Preoperative neuropsychological measurements also form a solid basis for evaluating the outcome of surgery with respect to cognitive function by comparing pre- to postoperative performance on the neuropsychological tests. This provides an objective determination of possible changes that can affect an individual's work, schooling or other activities. Knowledge gained from postoperative studies has also allowed the development of predictors as another application of preoperative evaluation: this includes prediction of surgery outcome in terms of seizure control and in terms of postoperative cognitive change/decline.

Determination of site of dysfunction

A thorough neuropsychological evaluation requires 6–8 h of direct contact between patient and examiner. A basic battery of tests should sample many different cognitive functions. If the battery were tailored for each patient from the outset, evaluations would be skewed to reflect the examiner's expectations. However, after exploring the whole brain with a comprehensive basic battery, findings or hypotheses for individual patients can be pursued with further tests aimed at delineating that patient's cognitive profile more precisely.

An exception to the rule of a lengthy evaluation applies to very low-functioning patients with diffuse abnormality. In those cases only limited testing is possible, and failure on even the easiest cognitive tests reflects a concomitant widespread brain dysfunction. However, cerebral dominance for language is frequently in question in such individuals, and this can be determined with intracarotid amobarbital testing [1,2] in almost any cooperative patient without respect to intellectual capacity.

A basic battery includes measures of intelligence, fronto-executive skills, memory, attention, visuospatial abilities and language. Some sensory functions and motor skills are also tested. Such an arsenal of tests taps function in the frontal and temporal lobes, and also parietal and more posterior regions. At its most fundamental level, the method underlying neuropsychological evaluation is to determine the dysfunctional hemisphere by comparing a patient's performance on verbal tasks to performance on visuospatial or visuoperceptual ones, and within the hemisphere to determine the dysfunctional region by comparing performance on various kinds of tasks. Results from this thorough, usually standardized, assortment of measures provide a reliable way of characterizing and quantifying the nature and degree of cognitive dysfunction arising from epilepsy. Candidates for corpus callosotomy or hemispherectomy most frequently have diffuse, or diffuse unilateral, abnormality and show depressed scores on most cognitive tests. In contrast, candidates for multiple subpial transsections [3] may have exquisitely focal abnormality in unresectable cortex, and show specific deficits on cognitive tests. In this chapter, the emphasis will be on testing methods that are useful in focal, surgically treatable epilepsy.

One approach to presurgical neuropsychological evaluation has been the so-called immediate postictal examination. Several studies comparing the interictal (standard) and immediate postictal evaluations (usually within 1 h of seizure) showed that a significant improvement in focus localization could be achieved if postictal evaluation is done (e.g. [4]). This approach may be particularly helpful in cases where interictal neuropsychological findings fall within the normal range [4].

Potential pitfalls in presurgical evaluation

Neuropsychological evaluation of unoperated epilepsy patients can be a challenge for a variety of reasons. Various demographic, medication and seizure-related variables have been shown to exert differential influences on performance. Some examples of demographic factors with a possible mediating role in neuropsychological functioning are gender and age, while seizure-related factors include age at onset of epilepsy, duration of disorder, seizure frequency, seizure spread, etc. These factors should not be ignored when interpreting results from an individual's preoperative evaluation. Potential problems that can affect findings and/or interpretation in neuropsychological practice will be introduced here and discussed further in the sections to follow.

First, as a cautionary note, one should be aware that some neuropsychological tests used in epilepsy may be based on findings from patients with other kinds of brain pathology. This application from one type of pathology to another arises from a logical assumption that patients with a same lesion localization will display the same or similar pattern of deficits (despite varying aetiologies underlying the brain damage). This assumption has been shown to be inaccurate in some cases [5]. Although the same principles of brain function and dysfunction apply generally, different pathological processes can vary, and extrapolating findings from one type of brain pathology to another may not always be appropriate. Traumatic brain injury, neoplasms, vascular disorders, brain damage due to different toxic conditions, degenerative disorders of the nervous system or infectious processes in the brain have specific features in terms of depth of lesion and involvement of cortical and/or subcortical structures, stability over time, presence of diffuse and/or distance effects and presence of diseased or dead brain tissue [6].

Furthermore, the pathological substrate of epileptogenic lesions is itself heterogeneous. For example, the most frequent structural abnormality found in temporal lobe epilepsy (TLE) is hippocampal sclerosis (HS). However, other neuropathological processes such as tumours, malformations, cerebrovascular accidents, trauma and infections are associated with epilepsy. It remains unclear whether HS and other seizure-inducing pathological processes at the same location may affect neuropsychological performance differently. Epileptic patients may or may not have discernible brain damage, and the existence of possible differential effects of lesional vs. non-lesional TLE on neuropsychological performance remains an open question. For example, whereas Hermann et al. [7] reported worse performance in TLE patients with HS than in those without it, others claimed no differences between TLE patients with vs. without visible morphological changes in the brain [8]. Related to these issues is the question of detecting dysfunction in subregions within the major brain lobes. Although some progress in such finer analyses has been made in experimental neuropsychology, attempts in clinical practice to demonstrate differential profiles associated with specific subregions within lobes of the brain have been either unsuccessful or inconsistent. As one example, Giovagnoli and Avanzini [8] were unable to demonstrate a difference between patient groups with left or right medial vs. lateral temporal epileptogenic lesions on several verbal and non-verbal memory measures, nor could they find any effects related to the presence or type of a visible lesion.

A second potential problem is that much of neuropsychological clinical practice derives from information gained from operated patients; preoperative studies, although increasing, are still uncommon. This generalization from operated patients to unoperated ones was based on the expectation that tests that demonstrate deficits in operated epilepsy patients should be sensitive also to focal dysfunction related to a discharging epileptic focus. However, the cognitive effects of surgical lesions are not directly comparable to the effects of brain pathology generating seizures. Cognitive deficits are often more difficult to demonstrate in unoperated than in operated patients, possibly owing to such factors as the size of the lesion (larger in the case of surgical lesions) and uniformity of surgical vs. heterogeneity of epileptogenic lesions. Fortunately, the number of studies providing data on unoperated epileptic patients is growing.

A third problem encountered in the field is a relative lack of analogous verbal and non-verbal tests. The concept of hemispheric specialization is widely accepted in neuropsychological practice, and therefore verbal and non-verbal tests are commonly used for assessment of the dominant and non-dominant hemispheres, respectively. However these tests have often been different in a variety of ways, introducing noise and interfering with direct comparisons of the functional abilities of the two hemispheres, especially in the clinical setting where it is most important to compare results from the various tests within an individual patient. A strategy of using matched verbal and non-verbal tasks to study analogous brain regions in left and right hemispheres adds power to the neuropsychologist's ability to localize dysfunction and to analyse the nature of a patient's deficits. We consider this idea particularly important and will discuss it in more detail later in the chapter. We are pleased to note that the concept is becoming more widespread in test development, resulting in a growing availability of such paired verbal/non-verbal neuropsychological tests.

Last but not least are the issues of clinical utility of neuropsychological instruments and the development and publication of norms for neuropsychological tests. The number of tests proven to be effective for presurgical evaluation of patients with epilepsy is not large. Even those demonstrated to distinguish between different clinical groups may be successful on the group but not on the individual level: when a test can distinguish among patient groups with epileptogenic lesions of different locations, the questions of its sensitivity and specificity need to be answered. Thus, a valuable diagnostic tool should be able not only to distinguish among groups, but also to classify individual subjects with a high degree of accuracy. Finally, the field needs published norms on its tests, to allow meaningful interpretation of results. Neuropsychological expertise depends on the use of sensitive tests and a solid database about those tests, and happily, this is an area of growth in recent years.

Despite these caveats, the field has matured well over the past several years and there are many instruments in current use to evaluate patients for epilepsy surgery. Our discussion of methods of evaluation will be organized primarily (but not solely) by brain region, beginning with that very large and heterogeneous expanse of cortex, the frontal lobes.

Evaluation of frontal lobe function

Contemporary characterizations of frontal lobe functioning have shifted the emphasis from anatomically based descriptions (i.e.

frontal or prefrontal lobe syndrome or signs) to functional ones, encompassing a variety of psychological constructs and with the concept of 'executive function' being a particularly prevalent descriptor. Although definitions of this concept vary from one author to another (e.g. [6,9]), most agree that a part of the known functions of this brain region has to do with planning, initiation, organization, self-monitoring, self-regulation and decision making. Among measures commonly used to explore possible damage in the frontal lobes are tests of problem-solving, fluency, susceptibility to interference, planning and motor skills. Among the earliest objective measures were formal word fluency tests, which documented the clinically known paucity of spontaneous speech in patients with severe frontal lobe damage, and a card sorting test, which tapped several aspects of frontal lobe damage including problem-solving, impulsivity and inability to use cues to guide behaviour. Some of the most frequent 'frontal lobe' tests now used for evaluation of patients with epilepsy will be described and roughly categorized in this section.

Problem-solving: WCST and MCST

In addition to the well-known Wisconsin Card Sorting test (WCST) as a problem-solving task [10], a modified and shorter version, called the Modified Card Sorting test (MCST), has been introduced [11]. In the MCST, the deck consists of 48 (instead of 128) cards, from which all cards that share more than one attribute with a stimulus card have been removed. A completed category consists of six (instead of 10) consecutive correct responses, after which the patient is told that the rule has changed. There has been much debate as to whether the two versions of this task are comparable in terms of their sensitivity to frontal lobe disturbance and in terms of the psychological functions they measure. However, it seems that both are being used for clinical purposes in neuropsychological assessments of patients with epilepsy. Therefore, findings from both tests will be considered here. In the first studies using the WCST with epileptic patients, Milner [12] reported that patients with resection from a frontal lobe, especially the left frontal lobe [13], show an impairment on this task. Since that time the literature has grown to contain many articles concerning the sensitivity or lack of sensitivity of this task to frontal lobe dysfunction (e.g. [14]). Furthermore, several studies have demonstrated that a significant proportion of patients with TLE display deficits on card sorting tests (e.g. [15–17]). We undertook a retrospective study of WCST performance in 50 patients with unilateral resection from a frontal lobe (25 left, 25 right) and 40 patients (20 left, 20 right) with unilateral resection from a temporal lobe. The temporal lobe cases were included as a lesion control group and were therefore selected randomly from the same time period as the frontal lobe patients [18]. Preoperatively, we found no differences in performance among our four groups of patients (unpublished results). Postoperatively, we found that the left frontal lobe group did significantly worse on all measures compared to the right frontal and left temporal lobe groups, but they did not differ from the right temporal lobe group. In fact, the right temporal lobe group performed worse than the left frontal lobe group on one measure. Clearly, poor performance on this task can occur in patients with dysfunction in the right [15,17,18] or left [16] temporal lobe, in addition to the traditionally expected deficit after left frontal lobe damage.

Despite the data pointing to a poor card sorting performance in patients with TLE, there is no agreement about the determinants of such performance. Some authors believe that structural damage of the temporal lobes, and HS in particular, may be the crucial factor [16–18]. Others suggest that functional disruption of extratemporal regions might be responsible [15,19,20].

Thus, although many still consider performance on card sorting tests to be a 'gold standard' and a 'marker of prefrontal pathology', the empirical evidence has failed to confirm its exclusive relationship with frontal lobe pathology in patients with epilepsy. This is consistent with findings obtained in patients with brain pathology of other aetiologies. Interpretation of results obtained from this test should be made cautiously, and should be viewed together with results obtained from other tests of frontal lobe function.

Generation of novel responses: word and design fluency

One implication from the card sorting data is that it may be difficult to detect deficits associated with right frontal lobe damage. One of the rare measures shown to be able to capture dysfunction of the non-dominant frontal lobe is the Design Fluency test (DFT) [21,22], which is used to measure fluency in the non-verbal mode. The task requirements are to create original abstract designs that do not represent anything and cannot be named, and to produce as many different designs as possible in 5 min. On average, healthy subjects produce about 16 acceptable drawings. Patients with right frontal lobe or right central lesions are impaired on this task, producing on average five or six acceptable designs, while patients with left frontal lesions, or left or right temporal lobe lesions are not impaired [22]. Patients with parietal lobe damage also perform normally according to a study [21] that included a small group of patients with parietal resection. The inability of patients with damage in the right frontal lobe to produce novel designs is manifested in some cases simply by a low output, which may also involve looking around the room for inspiration. Rule breaking, which in the 'free condition' of the test usually consists of making representational drawings, is also observed often in this group of patients. However, in some frontal lobe patients the deficit is characterized by perseveration: drawings are produced, but they are all alike. Figure 58.1 shows three examples of design fluency, one from a healthy subject (a) and two from patients with a right frontal lobe lesion. One patient (b) illustrates a low output, while the other (c) illustrates a highly perseverative output. In both cases, the score (acceptable drawings) is very low.

Different researchers have shown that DFT is characterized by very good intra- [23] and interrater reliability [23–25], and convergent and divergent validity [23]. Normative data for DFT have been published [25].

In contrast to their poor performance on the DFT, patients with a right frontal lobe lesion can do very well on verbal fluency tasks, and patients with a left frontal lobe lesion can perform well on figural fluency but poorly on word fluency. Comparing an individual's performance on paired verbal and visuoperceptual tasks that are as similar as possible except for the actual material (e.g. words vs. designs) of each task aids in teasing out subtle deficits. In this case, comparing verbal to figural fluency within an individual patient can help determine whether there is frontal lobe abnormality, and can also indicate the side of dysfunction. This is especially relevant given

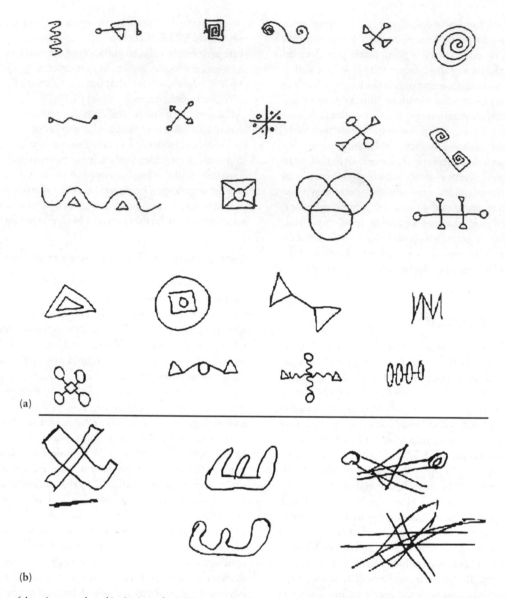

Fig. 58.1 Examples of drawings produced in 5 min in the DFT. (a) Productions made by a healthy control subject. This subject made three drawings that were discounted as perseverative (scoring not shown); producing a few such errors is normal [21]. (b, c) Drawings made by two patients with right frontal lobe resection. (b) The patient, a clerk, had a full-scale IQ of 112. The underlined drawing represented a sculpture in his town, as did the drawing that resembles a rotated E. In addition to these representational drawings, which are not allowed, the patient repeated one of the 'sculptures' (perseverative error), and the two remaining drawings were also highly similar to one another. This illustrates low output, rule-breaking and perseveration.

that discrimination between left and right frontal lobe damage may be difficult if based only on verbal fluency tasks, including letter-based and semantic (category) fluency [26]. Furthermore, some patients with left TLE may perform poorly on verbal fluency tasks [27], so it may be difficult to make distinctions between patients with TLE and frontal lobe epilepsy (FLE) based on word fluency tasks [17,28,29].

Susceptibility to interference: the Stroop test

In addition to requiring a capacity for generating or producing responses, fluency tasks require mental flexibility. Such flexibility is an important aspect of frontal lobe function, and it is often explored also with the Stroop test [30], which in its 'interference condition' requires that one inhibit a common or well-practised response and produce instead an uncommon one. In that condition, patients are shown words naming colours (e.g. the word 'red') printed in a colour other than what is written (e.g. 'red' written in yellow ink); they must name the colour of the ink and inhibit the more common response to read the words. Perret [31] demonstrated greatest impairment in patients with left frontal lobe lesions on this task. Mixed results are found with epilepsy patients. Richer *et al.* [32] showed that patients with surgical frontal lesions are slower than patients with temporal excisions or healthy control subjects on the Stroop task, and Upton and Thompson [29] reported the same finding in unoperated patients. However, Corcoran and Upton [17] did

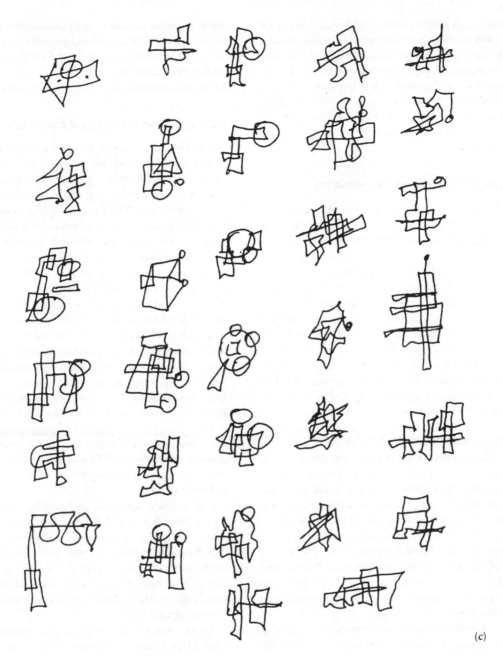

(c)

Fig. 58.1 *Continued.* (c) This patient, a geologist, had a full-scale IQ of 128. His output illustrates extreme perseveration: although he made many drawings, they are all alike.

not find significant differences between candidates for temporal vs. frontal lobe surgery, and Helmstaedter *et al.* [28] also reported impairments on this test in unoperated patients with either FLE or TLE. Thus it seems that the Stroop interference condition is sensitively to the effects of frontal surgical lesions, but may not consistently reveal dysfunction in preoperative epilepsy patients with frontal lobe seizure origin. In addition, lateralized effects on the Stroop test have not been demonstrated in epilepsy patients, although worse performance after left than after right frontal lesions has been documented in patients with brain damage of other aetiologies.

Planning: the Tower of London test

Tests of planning ability are among the staples for assessment of frontal lobe function; various versions of maze tests have been used for this purpose. One of the more recent tests measuring planning that has gained wide acceptance is the Tower of London test [33]. This test comprises a series of trials in which coloured beads must be moved from an initial position to a goal position in the smallest possible number of moves. For optimum performance, the sequence of moves should be planned before the first move is made. Initial studies showed that patients with predominantly left anterior lesions perform poorly on this test (e.g. [33]), but some later studies failed to confirm this finding in patients with lesions restricted to the frontal lobes [34]. Owen *et al.* [35] compared the performance of patients with aetiologically heterogeneous frontal lobe surgical lesions to that of healthy control subjects and patients with resection from a temporal lobe, and showed a clear impairment in those with frontal lobe resections. In contrast to the lateralized findings reported by Shallice [33] suggesting a specific role of the left frontal lobe, Owen *et al.* [35] did not find differences between unilateral left vs. right frontal lobe surgery.

Motor tasks: strength, dexterity and coordination

Many neuropsychologists include motor tasks as measures of frontal lobe function. Among these measures are strength tasks using hand or pinch dynamometer, manual dexterity tasks as measured by the Purdue or Grooved Pegboard tests, finger tapping tests and sequential unimanual and bimanual tapping (see [6]). The first factor to consider when interpreting results from motor tasks is gender. As women and men are known to differ significantly (e.g. [36,37]), separate norms should be used according to gender. In addition, a gender difference in the *pattern* of deficits has been noted on some motor tasks [38,39]. For example, women but not men with left frontal lobe damage display bilateral deficits on handgrip strength [38] or tapping in place [39]. This suggests that a different cortical organization of motor functions may exist in women vs. men (the notion being that functions are less focally organized in women). A second factor to be considered is age, as decline of performance on various motor tasks has been associated with advancing age [37]. A third important factor is hand dominance [37], as one expects performance to be superior using the dominant vs. non-dominant hand. If differences between the hands are unusually large or in an unexpected direction, dysfunction in the contralateral motor and/or premotor and prefrontal cortex is implicated. However, patients with either left or right frontal lobe lesions show impairments on simultaneous bimanual tapping [38]. Therefore a deficit on this complex bimanual task (which requires simultaneous coordination of different movements of the left and right hand) can be interpreted as a possible indicator of a frontal lobe dysfunction without respect to laterality.

There is ample evidence that motor performance is affected in patients with focal damage in motor and premotor cortex and also in patients who have prefrontal abnormalities that do not involve motor areas [28,39,40]. However, a relationship between the site of resection within the frontal lobe (lateral vs. premotor/supplementary motor area) and impaired motor coordination could not be demonstrated, except that frontal lobe resections with additional multiple subpial transections affecting the primary motor cortex tended to have a negative effect on motor coordination [40].

As we have pointed out for other tests, most of the data on motor tasks were obtained on patients who had undergone epilepsy surgery, and it remains unknown to what extent these motor tasks are sensitive to subtle damage in preoperative patients. The few reports that do exist, however, are positive: Upton and Thompson [29] showed that a deficit in copying gesture sequences is a discriminative feature in presurgical FLE vs. TLE. Similarly, Helmstaedter *et al.* [28] showed that motor coordination (as measured by uni- and bimanual alternating hand sequences, i.e. fist/edge/palm) was selec-

tively impaired in unoperated patients with FLE and not in those with TLE, although they found no laterality effects. Again, in individual cases a pattern of unilateral weakness or lack of dexterity and/or coordination on more than one of these tasks adds strength to the findings and allows one to make a diagnosis.

Concluding comments about frontal lobe function

There is still a scarcity of data on tests sensitive to a frontal lobe seizure focus in unoperated patients. Most of the clinical lore relies on deficits documented in patients who had surgical removals, a practice that we have already criticized in this chapter. For example, our comparison of WCST performance in unoperated patients with presumed lesions or dysfunction in frontal vs. temporal lobes revealed no differences [18], although differences would be expected based on findings obtained with operated patients. Similarly, no study to our knowledge showed a sensitivity of the Tower of London test in unoperated epilepsy patients. The Stroop test also seems to be sensitive to frontal lesions after surgery [32], while its value in localizing frontal lobe dysfunction before epilepsy surgery is inconsistent [17,28,29]. One study that used verbal and nonverbal fluency tasks failed to distinguish between frontal and temporal lobe seizure focus in unoperated patients [28], but the fluency tests used in that study were a letter-based task using three letters and a modified Five-Point test [41]. We would argue that the Five-Point test is more an attention task than a fluency task because patients are not required to generate responses, but only to manipulate stimuli provided for them and to monitor their responses. The question of whether the DFT and its verbal analogue can distinguish better between preoperative patients with left vs. right FLE remains to be addressed.

Only a few studies have analysed the neuropsychological profiles of patients with FLE before surgery. Among these, Upton and Thompson [29] were unable to show consistent deficits associated with frontal lobe epileptic dysfunction, motor coordination being an exception. Helmstaedter *et al.* [28,40] have suggested that a pattern of impaired motor coordination and/or response inhibition may be the profile that distinguishes unoperated patients with FLE from those with TLE.

An important factor in using and interpreting tests to assess frontal lobe function is the complexity of the cognitive operations that they measure. Most of them tap several important skills, and it is artificial to attempt to categorize them. For example, the Stroop test requires attention and naming in addition to mental flexibility and susceptibility to interference. Although the WCST has been in use for more than half a century, there does not seem to be agreement as to what functions are crucial for its execution: concept formation, set maintenance, set shifting, working memory, rule learning, problem-solving and use of feedback information have all been suggested as cognitive operations probed by this test. Similarly, an important aspect of fluency tests is the ability to produce or generate responses, but they also depend on mental flexibility and on an ability to sustain attention. In other words, neuropsychological tests in most cases do not measure single cognitive operations. This is why convergent qualitative and quantitative signs, suggesting coherent profiles, should be used rather than single indicators in making diagnostic hypotheses or conclusions.

Evaluation of parietal lobes

Traditional tests of parietal lobe function in patients with stroke, tumour or other large lesions are well known. Demonstration of parietal lobe dysfunction in patients with epilepsy arising from a parietal lobe focus is more difficult, and the frank impairments seen after extensive lesions are not seen or are attenuated. Salanova et al. [42] described a series of 82 patients with non-tumoural parietal lobe epilepsy treated surgically at the Montreal Neurological Hospital between 1929 and 1988. Preoperative neuropsychological evaluation was available in 30 patients from that series, and postoperative results were available in 27 of them. Preoperatively, impairment of spatial ability was reported in nine (30%) and was marked in four (13%) of these patients, as revealed by difficulties reproducing complex pictorial material, constructing block designs and/or by right–left confusion. Unilateral visuospatial neglect was observed in two patients with right parietal lesions, expressed through not completing the left side of drawings. Two others displayed a deficit in card sorting. New ($n = 7$) or exacerbated ($n = 2$) deficits appeared in some of these patients after focal parietal resection; those deficits included dressing apraxia and difficulty identifying faces, and disturbances in spatial orientation, visuoconstructive functions and body image. Two patients also showed acalculia, anomia, agraphia and partial auditory and verbal agnosia. The implications of this study were that patients with parietal lobe epilepsy constitute a neuropsychologically heterogeneous group, and that their focal lesions result in observable deficits in a significant minority of cases. A recently published study of two patients evaluated both pre- and postoperatively following parietal lobe resections failed to document any deficits in visuospatial perception or manipulation, nor was there any sign of unilateral neglect or body schema disturbance [43]. The authors interpreted these findings of preserved neuropsychological functioning as reflecting plasticity of this cortical region, suggesting that some other cortical regions might have taken over the organization of attentional and visuospatial processing in those patients.

A retrospective look at our own pre- and postoperative data on epileptic patients with neocortical epilepsies revealed some significant findings. A very poor or distorted copy of the complex Rey–Osterrieth Figure [44,45] is believed to arise from interference in parietal lobe function. As our sample included a small number of patients ($n = 13$, eight left and five right) with highly focal damage confined to the left or right parietal lobe, we were able to test that notion. Our analysis showed that this is true only of patients with a right parietal focus (unpublished data). In contrast, our results with the same sample of patients show the least efficient reading in the patients with left parietal focus. Somatosensory tests are also used to evaluate the parietal region [6,46]. In the same retrospective study we had data from a systematic test of two-point discrimination on the palms of the hands. The results showed raised thresholds contralateral to the focus in the right parietal group compared to the left. As with many other tasks, the difference was more pronounced after surgery.

To summarize, evaluation of parietal lobe function and dysfunction in epilepsy remains a challenge. A part of the difficulty in demonstrating deficits may be that most patients with a parietal epileptic focus have minor or subtle abnormalities that cannot be detected by neuropsychological tests. It is also likely that we have not yet developed the optimal instruments that will allow us to detect those subtle abnormalities. Among the measures currently available, those that test visuoconstructive and visuospatial functions, reading and somatosensory functions seem to be the best and to present the approach to be pursued in developing new instruments.

Evaluation of occipital lobes

An occipital lobe focus is rare in epilepsy. As a consequence, little effort has been made to develop special tests of occipital lobe dysfunction for epileptic patients. Tests of visual perception that are available include tests of visual (in)attention and scanning (cancellation tests, line bisection test), colour processing (perception, recognition, naming), face recognition and discrimination, visuospatial processing (Benton Judgment of Line Orientation, Hooper Visual Organization test) and visual interference (Hidden and Overlapping Figures tests) (see [6] for details on these tests). These instruments offer evaluation of visual and/or visuospatial functioning with minimal or no engagement of the motor system. Although deficits on some of these tests have been associated with right posterior cerebral lesions (e.g. [47]), the findings have not always been consistent. In particular, the clinical utility of these tests in preoperative evaluations of patients with epilepsy remains questionable given the lack, or inconclusiveness, of published findings.

Going beyond the paucity of information on individual tests sensitive to occipital lobe damage, information on full neuropsychological profiles of patients with occipital lobe epilepsy are also practically non-existent. Gülgönen et al. [48] published a study of neuropsychological functioning in 21 children with idiopathic occipital lobe epilepsy. Their results suggested subtle cognitive deficits in attention, memory and intellectual functioning (WISC-R full-scale IQ), but not in visuomotor and executive functioning, in patients with occipital lobe epilepsy compared with matched healthy control subjects. The clinical utility of these data remains unclear, however, because no other lesion groups were included in the study, leaving open the question of the discriminant value of the findings.

Fleischman et al. [49] reported a case study of a patient who had most of his right occipital lobe removed for the treatment of intractable epilepsy: he was found to have intact performance on standardized neuropsychological tests of attention, memory, language, perception and reasoning. However, a very specific deficit was found: this patient had intact visuoperceptual explicit memory (recall and recognition), but his visuoperceptual implicit (repetition priming) memory was impaired. This lack of superiority for previously presented visual stimuli on word identification and visual stem completion tasks (in the context of preserved visual recognition memory) was interpreted as indicating that visuoperceptual implicit memory processes may be subserved by the right occipital cortex [49].

As can be seen from the brevity of this section, patients with seizures originating in the occipital lobes are uncommon, resulting in a scarcity of information about their neuropsychological profiles.

Further studies are needed to address the question of cognitive deficits displayed by these patients.

Evaluation of temporal neocortex

Although memory is the hallmark of medial temporal lobe function, several other types of measures are used to assess the temporal neocortex. Among the most important of these are word retrieval tests (e.g. [50]). Word-finding difficulties are among the first complaints to be made by patients with a lesion or focus in the dominant hemisphere, and the importance of testing confrontation naming to document postsurgical decline is well established (e.g. [51,52]). Using the Boston Naming test, we demonstrated a difference between left and right temporal lobe focus in unoperated patients (unpublished data). Of particular interest in our study was a difference between anglophone and francophone healthy subjects on the task: the mean score of francophone subjects was about three points lower than that of the anglophone subjects. The same healthy subjects did not differ on a visuoperceptual task (Hooper Visual Organization Test, or VOT), making it unlikely that the difference on the naming test arose from a chance difference in basic cognitive level. This result underlines the importance of gathering norms after adapting a standardized test for a new population or translating it to another language. With respect to the findings for patients, anglophones and francophones were each compared to the appropriate language control group, and the left temporal lobe deficit was present in both language groups. Other authors also demonstrated a confrontation naming deficit preoperatively in patients with left, but not with right, TLE [50,51,53]. However, results are less clear regarding the existence of other language deficits in left TLE. Hermann et al. [53] reported that naming was impaired in left compared to right TLE, along with repetition, comprehension and reading, whereas Saykin et al. [51] demonstrated a left TLE naming deficit in the context of preserved verbal fluency, repetition, comprehension and reading.

Although naming has traditionally been considered a function of temporal neocortex, some studies suggest that hippocampal structures also play a role. Davies et al. [52] showed that among unoperated left TLE patients, confrontation naming was significantly worse in patients with HS than in those without it, indicating that the naming function may be associated with the pathological status of the hippocampus. This relationship was restricted to naming (and verbal memory), as other language functions such as verbal fluency and comprehension were not related to presence or absence of HS. This report is consistent with our finding of impaired naming in patients with severe anterograde amnesia: all patients in our series had hippocampal damage [54]. Hermann et al. [7] also found impaired naming in TLE patients with HS compared to those without it regardless of the side. The presence of impairment in both left and right HS groups led these authors to postulate that hippocampal pathology per se may not cause a naming deficit, but rather that HS is associated with earlier onset, and therefore longer duration, of epilepsy, leading to more long-standing and diffuse consequences.

One way that these issues might be resolved is to analyse naming decline after surgery encroaching on different temporal lobe structures. Hermann et al. [55] compared naming in patients with surgery from the left temporal lobe that either resected or spared the superior temporal gyrus, and reported no differences between the two groups. However, in another (multicentre) study, patients undergoing left anterior temporal lobectomy with varying degrees of lateral temporal neocortex either spared or resected were analysed: in this case Hermann et al. [56] reported that a decline in visual confrontation naming was associated with a more extensive resection of lateral temporal neocortex. Interestingly, Strauss et al. [57] showed that left temporal lobectomy impaired naming of living things more than of non-living things, providing support for the notion of category specificity and a somewhat differential role of more anterior (living things) vs. more posterior (non-living objects) temporal regions in naming.

Other verbal functions routinely assessed in preoperative evaluations are language comprehension and reading. One of the most widespread tests of language comprehension is the Token test [58]. Reports on Token test results in unoperated epilepsy patients are conflicting. For example, Hermann et al. [53] showed that patients with left TLE are impaired on this test compared with patients with right TLE. However, our own analysis of 131 patients with focal cortical resection from a left or right temporal, frontal, parietal or occipital lobe indicated that all preoperative patients with a left-sided focus showed an impairment compared to those with a right-sided focus: we found no difference among the sites within the left hemisphere (unpublished data). Giovagnoli [59] reported that patients with left or right temporal and extratemporal epilepsies all performed within a normal range on the Token test, and Hermann et al. [7] found no differences among unilateral TLE groups compared for absence or presence of HS.

Another language function that is usually tested is reading [60], although the specific instruments used to evaluate this function vary among centres. There is a dearth of literature on results of reading tests in patients with epilepsy despite the fact that reading is routinely assessed. Again, one study reported presence [53] and another an absence [51] of reading deficits in left TLE preoperatively.

For the non-dominant temporal neocortex, auditory and visuoperceptual functioning are most often investigated. Impairments in these skills are more difficult to document than are the naming deficits seen from the dominant hemisphere, except in the less frequent cases of patients with severe or bilateral damage. This difficulty in demonstrating subtle perceptual inefficiencies may simply reflect inadequacies in the traditional instruments used to assess these functions [60].

Auditory testing is not included in the basic neuropsychological test battery in the majority of centres. When audition is assessed, the Seashore test of musical talents seems to be the most frequently used instrument (see [60]). It measures several aspects of auditory function such as loudness, timbre, duration, rhythm and melodic discrimination. Milner [61] showed that patients with right but not left temporal lobectomy show impairments on tonal memory, timbre and duration in the context of preserved hearing. However, there is evidence that lesions in the primary auditory region of the left hemisphere affect performance on such auditory tasks as well (e.g. [62]). One should therefore be cautious when interpreting results from auditory tests as signs of non-dominant temporal damage, given the inconsistent laterality findings and also in light of the fact that these findings were reported in patients with surgical excisions and not in preoperative patients.

Visual association cortex is part of the temporal lobes, and therefore tests meant to tap complex visuoperceptual functions are frequently included to evaluate the functional integrity of this region. Such tasks use primarily non-verbal material, as their aim is to test function in the non-dominant hemisphere. The most widely used visuoperceptual tests include the Hooper Visual Organization test, the Benton Judgment of Line Orientation test and the Benton Face Recognition test. Some of these are mentioned above with reference to evaluating the parietal and occipital lobes. For these and similar tests, an association with a particular site (lobe) within the brain has not been consistently demonstrated. For example, patients with left vs. right TLE do not differ on the Benton Face Recognition test [63]. Hermann *et al.* [7] showed that TLE patients with HS perform worse than those without HS on tests of visuoperceptual function, regardless of the side of temporal lobe focus (tests included Hooper VOT, Judgement of Line Orientation and Face Recognition). In general, care should be taken when interpreting results from visual perception tests because of the lack of exclusive relationship between poor performance and dysfunction of a particular site and side within the brain.

In summary, assessment of temporal neocortical function includes evaluation of language skills (i.e. confrontation naming, language comprehension, reading) for the left, and auditory as well as visual perceptual tasks for the right temporal neocortex. Whereas language deficits, and naming in particular, seem to be a consistent finding in patients with left TLE, auditory and visuoperceptual tasks are less helpful in making diagnostic conclusions about the integrity of the right temporal neocortex. Hence, future research should focus particularly on the development of sensitive measures of abnormality in the non-dominant temporal neocortex.

Medial temporal lobe function: memory assessment

A thorough evaluation of memory is particularly important in the assessment of epileptic patients because the majority of surgical candidates have a temporal lobe focus, and memory is the most salient of temporal lobe functions. As with other neuropsychological tests, we expect memory test results to provide two kinds of information, one about the site of dysfunction—in this case deficient performance would suggest that one or both temporal lobes are not functioning adequately—and the other about the aspects of memory that are affected.

It is well known that bilateral lesions in the medial temporal lobe can result in severe global memory deficits (e.g. [64,65]). Such profound memory impairment, however, is rare, while a more restricted, material-specific deficit is frequent in patients with temporal lobe dysfunction. Therefore, a thorough memory assessment should address each hemisphere with tasks appropriate to its specialization.

The fundamental difference between the two temporal lobes is well known. The left (dominant) temporal lobe mediates memory for verbal material, such as names, word lists, stories or number sequences, and the right temporal lobe mediates memory for material that cannot be verbalized readily, such as faces, places, music or abstract designs. Because of this difference between the temporal lobes in the kind of material each mediates, memory tests ideally should be as purely verbal, or purely non-verbal, as possible. In this way we attempt to maximize differences between the hemispheres by using memory tasks that are polarized into the verbal or non-verbal domain, and in doing so we increase the probability that our tests tax primarily one temporal lobe.

Traditional memory tests

Most neuropsychologists working in epilepsy programmes use memory tests from published batteries [60], especially those in the Wechsler Memory Scales (WMS). The latest revision of the WMS [66] is greatly expanded compared to the older versions, but its efficacy with respect to diagnosis in patients with focal brain dysfunction has not yet been established. Also, almost without exception (the exception being a face memory test) the tasks remain for the most part dually encodable (containing both verbal and non-verbal elements), and the battery does not include matched verbal and non-verbal tasks that would allow comparison between the hemispheres.

Another test that is used by most neuropsychologists in epilepsy is the Rey–Osterrieth Complex Figure test [44,45]. This consists of a complex geometric design that patients must copy, followed by a free recall test that may occur immediately and/or after a delay. The copy task provides useful information (see parietal lobe section), but memory results are variable. There is a rather large literature about performance of epilepsy patients on this test and it could be summarized as providing contradictory results. Some group data show impairment after right temporal lobe damage, while other group data show no difference between left and right temporal lobe damage. The usefulness of the memory task for individual cases is thus very limited. One reason for this is that the task, while considered non-verbal, has a clear verbal component. Depending upon an individual's strategies, this can help or hinder recall.

Since these tasks are suboptimal, one might ask why they continue to be used so widely. One reason is that they are self-perpetuating: they have been used and reported upon for many years and therefore they continue to be used. Also, there is a large body of patient data accumulated on them to which, in principle, new patients can be compared. In the case of the Wechsler tests, people are also attracted by the fact that there are norms available.

Implied in the continued use of these tests is the expectation that they will give meaningful information about memory, and about brain function, and about the site of epileptic abnormality. We expect this because we have seen the reports that show groups of patients with left temporal lobe *resection* performing differently from groups of patients with right temporal lobe *resection* on these tasks. We have also seen papers arguing about the importance—or lack of importance, depending on the task—of a healthy hippocampus for adequate performance on different memory tasks. However, until recently the information available about extent of hippocampal removal in those patients was based primarily on the estimate made by the surgeon during the operation. Owing to high-resolution neuroimaging, we now know that there is a certain margin of error in such estimates [67]. This calls into question the strength of the conclusions made previously based solely on surgeons' reports.

Another important point is that most of the information available from earlier studies about memory performance of patients with temporal lobe epilepsy was based on postoperative results in patients who had undergone resection from a temporal lobe; as discussed above, those results do not necessarily generalize to the unoperated case. With the high resolution currently available in MRI scans, together with such techniques as volumetric measurements of specific brain structures and behavioural activation PET studies, we can now investigate brain–behaviour relationships with a degree of accuracy that was not possible before, and we can do so in unoperated patients. One result of this improved technology is that it allows us to confirm (or not) our expectations for the meaning of test results in unoperated patients. We have used this methodology to explore the efficacy of several memory tests [68], including three Wechsler Memory subtests (Logical Memory or prose passages, Associate Learning or word pairs, Visual Reproduction) [69] and the Rey–Osterrieth Complex Figure test described above. For those analyses, patients were grouped according to side of hippocampal atrophy (HA), which had been determined from volumetric measurements of MRI scans. Significant atrophy was defined, both in terms of the absolute volume of each hippocampus and in terms of the relative difference between the two hippocampi of a given individual, with respect to a group of healthy control subjects [70]. The patients studied had highly significant and strictly unilateral HA. All were surgical candidates, but were unoperated when testing took place.

Figure 58.2 shows the performance of left and right HA patients on the three Wechsler Memory subtests and on the Rey Figure memory task. The performance measure in all cases was mean recall score after a 90-min delay. There were no significant differences between the left- and right-sided atrophy groups on any of these measures [68].

Since these remain the most widely used memory tests in the evaluation of epilepsy surgery candidates, results from them are frequently reported in the literature. In a recent meta-analysis of studies reporting memory data in epilepsy, Lee *et al.* [71] were limited to analysing WMS findings because only WMS data were plentiful enough to allow a large analysis. The findings from the meta-analysis were not surprising, especially in the context of the

data we have just shown: the WMS tests did not differentiate left and right temporal lobe groups. In a recent multicentre (seven epilepsy centres) study, Barr *et al.* [72] analysed results of 757 left or right TL presurgical patients on the visual reproduction subtests from the Wechsler Memory Scales and on delayed recall of the Rey–Osterrieth Complex Figure test. Despite their large sample, they also found no differences between left and right presurgical patients on any of these measures.

These are rather sobering, but hardly surprising, findings. Those tests are outdated and psychometrically naïve, and not one of them is strongly polarized into the verbal or non-verbal domain. Furthermore, except for the WMS paired associates test, the recall tests shown in Fig. 58.2 occurred after a single exposure to the material to be remembered. Effects of attention, comprehension and individual strategies are probably most variable on a first trial, or on an only trial, and these effects can confound memory findings.

Matched verbal and non-verbal learning and memory tests

If these explanations are valid, do tests that are not subject to these criticisms yield more promising results? The same patients with severe left or right HA were compared on two tasks that tested learning over the course of four trials. The tasks [68,73] were matched, differing only in the type of material to be learned: the material in one consisted of 13 abstract words, and in the other, 13 abstract designs (Fig. 58.3). On each learning trial subjects copied the 13 items, which were shown one at a time, and immediately upon completion of the copy task they wrote (words) or drew (designs) as many items as they could remember. A delayed recall was obtained 24 h later.

On these tests there was a clear difference between patients with left HA compared to those with right HA in the pattern of results [68]. The patients with left HA were worse than those with right HA on the verbal task, in that they showed severe forgetting of the words after the delay interval (Fig. 58.4). In contrast, the patients

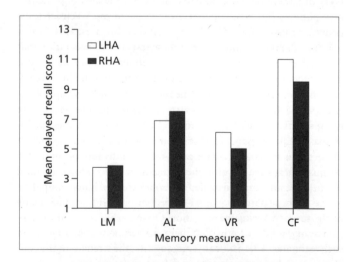

Fig. 58.2 Mean delayed recall scores of patients with left or right HA on three WMS tasks and on the Rey–Osterrieth Complex Figure (CF). LM, Logical Memory, maximum score 23; AL, Associate Learning, maximum score 10; VR, Visual Reproduction, maximum score 14; CF, Rey–Osterrieth Complex Figure, maximum score 36. LHA, left hippocampal atrophy group; RHA, right hippocampal atrophy group.

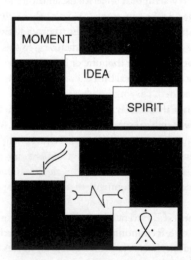

Fig. 58.3 Examples of stimuli from the matched learning tasks: Abstract Word List learning task (AWL) and Abstract Design List learning task (ADL). The ADL is administered before the AWL. During the learning phase, stimuli are shown one at a time while subjects copy them; each learning trial is followed by a free recall test, and an additional delayed recall test is obtained 24 h later.

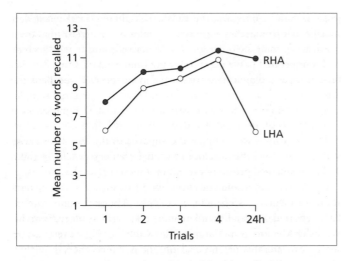

Fig. 58.4 Learning (four trials) and 24-h delayed recall of abstract words in patients with left or right HA. Maximum score on each trial is 13. LHA, left hippocampal atrophy group; RHA, right hippocampal atrophy group.

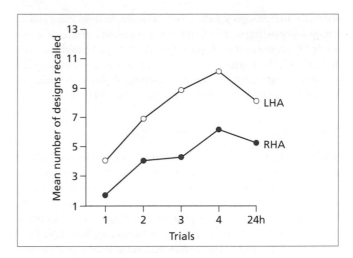

Fig. 58.5 Learning and delayed recall of abstract designs in patients with left or right HA. Maximum score on each trial is 13. LHA, left hippocampal atrophy group; RHA, right hippocampal atrophy group.

with right HA were worse than those with left HA on the non-verbal task, in that they were slow and inefficient during the learning phase (Fig. 58.5). In other words, patients with left HA were impaired in *retention* but not learning of words, while right HA patients showed deficient *learning* of designs but did not forget what they had learned.

Thus the results showed a double dissociation in unoperated patients for verbal vs. non-verbal material in two tasks that were identical except for the nature of the material. This finding contrasts sharply with the lack (or inconsistency) of effect in the four measures reported above, and emphasizes the importance of test selection. The critical features of these more sensitive tasks are as follows.

1 The material used is polarized—the abstract words are presumably as purely verbal as stimuli can be, and the abstract designs are highly non-verbal.

2 These are learning tasks, providing the possibility to improve with additional exposure to the material, increasing the difference between people with a true learning deficit and those who do poorly on a first trial for other reasons.

3 They are matched, varying only according to the verbal vs. non-verbal nature of the material. This allows direct comparison of the efficiency of the two hemispheres, even within individual patients.

These examples have been given to illustrate the importance of the choice of tasks in neuropsychological testing. Several matched memory tasks have been developed in recent years (e.g. [74,75]); this often represents development of a non-verbal analogue for a previously existing verbal test such as the Rey Auditory Verbal Learning Test [6,76], the California Verbal Learning Test [77], the Buschke Selective Reminding test [78] or the modified Brown–Peterson paradigm [79,80]. Although some results in presurgical epilepsy patients have been published and may be described as encouraging, these tests await further empirical confirmations. For example, Giovagnoli and Avanzini [8] tested unoperated epilepsy patients on a matched verbal and non-verbal selective reminding procedure that required learning of 10 words or designs over repeated trials with selective repeating of items that had not been re-called on the preceding trial. Verbal delayed recall successfully discriminated between patients with left and right TLE, but the non-verbal task did not. However, in a previous study using only the non-verbal test, Giovagnoli *et al.* [81] demonstrated a learning deficit in patients with right TLE compared to left TLE and healthy control subjects. These conflicting results remain unexplained. The same authors devised matched verbal and non-verbal versions of the Brown–Peterson interference task (the 'Memory Distracter' tests). Both tests measure recall of a presented stimulus (words or designs) after a distracting activity over delays of 5, 10, 15, 30 or 60 s. Again patients with left TLE performed worse than those with right TLE on the verbal task, while patients with right and left TLE did not differ on the non-verbal one [8].

The Warrington Recognition Memory test (WRM), which is a matched pair of tasks using words (verbal) and faces (non-verbal), was reported to be sensitive to the effects of temporal lobe lesions in patients with neoplasms and infarctions [82] and in resected TLE patients [83,84]. However, several studies showed that the test's clinical utility in distinguishing left from right presurgical epilepsy patients is very limited [83–86]. Furthermore, Baxendale [86] suggested that temporal lobe lesions that extend beyond hippocampus may be necessary to produce deficits on the WRM. Some properties of this instrument that may contribute to its lower diagnostic efficiency in focal epilepsy are first, that it uses an incidental memory paradigm and therefore consists of a single exposure to the stimuli rather than learning over repeated trials. Second, memory is tested immediately after presentation of the stimuli, and it may be that delayed memory tasks are more sensitive to dysfunction in medial temporal lobe structures.

The fact that the WRM does not reliably differentiate left and right temporal lobe dysfunction despite using paired tasks adds emphasis to the apparent sensitivity of the paired learning tasks illustrated above [68,73]. Those tasks alerted us to the difference in pattern as well as in material that distinguishes the left and right temporal lobe memory deficits. Some findings obtained by other authors and using different testing paradigms are consistent with the idea that deficits from unilateral temporal lobe lesions may be both material- and process-specific. For example, several independent groups reported impaired recall but not impaired learning of words in left TLE compared to those with right TLE and healthy control subjects [87,88]. Furthermore, some authors who examined non-verbal learning reported a deficit in learning of non-verbal material but not in its retention in right TLE patients [81,89].

Other verbal learning and memory tests

In addition to matched verbal and non-verbal memory tasks, there is a growing literature on single tasks that seem to be sensitive to memory deficits in unoperated epilepsy patients. In the verbal domain, the most frequently used tests (besides subtests from the Wechsler Memory Scales) are the Rey Auditory Verbal Learning Test (RAVLT) and the California Verbal Learning Test (CVLT). In both cases, lists of words are presented over several trials, a second (interference) list is presented once, and recall trials are obtained after interference and after a delay. Published results from these tests suggest that they can distinguish between left and right TLE, particularly on the measures of retention [87,88,90].

A relatively new and promising test that taps a more everyday life aspect of memory is the Story Learning test developed by Frisk and Milner [91]. The test consists of repeated presentation of a story until it is learned to a criterion: therefore it provides measures of learning and of immediate and delayed retention. In the original study, patients with left temporal lobe excisions were impaired on this test compared to those with right temporal lobe excisions and healthy control subjects [91]. We have used the test with unoperated patients for several years, with excellent results that differentiate patients with left TLE from those with right TLE and control subjects [92].

Non-verbal learning and memory tests

Since the old non-verbal memory measures had little success in detecting right temporal lobe damage, there have been a number of attempts at modifying the existing tests or developing new procedures to evaluate non-verbal memory. Helmstaedter et al. [93] introduced a six-trial learning test in which five-line designs had to be reconstructed using five wooden sticks. The authors reported learning deficits in patients with right but not left TLE [93]. More recently, Gleißner et al. [89] compared performance on this test in right TLE patients with and without HS or atrophy. They found impaired learning only in the patients with right HA, and interpreted their findings to mean that hippocampal damage is the major cause of non-verbal learning deficits in patients with right TLE.

Barr [63] tested unoperated TLE patients on two memory tasks and found an impairment in the right TLE cases on one of them, the Denman Face Recognition test [94]. To our knowledge, this finding has not been replicated, and we have been unable to replicate it in our TLE patients. This was not surprising, however, since that task tests memory after a single exposure. Recently we developed a face memory test using a learning paradigm ('the Twins test') [95]. Twelve unfamiliar faces are presented for learning over four trials, and a delayed recognition test is given 24 h after learning. Our patients with resection from the right temporal lobe were significantly worse at learning the faces than were patients with left temporal resections, and the latter performed identically to normal control sub-

jects. As with the design learning task, the right temporal deficit was specific to learning; they showed no greater forgetting of what they had learned than the other groups. We have begun to use this test with unoperated patients, and our preliminary data show it to be promising as a diagnostic tool for the evaluation of TLE patients [96].

Spatial memory has been tested in unoperated TLE patients by Baxendale et al. [97] and Abrahams et al. [98]. In both cases, the right TLE groups were impaired compared to the left. Thus these studies confirmed the presence of spatial memory deficits in right TLE, documented previously in patients with surgical lesions.

Let us summarize and comment upon this survey of the current status of memory assessment in epilepsy. Although some studies have reported that traditional memory tests such as those from the Wechsler Memory Scales and the Rey Complex Figure test can be sensitive to laterality of temporal lobe focus, many others show that they are not sensitive. Non-verbal memory deficits were particularly difficult to demonstrate with traditional tasks. On the other hand, some newer tests can demonstrate impairments in unoperated patients not only with a left, but also with a right temporal lobe focus. Furthermore, the results revealed that memory processes in the two hemispheres may differ in more ways than in the verbal or non-verbal nature of the material. A *learning* deficit seems to characterize memory dysfunction associated with a seizure focus in the non-dominant medial temporal lobe, whereas impaired *retention* is the most salient feature of the epileptic focus in the dominant medial temporal lobe. We argue that the development and validation of original testing procedures and replacement of the old ones with new and more sensitive ones is a desirable trend in the field. We recognize that there are disadvantages to having a wide variety of testing procedures in different centres because it means that results across centres cannot be compared directly. However, we believe that the possible gains outweigh the disadvantages. A search for better tools is more important than uniformity, and the development of efficient instruments will best enable the advancement of the field.

Intracarotid amobarbital procedure (IAP)

Nowhere is the sensitivity of neuropsychological measurement more important than in the intracarotid amobarbital test. This invasive procedure is part of the preoperative evaluation of most patients who are candidates for surgical treatment of epilepsy. In many institutions all patients undergo the IAP, especially when it is performed to aid in localizing the seizure focus [99]. In other institutions patients undergo the test only if they are shown to need it either for determination of cerebral dominance for language if atypical dominance is suspected, or to evaluate memory function in each hemisphere independently if bitemporal dysfunction is suspected. These decisions will also be influenced by the extent of routine resection in patients with mesial TLE.

Atypical language dominance is suspected in patients who are left-handed, who have a strong family history of left-handedness, who do not show the normal right-ear dominance on dichotic listening tests, and/or whose pattern on cognitive tests indicates dysfunction in the hemisphere opposite to a lesion or focus identified by clinical signs, neuroimaging or EEG. Bitemporal dysfunction may be suspected in several ways. Impairments on both verbal and non-verbal memory tests in the basic, non-invasive clinical memory evaluation suggest bitemporal abnormality. Evidence from EEG or neuroimaging pointing to bitemporal abnormality is also grounds for carrying out an IAP, as is conflicting evidence arising when an EEG focus is clearly in one temporal lobe but the opposite hippocampus is significantly abnormal according to MRI.

The IAP is performed differently at different centres, but the basic core is similar across institutions. For example, although most centres carry out a 'standard' test, injecting the drug through the internal carotid artery [100], some perform selective and superselective procedures into other vessels for selective inactivation of hippocampal structures [101,102].

Description of procedure

The basic procedure consists of injection of a barbiturate, almost always sodium amobarbital, into one hemisphere, usually through the internal carotid artery. This anaesthetizes the injected hemisphere and allows one to test the abilities of the awake hemisphere in isolation. The effect is short, and is usually dissipated after about 5–8 min. During the effect, simple speech and memory tests are performed. The injection is made by a radiologist, who has performed a $3\,cm^3$ angiogram before the test to verify that there is no serious vascular anomaly and to predict the distribution of the drug. In most institutions an EEG is obtained during the test; in some instances this is read on-line and in others it is recorded on a computer for playback and interpretation later by an electroencephalographer [103]. As it is becoming increasingly difficult to obtain sodium amobarbital, there is an accelerating movement toward using other agents (methohexital sodium and propofol).

Before injection, basic speech and memory tests are performed to establish a baseline. Upon injection, more speech and memory tests are carried out while one hemisphere is inactivated. Memory testing consists of showing new material while only one hemisphere is functional, and then testing memory for that material later, when the drug is no longer active and both hemispheres are back to baseline functioning. Speech tests are kept simple and usually include naming, serial or automatic speech (such as counting and reciting days of the week), comprehension, reading and repetition [104].

Interpretation of IAP results: language dominance

Interpretation of the speech tests is most often unambiguous: if the dominant hemisphere is injected the patient is aphasic while the drug is active, whereas if the non-dominant hemisphere is injected the patient continues talking without significant errors. However, several different patterns may be observed in bilateral speech representation. These include disruption of all speech functions after injection in one hemisphere with minor but significant disruption after injection in the other; dissociation of type of disruption (e.g. naming in one hemisphere and comprehension in the other); equal and significant disruption in both hemispheres; or no obvious disruption in either hemisphere (see especially [105]).

Interpretation of bilateral speech differs among institutions and individuals, consequently reports of the incidence of this type of atypical language organization varies (e.g. see [100]). This is of considerable theoretical interest but it does not impact significantly on patient management because the most critical practical question (is there significant language function in the hemisphere destined for surgery?) can almost always be answered.

Interpretation of IAP results: memory

Underlying the memory application of the IAP is a basic assumption that the patient will have to rely on the awake hemisphere to remember material shown while the drug is active. The patient will not remember the material if the awake, or non-injected, hemisphere is damaged in areas important for memory. The crucial test is after injection of the hemisphere destined for surgery, because it tests the memory function of the hemisphere that will be left intact. The premise is that the test should predict how well memory will function after resection from a temporal lobe. However, other important information is also obtained from injection opposite the hemisphere destined for surgery, as the result should confirm or disconfirm an expected dysfunction in that hemisphere.

One assumption underlying this aspect of the IAP is that the hippocampus is necessary for adequate memory function, and that the IAP memory test specifically addresses the adequacy of hippocampal function. Therefore, in some centres a limited resection, either sparing the hippocampus or encroaching modestly upon it, is performed in patients who show significant forgetting on amobarbital memory tests after injection into the hemisphere of a planned temporal lobe excision. In some other centres, surgery is denied altogether to such patients. Thus there are important consequences for patients who fail in the crucial test. There is no current standard for defining such failure; some centres have a cutting score and others compare performance from the two injections, making a relative rather than an absolute judgement [99]. It is important also to take language dominance into account when interpreting IAP memory results, because in most patients there is a bigger drug effect in the dominant than in the non-dominant hemisphere [106]. This results in smaller differences between ipsilateral-to-focus and contralateral-to-focus injections when the focus is in the dominant hemisphere than when it is in the non-dominant hemisphere.

A number of controversies and issues concerning the IAP have arisen in recent years. These include questions about the extent to which critical memory regions are affected by injection into the internal carotid artery, given that the posterior hippocampus is not irrigated by that artery, and questions about the true risk of amnesia in patients who fail an IAP memory test given that many of them undergo partial hippocampal resection and do not become amnesic. Other issues involve the timing of presentation of memory stimuli after injection, the number and type of stimuli used, determination of drug dosage and the effect of different dosages, and dealing with fluctuations in attention. Discussion of these questions cannot, for reasons of space, be included here, but interested readers are directed to a special issue of *Brain and Cognition* (volume 33, numbers 1 and 2, 1997); it is devoted entirely to the IAP, and several of the papers deal with these issues.

Present status and utility of IAP

Sufficient evidence exists showing that the IAP memory tests do tap the function of the hippocampal region, and it is inferred further that the test therefore can predict possible postoperative memory loss (e.g. [107]). However, postsurgical amnesia is extremely rare, and the IAP is increasingly used in a more general sense to predict postoperative memory performance, without reference to global amnesia. IAP results can add confirming evidence indicating the site of epileptic focus when injection opposite the supposed focus results in memory failure (e.g. [108]). Good memory after injection opposite a temporal lobe targeted for surgery is another meaningful result. It shows that that temporal lobe, and presumably the hippocampus planned for resection, functions well. Resection from a well-functioning hippocampus can result in a more marked postoperative memory loss than resection from a damaged one [109,110]. Thus IAP memory performance in both tests, ipsilateral and contralateral to proposed surgery, should be taken into account in decisions regarding hippocampal excision.

The question of seizure control is closely linked to questions of sparing hippocampus. Since at-risk patients who undergo surgery show poor memory but are not amnesic, and since most of them experience a significant postoperative reduction in their seizures [111], they both gain and lose from surgery. Thus surgical decisions concerning hippocampal excision weigh the negative effect of possible memory dysfunction against the positive effect of seizure control, but this issue is complex and must add the presurgical efficiency of the patient's memory and hippocampus into the equation. Furthermore, the memory efficiency itself can contribute to predicting outcome: IAP results that clearly lateralize dysfunction with a difference score comparing performance of the two hemispheres have been shown to be successful predictors of seizure control [112,113].

Non-invasive procedures

Information gained from the IAP is important in the surgical treatment of epilepsy, but a non-invasive alternative would be welcome. Paradigms have been developed using PET [114] and functional MRI (fMRI) [115,116] to determine language dominance. These paradigms are still experimental, and the PET methodology has been limited because only a restricted number of language aspects could be tested, unlike the IAP in which many language tasks are used. However, the fMRI is not limited in that way, and speech-activated neuroimaging is becoming an important tool that currently supplements and may eventually replace the role of IAP in determining cerebral dominance for language. A viable alternative to the IAP memory test remains more remote. It has been notoriously difficult to activate the medial temporal lobes in PET and fMRI, and only recently have a few studies succeeded in doing so [117–119]. We are working on this problem in our centre and have developed an fMRI memory paradigm that activates the hippocampal region bilaterally in healthy individuals [120]. Our preliminary results with patients are encouraging, suggesting that it may eventually be a viable alternative for some patients, and that such a task may provide information about reorganization and plasticity in the patient's memory systems as well as about regions of dysfunction.

Thus, fMRI seems to offer a possible means of testing memory, but the fMRI paradigms that are being developed must still be validated before eventually one can consider using them in place of the IAP. Once the methodology is considered reliable, there will still be the occasional problem of patients who are not capable of performing the cognitive tasks required in activation neuroimaging, and the

problem of individuals who cannot go into a scanner because of claustrophobia or metal parts in their bodies, or who cannot spend the necessary amount of time in the scanner because of frequent seizures. In addition, an important argument against an eventual total replacement of the IAP is that only the IAP mimics, and therefore predicts, the effects of surgery because it transiently disables most of one hemisphere.

Summary

Neuropsychological evaluation in epilepsy addresses cerebral function widely in its attempt to determine the dysfunctional region and predict the effect of surgery on postsurgical function. We have described the spectrum of tests used for this purpose and have emphasized what we consider to be the strengths and weaknesses among them. With the growth of surgical treatment for epilepsy has come an influx of information about tests used in this specialty, but we find that there is still a need for development in the field.

Too often we noted that tests being used did not reliably detect a lesion or a focus. This can indicate either that the epileptic focus did not produce a significant effect or that the tests used to measure it were inappropriate. However, we showed that an increasing number of tasks are succeeding in demonstrating neuropsychological deficits in focal epilepsy, suggesting that ineffective tests were probably responsible for the previous lack of effect. We recommend that clinicians and researchers make a concentrated effort to seek and/or develop appropriate instruments specifically for this field, and we have pointed out areas of greatest need for growth.

However, despite our calls for improvements, overall our evaluation of the contribution of neuropsychological assessment in the preoperative evaluation of patients with epilepsy is very positive. Results from these tests continue to contribute to decisions about patient management with respect to feasibility of surgery, extent of surgery and cognitive outcome after surgery.

Acknowledgements

This work was supported in part by grant MOP-53234 awarded to M. Jones-Gotman by the Canadian Institutes of Health Research. We thank Andre Olivier for the opportunity to study his patients, Fernando Cendes for volumetric measurements of MRI scans and Zia Lakdawalla for preparation of graphs and help with the literature search.

References

1 Branch C, Milner B, Rasmussen T. Intracarotid sodium Amytal for the lateralization of cerebral speech dominance: Observations in 123 patients. *J Neurosurg* 1964; 21: 399–405.

2 Wada J, Rasmussen T. Intracarotid injection of sodium Amytal for the lateralization of cerebral speech dominance: Experimental and clinical observations. *J Neurosurg* 1960; 17: 226–82.

3 Morrell F, Whisler W, Bleck T. Multiple subpial transsection: a new approach to the surgical treatment of focal epilepsy. *J Neurosurg* 1989; 70: 231–9.

4 Pegna AJ, Qayoom Z, Gericke CA, Landis T, Seeck M. Comprehensive postictal neuropsychology improves focus localization in epilepsy. *Eur Neurol* 1998; 40: 207–11.

5 Delaney RC. Screening for organicity: the problem of subtle neuropsychological deficit and diagnosis. *J Clin Psych* 1982; 38: 843–6.

6 Lezak MD. *Neuropsychological Assessment*, 3rd edn. New York: Oxford University Press, 1995.

7 Hermann BP, Seidenberg M, Schoenfeld J, Davies K. Neuropsychological characteristics of the syndrome of mesial temporal lobe epilepsy. *Arch Neurol* 1997; 54: 369–76.

8 Giovagnoli AR, Avanzini G. Learning and memory impairment in patients with temporal lobe epilepsy: Relation to the presence, type, and location of brain lesion. *Epilepsia* 1999; 40(7): 904–11.

9 Tranel D, Anderson SW, Benton A. Development of the concept of 'executive function' and its relationship to the frontal lobes. In: Boller F, Grafman J, eds. *Handbook of Neuropsychology*, Vol. 9. Amsterdam: Elsevier Science, 1994: 125–48.

10 Grant DA, Berg GA. A behavioral analysis of degree of reinforcement and ease of shifting to new responses in a Weigl-type card-sorting problem. *J Exp Psych* 1948; 38: 404–11.

11 Nelson HE. A modified card sorting test sensitive to frontal lobe defects. *Cortex* 1976; 12: 313–24.

12 Milner B. Effects of different brain lesions on card sorting. *Arch Neurol* 1963; 9: 90–100.

13 Milner B. Some effects of frontal lobectomy in man. In: Warren JM, Akert K, eds. *The Frontal Granular Cortex and Behavior*. New York: McGraw Hill, 1964: 313–34.

14 Anderson SW, Damasio H, Jones RD, Tranel D. Wisconsin Card Sorting Test performance as a measure of frontal lobe damage. *J Clin Exp Neuropsych* 1991; 13: 909–22.

15 Hermann BP, Wyler AR, Richey ET. Wisconsin Card Sorting Test performance in patients with complex partial seizures of temporal-lobe origin. *J Clin Exp Neuropsych* 1988; 10(4): 467–76.

16 Giovagnoli AR. Relation of sorting impairment to hippocampal damage in temporal lobe epilepsy. *Neuropsychologia* 2001; 39(2): 140–50.

17 Corcoran R, Upton D. A role for the hippocampus in card sorting? *Cortex* 1993; 29(2): 293–304.

18 Djordjevic J, Piazzini A, Jones Gotman M. Two scoring systems for the Wisconsin Card Sorting Test: same or different measures? *Epilepsia* 1997; 38 (Suppl. 8): 163.

19 Hermann B, Seidenberg M. Executive system dysfunction in temporal lobe epilepsy: Effects of nociferous cortex versus hippocampal pathology. *J Clin Exp Neuropsych* 1995; 17(6): 809–19.

20 Martin RC, Sawrie SM, Gilliam FG *et al*. Wisconsin Card Sorting performance in patients with temporal lobe epilepsy: clinical and neuroanatomical correlates. *Epilepsia* 2000; 41(12): 1626–32.

21 Jones-Gotman M, Milner B. Design fluency: the invention of nonsense drawings after focal cortical lesions. *Neuropsychologia* 1977; 15: 653–74.

22 Jones-Gotman M. Localization of lesions by neuropsychological testing. *Epilepsia* 1991; 32 (Suppl. 5): 41–52.

23 Sands KA. Nonverbal fluency: A neuropsychometric investigation. *Dissertation Abstracts International: Section B: the Sciences & Engineering* 1998; 58 (8-B): 4470.

24 Woodard JL, Axelrod BN, Henry RR. Interrater reliability of scoring parameters for the Design Fluency Test. *Neuropsychology* 1992; 6(2): 173–8.

25 Carter SL, Shore D, Harnadek MCS, Kubu CS. Normative data and interrater reliability of the Design Fluency Test. *Clin Neuropsychol* 1998; 12(4): 531–4.

26 Baldo JV, Shimamura AP. Letter and category fluency in patients with frontal lobe lesions. *Neuropsychology* 1998; 12(2): 259–67.

27 Martin RC, Loring DW, Meador KJ, Lee GP. The effects of lateralized temporal lobe dysfunction on formal and semantic word fluency. *Neuropsychologia* 1990; 28(8): 823–9.

28 Helmstaedter C, Kemper B, Elger CE. Neuropsychological aspects of frontal lobe epilepsy. *Neuropsychologia* 1996; 34(5): 399–406.

29 Upton D, Thompson PJ. General neuropsychological characteristics of frontal lobe epilepsy. *Epilepsy Res* 1996; 23: 169–77.

30 Stroop JR. Studies of interference in serial verbal reactions. *J Exp Psych* 1935; 18: 643–62.

31 Perret E. The left frontal lobe of man and the suppression of habitual responses in verbal categorical behaviour. *Neuropsychologia* 1974; 12: 323–30.

32 Richer F, Décary A, Lapierre MF, Rouleau I, Bouvier G, Saint-Hilaire JM. Target detection deficits in frontal lobectomy. *Brain Cognition* 1993; 21(2): 203–11.

33 Shallice T. Specific impairments of planning. *Phil Trans Roy Soc Lond* 1982; 298: 199–209.

34 Andrés P, Van der Linden M. Supervisory attentional system in patients with focal frontal lesions. *J Clin Exp Neuropsych* 2001; 23(2): 225–39.

35 Owen AM, Downes JJ, Sahakian BJ, Polkey CE, Robbins TW. Planning and spatial working memory following frontal lobe lesions in man. *Neuropsychologia* 1990; 28(10): 1021–34.

36 Mathiowetz V, Kashman N, Volland G, Weber K, Dowe M, Rogers S. Grip and pinch strength: normative data for adults. *Arch Phys Med Rehabil* 1985; 66: 69–74.

37 Mitrushina MN, Boone KB, D'Elia LF. *Handbook of Normative Data for Neuropsychological Assessment*. New York: Oxford University Press, 1999.

38 Leonard G, Jones L, Milner B. Residual impairment in handgrip strength after unilateral frontal-lobe lesions. *Neuropsychologia* 1988; 26(4): 555–64.

39 Leonard G, Milner B, Jones L. Performance on unimanual and bimanual tapping tasks by patients with lesions of the frontal or temporal lobe. *Neuropsychologia* 1988; 26(1): 79–91.

40 Helmstaedter C, Gleißner U, Zentner J, Elger CE. Neuropsychological consequence of epilepsy surgery in frontal lobe epilepsy. *Neuropsychologia* 1998; 36(4): 333–41.

41 Regard M, Strauss E, Knapp P. Children's production on verbal and non-verbal fluency tasks. *Percept Motor Skills* 1982; 55: 839–44.

42 Salanova V, Andermann F, Rasmussen T, Olivier A, Quesney LF. Parietal lobe epilepsy: Clinical manifestations and outcome in 82 patients treated surgically between 1929 and 1988. *Brain* 1995; 118: 607–27.

43 Morris RG, Feigenbaum JD, Binnie CD, Elwes RDC, Polkey CE. Plasticity of right parietal lobe functioning in focal cortical dysplasia. *Adv Neurol* 1999; 81: 363–70.

44 Rey A. L'examen psychologique dans les cas d'encéphalopathie traumatique. *Arch Psychol* 1942; 28: 112.

45 Osterrieth P. Le test de copie d'une figure complexe. *Arch Psychol* 1944; 30: 206–356.

46 Corkin S, Milner B, Rasmussen T. Somatosensory thresholds. Contrasting effects of post-central gyrus and posterior parietal-lobe excisions. *Arch Neurol* 1970; 22: 41–58.

47 Benton AL, Hannay HJ, Varney NR. Visual perception of line direction in patients with unilateral brain disease. *Neurology* 1975; 25: 907–10.

48 Gülgönen S, Demirbilek V, Korkmaz B, Dervent A, Townes BD. Neuropsychological functions in idiopathic occipital lobe epilepsy. *Epilepsia* 2000; 41(4): 405–11.

49 Fleischman DA, Vaidya CJ, Lange KL, Gabrieli JDE. A dissociation between perceptual explicit and implicit memory processes. *Brain Cognition* 1997; 35(1): 42–57.

50 Mayeux R, Brandt J, Rosen J, Benson FD. Interictal memory and language impairment in temporal lobe epilepsy. *Neurology* 1980; 30: 120–5.

51 Saykin AJ, Stafiniak P, Robinson LJ *et al*. Language before and after temporal lobectomy: Specificity of acute changes and relation to early risk factors. *Epilepsia* 1995; 36(11): 1071–7.

52 Davies KG, Bell BD, Bush AJ, Hermann BP, Dohan Jr FC, Jaap AS. Naming decline after left anterior temporal lobectomy correlates with pathological status of resected hippocampus. *Epilepsia* 1998; 39(4): 407–19.

53 Hermann BP, Seidenberg M, Haltiner A, Wyler AR. Adequacy of language function and verbal memory performance in unilateral temporal lobe epilepsy. *Cortex* 1992; 28: 423–33.

54 Guerreiro CAM, Jones-Gotman M, Andermann F, Bastos A, Cendes F. Severe amnesia in epilepsy: causes, anatomopsychological consideration, and treatment. *Epilepsy Behav* 2001; 2: 224–46.

55 Hermann BP, Davies K, Foley K, Bell B. Visual confrontation naming outcome after standard left temporal lobectomy with sparing versus resection of the superior temporal gyrus: a randomized prospective clinical trial. *Epilepsia* 1999; 40(8): 1070–6.

56 Hermann BP, Perrine K, Chelune GJ *et al*. Visual confrontation naming following left anterior temporal lobectomy: a comparison of surgical approaches. *Neuropsychology* 1999; 13(1): 3–9.

57 Strauss E, Semenza C, Hunter M et al. Left anterior lobectomy and category-specific naming. Brain Cognition 2000; 43(1–3): 403–6.

58 De Renzi E, Vignolo LA. The Token Test: A sensitive test to detect disturbances in aphasics. Brain 1962; 85: 665–78.

59 Giovagnoli AR. Verbal semantic memory in temporal lobe epilepsy. Acta Neurol Scand 1999; 99: 334–9.

60 Jones-Gotman M, Smith M-L, Zatorre RJ. Neuropsychological testing for localizing and lateralizing the epileptogenic region. In: Engel J Jr, ed. Surgical Treatment of the Epilepsies, 2nd edn. New York: Raven Press, 1993: 245–62.

61 Milner B. Laterality effects in audition. In: Mountcastle VB, ed. Interhemispheric Relations and Cerebral Dominance. Baltimore: Johns Hopkins Press, 1962: 177–95.

62 Samson S, Zatorre RJ. Melodic and harmonic discrimination following unilateral cerebral excision. Brain Cognition 1988; 7: 348–60.

63 Barr WB. Examining the right temporal lobe's role in nonverbal memory. Brain Cognition 1997; 35: 26–41.

64 Scoville W, Milner B. Loss of recent memory after bilateral hippocampal lesions. J Neurol Neurosurg Psychiatr 1957; 20: 11–21.

65 Press G, Amaral D, Squire L. Hippocampal abnormalities in amnesic patients revealed by high-resolution magnetic resonance imaging. Nature 1989; 341: 54–57.

66 Wechsler D. WMS-III. Administration and Scoring Manual. San Antonio: The Psychological Corporation, Harcourt Brace Jovanovich, 1997.

67 Awad IA, Katz A, Hahn JF, Kong AK, Ahl J, Lüders H. Extent of resection in temporal lobectomy for epilepsy. I. Interobserver analysis and correlation with seizure outcome. Epilepsia 1989; 30: 756–62.

68 Jones-Gotman M, Brulot M, McMackin D et al. Word and design list learning deficits related to side of hippocampal atrophy as assessed by volumetric MRI measurements. Epilepsia 1993; 34(6): 71.

69 Wechsler D. A standardized memory scale for clinical use. J Psych 1945; 19: 87–95.

70 Watson C, Andermann F, Gloor P et al. Anatomic basis of amygdaloid and hippocampal volume measurement by magnetic resonance imaging. Neurology 1992; 42: 1743–50.

71 Lee TMC, Yip JTH, Jones-Gotman M. Memory deficits after resection from left or right anterior temporal lobe in humans: A meta-analytic review. Epilepsia 2002; 43(3): 283–91.

72 Barr WB, Chelune GJ, Hermann BP et al. The use of figural reproduction tests and measures of nonverbal memory in epilepsy surgery candidates. J Int Neuropsychol Soc 1997; 3: 435–43.

73 Jones-Gotman M, Zatorre RJ, Olivier A et al. Learning and retention of words and designs following excision from medial or lateral temporal-lobe structures. Neuropsychologia 1997; 35(7): 963–73.

74 Glosser G, Goodglass H, Biber C. Assessing visual memory disorders. J Cons Clin Psychol 1989; 1: 82–91.

75 Majdan A, Sziklas V, Jones-Gotman M. Performance of healthy subjects and patients with resection from the anterior temporal lobe on matched tests of verbal and visuoperceptual learning. J Clin Exp NeuroPsych 1996; 18(3): 416–30.

76 Rey A. L'examen clinique en psychologie. Paris: Presses Universitaire de France, 1964.

77 Delis DC, Kramer J, Ober BA, Kaplan E. The California Verbal Learning Test. New York: Life Science Associates, 1993.

78 Buschke H, Fuld PA. Evaluating storage, retention, and retrieval in disordered memory and learning. Neurology 1974; 24: 1019–25.

79 Brown J. Some tests of the decay theory of immediate memory. Q J Exp Psych 1958; 10: 12–21.

80 Peterson LR, Peterson MJ. Short-term retention of individual verbal items. J Exp Psych 1959; 58: 193–8.

81 Giovagnoli AR, Casazza M, Avanzini G. Visual learning on a selective reminding procedure and delayed recall in patients with temporal lobe epilepsy. Epilepsia 1995; 36(7): 704–11.

82 Warrington EK. Recognition Memory Test. Berkshire: NFER-Nelson, 1994.

83 Naugle RI, Chelune GJ, Schuster J, Lüders H, Comair Y. Recognition memory for words and faces before and after temporal lobectomy. Assessment 1994; 1: 373–81.

84 Hermann BP, Connell B, Barr WB, Wyler A. The utility of the Warrington Recognition Memory Test for temporal lobe epilepsy: Pre- and postoperative results. Epilepsy 1995; 8: 139–45.

85 Miller LA, Munoz DG, Finmore M. Hippocampal sclerosis and human memory. Arch Neurol 1993; 50: 391–4.

86 Baxendale SA. The role of the hippocampus in recognition memory. Neuropsychologia 1997; 35(5): 591–8.

87 Helmstaedter C, Elger CE. Cognitive consequences of two-thirds anterior temporal lobectomy on verbal memory in 144 patients: A three-month follow-up study. Epilepsia 1996; 37(2): 171–80.

88 Mungas D, Ehlers C, Walton N, McCutchen CB. Verbal learning differences in epileptic patients with left and right temporal lobe foci. Epilepsia 1985; 26(4): 340–5.

89 Gleißner U, Helmstaedter C, Elger CE. Right hippocampal contribution to visual memory: a presurgical and postsurgical study in patients with temporal lobe epilepsy. J Neurol Neurosurg Psychiatr 1998; 65: 665–9.

90 Sziklas VG, Grunfeld D, Quintin G, Jones-Gotman M. The Rey Auditory Verbal Learning Test and the left temporal lobe: Different deficits before vs. after surgery. Epilepsia 2000; 41 (Suppl. 7): 150.

91 Frisk V, Milner B. The role of the left hippocampal region in the acquisition and retention of story content. Neuropsychologia 1990; 28(4): 349–59.

92 Jones-Gotman M, Smith ML, Frisk V, Routhier N. Learning and retention of connected prose before and after surgical resection from a temporal lobe. Epilepsia 1996; 37 (Suppl. 5): 120.

93 Helmstaedter C, Pohl C, Hufnagel A, Elger CE. Visual learning deficits in nonresected patients with right temporal lobe epilepsy. Cortex 1991; 27: 547–55.

94 Denman SB. Denman Neuropsychology Memory Scale. Charleston: Sidney B Denman, 1984.

95 Dade L, Jones-Gotman M. Face learning and memory: The Twins Test. Neuropsychology 2001; 15(4): 525–34.

96 Dade LA, Lakdawalla Z, Jones-Gotman M. Pegging right temporal lobe function: the Twins Test. Epilepsia 2001; 42(7): 235.

97 Baxendale SA, Thompson PJ, van Paesschen W. A test of spatial memory and its clinical utility in the pre-surgical investigation of temporal lobe epilepsy patients. Neuropsychologia 1998; 36(7): 591–602.

98 Abrahams S, Pickering A, Polkey CE, Morris RG. Spatial memory deficits in patients with unilateral damage to the right hippocampal formation. Neuropsychologia 1996; 35(1): 11–24.

99 Engel JJr, Rausch R, Lieb JP, Kuhl DE, Crandall PH. Correlation of criteria used for localizing epileptic foci in patients considered for surgical therapy of epilepsy. Ann Neurol 1981; 9: 215–24.

100 Rausch R, Silfvenius H, Wieser H-G, Dodrill C, Meador K, Jones-Gotman M. Intraarterial amobarbital procedures. In: Engel J Jr, ed. Surgical Treatment of the Epilepsies, 2nd edn. New York: Raven Press, 1993; 341–57.

101 Jack C, Nichols D, Sharbrough F, Marsh WR, Petersen R. Selective posterior cerebral artery amytal test for evaluating memory function before surgery for temporal lobe seizure. Neuroradiology 1988; 168: 787–93.

102 Jones-Gotman M, Smith ML, Wieser H-G. Intraarterial amobarbital procedures. In: Engel J Jr, Pedley T, eds. Epilepsy: A Comprehensive Textbook, Vol. 2. New York: Raven Press, 1998; 1767–75.

103 Gotman J, Bouwer MS, Jones-Gotman M. Intracranial EEG study of brain structures affected by internal carotid injection of sodium amobarbital. Neurology 1992; 42: 2136–43.

104 Ravdin LD, Perrine K, Haywood CS, Gershengorn J, Nelson PK, Devinsky O. Serial recovery of language during the intracarotid amobarbital procedure. Brain Cognition 1997; 33(2): 151–60.

105 Risse GL, Gates JR, Fangman MC. A reconsideration of bilateral language representation based on the intracarotid amobarbital procedure. Brain Cognition 1997; 33(1): 118–32.

106 McMackin D, Jones-Gotman M, Dubeau F et al. Asymmetry in regional cerebral blood flow in relation to language dominance: A study using co-registered SPECT and MRI during the intracarotid sodium amobarbital procedure. Neurology 1998; 50: 943–50.

107 Loring DW, Meador KJ, Lee GP et al. Wada memory asymmetries predict verbal memory decline after anterior temporal lobectomy. Neurology 1995; 45(7): 1329–33.

108 Powell G, Polkey C, Canavan A. Lateralization of memory functions in epileptic patients by use of the sodium amytal (Wada) technique. *J Neurol Neurosurg Psychiatr* 1987; 50: 665–72.

109 Hermann BP, Wyler AR, Somes G, Berry AD, Dohan FC Jr. Pathological status of the mesial temporal lobe predicts memory outcome from left anterior temporal lobectomy. *Neurosurgery* 1992; 31: 652–7.

110 Trenerry M, Jack C, Ivnik R *et al.* MRI hippocampal volumes and memory function before and after temporal lobectomy. *Neurology* 1993; 43: 1800–5.

111 Olivier A. Risk and benefit in the surgery of epilepsy: Complications and positive results on seizure tendency and intellectual function. *Acta Neurol Scand* 1988; 78 (Suppl.): 114–21.

112 Loring DW, Meador K, Lee G *et al.* Wada memory performance predicts seizure outcome following anterior temporal lobectomy. *Neurology* 1994; 44: 2322–4.

113 Sperling M, Saykin A, Glosser G *et al.* Predictors of outcome after anterior temporal lobectomy: The intracarotid amobarbital test. *Neurology* 1994; 44: 2325–30.

114 Hunter KE, Blaxton TA, Bookheimer SY *et al.* [15]O water positron emission tomography in language localization: a study comparing positron emission tomography visual and computerized region of interest analysis with the Wada test. *Ann Neurol* 1999; 45(5): 662–5.

115 Binder JR, Swanson SJ, Hammeke TA *et al.* Determination of language dominance using functional MRI: A comparison with the Wada test. *Neurology* 1996; 46(4): 978–84.

116 Lehericy S, Cohen L, Bazin B *et al.* Functional MR evaluation of temporal and frontal language dominance compared with the Wada test. *Neurology* 2000; 54(8): 1625–33.

117 Detre JA, Maccotta L, King D *et al.* Functional MRI lateralization of memory in temporal lobe epilepsy. *Neurology* 1998; 50(4): 926–32.

118 Dupont S, Van de Moortele PF, Samson S *et al.* Episodic memory in left temporal lobe epilepsy: a functional MRI study. *Brain* 2000; 123(8): 1722–32.

119 Killgore W, Glosser G, Casasanto DJ, French JA, Alsop DC, Detre J. Functional MRI and the Wada test provide complementary information for predicting post-operative seizure control. *Seizure* 1999; 8: 450–5.

120 Forster L, Jones-Gotman M, Pike B. Hippocampal activation during encoding of pictures of objects: an fMRI study. *Neuroimage* 2001; 13(6): S667.

59 The Role of Psychiatric Assessment in Presurgical Evaluation of Epilepsy

E.S. Krishnamoorthy

The widespread lack of agreement on the importance of psychiatric and social issues for the surgical treatment for epilepsy is well known [1]. While a number of studies have shown that considerable psychiatric comorbidity exists in patient populations being evaluated for surgery [2], it is not clear whether such presurgical psychiatric comorbidity has an impact on postsurgical psychiatric outcome [3]. On the one hand, the beneficial effects of surgery (particularly temporal lobe resection) on overall outcome have been demonstrated in a number of studies [4]. On the other, prospective studies have shown *de novo* psychiatric complications such as depression, psychosis and personality change following temporal lobectomy [5]. Further, there is considerable disagreement on what the psychiatric contraindications for epilepsy surgery are, if any, and concern has also been expressed that patients with comorbid psychiatric disorder may be denied potentially beneficial surgical intervention [6].

This lack of consensus is reflected in the limited attention paid to psychiatric assessment in the evaluation of patients for epilepsy surgery. It has been pointed out that different centres worldwide have markedly different protocols, ranging from detailed to cursory, and that there is a clear need for each centre to state its policy with regard to rejecting or accepting patients with comorbid psychiatric conditions for surgery [7]. While some consensus has emerged from meetings like the Palm Desert Conferences, this has not seen wide implementation.

With this in mind the First Commission on Psychobiology, established by the International League Against Epilepsy, set up a subcommission on 'psychiatric aspects of epilepsy surgery'. This subcommission has surveyed epilepsy surgery centres worldwide and conducted a wide-ranging consultation exercise with presurgical neuropsychiatric assessment as a focus of interest. The commission aimed to build consensus among experts on a range of issues including the assessment and role of psychiatric comorbidity in the selection of candidates for epilepsy surgery, the methods to be used in such assessment and their frequency of application, the psychiatric indications and contraindications for epilepsy surgery (if any), the identification of candidates at risk of poor psychiatric outcome, the measures to be chosen to assess psychiatric outcome after surgery and the optimal rehabilitation process to be implemented after surgery. A series of Delphi panel [8] focus groups involving experts from various specialities (neuropsychiatry, neuropsychology, neurology, neurosurgery and rehabilitation) were conducted in the UK, and these results are being drawn upon here in making recommendations.

What should we assess for?

From the perspective of presurgical assessment it would perhaps suffice to mention that both generic psychopathology as described in the major classificatory systems (DSM-IV [9] for example) and psychopathology specific to epilepsy must be assessed as part of the presurgical assessment process.

The Diagnostic and Statistical Manual of Mental Disorders (DSM-IV) [9] recognizes few classes of psychiatric disorders 'due to epilepsy', namely Depressive Disorders (293.83 Mood Disorder Due to Epilepsy, as a General Medical Condition), Psychotic Disorder (293.8x Psychotic Disorder Due to Epilepsy, as a General Medical Condition) and Personality Disorders (310.1 Personality Change Due to Epilepsy, as a General Medical Condition). Depression and anxiety, for example, are prevalent in epilepsy, and have been described in detail elsewhere [10,11]. A comprehensive discussion of psychiatric disorders, which are most clearly linked to epilepsy, including interictal [12], alternative [13] and postictal psychosis [14], affective-somatoform symptoms, which occur during the prodromal, interictal and postictal phases [15], phobic fears [16] and personality disorders [17,18], is provided in Chapter 20. It is not uncommon for these disorders to go unrecognized.

Who should be assessed and by whom?

It is widely recommended that all subjects being considered for epilepsy surgery undergo comprehensive neuropsychiatric evaluation. In many specialist centres like the National Hospital for Neurology and Neurosurgery in London, comprehensive assessment by an expert team is mandatory. The assessment team should be multidisciplinary and should include (apart from the electrophysiologist, neurologist and neurosurgeon and other such mandatory members) a neuropsychiatrist, preferably with an understanding of the special issues in epilepsy, a neuropsychologist (presurgical neuropsychological assessment is detailed elsewhere in Chapter 58) and an epilepsy counsellor/specialist nurse. The role of the specialist nurse/counsellor is important as they interact closely with the patient and the family during the course of this process, explore expectations of surgery, obtain detailed information from the general practitioner/referring physician and liaise with family and community services in assessing and developing psychosocial support structures.

It is recognized that smaller centres may not have sufficient resources available to perform such a detailed evaluation in every case. In these situations the consulting neurologist or neuropsychologist should screen the subject for neuropsychiatric disorders, perhaps aided by self-rating measures of psychological well-being, described here. Further, such screening could be done when suitability for surgery has been assessed, in order to avoid the extra burden of screening individuals who may not qualify for other reasons.

How should patients be assessed?

There is no instrument specifically designed to diagnose and assess psychiatric disorders in epilepsy. A standardized psychiatric interview modified for epilepsy is necessary, along with guidelines for training. Interview schedules such as the Structured Clinical Interview for DSM [19], which has been adapted for use in epilepsy, or Schedules for Assessment in Neuropsychiatry (SCAN) [20], may be useful. Other interview measures that have been used in research on psychiatry of epilepsy include the Clinical Interview Schedule (now revised) (CIS-R) [21] and the Composite International Diagnostic Interview (CIDI) [22].

In addition to the above tools, questionnaires may provide a structured, standardized and validated method of assessment that can be used in different centres. Information collected by questionnaires is very useful for research, as more data is needed on the long-term psychiatric sequelae of epilepsy surgery. The following questionnaires are suggested as useful adjuncts to the clinical evaluation.
1 The Neurobehavioral Inventory (NBI) [23] (a measure of epilepsy-specific psychopathology such as the Geschwind syndrome).
2 Hospital Anxiety and Depression Scale (HADS) [24] (a well-validated generic measure of anxiety and depression in the hospital setting).
3 State-Trait Anxiety Inventory [25].
4 The Beck Depression Inventory (BDI) [26] (a well-validated generic measure of depression based on Beck's cognitive theory of depression).
5 Subjective Handicap of Epilepsy Scale (SHE) [27].
6 Quality of Life in Epilepsy, QOLIE [28] (both SHE and QOLIE are reasonable measures of outcome. Of the two, QOLIE is the more widely used instrument).
7 Questionnaire for Expectations and Beliefs about Epilepsy Surgery (S. Baxendale, personal communication).
8 Minnesota Multiphasic Personality Inventory (MMPI) [29], Standardized Assessment of Personality (SAP) [30] or other well-validated instruments for the assessment of personality.

As far as other sources of information are concerned, input from the carer/family is very important for assessing both psychopathology and personality. The Neuropsychiatric Inventory (NPI) [31] is a widely used tool in neurological settings, and enables the documentation of a structured carer's report of psychopathology. It has been used in epilepsy settings and demonstrated to have acceptable psychometric properties [32]. Personality inventories such as the SAP also rely upon structured carers' reports.

The assistance of the general practitioner/referring physician should also be sought. A standardized letter asking for information on past psychiatric history/personality disorder and/or any evidence of somatization could be sent to the general practitioner/primary care physician, as going through the primary care medical notes for each patient would be time-consuming and impractical.

Finally, it has been pointed out [33] that assessment of frontal and parietal lobe neurobehavioural function is assuming greater impor-

tance. The assessment of these functions is specialized although excellent bedside test protocols are widely available [34] and may be followed. Close collaboration with the neuropsychologist may also yield valuable information correlating cognition and behavioural states in some individuals.

When should patients be assessed?

The neuropsychiatric evaluation is ideally performed early in the epilepsy surgery process and should form an integral part of the protocol, rather than being an 'add-on', for a number of reasons.
1 Early assessment is necessary to identify patients who are unsuitable for surgery, which would save time and resources. This would also avoid the trauma of being turned down after the long drawn-out process of presurgical evaluation.
2 Psychiatric assessment would be more acceptable to the patient if it were a part of the assessment protocol rather than a 'last test' or hurdle to clear.
3 A better understanding of the patient's epilepsy, and exploration of various treatment options, are also aims of presurgical evaluation, and surgery should not be considered the sole purpose of the process. Early assessment should not therefore be aimed at screening out patients, but at treating the problems in an attempt to make surgery a viable option.
4 Re-evaluation in the course of the assessment depends on the initial findings, the length of the process and the resources available. A reassessment closer to the time of surgery would be ideal.
5 Psychiatric problems may contribute to death in patients rejected for surgery—early presurgical psychiatric evaluation is therefore vital.

At around the time of surgery, a number of additional issues need to be considered.
1 It may be important to reassess patients for psychological preparedness just prior to surgery, independent of the family. Some patients, especially adolescents, may be pressurized by their families to have surgery, and surgery should be postponed if such problems are noted.
2 The neurologist or neurosurgeon sensitive to these issues should be in a position to assess preparedness for surgery, and refer the patient to the neuropsychiatrist if necessary. The specialist epilepsy nurse practitioner (nurse clinician) or the neuropsychologist are also ideally placed to alert the treating clinician on such issues.
3 If acute neuropsychiatric crises were to supervene around the time of surgery, a decision to delay surgery until this has been addressed will need to be made. This decision, however, will depend on how serious or life-threatening the seizures are.

Why should patients undergo presurgical neuropsychiatric assessment?

The aims of presurgical assessment include the following.
1 To identify the presence of psychiatric contraindications to surgery (Table 59.1).
2 To identify patients at risk of developing psychiatric complications after epilepsy surgery.
3 To ensure that the patient is fully capable of giving informed consent.

Table 59.1 Main psychiatric and psychosocial contraindications to epilepsy surgery

Ongoing interictal psychosis (absolute contraindication)
Personality disorders
Comorbid NEAD
Serious or disabling psychiatric disorder
Ongoing or recent alcohol/drug abuse
History of interictal psychosis or other disabling psychiatric disorder
Strong family history of psychiatric illness
Poor psychosocial supports
Poor understanding of the benefits vs. risks; unrealistic expectations
History of aggression, antisocial behaviour, alcohol or drug abuse

4 To identify and treat comorbid psychiatric disorders which would then make epilepsy surgery a more viable option.

There is, however, lack of consensus on how results of the psychiatric assessment can be used to select patients suitable for surgery.

Absolute neuropsychiatric contraindications to epilepsy surgery

An ongoing interictal psychosis is the only absolute contraindication to epilepsy surgery because such illness would preclude the subject from making an informed decision about surgery, and giving informed consent. It is recognized that psychosis may worsen after surgery, and a continuing psychotic illness postsurgery is likely to have an adverse impact on quality of life and outcome, even if seizures do not recur. However, there have been reports of patient series with epilepsy and psychoses treated with surgery in specialist settings, who have enjoyed good outcome, both from the seizure viewpoint and the psychopathology viewpoint [35]. It must however be recognized that the resources made available in these cases were exceptional, and the management team expert. Surgery for patients with active psychoses must therefore be approached with due caution and by teams with considerable expertise alone. Further, it must be recognized that the ability to give informed consent may be an issue here and, while the psychopathology (delusions for example) do not necessarily incorporate the surgical process, they may well begin to do so, later in the course of this process, or even postsurgically.

Relative neuropsychiatric contraindications to epilepsy surgery

Personality disorders are difficult to treat, and their very nature may in some cases predicate the likelihood of a poor outcome, even if the surgery were successful in stopping or reducing seizures. However, targeting these patients for intensive postsurgical rehabilitation may permit consideration for surgery, especially in those cases where the epilepsy is severe and life-threatening. One problem here is the need to distinguish between premorbid personality traits and comorbid psychopathology. This is particularly difficult in epilepsy, as in many subjects seizures begin in childhood or adolescence, before the personality has evolved. Enduring aberrant patterns of behaviour independent of mood states and psychopathology that characterize the person's life, and are a constant source of distress,

either to the person concerned or to those around him or both, may be considered relevant here. A reliable family member is an invaluable asset in these situations, as history taking may be both complex and confusing.

Comorbid non-epileptic attack disorder (NEAD) is another contraindication to be considered. The assessment of patients with epilepsy and comorbid NEAD is complicated by both the tenuous nature of non-epileptic events, and by comorbid psychopathology. Indeed, the history of comorbid NEAD often becomes apparent only after surgery, when subjects manifest with an event that is documented to be non-epileptic. More information is required before NEAD can be accepted as an absolute contraindication. Empirical evidence suggests that it may be considered a relative contraindication, as it is quite common for people with epilepsy and NEAD to continue having non-epileptic attacks postsurgically. However, if the NEAD component could be identified and treated before surgery, the patient may not be denied surgery for the epilepsy component. It is also important to ensure that patients with the first non-epileptic seizure during telemetry are not excluded from surgery, as they often are 'under pressure to perform'. Further, patients with NEAD that is difficult to treat should not be denied surgery if the epileptic seizures are life-threatening.

Other relative contraindications are the presence of a serious or disabling psychiatric disorder, such as major depression or obsessive–compulsive disorder; ongoing or recent history of alcohol or drug abuse; a history of interictal psychosis or other disabling psychiatric disorder; a strong family history of psychiatric illness; poor psychosocial supports (living alone, no identifiable next of kin, close friend or associate, unemployed); or history of aggression, antisocial behaviour, alcohol or drug abuse. Experts also agree [33] that patients with undue eagerness for surgery, unrealistic expectations and inability to assess risks vs. benefits, need to be approached with great caution. All these attributes must be relevant to the cultural context, and must be considered from that perspective. In all these situations a considered decision by a multidisciplinary team is necessary.

Neuropsychiatric indications for epilepsy surgery

Postictal psychosis could be considered as an indication for surgery as it is clearly precipitated by seizures. Further, the disorder may result in significant morbidity, even mortality, as patients tend on occasion to indulge in explosive/destructive behaviour that places themselves or others at serious risk. The prevention of postictal psychosis is through the prevention of seizures. In persons who otherwise are good candidates for epilepsy surgery, postictal psychosis (in the clear absence of any interictal psychopathology) may be an indication for surgery. However, more studies are required to determine how many patients with postictal psychoses go on to develop chronic psychoses after surgery.

The postsurgery period

While the focus of this chapter is on presurgical neuropsychiatric assessment, care in this regard does in practice spill over to the period after surgery. A number of issues need to be considered in neuropsychiatric assessment postsurgery, and some of these will be addressed here.

Immediate postsurgical crises

Acute psychological or psychiatric crises are not uncommon in the immediate postsurgical period. Acute anxiety and hypersexuality have been observed in the week following surgery, but more information is required on these issues. Anxiety in particular is aggravated by seizures occurring in the immediate postsurgical period, which is not an uncommon occurrence even though they are not generally perceived to be a predictor of poor long-term outcome. A specialist epilepsy nurse practitioner would be the ideal person to monitor patients for any problems during this period. Reassurance and support are often adequate, although in a small number of cases anxiolytic drugs may become necessary.

Neuropsychiatric follow-up post surgery

Neuropsychiatric reassessment is mandatory in the first year after epilepsy surgery. Patients should ideally be assessed within 3 months (preferably at 6 weeks), at 1 year and then 5 years after surgery. The late assessment at 5 years may depend on the resources available to the epilepsy surgery centre.

The same neuropsychiatry team based at the epilepsy surgery centre should ideally perform both pre- and postsurgical psychiatric assessments. If that is not possible due to lack of resources, the neuropsychologist who routinely sees the patient or a specialist nurse may be able to identify issues, which need to be addressed by a neuropsychiatrist. As most patients travel long distances to these referral centres, the decision about who should perform the assessment is likely to depend on availability of local resources and the link between local and specialist centres.

Rehabilitation

It is the responsibility of the epilepsy surgery centre to organize and coordinate rehabilitation. The epilepsy centre should set broad guidelines, as local health services may not be aware of the special issues in epilepsy. Rehabilitation protocols may be individualized rather than standardized as patients have different needs postoperatively.

The following are identified as responsibilities of the epilepsy group regarding rehabilitation.
1 Identifying before surgery those patients who will need intensive rehabilitation post surgery. Examples of such patients include those with affective disorders, personality disorders and NEAD, and those with inadequate psychological support from family and friends.
2 Goal setting, including the identification of priority issues that need to be addressed quickly, and the drawing up of a management plan.
3 Coordinating the rehabilitation process with the general practitioner/primary care physician and local community mental health teams/psychiatrists.

It is recommended that the rehabilitation process be engendered through teamwork involving the neuropsychiatrist, neuropsychologist, neurologist, specialist epilepsy nurse, epilepsy counsellor, general practitioner, community mental health team, cognitive behaviour therapist, occupational therapist and social worker.

A booklet for patients (preferably in the local language) explaining the problems that may arise after surgery and list of potential local resources for support would be very useful. The National Hospital for Neurology and Neurosurgery in London, one of the large epilepsy surgery centres, has such a booklet available. Self-help groups, Internet websites and help-lines may also be helpful. Unfortunately, there is always the issue of resource limitation and the need to prioritize, which impacts on these services.

Special groups

This chapter has focused mainly on the adult non-learning disabled subject with epilepsy. Adult non-learning disabled women do form a special group in that their seizures and comorbid behavioural disorders (usually affective somatoform in nature) can be catamenial and thus predictable in some way. This pattern may well be disturbed post surgery, especially if surgery is not successful, and this is important to keep in mind. Further, it is important to remember that some young women might want to have surgery in order to discontinue their medication and start planning a family. This might be a source of potential distress, especially if the seizures are not completely controlled by surgery, or indeed if medication cannot be discontinued for any reason.

Children are another special group, as indeed are the learning disabled. Psychiatric disorders in both these groups of epilepsy patients are quite different from those seen in adults, and both these groups of patients are best managed by professionals with special expertise. Equally, it is important with both these groups to consider family dynamics, and the decision to operate must be made only after ascertaining that there is no conflict between the parents/principal carers on this issue. Also, these groups are often pressurized by the family to have surgery, especially older children and adolescents, as well as those with mild learning disability; the professional must take care to assess the individual's real feelings and concerns. Further, families may have unrealistic expectations and therefore they should be interviewed separately from the patient to ascertain these issues.

Poor psychiatric outcome after epilepsy surgery: who is at risk?

While there is little information on long-term psychiatric/psychological outcome after epilepsy surgery, the problems in Table 59.2 have been reported and must be looked for, whether or not seizures have been controlled. However, the entire subject of postsurgery psychiatric comorbidity has been controversial and the identification of groups at risk remains difficult.

The Maudsley series established by Falconer [4,36] was the progenitor of many other epilepsy surgery series that followed, particularly with regard to neuropsychiatric aspects. Falconer showed that while aggression, sexual disorders and postictal psychoses could improve with good seizure control chronic psychosis did not. Falconer also reported in his series *de novo* schizophrenia-like psychosis postoperatively, which could run a chronic course independent of seizure control. These findings have been replicated in more recent series [5,37], with some patients demonstrating improvement in psychiatric status following surgery and others developing *de novo* psychopathology, often without any relation to change in seizure status. A strong association between the

Table 59.2 Main psychiatric and psychosocial complications of epilepsy surgery

Acute anxiety and depression, especially in the 3–6-month period
  following surgery
Psychoses, including schizophrenia-like and organic psychosis
Hypomania/lability of mood
Major depression
Anxiety and depersonalization
Irritability, anger and aggression
Non-epileptic events
Difficulties in adjusting to not having epilepsy any more, and
  subsequent changes in lifestyle/difficulties due to
  loss of benefits and carers
Feelings of abandonment that may arise from lack of medical
  attention after surgery

removal of ganglioglioma and *de novo* postoperative psychosis has emerged in some series [38]. It has also been suggested that patients with enduring seizures postoperatively are at risk of developing postictal psychosis [39]. Experts have commented that *de novo* psychosis in the absence of continuing seizures is rather exceptional [33], although it is widely recognized that exceptions to this rule exist [40,41].

Problems such as depression and anxiety have received much less scientific attention. The vast majority of series [4,5,36,37] have reported cases of postoperative depression, and while anxiety has been far less studied, there are reports of significant numbers of cases in the literature [42]. An early study by our group [43] in which 60 patients were interviewed pre- and postoperatively by an experienced neuropsychiatrist showed that half of those with no psychopathology preoperatively had developed *de novo* symptoms of anxiety or depression 6 weeks postoperatively, and 45% of all patients were noted to have emotional lability in addition. When patients were reassessed 3 months postoperatively, anxiety states and emotional lability had become less common, but more patients were depressed in all groups. Left hemisphere preponderance to the increase of anxiety was also demonstrated in this study.

We examined the predictors of psychiatric outcome after temporal lobectomy in a further study of 121 subjects [44] who had undergone epilepsy surgery at the National Hospital in London. Interestingly poor psychiatric outcome was positively associated with preoperative bilateral independent spike discharges at telemetry. The study clearly demonstrated that psychopathology was very common both pre- and postoperatively in subjects undergoing temporal lobectomy. Nearly 10% of subjects required hospitalization for psychiatric symptoms postoperatively and many more needed consultation and treatment. Patients with preoperative psychiatric history and *de novo* psychiatric symptoms had poorer surgical outcome in terms of seizure frequency, although this effect was marginal. While we found no evidence to suggest a link between pre- and postoperative psychopathology in general, preoperative mood disorder was linked with postoperative anxiety, a common complaint.

The size of surgical resection was correlated with the occurrence of emotional lability postoperatively. While no laterality differences were demonstrated, developmental lesions were associated with a good psychiatric outcome at a marginally significant level, although the number of patients with alien tissue lesions (gangliogliomas for example) was small in this series. This is relevant because it has been suggested that patients with alien tissue lesions are more at risk of developing *de novo* psychopathology than those with mesial temporal sclerosis [38,45].

Taken together, however, the results of various studies produce little consensus about risk, except perhaps the differences in psychiatric outcome between developmental and alien tissue lesions. In general patients with a strong past or family history of psychopathology must be approached with caution as they demonstrate inherent biological vulnerability. While it is not clear if comorbid psychopathology *per se* increases the risk of postoperative psychopathology, it must be borne in mind that the perceived burden of the surgical process is likely to be greater in someone who has an ongoing psychiatric illness. Also, candidates for surgery with poor psychosocial support, strained personal and familial circumstances, poor understanding of the process or unreasonable expectations must all be considered at greater risk of developing postoperative psychopathology. The link between bilateral spikes and poor psychiatric outcome in our study while being novel perhaps reflects the exponential relationship between the degree of brain insult or injury and liability to psychopathology, which is from an empirical viewpoint understandable. Finally, these risk factors must be considered in light of the contraindications to surgery identified herein (Table 59.1).

What do we tell our patients in clinical practice?

Counselling patients about the neuropsychiatric risks and benefits of epilepsy surgery is an essential part of the process (Table 59.1). There are no strict guidelines available and, while it is important to give patients accurate information, it is important not to frighten them or cause further confusion in what is already a very difficult process. What we tell patients is also dependent upon factors such as the cultural ethos of the society one lives in, the age and personality of the concerned individual and indeed to some extent the personal attributes of the physician in question. Presurgical counselling is thus very individualized, and we all have our own ways developed over years of experience. Table 59.1 is a summary of what this author communicates to his patients.

Conclusions

There is growing awareness of the importance of psychosocial well-being towards achieving favourable outcomes after epilepsy surgery. Psychiatric comorbidity should no longer be viewed as a contraindication for surgery. Instead, each patient should have a psychiatric and social care programme with set goals determined before surgery, with regular monitoring of the achievement of these plans and goals.

Presurgical neuropsychiatric assessment is a very important component of the epilepsy surgery process and particular attention needs to be paid to this. As detailed above, a comprehensive and multidisciplinary approach that employs standardized tools and outcome measures is necessary. Comorbid psychopathology must not be viewed as a deterrent to surgery except in exceptional situa-

Table 59.1 Emotion, behaviour and epilepsy surgery: advice to patients

Emotional difficulties are closely linked with this kind of operation, as it often involves parts of the brain that control emotion and behaviour. It is therefore important that the neuropsychiatry team sees you during the evaluation process and follows you up after surgery, if this were to go ahead

There are several reasons for this. First, people who have suffered from certain emotional difficulties may not do well after surgery, and it is important therefore that they are assessed for these problems. Second, even those people who have never suffered from emotional difficulties in the past may develop these after surgery, and it is desirable that a presurgical assessment be carried out by the neuropsychiatrist, so that they can help you effectively in the period after surgery, were this to become necessary

The most common problems are mood swings, and a combination of anxiety and depression. These are seen in 20–30% of people who undergo surgery for epilepsy. While this can be distressing, cause tiredness, loss of sleep, poor appetite and make the person feel on edge, these symptoms do tend to go away on their own in a few weeks (usually 4–6 weeks), although some people may need antidepressant medication or counselling

Less commonly, in about 10% of people, a more significant form of depression, with sustained mood change and negative thoughts about oneself, the world and the future occurs. This may require formal support, including antidepressant drugs and/or counselling, rarely admission to hospital, but usually responds to treatment over a 6-month period

A more serious psychiatric disorder called psychosis, can occur after surgery but is relatively uncommon, seen in perhaps 3 or 4% of patients. Here, the person may lose touch with reality, and harbour abnormal beliefs, which other people around him do not share. This illness does require considerable formal support including psychiatric admission, and can cause considerable distress and disability. Although uncommon, you need to be aware of this risk in making your decision about surgery

What can be done?

As mentioned above, most psychiatric complications of surgery are either self-remitting or respond well to treatment. Some of the drugs used do have the potential to provoke seizures and hence need to be chosen and monitored carefully. However, there are usually few interactions between these drugs and those that you take for epilepsy. Other supportive therapies that are helpful in managing these disorders include counselling, psychotherapy and behaviour therapy

How and where will I be managed?

Once you have been assessed by the neuropsychiatry service, you will have the support of that service all through the surgical process and this will continue as long as it is necessary. Members of our service will see you in clinic, liaise with your physician and other doctors in your hospital and make suitable referrals for therapy (either here or in your local area) as appropriate

How important are these emotional issues?

Psychiatric issues are rarely a contraindication for surgery and by themselves seldom prevent us from offering you the chance to have an operation. While they may affect outcome, most often the disability they cause is self-limiting or responds to appropriate treatment. Major psychiatric complications are uncommon, and even these can be managed successfully in most people. It is important to remember that the benefits of epilepsy surgery usually outweigh the psychiatric risks in most people

---

tions, and may well even be an indication to surgery if properly identified (for example postictal psychosis). In most situations, early detection and effective management of such comorbidity may result in epilepsy surgery becoming both possible and successful. Also, a team approach involving several disciplines working in tandem is the ideal. The role of family, friends, primary care services and support groups cannot be overemphasized.

It is evident that neuropsychiatric assessment for epilepsy surgery is not a single stage procedure, but a process that begins early in the surgical evaluation, continues right through actual surgery, and for months, even years afterwards. Indeed, neuropsychiatric units in major epilepsy surgery centres continue following up some patients long after neurosurgeons and even neurologists have discharged them from their services, following seizure cessation and successful discontinuation of antiepileptic drug therapy.

Acknowledgements

I acknowledge Dr S. Koch-Stoecker and Dr L. Vijayaraghavan for early data from the Delphi exercise conducted by the First ILAE Commission on Epilepsy and Psychobiology and the numerous experts who participated in this effort.

References

1 Engel J Jr. Update on the Second International Palm Desert Conference on the Surgical Treatment of the Epilepsies (1992). *Neurology* 1993; 43(8): 1612–7.

2 Manchanda R, Schaefer B, McLachlan RS *et al.* Psychiatric disorders in candidates for surgery for epilepsy. *J Neurol Neurosurg Psychiatr* 1996; 61(1): 82–9.

3 Anhoury S, Brown RJ, Krishnamoorthy ES, Trimble MR. Psychiatric outcome following temporal lobectomy: A predictive study. *Epilepsia* 2000; 41(12): 1608–15.

4 Falconer MA. Reversibility by temporal lobe resection of the behavioural abnormalities of temporal lobe epilepsy. *NEJM* 1973; 289: 451–5.

5 Blumer D, Wakhlu S, Davies K, Hermann B. Psychiatric outcome of temporal lobectomy for epilepsy: incidence and treatment of psychiatric complications. *Epilepsia* 1998; 39: 47S–86S.

6 Ferguson S *et al.* Postoperative psychiatric changes. In: Engel J Jr, ed. *Surgical Treatment of the Epilepsies*. New York: Raven Press, 1993.

7 Fenwick PB *et al.* Pre-surgical psychiatric assessment. In: In Engel J Jr, ed. *Surgical Treatment of the Epilepsies*. New York: Raven Press, 1993.

8 Linstone HA, Turoff M. Introduction. In: Linstone HA, Turoff M, eds. *The Delphi Method: techniques and applications*. New York: Addison Wesley, 1975: 3–12.

9 American Psychiatric Association. *Diagnostic and Statistical Manual of Mental Disorders*, 4th edn. Washington, DC: American Psychiatric Press, 1994.

10 Lambert M, Robertson MM. Depression in epilepsy: etiology, phenomenology, and treatment. *Epilepsia* 1999; 40 (Suppl. 10): S21–S47.

11 Goldstein MA, Harden CL. Epilepsy and anxiety. *Epilepsy Behav* 2000; 1: 228–34.

12 Trimble MR. *The Psychoses of Epilepsy*. New York: Raven Press, 1991.

13 Krishnamoorthy ES, Trimble MR. Forced normalization—clinical and therapeutic relevance. *Epilepsia* 1999: 40 (Suppl. 10): S57–S64.

14 Logsdail SJ, Toone BK. Post-ictal psychoses. A clinical and phenomenological description. *Br J Psych* 1988; 152: 246–52.

15 Blumer D. Dysphoric disorders and paroxysmal effects: recognition and treatment of epilepsy-related psychiatric disorders. *Harvard Rev Psychiatr* 2000; 8(1): 8–17.

16 Newsom-Davis I, Goldstein LH, Fitzpatrick D. Fear of seizures—an investigation and treatment. *Seizure* 1998; 7: 101–6.

17 Blumer D. Personality disorders in epilepsy. In: Ratey JJ, ed. *Neuropsychiatry of Personality Disorders*. Boston: Blackwell Science, 1995: 230–63.

18 Trimble M. Cognitive and personality profiles in patients with juvenile myoclonic epilepsy. In: Schmitz B, Sander T. *Juvenile Myoclonic Epilepsy—The Janz Syndrome*, Petersfield: Wrightson Biomedical Publishing, 2000: 101–11.

19 Spitzer RL, Williams JB. Revised diagnostic criteria and a new structured interview for diagnosing anxiety disorders. *J Psychiatr Res* 1988; 22 (Suppl. 1): 55–85.

20 World Health Organisation, Division of Mental Health, Geneva. *Schedules for Clinical Assessment in Neuropsychiatry (SCAN)*. Geneva: WHO, 1992.

21 Lewis G, Pelosi AJ, Araya R, Dunn G. Measuring psychiatric disorder in the community: a standardised assessment for use by lay interviewers. *Psychol Med* 1992; 22: 465–86.

22 Robins LN. The composite international diagnostic interview. *DIS Newsletter* 1985; Spring: 1–2 (DIS Training Faculty and Staff, Washington University School of Medicine, St Louis, Missouri).

23 Blumer D. Personality disorders in epilepsy. In: Ratey JJ, ed. *Neuropsychiatry of Personality Disorders*. Boston: Blackwell Science, 1995: 230–63.

24 Zigmond AS, Snaith RP. The Hospital Anxiety and Depression Scale. *Acta Psychiatr Scand* 1983; 67: 361–70.

25 Spielberger CD, Gorsuch RL, Luchene R, Vagg PR, Jacobs GA. *Manual for the State-Trait Anxiety Inventory*. Palo Alto: Consulting Psychologists Press, 1983.

26 Beck AT, Ward CH, Mendelson M, Mock J, Erbaugh J. An inventory for measuring depression. *Arch Gen Psychiatr* 1961; 4: 561–71.

27 O'Donoghue MF, Duncan JS, Sander JWAS. The subjective handicap of epilepsy—a new approach to measuring treatment outcome. *Brain* 1998; 121: 317–43.

28 Devinsky O, Vickrey BG, Cramer J *et al.* Development of the quality of life in epilepsy inventory. *Epilepsia* 1995; 36(11): 1089–104.

29 Pearson JS, Rome HP, Swenson WM, Mataya P, Brannick TL. Development of a computer system for scoring and interpretation of Minnesota Multiphasic Personality Inventories in a medical clinic. *Ann NY Acad Sci* 1965; 126(2): 684–95.

30 Mann AH, Jenkins R, Cutting JC, Cowen PJ. The development and use of a standardised assessment of abnormal personality. *Psychol Med* 1981; 11: 839–47.

31 Cummings JL, Mega M, Gray K *et al.* The Neuropsychiatric Inventory: comprehensive assessment of psychopathology in dementia. *Neurology* 1994; 44: 2308–14.

32 Samuel R, Krishnamoorthy ES, Trimble MR. Efficacy of the Neuropsychiatry Inventory in the behavioural assessment of patients with epilepsy and learning disability. *Epilepsia* 1999; 40 (Suppl. 2): 291.

33 Savard G, Manchanda R. Psychiatric assessment of candidates for epilepsy surgery. *Can J Neurol Sci* 2000; 27 (Suppl. 1): S44–S49.

34 Strub RL, Black FW. *The Mental Status Examination in Neurology*. Philadelphia: FA Davis Company, 1985.

35 Reutens DC, Savard G, Andermann F, Dubeau F, Olivier, A. Results of surgical treatment in temporal lobe epilepsy with chronic psychosis. *Brain* 1997; 120: 1929–36.

36 Falconer MA. Pathological substrates in temporal lobe epilepsy with psychoses. In: Latinen LV, Livingston KE, eds. *Surgical Approaches in Psychiatry*. Baltimore: University Park Press, 1973: 121–4.

37 Naylor AS, Rogvi-Hansen BA, Kessing L, Kruse-Larsen C. Psychiatric morbidity after surgery for epilepsy: short-term follow up of patients undergoing amygdalohippocampectomy. *J Neurol Neurosurg Psychiatr* 1994; 57(11): 1375–81.

38 Bruton CJ. *The Neuropathology of Temporal Lobe Epilepsy*. Oxford: Oxford University Press, 1988: 158.

39 Manchanda R, Miller H, McLachlan RS. Post-ictal psychosis after right temporal lobectomy. *J Neurol Neurosurg Psychiatr* 1993; 56(3): 277–9.

40 Stevens JR. Psychiatric consequences of temporal lobectomy for intractable seizures: a 20–30 year follow up of 14 cases. *Psychol Med* 1990; 20: 529–45.

41 Mace CJ, Trimble MR. Psychosis following temporal lobe surgery: a report of six cases. *J Neurol Neurosurg Psychiatr* 1991; 54: 639–44.

42 Bladin PF. Psychosocial difficulties and outcome after temporal lobectomy. *Epilepsia* 1992; 33: 898–907.

43 Ring HA, Moriarty J, Trimble MR. A prospective study of the early postsurgical psychiatric associations of epilepsy surgery. *J Neurol Neurosurg Psychiatr* 1998; 64: 601–4.

44 Anhoury S, Brown RJ, Krishnamoorthy ES, Trimble MR. Psychiatric outcome after temporal lobectomy: a predictive study. *Epilepsia* 2000; 41: 1608–15.

45 Taylor DC. Factors influencing the occurrence of schizophrenia-like psychosis in patients with temporal lobe epilepsy. *Psychol Med* 1975; 5: 249–54.

60 Surgery of Hippocampal Sclerosis

J.G. Ojemann and T.S. Park

Temporal lobectomy for mesial temporal sclerosis is the most commonly performed epilepsy operation. In practice, temporal lobectomy includes a variety of operations including resections for medial temporal lobe pathology (e.g. medial temporal sclerosis), lesions within the medial or lateral temporal lobe, or resections of lateral, neocortical temporal lobe. Hippocampal sclerosis can occur in adults or children [1,2], but in children it is often associated with other pathologies, especially cortical dysplasia [3]. Temporal lobectomy has been shown, in a randomized trial, to give improved seizure control compared to conservative management for patients with temporal lobe epilepsy [4]. Many technical variations have been proposed (Table 60.1)—all include resection of the hippocampal structures, with differences in approach to these structures and differences in the inclusion or exclusion of other temporal lobe structures (e.g. lateral temporal lobe, amygdala, basal temporal lobe). Although other structures may be additionally targeted in the setting of sclerosis, the common goal of all approaches is the resection of the hippocampus (Fig. 60.1). This chapter deals with the surgical method and outcome of hippocampal surgery. Presurgical evaluation is covered in Chapters 51–59 and the complications of surgery in Chapter 2.

Surgical methods

The anatomical relationship between the hippocampus and the rest of the temporal lobe permits various surgical approaches (Figs 60.2–60.5). A standardized anterior temporal lobectomy involves resection of the lateral aspect of the anterior temporal lobe, entering the temporal horn deep to the temporal gyri (Fig. 60.2) [5,6]. The ventricle forms the roof of the hippocampus which is visible once the ventricle is entered. The hippocampus is then resected posteriorly, at least 1.5–3.5 cm posterior from the pes, or anterior portion, of the hippocampus.

For most approaches to hippocampal resection, general neurosurgical issues are addressed similarly. Large-bore IV catheters are used; often radial artery catheters are used to monitor blood pressure and permit rapid serum laboratory testing. Large amounts of bleeding are uncommon, but proximity to major vessels makes haemorrhage a definite risk. Close attention to vital signs, with communication of any change to the surgeon, is critical. Monitoring for bradycardia and hypotension is especially important, as mesial temporal resections are adjacent to the brainstem. In some patients the dura is especially sensitive and coagulation or manipulation can also result in bradycardia.

For selective procedures, a smaller incision can be made, as a fairly small amount of bone removal is required. The dura is opened and lateral cortex is resected until the ventricle is entered. This may be done under stereotactic guidance. Alternatively, in a subtemporal approach, the basal temporal lobe is exposed and the ventricle is entered inferiorly. A relaxed brain is vital as some degree of temporal lobe manipulation and retraction is required for any selective procedure. Options to relax the brain include administration of mannitol prior to opening the dura, mild hyperventilation and diuretics. Cerebrospinal fluid (CSF) drainage usually provides adequate relaxation, so avoiding the need for other measures. Often we achieve sufficient CSF drainage from the convexities, or from gentle exposure of the basal temporal lobe. Certainly once the temporal horn is exposed, CSF drainage is sufficient to achieve relaxation. Lumbar drainage before positioning for the craniotomy can also be used, but we have abandoned that for routine use.

The important anatomical landmarks for hippocampal removal are its borders, namely the temporal horn of the lateral ventricle, the choroidal fissure and the medially placed structures, including the internal carotid artery, brainstem and oculomotor (III) nerve.

When the approach is taken through the lateral temporal lobe, the ventricle is typically found directly medial to the middle temporal gyrus. The lateral corticectomy is performed under direct vision and the white matter resected medially (Plate 60.6, shown in colour between pp. 670 and 671). By extending the resection inferiorly as it progresses medially, the ventricle will be entered without inadvertently entering the temporal stem superior to the ventricle. Indeed, in the superior direction, there are no boundaries between the temporal white matter and the midbrain. Therefore, on finding the ventricle, care must always be taken to resect in the inferior and anterior direction.

The collateral sulcus projects superiorly from the fusiform gyrus running along the inferior aspect of the temporal lobe. This structure usually points to the lateral ventricle, just posterior to the tip of the temporal horn of the ventricle. In a selective procedure, the collateral sulcus is not routinely exposed.

Once the ventricle is exposed, a cottonoid is placed in the temporal horn to prevent excessive blood from entering the ventricle. The ventricle wall often has small veins which should be coagulated. Care is taken to avoid excessive coagulation or manipulation of the posterosuperior medial wall of the ventricle, which includes the optic radiations and lateral geniculate. The ventricle is opened more widely and retractors are then advanced into the ventricle.

Once the ventricle is entered, the alveus is immediately visible as a smooth surface (Plate 60.7, shown in colour between pp. 670 and 671). The pes of the hippocampus will be seen anteriorly. The amygdala overhangs the ventricle from the anterior roof. The lateral amygdala protrudes into the ventricle to a variable degree, and, if large, may obstruct visualization of the medial head of the hippocampus.

Table 60.1 Surgical approaches to hippocampal resection

> *Selective approaches*
> Middle temporal gyrus (transventricular)
> Inferior temporal gyrus
> Transparahippocampal
> Sylvian fissure
>
> *Anterior temporal lobectomy*
>
> *Tailored resection*
> Guided by lateral and/or hippocampal ECoG
> Functional (language) mapping

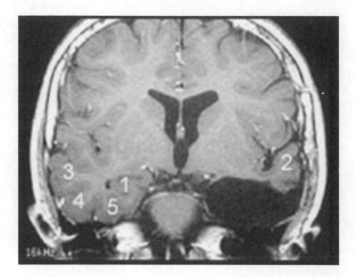

Fig. 60.2 Postoperative coronal T1-weighted MRI following a 'standard' temporal lobectomy. Extensive lateral temporal lobe is removed to expose the temporal horn of the lateral ventricle. The hippocampus has been resected (normal hippocampus labelled '1' on opposite side). The spared superior gyrus (2) is labelled. Resected structures (shown on the opposite side) also include middle temporal gyrus (3), inferior temporal gyrus (4) and fusiform gyrus (5).

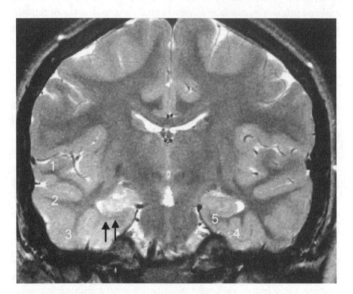

Fig. 60.1 Mesial temporal sclerosis. Coronal, T2-weighted MRI demonstrating increased signal in the hippocampus (arrows). This sclerotic hippocampus is the target of surgical resection for many cases of intractable seizures. Other structures noted are superior (1), middle (2) and inferior (3) temporal gyrus, fusiform gyrus (4) and parahippocampus (5). Cerebral peduncle is also evident along with the temporal horn of the lateral ventricle.

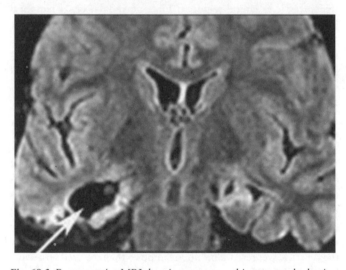

Fig. 60.3 Postoperative MRI showing a transparahippocampal selective amygdalohippocampectomy. The medial structures (arrow) are resected with sparing of lateral temporal lobe.

Posteriorly, the choroid plexus is seen overlying the posterior hippocampus (Fig. 60.7). The choroid plexus attaches to the tela choroidae, which runs parallel to the choroidal fissure. Thus the choroidal fissure, carrying the anterior choroidal artery, marks the medial border of the posterior aspect of the hippocampus. Anteriorly, the hippocampus courses medially, anterior to the cerebral peduncle, following the contour of the uncus of the temporal lobe.

Although the order of resection is not uniform, the hippocampus must be disconnected from surrounding structures, with special care medially to avoid the brainstem, vessels and cranial nerves. A certain amount of basal temporal lobe is resected. There is some suggestion that parahippocampus and basal temporal lobe (e.g. fusiform gyrus) may also contribute to epileptogenicity [7]. In any case, resection of the parahippocampus is performed in a subpial fashion with either suction and/or the ultrasonic aspirator. This is usually done under microscopic dissection, providing superior illumination and magnification when working near the brainstem. Re-

secting the mesial pia will protect the carotid and third nerve, which are visible medial to the edge of the tentorium. The fourth nerve is sometimes visible if it deviates slightly from its usual course inferior to the tentorial edge. The resection is executed from anterior to posterior and the hippocampus is thereby disconnected inferiorly.

The lateral amygdala is often removed prior to further work on the head of the hippocampus. Removal of the lateral amygdala provides a more extensive view of the hippocampal complex anteriorly. The amygdala is somewhat vascular and care is taken to remove only the lateral component. As there is no boundary between amygdala and midbrain/basal ganglia, the roof of the ventricle is

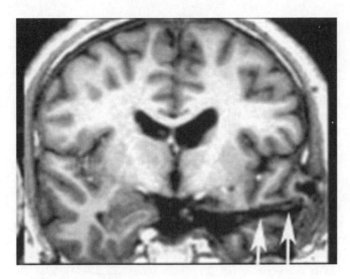

Fig. 60.4 Resection through the middle temporal gyrus (arrows) allows access to the medial structures (e.g. hippocampus) that have been removed.

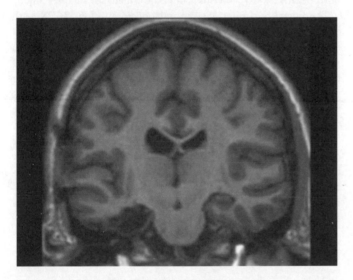

Fig. 60.5 Removing the inferior temporal gyrus decreases the potential for undercutting the fibres deep to the superior temporal gyrus. The medial structures can be accessed in this plane, with resection of basal temporal lobe.

typically used as the limit of amygdala resection; thus the amygdala is resected until flush with the remainder of the ventricular wall. If desired, the amygdala can be biopsied at this point as well.

At this point, the amygdalohippocampal connections are evident and can be resected down to the medial pia. The pia should be left intact and the carotid and third nerve are typically visualized at this point. Removal of the amygdala also exposes the uncus medially, which can be resected if desired.

The posterior resection of the hippocampus is then determined. In a standard resection, this is usually selected just where the tail of the hippocampus begins to curve medially behind the collicular plate. This will usually permit a resection of approximately 2.5 cm behind the hippocampal head. Some authors advocate intraoperative corticography to determine the posterior extent of resection [8].

At the posterior margin of the resection, the hippocampus is resected from the exposed hippocampal surface down to the choroidal fissure. The hippocampal fissure will arise medially. On the medial aspect, the hippocampus is resected back to the medial pia. The brainstem and/or colliculus are usually visible through the pia. Vessels in the hippocampal fissure can be coagulated, but coagulation of more medial pia can endanger perforating vessels from the internal carotid artery, posterior communicating artery and/or choroidal arteries and should thus be avoided. Gentle application of oxidized cellulose usually can control medial oozing.

At this point, the hippocampus is only connected to the choroidal fissure, the hippocampal fissure and any residual parahippocampal structures. If the border with the choroidal fissure is removed using aspiration, the hippocampus can often be gently dissected from the remaining pia. This allows for sufficient specimen to be sent for histopathology and completes the hippocampectomy. If additional hippocampus is resected posteriorly, this can be done with piecemeal aspiration of the truncated posterior hippocampus, following the hippocampal sulcus and choroidal fissure posteriorly. The hippocampal tail rapidly thins and resection back to the atrium of the ventricle is rarely indicated. Again, coagulation of the medial structures is avoided if possible.

Several other approaches to the ventricle have been advocated. Some surgeons have promoted the subtemporal, transparahippocampal approach [9,10]. Avoiding any involvement of lateral temporal cortex, the basal temporal lobe is gently elevated and the fusiform gyrus identified. Just medial to this, a corticectomy is made and the ventricle entered from inferiorly. Advancing the retractor exposes the hippocampus and amygdala as with a standard approach, from a more inferosuperior angle. The hippocampus and lateral amygdala can then be removed in the same subpial fashion, respecting the landmarks as with other mesial resections. The result (Fig. 60.3) is very precise in involving resection of only mesial structures and appears to lead to equivalent seizure outcome as other procedures, with theoretically less cognitive and visual field deficits.

An approach through the Sylvian fissure has been proposed, especially from groups familiar with this approach for surgery involving the circle of Willis. Deep within the Sylvian fissure, the resection can be carried out towards the temporal lobe. This allows for resection of the medial temporal structures. Although outcomes have been satisfactory [11,12], a steep learning curve with a high potential for hemiparesis [13] and increased manipulation of the vessels (such as the middle cerebral artery) have limited widespread use of this approach.

A common selective entry to the ventricle from the lateral cortex is the middle temporal gyrus approach [14]. This approach typically uses frameless stereotaxy, which requires a preoperative MRI prior to anaesthesia, with scalp fiducials placed on the patient that are visible on the MRI study. After the MRI and induction, the patient is fixed in a rigid head holder, the fiducials are coregistered with the MRI using an infrared localizer and approaches to the lateral ventricle can be planned and confirmed intraoperatively [12,14]. The extent of lateral cortical disruption can be minimized with this technology. The middle temporal gyrus is then resected medially until the ventricle is entered. The mesial temporal structures are then resected as described above (Fig. 60.4).

A further variation of this surgical approach is to resect the inferior temporal gyrus laterally and follow this plane, including the entire basal temporal lobe, until the inferior border of the ventricle is entered (Fig. 60.5). The mesial resection is then carried out in the standard fashion. This has the advantage over the subtemporal approach of limiting retraction of the temporal lobe and includes resection of basal temporal lobe which, in some cases, may be independently epileptogenic [7]. Unlike the middle temporal gyrus approach, resection of the inferior gyrus is much less likely to undercut white matter radiations from the superior gyrus which run just under the middle temporal gyrus as they travel out from the temporal stem (Fig. 60.5).

Certainly these methods vary in the extent of extrahippocampal structures that are resected, including both lateral neocortical and basal temporal regions. No evidence supports one method over another. Historic results have shown good outcome even when the amygdala is spared altogether [15].

Several variants of a standardized anatomical approach to the temporal lobectomy have been developed. In particular, a tailored resection has been advocated by several groups, tailoring the resection in regard both to epileptic foci and to language function [5]. These approaches involve surgery under local anaesthesia in order that language mapping can be performed. Short-acting agents are used to sedate the patient during the exposure of the dura; the patient is then allowed to awaken. Sites critical for language function are determined by stimulating the cortex while the patient performs an object naming task. These areas are then avoided during the temporal lobe resection. ECoG can also be used to tailor the resection. Placement of electrodes on the temporal lobe surface can identify lateral cortex with interictal spike activity, although the significance of this activity remains controversial [5,16]. Additionally, electrical recordings directly from the hippocampus can be used to guide the extent of hippocampal resection [8]. The inclusion of lateral cortex in the temporal lobe resection may be especially appropriate when it is not clear that the pathology is limited to medial temporal structures.

Outcome

The prognosis for seizure control following temporal lobectomy has improved over the last 10 years, probably largely due to advances in preoperative investigation [17]. Approximately 70% of patients achieve seizure freedom following temporal lobectomy [17]. In a given patient, the outcome from temporal lobectomy cannot be established until at least 1 year postoperatively, as seizure control will change over time [18], even over several years postoperatively. Although seizures in the immediate postoperative period do not predict long-term seizure control [19], recurrence of seizures within the first year postoperatively carries a worse prognosis [18,20]. Overall if seizure free at 1 year, there is a 70% chance of being seizure free at 10 years, and if seizure free by 2 years then there is a greater than 80% chance of being seizure free by 10 years [21]. A history of febrile seizures, MRI demonstrating hippocampal sclerosis and concordant EEG findings are all predictive of a good surgical outcome [17]. Indeed, in the subgroup of patients with mesial temporal lobe sclerosis and concordant EEG, resection leads to good outcome (seizure freedom) in the vast majority [3].

The complications of temporal lobe surgery are dealt with in more detail in Chapter 71; we will largely confine ourselves to the

complications that directly result from surgical approaches. Some degree of superotemporal quadrantanopia [22] is common following temporal lobe resection, as Meyer's loop fibres pass from the lateral geniculate to the occipital lobe via the temporal lobe white matter [23,24]. Anterior temporal lobectomy opens the ventricle wall, probably damaging visual fibres at that point. However, even selective procedures do not seem to change the risk of these deficits [22], so the exact mechanisms of visual field loss and the predictability of postoperative deficits remain unclear. Fortunately, such deficits are often neither noticed by patients nor identifiable on bedside examination [25]. In dominant temporal lobe resections, transient speech difficulties may result from postoperative oedema, especially when resections are taken close to language areas [25–27]. Some series have reported a small incidence of significant verbal performance loss after dominant temporal lobectomy especially in patients with normal preoperative MRI and patients with higher preoperative verbal memory scores [28,29–31]. Since the extent of lateral temporal resection has been correlated with verbal memory deficits [32], selective procedures that minimize lateral resection may be less prone to give memory problems postoperatively [10], but this is not established (see Chapter 58).

The mortality of anterior temporal lobectomy is low [26,28] with general neurosurgical risks including infection (less than 0.5% risk [26]), CSF leak and haemorrhage. Along with specific risks to visual and language function discussed above, the medial aspect of the temporal lobe resection puts other structures at risk, including the oculomotor nerve (III) and the cerebral peduncle which lies immediately medial to the temporal lobe. The incidence of damage to these structures is less than 1% [28].

Surgery of the hippocampus can be accomplished using a variety of approaches. All include resection of the hippocampus. All of the methods appear to be safe and effective for the treatment of intractable seizures, associated with MRI-identified hippocampal sclerosis, especially when this is congruent with ictal and interictal EEG findings.

References

1 Holmes G. Epilepsy surgery in children: when, why, and how. *Neurology* 2002; 58 (Suppl. 7): S13–S20.
2 Ojemann JG. Surgical treatment of pediatric epilepsy. *Semin Neurosurg* 2002; 13: 71–80.
3 Mohamed A, Wyllie E, Ruggieri P *et al*. Temporal lobe epilepsy due to hippocampal sclerosis in pediatric candidates for epilepsy surgery. *Neurology* 2001; 56: 1643–9.
4 Wiebe S, Blume WT, Girvin JP, Eliasziw M. Effectiveness and efficiency of surgery for Temporal Lobe Epilepsy Study Group. A randomized, controlled trial of surgery for temporal lobe epilepsy. *N Engl J Med* 2001; 345: 311–18.
5 Silbergeld DL, Ojemann GA. The tailored temporal lobectomy. *Neurosurg Clin N Am* 1993; 4(2): 273–81.
6 Spencer DD, Spencer SS, Mattson RH, Williamson PD, Novelly RA. Access to the posterior medial temporal lobe structures in the surgical treatment of temporal lobe epilepsy. *Neurosurgery* 1984; 15: 667–71.
7 Wennberg R, Arruda F, Quesney LF, Olivier A. Preeminence of extrahippocampal structures in the generation of mesial temporal seizures: Evidence from human depth electrode recordings. *Epilepsia* 2002; 43: 716–26.
8 McKhann GM II, Schoenfeld-McNeill J, Born DE, Haglund MM, Ojemann GA. Intraoperative hippocampal electrocorticography to predict the extent of hippocampal resection in temporal lobe epilepsy surgery. *J Neurosurg* 2000; 93: 44–52.

9 Park TS, Bourgeois BF, Silbergeld DL, Dodson WE. Subtemporal transparahippocampal amygdalohippocampectomy for surgical treatment of mesial temporal lobe epilepsy. *J Neurosurg* 1996; 85: 1172–6.

10 Robinson S, Park TS, Blackburn LB, Bourgeois BFD, Arnold ST, Dodson WE: Transparahippocampal selective amygdalohippocampectomy in children and adolescents: efficacy of the procedure and cognitive morbidity in patients. *J Neurosurg* 2000; 93: 402–9.

11 Wieser HG, Yasargil MG. Selective amygdalahippocampectomy as a surgical treatment of mediobasal limbic epilepsy. *Surg Neurol* 1982; 17: 445–57.

12 Wurm G, Wies W, Schnizer M, Trenkler J, Holl K. Advanced surgical approach for selective amygdalohippocampectomy through neuronavigation. *Neurosurgery* 2000; 46: 1377–83.

13 Barbaro NM. Comment on 'Advanced surgical approach for selective amygdalohippocampectomy through neuronavigation'. *Neurosurgery* 2000; 46: 1382–3.

14 Olivier A. Transcortical selective amygdalohippocampectomy in temporal lobe epilepsy. *Can J Neurol Sci* 2000; 27 (Suppl. 1): S68–S76.

15 Goldring S, Edwards I, Harding GW *et al*. Results of anterior temporal lobectomy that spares the amygdala with complex partial seizures. *J Neurosurg* 1992; 77: 185–93.

16 Schwartz TH, Bazil CW, Walczak TS, Chan S, Pedley TA, Goodman RR. The predictive value of intraoperative electrocorticography in resections for limbic epilepsy associated with mesial temporal sclerosis. *Neurosurgery* 1997; 40: 302–9.

17 McIntosh AM, Wilson SJ, Berkovic SF. Seizure outcome after temporal lobectomy: current research practice and findings. *Epilepsia* 2001; 42: 1288–307.

18 Engel J Jr, Van Ness PC, Rasmussen TB, Ojemann LM. Outcome with respect to epileptic seizures. In: Engel J Jr, ed. *Surgical Treatment of the Epilepsies*, 2nd edn. New York: Raven Press, 1993.

19 Ojemann GA, Bourgeois BF. Early postoperative management. In: Engel J Jr, ed. *Surgical Treatment of the Epilepsies*, 2nd edn. New York: Raven Press, 1993.

20 Armon C, Radtke RA, Friedman AH, Dawson DV. Predictors of outcome of epilepsy surgery: multivariate analysis with validation. *Epilepsia* 1996; 37: 814–21.

21 Foldvary N, Nashold B, Mascha E *et al*. Seizure outcome after temporal lobectomy for temporal lobe epilepsy. *Neurology* 2000; 54: 630–4.

22 Egan RA, Shults WT, So N, Burchiel K, Kellogg JX, Salinsky M. Visual field deficits in conventinoal anterior temporal lobectomy versus amygdalohippocampectomy. *Neurology* 2000; 55: 1818–22.

23 Marino R, Rasmussen T. Visual field changes after temporal lobectomy in man. *Neurology* 1968; 18: 825–35.

24 Van Buren JM, Baldwin M. The architecture of the optic radiation in the temporal lobe of man. *Brain* 1958; 81: 15–40.

25 Wyllie Luders H, Morris H, Lesser RP, Dinner DS, Hahn J, Estes ML. Clinical outcome after complete or partial cortical resections for intractable epilepsy. *Neurology* 1987; 37: 1634–41.

26 Pilcher WH, Rusyniak WG. Complications of epilepsy surgery. *Neurosurg Clin N Am* 1993; 4(2): 311–25.

27 Stafiniak P, Saykin AJ, Sperling MR *et al*. Acute naming deficits following dominant temporal lobectomy: prediction by age at first risk for seizures. *Neurology* 1990; 40: 1509–12.

28 Pilcher WH, Roberts DW, Flanigin HF *et al*. Complications of epilepsy surgery. In: Engel J Jr, ed. *Surgical Treatment of the Epilepsies*, 2nd edn. New York: Raven Press, 1993.

29 Gleissner U, Helmstaedter C, Schramm J, Elger CE. Memory outcome after selective amygdalohippocampectomy: a study in 140 patients with temporal lobe epilepsy. *Epilepsia* 2001; 43: 87–95.

30 Hermann BP, Wyler AR, Sones G, Clement L. Dysnomia after left anterior temporal lobectomy without functional mapping: frequency and correlates. *Neurosurgery* 1994; 35: 52–6.

31 Lee TMC, Yip JTH, Jones-Gotman M. Memory deficits after resection from left or right anterior temporal lobe in humans: a meta-analytic review. *Epilepsia* 2002; 43: 283–91.

32 Ojemann GA, Dodrill CB. Verbal memory deficits after left temporal lobectomy for epilepsy. Mechanism and intraoperative prediction. *J Neurosurg* 1985; 62: 101–7.

61 Resective Surgery of Neoplastic Lesions for Epilepsy

N.M. Wetjen, K. Radhakrishnan, A.A. Cohen-Gadol and G. Cascino

The association of brain tumours with epilepsy has been suspected since ancient times [1]. In the classic book of William Gowers, published in 1881 [2], a clear distinction between focal seizures due to a demonstrable pathological lesion and generalized seizures, constituting idiopathic epilepsies, was emphasized. However, Hughlings Jackson [3] was the first to provide a comprehensive understanding of the significance of focal seizures when he described uncinate seizures in patients with neoplastic and non-neoplastic lesions of the temporal lobe. He emphasized that epilepsy could be the initial and only clinical manifestation of a brain tumour [3]. Victor Horsley [4] reported his three landmark cases in which he surgically cured the patients of their focal epilepsy. More recently, various seizure patterns in patients with structural lesions and their surgical management were described by Penfield and Jasper [5], Ingraham and Matson [6], Falconer and Serafetinides [7], LeBlanc and Rasmussen [8], Spencer *et al.* [9], Boon *et al.* [10], Awad *et al.* [11] and Cascino *et al.* [12].

The remarkable development of neuroimaging during the past 20 years has allowed detection of various types of intracranial abnormalities in patients with medically intractable epilepsy with increasing frequency [9,13]. Primary brain tumours, hamartomas and vascular malformations are the underlying pathology in approximately 20–30% of patients with intractable epilepsy. MRI is the most sensitive and specific imaging modality to distinguish a mass lesion from other pathological entities in patients with epilepsy [14,15]. If a circumscribed lesion is responsible for intractable seizures and the relationship of the lesion to the seizures can be verified, surgical resection of the lesion and surrounding brain tissue can render the patient seizure free and improve the quality of life [8,9,10,11,16–18].

With accumulating experience, it has become evident that the neurological examination, electrophysiological studies, seizure types and response to antiepileptic medications may not be useful in predicting the nature of the underlying pathology. Long-standing partial epilepsy may be related to an indolent low-grade glioma with a clinical course indistinguishable from that of a non-neoplastic process. Lesional epilepsy can be associated with simple partial, complex partial or secondary generalized tonic-clonic seizures.

It is the purpose of this chapter to elaborate on the current concepts concerning the diagnosis and surgical management of patients with epilepsy associated with neoplastic mass lesions (Table 61.1). The lesion associated with epilepsy may warrant neurosurgical intervention because of mass effect, growth or haemorrhage. In other cases, the lesions are static and benign with the neurosurgical significance being related to the intractable epilepsy only; it is this latter group that is the subject of discussion in this chapter. The results of surgical resection of the lesion with respect to seizure frequency, surgical morbidity and psychosocial outcome will be discussed. Seizures specifically associated with cortical dysplasias and vascular and infective lesions are discussed elsewhere in this volume.

Mechanism of epileptogenesis associated with structural mass lesions

The pathophysiological mechanisms of ictogenesis associated with intracranial mass lesions are poorly understood. Early proposed mechanisms included impaired vascularization of the surrounding cerebral cortex and direct irritation of the brain and denervation hypersensitivity due to partial isolation and transection of a region of the cerebral cortex [19]. There is conflicting evidence regarding the contribution of hereditary predisposition in the development of epilepsy in patients with intracranial structural lesions [10].

The mechanisms of epileptogenesis for different pathological lesions must vary since some are extracerebral while others are intracerebral, some tumours are infiltrative into the brain and others distort it by mass effect. This suggests that the aetiology of seizures in various lesional pathologies is multifactorial involving factors intrinsic to the lesion itself, the location of the tumour and factors unique to the host harbouring the pathology.

Factors unique to a pathological lesion, particularly tumours, may be associated with the expression of various ion channels and receptors, and the relative proportion of different cell types within the tumour. Peritumoural amino acid disturbances, local metabolic imbalances, cerebral oedema, pH abnormalities, morphological changes in the neuropil, changes in neuronal and glial enzyme and protein expression and immunological activity are all thought to contribute to the pathogenesis of lesional epilepsy syndromes. Future studies from pathological specimens and the development of animal models may further characterize the relative contributions of each of these factors in the development of lesional epilepsy syndromes [20–25]. In addition to properties of the tumours themselves, numerous studies have investigated the role of various properties of peritumoural tissue [26]. These investigators have focused on how tumours located in the brain disrupt signal processing. These mechanisms propose that the tumour either infiltrates into brain tissue or exerts mass effect, and so transects inhibitory populations of neurones; this upsets the balance of excitatory and inhibitory output in favour of overstimulation, resulting in seizures.

In defining the area of resective surgery, Rasmussen [27] identifies a primary localization, which is the site of seizure initiation, and a

Table 61.1 Classification of structural mass lesions associated with intractable epilepsy

> *Neoplastic lesions*
> Neuronal/glial tumours
> Ganglioglioma
> Dysembryoplastic neuroepithelial tumour
> Glial tumours
> Pilocytic astrocytoma
> Low-grade astrocytoma
> Oligodendroglioma
> Mixed glial tumours
> Oligoastrocytoma
>
> *Development lesions*
> Glioneuronal hamartomas
> Focal cortical dysplasia
>
> *Vascular lesions*
> Arteriovenous malformation
> Cavernous angioma
>
> *Inflammatory/infectious lesions*
> Tuberculoma
> Cysticercosis
> Rasmussen's encephalitis

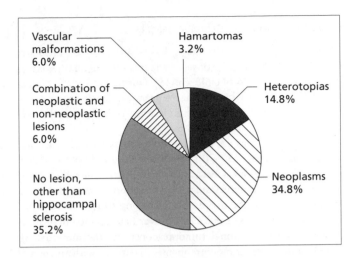

Fig. 61.1 The distribution of pathological findings among 216 surgical specimens of patients with medically intractable temporal lobe epilepsy. From [22].

secondary localization, which indicates the volume of tissue adjacent to the site of origin that must be recruited to produce a clinical seizure. The amygdala and hippocampus appear to be critical sites of secondary localization by providing synchronized output and amplifying an ictal discharge [28,29]. Seizures originating as far posteriorly as the occipital lobe may preferentially spread forward through the hippocampus [30]. Anterior temporal lobectomy can result in seizure relief despite the presence of a posteriorly located temporal lobe tumour [31–33]. This suggests that the effect of surgery need not depend on the excision of the primary epileptogenic focus, but on the elimination of the recruitment of other cells for full seizure development and interruption of the neuronal pathways required for seizure propagation.

Histological studies have demonstrated gliosis or sclerosis of the mesial temporal structures in patients with medically resistant complex partial seizures (CPS) and small vascular or neoplastic lesions in more posterior parts of the temporal lobe [34–38]. However, in 216 consecutive surgical specimens from patients with chronic, medically intractable temporal lobe epilepsy (TLE), Ammon's horn sclerosis was significantly more common in patients without focal mass lesions as compared to those with focal lesions [22]. Dual pathology, if present, may produce a combination of neocortical and temporolimbic epilepsies (TLME) that necessitates a precise definition of the true epileptogenic area(s) in order to achieve maximum benefit from surgery [39].

Pathology

An intracranial mass lesion may be diagnosed and surgically verified in 10–20% of patients with long-standing medically intractable partial epilepsy [8,9,40]. In patients with a mass lesion, neoplastic

lesions outnumber non-neoplastic lesions. In a recent report of 216 consecutive surgical specimens of patients with chronic medically intractable TLE, there were 75 (34.7%) with tumours and 51 (23.4%) with non-neoplastic focal lesions [22] (Fig. 61.1).

Neoplastic lesions

Epilepsy as a symptom of brain tumour

Seizures occur in approximately 50% of patients with intracerebral neoplasms [8]. The incidence of seizures among patients with primary brain tumour is related to the tumour pathology and cortical localization [8,41,42].

Slow-growing, low-grade and well-differentiated gliomas are the most epileptogenic lesions [8,41,42]. In the Montreal series of 230 patients with gliomas, seizures occurred in 70% of those with astrocytomas, in 92% of those with oligodendrogliomas and in 37% of those with glioblastomas [41]. The incidence of epilepsy is lower in patients with glioblastoma, perhaps because of the shorter duration of the disease. These more aggressive lesions, including cerebral metastasis, are associated with a risk of seizures in the range of 20–30% [41].

Tumours located in close proximity to the centrotemporoparietal region are more frequently associated with epilepsy [8,41]. Nearly 75% of the epileptogenic neoplastic lesions are located in or involve the temporal lobe [9,10]. Lesions in the frontal lobe are at least as frequent as lesions in the temporal lobe in patients with neoplasms who do not have seizures [43]. This discrepancy is possibly related to the lower seizure threshold of the temporal lobe, and also to the fact that patients with temporal lobe partial seizures are more likely to be referred for surgical treatment of epilepsy [10]. In a recent series from the Cleveland Clinic consisting of 133 patients who underwent operations for extratemporal epilepsy, tumours were identified in 27.8% of cases; these included, in order of decreasing frequency, astrocytoma, ganglioglioma, dysembryoplastic neuroepithelial tumours (DNET), glioneuronal hamartomas, oligodendrogliomas and oligoastrocytoma [44].

Brain tumour as a cause of chronic epilepsy

CT studies in patients with epilepsy have demonstrated a neoplasm in 10–25% of patients with onset of seizures after the age of 40 years and in fewer than 5% of children [45]. During presurgical evaluation of 190 patients with intractable partial epilepsy, Spencer et al. [9] detected 15% with a mass lesion, 10% of which were neoplasms.

Low-grade gliomas are the most frequent pathological lesions, accounting for nearly 50–70% of all lesions and 70–90% of neoplasms [10,22,23,46,47]. Because of differences in the selection and histopathological criteria used in the ascertainment of these lesions, the distribution of the neoplasms according to type have varied widely between series (Table 61.2). Nevertheless, indolent or slow-growing glial or neuronal tumours constitute the majority. Although tumours occur more frequently in patients with an onset of epilepsy during adulthood, brain tumours also remain an important cause of intractable epilepsy in children and adolescents as well [35,48,49]. In a series of 33 children who underwent temporal lobectomy at an average age of 8 years, 48% were diagnosed as having tumours [50].

Gangliogliomas

Gangliogliomas are mixed tumours that are composed of neoplastic glial and neuronal cell types [51]. They comprise 10–50% of the neoplasms associated with medically intractable partial epilepsy [22,23,47,52]. Seizures are the primary presenting symptom in 80–90% of patients with gangliogliomas [53,54]. Among 11 patients with gangliogliomas, the age at diagnosis ranged between 4 and 69 years [55]. Seizures often occur years before the tumour is detected [53].

These tumours are located within the temporal and frontal lobes in most cases [56,57]. Mesial temporal sclerosis was identified in the hippocampus of the excised temporal lobe in seven of 13 children

Table 61.2 Comparison of the histopathological diagnosis of neoplastic lesions associated with medically intractable temporal lobe epilepsy from three series.

Tumour type	Bonn series [22] (n = 75)	Maudsley series [52] (n = 30)	Mayo series [106] (n = 51)
Ganglioglioma	45.3	10	7.8
Pilocytic astrocytoma	22.7		11.8
Oligodendroglioma	12.0		29.4
Astrocytoma (WHO grades I and II)	8.0		23.5
Dysembryoplastic neuroepithelial tumour	8.0	90	7.8
Oligoastrocytoma	1.3		11.8
Anaplastic astrocytoma	1.3		2.0
Pleomorphic xanthoastrocytoma	1.3		2.0
Unspecified			3.9

with gangliogliomas and intractable seizures [57]. The surgical approach to resect gangliogliomas, therefore, requires careful preoperative evaluation to delineate the extent of the epileptogenic zone.

DNETs

These morphologically unique and surgically curable neuroepithelial tumours are included in the group of neuronal/glial tumours, grade I, in the new World Health Organization (WHO) classification [51]. The possibility that these are developmental abnormalities is discussed further in Chapter 63. In one recent series, DNET comprised 8% of the lesions in a sizeable number of patients with neoplasms and chronic medically intractable epilepsy [22]. By contrast, in a recent Maudsley Hospital series, 90% of the neoplasms were interpreted as DNET [52].

In a group of 39 patients with DNET, age at onset of seizures ranged from 1 to 19 years (mean 9 years), and the duration of seizure prior to surgery averaged 9 years (range 2–18 years) [58]. The tumour involved the temporal lobe in two-thirds of patients and the frontal lobe in one-third of patients; parietal and particularly occipital involvement was infrequent [51,58].

Hamartomas

Hamartomas and heterotopias comprise 15–20% of pathological findings in specimens removed from patients with uncontrolled TLE [22,23]. In the paediatric pathological material, one often finds unusual proliferation of glial and neuronal elements (hamartomas) in association with severe neocortical dysplasia [59,60]. The distinction between cortical dysplasia, hamartomas and relatively indolent neoplasms, such as DNET, may be somewhat arbitrary.

Tuberous sclerosis

The classic clinicopathological finding of tuberous sclerosis is the periventricular glial nodule or subependymal tuber, which can be demonstrated in nearly all patients with a clinical diagnosis of tuberous sclerosis [61]. Pathologically, tubers are hamartomas of the subependymal or subpial regions of the brain and consist of foci of gliosis, which include both glial cells and neurones, having both abnormal cell structure and tissue architecture [62]. Rarely, an intractable seizure focus can be localized to a particular cortical tuber and resection may be indicated to improve seizure control [63,64].

Meningiomas

In a retrospective series of 222 consecutive surgically treated meningiomas, 26.6% of patients presented initially with seizures [65]. Approximately 63% of these patients achieved relief from their seizure disorder following surgical excision of the tumour. Following removal of the meningioma, 20% of patients who did not have preoperative seizures developed a seizure disorder; 33% of these patients had evidence of a haematoma in the resection cavity postoperatively. Meningiomas that were more commonly associated with preoperative epilepsy were more likely to be located over the convexity or supratentorial, and had evidence of severe peritumoural oedema. The highest incidences of preoperative epilepsy were found in convexity, parasagittal/falx, and sphenoid ridge meningiomas abutting the temporal lobe. There was no relationship to histological type, left or right hemisphere, or sex of the patient. Review of the literature suggests that epilepsy is the first symptom of meningioma in 20–50% of cases and that epilepsy is cured in 19–63% of patients following resection of the tumour [65–68].

Presurgical evaluation

Finding an intracerebral lesion in a patient with recurrent seizures does not necessarily mean that this structural abnormality is producing the seizure activity. The main purpose of the presurgical evaluation in patients with intracranial lesions and intractable seizures is to confirm the relationship between the lesion and the seizure foci. In some patients, the epileptogenic focus is contiguous with but extends beyond the structural lesion [9,11,27,35]. The lesion may occasionally be incidental and bear no causal relationship to the epileptogenic focus. Therefore, the understanding of spatial and causal relationship between structural lesions of the brain and intractable epilepsy is essential in planning therapeutic strategies. The preoperative evaluation in patients with substrate-directed partial epilepsy is designed to determine the epileptogenicity of structural abnormalities identified by MRI or other imaging modalities.

History and examination

A careful history should be taken in all patients, with particular attention to a history of febrile seizures, developmental milestones, head trauma and previous neurological problems. Boon et al. [10] noted no significant difference in the frequency of febrile seizures in patients with intra-axial space-occupying lesions and intractable seizures when compared to the general population. Sixteen per cent of the patients with space-occupying lesions and intractable epilepsy had a positive family history of epilepsy, which may indicate an increased susceptibility to seizures in these patients [10].

A thorough neurological examination can detect abnormalities such as a mild hemiparesis or visual field defect that may assist in clinically lateralizing the epileptogenic zone. Facial weakness, especially during emotional expression, may occur in patients contralateral to the epileptic temporal lobe and is uncommon in normal subjects [69,70]. However, since a majority of the lesions are small and are detected before any gross mass effect appears, clinical examination is non-contributory in most of these patients.

Age at onset of seizures

Although earlier studies found a low incidence of tumours in patients with onset of seizures before the age of 20 years [71–73], more recent data suggest that refractory partial seizures, even before the age of 20, should raise suspicion of an intracranial mass lesion [9,10,48]. Blume et al. [48] found tumours in 46% of patients under the age of 21 who had undergone surgery for chronic uncontrolled seizures. Among a group of 27 patients with intracranial mass lesions and medically refractory partial epilepsy, age at onset of seizures was the same for neoplastic and non-neoplastic lesions

[9]. In a selected series of operated cases, Boon et al. [10] found 78% of their patients who had a neoplasm had seizure onset after the age of 20; however, 70% of patients with seizure onset before the age of 20 also had a neoplasm.

Duration of seizure disorder

Douglas [74] found that the risk of neoplasm declined precipitously with duration of the epilepsy, whereas Vignaedra et al. [73] found no differences in epilepsy duration among patients with and without neoplasms. The majority of patients with lesional epilepsy previously considered for surgery have had seizures for more than 10 years [8–10,75]; however, today, with the availability of MRI, patients with lesional epilepsies are operated on earlier [12]. No significant difference in the duration of seizures has been observed between patients with neoplastic and non-neoplastic lesions [9,10].

Clinical seizure characteristics

Lesional epilepsy may be associated with simple partial, complex partial or secondary generalized tonic-clonic seizures [8–10,12]. There is an established association between gelastic seizures and hypothalamic hamartomas [76–78]. Isolated reports of patients with electroclinical characteristics of Landau–Kleffner syndrome [79], West's syndrome [80,81] and Lennox–Gastaut syndrome [82] associated with benign brain tumours successfully treated by lesion resection have been documented.

Thirty-four of the 50 patients with intractable seizures associated with space-occupying lesions reported by Boon et al. [10] had auras, most frequently epigastric sensations. With the exception of visual auras in patients with occipital lesions, the characteristics of the aura did not help in the localization of the lesion [10].

The most frequent seizure type associated with lesional epilepsy is the complex partial seizure. Williamson [83] has described ictal features of CPS arising from different lobes. Among 50 patients with lesional epilepsy, all of them with a temporal lobe lesion had CPS; however, 74% of extratemporal lesions also had CPS [10]. Seventy-five per cent of patients with temporal lobe lesions had typical temporal lobe seizures [10]. An equally good correlation was shown in patients with frontal and occipital lobe lesions but not in patients with parietal lobe lesions [10]. Seizures originating in the parietal lobe can mimic frontal and temporal lobe seizures [84]. A simple partial seizure as a manifestation of a lesional syndrome, either alone or with CPS or tonic-clonic seizures, was found to be nearly always associated with neoplasms by several workers [9,10]. Contrary to previous statements [75], a change in seizure frequency was not found to be a reliable indicator of a cerebral neoplasm [9]. However, after successful treatment, return of seizures has been an indicator of tumour recurrence that may not be detected radiologically for several months [8,9].

Scalp EEG recording

The occurrence of interictal focal sharp and/or focal slow activity in patients with an intracranial space-occupying lesion has been extensively documented [85]. In patients who presented with intractable epileptic seizures as the main feature of an intracerebral mass, nearly two-thirds had an abnormal EEG, and epileptiform activity is more common than slow waves [85]. The absence of prominent focal slow-wave activity in this patient population is mainly due to the limited circumscribed character of most of these lesions. However, when present, a unilateral focal interictal abnormality was a reliable predictor of, at least, the side of the lesion.

The spatial distribution of the focus coincided with the lesion localization in only 30% of the patients, especially with occipital lesions [86,87]. Epileptiform activity localized by scalp EEG distant from the site of a structural lesion is not uncommon. Salanova *et al.* [88] found that, in a group of patients with frontal lobe epilepsy, scalp EEG provided misleading localizing features in nearly one-third of cases. Patients with temporal lobe lesions were not significantly more likely than extratemporal patients to have an ipsilateral temporal spike or sharp wave focus. Extracranial, interictal and ictal EEG changes were found to be unreliable markers of parietal lobe origin of seizure activity [84,89]. Poor interictal scalp localization has been attributed to the fact that the recorded focal abnormality may only be a part of a deeply localized, more extended focus that propagates to the surface.

The occurrence of bilateral independent sharp waves and spikes in patients with epilepsy has been well recognized [90,91]. In the absence of a detectable lesion, this finding can lead to a decision not to operate on a patient with intractable partial seizures. However, it has been demonstrated that this EEG finding does not correlate with a poor outcome [91,92]. Nearly 20% of the patients with unilateral structural temporal lobe lesions may show this EEG abnormality, and bilateral independent temporal paroxysmal activity has been observed in patients with extratemporal lesions as well [12].

Intensive video scalp EEG monitoring

Intensive monitoring with simultaneous close circuit television (CCTV) and scalp EEG recording may reveal interictal focal paroxysmal epileptiform activity but may be normal or show non-specific changes. Continuous video-EEG monitoring with recording of habitual seizures and careful analysis of the recorded seizures and the simultaneous recorded EEG allows good correlation of clinical events with electrical phenomena. Proper classification of seizure type can be made on the basis of specific, stereotyped signs and symptoms during the attack and the findings on the scalp EEG. In most patients with intracranial lesions detected with neuroimaging, the additional information gathered by scalp EEG-video monitoring is sufficient to consider the lesion as the cause of the epilepsy, and those patients can proceed to surgery without invasive monitoring.

Lesion detection

Advanced neuroimaging is arguably the most important aspect of the presurgical evaluation of patients with lesional epilepsy because it provides information about the exact location and extent of the lesion. Two structural neuroimaging modalities are used in the identification of potential candidates with intractable partial epilepsy for resective surgery: CT and MRI. The diagnostic yield of the neuroimaging studies depends on the underlying pathology and the anatomical localization of the epileptogenic area. The selection of patients for epilepsy surgery, the presurgical evaluation and the surgical strategy will be greatly influenced by the neuroimaging-identified lesion [15].

CT

The importance of imaging patients with intractable epilepsy was obvious shortly after the introduction of CT [93]. However, the limitations of CT in detecting small, benign lesions usually associated with long-standing medically intractable epilepsy soon became apparent [94]. A normal CT scan may not exclude a low-grade glioma, cryptic arteriovenous malformation (AVM), hamartoma or cortical dysplasia.

In the absence of MRI, CT is a valuable part of the presurgical evaluation of patients with partial seizure disorders. All patients should have a non-contrast and contrast CT study on a third- or fourth-generation CT scanner if MRI is not available or cannot be performed [95]. The use of reverse-axial images to enhance CT abnormalities within the temporal lobe was associated with a high yield of positivity in tumour-related epilepsy [52]. CT may complement MRI in selected patients with bony lesions and calcified intracranial abnormalities.

In developing countries, where the availability of MRI is very limited, CT remains the radiological investigation of choice in lesional syndromes.

MRI

Investigators at Nottingham University first applied MRI to the study of the brain in 1980 [96]. MRI is the structural neuroimaging modality of choice in patients with intractable partial epilepsy. MRI has been shown to be superior in sensitivity and specificity to CT in identifying the intra-axial structural abnormalities associated with partial epilepsy [97,98]. Neoplastic, vascular and infective mass lesions are almost always associated with an MRI-identified abnormality [15,99,100,101]. In addition, particular MRI characteristics may help identify the underlying pathology and can demonstrate associated features of calvarial moulding, focal atrophy/encephalomalacia or mass effect (Table 61.3). In essence, MRI has been the

Table 61.3 MRI in substrate-directed partial epilepsy

Pathology[a]	Structural MRI findings[b,c]				
	T1	T2	FLAIR	Gad-DTPA	MRIVol
MTS	++	+	++	0	++
Tumour	+	++	++	0 to ++	0
Vascular anomaly	++	++	++	+	0

Adapted from [102].
[a] Mesial temporal sclerosis (MTS), primary brain tumour (tumour), cavernous haemangioma and arteriovenous malformation (vascular anomaly) and focal cortical dysplasia (FCD).
[b] T1-weighted image (T1), T2-weighted image (T2), fluid attenuated inversion recovery (FLAIR), gadolinium-DTPA enhanced (Gad-DTPA) study and MRI-based hippocampal formation volumetric studies (MRIVol).
[c] No consistent alteration (0), usually abnormal (may be difficult to identify pathological substrate) (+), major abnormality of diagnostic importance (++).

most successful modality in separating patients with intractable partial epilepsy to be separated into two groups: those with substrate-directed and those with non-substrate-directed disease [102]. Patients with substrate-directed or lesional disease have one or more potentially epileptogenic structural abnormalities that may be coexistent with the epileptogenic zone [103].

In an evaluation of 23 patients who had both MRI and CT of the head prior to surgery for medically intractable epilepsy, patients with normal MRI all had non-neoplastic lesions [97]. In contrast, in this selected series, all patients with foci of increased signal on T2-weighted MRI images had neoplasms, even when the CT was negative. MRI studies are useful for surgical localization and have variable sensitivity and specificity for the major pathological entities but both are usually greater than 90% and the diagnostic yield of these lesions has been confirmed in surgical series [97,98,103,104]. MRI studies may also be performed to confirm the extent of corticectomy and lesion resection postoperatively.

As stated above, the most common presenting symptom in patients with low-grade and slow-growing primary brain tumours is epilepsy. MRI will reveal a structural intra-axial abnormality in the majority of these patients [105]. Imaging features common to all these tumours include the presence of a cortically based lesion, with sharply defined borders, little or no surrounding oedema and, with the exceptions of pilocytic or gangliogliomas, little or no contrast enhancement. Some lesions may have characteristic, distinguishing features. For example, gangliogliomas are often associated with a cystic lesion and a mural nodule. Although MRI is highly sensitive in detecting neoplasms, it is not specific to particular histopathology. Primary resection of these MRI-identified lesions is associated with a seizure remission in 80–90% of patients [10,11,106].

MRI-based volumetric measurement of the hippocampal formation [107] may provide additional information about the possible sites of epileptogenesis in patients with mass lesions. In a recent study, MRI-based volumetric measurements of the hippocampal formations were correlated with seizure outcome after temporal lobectomy [108]. Trenerry et al. [109,110] found a number of correlations between preoperative hippocampal volumetric measurements and the effect of temporal lobectomy on a variety of neuropsychological performance criteria. Volumetric measurements of the hippocampi should now be routine in lesional epilepsy in order to characterize the possible extent of the epileptogenic zone(s), especially given the possibility of dual pathology.

Several centres have incorporated MRI-compatible implantation frames to provide accurate anatomical information for use with intracranial depth electrodes [111,112]. Quantitative MRI-based techniques to assess the extent of cortical resection, and thereby to correlate the extent of resection and patient outcome, have been developed [113,114].

Neuropsychological assessment

A battery of standard neuropsychological tests, aimed to lateralize and localize the area(s) of functional abnormality, are administered during preoperative evaluation of patients with intractable seizures [115,116]. In a recent study of patients with intra-axial space-occupying lesions with intractable partial seizures, lateralized neuropsychological findings were congruent with the lesion in 56% but incongruent in 14%; furthermore, localization corresponded with

the lobe of the lesion localization in 26% but did not correspond in 30% [10]. Incorrect localizing findings from neuropsychological testing were more frequent when lesions were extratemporal [10]. Preoperative neuropsychological evaluation forms a baseline with which postoperative psychological outcome can be compared.

Invasive monitoring

Patients may require invasive monitoring if the results from all previous procedures are conflicting [117]. Invasive monitoring is defined as the long-term recording of EEG from subdural and/or intraparenchymal brain areas using intracranial electrodes. This recording technique is generally required in patients with stereotyped partial seizures in whom no consistent epileptiform focus could be demonstrated during the non-invasive monitoring. In patients with known lesions, a subdural or epidural grid consisting of a thin layer of silastic with numerous embedded electrodes is laid over the cerebral cortex in proximity to the neuroimaging-identified lesion [11,118].

However, in addition to morbidity, the apparent lack of sensitivity in localization, especially when subdural grids are placed directly over the epileptogenic lesion, is well documented [12]. Several authors have reported the poor yield of extracranial and intracranial EEG recordings in patients with an epileptic lesion in the parietal lobes [36,84,89]. Cascino et al. [84] studied a group of 11 patients with seizures associated with lesions in the parietal lobe. Out of five patients with a parietal lesion who underwent intracranial monitoring with depth and/or subdural electrodes in an attempt to localize the region of ictogenesis, parietal lobe origin was documented in only two. MRI detected the lesion in all. The authors recommended lesionectomy without chronic intracranial monitoring as an effective and safe surgical procedure in patients with partial epilepsy related to parietal lobe lesions [84].

Functional mapping

The importance of physiological identification of functionally important areas is being increasingly recognized in neurosurgery. Functional imaging of the brain may provide information which may be complementary to that provided by EEG and structural neuroimaging studies. In addition, when neurosurgical procedures are planned in neocortical sensory, motor or speech areas, functional mapping is performed to circumscribe these areas and avoid an unacceptable neurological deficit post surgically. Functional imaging proves most useful when structural pathology cannot be visualized on MRI.

Non-invasive mapping procedures

SPECT

Cerebral blood flow changes associated with cerebral metabolism can be studied by SPECT as well as by PET. Unlike PET, SPECT does not require a cyclotron to be on site for the production of radioisotopes; SPECT has radioisotopes of longer half-life and retention in brain than PET and can be performed up to 4 h after the radiotracer is injected. This allows for the injection of SPECT radiotracers during a seizure and subsequent transportation to the scanner within a clinically practical timeframe. Newer radiotracers (^{99m}Tc-ECD) are more stable than those used in earlier studies and have longer half-lives, thus enabling the localization of abnormalities during seizure activity.

There are several inherent limitations in the interpretation of ictal SPECT to identify the partial seizure focus. The pattern of perfusion activity must be visually compared to the baseline interictal SPECT and relies on subjective judgement of perfusion intensities in the corresponding brain regions on the different scans. If the focus is hypoperfused interictally, an ictal focus of increased perfusion may not stand out against the background. The time between injection and image acquisition as well as the amount of radiotracer injected in the two scans may affect the overall intensity using this method of comparison. The differences in head position may vary in the level of image slices compared. It has less spatial resolution and provides less anatomical detail than provided by structural MRI.

Peri-ictal SPECT appears to be more useful than interictal SPECT [119]. In a group of 28 patients with medically intractable epilepsy, ictal/postictal HMPAO-SPECT showed changes from interictal in 29 cases (93%) [120]. However, in a recent study involving 15 patients using ^{99m}Tc-HMPAO, interictal SPECT showed hypoperfusion at the site of the lesion in all five patients with tumours [121].

Grunwald *et al.* [122] evaluated the predictive value of interictal ^{99m}Tc-HMPAO SPECT on outcome after temporal lobectomy for intractable seizures. SPECT results correlated with temporal lobectomy in 68% of patients. In patients who underwent left-side lobectomy, the presence of SPECT identified hypoperfusion on the right side correlated with the degree of verbal and memory impairment. No relationship between SPECT concordance with the side of temporal lobectomy and postoperative seizure frequency and nonverbal memory was noted.

Because of the small number of patients studied by each author and the heterogeneity of the patient population and the methods used in studying them, the value of SPECT for presurgical evaluation of lesional syndromes remains uncertain at present. For an extensive review of the relative contributions of various imaging modalities in the evaluation of epilepsy consult So and Spencer [123,131].

Computer-aided subtraction ictal and postictal imaging SPECT coregistered to MRI (SISCOM)

SISCOM is a recently developed neuroimaging technique that localizes cerebral blood flow abnormalities and may identify the epileptogenic region, minimizing some of the inherent limitations of direct side-by-side visual comparison of the SPECT and MRI separately [123–126]. The technique utilized at the Mayo Clinic consists of computer-aided subtraction of the coregistered normalized interictal SPECT from the normalized ictal SPECT, followed by the coregistration of the image difference to the MRI (Plate 61.2, shown in colour between pp. 670 and 671). This provides a more sensitive and specific, semiquantitative map of the cerebral blood flow during a seizure. The method for image registration is described in more detail in another review [123].

In a study by O'Brien *et al.* [125] interictal and ictal side-by-side visual interpretation was compared with SISCOM in 51 patients with intractable epilepsy. SISCOM revealed a localized alteration in cerebral perfusion in 88.2% of patients compared to 39.2% of pa-

tients using side-by-side visual interpretation. This method has also been shown to be more specific, as determined by concordance with long-term EEG monitoring. The functional change is concordant with the ictal onset zone in approximately 80% of patients [123,125,127].

Patients with non-lesional extratumour syndrome have recently been found to have a localized SISCOM alteration in 75%. Many patients with extratemporal epilepsy have inconclusive long-term video-EEG monitoring and no lesion on the MRI. SISCOM has its greatest potential in these more difficult cases for localization of the seizure onset.

Detection of peri-ictal hypo- or hyperperfusion localized abnormalities has been shown to reliably locate an epileptogenic focus and select the patients for operative resection. A localized cerebral blood flow abnormality at this potential epileptogenic focus provides a preliminary map and guides the placement of subdural grids/electrodes. Furthermore, the SISCOM images can be transferred across a computer network to the surgical suite where a frameless stereotactic surgical navigation system can be used to localize the SPECT activation in the surgical field intraoperatively. This technique may potentially play an important role in identifying the optimal amount of cortical resection related to epileptogenic lesions.

A recent study from the Mayo Clinic investigated (a) whether the localization of extratemporal epilepsy with the SISCOM technique is predictive of outcome after resective epilepsy surgery; (b) if the SISCOM images provide prognostically important information in addition to those provided by the standard tests; and (c) whether the area of blood flow change on SISCOM images is useful in determining the site and the extent of the excision required for successful postoperative seizure control [127]. The concordance of the SISCOM focus with the site of surgery was predictive of an excellent postoperative outcome. Overall, 38.9% had an excellent postoperative outcome and 72.2% had at least a favourable outcome. All patients with excellent outcome except one were seizure free. The exception was a patient who had rare nocturnal seizures.

SISCOM localization was concordant with the site of the surgical excision in 52.8%, non-concordant in 13.9% and non-localizing in 33.3%. The concordant SISCOM group had significantly higher rates of excellent and favourable outcome than the other groups. This study also found that one-half of the patients whose ictal scalp EEG was non-localizing had localizing SISCOM abnormalities. These results strongly argue that SISCOM provides localizing information that is in addition to and not redundant for that provided by the more standard tests.

The importance of SISCOM localization in determining surgical outcome has been confirmed in intractable extratemporal epilepsy. Further analysis of this data revealed that the extent of excision of the SISCOM focus is predictive of the success of the surgery. Concordance of the SISCOM focus with the surgical site and the extent of the excision are the only two predictors of the excellent outcome. Many of the patients in this study had SPECT studies because their seizures were not well localized with more standard tests.

PET

Interictal or peri-ictal PET using 2-[^{18}F] fluoro-2-deoxyglucose (FDG-PET) is included routinely in the presurgical evaluation protocols of many adult and paediatric epilepsy surgery programmes [128,129]. However, PET findings, characterized by the increased or decreased uptake of FDG, reflect not only the neuronal activity at the site of the ictal onset but also in areas of ictal spread and postictal depression.

PET when used in the presurgical evaluation of patient with epilepsy employs either measurements of tissue oxygen consumption (radionuclide ^{18}FDG) and/or blood flow (radionuclides $H_2^{15}O$ or ^{15}O). Tomographic reconstruction locates the sources of gamma ray photons produced after annihilation of the oppositely charged electron and positron that are emitted by the radionuclide. Interictal PET scans may reveal areas of reduced glucose uptake (hypometabolic foci) that correspond to potentially epileptogenic zones.

During a seizure, glucose uptake increases in the area of reduced uptake identified during the interictal scan. The localization of these zones of increased metabolic activity during a seizure is difficult to the point of being impractical. FDG uptake takes place 30–45 min after its injection. The seizure must occur early in this period of radionuclide uptake for the focus to be identified. Additionally, FDG has a short half-life requiring a continuous supply of the isotope during this time. Since seizures are unpredictable, timing limits the utility of ictal PET in localizing seizure foci.

Interictal PET has been shown to be more sensitive than MRI in detecting foci of gliotic tissues with decreased metabolic uptake of FDG. However, gliotic tissue does not necessarily correlate with an epileptogenic region. Only one-third of patients with extratemporal seizures have relevant hypometabolic abnormalities concordant with an abnormal EEG focus [130,131]. These regions of hypometabolic activity are frequently widely distributed and poorly localized [132].

Overall, published clinical series indicate that FDG-PET does not appear to provide additionally clinically useful information in the majority of patients with epilepsy. The continuing development of PET technology may enhance its utility in the evaluation of patients undergoing surgery. The development of receptor-specific ligands (such as ^{11}C flumazenil) to improve the accuracy of defining seizure foci may lead to future studies relating PET localization to seizure outcome following surgical resection [133–135]. The usefulness of PET in the presurgical evaluation of lesional syndromes will be judged by its sensitivity, specificity and cost compared with other procedures, and how the information provided by PET contrasts with other relatively inexpensive techniques used in presurgical evaluation and in predicting the postsurgical outcome. Since PET and other diagnostic technologies are in the process of continuous evolution and improvement, the role of PET in the evaluation of medically intractable lesional epileptic syndromes is unlikely to be settled in the near future.

Magnetic resonance spectroscopic imaging (MRSI)

Whole-brain MRSI is being developed as a functional neuroimaging modality. The usefulness of this imaging technique in the assessment of patients with focal epilepsy is being assessed. In a recent study, phosphorus MRSI correctly lateralized the epileptogenic foci in all eight patients, including a patient with a medial frontal focus [136].

MEG

The MEG requires complex and costly recording methodology but allows simple interpretation of the field of brain electrical activity [137]. This technique has been shown to map human auditory cortex [138], locations of cortical response to pain and primary and sensory somatosensory cortex [139,140]. With improvement in technology and the availability of simple and less expensive equipment, such localization and quantification of the brain region by non-invasive field measurement may have a major impact in the presurgical evaluation of mass lesions located close to the vital cortical areas.

Invasive cortical mapping

Since the pioneering studies of Penfield and Jasper [5], it has been demonstrated that cortical stimulation of discrete brain areas during neurosurgical procedures is a useful technique for mapping brain areas close to the epileptogenic foci [11,141,142]. Cortical mapping before tumour resection may be required to identify regions involved in critical functions. Because lesions distort the normal topography of the cerebral cortex and vascular landmarks may vary between individuals, cortical mapping may be required to identify regions involved in critical functions. Cortical stimulation techniques have been applied during resection of AVMs and tumours within the language-dominant hemisphere of patients with medically intractable epilepsy [11,142].

Mapping can be done intraoperatively, but this requires that the surgical procedure be carried out under local anaesthesia [141,142]. Alternatively, mapping can be done preoperatively using an implanted subdural electrode array to record both interictal and ictal EEG and to stimulate the cortex at different contact points [11,118,143]. A major advantage of the grid system is that the patient can fully cooperate in a non-surgical environment and a more elaborate series of functional tasks can be evaluated. Subdural grids of electrodes have also been used for recording cortical somatosensory evoked potentials by stimulating a peripheral nerve to locate the primary somatosensory cortex and to delineate the location of the central fissure.

ECoG

Controversy exists regarding the usefulness of intraoperative ECoG to identify and resect the seizure foci vs. tumour removal alone. Berger et al. [144] analysed 45 patients with low-grade gliomas and intractable epilepsy who underwent ECoG during surgery. Multiple vs. single seizure foci were more likely to be associated with a longer preoperative duration of epilepsy. Postoperatively, 41% of the adults and 85% of the children were seizure free without any antiepileptic medication, with a mean postoperative follow-up of over 50 months. Based on their experience, Berger et al. [144] advocate ECoG as a useful predictor of seizure outcome in patients with a long-standing seizure disorder. In contrast, among the Maudsley Hospital series of 31 patients who underwent temporal lobectomy for tumour-related epilepsy, postoperative relief of seizures could not be predicated by intraoperative ECoG [52]. The authors routinely perform intraoperative ECoG during resection surgery for epilepsy.

Treatment

Indications for surgery

The widespread and increasing availability of sensitive, non-invasive and neuroimaging techniques means that patients with epilepsy are more likely to be imaged for a structural lesion. The identified lesion may require resective surgery either because of the epileptic seizures refractory to antiepileptic drugs (AEDs) or for pathological verification before additional treatment, such as radiotherapy, can be administered.

Patients with medically intractable epilepsy

All patients with medically intractable epilepsy and neuroimaging-detected lesions should be referred to comprehensive centres for surgical consideration. Several years of polypharmacy with AEDs is not required to define intractability of the seizures. Although a period of 2 years of observation on adequate AED coverage is advocated prior to consideration of epilepsy surgery, socially disabling seizures, even of a 1-year duration, may necessitate a referral for surgery. Unnecessary AED toxicity and delay in initiating a surgical evaluation may increase a patient's psychosocial debilitation. In contrast, a lesion involving functional cortex may be associated with increased neurosurgical morbidity and surgical management may be deferred.

Patients with well-controlled recent onset or infrequent seizures

Seizure was the first symptom in 164 of 560 patients with a CT diagnosis of supratentorial intra-axial brain tumours [145]. Patients presenting with epilepsy are more likely to have a low-grade tumour associated with a prolonged survival [8,145]. In these instances, surgery is not performed for the management of epilepsy but to establish a histological diagnosis. It remains controversial whether resection of the tumour either reduces the risk of mortality or improves long-term survival or the control of epilepsy [145]. The controversies in the management of low-grade intracranial neoplasms [146] and the role of radiotherapy [147,148] are beyond the scope of this chapter.

Role of biopsy

It has been suggested that all patients with CT/MRI-identified mass lesions and seizures should be biopsied to avoid missing a curable condition and to predict the prognosis [149]. However, biopsy is not without risk and histological confirmation of the diagnosis will not necessarily alter the management. Availability of stereotactic techniques [64,150] has significantly reduced the morbidity of biopsy. In a recent study of 419 image-guided stereotactic biopsies, the diagnostic yield was over 94% in gliomas [151]. It is the authors' practice to investigate a majority of the neuroimaging-identified mass lesions by stereotactic biopsy. If resective surgery is being planned, as for chronic intractable seizures, biopsy obviously would not be required.

Surgical methods

Resection of the lesion and the surrounding epileptogenic cortex may be carried out by a conventional neurosurgical approach or by stereotactic extirpation of the lesion [40,64,152,153]. There have been conflicting results regarding the therapeutic efficacy of stereotactic lesionectomy in patients with partial epilepsy [11,46].

A follow-up study of the outcome of stereotactic lesionectomy in 23 patients with mass lesions and intractable partial epilepsy was recently reported [103]. Sixteen lesions involved functional or eloquent cortex as determined by anatomical localization. The mean duration of follow-up was 48.5 months. Of the 23 patients, 17 (74%) had a significant reduction in seizures and five of them were successfully discontinued from AEDs.

Moore *et al.* [154] compared the surgical outcome of anterior temporal lobectomy and stereotactic lesionectomy in 20 and 14 patients, respectively, with intractable seizures operated on at the Mayo Clinic. Seventy-one per cent of lesionectomy patients and 90% of lobectomy patients experienced a worthwhile reduction in seizure tendency.

Outcome

Seizure outcome

The beneficial effect of epilepsy surgery in patients with medically refractory partial seizures associated with structural lesions is well established [8,9,11,12]. Postoperative seizure-free rates of up to 83% have been reported, with many of the remaining patients showing a significant improvement in seizure control [12].

The outcome of the surgical treatment of lesional epilepsy is influenced by the nature of the underlying pathology, the completeness of resection of the structural lesion and the extent of the removal of the functionally defined associated epileptic focus [11,12,155]. The relative contributions of these factors and their interactions are difficult to delineate. Moreover, the outcome results from the published series are difficult to compare because of different methods of patient selection, pathological classification, surgical technique and follow-up.

Pathology

Neoplastic lesions

LeBlanc and Rasmussen [8] observed in their 108 patients with astrocytomas and other low-grade primary intracranial neoplasms that 70% became seizure free or had a marked reduction in seizures, whereas complete seizure control was unlikely in malignant astrocytomas. Tumour recurrence was often heralded first by a recurrence of seizures after a seizure-free period of variable length [8].

Surgical excision of indolent intra-axial tumours such as gangliogliomas and DNETs are associated with a likelihood of complete or near-complete relief of seizures in nearly 90% of patients [52,58]. Out of 15 children, 11 operated for ganglioglioma and intractable seizures were seizure free over a mean follow-up period of 4 years [156]. These tumours constitute the majority of lesional cases [22,46]. There is a higher incidence of more benign lesional pathology in intractable temporal rather than extratemporal epilepsy [9].

Single small CT lesions associated with seizures

A series of patients with seizures who showed single, small, enhancing CT lesions with or without perifocal oedema has been reported from India [157–159]. Isolated reports of patients with similar clinical and CT features have appeared from all over the world [160]. Most of these lesions resolve spontaneously with no treatment other than AEDs [160]. Chandy *et al.* [161] carried out stereotactic or excision biopsy in 25 consecutive patients with these lesions, and a majority of them were found to be caused by cysticercosis. The authors recommended symptomatic treatment with AEDs and monitoring with CT scan examination 8–12 weeks after the initial presentation, with the lesions which increased in size requiring stereotactic biopsy and/or surgical excision [160,161].

Completeness of lesion resection

The relationship between outcome and extent of the resection of the lesion is complex and is influenced by the pathology and the extent of the removal of a coexisting epileptic focus. Awad *et al.* [11] studied the effects of the extent of the resection of the structural lesion and the epileptic focus in 47 patients with intractable epilepsy and structural lesions. Complete lesion resection with or without the epileptic focus was associated with a higher chance of a seizure-free outcome than incomplete removal of the lesion [11]. In contrast, despite incomplete tumour removal, 81% of 22 patients from the Maudsley Hospital were completely free of seizures and 10% were almost seizure free during a mean follow-up period of 5.8 years (in this series, DNETs were the most common pathology) [53].

Completeness of epileptic focus resection

Many patients undergoing resective surgery for mass lesions have congruent epileptic foci. Wyllie *et al.* [155] reported better results in those patients in whom the epileptic lesion was fully excised. Extrahippocampal lesions may be associated with cell loss and sclerotic changes in the hippocampus [35,36,39]. Nayel *et al.* [162] reported that the extent of anterior temporal lobe resection may influence the outcome of surgery in patients with posterior temporal and extratemporal lesions.

The factors predictive of a good prognosis in resective surgery for intractable epilepsy guided by subdural electrode arrays and operative ECoG were reported for 64 patients [163]. After 1 year, 70% of the patients with a temporal ictal focus were seizure free compared to 55% of patients with an extratemporal focus. Patients with no postresection spikes had a better prognosis than patients with residual postresection spikes evaluated by operative ECoG. Other factors such as age, gender, duration of epilepsy prior to surgery, extent of temporal lobe resection and structural abnormalities as determined by MRI were not correlated with a favourable seizure outcome after surgery [163]. However, there are several case reports or small series of patients with congruent epileptogenic foci who became seizure free after surgery limited to the site of structural lesion [7,11,52].

The goal of epilepsy surgery is to render the individual seizure free without producing surgical morbidity. The primary aim of the treatment should be the removal of the lesion. If complete removal of the lesion cannot be achieved without added risk and morbidity, incomplete lesion removal may provide equally satisfactory results. Many of the tumours associated with medically intractable epilepsy are indolent, with no tendency to progress, and in these cases adjuvant tumour therapy does not appear to be necessary. The relative merits of simple lesionectomy vs. additional removal of the epileptic focus in patients with lesional syndromes need further investigation.

Functional outcome

Psychosocial outcomes of epilepsy surgery is a largely neglected field. Little shift in the emphasis of reporting outcome following surgery, other than the seizure frequency, has occurred in recent years. Awad *et al.* [11] reported 47 patients with lesional medically intractable epilepsy showing an association between the extent of the resection of the lesion and seizure control without concomitant indication of whether or how these factors influenced the psychosocial and occupational performance. In a case–control analysis, Gulgvog *et al.* [164] were unable to show any benefit in psychosocial performance in a group of operated patients, in spite of significant reduction of seizures. In children with intractable epilepsy due to brain tumours treated by surgery, Berger *et al.* [165] reported optimal seizure control in 14 children, but postoperative psychosocial or educational performance was not mentioned.

Psychiatric outcome

Much of the early work in this area came from the surgical series of the Maudsley Hospital in the UK, which has a large psychiatric referral base, thereby biasing the cohort towards behavioural disorders in addition to epilepsy [166]. Falconer [16] reported seven out of 12 patients from this series with psychosis who benefited from temporal lobectomy. When a schizophreniform psychosis supervened, hamartoma was the most frequent pathological substrate [16]. While it is a universal practice to obtain neuropsychological studies before and after temporal lobectomy, many epilepsy centres only obtain psychiatric evaluation for extratemporal lesional syndromes when pertinent symptoms exist. Moreover, psychiatric and psychosocial improvement postoperatively may be due to fewer seizures, medication changes and placebo effect due to patient expectations, rather than tissue resection *per se*. In contrast, development of new psychiatric symptoms is more likely to be related to the removal of the brain tissue.

In a 1987 survey of 53 epilepsy centres, at which a total of over 250 operations were performed annually, 10% of the temporal lobectomy patients developed significant psychiatric complications within 3 months of surgery, but 93% of these had pre-existing psychiatric illness, leaving only 0.7% of cases with new psychiatric symptoms of any type [167]. In a recent review of postoperative psychiatric disease after temporal lobectomy, it was reported that 10% of patients developed a postoperative affective disorder, and up to 5% committed suicide [168]. These observations contrast with a 1979 estimate of 15–27% increases in psychosis rates from preoperative to postoperative assessments [169]. The decreases in the rate of new psychosis in recent series may reflect a change in selection criteria that excludes patients with significant psychiatric disease from consideration for epilepsy surgery.

Psychological outcome

At most epilepsy centres, a comprehensive neurophysiology battery is administered preoperatively and repeated 1 year postoperatively. New material-specific memory deficits are often noted after temporal lobectomy [109,110,170]. These abnormalities are usually subtle, asymptomatic and detected only by neuropsychological testing. Dominant temporal lobectomies impair verbal memory, while non-dominant temporal lobectomies impair visuospatial memory [171,172]. This observation indicates that the presence of a contralateral, normal, non-operated temporal lobe is a determinant of the functional outcome. In fact, many patients can show improvement in verbal and visuospatial memory following epilepsy surgery [173,174]. These improvements may be attributed to significantly reduced postoperative seizure rates and fewer antiepileptic medications.

References

1 Temkin O. *The Falling Sickness*. Baltimore: The Johns Hopkins Press, 1945: 380.

2 Gowers WR. *Epilepsy and Other Chronic Convulsive Diseases*. London: J and A Churchill, 1881: 309.

3 Jackson JH. Localized convulsions from tumour of the brain. *Brain* 1882; 5: 364–74.

4 Horsley V. Brain surgery. *Br Med J* 1886; 2: 670–5.

5 Penfield WS, Jasper H. *Epilepsy and the Functional Anatomy of the Human Brain*. Boston: Little, Brown, 1954: 281–349.

6 Ingraham FD, Matson DD. *Neurosurgery of Infancy and Childhood*. Springfield: Charles C. Thomas, 1954: 88–422.

7 Falconer MA, Serafetinides EA. A follow-up study of surgery in temporal lobe epilepsy. *J Neurol Neurosurg Psychiatr* 1963; 26: 154–65.

8 LeBlanc FE, Rasmussen T. Cerebral seizures and brain tumours. In: Vinken PJ, Bruyn GW, eds. *Handbook of Clinical Neurology*, Vol. 15. Amsterdam: North-Holland Publishing Co., 1974: 295–301.

9 Spencer DD, Spencer SS, Mattson RH, Williamson PD. Intracerebral masses in patients with intractable partial epilepsy. *Neurology* 1984; 34: 432–6.

10 Boon PA, Williamson PD, Fried I *et al*. Intracranial, intra-axial, space-occupying lesions in patients with intractable partial seizures: an anatomoclinical, neuropsychological and surgical correlation. *Epilepsia* 1991; 32: 467–76.

11 Awad IA, Rosenfeld J, Ahl J, Hahn JF, Lüders H. Intractable epilepsy and structural lesions of the brain: mapping, resection strategies and seizure outcome. *Epilepsia* 1991; 32: 179–86.

12 Cascino GD, Boon PA, Fish DR. Surgically remediable lesional syndromes. In: Engel J Jr, ed. *Surgical Treatment of the Epilepsies*, 2nd edn. New York: Raven Press, 1993: 77–86.

13 Cascino GD. Intractable partial epilepsy: evaluation and treatment. *Mayo Clin Proc* 1990; 65: 1578–86.

14 Cascino GD, Jack CR Jr, Hirschorn KA, Sharbrough FW. Identification of the epileptic focus: magnetic resonance imaging. In: Theodore WH, ed. *Surgical Treatment of Epilepsy*. New York: Elsevier, 1992: 95–100.

15 Kuzniecky RI, Cascino GD, Palmini A *et al*. Structural neuroimaging. In: Engel J Jr, ed. *Surgical Treatment of the Epilepsies*. New York: Raven Press, 1993: 197–209.

16 Falconer MA. Reversibility by temporal-lobe resection of the behavioral abnormalities of temporal-lobe epilepsy. *N Engl J Med* 1973; 289: 451–5.

17 Engel J Jr, Driver M'V, Falconer MA. Electrophysiological correlates of pathology and surgical results in temporal lobe epilepsy. *Brain* 1975; 87: 129–56.

18 Cascino GD. Epilepsy and brain tumors: implications for treatment. *Epilepsia* 1990; 31 (Suppl. 3): S37–S44.

19 Echlin FA. The supersensitivity of chronically isolated cerebral cortex as a mechanism in focal epilepsy. *Electroencephalogr Clin Neurophysiol* 1959; 11: 697–722.

20 Kim JH, Guimaraes PO, Shen MY, Masukawa LM, Spencer DD. Hippocampal neuronal density in temporal epilepsy with and without gliomas. *Acta Neuropathol Berl* 1990; 80: 41–5.

21 Vezzani A, Gramsbergen JB, Speciale C, Schwarcz R. Production of quinolinic acid and kyurenic acid by human gliomas. *Adv Exper Med Biol* 1991; 294: 691–5.

22 Wolf HK, Campos MG. Zentner J *et al*. Surgical pathology of temporal lobe epilepsy. Experience with 216 cases. *J Neuropathol Exp Neurol* 1993; 52: 499–506.

23 Wolf HK, Wiestler OD. Surgical pathology of chronic epileptic seizure disorders. *Brain Pathol* 1993; 3: 371–80.

24 Patts S, Labrakakis C, Bernstein M *et al*. Neuron-like physiological properties of cells from human oligodendroglial tumors. *Neuroscience* 1996; 71: 601–11.

25 Labrakakis C, Patt S, Weydt P *et al*. Action potential generating cells in human glioblastoma. *J Neuropath Exp Neurol* 1997; 56: 243–54.

26 Beaumont A, Whittle IR. The pathogenesis of tumor associated epilepsy. *Acta Neurochir Wien* 2000; 142: 1–15.

27 Rasmussen TR. Surgical treatment of complex partial seizures: results, lessons, and problems. *Epilepsia* 1983; 24 (Suppl. 1): S65–S76.

28 Babb TL, Brown WJ. Neuronal, dendritic, and vascular profiles of human temporal lobe epilepsy correlated with cellular physiology *in vivo*. In: Delgado-Escueta AV, Ward AA Jr, Woodbury DM, Porter RJ, eds. *Basic Mechanisms of the Epilepsies. Molecular and Cellular Approaches. Advances in Neurology*, Vol. 44. New York: Raven Press, 1986: 949–66.

29 Lieb JP, Hogue K. Skomer CE, Song XW. Inter-hemispheric propagation of human mesial temporal lobe seizures. *Electroencephalograph Clin Neurophysiol* 1987; 67: 101–19.

30 Putsch H, Proshaska O, Rappelsberger P, Kaizer A. Cortical seizure patterns in multidimensional view: the informational content of equipotential maps. *Epilepsia* 1974; 15: 439–63.

31 Falconer MA, Driver MV, Serafetinides EA. Temporal lobe epilepsy due to distant lesions: two cases relieved by operation. *Brain* 1962; 85: 521–34.

32 Olivier A, Gloor P, Andermann F. Occipitotemporal epilepsy studied with stereotactically-implanted depth electrodes and successfully treated by temporal resection. *Ann Neurol* 1982; 11: 428–32.

33 Sperling MR, Cahan LD, Brown WJ. Relief of seizures from a predominantly posterior temporal tumor with anterior temporal lobectomy. *Epilepsia* 1989; 30: 559–63.

34 Cavanagh JB. On certain small tumors encountered in the temporal lobe. *Brain* 1958; 81: 389–405.

35 Drake J, Hoffman HJ, Kohayashi J. Hwang P, Becker LE. Surgical management of children with temporal lobe epilepsy and mass lesions. *Neurosurgery* 1987; 21: 792–7.

36 Fish D, Andermann F, Oliver A. Complex partial seizures and small posterior temporal or extratemporal structural lesions: surgical management. *Neurology* 1991; 41: 1781–4.

37 Fried I, Kim JH, Spencer DD. Hippocampal pathology in patients with intractable seizures and temporal lobe masses. *J Neurosurg* 1992; 76: 735–40.

38 Nakasato N, Levesque MF, Babb TL. Seizure outcome following standard temporal lobectomy: correlation with hippocampal neuron loss and extrahippocampal pathology. *J Neurosurg* 1992; 77: 194–200.

39 Levesque MF, Nakasato N, Vinters HV, Babb TL. Surgical treatment of limbic epilepsy associated with extra-hippocampal lesions: the problem of dual pathology. *J Neurosurg* 1991; 75: 364–70.

40 Cascino GD, Kelly PJ, Hirschorn NA, Marsh WR, Sharbrough FW. Stereotactic lesion resection in partial epilepsy. *Mayo Clin Proc* 1990; 65: 1053–60.

41 Penfield W, Erickson TC, Tarlov I. Relation of intracranial tumors and symptomatic epilepsy. *Arch Neurol Psychiatr* 1940; 44: 300–15.

42 Lund M. Epilepsy in association with intracranial tumor. *Acta Neuro Psychiatr Scand* 1952; 81 (Suppl.): 87–106.

43 Laws ER, Taylor WF, Clifton MB, Okazaki NI. Neurosurgical management of low grade astrocytoma of the cerebral hemisphere. *J Neurosurg* 1984; 61: 665–73.

44 Frater JL, Prayson RA, Morris III HH, Bingaman WE. Surgical pathologic findings of extratemporal-based intractable epilepsy: a study of 133 consecutive resections. *Arch Pathol Lab Med* 2000; 124: 545–9.

45 Shorvon S. Imaging in the investigation of epilepsy. In: Hopkins A, ed. *Epilepsy*. New York: Demos, 1987: 201–28.

46 Goldring S, Rich KM, Picker S. Experience with gliomas in patients presenting with a chronic seizure disorder. *Clin Neurosurg* 1986; 33: 15–42.

47 Armstrong DD. The neuropathology of temporal lobe epilepsy. *J Neuropathol Exp Neurol* 1993; 52: 433–43.

48 Blume WT, Girvin JP, Kaufman JCE. Childhood brain tumors presenting as chronic uncontrolled focal seizure disorders. *Ann Neurol* 1982; 12: 538–41.

49 Suarez JC, Sfaello ZM, Guerrero A *et al*. Epilepsy and brain tumors in infancy and adolescence. *Child Nerv Syst* 1986; 2: 169–74.

50 Adelson PD, Peacock WJ, Chugani HT *et al*. Temporal and extended temporal resection for the treatment of intractable seizures in early childhood. *Ped Neurosurg* 1992; 18: 169–78.

51 Kleihues P, Burger PC, Scheithauer BW. The new WHO classification of brain tumors. *Brain Pathol* 1993; 3: 255–68.

52 Kirkpatrick PJ, Honavar M, Janota I, Polkey CE. Control of temporal lobe epilepsy following en bloc resection of low grade tumors. *J Neurosurg* 1993; 78: 19–25.

53 Silver JM, Rawling CE, Rossitch ER, Zeidman SM, Friedman AH. Ganglioglioma: a clinical study with long-term follow-up. *Surg Neurol* 1991; 35: 261–6.

54 Zentner J, Wolf HK, Osterun B *et al*. Gangliogliomas: clinical, radiological, and histopathological findings in 51 patients. *J Neurol Neurosurg Psychiatr* 1994; 57: 1497–502.

55 Isla A, Alvarez F, Gutierrez M, Paredes E, Blazquez MG. Gangliogliomas: clinical study and evolution. *J Neurosurg Sci* 1991; 35: 193–7.

56 Casazza M, Avanzini G, Broggi G, Fornari M, Franzini A. Epilepsy course in cerebral gangliogliomas: a study of 16 cases. *Acta Neurochir* 1989; 46 (Suppl.): 17–20.

57 Hwang PA, Becker LE, Chuang SH. Evaluation, surgical approach and outcome of seizure in patients with gangliogliomas. *Pediatr Neurosurg* 1990–1991; 16: 208–12.

58 Daumas-Duport C, Scheithauer BW, Chodkiewicz JP, Laws ER Jr, Vedrenne C. Dysembryoplastic neuroepithelial tumor: a surgically curable tumor of young patients with intractable partial seizures. Report of thirty-nine cases. *Neurosurgery* 1988; 23: 545–56.

59 Taylor DC, Falconer MA, Burton CJ, Corsellis JAN. Focal dysplasia of the cerebral cortex in epilepsy. *J Neurol Neurosurg Psychiatr* 1971; 34: 369–87.

60 Vinters HV, Mah V, Shields WD. Neuropathologic correlates of pediatric epilepsy. *J Epilepsy* 1990; 3 (Suppl.): 227–35.

61 Altman NR, Purser RK, Post MJD. Tuberose sclerosis. Characteristics of CT and MR imaging. *Radiology* 1988; 167: 527–32.

62 Russell DS, Rubinstein U. *Pathology of Tumors of the Nervous System*, 5th edn. Williams and Wilkins, Baltimore, 1989: 767–8.

63 Nagib MG, Haines SJ, Erickson DL, Mastri AR. Tuberous sclerosis: a review for the neurosurgeon. *Neurosurgery* 1984; 14: 93–8.

64 Al-Rodhan NRF, Kelly PJ. Stereotactic surgery in the diagnosis and treatment of brain tumors. In: Morantz RA, Walsh JW, eds. *Brain Tumors: A Comprehensive Text*. New York: Marcel Dekker, 1994: 493–511.

65 Lieu AA, Howng SL. Intracranial meningiomas and epilepsy: incidence, prognosis and influencing factors. *Epilepsy Res* 2000; 38: 45–52.

66 Ramamurthi B, Ravi R, Ramachandran V. Convulsions with meningiomas: incidence and significance. *Surg Neurol* 1980; 14: 415–16.

67 Chan RC, Thompson GB. Morbidity, mortality, and quality of life following surgery for intracranial meningiomas. A retrospective study of 257 cases. *J Neurosurg* 1984; 60: 52–60.

68 Rohringer M, Sutherland GR, Louw DF, Sima AAF. Incidence and clinicopathologic features of meningioma. *J Neurosurg* 1989; 71: 665–72.

69 Remillard GM, Andermann F, Rhi-Sausi A, Robbins NM. Facial asymmetry in patients with temporal lobe epilepsy. *Neurology* 1977; 27: 109–14.

70 Cascino GD, Luckstein RB., Sharbrough FW, Jack CR Jr. Facial asymmetry, hippocampal pathology, and remote symptomatic seizures: a temporal lobe epileptic syndrome. *Neurology* 1993; 43: 725–7.

71 Page LK, Lombroso CT, Matson DD. Childhood epilepsy in the late detection of cerebral glioma. *J Neurosurg* 1969; 31: 253–61.

72 Bachman DS, Hodges FJ III, Freeman JM. Computerized axial tomography in chronic seizure disorders in childhood. *Pediatrics* 1976; 58: 828–32.

73 Vignaedra V, Ng KK, Lim CL, Loh TL. Clinical and electroencephalographic data indicative of brain tumors in a seizure population. *Postgrad Med J* 1978; 54: 1–5.

74 Douglas DB. Interval between first seizure and diagnosis of brain tumour. *Dis Nerv Syst* 1971; 32: 255–9.

75 Fincham RW, Adams HP Jr. Brain tumor as a cause of epilepsy. *Am Fam Phys* 1977; 6: 165–7.

76 Berkovic SF, Andermann F, Melanson D, Ethier RE, Feindel W, Gloor P. Hypothalamic hamartomas and ictal laughter: evolution of a characteristic epileptic syndrome and diagnostic value of magnetic resonance imaging. *Ann Neurol* 1988; 23: 429–39.

77 Machado HR, Hoffman HJ, Hwang PA. Gelastic seizures treated by resection of a hypothalamic hamartoma. *Childs Nerv Syst* 1991; 7: 462–5.

78 Cascino GD, Andermann F, Berkovic SF *et al*. Gelastic seizures and hypothalamic hamartomas: evaluation of patients undergoing chronic intracranial EEG monitoring and outcome of surgical treatment. *Neurology* 1993; 43: 747–50.

79 Solomon GE, Carson D, Pavlakis S, Fraser R, Labar D. Intracranial EEG monitoring in Landau–Kleffner syndrome associated with left temporal astrocytoma. *Epilepsia* 1993; 34: 557–60.

80 Morimoto K, Aberkura M, Nii Y, Nakatani S, Hayakawa T, Mogami H. Nodding attacks. Infantile spasms; associated with temporal lobe astrocytoma – case report. *Neurol Med Chir Tokyo* 1989; 29: 610–13.

81 Ruggieri V, Caraballo R, Fejerman N. Intracranial tumors and West syndrome. *Pediatr Neurol* 1989; 5: 327–9.

82 Angelini L, Broggi G, Riva D, Lazzaro-Solero C. A case of Lennox—Gastaut syndrome successfully treated by removal of a parieto-temporal astrocytoma. *Epilepsia* 1979; 20: 665–9.

83 Williamson PD. Intensive monitoring of complex partial seizures: diagnosis and subclassification. In: Gumnit RJ, ed. *Intensive Neurodiagnostic Monitoring. Advances in Neurology*, Vol. 46. New York: Raven Press, 1986: 69–89.

84 Cascino GD, Hulihan JF, Sharbrough FW, Kelly PJ. Parietal lobe lesional epilepsy: electroclinical correlation and operative outcome. *Epilepsia* 1993; 34: 522–7.

85 Fischer-Williams M. Brain tumors and other space-occupying lesions with a section on oncological CNS complications. In: Niedermeyer E, Lopes Da Silva F, eds. *Electroencephalography — Basic Principles, Clinical Application, and Related Fields*, 3rd edn. Baltimore: Williams and Wilkins, 1993: 263–89.

86 Salanova V, Andermann F, Olivier A, Rasmussen T, Quesney LF. Occipital lobe epilepsy: electroclinical manifestations, electrocorticography, cortical stimulation and outcome in 42 patients treated between 1930 and 1991. Surgery of occipital lobe epilepsy. *Brain* 1992; 115: 1655–80.

87 Williamson PD, Thadani VM, Darcey TM, Spencer DD, Spencer SS, Mattson RH. Occipital lobe epilepsy: clinical characteristics, seizures spread patterns and results of surgery. *Ann Neurol* 1992; 31: 3–13.

88 Salanova V, Morris HH III, Van-Ness PC, Lüders H, Dinner D, Wyllie E. Comparison of scalp electroencephalogram with subdural electrocorticogram recordings and functional mapping in frontal lobe epilepsy. *Arch Neurol* 1993; 50: 294–9.

89 Williamson PD, Boon PA, Thadani VM *et al*. Parietal lobe epilepsy: diagnostic considerations and results of surgery. *Ann Neurol* 1992; 31: 193–201.

90 Lieb JP, Engel J Jr, Brown WJ, Gevins AS, Crandall PH. Neuropathological finding following temporal lobectomy related to surface and deep EEG patterns. *Epilepsia* 1981; 22: 539–49.

91 So N, Olivier A, Andermann F, Gloor P, Quesney LF. Results of surgical treatment in patients with bitemporal epileptiform abnormalities. *Ann Neurol* 1989; 25: 432–9.

92 Sammaritano M, deLotbiniere A, Andermann F, Olivier A, Gloor P, Quesney LF. False lateralization by surface EEG of seizure onset in

patients with temporal lobe epilepsy and gross focal cerebral lesions. *Ann Neurol* 1987; 21: 361–9.

93 Gastaut H, Gastaut JL. Computerized transverse axial tomography in epilepsy. *Epilepsia* 1976; 17: 325–36.

94 Blom RJ, Vinuela F, Fox AJ *et al.* Computed tomography in temporal lobe epilepsy. *J Comput Assist Tomogr* 1984; 8: 401–5.

95 Molyneux AJ, Anslow P, Easterbrook P, Oxbury JM, Adams CB, Hughes JT. The radiologic investigation of temporal lobe epilepsy. Value of high resolution CT with temporal oriented sections. *Acta Radiol Suppl* 1986; 369: 400–2.

96 Holland RC, Hawkes GN, Moore WS. Nuclear magnetic resonance; tomography of the brain: Coronal and sagittal sections. *J Compt Assist Tomgr* 1980; 4: 429–33.

97 Bergen D, Bleck T, Ramsey R *et al.* Magnetic resonance imaging as a sensitive and specific predictor of neoplasms removed for intractable epilepsy. *Epilepsia* 1989; 30: 318–21.

98 Cascino GD. Commentary: How has neuroimaging improved patient care? *Epilepsia* 1994; 35 (Suppl. 6): S103–107.

99 Heinz ER, Cram BJ, Radtke *et al.* MR imaging in patients with temporal lobe seizures: correlation of results with pathologic findings. *Am J Neuroradiol* 1990; 11: 827–32.

100 Dowd CF, Dillon WP, Barbaro NM, Laxer ND. Intractable complex partial seizure: correlation of magnetic resonance imaging with pathology and electroencephalography. *Epilepsy Res Suppl* 1992; 5: 101–10.

101 Kuznicky R, Murro A, King D *et al.* Magnetic resonance imaging in childhood intractable partial epilepsies: pathologic correlations. *Neurology* 1993; 43: 681–7.

102 Cascino GD. Advances in neuroimaging: Surgical localization. *Epilepsia* 2001; 42: 3–12.

103 Cascino GD, Kelly PJ, Sharbrough FW, Hulihan JF, Hirschorn KA, Trenerry MR. Long-term follow-up of stereotactic lesionectomy in partial epilepsy: predictive factors and electroencephalographic results. *Epilepsia* 1992; 33: 639–44.

104 Friedland RJ, Bronen RA. Magnetic resonance imaging of neoplastic, vascular and indeterminant substrates. In: Cascino GD, Jack CR Jr, eds. *Neuroimaging in Epilepsy: principles and practice.* Boston: Butterworth-Heinemann, 1996: 29–50.

105 Wetjen NM, Cohen-Gadol AA, Maher CO *et al.* Frontal lobe epilepsy: diagnosis and surgical treatment. *Neurosurg Rev* 2002; 25: 119–38.

106 Britton JW, Cascino GD, Sharbrough FW, Kelly PJ. Low grade glial neoplasms and intractable partial epilepsy. Efficacy of surgical treatment. *Epilepsia* 1994; 35: 1130–5.

107 Jack CR Jr. Bentley MD, Twomey CK, Zinsmeister AR. MR-based volume measurements of the hippocampal formation and anterior temporal lobe: validation studies. *Radiology* 1990; 175: 205–9.

108 Jack CR Jr, Sharbrough FW, Cascino GD. MRI-based hippocampal volumetry: correlation with outcome after temporal lobectomy. *Ann Neurol* 1992; 31: 138–46.

109 Trenerry MR, Jack CR Jr, Ivnik RJ *et al.* MRI hippocampal volumes and memory function before and after temporal lobectomy. *Neurology* 1993; 43: 1800–5.

110 Trenerry MR, Jack CR Jr, Sharbrough FW *et al.* Quantitative MRI hippocampal volumes: association with onset and duration of epilepsy, and febrile convulsions in temporal lobectomy patients. *Epilepsy Res* 1993; 15: 247–52.

111 Duckwiler G, Levesque M, Wilson C, Behnke E, Babb T, Lufkin R. Imaging of MR-compatible intracerebral depth electrodes. *Am J Neuroradiol* 1990; 11: 353–4.

112 Katz A. Inserni J, Marks D, McCarthy G, Spencer D. MRI of intracranial electrodes. *Epilepsia* 1990; 31: 669.

113 Jack CR Jr, Sharbrough FW, Marsh WR. Use of MR imaging for quantitative evaluation of resection for temporal lobe epilepsy. *Radiology* 1988; 169: 463–8.

114 Awad I, Katz A, Hahn J, Kong A, Ahl J, Lüders H. Extent of resection in temporal lobectomy for epilepsy. *Epilepsia* 1989; 30: 756–62.

115 Dodrill CB. A neuropsychological battery for epilepsy. *Epilepsia* 1978; 27: 1023–8.

116 Novelly RA, Schumartz HM, Mattson RH, Cramer JA. Behavioral toxicity associated with antiepileptic drugs: concepts and methods of assessment. *Epilepsia* 1986; 27: 331–40.

117 Spencer DD. Strategies for focal resection in medically intractable epilepsy. *Epilepsy Res Suppl* 1992; 5: 157–68.

118 Boon PA, Williamson PD. Presurgical evaluation of patients with intractable partial seizures, indications and evaluation techniques for resective surgery. *Clin Neurol Neurosurg* 1989; 91: 3–11.

119 Lee BI. Markand ON, Wellman HN *et al.* HIPDN1 single photon emission computer tomography brain imaging in partial onset secondary generalized tonic-clonic seizures. *Epilepsia* 1987; 28: 305–11.

120 Duncan B., Patterson J, Roberts R., Hadley DM, Bone I. Ictal/postictal SPECT in the presurgical localization of complex partial seizures. *J Neurol Neurosurg Psychiatr* 1993; 56: 141–8.

121 Buchpiquel CA, Cukiert A, Hironaka FH, Cerri GG, Magalhaes AE, Marino R Jr. Brain SPECT in the presurgical evaluation of epileptic patients. Preliminary Results. *Arq Neuro-Psiquiatr* 1992; 50: 37–42.

122 Grunwald F, Durwen HF, Bolkisch A *et al.* Technetium-99-M-HMPAO brain SPECT in medically intractable temporal lobe epilepsy: a postoperative evaluation. *J Nuclear Med* 1991; 32: 388–94.

123 So EL. Integration of EEG, MRI and SPECT in localizing the seizure focus for epilepsy surgery. *Epilepsia* 2000; 41 (Suppl. 3): S48–S54.

124 Brinkmann BH, O'Brien TJ, Mullan BP, O'Connor MK, Robb RA, So EL. Subtraction ictal SPECT coregistered to MRI for seizure focus localization in partial epilepsy. *Mayo Clin Proc* 2000; 75: 615–24.

125 O'Brien TJ, O'Connor MK, Mullan BP *et al.* Subtraction ictal SPECT coregistered to MRI in partial epilepsy: Description and technical validation of the method with phantom and patient studies. *Nuclear Med Commun* 1998; 19: 31–45.

126 O'Brien TJ, So EL, Mullan BP *et al.* Subtraction SPECT co-registered to MRI improves postictal SPECT localization of seizure foci. *Neurology* 1999; 52: 137–46.

127 O'Brien TJ, So EL, Mullan BP *et al.* Subtraction peri-ictal SPECT is predictive of extratemporal epilepsy surgery outcome. *Neurology* 2000; 55: 1448–77.

128 Engel J Jr. PET scanning in partial epilepsy. *Can J Neurol Sci* 1991; 18: 588–92.

129 Henry TR, Chugani HT, Abon-Khalil BW, Theodore WH, Schartz BE. Positron emission tomography. In: Engel J Jr, ed. *Surgical Treatment of the Epilepsies*, 2nd edn. New York: Raven Press, 1993: 211–32.

130 Radtke R, Hanson M, Hoffman J. Positron emission tomography: comparison of clinical utility in temporal lobe epilepsy and extratemporal epilepsy. *J Epilepsy* 1994; 7: 27–33.

131 Spencer SS. The relative contributions of MRI, SPECT, and PET imaging in epilepsy. *Epilepsia* 1994; 35 (Suppl. 6): S72–S89.

132 Swartz BE, Delgado-Escueta AV, Mandelkern M *et al.* Neuroimaging in patients with seizures of probable frontal lobe origin. *Epilepsia* 1989; 30: 547–58.

133 Koepp MJ, Richardson MP, Brooks DJ *et al.* Central benzodiazepine receptors in hippocampal sclerosis: an objective in vivo analysis. *Brain* 1996; 119: 1677–87.

134 Frost J. Receptor imaging by PET and SPECT: focus on the opiate receptor. *J Receptor Res* 1993; 13: 39–53.

135 Henry T. Functional neuroimaging with positron emission tomography. *Epilepsia* 1996; 37: 1141–54.

136 Laxer KD, Rowley HA, Novotny EJ Jr. Experimental technologies. In: Engel J Jr, ed. *Surgical Treatment of Epilepsies*, 2nd edn. New York: Raven Press, 1993: 291–308.

137 Sato S, Balish NI, Niuratore R. Principles of magnetoencephalography. *J Clin Neurophysiol* 1991; 8: 144–56.

138 Romani GL, Williamson SJ, Kaufman L. Tonotopic organization of the human auditory cases. *Science* 1982; 216: 1339–40.

139 Hari R, Reinikainen K, Kaukoranta *et al.* Somatosensory evoked cerebral magnetic fields from SI and SII in man. *Electroencephalogr Clin Neurophysiol* 1984; 57: 254–63.

140 Hari R, Hamalainen M, Ilmoniemi R, Lounsmaa OV. MEG versus EEG localization test. Letter. *Ann Neurol* 1991; 30: 222–3.

141 Black PM, Ronner SF. Cortical mapping for defining the limits of tumour resection. *Neurosurgery* 1987; 20: 914–19.

142 Ojemann G. Comment: Cortical mapping for defining the limits of tumor resection. *Neurosurgery* 1987; 20: 918–19.

143 Morris HH III, Lüders H, Hahn JF, Lesser BY, Dinner DS. Surgical treatment of primary brain tumors. *Ann Neurol* 1986; 19: 559–67.

144 Berger MS, Ghatan S, Haglund MM, Dobbins J, Ojemann GA. Low grade gliomas associated with intractable epilepsy: seizure outcome utilizing electrocorticography during tumor resection. *J Neurosurg* 1993; 79: 62–9.

145 Smith DF, Hutton JL, Sandemann D *et al.* The prognosis of primary intracerebral tumors presenting with epilepsy: the outcome of medical and surgical management. *J Neurol Neurosurg Psychiatr* 1991; 54: 915–20.

146 Cairncross JG, Laperriere NJ. Low-grade glioma: to treat or not to treat. *Arch Neurol* 1989; 46: 1238–9.

147 Marks JE, Baglan RJ, Prassad SC, Blank WF. Cerebral necrosis: incidence and risk in relation to dose, time, fractionation and volume. *Int J Radiat Oncol Biol Phys* 1981; 7: 243–52.

148 Sandeman DR, Sandeman AP, Buxton P *et al.* The management of patients with an intrinsic supratentorial brain tumor. *Br J Neurosurg* 1990; 4: 299–312.

149 Choksey MS, Valentine A, Shawdon H *et al.* Computed tomography in the diagnosis of malignant brain tumors: do all patients require biopsy? *J Neurol Neurosurg Psychiatr* 1989; 52: 821–5.

150 Wilden JN, Kelly PJ. Computerized stereotactic biopsy for low density CT lesions presenting with epilepsy. *J Neurol Neurosurg Psychiatr* 1987; 50: 1302–5.

151 Revesz T, Scaravilli F, Coutinho I, Cockburn H, Sacares P, Thomas DGT. Reliability of histological diagnosis including grading in gliomas biopsied by image-guided stereo-tactic technique. *Brain* 1993; 116: 781–93.

152 Heikkinen ER. Stereotactic neurosurgery: new aspects of an old method. *Ann Clin Res* 1986; 18 (Suppl. 47): 73–83.

153 Kelly PJ. Volumetric stereotactic surgical resection of intra-axial brain mass lesions. *Mayo Clin Proc* 1988; 63: 1186–98.

154 Moore JL, Cascino GD, Trenerry MR, Kelly PJ, Marsh WR. A comparative study of lesionectomy versus corticectomy in patients with temporal lobe lesional epilepsy. *J Epilepsy* 1993; 6: 239–42.

155 Wyllie E, Lüders H, Morris HH III *et al.* Clinical outcome after complete or partial cortical resection for intractable epilepsy. *Neurology* 1987; 37: 1634–41.

156 Otsubo H, Hoffman HJ, Humphreys HJ, Hendrick EB, Drake JM. Evaluation, surgical approach and outcome of seizure patients with gangliogliomas. *Pediatr Neurosurg* 1990–1991; 16: 208–12.

157 Sethi PK, Kumar BR, Madan VS, Mohan V. Appearing and disappearing CT abnormalities and seizures. *J Neurol Neurosurg Psychiatr* 1985; 48: 866–9.

158 Goulatia RK, Verna A, Mishra NK, Ahuja GK. Disappearing CT lesions in epilepsy. *Epilepsia* 1987; 28: 523–7.

159 Rajshekar V, Haran RP, Prakash GS, Chandy MJ. Differentiating solitary – small cysticercus granulomas and tuberculomas in patients with epilepsy. Clinical and computerized tomographic criteria. *J Neurosurg* 1993; 78: 402–7.

160 Rajshekar V. Etiology and management of single small CT lesions in patients with seizures: understanding a controversy. *Acta Neurol Scand* 1991; 84: 465–70.

161 Chandy MJ, Rajshekar V, Ghosh S *et al.* Single small enhancing CT lesions in Indian patients with epilepsy: clinical, radiological and pathological considerations. *J Neurol Neurosurg Psychiatr* 1991; 54: 702–5.

162 Nayel MH, Awad IA, Lüders H. Extent of mesiobasal resection determines outcome after temporal lobectomy for intractable complex partial seizures. *Neurosurgery* 1991; 29: 55–61.

163 Jennum P, Dhuna A, Davis K, Frol M, Maxwell R. Outcome of resective surgery for intractable partial epilepsy guided by subdural electrode arrays. *Acta Neurol Scand* 1993; 87: 434–7.

164 Gulgvog B, Loyning V. Hauglie-Hanssen E, Flood S, Bjornaes H. Surgical versus medical treatment for epilepsy. II. Outcome related to social areas. *Epilepsia* 1991; 32: 477–86.

165 Berger MS, Ghatan S, Geyer JR, Keles GE, Ojemann GA. Seizure outcome in children with hemispheric tumors and associated intractable epilepsy: the role of tumor removal combined with seizure foci resection. *Pediatr Neurosurg* 1991–92; 17: 185–91.

166 Taylor D. Psychiatric and social issues in measuring the input and output of epilepsy surgery. In Engel J Jr, ed. *Surgical Treatment of Epilepsies.* New York: Raven Press, 1987: 485–504.

167 Fenswick P. Postscript: What should be included in a standard psychiatric assessment? In: Engel J Jr, ed. *Surgical Treatment of Epilepsies.* New York: Raven Press, 1987: 505–10.

168 Trimble NI. Behavior changes following temporal lobectomy with special reference to psychosis. *J Neurol Neurosurg Psychiatr* 1992; 55: 89–91.

169 Jensen I, Larson K. Mental aspects of temporal lobectomy. *J Neurol Neurosurg Psychiatr* 1979; 42: 256–65.

170 Naugle R. Neuropsychological effects of surgery of epilepsy. In: Lüders H, ed. *Epilepsy Surgery.* New York: Raven Press, 1991: 637–46.

171 Penfield W, Mathieson G. Memory, autopsy findings, and comments on the role of the hippocampus in experimental recall. *Arch Neurol* 1974; 31: 145–54.

172 Katz A *et al.* Extent of resection in temporal lobectomy for epilepsy. II. Memory changes and neurological complications. *Epilepsia* 1989; 30: 763–71.

173 Rausch R, Crandall P. Psychosocial status related to surgical control of temporal lobe seizures. *Epilepsia* 1982; 23: 191–202.

174 Novelly RA, Augustine EA, Mattson RH *et al.* Selective memory improvement and impairment in temporal lobectomy for epilepsy. *Ann Neural* 1984; 15: 64–7.

62 Resective Surgery of Vascular and Infective Lesions for Epilepsy

N.D. Kitchen, A. Belli and J.A. Sen

Vascular and infective lesions of the brain are non-neoplastic pathologies with a high propensity to induce seizures. Epilepsy may be the sole or main manifestation and, in some cases, recognizing the underlying lesion can be difficult.

Beside their epileptogenic potential, these lesions also pose other risks and raise treatment issues which differently influence their medical and surgical management. Whilst the presence of intractable epilepsy may strengthen the indications for surgical treatment, careful consideration must be paid to other aspects of the pathology, such as location of the lesion, age of the patient, availability and efficacy of alternative treatment, natural history, etc. Often the complexity of the problem demands a multidisciplinary approach with strict cooperation between the neuroradiologist, neurologist, neurosurgeon and microbiologist. Vascular malformations, for example, have been recognized for hundreds of years, yet many aspects of their natural history are still unclear. Whilst many surgeons in the past would see these lesions, particularly if associated with epilepsy, as clear targets for resection, recent studies on the outcome of operative series and the emergence of new medical and radiological treatment have made the surgical selection criteria increasingly stringent. Yet, the refinement of radiological techniques has led to an upsurge in the number of cases referred for surgery in recent years, and the detection of 'incidental' or causative structural lesions during the course of investigations for epilepsy has become a frequent occurrence.

In parallel, there has been a definite increase in the number of infective lesions of the central nervous system (CNS) worldwide; it is now recognized that infection is one of the major causes of acquired epilepsy in the world [1]. In a recent study of 100 cases of intractable epilepsy in a low economy country, CNS infection was found to be the leading aetiological factor [2]. Approximately 75% of the world's 50 million epilepsy sufferers live in poor countries and up to 94% of these cases go untreated. This is largely because of lack of access to appropriate management [3]. Provision of the necessary services to these people will be a major public health undertaking from the point of view of economy and logistics, but also because — despite great research efforts — little is really known about the causes of epilepsy in developing countries [4]. Further aetiological and epidemiological studies will be required to develop a good evidence base for treatment approaches.

Increasingly sophisticated neuroimaging has, however, improved detection rates of intracranial abnormalities in patients with epilepsy [5] (see Table 62.1 for classification of intracranial abnormalities associated with intractable epilepsy). In particular, MRI is sensitive and specific in distinguishing mass lesions from other pathological entities in patients with epilepsy [6]. If an operable lesion is considered to be responsible for intractable seizures and the relationship between the lesion and seizures is verified, resective surgery can render the patient seizure free and improve quality of life [7]. Such lesions may also warrant neurosurgical intervention because of mass effect, haemorrhage or growth. In other cases, where the lesion is static or sited in eloquent or inaccessible areas, surgery may increase morbidity and is best deferred. In this chapter, current concepts regarding the diagnosis and management of patients with epilepsy associated with infective and vascular mass lesions will be discussed.

Vascular lesions

Arteriovenous malformations (AVMs)

AVMs are racemose networks of arterial and venous channels that communicate directly rather than through a capillary bed. Despite the fact that these lesions have been recognized for at least 300 years, their natural history is still not clearly understood. The propensity of cerebral AVMs to haemorrhage has convinced many neurosurgeons that they should be treated whenever possible. For this reason untreated lesions have been subjected to selection and the natural history of these is probably not representative of the natural history of the entire group.

Several studies highlight the benefit of surgical resection for accessible cerebral AVM [8–12] in terms of rebleeding and overall morbidity and mortality, although this view is not universally accepted [13]. The effect of surgery on long-term control of seizures associated with cerebral AVMs is even more controversial.

It is estimated that between 17% and 36% [14–16] of supratentorial AVMs will present with seizures, with or without associated neurological deficits. By contrast, between 42% and 50% present with haemorrhage [17,18]. It is generally thought that small AVMs (<3 cm diameter) tend to manifest themselves more often with haemorrhage than large ones [19,20]. This is probably because smaller AVMs tend to have higher pressures in the feeding arteries [20].

Irrespective of the initial presentation, a significant proportion of patients with cerebral AVMs will develop epilepsy after diagnosis. The risk of seizures seems to be higher the younger the patient at the time of diagnosis. Crawford *et al.* estimated that patients aged between 10 and 19 years had a 44% risk of epilepsy by 20 years; this risk declined to 31% for patients aged 20–29 years and to 6% for patients aged 30–60 years [19]. In another paper the same authors suggested that surgery was the most important risk factor for subsequent development of epilepsy. In their series of 234 patients, the surgically treated group (96 patients) had a 57% risk of seizures by 20 years, as compared with 19% risk for those managed conserva-

Table 62.1 Classification of structural mass lesions associated with intractable epilepsy

Neoplastic lesions
Neuronal/glial tumours
    Ganglioglioma
    Dysembryoplastic neuroepithelial tumour
Glial tumours
    Pilocytic astrocytoma
    Low-grade astrocytoma
    Oligodendroglioma
Mixed glial tumours
    Oligoastrocytoma

Developmental lesions
Glioneuronal hamartomas
Focal cortical dysplasia

Vascular lesions
Arteriovenous malformation
Cavernous angioma

Inflammatory/infectious lesions
Tuberculoma
Cystercosis
Rasmussen's encephalitis

tively (138 patients). The 10-year risk was 47% vs. 11% for the same groups, respectively [21]. Interestingly, in this series, no patient with either initial neurological signs or in whom the AVM was a coincidental finding developed epilepsy when treated conservatively. Foy *et al.* found that epilepsy was present in 50% of patients operated on for AVMs after surgery, as compared with an overall incidence of 17% for all patients undergoing supratentorial craniotomies [22]. In other series the incidence of postoperative epilepsy has ranged from 4% [8] to 22% [9].

In contrast to these observations, other authors have reported a beneficial effect of surgery on epilepsy associated with cerebral AVMs. Guidetti and Delitala reported that in their series of 130 patients (86 treated surgically and 44 treated conservatively) with follow-up for a minimum of 2 years, 53% of the surgically treated cases improved while only 36% of the conservatively managed group did [8]. Pool found the incidence of epilepsy to range between 30% and 50% in 187 patients who underwent surgical resection, whereas the same incidence was 64% among patients treated conservatively [18]. Trumpy and Eldevik reported that five patients in their series of surgically treated AVMs had no epilepsy following the operation, but five patients developed seizures after surgery [23]. Finally Murphy found no statistical difference between the percentage of seizure-free patients in the medically treated group and those in the surgical group in his series of 46 patients followed up for a mean of 13 years [15].

A possible explanation of this apparent lack of substantial improvement in seizure control following surgical resection could be made on the basis of pathological studies of AVMs. The tissue adjacent to AVMs is characterized by neuronal loss, gliosis, demyelination and haemosiderin deposits, which are probably the structural substratum of the epileptic focus [24,25]. In all the series examined, no mention has been made of any effort by the surgeon to remove surrounding or intervening areas of abnormal brain tissue along with the malformation. Although the importance of preserving normal tissue at surgery is paramount, this approach also has the theoretical disadvantage of leaving the epileptic focus undisturbed.

Beside the issue of long-term seizure control, the aim of treatment of AVMs should be to prevent bleeding and reduce overall morbidity and mortality. It is estimated that the average risk of bleeding from an AVM is around 2–4% per year [26]. In a study of 166 symptomatic AVMs with long mean follow-up (23.7 years) Ondra *et al.* found that the risk of haemorrhage was constant at 4%, irrespective of whether the malformation presented with or without haemorrhage [27]. In the same study, the mortality rate was 1% per year, with a combined major morbidity and mortality of 2.7% per year. Of the patients with cerebral AVMs who survived long enough after the initial haemorrhage to be entered into the Cooperative Study, 53% were reported to have a neurological deficit attributable to the bleeding. Approximately 10% of these patients died as a direct result of their first known haemorrhage [14]. Twenty-three per cent of the survivors suffered recurrent haemorrhages, with a mortality rate of 12%.

Evaluation

MRI followed by cerebral angiography is currently considered the gold standard in the evaluation of AVMs. An MRI scan can reveal flow void on T1- and T2-weighted images and show the characteristics of feeding arteries and draining veins (Fig. 62.1). It can also help to differentiate between AVM and neoplasm, and provide the surgeon with vital information in the case of angiographically occult vascular malformations. In all cases a cerebral angiogram will better outline the characteristics of feeding arteries and draining veins and reveal any associated aneurysms (present in 7% of AVMs) [19] (Fig. 62.2).

CT of the brain may show presence of blood around the AVM, as well as possible areas of calcification related to the malformation. It may also reveal pathological contrast enhancement in the area of the AVM itself.

If surgery is considered for the treatment of epilepsy associated with an AVM, rather than to reduce or abolish the bleeding potential of the lesion, every effort should be made to establish the congruence between the area targeted for resection and the epileptic focus. In the majority of patients scalp EEG alone may not localize or even lateralize the seizure focus. Prolonged EEG monitoring with video correlation of seizures, interictal and ictal PET, as well as meticulous history taking and neurological examination, may yield convergent data and therefore augment the accuracy of localization.

Treatment

Surgery

At present surgery is considered the treatment of choice for cerebral AVMs. Although, as discussed above, the results on long-term seizure control are uncertain, surgery abolishes the risk of rebleeding with immediate effect. As the risk of haemorrhage is higher for small AVMs, Luessenhop and Rosa in 1985 stated that surgical mortality and morbidity for this group are lower than a reasonably

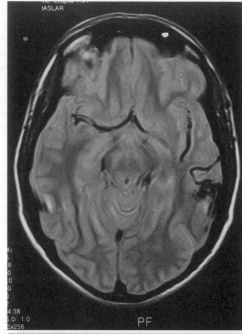

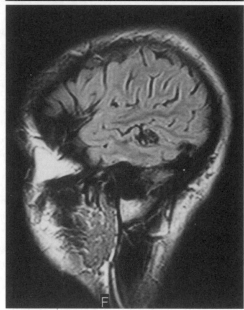

Fig. 62.1 (a) Coronal view of a MRI scan of a 21-year-old man who presented with generalized seizure activity, showing a left temporal AVM with a large draining vein. There is flow void within the lesion and in the draining vessel. (b) Sagittal view of the same. The scan shows no evidence of previous haemorrhage.

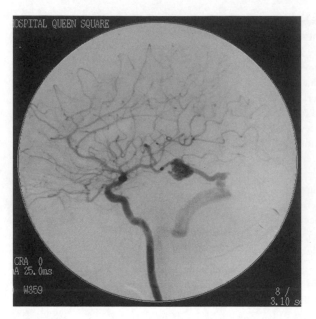

Fig. 62.2 Cerebral angiography of the same AVM (lateral view). The exam shows a single arterial feeder and a single draining vein discharging into the proximal sigmoid sinus. After a failed attempt at embolization the AVM was successfully excised surgically. The patient remains seizure-free on phenytoin.

of life are probably less than the surgical risks by present operative techniques. They based these considerations on an overall operative mortality rate of 10% and morbidity rate of 30% for AVMs. In 1980 Pellittieri presented his surgical results in 166 consecutive patients and defined the characteristics of the most favourable operative risk profile as age below 40 years, absence of a neurological deficit, a superficial and small AVM in a silent area, female sex and subarachnoid haemorrhage at presentation.

Radiotherapy

Radiation treatment is also available for AVMs. Conventional radiotherapy is only successful in 20% or less of cases and therefore is not considered effective [29,30]. Stereotactic radiosurgery (SRS) is accepted for small lesions, with a compact nidus measuring less than 2.5–3 cm diameter. This technique induces endothelial proliferation and ultimately causes obliteration of the lumen over a period of 1–2 years. SRS is non-invasive and can be administered on an outpatient basis, but the length of time it takes to work leaves the patient exposed to the risk of rehaemorrhage for the same duration. Haemorrhages have been documented to occur during the incubation period, even in AVMs that had not previously bled, raising the question of whether a partially thrombosed AVM is more likely to bleed due to increased outflow resistance [34]. Several authors suggest that this modality is the best treatment for small malformations located deeply in eloquent areas of the brain [31–33]. It is estimated that between 46% and 61% of AVMs appear obliterated on angiography 1 year after treatment and 86% will be obliterated at 2 years [34]. The likelihood of success depends on the diameter of the nidus; SRS will obliterate all lesions <2 cm diameter 3 years after

projected natural risk [28]. For more extensive AVMs, consideration of anticipated future years of exposure to the natural risk and the location of the AVM in the brain are necessary to determine operability. The same authors also state that neither seizures nor incipient focal neurological dysfunction alone are indications for surgery and that the risks of disability or death after the fifth decade treatment, whilst it will only obliterate 50% of lesions with a diameter greater than 2.5 cm. In a study of 462 cases of cerebral AVM treated with gamma-radiosurgery, 68% of which presented with haemorrhage and 12.8% with epilepsy, the overall results indicated that seizures improved in 85.5%, were unchanged in 11.6% and deteriorated in 2.9% of patients [35]. In the same study, of the 79 cases (17.1%) who had had a convulsive seizure before radiosurgery, 58 presented with seizure as an initial symptom and the other 21 cases mostly had seizures following intracranial haemorrhage. Seizures were either decreased or had disappeared in 91.6% of the former group and in 62.5% of the latter. The authors concluded that radiosurgery is effective not only for the obliteration of the nidus of cerebral AVM, but also for seizure control, even before complete occlusion of the nidus. In another study of 100 patients with AVMs, 33 presented with seizures (11 generalized tonic-clonic seizures, eight simple partial seizures and 14 complex partial seizures with or without secondary generalization); following radiosurgery 59% of these were seizure free and 19% had marked reduction of seizure frequency [36]. Interestingly, four out of the five patients in this study who had not had obliteration of the AVM on angiography 2 years afters SRS, also became seizure free. This suggests that structural or biochemical alterations of epileptogenic neurones following radiosurgery may reduce epileptogenicity. Similar results have also been reported by other authors [37–39], but new onset of seizures in 1–3% of patients treated with this technique has also been reported [40–42].

Endovascular treatment

Embolization is also available for the treatment of cerebral AVMs. Whilst this technique usually facilitates surgery, it is generally accepted that it may not achieve permanent obliteration of the malformation due to the high rate of recanalization [43]. It can also induce acute haemodynamic changes in the treated region and multiple procedures may be required to complete the treatment. The complication rate reported by Jafar *et al.* in 1993 for this procedure included a 1.5% risk of severe deficit, a 1–2% risk of death, a 10% risk of haemorrhage (including 3% first time haemorrhage) and a 3% risk of new onset seizures [43].

Cavernous haemangioma (cavernoma)

Cavernous haemangiomas are hamartomatous well-circumscribed vascular lesions consisting of irregular-walled sinusoidal vascular channels, located within the brain but without intervening neural tissue, large feeding arteries or draining veins. They have the potential to haemorrhage, calcify or thrombose and are multiple in 50% of cases [44]. It is estimated that they constitute 5–13% of vascular malformations of the CNS and have been found to be present in 0.02–0.13% of autopsy series [45]. The majority of these lesions present in the third and fourth decades of life and between a quarter and a third of them in the first and second decades [46,47]. Familial clustering can be found in 10–30% of cavernous haemangiomas [48]. These lesions are usually diagnosed on CT or MRI, whereas cerebral angiography often shows no abnormality. Typical CT appearances are those of a well-circumscribed hyperdense area with moderate enhancement and variable mass effect [47]. CT may also

show previous bleeding, calcification, oedema or cystic areas associated with the lesion [49]. MRI is the most sensitive investigation. On T2-weighted images the typical appearance of cavernomas is that of a reticulated core of mixed signal representing blood in various states of degradation surrounded by a hypointense haemosiderin halo (Fig. 62.3). T1 images show a similar pattern but they are less sensitive. There is slight contrast enhancement in some cases [44].

In 1978 Giombini and Morello published a series of 51 cases of cavernous haemangioma. In 19 of these the first symptom was epilepsy, whereas haemorrhage was the presenting symptom in 12 of them [50]. In another series of 25 cavernous haemangiomas published in 1987, 70% of lesions located within the cerebral hemi-

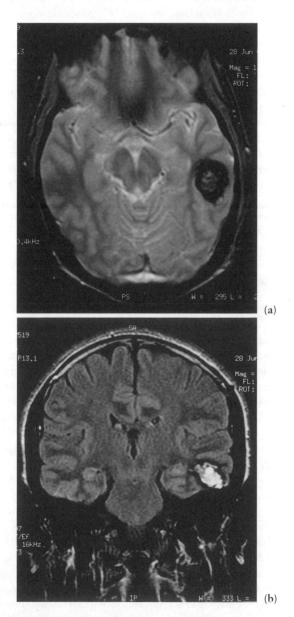

Fig. 62.3 (a) MRI of a left temporal cavernous angioma causing complex partial seizures in a 27-year-old man. The scan shows the typical appearances of a hypo-intense haemosiderin halo with a mixed-signal core on a T2-weighted image. (b) Same cavernoma on a T1-weighted coronal view.

spheres presented with seizures as the only complaint, 20% had symptoms or signs of raised intracranial pressure and 10% presented with a haemorrhagic syndrome [51]. The bleeding potential of such lesions is uncertain. In a study of 62 patients with a short follow-up (mean 22.4 months), the haemorrhage risk was estimated to be 1.4% per lesion per annum [52]. In a similar study of 122 patients followed up for a mean time of 34 months the bleeding rate was 4.5% for patients with a prior haemorrhage and 0.6% for patients that presented in another fashion [53]. The authors also found that presence of seizures had no significant association with the risk of haemorrhage.

Cavernous malformations are twice as likely to be associated with seizures as other vascular lesions, such as AVMs, or tumours with similar volume and location. In a study of 27 vascular lesions associated with intractable epilepsy, 74% were cavernous haemangiomas and only 14.8% were AVMs [54]. Considering that the prevalence of AVMs is at least 50% greater than that of cavernous haemangiomas, this finding suggests a greater epileptogenic potential of cavernous malformations.

The pathophysiological mechanisms underlying the association between cavernous malformations and seizures are still unclear. It has been postulated that these lesions exert a compressive and irritative effect on the surrounding brain by producing mass effect and multiple local haemorrhages. This results in deposition of blood breakdown products, notably iron, which can elicit a local gliomatous reaction [44,55,56]. Iron has been shown to have an epileptogenic effect in animal studies [55,57,58]. Other mechanisms may include oxygen free radical formation, imbalance of excitatory and inhibitory neurotransmitters, calcium influx and cytotoxicity [59].

Treatment

Surgery

Although the per annum risk of haemorrhage from cavernous haemangiomas is lower than that of AVMs, the cumulative lifetime risk for younger patients may not be insubstantial. It is generally acknowledged that such risk is higher for patients with documented previous haemorrhage. Several published series show that excisional surgery can be accomplished with low morbidity, with excellent or good results achieved in 82.2–100% of cases [50,51,59]. Unlike AVMs, the results in terms of epilepsy control in surgical series are generally favourable. A meta-analysis of surgical results for 268 supratentorial cavernous haemangiomas showed that 84% of patients were seizure free and 21% were improved; there was no change in only 6% and 2% were worse [60]. Lesionectomy alone yielded seizure control in 92% of cases. The same authors also reported their own surgical results in 17 patients with a mean follow-up of 3.2 years: improvement occurred in the thirteen cases, whilst four patients remained unchanged. No deterioration of seizures was reported. It was also noted that duration of epilepsy negatively affected the outcome of surgery, suggesting that resection should be performed sooner rather than later. A similar suggestion has been made for AVMs [61]. In another study of 122 patients who all had operations for cavernous haemangiomas, 1 year after surgery 85% of patients that presented with seizures were symptom free and taking no antiepileptic drugs (AEDs) [53].

Radiotherapy

The treatment of cavernous malformations by radiotherapy has been largely confined to brainstem lesions. Some authors have reported good results but others have found the rebleed rate to be as high as 33%, with a particularly significant incidence of radiation-related complications [62–64]. In a histological study, no significant changes were found in cavernous malformations following irradiation [65].

A more recent multicentre study on the use of gamma knife for cavernous malformations suggested that, despite the failure of this treatment to protect against risk of rehaemorrhage, there was a beneficial effect on epilepsy. Out of 49 patients treated with radiosurgery 26 (53%) were seizure free, two had occasional auras (4%) and 10 (20%) had a significant decrease in the number of seizures; the remaining 13 patients (26%) were unchanged [66]. The authors found that sex, age and duration of epilepsy had no prognostic value, but the outcome was better for patients with simple partial seizures than for those with complex partial seizures. Location in the mesiotemporal region was associated with a poor outcome, whereas location in the laterotemporal and central regions was associated with significantly better results. It should be noted that some studies also report excellent results for the treatment of mesial temporal lobe epilepsy associated with hippocampal sclerosis by gamma knife [67,68]. Although further evaluation of effects of radiosurgery on seizures associated with cavernous malformation is necessary, ideally with a prospective study, this form of treatment may be useful for intractable epilepsy related to lesions situated in eloquent or inaccessible areas of the brain.

Other vascular lesions

Venous malformations

Venous malformations, also known as developmental venous abnormalities (DVA), are thought to be congenital anomalies of normal venous drainage. They represent the most commonly documented intracranial vascular malformation by either brain imaging or autopsy, with a prevalence as high as 3% [69]. They can be associated with cavernous malformations or, more rarely, with AVMs. On MRI they appear as a stellate vascular or contrast enhancing mass [70]. Angiography typically shows a caput medusae appearance in the late venous phase [71].

The haemorrhage risk associated with venous malformations is thought to be low. In a prospective study of 80 patients the bleeding rate per year was calculated to be 0.61%, although the risk of symptomatic haemorrhage was considerably lower (0.34%) [72]. In an older retrospective MRI study, the risk of haemorrhage was estimated to be 0.22% [73].

The risk of epilepsy associated with venous malformation is uncertain. In a retrospective review of MRI scan performed on 1020 epileptic patients, only four had venous malformations [74]. It is also interesting to note that in only two of these cases there was concordance between the vascular lesion and the EEG focus. In another study by Topper et al. on 67 patients with venous angiomas, the concordance was even lower. In their analysis only in one case out of 15 that presented with seizures was the EEG found to be congruent with the topography of the lesion [75]. In fact, none of the 67 patients showed an association between the complaints that led to the MRI and the location of the venous malformation, supporting the view that these are a congenital abnormality of venous drainage of no clinical significance.

Resection of these lesions is generally associated with high morbidity and mortality [76–78]. This is probably because the venous anomaly is a functioning venous channel that drains normal parenchyma; the surgical removal of such channels can thus lead to venous infarction [72]. Similarly, radiosurgery is thought to carry a 30% risk of radiation complications or venous infarctions and may not achieve total obliteration [79].

Capillary malformations

Capillary malformations are often dictated as incidental findings at autopsy. They appear as poorly demarcated pink or reddish discoloured lesions with dilated capillaries and may look like a petechial haemorrhage. The intervening parenchyma between the vessels is usually normal and gliosis and microhaemorrhages are usually absent, distinguishing these anomalies from other vascular malformations [80].

These lesions are extremely rare. In a series of 30 000 autopsies, telangiectasias were identified in 0.06% of the cases [81]. They probably represent less than 4% of all angiographically occult vascular lesions [77]. These malformations are usually seen in hereditary haemorrhagic telangiectasias, such as Rendu–Osler–Weber syndrome or associated with other vascular anomalies, e.g. cavernous angiomas. Non-hereditary cases are rare and usually remain asymptomatic [82]. The usual presentation of symptomatic lesions is a haemorrhagic syndrome or epilepsy [83]. In a study of 21 symptomatic patients, seizures occurred in nine cases [83]. During the follow-up period, eight patients developed haemorrhagic syndromes.

MRI studies are increasingly detecting capillary telangiectasias. Typical MRI features include a variable T1 appearance, high signal intensity on T2-weighted images, contrast enhancement and lack of mass effect. Macroscopic haemorrhage and calcifications are rare in capillary telangiectasia, suggesting that the findings on T2-weighted images are probably related to the presence of deoxyhaemoglobin in the slow-flowing blood. After administration of contrast they enhance faintly in a 'brush-like' or 'stipple' pattern [84].

The presence of an enlarged vessel in about two-thirds of capillary telangiectasias, thought to represent a draining vein, has led some authors to consider these lesions 'transitional malformations' [85]. The brainstem seems to be the most common location [84].

Although seizures may be present in a high percentage of these [77], the number of reported cases is so small that the possibility that these may be purely serendipitous findings in radiological investigations performed for epilepsy cannot be discounted.

The exiguity of cases reported in the literature does not allow us to draw any firm conclusions on the epileptogenic or bleeding potential of capillary malformations.

On the strength of the medical evidence currently available, the discovery of one or more of these lesions during investigations for epilepsy or haemorrhage should not alter the routine surgical or medical management of the underlying pathology.

Infective lesions

In this section, current concepts regarding the diagnosis and management of patients with epilepsy associated with infective mass lesions will be discussed. Emphasis will be on pyogenic brain abscesses, neurocysticercosis (NCC), cerebral hydatid disease and cerebral tuberculoma. A full treatment including schistosomiasis, toxocariasis, toxoplasmosis, paragonomiasis and gnathostomiasis is beyond the scope of this chapter. There is now good evidence that Rasmussen's encephalitis, previously thought to be usually of viral origin by some, has an autoimmune basis [86].

Pyogenic cerebral abscess

Background

Pyogenic brain abscess, although uncommon, has enormous clinical significance. Its relative rarity and frequent delays in diagnosis make it a very challenging condition for the clinician in general, and particularly for the neurosurgeon.

Brain abscess can be defined as a focal suppurative process within the brain parenchyma usually without accompanying parameningeal infection or meningitis. Brain abscesses can range in size from microscopic foci of inflammatory cells to major encapsulated necrotic areas of a cerebral hemisphere exerting significant mass effect. Unless adequately treated, bacterial abscesses produce major morbidity and mortality by destroying cerebral tissue; this occurs through mass effect and through the effect of raised intracranial pressure related to both the abscess and associated cerebral oedema. However, recent advances in the diagnosis and management of brain abscesses have led to improved survival rates. In the 1950s, the mortality rate associated with brain abscess in the USA was estimated to be 38%. By the 1980s this had fallen to 25%. The current figure is between 5 and 10% [87]. This reduction has been attributed to improved diagnostic imaging (especially CT), neuro-anaesthesia and critical care and the evolution of neurosurgical techniques. A better understanding of the pathophysiology and management of raised intracranial pressure and the development of new and more effective antibiotics have also helped to improve outcome [88]. The major progress in brain abscess treatment has been reducing the time to diagnosis; CT and MRI have greatly facilitated speed of diagnosis, markedly improving the prognosis of brain abscess. Despite these improvements, brain abscess remains a serious and potentially fatal condition.

The estimated annual incidence of brain abscess in the USA is 1 in 10 000 hospital admissions. It occurs approximately one-sixth as frequently as bacterial meningitis and accounts for 0.7% of all neurosurgery operations. Large postmortem series report brain abscess occurrence rates of 0.18–1.3%. Nicolosi et al. [89] evaluated brain abscess incidence in Minnesota from 1935 to 1981. Thirty-eight cases were identified and followed; they estimated the incidence to be 1.3 per 100 000 person years (1.9 in males and 0.6 in females). This decreased from 2.7 during the period 1935–44 to 0.9 during 1965–81. Several papers have demonstrated a higher incidence in males, the ratio varying from 3 : 1 [89] to 2 : 1 [90]. However others suggest this finding is inaccurate and that currently male and female incidences are equivalent [91].

Brain abscess may occur at any age, but the median age is between

30 and 45 years. The age at which an abscess occurs is related to the aetiology of the abscess. For example brain abscess due to otitis media has a bimodal age distribution, with peaks in childhood and above 40 years of age. Abscess secondary to paranasal sinusitis commonly occurs between 10 and 30 years of age; 25% of all brain abscesses occur in children below 15 years of age.

Predisposing factors

Brain abscesses develop in four main ways—in association with a contiguous suppurating process (50%), due to haematogenous spread from a distant focus (25%), as a complication of intracranial surgery (15%) and due to trauma (10%).

Contiguous spread

Examples of this include otitis media and mastoiditis. Chronic middle ear infection remains the single most common cause leading to intracranial extension 4–8 times more frequently than occurs with acute disease. Cholesteatoma is an additional risk factor, increasing intracranial extension of infection from 23.2% to 74%. Brain abscesses related to middle ear infection are most often solitary, developing in the inferior portion of the ipsilateral temporal lobe. Abscess formation may be due to direct invasion through the dura, by bacterial transmission through diploic or emissary veins, or by spread through existing channels (e.g. internal auditory meatus, cochlear and vestibular aqueducts, temporal suture lines). In contrast to middle ear infections which usually result in middle cranial fossa spread and temporal lobe abscess, mastoid infections typically result in abscess formation in ipsilateral cerebellum.

Paranasal sinus and periodontal infection can also lead to brain abscess formation. A 1984 report showed that sinusitis was the underlying cause in 15% of patients [92]. However, this figure is likely to be decreasing because of earlier diagnosis and treatment of purulent sinusitis and the development of more effective antibiotics for sinus infection. The majority of abscesses complicating infection in frontal, ethmoidal or maxillary sinuses occur in the frontal lobe. Indeed frontal lobe abscesses are almost always the result of a complication of an underlying sinus infection. Sphenoid sinusitis is the least common of the paranasal infections but must be treated with great caution as its complications tend to be more frequent and more severe. This stems from difficulty in diagnosing sphenoidal sinusitis and the lack of suitably aggressive therapies for this condition. Cocaine abuse has been suggested as a risk factor for sphenoidal sinusitis and subsequent brain abscess development [93]. Intracranial abscesses resulting from sphenoid sinusitis tend to occur in either the pituitary fossa or the temporal lobe.

Brain abscess is less likely to be related to periodontal infection than to middle ear or paranasal sinus infection. Periodontal infection is implicated in 6–13% of cases of brain abscess [94]. Organisms spread by either contiguous extension of the dental focus or by haematogenous seeding. Infection of a molar tooth is more likely to metastasize since it can spread between the muscles of mastication along fascial planes to the skull, most commonly to the frontal lobe, but temporal lobe abscesses can also occur by direct extension. Unlike abscesses that complicate otogenic infections, most odontogenic cranial abscesses occur as sequelae of acute rather than chronic infections [95].

Finally brain abscess is a rare complication of bacterial meningitis in adults; it is, however, commoner in infants, particularly those with gram negative meningitis. Cerebral abscesses have been associated with over 70% of cases of *Citrobacter diversus* in infants. On this basis it is arguable that all those from whom this organism is isolated from blood or CSF, should undergo neuroimaging to exclude an intracranial abscess.

Haematogenous spread

The metastatic spread from distant parts of the body frequently leads to development of brain abscesses. The most common sites of origin is a pyogenic lung infection, such as lung abscess, bronchiectasis, empyema, cystic fibrosis and acute endocarditis. Other potential primary foci include osteomyelitis, wound and skin infections, cholecystitis, pelvic infection and other forms of intra-abdominal sepsis. Irrespective of the focus of origin, haematogenous brain abscesses have certain features in common. Because their final location is based on the relative distribution of cerebral blood flow to various brain regions, most will occur in the frontal and parietal lobes, i.e. in middle cerebral artery territory. Furthermore, they usually form at the grey–white matter junction, where brain capillary flow is slowest; they tend to be less well encapsulated than those which have spread contiguously and are more frequently multifocal and multiloculated. Finally, metastatic abscesses are associated with a higher mortality rate, although this may be at least in part related to comorbid conditions. The formation of these abscesses appears to depend on the combination of bacteraemia and the presence of the appropriate environment. Areas of infection, ischaemia and contusion provide a fertile territory for bacterial seeding and abscess formation. Brain abscesses secondary to infective endocarditis are often accompanied by cardiovascular disease or microemboli, resulting in reduced tissue perfusion and oxygenation. In watershed zones with reduced collateral flow, stasis or sludging associated with hypercoagulable states or altered red blood cell rheology may also create an ideal environment for bacterial seeding.

Postoperative abscess

Factors that may increase the risk of a postoperative abscess include cranial bone flap infections, deep wound infections and CSF leak. If the cause of a postoperative abscess remains uncertain, this should raise suspicion of an unusual source of bacteraemia or a microscopic communication between the ears, mastoid or paranasal sinuses and the cranial vault.

Trauma

Brain abscess complicates approximately 3% of penetrating craniocerebral injuries, especially those caused by gunshot injuries. In general, metal fragments do not pose a significant risk for the development of an abscess and therefore tend not to be removed. Bone fragments, on the other hand, tend to require removal, as they have consistently been recognized as an important factor in brain abscess development. Several studies of penetrating head injuries (combat related) reveal a brain abscess incidence of 3–17% [96] with a mortality rate of 54% [97]. It should be noted that post-traumatic abscess development can be significantly delayed: a brain abscess due to *Clostridium bifermentans* occurred as a result of a metal fragment from a Vietnam war mortar that had been in place for 15 years [98]. In another case, a brain abscess formed 10 years after traumatic head injury with retained glass fragments [99].

Microbiology

The species of bacteria responsible for brain abscess depends on the pathogenic mechanism involved. Commonly isolated organisms are streptococci, including aerobic, anaerobic and microaerophilic types. These are found in 60–70% of non-traumatic brain abscesses and many, particularly *Streptococcus milleri* are part of the normal bacterial flora of the oral cavity, appendix and female genital tract. *Strep. pneumoniae* is a rarer cause of brain abscesses, which are often the sequel to occult CSF rhinorrhoea and also to pneumococcal pneumonia in elderly patients. Enteric bacteria and *Bacteroides* are isolated in 20–40% of cases and often in mixed culture. Anaerobic organisms have become increasingly important organisms and in many instances more than a single bacterial species is recovered. Gram-negative bacilli rarely occur alone. Staphylococcal abscesses account for 10–15% of cases and are usually caused by penetrating head injury or bacteraemia secondary to endocarditis. Clostridial infections are most often post-traumatic. Rarely *Actinomyces* or *Nocardia* are found to be the causative agent in a brain abscess. Actinomycotic abscess can occur secondary to distant infection particularly in the chest or oropharynx. *N. asteroides* is an unusual cause of brain abscesses which are often multiple, multilobular and thick walled. Almost invariably they are associated with pulmonary infection and are often seen in patients with defects in cell-mediated immunity.

Diagnosis

The clinical presentation, laboratory findings and neuroimaging all contribute useful diagnostic information. The clinical presentation of patients with brain abscess depends on the size, location and number of lesions, the virulence of the microorganism, the host response and the severity of cerebral oedema. No particular pattern of features is pathognomonic of brain abscess. Parenchymal destruction combined with oedema most often results in generalized signs of raised intracranial pressure and focal neurological deficit. The classical clinical triad of headache, fever and focal neurological deficit is present in fewer than 50% of patients with brain abscess. A constant progressive headache, which is refractory to treatment, is the most common symptom of brain abscess, occurring in 70–97% of patients [100]. The headache may be localized to the side of the abscess, but it is often generalized and increases in severity as the abscess expands. Abscesses that are adjacent to meningeal surfaces may provoke meningeal irritation.

Symptoms of acute infection can be lacking unless there is an active systemic focus of infection. Only around 50% of adult patients are febrile at time of diagnosis, and this is usually a low-grade fever [101]. In children fever occurs in up to 80%. High-grade temperature of up to 38.6C or more is less common and frequently indicates the presence of systemic infection or meningitis [102]. A reduced Glasgow Coma Score is seen in up to two-thirds of patients and ranges from mild confusion and drowsiness to coma [100]. A rela-

tively late event is papilloedema which is seen in approximately 50% of patients. Third and sixth cranial nerve palsy may likewise reflect raised intracranial pressure. In most large series, over 60% of patients present with focal neurological deficit [100]. In a recent analysis of the clinical features of 20 patients with streptococcal brain abscess, nine presented with hemiparesis [103]. All of these were supratentorial. Whilst the majority of supratentorial abscesses (especially parietal) tend to result in hemiparesis, those in temporal lobe cause varying degrees of dysphasia and visual field deficit. Cerebellar abscesses can lead to ataxia and nystagmus. Seizures occur in 30–80% of patients preoperatively in larger series, but are a clinical manifestation in only one of a series of 20 streptococcal brain abscesses analysed by Su *et al*. [103].

Occasionally, brain abscess may mimic a cerebrovascular event. Shintani *et al*. [104] reported a patient in whom sudden onset homonymous hemianopia was later found to be caused by bacterial brain abscess. Initial CT scan had suggested stroke, but later CT and MRI demonstrated an abscess and this was proved at surgery.

Adults with a normal immune response frequently show a rapid onset and progression of symptoms. Conversely, patients with immunodeficiency may have an insidious onset of symptoms, in which case a high index of suspicion is necessary to make an early diagnosis. Infants usually present with a combination of features such as bulging fontanelle, enlarging head circumference, cranial suture separation, seizures, irritability, nausea and vomiting.

Untreated, brain abscess is usually fulminant, ending in death in 5–15 days. If the initial picture is suggestive of a focal lesion and then rapid deterioration occurs with fever, headache and stiff neck, then rupture of an abscess into the intraventricular or subarachnoid space should be seriously considered. Abscess rupture is a true neurosurgical emergency; despite diagnostic and treatment advances, the mortality associated with intraventricular rupture has remained consistently high, exceeding 80% [104].

Laboratory diagnosis

Routine laboratory studies are of limited value in establishing a diagnosis of brain abscess. The peripheral white cell (WBC) count is frequently normal or only mildly elevated in up to 60–70% of patients [105]. Blood cultures are likely to be negative unless the abscess is associated with septic embolization from an intravascular endothelial infection, e.g. infective endocarditis or mycotic aneurysm. The erythrocyte sedimentation rate (ESR) is raised in approximately 90% of patients in whom it is measured but is a nonspecific indicator of inflammation. Serum C-reactive protein (CRP) has use in differentiating brain abscess from other intracranial mass lesions [106]. CRP levels were shown to return to normal after successful treatment in this study and persistently increased CRP correlated with incomplete treatment. Based on these observations, it was suggested that the return of the CRP to normal coupled with improved clinical condition and CT evidence of abscess resolution should be used as guidelines for early discontinuation of antibiotics. CSF studies are also non-specific. Opening pressure is usually high indicating increased intracranial pressure. There is generally a mild pleocytosis with WBC count of less than $100/cm^3$ unless there is concomitant meningitis [105]. However, in another study, one-third of patients with well-established abscesses had no evidence of pleocytosis. CSF protein is mildly elevated (usually below

100 mg/dL) and cultures are usually sterile, especially in patients on antibiotics. Given the limited use of CSF analysis and the presence of an intracranial mass, lumbar puncture should not usually be performed.

Radiological diagnosis

Advances in neuroimaging, particularly the routine use of CT scanning, have dramatically improved diagnosis and management of brain abscesses. More recently, MRI, magnetic resonance spectroscopy (MRS) and diffusion-weighted imaging (DWI) have emerged as useful tools in the evaluation of patients with suspected brain abscess.

Plain radiography

Skull X-ray is frequently normal in patients with brain abscess. Some plain films may demonstrate inflammatory disease of the paranasal sinuses and mastoid air cells, but these findings are better illustrated on CT. Intracranial air may be demonstrated radiographically especially in abscesses resulting from trauma. However, pneumocephalus most commonly indicates persisting extracranial communication and the need for surgery rather than local gas formation within an abscess by gas-forming organisms. Generally, plain skull films are not particularly helpful or cost-effective.

CT

CT allows early diagnosis, localization and staging of the abscess according to criteria developed by Enzmann *et al.* [107] who classified abscesses as cerebritis or capsule stage according to patterns of contrast enhancement. Furthermore, they showed that CT classification corresponds well with histopathological stage as confirmed at surgery or postmortem. They noted that the early and late cerebritis phase is characterized by a poorly defined area of low density on non-contrast scans, indicating development of the necrotic centre of the abscess. As the early capsule phase is reached, non-contrast scans demonstrate a faint ring of slightly higher density compared to the necrotic lucent centre and the surrounding oedematous brain. This ring correlates histologically with the developing collagen capsule. Use of corticosteroids significantly reduces peripheral enhancement during the cerebritis stage but has little effect on a mature encapsulated lesion [107]. The characteristic features of the capsule help distinguish ring enhancement due to abscess from that caused by neoplasm. Other features indicative of brain abscess include multiplicity, multiloculation and location at the corticomedullary junction. Ependymal or leptomeningeal enhancement also favours a diagnosis of brain abscess. With no history of penetrating head injury or craniotomy, the finding of gas within an intracranial lesion is highly suspicious of an abscess involving a gas-forming organism.

It is important to note that these CT findings are characteristic but not pathognomonic of brain abscess. The differential diagnosis of a ring-enhancing lesion is very broad, including entities such as malignant glioma, metastatic tumour, infarction, radiation necrosis and resolving haematoma. With an increasing population of

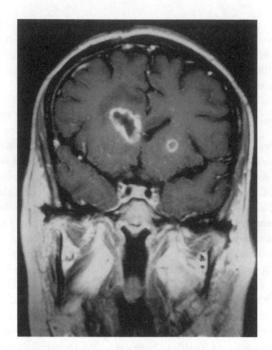

Fig. 62.4 *Aspergillus* abscesses in 38-year-old-immunocompromised man.

immunocompromised patients, there has been a corresponding increase in the number of abscesses caused by opportunistic infections. Parasites, fungi and atypical bacteria cause a variety of diseases such as brain abscess (Fig. 62.4), meningitis, meningoencephalitis and granuloma. Because of compromised host defence mechanisms, parenchymal infections may be poorly localized and may fail to become encapsulated [108].

MRI

MRI is a more powerful tool than CT for the identification of brain abscesses. It is now the gold standard, having greater sensitivity than CT and being capable of detecting brain abscesses in the earliest stages of development [109]. Some investigators have suggested that, even without the benefit of contrast enhancement, the MRI characteristics of brain abscess are specific enough to make an accurate diagnosis [110]. In addition, MRI can better demonstrate anatomical detail and multiple imaging planes. The MRI features of brain abscess, like CT features, are related to the pathological phase of the abscess. On T1-weighted images, a peripheral zone of mild hypointensity relative to adjacent brain is seen, representing oedema formation. This surrounds a core of more marked signal hypointensity, which equates to the necrotic centre of the abscess. Between these two regions is the capsule, which appears as a discrete rim that is isointense to mildly hyperintense. On T2-weighted images, the signal intensity of the oedematous region increases markedly compared with adjacent brain, while the centre is isointense to hyperintense compared with grey matter. The capsule has better definition and is seen as a hypointense rim at the margin of the abscess. Finally, one author has suggested that MRI is more specific than CT in differentiating oedema from liquefactive necrosis, which is valuable for planning the timing of aspiration [111].

MRS

MRS has emerged as a useful technique for the differentiation of brain abscess from neoplasm [112]. It is non-invasive and complements MRI. It can be added to routine MRI examinations with only minimal increase in cost and time [113]. *In vivo* MRS, when combined with MRI, can help to characterize cystic intracranial mass lesions [114]. Lesion specific spectral patterns may assist in tissue characterization, for example they permit differentiation of brain abscess from necrotic or cystic tumours [115]. Compounds seen in MRS spectra of abscesses are often absent from tumour spectra. Intracranial tumours demonstrate resonance lines from compounds such as lactate, choline and lipids, whereas abscesses demonstrate resonance lines from infection markers such as succinate, acetate and several amino acids derived from extracellular proteolysis or bacterial metabolism.

DWI

CT and/or MRI can sometimes be inconclusive in which case DWI can help clarify the diagnosis. Ebisu *et al.* [116] examined the diagnostic ability of DWI to differentiate brain abscess from necrotic or cystic tumours. In previous studies, necrotic or cystic tumours showed low signal intensity on DWI, indicating a high apparent diffusion coefficient (ADC). Ebisu *et al.*, in contrast, observed high signal intensity in the abscess fluid, associated with low ADC.

Surgical management

Until the early 1970s, surgery (aspiration, drainage, excision) was considered the method of choice in the management of brain abscess. Later evidence, however, suggested that selected patients, especially those in the early cerebritis stages could be managed successfully with antibiotics alone, plus careful monitoring and follow-up [117,118]. Heineman and Braude were the first to suggest that brain abscess can be treated successfully without surgery. They reported six patients with brain abscesses who were cured with antibiotics alone. Following this, several similar reports were published. Rousseaux *et al.* [117] reported a series of 31 patients with apparently well-encapsulated abscesses. Fifteen patients received antibiotics alone, four received antibiotics after aspiration and 12 underwent surgical excision followed by antibiotics. All had comparable neurological status on admission. The outcomes in medically treated patients were similar to those in patients who underwent either aspiration or excision and so the authors suggested that most abscesses can be managed successfully with antibiotics alone. However, closer scrutiny reveals diagnostic differences between the groups, which may have affected the results. Medically managed patients had smaller abscesses (average diameter 2.1 cm) compared to those managed by aspiration and excision (4.5 and 3.7 cm diameter, respectively). Also, almost half the patients managed with antibiotics alone had deep seated lesions that may not have been amenable to surgery. Rosenblum *et al.* [118] reviewed five large series concerning non-operative management of brain abscess, including that of Rousseaux *et al.* [117]. Overall success rate was 74%, with a mortality rate of 4% among 50 patients.

However, despite the apparent success of medical management,

there are pitfalls associated with this approach. Multiple antibiotics tend to be empirically prescribed to cover all possible causative organisms. This may unnecessarily commit the patient to long-term treatment with multiple agents when a single drug specific to the organism could suffice. Given the ease and safety with which many abscesses can be aspirated through a single burr hole, it would seem preferable to obtain cultures in most cases. Furthermore, in Rosenblum *et al.*'s study, it was found that no abscesses over 2.5 cm in diameter resolved without surgical intervention. Black *et al.* [119] found complete failure of antibiotic therapy alone for large abscesses despite adequate concentrations of antibiotics in the abscess cavity. Moreover, because other pathological entities can mimic brain abscess (e.g. primary or secondary tumours, infarction, resolving haematoma), aspiration provides confirmation of the diagnosis. This is of particular relevance to immunocompromised patients who may harbour opportunistic infections not responsive to conventional antibiotic therapy. Removal of purulent matter provides the additional benefits of immediate reduction in mass effect and intracranial pressure and a more favourable environment in which antibiotics can work (many antibiotics are rendered ineffective by the acidic milieu within an abscess cavity). Non-operative management without an attempt to culture abscess material directly therefore has a limited role, especially given that there are relatively few instances in which aspiration of a suspected abscess for culture is not feasible or possible. The only absolute contraindication to aspiration is a bleeding diathesis, but even in this situation, close involvement of a haematologist can allow stereotactic or even open procedures to be performed safely after appropriate factor replacement.

The optimal surgical management of brain abscess remains a subject of great controversy. Various procedures have been utilized, the most common being continuous tube drainage, stereotactic or open aspiration, marsupialization of the abscess and craniotomy with complete excision [120]. At present, drainage and marsupialization are rarely used; aspiration and excision are the mainstay of surgical treatment. There continues to be controversy regarding whether aspiration or excision represents optimal treatment. Whilst many surgeons have particular preferred methods, choice of one procedure over another may also be influenced by patient factors such as age, neurological and general condition, stage and type of abscess, and whether multiple lesions are present. Aspiration alone has led to excellent outcomes in several reports [121,122] and in combination with appropriate antibiotics is considered by many to be the procedure of choice [105]. The advantages of aspiration are that it can be performed quickly and safely through a single burr hole under local anaesthetic. Multiple lesions can frequently be aspirated through a single burr hole. In the majority of cases aspiration can confirm the diagnosis and provide culture material to deduce sensitivities. Large abscesses can be completely decompressed with minimal trauma and immediate reduction in mass effect and intracranial pressure. Accurate localization is possible with use of stereotactic CT- or MRI-guided imaging or real-time ultrasound (particularly useful for supratentorial lesions over 15 mm in diameter and in infants through an open fontanelle) [123]. CT-guided aspiration is useful in the management of deep-seated abscesses, multiple abscesses and abscesses situated in eloquent areas of the brain where excision would be inappropriate. Factors shown to be related to failure of this approach include inadequate aspiration, lack of catheter drainage of larger abscesses, chronic immunodeficiency and insufficient antibiotic therapy.

Direct instillation of antibiotics into the abscess cavity during aspiration has frequently been employed, but the benefits of this practice are ill-defined. There is as yet no direct evidence that this practice hastens abscess resolution, although it is argued to be a useful adjunct in cases of recurrent refractory abscesses. Instillation during the early cerebritis phase may be deleterious in that the irrigating fluid can promote spread of infection to surrounding tissues [119]. Also, high local concentrations of some antibiotics, notably the β-lactams, can cause seizures.

The most common complication of aspiration is intracranial haemorrhage. This seems to occur from the region of the developing collagen capsule, which is friable and vascular; haemorrhage is a more common event in patients with cyanotic congenital heart disease.

Whilst aspiration has clearly proved successful, some surgeons favour excision via formal craniotomy, especially for cerebellar abscesses. The main disadvantage is that it is inappropriate for lesions in the cerebritis phase, a time during which aspiration can be performed with relative ease. For deep abscesses and those located in eloquent regions, excision carries the serious risk of neurological deficit. Multiple lesions are not amenable to excision. However, in certain conditions abscess resection is the favoured option, such as retained foreign bodies from traumatic abscess (e.g. bone fragments) which may lead to recurrence if not removed [124]. Excision is more likely to result in cure in these cases. Patients with fungal abscesses may also require excision rather than aspiration—many fungi are resistant to conventional antibiotics and, as they tend to aggregate within the substance of the capsule, eradication can be difficult.

Some authors recommend that all gas-containing abscesses be excised on the basis that, although gas-forming bacteria can occasionally be responsible, the gas or air is more often an indication of a dural fistula. One study examined five patients in whom gas was found in the abscess cavity. All five were eventually found to have an extracranial communication which required repair [125].

Finally, multiloculated abscesses may be appropriate for excision owing to the difficulty in completely aspirating these lesions.

The role of surgery is slightly different in cases of multiple abscesses. These are most commonly encountered in patients with cyanotic heart disease and in those where the abscess results from haematogenous, metastatic spread. In one series the incidence was said to approach 50% [126] with a mortality of approximately 32%; failure to control intracranial and systemic infection being the main source of mortality. Because multiple abscesses tend to be smaller on average, the role of surgery is primarily diagnostic rather than curative—identification of the organism being the principal aim. Nevertheless, in patients who have one or more larger abscesses, surgery can still significantly reduce intracranial pressure and improve neurological function. In some patients with multiple abscesses, aspiration of pus can be a life-saving measure [126]. Multiple abscesses represent a potentially curable condition. Mamelak et al. [91] suggest that the combined approach of appropriate antibiotics, elimination of the primary septic focus and liberal use of CT to anticipate intracranial complications should yield cure rates of over

90%—a result comparable to that expected when treating patients with solitary lesions.

As an adjunct to surgery, corticosteroids have been used to attempt to reduce the cerebral oedema and mass effect that accompany an abscess. However, in some studies, steroids have been found to inhibit leukocyte migration and impair host defence mechanisms that help to contain the infection. In experimental animal models of brain abscess, the collagen capsule in dexamethasone-treated animals did not develop [127] or development was delayed [128]. In addition, corticosteroids appear to reduce the degree of contrast enhancement on CT scan, especially in the early cerebritis stage [129]. Therefore, in patients treated with steroids, reduction in contrast enhancement cannot be assumed to be evidence of abscess resolution. In these cases, a decrease in the ring diameter should be taken as the indicator of abscess regression. In most centres, steroids are currently used only in those patients in whom significant mass effect is thought to be responsible for neurological deficit. Steroid treatment should be continued until the neurological condition stabilizes and then tapered.

Despite the reported success with non-operative management as well as various forms of surgery, there is no consensus as to what constitutes optimal management of brain abscess. No strict protocols can be devised; each case must be treated individually, on its own merits, taking account of the factors described above.

Outcome

This will be described with particular reference to epilepsy. A full treatment of all potential complications and outcomes is beyond the scope of this chapter.

Despite the best efforts, even successfully treated brain abscesses can result in long-term neurological sequelae and morbidity [130,131]. Long-term morbidity is most frequently related to seizures, cognitive dysfunction and focal neurological deficit. Up to 50% of patients have permanent neurological deficit after brain abscess [132]. The single most important factor that influences mortality is the neurological condition of the patient at the time of diagnosis [105]. Patients who are alert with minimal deficits tend to have a good outcome. Mortality rates are much higher in patients who present in obtunded or comatose states. Delay in diagnosis and/or poor access to services are clearly pivotal factors in determining outcome.

The reported incidence of epilepsy following brain abscess is between 30% and 80% in most studies. One study [133] showed that late epilepsy developed in 51 of 70 observed patients (72%). All the patients who had seizures preoperatively went on to develop late epilepsy. The mean onset time of seizures for patients in this group was approximately 3.5 years after diagnosis, although this was age dependent. In the 20–40-year age group, seizures began on average 1.7 years after diagnosis compared with 4.4 years for patients below 20 years of age. In fact 50% of patients in the older group had their first seizure during the first year after diagnosis compared with only 20% in the younger group. Analysis of seizure frequency showed that the maximum frequency occurred during the fourth and fifth years postdiagnosis. This peak correlated well with the occurrence of epileptogenic EEG patterns [133].

Some reports suggest that the risk of developing late seizures is related to the location of the abscess. Nielsen et al. [131] found a higher incidence of seizures with frontal lobe abscesses. Others, however, reported no such relationship [133]. Significantly, some report a trend towards reduction in seizures among patients treated with aspiration as opposed to excision [105,134].

The majority of seizure disorders occurring after brain abscess are relatively well controlled with AEDs. For those that remain intractable to maximal medical therapy, seizure focus resection may be considered [105]. Given the high likelihood of development of seizures, all patients with supratentorial brain abscesses should routinely be placed on prophylactic AEDs to continue for 1–2 years as directed. They may then be tapered, providing that the EEG shows no epileptogenic activity.

Neurocysticercosis

Background

There is a voluminous literature on cysticercosis. Despite this, it is a disease that is unlikely to be familiar to most clinicians in the UK and Western Europe [135]. Worldwide, it is the most common parasitic disease of the CNS and a major cause of epilepsy and death in endemic areas such as Mexico, India and China [136]. Indeed, epilepsy is the commonest clinical manifestation and presenting feature of NCC [137]. With the exception of the south-west USA, it is very rare for it to present in industrialized nations [138]. Prevalence is highest in Latin America and South-East Asia, particularly in areas of poverty, poor hygiene and poor living conditions. It may also be endemic in sub-Saharan Africa, although few studies have been carried out [139]. Recent reports have confirmed that NCC is still a significant cause of epilepsy in Ecuador [140], Honduras [141], Brazil [142], Cuba [143], Colombia [144] and Peru [145]. A resurgence of cases of epileptic seizures associated with NCC has been reported in Indonesia [146]. Furthermore, it would appear that the disorder is now more frequently diagnosed in developed countries as a result of carriers travelling from countries where the disease is endemic [147]. All told, NCC causes enormous human and economic cost due to medical resources, AEDs and lost production. It has recently been proposed that NCC should be an internationally reportable disease [148]. New cases should be notified to health ministries in order that epidemiological interventions are set up to interrupt the chain of transmission. Accurate quantification of the incidence and prevalence of NCC at regional level permits the rational use of resources in eradication campaigns. As for most infectious diseases, tackling the underlying cause is paramount—prevention is the best form of treatment. Until this is possible, medical and surgical treatments must continue to develop.

NCC is a helminthiasis caused by the encysted larval stage, *Cysticercus cellulosae*, of the pork tapeworm *Taenia solium*. In the first stage, the human (definitive) host ingests undercooked diseased pork containing viable cysticerci from within which the scolex (head) of the organism evaginates in the gut and attaches to the intestinal mucosa. Over 3 months, the tapeworm matures to a length of 2–7 m. Gravid segments containing eggs are released into the faeces, often unknown to the host. Following ingestion, eggs hatch and activate in the pig (intermediate host) small intestine and develop in the CNS and striated muscle. When humans become intermediate hosts by accidental ingestion of eggs, the lifecycle is completed in a similar way in the CNS, skin and muscle [135]. Postmortem data

studies of expatriates from endemic zones have improved our knowledge of natural human infection. It is now known that parenchymal cysts usually lie dormant for many years and symptoms usually coincide with larval death and an intense inflammatory response caused by the release of larval antigens. The solitary parenchymal lesion is the most common form and seizures are the most common symptom in 70–90% of patients, but the lesions may be multiple and cause mass effect, hydrocephalus, basal arachnoiditis and cerebral infarction. The cysts tend to shrink, resulting in a granuloma which either calcifies or disappears completely [138]. This pattern of spontaneous resolution has important implications for the correct diagnosis and treatment of the disease.

Diagnosis

Thorough history and neurological examination may yield clues, but there is a wide variation in the clinical manifestation of NCC. Seizures are the commonest symptom and may occur when a cyst is degenerating or around a chronic, calcified lesion [137]. Other common presentations include symptoms of raised intracranial pressure. CSF in NCC usually shows mild abnormalities such as increased protein or pleocytosis; eosinophils are not always raised. EEG shows focal or generalized abnormality or no abnormality in NCC-associated epilepsy. A recent study of the interictal EEG of 50 patients with epilepsy and with CT/MRI and CSF evidence of NCC has shed more light on the use of EEG [149]. Twenty-two patients had parenchymal calcifications (inactive form), 21 had parenchymal cysts (active form) and seven had both. The EEG was normal in patients with inactive forms of NCC. It was abnormal in 50% of patients with active and mixed forms of NCC and in 48% of patients with active forms only. Thus, active forms of NCC should be suspected in the presence of an abnormal EEG. Furthermore, EEG abnormality was not seen to depend on the number of lesions but rather on the viability and location of the cysts and on host response.

Approximately 10–20% of patients present with ventricular cysts, accompanied by symptoms such as nausea and vomiting, headache, ataxia and confusion. Focal neurological deficits are uncommon. Basal cistern cysts can present with meningeal signs, hydrocephalus, vasculitis and stroke. Rarer neurological manifestations such as altered mental state, spinal NCC with radicular pain or paraesthesiae, cord compression, migraine headache, ophthalmic cysticercosis and neurocognitive deficits, have also been reported. Cysticercal encephalitis with multiple parenchymal inflammatory cysts and diffuse cerebral oedema has been described in young girls: such patients are at risk of severe neurological sequelae. Intracranial hypertension and meningeal NCC have been described, but with lower frequency in India [150]. Solitary enhancing CT lesions, on the other hand, are particularly common in India—why this is so remains unclear.

Cerebral tuberculoma is the main differential diagnosis, criteria for differentiation being set out by Rajshekar *et al.* [151]. In a series of histopathologically diagnosed cases, intracranial hypertension and progressive neurological deficit were not seen with NCC. NCC lesions were well circumscribed, less than 20 mm in size and not associated with midline shift. Tuberculomas are, by contrast, usually irregular, solid, greater than 20 mm in size and present with a progressive deficit. This distinction is very significant to management, since parenchymal cysticercosis is a benign and mostly self-limiting condition whereas a tuberculoma is an active infection that requires prolonged therapy with potentially toxic drugs.

Neuroimaging is crucial to diagnosis, CT being particularly useful for showing calcified inactive lesions; MRI is superior for demonstrating subarachnoid or intraventricular cysts and for showing inflammation around a cyst [152]. Cysts may be single or multiple and at different pathological stages at any given time. A classification system that corresponds to parasite viability has been proposed by Carpio et al. [153]: active, transitional and inactive. In the active stage (cyst asymptomatic) the CT appearance is that of a rounded, hypodense area or there may be a CSF-like signal on MRI. The 'starry night' effect—the presence of multiple eccentric mural nodules—is characteristic of NCC, although it may also be seen in cases of Toxoplasma infection. The transitional stage is due to cystic degeneration. This appears on CT as a diffuse hypodense area with an irregular border which enhances with contrast. They appear as low signal areas on T2-weighted MRI. Lastly, with the death of the cyst, it either disappears or becomes a calcified inactive nodule of low intensity on proton-weighted MRI or homogenous high density on CT scan.

Standard enzyme-linked immunosorbent assay (ELISA) diagnostic techniques have proved less useful than hoped because of high false negative and false positive rates. Newer enzyme-linked immunoelectron transfer blot (EITB) assays on CSF or serum appear to have higher sensitivity (98%) and specificity (100%) in Latin American samples [154] but are less accurate for solitary enhancing CT lesions in India [155], Ecuador [156] and Honduras [140]. Its superiority to ELISA is due to its ability to detect up to seven glycoproteins specific to T. solium. It is visualized like a western blot, so that non-specific bands can be ignored thereby ruling out crossreactivity. Recently, an antigen detection ('capture') assay specific for viable metacestodes in CSF has been designed [157]. So far, this has proved to be perhaps the most reliable method of detecting active cases of NCC in epidemiological studies. Unfortunately, immunodiagnostic kits are difficult to obtain in endemic countries where they are most needed, so the use of special assays has thus far been restricted to research studies.

A satisfactory international diagnostic protocol has yet to be agreed upon [158], although this was addressed recently by a panel led by Del Brutto et al. [159] who have summarized diagnostic criteria and degrees of diagnostic certainty (Tables 62.2, 62.3). Criteria are divided into categories based on the weight attached to each feature, absolute, major, minor or epidemiological. Data interpretation allows the calculation of three degrees of diagnostic certainty—definitive, probable and possible. Since spontaneous cyst resolution is typical of NCC, it has been suggested by another group that this is also included as a minor criterion [135].

The most effective approach to NCC infection is prevention and this should be a primary public health focus for all developing countries [153].

With the advent of modern neuroimaging, the natural history and true prevalence of this disease is being realized. Once these small enhancing lesions are identified, the main concern is that they might represent malignancy. This is why stereotactic biopsy or excision may initially be advocated unless consideration is given to the possibility of other conditions, such as cerebral tuberculoma, bacterial abscess, hydatid cyst, toxoplasmosis, mycotic granuloma, sar-

Table 62.2 Diagnostic criteria

Absolute
Histological demonstration of parasite
Fundoscopic visualization of parasite
Cystic lesions with scolex on CT or MRI

Major
Lesions suggestive of neurocysticercosis on CT or MRI
Positive anticysticercal antibodies in serum or CSF
Calcifications on plain X-rays of thigh

Minor
Subcutaneous nodules
Clinical manifestations suggestive of cysticercosis
Disappearance of brain lesions with anticysticercal therapy

Epidemiological
Immigration from or living in endemic area
Travel to endemic area
Household contact with T. solium infection

After [159].

Table 62.3 Degrees of certainty for diagnosis

Definitive diagnosis
One absolute criterion
Two major criteria
One major, two minor and one epidemiological criteria

Probable diagnosis
One major and two minor criteria
One major, one minor and one epidemiological criteria
Three minor and one epidemiological criteria

Possible diagnosis
One major criterion
Two minor criteria
One minor and one epidemiological criteria

After [159].

coidosis or larva migrans. If one of the above can be diagnosed on the strength of clinical, radiological and laboratory findings, medical treatment should be initiated and biopsy only considered if the patient fails to respond. Likewise, if malignancy is unlikely and there is high index of suspicion or diagnosis of NCC, medical therapy should be commenced straight away. The mainstay of treatment in this patient group during observation has been control of seizures with AEDs. Seizures caused by a single cysticercus are usually very well controlled. Two anticysticercal drugs are in wide use in endemic areas—albendazole and praziquantel—although no controlled trials exist that establish specific indications, definitive doses and treatment duration. It is not general policy to use these drugs with single lesions since the enhancing cysticerci shown on imaging are by definition dying away and will resolve spontaneously [138].

The management of NCC depends upon cyst location, magnitude of cyst burden, the degree of neurological impairment, viability of the cysticerci and the extent of the immune response [160]. Treatment in individual cases is based on the anatomical form of the disease (parenchymal, subarachnoid, intraventricular, ocular or spinal). Mixed forms of NCC constitute more than 50% of cases. Therapy for mixed forms should address the most serious or life-threatening type first. These forms include hydrocephalus (of any mechanism), subarachnoid or intraventricular NCC with chronic meningitis, cysticercal encephalitis, spinal NCC with myelopathy and raised intracranial pressure. They have been designated 'malignant' as this reflects their high morbidity and mortality. Benign forms of NCC include parenchymal cysts or calcifications without associated hydrocephalus and chronic meningitis. Surgical excision is occasionally indicated for large solitary parenchymal cysts that exert local mass effect or cause raised intracranial pressure or both [161]. It is also indicated in cases of focal, medically intractable epilepsy which can be localized on EEG to a parenchymal cyst or granuloma. Cysticidal therapy alone could potentially lead to herniation or permanent neurological injury to eloquent cortex.

Giant convexity subarachnoid cysts have been treated surgically since they were often misdiagnosed as arachnoid cysts or subdural haemorrhages on CT scans. Surgical intervention has been advocated for subarachnoid cysts because of the poor CSF penetration of praziquantel and its lack of effect on these cysts [162]. Since 1990, reports have appeared of successful treatment of subarachnoid cysts with albendazole [163]. Although surgery may still be indicated for subarachnoid cysts refractory to albendazole, anticysticercal therapy is now clearly the initial treatment of choice. However, this rule does not apply in certain anatomical situations. For example, cysts in the parasellar region excite an intense inflammatory response when treated with cysticidal drugs and in some cases this will lead to optichiasmatic arachnoiditis and endarteritis with occlusion of the supraclinoid internal carotid artery. Surgery may be preferable to medical treatment for cysts in this territory. Similarly, surgical resection may be preferred for removal of large racemose cysts in the Sylvian fissure for prevention of endarteritis and middle cerebral artery occlusion [164]. A large cerebellopontine cyst causing brainstem compression would be a further situation in which surgery would be indicated prior to anticysticercal treatment.

Surgical resection has been suggested as the treatment of choice for intraventricular lesions by several authors [165]. This was based on evidence from cases of sudden death related to CSF obstruction. Although standard open procedures provide acceptable access to most cysts, recent advances in neuroendoscopy (ventriculoscopy) have made removal of freely mobile, lateral and third ventricle cysts popular and even preferable to open craniotomy [166]. For fourth ventricle cysts, treatment of hydrocephalus is clearly the first priority [165]. The next decision is whether to surgically resect the cyst or to treat it with cysticidal drugs. Cyst excision may be warranted because of the potential for acute clinical deterioration due to cyst expansion with brainstem compression, cyst migration and formation of granular ependymitis requiring permanent ventriculoperitoneal shunt placement. Two surgical series of 27 and 21 patients with fourth ventricular cysts showed good or excellent initial clinical outcomes in 81% and 71% of patients, respectively. The morbidity in these two series was 15% and 26%, respectively [167,168].

A study of 10 patients with combined praziquantel and albendazole treatment showed complete disappearance of 80% of fourth ventricular cysts by MRI. Of the other two cysts, one decreased significantly in size and the other remained unchanged. Six out of the 10 patients presented with hydrocephalus and underwent shunting

before anticysticercal therapy. This drug combination, therefore, may obviate the need for surgical excision of most fourth ventricle cysts in the future [169]. However, studies on the effectiveness of albendazole on lateral ventricle cysts are yet to be carried out.

A paper describing the experience of eight patients with NCC in the UK has demonstrated the value of a general conservative approach to treatment [135] and the development of a useful management protocol in part based on the diagnostic criteria of Del Brutto et al. [159]. Seven of these patients presented with epilepsy and single or multiple small enhancing parenchymal lesions and one with hydrocephalus caused by a midbrain lesion. One lesion was stereotactically excised after it had persisted but in five other cases spontaneous cyst resolution was observed during expectant management with AEDs. Two patients with multiple lesions were free of active infection. The authors' view was that small cortical granulomas such as those in their series should not be biopsied or removed since the parasite is dying and will disappear spontaneously. This view is corroborated by other authors [151,159]. A conservative approach is also beneficial in that stereotactic biopsy may be complicated by the toughness and mobility of the cysticercus and hazardous owing to the usual site of lesions at the grey–white matter junction with the subsequent risk of haemorrhage [170]. In the unlikely event of a cyst enlarging or causing increasing neurological deficit, treatment with anticysticercal therapy should be initiated in the first instance. If the diagnosis is definite and if the lesion remains refractory to treatment, then surgery is inevitable [135]. In all cases in the series of eight described by Wadley et al. a definitive diagnosis was made as per the diagnostic criteria outlined in Tables 62.2 and 62.3. During the course of treatment and observation of these patients, a coherent management strategy for patients presenting with epilepsy was produced (Fig. 62.5). It is recommended that for patients with a definitive or probable diagnosis after investigation, management should be expectant with AEDs alone and imaging should be repeated at 8–10 weeks. Stereotactic or image-guided excision should be reserved for lesions that enlarge or persist despite additional anticysticercal treatment or when there is diagnostic uncertainty. Indeed, correct differential diagnosis with other ring-enhancing lesions is crucial to avoid mistaken biopsy or excision of lesions thought to be tuberculoma or malignant. This conservative approach is corroborated by other authors. Proano et al. recently described their treatment of 33 patients with large subarachnoid cysticercal cysts, for whom the usual recommendation would be surgical treatment. All of the patients in this series improved with albendazole and dexamethasone at 59-month follow-up. In most patients, improvement was rapid after the initiation of treatment [169]. Reports such as these may change the standard of care for patients with NCC. NCC with a solitary or small number of cerebral lesions is a self-limiting infestation with a pattern of spontaneous resolution. Unnecessary surgery or therapy with potentially toxic drugs should be avoided.

Cerebral tuberculoma

Background

Tuberculosis remains a major problem in developing countries; the incidence is rising in many industrialized countries with increasing migration and spread of human immunodeficiency virus (HIV).

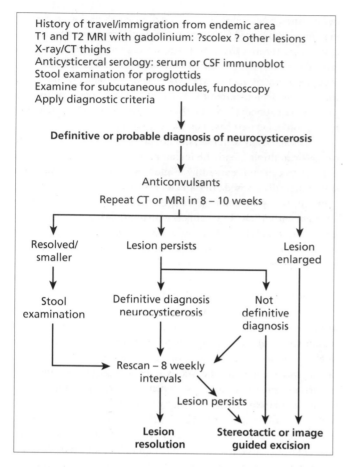

History of travel/immigration from endemic area
T1 and T2 MRI with gadolinium: ?scolex ? other lesions
X-ray/CT thighs
Anticysticercal serology: serum or CSF immunoblot
Stool examination for proglottids
Examine for subcutaneous nodules, fundoscopy
Apply diagnostic criteria

↓

Definitive or probable diagnosis of neurocysticerosis

↓

Anticonvulsants
Repeat CT or MRI in 8 – 10 weeks

| Resolved/ smaller | Lesion persists | Lesion enlarged |

Stool examination

Definitive diagnosis neurocysticerosis

Not definitive diagnosis

Rescan – 8 weekly intervals

Lesion persists

Lesion resolution

Stereotactic or image guided excision

Fig. 62.5 Management protocol of a patient presenting with epilepsy and small enhancing lesion(s).

While the most common form of tuberculosis is pulmonary infection, one of the most serious forms is that affecting the CNS. However, the incidence of intracranial tuberculoma (tuberculous abscess) has decreased, particularly in Western countries, and CNS involvement is less frequent than in countries where TB is endemic. This is mainly due to the BCG vaccination programme. In an autopsy study of intracranial space-occupying lesions (SOLs) conducted early in the 20th century, Garland and Armitage found that tuberculomas represented 34% of all the SOLs [171]. In 1940, tuberculomas were said to account for 3.6% of 2190 brain tumours [172]. In 1959, a study by Obrador [173] showed that cerebral tuberculoma was a common lesion, accounting for 20–40% of all intracranial masses. In 1972, the incidence was put at 0.15% of 2200 intracranial masses [174]. In 1987, a study in Saudi Arabia showed that tuberculoma constitutes approximately 5% of intracranial SOLs [175] and a further report in 1993 estimated that cerebral tuberculoma in children constitutes 5–10% of intracranial SOLs in developing countries [176]. Reports of brain tuberculoma have appeared in the West among immigrants [177] and patients with acquired immune deficiency syndrome (AIDS) [178]. In a recent study of 455 HIV cases in India, 23 patients had new onset seizures and 13% of these were caused by cerebral tuberculoma [2]. Gulati *et al.* in 1991 studied 170 Indian children with chronic seizures and a high index of suspicion of an underlying SOL. MRI indicated tuberculoma in 64 of them [179]. A study by Rebai *et al.* over 16 years

examined 1015 cases of intracranial SOLs. Twenty-four of these (2.4%) were found to be tuberculomas [180]. Because of their rarity, tuberculomas are not always considered in the differential diagnosis of intracranial SOLs. Furthermore, the exact pathophysiology is still not clear, partly because of the impossibility of reproducing tuberculoma in animals.

Tuberculous abscesses form with infection of the brain parenchyma. Tuberculomas are typically firm, lobulated masses of granulomatous inflammation with central caseous necrosis up to several centimetres in diameter and walled off by fibrous tissue. Lesions can occur within the cerebellum but are most common in the cerebral hemispheres [180].

Diagnosis

The diagnosis of intracranial tuberculoma should rest on the proper integration of data from clinical manifestations, CSF analysis and neuroimaging studies [181]. The tuberculoma should be distinguished from infection of the leptomeninges, although the two may sometimes coexist and rupture of a parenchymal lesion into the CSF has been implicated in the initiation of tuberculous meningitis [182].

The two main structural imaging modalities used for diagnosis and identification of potential candidates for resective surgery are CT and MRI. These modalities were directly compared in a study of six patients [181]. While both CT and MRI were equally sensitive in visualizing the intracranial tuberculoma in every patient, MRI was superior in demonstrating the extent and maturity of the lesion, especially for brainstem lesions. Nevertheless, the diagnostic role for MRI in intracranial tuberculomas is limited for two reasons. Firstly, other infections or neoplastic lesions may present with similar findings. Secondly, the availability of MRI in developing countries is very limited. In this scenario, CT remains the radiological investigation of choice in lesional syndromes. The identification of a 'target lesion' in an enhanced CT scan is considered to be characteristic of tuberculoma, although this sign may also be produced by cerebral toxoplasmosis. The difficulty of distinguishing NCC from tuberculoma has been mentioned; the criteria for differentiation using CT were described by Rajshekar *et al.* [151]. This difficulty has again been highlighted recently by Garg *et al.* [183] who describe an NCC-like presentation in a case of CNS tuberculosis in India. Here, a clinical picture of seizures, multiple non-tender subcutaneous nodules and multiple ring-enhancing lesions on brain CT was seen in a patient in an area endemic for NCC. Serological tests and histopathology established tuberculosis as the cause.

Diagnosis is further made difficult by the fact that many patients with tuberculoma have no preceding history of tuberculosis infection. In the series of Rebai *et al.* only 29% of patients with tuberculoma had a history of tuberculous infection (although bacterial examination is not conclusive even if negative). In areas where tuberculosis is endemic, the value of this factor as a diagnostic indicator further declines.

The finding of tuberculoma in the brain is rare—its location in the cavernous sinus is exceptional. Only four cases have been described [180,184–186]. In the latter case of a 44-year-old female with persistent headache and right cavernous sinus syndrome, this was a solitary lesion initially mimicking a meningioma. Although solitary lesions are generally more common, the diagnosis has been stated to be easier in cases with numerous intracerebral lesions. Boucetta *et al.* reported solitary lesions in 84% of their patients [187] and 19% of the patients in the series by Rodat *et al.* had multiple tuberculomas [188]. In such a case, with location in the cavernous sinus, no sign of extracerebral tuberculosis, a solitary brain lesion, negative laboratory examination, non-specific imaging and negative angiography, confirmation of the diagnosis by surgical exploration and biopsy is clearly warranted, so that antituberculous therapy may be started. In this case, the results were favourable and the lesion regressed.

Management

Management of tuberculomas in the past was mainly surgical but medical treatment has been emphasized more recently [189]. Identified lesions may, however, require exploration or resective surgery for pathological verification to allow antituberculous chemotherapy to be initiated or because of intractable epilepsy. Surgery is still indicated for larger, symptomatic mass lesions causing midline shift and severe intracranial hypertension, especially considering the increasing numbers of reports describing paradoxical expansion of intracranial tuberculomas during chemotherapy [190]. Decision to refer for surgery must be taken with care. Prolonged polypharmacy with AEDs is not required to define intractability of seizures and may lead to toxicity. Although a period of up to 2 years medical coverage is deemed suitable prior to consideration of epilepsy surgery, occasional debilitating seizures may warrant much earlier referral and the patient's psychological state must be taken into account in this respect. Delay in definitive treatment can indeed be devastating. In one case [194], rupture of the parenchymal lesion into the CSF led to the fulminating and fatal intracranial spread of the tuberculosis. However, lesions involving eloquent or functional cortical areas are likely to lead to increased neurological morbidity and it may be prudent in such cases to defer surgical referral. It has been argued that, if diagnosis is considered probable, a trial of antituberculous therapy should be begun without biopsy confirmation [167]. Others [190] favour early open brain biopsy as soon as intracranial tuberculoma is suspected, especially in more rapidly progressing cases. Certainly, primary medical treatment with frequent monitoring is reserved for lesions in the pons and brainstem or for multiple forms that are impossible to approach surgically. Cerebral tuberculomas with coexistant extracranial disease should also have primary medical treatment. Cerebral tuberculomas tend to decrease in size within 8 weeks of medical therapy and this is accompanied by improved neurological status. Diagnosis should be reviewed if the anticipated improvement in clinical and CT picture is not forthcoming [175]. Furthermore, one should avoid the use of corticosteroids during the therapeutic trial as regression of an underlying lymphoma can be misinterpreted as a favourable response to antituberculous chemotherapy [191]. With early diagnosis and a balanced combination of surgical and medical management, tuberculomas must be viewed as potentially curable.

Hydatid disease

Background

Echinococcus is a parasitic disease endemic to Eastern Europe, the Middle East, Argentina, Chile, Uruguay, South Africa, Australia and New Zealand, although its distribution is worldwide. Hydatid or 'drop of water' is a term which describes the fluid-filled cysts created by the parasite. The canine tapeworm *E. granulosus* accounts for the majority of hydatid disease and tends to cause cystic brain lesions. *E. multilocularis* is a rarer cause of hydatid disease which produces alveolar brain lesions. Domesticated dogs are the definitive hosts for the parasite and acquire the tapeworm when ingesting parasite-infested viscera of sheep and cattle (which function as intermediate hosts). The adult worm resides in the intestinal villi and has a lifespan of approximately 6 months. Sheep typically become intermediate hosts by ingesting parasite ova discharged in dog faeces harbouring the adult tapeworm. Humans interrupt the cycle and become intermediate hosts by ingesting parasite ova excreted in the faeces of dogs carrying the intestinal tapeworm. On ingestion of the parasitic ova, larvae are released and penetrate the intestinal mucosa. Haematogenous dissemination leads to the formation of brain and spinal cord cysts which constitute 2–3% of all hydatid cysts [192].

Two different histological types of cerebral hydatid cyst have been described: embryonal (primary) and scolical (metastatic or secondary) [193]. Primary cerebral hydatidosis is caused by embryos that escape filtration by the liver, lungs or heart and become implanted in the brain parenchyma. Due to their embryonal origin, primary cysts are usually fertile since they contain many scolices. Primary cysts are almost always solitary, reports of multiple primary cerebral hydatid cysts being very rare [194]. In contrast, secondary or metastatic cerebral hydatid cysts originate from infertile scolices of ruptured fertile cysts and therefore are usually infertile. Cerebral cysts have a variable rate of growth (1–5 cm/year) but may expand relatively quickly due to the immunological quiescence of the brain and a scant fibroblastic response. Cystic expansion may lead to compression and sometimes necrosis of surrounding tissues. In a series of 120 patients 6% of the cysts measured between 6 and 10 cm in diameter and six cysts measured more than 20 cm [193].

Diagnosis

A thorough history, clinical manifestations, laboratory and neuroimaging investigations are crucial to making a correct diagnosis. Cerebral hydatid cysts can occur at any age, but are most common in children. In a recent series of 155 cases, 117 were children, with a mean age of 7.2 years and a slight male predominance [195]. The commonest mode of presentation in children is with symptoms and signs of raised intracranial pressure. In adults, focal motor deficits are the most common presenting clinical feature with signs and symptoms of raised intracranial pressure usually occurring later in the course of the disease. The presenting symptoms and signs in reducing order of frequency in a group of 120 patients with cerebral hydatid disease were: headache (80%), papilloedema (74%), emesis (70%), hemiparesis (60%), facial paresis (42%), cerebellar dysfunction (42%), hemianopsia (40%), seizures (36%), reduced visual acuity (35%), ataxia (20%), somnolence (20%) and speech disturbance (15%) [193].

Laboratory tests are not particularly helpful in establishing the diagnosis, although serological tests can be useful. ELISA, latex fixation and haemagglutination are acceptably sensitive and specific, but all are limited by crossreactivity with *T. solium* and alone are not sufficient to establish the diagnosis [196]. IgG ELISA, however, is useful as it has a sensitivity of up to 94% and a specificity of up to 99%. The most important test in the diagnostic evaluation of patients with echinococcosis is CT. The classic CT appearance of a cerebral hydatid cyst is a large rounded intraparenchymal lesion with a well-circumscribed border containing fluid with a density equivalent to or slightly greater than CSF [197]. Lack of rim enhancement, absence of perilesional oedema and, occasionally, calcification of the cyst rim are seen. These appearances are, however, not pathognomonic. Studies have shown significant variability in CT and MRI features of these cysts, such as irregularity in shape and contour of the cyst wall, cyst contents isodense to brain, heterogeneity of cyst fluid density, enhancement of the rim, surrounding brain oedema and globular calcification of the cyst margin [198].

Differential diagnosis should include NCC, arachnoid cysts, cerebral abscess and cystic tumours such as metastasis, haemangioblastoma and gliomas. Features distinguishing NCC from hydatid cyst include size of the lesion and the presence of calcifications. Most parenchymal cysts of NCC are less than 2 cm in diameter whereas hydatid cysts are usually much larger. Calcified parenchymal granulomas are seen in 58% of NCC patients, whereas calcification of the cyst rim is seen in fewer than 20% of hydatid cyst cases [193]. Brain abscesses and many neoplasms may produce perilesional oedema and also demonstrate significant contrast enhancement. A recent case report of solid cerebral *Echinococcus* mimicking primary brain tumour has been described. A 35-year-old female presented with tonic-clonic seizures due to a right-sided frontal partially cystic SOL. Preoperative CT and MRI were suggestive of cystic astrocytoma. However, histological examination yielded a diagnosis of 'chitinoma', a very rare subtype of solid cerebral hydatid disease. This mimicking of primary brain tumour poses diagnostic and therefore management difficulties [199]. However, arachnoid cysts are probably the most difficult lesions to differentiate from hydatid cysts; arachnoid cysts typically are less spherical than hydatid cysts, but this is not always the case.

Management

Establishment of the preoperative diagnosis is crucial as this guides surgical technique. Resective surgery remains the primary treatment of the disease. The standard surgical technique used for excision of large tumours containing cysts, i.e. aspiration and deflation of the cyst before resection of the tumour itself, is contraindicated. This practice risks turning a potentially curable condition into a chronic ongoing disease characterized by repetitive cyst recurrence. This is because the outer layer of the cyst is easily ruptured unless a very delicate surgical technique is used. If the primary cyst ruptures, the enclosed protoscolices spill into the surrounding parenchyma and each protoscolex is able to transform into a secondary cyst. Most hydatid cysts are located at the grey–white matter junction as a result of haematogenous spread, typically in the distribution of the middle cerebral arteries. However, deep brain or intraventricular lesions are virtually impossible to resect without them rupturing. One accepted method of cyst removal is the Dowling technique [192]. Rather than using sharp dissection, this method relies on gravity to deliver the cyst from the surrounding brain. The patient is positioned on the operating table such that the cyst is in a dependent position. A large bone and dural flap are reflected and a cortical in-

cision is made over the thinnest area overlying the cyst. Saline irrigation is used to dissect a tissue plane between the cyst and surrounding parenchyma. If the lesion is deep to the cortical surface and complete resection is not feasible, careful cyst aspiration is recommended, with hypertonic saline or silver nitrate solution used to destroy protoscolices [192].

The antihelminthic drug albendazole is effective in the treatment of cerebral forms of *Echinococcus* [200]. Indeed, its success in a limited number of these patients suggests that it may eventually be preferred to surgery in certain clinical settings. Albendazole can achieve cyst concentrations of up to 40% of serum concentrations, causing disruption of the cyst wall and death of the protoscolices. It could be used adjunctively to shrink large superficial cortical cysts, as this would facilitate removal and reduce risk of rupture during resective surgery. Furthermore, albendazole prevents the formation of secondary cysts in case of inadvertent rupture. For cysts in eloquent brain or those in deep areas, the risks of surgery may be substantial. In such cases, albendazole alone may be able to resolve the cyst and obviate the need for surgery. It is also useful in the treatment of secondary cysts that recur after surgery at the original site. Hepatotoxicity is a major limitation of albendazole use and hepatic enzyme levels must be monitored closely. Surgery remains the best option for large lesions. It produces immediate clinical improvement compared with drug therapy where cyst resolution may take several months or even years.

Cyst rupture during attempted resection significantly affects prognosis. This is because the cyst contents are highly antigenic and rupture may lead to severe anaphylaxis with circulatory shock and death [201,202]. In a 1992 study, 10 (24%) of 41 patients in whom cyst rupture occurred during surgery died within 36 days of surgery. However, no deaths occurred among the 79 patients without cyst rupture.

Cyst rupture has also been seen to occur spontaneously in some patients. A rapid clinical deterioration is seen and severe pericystic oedema is seen on CT. This is a surgical emergency: removal of cyst contents must be carried out immediately, with copious saline irrigation and administration of antihelminthic drugs.

References

1 Gonzalez AE, Gavidia C, Falcon N et al. Protection of pigs with cysticercosis from further infection after treatment with oxfendazole. Am J Trop Med Hyg 2001; 65: 15–18.
2 Singhvi JP, Sawhney IM, Lal V et al. Profile of intractable epilepsy in a tertiary referral centre. Neurol India 2000; 48 (4): 351–6.
3 Pal DK, Carpio A, Sander JWAS. Neurocysticercosis and epilepsy in developing countries. J Neurol Neurosurg Psychiatr 2000; 68: 137–43.
4 Sander JW, Shorvon SD. Epidemiology of the epilepsies. J Neurol Neurosurg Psychiatr 1996; 61: 433–43.
5 Cascino GD. Intractable partial epilepsy: evaluation and treatment. Mayo Clin Proc 1990; 65: 1578–86.
6 Kuzniecky RI, Cascino GD, Palmini A et al. Structural neuroimaging. In Engel J Jr, ed. Surgical Treatment of the Epilepsies. New York: Raven Press, 1993: 197–209.
7 Boon PA, Williamson PD, Fried I et al. Intracranial, intraaxial, space occupying lesions in patients with intractable partial seizures: anotomoclinical neuropsychological and surgical correlation. Epilepsia 1991; 32: 467–76.
8 Guidetti B, Delitala A. Intracranial arteriovenous malformations: Conservative and surgical treatment. J Neurosurg 1980; 53: 149–52.

9 Forster DM, Steiner L, Hakanson S. Arteriovenous malformations of the brain: A long-term clinical study. *J Neurosurg* 1972; 37: 562–70.

10 Troupp H, Marttila I, Halonen V. Arteriovenous malformations. *Acta Neurochir* 1970; 22: 125–8.

11 Abad JM, Alvarez F, Manrique M, Garcia-Blazquez M. Cerebral arteriovenous malformations. Comparative results of surgical vs. conservative treatment in 112 cases. *J Neurosurg Sci* 1983; 27: 203–10.

12 Moody R, Poppen JL. Arteriovenous malformations. *J Neurosurg* 1970; 32: 503–11.

13 Fults D, Kelly D. Natural history of arteriovenous malformations of the brain: a clinical study. *Neurosurgery* 1984; 5(15): 658–62.

14 Perret G, Nishioka H. Arteriovenous malformations: an analysis of 545 cases of cranio-cerebral arteriovenous malformations and fistulae reported to the Cooperative Study. *J Neurosurg* 1966; 25: 467–90.

15 Murphy MJ. Long-term follow-up of seizures associated with cerebral arteriovenous malformation. Results of therapy. *Acta Neurol* 1985; 42: 477–9.

16 Leblanc R, Feindelm W, Ethier R. Epilepsy from cerebral arteriovenous malformations. *Can J Neurol Sci* 1983; 10: 91–5.

17 Drake CG. Cerebral AVMs: considerations for and experience with surgical treatment in 166 cases. *Clin Neurosurg* 1979; 26: 145–208.

18 Pool JL. Treatment of arteriovenous malformations of the cerebral hemispheres. *J Neurosurg* 1962; 19: 136–41.

19 Crawford PM, West CR, Chadwick DW *et al*. AVM of the brain natural history in unoperated patients. *J Neurol Neurosurg Psychiatr* 1986; 49: 1–10.

20 Spetzler RF, Hargraves RW, McCormick PW *et al*. Relationship of perfusion pressure and size to risk of haemorrhage from arteriovenous malformations. *J Neurosurg* 1992; 76: 918–23.

21 Crawford PM, West CR, Shaw MDM *et al*. Cerebral arteriovenous malformations and epilepsy: factors in the development of epilepsy. *Epilepsia* 1986; 27(3): 270–5.

22 Foy PM, Copeland GP, Shaw MDM. The incidence of post-operative seizures. *Acta Neurosurg* 1981; 55: 253–64.

23 Trumpy JH, Eldevik P. Intracranial arteriovenous malformations: Conservative or surgical management? *Surg Neurol* 1977; 8: 171–5.

24 McCormick WF. The pathology of vascular ('arteriovenous') malformations. *J Neurosurg* 1966; 24: 807–16.

25 Takashima S, Becker LE. Neuropathology of cerebral arteriovenous malformations in children. *J Neurol Neurosurg Psychiatr* 1980; 43: 380–5.

26 Kondziolka D, McLaughlin MR, Kestle JRW. Simple risk predictions for arteriovenous malformation hemorrhage. *Neurosurgery* 1995; 37: 851–5.

27 Ondra SL, Troupp H, George ED *et al*. The natural history of symptomatic arteriovenous malformations of the brain. A 24-year follow-up assessment. *J Neurosurg* 1990; 73: 387–91.

28 Luessenhop AJ, Rosa L. Cerebral arteriovenous malformations: Indications for and results of surgery, and the role of intravascular techniques. *J Neurosurg* 1985; 60: 14–22.

29 Laing RW, Childs J, Brada M. Failure of conventionally fractionated radiotherapy to decrease the risk of haemorrhage in inoperable arteriovenous malformations. *Neurosurgery* 1992; 30: 872–6.

30 Redekop GJ, Elisevich KV, Gaspar LE *et al*. Conventional radiation therapy of intracranial arteriovenous malformations: long-term results. *J Neurosurg* 1993; 78: 413–22.

31 Poulsen MG. Arteriovenous malformations: A summary of 6 cases treated with radiation therapy. *Int J Radiation Oncol Biol Phys* 1987; 13: 1553–7.

32 Kjellberg RN, Hanamura T, Davis KR *et al*. Bragg-Peak proton-beam therapy for arterio-venous malformations of the brain. *N Engl J Med* 1983; 309: 269–74.

33 Saunders WM, Winston KR, Siddon RL *et al*. Radiosurgery for arteriovenous malformations of the brain using a standard linear accelerator: rationale and technique. *Int J Radiation Oncol Bio Phys* 1988; 13: 441–7.

34 Steinberg GK, Fabrikant JI, Marks MP *et al*. Stereotactic heavy-charged-particle Bragg-Peak radiation for intracranial arteriovenous malformations. *N Engl J Med* 1990; 323: 96–101.

35 Kida Y, Kobayashi T, Tanaka T *et al*. Seizure control after radiosurgery on cerebral arteriovenous malformations. *J Clin Neurosci* 2000; 7 (Suppl. 1): 6–9.

36 Eisenschenk S, Gilmore RL, Friedman WA, Henchey RA. The effect of LINAC stereotactic radiosurgery on epilepsy associated with arteriovenous malformations. *Stereotact Funct Neurosurg* 1998; 71(2): 51–61.

37 Kurita H, Kawamoto S, Suzuki I, Sasaki T, Tago M, Terahara A, Kirino T. Control of epilepsy associated with cerebral arteriovenous malformations after radiosurgery. *J Neurol Neurosurg Psychiatr* 1998; 65(5): 648–55.

38 Falkson CB, Chakrabarti KB, Doughty D *et al*. Stereotactic multiple arc radiotherapy. Influence of treatment of arteriovenous malformations on associated epilepsy. *Br J Neurosurg* 1997; 11(1): 12–15.

39 Heikkinen ER, Konnov B, Melnikov L *et al*. Relief of epilepsy by radiosurgery of cerebral arteriovenous malformations. *Stereotact Funct Neurosurg* 1989; 53(3): 157–66.

40 Flickinger JC, Kondziolka D, Lunsford LD *et al*. Multi-institutional analysis of complication outcomes after arteriovenous malformation radiosurgery. *Int J Radiat Oncol Biol Phys* 1999; 44(1): 67–74.

41 Schlienger M, Atlan D, Lefkopoulos D *et al*. Linac radiosurgery for cerebral arteriovenous malformations: results in 169 patients. *Int J Radiat Oncol Biol Phys* 2000; 46(5): 1135–42.

42 Gerszten PC, Adelson PD, Kondziolka D *et al*. Seizure outcome in children treated for arteriovenous malformations using gamma knife radiosurgery. *Pediatr Neurosurg* 1996; 24(3): 139–44.

43 Jafar JJ, Davis AJ, Berenstein A *et al*. The effect of embolization with N-butyl cyanoacrilate prior to surgical resection of cerebral arteriovenous malformations. *J Neurosurg* 1993; 78: 60–9.

44 Rigamonti D, Drayer BP, Johnson PC *et al*. The MRI appearance of cavernous malformations (angiomas). *J Neurosurg* 1987; 67(4): 518–24.

45 Simard JM, Garcia-Bengochea F, Ballinger WE *et al*. Cavernous angioma: a review of 126 collected and 12 new clinical cases. *Neurosurgery* 1986; 18: 162–72.

46 McCormick WF, Nofzinger JD. 'Cryptic' vascular malformations of the central nervous system. *J Neurosurg* 1966; 24: 865–75.

47 Ferrante L, Palma L, D'Addetta R *et al*. Intracranial cavernous angioma. *Neurosurg Rev* 1992; 15: 125–33.

48 Maraire JN, Awad IA. Intracranial cavernous malformations: lesion behavior and management strategies. *Neurosurgery* 1995; 37: 591–605.

49 Ishikawa M, Handa H, Moritake K *et al*. Computed tomography of cerebral cavernous hemangiomas. *J Comput Assist Tomogr* 1980; 4: 587–91.

50 Giombini S, Morello G. Cavernous angiomas of the brain: Account of 14 personal cases and review of the literature. *Acta Neurochir (Wien)* 1978; 40: 61–82.

51 Vaquero J, Salazar J, Martinez R *et al*. Cavernomas of the central nervous system: clinical syndromes, CT scan diagnosis, and prognosis after surgical treatment in 25 cases. *Acta Neurochir (Wien)* 1987; 85: 29–33.

52 Kim DS, Park YG, Choi JU *et al*. An analysis of the natural history of cavernous malformations. *Surg Neurol* 1997; 48(1): 9–17.

53 Kondziolka D, Lunsford LD, Kestle JR. The natural history of cerebral cavernous malformations. *J Neurosurg* 1995; 83(5): 820–4.

54 Awad IA, Robinson J. Cavernous malformations and epilepsy. In: Awad IA, Barrow DL, eds. *Cavernous Malformations*. Park Ridge: AANSS, 1993: 49–63.

55 Kraemer DL, Awad IA. Vascular malformations and epilepsy: clinical considerations and basic mechanisms. *Epilepsia* 1994; 35 (Suppl. 6): S30–S43.

56 Weber M, Vespignani H, Bracard S *et al*. Intracerebral cavernous angioma. *Rev Neurol (Paris) MDN* 1989; 145: 429–36.

57 Moriwaki A, Hattori Y, Nishida N *et al*. Electrocorticographic characterization of chronic iron induced epilepsy in rats. *Neurosci Lett* 1990; 110: 72–6.

58 Willmore L, Sypert G, Munson J. Chronic focal epileptiform discharge induced by injection of iron into rat and cat cortex. *Science* 1978; 200: 1501–3.

59 Maraire JN, Awad IA. Intracranial cavernous malformations: lesion behavior and management strategies. *Neurosurgery* 1995; 37: 591–605.

60 Moran NF, Fish DR, Kitchen N *et al*. Supratentorial cavernous heaemangiomas and epilepsy: a review of the literature and case series. *J Neurol Neurosurg Psychiatr* 1999; 66: 561–8.

61 Yeh H, Privitera MD. Secondary epileptogenesis in cerebral arteriovenous malformations. *Arch Neurol* 1997; 48: 1122–4.

62 Kondziolka D, Lunsford LD, Flickinger JC. Reduction of hemorrhage risk after stereotactic radiosurgery for cavernous malformations. *J Neurosurg* 1995; 83: 825–31.

63 Stea RA, Schilker L, King GA *et al.* Stereotactic linear radiosurgery for cavernous angiomas. *Acta Neurochir Suppl (Wien)* 1995; 63: 68–72.

64 Karlsson B, Kihlstom L, Lindquist C *et al.* Radiosurgery for cavernous malformations. *J Neurosurg* 1988; 88: 293–7.

65 Gewirtz RJ, Steinberg GK, Crowley R *et al.* Pathological changes in surgically resected angiographically occult vascular malformations after radiation. *Neurosurgery* 1998; 42: 738–42.

66 Regis J, Bartolomei F, Yoshihisa K *et al.* Radiosurgery for epilepsy associated with cavernous malformations: Retrospective study in 49 patients. *Neurosurgery* 2000; 47: 1091–7.

67 Regis J, Bartolomei F, Rey M *et al.* Gamma knife surgery for mesial temporal lobe epilepsy. *Epilepsia* 1999; 40: 1551–6.

68 Regis J, Semah F, Bryan RN *et al.* Early and delayed MR and PET changes after selective temporomesial radiosurgery in mesial temporal lobe epilepsy. *Am J Neuroradiol* 1999; 20: 213–16.

69 Sarwar M, McCormick WF. Intracerebral venous angioma: Case Report and Review. *Arch Neurol* 1978; 35: 323–5.

70 Riagamonti D, Spetzler RF, Medina M *et al.* Appearance of venous malformations on magnetic resonance imaging. *J Neurosurg* 1988; 69: 535–9.

71 Fierstien SB, Pribram HW, Hieshima G. Angiography and computed tomography in the evaluation of cerebral venous malformations. *Neuroradiology* 1979; 17: 137–48.

72 McLaughlin MR, Kondziolka D, Flickinger JC *et al.* The prospective natural history of cerebral venous malformations. *Neurosurgery* 1998; 43: 195–201.

73 Garner TB, Curling OD, Kelly DL *et al.* The natural history of intracranial venous angiomas. *J Neurosurg* 1991; 75: 715–22.

74 Striano S, Nocerino C, Striano P *et al.* Venous angiomas and epilepsy. *Neurol Sci* 2000; 21(3): 151–5.

75 Topper R, Jurgens E, Reul J *et al.* Clinical significance of intracranial developmental venous anomalies. *J Neurol Neurosurg Psychiatr* 1999; 67(2): 234–8.

76 Biller J, Toffol GJ, Shea JF *et al.* Cerebellar venous angiomas. *Arch Neurol* 1985; 42: 367–70.

77 Lobato RD, Perez C, Rivas JJ *et al.* Clinical, radiological, and pathological spectrum of angiographically occult intracranial vascular malformations. *J Neurosurg* 1988; 68: 518–31.

78 Meyer B, Stangl AP, Schramm J. Association of venous and true arteriovenous malformation: A rare entity among mixed vascular malformations of the brain. *J Neurosurg* 1995; 83: 141–4.

79 lindquist C, Guo WY, Karlsson B *et al.* Radiosurgery of venous angiomas. *J Neurosurg* 1993; 78: 531–6.

80 Wilkins RH. Natural history of intracranial vascular malformations. A review. *Neurosurgery* 1985; 16: 421–30.

81 Courville CB. *Pathology of the Central Nervous System.* Mountain View, CA: Pacific Press Publishing Association.

82 McCormick WF, Hardman JM, Boulter TR. Vascular malformations ('angiomas') of the brain, with special reference to those occurring in the posterior fossa. *J Neurosurg* 1968; 28: 241–51.

83 Milandre L, Pellissier JF, Bourdouresques G *et al.* Non-hereditary multiple telangiectasias of the central nervous system. Report of two clinicopathological cases. *J Neurol Sci* 1987; 82: 291–304.

84 Castillo M, Morrison T, Shaw JA, Bouldin TW. MR imaging and histologic features of capillary telangiectasia of the basal ganglia. *Am J Neuroradiol* 2001; 22(8): 1553–5.

85 Rigamonti D, Johnson PC, Spetzler RF, Hadley MN, Drayer BP. Cavernous malformation and capillary telangiectasia: a spectrum within a single pathological entity. *Neurosurgery* 1991; 28: 60–4.

86 Whitney KD, McNamara JO. GluR3 autoantibodies destroy neural cells in a complement dependent manner modulated by complement regulatory proteins. *J Neurosci* 2000; 20 (19): 7307–16.

87 Levy RM. Brain abscess and subdural empyema. *Curr Opin Neurol* 1994; 7: 223–8.

88 Zeidman SM, Geisler FH, Olivi A. Intraventricular rupture of a purulent brain abscess: case report. *Neurosurgery* 1995; 36: 189–93.

89 Nicolosi A *et al.* Incidence and prognosis of brain abscess in a defined population: Olmsted County, Minnesota, 1935–1981. *Neuroepidemiology* 1991; 10: 122–31.

90 Seydoux C, Francioli P. Bacterial brain abscesses: factors influencing mortality and sequelae. *Clin Infect Dis* 1992; 15: 394–401.

91 Mamelak *et al.* Improved management of multiple brain abscesses: a combined surgical and medical approach. *Neurosurgery* 1995; 36: 76–85.

92 Bradley P, Manning K, Shaw M. Brain abscess secondary to paranasal sinusitis. *J Laryngol Otol* 1984; 98: 719–25.

93 Rao A. Brain abscess as a complication of cocaine inhalation. *N Y State J Med* 1988; 88: 548–50.

94 Matthews T, Marcus G. Otogenic intradural complications. *J Laryngol Otol* 1988; 102: 121–4.

95 Hollin S, Hayashi H, Gross S. Intracranial abscesses of odontogenic origin. *Oral Surg* 1967; 23: 277–93.

96 Patir R, Sood S, Bhatia R. Post-traumatic brain abscess: experience of 36 patients. *Br J Neurosurg* 1995; 9: 29–35.

97 Rish B *et al.* Analysis of brain abscess after penetrating craniocerebral injuries in Vietnam. *Neurosurgery* 1981; 9: 535–41.

98 Panek T, Burchiel K. Delayed brain abscess related to a retained foreign body with culture of *Clostridium bifermentans.* *J Neurosurg* 1986; 64: 13.

99 Gordon SB *et al.* Brain abscess ten years after penetrating glass injury to the skull. *Ulster Med J* 1992; 61: 116–18.

100 Yang S. Brain abscess: a review of 400 cases. *J Neurosurg* 1981; 55: 794–9.

101 Saex-Lorens X *et al.* Brain abscess in infants and children. *Paed Infect Dis J* 1989; 8: 449–58.

102 Carey M, Shou S, French L. Long term neurological residua in patients surviving brain abscess with surgery. *J Neurosurg* 1971; 34: 652–6.

103 Su TM *et al.* Streptococcal brain abscess: analysis of clinical features in 20 patients. *Surg Neurol* 2001; 56: 189–94.

104 Shintani S *et al.* Sudden 'stroke like' onset of homonymous hemianopsia due to bacterial brain abscess. *J Neurol Sci* 1996; 143: 190–4.

105 Morgan H, Wood M, Murphy F *et al.* Experience with 88 consecutive cases of brain abscess. *J Neurosurg* 1973; 38: 698–704.

106 Jamjoom AB. Short course antimicrobial therapy in intracranial abscess. *Acta Neurochir (Wien)* 1996; 138: 835–9.

107 Enzmann D, Britt R, Placone R. Staging of human brain abscess by Computed Tomography. *Radiology* 1983; 146: 703–8.

108 Britt R. Brain abscesses. In: Wilkins R, Rengachary S, eds. *Neurosurgery.* New York: McGraw-Hill, 1985: 1928–56.

109 Adachi J *et al.* Diagnosis of brainstem abscess in the cerebritis stage by MRI-case report. *Neurol Med Chir (Tokyo)* 1995; 35: 467–70.

110 Sze G, Zimmerman R. The MRI of infections and inflammatory diseases. *Radiol Clin North Am* 1988; 26: 839–59.

111 Brant-Zawadzki, Enzmann D, Placone R *et al.* NMR imaging of experimental brain abscess: comparison with CT. *Am J Neuroradiol* 1983; 4: 250–3.

112 Remy C, Grand S, Lai ES *et al.* 1H MRS of human brain abscesses in vivo and in vitro. *Magn Reson Med* 1995; 34: 508–14.

113 Martinez PI, Moreno A, Alonso J *et al.* Diagnosis of brain abscess by MRS: report of two cases. *J Neurosurg* 1997; 86: 708–13.

114 Miller E, Dias P, Uttley D. CT scanning in the management of intracranial abscess: a review of 100 cases. *Br J Neurosurg* 1988; 2: 439–46.

115 Kim SH, Chang KH, Song IC *et al.* Brain abscess and brain tumor: discrimination with 1H MR spectroscopy. *Radiology* 1997; 204: 239–45.

116 Ebisu T, Tanaka C, Umeda M *et al.* Discrimination of brain abscess from necrotic or cystic tumors by diffusion-weighted echo planar imaging. *Magn Reson Imaging* 1996; 14: 1113–16.

117 Rousseaux M, Lesoin F, Destee A *et al.* Developments in the treatment and prognosis of multiple cerebral abscesses. *Neurosurgery* 1985; 16: 304–8.

118 Rosenblum M, Hoff J, Norman D *et al.* Nonoperative treatment of brain abscesses in selected high risk patients. *J Neurosurg* 1980; 52: 217–25.

119 Black P, Graybill J, Charache P. Penetration of brain abscess by systemically administered antibiotics. *J Neurosurg* 1973; 38: 705–9.

120 Stephanov S, Joubert M. Large brain abscess treated by aspiration alone. *Surg Neurol* 1982; 17: 338–40.

121 Alderson D, Strong A, Ingham H *et al*. Fifteen year review of the mortality of brain abscess. *Neurosurgery* 1981; 8: 1–6.

122 Dyste G, Hitchon P, Menezes A *et al*. Stereotaxic surgery in the treatment of brain abscesses. *J Neurosurg* 1988; 69: 188–94.

123 Nagle R, Takeman M, Shallat R *et al*. Brain abscess surgery in nursery with ultrasound guidance. *J Neurosurg* 1986; 65: 557–9.

124 Hagan R. Early complications following penetrating wounds of the brain. *J Neurosurg* 1971; 34: 132–41.

125 Young R, Frazee J. Gas within intracranial abscess cavities: an indication for surgical excision. *Ann Neurol* 1984; 16: 35–9.

126 Sharma BS, Khosla VK, Kak VK *et al*. Multiple pyogenic brain abscesses. *Acta Neurochir (Wien)* 1995; 133: 36–43.

127 Quartey G, Johnston J, Rozdilsky B. Decadron in the treatment of cerebral abscess: an experimental study. *J Neurosurg* 1976; 45: 301–10.

128 Schroeder K, McKeever P, Schaberg D *et al*. Effect of dexamethasone on experimental brain abscess. *J Neurosurg* 1987; 66: 264–9.

129 Britt R, Enzmann D. Clinical stages of human brain abscesses on serial CT scans after contrast infusion: CT, neuropathological and clinical correlations. *J Neurosurg* 1983; 59: 972–89.

130 Carey M, Shou S, French L. Experience with brain abscesses. *J Neurosurg* 1972; 36: 1–9.

131 Nielsen H, Harmsen A, Gyldensted C. Cerebral abscesses: a long term follow up. *Acta Neurol Scand* 1983; 67: 330–7.

132 Beller A, Sahar A, Praiss I. Brain abscess: review of 89 cases over a period of 30 years. *J Neurol Neurosurg Psychiatr* 1973; 36: 757–68.

133 Legg N, Gupta P, Scott D *et al*. Epilepsy following cerebral abscess: a clinical and EEG study of 70 patients. *Brain* 1973; 96: 259–68.

134 Samson D, Clark K. A current review of brain abscesses. *Am J Med* 1973; 54: 201–10.

135 Wadley JP, Shakir RA, Rice-Edwards JM. Experience with neurocysticercosis in the UK: correct diagnosis and neurosurgical management of the small enhancing brain lesion. *Br J Neurosurg* 2000; 14 (3): 211–18.

136 Shakir RA, Pfister HW. Parasitic infections. In: Brandt T, ed. *Neurological Disorders: course and treatment*. San Diego: Academic Press, 1996: 433–42.

137 Del Brutto OH, Santibanez R, Noboa CA *et al*. Epilepsy due to neurocysticercosis: analysis of 203 patients. *Neurology* 1992; 42: 389–92.

138 Wadia NH. Neurocysticercosis. In: Shakir RA, Newman PK, Poser CM, eds. *Tropical Neurology*. London: WB Saunders, 1996: 247–73.

139 Balogou AA, Grunitzky KE, Bekiti KA *et al*. Cysticercosis and epilepsy in the city of Tone, North of Togo. *Rev Neurol (Paris)* 2000; 156 (3): 270–3.

140 Cruz ME, Schantz PM, Cruz I *et al*. Epilepsy and neurocysticercosis in an Andean community. *Int J Epidemiol* 1999; 28 (4): 799–803.

141 Sanchez AL, Lindback J, Schantz PM *et al*. A population based, case control study of *Taenia solium* taeniasis and cysticercosis. *Ann Trop Med Parasitol* 1999; 93 (3): 247–58.

142 Gomes I, Veiger M, Correa D *et al*. Cysticercosis in epileptic patients of Mulungu do Morro, Northeastern Brazil. *Arq Neuropsiquiatr* 2000; 58 (3A): 621–4.

143 Hernandez-Cossio O, Hernandez-Fustes OJ. Neurocysticercosis and epilepsy in Cuba. *Rev Neurol* 1999; 29 (11): 1003–6.

144 Palacio LG, Jimenez I, Garcia HH *et al*. Neurocysticercosis in persons with epilepsy in Medellin, Columbia. The Neuroepidemiological Research Group of Antioquia. *Epilepsia* 1998; 39 (12): 1334–49.

145 Garcia HH, Gilman RH, Tsang VC *et al*. Clinical significance of neurocysticercosis in endemic villages. The Cysticercosis Working Group of Peru. *Trans R Soc Trop Med Hyg* 1997; 91 (2): 176–8.

146 Wandra T, Nakaya K, Simanjuntak GM *et al*. Resurgence of cases of epileptic seizures and burns associated with cysticercosis in Assologaima, Indonesia. *Trans R Soc Trop Med Hyg* 2000; 94 (1): 46–50.

147 Garcia HH, Del Brutto OH. *Taenia solium* cysticercosis. *Infect Dis Clin North Am* 2000; 14 (1): 97–119.

148 Roman G, Sotelo J, Del Brutto OH *et al*. A proposal to declare neurocysticercosis an internationally reportable disease. *Bull World Health Organ* 2000; 78 (3): 399–406.

149 Chayasivisobhan S, Menoni R, Chayasivisobhan W *et al*. Correlation of EEG and the active and inactive forms of neurocysticercosis. *Clin Electroencephalogr* 1999; 30 (1): 9–11.

150 Singh G. Neurocysticercosis in South Central America and the Indian Subcontinent; a comparative evaluation. *Arq Neuropsiquiatr* 1997; 55: 349–56.

151 Rajshekar V, Haran RP, Prakash S *et al*. Differentiating solitary small cysticercus granulomas and tuberculomas in patients with epilepsy. Clinical and CT criteria. *J Neurosurg* 1993; 78: 402–7.

152 Rosenfeld EA, Byrd SE, Schulman ST. Neurocysticercosis among children in Chicago. *Clin Infect Dis* 1996; 23: 262–8.

153 Carpio A, Escobar A, Hauser W. Epilepsy and cysticercosis: a critical review. *Epilepsia* 1998; 39: 1025–40.

154 Tsang V, Brand A, Boyer A. An enzyme linked immunoelectrotransfer blot assay by glycoprotein antigens for diagnosing human cysticercosis (*Taenia solium*). *J Infect Dis* 1989; 159: 50–9.

155 Rajshekar V, Wilson M, Schantz PM. Cysticercus immunoblot assay in Indian patients with single, small enhancing CT lesions. *J Neurol Neurosurg Psychiatr* 1991; 54: 561.

156 Goodman K, Ballagh SA, Carpio A. A case control study of seropositivity for cysticercosis in Cuenca, Ecuador. *Am J Trop Med Hyg* 1999; 60: 70–4.

157 Garcia HH, Harrison LJS, Parkhouse RME *et al*. A specific antigen detection ELISA for the diagnosis of human neurocysticercosis. *Trans Med Soc Trop Med Hyg* 1998; 92: 411–14.

158 Carpio A. Diagnostic criteria for human cysticercosis. *J Neurol Sci* 1999; 161: 185–8.

159 Del Brutto OH, Wadia NH, Dumas M *et al*. Proposal of diagnostic criteria for human cysticercosis and neurocysticercosis. *J Neurol Sci* 1996; 142: 1–6.

160 Stern WE. Neurosurgical considerations of cysticercosis of the central nervous system. *J Neurosurg* 1981; 55: 382–9.

161 Rueda-Franco F. Surgical considerations in neurocysticercosis. *Childs Nerve Syst* 1987; 3: 212.

162 Colli BO, Martelli N, Assirati JA *et al*. Results of surgical treatment of neurocysticercosis in 69 cases. *J Neurosurg* 1986; 65: 309–15.

163 Del Brutto OH, Sotelo J. Albendazole therapy for subarachnoid and ventricular cysticercosis: case report. *J Neurosurg* 1990; 72: 816–17.

164 Rodriguez-Carbajal J, Del Brutto OH, Penagos P *et al*. Occlusion of the middle cerebral artery due to cysticercotic angiitis. *Stroke* 1989; 20: 1095–9.

165 Apuzzo ML, Dobkin WR, Zee CS *et al*. Surgical considerations in treatment of intraventricular cysticercosis: analysis of 45 cases. *J Neurosurg* 1984; 60: 400–7.

166 Couldwell WT, Apuzzo ML. Management of cysticercosis cerebri. *Contemp Neurosurg* 1989; 19: 1–6.

167 Loyo M, Kleriga E, Estanol B. Fourth ventricular cysticercosis. *Neurosurgery* 1980; 7: 456–8.

168 Madrazo I, Renteria JA, Sandoval M *et al*. Intraventricular cysticercosis. *Neurosurgery* 1983; 12: 148–52.

169 Proano JV, Madrazo I, Garcia L *et al*. Albendazole and praziquantel treatment in neurocysticercosis of the 4th ventricle. *J Neurosurg* 1997; 87: 29–33.

170 Chandy MJ, Rajshekar V, Ghosh S *et al*. Single small enhancing CT lesions in Indian patients with epilepsy: clinical, radiological and pathological considerations. *J Neurol Neurosurg Psychiatry* 1991; 54: 702–5.

171 Garland HG, Armitage G. Intracranial tuberculoma. *J Path Bact* 1933; 37: 461–71.

172 Wilson SAK. Neurotuberculosis. In: Bruce AN, ed. *Neurology*, Vol. 1. Baltimore: Williams and Wilkins, 1941.

173 Obrador S. Intracranial tuberculomas: review of 47 cases. *Neurochirurgica* 1959; 1: 150–7.

174 Maurice-Williams RS. Tuberculomas of the brain in Britain. *J Postgrad Med* 1972; 48: 678–81.

175 Naim-Ur-Rahman. Intracranial tuberculomas: diagnosis and management. *Acta Neurochirurgica (Wien)* 1987; 88: 109–15.

176 Leary PM, Cremin BJ, Daubentow JD *et al*. A study of African children into prolonged focal seizure and a specific CT scan finding. *J Tropical Paediatr* 1993; 39: 176–8.

177 Traub M, Colchester AC, Kingsley DP *et al*. Tuberculosis of the nervous system. *Q J Med* 1984; 53 (209): 81–100.

178 Abos J, Graus F, Miro JM *et al*. Intracranial tuberculosis in patients with AIDS. *AIDS* 1991; 5: 461–2.

179 Gulati P, Jena A, Tripathi RP *et al*. MRI in childhood epilepsy. *Indian Pediatr* 1991; 28: 761–5.

180 Rebai R, Boudawara MZ, Kamel B *et al*. Cavernous sinus tuberculoma: diagnostic difficulties in a personal case. *Surg Neurol* 2001; 55: 372–5.

181 Salgado P, Del Brutto OH, Talamas O *et al*. Intracranial tuberculoma: MR imaging. *Neurorad* 1989; 31: 299–302.

182 Rich AR. *The Pathogenesis of Tuberculosis*. Oxford: Blackwell, 1951.

183 Garg RK, Kar AM, Kumar T. Neurocysticercosis like presentation in a case of CNS tuberculosis. *Neurol India* 2000; 48 (3): 260–2.

184 Morris JT. CNS tuberculoma presenting as cavernous sinus tumor (letter). *Clin Infect Dis* 1992; 15: 181–2.

185 Phookan G. Tuberculoma of the cavernous sinus: case report. *Br J Neurosurg* 1995; 9: 205–7.

186 Grayeli AB. Tuberculoma of the cavernous sinus: case report. *Neurosurgery* 1998; 42: 179–82.

187 Boucetta M, Sami A, Choukri M *et al*. Les tuberculomes encephaliques: 40 cases. *Neurochirurgie* 1993; 39: 42–6.

188 Rodat O, Resch F, Lajat Y *et al*. Absec tuberculeux du nevraxe: revue de la literature sur dix ans. *Sem Hop Paris* 1980; 56: 38–42.

189 Harder E, Al-Kawi MZ, Carney P. Intracranial tuberculoma: conservative management. *Am J Med* 1983; 74: 570–6.

190 Nakamura H, Tanaka H, Ibayashi S *et al*. A case of intracranial tuberculoma early diagnosed by open brain biopsy. *No-to-shinkei* 2001; 53(4): 387–90.

191 Bouchama A, Al-Kauri MZ, Coates R *et al*. Brain biopsy in tuberculoma: the risks and benefits. *Neurosurgery* 1991; 28: 405–9.

192 Carrea R, Dowling E, Guevara JA. Surgical treatment of hydatid cysts of the central nervous system in the pediatric age (Dowling's technique). *Childs Brain* 1975; 1: 4–21.

193 Cataltape O, Colak A, Ozcan OE *et al*. Intracranial hydatid cysts: experience with surgical treatment in 120 patients. *Neurochirurgie* 1992; 35: 108–11.

194 Sharma A, Abraham J. Multiple giant hydatid cysts of the brain: a case report. *J Neurosurg* 1982; 57: 413–15.

195 Khaldi M, Mohamed S, Kallel J *et al*. Brain hydatidosis: report on 117 cases. *Child's Nerv Syst* 2000; 16(10–11): 765–9.

196 Feldman M, Plancarte A, Sandoval M *et al*. Comparison of two assays (EIA and EITB) and two saliva samples (saliva and serum) for the diagnosis of neurocysticercosis. *Trans R Soc Trop Med Hyg* 1990; 84: 559–62.

197 Ruttinger P, Hadidi H. MRI in cerebral toxocaral disease. *J Neurol Neurosurg Psychiatry* 1991; 54: 361–2.

198 Peter JC, Domingo Z, Sinclair-Smith C *et al*. Hydatid infestation of the brain: difficulties with CT diagnosis and surgical treatment. *Pediatr Neurosurg* 1994; 20: 78–83.

199 Nanassis K, Alexiadou-Rudolf C, Tsitsopolous P *et al*. Solid cerebral echinococcus mimicking a primary brain tumor. *Neurosurg-Rev* 1999; 22(1): 58–61.

200 Morris DL, Dykes PW, Marriner S *et al*. Albendazole: objective evidence of response in human hydatid disease. *JAMA* 1985; 253: 2053–7.

201 Kaya U, Ozden B, Turker K *et al*. Intracranial hydatid cyst: study of 117 cases. *J Neurosurg* 1975; 42: 580–4.

202 Lunardi P, Missori P, Lorenzo N *et al*. Cerebral hydatidosis in childhood: a retrospective survey with emphasis on long term follow up. *Neurosurgery* 1991; 29: 515–17.

63 Surgery of Cortical Dysgenesis for Epilepsy

S.M. Sisodiya

Brain malformations are a significant cause of epilepsy, particularly epilepsy that is refractory to drug treatment. Neuroimaging detects brain malformations in 8–12% of patients with refractory epilepsy [1,2], and up to 14% of children with refractory epilepsy and retardation [3,4]. A prospective incident study using high-resolution MRI in patients having their first seizure identified brain malformations in 3% of cases with partial onset seizures [5]. These figures are, however, likely to underestimate the true incidence. Brain malformations can remain undetected by high-resolution MRI preoperatively, only to be found at histology after surgery [6,7]. Thus a proportion of the 25% of cases with refractory epilepsy and normal conventional MRI [8] could harbour brain malformations. The management of epilepsy due to brain malformations thus presents a significant clinical issue. Most cases are refractory to medical treatment [2,9], and alternative treatment strategies are needed. This chapter considers the indications and prognosis of surgery for epilepsy in patients with specific brain malformations, but will not deal with technical details. Although psychological, psychiatric and social aspects are also important, these will not be addressed here.

The thesis underpinning epilepsy surgery is that it is possible to identify a critical area which when resected results in cessation of the seizures. As has been stated ' . . . the objective of presurgical evaluation is to identify the area of brain most responsible for generating habitual seizures and to demonstrate that it can be removed without causing additional unacceptable neurologic or cognitive deficits. There is no simple test to delineate the epileptogenic zone, defined as the volume of brain tissue necessary and sufficient for the generation of seizures' [10]. This statement does not imply that the epileptogenic zone in partial epilepsy is necessarily focal, but that in cases when it is *effectively* focal and when that focus can be resected, then seizure freedom may follow. There is a growing school of thought that epileptogenesis is a distributed process. Even in temporal lobe epilepsy attributed to hippocampal sclerosis (HS), the diversity of aura, varieties of autonomic and psychomotor ictal manifestations and often widespread neuropsychological deficits suggest involvement of other brain structures (e.g. [11,12]). Moreover, neuroimaging studies have revealed a variety of subtle abnormalities in addition to atrophy of the hippocampus; additional extrahippocampal temporal, extratemporal, basal ganglia and ipsilateral hemispheric changes have all been detected [13–15], though whether these are present *ab initio* or develop secondarily remains to be determined. In most (70%) HS cases, the presence of more widespread structural change is unimportant for the outcome—patients become seizure free, with good psychosocial outcomes. Persistent extrahippocampal or extratemporal epileptogenic abnormalities could, however, undoubtedly contribute to the poorer

outcome of the 30% of HS cases who do not become seizure free despite being ostensibly good candidates. The distributed nature of epileptogenesis, whether on a structural or functional basis, is even more relevant when considering surgery for brain malformations, and may be the key issue in management as I will discuss. Surgery for malformations not only has therapeutic implications, but also contributes to our understanding of the processes of epileptogenesis.

There are many types of brain malformation. In children and adults, the brain malformations of importance from the surgical perspective are: focal cortical dysplasia (FCD), periventricular heterotopia (PVH), subcortical heterotopia (SH), polymicrogyria and schizencephaly, and lissencephaly. Some of these brain malformations may occur as part of a more widespread disease entity or syndrome (e.g. Aicardi syndrome; muscle–eye–brain disease, etc.). A variety of other brain malformations are recognized that can cause epilepsy but are not considered in this chapter; these include definite hippocampal malformations, callosal agenesis and holoprosencephaly (rare); microdysgenesis (probably relatively common, but not identifiable currently on preoperative MRI, precluding presurgical assessment of this pathology specifically). I have also included a section on dysembryoplastic neuroepithelial tumours (DNT) for completeness. There is some debate as to their exact classification, so I have considered them separately from brain malformations. Whilst brain malformations are usually grouped together, and have been known variously as 'cortical dysgeneses', 'neuronal migration disorders' and 'malformations of cortical development', these terms carry descriptive or aetiological implications that may not be correct. In addition, whilst the grouping of these disorders is convenient and has helped to bring the conditions to wider attention, it is no more valid biologically to analyse their treatment as a group than it is to consider the treatment of epilepsy itself as a single condition. In this chapter, the literature will first be reviewed, followed by an analysis of the individual brain malformations from a biological viewpoint and suggestions for presurgical assessment of patients with brain malformations in the final section.

Outcome of surgery in brain malformation: the literature

There are a number of confounding factors that make it more difficult to assess the results of surgical treatment for brain malformations than for HS: (a) there are very few adequate surgical series of 'pure cultures' of a given brain malformation, because of variations in anatomy, localization, pathology and seizure characteristics; (b) management strategies, involving such issues as the relevance of epileptic discharges distant from the structural lesion, differ from

Table 63.1 Outcome of surgery for brain malformations: review of adequate literature published since 1971 to June 2001

Minimum duration of follow-up	Numbers	All brain malformation pathologies		FCD only or main pathology FCD	
		Series only	Series and single cases	Series only	Series and single cases
1 year	All	510	532	305	326
	Seizure free (%)	233 (46%)	250 (47%)	137 (45%)	149 (45%)
2 years	All	273	302	158	175
	Seizure free (%)	129 (47%)	142 (47%)	71 (45%)	81 (46%)

FCD, focal cortical dysplasia. Seizure free is Engel grade I or equivalent.

centre to centre; and (c) outcome parameters are very variable and sometimes inadequate: for example, many studies report postoperative follow-up for less than 1 year, whilst the most rigorous current series favour a minimum of 2 years [16–18]. Curiously some of the largest surgical series give no follow-up at all. Individual patient data are not always given, follow-up outcome scales are not universal and are often not widely-used measures, but rather parochial ones. Pathological diagnoses are often unclear or outmoded. Patients are frequently included inextricably in more than one series. For series with longer follow-up, neuroimaging data may inevitably be unavailable. In many reports details are simply insufficient to allow meaningful interpretation. Of these problems, that of inadequate duration of postsurgical follow-up is undoubtedly most important. For refractory epilepsy due to HS, 96% of seizure recurrences after surgery occur within the first 2 years of follow-up [19]. Late recurrences can develop irrespective of pathology; Paillas *et al.* [20] documented recurrence in a higher proportion of patients over a longer follow-up. Bruton [21], Gilliam *et al.* [22] and Döring *et al.* [23] report late recurrence for brain malformations specifically. The basis of recurrence may—or may not—differ between HS and brain malformations, but a minimum duration of follow-up of at least a year is essential when reporting outcome. Considering all these issues, data are limited. Whilst several thousand HS cases are now documented in the literature, allowing sophisticated analyses, fewer than 1000 brain malformations cases in total, including all variety of pathologies, are adequately documented.

A summary of surgical results in the English language literature is given in Table 63.1. Tables 63.2 and 63.3 give outcome data according to age at surgery and location of resection. About 45% of patients become seizure free postoperatively at 1 or 2 years follow-up, whether considering all brain malformation varieties together, or solely FCD, which is the most common brain malformation reported. This compares with 70% seizure freedom for those with unilateral HS. Psychosocial outcomes are critical, but rarely reported and cannot be considered in this analysis. The potential benefit of seizure freedom or reduction in seizure frequency even for a limited period during childhood should not be underestimated, but neither should the adverse effects of neurological, cognitive or psychiatric deficits: not to report the entire outcome is to do patients a disservice.

The figure of 45% of patients with brain malformations seizure free is likely to be a realistic reflection of modern outcomes, as many of the studies are recent, since the detection of the abnormalities are dependent upon the availability of high-resolution MRI.

Table 63.2 Outcome by age at surgery: adequately documented cases only (series and single reports)

Engel class I outcome only		All brain malformation pathologies		
Minimum duration of follow-up	Numbers	Age (years)		
		<1	1–16	>16
1 year	All	39	132	155
	Seizure free (%)	22 (56)	58 (45)	60 (30)
2 year	All	14	53	76
	Seizure free (%)	8 (57)	21 (40)	34 (36)

The comparatively poorer outcome of surgery in brain malformations compared with HS must reflect a higher percentage of brain malformation cases in which epileptogenic tissue persists after focal resection. In fact, the issues are likely to be more involved still—what constitutes the epileptogenic tissue? Recent genetic and pathological studies suggest that the biology of malformations is much more complex than previously considered, even from what little is known currently. Whilst detailed clinical, imaging and pathological aspects of these varied malformations are described in a number of excellent monographs (e.g. [24,25]), I have selected some key aspects for each of the brain malformations in the sections below.

Outcome of surgery in brain malformation: biological limitations

Although surgery for brain malformations may be limited by the location of brain malformations within or adjacent to normally eloquent cortex, the functions normally ascribed to a given cortical area may be completely displaced, or lost, and thus not impede surgery [26]. Specific function normally ascribed to an affected region may, however, persist in a modified fashion. Raymond *et al.* [27] recorded distorted somatosensory evoked potentials in five of 13 patients with brain malformations affecting the appropriate central regions. Leblanc *et al.* [28] demonstrated that electrocortical stimulation over a malformed posterior temporal gyrus led to interference with speech. Duchowny *et al.* [29] found cortical language representation overlapping brain malformations, and there have

Table 63.3 Outcome by location of surgery: adequately documented cases only (series and single reports)

Engel class I outcome only		All brain malformation pathologies			FCD only or main pathology FCD		
Minimum duration of follow-up	Numbers	Temporal[a]	Extratemporal	H'tomy	Temporal[a]	Extratemporal	H'tomy
1 year	All	146	194	60	85	151	13
	Seizure free (%)	51 (32)	78 (35)	35 (58)	37 (42)	58 (34)	5 (38)
2 years	All	65	83	43	40	47	8
	Seizure free (%)	22 (32)	33 (34)	25 (58)	14 (35)	19 (38)	2 (25)

[a] Some component of surgery involved temporal lobe (exact extent may be undefined).

H'tomy: hemispherectomy or hemispherotomy. Included in this category are patients who had partial resections initially but went on to have hemispherectomy.

been similar observations concerning neuronal activity [30] and motor function [31,32]. In some cases, normal function is reorganized but abuts brain malformations [33], limiting resection margins. The complexities of the mixture of normal and abnormal neurones within brain malformations [34], of neuronal connections and of the timing of maldevelopment with respect to synaptogenesis and functional commitment, may explain why cortical function is not always reallocated to other regions. ECoG, with stimulation, is currently the best means of identifying eloquent cortex *in vivo*, and in cases where brain malformations abut such cortex, corticography can delimit the boundaries of resection. Clearly, this biological feature of some cases of brain malformation cannot be overcome by current surgical techniques. In addition, the structural substrate of normal function (and indeed, epileptogenesis) may be more dispersed than suggested by investigations dependent on changes in spatial density of information (e.g. functional MRI, PET studies). In some circumstances, when brain malformations are responsible for disabling convulsive or focal motor status epilepticus, eloquent cortex may need to be sacrificed to stop seizures, even at the cost of a hemiplegia [35].

Focal cortical dysplasia

Identified in 1971 by Taylor *et al.* FCD is the most common brain malformation reported in surgical resection specimens [36]. There is strong evidence that FCD is intrinsically epileptogenic. FCD occurring independently of epilepsy has not been reported in neuroimaging studies, despite the large number of normal individuals scanned across the world in a range of MRI studies. Electrophysiological evidence, from scalp and intracranial recordings (e.g. [37,38]), even when such FCD is not visible to the naked eye [28,39,40], and *in vitro* studies of resection specimens containing FCD [41], confirm its abnormal electrical behaviour. In one case, intralesional EEG demonstrated epileptiform activity within FCD; in this report, magnetic source imaging localized dipoles within the FCD in three out of four cases [42]. In the remaining case, multiple dipoles were calculated, some of which lay outside the visualized abnormality. This patient did not become seizure free after resection of the visualized abnormality, even with guidance by ECoG and depth electrode study. Histopathological changes that are likely to contribute to intrinsic hyperexcitability have also been shown in

FCD [25,38,43]. Of all the brain malformations considered, the case for intrinsic epileptogenicity is best supported for FCD.

Following the basic thesis of epilepsy surgery, completeness of excision of FCD is thus likely to be important for seizure freedom. Overall, with no comment possible on the extent of resection, 46% of cases of FCD become seizure free with surgery (see Table 63.1). Not all FCD cases reported to have undergone complete excision become seizure free [18,37]. The means of assessment of completeness of excision have, however, not always been clear, though the most detailed and recent study determined completeness of excision on postoperative MRI [18]. The failure of surgery to render patients seizure free despite apparent complete resection on MRI has a number of possible causes. For FCD, persistent primary epileptogenic pathology must be the most likely cause. Even in their seminal paper, Taylor *et al.* recognized that FCD is probably not a discrete abnormality: 'There is some reason, therefore, to suspect that the operation had removed the main, if not the only, lesion . . . it may well be that other, if less ostentatious, areas of cortical dysplasia have been left behind. This possibility is supported by the fact that even within the limits of the resected lobes the abnormality was sometimes disseminated rather than confined to a single patch. The degree, therefore, to which the brain as a whole may be affected remains uncertain. It will probably vary greatly from one case to another' [36].

Because FCD may cause little apparent disruption of normal cortical architecture, even on macroscopic pathology, and because FCD usually consists of a mixture of normal and dysplastic tissue, not only may it be difficult to establish lesional boundaries microscopically, but it may also be impossible to identify the full extent of FCD preoperatively even using the best means of detecting structural abnormalities (high-resolution MRI). Though a number of methods have been devised to increase the detection rate of FCD preoperatively, including new MRI sequences [44] and qualitative [45] and quantitative postprocessing of conventional MRI [15,46,47], few are directed to the detection of widespread structural abnormalities, and none has yet been widely taken up by the majority of epilepsy centres. There is a pressing need for a reliable and robust means of detecting the entire extent of FCD preoperatively. Conversely, cases exist in which incomplete resection is associated with prolonged freedom from seizures [18,48]. Indeed, what is critical is not simply detecting the full extent of structural change in FCD, but the identification of the full extent of epileptogenic FCD. There are currently no proven means of achieving this, a problem that I will address in the discussion. The lack of good animal models of the precise histological abnormalities found in FCD with dysplastic neurones and balloon cell glia further limits understanding the biology of FCD.

Therefore, as judged by surgical results, the biology of FCD evades current means of delineating the epileptogenic zone in over half of surgically treated cases. These same considerations might be applied to each of the pathobiologies to be considered in the rest of this chapter, but to perhaps an even greater extent, as there are even less extensive data available for each of the other pathologies.

Periventricular heterotopia

PVH is the second most commonly detected brain malformation, and the second most commonly reported to have been treated surgically. Unfortunately, surgery is almost always ineffective: indeed, the presence of PVH is considered by some a 'red flag' for surgery [49].

There is direct evidence for the intrinsic epileptogenicity of PVH in humans undergoing invasive electrical recordings [15,49–51]. This is underpinned by histological evidence of an imbalance between excitation and inhibition within nodules and of their connectivity to extranodular structures [52,53]. However, nodules are rarely localized [54], so that complete excision is rarely feasible.

Neuroimaging and resulting genetic linkage studies have now established that mutations in the X-linked *filamin 1* gene underlie most cases of familial bilateral nodular PVH [55], though only a small proportion of sporadic nodular PVH. Recent studies suggest that the mutation results in an altered facility for migration in the developmental fields containing the neurones that express the mutant *filamin* allele. It is possible that neurones beyond the most obvious manifestation of the mutation, the periventricular nodules, also express the mutant allele, with untold structural and functional consequences, as *filamin* interacts with a large number of proteins. Perhaps not surprisingly, therefore, additional structural abnormalities are often seen on neuroimaging in patients with PVH; these include SH and overlying gyral abnormalities. PVH is the most common developmental change seen in association with HS in patients with so-called 'dual pathology' [54,57,58]. In addition, occult structural abnormalities in the overlying cortex have been described both histologically and on imaging and these may be of epileptogenic significance [7,53]. Males in particular may have widespread cortical changes [15]. These factors all suggest that the 'epileptogenic zone' in patients with PVH is probably more widespread and disparate, even though many patients with PVH appear neurologically and cognitively intact.

Insults during development can cause the formation of both periventricular and subcortical heterotopic nodules in animal models [59]. The nodules are epileptogenic, and contain hyperexcitable neurones that can sustain repetitive bursts of action potentials. These studies show nodules are intrinsically epileptogenic, but do not exclude other regions of epileptogenicity. It would be of interest to determine whether surgical treatment can be effective in these models, bearing in mind the limited applicability such studies have to human epilepsy.

Therefore, apart from *filamin* mutation-negative females with visually isolated, unifocal, completely resectable PVH, the theoretical chances of rendering a patient with PVH seizure free surgically must be small. This is supported by the literature, notwithstanding that PVH has only recently been easily diagnosed on neuroimaging. In the largest series, epileptogenic activity was recorded from co-existent HS using intracranial electrodes, leading to temporal lobectomy in nine patients [49]. This was uniformly unsuccessful, the best result being obtained when the majority of the PVH was also excised. This provides perhaps the clearest example of dual pathologies both being capable of ictogenesis, perhaps explaining persistent seizures post surgery. Though probably widely applicable, this principle is rarely so dramatically demonstrated. The limitation of intracerebral recordings is highlighted by these findings: *de facto*, coverage is limited to the areas sampled and results may be deceptive or incomplete.

PVH thus well illustrates the difficulties in surgical treatment of specific classes of brain malformations, leaving aside technical issues such as access to periventricular structures: important abnormalities are probably widespread, may not all be identifiable preoperatively, usually cannot all be sampled electrophysiologically and can rarely be completely resected at surgery. In addition, follow-up is often poor, and cases that do badly are less likely to be published. But with advancements from molecular biological studies, and with continuing improvements in structural and functional imaging studies, it is likely that our understanding will continue to improve, and possibly with that our ability to select and manage cases for surgery.

Subcortical heterotopia

SH describes a variety of different phenotypes, ranging from relatively rare isolated unilateral small heterotopic nodular masses, through massive unilateral SH with additional PVH and overlying gyral changes, to bilateral laminar SH. This may or may not represent a biological continuum. Thus whilst bilateral laminar SH may be sporadic or familial, and in either case may be due to mutations in a novel X-linked gene called *doublecortin* (*DCX* [60]), the relevance of *doublecortin* mutations in other SH phenotypes has not been reported. The detection of a mutation is important: it probably increases the likelihood of more spatially disseminated phenotypic abnormalities, with possible functional consequences for epileptogenesis and surgical management.

There are few adequately reported cases in the literature. Limited electrophysiological studies in man imply that nodules have the capacity for independent generation of epileptogenesis [61], though acute recordings have not always established this [34]. Histology suggests an imbalance between excitation and inhibition [53]. Unsurprisingly, incomplete excision of SH is associated with a poor outcome [34,50], whilst complete excision, as guided by intracerebral EEG, may lead to seizure freedom [61]. Recently, a structural animal model of the bilateral laminar form of SH has been generated: the *tish* rat (telencephalic internal structural heterotopia [62]). It is not a genetic model of the human condition but, given the poverty of human literature, study of the model may give further insights into the epileptogenic characteristics of such malformed brains; in particular it offers the chance of widespread examination of both structural and functional aspects, and the testing of hypotheses regarding seizure generation and propagation in SH. Neurones within the band heterotopia are known to be connected [63], and *tish* mice have spontaneous seizures. Epileptogenesis is probably widespread; although it may involve the SH masses, seizure generation appears to be initiated in overlying normotopic cortex [64].

Most human cases of SH have not been studied in sufficient detail to consider these possibilities, but it is certainly the case that many, if not most, cases of SH have additional extra-SH abnormalities likely to contribute to epileptogenesis. Whether this abnormality should also be considered a 'red flag' in presurgical assessment cannot yet be determined.

Lissencephaly

There are few reports in the literature of focal surgery for lissencephaly or pachygyria, and none give adequate histological details. Lissencephaly is usually too extensive an abnormality, associated with too severe a phenotype, to allow focal resection. No data are available from *in vivo* depth recordings from lissencephaly, and animal models have not been studied from this viewpoint. Given the recent discovery of genetic mutations underlying lissencephaly [65,66], suggesting widespread neuronal involvement by the mutation, it would not be surprising if epileptogenicity, or at least extensive secondary connectional involvement, were not widespread. Pathophysiological parallels with other brain malformations are therefore likely.

Polymicrogyria and schizencephaly

There are few published cases of surgical treatment of epilepsy in polymicrogyric brain malformations. Brodtkorb *et al.* [67] report on excision of a region of polymicrogyria (the completeness of excision was not stated). Over the 10-month follow-up period, the seizures continued unchanged, as did the specific scalp EEG picture, leading the authors to question whether the histologically abnormal, resected brain malformation was indeed the source of the seizures. Hashizume *et al.* [68] raise similar issues in a child with localized pachygyria and polymicrogyria. As with FCD, the possibility exists that the surrounding cortex is not entirely normal, even if it appears to be so on high-resolution neuroimaging. Thus, in a childhood hemispherectomy specimen with polymicrogyria as the dominant pathology, non-contiguous, distant occult brain malformations have also been demonstrated. The extraordinary connectivity in the human brain makes this likely to be a common phenomenon in brain malformations, as it is in animal studies.

In the best animal model of polymicrogyria, the abnormal cortex has excitability changes compatible with intrinsic epileptogenesis [69], but transaction experiments demonstrate that it is the apparently normal-appearing cortex surrounding a microgyrus, rather than the malformed cortex, that is epileptogenic [70]. In some cases, identical excitability changes in surrounding histologically normal cortex, with extensive molecular changes, have also been shown suggesting that 'cortical dysplastic lesions induce long-term functional alterations in structurally normal brain regions'. Thus polymicrogyria may be the mark of a brain that has suffered an insult, and may help localize a visually occult epileptogenic region,

but may not itself be epileptogenic. A poor outcome with resection of the MRI-visible abnormality should therefore not be entirely surprising. If adjacent functional regions are normal on imaging and inspection, and not studied by ECoG, or are suppressed by more active regions, then poor outcome might be explained even when the visible abnormality and regions harbouring abnormal corticographic activity are excised.

Schizencephaly is amongst the rarest of brain malformations. It is characterized by a cleft extending through the thickness of the cortex, lined by polymicrogyria. Its aetiology may be genetic [71]. There are currently no functional animal models of schizencephaly, but by inference from polymicrogyria, schizencephaly may not be intrinsically epileptogenic. Other areas of the brain may be histologically abnormal [72]. It is intriguing that of the few cases reported in the literature, in most the cleft itself was not completely excised. Significantly improved seizure control was achieved in four cases by excision of adjacent epileptogenic tissue identified by ECoG or extraoperative intracranial studies [73,74]; another case remained seizure free for 5 years after extralesional temporal lobectomy [75]. In another case [76], the lips of the cleft were excised, under electrocorticographic guidance, and a seizure-free outcome achieved over the 1 year follow-up period. In Hashizume *et al.*'s case [68], the implication is that the epileptogenic zone may have been distant from the schizencephaly, though this is not stated explicitly.

Therefore, visible polymicrogyria and schizencephaly may indicate, rather than contain, the critical part of the epileptogenic zone. However, even with local exploration using corticography, the entire extent of the brain malformation may not be revealed, and other means are still required to identify the true extent.

Dysembryoplastic neuroepithelial tumour

DNTs are cortically based lesions, with specific histological and radiological features, responsible for refractory epilepsy, and considered by some to be a 'neoplastic derivative from cortical matrix' rather than purely a hamartoma. However, published imaging and pathological features leave the origin of DNTs obscure. That they are probably developmental is supported by their existence as early as 2 weeks of life [77], thinning or indenting of the calvarium and the association with reorganized cortical function [78]. The coexistence of FCD (in most cases, [79–87]), neuronal heterotopia [86], microdysgenesis [88] and neurofibromatosis [89] support a developmental origin. The variety of positions in which DNTs have been detected (hippocampus alone, basal ganglia, third ventricle, pons, cerebellum [81, 86, 90–93]) supports the suggestion that they probably originate from secondary germinal layers [87]. However, the condition is included in this chapter as its study may contribute to an understanding of epilepsy surgery in brain malformations in general. Marked in general by benignity, surgery offers effective epilepsy treatment; adjunctive chemotherapy or radiotherapy are unnecessary [79]. There are some 200 cases published, most conforming to this stereotype. The diagnostic spectrum has been widened, criteria emphasizing clinical rather than histological aspects [87]. Most cases, however, probably remain unreported, because recognition is simple and treatment effective.

DNTs usually cause localization-related epilepsy before the age of 20 years. Neurological signs are absent, or minor and stable (e.g. [80,94]). The epilepsy is almost always refractory to drug treatment, notwithstanding reporting bias. There are characteristic findings on neuroimaging [87]. DNTs may be associated with other epileptogenic abnormalities.

Findings with respect to epileptogenesis are variable. Surgical treatment very commonly renders patients seizure free (158/187 cases seizure free at 1 year; 53/60 cases free at 2 years; review of English language literature to 2001), suggesting the DNT is necessary for epileptogenesis. However, EEG, electrocorticographic and magnetoencephalographic findings are contradictory [85,99], with at least one reported case in which DNT resection failed to render a patient seizure free, and in whom postoperative studies suggested perilesional seizure onset [96]. These are incomplete and unexplained findings. Remarkably, the extent of resection of the DNT and the presence of additional pathologies appear not to influence outcome, in stark contrast to outcome for other malformations treated surgically [15,80,86,97–99]. The reason for this intriguing finding is unknown, but merits further study, particularly as a variable finding in some studies has been the identification of malformation (microdysgenesis, glioneuronal hamartia or microdysgenetic nodules) and occasionally grey matter heterotopias and cortical dysplasia with giant neurones [86,87] in the adjacent resected cortex. Overall, surgery remains an effective treatment for DNT causing refractory epilepsy. Resection should be as complete as anatomy allows, not least because of reports of haemorrhagic transformation [100] and one reported case of late malignant transformation [101].

Discussion

Epileptogenesis is a complex and largely mysterious process. The basis of epileptogenesis even in HS remains unclear. Undoubtedly, the sclerosed hippocampus itself is involved in the disease process. Hippocampal resection is associated with cessation of seizures in approximately 70% of patients, but this does not imply that epileptogenesis and the epileptogenic zone are encapsulated within the diseased hippocampus. Indeed, the clinical manifestations of epilepsy associated with HS argue against a strictly localized disease process. Moreover, neuroimaging reveals a variety of subtle abnormalities in addition to atrophy of the hippocampus alone. The presence of these unsuspected additional changes may be associated with a poorer outcome after surgery. These additional changes may be part of the underlying primary disease process or its consequence. There is, of course, the possibility that at least some component of HS itself is developmental rather than acquired in origin [51,102], and that the visualized hippocampal atrophy is just the most visible part of a more widespread abnormality [103]. Therefore, dysfunction, including epileptogenesis, may be distributed in some patients with HS. Gloor [104] hypothesized that persistent experiential auras after temporal lobectomy might be due to 'distributed matrices' capable of maintaining the substance of an aura even after resection of part of a network responsible for its generation. Using stimulation experiments in patients undergoing preoperative intracranial recordings, Fish et al. [11] rigorously confirmed that the same aura could be generated by stimulation in physically disparate and electrically distinct sites. That seizures might also be generated in a similarly distributed network was not discussed, but remains possible. A network of neurones, distributed non-contiguously in the brain, may be involved in the generation of seizures. The evidence is, however, circumstantial, and there is little direct proof. Surprisingly little is written about postoperative findings in patients who fail to become seizure free after surgery.

The conceptual link between surgical failure blamed on a distributed epileptogenic zone and widespread structural abnormalities is easily made. Mesial temporal resection might be sufficient to inactivate a distributed epileptogenic zone without complete resection of the entire zone in most cases but may not be sufficient to inactivate a more distributed epileptogenic zone. Indeed, many patients who have mesial temporal resection remain antiepileptic drug dependent. Time, too, may be a variable. Resection may remove enough of the epileptogenic zone to render a patient seizure free for a certain period, but given sufficient time, the remainder of a distributed epileptogenic zone may reorganize, causing seizure recrudescence [45]. The epileptogenic zone should be conceptualized as having both spatial and temporal dimensions.

There is obvious spatially distributed pathology in cases of HS with dual pathology. In general, it is known that when lesions are present, their removal is fundamental to a successful outcome (e.g. [58,105]. For dual pathology cases, removal of one lesion is not usually sufficient to render that patient seizure free [49]; removal of both abnormalities, where possible, is a better option [58]. Raymond et al. [56] identified localized areas of brain malformations in 15% of patients with MRI or histological evidence of hippocampal sclerosis. In 25% of patients with MRI-identified brain malformations significant hippocampal asymmetry was found [57], whilst in a large retrospectively studied pathological series, 15% had brain malformations and a second pathology [106]. Ho et al. [107], studying patients with temporal lobe brain malformations, demonstrated a very high proportion (87%) of patients with either unilateral or bilateral dual pathologies. The possibility of dual pathology makes hippocampal volume and T2 measurements necessary for all patients with brain malformations being assessed for epilepsy surgery.

In terms of epileptogenesis, the distinction between overt 'dual pathology' and occult widespread pathology is artificial. Distributed occult brain malformations in addition to overt brain malformations could thus account for poor seizure outcome in some instances. This returns to the issue of what actually constitutes the epileptogenic zone in brain malformations. The most parsimonious working definition is that the epileptogenic zone in brain malformations is that region which when excised leads to freedom from seizures over a defined period of follow-up. The latter addition to the definition is important: some patients who are initially seizure free may develop seizures without a second precipitating factor after some years. The dynamic and distributed properties of epileptogenesis in brain malformations can be reflected in the results of tests currently used to identify the epileptogenic zone, can manifest as non-concordant or widespread abnormalities at one time (e.g. [15,42,108–110]), or can manifest as changing abnormalities over time (e.g. [23,111]). The epileptogenic zone in brain malformations may also be a changing spatiotemporal entity—possibly with different properties in different brain malformations. Spatially distributed epileptogenesis may form a hierarchical network: the most active part, the 'pacemaker', may also be the most visually apparent, whilst other occult components form the rest of the network, and may be normally entrained by the pacemaker, as suggested by Awad *et al.* [112]. Excision of the most active area of a brain malformation may release the rest of an epileptogenic network. The human cardiac conducting system is, of course, an excellent example of this behaviour. In summary, for many types of brain malformations, at any one time the complete epileptogenic zone may be more widespread than the visualized abnormality, even if the most active part of the epileptogenic zone is for most of the time contained within the visualized abnormality. The structural basis of such systems may be the widespread histological change reported in some brain malformations (see above).

If the epileptogenic zone in brain malformations is a distributed spatiotemporal entity, how can its true extent be determined? How also can the proportion of the epileptogenic zone that needs to be removed to stop seizures be established? To date, the presence of persistent epileptogenic brain malformation tissue has been *assumed* in cases of surgical failure (e.g. [36,112–115]). Widespread histological examination of the brain is rarely feasible, as resections are necessarily minimized. Only in a few cases has there been histological proof of extensive abnormalities—and this is usually by chance [116].

History, seizure semiology and clinical examination are not able to identify the full extent of brain malformations in most cases. Investigations are required. These include EEG, MRI, PET and SPECT. Scalp EEG findings in patients with brain malformations are diverse [110], often showing widespread or multifocal interictal spiking, and tend to poorly localize ictal onset. Raymond *et al.* [9] reported focal or lateralized interictal epileptiform discharges on scalp EEG in only 51/100 patients with localized brain malformations. Epileptiform discharges were often more widespread and sometimes only evident at sites separate from that anticipated by clinical features or imaging. Palmini *et al.* [113] reported preoperative scalp EEGs in 30 patients with focal brain malformations. Only one-third had EEG findings suggesting abnormalities confined to one lobe. Half the patients had multilobar interictal spiking, three patients had bitemporal and two generalized interictal abnormalities. Of 12 patients with apparently localized brain malformations reported by Hirabayashi *et al.* [117], only four showed localized interictal spiking. Kuzniecky *et al.* [118] reported predominantly unilateral spiking in eight of 10 patients with temporal lobe brain malformations. However in patients with frontal lobe brain malformations, only two of 11 showed focal spiking. These scalp EEG studies therefore demonstrate a high incidence of widespread interictal spiking in patients with focal brain malformations. Scalp EEG changes in some patients demonstrating recurrent, reasonably well localized or at least lateralized, continuous or near-continuous runs of interictal spikes [9,119,120] presumably reflect hyperexcitability of underlying cortex, but do not exclude more widespread abnormalities.

The worrying non-congruence of EEG abnormalities and structural changes may be due to the limitations of scalp EEG, or the complex anatomy of brain malformations, with modulation of epileptiform discharges before reaching the surface. Focal ictal or interictal scalp EEG changes have rarely been used as the sole guide to the identification of the epileptogenic zone in brain malformations. Most authors have concluded that scalp EEG studies do not correlate significantly with outcome [23,49,117] particularly with regard to ictal scalp EEG in brain malformations in infants [121].

As some patients have become seizure free despite extensive scalp EEG changes, such findings should not preclude further presurgical evaluation. Thus some authors have altogether stopped attempting to relate outcome to scalp EEG results [18].

The role of intracranial recordings remains uncertain and in need of clarification. As some brain malformations show intrinsic epileptogenicity ([37,41]; see below), detailed neurophysiological investigations should theoretically be helpful. Though many authors suggest that chronic subdural findings do not correlate with outcome (e.g. [117,121,122]), there are insufficient published data to determine the place of chronic subdural recordings alone in management. ECoG is widely used to guide resections intraoperatively [35,44,48,121–125]. Most centres employ ECoG in locations identified by preoperative clinical and MRI findings, precluding evaluation of ECoG alone. Palmini *et al.* [37] recorded 'ictal/continuous epileptogenic discharges (I/CEDs)' from the surface of brain malformation cortex, and in some cases from surrounding cortex that appeared normal on inspection, but was subsequently proven histologically to harbour brain malformations. Completeness of resection of the cortex evincing I/CEDs, as demonstrated by disappearance of the I/CEDs on postoperative ECoG, was correlated with a significantly better outcome. However, 9/12 patients showing disappearance of such ECoG abnormalities did not have an excellent (Engel class I) outcome, and the disappearance of interictal spiking on ECoG did not predict a seizure free outcome. The value of I/CEDs in defining the epileptogenic zone thus remains unclear. Ferrier *et al.* [48], studying pathologies including FCD, confirmed that ECoG-detected spikes and loss of spikes after surgery is not predictive of good outcome, whereas abolition of ECoG-detected 'seizure patterns' is. The authors suggest ECoG may thus help in the identification of epileptogenic regions intraoperatively. Similarly, ECoG studies in some patients with schizencephaly actually guided resections away from the visualized brain malformations to electrically more active regions, with, in all cases, more than 80% reduction in seizure frequency for at least a year of follow-up [68,73,74].

Chronic intracranial recordings may show independent epileptiform activity in brain malformations and, in addition, spreading activity from other epileptogenic tissue (e.g. coexistent HS), and changes emanating from normal-appearing regions (e.g. [50,51,61]). Bautista *et al.* [40] raise the possibility that chronic interictal recordings might better predict outcome than other measures in extratemporal epilepsy, on the basis that even modern neuroimaging methods do not necessarily reveal all the pathology present. Although seizure-free rates following the use of intracranial EEG for localization have thus in a few reports been associated with a high seizure-free rate postoperatively (e.g. 64% in [126]: 18/28 of 500 corticectomy patients), such recording cannot access large areas of the brain, and an epileptogenic zone might thus not be completely revealed. Intracranial recording obviously is also limited by risks of associated morbidity and mortality. All intracranial recordings suffer from limited spatial sampling: they can only provide information from recorded regions, not from unsampled areas. Thus in the report of Li *et al.* [49], intracranial electrode studies were in fact deceptive, leading to unsuccessful temporal resections whilst associated brain malformations were rarely recorded from and consequently usually left unresected. These findings suggest the presence in some cases of more than one epileptogenic focus.

MRI permits the detection of brain malformations in many cases, and has obvious potential in identifying the true extent of brain malformations—and the degree of their resection. However, it is difficult to judge the impact of modern MRI techniques on outcome, as few studies address this question specifically. Some studies state that completeness of resection was judged using postoperative imaging [18,127]. There are reports of complete excision according to MRI not being associated with a seizure-free outcome (e.g. [7]), attributed variously to 'inaccuracy in method of quantitating lesion resection' [127], or the presence of MRI-occult pathology [37,114]. In the most comprehensive series (from the Cleveland Clinic [18]), extent of completeness of resection was judged by comparison of pre- and postoperative MRI data. A seizure-free outcome was achieved in 58% with complete resection, *and* in 27% of those with incomplete resection. This is the first large series using modern MRI methods to report on outcome with respect to completeness of resection in brain malformations. The benefit to patients of a good outcome, including possibly rare, non-disabling seizures, cannot be denied, and it is of great interest that some patients with multilobar involvement became seizure free. However, long-term follow-up is essential. In particular, it would appear that there remain patients (42% in this report) with apparently complete resection as judged by MRI who failed to become seizure free, and patients with incomplete resection who became seizure free, and it is from these groups that most stands to be learnt. Whilst the postoperative findings in the complete resection group will be of interest, it remains possible that even standard high-resolution MRI may fail to reveal the entire extent of a brain malformation, so that in some cases not all the pathology is resected. In addition, current structural MRI methods cannot identify which structural changes are actually epileptogenic.

There is little doubt that PET can identify brain malformations [8]: this has often been histologically verified (e.g. [121,128]). In paediatric practice PET may have a clinical role, revealing abnormalities that are otherwise difficult to detect, and leading to successful surgical intervention in a number of cases [121,128]. MRI was reported to be normal in many of these cases. It is not clear to what extent this would still be the case if state-of-the-art high-resolution scanners were employed, though, in a limited number of cases, it appears that flumazenil PET may support these findings in patients who have had high-resolution MRI [96]. In adults, there has been very little work demonstrating the utility of PET in presurgical evaluation. Most patients studied by PET have not proceeded to surgery. In a recent large series [108], both flumazenil and fluorodeoxyglucose (FDG) PET were normal in two patients with minute or subcortical brain malformations, and both PET scans showed multilobar involvement in a case with FCD, who was seizure free over a 2-year follow-up after a simple lesionectomy. In two other unoperated patients with mesial occipital brain malformations, both flumazenil and FDG-PET results were concordant with MRI and intracranial studies. Only more detailed flumazenil PET studies, of the type undertaken by Juhasz *et al.* [96] correlated with MRI and surgical outcome, can determine whether PET can identify a distributed epileptogenic zone.

SPECT has been shown to aid in the localization of the seizure focus in presurgical evaluation for epilepsy surgery (e.g. [129]). Though patterns of cerebral blood flow have been well documented in mesial temporal lobe epilepsy (MTLE) [130], studies may not be so reliable in extratemporal epilepsy, particularly if the injection is not truly ictal [130]. It can be more difficult to achieve ictal injections in extratemporal epilepsy because there may not be an aura of useful length, and the seizures themselves may be shorter. It is imperative that such studies are performed with concomitant video-EEG monitoring, as any delay in injection may mean the results show seizure spread rather than seizure onset. Few patients with brain malformations have been studied. Series to date concentrate more on localization of seizure onset than on underlying pathology. However, where data are available, seizures arising from brain malformations usually demonstrate an area of hyperperfusion concordant with the lesion following an ictal injection [123,131]. SPECT may be particularly useful if MRI is normal or inconclusive, ictal hyperperfusion compared to interictal hypoperfusion raising the possibility of brain malformations. In extratemporal epilepsy, SPECT may provide a guide to invasive monitoring. Data available from SPECT may be enhanced by the use of computerized subtraction and MRI-coregistration techniques (SISCOM; [109]). SPECT data must be examined in conjunction with data from other investigations, with an awareness of the spatial resolution of SPECT. SPECT is a complementary method, helping to define the epileptogenic zone rather than being of critical importance. In O'Brien *et al.*'s series [109], three patients with brain malformations are reported; in two SISCOM results were concordant with MRI, but in another patient, the SISCOM results were discordant with both scalp EEG and MRI. As with all new methods, it is not always clear what the results mean, and whether they identify the epileptogenic zone or reflect epiphenomena.

No current technique defines the epileptogenic zone in brain malformations reliably enough to guarantee a successful surgical outcome, echoing Engel's general statement [10]. Even with the best current guide, high-resolution structural imaging with intraoperative ECoG, it is evident that apparent complete resection, though probably necessary for a good outcome, does not guarantee such an outcome, probably reflecting still more widespread distribution of the epileptogenic zone, which it may not be possible to sample at operation.

More work thus needs to be undertaken to detect the full extent of brain malformations for surgery, but with the biology of brain malformations in mind. There are many ways of examining the whole extent of the cortex preoperatively. Some methods may allow detection of a potentially distributed epileptogenic zone. The widespread nature of scalp EEG changes in a high proportion of patients with brain malformations has been discussed. Though a few papers suggest that widespread changes are associated with a poor outcome, a thorough analysis, for example on all the cases in Table 63.1, is not currently possible, but would seem worthwhile. New tools for the determination of potential coherence of multifocal interictal and ictal changes are becoming available, both for the temporal [132] and spatial aspects of distribution (e.g. objective quantitative neuroimaging methods). Detailed analysis of single cases may show that such phenomena do exist and may stimulate more extensive study. The spatial resolution of scalp EEG can be enhanced by the use of a 64-channel systems. Ideally, EEG or functional imaging would be performed after reversible presurgical inactivation of the postulated focus alone. This cannot currently be achieved, but intracarotid amylobarbital tests offer the chance of studying with EEG other parts of postulated networks—without the influence of the dominant lesion and other brain regions supplied by either the middle or posterior cerebral arteries. Neuroimaging methods alone may demonstrate widespread changes and rarely these have been shown to be of biological relevance. Though PET may demonstrate MRI-occult subtle abnormalities (e.g. [128]), and the role of PET has not yet been fully considered, the increasing expense and limited availability of PET, even in epilepsy surgery centres, may mean that its role will never become fully defined.

The recent development of *in vivo* imaging of interictal epileptiform activity may provide further information [133], especially if data are continuously acquired and analysed, bearing the possibility of distributed malfunction in mind. Magnetic source imaging can provide another means of examining distributed hierarchical networks [42], especially if preconceived models of focal onset are not used to study real data. Although many of these methods are not widely available, a period of comprehensive evaluation in a cohort of patients might establish which test is most discriminatory in specific types of brain malformations. Sugimoto *et al.* [134] report that in some cases, reoperation for brain malformations can improve outcome: it may be that additional investigative methods can be used on cases that have failed to become seizure free with a view to more complete excision of epileptogenic pathology, and a better understanding of epileptogenesis.

The operational significance of additional abnormalities shown by these tests can only be determined by correlation with prolonged outcome measures. Perhaps only a proportion of patients with brain malformations can ever be helped by surgery, if for example the distribution of changes is too widespread for current surgical methods to tackle. In this case, the purpose of further study must be to identify the patients who will actually benefit from surgery. If newer surgical methods are developed, such studies might also help to direct their application. The importance of prolonged follow-up is clear. A central registry of cases might fulfil this need, facilitating assiduous reporting that need not depend on either follow-up at a tertiary referral facility or limited reporting opportunities. There are too few cases in the literature: a central registry would also help to build up the numbers of patients being studied.

Despite all these factors, surgery for epilepsy associated with brain malformations can render about half of patients currently seizure free, at least as judged by the literature. Questions remain of whether selection could be improved so that surgery can be offered to those most likely to benefit and perhaps to more people with brain malformations overall. Recent advances in the biological understanding of brain malformations, particularly at pathological and genetic levels, should contribute significantly to improved surgical management.

Recommendations

In order to improve surgical outcome, the following will eventually need to be considered.

1 Identification of the true extent of the epileptogenic components—this is likely to necessitate a combined structural and functional imaging approach, with initial correlation with surgical and pathological findings.

2 Determination of what fraction of the epileptogenic network needs removal or disconnection to stop the epilepsy.

3 Continue long-term complete data collection—we know relatively little about its long-term postoperative history.

Detailed postoperative study of cases that have not become seizure free is vital to achieve these aims. These cases receive the least attention, yet may have the most to offer in terms of extending our understanding.

For current practice, the following recommendations can be made.

1 For all patients undergoing surgical treatment, the minimum presurgical assessment necessitates: a detailed personal and family history; clinical examination; characterization of seizure semiology; scalp EEG recordings, including ictal videotelemetric recordings, and high-resolution multisequence MRI—at our institution: on a 1.5 T scanner: 256×192 matrix on a 24.0/18.0 cm field of view: sagittal T1-weighted (TE/TR 14/620 ms, 5.0/2.5 mm slices); coronal VEMP (TE1/TE2/TR 30/120/2000, 5.0/0.0 mm slices); coronal FSPGR (TE/TI/TR 4.2/450/15.5, flip 20 degrees, 1.5/0.0 mm slices); coronal Fast FLAIR (TE/TI/TR 144/260/11000, 5.0/0.0 mm slices). Hippocampal volumetry and T2 measures in all patients being considered for surgery.

2 Identification of the type of brain malformation by detailed scrutiny of high-resolution images, including multiplanar reformatting and three-dimensional rendering of cortical surface.

3 Additionally, for specific types of brain malformations:

(a) FCD: quantitative MRI analyses of the cerebral hemispheres; functional imaging (EEG-fMRI, fMRI activation studies; flumazenil PET); intraoperative ECoG;

(b) PVH: as above, with particular emphasis on identification of additional abnormalities and *filamin 1* mutation analysis in sporadic or familial bilateral nodular PVNH. Genetic counselling will be necessary before any genetic testing is undertaken;

(c) SH: as above, but with special attention paid to the total extent of heterotopia, using high-resolution MRI and postprocessing tools (e.g. three-dimensional reformatting); genetic counselling, genetic testing and MRI scans of appropriately selected relatives may be necessary. Intracranial EEG studies may be required and false localization should be considered—the heterotopia should be included in the study, as should overlying cortex even if it appears normal on imaging;

(d) polymicrogyria, schizencephaly: as for FCD. The perilesional area requires careful examination as it may be a more important component of the epileptogenic zone; and

(e) DNT: adequate definition of the extent of DNT by high-resolution MRI.

In addition, for all cases, histological examination of the resection specimen and careful study of the resection margins is essential. Follow-up extending over at least 2 years is required. Detailed study of cases not rendered seizure free may be most informative, and reporting to a central registry may facilitate comprehensive follow-up and the study of more cases.

References

1 Li LM, Fish DR, Sisodiya SM, Shorvon SD, Alsanjari N, Stevens JM. High resolution magnetic resonance imaging in adults with partial or second-

ary generalised epilepsy attending a tertiary referral unit. *J Neurol Neurosurg Psychiatr* 1995; 59: 384–7.

2 Semah F, Picot MC, Adam C *et al*. Is the underlying cause of epilepsy a major prognostic factor for recurrence? [see comments]. *Neurology* 1998; 51: 1256–2.

3 Brodtkorb E, Nilsen G, Smevik O, Rinck PA. Epilepsy and anomalies of neuronal migration: MRI and clinical aspects. *Acta Neurol Scand* 1992; 86: 24–32.

4 Steffenburg U, Hedstrom A, Lindroth A, Wiklund LM, Hagberg G, Kyllerman M. Intractable epilepsy in a population-based series of mentally retarded children. *Epilepsia* 1998; 39: 767–75.

5 Everitt AD, Birnie KD, Stevens JM, Sander JW, Duncan JS, Shorvon SD. The NSE MRI study: structural brain abnormalities in adult epilepsy patients and healthy controls. *Epilepsia* 1998; 39 (Suppl. 6): 140.

6 Ying Z, Babb TL, Comair YG, Bingaman W, Bushey M, Touhalisky K. Induced expression of NMDAR2 proteins and differential expression of NMDAR1 splice variants in dysplastic neurons of human epileptic neocortex. *J Neuropathol Exp Neurol* 1998; 57: 47–62.

7 Spreafico R, Pasquier B, Minotti L *et al*. Immunocytochemical investigation on dysplastic human tissue from epileptic patients. *Epilepsy Res* 1998; 32: 34–48.

8 Duncan JS. Imaging and epilepsy. *Brain* 1997; 120 (Pt 2): 339–77.

9 Raymond AA, Fish DR, Sisodiya SM, Alsanjari N, Stevens JM, Shorvon SD. Abnormalities of gyration, heterotopias, tuberous sclerosis, focal cortical dysplasia, microdysgenesis, dysembryoplastic neuroepithelial tumour and dysgenesis of the archicortex in epilepsy. Clinical, EEG and neuroimaging features in 100 adult patients. *Brain* 1995; 118 (Pt 3): 629–60.

10 Engel J Jr. Surgery for seizures. *N Engl J Med* 1996; 334: 647–52.

11 Fish DR, Gloor P, Quesney LF, Olivier A. Clinical responses to electrical brain stimulation of the temporal and frontal lobes in patients with epilepsy. Pathophysiological implications. *Brain* 1993; 116: 397–414.

12 Baxendale SA, Sisodiya SM, Thompson PJ *et al*. Disproportion in the distribution of gray and white matter: neuropsychological correlates. *Neurology* 1999; 52: 248–52.

13 DeCarli C, Hatta J, Fazilat S, Fazilat S, Gaillard WD, Theodore WH. Extratemporal atrophy in patients with complex partial seizures of left temporal origin. *Ann Neurol* 1998; 43: 41–5.

14 Lee JW, Andermann F, Dubeau F *et al*. Morphometric analysis of the temporal lobe in temporal lobe epilepsy. *Epilepsia* 1998; 39: 727–36.

15 Sisodiya SM, Moran N, Free SL *et al*. Correlation of widespread preoperative magnetic resonance imaging changes with unsuccessful surgery for hippocampal sclerosis. *Ann Neurol* 1997; 41: 490–6.

16 Engel J Jr, Van Ness PC, Rasmussen TB, Ojemann LM. Outcome with respect to epileptic seizures. In: Engel J Jr, ed. *Surgical Treatment of the Epilepsies*. New York: Raven Press, 1993: 609–21.

17 Berkovic SF, McIntosh AM, Kalnins RM *et al*. Preoperative MRI predicts outcome of temporal lobectomy: an actuarial analysis. *Neurology* 1995; 45: 1358–63.

18 Edwards JC, Wyllie E, Ruggeri PM *et al*. Seizure outcome after surgery for epilepsy due to malformation of cortical development. *Neurology* 2000; 55: 1110–14.

19 Sperling MR, O'Connor MJ, Saykin AJ, Plummer C. Temporal lobectomy for refractory epilepsy. *JAMA* 1996; 276: 470–5.

20 Paillas JE, Gastaut H, Sedan R, Bureau M. Long-term results of conventional surgical treatment for epilepsy. Delayed recurrence after a period of 10 years. *Surg Neurol* 1983; 20: 189–93.

21 Bruton CJ. *Neuropathology of Temporal Lobe Epilepsy*. Oxford: Oxford University Press, 1988.

22 Gilliam F, Wyllie E, Kashden J *et al*. Epilepsy surgery outcome: comprehensive assessment in children. *Neurology* 1997; 48: 1368–74.

23 Döring S, Cross H, Boyd S, Harkness W, Neville B. The significance of bilateral EEG abnormalities before and after hemispherectomy in children with unilateral major hemisphere lesions. *Epilepsy Res* 1999; 34: 65–73.

24 Guerrini R, Andermann F, Canapicchi R, Roger J, Zifkin BG, Pfanner P eds. *Dysplasias of Cerebral Cortex and Epilepsy*. New York: Lippincott-Raven, 1996.

25 Spreafico R, Tassi L, Colombo N *et al*. Inhibitory circuits in human dysplastic tissue. *Epilepsia* 2000; 41 (Suppl. 6): S168–S173.

26 Brown MC, Levin BE, Ramsay RE, Landy HJ. Comprehensive evaluation of left hemisphere type I schizencephaly. *Arch Neurol* 1993; 50: 667–9.

27 Raymond AA, Jones SJ, Fish DR, Stewart J, Stevens JM. Somatosensory evoked potentials in adults with cortical dysgenesis and epilepsy. *Electroencephalogr Clin Neurophysiol* 1997; 104: 132–42.

28 Leblanc R, Robitaille Y, Andermann F, Ptito A. Retained language in dysgenic cortex: case report. *Neurosurgery* 1995; 37: 992–7.

29 Duchowny M, Jayakar P, Harvey AS *et al*. Language cortex representation: effects of developmental versus acquired pathology. *Ann Neurol* 1996; 40: 31–8.

30 Hatazawa J, Sasajima T, Shimosegawa E *et al*. Regional cerebral blood flow response in gray matter heterotopia during finger tapping: an activation study with positron emission tomography. *Am J Neuroradiol* 1996; 17: 479–82.

31 Richardson MP, Koepp MJ, Brooks DJ, Duncan JS. ^{11}C-flumazenil PET in neocortical epilepsy. *Neurology* 1998; 51: 485–92.

32 Pinard J, Feydy A, Carlier R, Perez N, Pierot L, Burnod Y. Functional MRI in double cortex: functionality of heterotopia. *Neurology* 2000; 54: 1531–3.

33 Gondo K, Kira H, Tokunaga Y *et al*. Reorganization of the primary somatosensory area in epilepsy associated with focal cortical dysplasia. [In Process Citation]. *Dev Med Child Neurol* 2000; 42: 839–42.

34 Preul MC, Leblanc R, Cendes F *et al*. Function and organization in dysgenic cortex. Case report. *J Neurosurg* 1997; 87: 113–21.

35 Desbiens R, Berkovic SF, Dubeau F *et al*. Life-threatening focal status epilepticus due to occult cortical dysplasia. *Arch Neurol* 1993; 50: 695–700.

36 Taylor DC, Falconer MA, Bruton CJ, Corsellis JA. Focal dysplasia of the cerebral cortex in epilepsy. *J Neurol Neurosurg Psychiatr* 1971; 34: 369–87.

37 Palmini A, Gambardella A, Andermann F *et al*. Intrinsic epileptogenicity of human dysplastic cortex as suggested by corticography and surgical results. *Ann Neurol* 1995; 37: 476–87.

38 Ying Z, Babb TL, Mikuni N, Najm I, Drazba J, Bingaman W. Selective co-expression of NMDAR2A/B and NMDAR1 subunit proteins in dysplastic neurons of human epileptic cortex. *Exp Neurol* 1999; 159: 409–18.

39 Rosenow F, Luders HO, Dinner DS *et al*. Histopathological correlates of epileptogenicity as expressed by electrocorticographic spiking and seizure frequency. *Epilepsia* 1998; 39: 850–6.

40 Bautista RE, Cobbs MA, Spencer DD, Spencer SS. Prediction of surgical outcome by interictal epileptiform abnormalities during intracranial EEG monitoring in patients with extrahippocampal seizures. *Epilepsia* 1999; 40: 880–90.

41 Avoli M, Bernasconi A, Mattia D, Olivier A, Hwa GG. Epileptiform discharges in the human dysplastic neocortex: in vitro physiology and pharmacology. *Ann Neurol* 1999; 46: 816–26.

42 Morioka T, Nishio S, Ishibashi H *et al*. Intrinsic epileptogenicity of focal cortical dysplasia as revealed by magnetoencephalography and electrocorticography. *Epilepsy Res* 1999; 33: 177–87.

43 White R, Hua Y, Scheithauer B, Lynch DR, Henske EP, Crino PB. Selective alterations in glutamate and GABA receptor subunit mRNA expression in dysplastic neurons and giant cells of cortical tubers. *Ann Neurol* 2001; 49: 67–78.

44 Chan S, Chin SS, Nordli DR, Goodman RR, DeLaPaz RL, Pedley TA. Prospective magnetic resonance imaging identification of focal cortical dysplasia, including the non-balloon cell subtype. *Ann Neurol* 1998; 44: 749–57.

45 Barkovich AJ, Rowley HA, Andermann F. MR in partial epilepsy: value of high-resolution volumetric techniques. *Am J Neuroradiol* 1995; 16: 339–43.

46 Bastos AC, Comeau RM, Andermann F *et al*. Diagnosis of subtle focal dysplastic lesions: curvilinear reformatting from three-dimensional magnetic resonance imaging. *Ann Neurol* 1999; 46: 88–94.

47 Bernasconi A, Antel SB, Collins DL *et al*. Texture analysis and morphological processing of magnetic resonance imaging assist detection of focal cortical dysplasia in extra-temporal partial epilepsy. *Ann Neurol* 2001; 49(6): 770–5.

48 Ferrier CH, Alarcon G, Engelsman J *et al*. Relevance of residual histologic and electrocorticographic abnormalities for surgical outcome in frontal lobe epilepsy. *Epilepsia* 2001; 42: 363–71.

49 Li LM, Dubeau F, Andermann F *et al*. Periventricular nodular heterotopia and intractable temporal lobe epilepsy: poor outcome after temporal lobe resection. *Ann Neurol* 1997; 41: 662–8.

50 Dubeau F, Tampieri D, Lee N *et al*. Periventricular and subcortical nodular heterotopia. A study of 33 patients. *Brain* 1995; 118 (Pt 5): 1273–87.

51 Kothare SV, VanLandingham K, Armon C, Luther JS, Friedman A, Radtke RA. Seizure onset from periventricular nodular heterotopias: depth-electrode study. *Neurology* 1998; 51: 1723–7.

52 Colacitti C, Sancini G, Franceschetti S *et al*. Altered connections between neocortical and heterotopic areas in methylazoxymethanol-treated rat. *Epilepsy Res* 1998; 32: 49–62.

53 Hannan AJ, Servotte S, Katsnelson A *et al*. Characterization of nodular neuronal heterotopia in children. *Brain* 1999; 122 (Pt 2): 219–38.

54 Raymond AA, Fish DR, Stevens JM *et al*. Subependymal heterotopia: a distinct neuronal migration disorder associated with epilepsy. *J Neurol Neurosurg Psychiatr* 1994; 57: 1195–202.

55 Fox JW, Lamperti ED, Eksioglu YZ *et al*. Mutations in filamin 1 prevent migration of cerebral cortical neurons in human periventricular heterotopia. *Neuron* 1998; 21: 1315–25.

56 Raymond AA, Fish DR, Stevens JM *et al*. Association of hippocampal sclerosis with cortical dysgenesis in patients with epilepsy. *Neurology* 1994; 44: 1841–5.

57 Cendes F, Cook MJ, Watson C *et al*. Frequency and characteristics of dual pathology in patients with lesional epilepsy. *Neurology* 1995; 45: 2058–64.

58 Li LM, Cendes F, Andermann F *et al*. Surgical outcome in patients with epilepsy and dual pathology. *Brain* 1999; 122 (Pt 5): 799–805.

59 Colacitti C, Sancini G, DeBiasi S *et al*. Prenatal methylazoxymethanol treatment in rats produces brain abnormalities with morphological similarities to human developmental brain dysgeneses. *J Neuropathol Exp Neurol* 1999; 58: 92–106.

60 Gleeson JG, Minnerath SR, Fox JW *et al*. Characterization of mutations in the gene *doublecortin* in patients with double cortex syndrome [see comments]. *Ann Neurol* 1999; 45: 146–53.

61 Francione S, Kahane P, Tassi L *et al*. Stereo-EEG of interictal and ictal electrical activity of a histologically proved heterotopic grey matter associated with partial epilepsy. *Electroencephal Clin Neurophysiol* 1994; 90: 284–90.

62 Lee KS, Schottler F, Collins JL *et al*. A genetic animal model of human neocortical heterotopia associated with seizures. *J Neurosci* 1997; 17: 6236–42.

63 Schottler F, Couture D, Rao A, Kahn H, Lee KS. Subcortical connections of normotopic and heterotopic neurons in sensory and motor cortices of the tish mutant rat. *J Comp Neurol* 1998; 395: 29–42.

64 Chen ZF, Schottler F, Bertram E, Gall CM, Anzivino MJ, Lee KS. Distribution and initiation of seizure activity in a rat brain with subcortical band heterotopia. *Epilepsia* 2000; 41: 493–501.

65 Reiner O, Carrozzo R, Shen Y *et al*. Isolation of a Miller-Dieker lissencephaly gene containing G protein beta-subunit-like repeats. *Nature* 1993; 364: 717–21.

66 Gleeson JG. Classical lissencephaly and double cortex (subcortical band heterotopia): LIS1 and doublecortin. *Curr Opin Neurol* 2000; 13: 121–5.

67 Brodtkorb E, Andersen K, Henriksen O, Myhr G, Skullerud K. Focal, continuous spikes suggest cortical developmental abnormalities. Clinical, MRI and neuropathological correlates. *Acta Neurol Scand* 1998; 98: 377–85.

68 Hashizume K, Kiriyama K, Kunimoto M *et al*. Correlation of EEG, neuroimaging and histopathology in an epilepsy patient with diffuse cortical dysplasia. *Child's Nerv Syst* 2000; 16: 75–9.

69 Redecker C, Lutzenburg M, Gressens P, Evrard P, Witte OW, Hagemann G. Excitability changes and glucose metabolism in experimentally induced focal cortical dysplasias. *Cereb Cortex* 1998; 8: 623–34.

70 Jacobs KM, Kharazia VN, Prince DA. Mechanisms underlying epileptogenesis in cortical malformations. *Epilepsy Res* 1999; 36: 165–88.

71 Brunelli S, Faiella A, Capra V *et al*. Germline mutations in the homeobox gene EMX2 in patients with severe schizencephaly. *Nat Genet* 1996; 12: 94–6.

72 Packard AM, Miller VS, Delgado MR. Schizencephaly: correlations of clinical and radiologic features. *Neurology* 1997; 48: 1427–34.

73 Leblanc R, Tampieri D, Robitaille Y, Feindel W, Andermann F. Surgical treatment of intractable epilepsy associated with schizencephaly. *Neurosurgery* 1991; 29: 421–9.

74 Landy HJ, Ramsay RE, Ajmone-Marsan C *et al*. Temporal lobectomy for seizures associated with unilateral schizencephaly. *Surg Neurol* 1992; 37: 477–81.

75 Silbergeld DL, Miller JW. Resective surgery for medically intractable epilepsy associated with schizencephaly. *J Neurosurg* 1994; 80: 820–5.

76 Maehara T, Shimizu H, Nakayama H, Oda M, Arai N. Surgical treatment of epilepsy from schizencephaly with fused lips. *Surg Neurol* 1997; 48: 507–10.

77 Neville BG, Harkness WF, Cross JH *et al*. Surgical treatment of severe autistic regression in childhood epilepsy. *Pediatr Neurol* 1997; 16: 137–40.

78 Devaux B, Chassoux F, Landre E *et al*. Chronic intractable epilepsy associated with a tumor located in the central region: functional mapping data and postoperative outcome. *Stereotact Funct Neurosurg* 1997; 69: 229–38.

79 Daumas-Duport C, Scheithauer BW, Chodkiewicz JP, Laws ER Jr, Vedrenne C. Dysembryoplastic neuroepithelial tumor: a surgically curable tumor of young patients with intractable partial seizures. Report of thirty-nine cases. *Neurosurgery* 1988; 23: 545–56.

80 Raymond AA, Fish DR, Boyd SG, Smith SJ, Pitt MC, Kendall B. Cortical dysgenesis: serial features in 16 patients. *Brain* 1994; 117 (Pt 3): 461–75.

81 Gottschalk J, Korves M, Skotzek-Konrad B, Goebel S, Cervos-Navarro J. Dysembryoplastic neuroepithelial micro-tumor in a 75-year-old patient with long-standing epilepsy. *Clin Neuropathol* 1993; 12: 175–8.

82 Prayson RA, Estes ML. Dysembryoplastic neuroepithelial tumor. *Am J Clin Pathol* 1992; 97: 398–401.

83 Prayson RA, Estes ML, Morris HH. Coexistence of neoplasia and cortical dysplasia in patients presenting with seizures. *Epilepsia* 1993; 34: 609–15.

84 Becker LE. Central neuronal tumors in childhood: relationship to dysplasia. *J Neurooncol* 1995; 24: 13–19.

85 Shimbo Y, Takahashi H, Hayano M, Kumagai T, Kameyama S. Temporal lobe lesion demonstrating features of dysembryoplastic neuroepithelial tumor and ganglioglioma: a transitional form? *Clin Neuropathol* 1997; 16: 65–8.

86 Honavar M, Janota I, Polkey CE. Histological heterogeneity of dysembryoplastic neuroepithelial tumour: identification and differential diagnosis in a series of 74 cases. *Histopathology* 1999; 34: 342–56.

87 Daumas-Duport C, Varlet P, Bacha S *et al*. Dysembryoplastic neuroepithelial tumors: nonspecific histological forms—a study of 40 cases. *J Neurooncol* 1999; 41: 267–80.

88 Rojiani AM, Emery JA, Anderson KJ, Massey JK. Distribution of heterotopic neurons in normal hemispheric white matter: a morphometric analysis. *J Neuropathol Exp Neurol* 1996; 55: 178–83.

89 Lellouch-Tubiana A, Bourgeois M, Vekemans M, Robain O. Dysembryoplastic neuroepithelial tumors in two children with neurofibromatosis type 1. *Acta Neuropathol (Berl)* 1995; 90: 319–22.

90 Leung SY, Gwi E, Ng HK, Fung CF, Yam KY. Dysembryoplastic neuroepithelial tumor. A tumor with small neuronal cells resembling oligodendroglioma. *Am J Surg Pathol* 1994; 18: 604–14.

91 Kuchelmeister K, Demirel T, Schlorer E, Bergmann M, Gullotta F. Dysembryoplastic neuroepithelial tumour of the cerebellum. *Acta Neuropathol (Berl)* 1995; 89: 385–90.

92 Cervera-Pierot P, Varlet P, Chodkiewicz JP, Daumas-Duport C. Dysembryoplastic neuroepithelial tumors located in the caudate nucleus area: report of four cases. *Neurosurgery* 1997; 40: 1065–9.

93 Yasha TC, Mohanty A, Radhesh S *et al*. Infratentorial dysembryoplastic neuroepithelial tumor (DNT) associated with Arnold–Chiari malformation. *Clin Neuropathol* 1998; 17: 305–10.

94 Wolf HK, Wiestler OD. Surgical pathology of chronic epileptic seizure disorders. *Brain Pathol* 1993; 3: 371–80.

95 Taratuto AL, Pomata H, Sevlever G, Gallo G, Monges J. Dysembryoplastic neuroepithelial tumor: morphological, immunocytochemical, and deoxyribonucleic acid analyses in a pediatric series. *Neurosurgery* 1995; 36: 474–81.

96 Juhasz C, Chugani DC, Muzik O *et al*. Relationship of flumazenil and glucose PET abnormalities to neocortical epilepsy surgery outcome. *Neurology* 2001; 56: 1650–8.

97 Kirkpatrick PJ, Honavar M, Janota I, Polkey CE. Control of temporal lobe epilepsy following en bloc resection of low-grade tumors. *J Neurosurg* 1993; 78: 19–25.

98 Hirose T, Scheithauer BW. Mixed dysembryoplastic neuroepithelial tumor and ganglioglioma. *Acta Neuropathol (Berl)* 1998; 95: 649–54.

99 Lee DY, Chung CK, Hwang YS *et al*. Dysembryoplastic neuroepithelial tumor: radiological findings (including PET, SPECT, and MRS) and surgical strategy. *J Neurooncol* 2000; 47: 167–74.

100 Thom M, Gomez-Anson B, Revesz T *et al*. Spontaneous intralesional haemorrhage in dysembryoplastic neuroepithelial tumours: a series of five cases. *J Neurol Neurosurg Psychiatr* 1999; 67: 97–101.

101 Hammond RR, Duggal N, Woulfe JM, Girvin JP. Malignant transformation of a dysembryoplastic neuroepithelial tumor. Case report. *J Neurosurg* 2000; 92: 722–5.

102 Fernandez G, Effenberger O, Vinz B *et al*. Hippocampal malformation as a cause of famial ferile convulsions and subsequent hippocampal sclerosis. *Neurology* 1998; 50: 909–17.

103 Baulac M, De Grissac N, Hasboun D *et al*. Hippocampal developmental changes in patients with partial epilepsy: magnetic resonance imaging and clinical aspects. *Ann Neurol* 1998; 44: 223–33.

104 Gloor P. Experiential phenomena of temporal lobe epilepsy. Facts and hypotheses. *Brain* 1990; 113 (Pt 6): 1673–94.

105 Fish DR, Smith SJ, Quesney LF, Andermann F, Rasmussen T. Surgical treatment of children with medically intractable frontal or temporal lobe epilepsy: results and highlights of 40 years' experience. *Epilepsia* 1993; 34: 244–7.

106 Frater JL, Prayson RA, Morris III HH, Bingaman WE. Surgical pathologic findings of extratemporal-based intractable epilepsy: a study of 133 consecutive resections. *Arch Pathol Lab Med* 2000; 124: 545–9.

107 Ho SS, Kuzniecky RI, Gilliam F, Faught E, Morawetz R. Temporal lobe developmental malformations and epilepsy: dual pathology and bilateral hippocampal abnormalities. *Neurology* 1998; 50: 748–54.

108 Ryvlin P, Bouvard S, Le Bars D *et al*. Clinical utility of flumazenil-PET versus [18F]fluorodeoxyglucose-PET and MRI in refractory partial epilepsy. A prospective study in 100 patients. *Brain* 1998; 121 (Pt 11): 2067–81.

109 O'Brien TJ, So El, Mullan BP *et al*. Subtraction ictal SPECT coregistered to MRI improves clinical usefulness of SPECT in localising the surgical seizure focus. *Neurology* 1998; 50: 445–54.

110 Raymond AA, Fish DR. EEG features of focal malformations of cortical development. *J Clin Neurophysiol* 1996; 13: 495–506.

111 Raymond AA, Fish DR, Boyd SG *et al*. Cortical dysgenesis: serial EEG findings in children and adults. *Electroencephal Clin Neurophysiol* 1995; 94: 389–97.

112 Awad IA, Rosenfeld J, Ahl J, Hahn JF, Luders H. Intractable epilepsy and structural lesions of the brain: mapping, resection strategies, and seizure outcome. *Epilepsia* 1991; 32: 179–86.

113 Palmini A, Andermann F, Olivier A *et al*. Focal neuronal migration disorders and intractable partial epilepsy: a study of 30 patients. *Ann Neurol* 1991; 30: 741–9.

114 Aykut-Bingol C, Bronen RA, Kim JH, Spencer DD, Spencer SS. Surgical outcome in occipital lobe epilepsy: implications for pathophysiology. *Ann Neurol* 1998; 44: 60–9.

115 Mukahira K, Oguni H, Awaya Y *et al*. Study on surgical treatment of intractable childhood epilepsy. *Brain Dev* 1998; 20: 154–64.

116 Jahan R, Mischel PS, Curran JG, Peacock WJ, Shields DW, Vinters HV. Bilateral neuropathologic changes in a child with hemimegalencephaly. *Pediatr Neurol* 1997; 17: 344–9.

117 Hirabayashi S, Binnie CD, Janota I, Polkey CE. Surgical treatment of epilepsy due to cortical dysplasia: clinical and EEG findings. *J Neurol Neurosurg Psychiatr* 1993; 56; 765–70.

118 Kuzniecky R, Garcia JH, Faught E, Morawetz RB. Cortical dysplasia in temporal lobe epilepsy: magnetic resonance imaging correlations. *Ann Neurol* 1991; 29: 293–8.

119 Guerrini R, Dravet C, Raybaud C *et al*. Epilepsy and focal gyral anomalies detected by MRI: electroclinico-morphological correlations and followup. *Dev Med Child Neurol* 1992; 34: 706–18.

120 Ambrosetto G. Treatable partial epilepsy and unilateral opercular neuronal migration disorder. *Epilepsia* 1993; 34: 604–8.

121 Wyllie E, Comair YG, Kotagal P, Raja S, Ruggieri P. Epilepsy surgery in infants. *Epilepsia* 1996; 37: 625–37.

122 Wyllie E, Comair YG, Kotagal P *et al*. Seizure outcome after epilepsy surgery in children and adolescents. *Ann Neurol* 1998; 44: 740–8.

123 Kuzniecky R, Gilliam F, Morawetz R *et al*. Occipital lobe developmental malformations and epilepsy: clinical spectrum, treatment and outcome. *Epilepsia* 1997; 38: 175–81.

124 Shaver EG, Harvey AS, Morrison G *et al*. Results and complications after reoperation for failed epilepsy surgery in children. *Pediatr Neurosurg* 1997; 27: 194–202.

125 Keene DL, Jimenez CC, Ventureyra E. Cortical microdysplasia and surgical outcome in refractory epilepsy of childhood. *Pediatr Neurosurg* 1998; 29: 69–72.

126 Chassoux F, Devaux B, Landre E *et al*. Stereoelectroencephalography in focal cortical dysplasia: a 3D approach to delineating the dysplastic cortex. *Brain* 2000; 123 (Pt 8): 1733–51.

127 Palmini A, Andermann F, Olivier A, Tampieri D, Robitaille Y. Focal neuronal migration disorders and intractable partial epilepsy: results of surgical treatment. *Ann Neurol* 1991; 30: 750–7.

128 Chugani HT, Shewmon DA, Shields WD *et al*. Surgery for intractable seizures. *Epilepsia* 1993; 34: 764–71.

129 Cross JH, Boyd SB, Gordon I, Harper A, Nebille BGR. Ictal cerebral perfusion related to EEG in intractable focal epilepsy of childhood. *J Neurol Neurosurg Psychiatr* 1997; 62: 377–84.

130 Newton MR, Berkovic SF, Austin MC *et al*. SPECT in the localisation of extratemporal and temporal seizure foci. *J Neurol Neurosurg Psychiatr* 1995; 59: 26–30.

131 Aihara M, Hatakeyama K, Koizumi K, Nakazawa S. Ictal EEG and single photon emission computed tomography in a patient with cortical dysplasia presenting with atonic seizures. *Epilepsia* 1997; 38: 723–7.

132 Martinerie J, Adam C, Le Van QM *et al*. Epileptic seizures can be anticipated by non-linear analysis. *Nat Med* 1998; 4: 1173–6.

133 Krakow K, Woermann FG, Symms MR *et al*. EEG-triggered functional MRI of interictal epileptiform activity in patients with partial seizures. *Brain* 1999; 122 (Pt 9): 1679–88.

134 Sugimoto T, Otsubo H, Hwang PA, Hoffman HJ, Jay V, Snead OC, III. Outcome of epilepsy surgery in the first three years of life. *Epilepsia* 1999; 40: 560–5.

64 Surgery of Post-Traumatic Epilepsy

K.S. Firlik and D.D. Spencer

Post-traumatic medically refractory epilepsy poses particular challenges for neurologists and epilepsy surgeons. This chapter is concerned with the surgery of late epilepsy in cases without evidence of extensive cerebral damage due to trauma. The surgery of acute trauma (with or without early epilepsy) is covered in general neurosurgical texts. The resective surgery of post-traumatic epilepsy with overt extensive cerebral damage is usually only palliative and this too will not be considered here. For patients who are considered for surgical intervention, accurate localization can be difficult, especially given the often diffuse nature of traumatic brain injury. Imaging studies frequently fail to disclose focal pathology and neuropsychological testing often reveals diffuse deficits. Despite these challenges surgery can be helpful in carefully selected patients.

Association between trauma and epilepsy

Post-traumatic seizures are traditionally divided into early and late seizures, depending upon their onset in relation to the trauma. Early seizures occur within the first week. Late seizures occur after 1 week. A further designation—immediate seizures—typically refers to seizures that occur within the first 24h after injury. Whereas children more frequently exhibit early seizures, adults are more likely to develop late seizures [1]. Late seizures can develop years after the trauma, although the risk tends to decline over time [2,3].

The investigation of predictive factors in the development of late seizures has been undertaken by many groups, with varied results. Many would agree, however, that significant risk factors include a penetrating injury or focal haematoma [3,4]. In addition, the more severe the injury, the more likely late seizures are to occur [2]. It is unclear whether or not early seizures represent an independent risk factor for late seizures [4–6].

Accurate determination of the incidence of late trauma-related epilepsy is complicated. Minor head injuries are common in the general population, especially during childhood, and it is impossible to know whether a minor remote childhood injury was causative or incidental. Furthermore, the grading of injury, the severity and definition of post-traumatic epilepsy are not consistent in the literature. To offer a benchmark, however, post-traumatic epilepsy accounted for 5.5% of all epilepsy cases from 1935 to 1984 in Rochester, Minnesota [7].

More pressing than the issue of defining incidence is the quest to prevent late seizure occurrence. Based on a meta-analysis of studies that investigated phenytoin therapy, it is clear that *early* seizures can be reduced by approximately 57%, but there is no clear benefit in terms of preventing *late* seizures [8]. For that reason, most trauma centres advocate phenytoin prophylaxis for only 1 week following severe head injuries. Although present antiepileptic drugs are not proven to be effective as prophylaxis for late seizures [9], there are other neuroprotective strategies, such as antioxidants, that may prevent secondary brain injury and so prove to be antiepileptogenic [10].

Proposed mechanisms for post-traumatic epilepsy

Which pathological changes following traumatic brain injury predispose a patient to delayed epileptogenesis? Many authors have focused on the role of blood products, such as the deposition of haemosiderin or iron that may occur with the shearing of vessels at the time of impact—a plausible mechanism [5,11–16]. Others have emphasized that head injury can result in white matter lesions and cavitation that can effectively undercut the cortex resulting in hyperexcitability [17,18].

Theories regarding the role of hippocampal damage following head injury have been equally compelling. In a series of 112 cases of 'fatal non-missile' head injuries, hippocampal damage was found on histopathology in 84% of cases. In 58% of these cases, the damage was focal and, in all cases, the pathological changes of neuronal loss and gliosis involved the CA1 region [19]. The authors disclose that in only 18 cases, there was specific documentation of no hypoxia or hypotension. In many cases, then, global ischaemic insults rather than the trauma *per se* may have contributed to the hippocampal damage. However, enhanced excitability secondary to death of inhibitory dentate hilar neurones has been demonstrated in animal models of head injury, under more controlled circumstances [20,21]. Indeed such hyperexcitability can last for months following the trauma with reorganization of excitatory pathways such as mossy fibre sprouting [22].

At least one author has postulated that very early head injury can induce cortical dysplasia [23], an idea that has been investigated in animal models. The author described two children who sustained a head injury within 4 days of birth, developed delayed intractable epilepsy and underwent surgery. Histopathological examination of resected cortex demonstrated microdysplastic changes adjacent to regions of meningeal fibrosis, which were assumed to be secondary to the trauma. This interesting theory has yet to be further substantiated in the human literature.

Surgery for post-traumatic epilepsy

Because patients with post-traumatic epilepsy represent a relatively small subset of patients evaluated at epilepsy centres, the literature focusing on surgery for this group is less plentiful than for other aetiologies, such as tumour-related epilepsy. Two studies considered all trauma-related epilepsy [24,25], and three others focused exclusively on temporal lobe epilepsy [26–28].

Marks *et al.* [24] studied 25 patients with post-traumatic intractable epilepsy, not specifically restricted to the temporal lobe, who were evaluated for potential surgery. Of those, 21 patients required invasive monitoring. As a testament to the difficulties in localizing all-comers with post-traumatic epilepsy, only a putative focus was successfully localized in nine patients. All nine underwent surgery and remained seizure free at least 1 year after surgery. In six of these nine surgical patients, a mesial temporal focus was identified, five of whom were diagnosed as having mesial temporal sclerosis on pathology. The authors pointed out that for all five of the mesial temporal sclerosis cases, the inciting head injury occurred by the age of 5 years. They thus concluded that early trauma, in contrast to trauma after the age of 5 years, is associated with mesial temporal sclerosis. One element of concern regarding this study, however, is that three of the six patients with a mesial temporal focus had only a 'mild' head injury. The causative role of such head injuries in the later development of chronic refractory epilepsy is questionable.

Diaz-Arrastia *et al.* [25] investigated the issue of age at trauma and the finding of mesial temporal versus neocortical epilepsy. They studied 23 patients with medically intractable epilepsy who sustained a head injury after 10 years of age (mean 22.9 years). Based upon comprehensive epilepsy evaluations, eight patients (35%) were found to have mesial temporal lobe seizures, whereas 11 had neocortical epilepsy (three could not be localized and one was primarily generalized). Two patients underwent anterior temporal lobectomy and were found to have hippocampal sclerosis (one became seizure free and the other had a significant improvement). This study stands in contrast to the study by Marks *et al.* [24] by revealing that injury at an older age can also result in a mesial temporal focus (although the diagnosis of mesial temporal sclerosis was confirmed in only two patients). This study, however, is limited by the fact that seizure localization was based on non-invasive data only.

Mathern *et al.* [26] studied a group of 120 patients who were operated on for non-lesional temporal lobe epilepsy who had a history of 'injury'. Injury was widely defined and included, in addition to trauma: birth injury, prolonged seizure and others, such as hypoxia and encephalitis or meningitis. Of the 120 patients, 26 (15%) had had a traumatic head injury. Of these 26 patients, 15 were classified as having had a severe head injury, six had a moderate injury and five had a mild injury. In terms of hippocampal neuronal cell loss, the trauma group demonstrated a mean loss of 60.6% (which was within the range of means for the other injury groups: 54.5–68.3%). In terms of seizure outcome, the trauma group fared better than the other injury groups. Approximately 80% were seizure free and 12% had fewer than six seizures per year (at least 1 year after surgery). It should, however, be noted that this was a study of selected patients who had epilepsy localized to one temporal lobe.

The same group group [27] published another study on temporal lobe epilepsy after injury, this time focusing on only 20 more recent patients. Again, injury was widely defined and included non-traumatic aetiologies. The group of 20 patients included three with a history of head trauma, and these three were not analysed separately. Despite considering trauma along with other types of injury, their findings are of interest. The authors found that hippocampal atrophy was more common in patients who suffered an injury prior to the age of 5 years. In addition, patients with injuries at an early age demonstrated significantly longer latent periods and had worse postoperative outcomes in terms of seizure control. These results, however, are based on a small sample size (the 20 patients were divided into five smaller groups for the purposes of analysis).

Schuh *et al.* [28] examined the influence of prior head injury, and other risk factors, on seizure outcome after anterior temporal lobectomy. They studied a consecutive series of 102 patients who had undergone anterior temporal lobectomy. A total of 29 patients had a history of head injury, although only 10 of these had trauma alone as a risk factor (the others had additional risk factors, including febrile seizures, family history of epilepsy, perinatal insult or a lesion on MRI). The authors concluded that the history of a significant head injury correlated with worse outcome after surgery, regardless of age at the time of trauma. No other risk factor showed a statistically significant correlation with poor outcome.

Several other findings from this study are of interest [28]. Patients with head injury as a risk factor were not more likely to have bitemporal epilepsy or require invasive studies. Furthermore, selected patients with post-traumatic epilepsy who had evidence of haemosiderin deposition on MRI tended to have better outcomes. Finally, 20 of the 29 patients with post-traumatic epilepsy had histopathologically confirmed mesial temporal sclerosis. This ratio was similar to that for other risk factors except for meningitis (for which all cases showed mesial temporal sclerosis).

Illustrative cases

Case 1: head injury as an adult

M.M. is a 47-year-old right-handed man who was evaluated and treated for post-traumatic medically intractable complex partial seizures.

The patient was the product of a normal pregnancy and uncomplicated spontaneous vaginal delivery. He had no history of a central nervous system infection or febrile seizures. There was no family history of epilepsy. At the age of 21 he fell from a horse, struck his occiput and suffered a loss of consciousness that lasted several minutes. After regaining consciousness, he had a generalized tonic-clonic seizure that lasted between 5 and 10 min. As a result of the fall, he reportedly suffered a right temporal contusion and skull fracture (his original films were not available for review at the time of his evaluation). While in the intensive care unit, he had a second generalized seizure.

The patient was discharged from the hospital without antiepileptic drugs and had no further seizures until 16 years later, at the age of 37, when he had two more generalized seizures. During this long intervening period, he attended and graduated from law school, and had been practising trial law. He was started on carbamazepine, later switched to phenytoin and again enjoyed a long seizure-free period lasting approximately 4 years.

In his early 40s, the patient began to experience complex partial seizures refractory to antiepileptic medication. His seizures began with an aura of a feeling of 'loss of control' associated with making grammatical or syntactic errors. This would then be followed by a loss of contact, staring and speech difficulties lasting a few minutes. The postictal period was characterized by confusion, lethargy and amnesia for the event. His seizures tended to occur in clusters during which he would have several per week, typically followed by several weeks without seizures.

At the age of 44 he underwent a comprehensive epilepsy evaluation at Yale University. His continuous audiovisual scalp EEG monitoring captured six stereotypical seizures; all appeared to arise from the left temporal region. His neuropsychological testing revealed a verbal IQ of 130, a performance IQ of 126 and a full-scale IQ of 132. He demonstrated specific difficulties with receptive language and verbal memory. His MRI was normal. Wada testing showed left-dominant speech, normal right memory and adequate left memory.

Due to the consistent character of his seizures and the concordant non-invasive data that implicated the left temporal lobe, the patient was felt to be a potential surgical candidate. He underwent a craniotomy for placement of intracranial electrodes, including subdural and bilateral hippocampal depth electrodes. Three typical seizures were recorded, all arising from the left anterior hippocampus and amygdala.

The patient then underwent a left anteromedial temporal lobectomy with resection of approximately one-third of the hippocampus, anteriorly. The pathology revealed minimal hippocampal neuronal loss and focal moderate to severe gliosis.

Postoperatively, the patient remained seizure free for approximately 2 years on carbamazepine monotherapy. Unfortunately, however, his seizures then returned at a rate of one or two per month, with rare secondary generalizations. In addition to his recurrent epilepsy, he also suffered from depression and irrational outbursts of anger. Phenobarbital was added to his anticonvulsant regimen, and he was able to continue teaching law despite his seizures. He was re-evaluated by continuous audiovisual scalp EEG that again implicated the left temporal lobe. It was decided to continue trials of antiepileptic medication rather than to consider further surgery.

Case 2: head injury as a child

D.T. is a 38-year-old right-handed man who was in a motor vehicle accident at the age of 2 years. He suffered a skull fracture and had an immediate post-traumatic generalized seizure. He was otherwise healthy, the product of a normal pregnancy and delivery and had no history of febrile seizures or central nervous system infections. There was no family history of epilepsy.

The patient did well and remained seizure free, without medications, until 17 years later. At the age of 19, he had a generalized seizure and subsequently developed medically refractory complex partial seizures. His seizures began without an aura and consisted of a loss of contact, blank stare, mumbling and hand automatisms. Postictal lethargy was common. On occasion, a postictal expressive aphasia was noted as well. These seizures lasted anywhere from 30s to several minutes and occurred once every 1–2 weeks. Secondary generalization was rare.

At the age of 31 he was evaluated at Yale University. His MRI demonstrated left hippocampal atrophy. Continuous audiovisual monitoring captured seven typical seizures, four of which lateralized to the left. The remaining two seizures could not be lateralized.

His neuropsychological testing revealed a verbal IQ of 90, performance IQ of 110 and full-scale IQ of 97. Although his verbal memory was specifically diminished, other tests suggested more diffuse bilateral cognitive difficulties. A Wada examination revealed left-hemispheric speech dominance, marginally adequate right memory and poor left memory. A subsequent SPECT scan demonstrated decreased perfusion of the left temporal lobe.

An intracranial electrode study was performed, including bilateral subdural and hippocampal depth electrodes. Several seizures were recorded. His typical seizures arose from the left hippocampal depth electrode. The patient then underwent a left anteromedial temporal lobectomy, including a complete hippocampectomy. Pathology revealed severe hippocampal neuronal loss.

The patient has had 6 years of postoperative follow-up. He has been seizure free on carbamazepine monotherapy, except for a single seizure that occurred in the context of abrupt medication withdrawal. His major complaint was of poor impulse control, outbursts of anger and depression. Prior to surgery, the patient was a high school graduate and was working as a carpenter. Postoperatively, he decided to further his education and enrolled in college courses.

Comments

Both cases are illustrative of the long seizure-free interval that can be observed following the inciting head injury. In addition, both patients suffered from psychological disturbances—depression and impulsivity—which is not unexpected, given the potentially diffuse nature of closed head injuries, compounded by years' worth of uncontrolled epilepsy. Both patients were considered to be surgical candidates as they had predominantly one consistent seizure type and location: complex partial seizures of temporal lobe origin.

Case 1 differed from case 2 in that the patient's injury occurred in adulthood and was associated with a normal-appearing hippocampus on MRI. Despite this, the resected hippocampus demonstrated mild to moderate pathology; this emphasizes the insensitivity of MRI to subtle pathological change that may be epileptogenic. In addition, postoperative seizure control was inadequate for case 1 and excellent for case 2. It is unclear whether or not a complete, rather than a partial, hippocampectomy would have resulted in better seizure control in case 1.

Conclusions

Based on the small number of operative series in the literature, it is evident that patients with well-localized post-traumatic epilepsy can be treated with surgery, leading to satisfactory outcomes in many cases. The major difficulty in managing this group of patients, however, is that adequate localization is not possible for a significant subset. Many studies have emphasized the correlation between head trauma and the development of mesial temporal sclerosis, although there is no clear consensus regarding the influence of age at the time of trauma. We can assume that seizures well localized to the mesial temporal lobe should respond favourably to anteromedial temporal lobectomy, despite the history of trauma as a risk factor. In addition, focal neocortical injuries from direct trauma, such as depressed skull fractures, intracerebral haematomas or contusions, can lead to focal epileptogenesis which can respond to resection.

Most of these patients, however, should undergo invasive recordings, given the possible heterogeneous nature of the pathology, and the possibility that the epileptogenic zone extends beyond the area of pathology detected by MRI. For patients who cannot be localized, or who have multifocal disease, recent technical innovations, such as vagus nerve stimulation [29], may offer some hope in drug-resistant cases.

References

1 Asikainen I, Kaste M, Sarna S. Early and late posttraumatic seizures in traumatic brain injury rehabilitation patients: brain injury factors causing late seizures and influence of seizures on long-term outcome. *Epilepsia* 1999; 40: 584–9.

2 Annegers JF, Grabow JD, Groover RV *et al*. Seizures after head trauma: a population study. *Neurology* 1980; 30: 683–9.

3 Salazar AM, Jabbari B, Vance SC *et al*. Epilepsy after penetrating head injury. I. Clinical correlates: a report of the Vietnam Head Injury Study. *Neurology* 1985; 35: 1406–14.

4 Temkin NR, Haglund M, Winn HR. Post-traumatic seizures. In: Narayan RK, Wilberger JE, Povlishock JT, eds. *Neurotrauma*. New York: McGraw Hill Companies, Inc., 1996: 611–19.

5 Yablon SA. Posttraumatic seizures (review). *Arch Phys Med Rehab* 1993; 74: 983–1001.

6 Schweitzer JS, Spencer DD. Surgery of congenital, traumatic and infectious lesions and those of uncertain aetiologies. In: Shorvon S, Dreifuss F, Fish D, Thomas D, eds. *The Treatment of Epilepsy*. Oxford: Blackwell Science Ltd, 1996: 669–88.

7 Hauser WA, Annegers JF, Kurland LT. Incidence of epilepsy and unprovoked seizures in Rochester, Minnesota: 1935–1984. *Epilepsia* 1993; 34: 453–68.

8 Tempkin NR, Dikmen SS, Winn HR. Posttraumatic seizures. *Neurosurg Clin North Am* 1991; 2: 425–35.

9 Temkin NR. Antiepileptogenesis and seizure prevention trials with antiepileptic drugs: meta-analysis of controlled trials. *Epilepsia* 2001; 42(4): 515–24.

10 Willmore LJ. Posttraumatic epilepsy. *Neurol Clin* 1992; 10: 869–78.

11 Payan H, Toga M, Berard-Badier M. The pathology of post-traumatic epilepsies. *Epilepsia* 1970; 11: 81–94.

12 Jennett B. Epilepsy and acute traumatic intracranial hematoma. *J Neurol Neurosurg Psychiatry* 1975; 38: 378–81.

13 Willmore LJ. Recurrent seizures induced by cortical iron injection: a model of posttraumatic epilepsy. *Ann Neurol* 1978; 4: 329–36.

14 Reid SA, Sypert GW. Acute FeC13-induced epileptogenic foci in cats: electrophysiological analyses. *Brain Res* 1980; 188: 531–42.

15 Willmore LJ. Post-traumatic epilepsy: cellular mechanisms and implications for treatment (review). *Epilepsia* 1990; 31: S67–S73.

16 Moriwaki A, Hattori Y, Hayashi Y *et al*. Development of epileptic activity induced by iron injection into rat cerebral cortex: electrographic and behavioral characteristics. *Electroencephalogr Clin Neurophysiol* 1992; 83: 281–8.

17 Echlin F, Battista A. Epileptiform seizures from chronic isolated cortex. *Arch Neurol* 1963; 9: 154–70.

18 Sharpless S, Halpern L. The electrical excitability of chronically isolated cortex studied by means of chronically implanted electrodes. *Electroencephalogr Clin Neurophysiol* 1962; 14: 244–55.

19 Kotapka MJ, Graham DI, Adams JH *et al*. Hippocampal pathology in fatal non-missile human head injury. *Acta Neuropathol* 1992; 83: 530–4.

20 Lowenstein DH, Thomas MJ, Smith DH *et al*. Selective vulnerability of dentate hilar neurons following traumatic brain injury: a potential mechanistic link between head trauma and disorders of the hippocampus. *J Neurosci* 1992; 12: 4846–53.

21 Coulter DA, Rafiq A, Shumate M *et al*. Brain injury-induced enhanced limbic epileptogenesis: anatomical and physiological parallels to an animal model of temporal lobe epilepsy. *Epilepsy Res* 1996; 26: 81–91.

22 Santhakumar V, Ratzliff AD, Jeng J, Toth Z, Soltesz I. Long-term hyperexcitability in the hippocampus after experimental head trauma. *Ann Neurol* 2001; 50: 708–17.

23 Lombroso CT. Can early postnatal closed head injury induce cortical dysplasia? *Epilepsia* 2000; 41: 245–53.

24 Marks DA, Kim J, Spencer DD *et al*. Seizure localization and pathology following head injury in patients with uncontrolled epilepsy. *Neurology* 1995; 45: 2051–7.

25 Diaz-Arrastia R, Agostini MA, Frol AB *et al*. Neurophysiologic and neuroradiologic features of intractable epilepsy after traumatic brain injury in adults. *Arch Neurol* 2000; 57: 1611–16.

26 Mathern GW, Babb TL, Vickrey BG *et al*. Traumatic compared to nontraumatic clinical–pathologic associations in temporal lobe epilepsy. *Epilepsy Res* 1994; 19: 129–39.

27 Mathern GW, Pretorius JK, Babb TL. Influence of the type of initial precipitating injury and at what age it occurs on course and outcome in patients with temporal lobe seizures. *J Neurosurg* 1995; 82: 220–7.

28 Schuh LA, Henry TR, Fromes G *et al*. Influence of head trauma on outcome following anterior temporal lobectomy. *Arch Neurol* 1998; 55: 1325–8.

29 Morris GL, Mueller WM. Long-term treatment with vagus nerve stimulation in patients with refractory epilepsy. The Vagus Nerve Stimulation Study Group E01-E05. *Neurology* 1999; 53: 1731–5.

65 Paediatric Epilepsy Surgery

J.A. Lawson and M.S. Duchowny

Increasing attention has been given to the potential benefits of performing epilepsy surgery earlier in life, to improve social and quality of life outcomes. This chapter reviews the surgical treatment of epilepsy in children and presents the reasons why surgery should not be considered as a last resort. Children are not 'little adults' and many of the principles that guide adult surgical decision-making are not applicable to paediatrics. Our understanding of the wide spectrum of disorders that result in epilepsy and the effects of seizures and their treatment on the developing brain is in its infancy. It is the aim of this chapter to review the current level of our understanding and perhaps to stimulate further advances in the management of this potentially devastating condition.

Rationale for paediatric epilepsy surgery

Epidemiology of intractable childhood epilepsy

Childhood epilepsy is a common disorder. Epidemiological studies [1,2] demonstrate an annual incidence of epilepsy in children of up to four cases per 1000 population. An estimated [3] 10% of these children are resistant to medical treatment. Only 11% of patients who fail to respond to an initial anticonvulsant drug will achieve seizure freedom after the addition of a second medication [4]. There are thus a large body of patients who carry the burden of intractable epilepsy and its treatment. Unfortunately, only a small percentage of these children will be evaluated for surgery.

Early identification of epilepsy surgery candidates

Early and accurate identification of children with surgically remediable epilepsy syndromes is essential. Several key adult studies [4,5] suggest that for patients with correctable structural abnormalities, surgery should be considered as soon as treatment with two first-line drugs fails. Table 65.1 summarizes the factors identified by prospective paediatric studies that are predictive of medical intractability. The age of onset data appears contradictory, but delineates a window between infancy and adolescence when benign age-related syndromes with good prognosis are prevalent. The most recent of these predictive studies [3] reports that the most significant predictor of intractability was a high seizure frequency occurring immediately from epilepsy onset. Recognition of these negative prognostic factors should facilitate early referral for consideration of epilepsy surgery.

The argument for earlier surgery

The impact of epilepsy is much greater than simply the effects of seizures. This section reviews these broader aspects of epilepsy: behaviour, cognition, psychosocial disorders, increased morbidity and mortality. That epilepsy surgery offers an opportunity for freedom from seizures is beyond doubt. The potential for significant improvement in these broader areas is a major argument for earlier surgery, but the evidence for the existence of this 'magic bullet' is scanty, particularly in children.

Psychosocial effects of intractable epilepsy

Children with intractable epilepsy commonly manifest behavioural and educational problems related to the seizure disorder or medications. It is often the major concern of the parent, overshadowing anxiety expressed about seizures. The social morbidity resulting from the stigma of epilepsy is also a common problem. Given the pervasive effect of epilepsy on many aspects of daily living, it is no surprise that problems arise in the long term.

Early consideration for surgery or other alternative therapies in those who are refractory to medical treatment is imperative, as serious long-term problems are inevitable. Significant proportions of those with childhood epilepsy have persistent social problems as adults. A prospective 30-year study [6] of childhood onset epilepsy showed significantly more patients had limited schooling, were unemployed, not married and had no children.

Evidence that epilepsy surgery improves behavioural and long-term social outcomes

Improvements in behavioural disorders following epilepsy surgery have been reported in short-term studies. A prospective comparative study [7] of 28 children undergoing epilepsy surgery with 28 epilepsy controls found that behavioural problems were present in half of the group preoperatively. At 6 months follow-up significant improvements in behaviour were noted only in the surgery group, predicted solely by a good seizure outcome.

The long-term psychosocial effects of intractable childhood epilepsy are clearly of concern, but is there evidence that epilepsy surgery performed earlier in life arrests this process? A study [8] of the long-term outcomes of 64 patients who had epilepsy surgery prior to 18 years of age found significantly higher levels of education and employment in patients who became seizure free compared to lesser outcomes. Several other studies in adults [9–11] have also shown improvement in socioeconomic outcome when surgery is performed in younger patients.

Table 65.1 Factors predictive of intractable epilepsy

Predictors of medical intractability
Neonatal seizures [86]
Infantile spasms [83]
Earlier age of epilepsy onset [83]
Symptomatic epilepsy [83,87]
Acute symptomatic status epilepticus at onset [3]
Initial high seizure frequency [3]
Focal slowing on EEG [3]
Type of MRI lesion [88]

Predictors of long-term seizure freedom
Rapid response to therapy [6]
Idiopathic epilepsy [6]
Age of onset <12 years [86]
Normal intelligence [86]
Small number of seizures prior to diagnosis [86]

Quality of life outcomes

There is a clear recognition that the patient's perceived adequacy of functioning adds new and important information to other traditional surgical outcome measures such as seizure control and cognitive improvement. A number of instruments have been developed to measure the health-related quality of life (HRQOL) of adult epilepsy patients. Prospective surgical data are available only for adults [12,13] with significant improvements reported in emotional well-being, attention, language, social isolation, health perception, physical/work/drive/social limitations and anxiety. In one study [13], patients with continuing auras and/or seizures had no significant improvement in their overall HRQOL scores. The HRQOL improvement was confined to those who achieved an entirely seizure-free state.

Long-term social disabilities are likely to have their genesis in childhood, an age group inadequately studied because of limitations in the current instruments available to assess HRQOL. The lack of data on HRQOL outcomes for paediatric epilepsy surgery is of concern. Major methodological problems exist such as the need for assessment by proxy, usually the parent. Several groups have developed measures [14–16] that are promising and their application in a prospective surgical study is awaited.

Effect of epilepsy surgery on neuropsychological outcome

Effects on overall intelligence scores

There are several unresolved questions regarding the effect of successful epilepsy surgery in childhood on neuropsychological status. Unfortunately, only limited studies have been performed using small sample sizes. Studies of infants and preschool children are non-existent. The largest study [17] of the effect of surgery on intelligence was a multicentre collaboration that examined 82 patients with temporal lobe epilepsy from 6 to 17 years of age. Following surgery, approximately 10% of the sample experienced a significant decline in verbal IQ while a similar proportion showed significant improvement. Risk factors for significant decline included older age at the time of surgery and the presence of a structural lesion other than hippocampal sclerosis.

Specific cognitive effects of focal resections

The few small studies of specific cognitive effects of the various surgery types are summarized in an excellent review [18]. In the review of paediatric temporal lobe resections, there was no significant decrease in memory function, especially in the preadolescent age group. Overall improvements were noted in attention and language. For extratemporal focal resections, deficits in language have been observed following left frontal resection while improved language has been noted after right frontal resection. Again, greater deficits correlated with a later age at surgery.

For hemispherectomy, most studies report no change in global IQ, but language outcomes are directly related to age at operation and side of surgery. The language outcome of a subset of patients from the Johns Hopkins series [19] with onset of Rasmussen's encephalitis (RE) after the age of 5 years treated with left hemispherectomy was disconcerting. By 12 months postsurgery, speech was limited largely to production of single words with no receptive language deficit. Study of larger series of patients utilizing the newer technologies such as functional MRI (fMRI) could help clarify the short- and long-term neuropsychological risks and benefits of epilepsy resection in childhood.

Other risks of intractable epilepsy

Patients whose epilepsy does not remit have an increased risk of death [6,20]. The primary causes of death include accidents while driving or swimming, status epilepticus or sudden unexpected death (SUDEP).

The potential adverse effects of repetitive seizures and anticonvulsant use [21–23] on the developing brain is of special concern that is beyond the scope of this discussion.

Cost-effectiveness of epilepsy surgery in children

The increasingly stringent fiscal situation in industrialized nations requires assessment of the health economics of medical procedures. Several studies [24,25] have examined the cost-effectiveness of epilepsy surgery. The benefits would be expected to be even greater in the paediatric population. One paediatric study [25] over 25 years found that the initial costs for the surgically treated group were significantly higher than those in the medical treatment arm. Beyond 10 years, surgery ultimately became more cost-effective due to reduced medication costs and decreased social morbidity such as increased employment in the surgically treated group.

Surgically amenable epilepsy syndromes and pathologies common or unique to the paediatric age group

These are detailed in Table 65.2.

Malformations of cortical development (MCD)

The descriptive radiological term MCD is an increasingly accepted, all-inclusive term to denote non-neoplastic lesions that result from anomalies during cortical development. MCD is meant to encompass terms such as cerebral dysgenesis and neuronal migration

Table 65.2 Surgically amenable brain pathologies/epilepsy syndromes common or unique to children

---

Malformations of cortical development
Developmental tumours
Tuberous sclerosis
Sturge–Weber syndrome
Hypothalamic hamartoma
Rasmussen's encephalitis
Infantile spasms
Ohtahara syndrome
Landau–Kleffner syndrome

---

disorder. Well-described histopathological patterns of MCD include focal cortical dysplasia of Taylor type, nodular heterotopia, polymicrogyria, schizencephaly and hemimegalencephaly. Not all subtypes of MCD are suitable for surgery, as borne out by the poor results obtained for focal cortical resections in patients with periventricular nodular heterotopia [26].

MCD are a frequent cause of intractable epilepsy with an incidence estimated at 28–56% [27,28] of paediatric surgical candidates. Characteristic clinical features include very early onset of seizures, intractability with multiple daily seizures and frequently a focal neurological or generalized cognitive deficit [29]. MRI features are varied, ranging from normal to cortical thickening, blurring of the grey–white junction and increased subcortical T2 signal depending on the underlying pathology [30].

Epilepsy surgery in children or adults with MCD has been less successful compared to surgery in other pathologies. Seizure-free outcomes are obtained in 49–64% of operated cases [27,29–31]. The main explanation given for surgical failure in the paediatric series is incomplete resection of the lesion. Cortical resections are limited by the predilection of MCD for involving the eloquent cortex of the central regions. In addition, the true extent of the malformative changes may not be apparent on MRI necessitating other methods to define the epileptogenic zone.

Functional neuroimaging (PET or SPECT), extraoperative subdural EEG and intraoperative ECoG have been used in paediatric series of MCD in an attempt to improve the demarcation of the epileptogenic zone. In the Cleveland Clinic series [30], neither PET nor subdural EEG were shown to improve surgical outcome, but the techniques were not examined in a controlled fashion.

Brain tumours and epilepsy

In a childhood epilepsy population, the overall incidence of brain tumours is low and the majority of the tumours have a low grade of malignancy. In large paediatric epilepsy surgery series [27,28,32] brain tumours are common, representing from a third to over half of all surgical cases. Clinically, children often present with epilepsy at an age significantly later than children with other pathologies. Because of the benign nature of most of these lesions, it is uncommon or rare for children to present with focal neurological signs or raised intracranial pressure.

Investigations in this population differ very little from the routine presurgical evaluation. CT is less sensitive than MRI and misses a significant proportion of low-grade lesions. The additional value of ancillary studies such as SPECT and PET is questionable if there is a well-defined lesion on MRI and confirmatory video-EEG studies. The role of ECoG is controversial. Defining the location of eloquent cortex in relation to the lesion is an absolute requirement. Complete tumour resection is of paramount importance but whether additional resection of neighbouring tissue identified as potentially epileptogenic on ECoG is of benefit remains an open question. Paediatric studies [33,34] addressing this aspect have reached opposing conclusions. Until a randomized study of the benefits of ECoG is performed, the policy of epilepsy centres will continue as their experience dictates.

Seizure-free outcomes for tumour-related epilepsy are amongst the highest of any pathology with reported rates above 80% [33,34]. Predictors of excellent outcomes include low preoperative seizure frequency and complete removal of the lesion. The most frequent histological tumour type is ganglioglioma, representing over 40% of cases in most series. Other common examples include low-grade astrocytoma and dysembryoblastic neuroepithelial tumours. In childhood, the majority of epileptogenic neoplasms arise from the temporal lobe and, occasionally, local infiltration of the insula or nearby basal ganglia can be a major limiting factor for resection.

Tuberous sclerosis (TS)

Children with TS have a high rate of epilepsy with onset usually in the first decade of life. Although classically associated with infantile spasms (IS), partial seizures in fact represent a higher proportion of the clinical presentations.

The successful outcomes obtained from resection of a single tuber in this multilesional disease have greatly extended the potential for epilepsy surgery. The largest reported paediatric series [35] was from Miami Children's Hospital (MCH) where a 69% seizure-free outcome was obtained following focal resection. The challenges that are unique to the presurgical evaluation of TS include multiple regions of abnormality on MRI and PET and multifocal, interictal, epileptiform discharges. In contrast, ictal EEG onsets are usually well localized with concordant hyperperfused regions on ictal SPECT. The presence of calcification and the largest discrete tuber on MRI also correlate well with the epileptogenic region. The main reason for surgical failure was incomplete resection of the tuber and surrounding epileptogenic zone with only one case showing activation of another region.

The long-term prognosis for seizure recurrence in TS after successful epilepsy surgery is unknown. The theoretical potential for other tubers to activate later in life remains, but this risk is not unique to TS. There is a definite correlation between seizures and lower intelligence in TS. The evidence from antiepileptic drug and surgical therapies is that seizure freedom can result in marked developmental gains.

Sturge–Weber syndrome (SWS)

SWS is a rare neurocutaneous disorder consisting of a congenital haemangioma of the upper face, with associated, usually ipsilateral, venous angioma of the leptomeninges. Associated features include mental retardation in over half of affected children and seizures occurring in up to 80% with a median age of onset of 6 months [36].

SWS represents a classic example of the question of the indications and timing for paediatric epilepsy surgery. An estimated 50% of cases can be well controlled on antiepileptic drugs [36]. A further problem is the unpredictable natural course of the seizures with prolonged periods of remission seen in some patients. Progressive cognitive deterioration with focal neurological signs is a common feature of the disease with difficulty in separating the relative contribution of seizures and ongoing cerebral atrophy.

Optimal presurgical evaluation relies on gadolinium-enhanced MRI to confirm that the pial angioma is indeed unilateral and to define the extent of the lesion. The scalp EEG can show bilateral epileptiform discharges that are not a contraindication to surgery. The extent of the lesion is essential to guide the type of operation—focal resection or hemispherectomy. Intraoperative ECoG indicates that the most active epileptogenic regions are usually adjacent to the angioma, but ECoG has not been shown to improve outcome. Extraoperative subdural recording is rarely required with visually guided lesionectomy usually sufficient for seizure freedom [37]. Two large surgical series [37,38] have reported rates of seizure freedom of 65–85%. Both studies indicate improved cognitive outcomes in children operated on earlier, especially less than 2 years of age.

Infantile spasms (IS)

IS is a 'catastrophic' epilepsy syndrome that begins in infancy and is accompanied by cognitive regression. The reported neurodevelopmental outcome of children with symptomatic IS treated medically is generally poor [39] which raises the question of surgery for intractable cases. A general principle of epilepsy treatment is that patients with generalized syndromes are not amenable to focal resection. This rule is broken by IS; although classified as a generalized symptomatic epilepsy syndrome, it is clear that the underlying aetiology may still be focal, and that removal of the epileptogenic region can arrest the spasms. Features indicating focality include a history of partial seizures, asymmetric spasms, hemihypsarrhythmia and hemiparesis [40]. These need to be thoroughly looked for, preferably using video-EEG telemetry and functional neuroimaging. In surgically treated cases, the common underlying focal pathologies include malformations of cortical development and encephalomalacia [41].

A large paediatric series from UCLA [41] reported short-term seizure freedom rates of 65% postmultilobar resection or hemispherectomy, although, in the long term, the success rate drops significantly [42]. A primary objective of surgery for IS, in addition to seizure control, is to improve cognitive outcome. Short-term follow-up of the UCLA cohort [39] revealed that post surgery only one of the 24 children achieved normal cognitive development and that, as a group, the standardized developmental scores were significantly lower at 2 years postoperatively than preoperatively. The authors argued that overall the group remained significantly better functioning than historical controls. An earlier age at surgery was associated with higher developmental scores, suggesting a need for early intervention to prevent regression of cognitive abilities.

The question of timing of surgery has not been resolved; this involves balancing the risks of cognitive regression versus unnecessary surgery for a child whose epilepsy may come under control [43]. Confusing semiology, multifocal EEG abnormalities and possibly a lower sensitivity of routine MRI for cortical lesions in the first 12 months of life hamper early identification of a surgical candidate. More prospective trials of epilepsy surgery for IS need to be conducted in order to delineate more clearly those who are suitable for surgery and the optimal timing that maximizes both seizure and developmental outcomes.

Landau–Kleffner syndrome (LKS)

LKS, first described in 1957 [44], is an age-related disorder of acquired aphasia with auditory verbal agnosia and a concomitant seizure disorder. Children with LKS present with a diverse epilepsy phenotype of generalized and/or partial seizures with a seizure frequency that varies from rare to intractable. Attempts to reverse this process using various medical therapies have been generally disappointing [45].

Morrell et al. [46] reported a series of LKS patients in 1995 who underwent a new surgical technique, multiple subpial transection (MST). The theoretical rationale for the use of MST is the selective severance of tangential intracortical pathways with minimal injury to the radially aligned neuronal functional unit. The intended result is the elimination of the epileptogenic capacity of the treated cortex without substantially compromising the physiological activity.

Unique to epilepsy surgery, the major aim of MST for LKS is to improve language outcome. Few centres have published their experience with sufficient sample size to draw definitive conclusions [47,48]. The largest reported series [47] is from Chicago where criteria for surgical candidacy included: (a) history of acquired aphasia, including auditory verbal agnosia, in the context of previously normal language abilities; (b) severe epileptiform EEG abnormality characterized by bilateral spike-wave discharges in slow-wave sleep; (c) neuropsychological test findings indicating relative preservation of non-verbal skills; and (d) electrophysiological evidence of a unilateral origin of the bilateral epileptiform discharge. Methods for determining the fourth criterion include the methohexital suppression test (described in detail in Morrell's study [46]) and MEG. MEG studies [49] have localized the interictal spike wave discharges to the posterior perisylvian cortex, but this finding is bilateral in the majority of patients with LKS.

The Chicago group reported that, of the 14 patients who underwent MST, the majority had significant improvements in receptive and expressive vocabulary. Children with a longer history of language impairment prior to surgery were less likely to show significant postoperative improvements. Serial testing indicated that children did not show significant gains on language testing until at least 6 months after surgery. As the authors acknowledge, the absence of a control group makes the effects of surgery difficult to extract from the natural course of the disease.

Although other small series have been published [48], further work is required before MST for LKS can be advocated for more widespread use.

Hypothalamic hamartoma and gelastic epilepsy

A hypothalamic hamartoma can be demonstrated on MRI in a proportion of children who present with gelastic seizures (ictal laughter). This rare syndrome presents typically in the first decade of life but has been reported in neonates. Comorbid problems include precocious puberty, severe behavioural disturbances and cognitive regression.

The initial surgical approach was based on the identification of apparent abnormal cortical epileptogenic activity on intracranial monitoring most frequently in the temporal lobes. Unfortunately focal cortical resection of these regions was uniformly unsuccessful [50]. Ictal SPECT studies and direct EEG recording from the hypothalamus revealing focal spiking were evidence that a subcortical grey matter structure could be responsible for epilepsy. Several surgical approaches have been advocated to attempt to resect this difficult region with varying degrees of success [51,52]. The most recent surgical series [51] advocates an approach via the corpus callosum between the fornices to the third ventricle using a microsurgical technique and frameless stereotaxy. In these five patients, complete or nearly complete resection of greater than 95% of the lesion was obtained in all with no long-term neurological or endocrine sequelae. Three patients achieved seizure freedom, with two markedly improved. In addition, a subjective assessment indicated that behaviour and overall quality of life also improved.

Alternatives to open surgery have included radiofrequency ablation and gamma-knife surgery (GKS). In a multicentre trial [53] 10 patients with severe epilepsy had GKS to their hypothalamic hamartoma at an average age of 13 years. Six of the 10 achieved either seizure freedom or rare seizures only, those being the patients who received higher doses to the lesion. No significant side-effects were reported, but follow-up was relatively short at just over 2 years.

Rasmussen's encephalitis (RE)

RE is characterized by intractable focal seizures (characteristically epilepsia partialis continua), progressive hemiplegia and cerebral inflammation typically confined to one hemisphere. Evidence for an immunological basis for this disease includes the presence in the serum and cerebrospinal fluid (CSF) of glutamate receptor subunit (Glu-R3) autoantibodies and focal immunoglobulin G (IgG)-dependent classical complement cascade activation in brain tissue of RE patients [54]. The use of anti-inflammatory agents produces only short-term reductions in seizure frequency [55,56].

The largest reported [57] surgical experience in RE consisted of 27 children at the Johns Hopkins Medical Institute. Surgical candidacy was based on a definite diagnosis of RE with the progressive nature of the disease firmly established and all other diagnoses excluded. In practical terms, this means a consistent clinical history with progressive unilateral hemisphere atrophy on MRI. Ancillary studies such as PET or SPECT often show a large region of decreased function beyond the obvious MRI change. Focal resections or biopsies were not considered part of the routine diagnostic work-up. Intractability to medical therapy was not a requirement for surgery.

Seizure freedom, or rare seizures, was achieved after hemispherectomy in 89% of the patients. The authors [57] proposed that these impressive results could be improved with careful attention to removal of residual grey matter along the mesial structures and the insula. Many children were operated on early in their illness, often when only a mild hemiparesis was present. Heminopia and a dense hemiplegia are an expected result of this procedure and are very disabling, although all children remain able to walk. In this series [57],

no child showed deterioration in overall health status, measured on a subjective 'burden of illness' scale. A major concern arises for children who have dominant hemisphere disease with the risk of severe language impairment following hemispherectomy. This is discussed in more detail in the neuropsychological outcomes section.

Early infantile epileptic encephalopathy (EIEE; Ohtahara syndrome)

EIEE is a rare, catastrophic epilepsy syndrome characterized by neonatal onset of frequent tonic seizures and a continuous burst-suppression pattern on EEG. Malformations of cortical development or metabolic disorders underlie the majority of cases [58]. The long-term prognosis is extremely poor with severe mental retardation and commonly progression to IS and/or Lennox–Gastaut syndrome [59].

Similar to IS, the apparently generalized nature of EIEE can be associated with a localized pathology such as focal cortical dysplasia. There are several case reports of elimination of seizures following a limited resection [58] with short-term improvements noted in psychomotor development.

Preoperative evaluation: current practice and future directions

Video-EEG telemetry and MRI, the current standard for presurgical evaluation

Video-EEG monitoring of clinical events remains the cornerstone of paediatric surgical evaluation. Epilepsy surgery can be considered after only limited investigations if localization by neuroimaging and electrophysiology converge. Certain adult centres have argued that in highly selected cases, surgical candidacy can be decided on the basis of interictal EEG and MRI without prolonged video-EEG telemetry. This approach, even if correct, is best suited to patients with mesial temporal lobe epilepsy, a minority of the cases in paediatric epilepsy series. A summary of the pitfalls and limitations of interpretation of EEG in seizure localization is given in an excellent review [60].

Invasive EEG monitoring (IEM)

The accurate definition of the epileptogenic region is the primary goal of the presurgical evaluation. IEM can delineate the epileptogenic region and its location relative to eloquent cortex more accurately than other technologies. The proportion of patients undergoing invasive EEG recording for seizure localization is declining primarily because of the increased sensitivity of non-invasive methods to detect focal abnormalities.

Extraoperative IEM entails increased costs and a small risk of morbidity from infection and haemorrhage; a cooperative family is a prerequisite. One must balance this with the potential benefits to the individual patient. Completeness of resection is crucial and IEM may be needed to guide resection by mapping eloquent cortex and by determining the extent of the epileptogenic area. Guidelines for invasive testing are given in Table 65.3. Patients with specific lesions on MRI (hippocampal sclerosis, tumours) and concordant non-invasive data can have excellent outcomes obtained without IEM. In

Table 65.3 General guidelines for considering invasive EEG monitoring (IEM)

Case scenario	IEM indicated	One stage resection
CT/MRI scans		
Normal	+	
Lesion		
Tumour/vascular		+
Hippocampal sclerosis		+
Sturge–Weber syndrome		+
Tuberous sclerosis	+	
MCD	+	
ER location and extent		
Anterior temporal		+
Extratemporal	+	
Multilobar		+
Divergent non-invasive data	+	
Encroachment on eloquent cortex	+	

Adapted with permission from the author [62].

contrast, surgical studies [30] of MCD suggest that the epileptogenic region is more extensive than the MRI abnormality and IEM is often indicated. Cases with no lesion on MRI but concordant non-invasive data should be candidates for extraoperative IEM. In these cases, the current precision of non-invasive methods is too low to contemplate resection without IEM.

The role of intraoperative ECoG in tailoring the size of cortical resection is limited by the reliance on interictal data, and its value has been a matter of debate [61]. In addition, intraoperative functional mapping of language is nearly impossible in children because it requires awake testing, and fine motor mapping is even less precise [62].

The place of IEM in the presurgical evaluation is changing as experience with non-invasive techniques increases. There is no doubt that the proportion of children requiring extraoperative IEM will continue to diminish. Experience and training in the interpretation of these complex EEG data will also decline, an unfortunate consequence that may result in its use being confined to highly specialized epilepsy centres.

MRI

The advent of MRI was a revolutionary step in the surgical treatment of epilepsy. MRI provides structural localization and accurate identification of the pathology. The greatest advantage over CT is in the assessment of mesiobasal structures such as the hippocampus and in malformations of cortical development where subtle differences in tissue characteristics and gyral pattern cannot be appreciated with CT. The majority of paediatric surgical candidates will have a lesion identified by MRI.

In addition to the basic T1- and T2-weighted images, additional imaging sequences should be tailored to the individual patient. All epilepsy surgery candidates should have their mesial temporal structures assessed with contiguous fine slice T1- and T2-weighted coronal images acquired in the hippocampal plane. T2-weighted images and particularly inversion recovery sequences (FLAIR) have a high sensitivity for detecting signal abnormality associated with malformations of cortical development. There are numerous other methods for increasing the yield from standard MRI in the paediatric surgical evaluation that are beyond the extent of this chapter.

Other MRI-based technologies

Several advances in MRI technology have contributed to improvements in localization of the epileptogenic zone. One of the first technologies was quantitative MRI, the computer-assisted volume measurement of brain structures, with the hippocampus being the main region of interest. Demonstration of unilateral or bilateral hippocampal volume reduction in adults with temporal lobe epilepsy is highly predictive of the epileptogenic zone, seizure freedom and memory outcomes after surgical resection [63]. Quantitative MRI studies [22,64] in paediatrics are few in number. In summary, because hippocampal sclerosis is an uncommon pathology in children and the logistical commitment is significant, the application of quantitative MRI in paediatrics is mainly limited to research.

Proton magnetic resonance spectroscopic imaging (^{1}H MRSI) is a technique that measures the spectra of the molecules that contribute to the proton signal in cerebral tissue. The major compounds identified include choline, creatine and N-acetylaspartate. The primary use has been in temporal lobe epilepsy in adults where, in general, unilateral abnormalities are concordant with EEG and other imaging methods. A recent ^{1}H MRSI study [65] in adults with bilateral hippocampal atrophy reported features associated with favourable surgical outcome including concordant ^{1}H MRSI lateralization with an absence of contralateral abnormality.

In children, few ^{1}H MRSI studies [66] have been performed; this is especially so in preadolescent children. A major limitation is the need for child control values as the developing brain has higher rates of myelination that results in alterations in the ratios of the molecules measured. The low molecular concentration necessitates sampling of larger regions; this reduces spatial resolution and increases signal contamination. Before ^{1}H MRSI can be recommended in the routine presurgical evaluation clearly more work needs to be done to determine the indications and limitations.

Diffusion-weighted imaging (DWI) is used mainly in acute stroke and is an MRI method that accentuates the appearance of cytotoxic oedema. A recent small adult study [67] found a low sensitivity of DWI following single brief seizures with some suggestion of a higher yield following prolonged focal seizures. Formal paediatric studies have not been performed, but our own experience has been similar to the above.

Functional neuroimaging studies

The current foundation for selection of candidates for epilepsy surgery is clearly the video-EEG and MRI. Several new imaging techniques have been developed to improve further localization of the epileptogenic region and to enhance surgical outcomes. A great potential for these methods is in patients with no lesion on MRI. It is unclear whether these new techniques add important information to surgical planning and decrease invasive EEG monitoring sufficient to justify the additional costs and time involved.

SPECT

Focal seizures produce regional increases in cerebral blood flow. Injection of radioligands during the ictal phase results in accumulation of the isotope in a pattern that mirrors cerebral blood flow. Large adult series [68] reveal that ictal SPECT has a high sensitivity and specificity for detecting temporal and extratemporal foci. Further processing by subtracting the interictal from the ictal scan with MRI coregistration (SISCOM) has been reported [69] to increase the yield. SISCOM localization was predictive of postsurgical outcome in extratemporal cases, independent of MRI or EEG findings. The extent of resection of the cortical region of the SISCOM focus was significantly associated with an excellent outcome.

Fewer paediatric SPECT studies have been performed with the important principles of methodology covered in a review article [70]. One paediatric series [71] addressed the question of whether ictal SPECT provided localizing data independent from EEG and MRI. Not surprisingly, SPECT was concordant in most children whose lesions were already localized by MRI and video-EEG and provided localizing data in more than half not localized by these modalities. In the small subgroup who had epilepsy surgery, SPECT provided no additional prognostic benefit in patients who already had an MRI lesion. In patients without lesions, however, ictal SPECT provides useful additional localization that can be used as a guide to intracranial implantation.

Limitations of SPECT are mainly logistical, requiring specially trained staff, a cooperative nuclear medicine department with sedation facilities for children. Additional problems include the brevity of extratemporal seizures and the comparatively poor spatial resolution of the images.

PET

Hypometabolic cerebral regions are identified by PET utilizing isotope-labelled glucose, the major ligand used in epilepsy studies. Published experience with PET in childhood epilepsy is relatively small. In adults, the major role has been in temporal lobe epilepsy and is perhaps most beneficial when no lesion is detected on MRI. The benefit of PET in paediatric epilepsy was first demonstrated in an infantile spasm series [72]. Five of 13 cases with a normal MRI had focal regions of hypometabolism identified on PET. Surgical resection of the PET-identified region resulted in seizure freedom.

This reliance on PET without extraoperative subdural recording was later challenged in a series [73] of 56 children with partial epilepsy who had a PET scan as part of their preoperative evaluation. These authors reached several conclusions: a normal PET did not exclude a child as a surgical candidate and an abnormal PET was an additional piece of data that, only when combined with concordant MRI and EEG data, could prevent chronic invasive intracranial monitoring.

PET is a more expensive technology than SPECT and is available in only a few centres. The lengthy scanning times mean that sedation is often required for children.

fMRI

In fMRI, regional brain activation is elicited by means of a specific task. Focal brain activation results in regional increases of cerebral blood flow and oxygen delivery, with a modest increase in oxygen extraction. The ratio between oxy- and deoxyhaemoglobin in venous blood actually increases. Signal production is due to the reduced paramagnetic effect of deoxyhaemoglobin with more signal observable on T2-weighted images. This is termed the blood oxygen level dependent (BOLD) effect.

A role for fMRI in the presurgical evaluation of childhood epilepsy holds promise [74]. Localization of a seizure focus by correlation of blood flow changes with interictal and ictal EEG abnormality is logistically difficult but possible. Identification of the language-dominant hemisphere is well validated in normal volunteers and left hemisphere dominant epilepsy patients. Mapping of sensory and motor functions is well established. Localization of higher cognitive functions such as memory and executive skills are yet to be developed.

Paradigms designed for adults cannot as easily be applied to children because of decreased compliance, frequent need for sedation and higher rates of intellectual disability. Passive stimuli paradigms, requiring no patient interaction (including while asleep) have been developed [75] for assessing visual, sensorimotor and language functions.

The clinical use of fMRI in epilepsy, although potentially revolutionary, remains in its infancy. Large epilepsy populations will need to be sampled to ensure the high sensitivity and specificity required for surgical decision-making. Those centres that have fMRI available will continue to rely on established multimodal techniques.

Intracarotid amobarbital procedure (IAP)

The IAP or Wada test remains in use in epilepsy centres to assist in hemispheric lateralization of memory and language. The main clinical role of the IAP has been to assess the risk of memory decline following temporal lobectomy. In paediatrics, an additional role for unilateral IAP has been in assessment of language dominance prior to hemispherectomy

A recent report [76] from the Cleveland Clinic discusses their experience with the IAP in 42 preadolescent children with the youngest child tested at 5 years of age. The IAP was technically possible in 40 children. Failure to complete the study occurred in 30% of those language tested and 36% of the memory tests because of either obtundation or agitation. The IAP successfully established hemispheric language dominance and memory representation in just under two-thirds of the group. The younger the child and the lower the IQ, the greater the likelihood of the study being unsuccessful.

Whether recent advances in functional imaging with MRI and PET will replace the Wada test is unknown. The principle difference is that the IAP results in cerebral hypofunction, which most closely resembles the effect of surgical removal. This is distinct from fMRI and PET that display a network of activated regions. The inability to determine whether these activated regions are either necessary or sufficient to support the task tested limits their role in surgical planning.

Specific issues related to epilepsy surgery in children

Surgery in infants with partial epilepsy

Several paediatric centres [77–79] have reported the unique challenges of epilepsy surgery in infancy. Partial epilepsy in infancy and early childhood is often a catastrophic disorder; very frequent seizures refractory to medical treatment can result in coincident developmental stagnation or regression. Long-term prognosis is poor, emphasizing the need for alternative therapies. Table 65.4 lists some of the clinical features that distinguish this age group from older patients.

The largest published surgical experience [77] in the age range of less than 3 years is from MCH. Of the 31 patients, 61% were seizure free at 12 months follow-up, similar to other reported series. The common pathologies seen from this and other series [78] were usually prenatal in origin with a high prevalence of malformations of cortical development. A higher proportion of multilobar resection or hemispherectomy in this age group reflects the more widespread pathology. No difference in seizure-free outcomes for temporal versus extratemporal resections illustrates the predominantly neocortical location of the pathology.

Data suggest that invasive monitoring may have been responsible for a lower need for reoperation in the MCH [77] and Cleveland series [78]. Functional cortical mapping can be problematic in infants because of a lower threshold for inducing epileptic after-discharges and higher amplitudes required to evoke normal cortical responses. A modified paradigm is often required [80] utilizing dual electrode stimulation with increased output intensities and duration. On a cautionary note, higher mortality rates are reported [77,78] particularly in patients under 12 months of age.

Epilepsy surgery in children with developmental and intellectual disabilities

Patients with intellectual and developmental disabilities have traditionally been considered poor candidates for focal resective epilepsy surgery. This was based on the concept that a low IQ was an indicator of bilateral widespread pathology. This hypothesis was supported in a large multicentre adult series [81] of over 1000 temporal lobectomies. Among patients with an IQ less than 75, one-third continued to have seizures following surgery compared to seizure-free rates of 76% in those with average intelligence and 83% in the above average IQ group. The authors recommended

that intelligence should not be used to exclude patients as surgical candidates but that the prognosis was less favourable. A paediatric temporal lobe series [82] indicated that predictors of outcome of temporal lobectomy in adults might not apply to children; no significant effect was found for factors such as mental retardation or focal temporal lesions. This result reflects the inherent neurobiological differences in the aetiology and expression of temporal lobe epilepsy in children. Adult data cannot thus be directly extrapolated to children.

Some degree of intellectual disability (ID) is present in up to 60% of paediatric intractable epilepsy patients. The natural history of epilepsy in children with ID is that seizures are much less likely to remit spontaneously [6,83]. Attempting to separate the functional effects of seizures from the underlying structural abnormality and thus predicting the long-term intellectual outcome of infants and young children is notoriously difficult. This group is where earlier surgery is likely to have the greatest benefit.

It is always essential to search for a neurodegenerative, metabolic or chromosomal disorder. One needs to be wary of diagnoses such as perinatal asphyxia and 'presumed viral encephalitis' to explain intractable epilepsy, as an undiagnosed metabolic disease remains a possibility. Table 65.5 is a partial list of diseases and syndromes associated with intractable epilepsy that are unlikely to benefit from epilepsy surgery. In addition to those diseases listed in the table, one should examine the MRI carefully for evidence of lesions that are also markers of a poor surgical prognosis such as periventricular nodular heterotopia [26].

The presurgical evaluation of children with ID does not differ greatly from the usual protocol. Video-EEG monitoring can be challenging as keeping electrodes in place on a child confined to a small room can be difficult in even the most attentive of children. Motor stereotypies, self-stimulatory behaviour and abnormal postures of spasticity are not infrequent presentations as non-epileptic events and need clear differentiation from true seizure episodes.

Functional brain investigations such as fMRI, Wada and extraoperative cortical mapping rely on a sufficient degree of cooperation and cognitive ability. There are paradigms that have been designed for fMRI and cortical mapping to map receptive language areas for non-verbal patients. Despite this, inability to localize eloquent cortex accurately can result in a conservative approach, ultimately limiting the extent of cortical resection.

Despite the hypothetical concerns and the limitations detailed above, children with intellectual disability represent a large proportion of a paediatric epilepsy surgery cohort, with over 40% of cases in one series [27]. Several studies [27,28] reveal that children with lower intelligence scores had similar surgical outcomes to others.

Table 65.4 Epilepsy surgery on infants

Distinctive features of epilepsy surgery in infants
Clinical semiology: often bilateral or non-localizing
Very frequent, often multiple, daily seizures
High incidence of intellectual disability
Requires a modified paradigm for functional cortical mapping
Predominance of malformations of cortical development
Higher rate of hemispherectomy or multilobar resection
No difference in outcome for temporal vs. extratemporal resections
Higher surgical mortality rate

Table 65.5 Disorders not amenable to epilepsy surgery

Neuronal ceroid lipofuscinosis
Peroxisomal disorders
Mitochondrial diseases (MERRF, MELAS, Alpers)
Pyridoxine dependency
Angelman's syndrome
Rett's syndrome
Progressive myoclonic epilepsies

Table 65.6 Results from major paediatric epilepsy surgical series

Paediatric epilepsy centre	Age range (mean)	Ix. in addition VEEG/MRI	Site of surgery	Pathology	Invasive EEG monitoring	Class I–II outcomes (mean years F/U)
MCH [27] (n = 75) 1988–97	0–12 years (8 years)	SPECT	T 39% E 61%	MCD 56% NEO 33% HS 8%	73%	I 59% II 19% (5 years)
UCLA [85] (n = 198) 1986–97	0–18 years	PET	H 42% M 23% T 19% E 15%	MCD 32% NEO 7% HS 7%	Nil	I 59% (2 years)
CCF [28] (n = 136) 1990–96	0–20 years (12 years)	PET	T 53% E 35% H 12%	NEO 37% MCD 26% HS 15%	29%	I 68% II 13% (3.6 years)
Paris [32] (n = 171) 1981–96	0–15 years (9 years)	Nil	T 39% E 61%	NEO 58% MCD 13%	Nil	I 82% II 8% (5 years)
MNI [84] (n = 118) 1940–80	0–15 years (12 years)	CT	F 37% T 62%	NR	NR	Good 47%

E, extratemporal; F, frontal; H, hemispherectomy; HS, hippocampal sclerosis; M, multilobar; MCD, malformations of cortical development; NEO, neoplasia; NR, not reported; T, temporal lobe.

Even children with moderate to severe intellectual disability can be successfully rendered seizure free and their quality of life improved.

Lessons from large paediatric surgical cohorts

A summary of the large paediatric surgical series is presented in Table 65.6 and highlights some of the major clinical differences from adult centres. A number of features are highly characteristic of childhood epilepsy. Malformations of cortical development and developmental tumours are the common pathologies in contrast to adult series where hippocampal sclerosis is predominant. The higher rates of extratemporal surgery and hemispherectomy are also a feature of the paediatric population.

These centres all had differing approaches to the selection of surgical candidates but had in common VEEG telemetry and structural imaging as the foundation. The unique feature of the Parisian series [32] was that all cases had a lesion demonstrated on CT or MRI, the majority of which proved to be neoplastic on pathology. No additional investigations were performed such as SPECT, PET or invasive EEG monitoring. Despite this, remarkable outcomes were obtained in this series with an Engel class 1 outcome obtained in 82% of cases with an average follow-up time of nearly 6 years. This highlights the excellent outcomes obtainable in selected subgroups, similar to adult data for lesionectomy of low-grade tumours. In stark contrast, only 24% of patients who had incomplete resection of their lesion achieved seizure freedom.

Across the paediatric series a seizure-free outcome was obtained in the majority of cases. A number of factors were identified as predictive of a good outcome. Common to all of these studies was the importance of completeness of resection. In fact, this variable was the only significant predictor of outcome after multivariate analysis in the MCH series [27] with 92% improved with complete resection compared to 50% if incomplete. Definition of completeness varies; one invasive EEG study [27] used prominent interictal activity, focal attenuation of background and ictal onset zones with intraictally activated regions as evidence of the epileptogenic zone.

The Montreal (MNI) series [84] reported extremely poor outcomes in non-lesional cases, with only one of 11 frontal lobe cases seizure free. The Cleveland (CCF), University of California (UCLA) and Paris cohorts were almost entirely lesional cases. Children with a normal MRI (n = 35) in the MCH series showed a 56% seizure-free rate, not significantly below the overall outcome figures. Malformations of cortical development uniformly had lower rates of seizure freedom compared to other pathologies.

Other factors associated with poorer outcomes included a longer duration of epilepsy, multilobar resections and an injury resulting from the surgery. The Paris group reported [32] that 15/16 patients (94%) with vascular insults or local contusions as a result of surgery had seizure recurrence, an important factor not identified in the other series. Late recurrences are not uniformly detailed except for UCLA [85] reporting that 25% of their MCD cases had a recurrence of seizures after 2 years.

Morbidity and mortality was uniformly low with a mortality rate of 0–1.3% predominantly in younger children. The major morbidity was from perioperative haemorrhage and wound infection, which occurred in a few patients.

Future directions

It is clear from the above review that an enormous amount of research is still required in the field of paediatric epilepsy surgery. This research is hampered by the broad spectrum of aetiologies and pathologies, the vast differences between infants and adolescents and the persistent problem of failure of early referral for presurgical evaluation in intractable cases. The resultant small sample sizes limit the power of studies to address important questions such as the appropriate timing of surgery to maximize developmental outcomes.

Paediatric epilepsy surgery will likely benefit from advances in several unrelated disciplines. Techniques in brain imaging and functional brain mapping will increasingly permit more precise definitions of the neuronal events underlying epilepsy and cognition, and facilitate more definitive surgical planning. The list of new technologies is growing and already includes fMRI, MEG, magnetic source imaging, optical source imaging and transcranial magnetic stimulation. Delineation of gene expression through techniques such as PET reporter genes may soon have direct clinical applications.

Future experimental models of neuroembryological events should also foster an understanding of the aetiology and pathogenesis of medically resistant childhood epilepsy. A variety of pathological and environmental factors in the embryo alter neurotransmitter signalling and interfere with normal developmental processes. It will be increasingly important to understand how these factors modify structural and functional brain organization, and to define the general principles and mechanisms of neural circuit dysfunction.

Lastly, emerging surgical therapies such as gamma-knife and targeted deep brain stimulation should increase the number of potential cases to include those that might otherwise have been judged inoperable.

References

1 Hauser WA, Annegers JF, Kurland LT. Incidence of epilepsy and unprovoked seizures in Rochester, Minnesota: 1935–1984. *Epilepsia* 1993; 34: 453–68.
2 Kurtz Z, Tookey P, Ross E. Epilepsy in young people: 23 year follow up of the British national child development study. *Br Med J* 1998; 316: 339–42.
3 Berg AT, Shinnar S, Levy SR, Testa FM, Smith-Rapaport S, Beckerman B. Early development of intractable epilepsy in children: A prospective study. *Neurology* 2001; 56(11): 1445–52.
4 Kwan P, Brodie MJ. Early identification of refractory epilepsy. *N Engl J Med* 2000; 342: 314–19.
5 Engel J. Surgery for seizures. *N Engl J Med* 1996; 334: 647–52.
6 Sillanpaa M, Jalava M, Kaleva O, Shinnar S. Long-term prognosis of seizures with onset in childhood. *N Engl J Med* 1998; 338: 1715–22.
7 Lendt M, Helmstaedter C, Kuczaty S, Schramm J, Elger CE. Behavioural disorders in children with epilepsy: early improvement after surgery. *J Neurol Neurosurg Psychiatr* 2000; 69: 739–44.
8 Keene DL, Loy-English I, Ventureyra EC. Long-term socioeconomic outcome following surgical intervention in the treatment of refractory epilepsy in childhood and adolescence. *Childs Nervous System* 1998; 14: 362–5.
9 Sirven JI, Malamut BL, O'Connor MJ, Sperling MR. Temporal lobectomy outcome in older versus younger adults. *Neurology* 2000; 54: 2166–70.
10 Mihara T, Inoue Y, Matsuda K *et al*. Recommendation of early surgery from the viewpoint of daily quality of life. *Epilepsia* 1996; 37 (Suppl. 3): 33–6.
11 Lendt M, Helmstaedter C, Elger CE. Pre- and postoperative socioeconomic development of 151 patients with focal epilepsies. *Epilepsia* 1997; 38: 1330–7.
12 Selai CE, Elstner K, Trimble MR. Quality of life pre and post epilepsy surgery. *Epilepsy Res* 2000; 38: 67–74.
13 Markand ON, Salanova V, Whelihan E, Emsley CL. Health-related quality of life outcome in medically refractory epilepsy treated with anterior temporal lobectomy. *Epilepsia* 2000; 41: 749–59.
14 Sabaz M, Cairns DR, Lawson JA, Nheu N, Bleasel AF, Bye AM. Validation of a new quality of life measure for children with epilepsy. *Epilepsia* 2000; 41: 765–74.
15 Camfield C, Breau L, Camfield P. Impact of pediatric epilepsy on the family: a new scale for clinical and research use. *Epilepsia* 2001; 42: 104–12.
16 Devinsky O, Westbrook L, Cramer J, Glassman M, Perrine K, Camfield C. Risk factors for poor health-related quality of life in adolescents with epilepsy. *Epilepsia* 1999; 40: 1715–20.
17 Westerveld M, Sass KJ, Chelune GJ *et al*. Temporal lobectomy in children: cognitive outcome. *J Neurosurg* 2000; 92: 24–30.
18 Lassonde M, Sauerwein HC, Jambaque I, Smith ML, Helmstaedter C. Neuropsychology of childhood epilepsy: pre- and postsurgical assessment. *Epileptic Dis* 2000; 2: 3–13.
19 Boatman D, Freeman J, Vining E *et al*. Language recovery after left hemispherectomy in children with late-onset seizures. *Ann Neurol* 1999; 46: 579–86.
20 Olafsson E, Hauser WA, Gudmundsson G. Long-term survival of people with unprovoked seizures: a population-based study. *Epilepsia* 1998; 39: 89–92.
21 Holmes GL. Epilepsy in the developing brain: lessons from the laboratory and clinic. *Epilepsia* 1997; 38: 12–30.
22 Lawson JA, Vogrin S, Bleasel AF *et al*. Predictors of hippocampal, cerebral, and cerebellar volume reduction in childhood epilepsy. *Epilepsia* 2000; 41: 1540–5.
23 Stafstrom CE, Lynch M, Sutula TP. Consequences of epilepsy in the developing brain: implications for surgical management. *Semin Pediatr Neurol* 2000; 7: 147–57.
24 Silfvenius H. Cost and cost-effectiveness of epilepsy surgery. *Epilepsia* 1999; 40 (Suppl. 8): 32–9.
25 Keene D, Ventureyra EC. Epilepsy surgery for 5- to 18-year old patients with medically refractory epilepsy – is it cost efficient? *Childs Nervous System* 1999; 15: 52–4.
26 Dubeau F, Tampieri D, Lee N *et al*. Periventricular and subcortical nodular heterotopia. A study of 33 patients. *Brain* 1995; 118: 1273–87.
27 Paolicchi JM, Jayakar P, Dean P *et al*. Predictors of outcome in pediatric epilepsy surgery. *Neurology* 2000; 54: 642–7.
28 Wyllie E, Comair YG, Kotagal P, Bulacio J, Bingaman W, Ruggieri P. Seizure outcome after epilepsy surgery in children and adolescents. *Ann Neurol* 1998; 44: 740–8.
29 Chassoux F, Devaux B, Landre E *et al*. Stereoelectroencephalography in focal cortical dysplasia: a 3D approach to delineating the dysplastic cortex. *Brain* 2000; 123: 1733–51.
30 Edwards JC, Wyllie E, Ruggeri PM *et al*. Seizure outcome after surgery for epilepsy due to malformation of cortical development. *Neurology* 2000; 55: 1110–14.
31 Keene DL, Jimenez CC, Ventureyra E. Cortical microdysplasia and surgical outcome in refractory epilepsy of childhood. *Pediatr Neurosurg* 1998; 29: 69–72.
32 Bourgeois M, Sainte-Rose C, Lellouch-Tubiana A *et al*. Surgery of epilepsy associated with focal lesions in childhood. *J Neurosurg* 1999; 90: 833–42.
33 Khajavi K, Comair YG, Wyllie E, Palmer J, Morris HH, Hahn JF. Surgical management of pediatric tumor-associated epilepsy. *J Child Neurol* 1999; 14: 15–25.
34 Berger MS, Ghatan S, Geyer JR, Keles GE, Ojemann GA. Seizure outcome in children with hemispheric tumors and associated intractable epilepsy: the role of tumor removal combined with seizure foci resection. *Pediatr Neurosurg* 1991; 17: 185–91.
35 Koh S, Jayakar P, Dunoyer C *et al*. Epilepsy surgery in children with tuberous sclerosis complex: presurgical evaluation and outcome. *Epilepsia* 2000; 41: 1206–13.
36 Sujansky E, Conradi S. Sturge–Weber syndrome: age of onset of seizures and glaucoma and the prognosis for affected children. *J Child Neurol* 1995; 10: 49–58.
37 Arzimanoglou AA, Andermann F, Aicardi J *et al*. Sturge–Weber syndrome: indications and results of surgery in 20 patients. *Neurology* 2000; 55: 1472–9.
38 Ogunmekan AO, Hwang PA, Hoffman HJ. Sturge-Weber-Dimitri disease: role of hemispherectomy in prognosis. *Canad J Neurol Sci* 1989; 16: 78–80.
39 Asarnow RF, LoPresti C, Guthrie D *et al*. Developmental outcomes in children receiving resection surgery for medically intractable infantile spasms. *Dev Med Child Neurol* 1997; 39: 430–40.

40 Kramer U, Sue WC, Mikati MA. Focal features in West syndrome indicating candidacy for surgery. *Pediatr Neurol* 1997; 16: 213–17.

41 Chugani HT, Shewmon DA, Shields WD *et al*. Surgery for intractable infantile spasms: neuroimaging perspectives. *Epilepsia* 1993; 34: 764–71.

42 Shewmon DA, Shields WD, Sankar R. Follow-up on infants with surgery for catastrophic epilepsy. In: Tuxhorn I, Holthausen H, Boenigk H, eds. *Pediatric Epilepsy Syndromes and their Surgical Treatment*. London: John Libbey, 1997: 513–25.

43 Shields WD, Shewmon DA, Peacock WJ, LoPresti CM, Nakagawa JA, Yudovin S. Surgery for the treatment of medically intractable infantile spasms: a cautionary case. *Epilepsia* 1999; 40: 1305–8.

44 Landau WM, Kleffner FR. Syndrome of acquired aphasia with convulsive disorder in children. 1957. *Neurology* 1998; 51: 1241–9.

45 Robinson RO, Baird G, Robinson G, Simonoff E. Landau–Kleffner syndrome: course and correlates with outcome. *Dev Med Child Neurol* 2001; 43: 243–7.

46 Morrell F, Whisler WW, Smith MC *et al*. Landau–Kleffner syndrome. Treatment with subpial intracortical transection. *Brain* 1995; 118: 1529–46.

47 Grote CL, Van Slyke P, Hoeppner JA. Language outcome following multiple subpial transection for Landau–Kleffner syndrome. *Brain* 1999; 122: 561–6.

48 Irwin K, Birch V, Lees J *et al*. Multiple subpial transection in Landau–Kleffner syndrome. *Dev Med Child Neurol* 2001; 43: 248–52.

49 Lewine JD, Andrews R, Chez M *et al*. Magnetoencephalographic patterns of epileptiform activity in children with regressive autism spectrum disorders. *Pediatrics* 1999; 104: 405–18.

50 Cascino GD, Andermann F, Berkovic SF *et al*. Gelastic seizures and hypothalamic hamartomas: evaluation of patients undergoing chronic intracranial EEG monitoring and outcome of surgical treatment. *Neurology* 1993; 43: 747–50.

51 Rosenfeld JV, Harvey AS, Wrennall J, Zacharin M, Berkovic SF. Transcallosal resection of hypothalamic hamartomas, with control of seizures, in children with gelastic epilepsy. [Review] [43 refs]. *Neurosurgery* 2001; 48: 108–18.

52 Valdueza JM, Cristante L, Dammann O *et al*. Hypothalamic hamartomas: with special reference to gelastic epilepsy and surgery. *Neurosurgery* 1994; 34: 949–58; discussion 958.

53 Regis J, Bartolomei F, de Toffol B *et al*. Gamma knife surgery for epilepsy related to hypothalamic hamartomas. *Neurosurgery* 2000; 47: 1343–51.

54 Whitney KD, Andrews PI, McNamara JO. Immunoglobulin G and complement immunoreactivity in the cerebral cortex of patients with Rasmussen's encephalitis. *Neurology* 1999; 53: 699–708.

55 Andrews PI, Dichter MA, Berkovic SF, Newton MR, McNamara JO. Plasmapheresis in Rasmussen's encephalitis. *Neurology* 1996; 46: 242–6.

56 Hart YM, Cortez M, Andermann F *et al*. Medical treatment of Rasmussen's syndrome (chronic encephalitis and epilepsy): effect of high-dose steroids or immunoglobulins in 19 patients. *Neurology* 1994; 44: 1030–6.

57 Vining EP, Freeman JM, Pillas DJ *et al*. Why would you remove half a brain? The outcome of 58 children after hemispherectomy – the Johns Hopkins experience: 1968–1996. *Pediatrics* 1997; 100: 163–71.

58 Komaki H, Sugai K, Sasaki M *et al*. Surgical treatment of a case of early infantile epileptic encephalopathy with suppression-bursts associated with focal cortical dysplasia. *Epilepsia* 1999; 40: 365–9.

59 Verrotti A, Domizio S, Sabatino G, Morgese G. Early infantile epileptic encephalopathy: a long-term follow-up study. *Childs Nervous System* 1996; 12: 530–3.

60 Jayakar P, Duchowny M, Resnick TJ, Alvarez LA. Localization of seizure foci: pitfalls and caveats. [Review] [75 refs]. *J Clin Neurophysiol* 1991; 8: 414–31.

61 Keene DL, Whiting S, Ventureyra EC. Electrocorticography. *Epileptic Dis* 2000; 2: 57–63.

62 Jayakar P. Invasive EEG monitoring in children: when, where, and what? *J Clin Neurophysiol* 1999; 16: 408–18.

63 Watson C, Jack CR Jr, Cendes F. Volumetric magnetic resonance imaging. Clinical applications and contributions to the understanding of temporal lobe epilepsy. *Arch Neurol* 1997; 54: 1521–31.

64 Lawson JA, Nguyen W, Bleasel AF *et al*. ILAE–defined epilepsy syndromes in children: correlation with quantitative MRI. *Epilepsia* 1998; 39: 1345–9.

65 Li LM, Cendes F, Antel SB *et al*. Prognostic value of proton magnetic resonance spectroscopic imaging for surgical outcome in patients with intractable temporal lobe epilepsy and bilateral hippocampal atrophy. *Ann Neurol* 2000; 47: 195–200.

66 Cross JH, Connelly A, Jackson GD, Johnson CL, Neville BG, Gadian DG. Proton magnetic resonance spectroscopy in children with temporal lobe epilepsy. *Ann Neurol* 1996; 39: 107–13.

67 Diehl B, Najm I, Ruggieri P *et al*. Postictal diffusion-weighted imaging for the localization of focal epileptic areas in temporal lobe epilepsy. *Epilepsia* 2001; 42: 21–8.

68 Newton MR, Berkovic SF, Austin MC, Rowe CC, McKay WJ, Bladin PF. SPECT in the localisation of extratemporal and temporal seizure foci. *J Neurol Neurosurg Psychiatr* 1995; 59: 26–30.

69 O'Brien TJ, So EL, Mullan BP *et al*. Subtraction peri-ictal SPECT is predictive of extratemporal epilepsy surgery outcome. *Neurology* 2000; 55: 1668–77.

70 Harvey AS, Berkovic SF. Functional neuroimaging with SPECT in children with partial epilepsy. *J Child Neurol* 1994; 9 (Suppl. 1): S71–81.

71 Lawson JA, O'Brien TJ, Bleasel AF *et al*. Evaluation of SPECT in the assessment and treatment of intractable childhood epilepsy. *Neurology* 2000; 55: 1391–3.

72 Chugani HT, Shields WD, Shewmon DA, Olson DM, Phelps ME, Peacock WJ. Infantile spasms: I. PET identifies focal cortical dysgenesis in cryptogenic cases for surgical treatment. *Ann Neurol* 1990; 27: 406–13.

73 Snead OC, Chen LS, Mitchell WG *et al*. Usefulness of [18F]fluorodeoxyglucose positron emission tomography in pediatric epilepsy surgery. *Pediatr Neurol* 1996; 14: 98–107.

74 Bookheimer SY, Dapretto M, Karmarkar U. Functional MRI in children with epilepsy. *Dev Neurosci* 1999; 21: 191–9.

75 Souweidane MM, Kim KH, McDowall R *et al*. Brain mapping in sedated infants and young children with passive-functional magnetic resonance imaging. *Pediatr Neurosurg* 1999; 30: 86–92.

76 Hamer HM, Wyllie E, Stanford L, Mascha E, Kotagal P, Wolgamuth B. Risk factors for unsuccessful testing during the intracarotid amobarbital procedure in preadolescent children. *Epilepsia* 2000; 41: 554–63.

77 Duchowny M, Jayakar P, Resnick T *et al*. Epilepsy surgery in the first three years of life. *Epilepsia* 1998; 39: 737–43.

78 Wyllie E, Comair YG, Kotagal P, Raja S, Ruggieri P. Epilepsy surgery in infants. *Epilepsia* 1996; 37: 625–37.

79 Sugimoto T, Otsubo H, Hwang PA, Hoffman HJ, Jay V, Snead OC. Outcome of epilepsy surgery in the first three years of life. *Epilepsia* 1999; 40: 560–5.

80 Jayakar P, Alvarez LA, Duchowny MS, Resnick TJ. A safe and effective paradigm to functionally map the cortex in childhood. *J Clin Neurophysiol* 1992; 9: 288–93.

81 Chelune GJ, Naugle RI, Hermann BP *et al*. Does presurgical IQ predict seizure outcome after temporal lobectomy? Evidence from the Bozeman Epilepsy Consortium. *Epilepsia* 1998; 39: 314–18.

82 Goldstein R, Harvey AS, Duchowny M *et al*. Preoperative clinical, EEG, and imaging findings do not predict seizure outcome following temporal lobectomy in childhood. *J Child Neurol* 1996; 11: 445–50.

83 Berg AT, Levy SR, Novotny EJ, Shinnar S. Predictors of intractable epilepsy in childhood: a case-control study. *Epilepsia* 1996; 37: 24–30.

84 Fish DR, Smith SJ, Quesney LF, Andermann F, Rasmussen T. Surgical treatment of children with medically intractable frontal or temporal lobe epilepsy: results and highlights of 40 years' experience. *Epilepsia* 1993; 34: 244–7.

85 Mathern GW, Giza CC, Yudovin S *et al*. Postoperative seizure control and antiepileptic drug use in pediatric epilepsy surgery patients: the UCLA experience, 1986–1997. *Epilepsia* 1999; 40: 1740–9.

86 Camfield C, Camfield P, Gordon K, Smith B, Dooley J. Outcome of childhood epilepsy: a population-based study with a simple predictive scoring system for those treated with medication. *J Pediatr* 1993; 122: 861–8.

87 Rantala H, Ingalsuo H. Occurrence and outcome of epilepsy in children younger than 2 years. *J Pediatr* 1999; 135: 761–4.

88 Van Paesschen W, Duncan JS, Stevens JM, Connelly A. Etiology and early prognosis of newly diagnosed partial seizures in adults: a quantitative hippocampal MRI study. *Neurology* 1997; 49: 753–7.

Hemispherectomy for Epilepsy

J.-G. Villemure and V. Bartanusz

While hemispherectomy was introduced in neurosurgery by Walter Dandy in 1928 [1] for the treatment of infiltrating glioma, this indication was abandoned and hemispherectomy has over the past 30 years been performed exclusively for the control of pharmacologically refractory seizures. The term 'hemispherectomy' is used to describe the surgical procedure by which a cerebral hemisphere is either anatomically excised or made non-functional by disconnection. Indeed, in this chapter, we will include under the heading 'hemispherectomy' the different methods available to achieve the removal or disconnection of one cerebral hemisphere.

Indications

The success of hemispherectomy in controlling seizures critically depends on the criteria for patient selection. Two groups of criteria have to be considered in the decisional process for hemispherectomy: (a) general considerations regarding the indication of surgery in patients with epilepsy such as the intractability of the epilepsy; and (b) specific criteria relating to the severity of the damage of the diseased hemisphere from which the epileptic activity originates (Table 66.1) [2]. The psychological and social assessments are also important for determining the global impact of the operation but are not considered essential criteria for hemispherectomy (see below).

Seizures: intractability and types

Patients who are candidates for hemispherectomy usually present with seizures which have not responded adequately to multiple antiepileptic drugs or combinations of antiepileptic drugs. Typically, the seizure frequency is not satisfactorily controlled by optimal medical therapy, and the side-effects of adequate therapy may be psychosocially unacceptable and indeed may be worse than the seizures themselves. The lack of seizure control is thus the first element to consider in the decision to proceed to hemispherectomy.

Seizure frequency can vary from 5 to 150 seizures per day according to seizure types and underlying pathology. Since most hemispherectomy candidates suffer from unilateral cerebral pathology, over 80% of patients will have as their predominant seizure pattern a focal motor component affecting the contralateral side; this can either be purely focal or can progress as a jacksonian march. The condition in which focal motor seizures are most frequently seen is epilepsia partialis continua, usually secondary to Rasmussen's encephalitis. Only rarely do patients considered for hemispherectomy have a single seizure type; more commonly they exhibit a combination of seizures consisting of generalized, drop and focal motor seizures. Complex partial seizures are generally rare. The clinical

semiology can be helpful in confirming the lateralization, and also in determining if the seizures have a more focal onset.

Neurological examination

A detailed preoperative neurological assessment is necessary in all patients considered for hemispherectomy in order to predict outcome. Neurological examination of patients who are candidates for hemispherectomy usually reveals a neurological deficit that reflects the degree of hemispheric damage. The severity of the neurological deficits will, however, vary according to the aetiology responsible for the intractable seizures and, in progressive conditions, according to the natural history of the disease.

The neurological deficits are a severe hemiparesis, hemianopsia, altered sensory examination and some degree of psychomotor retardation.

Severe hemiparesis

The severe hemiparesis is manifest by an inability of the patient to perform individual finger movements and foot tapping. There is usually increased tone and hyperreflexia. Patients are, however, able to voluntarily perform movements at major joints such as the shoulder, elbow, hip or knee and even in some instances able to open and close their affected hand. Hemispherectomy does not aggravate this level of motor performance in the long term. It may, however, temporarily (weeks) aggravate the deficit, create a flaccid hemiplegia or decrease the tone of the affected limbs (possibly chronically), but patients should rapidly recover to their preoperative motor status within a few weeks.

Sometimes, in progressive conditions, the motor deficit prior to operation is moderate or even mild. In these cases, the benefit of early surgery and seizure control has to outweigh the aggravation of the neurological status. In some cases the natural history of the condition would be one of rapid progression of the motor deficit, and thus little is lost by acutely aggravating the deficit with surgery. In instances of incomplete motor deficit prior to surgery, one should expect a worsening of the hemiparesis with loss of fine movements, but recovery of gross movements and walking. In children, social and intellectual development will be accelerated with improved seizure control resulting from the operation, so that early hemispherectomy should be considered despite the known worsening of motor function [3,4].

Hemianopsia

Hemianopsia in these patients usually accompanies the motor

Table 66.1 Considerations in patient selection for hemispherectomy

General considerations
Medically intractable epilepsy
Resectable structural abnormality
Seizures arising from the diseased hemisphere
No medical contraindication

Specific considerations
Maximum hemiplegia
Somatosensory deficit
Homonymous hemianopsia
Psychomotor deterioration
Deficit in language functions
Diffuse hemispheric abnormalities on EEG
Radiological findings confirming hemispheric involvement
Partial hemispheric syndrome secondary to progressive pathology
(Rasmussen's encephalitis, Sturge–Weber syndrome)
Partial hemispheric syndrome with functional incapacity despite
preservation of some neurological function from the diseased
hemisphere

Table 66.2 Underlying aetiologies in the author's series of 70 disconnective hemispherectomies

	Aetiologies
Perinatal insult	22
Hemimegalencephaly	8
Migrational disorder	5
Sturge–Weber syndrome	2
Infection (viral, bacterial)	1
Chronic encephalitis	21
Head trauma	6
Vascular accident	4
Anoxia	1
Total	70

deficit. In some, the visual field is unaltered or only partially impaired due to the relative preservation of the anatomical and physiological integrity of the visual pathways. The absence of hemianopsia needs to be considered in context and should not be considered an absolute contraindication to hemispherectomy; patients can often adapt easily to a visual field defect.

Sensory examination

The sensory examination does not have an important impact on the decision to perform hemispherectomy. Most patients have preserved but altered sensation; stereognosis is usually severely impaired. Surgery results in little if any change in sensory performance.

Degree of psychomotor retardation

The degree of psychomotor retardation varies according to the severity of the seizures (generalized vs. focal), the extent of the disease process, social milieu, the age at onset of the cerebral insult responsible for the seizures and the age at time of surgery. The early occurrence of focal pathology is associated with better preservation of function due to compensation by the other hemisphere. The same observation applies to the timing of hemispherectomy; the best psychomotor development following hemispherectomy is in patients who had surgery performed early in life.

The degree of psychomotor retardation may be a very good index of the integrity of the good hemisphere. A proportion of hemispherectomy candidates exhibit evidence of some degree of bilateral cerebral damage or bilateral seizure activity. Severe psychomotor retardation should be interpreted as reflecting bilateral cerebral damage; although this is not a contraindication to hemispherectomy, the outcome is likely to be poorer, but still often worthwhile.

Language

Language is located in most right-handed individuals in the left hemisphere, and it seems that the process of lateralization is completed by 5 years of age — the end of the critical period for language acquisition. When hemispherectomy is carried out before the end of the critical period, the outcome is usually excellent, with no major impairment in language functions. This is also the case in congenital conditions involving the left hemisphere in which language does not develop at all in the left hemisphere. Recovery after left hemispherectomy in children with later onset seizures (after the age of 5 years) is, however, rarely completely normal. Nevertheless, speech following left hemispherectomy after that age is usually sufficient for communication, but remains definitively abnormal [5,6]. Chronic dominant hemispheric damage causes transfer of language functions to the other hemisphere at least up to adolescence. Language localization can be confirmed preoperatively by the intracarotid amytal test, but this is rarely necessary.

Aetiology

The aetiological factors underlying seizures in these cases can be divided into congenital or acquired. Congenital disorders comprise these conditions genetically determined (e.g. Sturge–Weber disease) and those resulting from a disorder during pregnancy or perinatally. *In utero* or perinatal cerebral vascular occlusion can result in large porencephaly or migrational and maturation disorders. Acquired conditions are usually secondary to cerebral bacterial or viral infection, Rasmussen's encephalitis, head trauma or vascular accident in childhood. Table 66.2 summarizes the aetiological findings in 70 consecutive patients who underwent functional hemispherectomy (senior author's series) (Plate 66.1, shown in colour between pp. 670 and 671).

In assessing the aetiological factors, it is important to appreciate whether the condition responsible for the brain damage has created a focal (unilateral) insult or a more diffuse one which may affect both hemispheres. This may be helpful in predicting the outcome of hemispherectomy. Diffuse infectious process, prolonged periods of anoxia, head injury with bilateral cerebral involvement, prolonged coma following haemorrhage or trauma may predict a less than excellent outcome, since these pathologies can be associated with bilateral cerebral involvement.

EEG

EEG usually confirms diffuse unilateral cerebral involvement. The EEG demonstrates low-amplitude slow activity accompanied by multifocal independent epileptic spikes that should ideally be lateralized to the diseased hemisphere. In about 50% of hemispherectomy candidates, epileptic activity is also recorded from the good hemisphere; the activity is either secondary or independent. The presence of independent activity should alert the clinician to the possibility of a bilateral process, but is in itself not a contraindication to the operation. Even apparently independent epileptic spikes originating from the 'good' hemisphere usually disappear after hemispherectomy.

Radiological investigation

The radiological findings on skull X-ray, CT or MRI are characterized by evidence of atrophy; this is usually unilateral, or predominantly involves one hemisphere (Fig. 66.2). The atrophy is characterized by increased skull thickness, a smaller hemisphere with enlarged sulci and ventricles and the presence of a smaller cerebral peduncle. Anomalies of the parenchyma may be found according to the underlying condition: grey and white matter abnormalities in migrational disorder, calcification in Sturge–Weber syndrome, gyri–sulci malformations in hemimegalencephaly, porencephaly following a vascular event and gradual diffuse unilateral atrophy in chronic encephalitis. The radiological findings may be minor in early life or at the onset of a disorder that is progressive such as chronic encephalitis. They are, however, obvious in most clinical situations. Gross abnormality of one

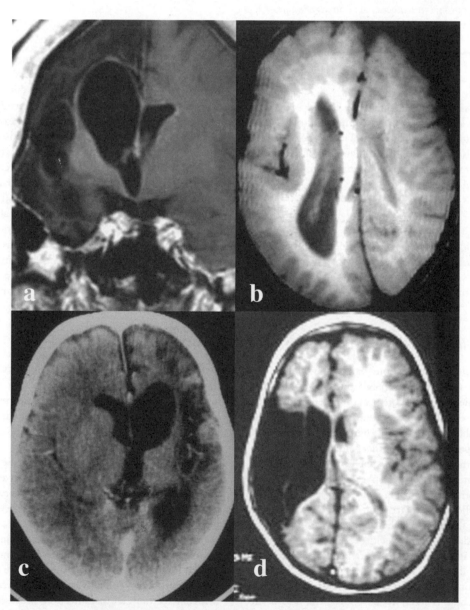

Fig. 66.2 (a) MRI, coronal, T1. Right hemispheric atrophy in infantile hemiplegia. (b) MRI, axial, T1. Enlarged right hemisphere in hemimegalencephaly. (c) CT, axial. Left hemispheric atrophy in Rasmussen's chronic encephalitis. (d) MRI, axial, T1. Right porencephaly.

hemisphere should not distract the clinician from assessing the other.

The suitability of any individual for hemispherectomy depends upon evidence based on the assessment of the seizure frequency and types, the neurological examination, the aetiology of the cerebral condition, the EEG and the results of neuroimaging. All these elements not only contribute to the assessment of the diseased hemisphere, but also help to determine the integrity of the 'good' hemisphere.

Surgical methods

Many hemispherectomy techniques have been developed over the past three decades; these aim to eliminate the complications seen following anatomical hemispherectomy while providing the patient with the same degree of seizure control. Table 66.3 summarizes the different hemispherectomy techniques. These involve either excision or disconnection.

Anatomical hemispherectomy

Anatomical hemispherectomy consists of complete removal of the cerebral hemisphere with or without the basal ganglia. Dandy described the original technique in 1928 and used it in the treatment of some tumours. Despite modifications [7] to the technique over the subsequent three decades, the end result of this operation has been the same, with the creation of a large subdural cavity. Use of the operation for seizures was popularized in the early 1950s following a report of 12 cases by Krynauw [8]. By 1961, over 260 cases of hemispherectomy had been documented in the literature [9].

Some technical variations have been reported. The hemispherectomy can be carried out either *en bloc* [10,11] or in fragments [1,8,12]. The basal ganglia can be removed or spared; this latter variation does not, however, have any long-term effect on motor function [13,14].

Modified hemispherectomy

Modified hemispherectomy originated in Oxford [15] and was popularized by Adams [16]. The operation consists of anatomical hemispherectomy followed by blocking the cerebrospinal fluid communication with the hemispherectomy cavity, and then reduction of the cavity. This is accomplished by obstructing the ipsilateral foramen of Monro with a piece of muscle; the volume of the hemispherectomy cavity is then reduced, at the expense of creating a large extradural space, by stripping the dura of the bone and tacking it to the basal dura and falx.

Table 66.3 Hemispherectomy techniques

Anatomical hemispherectomy
Modified hemispherectomy
Hemidecortication
Hemicorticectomy
Functional hemispherectomy
Hemispherotomy
Peri-insular hemispherotomy

Hemidecortication

Hemidecortication proposed by Ignelzi and Bucy [17] and popularized by Hoffman [18] consists of excising the whole cerebral cortex of the affected hemisphere; a temporal lobectomy allows the removal of the medial temporal structures. As much white matter as possible is preserved, thus avoiding unnecessary opening of the ventricle and so reducing the volume of the hemispherectomy cavity.

Hemicorticectomy

Hemicorticectomy technique developed by K. Welch and published by Winston *et al.* [19] shares the principle of hemidecortication [17], in which the white matter around the ventricle is preserved. The grey matter of the frontoparietal region is undercut in large slabs and removed; the white matter surrounding the ventricle is spared thus decreasing the risk of blood mixing with cerebrospinal fluid. Medial cortex is removed piecemeal.

Functional hemispherectomy

Functional hemispherectomy consists of a subtotal anatomical removal of the hemisphere, but complete physiological disconnection (Fig. 66.3a). The classical technique first reported by Rasmussen [11] involves a large central removal including parasagittal tissue, exposing the whole length of the corpus callosum. All fibres entering the corpus callosum are then interrupted from within the lateral ventricle in a parasagittal plane. The residual frontal and parieto-occipital lobes are then disconnected by aspiration of white and grey matter in the posterior frontal region to the level of the sphenoid wing, and in the parieto-occipital region down to the tentorium. A large temporal lobectomy including excision of medial structures is then carried out. Modifications to this original technique consist of smaller brain resection that permits complete hemispheric disconnection with minimal brain removal.

Hemispherotomy

In 1992, Delalande *et al.* [20] coined the term hemispherotomy to describe a technique of cerebral disconnection. This is performed through a central vertex cortical window which allows access to the lateral ventricle. Once in the ventricle, the neurosurgeon carries out a callosotomy and section of the fornix. The rest of the hemisphere is disconnected by section through the basal ganglia, entering the temporal horn.

Peri-insular hemispherotomy

Peri-insular hemispherotomy developed by Villemure [21,22] represents an extension of the principle of functional hemispherectomy (Fig. 66.3b). The procedure is carried in two major stages via the supra and infrainsular windows. In the suprainsular window, the body of the lateral ventricle is accessed by removing the frontoparietal opercular cortex and sectioning perpendicular to the underlying white matter. Once the lateral ventricle is reached, a functional hemispherectomy is achieved by callosotomy and frontobasal disconnection from within the lateral ventricle. In the infrainsular window, the temporal opercular cortex (T1) is excised, and the tem-

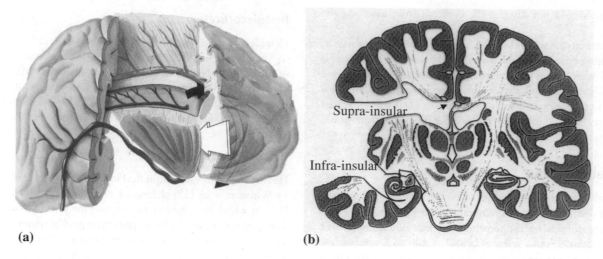

(a) **(b)**

Fig. 66.3 (a) Representation of right functional hemispherectomy. (b) Diagrammatic representation of right peri-insular hemispherotomy (supra- and infrainsular windows; arrow indicates the site of transventricular callosotomy).

poral horn is exposed from the tip to the trigone by sectioning of the temporal stem. The amygdala is excised by aspiration, and the anterior hippocampus is removed back to the choroidal fissure. The hippocampus need not be removed, but instead its output through the fimbria–fornix can be interrupted just opposite the splenium of the corpus callosum. This technique allows disconnection of the hemisphere with minimal brain removal. Sylvian arteries and veins should be preserved to avoid postoperative swelling of the residual brain.

Regardless of which surgical technique is chosen, the insular cortex may or may not be excised. There is no clear evidence from the literature that removal of the insula is necessary for the operation to be successful. However, there are reports of continued seizures in patients in whom the insula is preserved, and we thus recommend that the insula be either removed or undercut systematically [23,24].

Surgical morbidity

In the mid 1960s, superficial cerebral haemosiderosis (SCH) was recognized as a late complication of anatomical hemispherectomy. This provided the incentive to develop new methods of hemispherectomy in order to decrease the rate of complications [25].

Surgical morbidity of hemispherectomy is classified either as 'early', if it occurs within 30 days of surgery, or 'late' when it occurs 1 month to many years postoperatively. Morbidity may be further subdivided into side-effects (expected) and complications (unexpected) [26].

Early morbidity

Early side-effects of the operation that are common, expected or self-limiting have to be differentiated from complications. Immediate postoperative low-grade fever lasting up to 10–12 days is seen quite frequently following large brain removal; it is suspected to arise from aseptic meningitis due to blood products in the cerebrospinal fluid. Isolated postoperative seizures have rarely been ob-

served to occur within 48 h of surgery. These are usually generalized and do not necessarily recur. Their aetiology is unclear; they may be drug-related secondary to medications and anaesthesia, or in some cases indicate epileptogenicity of the 'normal' hemisphere.

Non-specific complications, such as haemorrhage [27] and infection, inherent to any surgical procedure, are relatively rare and are not specifically secondary to the hemispherectomy.

The incidence of early postoperative hydrocephalus is related to the surgical technique used. It is likely to result from three factors solely or in combination: (a) the nature of the disease process underlying the brain pathology, inflammatory processes or head injury may interfere with cerebrospinal fluid flow and absorptive mechanisms; (b) the presence of blood in the cerebrospinal fluid following surgery; or (c) the reduction in the surface of the subarachnoid space resulting from surgery; this varies from half the supratentorial subarachnoid space in anatomical hemispherectomy and hemidecortication, to minimal removal in hemispherotomy.

The incidence of hydrocephalus varies from 5% to 30% according to several series using different surgical techniques, but it is not always divided into early and late occurrence [18,19]. A cerebrospinal fluid shunt procedure is indicated for treatment of hydrocephalus.

Early postoperative brain herniation and death have been reported [28]. This is thought to be secondary to brain shift towards the hemispherectomy side following anatomical hemispherectomy. Early hydrocephalus of the remaining hemisphere is also a contributory factor. Diffuse hemispheric swelling following peri-insular hemispherotomy can occur, secondary to the sacrificing of arteries and veins around the insula when there is minimal brain atrophy.

Late morbidity

Infection, haemorrhage and brain shift can occur late, but more specific late complications consist of superficial cerebral haemosiderosis (SCH) and late hydrocephalus. The reported incidence of these late complications is naturally related to the duration of follow-up.

SCH was recognized in the mid 1960s as a late complication of anatomical hemispherectomy. Oppenheimer and Griffith [25] gave a clinical and pathological description of this condition which may be summarized as follows. At an average interval of 8 years following surgery, patients who otherwise have been well since hemispherectomy then present with an insidious neurological deterioration that can lead to death. The pathological findings are those of obstructive hydrocephalus secondary to aqueductal stenosis, due to gliosis and ependymitis. The hemispherectomy cavity and the ventricular walls are lined by a membrane similar to the one found in chronic subdural haematoma. The fluid entrapped in the ventricle is brownish and described as machinery oil. The authors postulated that these findings were secondary to repeated small subclinical haemorrhages occurring following minor trauma, with secondary bleeding into the hemispherectomy cavity. Descriptions of this late complication have led to more widespread recognition; the incidence has varied from 15% to 35% [27,29–32]. The severity and frequency of this complication has led many leading centres to abandon anatomical hemispherectomy, and to employ less extensive brain removals. This complication has also resulted in the development of new surgical methods of hemispherectomy (Table 66.3). SCH following hemispherectomy has not been reported over the past 25 years.

The late complication of hydrocephalus is secondary to the same mechanisms postulated for the appearance of early hydrocephalus [26]. The late appearance can be explained by the presence of compensatory mechanisms during the early postoperative period or that there was early hydrocephalus that was asymptomatic and so was not investigated. Routine radiological examination by CT or MRI is useful to detect hydrocephalus and instigate early treatment [26,33].

Death following hemispherectomy has been reported to occur in 6–7% of patients [9]. Wilson [15] reported a mortality rate of 30% following hemispherectomy, taking into account immediate surgical death and the complications of hemispherectomy.

Outcome

As in all operations, understanding the balance of risk vs. benefit is essential. The morbidity of hemispherectomy has been discussed; we now turn our attention to the potential benefits, including seizure control and the consequent improvement in psychosocial development.

Seizure control

In patients selected according to the criteria discussed earlier, hemispherectomy is one of the most successful operations for the treatment of refractory seizures. Factors that could influence outcome include: the surgical method used, the aetiology and the surgical group performing the operation. In theory, in the same situation, the seizure control obtained with each operation should be identical, since all the techniques achieve the same physiological result—elimination of the seizure foci by excision or disconnection. However, the published results vary according to the different techniques of hemispherectomy [22].

Long-term improvement in seizure control (at least an 80% reduction in seizure frequency) is obtained in over 90–95% of appropriately selected operated patients. About 70–80% of patients undergoing hemispherectomy will become seizure free postoperatively and remain so. Despite careful preoperative evaluation, about 5% of patients will not show any worthwhile benefit from hemispherectomy. These figures provide general guidelines for the purpose of discussion with patients and their family [3,18,19].

Patients who continue to have seizures post-hemispherectomy represent a special category that requires further discussion. Why do the seizures continue and from where do they originate? The answers may not be as clear as one would like, but the following factors have to be considered: (a) the completeness of the hemispherectomy; and (b) the nature of the underlying condition responsible for the brain damage and subsequently the seizures. Bilaterality of cerebral damage is sometimes the cause of continuing seizures. Some conditions are purely unilateral such as chronic encephalitis, vascular events after birth, Sturge–Weber syndrome, perinatal insult with resultant porencephaly, while others such as viral encephalitis, bacterial meningitis, head injury or cerebral haemorrhage with period of coma may have created bilateral cerebral damage with one side being predominantly affected.

Psychosocial development

Patients who show improvement in their seizure control following hemispherectomy benefit from secondary gains in psychosocial development and improvement in behaviour. These benefits have been gauged by psychological assessment and by observations from health professionals and the patients' families. While improvement in behaviour is not considered today an indication in itself, Krynauw [8], in his original report, described performing hemispherectomy in two children with infantile hemiplegia for the sole indication of behavioural improvement. The exact mechanisms underlying preoperative abnormalities of behaviour (often characterized by aggression and non-cooperation) are unclear, but probably involve some combination of repeated seizures and bilateral hemispheric disturbance.

Patients who obtain complete or improved seizure control with hemispherectomy, integrate better into their family, school and other social milieu. An improvement in seizures increases their confidence and allows them to perform better; when behaviour is improved following surgery, the patients are more able to integrate socially.

The capacity to concentrate and learn may also increase tremendously following surgery. Repeated seizures can result in intellectual deterioration [34]. This decline not only stabilizes after surgery, but, as documented by Beardsworth and Adams [35], there might also be continued intellectual improvement postoperatively. Lowering of anticonvulsant medication dosages may also influence this improvement.

Hemispherectomy and brain plasticity

An increasing body of evidence has demonstrated that the brain is able to reorganize and reallocate its psychological and neurological functions after injury. Hemispherectomy represents such an insult. Long-term follow-up of patient's language [5,6], sensorimotor [36,37] and visual [38] capacities reveal an important reorganization of functional areas in the remaining hemisphere, as demonstrated by functional MRI or H$_2$^{15}O PET scans [39]. This is paralleled by a surprisingly good or even improved neurological status of the patient following operation.

Two main mechanisms are considered in the recuperation of lost functions: (a) the unmasking of inactive neuronal populations; or (b) the taking over of function by the remaining hemisphere. So far it is not clear which of these two mechanisms is responsible for language recovery after left hemispherectomy, or how to explain the residual vision in the field contralateral to hemispherectomy [5,38]. With respect to preserved sensorimotor functions, it seems that associative motor and sensory areas that do not include the primary sensorimotor cortex of the remaining hemisphere are activated [36,39]. The long-term follow-up of hemispherectomized patients, using functional neuroimaging, represents a unique opportunity in the understanding of brain plasticity.

Conclusions

Hemispherectomy is a very effective operation for the control of pharmacologically refractory seizures. Its indication is based on the critical analysis of the seizures, the neurological examination, the aetiology and radiological and EEG investigations. In well-selected cases, it provides complete seizure control in 70–80% of patients. Altogether, about 95% of the patients will show a worthwhile benefit. These results should be independent of the surgical technique applied, since all these operations, in theory, have the same physiological effect on the seizure focus by either removal or disconnection of the hemisphere. However, different techniques have distinctive outcomes. All the techniques, except anatomical hemispherectomy, have in common reduction of the hemispherectomy cavity. The Oxford–Adams modification consists of reducing the subdural space of the hemispherectomy cavity at the expense of a large extradural space. Techniques preserving white matter also reduce the cavity but aim predominantly to avoid ventricular exposure. Functional hemispherectomy and hemispherotomy are predominantly disconnective rather than resective procedures. These latter techniques also preserve a greater amount of undisturbed subarachnoid space; this should, in theory, reduce the incidence of hydrocephalus.

When hemispherectomy is indicated, it should be offered to patients as early as possible to allow them to achieve maximum psychosocial benefit. The choice of surgical method should be guided by the least invasive approach providing the lowest rate of early and late complications. The disconnective techniques of functional hemispherectomy or hemispherotomy appear to be the techniques of choice.

Acknowledgements

We are grateful to Professor G. Broggi, Dr J.P. Farmer, Dr C. Mercier, Dr J.L. Montes and Dr A. Turmel for allowing us to share some data.

References

1 Dandy W. Removal of right cerebral hemisphere for certain tumors with hemiplegia. *JAMA* 1928; 90: 823–5.
2 Villemure JG. Hemispherectomy. In: Resor SR, Kutt H, ed. *The Medical Treatment of Epilepsy*. New York: Marcel Dekker Inc, 1992: 243–49.
3 Vining EPG, Freeman JM, Brandt J, Carson BS, Uematsu S. Progressive unilateral encephalopathy of childhood (Rasmussen's syndrome): A reappraisal. *Epilepsia* 1993; 34 (4): 639–50.
4 Villemure JG. Hemispherectomy techniques. In: Luders HO, ed. *Epilepsy Surgery*. New York: Raven Press, 1992: 569–78.
5 Boatman D, Freeman J, Vining E et al. Language recovery after left hemispherectomy in children with late-onset seizures. *Ann Neurol* 1999; 46: 579–86.
6 Vargha-Khadem F, Mishkin M. Speech and language outcome after hemispherectomy in childhood. In: *Paediatric Epilepsy Syndromes and their Surgical Treatment*. London: John Libbey, 1997: 774–84.
7 Gardner WJ. Removal of the right cerebral hemisphere for infiltrating glioma. *JAMA* 1933; 12: 154–64.
8 Krynauw RA. Infantile hemiplegia treated by removing one cerebral hemisphere. *J Neurol Neurosurg Psychiatr* 1950; 13: 243–67.
9 White HH. Cerebral hemispherectomy in the treatment of infantile hemiplegia: review of the literature and report of two cases. *Confin Neurol* 1961; 21: 1–50.
10 Obrador A. About the surgical technique of hemispherectomy in cases of cerebral hemiatrophy. *Acta Neurochir* 1952; 3: 57–63.
11 Rasmussen T. Hemispherectomy for seizures revisited. *Can J Neurol Sci* 1983; 10: 71–8.
12 Griffith HB. Cerebral hemispherectomy for infantile hemiplegia in the light of late results. *Ann R Coll Surg Engl* 1967; 41: 183–201.
13 Laine E, Pruvot P, Osson D. Résultats éloignés de l'hémisphérectomie dans les cas d'hémiatrophie cérébrale infantile génératrice d'épilepsie. *Neurochirurgie* 1964; 10: 507–22.
14 French LA, Johnson DR, Brown IA, Van Bergen FB. Cerebral hemispherectomy for control of intractable convulsive seizures. *J Neurosurg* 1955; 12: 154–64.
15 Wilson PJE. Cerebral hemispherectomy for infantile hemiplegia. *Brain* 1970; 93: 147–80.
16 Adams CBT. Hemispherectomy: a modification. *J Neurol Neurosurg Psychiatry* 1983; 46: 617–19.
17 Ignelzi RJ, Bucy PC. Cerebral hemidecortication in the treatment of infantile cerebral hemiatrophy. *J Nervous Mental Dis* 1968; 147: 14–30.
18 Villemure JG, Adams CBT, Hoffman HJ, Peacock WJ. Hemispherectomy. In: Engel J, ed. *Surgical Treatment of the Epilepsies*. New York: Raven Press, 1993: 511–18.
19 Winston KR, Welch K, Adler JR, Erba G. Cerebral hemicorticectomy for epilepsy. *J Neurosurg* 1992; 77: 889–95.
20 Delalande O, Pinard JM, Basdevant C, Gauthe M, Plouin P, Dulac O. Hemispherotomy: a new procedure for central disconnection. *Epilepsia* 1992; 33 (Suppl. 3): 99–100.
21 Villemure JG, Mascott C. Hemispherotomy: The peri-insular approach. Technical aspects. *Epilepsia* 1993; 34 (Suppl. 6): 48.
22 Villemure JG, Mascott C. Peri-insular hemispherectomy: surgical principles and anatomy. *Neurosurgery* 1995; 37: 975–81.
23 Villemure JG, Mascott C, Andermann F, Rasmussen T. Is removal of the insular cortex in hemispherectomy necessary? *Epilepsia* 1989; 30: 728.
24 Freeman JM, Arroyo S, Vining EP et al. Insular seizures: a study in Sutton's law. *Epilepsia* 1994; 35 (Suppl. 8): 49.
25 Oppenheimer DR, Griffith HB. Persistent intracranial bleeding as a complication of hemispherectomy. *J Neurol Neurosurg Psychiatry* 1966; 9: 229–40.
26 Villemure JG. Hemispherectomy: Techniques and complications. In: Wyllie E, ed. *The Treatment of Epilepsy: Principles and Practice*. Philadelphia: Lea and Febiger, 1993: 1116–19.
27 Falconer MA, Wilson PJE. Complications related to delayed hemorrhage after hemispherectomy. *J Neurosurg* 1969; 30: 413–26.
28 Cabiese F, Jeni R, Landa R. Fatal brain-stem shift following hemispherectomy. *J Neurosurg* 1957; 14: 74–91.
29 Ransohoff J, Hess W, in discussion with Rasmussen T. Post-operative superficial hemosiderosis of the brain, its diagnosis, treatment and prevention. *Ann Neurol Assoc* 1973; 98: 133–7.
30 Rasmussen T. Hemispherectomy. In: Schmidek HH, Sweet WH, eds. *Operative Neurosurgical Techniques*, 2nd edn. Philadelphia: WB Saunders, 1988.
31 Rasmussen T, Villemure JG. Cerebral hemispherectomy for seizures with hemiplegia. *Clev Clin J Med* 1989; 56 (Suppl. 1): S62–S83.

32 Davies KG, Maxwell RE, French LA. Hemispherectomy for intractable seizures: long-term results in 17 patients followed for up to 38 years. *J Neurosurg* 1993; 78: 733–40.

33 Villemure JG. Anatomical to functional hemispherectomy from Krynauw to Rasmussen. *Epilepsy Res* 1992; (Suppl. 5): 209–15.

34 Lindsay J, Ounsted C, Richards P. Hemispherectomy for childhood epilepsy: a 36 years study. *Dev Med Child Neurol* 1987; 29: 592–600.

35 Beardsworth ED, Adams CBT. Modified hemispherectomy for epilepsy: early results in 10 cases. *Br J Neurosurg* 1988; 2: 73–84.

36 Graveline C, Mikulis D, Crawley AP, Hwang P. Regionalized sensorimotorplasticity after hemispherectomy fMRI evaluation. *Pediatr Neurol* 1998; 19: 337–42.

37 Wieser GH, Henke K, Zumsteg D, Taub E, Yonekawa Y, Buck A. Activation of the left motor cortex during left leg movements after right central resection. *J Neurol Neurosurg Psychiatr* 1999; 67: 487–91.

38 Wessinger CM, Fendrich R, Ptito A, Villemure J-G, Gazzaniga MS. Residual vision with awareness in the field contralateral to a parietal or complete functional hemispherectomy. *Neuropsychologia* 1996; 34: 1129–37.

39 Bernasconi A, Bernasconi N, Lassonde M *et al*. Sensorimotor organization in patients who have undergone hemispherectomy: a study with (15)O-water PET and somatosensory evoked potentials. *Neuroreport* 2000; 11 (14): 3085–90.

Corpus Callosum Section for Epilepsy

J.R. Gates and L. De Paola

In 1764, Thomas Southwell expressed an interesting collective belief of the scientific community: 'all anatomists are now agreed that the soul is seated in the brain, but are not agreed as to the particular part . . .' [1]. At that point in time the 'hard part of the brain' or corpus callosum was seriously considered to play such a role. In 1863, T.H. Huxley called the corpus callosum 'the greatest leap anywhere made by Nature in her brain work' [2]. The passionate tone of those early descriptions certainly planted the necessary enthusiasm for almost two centuries of dedicated research on this structure of 180 million axons.

Curiously, at a time when we barely understood its properties, Dandy [3] decided to approach a congenital cyst of a cavum septi pellucidi and cavum vergae in a 4-and-a-half year old boy by sectioning the corpus callosum, not knowing that by doing so he would, in addition to his original intention, free his patient from a seizure disorder and set the stage for a new treatment modality for epilepsy [3]. Van Wagenen and Aird [4] discussed the surgical options for the dilatations of the cavity of the septum pellucidum and cavum vergae. They bluntly discouraged the use of a transcallosal approach. Only a few years later the same Van Wagenen, then working with Herren [5], started the era of commissurotomy for the treatment of clinically refractory epilepsy. As the procedure completed 60 years in 2000, its indications, the surgical techniques used, results and consequences are still the object of continuous clinical and experimental research. This chapter discusses the more prominent contributions to the field of each of the above aspects.

The essentials in the anatomy and physiology of the corpus callosum

Anatomical aspects

The anatomy of the corpus callosum differs significantly between different species, and within the same species it varies according to the evolutionary stage. In mammals, it develops in proportion to the neocortex and therefore reaches its maximal volume in adult humans, where it measures approximately 10 cm in length [6]. Figure 67.1 demonstrates the different anatomical components of the corpus callosum and their relation to the other inter-hemispherical commissures.

The most important of the forebrain commissures, the callosal structure, is composed of 180 million axons [7]. A fundamental concept is that the connections established between the cerebral hemispheres can be homotopic or heterotopic, as elaborated by Pandya in the rhesus monkey [8]. In this animal the primary auditory cortex sends projections mainly to the opposite auditory cortex, whereas the primary somatosensory cortex sends projections not only to the opposite somatosensory cortex, but also to second-ary and supplementary sensory cortex. Furthermore, it is now known that different sets of neurones may project ipsilaterally [9]. As expected, the callosal connections between the cerebral hemispheres are roughly organized in a rostral-caudal manner, with the frontal lobes occupying the rostral portion of the callosum and the other lobes following the anterior-posterior anatomy (i.e. parietal, temporal and occipital). Studying the transcallosal response, Grafstein [10] concluded that the callosal axons of homotopic connections terminate at the same cortical depth as they arose in the opposite hemisphere. As emphasized by Jones [2], there are few neurophysiological studies of synaptic organization. There is evidence suggesting that electrical stimulation of callosal axons can lead to both excitatory and inhibitory responses, varying according to the relative latency involved. Nevertheless, such data fully support the anatomical hypothesis that the corpus callosum plays a principal role in the propagation of electrical discharges from one hemisphere to the other. The extrapolation of these findings to the epileptogenic state was inevitable.

In 1993, Gates *et al.* [11] speculated about the pathological preservation of ontogenic exuberance as a predisposing factor to secondarily generalized seizures. Exuberance was the term used by Innocenti [9] to describe the widespread distribution of callosal projection neurones in the visual cortex of the neonatal cat. Subsequent studies demonstrated that such projections are not only seen in different mammalians but are also subject to substantial changes in the mature brain of the primate. Kass [12], studying patterns of inter-hemispheric connections in prosimian galagos, a different species of New World monkeys, and Old World macaque monkeys, has demonstrated 'significant reduction of density and distribution of callosal connections to some cortical fields, particularly those early in processing hierarchies, as if the transfer of information is being delayed until some initial processing is complete'. It was suggested that the alteration in the connections is part of a pattern related to the evolution of more complex processing systems with more cortical fields. In other words, with few fields, each field is more general and has more connections; with more fields, each field becomes more specialized and has fewer connections, with the emphasis on thalamic, rather than callosal, inputs. Thus, a pathological preservation of ontogenic exuberance could, theoretically, work as a facilitator to rapid secondary generalized events, potentially prevented by the callosal section [11].

Neurophysiological aspects

The experimental data

At the second Dartmouth International Conference in Epilepsy and the Corpus Callosum, Wada [13] commented on two important

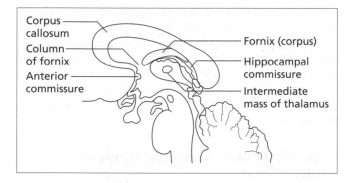

Fig. 67.1 Diagram of a sagittal cut through the corpus callosum showing its relation to the other brain commissures.

limiting factors in corpus callosum research: (a) the simple extrapolation of findings in animal models to humans involves a significant risk, as anatomical and physiological differences make human epilepsy far more complex than the animal models; and (b) although the corpus callosum constitutes the largest commissural pathway, other commissural pathways are present. A number of pathways ensure the transmission of information between the hemispheres, including the hippocampal commissure, anterior commissure, massa intermedia, habenular commissure, posterior commissure, supramammillary commissure, collicular commissure, brainstem and cerebellum, not to mention the diencephalic structures. Not all of these are fully understood but they likely play a significant role in transhemispheric epileptic phenomena.

The following discussion targets some of the aspects described above. Musgrave and Gloor [14], when studying feline generalized penicillin epilepsy, assessed the role of the corpus callosum in bilateral interhemispherical synchrony of spike-and-slow wave discharges. They used four different groups of cats, which were subjected to: complete section of the corpus callosum and anterior commissure, division of the massa intermedia alone, partial section of the massa intermedia and a last group where a slab of cortex (17 mm of the lateral and suprasylvian gyri) was disconnected from all its subcortical inputs. The results clearly demonstrated persistence of generalized discharges in all experimental groups except the first, i.e. the complete callosum section. Therefore, in the feline generalized epilepsy model the corpus callosum is the main, if not exclusive, pathway ensuring bilateral synchrony of the epileptic discharges.

The genetic absence rats of Strasbourg (GAERS) spontaneously have generalized non-convulsive seizures, correlated to 7–10 Hz generalized synchronous spike and wave discharges on the EEG. This model was described by Vergnes et al. in 1982 [15] and revisited later [16] to assess the role of corpus callosum section in disrupting the interhemispherical synchronization of discharges. They demonstrated the presence of 'a few bilateral spike-and-wave discharges' after the callosum division. The persistence of generalized discharges suggested that although the callosum plays a major role it may not be the only structure involved in bilateral synchronization in this Wistar rat model.

Wada and Komai [17], and subsequently Naquet and Wada [18], have discussed the effects of callosal section in the photosensitive Senegalese baboon, Papio papio. The animals respond to intermittent photic stimulation at 25 Hz with photomyoclonic and photoconvulsive discharges. Furthermore, some have spontaneous generalized tonic-clonic seizures and when submitted to kindling from the amygdala or frontal cortex eventually develop bisymmetrical and bisynchronous convulsions. After callosal section, the synchronization of paroxysmal discharges and seizures induced by photic stimulation is diminished. The EEG shows what was described by the researchers as 'almost generalized onset which would terminate predominating in one hemisphere or the other', thus demonstrating the importance of the callosal fibres in bilateral synchrony.

The overall results on the three species (i.e. cat, rat, baboon) imply that the corpus callosum sustains a facilitatory role in the interhemispherical spread of epileptic discharges. From the rhesus monkey model we have learned a different lesson. When these animals have the anterior two-thirds of their corpus callosum severed, they develop partial motor seizures five times faster than non-bisected monkeys, and the seizures spread twice as fast as in non-operated animals. All of the above suggests that the corpus callosum sustains an inhibitory role in this particular model.

Therefore, it is clear that extrapolations from the animal models to the human should be made with care.

The clinical data

Van Wagenen and Herren [5] subjected 10 patients to corpus callosotomy; three of them were performed in two stages, and the effects of the division were described. Historically, it is of interest that they attempted the procedure based on their own observations, with no reference to a great deal of experimental data available at that point, including the contemporary study by Erickson on the spread of epileptic discharges [19]. Although their results seemed promising, the small population, lack of neurophysiological assessment and short follow-up suggested a need for further studies. This was addressed a few years later by Hursch [20], who described the EEG features in two postcallosotomy patients of Van Wagenen's series. Since the patients had been subjected to partial callosotomies, not surprisingly the persistence of bilateral synchronous discharges was noticed in spite of the clinical improvement.

Curiously, it took a decade before the subsequent wave of reports on corpus callosotomy became available; this finally happened with contributions from Bogen et al. [21–23] who addressed the seizure results as well as neuropsychological outcome, and from Luessenhop et al. [24,25], discussing the callosotomy as an alternative to hemispherectomy. The EEG aspects of complete corpus callosotomy were briefly and quite subjectively described by Mann et al. [26], who studied patients from Bogen's series and observed 'the tendency of the two hemispheres to follow separate courses of subsidence' after callosotomy. Up to this point, most of the literature was characterized by small series and case reports. More substantial data appeared in the 1970s with the first Dartmouth series, endorsing the benefits of the procedure [27–29].

Although the ultimate goal of callosal bisection is to prevent bilateral synchrony of epileptiform activity, most of the human data are focused on the seizure results, with the neurophysiological aspects being somewhat less emphasized. This is partly due to the fact that research in the field is limited by obvious ethical implications. Indeed, as a consequence, most of the observations are based on simple interpretations of the surface pre- and postoperative

EEGs, with fewer reports on intraoperative recordings. Furthermore, the majority of the literature involves interictal epileptiform activity, with the ictal phenomenon receiving significantly less attention. Nevertheless, there is important literature on the subject, as demonstrated by the following review.

Although a number of papers have attempted to address the issue of persistence of bilateral synchronous interictal discharges after complete callosotomy [7,30,31], this was first specifically reviewed by Spencer et al. [32]. They described 13 patients who presented with bilateral synchronous interictal discharges on preoperative EEG. After complete corpus callosotomy, such activity remained present, although significantly reduced in 12/13 patients. It was then suggested that bisynchrony could also be mediated by diencephalic or mesencephalic structures. Gates et al. [33] also noticed the persistence of generalized bisynchronous spike and wave discharges on the surface recordings from 14 patients subjected to partial callosotomies. Another interesting piece of evidence in the role of the corpus callosum in human epilepsy comes from Pinard et al. [34], who described two children with West syndrome subjected to callosal section. Although variations of hypsarrhythmia were well described [35], the patients presented with the typical bilateral epileptiform pattern. After surgery both showed unilateral hypsarrhythmia during asymmetrical spasms [34].

The above re-emphasizes the role of the corpus callosum as the main pathway underlying bilateral synchrony of epileptiform discharges, thus justifying the callosum division as an approach to intractable epilepsy. It is also true that most of the data so far presented is limited to the observation of interictal epileptiform discharges.

The ictal phenomenon postcallosotomy has received little attention in the literature. Spencer et al. [36] described the issue of dissociation between the persistence of bilateral synchronous interictal discharges and the somewhat unexpected lateralization of clinical seizures after corpus callosotomy. The effect of corpus callosotomy on ictal discharges was analysed in 18 patients subjected to anterior two-thirds section and 10 patients subjected to complete section. Of these, 11/18 anterior section and 5/10 complete section patients showed bilateral synchronous seizure onset before corpus callosotomy. This pattern was abolished in 5/11 anterior section and 5/5 complete section patients. The fact that they were unable to demonstrate the presence of generalized ictal onset after complete corpus callosotomy led the authors to state that 'the corpus callosum may be the only pathway used in the production of bilateral synchronous seizure onset'. Some 7/13 patients showed an increase in focal epileptiform discharges on EEG, with 5/17 patients from the Yale series showing more intense or frequent partial seizures after partial or complete callosotomy. In other series [31,37] this apparent exacerbation of focal seizures postcallosotomy has been attributed to amelioration of the preoperative secondary generalized, predominantly tonic or atonic, seizures.

The authors published reports on two patients (out of a series of 59 callosotomies reported [38,39]) who underwent complete callosotomy, as demonstrated by MRI, but nonetheless still presented with ictal discharges which were bilateral and synchronous [40]. Our findings challenge the theory that the corpus callosum is the only responsible pathway for bisynchronous EEG ictal expression. It appears that pathways for secondary epileptogenesis continue to exist postoperatively, even after complete corpus callosotomy.

Diencephalic, brainstem or anterior commissure participation in such expression must be considered.

Maehara and Shimizu [41] reported the most recent series of 52 patients with drop attacks. They found callosotomy, especially total, effective (defined as a >90% reduction) in 85% of patients with drop seizures. A younger age was independently predictive of an overall improvement in daily function and family satisfaction with outcome.

Presurgical evaluation: indications and seizure effects

Trying to define accurately the candidacy for corpus callosotomy by means of reviewing the relatively vast literature in the field can be potentially problematic. As expected in surgery, once the first cases are operated on, the future surgical recommendations are based on the outcome of these patients. In attempting to gather the data available from different institutions one invariably faces many challenges.

1 The surgical procedures are not uniform and it is intrinsically difficult to assess the exact extent of the surgery.

2 The terminology varies from series to series and when reading 'akinetic seizures' it is not clear if the falls described are the results of tonic or atonic events; furthermore, although seizures are usually well described preoperatively, clear discrimination of the remaining seizure types after surgery is often not available.

3 Not infrequently, the same population of patients is repeatedly used, in different publications, to describe results on distinct aspects of the procedure; this is aggravated by the failure to disclose such repetitive use of patient data in the text.

4 Results are rated differently, from 'poor' to 'excellent', as well as 'satisfactory' and 'unsatisfactory', with successful outcomes variably expressed as 'over 50%' of seizure reduction or 'over 80%' of seizure reduction.

Engel's four-part classification for outcome with respect to epileptic seizures, discussed at the first Palm Desert Conference, although useful for focal resections, does not apply to patients where surgery is indicated as a palliative procedure, rarely rendering seizure-free outcome [42].

Despite these problems, the following is an attempt to bring together the experience from different centres, defining the target population, based on surgical results. Tables 67.1–67.3 show results from different series in adult and paediatric populations, some of which are reviewed below.

As a general principle, epilepsy surgery involves the resection of cerebral cortex held responsible for the genesis of epileptic activity. This does not apply in corpus callosotomy. Nonetheless, the significant decrease in the generalized seizure frequency and the overall improved quality of life appear to justify the procedure. A number of publications have specifically outlined the indications for corpus callosotomy [37,43–46]. Several workers also have touched upon the subject when discussing other aspects in the field or as part of general reviews [11,47–52].

Corpus callosotomy in the paediatric population does have a few special features. Gates et al. [53], when focusing on callosotomy in children, found only 21 cases in the peer-reviewed literature. More recently, a significant number of patients have been added to this group [54–57].

Table 67.1 Outcome after corpus callosotomy in patients under 16 years of age

Reference	Number	Number/type of CC	Seizure types	Satisfactory outcome (%)	Comments
Amacher [101]	1	1 C	Akinetic Focal Major	100	(*)
Geoffroy et al. [65]	9	9 C	AB, TC, T, MY, AK	67	(*)
Murro et al. [60]	2	2 AC	TC CP T, AB, A	50 100 100	
Makari et al. [102]	6	6 AC	TC CP A T	50 100 100 0	
Black et al. [55]	10	2 AC 4 C 4 TS	T, A T, TC, A TC, MY, drops	50 50 67	1/2 = MR 3/4 = MR 3/4 = MR
Raffel et al. [56]	3	3 TS	T, MY	67	(*)
Cendes et al. [57]	34	21 partial 13 complete	A, TC, T, AB A, TC, T, AB	67 77	Moderate MR = 75% Severe MR = 67%
Mamelak et al. [63]	2	2 TS	TC, A, CP, SP	50	(*)
Gates et al. [39]	33	16 A	T, A	61	
Courtney et al. [38]		7 TS 10 C			

Satisfactory outcome, over 50% reduction of main seizure types.

* Seizure type is not specified/results are grouped.

'Partial' and 'complete' are used when specific data are not clearly described.

A, atonic; AB, absence; AC, anterior callosotomy; AK, akinetic; C, complete callosotomy; CC, corpus callosotomy; CP, complete partial; MR, mental retardation; MY, myoclonic; T, tonic; TC, tonic-clonic; TS, two-staged callosotomy.

From the various series, the following general principles pertaining to the indications for corpus callosotomy appear accepted and self-explanatory: (a) proven medically refractory epilepsy (with most of the literature reporting periods from 2 to 3 years of thorough trials with various antiepileptic drugs, including detailed documentation of the blood levels); and (b) lack of evidence of surgically approachable focal disease.

From this point a clear dichotomy is evident in the literature, with the indications for surgery based either on (a) the seizure type (with the associated EEG input); or, less frequently, on (b) the category of disease, i.e. the type of epilepsy or epileptic syndrome. The latter form was presented by Williamson [43], who reviewed the literature and found six categories of patient potentially considered for commissurotomy. These included patients with infantile hemiplegia, forme-fruste infantile hemiplegia, progressive hemiplegic encephalopathy (Rasmussen syndrome), epilepsy with bilateral dependent and independent sharp and slow paroxysms (Lennox–Gastaut syndrome), frontal epilepsy and focal/multifocal epilepsy.

Among the limitations of the study were the short follow-up and the inconsistency in the exact type of surgery performed between different groups. Results were rated as: excellent (greater than 80% seizure reduction), good (greater than 50% seizure reduction), poor (no change) and worse (more seizures or significant neurological deficit). The overall results showed clear predominance of excellent and good outcomes in all groups, with the exception of Rasmussen syndrome patients (one excellent, two good and two poor results in five patients). It is likely, as discussed by Andermann [46], that hemispherectomy (particularly functional hemispherectomy) is the procedure of choice in that unfortunate population, so that these less good results are not necessarily surprising [58].

However, the analysis of seizure type appears to be the most popular criterion in determining candidacy for callosotomy. Although the types of seizures that respond to corpus callosotomy are still being elucidated, there is enough evidence to support the view that atonic, tonic and, less predictably, generalized tonic-

Table 67.2 Outcome after corpus callosotomy in patients over 16 years of age

Reference	Number	Number/type of CC	Seizure types	Satisfactory outcome (%)	Comments
Amacher [101]	3	3 C	Major Akinetic Focal	100	(*)
Murro et al. [60]	23	23 AC	TC CP SP, A, T, AB	67 40 0	6/10 MR = sat 1/5 MR = sat
Purves et al. [61]	24	24 AC	CP 2 general AB, MY, falls	62 50 75	(*)
Black et al. [55]	4	2 AC 2 TS	T, A T, MY, drops	100 50	1/2 = MR 2/2 = MR
Mamelak et al. [63]	13	9 AC 3 TS 1 C	TC, A, CP, SP TC, A, CP, SP TC, A, SP	89 67 0	(*)
Spencer [49]	50	41 AC	SP/CP TC T A MY HEM	46 83 60 100 100 30	
		14 TS	SP/CP TC T A MY HEM	14 60 50 40 100 0	
		22 C	SP/CP TC T A MY HEM	47 68 57 50 100 22	
Courtney et al. [38] Gates et al. [39]	26	16 AC 4 TS 6 C	T, A	76	

Satisfactory outcome, over 50% reduction of main seizure types.
* Seizure type is not specified/results are grouped.
A, atonic; AB, absence; AC, anterior callosotomy; C, complete callosotomy; CC, corpus callosotomy; CP, complex partial; HEM, hemiclonic; MY, myoclonic; SP, simple partial; T, tonic; TC, tonic-clonic; TS, two-staged callosotomy.

clonic seizures constitute primary indications for the procedure, regardless of age group. The indication of the first two seizure types (atonic and tonic) seems to be universally endorsed, with favourable outcome varying from 60 to 100% in most of the series. The seizure outcome when the main type is generalized tonic-clonic is more controversial. Satisfactory results are usually found when tonic-clonic seizures are associated with either atonic or tonic events. Gates et al. [59] described 12/17 patients who became free of the associated tonic-clonic seizures after surgery, but their primary indication for the procedure was tonic or atonic seizures. A review of seven recent series [38,39,57,60–63] demonstrated that in 203 patients only 30 (or 15%) had generalized tonic-clonic seizures not associated with tonic or atonic events as their main indication. Under these circumstances, satisfactory outcome varied from 21 to 67%. Even the higher percentage is still significantly below the 83% of satisfactory outcome claimed by the Yale group [64]. Such a wide range may be explained by different criteria for recommending surgery. Myoclonic seizures also seem to respond well, but they are usually not considered a primary indication, being more commonly associated with other seizure types.

Table 67.3 Outcome after corpus callosotomy. Seizure effect not specifying the age group

Reference	Number	Number/type of CC	Seizure types	Satisfactory outcome (%)
Oguni *et al.* [62]	43 (7.8–60 years)	43 A	Drops	65
			TC	38
			AB	42
			T	60
			CP	50
			SP	60
Fuiks *et al.* [68]	80 (4–53 years)	70 A	TC	86
			CP	88
			A	83
			T	50
		10 TS	TC, CP, A, T	Not improved
Reutens *et al.* [66]	64 (3–47 years)	49 A	TC	49
			T	47
			Drops	60
			CP	55
		5 C		
		10 TS	TC	50
			T	43
			Drops	71
			CP	51
Maehara & Shimizu *et al.* [41]	52	A, C	Drops	85 > 90%
			T	32 > 90%
			TC	31% > 90%

Satisfactory outcome, over 50% of reduction of the main seizure types.
A, anterior callosotomy; AB, absence; C, complete callosotomy; CP, complex partial; SP, simple partial; T, tonic; TC, tonic–clonic; TS, two-staged callosotomy.

The authors have presented their results on 59 patients subjected to partial and complete callosotomies [38,39]. Thirty-seven patients were older than 10 years. The prevalent seizure types in this population were atonic, tonic and generalized tonic-clonic episodes, although other seizure types were included. Satisfactory outcome (i.e. 80% reduction in the primary seizure type) was achieved in 75% of the patients. Seventy-five per cent of the patients with tonic seizures had successful outcomes as compared to only 25% of the generalized tonic-clonic patients ($P < 0.05$). The EEG ictal pattern more often associated with successful outcome was electrodecremental epileptiform fast (EEF) activity (Fig. 67.2). When both factors were combined on presentation they were associated with a successful outcome in 92% of the patients ($P < 0.001$). In the paediatric population (22 patients below 10 years of age), in spite of a successful outcome being observed in 50% of the patients with atonic or tonic seizures, neither seizure type, nor ictal EEG pattern predicted outcome.

Tables 67.1–67.3 summarize the work of several different institutions between 1976 and 1993; some modifications were necessary in bringing the available data to a common format.

The role of corpus callosotomy in children resembles that in the adult, although the nature of the age-related syndromes may generate more specific indications. For instance, 70–80% of the patients with the Lennox–Gastaut syndrome show favourable effects on seizures after the procedure [44]. Patients under 16 years of age could be individually analysed in nine series (see Table 67.1). From the total group of 100 patients, 53 were subjected to complete callosotomy, either in one or two stages and 47 to anterior callosotomy. No major differences were seen in the indication for surgery between the two groups. The two series tend to parallel each other in terms of seizure outcome, with an overall satisfactory effect between 50 and 77% in the larger series. Isolated seizure-free patients were reported.

An interesting aspect in terms of indication for the procedure rests in the issue of patients with cognitive impairment. This is particularly so in the paediatric population, although given the nature of most of the seizures, it certainly applies to older groups. The origin of this question dates back to when Wilson *et al.* [47] described results on the initial Dartmouth series of 20 patients in which two severely retarded patients (IQ lower than 70) were 'not measurably improved by commissurotomy'. Geoffroy *et al.* [65] were among the first rejecting this hypothesis, less than 1 year after Wilson's observation, when they described satisfactory outcome (67% of the patients with greater than 50% seizure reduction) in a small series of nine mentally retarded children. Similar findings were later stressed by Black *et al.* [55] with similar results. Drop attacks improved in 60% of Reuten's population, in which 54% were mentally retarded [66]. Finally, Cendes *et al.* [57] presented a series

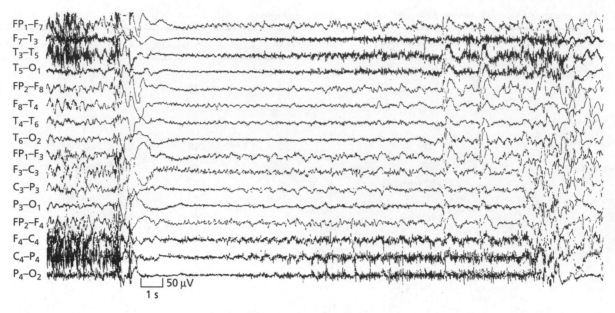

Fig. 67.2 EEG obtained from a 6-year-old patient, prior to a corpus callosotomy. The main seizure type was a brief tonic event consistently correlated with a high-amplitude burst with subsequent generalized electrodecremental changes and epileptiform fast pattern, as demonstrated in this template.

of 29/34 patients who were mentally retarded (20/29 had moderate mental retardation and 9/29 severe mental retardation). Their results show satisfactory outcome in 67–75% of this population. These percentages are not significantly lower than the 80% of satisfactory outcome on the normal intelligence or mild mentally retarded population (5/34 patients) in the same study [57].

Table 67.2 shows results in 143 adult patients from seven distinct institutions. A favourable response to atonic (50–100% of the patients) and tonic (60–100% of the patients) seizures was consistently seen in most of the series. The Yale series shows a good response of tonic-clonic seizures to anterior callosotomy alone in their most recent review, in which over 80% of the patients experienced a good outcome. Curiously, this is also the seizure type that shows the more significant incremental response upon completion of the callosotomy in at least 60% of the patients [64]. The fact that these results are significantly different from the other series may be due to differences in selection of patients.

Table 67.3 shows data pooled from series that did not distinguish age groups. Altogether almost 200 patients are included. Of these patients, 50–60% had a satisfactory outcome for the primary indications, which is consistent with data reviews of the overall outcome of corpus callosotomy [42,67].

At present, the issue of anterior vs. complete callosotomy remains a source of potential controversy, due to the different results obtained from various institutions. The Tennessee group reviewed a series of 80 patients, and in their hands over 80% satisfactory outcome was achieved after anterior callosotomy, with no significant benefit obtained upon completion [68]. Similar results are found by the Vancouver group, with 75% good outcome [61] and the Montreal series with 65% good outcome after partial callosal section [62]. The Yale group, however, reports elimination of secondary generalized seizures in only 33% of their patients after anterior callosotomy, whereas 77% benefited by complete callosotomy [69].

Intermediate results were reported by the Australian group with 47–60% satisfactory outcome after anterior section, but with no significant change upon completion [66]. At the Minnesota Epilepsy Group 20/30 (66%) patients subjected to anterior callosotomy showed a satisfactory outcome. Where completion of the callosotomy was performed, 8/11 (73%) patients had a better than 50% reduction in their seizure frequency [38,39].

Few papers have specifically addressed complex partial seizures as a primary indication for callosal section. Purves et al. [61] reported optimistic results in three patients, originally taken to callosotomy with the intention of pursuing better lateralization and avoiding depth electrodes. An epileptic syndrome characterized by bilateral co-ordinated limb movements, vocalization and non-masticatory oral activity was described by Waterman et al. [70] in 12 patients. The syndrome is associated with discharges in the mesial frontal lobe. Three patients were improved after anterior callosotomy. Whenever complex partial seizures are associated with other seizure types, satisfactory improvement is noticed in as low as 14% to as high as 88% of the patients. The current thoughts in corpus callosotomy for complex partial seizures were summarized by Purves et al. [71] at the Second Dartmouth International Conference on Epilepsy and the Corpus Callosum, and narrowed the indications for the procedure to patients with frontal lobe epilepsy, who present with such rapid interhemispheric spread that their seizures are classified as generalized [71]. Nevertheless, the data available are anecdotal and require further clarification. Moreover, newer techniques for frontal localization [37] now allow lateralization/localization of a focus that was not previously possible.

The role of cortical heterotopias and corpus callosotomy was the object of at least two case reports [72,73]. Both patients did improve after surgery, suggesting that callosal section might be useful in carefully selected patients with intractable epilepsy and severe neuronal migration disorders.

Most series in the last 10 years have essentially been 'me too' experiences, with no real breakthroughs in outcomes.

Surgical aspects: variations on technique

Since Van Wagenen and Herren's first efforts [5], over 50 years have passed. A better understanding of the neurophysiological issues, along with growing experience and more sophisticated techniques, have effected profound changes in the procedure. In the pioneering series from Bogen, Luessenhop and Wilson, other structures, such as the anterior commissure, hippocampal commissure and massa intermedia [21–23], the anterior commissure and the right fornix [24,25] and combinations of the above [27,28] were severed along with variable portions of the corpus callosum. Since then, the number of structures involved in the section has significantly decreased. Van Wagenen and Herren [5] performed a version of the two-stage surgery technique that was popularized in the second series from Dartmouth [47].

A number of publications have outlined the current approach to callosal section. Some groups such as those from Tennessee [74] and New Hampshire [75–79] use basically the same technique with only minor variations. They all share the preference for staging the callosal section. The issue of anterior vs. complete callosotomy has generated both considerable controversy and a generous number of reviews. Unfortunately, when comparing series, one faces the problem of not knowing the exact amount of section during the first procedure. Nevertheless, fairly large series have shown 75–80% successful outcome after anterior corpus callosotomy [61,68]. An earlier report by the Yale group [69] did suggest more beneficial results upon completion of the callosotomy. The same group reanalysed their series of 50 callosotomies, with thorough characterization of the seizure effects after the different procedures. They demonstrated that different surgical procedures apparently suit distinct seizure patterns, e.g. anterior callosotomy in atonic, myoclonic and tonic-clonic seizures, total callosotomy (for tonic-clonic, with less impressive responses for tonic and atonic seizures) and two-staged callosotomy with incremental responses in tonic-clonic and tonic seizures [64]. In addition, the two-stage procedure facilitated postoperative recovery.

Surgery

There follows a brief description of the surgery, as performed in the above centres. Subtle differences in the technique do exist and are pointed out.

As a general rule, for anterior corpus callosotomy, the patient is operated on under general anaesthesia, in the supine position with the head fixed in a neutral position. A variation of this set-up is used by the Tennessee and Connecticut groups, which use the lateral decubitus position, facilitating the callosal exposure. The rationale for this position is that it would provide gravity retraction to the dependent hemisphere and eliminate manual retraction [68]. The incision is made anterior to the coronal suture, with most of its length over the non-dominant hemisphere. Once the bone flap is removed, the dura is opened. The exploration between the hemispheres begins, with special attention to the presence of bridging veins and arachnoidal adhesions. Once the corpus callosum is iden-

tified, the section takes place, usually performed with a blunt instrument, although microsuction with fine tip, microscissors and laser beam could also be used [80]. Most surgeons use anatomical references to determine when the anterior portion of the corpus callosum has been adequately severed. The best landmarks, as described by Roberts [78], are the thinning seen at the junction of the posterior body and the splenium and the apposition of the fornices to the ventral aspect of the posterior corpus callosum. This may also be accomplished by comparison with the preoperative MRI measurements. Awad et al. [81] have described a technique combining preoperative MRI findings and intraoperative skull X-ray, in order to assess the extension of the callosotomy. Some centres used a small clip in a piece of gelfoam to mark the posterior limit of the callosotomy, although this is not essential [80].

The division of the posterior callosum follows basically the same principles, using an incision at the parietal eminence. The section is usually performed from the posterior portion of the callosum and carried anteriorly to meet the end of the anterior callosotomy.

In the authors' institution the surgery is performed with the patient in a prone position. The rationale behind this position is twofold: (a) prevention of embolism; and (b) to provide a technically more comfortable posture for the surgeon (M.E. Dunn, personal communication).

MRI preoperatively, as well as after partial and complete callosotomies, respectively, is shown in Fig. 67.3.

Gates et al. [30] and Spencer et al. [69] analysed the pre- and postoperative EEG in their series as an attempt to predict the surgery outcome in terms of seizure effects. Neither of the studies succeeded in reaching statistical significance, although better results did tend to occur in patients displaying bilateral synchronous discharges or lateralized abnormalities as opposed to independent multifocal epileptiform activity on the preoperative study. The value of intraoperative EEG during corpus callosotomy remains controversial.

Torres and French [82] were the first to describe the acute effect of callosal section in one case when both focal and generalized epileptiform discharges were disrupted. In some centres EEG monitoring is routinely used, and when generalized discharges are present the section proceeds until bilateral synchrony is significantly disrupted [80].

Fiol et al. [83] demonstrated lateralization of epileptiform discharges in 78% of patients during partial and complete callosotomies, but this finding was not statistically correlated with the seizure outcome after surgery. Although this issue certainly demands further study, it appears that EEG monitoring cannot yet guide the extent of the callosotomy.

Nevertheless, intraoperative EEG recording can assist the surgeon in retractor placement and adjustment during the procedure as shown by changes in focal slowing or α-activity suppression (J.R. Gates, personal observation). The Sao Paulo group has described a unique approach to callosal section [84,85]. Selective microsurgical callosotomy is performed, guided by intraoperative electrocorticography, i.e. the callosal section is conducted only in the portions of the corpus callosum associated with the presence of bilateral and synchronous epileptiform discharges. In 28 patients followed up for 4–11 years, 94% showed a 'marked decrease in the frequency of generalized seizures'. Furthermore, the same group has performed stereotactic segmental callosotomies, by means of producing

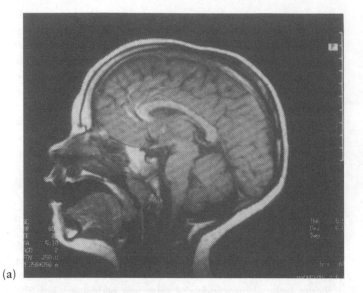

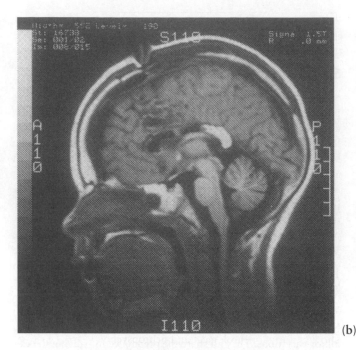

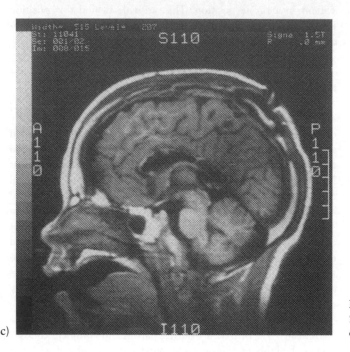

Fig. 67.3 MRI showing sagittal cuts through the corpus callosum in a 9-year-old patient. (a) Preoperative, (b) after anterior two-thirds corpus callosotomy and (c) after callosotomy completion.

radiofrequency lesions on selected areas of the corpus callosum. Eleven out of 12 patients subjected to this technique showed 'marked decrease in the frequency of generalized seizures' [86]. In spite of the tendency to develop more restricted sections, as discussed by Wyler [51], this technique has not been widely duplicated as yet, and therefore further studies are necessary.

Role of vagus nerve stimulation

With the advent of vagus nerve stimulation, the role of callosotomy in most developed countries has been significantly reduced. Most centres essentially limit the technique to those patients with drop seizures, in particular, those who fail vagus nerve placement. Figure 67.4 demonstrates the extraordinary results of vagus nerve treatment for drop seizures, especially in Lennox–Gastaut syndrome,

from a multicentre collaborative study [87]. With over a 90% reduction in drops by vagus nerve stimulation alone, our institution has reduced callosotomies from 25 to 30 per year to just over five, which are typically vagus nerve stimulation failures.

Neurological, neuropsychological and psychiatric aspects after corpus callosum section

Fifty years of commissural sections have generated a wealth of data on the neurological and neuropsychological consequences of the procedures. Analysing this information, however, constitutes a difficult task since factors other than the commissurotomy itself may be held responsible for undesirable results after the surgery. The surgical trauma and the fact that the epileptic population might already

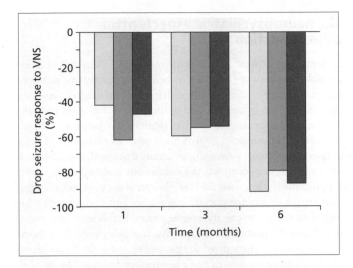

Fig. 67.4 Drop seizure response to vagus nerve stimulation.

show abnormal neurological and neuropsychological profiles are among such factors. Nevertheless, a few observations, due to their consistency, have become classic and certainly merit discussion.

Gazzaniga *et al.* [88] have commented upon the historical aspects pertaining to the consequences of the commissurotomies. They elegantly described how Akelaitis, a pioneer in assessing the neuropsychological consequences of the procedure, had been misled in assuming that callosal section would not cause major sequelae. Although imbued with the best intentions, he simply did not ask the right questions to Van Wagenen's patients in the early 1940s. Gazzaniga subsequently described how Roger Sperry was invited by Joseph Bogen (who was willing to revive the procedure) to study the unknown consequences of the callosal section in humans. Gazzaniga was assigned to the project and subsequently became involved with the first Dartmouth series [27,28].

From these studies to the more recently published data supported by MRI [88–91] we have learned that the incidence of long-term deficits consequent to callosotomy is decreasing. It has been informally discussed among different centres that, as surgeons become more experienced with the procedure, postoperative consequences dramatically decrease [11]. Whenever existent, the deficits are usually transient and only rarely long lasting. The type of surgery (i.e. anterior, complete, one or two stages) may also influence the outcome.

Much of the literature gathered under the label 'disconnection syndromes' is based on individual case reports, therefore concentrating on the minority of unusual cases in the large series. In addition, some of the classic 'syndromes' have been associated with aetiologies other than the pure callosal section. For example, the ultimate 'disconnection syndrome' (the 'alien hand') has been described as acute (associated with callosal section) or chronic (associated with frontomesial lesions), affecting the dominant hand (associated with left frontal lesions) or the non-dominant hand (associated with callosal section), implying different causes for the phenomenon. Trojano *et al.* [92] recently described a case of 'chronic alien hand' where the aetiology was an ischaemic lesion in the right frontomesial region extending to the anterior cingulate

gyrus, supplementary motor area and anterior fibres of the callosum. The acute postoperative consequences of corpus callosotomy will be reviewed.

Anterior callosotomy

Early complications of anterior callosotomy are characterized by paresis of the non-dominant leg, incontinence and decrease of spontaneous speech. These features were seen in the majority of the Yale patients [49] and were demonstrated in virtually all patients in Wilson's earlier series with complete sections [29]. After anterior callosotomy, as explained by Reeves [93], the major finding is a transient decrease in the spontaneity to speech, which may be mild (slowness in initiating speech) or severe (mutism). Whether this may be due to retraction over the supplementary motor area or to another mechanism remains unclear [94]. Other features include variable degrees of paresis of the non-dominant leg, a disinhibited forced grasping reflex in the non-dominant hand and urge incontinence [93]. The syndrome lasts days or weeks, rarely months [48]. More modern series are not reporting these effects, strongly indicating they are probably due to technique, more specifically, damage to the non-dominant cingulate gyrus.

Risse *et al.* [91] have conducted tests of interhemispheric transfer in six modalities on a group of seven patients subjected to partial callosotomies, verified by MRI. The results obtained were consistent with anatomical studies describing the projection areas for fibres in the posterior callosum, and re-emphasize the importance of this region for the interhemispheric transfer of sensory motor information (i.e. visual, kinaesthetic and complex motor information). In two patients, where the callosal section was carried out more posteriorly (only the posterior splenium left unsectioned), disconnection was demonstrated in all modalities except vision. Interestingly, however, left limb apraxia, classically described as a result of the anterior callosotomy, was not verified in this series. The absence of complications in epileptic patients undergoing uncomplicated callosotomies may be secondary to either a gradual attainment of ipsilateral motor control or increased language comprehension in the right hemisphere. This finding, therefore, suggests the critical importance of the posterior callosal fibres in the maintenance of the sensory motor integration. Furthermore, reports of left limb apraxia attributable to anterior callosal lesion alone must be accompanied by anatomical verification of integrity of the posterior callosal region, as well as ruling out the possibility that such deficits are not secondary to lesions involving the frontal or parietal regions.

Posterior callosotomy

The role of the posterior corpus callosum in mediating the interhemispherical sensory, sensory/motor and visual transfer is now well established [91,93]. Therefore, the fact that after posterior callosotomy the non-dominant hand is able to recognize objects but the patient is not able to name them (since the language-dominant hemisphere has no access to the information and the non-dominant hemisphere has no verbal ability to report it) is not surprising. A similar situation, with the same explanation, occurs with tachistoscopical input presented to the non-dominant occipital lobe. In practical terms, this latter situation might not be a problem since the dominant hemisphere can always scan the visual world and process the information.

Gazzaniga *et al.* [94] presented a patient subjected to complete two-staged callosotomy (posterior first) who, under special testing situations, was able to name and write about information presented to his right hemisphere. This was interpreted to imply that somehow the right hemisphere was able to feed the left information, although the latter was not aware it was being informed. Thus, even though the changes appear to be permanent, they are not significantly disabling [52]. However, Spencer *et al.* [69] have proposed that, if the patient presented a pre-existing complete dominant visual field deficit, posterior callosotomy would effect a devastating result.

Complete callosotomy

At this point, the vast majority of centres performing corpus callosotomy have agreed on the benefits of performing the procedure in two stages. Avoiding the classic 'split-brain' (retraction injured?) syndrome, which may follow single-staged procedures, is probably the strongest reason behind this approach. Pilcher and Ojemann [52] have established the occurrence of this syndrome transiently in 30% and permanently in 5% of the patients. Basically, both sensory and motor connections between the cerebral hemispheres are interrupted. As a consequence, the non-dominant hand is no longer responsive to verbal commands ('alien hand') and may actually display antagonistic function to the dominant hand [69]. Interestingly enough, as described by Reeves [93], each hemisphere is capable of co-ordinating some proximal movements, due to ipsilateral uncrossed pathways.

Lassonde *et al.* [95] studied the developmental aspects of callosal plasticity, comparing four acallosal subjects, five epilepsy patients subjected to corpus callosotomy at different ages and matched controls. Patients operated on at an early age were initially inferior to their matched controls but recovered and eventually reached the same level of proficiency. The patients operated on later in life showed a 'disconnection effect'. Interestingly, however, the acallosal patients did as well as or better than their peers in the transfer tasks. Among other conclusions it appeared that the compensatory mechanisms do occur, but tend to become more limited in late adolescence.

Spencer [49] estimated the possibility of memory deficits after callosotomy: 2% after partial and 8% after complete sections. Reeves [93] made reference to the work of Novelly and Lifrak [96], that a deficit in learning new material may be a consequence of disconnecting two damaged and interdependent hippocampal formations. Other scattered reports are available in the literature. Beniak *et al.* [97] have suggested that at least part of the explanation may be associated with deficits in attention and concentration. Both Ferrel *et al.* [98], studying eight cases, and more recently Provinciali *et al.* [99] with 15 cases failed to demonstrate significant cognitive impairment in their patients. In their review of anterior callosotomy, Risse *et al.* [91] made reference to possible involvement of the anterior corpus callosum with higher order cognitive functions and advised that it would be injudicious to conclude that anterior corpus callosum section has no neuropsychological significance. Further investigation of this particular aspect is certainly necessary.

The neuropsychiatric aspects after callosal section

In resective epilepsy surgery it is not conceptually difficult to accept possible changes in personality or behaviour simply due to the removal of brain tissue, especially with frontal lobe surgery. Assessing such change may be complicated by the fact that the consequent improvement in seizure frequency may mask the psychiatric consequences of the surgery [100]. This is probably partially true for corpus callosotomy, although, as already discussed, the scenario is totally different concerning the indications and expectancy from the procedure. Reviewing the literature turns out to be a challenging task, mainly due to the unclear boundaries between neuropsychological and neuropsychiatric consequences. In this sense, and trying to focus on the psychiatric perspective, it would probably be better to quote the conclusions of Ferguson's reviews: (a) 'callosotomy produced no alterations of basic personality and had beneficial effects on behaviour as a result of case-specific changes in seizure characteristics or frequency' [100]; and (b) 'gains outweighed the negative consequences of callosal transection in most cases. Improvement occurred in the areas of independence, scope of daily activities, and reduction of difficult preoperative behavior' [100].

Summary and conclusions

1 Extrapolations from animal models to the human should be carefully approached. Significant differences do exist between species, with the corpus callosum sustaining either a facilitatory or inhibitory role in the inter-hemispherical spread of epileptic discharges; in fact, *different* distributions of the callosal projection neurones between species are well described. It is further proposed that a pathological preservation of the ontogenic 'exuberance' could work as a facilitator to rapid secondary generalized events, potentially prevented by callosal section.
2 The indications for callosotomy certainly include tonic and atonic seizures not unifocal in origin. Satisfactory outcomes are reported in 60–100% of the patients undergoing surgery under such indications.
3 Generalized tonic-clonic seizures, as the main indication for callosal section, constitute a somewhat more controversial issue, as demonstrated by lower rates of successful outcome (21–67%) verified in the majority of the series reviewed. Different criteria for surgical recommendation could explain the diversity in results.
4 The surgical indication for other seizure types is unclear. Complex partial seizures, as well as myoclonic seizures, when associated with tonic or atonic seizures, appear to improve after callosal section, but their role as main indications has not been proved.
5 A substantial volume of literature supports the indication of corpus callosotomy for patients with low IQs, especially those with Lennox–Gastaut syndrome. The percentage of satisfactory outcome observed in the moderate and severely cognitively impaired population is not significantly lower than the results on the mildly improved or normal functioning patients.
6 The issue of anterior vs. complete callosotomy is also controversial. For patients with tonic or atonic seizures as a primary indication, most will substantially benefit from the anterior two-thirds section, and 75% of the failures of the two-thirds section will improve after completion of the section.

7 Modern series report significantly fewer complications after corpus callosotomy, particularly from the neuropsychological perspective. It is the authors' impression that this observation is associated with improvement in the surgical technique and consequent decrease in the trauma to the cortex during callosotomy.

8 Corpus callosotomy is essentially a palliative procedure, rarely rendering patients seizure free; therefore, the available classifications for seizure outcome do not apply in this particular situation. There is considerable discrepancy in the definition of 'satisfactory seizure outcome' among the different institutions preventing meaningful comparisons between series. A consensus must be developed aiming at uniformity of reporting between different epilepsy centres.

9 With an efficacy in reducing drop seizures by over 90%, vagus nerve stimulation has essentially replaced the more invasive callosotomy procedure as the procedure of first choice. The role of vagus nerve stimulation and callosotomy for particularly difficult cases remains to be clarified.

References

1 Collonier M. Notes on the early history of the corpus callosum with an introduction to the morphological papers published in this Festschrift. In: Leporé F, Ptito M, Jasper HH, eds. *Two Hemispheres—One Brain: Functions of the Corpus Callosum*. New York: Alan R Liss, 1986: 37–45.

2 Jones EG. Anatomy, development and physiology of the corpus callosum. In: Reeves AE, ed. *Epilepsy and the Corpus Callosum*. New York: Plenum Press, 1985: 3–20.

3 Dandy WE. Congenital cerebrae cysts of the cavum septi pellucidi (fifth ventricle) and cavum vergae (sixth ventricle). Diagnosis and treatment. *Arch Neurol Psychiatr* 1931; 25: 44–66.

4 Van Wagenen WP, Aird RB. Dilatations of the cavity of the septum pellucidum and cavum vergae. Report of cases. *Am J Cancer* 1934; 20(3): 539–57.

5 Van Wagenen WP, Herren RY. Surgical division of commissural pathways in the corpus callosum in relation to spread of an epileptic attack. *Arch Neurol Psychiatr* 1940; 44: 740–59.

6 Williams PL, Warwick R. The corpus callosum. In: Williams PL, Warwick R, eds. *Functional Neuroanatomy of the Man*. Philadelphia: WB Saunders Company, 1975: 965–7.

7 Blume WT. Corpus callosum section for seizure control: rationale and review of experimental and clinical data. *Cleveland Clin Quart* 1984; 51: 319–32.

8 Pandya DN, Seltzer B. The topography of commissural fibers. In: Leporé F, Ptito M, Jasper HH, eds. *Two Hemispheres—One Brain: Functions of the Corpus Callosum*. New York: Alan R Liss, 1986: 47–73.

9 Innocenti GM. What is so special about callosal connections? In: Leporé F, Ptito M, Jasper HH, eds. *Two Hemispheres—One Brain: Functions of the Corpus Callosum*. New York: Alan R Liss, 1986: 75–81.

10 Grafstein B. Organization of callosal connections in suprasylvian gyrus of cats. *J Neurophysiol* 1959; 22: 504–15.

11 Gates JR, Wada JA, Reeves AG *et al*. Reevaluation of corpus callosotomy. In: Engel J Jr, ed. *Surgical Treatment of the Epilepsies*, 2nd edn. New York: Raven Press Ltd, 1993: 637–48.

12 Kass JH. Organization of callosal projections in primates. *The 2nd Dartmouth International Conference on Epilepsy and the Corpus Callosum*, Dartmouth College, Hanover, New Hampshire, 1991.

13 Wada J. Midline structures for transhemispheric ictal and interictal transmission. *The 2nd Dartmouth International Conference on Epilepsy and the Corpus Callosum*, Dartmouth College, Hanover, New Hampshire, 1991.

14 Musgrave J, Gloor P. The role of the corpus callosum in bilateral interhemispheric synchrony of spike and wave discharge in feline generalized penicillin epilepsy. *Epilepsia* 1980; 21: 369–78.

15 Vergnes M, Marecaux C, Micheletti G *et al*. Spontaneous paroxysmal electroclinical patterns in rat: a model of generalized non-convulsive epilepsy. *Neurosci Lett* 1982; 33: 97–101.

16 Vergnes M, Marescaux C, Lannes B, Depaulis A, Micheletti G, Warter JM. Interhemispheric desynchronization of spontaneous spike and wave discharges by corpus callosum transection in rats with petit mal-like epilepsy. *Epilepsy Res* 1989; 4: 8–13.

17 Wada JA, Komai S. Effect of anterior two-thirds callosal bisection upon bisymmetrical and bisynchronous generalized convulsions kindled from amygdala in epileptic baboon, *Papio papio*. In: Reeves AG, ed. *Epilepsy and the Corpus Callosum*. New York: Plenum Press, 1985: 75–97.

18 Naquet R, Wada JA. Role of the corpus callosum in photosensitive seizures of epileptic baboon *Papio papio*. *Adv Neurol* 1992; 57: 579–87.

19 Erickson TE. Spread of the epileptic discharge: an experimental study of the after discharge induced by electrical stimulation of the cerebral cortex. *Arch Neurol Psychiatr* 1940; 43: 429.

20 Hursch JB. Origin of the spike and wave pattern of petit mal epilepsy: an electroencephalographic study. *Arch Neurol Psychiatr* 1945; 53: 274–82.

21 Bogen JE, Vogel PJ. Cerebral commissurotomy in man: preliminary case report. *Bull LA Neurol Soc* 1962; 27: 169–72.

22 Bogen JE, Fisher ED, Vogel PJ. Cerebral commissurotomy: a second case report. *J Am Med Assoc* 1965; 194(2): 1328–9.

23 Bogen JE, Sperry RW, Vogel PJ. Addendum: commissural section and the propagation of seizures. In: Jasper HH, Ward AA, Pope A, eds. *Basic Mechanisms of Epilepsy*. Boston: Little Brown, 1969: 439.

24 Luessenhop AJ. Interhemispheric commissurotomy (the split brain operation) as an alternative to hemispherectomy for control of intractable seizures. *Am Surg* 1970; 36: 265–8.

25 Luessenhop AJ, de la Cruz TC, Fenichel GM. Surgical disconnection of the cerebral hemispheres for intractable seizures. *J Am Med Assoc* 1970; 213(10): 1630–6.

26 Mann LB, Bogen JE, Vogel PJ, Saul R. Cerebral commissurotomy in man: EEG findings. *Electroencephalogr Clin Neurophysiol* 1969; 27: 660.

27 Wilson DH, Culver C, Waddington M, Gazzaniga M. Disconnection of the cerebral hemispheres. *Neurology* 1975; 25: 1149–53.

28 Wilson DH, Reeves AG, Gazzaniga M, Culver C. Cerebral commissurotomy for control of intractable seizures. *Neurology* 1977; 27: 708–15.

29 Wilson DH, Reeves AG, Gazzaniga M. Division of the corpus callosum for uncontrollable seizures. *Neurology* 1978; 28: 649–53.

30 Gates JR, Leppik IE, Yap J, Gumnit RJ. Corpus callosotomy: clinical and electroencephalographic effects. *Epilepsia* 1984; 25(3): 308–16.

31 Gates JR, Maxwell R, Leppik IR, Fiol M, Gumnit RJ. Electroencephalographic and clinical effects of total corpus callosotomy. In: Reeves AG, ed. *Epilepsy and the Corpus Callosum*. New York: Plenum Press, 1986: 315–28.

32 Spencer SS, Spencer DS, Williamson PD, Mattson R. Effects of corpus callosum section on secondary bilaterally synchronous interictal EEG discharges. *Neurology* 1985; 35: 1689–94.

33 Gates JR, Ritter FJ, Ragazza PC *et al*. Corpus callosum section in children: seizure response. *J Epilepsy* 1990; Suppl.: 271–8.

34 Pinard JM, Delalande O, Plouin P, Dulac O. Callosotomy in West syndrome suggests a cortical origin of hypsarrhythmia. *Epilepsia* 1993; 34(4): 780–7.

35 Hrachovy RA, Frost JD, Kellaway P. Hypsarrhythmia revisited: variations on the theme. *Epilepsia* 1984; 25: 317–25.

36 Spencer SS, Katz A, Ebersole J, Novotny E, Mattson R. Ictal EEG changes with corpus callosotomy section. *Epilepsia* 1993; 34(3): 568–73.

37 Gates JR. Presurgical evaluation for epileptic surgery in the era of long term monitoring for epilepsy. In: Apuzzo MLJ, ed. *Neurosurgical Aspects of Epilepsy*. Illinois: AANS Publications, 1991: 59–72.

38 Courtney W, Gates JR, Ritter FJ *et al*. Prediction of seizure outcome after corpus callosotomy in patients ten years or older. *Epilepsia* 1993; 34 (Suppl. 6): 43.

39 Gates JR, Courtney W, Ritter FJ *et al*. Prediction of seizure outcome after corpus callosotomy among young children. *Epilepsia* 1993; 34 (Suppl. 6): 111.

40 De Paola L, Gates JR, Ritter FJ *et al*. Persistence of generalized ictal electroencephalographic onset after total corpus callosotomy. *Neurology* 1995; (from an unpublished manuscript by De Paola *et al*.).

41 Maehara T, Shimizu H. Surgical outcome of corpus callosotomy in patients with drop attacks. *Epilepsia* 2001; 42(1): 67–71.

42 Engel J Jr, Van Ness PC, Rasmussen TB, Ojemann LM. Outcome with respect to epileptic seizures. In: Engel J Jr, ed. *Surgical Treatment of the Epilepsies*, 2nd edn. New York: Raven Press Ltd, 1993: 609–22.

43 Williamson PD. Corpus callosum section for intractable epilepsy: criteria for patient selection. In: Reeves AG, ed. *Epilepsy and the Corpus Callosum*. New York: Plenum Press, 1985: 243–57.

44 Gates JR. Candidacy for corpus callosotomy. In: Lüders H, ed. *Epilepsy Surgery*. New York: Raven Press Ltd, 1991: 140–50.

45 Gates JR. EEG selection for corpus callosotomy. *Epilepsy Res* 1992; Suppl. 5: 201–4.

46 Andermann F. Clinical indications for hemispherectomy and callosotomy. *Epilepsy Res* 1992; Suppl. 5: 189–99.

47 Wilson DH, Reeves AG, Gazzaniga M. Central commissurotomy for intractable generalized epilepsy: series two. *Neurology* 1982; 32: 687–97.

48 Spencer SS, Gates JR, Reeves AG, Spencer DS, Maxwell RE, Roberts D. Corpus callosum section. In: Engel J Jr, ed. *Surgical Treatment of the Epilepsies*. New York: Raven Press, 1987: 425–44.

49 Spencer SS. Corpus callosum section and other disconnection procedures for medically intractable epilepsy. *Epilepsia* 1988; 29 (Suppl. 2): S85–S99.

50 Wyllie E. Corpus callosotomy for intractable generalized epilepsy. *J Pediatr* 1988; 113: 255–61.

51 Wyler AR. Corpus callosotomy. *Epilepsy Res* 1992; Suppl. 5: 205–8.

52 Pilcher WH, Ojemann GA. Presurgical evaluation and epilepsy surgery. In Apuzzo MLJ, ed. *Brain Surgery, Complication Avoidance and Management*. New York: Churchill Livingstone 1993: 1525–55.

53 Gates JR, Ritter FJ, Ragazzo PC, Reeves AG, Nordgen RE. Corpus callosum section in children: seizure response. *J Epilepsy* 1990: 3 (Suppl.): 271–8.

54 Spencer DD, Spencer SS. Corpus callosotomy in the treatment of medically intractable secondarily generalized seizures in children. *Cleve Clin Med J* 1989; 56 (Suppl. 1): S69–S78.

55 Black PM, Holmes G, Lombroso C. Corpus callosum section for intractable epilepsy in children. *Pediatr Neurosurg* 1992; 18: 298–304.

56 Raffel C, Kongelbeck SR, Snead OC III. Corpus callosotomy for intractable epilepsy in children. *Pediatr Neurosurg* 1992; 18: 305–9.

57 Cendes F, Ragazzo PC, da Costa V, Martins LF. Corpus callosotomy in treatment of medically resistant epilepsy: preliminary results in a pediatric population. *Epilepsia* 1993; 34(5): 910–17.

58 Tinuper P, Andermann F, Villemure JG, Rasmussen TB, Quesney LF. Functional hemispherectomy for treatment of epilepsy associated with hemiplegia: rationale, indications, results, and comparison with callosotomy. *Ann Neurol* 1988; 24: 27–34.

59 Gates JR, Rosenfeldt WE, Maxwell RE, Lyons RE. Response of multiple seizure types to corpus callosum section. *Epilepsia* 1987; 28(1): 28–34.

60 Murro AM, Flanigin HF, Gallagher BB, King DW, Smith JR. Corpus callosotomy for the treatment of intractable epilepsy. *Epilepsy Res* 1988; 2: 44–50.

61 Purves SJ, Wada JA, Woodhurst WB *et al*. Results of anterior corpus callosum section in 24 patients with medically intractable seizures. *Neurology* 1988; 38: 1194–201.

62 Oguni H, Olivier A, Andermann F, Comair J. Anterior callosotomy in the treatment of medically intractable epilepsies: a study of 43 patients with a mean follow-up of 39 months. *Ann Neurol* 1991; 30: 357–64.

63 Mamelak AN, Barbaro NM, Walker JA, Laxer KD. Corpus callosotomy: a quantitative study of the extent of resection, seizure control, and neuropsychological outcome. *J Neurosurg* 1993; 79: 688–95.

64 Spencer SS, Spencer DD, Sass K, Westerveld M, Katz A, Mattson R. Anterior, total, and two-staged corpus callosum section: differential and incremental seizure responses. *Epilepsia* 1993; 34(3): 561–7.

65 Geoffroy G, Lassonde M, Delisle F, Decarie M. Corpus callosotomy for control of intractable epilepsy in children. *Neurology* 1983; 33: 891–7.

66 Reutens DC, Bye AM, Hopkins IJ *et al*. Corpus callosotomy for intractable epilepsy: seizure outcome and prognostic factors. *Epilepsia* 1993; 34(5): 904–9.

67 Wyllie E. Corpus callosotomy: outcome with respect to seizures. In: Lüders H, ed. *Epilepsy Surgery*. New York: Raven Press Ltd, 1991: 120–35.

68 Fuiks K, Wyler AR, Hermann BP, Somes G. Seizure outcome from anterior and complete corpus callosotomy. *J Neurosurg* 1991; 74: 573–8.

69 Spencer SS, Spencer DD, Williamson PD, Sass K, Novelly RA, Mattson RH. Corpus callosotomy for epilepsy. I. Seizure effects. *Neurology* 1988; 38: 19–24.

70 Waterman K, Purves SJ, Kosaka B, Strauss E, Wada JA. An epileptic syndrome caused by mesial frontal lobe seizure foci. *Neurology* 1987; 37: 577–82.

71 Purves SJ, Wada JA, Woodhurst WB. Anterior callosotomy for complex partial seizures. *The 2nd Dartmouth International Conference on Epilepsy and the Corpus Callosum*, Dartmouth College, Hanover, New Hampshire, 1991.

72 Stearns M, Wolf AL, Barry E, Bergey G, Gellad F. Corpus callosotomy for refractory seizures in a patient with cortical heteropia: case report. *Neurosurgery* 1989; 25(4): 633–6.

73 Landy JH, Curless PG, Ramsay RE, Slater J, Ajmone-Marsan C, Quencer RM. Corpus callosotomy for seizures associated with band heterotopia. *Epilepsia* 1993; 34(1): 79–83.

74 Wyler AR. Corpus callosotomy. In: Wyllie E, ed. *The Treatment of Epilepsy: Principles and Practice*. Philadelphia: Lea, Febiger, 1993: 1120–5.

75 Roberts DW. Corpus callosotomy—surgical technique. In: Reeves AG, ed. *Epilepsy and the Corpus Callosum*. New York: Plenum Press, 1985: 259–67.

76 Roberts DW. Section of the corpus callosum for epilepsy. In: Schmidek HH, Sweet WH, eds. *Operative Neurosurgical Techniques, Indications, Methods and Results*. Philadelphia: WB Saunders Company, 1988: 1243–50.

77 Roberts DW. Corpus callosum section. In: Spencer SS, Spencer DD, eds. *Surgery for Epilepsy*. Oxford: Blackwell Scientific Publications, 1990: 168–78.

78 Roberts DW. The role of callosal section in the surgical treatment of epilepsies. *Neurosurg Clin N Am* 1993; 4(2): 293–300.

79 Roberts DW, Rayport M, Maxwell RE, Olivier A, Marino R Jr. Corpus callosotomy. In: Engel J Jr, ed. *Surgical Treatment of the Epilepsies*, 2nd edn. New York: Raven Press Ltd, 1993: 519–26.

80 Maxwell RF, Gates JR. Evaluation of patients for the surgical management of epilepsy. *Minn Med* 1985; July.

81 Awad IA, Wyllie E, Lüders H, Ahl J. Intraoperative determination of the extent of corpus callosotomy for epilepsy: two simple techniques. *Neurosurgery* 1990; 26(1): 102–6.

82 Torres F, French LA. Acute effect of the section of the corpus callosum upon independent epileptiform activity. *Acta Neurol Scand* 1973; 49: 47–62.

83 Fiol ME, Gates JR, Mireles R, Maxwell RE, Erickson DM. Value of intraoperative EEG changes during corpus callosotomy in predicting surgical results. *Epilepsia* 1993; 34(1): 74–8.

84 Marino R Jr, Ragazzo PC. Selective criteria and results of partial callosotomy. In: Reeves AG, ed. *Epilepsy and the Corpus Callosum*. New York: Plenum Press, 1985: 281–301.

85 Marino R Jr, Radvany J, Huck F, De Camargo CHP, Gronich G. Selective electroencephalograph-guided microsurgical callosotomy for refractory generalized epilepsy. *Surg Neurol* 1990; 34: 219–28.

86 Marino R Jr, Cukiert A, Gronich G. Open and stereotactic segmental callosotomy: effects on seizure frequency. *The Second Dartmouth International Conference on Epilepsy and the Corpus Callosum*, Hanover, New Hampshire, 1991.

87 Frost MD, Gates JR, Conry JA *et al*. Vagus nerve stimulation (VNS) in Lennox–Gastaut syndrome (LGS). *Epilepsia* 1999; 40(7): 95.

88 Gazzaniga MS, Holtzman JD, Deck MDF, Lee BCP. MRI assessment of human callosal surgery with neuropsychological correlates. *Neurology* 1985; 35: 1763–6.

89 Gazzaniga MS, Kutas M, Van Petten C, Fendrich R. Human callosal function: MRI-verified neuropsychological functions. *Neurology* 1989; 39: 942–6.

90 Gates JR, Mireles R, Maxwell R, Sharbrough F, Forbes G. Magnetic resonance imaging, electroencephalogram, and selected neuropsychological testing in staged corpus callosotomy. *Arch Neurol* 1986; 43: 1188–91.

91 Risse GL, Gates JR, Lund G, Maxwell R, Rubens A. Interhemispheric transfer in patients with incomplete section of the corpus callosum—

anatomic verification with magnetic resonance imaging. *Arch Neurol* 1989; 46: 437–43.

92 Trojano L, Crisci C, Lanzillo B, Elefante R, Caruso G. How many alien hand syndromes? Follow-up of a case. *Neurology* 1993; 43: 2710–12.

93 Reeves AG. Behavioral changes following corpus callosotomy. *Adv Neurol* 1992; 55: 293–300.

94 Gazzaniga MS, Holtzmann JD, Smylie CS. Speech without conscious awareness. *Neurology* 1987; 37: 682–5.

94 Sussman NM, Ruben CG, Gur RE, O'Connor MJ. Mutism as a consequence of callosotomy. *J Neurosurg* 1983; 59: 514–19.

95 Lassonde M, Sauerwein H, Chicoine AJ, Geoffroy G. Absence of disconnexion syndrome in callosal agenesis and early callosotomy: brain reorganization or lack of structural specificity during ontogeny? *Neuropsychologia* 1991; 29(6): 481–95.

96 Novelly RA, Lifrak MD. Forebrain commissurotomy reinstates effects of preexisting hemisphere lesions: an examination of the hypothesis. In: Reeves AG, ed. *Epilepsy and the Corpus Callosum*. New York: Plenum Press, 1985: 467–500.

97 Beniak TE, Gates JR, Risse GL. Comparison of selected neuropsychological test variables pre and post operatively on patients subjected to corpus callosotomy. *Epilepsia* 1985; 26: 534.

98 Ferrel RB, Culver CM, Tucker GJ. Psychosocial and cognitive function after commissurotomy for intractable seizures. *J Neurosurg* 1983; 58: 374–80.

99 Provinciali L, Del Pesce M, Censori B *et al*. Evolution of neuropsychological changes after partial callosotomy in intractable epilepsy. *Epilepsy Res* 1990; 6: 155–65.

100 Ferguson SM, Rayport M, Blumer DP, Fenwick PBC, Taylor DC. Postoperative psychiatric changes. In: Engel J Jr, ed. *Surgical Treatment of the Epilepsies*. New York: Raven Press Ltd, 1993: 649–62.

101 Amacher AL. Midline commissurotomy for the treatment of some cases of intractable epilepsy. Preliminary report. *Child Brain* 1976; 2: 54–8.

102 Makari GS, Holmes GL, Murro AM. Corpus callosotomy for the treatment of intractable epilepsy in children. *Epilepsy Res* 1988; 2: 44–50.

68 Multiple Subpial Transection for Epilepsy

R. Selway and R. Dardis

One of the central tenets of epilepsy surgery is that resection of the epileptogenic zone is generally associated with an excellent outcome [1]. There are not infrequent situations, however, where this zone is either rather extensive or situated in eloquent cortex, such that resection would lead to significant morbidity. Multiple subpial transection (MST) is a technique developed to address such problems.

The cerebral cortex is organized in such a way that the functional units are arranged in columns, radially to the gyrus surface. However, epileptic discharges are thought to spread in a tangential direction, relying on the cortical connections between the columns. MST creates numerous interruptions in the surface spread of discharges while apparently leaving the function of that cortex unaffected. Using this technique it has proved possible to undertake surgery with low rates of morbidity in patients whose seizure onset occurs in regions such as the primary motor cortex or in an area essential for speech. There are relatively few large published series and many of these include patients who underwent combined cortical resection and MST. Results, therefore, are often difficult to interpret; they do, however, appear to demonstrate that MST is a valuable technique applicable to such difficult presentations. MST has a particular role in the treatment of acquired epileptic aphasia (Landau–Kleffner syndrome or LKS), where it may be the treatment of choice in medically resistant patients, and has also been applied to multifocal epilepsies.

Physiology

The late Frank Morrell was largely responsible for the coalescence of thought required to develop MST. He had a long and distinguished career not only in the development of experimental models of epilepsy and behaviour but also as an astute neurologist with a special interest in epilepsy. His experimental work led to a refinement of the understanding of the pathways by which seizures spread [2–15]. From this appreciation of basic mechanisms, he suggested and developed the technique of MST for use in areas of eloquent cortex that produced epileptic discharges. Somewhat later on, after observing how epileptic foci in an experimental model can produce distant foci, a process he described as secondary epileptogenesis, he also applied MST to LKS.

The concept of MST arose from three independent sets of laboratory experiments, none of which was designed with a clinical purpose in mind.

The first set involved the concept that the functional unit of cortical architecture is the column [16]. A column is a group of radially orientated incoming and outgoing fibres, and associated neurones, which form the anatomical keystone on which the bulk of functional attributes are built. That function within the cortex depends on columns rather than transverse connections has been confirmed in numerous subsequent models, most notably the Nobel Prize winning work of Hubel and Wiesel in the visual cortex [17]. Interestingly the existence of the vertical connections of neurones was first proposed by Lorente de No from his histological studies [18] but the later functional studies, notably by Asanuma [19,20], have confirmed this physiologically.

This concept has been refined more recently into the 'minicolumn' [21]. The mini-column is a narrow chain of neurones extending radially across cellular layers II–VI of the six-layered neocortex, perpendicular to the pial surface. Each mini-column in primates contains about 80–100 neurones except in the striate cortex where they contain, perhaps, 200 neurones. The mini-columns are bound together by short-range transverse connections forming cortical columns. Central to all this work is the premise that function depends principally on radial architecture and very local transverse connections (up to about 0.5 mm across) within layers II and upper III of the cortex [20].

The second set of observations was based on studies of the anatomical organization of an epileptic 'spike'. Each neurone within a seizure focus has a stereotypic and synchronized electrical response know as the paroxysmal depolarizing shift (PDS). PDS synchrony is thought, from experimental studies in many animal models of focal epilepsy, to be of critical importance in generating the epileptic spike and hence possibly partial seizures. The generation and spread of such epileptiform activity in the neocortex is dependent on horizontal connections in all layers of the cortex, but especially in layer V, in which pyramidal cells can act as both the initiators and propagators of hypersynchronous activity [22,23].

A third series of experiments investigated the role of electrical fields in the brain. Sperry and colleagues, using complex perception models, performed various manoeuvres to isolate these electrical fields [24,25]. These experiments involved isolation of the cortex using strips of mica, tantalum wires and cortical incisions. All of these interrupted the transverse neuronal connections. None of the experiments produced impairment of behaviour. The extent of side-to-side interaction necessary to produce a spike was then investigated. It was presumed that the larger the cortical 'island' the more likely it could support epileptiform activity. A contiguous surface area of 12–25 mm^2 of cerebral cortex seems necessary to produce an epileptic spike [23,26].

On the basis of the above observations, Morrell and colleagues attempted to extinguish epileptic foci in animal models using multiple transections, so reducing the contiguous areas of cortex below that required for spike production. They found that sectioning horizontal cortical fibres at 5 mm intervals in an epileptic focus in the precentral cortex of a monkey abolished the spontaneous epileptic discharges from this area. Moreover the animals were seen to have no gross weakness of the limb [9]. The monkeys were observed for up to 1 year after such transection without recurrence of the discharges.

Such promising early work led to further examination of the size of the cortical island required to produce a spike and the separation of transections required to ensure function is maintained.

Epileptic foci produced experimentally at an interval of 4 mm produce a single dependent spike focus [23]. At an interval of 6 mm, the activity could be independent. However there do appear to be significant differences between deafferented *in vitro* preparations and the *in vivo* situation. Similarly there are species differences. Morrell proposed, on the basis of much laboratory work, that the transection interval should be 5 mm.

It was by good fortune that these manoeuvres did not disrupt the blood supply. Subsequent work has shown that, in general, the blood supply to the gyrus enters perpendicular to the long axis. A transverse transection therefore will (fortunately) tend to spare the vascular supply whereas a transection parallel to the long axis will cut across some of the feeding vessels. It has been shown that such parallel transections do result in impairment of function in animal models of spatial learning, probably by compromising blood supply [25].

Indications

Resections involving eloquent cortex

Victor Horsley recognized the inevitable consequences of resection of eloquent cortex in his 1886 report of the resection of a scar from the region of the motor cortex for epilepsy [27]. Penfield employed local anaesthetic surgery with intraoperative cortical stimulation to map these areas and hence avoid damaging them [28]. Many other techniques now allow cortical mapping to be performed, such as implantation of grid electrodes, functional MRI (fMRI) and magnetic source imaging (MSI) (Plate 68.1, shown in colour between pp. 670 and 671). In some circumstances preoperative investigations demonstrate that seizure onset directly involves regions of cortex which, if resected, would lead to significant morbidity. There is a wealth of evidence to show that complete resection of epileptogenic lesions, such as an area of focal cortical dysplasia, is required for a sustained seizure-free outcome. In these circumstances a resection sparing the 'absolutely eloquent' regions is likely to fail. MST is particularly useful in such cases, often combined with resection of the less eloquent brain. A typical example would include a dominant temporal resection when the pathology extends posteriorly along the superior temporal gyrus. If preoperative or intraoperative investigations suggest that this includes a region essential for language, then this area could be subjected to MST after a conventional anterior temporal resection. Similar approaches can be used in motor, somatosensory or visual cortex. If epilepsy results from a relatively long-standing lesion, then the eloquent cortex may have been displaced from its expected position. The displacement of language function to the contralateral side is well documented in cases where a lesion is present in childhood. The shift of primary motor or sensory cortex may be more subtle but is nevertheless described [29].

It should be emphasized that the preoperative assessments for such patients are rarely straightforward. If a lesion is visible on an MRI scan in a region suggesting close relationship with eloquent cortex, standard presurgical assessment with scalp videotelemetry will be insufficient. It will be necessary to demonstrate the relationship with the eloquent cortex. Investigations can be aided with MSI, fMRI and PET, but intracranial cortical mapping is often necessary. Chronic recording with grid electrode arrays allows both the mapping of functional cortex and also the recording of the ictal onset zone, the resection of which is associated with favourable outcome. Alternatively in selected patients craniotomy under local anaesthesia can allow accurate real-time mapping and assessment of the functionally abnormal area using electrocorticography (ECoG). Evoked potentials can also be used intraoperatively. The non-lesional cases are those with no concordant abnormality visible on the MRI. They present even greater difficulties during preoperative assessment. Although combining the newer imaging technologies (e.g. ictal SPECT and fMRI) may one day replace more invasive techniques, these still require further evaluation.

Many lesions involving eloquent cortex also extend considerably beyond these regions. Resection of these less eloquent areas may frequently be combined with MST.

MST has a particularly important role in the treatment of Rasmussen's chronic focal encephalitis. This is an inflammatory disease, thought to have an autoimmune basis in which there is a progressive unihemispheric epileptic disorder frequently leading to loss of all functions of that hemisphere and epilepsia partialis continua. Constant epileptic discharges may lead to dysfunction of the other hemisphere and to intellectual decline. If, despite medical treatment, the condition progresses to this most severe stage then a hemispherectomy is appropriate [30]. However, Rasmussen's disease does not always progress to this extent and the speed of progression is variable. There is sometimes an intermediate stage, in which, for example, there is only a mild hemiparesis, when such radical surgery may be undesirable. In this situation many authors have used a combination of resection of the most electrically active areas with MST over eloquent regions such as the primary motor and sensory strips. Such surgery would usually be palliative, aimed at controlling the worst of the clinical features and holding the hemispherectomy in reserve for a time when the disease has already caused a hemiplegia.

Landau–Kleffner syndrome (LKS)

LKS or acquired epileptic aphasia is a rare condition of childhood in which there is a progressive loss of normal speech [31]. It typically affects children of about 5 years of age and has a rather variable course of relapse and remission. Associated with the speech disturbance is an epileptic disorder, which usually is not the prominent clinical feature and may be well controlled medically. Usually speech comprehension is affected more severely than production and this may underlie the behavioural disorders common in this condition. While not a diagnostic criterion, sleep EEG characteristically reveals almost continuous spike-and-wave activity during slow wave sleep that may occur for more than 90% of the sleep record. While there are occasional case reports of structural lesions of the temporal lobe producing the syndrome, MRI is generally normal and biopsy results are non-specific.

There is now good evidence that there is a causal relationship between the prominent spike focus and the language disorder [32]. The patients appear to have a focus arising in one sylvian region that results in secondary spiking in the contralateral homotopic region. LKS has many features that are similar to more common conditions in which autistic behaviour and epilepsy overlap; however the normal early development and acquisition of speech appears central to the condition.

MST has been used now in many centres for the treatment of LKS. Diagnostic criteria and procedures for selection for surgery seem to vary considerably between units. Timing of surgery is another challenging dilemma. The condition has a variable course and improvements can occur spontaneously or following treatment, particularly with corticosteroids. However once aphasia has become established, surgery is probably the treatment of choice. The associated epilepsy is usually not difficult to control, although antiepileptic drugs seem to have little impact on the behavioural and language disturbance [33]. Whether surgery should be offered earlier in the disease has yet to be established.

Specific investigations seek to identify the region giving rise to the leading spikes on the EEG. This region is thought to drive the similar EEG abnormality in the opposite hemisphere. Morrell *et al.* described the use of the methohexital suppression test to detect the driving hemisphere [34]. When methohexital is administered intravenously at sufficiently high doses, it progressively abolishes excitatory synaptic transmission. He found that independent epileptogenic lesions showed great resistance to this increased inhibition. If, however, EEG spiking was not autonomous but depended upon synaptic activation from another region, then methohexital abolished this activity along with the other ongoing EEG rhythms. Thus, increasing intravenous doses of methohexital eventually reveal a region that demonstrates the last remaining spikes before electrocerebral silence. Similarly as the barbiturate wears off the driving region regains its electrical activity first. Deep levels of anaesthesia may be obtained during this test and ventilatory support and airway protection may be required. Although this test was central to Morrell's assessment of LKS, other authors have found it less reliable [35]. An alternative assessment is the electrical intracarotid amobarbital test. This is a variant of the Wada test that may be carried out under sedation or indeed under general anaesthetic [36]. Sodium amobarbital (amytal) is injected into one internal carotid artery through a catheter percutaneously placed via the femoral artery under radiological control. Injection on the 'driving' side will result in abolition of spiking in both hemispheres (Fig. 68.2). The procedure is repeated on the opposite side following electrical recovery of the bilateral spike discharges, typically about 10 min later. When the injection is contralateral to the driving hemisphere, only unilateral suppression occurs. The main difficulty with this test is obtaining the appropriate level of sedation. It may need careful adjustment to ensure that the bilateral spike-wave discharge is apparent on scalp recordings. Morrell used amitriptyline sedation, which did not suppress the activity; this approach is now, however, limited by the manufacturer's withdrawal of the intravenous preparation. Sleep deprivation the night before the test may help provoke the activity [33].

Although conventional scalp EEG generally shows bilateral synchronous activity in sleep, careful analysis can demonstrate that one side is leading the other. Morrell assessed this during the methohexital test and showed a typical phase difference of about 20 ms. The same assessment can be made on routine sleep EEG or intracranial recordings [37]. Similarly, scalp EEG data has been used to model dipole localization using linear inverse solution methods [38].

With the increasing availability of magnetoencephalography, MSI has proved to be a good and non-invasive alternative for detecting the laterality and anatomical position of the leading dipoles (see Plate 68.1, shown in colour between pp. 670 and 671). It is generally well tolerated by children of this age. Such dipoles generally appear within the sylvian fissure and are orientated parallel to the temporal convexity. Such a dipole is often difficult to detect with surface EEG because of its orientation.

This technique allows simultaneous display of EEG spike localization and the position of auditory evoked potentials [39,40]. Phase analysis can also be carried out on the MEG data to determine the leading area. These sophisticated tests are required to determine the side of surgery in LKS. A sizeable minority of cases are driven by right-sided discharges and only with surgery on this side are the bilateral EEG abnormalities abolished [34].

Multilobar or bihemispheric foci

A further group of patients who are not generally considered amenable to conventional epilepsy surgery are those with very extensive foci, either involving more than one lobe and including eloquent cortex, or involving foci in both hemispheres. There are, at present, very limited data on the management of such patients with MST, almost all of which comes from Patil's unit in Nebraska [41].

Within his group of patients were those with a variety of seizure types including Lennox–Gastaut syndrome and myoclonic seizures with hypsarrhythmia. Most, however, had complex partial seizures with or without secondary generalization. The patients were investigated with a combination of MRI, PET scanning and MSI. All had multiple apparent seizure foci. It is not entirely clear whether more intensive investigation, perhaps with intracranial ictal recording, may have demonstrated that not all these foci were primary. Indeed, some are likely to have been secondary to a single leading focus. However it is clear that at least some successfully treated patients in Patil's series would not have been regarded as surgical candidates in most units. His impressive results were obtained by very extensive MST, sometimes including homotopic regions of both frontal lobes, combined with limited topectomies. A topectomy is the excision of a small cortical region, in this case one with persistent ECoG spiking despite MST. Such areas generally prove to have histological abnormalities such as cortical dysplasia [42].

More recently Zhai from China has published a series of a hundred cases, many also suffering from multilobar or even apparently generalized epilepsy [43]. These were treated by extensive MST, together with either focal resection or anterior corpus callosotomy. The application of MST to these patient groups has not yet achieved general acceptance.

Surgical technique

Once the preoperative investigations described above have defined the region to be transected the surgical strategy can be refined. If a combination of resection and MST is planned, then the limits of re-

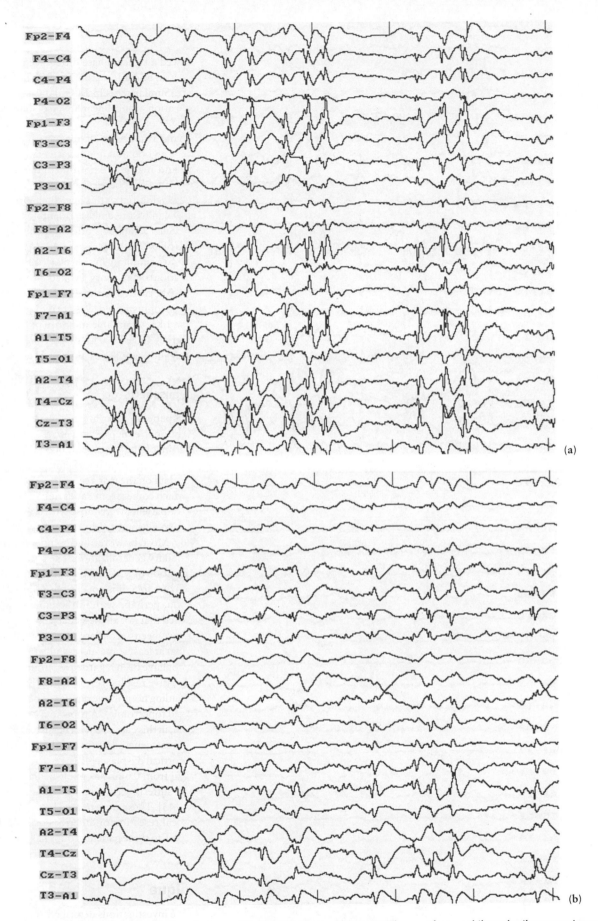

Fig. 68.2 The electrical intracarotid amobarbital test in a case of Landau–Kleffner syndrome. (a) There are frequent bilateral spikes occurring at the start. (b) After the right-sided injection the ipsilateral activity is abolished but the left-sided spikes continue.

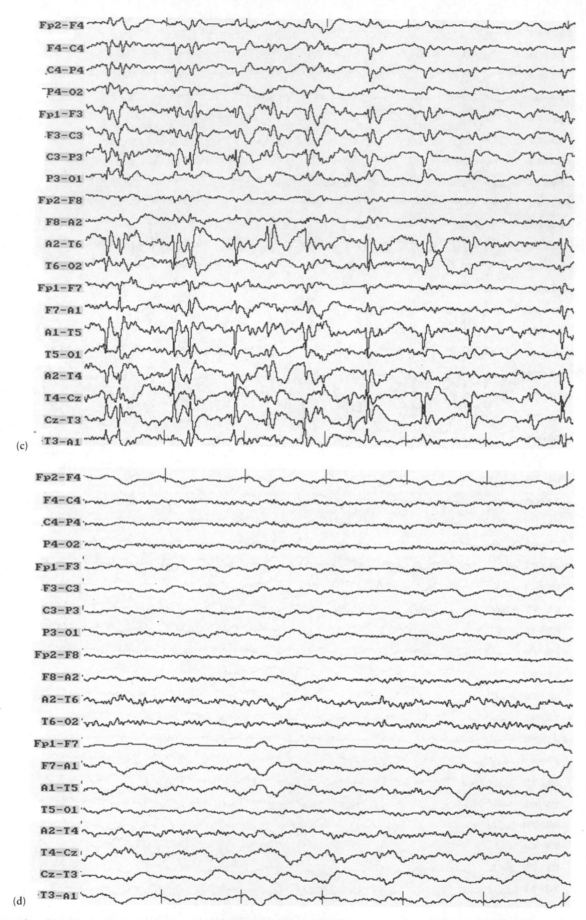

Fig. 68.2 (c) After about 10 min the recording returns to bilateral spike activity. (d) A left-sided injection promptly produces bilateral suppression. This confirms that the left side is driving the bilateral EEG abnormality.

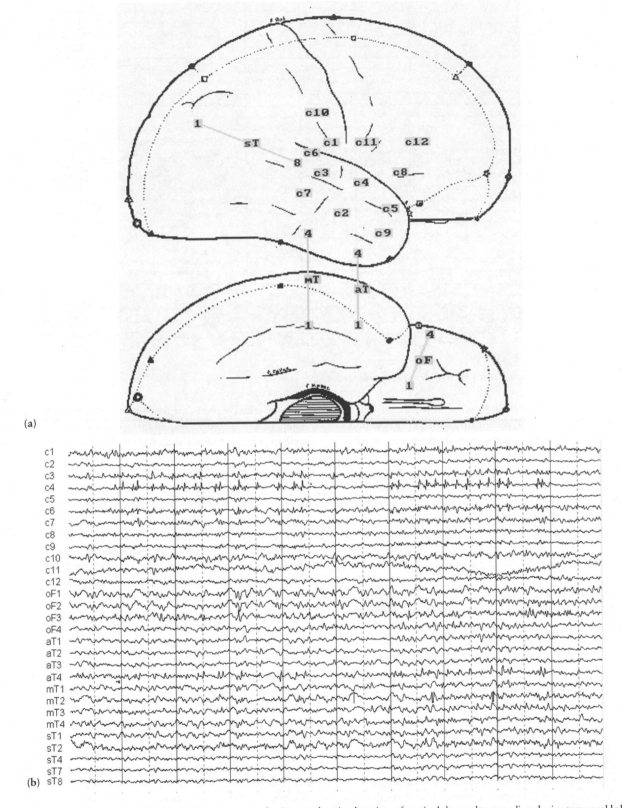

(a)

(b)

Fig. 68.3 Pre- and post-transection ECoGs. (a) Intra-operative brain map showing location of cortical electrodes recording during temporal lobe MST. (b) The pre-transection record shows frequent spikes over the lateral temporal cortex.

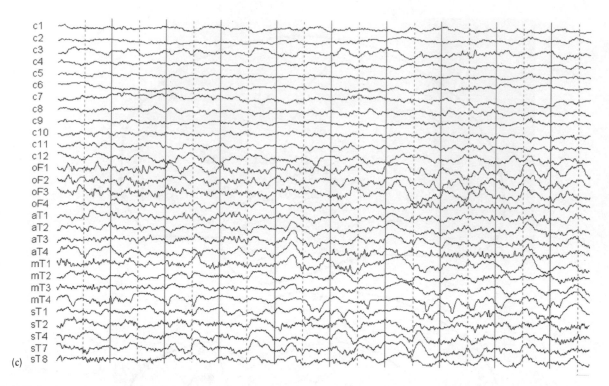

Fig. 68.3 (c) Following transection, the spikes have been substantially reduced.

section need to be decided preoperatively, usually on the basis of the mapping of eloquent cortex. Typically surgery is performed under general anaesthesia; if intraoperative cortical mapping is required, then local anaesthesia procedures may be necessary [11]. It is useful to position the surgical field so that the surface to be transected is approximately horizontal. This is not always possible, particularly if one is approaching large areas or inaccessible regions such as within the sylvian fissure or the parafalcine cortex.

The craniotomy and cortical exposure should be generous as the exact extent of the transection is guided by intraoperative ECoG which can occasionally indicate a wider field than originally expected (Fig 68.3).

The first manoeuvre is to perform the ECoG. This confirms the area to be transected. Each transection is performed by using a combination of steel wire hooks specifically designed for the purpose by Morrell and Whisler (Fig. 68.4). Each wire is mounted on a handle which is square in cross-section allowing the surgeon to know precisely the position of the tip even when it is out of sight. At the other end of each wire is a short hook, 4 mm in length and turned up at an angle of 105–110 degrees. The hook is flat and blunt. The underlying principle is that as the hook is introduced such that the tip is just below the pia, the 4 mm length is sufficiently short that the hook is confined to the cortex and spares the white matter tracts that are leaving the gyrus.

It is best to start at the most dependent gyri, moving progressively to the higher regions of the exposed brain. This means that any blood oozing from the operated areas does not obscure the working region. As discussed above, the transections are made at right angles to the long axis of the gyrus. With the aid of an operating microscope, a tiny puncture is made with a Beaver knife through the pia–arachnoid at one edge of the selected gyrus. A transection hook is then inserted through this hole and passed across the gyrus to the opposite sulcal border. Care is needed to ensure that the hooked end is kept perpendicular to the pial surface to avoid undercutting a segment of cortex. The hook is then gently lifted until the tip is just visible beneath the pia and then brought back towards the entry point sparing the pial membrane. This manoeuvre will create a thin red line across the gyrus and may result in a small amount of bleeding as the hook is extracted through its entry hole. Such bleeding is usually easily controlled with a microcottonoid. Using another hook of appropriate shape the vertical part of the gyrus adjacent to the pial incision is then transected. This hook is passed through the hole and allowed to sink under gravity towards the depth of the sulcus. It is then brought up towards the surface again ensuring the hook is perpendicular to the pia (Fig. 68.5).

As the transection is being performed it is common to feel a slight resistance as a vessel is encountered. The angle of the hook is designed to minimize this snagging but if it is encountered then advancing the hook and withdrawing again by a slightly different path will usually avoid tearing the vessel. The blunted edges of the hooks are designed to prevent vascular injury.

It should be noted that the surface regions of each gyrus are transected under direct vision and the resulting red subpial line acts as a marker for planning the next transection. The depth of each sulcus is identified entirely by feel, and can be very difficult to gauge. Moreover, there are regions of the brain where access is even more difficult. Despite the variety of curved hook designs, it is technically much more difficult to transect a gyrus that is not facing the surgeon. The planum temporale in the sylvian fissure is the most frequently encountered difficult area, but the parasagittal region is even more challenging. Areas such as the posteriomedial orbitofrontal cortex or the inferior surface of the temporal lobe are probably not amenable to this technique because of difficulty of visualization and instrument access.

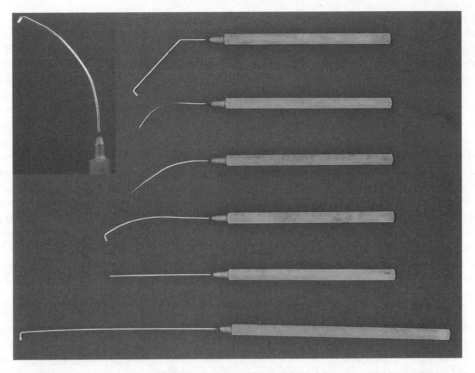

Fig. 68.4 Morrell hooks. The set comprises 4 mm hooks mounted on a variety of wire shafts. The choice of shaft depends on the orientation of the transection. The square-shaped handle allows the surgeon to know the orientation of the hook even when it is out of view within a gyrus.

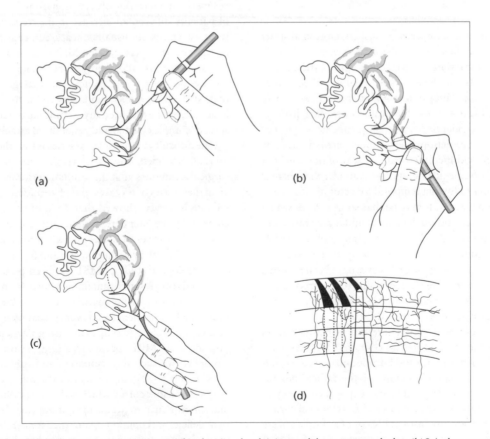

Fig. 68.5 Technique of MST. (a) After a timy incision is created in the pia, a hook is inserted down one gyral edge. (b) It is then swept across the full width of the gyrus. (c) The hook is brought back to its starting point such that the tip is just visible under the pia as it crosses the gyrus. (d) The procedure is repeated at less than 5 mm intervals along the gyrus leaving thin but visible scars. Thus, the transverse fibres only are sectioned, preserving the columnar organization.

Each transection is made 5 mm or less from the previous one along the gyrus. As a curve in the gyrus is encountered each transection is still made perpendicular to the long axis. This means that they are not parallel to one another and at sharp bends it may be easiest to complete two or more transections radially from the same pial incision.

Having completed multiple transections over the area defined by ECoG at the start of the procedure, a second cortical recording is made (Fig. 68.3). This will usually demonstrate a considerable reduction in spiking and an excess of slow activity. It may however show residual spiking, or spiking which has appeared outside the area which has been treated. A second passage of transections is frequently needed to address these, again followed by another recording. Persistence is required to ensure complete abolition of spiking. It is our impression that very low amplitude sparse spikes may be left, and in LKS a 10-fold reduction in the number of spikes seems to be associated with good outcome. If a particularly persistent spiking region is encountered, then a small topectomy may be effective although additional transections may also abolish them [41,44].

Once a satisfactory ECoG is obtained, surgical closure is performed in the usual fashion. There is little in the literature about repeat surgery with MST following initial suboptimal results [45,46]. Such surgery is feasible although the reflection of the dura from the previously transected cortex requires slow and painstaking work.

Results

There are a large number of case series published, most in abstract form only, and most including only small numbers of cases. The literature is probably substantially skewed due to publication bias—those with poorer results may be less likely to submit their figures and those that are submitted may be less likely to be accepted. There are a few substantial series in the literature concerning patients undergoing MST for an epileptic focus in eloquent cortex. Most of these patients underwent resection of less eloquent areas at the same procedure. It is therefore difficult to be quite clear of the benefit of the MST itself. It is a frequent finding, for example, that there is some spiking on ECoG following temporal lobectomy, situated at the posterior resection margin. It may be that some centres would perform MST over this area although many would regard this as unnecessary in most circumstances. The results in terms of seizure frequency of such procedures are therefore likely to be excellent. Similarly it is likely that many of the early cases have been reported in more than one publication. Hence combining results from several publications is also likely to create bias. Such difficulties make interpretation of surgical series extremely difficult.

By far the largest series is a collection of results from four centres and published by Spencer et al. [47]. This contains 211 cases operated in six centres in North America and Europe and is the only publication of this type. The specific details of the indications for surgery are only summarized in the paper and it appears that they all relate to cases of intractable seizures with a focus in eloquent cortex. It is not clear that there were any cases of LKS or of multiple seizure foci. Around three-quarters of the cases involved a combination of resection and MST and the age at surgery ranged from 1 to 75 years (mean 26 years).

The paper does not give a seizure-freedom rate but includes a category for patients with a greater than 95% reduction in frequency. Such a response was obtained for both simple and complex partial seizures in 68% of those undergoing MST plus resection and in 62–63% of those having MST alone. Such a response was also achieved for generalized seizures in 87% (46/53) including resection and 71% (10/14) without. The similarity of outcome between those with or without resection suggests that the efficacy of MST may approach that of resection. The outcome may depend more on the accuracy of target selection than on the method of surgical treatment. However, there may be a very large clinical difference between rendering a patient seizure free and simply reducing the frequency by 95%. Most resective surgical series report seizure-freedom rates and this paper does not provide information on such an outcome. Other substantial series (>20 patients) which quote seizure-freedom rates produce widely varying results from 0 to 64% for MST [48,49]. Most surgeons would regard MST, however, as less efficacious than resective surgery and reserve MST for situations in which resection could be associated with significant risk of morbidity.

Analysis of adverse effects of MST in this series, as with other series of any size that appear in the literature, is again complicated by the fact that many underwent simultaneous resection. The rates were 19% neurological deficit (severity unspecified) with MST alone and 23% when combined with resection. Interestingly there were no cases of language or sensory deficits after MST alone, although the denominator for these figures is not given.

One other interesting observation from this series is that 15–20% of patients suffered an increase in the frequency of simple partial seizures. This is not usually a feature of resective procedures, suggesting that it is related to the MST itself. Such findings may occur following corpus callosotomy and this suggests that these two 'disconnection' operations may act in an analogous way. It is suggested that MST could reduce inhibitory input to the abnormal cortex, hence increasing focal activity (simple partial seizures) but reducing spread (complex partial and generalized attacks).

One difficulty with this large series is that the duration of follow-up is not specified. There is certainly some evidence, as with other surgical techniques, that the results deteriorate with time. Orbach et al. in their series of 65 cases (only five undergoing MST without resection, however) showed that 16% of those with excellent outcome at 2 years later deteriorated [50]. This has particularly been a feature of the series from this unit when considering patients undergoing MST (with or without resection) for cortical dysplasia [51].

A histological study of MST has been performed acutely in humans and reveals significant impact not just on the horizontal fibres but also on some white matter tracts in a large minority of cases [52]. The low incidence of adverse local neurological deficits that occurs is therefore perhaps surprising particularly in view of the postoperative MRI appearances (Fig. 68.6). However, although major deficits (such as monoparesis and aphasia) appear rarely (approximately 5–7%) and many of these relate to surgery in the foot motor or sensory cortex which is the most difficult region of the primary motor strip to access [53], it appears that minor often transient deficits are common if examined for carefully. This seems to be particularly so in the sensory cortex subserving hand function [54].

A functional assessment of the hand using PET imaging in patients with apparently good outcome from MST showed preserved activation in the transected region but, compared with controls, substantial additional areas become activated. This suggests that there is indeed some minor alteration in function in eloquent cortex following MST [55]. However this reorganization appears to be transient with fMRI activation in the motor hand area returning to preoperative patterns by 16 weeks following surgery [56].

In most circumstances, MST is performed in the context of stable pathology. In the case of Rasmussen's encephalitis there is some experience of its use for progressive disease to stabilize the clinical course. Patients often present with epilepsia partialis continua but retain useful hemisphere functions. In such circumstances hemispherectomy may be unacceptable, but MST over the motor cortex perhaps together with resection of less eloquent areas has been reported in a few cases. Combining Morrell and Polkey's series, there are altogether nine such cases [13,57]. Surprisingly, two were rendered seizure free for prolonged periods and required no additional surgery. Five cases gained significant palliation for periods up to 2 years before hemispherectomy was needed and, in two, no benefit was derived and hemispherectomy was carried out on the same admission. MST therefore appears to be a satisfactory option when combined with resection of less eloquent cortex in the management of Rasmussen's encephalitis before the onset of severe permanent deficits. It is most likely to simply delay the need for hemispherectomy, but such a delay may be very valuable in the developing child.

The outcome with respect to LKS is less easy to define. Epilepsy is usually not the predominant symptom and overt seizure freedom may often be obtained with drug therapy. The natural history of the disease is little understood; in particular the long-term outcome has only rarely been reported [58].

Irwin et al. attempt to put the results of MST in LKS into appropriate context in their series of five surgically treated patients showing relative, but incomplete, improvements in EEG, behaviour and language function in all patients [46]. One required a repeat MST for a delayed deterioration, which yielded a good result. Similarly Morrell et al.'s series of 14 patients produced good results in terms of language function in 11 (79%). Indeed seven (50%) achieved age appropriate speech and returned to mainstream school [44].

The timing of surgery remains controversial and its place in relation to steroid therapy is also debated. These questions have been addressed by Robinson et al. [59] who showed that the duration of continuous spike-and-wave activity in sleep correlates with outcome. None of their 18 patients achieved age appropriate speech if they had continuous spike-and-wave activity in sleep for over 3 years. MST should therefore be considered fairly early in patients who are steroid resistant or intolerant and in whom laterality of driving spikes can be established (see above).

Much of the difficulty in the management of these patients surrounds the precision of diagnosis. There is a rather larger group of patients with epileptiform EEGs and more global deficits, either appearing after normal early development or on a background of developmental delay. The role of MST in this less well-defined group is little understood, although there may be scope for widening the application of MST to include what has been described as autistic epileptiform regression [60]. The role of MST in syndromes associated with continuous spike-and-wave activity in sleep but not clinically consistent with LKS is entirely undefined; MST does, however, remain a possible therapeutic approach for these syndromes [61].

Finally the results of MST for multifocal or poorly defined seizure foci have been examined by Patil and more recently by Zhai in

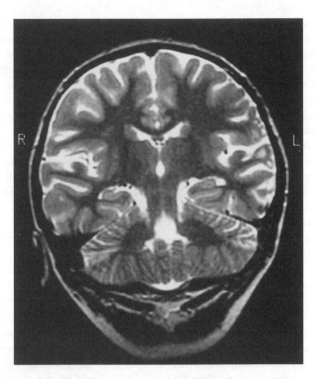

Fig. 68.6 Postoperative T2-weighted coronal MRI following MST over the left frontotemporal cortex, displaying multiple high-signal cortical lesions.

China [41,43]. In some of Patil et al.'s cases there is a widespread region of abnormal epileptiform discharge which becomes far better defined following extensive MST. This leaves a small 'dominant seizure focus' which may then be resected. Such a focus appears refractory to MST [42]. An impressive nine of 15 cases treated in this way were seizure free with median follow-up of 21 months, and all cases were at least 70% improved. In patients with multilobar or bilateral activity treated with extensive MST and topectomy, they report nine of 19 (47%) seizure free and an additional eight (41%) who were more than 90% improved with median follow-up of 33 months. It is not clear if some of these patients have been reported in both series. The Chinese approach apparently includes aggressive use of MST in a wider variety of cases than has been included by other groups, including those apparently with intractable generalized epilepsy. In this group they combined extensive bifrontal MST together with anterior corpus callosotomy. Their overall results for 100 patients with a wide mixture of epilepsies is said to be seizure freedom in 62%, and no improvement in only 6%. It is clear that the role of MST in patients with apparent multifocal epilepsy, either in better defining the dominant focus or in allowing very extensive areas of coverage, is something that requires much further investigation.

Conclusions

MST has been developed on the basis of extensive investigations of the mechanisms underlying cortical function and seizure spread, but its application has only gradually become widespread. The surgical series are generally small and, because MST procedures are often associated with cortical resection, the specific benefit of MST has not been firmly established.

MST does appear to have an excellent safety record considering it usually is applied to the most eloquent areas of cortex. Severe complications such as monoparesis occurred in fewer than 10% of cases and there appear to be no reports of mortality. In the management of epilepsy arising in eloquent cortex some, including Morrell, have claimed that MST is as effective as resection. Most surgeons however would feel that resection of the epileptic focus remains the 'gold standard', but that MST is much safer.

In Rasmussen's encephalitis, MST provides a useful method of seizure control at a stage before hemispherectomy would be appropriate. It may abolish epilepsia partialis continua and allow more normal function in the other hemisphere during childhood years; more radical surgery may thus be delayed or even avoided.

In LKS, MST undoubtedly has a beneficial effect although the comparison with medical therapy and with the natural history of the disease has not been rigorously assessed. It is probably the treatment of choice for those patients who have failed to respond to steroids. There may be scope for extending the indications to those with continuous slow wave status epilepticus in sleep without classical clinical features of LKS.

The benefits of MST in multifocal epilepsies, those with bihemispheric involvement or generalized epilepsies has only been reported by two centres but with extremely promising results. These indications undoubtedly require more widespread examination.

References

1 Palmini A, Andermann F, Oliver A et al. Neuronal migration disorders: Extent of lesion removal is the main predictor of seizure control in the surgical treatment of epilepsy. Neurology 1991; 41 (Suppl. 1): 403.

2 Morrell F. Secondary epileptogenic lesions. Epilepsia 1959; 1: 538–60.

3 Morrell F. Micro electrode and steady potential studies suggesting a dendritic locus of closure. In: Smirnov GD, Jasper HH, eds. The Moscow Colloquium on Electroencephalography of Higher Nervous Activity. Electroencephalogr Clin Neurophysiol 1960; (Suppl. 13): 65–80.

4 Morrell F. Microelectrode studies in chronic epileptic foci. Epilepsia 1961; 2: 81–8.

5 Morrell F. Electrical signs of sensory coding. In: Querton GC, Melnechnik T, Schmidt FO, eds. The Neurosciences. A Study Program. New York: Rockefeller University Press, 1967: 452–69.

6 Morrell F. Cellular pathophysiology of focal epilepsy. Epilepsia 1969; 10: 495–505.

7 Morrell F. Neuronal integrations in visions. In: Marois M, ed. Proceedings of the Second International Conference on Theoretical Physics and Biology. Paris: Editions du Centre National de la Recherche Scientifique, 1971: 365–400.

8 Morrell F. Electrophysiology of CSWS in Landau—Kleffner syndrome. In: Majno M, ed. Continuous Spikes and Waves during Slow Sleep. Electrical Status During Slow Sleep Acquired Epileptic Aphasia and Related Conditions. Milan: Mariani Foundation Paediatric Neurology, 1995.

9 Morrell F, Hamberg JW. A new surgical technique for the treatment of focal cortical epilepsy. Electroencephalog Clin Neurophysiol 1969; 26: 120.

10 Morrell F, Whisler WW. Multiple subpial transection for epilepsy eliminates seizures without destroying the function of the transectal zone. Epilepsia 1982; 23: 440.

11 Morrell F, Whisler WW. Multiple subpial transection, technique, results and pitfalls. Jpn J Neurosurg 1993; 12: 101–7.

12 Morrell F, Whisler WW, Bleck T. Multiple subpial transection; a new approach to the surgical treatment of focal epilepsy. J Neurosurg 1989; 70: 231–9.

13 Morrell F, Whisler WW, Smith MC. Multiple subpial transection in Rasmussens encephalitis. In: Andermann F, ed. Chronic Encephalitis and Epilepsy Rasmussen's Syndrome. Boston: Butterworth-Heinemann, 1991: 219–34.

14 Morrell F, Whisler WW, Smith MC et al. Clinical outcome in Landau–Kleffner syndrome treated by multiple subpial transection. Epilepsia 1992; 33 (Suppl. 3): 100.

15 Morrell F, Kanner AM, de Toledo-Morrell L et al. Multiple subpial transection. Adv Neurol 1991; 81: 259–70.

16 Mountcastle VB. Modality and topographic properties of single neurons of cat's somatic sensory cortex. J Neurophysiol 1957; 20: 408–34.

17 Hubel DH, Wiesel TN. Receptive fields, binocular interactions and functional architecture in the cat's visual cortex. Physiology 1962; 160: 106–54.

18 Lorente De No R. Cerebral cortex: architecture, intercortical connections, motor projection. In: Fulton JF, ed. Physiology of the Nervous System, 3rd edn. New York: Oxford University Press, 1949.

19 Asanuma H. Recent developments in the study of the columnar arrangement of neurons within the motor cortex. Physiol Rev 1975; 55: 143–56.

20 Asanuma H, Rosen I. Spread of mono and polysynaptic connections within cat's motor cortex. Exp Brain Res 1973; 16: 507–20.

21 Mountcastle VB. The columnar organisation of the neocortex. Review Article. Brain 1997; 120: 701–22.

22 Connors BW, Pinto DJ, Telfeian AE. Local pathways of seizure propagation in neocortex. Int Rev Neurobiol 2001; 45: 527–46

23 Lueders H, Busamante A, Zablow L, Goldensohn E. The independence of closely spaced discrete experimental spike foci. Neurology 1981; 31: 846–51.

24 Sperry RW, Miner N. Pattern perception following insertion of mica plates into the visual cortex. J Comp Physiol Psychol 1955; 48: 463–9.

25 Sperry RW, Miner N, Myers RE. Visual pattern perception following subpial slicing and tantulum wire implantation in visual cortex. J Comp Physiol Psychol 1955; 48: 50–8.

26 Reichental E, Hochermann S. The critical cortical area for development of penicillin-induced epilepsy. Electroenceph Clin Neurophysiol 1977; 42: 248–51.

27 Horsley V. Brain surgery. Br Med J 1886; 5 2: 670–5.

28 Penfield W, Jasper H. Epilepsy and the Functional Anatomy of the Human Brain. Boston: Little, Brown and Co, 1954.

29 Bittar RG, Olivier A, Sadikot A et al. Cortical motor and somatosensory representation: effect of cerebral lesions. J Neurosurg 2000; 92: 242–8.

30 Engel J. Outcome with respect to epileptic seizures. In: Engel J, ed. Surgical Treatment of Epilepsies. New York: Raven Press, 1987: 553–71.

31 Landau W, Kleffner F. Syndrome of acquired aphasia with convulsive disorder in children. Neurology 1957; 7: 523–30.

32 Deonna T, Roulet E. Epilepsy and language disorder in children. In: Fuikuyama Y et al., ed. Modern Perspectives of Child Neurology. Tokyo: The Japanese Society of Child Neurology, 1991.

33 Marescaux C, Hirsch E, Finck S et al. Landau–Kleffner syndrome: a pharmacologic study of five cases. Epilepsia 1990; 31: 768–77.

34 Morrell F, Whisler W, Smith M et al. Landau–Kleffner syndrome. Treatment with subpial intracortical transection. Brain 1995; 118: 1529–46.

35 Polkey CE. Multiple subpial transection. In: Cohadon F, ed. Advances and Technical Standards in Neurosurgery. Vienna: Springer–Verlag, 2000.

36 Wada J, Rasmussen T. Intracortical injection of sodium amytal for the lateralisation of cerebral speech dominance: experience and clinical observations. J Neurosurg 1960; 17: 266–82

37 Alarcon G, Garcia Seoanne J, Binnie C et al. Origin and propagation of interictal discharges in the acute electrocorticogram. Implications for pathophysiology and surgical treatment of temporal lobe epilepsy. Brain 1997; 120: 2259–82.

38 Seri S, Walsh A, Cerguiqlini A, Sgouros S. Extracranial localisation of interictal abnormalities in Landau–Kleffner syndrome, EEG—MRI fusioning and intraoperative validation. Epilepsia 1999; 40: 172.

39 Paetau R. Sounds trigger spikes in the Landau–Kleffner syndrome. J Clin Neurophysiol 1994; 11: 231–41.

40 Paetau R, Kajola M, Korkman M. Landau–Kleffner syndrome: epileptic activity in the auditory cortex. Neuroreport 1991; 2: 201–4.

41 Patil A, Andrews R, Torkelson R. Surgical treatment of intractable

seizures with multilobar bihemispheric seizure foci (MLBHSF). *Surg Neurol* 1997; 47: 72–8.

42 Patil A, Andrews R, Torkelson R. Isolation of dominant seizure foci by multiple subpial transections. *Stereotact Funct Neurosurg* 1997; 69: 210–15.

43 Zhai Q, Liu Z, Li S *et al*. Multiple subpial transection in surgical treatment of intractable epilepsy. *Zhonghia Wai Ke Za Zhi* 1998; 36(5): 304–6.

44 Morrell F, Whisler W, Smith M *et al*. Landau–Kleffner syndrome, treatment with subpial intracortical transection. *Brain* 1995; 118: 1529–46.

45 Grote C, Van Slyke P, Hoeppner J. Language dominance following multiple subpial transection for Landau–Kleffner syndrome. *Brain* 1999; 122: 561–6.

46 Irwin K, Birch V, Lees J *et al*. Multiple subpial transection in Landau–Kleffner syndrome. *Dev Med Child Neurol* 2001; 43: 248–52.

47 Spencer SS, Schramm J, Wyler A *et al*. Multiple subpial transection for intractable partial epilepsy: an international meta-analysis. *Epilepsia* 2002; 43(2): 141–5.

48 Hufnagel A, Zentner J, Fernandez G. Multiple subpial transection for control of epileptic seizures: efficacy and safety. *Epilepsia* 1997; 38: 678–88.

49 Liu Z, Zhao Q, Li S *et al*. Multiple subpial transection for the treatment of intractable epilepsy. *Chinese Med J* 1995; 108: 539–41.

50 Orbach D, Romanelli P, Devinsky O. Late seizures recurrence after multiple subpial transections. *Epilepsia* 2001; 42: 1316–19.

51 Selway R, Polkey C. Multiple subpial transections, clinical outcome in 34 patients. *Epilepsia* 2000; 41 (Suppl. 7): 145–6.

52 Kaufmann WE, Krauss GL, Vematsu S, Lesser RP. Treatment of epilepsy with multiple subpial transactions: an acute histologic analysis in human subjects. *Epilepsia* 1996; 37: 342–52.

53 Byrne R, Whisler W. Multiple subpial transections for epilepsy. In Schmidek A, ed. *Operative Neurosurgical Techniques. Indications methods and results*. Philadelphia: W.B. Saunders, 2000.

54 Morrell F, Helmstaedter C, Gleissner U *et al*. Neuropsychological consequences of epilepsy surgery in frontal lobe epilepsy. *Neuropsychologia* 1998: 36: 681–9.

55 Leonhardt G, Spiekermann G, Muller S *et al*. Cortical reorganisation following multiple subpial transection in human brain—a study with positron emission tomography. *Neurosci Lett* 2000; 292: 63–5.

56 Moo L, Slotnick S, Krauss G *et al*. A prospective study of motor recovery following multiple subpial transections. *Neuroreport* 2002; 13 (5): 665–9.

57 Sawhney I, Robertson I, Polkey C *et al*. Multiple subpial transection: a review of 21 cases. *J Neurol Neurosurg Psych* 1995; 58: 344–9.

58 Deonna T, Peter C, Ziegler A. Adult follow-up of the acquired aphasia—epilepsy syndrome in childhood. Report of seven cases. *Neuropediatrics* 1989; 20: 132–8.

59 Robinson R, Baird G, Robinson G *et al*. Landau–Kleffner syndrome: course and correlates with outcome. *Dev Med Child Neurol* 2001; 43: 243–7.

60 Nass R, Gross A, Wisoff J. Outcome of multiple subpial transection for autistic epilepiform regressions. *Paediatr Neurol* 1999; 21: 464–70.

61 Albaradie R, Bourgeois B, Thiele E *et al*. Treatment of continous spike and wave during slow wave sleep. *Epilepsia* 2001; 42 (Suppl. 7): 46–7.

Awake Surgery for Epilepsy

A.N. Miles and G.A. Ojemann

Surgery for epilepsy has two main aims. The primary objective is the removal of the epileptogenic zone, defined as the total area of brain that is necessary and sufficient to generate seizures and which must be removed to abolish seizures [1]. However, the second aim is to achieve this without producing new neurological and/or cognitive deficits. Tailored resections for epilepsy utilize data derived from ECoG in an attempt to identify the epileptogenic zone and data derived from functional mapping to identify eloquent cortex. Such data can be derived intra- or extraoperatively and thus place varying amounts of emphasis on interictal or ictal recordings. This chapter describes an approach where the resection is tailored based on findings derived when the patient is awake under local anaesthesia during a portion of the resective operation and will focus on the most common procedure performed by epilepsy surgeons, temporal lobe resection for temporal lobe epilepsy (TLE).

The classic form of the tailored resection for epilepsy appeared with the development of EEG in the 1930s. Scalp EEG identified interictal epileptiform abnormalities in medically refractory patients, particularly in the temporal lobe. Resections in the temporal lobe were tailored to the location of interictal epileptiform abnormalities on the ECoG recorded intraoperatively. Resections were also tailored to avoid 'eloquent' areas in the individual patient, as identified by electrical stimulation mapping, initially of motor and sensory cortex, and later of language [2]. These techniques were especially well developed at the Montreal Neurological Institute in the 1940s and 1950s, with an extensive experience reported by Penfield and Jasper [3]. However, the recognition that many patients with medically refractory TLE had pathological abnormalities in mesial temporal structures, especially hippocampus [4], provided the basis for developing anatomically standardized operations for TLE; these emphasize resection of specific anatomical structures, rather than tailoring the resection to the pathophysiological abnormalities present in an individual patient's ECoG. The original anatomically standardized resection for medically refractory TLE was the *en bloc* anterior temporal lobectomy first developed by Falconer [5]. This has subsequently been modified by varying the extent of medial temporal and lateral neocortical resection with the aim of reducing the risk of postoperative cognitive deficits [6].

The anatomically standardized procedures for medically refractory TLE are based on the premise that inclusion of structural pathology identified on imaging studies within a standardized resection will include the epileptogenic zone. It is also assumed that eloquent areas, such as language cortex, are sufficiently uniformly located that they can be avoided by conforming to the anatomical landmarks defining the standardized resection. Tailored resections for TLE, on the other hand, emphasize the importance of a patient's individual pathophysiology by altering the degree of resection based on the location of interictal epileptiform discharges and location of eloquent cortex determined by functional mapping. Tailored resections are based on the premise that there is considerable individual variability in the extent and location of both the epileptogenic zone and eloquent cortex, and that this variability can be identified utilizing interictal epileptiform discharge data from ECoG and functional mapping.

There are thus two major areas of controversy in the use of tailored resections for medically refractory TLE that derive from the two main aims of epilepsy surgery stated in the first paragraph of this chapter, i.e. removal of the epileptogenic zone without producing neurological or cognitive deficit. The first point of contention is the use of interictal epileptiform discharges on the intraoperative ECoG to identify the epileptogenic zone. While there is general agreement that, in the setting of TLE, identification of ictal onset zone using chronic extraoperative ECoG is not required if seizure semiology, interictal and/or ictal scalp EEG and MRI data are concordant [7], it is controversial whether interictal intraoperative ECoG adds any additional information to identify more accurately the epileptogenic zone and so tailor extent of resection. The second point of contention in surgery for TLE is the use of functional mapping techniques to identify temporal lobe cortex essential for language and memory prior to resection, with the aim of tailoring the resection to minimize risk of disturbance to this eloquent cortex.

Intraoperative ECoG

In tailoring a temporal lobe resection to a patient's individual pathophysiology, the surgeon uses: (a) data from the intraoperative interictal ECoG obtained preresection to guide the extent of resection; and (b) data from the postresection ECoG to assess the adequacy of resection. However, the literature that examines the relationship between pre- and post-temporal lobe resection ECoG and seizure outcome is contradictory. Early reports suggested a better outcome when all spike foci identified on preresection interictal ECoG were resected. Jasper *et al.* documented a good seizure outcome in 59% of patients with complete excision of cortex producing interictal spikes and in only 37% of patients with partial excision [8]. More recently, Binnie *et al.* also demonstrated that preresection ECoG findings were predictive of outcome [9]. They found that the presence of epileptiform spikes maximal in extratemporal regions on preresection ECoG was associated with only 30% good seizure outcome compared with a 71% good seizure outcome when the region of maximal epileptiform discharges was located within the temporal lobe. When patients with extratemporal discharges were excluded in this study, the presence of discharges maximal in posterior temporal regions was associated with a worse seizure outcome, only 47% of patients having good seizure outcomes compared with 76% of patients without posterior temporal maximal discharges. It remains unknown whether tailoring of the resection to include maximal discharges in posterior temporal regions would have improved seizure outcome, as this group performs only anatomically standardized *en bloc* resections. Other reports that have examined preresection ECoG findings as a predictor of seizure outcome have not found a correlation between features of the preresection ECoG, such as location of maximal spike amplitude or spike frequency, and outcome [10–13]. This is consistent with an earlier report demonstrating that the area of cortex defined by the presence of interictal spikes on ECoG/EEG, defined as the irritative zone [1], often markedly exceeds the area of cortex that must be excised to achieve a satisfactory outcome [14].

Reports examining postresection ECoG findings as a predictor of seizure outcome are also conflicting, with the majority not finding a correlation between the presence of residual spikes on postresection interictal ECoG and seizure outcome [9,12–22]. Others have, however, suggested that the presence of interictal epileptiform discharges on postresection ECoG portend a poor seizure outcome [8,23–26]. Bengzon *et al.* reported that 72% of patients with a poor seizure outcome and 36% of patients with a good seizure outcome had persistent epileptiform abnormalities on the postresection ECoG [23]. Similarly, Fiol *et al.* found that the presence of spontaneous residual ECoG spikes was significantly associated with a less favourable prognosis, with 47% of patients seizure free with residual spikes compared with 72% without [24].

In almost all published reports, the intraoperative ECoG is analysed by visual inspection to determine the features of the ECoG, such as location of maximal spike frequency or amplitude, that are assumed to correlate with the presumed epileptogenic zone. It has been suggested, however, that computer analysis of the ECoG can facilitate identification of the epileptogenic zone [15]. Alarcon *et al.* have hypothesized that regions where the earliest interictal spikes are found, which they have defined as 'leading regions', are located in the epileptogenic zone [27]. They propose that the leading regions behave as pacemakers for interictal spike activity in surrounding and even relatively remote cortex, and that sites in which secondary propagated activity occurs (equivalent to Luders' irritative zone [1]) have less epileptogenic potential and do not need to be excised. However, as the latency between interictal spikes recorded at different sites is usually <200 ms [28], which is too short to be easily detected by visual assessment of the ECoG, computer analysis of digital ECoG recordings is required to rapidly detect very short latencies between spikes recorded at different sites. Alarcon's group has developed a computer algorithm for automatic identification of interictal spikes on ECoG; this identifies the latency between spikes in all channels where the spike is detected. This algorithm has been evaluated retrospectively on 42 patients from their series who underwent anatomically standardized temporal lobectomies for medically refractory seizures [9,29]. Using the algorithm to identify leading regions revealed a significant relationship between surgical removal of leading regions and seizure outcome. Eighty-six per cent of patients with a good outcome (Engel class I and II [30]) had all leading regions excised and 83% of patients with a poor outcome (Engel class III and IV [30]) had at least one leading region remaining. Based on these results, the authors calculate that if they had tailored their resections to the location of leading regions instead of

performing standardized resections and were able to remove all identified leading regions, the proportion of good outcomes in their series would have increased from 71% to 95%. These results are currently being evaluated both retrospectively and prospectively in a larger series of patients [9].

An additional confounding issue in attempting to interpret the literature on intraoperative ECoG is the fact that the majority of reports have focused on ECoG recordings obtained from subtemporal and lateral temporal neocortex to guide the extent of temporal neocortical resection rather than direct hippocampal recordings to guide the extent of mesial resection. It has been suggested that an optimal seizure outcome depends upon an extensive hippocampal resection [6,31]. This is based upon reports demonstrating that patients with less complete hippocampal resections had worse seizure outcomes [31–33], and that reoperation of residual mesial temporal structures in those with recurrent seizures after initial temporal resection had a good seizure outcome [34,35]. However, several reports have compared direct intraoperative interictal ECoG recordings from the hippocampus as a guide to the extent of resection with seizure outcome and challenged the view that a maximal hippocampal resection is a necessary requirement for good seizure outcome in all patients [36–41]. Jooma *et al.* utilized direct intraoperative recordings from the hippocampus to guide the extent of mesial resection and analysed their results retrospectively in 70 patients [37]. They found no difference in seizure outcome between patients who underwent very limited mesial resections (corticoamygdalectomy) due to the presence of spiking restricted to only the amygdala region and those who underwent, in addition, varying degrees of hippocampal resection based on the extent of interictal hippocampal spiking on ECoG. Reviewing the Montreal experience, Rasmussen and Feindel also found no significant difference in seizure outcome in patients undergoing corticoamygdalectomy only versus the additional resection of at least 50% of the hippocampus [36,40]. Most recently, McKhann *et al.* reported on the University of Washington experience [39]. Similar to Jooma *et al.* [37], they found no correlation between the extent of hippocampal resection and seizure outcome, provided there were no spikes on postresection hippocampal ECoG recordings. There was a significant correlation between presence of spikes on postresection hippocampal ECoG and seizure outcome. Only 29% of patients who had postresection spikes in the hippocampus were seizure free compared with 73% seizure free with no hippocampal postresection spikes. These results suggest that intraoperative hippocampal ECoG recordings can be used to tailor the extent of hippocampal resection without compromising seizure outcome.

None of the reports that have found an association between smaller hippocampal resections and worse seizure outcome have utilized intraoperative direct hippocampal recording of interictal epileptiform activity to tailor the extent of hippocampal resection [31,42–44]. The finding that excellent seizure-free outcomes can be achieved with smaller hippocampal resections, tailored to the extent of interictal epileptiform spikes recorded directly from the hippocampus [37,39,41,45–47], suggests that some limited hippocampal resections fail not because of the size of the resection *per se* but rather because not all of the electrophysiologically abnormal hippocampus has been removed. Conversely, larger hippocampal resections do better in the absence of guidance from direct hippocampal ECoG because this ensures that all potential electrophysiologically abnormal hippocampus is removed, but at the cost of removing more hippocampus than is actually required to achieve a good seizure outcome.

An additional controversy in the use of intraoperative ECoG is the necessity for local anaesthesia. Resections tailored to the location of interictal epileptiform discharges on ECoG can be conducted with the patient under general anaesthesia. However, the majority of the drugs used in modern general anaesthesia, including barbiturates, benzodiazepines, opioid analgesics and volatile anaesthetics, can modify intraoperative ECoG recordings making the identification of electrically active cortex more difficult [48,49]. The intravenous sedative propofol has been increasingly used for sedation during awake craniotomies for epilepsy [50,51]. Propofol's sedative effects are rapid in onset and of short duration. As a result, awakening from propofol is rapid with minimal patient confusion. These characteristics and its additional anxiolytic and antiemetic properties make propofol an ideal intravenous sedative for craniotomies under local anaesthesia [50]. Propofol has been shown to affect the ECoG, producing a high-frequency background rhythm and has pro- and anticonvulsant effects [49,52]. However, its rapid metabolism allows the recording of the intraoperative ECoG in an awake and comfortable patient without the adverse effects of drugs on the ECoG. While there has never been a study comparing seizure outcome following temporal lobe resections tailored to intraoperative ECoG recorded with the patient under general anaesthesia versus local anaesthesia with intermittent propofol sedation, it is our view that tailored resections should be based on a spontaneous drug-free ECoG particularly given the possibility of 'false activation' of the interictal ECoG with pharmacological agents [53].

Functional mapping

In TLE surgery, the functionally essential areas that must be avoided are those for language and memory, particularly material-specific memory (verbal memory in dominant and visuospatial memory in non-dominant temporal lobes). Cortical stimulation mapping of language suggests significant individual variability in location of dominant hemisphere perisylvian sites essential for language [54–58]. In an electrical stimulation mapping investigation of 117 patients undergoing dominant temporal lobe resections, Ojemann *et al.* demonstrated stimulation evoked naming errors within 3–4 cm of the temporal pole along the middle temporal gyrus in 5% of cases and along the superior temporal gyrus in 14% of cases [56]. These sites are within the boundaries of an anatomically standardized temporal lobe resection. Similar individual variability and location of sites essential for language within the anatomically defined boundaries of a standard dominant temporal lobe resection have been found by others [59]. The utility of cortical stimulation language mapping as a technique to minimize the risk of postoperative language deficits following dominant hemisphere resections has been demonstrated by Haglund *et al.* and Ojemann [60,61]. In their series, no patient with a resection margin >1 cm away from a language site, identified by intraoperative cortical stimulation evoked naming errors, had permanent language deficits postoperatively. In contrast, all patients with resections < 0.7cm away from such sites had postoperative language deficits persisting 1–4 weeks and in 43% the deficits were permanent [60]. A number of risk

factors for atypical sites essential for language (particularly anteriorly in the dominant temporal lobe potentially within the boundaries of a standardized dominant temporal lobe resection) have been identified. These include late age of seizure onset, low preoperative verbal IQ scores, left handedness, right hemisphere memory dominance and absence of early risk factors for subsequent development of epilepsy [56,59,62–65].

The relative risk of postoperative language deficits following a tailored dominant temporal resection in an awake patient versus that following an anatomically standardized dominant temporal resection under general anaesthesia has been debated in the literature [66–70]. From a historical perspective, Penfield, performing awake craniotomies with language mapping at the Montreal Neurological Institute in the 1950s, reported transient postoperative language deficits in 8% and permanent deficits in 1% of his dominant temporal resections [2]. At the same time Falconer, performing anatomically standardized temporal resections under general anaesthesia at the Maudsley Hospital, London, reported transient postoperative language deficits in 52% and permanent deficits in 9% of his dominant temporal resections [71]. However, the standard dominant temporal resection as performed by Falconer included the anterior 2 cm of superior temporal gyrus and up to 8 cm (mean 6 cm) of middle temporal gyrus [5,71], which is a much larger standardized temporal resection than is currently performed [6]. Several recent reports have examined the incidence of postoperative language deficits following typical anatomically standardized dominant temporal resections that include 4–4.5 cm of lateral temporal neocortex sparing most of the superior temporal gyrus [68,69]. These studies identify a subgroup of patients (7%) who experience a significant language decline following an anatomically standardized dominant temporal resection [69,72]. This subgroup of patients was predicted by the cortical stimulation mapping studies of Ojemann and co-workers, which suggest that if 4–4.5 cm of middle temporal gyrus were removed without language mapping, 5% of patients would be expected to experience a significant language decline postoperatively and if 4–4.5 cm of superior temporal gyrus were also removed, then this would increase to 19% [56–58]. Language mapping during an awake dominant temporal resection in all patients, therefore, aims to minimize the risk of language deficits in this small subgroup. The lower incidence of postoperative language deficits following an awake dominant temporal resection with language mapping reported by Penfield [2], Haglund *et al.* and Ojemann [60,61] supports the use of this approach.

The second role of functional mapping in an awake dominant temporal resection is the identification and preservation of cortex eloquent for material-specific memory function. A relationship between temporal lobe resections and memory deficits was first established by Penfield, Scoville and Milner in the 1950s [73,74]. They observed that bilateral removal of uncus, amygdala and anterior hippocampus was associated with persistent global impairment of recent memory. Subsequently, Milner demonstrated verbal memory deficits following dominant temporal lobe resection and visuospatial memory deficits following non-dominant temporal lobe resection. The severity of these deficits was related to the extent of unilateral hippocampal removal [75]. More recent reports have documented substantial verbal memory deficits after dominant anterior temporal lobectomies [76–81].

A number of reports have suggested that larger hippocampal

resections are associated with greater postoperative memory deficits in verbal memory following dominant resections and visuospatial memory following non-dominant resections [75,76, 82–88]. Several variables have been identified that are associated with increased risk of postoperative verbal memory decline following dominant temporal lobe resection. These include high preoperative verbal memory scores, absence of ipsilateral hippocampal atrophy on MRI, absence of ipsilateral mesial temporal sclerosis (MTS) on pathological analysis of operative specimen, results of preoperative intracarotid amobarbital procedure (IAP), late age of seizure onset and male sex [79,89–98]. Analysis of our own data supports the association between larger hippocampal resections and greater postoperative verbal memory deficits following dominant temporal resections (submitted for publication). Specifically, when subgroups with either normal hippocampus/mild MTS or moderate/severe MTS were examined separately for the effect of the extent of dominant medial temporal resection on postoperative memory decline, a statistically significant correlation was seen only in the normal hippocampus/mild MTS subgroup. Further subgroup analysis, based on the presence or absence of a normal hippocampus on preoperative MRI, also revealed a significant correlation between the extent of dominant medial temporal resection and postoperative memory decline in the subgroup with a normal appearing hippocampus on preoperative MRI but not in the subgroup with MRI evidence of hippocampal atrophy.

Three reports have not found an association between extent of medial resection and postoperative memory outcome [31,99,100]. One of the reasons for these conflicting reports may be that, in addition to extent of hippocampal resection, other factors have also been shown to impact on the degree of postoperative memory loss following temporal lobectomy, in particular, the degree of hippocampal neuronal loss. Patients having mild MTS experience the most significant verbal memory decreases postoperatively [95,101], whereas patients with severe MTS have worse preoperative verbal memory function but actually experience less postoperative decline from their preoperative baseline [95,101,102]. Subgroup analysis of the University of Washington series (submitted for publication) suggests that if the majority of patients undergoing dominant temporal lobe resections have moderate to severe MTS, minimal pre- to postoperative change would be expected, making it difficult to show an effect of the extent of resection.

Of the three reports not finding an association between the extent of hippocampal resection and memory outcome, in two it is not possible to determine from the data provided by the authors what proportion of their patients had MTS [99,100]. This makes it difficult to assess to what extent the presence of large numbers of patients with severe MTS might impact on the effect of extent of hippocampal resection on memory decline. The third report did show a greater pre- to postoperative decline in measures of verbal memory following dominant total hippocampectomy as compared to partial hippocampectomy, although the difference did not achieve statistical significance [31]. Failure to achieve statistical significance for the observed decline in measures of verbal memory may reflect lower numbers of patients with either histologically normal resected hippocampi or mild MTS in this report as compared to our series (submitted for publication).

Evidence from cortical stimulation mapping of verbal memory in the dominant temporal lobe suggests that, in addition to the role played by the hippocampus, the lateral temporal neocortex has a significant role in the mediation of verbal memory, particularly in input and storage aspects of verbal memory [103–106]. Ojemann and co-workers have shown that there is considerable variability in the exact lateral temporal location of sites related to memory, with a significant minority of sites being identified within the boundaries of lateral resection in anatomically standardized operations [104,105,107]. There are thus two variables that must be considered in tailoring the extent of resection of the temporal lobe to minimize the risk of postoperative memory deficits, the extent of medial hippocampal resection and the extent of lateral temporal neocortex resection. In contrast to hippocampal memory function, lateral temporal neocortical memory function can be tested using standard techniques of cortical stimulation during an awake craniotomy. Utilizing a previously described technique for intraoperative mapping of language and verbal memory by direct cortical stimulation in the awake patient [107], Ojemann and Dodrill demonstrated a significant correlation between postoperative verbal memory scores and the extent of lateral temporal lobe resection [104,105]. The presence of intraoperative stimulation-evoked memory errors within the anterior temporal resection, or within 2 cm of its margin, identified 90% of cases with subsequent postoperative memory deficits. The absence of errors identified 70% of cases without such deficits [105]. Similar findings have been observed by others [106].

Technical aspects of resection tailored to intraoperative recording and stimulation at the University of Washington

The advent of propofol intravenous anaesthesia has made awake craniotomy much easier for both the patient and the surgeon [51]. About the only demand now made on patients is that they should hold still for 1–2 h while awake. Thus, the technique can be easily used in children of 12 years or older, and in most adolescents and adults. It can also be safely used in the presence of an intracranial mass, although the brain will be slightly tighter than is usually observed with modern endotracheal anaesthesia and it may be necessary to be slightly more aggressive with the use of intravenous osmotic agents.

We now use only the lateral position with propofol. In that position, we have not had difficulties maintaining an airway. Problems with maintaining the airway have occurred in patients in the supine position. The patient is positioned while awake with particular attention to their comfort. The head rests on a foam ring and skeletal fixation is not used. Propofol anaesthesia is then induced intravenously. Once the patient is asleep, a local anaesthetic field block is placed, using a mixture of equal volumes of 0.5% lidocaine and 0.25% bupivicaine, both with 1:200 000 epinephrine. Propofol is not a particularly good analgesic, so the patient under propofol anaesthesia will often show some reaction to the placement of this block. The block is performed by first making injections slowly through a needle, initially 30-gauge, at sites near the major scalp nerves and then completing the block around the entire area of the planned incision. Use of small amounts of intravenous fentanyl is of value in reducing responses to placement of the block. If the incision is to extend to the root of the zygoma, the temporalis muscle is also infiltrated. The scalp incision and craniotomy then proceed in the usual manner. Once the dura is exposed, dural pain sensation is blocked by intradural injection of small quantities of local anaesthetic around the middle meningeal artery, using the 30-gauge needle. A clamp is placed on the skull at the edge of the craniotomy to provide a place to attach ECoG recording equipment and also to provide a handle to control the head if the patient becomes restless and a place to attach the arc on a neuronavigation system if an MRI visible lesion is present.

At this point, all pain-sensitive structures have been blocked with local anaesthetic, and the bone removal completed with the patient asleep. The lateral surface of the brain, of course, is insensitive to pain or touch. We usually awaken the patient before opening the dura, unless that opening is expected to be very tedious, for example when extensive pial–dural adhesions are anticipated. Patients are usually conversant within 7–12 min of stopping the propofol. At that time, they are reminded that they are in the operating room and should not move their head without first asking. The longest period before awakening in our experience has been 45 min. The patient usually awakens abruptly, which is a major advantage of propofol, and there is commonly no period of confusion. Very rarely, patients may have seizures when awake. Short-acting benzodiazepines or a bolus of propofol may be needed to control them.

Intraoperative ECoG to identify epileptic areas

After the patient is awakened and the dura opened, ECoG recording is undertaken. As the patient recovers from the propofol anaesthesia a typical burst-suppression ECoG pattern is seen, which changes to a continuous recording once the patient is awake. An additional advantage of propofol, in our view, is in recording interictal ECoG in the small number of patients who predominantly have interictal epileptiform activity during sleep. It is our impression that rapidly awakening and then resedating these patients with propofol allows the identification of interictal discharges during this period that would not otherwise be seen during recording with the patient fully awake. The goal of the ECoG recording is to delineate the full extent of interictal spikes. To this end, subdural strip electrodes are placed over cortical areas not immediately under the craniotomy, such as basal temporal cortex, orbital frontal surface or the medial face of a hemisphere. Recordings are obtained from the lateral surface through carbon-tipped ball electrodes. The authors use referential ECoG recordings to a linked neck; 10–15 min of continuous ECoG recording is observed before the next phase of the procedure.

While the majority of cases undergoing resection for TLE at this institution have predominant interictal epileptiform discharges on intraoperative ECoG arising from the medial basal portion of the temporal lobe, a significant minority of patients have interictal discharges maximal from both basal and lateral temporal surfaces [108]. In these cases the extent of lateral resection is tailored to the location of interictal discharges on the lateral temporal surface, reflecting our contention that, at least in some patients, the lateral temporal neocortex contributes to the temporal lobe epileptic process and that localized lateral temporal interictal discharges are an indicator of this contribution. This is supported by previous published data from the University of Washington [109–112]. In a chronic primate experimental epilepsy model, excision of the area of interictal epileptiform activity was required to control seizures [110]. Clinically, localized interictal epileptiform discharges on

scalp EEG have been identified as a predictor of good seizure outcome [109,111,112].

The initial resection is designed to remove all tissue with interictal spikes identified during the ECoG and any grossly evident lesion, unless the tissue is functionally important. The resection is usually undertaken after completion of ECoG and functional mapping and after restarting propofol anaesthesia, unless tissue very close to an area essential for language or motor functions is to be removed. Then that portion of the resection is performed while testing the patient's function, stopping the resection when the function begins to fail. If stopped at that point, any postoperative deficit is only transient. This technique is particularly important for the occasional patient in whom no language sites are identified during cortical stimulation in the region of the proposed resection. This may be because there is no eloquent cortex for language in the area stimulated. For example, in the senior author's series, naming sites were identified only in the frontal lobe in 17% and only in the temporoparietal lobe in 15% of patients despite the classical model of language localization describing a frontal and temporoparietal site in all patients [56]. Alternatively, absence of language sites in the expected areas may reflect such high after-discharge thresholds that the stimulating current chosen is below that required to disrupt naming tasks. In this setting, the initial cortical resection is performed with the patient awake and performing naming tasks.

In temporal lobe resections, the authors repeat the ECoG recording after removal of the lateral cortex and opening the ventricle, placing a four-contact strip electrode directly on the hippocampus, and another parallel to it on the parahippocampal gyrus. Hippocampal surface interictal epileptiform spikes are typically positive, whereas those recorded from the parahippocampal gyrus are typically negative. The extent of hippocampal resection is tailored to the extent of interictal epileptiform discharges recorded from the hippocampus. The University of Washington experience is that hippocampus can be spared without sacrificing seizure control provided the hippocampal resection includes all ECoG-identified electrophysiologically abnormal tissue [39]; this further supports the role of localized interictal epileptiform discharges as an indicator of the epileptogenic zone. While this approach has not been associated with better seizure outcomes than those reported by other groups, our data suggest that preserving electrophysiologically normal hippocampus, particularly if it is also radiologically and/or histologically normal, may potentially reduce the risk of postoperative memory loss (submitted for publication). Propofol is briefly turned off for this recording, restarted for the mesial resection and then stopped again for a final ECoG recording performed after completion of the resection. The presence of interictal spikes in some locations on this postresection ECoG, such as discharges in the insula, is not an indication for further resection. Following a resection, interictal spikes sometimes appear at lateral cortical sites where they were previously absent. Whether or not this finding is an indication for further resection is still controversial. The authors do not perform further resection in this setting. Propofol anaesthesia is restarted for closure of the craniotomy.

Identifying eloquent cortex with electrical stimulation mapping

The standard technique for intraoperative identification of functionally important areas is electrical stimulation mapping, where an electric current is applied to the cortical surface. This procedure produces a variety of effects, both exciting neurones and *en passage* fibres as well as blocking their function. These effects can produce excitation and inhibition locally or at a distance [113]. Thus, the physiological effects of stimulation cannot be easily predicted but rather must be determined empirically. In the quiet patient, responses are readily evoked from primary motor and somatosensory cortex (localized movements or dysaesthesias), somewhat more rarely from primary visual cortex (localized phosphenes) and infrequently from primary auditory cortex. Stimulation of other cortical areas produces no response at currents below the threshold for after-discharges, although in patients with TLE larger currents associated with after-discharge occasionally evoke the interpretive and experiential responses observed by Penfield and co-workers [114–116]. However, if the patient engages in an ongoing measure of language, stimulation of some dominant hemisphere cortical areas outside primary cortices will disrupt language performance. Presumably, the predominant effect of stimulation at these sites is a disruption of function, probably by depolarization blockade. This is the technique of stimulation mapping of language initially developed by Penfield and Roberts [2]. The choice of language measure to use with stimulation mapping is somewhat controversial. Penfield used object naming, which has an advantage as a screening measure for language function because all perisylvian aphasic syndromes include deficits in naming. This is the language measure most often used at the University of Washington [56]. However, others have used reading measures as a screening test [117,118].

For the surgeon, the important aspects of stimulation mapping are how localized the effects are and how reliably those effects predict the outcome of cortical resection. Optical imaging of intrinsic signals from neurones has demonstrated that bipolar cortical surface stimulation, as used at the University of Washington, results in neuronal changes that are confined to tissue between the electrodes in both humans [119] and animals [120]. Behaviourally, both sensorimotor and language effects of stimulation are usually localized on a scale of millimetres to a few centimetres. Threshold sensorimotor effects with direct cortical stimulation are usually confined to a few millimetres on each side of the central sulcus, showing the classic homuncular pattern of localization. Sites where stimulation repeatedly evokes naming errors are often confined to several separate cortical sites, each 1–2 cm^2 in extent, often with sharp boundaries [56]. However, although they are often localized in an individual patient, there is significant interpatient variation [56]. Only the most posterior portion of the inferior frontal gyrus, immediately in front of face motor cortex, is essential in a large proportion of patients. Specific areas elsewhere, including within Wernicke's area, subserve language in less than one-third of patients. This substantial variability is one of the strongest arguments for using mapping function in each patient rather than depending on anatomical landmarks derived from population studies. Examination of the effects of perisylvian stimulation on varying aspects of language areas reveals that different cortical areas are essential for different language dimensions. Different sites seem to be essential for naming in two different languages [121–123], including sign and oral languages [124,125]. Different sites are often essential for naming or reading [122], or for recent verbal memory [104]. In a few special settings, it may be useful to map localization of some of these other language and memory functions, for example in a patient heavily dependent on a second language or on reading skill, or in patients who fail intracarotid amytal assessment of memory function and have other risk factors for significant memory loss [104].

Several technical factors are important to successful stimulation mapping.

1 Mapping is difficult beyond the edges of the craniotomy. The exposure should thus be generous and should include likely locations of functionally important areas.

2 Sites where language is located must be identified, because only then does the absence of language changes indicate cortex that can be resected with a low risk of aphasia. This also requires that the exposure include areas that are likely sites for language.

3 The stimulating current must be sufficiently large to alter function in cortex, but not so large as to evoke a seizure.

4 The patient must make few errors on the language measure in the absence of stimulation. Only a few samples of stimulation effect at any one site can be obtained. If there are many errors in the absence of stimulation, errors during stimulation may be random events and not related to stimulation effects at that site. The authors regularly obtain three samples of stimulation effect at each site. For errors on all samples to have less than a 5% probability of being random events, the error rate in the absence of stimulation must not exceed 20%. Thus, stimulation mapping is of limited value in severely aphasic patients. Patients with mild aphasias may not be able to name with a low enough control error rate, but they may be able to read single words or can be continuously engaged in conversation during stimulation, although neither technique seems to be as satisfactory as naming for localizing language.

The only parameters of stimulation varied at the University of Washington are the current level and train duration. All stimulations use 60-Hz trains of biphasic pulses, each phase 1 ms in duration, delivered from a constant current stimulator across 1 mm stainless steel bipolar ball electrodes placed 5 mm apart. Most other contemporary stimulation techniques use shorter pulses, often 0.3 ms for each phase, and some use 30-Hz frequency but are otherwise similar. Levels of electrical charge that produce histological changes in tissue have been extensively studied in animals [126]. Histological examination of stimulation sites in resected human cortex does not show any changes at the light microscopy level consistent with structural damage attributable to the electrical stimulation [127]. Moreover, patients' performance in the absence of stimulation does not deteriorate after repeated stimulations (unpublished observations). Both these findings indicate that stimulation at the indicated parameters does not permanently alter cortex.

At the completion of ECoG to identify the location of interictal epileptiform discharges, sensorimotor cortex is first identified. The authors use stimulus trains beginning at 2 mA, asking the patient for any evoked sensory responses, while an assistant looks for any overt movements. Current is increased at 1 mA intervals until responses are obtained. The site of each positive response is identified with a sterile numbered ticket. Motor cortex can also be identified with stimulation of the patient under general anaesthesia, so long as the patient is not paralysed. However, patient responses under general anaesthesia are much less focal, no sensory information is available and tongue movements are difficult to identify. Recording of somatosensory evoked responses provides an alternative technique for identifying sensory cortex while the patient is under general anaesthesia, but in patients who are awake, that procedure requires more time and provides less information than stimulation mapping.

Following identification of the rolandic cortex, sterile numbered tickets are placed across the remaining cortex that is to be mapped for language sites. Prior to commencing naming tasks, the after-discharge threshold is established for the area of cortex that will undergo language mapping. A small current, commonly 2 mA between pulse peaks, is applied for 4 s to cortex adjacent to an ECoG electrode. In the case of temporal exposures, thresholds are first determined for more posterior electrodes. This stimulation is repeated at increasing currents until after-discharges are evoked, the patient reports a response, or an arbitrary upper limit on current is reached, usually 10 mA between pulse peaks for direct cortical stimulation. The current is then reduced 1 mA below the after-discharge threshold, and the threshold at the next most anterior electrode is determined. After all electrodes are sampled, a process that requires 5–10 min, a current is selected for mapping that is at the lowest threshold for after-discharge. The main reason for establishing the after-discharge threshold is to avoid evoking a seizure. In addition, utilizing the maximal current that can be applied without inducing a seizure minimizes the risk that failure to elicit speech arrest or a speech error at a given cortical site is in fact due to an inadequate stimulating current rather than the stimulated cortical site being non-eloquent for language.

The patient then begins the naming task. The authors use slide pictures of common objects to elicit naming, showing each slide at 4-s intervals on a slide projector. A 4-s stimulation train is applied to one of the sites identified by a numbered ticket at the appearance of the second or third slide. An assistant records the patient's responses and the number of the site stimulated. Another site is stimulated two or three slides later, until all sites have been sampled once. The process is then repeated in a different order two more times, so that stimulation effects on naming have been determined three times for each site. Sites with repeated naming errors are considered essential for language. With this technique, stimulation effects on naming can be determined for 20 sites in ~20 min. Language mapping is performed in all patients undergoing dominant temporal resections, whereas verbal memory mapping is restricted to patients with pre-operative risk factors for a significant postoperative verbal memory decline such as a normal hippocampus on preoperative MRI, high preoperative verbal memory function on neuropsychological assessment and memory failure following ipsilateral IAP. Stimulation mapping for other language measures and memory follows this same general plan, although the relation of applying the current to the behavioural measures may vary, especially when assessing memory. The senior author's protocol for assessing cortical stimulation effects on the input, storage or retrieval phases of recent verbal memory and on reading has been published [104,122].

References

1 Luders H, Awad I. Conceptual considerations. In: Luders HO, ed. *Epilepsy Surgery*. New York: Raven Press, 1992: 51–62.
2 Penfield W, Roberts L. *Speech and Brain Mechanisms*. Princeton, N.J.: Princeton University Press, 1959.
3 Penfield W, Jasper H. *Epilepsy and the Functional Anatomy of the Human Brain*. Boston: Little, Brown & Co, 1954.
4 Margerison JH, Corsellis JAN. Epilepsy in the temporal lobes. *Brain* 1966; 89: 499–530.
5 Falconer MA. Discussion on the surgery of temporal lobe epilepsy. *Proc R Soc Med* 1953; 46: 971–5.
6 Fried I. Anatomic temporal lobe resections for temporal lobe epilepsy. *Neurosurg Clin N Am* 1993; 4: 233–42.
7 Diehl B, Luders HO. Temporal lobe epilepsy: when are invasive recordings needed? *Epilepsia* 2000; 41 (Suppl. 3): S61–S74.
8 Jasper H, Pertuisset B, Flanigin HF. EEG and cortical electrograms in patients with temporal lobe seizures. *Arch Neurol Psychiatr* 1951; 65: 272–90.
9 Binnie CD, Alarcon G, Elwes RD *et al*. Role of ECoG in 'en bloc' temporal lobe resection: the Maudsley experience. *Electroencephalogr Clin Neurophysiol Suppl* 1998; 48: 17–23.
10 Cascino GD, Trenerry MR, Jack CR Jr *et al*. Electrocorticography and temporal lobe epilepsy: relationship to quantitative MRI and operative outcome. *Epilepsia* 1995; 36: 692–6.
11 McBride MC, Binnie CD, Janota I *et al*. Predictive value of intraoperative electrocorticograms in resective epilepsy surgery. *Ann Neurol* 1991; 30: 526–32.
12 Schwartz TH, Bazil CW, Walczak TS *et al*. The predictive value of intraoperative electrocorticography in resections for limbic epilepsy associated with mesial temporal sclerosis. *Neurosurgery* 1997; 40: 302–9.
13 Tran TA, Spencer SS, Marks D *et al*. Significance of spikes recorded on electrocorticography in nonlesional medial temporal lobe epilepsy. *Ann Neurol* 1995; 38: 763–70.
14 Engel J Jr, Driver MV, Falconer MA. Electrophysiological correlates of pathology and surgical results in temporal lobe epilepsy. *Brain* 1975; 98: 129–56.
15 Chatrian GE, Tsai ML, Temkin NR *et al*. Role of the ECoG in tailored temporal lobe resection: the University of Washington experience. *Electroencephalogr Clin Neurophysiol Suppl* 1998; 48: 24–43.
16 Devinsky O, Canevini MP, Sato S *et al*. Quantitative electrocorticography in patients undergoing temporal lobectomy. *J Epilepsy* 1992; 5: 178–85.
17 Fenyes I, Zoltan I, Fenyes G. Temporal lobe epilepsies with deep seated epileptogenic foci. *Arch Neurol* 1961; 4: 103–15.
18 Graf M, Niedermeyer E, Schiemann J *et al*. Electrocorticography: information derived from intraoperative recordings during seizure surgery. *Clin Electroencephalogr* 1984; 15: 83–91.
19 Kanazawa O, Blume WT, Girvin JP. Significance of spikes at temporal lobe electrocorticography. *Epilepsia* 1996; 37: 50–5.
20 Rasmussen TB. Surgical treatment of complex partial seizures: results, lessons, and problems. *Epilepsia* 1983; 24 (Suppl. 1): S65–S76.
21 Tuunainen A, Nousiainen U, Mervaala E *et al*. Postoperative EEG and electrocorticography: relation to clinical outcome in patients with temporal lobe surgery. *Epilepsia* 1994; 35: 1165–73.
22 Wyllie E, Luders H, Morris HH, III *et al*. Clinical outcome after complete or partial cortical resection for intractable epilepsy. *Neurology* 1987; 37: 1634–41.
23 Bengzon AR, Rasmussen T, Gloor P *et al*. Prognostic factors in the surgical treatment of temporal lobe epileptics. *Neurology* 1968; 18: 717–31.
24 Fiol ME, Gates JR, Torres F *et al*. The prognostic value of residual spikes in the postexcision electrocorticogram after temporal lobectomy. *Neurology* 1991; 41: 512–16.
25 Stefan H, Quesney LF, Abou-Khalil B *et al*. Electrocorticography in temporal lobe epilepsy surgery. *Acta Neurol Scand* 1991; 83: 65–72.
26 So N, Olivier A, Andermann F *et al*. Results of surgical treatment in patients with bitemporal epileptiform abnormalities. *Ann Neurol* 1989; 25: 432–9.
27 Alarcon G, Garcia Seoane JJ, Binnie CD *et al*. Origin and propagation of interictal discharges in the acute electrocorticogram. implications for pathophysiology and surgical treatment of temporal lobe epilepsy. *Brain* 1997; 120: 2259–82.
28 Alarcon G, Guy CN, Binnie CD *et al*. Intracerebral propagation of interictal activity in partial epilepsy: implications for source localisation. *J Neurol Neurosurg Psychiatr* 1994; 57: 435–49.
29 Clark DL, Rosner BS. Neurophysiologic effects of general anesthetics. I. The electroencephalogram and sensory evoked responses in man. *Anesthesiology* 1973; 38: 564–82.
30 Engel J Jr. Outcome with respect to epileptic seizures. In: Engel J Jr, ed.

Surgical Treatment of the Epilepsies. New York: Raven Press, 1987: 553–71.

31 Wyler AR, Hermann BP, Somes G. Extent of medial temporal resection on outcome from anterior temporal lobectomy: a randomized prospective study. *Neurosurgery* 1995; 37: 982–90.

32 Nayel MH, Awad IA, Luders H. Extent of mesiobasal resection determines outcome after temporal lobectomy for intractable complex partial seizures. *Neurosurgery* 1991; 29: 55–60.

33 Awad IA, Katz A, Hahn JF *et al.* Extent of resection in temporal lobectomy for epilepsy. I. Interobserver analysis and correlation with seizure outcome. *Epilepsia* 1989; 30: 756–62.

34 Awad IA, Nayel MH, Luders H. Second operation after the failure of previous resection for epilepsy. *Neurosurgery* 1991; 28: 510–18.

35 Germano IM, Poulin N, Olivier A. Reoperation for recurrent temporal lobe epilepsy. *J Neurosurg* 1994; 81: 31–6.

36 Feindel W, Rasmussen T. Temporal lobectomy with amygdalectomy and minimal hippocampal resection: review of 100 cases. *Can J Neurol Sci* 1991; 18: 603–5.

37 Jooma R, Yeh HS, Privitera MD *et al.* Seizure control and extent of mesial temporal resection. *Acta Neurochir (Wien)* 1995; 133: 44–9.

38 Kanner AM, Kaydanova Y, Toledo-Morrell L *et al.* Tailored anterior temporal lobectomy. Relation between extent of resection of mesial structures and postsurgical seizure outcome. *Arch Neurol* 1995; 52: 173–8.

39 McKhann GM, Schoenfeld-McNeill J, Born DE *et al.* Intraoperative hippocampal electrocorticography to predict the extent of hippocampal resection in temporal lobe epilepsy surgery. *J Neurosurg* 2000; 93: 44–52.

40 Rasmussen T, Feindel W. Temporal lobectomy: review of 100 cases with major hippocampectomy. *Can J Neurol Sci* 1991; 18: 601–2.

41 Son EI, Howard MA, Ojemann GA *et al.* Comparing the extent of hippocampal removal to the outcome in terms of seizure control. *Stereotact Funct Neurosurg* 1994; 62: 232–7.

42 Awad IA, Katz A, Hahn JF *et al.* Extent of resection in temporal lobectomy for epilepsy. I. Interobserver analysis and correlation with seizure outcome. *Epilepsia* 1989; 30: 756–62.

43 Germano IM, Poulin N, Olivier A. Reoperation for recurrent temporal lobe epilepsy. *J Neurosurg* 1994; 81: 31–6.

44 Nayel MH, Awad IA, Luders H. Extent of mesiobasal resection determines outcome after temporal lobectomy for intractable complex partial seizures. *Neurosurgery* 1991; 29: 55–60.

45 Feindel W, Rasmussen T. Temporal lobectomy with amygdalectomy and minimal hippocampal resection: review of 100 cases. *Can J Neurol Sci* 1991; 18: 603–5.

46 Kanner AM, Kaydanova Y, Toledo-Morrell L *et al.* Tailored anterior temporal lobectomy. Relation between extent of resection of mesial structures and postsurgical seizure outcome. *Arch Neurol* 1995; 52: 173–8.

47 Rasmussen T, Feindel W. Temporal lobectomy: review of 100 cases with major hippocampectomy. *Can J Neurol Sci* 1991; 18: 601–2.

48 Modica PA, Tempelhoff R, White PF. Pro- and anticonvulsant effects of anesthetics (Part I). *Anesth Analg* 1990; 70: 303–15.

49 Modica PA, Tempelhoff R, White PF. Pro- and anticonvulsant effects of anesthetics (Part II). *Anesth Analg* 1990; 70: 433–44.

50 Herrick IA, Gelb AW. Anaesthesia for temporal lobe epilepsy surgery. *Can J Neurol Sci* 2000; 27 (Suppl. 1): S64–S67.

51 Silbergeld DL, Mueller WM, Colley PS *et al.* Use of propofol (Diprivan) for awake craniotomies: technical note. *Surg Neurol* 1992; 38: 271–2.

52 Herrick IA, Craen RA, Gelb AW *et al.* Propofol sedation during awake craniotomy for seizures: electrocorticographic and epileptogenic effects. *Anesth Analg* 1997; 84: 1280–4.

53 Fiol ME, Torres F, Gates JR *et al.* Methohexital (Brevital) effect on electrocorticogram may be misleading. *Epilepsia* 1990; 31: 524–8.

54 Burnstine TH, Lesser RP, Hart J Jr *et al.* Characterization of the basal temporal language area in patients with left temporal lobe epilepsy. *Neurology* 1990; 40: 966–70.

55 Davies KG, Maxwell RE, Jennum P *et al.* Language function following subdural grid-directed temporal lobectomy. *Acta Neurol Scand* 1994; 90: 201–6.

56 Ojemann G, Ojemann J, Lettich E *et al.* Cortical language localization in left, dominant hemisphere. An electrical stimulation mapping investigation in 117 patients. *J Neurosurg* 1989; 71: 316–26.

57 Ojemann GA, Whitaker HA. Language localization and variability. *Brain Lang* 1978; 6: 239–60.

58 Ojemann GA. Individual variability in cortical localization of language. *J Neurosurg* 1979; 50: 164–9.

59 Schwartz TH, Devinsky O, Doyle W *et al.* Preoperative predictors of anterior temporal language areas. *J Neurosurg* 1998; 89: 962–70.

60 Haglund MM, Berger MS, Shamseldin M *et al.* Cortical localization of temporal lobe language sites in patients with gliomas. *Neurosurgery* 1994; 34: 567–76.

61 Ojemann GA. Electrical stimulation and the neurobiology of language. *Behav Brain Sci* 1983; 6: 221–30.

62 Devinsky O, Perrine K, Llinas R *et al.* Anterior temporal language areas in patients with early onset of temporal lobe epilepsy. *Ann Neurol* 1993; 34: 727–32.

63 Devinsky O, Perrine K, Hirsch J *et al.* Relation of cortical language distribution and cognitive function in surgical epilepsy patients. *Epilepsia* 2000; 41: 400–4.

64 Saykin AJ, Stafiniak P, Robinson LJ *et al.* Language before and after temporal lobectomy: specificity of acute changes and relation to early risk factors. *Epilepsia* 1995; 36: 1071–7.

65 Stafiniak P, Saykin AJ, Sperling MR *et al.* Acute naming deficits following dominant temporal lobectomy: prediction by age at 1st risk for seizures. *Neurology* 1990; 40: 1509–12.

66 Barbaro NM, Walker JA, Laxer KD. Temporal lobectomy and language function. *J Neurosurg* 1991; 75: 830–1.

67 Buchtel HA, Kluin KJ, Ross DA *et al.* Language mapping in epilepsy patients undergoing dominant hemisphere anterior temporal lobectomy. *Epilepsia* 1995; 36: 1164–5.

68 Davies KG, Maxwell RE, Beniak TE *et al.* Language function after temporal lobectomy without stimulation mapping of cortical function. *Epilepsia* 1995; 36: 130–6.

69 Hermann BP, Wyler AR, Somes G. Language function following anterior temporal lobectomy. *J Neurosurg* 1991; 74: 560–6.

70 Hermann BP, Perrine K, Chelune GJ *et al.* Visual confrontation naming following left anterior temporal lobectomy: a comparison of surgical approaches. *Neuropsychology* 1999; 13: 3–9.

71 Falconer MA, Serafetinides EA. A follow-up study of surgery in temporal lobe epilepsy. *J Neurol Neurosurg Psychiatr* 1963; 26: 154–65.

72 Hermann BP, Wyler AR, Somes G *et al.* Dysnomia after left anterior temporal lobectomy without functional mapping: frequency and correlates. *Neurosurgery* 1994; 35: 52–6.

73 Penfield W, Milner B. Memory deficit produced by bilateral lesions in the hippocampal zone. *AMA Arch Neur Psychiatr* 1958; 79: 475–97.

74 Scoville WB, Milner B. Loss of recent memory after bilateral hippocampal lesions. 1957 [Classical Article]. *J Neuropsychiatr Clin Neurosci* 2000; 12: 103–13.

75 Milner B. Brain mechanisms suggested by studies of temporal lobes. In: Millikan CH, Darley FL, eds. *Brain Mechanisms Underlying Speech and Language.* New York: Grune and Stratton, 1967: 122–45.

76 Helmstaedter C, Elger CE. Cognitive consequences of two-thirds anterior temporal lobectomy on verbal memory in 144 patients: a three-month follow-up study. *Epilepsia* 1996; 37: 171–80.

77 Hermann BP, Wyler AR, Bush AJ *et al.* Differential effects of left and right anterior temporal lobectomy on verbal learning and memory performance. *Epilepsia* 1992; 33: 289–97.

78 Ivnik RJ, Sharbrough FW, Laws ER, Jr. Effects of anterior temporal lobectomy on cognitive function. *J Clin Psychol* 1987; 43: 128–37.

79 Martin RC, Sawrie SM, Roth DL *et al.* Individual memory change after anterior temporal lobectomy: a base rate analysis using regression-based outcome methodology. *Epilepsia* 1998; 39: 1075–82.

80 Novelly RA, Augustine EA, Mattson RH *et al.* Selective memory improvement and impairment in temporal lobectomy for epilepsy. *Ann Neurol* 1984; 15: 64–7.

81 Powell GE, Polkey CE, McMillan T. The new Maudsley series of temporal lobectomy. I: Short-term cognitive effects. *Br J Clin Psychol* 1985; 24: 109–24.

82 Baxendale SA, Thompson PJ, Kitchen ND. Postoperative hippocampal remnant shrinkage and memory decline: a dynamic process. *Neurology* 2000; 55: 243–9.

83 Katz A, Awad IA, Kong AK *et al.* Extent of resection in temporal

84 Kim HI, Olivier A, Jones-Gotman M *et al.* Corticoamygdalectomy in memory-impaired patients. *Stereotact Funct Neurosurg* 1992; 58: 162–7.

85 Milner B. Disorders of learning and memory after temporal lobe lesions in man. *Clin Neurosurg* 1972; 19: 421–46.

86 Nunn JA, Polkey CE, Morris RG. Selective spatial memory impairment after right unilateral temporal lobectomy. *Neuropsychologia* 1998; 36: 837–48.

87 Nunn JA, Graydon FJ, Polkey CE *et al.* Differential spatial memory impairment after right temporal lobectomy demonstrated using temporal titration. *Brain* 1999; 122: 47–59.

88 Pauli E, Pickel S, Schulemann H *et al.* Neuropsychologic findings depending on the type of the resection in temporal lobe epilepsy. *Adv Neurol* 1999; 81: 371–7.

89 Baxendale SA, Van Paesschen W, Thompson PJ *et al.* Hippocampal cell loss and gliosis: relationship to preoperative and postoperative memory function. *Neuropsychiatr Neuropsychol Behav Neurol* 1998; 11: 12–21.

90 Bell BD, Davies KG, Haltiner AM *et al.* Intracarotid amobarbital procedure and prediction of postoperative memory in patients with left temporal lobe epilepsy and hippocampal sclerosis. *Epilepsia* 2000; 41: 992–7.

91 Bell BD, Davies KG. Anterior temporal lobectomy, hippocampal sclerosis, and memory: recent neuropsychological findings. *Neuropsychol Rev* 1998; 8: 25–41.

92 Hermann BP, Wyler AR, Somes G *et al.* Pathological status of the mesial temporal lobe predicts memory outcome from left anterior temporal lobectomy. *Neurosurgery* 1992; 31: 652–6.

93 Kneebone AC, Chelune GJ, Dinner DS *et al.* Intracarotid amobarbital procedure as a predictor of material-specific memory change after anterior temporal lobectomy. *Epilepsia* 1995; 36: 857–65.

94 Sass KJ, Sass A, Westerveld M *et al.* Specificity in the correlation of verbal memory and hippocampal neuron loss: dissociation of memory, language, and verbal intellectual ability. *J Clin Exp Neuropsychol* 1992; 14: 662–72.

95 Sass KJ, Westerveld M, Buchanan CP *et al.* Degree of hippocampal neuron loss determines severity of verbal memory decrease after left anteromesiotemporal lobectomy. *Epilepsia* 1994; 35: 1179–86.

96 Seidenberg M, Hermann B, Wyler AR *et al.* Neuropsychological outcome following anterior temporal lobectomy in patients with and without the syndrome of mesial temporal lobe epilepsy. *Neuropsychology* 1998; 12: 303–16.

97 Trenerry MR, Jack CR Jr, Cascino GD *et al.* Gender differences in post-temporal lobectomy verbal memory and relationships between MRI hippocampal volumes and preoperative verbal memory. *Epilepsy Res* 1995; 20: 69–76.

98 Wyllie E, Naugle R, Awad I *et al.* Intracarotid amobarbital procedure: I. Prediction of decreased modality-specific memory scores after temporal lobectomy. *Epilepsia* 1991; 32: 857–64.

99 Loring DW, Lee GP, Meador KJ *et al.* Hippocampal contribution to verbal recent memory following dominant-hemisphere temporal lobectomy. *J Clin Exp Neuropsychol* 1991; 13: 575–86.

100 Wolf RL, Ivnik RJ, Hirschorn KA *et al.* Neurocognitive efficiency following left temporal lobectomy: standard versus limited resection. *J Neurosurg* 1993; 79: 76–83.

101 Baxendale SA, Van Paesschen W, Thompson PJ *et al.* Hippocampal cell loss and gliosis: relationship to preoperative and postoperative memory function. *Neuropsychiatr Neuropsychol Behav Neurol* 1998; 11: 12–21.

102 Hermann BP, Wyler AR, Somes G *et al.* Pathological status of the mesial temporal lobe predicts memory outcome from left anterior temporal lobectomy. *Neurosurgery* 1992; 31: 652–6.

103 Helmstaedter C, Grunwald T, Lehnertz K *et al.* Differential involvement of left temporolateral and temporomesial structures in verbal declarative learning and memory: evidence from temporal lobe epilepsy. *Brain Cogn* 1997; 35: 110–31.

104 Ojemann GA, Dodrill CB. Verbal memory deficits after left temporal lobectomy for epilepsy. Mechanism and intraoperative prediction. *J Neurosurg* 1985; 62: 101–7.

105 Ojemann GA, Dodrill CB. Intraoperative techniques for reducing language and memory deficits with left temporal lobectomy. In: Wolf P, Dam M, Janz D *et al.*, eds. *Advances in Epileptology*. New York: Raven Press, 1987: 327–30.

106 Perrine K, Devinsky O, Uysal S *et al.* Left temporal neocortex mediation of verbal memory: evidence from functional mapping with cortical stimulation. *Neurology* 1994; 44: 1845–50.

107 Ojemann GA. Organization of short-term verbal memory in language areas of human cortex: evidence from electrical stimulation. *Brain Lang* 1978; 5: 331–40.

108 Ojemann GA. Different approaches to resective epilepsy surgery: standard and tailored. *Epilepsy Res Suppl* 1992; 5: 169–74.

109 Dodrill CB, Wilkus RJ, Ojemann GA *et al.* Multidisciplinary prediction of seizure relief from cortical resection surgery. *Ann Neurol* 1986; 20: 2–12.

110 Harris AB. Absence of seizures or mirror foci in experimental epilepsy after excision of alumina and astrogliotic scar. *Epilepsia* 1981; 22: 101–22.

111 Holmes MD, Dodrill CB, Wilensky AJ *et al.* Unilateral focal preponderance of interictal epileptiform discharges as a predictor of seizure origin. *Arch Neurol* 1996; 53: 228–32.

112 Holmes MD, Kutsy RL, Ojemann GA *et al.* Interictal, unifocal spikes in refractory extratemporal epilepsy predict ictal origin and postsurgical outcome [in process citation]. *Clin Neurophysiol* 2000; 111: 1802–8.

113 Ranck JB. Which elements are excited in electrical stimulation of mammalian central nervous system: a review. *Brain Res* 1975; 98: 417–40.

114 Mullan S, Penfield W. Illusions of comparative interpretation and emotion; production by epileptic discharge and by electrical stimulation in the temporal cortex. *AMA Arch Neur Psychiatr* 1959; 81: 269–84.

115 Penfield W, Mullan S. Illusions of perception and the temporal cortex. *Trans Am Neur Ass* 1957; 82nd Meeting: 6–8.

116 Penfield W. The interpretive cortex; the stream of consciousness in the human brain can be electrically reactivated. *Science* 1959; 129: 1719–25.

117 Luders H, Lesser RP, Hahn J *et al.* Basal temporal language area demonstrated by electrical stimulation. *Neurology* 1986; 36: 505–10.

118 Luders H, Hahn J, Lesser RP *et al.* Basal temporal subdural electrodes in the evaluation of patients with intractable epilepsy. *Epilepsia* 1989; 30: 131–42.

119 Haglund MM, Ojemann GA, Hochman DW. Optical imaging of epileptiform and functional activity in human cerebral cortex. *Nature* 1992; 358: 668–71.

120 Haglund MM, Ojemann GA, Blasdel GG. Optical imaging of bipolar cortical stimulation. *J Neurosurg* 1993; 78: 785–93.

121 Ojemann GA, Whitaker HA. The bilingual brain. *Arch Neurol* 1978; 35: 409–12.

122 Ojemann GA. Brain organisation for language from the perspective of electrical stimulation mapping. *Behav Brain Sci* 1983; 6: 189–230.

123 Rapport RL, Tan CT, Whitaker HA. Language function and dysfunction among Chinese- and English-speaking polyglots: cortical stimulation, Wada testing, and clinical Studies. *Brain Lang* 1983; 18: 342–66.

124 Haglund MM, Ojemann GA, Lettich E *et al.* Dissociation of cortical and single unit activity in spoken and signed languages. *Brain Lang* 1993; 44: 19–27.

125 Mateer CA, Polen SB, Ojemann GA *et al.* Cortical localization of finger spelling and oral language: a case study. *Brain Lang* 1982; 17: 46–57.

126 Yuen TG, Agnew WF, Bullara LA *et al.* Histological evaluation of neural damage from electrical stimulation: considerations for the selection of parameters for clinical application. *Neurosurgery* 1981; 9: 292–9.

127 Gordon B, Lesser RP, Rance NE *et al.* Parameters for direct cortical electrical stimulation in the human: histopathologic confirmation. *Electroencephalogr Clin Neurophysiol* 1990; 75: 371–7.

70 Stereotactic Surgery for Epilepsy

A. W. McEvoy, B. M. Trivedi and N. D. Kitchen

The evolution of surgical treatment for epilepsy in the last century has been critically dependent on technical developments [1]. Conventional (i.e. resective) surgery for medically refractory epilepsy has a long tradition, and is effective in stopping or ameliorating seizures in 55–80% of patients depending on case selection. Stereotaxy is a navigational technology that allows neurosurgeons to determine accurately their location and direction during surgery. Stereotactic procedures offer the possibility of being more accurate, more economical and better tolerated than conventional craniotomy and resective surgery, and hence are being used more frequently in the management of medically refractory epilepsy.

During the past decade, technological advances have revolutionized the art of neurosurgical navigation, with frameless stereotaxy perhaps the most elegant. More recently, there has been a trend towards using radiosurgery; the gamma knife can make highly selective, discrete lesions in areas of the brain responsible for epilepsy.

The word stereotactic, derived from the Greek *stereos*, meaning 'three-dimensional', and *tactus*, meaning 'to touch', was coined by Horsley and Clarke in 1906 [2]. The technique involves the use of neuroradiological imaging modalities, linked to a three-dimensional coordinate system, in order to guide the surgeon to a chosen target with an accuracy of 1–2 mm.

Traditionally, registration of the radiological images to the patient in the operating theatre has involved the use of a stereotactic head-frame. This is fixed to the patient's head with screws, is visible on the imaging modality employed and remains on the patient's head during surgery. This rigid head-frame has the major advantage of maintaining a fixed three-dimensional coordinate system. Unfortunately, this bulky frame is also the system's main limitation, as it puts a constraint on head positioning and physically interferes with the execution of the craniotomy. Consequently, frame-based systems tend now to be reserved for procedures such as needle biopsy or placement of depth electrodes.

The next step was the development of image-based, intracranial navigation that is independent of an external frame. There are several such systems, each based on a combination of three fundamental concepts: (a) correlating physical space with image space; (b) using a pointing device for interactive localization; and (c) obtaining image-guided feedback through a computer-based interface. Frameless stereotaxy is based on the creation of a mathematical relationship between radiographic images and physical space. This process, termed 'registration', involves the precise mapping of every location in an image to the corresponding physical anatomy of the patient [3].

At present, stereotactic neurosurgery is increasing in popularity due to a number of developments in multimodality neuroradiological imaging. Thus, the advent of high-resolution MRI and its crucial role in the management of epilepsy, together with functional imaging modalities such as PET and SPECT, and advances in computer and stereotactic instrument technology, have introduced new possibilities in epilepsy treatment.

The use of preoperative high-resolution volumetric MRI has had an enormous impact on epilepsy surgery planning [4–9]. The responsible pathological substrate is now frequently identifiable using such methodologies [10,11]. In the epilepsy surgery programme at the National Hospital for Neurology and Neurosurgery, London, UK, the number of such abnormalities visualized on preoperative imaging of epilepsy surgery candidates has risen from less than 10% to over 90% with the routine use of volumetric MRI. In this way, epilepsy surgery is becoming increasingly image guided, with less reliance placed on electrophysiological localization. Frameless stereotactic neurosurgery is frequently the method by which this image guidance is best achieved.

In this chapter, we will discuss the principles of stereotaxy and their application to the basics of 'frame-based' and 'frameless' systems. We will show how the increasing use of multimodality imaging and its integration into image-directed neuronavigational systems has led to these techniques becoming an essential part of epilepsy surgical practice.

We will discuss the current status of stereotactic neurosurgery in the surgical management of epilepsy with reference to its role:

1 As an aid to conventional (i.e. resective) epilepsy surgery:

(a) diagnosis—the use of stereotactic methods to place depth electrodes for invasive EEG monitoring in the evaluation of epilepsy cases where there are diagnostic and management difficulties concerning lateralization and localization;

(b) treatment—selective stereotactic amygdalohippocampectomy which has been used as a method of minimizing the resection of the lateral temporal neocortex, while permitting the resection to the relevant part of the mesial temporal structures in cases of temporal lobe epilepsy, in which there is concern over the neuropsychological status of the patient (particularly with regard to postoperative memory function).

2 A second, very important use of stereotaxy is to guide the surgeon towards small epileptogenic lesions using the techniques of image-directed craniotomy, and also stereotactic lesioning of the central nervous system (CNS) (i.e. non-resective surgery).

However, it must be appreciated that image-directed surgery is now an inherent part of neurosurgical practice. Its use has become widespread and it is easily applied to almost all neurosurgical procedures.

Frame-based stereotactic neurosurgery

Traditional frame-based stereotaxy offers a high degree of point target localization, but unfortunately the identical stereotactic space is not easily reproducible in the same patient on different occasions (Plate 70.1a, b, shown in colour between pp. 670 and 671). Furthermore, skull fixation using either screws or pins is invasive, and uncomfortable for the patient. As a result, with traditional head-frames, the two phases of stereotaxy (i.e. image acquisition and surgery) need to be closely related to one another in time; usually one follows directly after the other [12,13]. Frameless stereotactic methodologies offer the potential for comprehensive image guidance not seen with frame-based stereotaxy.

Frameless stereotactic neurosurgery

Frameless stereotaxy is uniquely suited to intracranial surgery. The relatively fixed position of the brain within the skull facilitates the referencing of preoperative data with the real-time position of the head.

The main advantages of frameless stereotaxy are that it provides real-time, updated information to the surgeon, about location and trajectory. It can be helpful in localizing lesions, increasing the chances of complete lesion resection and helping to identify normal structures surrounding a lesion. Typically the result is faster, more complete and often safer neurosurgical procedures.

Frameless stereotaxy is invaluable at all stages of image-directed epilepsy surgery, including selection of the preoperative approach, sizing of the scalp incision, placement of the craniotomy and selection of the trajectory through or around cerebral structures. Resection of tumours is improved, with corticotomies precisely placed. In tumours with poorly defined margins, the constant feedback on location can be invaluable for maximizing tumour resection while minimizing brain injury. With frameless stereotactic neurosurgery, the surgeon can be accurately and easily guided to the area(s) in the brain responsible for the epilepsy [3].

There are four components to a frameless stereotactic neurosurgical system.

1 A pointing device (e.g. a wand).
2 A tracking system that is constantly locating the position of the localizing device in space.
3 A hardware system represented by a computer processing unit (CPU) and an output device (monitor).
4 Software that is able to reconstruct the data from the tracking system into a three-dimensional image, and is able to register the preoperative image data set onto physical space [14].

Image space is the three-dimensional volume represented by the series of multimodality neuroradiological images that are acquired preoperatively and which make up the imaged anatomy of the patient. Anatomical images obtained from CT and MRI scans are frequently defined in the image space and are of high resolution; images from other functional imaging modalities (fMRI, PET and

(a)

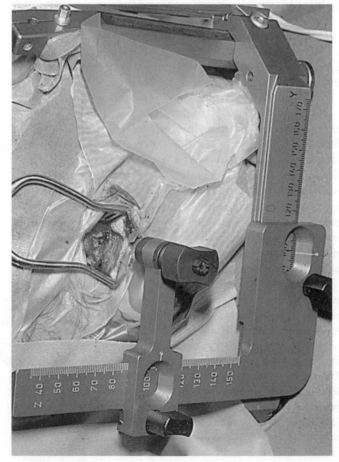

(b)

Fig. 70.1 Following electrode placement confirmatory radiological imaging is used to show the final position achieved, since it is critical to know precisely where the EEG recordings are emanating from in order to obtain an accurate three-dimensional picture of seizure activity. Usually, disposable multiple contact platinum electrodes are used. (a) The Lexell stereotactic frame. (b) The Lexell frame being used intraoperatively for the insertion of depth electrodes.

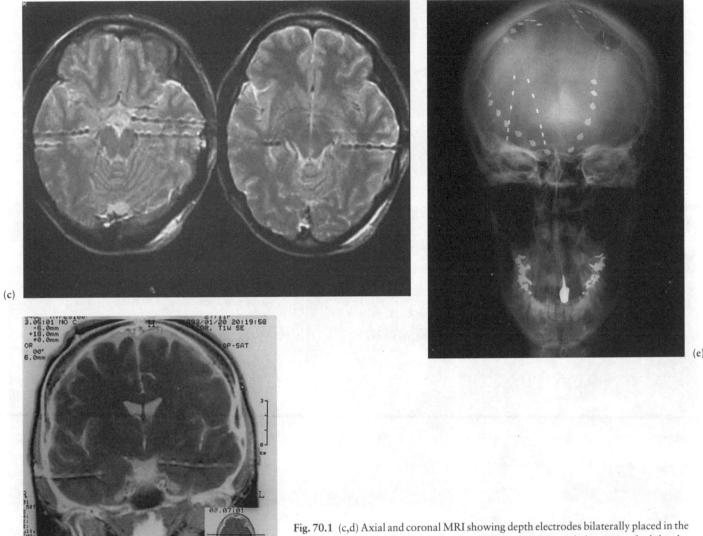

(c)

(d)

(e)

Fig. 70.1 (c,d) Axial and coronal MRI showing depth electrodes bilaterally placed in the temporal lobes. (e) AP radiograph of the skull showing bilateral placement of subdural grid electrodes and right-sided frontal depth electrodes. (Parts (a) and (b) shown in colour between pp. 670 and 671.)

SPECT) can be integrated and also used in image space [15]. As each point in either the CT or MRI image data set is defined in terms of a three-dimensional coordinate (x, y and z) relative to the origin of the Cartesian frame of reference [16], and as each coordinate has an intensity value, these imaging modalities have an already established three-dimensional coordinate system which relates each point in the image to the anatomy. Physical space is the three-dimensional volume represented by the real physical anatomy of the patient, and as such does not have an obvious coordinate system.

Frameless stereotaxy aims to define a three-dimensional coordinate system for the physical space, and superimpose the images of the anatomy of the patient from the CT or MRI data (i.e. the image space) onto the actual anatomy of the patient in the operating theatre (i.e. the physical space), and thus create a real-time navigational map, which the surgeon will use throughout the surgical procedure. This process is called registration.

One of the earliest technologies used to localize a point in space consisted of an articulated arm [17–24]. The ISG viewing wand

frameless stereotactic guidance system (ISG Technologies, Mississauga, Ontario, Canada) is an excellent example and was used extensively in neurosurgery because of its accuracy to less than 2 mm (Fig. 70.1c,d). The wand consists of two segments: a sterile surgical probe and a multijointed, articulated arm with six joints, which give it a 60-cm reach and six degrees of freedom. Electrical signalling from the joints are relayed to and processed by the CPU to give an accurate location of the probe tip in physical space.

The more recent technologies use a system to localize a point in physical space using less bulky and obstructive pointing devices (Fig. 70.2). These systems employ a 'free-hand' pointing tool. The methods of data acquisition between these free-hand pointing tools are similar. Essentially the free-hand pointing tool is capable of sending data to a receiver (a microphone or a camera) that will send the received signals to the main CPU without there being a direct physical connection between the tool and the CPU. The CPU will then be able to compute the precise location and three-dimensional coordinates for the pointing tool.

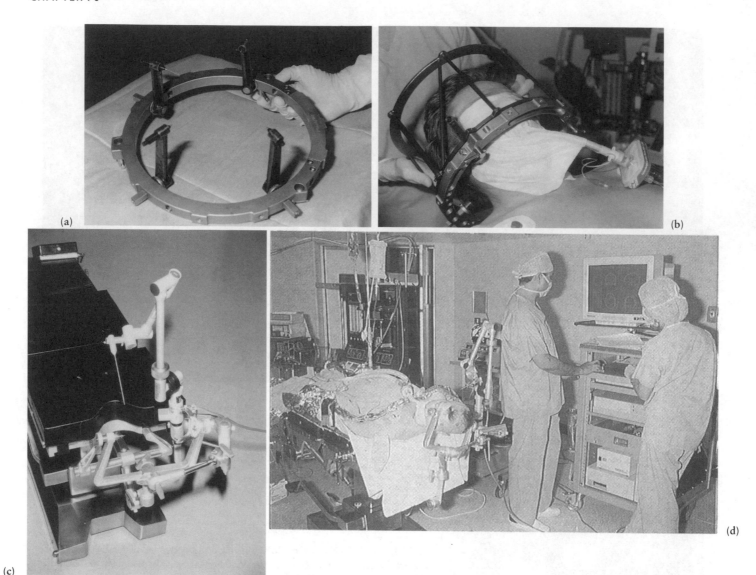

Fig. 70.2 (a) The Cosman–Roberts–Wells base ring. (b) The Cosman–Roberts–Wells base ring and fiducial system being used intraoperatively. (c,d) The ISG 'viewing wand' uses a passive mechanical arm for registration and pointing during surgery.

The first examples of these used an ultrasonic triangulating system [25,26]. The more recent systems rely upon the pointing device emitting infrared light from emitting diodes (iLEDs) to cameras located around the operating theatre [27,28]. This information is then processed by the CPU, in a similar way to the ultrasound triangulating system. Although the path between the iLEDs and the camera must be clear, this system does not suffer the disadvantage of interference or of temperature dependence. The accuracy of the pointing device is continually assessed during the surgical procedure with known anatomical landmarks. These systems have the advantage that almost any surgical instrument can be converted to the pointing device.

The latest development, and perhaps the most elegant, incorporates the localizing function into the operating microscope. Several systems have been developed, one example being the Leica Viewscope (Leica, Inc., Deerfield, IL), in which the pointing function is performed by two low-energy lasers designed to converge at a single point at the focal length of the microscope. After mapping this point to image space, the corresponding location on the imaging studies can be visualized. These systems have the advantage of continuous update, without the need for a separate pointing device. Although most systems require the surgeon to look away temporarily from the operating field to the computer display, some newer systems incorporate heads-up display of the frameless stereotactic data.

Registration of the image space onto the physical space is required for the navigational map to be produced. The precise way in which this is achieved is beyond the scope of this chapter. Briefly, there are two basic systems: paired point registration and surface registration.

Paired point registration uses natural landmarks, e.g. external auditory meatus, nasion or lateral canthus [20,28–30], or artificial landmarks (fiducial markers placed on the head) visible on CT and MRI scans [22,25–27,31,32]. Registration error is theoretically minimized at the epicentre of the registered points, so fiducials should be placed on the scalp so they 'surround' the lesion. The most precise landmarks for registration are either bolts or screws in the skull [30].

Surface-based registration systems match numerous points extracted from natural contours. They attempt to align the contour of a physical surface (such as the scalp) with a corresponding image surface.

The corresponding landmarks in the physical space are identified in the image space. With both data sets stored in the CPU, a 'best-fit' transformation matrix is applied by the CPU, transforming and superimposing image space onto physical space as accurately as possible. The surgeon can hence readily determine location and trajectory throughout the surgical procedure and the result is navigation.

The disadvantages of image-directed guidance systems are the learning time required to become fully confident with using the device, the preoperative set-up time and the space required for the system in the operating theatre [19]. In addition, changes in the cerebral blood volume, mechanical ventilation, cerebrospinal fluid (CSF) withdrawal, unopposed gravity and patient positioning can all affect registration. Other problems are brain shift once the skull has been opened or a mass lesion removed. In this case, the preoperative images will no longer provide an accurate anatomy of the contents inside the skull. The most definitive solution to this problem is the use of intraoperative MRI and frameless stereotaxy [33–43]. The neurosurgeon can then periodically update the reference images and re-register physical space to updated image space in 'real-time'. In other words, the images directing the surgery are not 'historical', but rather are providing information about what is actually occurring during the surgical procedure.

Multimodality imaging and image-directed neurosurgery

The last decade has seen neuroimaging take an increasingly important role in the management of epilepsy. New techniques and imaging sequences have appeared that give increasing sensitivity for detecting abnormalities of brain structure. Neuroimaging has become a powerful functional tool of high spatial resolution that has increased in temporal resolution to the point where it has become an important physiological probe of functions that were previously considered entirely the domain of electrophysiology.

A number of imaging modalities are now in common use for the localization of seizure foci as part of the preoperative investigation of patients with intractable epilepsy. In addition, non-invasive methods of mapping brain function, such as functional MRI (fMRI) [44–50] and PET with tracers such as [^{15}O]H$_2$O, are playing an increasing role in presurgical planning and in intraoperative surgical guidance [15,51,52] (Plate 70.3; part (d) also shown in colour between pp. 670 and 671).

Multimodality imaging is used widely in image-directed surgery. CT, MRI, PET, SPECT and fMRI contain complementary anatomical and physiological information.

CT and MRI scans provide images of the anatomy of the patient. These have good spatial resolution, with MRI giving the best spatial resolution. Functional brain mapping gives information on the location of the main functional areas of the cortex (somatosensory, somatomotor and language) but this imaging has lower spatial res-

olution. The anatomical location of the functional abnormality can be determined with greater certainty by aligning the functional images with the anatomical images.

Thus, there are two main areas in which multimodality imaging has been used in the investigation and surgical treatment of patients with intractable epilepsy: for functional mapping as an aid to surgical planning and guidance and for localization of the seizure focus.

Functional cortical mapping can have an essential role in resections in eloquent areas of the brain, to assess the surgical risks to normal cortical function and thus to plan the extent of surgical resection. The lesions that cause epilepsy often distort normal cerebral functional anatomy [1]. However, the place of functional imaging as a replacement for intraoperative EEG, somatosensory evoked potentials and awake craniotomy and stimulation is still to be established. In theory, functional imaging has the advantage that it can be used for preoperative planning, the patient does not need to be awake, operation time is reduced and there is no need for interactive patient cooperation during the procedure.

The integration of functional imaging information can help to localize and delineate accurately the seizure focus [44,53,54]. This offers the surgeon an extensive and more precise stereotactic navigational map that can be used to guide the neurosurgeon safely, accurately and optimally to the focus, with little or no damage to normal brain tissue.

However, in most situations, SPECT presently offers little new information in terms of localizing seizure foci. And while PET and fMRI do have their proponents, they presently have no firm place in routine practice in most situations [1].

In the future, as techniques evolve and registration improves, the incorporation of SPECT [10,55,56], PET [52], fMRI [44,53,54], MRI spectroscopy [57–60] and magnetoencephalographic data [61] into the evaluation and surgical planning of an epilepsy patient may become routine [62–65].

Stereotactic surgery as an aid to conventional surgery

Diagnosis — depth electrodes and stereotactic EEG

The role of invasive electrophysiological monitoring using depth electrodes (and other methods such as subdural grid electrodes and epidural pegs) is diminishing [4]. These changes are due to the increasing ease with which the structural changes within the brain responsible for the epileptic phenomena can now be identified using multimodality imaging techniques.

Intraparenchymal EEG monitoring began with the stereoencephalographic method introduced by Talairach et al. [66] and has progressed through stereotactic angiography [67], CT-guided stereotactic techniques [68–70] to multimodal stereotactic imaging using CT, MRI, PET and angiography [71] (Fig. 70.4). As stereotactic imaging has improved, so has the safety of the procedure [72].

Thus, in 1974 Talairach et al. described 400 instances of 'stereoencephalographie' in 300 patients over a 14-year period; 20–30% of the patients studied were subsequently operated upon, of whom 80% had a good or worthwhile result. These authors were therefore using stereoencephalography as the routine by which to localize accurately the epileptic focus in all their surgical candidates. By 1993

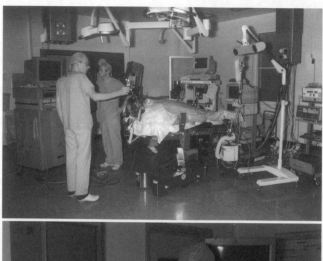

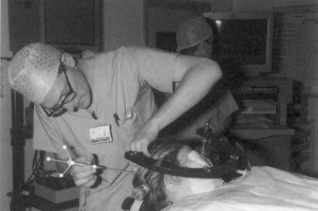

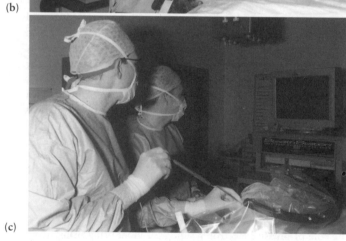

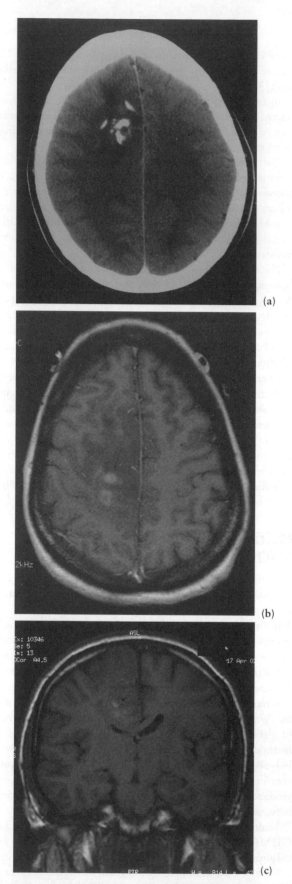

Fig. 70.3 Modern frameless stereotaxy. The Stealth neuronavigation system in use for tumour resection. (a) The patient's head must be fixed in Mayfield pins throughout the procedure. There must be unrestricted lines of sight between the exploratory probe and the camera receiver. (b) The fiducial points are carefully loaded into the computer so that image space can be accurately mapped to patient space. (c) The system is then ready for neuronavigation with a light-emitting diode probe. (d) The position of the probe tip is demonstrated relative to multiplanar pre-operative imaging enabling the margins of the lesion to be accurately delineated and an accurate trajectory taken (shown in colour between pp. 670 and 671).

Fig. 70.4 (a) CT, (b) axial and (c) coronal MRI of an epileptogenic, right-sided, calcified, posterior frontal tumour. Including functional MRI data from the right hand (d) into the image-guided operative data enabled the surgeon to know it was possible to resect the tumour anterior to the motor strip.

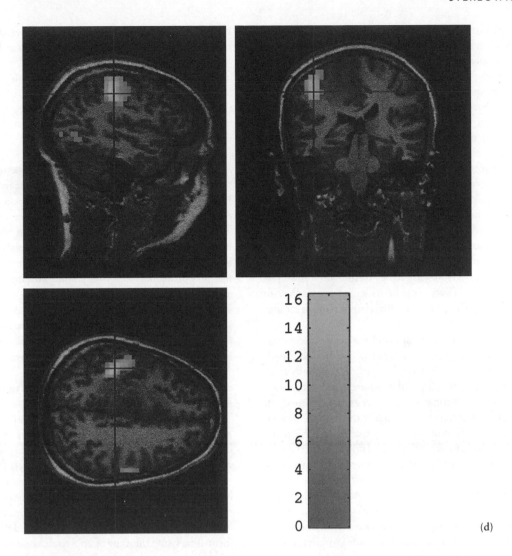

(d)

Fig. 70.4 *Continued.*

at the National Hospital for Neurology and Neurosurgery, London, UK, less than 10% of patients within the epilepsy surgery programme underwent depth electrode insertion [73]. This group [74,75] and others [22] have also described various computer-assisted methods to register the EEG epileptic focus accurately in stereotactic space, integrated both with MRI and CT.

Other non-invasive imaging modalities can also supply information traditionally obtained from depth studies. In Engel's study from UCLA [76], 153 cases were reviewed in which depth electrodes had been used alongside ictal telemetry and fluorodeoxyglucose (FDG)-PET. The conclusion drawn was that where PET and telemetry information were concordant (and this was the case in over 80% of patients), stereotactic EEG (i.e. EEG recordings from depth electrodes which can be localized highly accurately within the three-dimensional stereotactic space) did not supply further information that would have changed clinical management decisions.

With modern MRI protocols, depth electrode recording should be unnecessary in over 95% of patients with hippocampal sclerosis being evaluated for temporal lobe surgery [1].

Depth EEG records from otherwise functionally inaccessible cortex. Currently depth electrode implantation is used in three main

areas. First, to determine from which temporal lobe seizures are arising in patients with MRI evidence of bilateral hippocampal sclerosis. Secondly, to determine whether or not seizures are arising from the temporal lobe in patients in whom MRI shows dual pathology and the scalp EEG is indeterminate. Finally, it is used to localize the seizure discharge in patients with discordant MRI and functional data [1]. In this way, depth electrode studies continue to play a small but important defining role in the investigation of potential surgical candidates.

While depth electrode studies continue, they provide basic science with data concerning epilepsy. However, not only are other modern techniques perhaps more suitable for the investigation of the majority of surgical candidates, but depth electrode insertion also has the inherent disadvantage of being invasive and therefore not without risk.

In 1987, Van Buren [77] described the complications arising from 2674 electrode implantations from 14 centres in the pre-MRI era. There was no mortality, but there were 12 intracranial infections and seven intracranial haemorrhages with permanent neurological sequelae. In addition, there were two cases of Creutzfeldt–Jakob disease, where electrodes had been reused. Other groups have reported complications such as extra-axial haematoma and grid electrode placement within the white matter or within a cerebral sulcus [72]. One further disadvantage is expense, with each study costing at least £10 000 in the UK (including disposable platinum electrodes, 1–2 weeks' hospital stay with continuous telemetry, theatre time and other workforce implications). However, it is likely that invasive monitoring will retain a place in the minority of patients whose presentation is not straightforward but where it is worth considering surgical treatment.

Stereotactic neurosurgical techniques provide the means of performing such invasive monitoring as safely as possible. Using CT [73] or MRI [72,78] guidance, the desired position and trajectory of each electrode within the brain can be accurately calculated and insertion then safely performed. Occasionally, stereotactic angiography or MRA is integrated within the planning procedure in order to avoid major blood vessels during surgery. This is particularly useful where large numbers of electrodes are to be inserted into the anterior temporal region, sylvian fissure area or insular cortex, as the risk of haemorrhage is directly related to the number of electrodes inserted.

When investigating a possible temporal lobe onset of epileptiform activity most centres performing depth EEG studies have tended to use two to four temporal electrodes passed orthogonally from lateral to medial through the temporal neocortex and deep white matter to the hippocampal formation. Spencer et al. [79] however, generally pass just one electrode longitudinally through the temporal lobe from the posterior temporal region, in order to achieve the same end. The electrodes are not totally rigid, and although they can generally be placed to within 5 mm of the intended target, accuracy is inevitably limited by their flexible nature, and therefore it is advisable to check postoperatively the electrode positions that have actually been achieved. Although exact electrode position is not usually critical for recording purposes, it is essential that the neurophysiologist knows where they are placed in order to interpret the EEG correctly. Therefore, postoperative plain radiographs under stereotactic conditions or MRI may be performed. This makes it possible to determine the exact electrode position and then to translate this corrected position to the planning neuroradiological imaging modalities such as MRI and CT. The disposable platinum electrodes currently in use also have the added advantage of being MRI compatible, which allows postoperative MRI studies to be performed with the electrodes in situ.

Depth electrodes are still commonly placed with frame-based systems [72]. The added fixation and support that this provides is seen as its major advantage. However, exact electrode placement is less critical, and depth electrodes can be placed using a frameless technique, with the use of flexible guide arms to stabilize the drill and the electrode as it is advanced [80]. This technique can thus decrease the operative time and potential risks to the patient.

The advent of frameless image-directed systems has led relocatable head-frame devices to become obsolete in this regard [81,82].

Treatment

Stereotactic amygdalohippocampectomy

Although anterior temporal lobectomy remains the standard operation in most neurosurgical centres performing epilepsy surgery for hippocampal sclerosis, there is a trend towards more focal procedures (in part reflecting the neurosurgical trend towards minimally invasive surgery) [12].

Anterior temporal lobectomy is well tolerated, but sometimes leads to a bony defect, and atrophy of the temporalis muscle. Patients also experience discomfort after surgery whilst chewing. In addition, neurological deficits, including visual field defects, memory impairment and language problems have also been attributed to this approach [80].

The concept of a selective resection of the mesiobasal temporal structures was introduced by Niemeyer et al. in the mid-1950s [83]. He described a transcortical, transventricular approach through the second temporal gyrus to reach the hippocampus at the amygdala. Several methods have now been described for selective mesiobasal resections, on the basis that lateral neocortical resection is unnecessary for seizure control and can cause postoperative memory problems [79,84–92]. Some authors argue that the lateral aspect of the temporal lobe, which is typically normal on pathological evaluation, does not need to be resected. Furthermore, there is some evidence to suggest that resection of the lateral temporal structures may be responsible for postoperative neurological deficits, and only the mesial temporal structures harbour the epileptogenic focus [93]. It is suggested that stereotactic selective amygdalohippocampectomy can be used as an alternative to anterior temporal lobectomy.

Wieser and Yasargil [85,94] described a pterional trans-sylvian approach to the mesial temporal structures, which they suggested improved outcomes. Others use a trans-sulcal approach, usually between the middle and inferior temporal gyri [80,84]. When Kelly et al. initially described their technique for stereotactic amygdalohippocampectomy using the Compass stereotactic equipment [89], their approach was first via the occipital lobe and then suboccipitally because of the field defects which occurred through using the former route. Using this type of approach, the hippocampal formation is met along its axis and is entirely suitable for maximal resection. However, most authors have preferred the lateral approach in order to reach the anterior hippocampus and amygdala without damage to the posterior hippocampal structures. Inevitably there is some sacrifice of the lateral neocortical structures using the lateral approach, but much less than in a standard temporal lobe resection and without the risk of incurring visual field defects. Yasargil and others have also described selective amygdalohippocampectomy, but using solely microsurgical techniques and not stereotaxy [85,95].

In 1994, Olivier et al. [19] reported using the Viewing Wand (Elekta/ISG, Stockholm, Sweden) to perform selective mesial resections. The Montreal group successfully applied this device to selective mesial resections in a number of patients and found it useful not only in guiding the surgeon, but also in estimating the extent of the hippocampal resection. This paper also documented the successful use of this device in assisting lesionectomy, corpus callosotomy, neocortical resection and the placement of depth electrodes.

Because sulcal anatomy varies among individuals, frameless stereotactic guidance allows a small incision and craniotomy to be placed in the optimal location. This aids complete hippocampal resection through a key-hole approach. The image guidance and trajectory views are critical for gaining access to the temporal horn of the lateral ventricle and allowing visualization of the amygdala and hippocampus [96]. Successful surgery relies on adequate exposure. The most common mistake is inadequate inferior and anterior temporal exposure. The lower extent of the central sulcus must be reliably identified, and this is easily achieved with the aid of image guidance. On the dominant side, the cortical incision must be made in front of the central sulcus and preferably in front of the precentral sulcus. An errant trajectory can lead the surgeon to miss the temporal horn in the dissection through the white matter. A too anterior trajectory will pass by the anterior extent of the ventricle and a too dorsal one could lead into the insula or temporal stem [84]. The extent of resection is also demonstrated intraoperatively with the use of neuronavigation.

Neuropsychiatric evaluations performed after this minimally invasive procedure have documented no new language impairment [80]. Selective operations are more difficult technically and there is a higher reported risk of vascular disturbance and hemiplegia, but a lower risk of dysphasia and visual field defect [1]. Seizure control in these patients is encouraging [84,85,91,94], though so far not adequately studied.

Stereotactic craniotomy and lesionectomy

Perhaps the most common way in which stereotactic neurosurgery is currently utilized in the treatment of epilepsy is in the removal of epileptogenic lesions [97–100]. Many of those lesions that cause chronic epilepsy (as opposed to those high-grade brain tumours with a short history and mass effect, which have seizures as part of the clinical syndromes) are cortically based, small and would be difficult to find without some form of stereotactic image guidance.

Just as with tumours, certain vascular lesions (arteriovenous malformations (AVMs), cavernomas) may be difficult to localize if they are situated within deep brain structures. Stereotaxy may allow direct localization of the lesion as well as associated vascular structures feeding or draining the lesion. With AVMs, stereotaxy helps define both the superficial and deep limits of the nidus, and can help assure its complete removal [14].

Traditional frame-based stereotaxy has allowed stereotactic craniotomy to become a standard operation for epilepsy management, allowing epileptic lesions to be removed in minimally invasive ways (i.e. with 'mini' skull flaps and with minimal brain retraction, dissection and, hence, trauma). However, such methods are at odds with the techniques of traditional lesional epilepsy surgery where electrocorticography and cortical stimulation are employed with a view to *en bloc* resection of the surrounding cortex when this is considered to be epileptogenic. A basic principle of surgery for extratemporal neocortical epilepsy is that the wider the excision around an epileptic focus, the more likely complete seizure control will be achieved [1]. Clearly in this situation, a large craniotomy with a wide cortical exposure is necessary. Stereotactically guided lesionectomy therefore entails a simple lesionectomy without removal of surrounding brain tissue in an *en bloc* fashion. The comparative efficacy between simple lesionectomy and larger *en bloc* brain resections is currently controversial, and the issue must be considered unresolved at the present time [97,98,100–102]. Certainly, methods that maximize total lesion excision must be advantageous not only neuro-oncologically, but also in terms of seizure control.

In considering the practical surgical issues, when a lesion is ex-plored under the operating microscope following image guidance, a border between it and surrounding brain has to be determined. Sometimes direct inspection will reveal a clear-cut margin or even a pseudocapsule. However, on other occasions, the boundary will be less definite, and in these cases the trend is to remove more rather than to leave suspect or reactive tissue. Image-directed surgery can aid in directing this process.

A further diagnostic and also technical issue for the surgeon is the fact that a large proportion of lesions causing chronic epilepsy (cavernous angiomas, dysembryoplastic neuroepithelial tumours, low-grade gliomas) are poorly defined on CT and often visualized solely on MRI. In these instances image-directed surgery using MRI may be invaluable.

While we have detailed above specific instances where stereotaxy can be employed, its use may be applied to virtually all branches of epilepsy surgery. These include in addition non-lesional focal resections, multilobar resections (including hemispherectomy) and functional procedures such as multiple subpial transections and corpus callosectomy.

Stereotactic ablation and stimulation for epilepsy

Lesion-making in the CNS may be performed using a variety of methods which, except in one instance, require the opening of the skull, and the passage of some sort of needle into the brain substance. The actual method for producing focal brain necrosis can be chemical (absolute alcohol), freezing (using a cryoprobe) or by heating. Radiofrequency thermocoagulation is the most widely used method as it is flexible yet repeatable, and quick to use.

The one closed method of lesion-making in the CNS which is completely non-invasive (in a surgical respect at least, since there is a small but definite risk of radiation-induced necrosis of the surrounding normal brain) is stereotactic radiotherapy or radiosurgery (Plate 70.5, shown in colour between pp. 670 and 671).

Both stereotactic ablation and stimulation have been used for many years, in small numbers of patients, in an attempt to control or modify seizures. Targets have included the amygdala, various thalamic nuclei, the fields of Forel, the anterior commissure, the fornix and the posterior limb of the internal capsule [103–112].

While there are numerous articles in the literature describing stereotactic procedures in the management of epilepsy, analysis of these is complicated by a number of factors.

1 Most studies were done prior to the establishment of a uniform classification of seizures, making it difficult to determine the seizure disorder treated by a particular lesion.

2 Often multiple subcortical targets were used in individual patients, making it difficult to assess the role of a specific target for a specific condition.

3 There is sufficient variability in the location of subcortical nuclei with respect to internal reference points, so that in many cases it is uncertain whether unsuccessful surgery was a result of inaccurate localization, incomplete destruction or inappropriate selection of target.

4 There has been a tendency to reserve stereotactic surgery for particularly complex intractable seizure and behavioural problems. This philosophy may have eliminated some of the more straight-

forward disorders for which the procedures may have been more effective [93].

In 1970 Narabayashi and Mizutani [113] described the use of radiofrequency stereotactic amygdalotomy (i.e. a direct but very focal ablation of the epileptic focus) in 25 patients with 1–6 years follow-up. Some had unilateral and some bilateral lesions performed mainly for behavioural problems as the primary indication for surgery. Nine patients (36%) had complete abolition of EEG and clinical seizures, nine had reduction in seizures (36%) and seven had no change (28%). Several other authors have described their experience with stereotactic radiofrequency amygdalotomy [114–121].

Talairach and Szikla [122] used stereoencephalography to localize the amygdalohippocampal complex and then ablated these structures with yttrium-90. Fifteen cases were described in which an epileptic focus was ablated using stereotactically implanted yttrium-90 pellets to cause a localized necrotizing lesion. Pellets were routinely placed in the anterior commissure with the rationale of preventing spread to the contralateral temporal lobe. Using this regimen, nine patients were rendered seizure free (with short follow-up of 7–14 months), two were improved, while four showed no change.

There are few reports in the recent literature regarding stereotactic surgery for the treatment of epilepsy. Patil and Torkelson [123] described multiple interventions for epilepsy in 24 patients with seizures of multilobar origin. Their technique involved a combination of topectomy, multiple subpial transection and/or amygdalohippocampal radiofrequency ablation (amygdalohippocampotomy). Three of their patients with seizures of medial temporal origin underwent stereotactic amygdalohippocampotomy with good results (seizure free or rare seizures). This procedure involved CT-guided identification of the amygdala and hippocampus for stereotactic targeting. A radiofrequency lesion measuring 11×15 mm was then made in each of these structures [115].

Parrent and Blume [124] performed stereotactic amygdalotomy in 19 patients with temporal lobe epilepsy. All patients were shown to have mesial temporal originating seizures by continuous EEG monitoring ± subdural electrography, and all recorded seizures originated from the temporal lobe that was ultimately subject to the ablation. Surgical planning involved the identification of the amygdala and hippocampus on stereotactically acquired MRI scans, and postoperative MRI confirmed the accuracy of targeting. In five patients who underwent limited lesioning (mean 6.4 lesions, range 4–9) a favourable seizure outcome (defined as seizure free, auras only, or >90% seizure reduction) was obtained in only one patient (20%). However, 15 patients underwent extensive lesioning designed to produce a large confluent area of ablation (mean 26 lesions, range 12–54). In this group, nine (60%) achieved a favourable outcome and postoperative MRI demonstrated extensive ablation of the amygdala and hippocampus, sparing the parahippocampal gyrus.

The results of these operations have in general been disappointing, and this type of surgery has been, until recently, largely abandoned. The outcomes were not as good as one would expect following temporal lobectomy or selective amygdalohippocampectomy in a similar group of patients. Therapeutic success was unpredictable and often not without a significant risk of complications. Hence, the overall clinical impression of these procedures was that good outcomes were patchy, difficult to predict and the improvements not sustained.

Several strategies can be pursued with stereotactic and functional surgery. The first is to destroy the seizure focus in a minimally invasive manner. Such a targeted approach requires strong physiological evidence of the seizure focus together with as precise as possible anatomical delineation with modern imaging. A second strategy is to decrease the epileptogenic volume, in this way reducing seizure burden and, at least in theory, putting intrinsic brain mechanisms as well as antiepileptic drugs in a better position to deal with the epileptic tendency. A third use of stereotaxy is for the interruption of the pathways of seizure propagation. Because of the high precision of these techniques, discrete axonal projections can be interrupted, thereby disconnecting the seizure source from adjacent or remote brain structures. Further strategies that are possible with stereotactic neurosurgery are the destruction or modulation of brain structures which may have an influence on seizure tendency; thalamic lesioning/stimulation may reduce cortical excitability and thus epileptogenesis [125].

A recent resurgence of interest has occurred, encouraged by both the improved anatomical precision of stereotaxy made possible by MRI and better surgical stereotactic instrumentation, and also by the success of these procedures in other conditions, such as for Parkinson's disease and pain [126].

Traditionally, functional neurosurgery has relied upon frame-based stereotactic techniques. Recent developments in this field have included the incorporation of brain atlases and microelectrode recording devices into the registration of radiological data of image guidance systems to aid target identification.

The improvements in imaging have worked in concert with an increased understanding of the pathophysiology of epilepsy disorders, such that the identification and selection of targets has a stronger scientific rationale than was previously available. There is also research interest in the possibility of stem cell transplantation and stereotactic drug implantation [1]. The trend towards minimally invasive surgery has led to a re-examination of stereotactic functional procedures. Stereotactic procedures have the possibility of being highly accurate, more economical and better tolerated than conventional craniotomy and resective surgery.

Stereotactic radiosurgery

Radiosurgical techniques are used to create image-guided, physiological inactivity or focally destructive brain lesions without neurophysiological guidance [127]. They allow, in a single session, precise and complete destruction of chosen target structures containing healthy and/or pathological cells [128].

Leksell originally designed his gamma knife (in which multiple beams of gamma rays are focused to a single target using traditional stereotactic methods) for functional neurosurgery [129–131]. He realized that deep epileptic foci could become targets, especially with future advances in functional imaging.

At present, however, little functional radiosurgery is performed worldwide, probably less that 2% of all radiosurgical procedures, the vast majority of which are carried out for arteriovenous malformations, for benign tumours such as acoustic neuromas or in treatment of solitary cerebral metastases. The availability of high-quality, three-dimensional imaging with MRI (for precise targeting of normal structures), and evidence of some limitations regarding drug efficacy, has prompted a reappraisal of gamma knife surgery for functional disorders [132–137]. In the past decade, the number of studies in which radiosurgery has been described in experimental epilepsy and in clinical situations has increased significantly.

Heikkinen et al. [138] illustrated that although 16/29 AVM patients (55%) had improvement in their seizures following proton beam irradiation, only 17% of these demonstrated angiographic obliteration. Furthermore, 3/5 patients with complete obliteration, 5/7 partially obliterated and 8/17 non-obliterated patients became seizure free.

Between 1970 and 1984, Steiner et al. [139] treated 247 AVM patients with gamma knife surgery. Of the 247 patients, 59 had epilepsy. In the majority of these patients (52), their seizures improved significantly. The cessation of the seizures appeared to occur commonly several months prior to the occlusion of the arteriovenous malformation.

The Sheffield radiosurgical group have described the effect of radiosurgery on 160 of their 507 AVM patients who had been followed for 2 years [140]. In this group, 48 (30%) had epilepsy on presentation. On follow-up, 38% of these patients were seizure free, 22% had improved seizure control and 6% had increased seizures.

The results from most other centres performing radiosurgery for AVMs are similar, i.e. that radiosurgery to prevent rebleeding from AVMs does have some beneficial effect on seizures in a proportion of cases, and that the effect may well be independent of any obliteration of the AVM itself [139,141–144].

Cavernous haemangioma is a form of an arteriovenous malformation which most frequently presents with epilepsy [145]. Some authors have reported decreased bleeding after gamma knife surgery [146], while others have reported no effect [147,148]. Bartolomei et al. [149] conducted a retrospective multicentre study to evaluate the effectiveness of gamma knife radiosurgery in the treatment of drug-resistant epilepsy associated with cavernous haemangiomas. A total of 49 patients were studied (26 male and 23 female), with a mean age of 36 ± 10 years. The mean duration of epilepsy before gamma knife radiosurgery was 7.5 ± 9.3 years. The mean frequency of seizures prior to gamma knife radiosurgery was 6.9 episodes per month. The cavernous haemangioma was located in the temporal lobe in 23 cases, and in the extratemporal cortex in the remaining 26 cases. The mean margin dose to the lesion was 19.2 ± 4.4 Gy (range 11.3–36 Gy). The volume was 2370 ± 2211 mm^3 (range 110–10296 mm^3). No complications were reported on the day of the radiosurgical procedure. With a mean follow-up of 24 ± 13 months, 26 patients (53%) were seizure free (Engel class I). Of these, 24 patients were in class IA, and two patients with occasional auras in class IB. A highly significant decrease in the number of seizures was achieved in 10 patients (20%), and class IIB status. The remaining 13 patients (26%) showed little or no improvement in their seizures.

In the seizure-free group, the mean delay between gamma knife treatment and complete remission was 4 months (range from 0 to 9 months, median 6 months). This study demonstrated that the prognosis for seizure control depended on the type of epilepsy, and location of the cavernous haemangioma. The outcome was better for patients with simple partial seizures than for those with complex partial seizures. The location of the lesion was the most significant.

In the 14 patients whose lesion was located in the mesial temporal region, 12 showed a poor outcome of treatment. Lesions in the laterotemporal region were associated with a good outcome (six out of seven patients). A location in the central region was associated with an excellent outcome; all four patients in this group remained seizure free. For other locations, results were unpredictable. A possible explanation for the difference in prognosis is that the epileptic network in the medial temporal region is more complex and diverse and hence more difficult to ablate completely and accurately than in the extratemporal region and indeed in the more central regions.

The disappearance of seizures following conformal radiotherapy [150], and conventional radiotherapy [151,152], for tumours has also been reported.

In March 1993, Regis et al. [153] in Marseilles used gamma knife surgery to treat the first patient with medically refractory mesial temporal lobe epilepsy with hippocampal sclerosis. The group described that the entorhinoamygdalohippocampectomy was performed with the gamma knife at low marginal dose (25 Gy), a dose that later caused target necrosis. The 7000 mm^3 approximate volume represented the largest functional target irradiated until that time. This patient has remained seizure free with no associated complications.

This group has also studied the optimal parameters for the treatment of epilepsy without space-occupying lesions using the gamma knife [128,154]. In this study, they recruited seven patients, four male and three female who had medication-resistant mesial temporal lobe epilepsy. The mean duration of this disease was 27 years (range 16–35 years), and mean age at gamma knife surgery was 33 years (range 25–40 years). They used MRI for target localization. The mean calculated volume of the target was 6500 mm^3 (range 6350–6900 mm^3). According to the volume of the target, they used a dose margin of 25 Gy at the 50% isodose line. The range of patient follow-up was 24–61 months. There was a dramatic effect on seizure frequency around postoperative month 10 (range 8–15, mean 10.2). This was coincident with the development of MRI signal changes, and then atrophy in the related structures. All but one patient became seizure free. The authors suggested that there was a direct relationship between the quality of the results from gamma knife surgery and the dose and volume of the procedure.

In their current protocol, Regis et al. [155] describe the target being covered by two 18 mm collimators, with a dose of 20–25 Gy at the 50% marginal isodose line, the target volume being 6500–7000 mm^3. In this study, 25 patients were treated according to this protocol, and the follow-up of the entire group varied between 6 and 72 months. The median latency for seizure cessation was 10.5 months (range 6–21). Except for two patients who immediately became seizure free, the medial latency for aura cessation was 15.5 months. There was a gradual decrease in the frequency, intensity and duration of seizures in the other 23 patients. Low-dose steroids reduced reported side-effects, such as headaches, nausea and vomiting.

In 1994, Barcia-Salorio et al. [156] provided a long-term analysis of a series of 11 patients with temporal lobe epilepsy treated with stereotactic radiosurgery using a dose range of 10–20 Gy. Of these, five patients experienced complete cessation of seizures, and an additional five were improved. Seizures began to decrease gradually 3–12 months after radiosurgery. These authors noted that the main difficulty encountered was the correct localization of the epileptogenic focus.

Lindquist *et al.* [137] have also described the use of the gamma knife for the radiosurgical treatment of epilepsy. They report six patients with complex partial seizures, all of whom had a reduction in seizure frequency.

Heikkinen *et al.* [157] treated a single patient with temporal seizures by stereotactically irradiating the pes hippocampus. A lower radiation dose of 10 Gy was used and the MRI scan at 30 months showed no change to the radiated structures. Seizures ceased 7 months following treatment and had not recurred by 27 months.

In addition, there have been promising isolated reports for the use of radiosurgery to treat gelastic seizures associated with hypothalamic hamartomas [132,136,155] and to achieve a functional callosotomy in the management of Lennox–Gastaut syndrome [158].

Radiosurgery at doses that produce atrophy presumably works through destruction of the epileptogenic target. However, the mechanisms underlying the efficacy of lower dose radiosurgery is not known. This must involve changes in the neuronal network involved in seizure generation [93].

Potential advantages of stereotactic radiosurgery

1 No surgical incision.
2 Decreased morbidity and increased patient comfort.
3 High accuracy.
4 Accessibility of deep sites.
5 Potential efficacy in non-lesional surgery.
6 Single day stay in hospital.

Limitations of stereotactic radiosurgery

1 Delayed response.
2 Volume constraints.
3 Less predictable outcome than resective surgery.
4 Uncertain long-term effects.

The current evidence suggests that stereotactic radiosurgery can be effective in treating focal epilepsy. This form of treatment is closed, tractless and bloodless [159]. More importantly, the current advances in both diagnostic and functional imaging, and improvement of the therapeutic rationale (i.e. directing the radiosurgery towards the epileptogenic lesion itself rather than interrupting perceived pathways of seizure spread), may improve results further.

The optimal dose selection (necrotizing vs. non-necrotizing), methods for non-lesional epilepsy localization, and target volume for irradiation have still to be determined [127,133,135,160]. It is not known what type of tissue effect is required to stop the generation or propagation of seizures. Some studies have shown that low doses (below 20 Gy) are ineffective for the radiosurgical treatment of epilepsy [133,135]. On the other hand, high doses (as much as 100 Gy) can cause target necrosis and regional brain oedema [161].

Summary

Lesion-making in the CNS has a limited role at present, but it is anticipated that the use of stereotactic radiosurgery will become more

attractive in the future. Stereotactic lesioning in the medial temporal lobe has produced favourable results in a number of patients. However, the decrease in seizure frequency is not as dramatic as that following temporal lobectomy in properly selected cases. These techniques continue to undergo modification and will require further review in the future. The use of radiosurgery for lesion production is less invasive than radiofrequency ablation, and may prove to be safer. Radiosurgical trials in selected epileptic syndromes have shown highly promising although still preliminary results. If focal hippocampal (or any other brain tissue) irradiation can eliminate seizures without the need for complete tissue destruction, then radiosurgery will become an important therapy for patients with intractable epilepsy.

The future of frameless stereotaxy will include better registration techniques and more accurate positioning of the probe tips in space, and the integration of further functional imaging modalities. Video and heads-up displays within the surgical microscope will offer increasingly direct and accurate feedback to surgeons. The development of intraoperative imaging techniques will allow real-time anatomical updates to be performed to compensate for brain shifts associated with the surgical procedure. Intraoperative MRI will facilitate resection of abnormal brain tissue and brain tumours, by allowing residual tissue to be identified before closing the craniotomy.

The power of computers to generate three-dimensional renderings will also continue to improve. The inclusion of 'picture in a picture' technology in head-mounted displays will allow computer-generated three-dimensional images to be displayed adjacent to the surgeon's field of view, providing simultaneous projection of the surgical field and stereotactic images. The merging of CT, functional MRI, ultrasonography and MR spectroscopy into image-guided systems will allow neurosurgeons to treat increasingly complex lesions through smaller incisions [80].

Although stereotaxy and neuronavigation will never be a replacement for surgical skill, it is a powerful weapon in the armamentarium of contemporary neurosurgeons.

References

1 Shorvon SD. Surgical treatment of epilepsy. In: Shorvon SD, ed. *Handbook of Epilepsy Treatment*, 1st edn. Oxford: Blackwell Science, 2000: 195–226.
2 Clarke RH, Horsley V. On a method of investigating the deep ganglia and tracts of the central nervous system. *BMJ* 1906; 2: 1799–800.
3 Henn JS, Lemole GM, Gerber M, Spetzler RF. Theory and development of frameless stereotaxy. *BNI Q* 2001; 17(1): 4–15.
4 Diehl B, Luders HO. Temporal lobe epilepsy: When are invasive recordings needed? *Epilepsia* 2000; 41(3): S61–S74.
5 Cascino GD, Jack CR Jr, Parisi JE. Magnetic resonance imaging-based volume studies in temporal lobe epilepsy: pathological correlation. *Ann Neurol* 1991; 30: 31–6.
6 Jack CR Jr, Sharbrough FW, Cascino GD, Hirschorn KA, O'Brien PC, Marsh WR. Magnetic resonance imaging-based hippocampal volumetry: Correlation with outcome after temporal lobectomy. *Ann Neurol* 1992; 31: 138–46.
7 Cook MJ, Fish DR, Shorvon SD, Straughan K, Stevens JM. Hippocampal volumetric and morphometric studies in frontal and temporal lobe epilepsy. *Brain* 1992; 115 (Pt 4): 1001–15.
8 Jackson GD, Berkovic SF, Tress BM, Kalnins RM, Fabinyi GC, Bladin PF. Hippocampal sclerosis can be reliably detected by magnetic resonance imaging. *Neurology* 1990; 40(12): 1869–75.

9 Kuzniecky R, Burgard S, Faught E, Morawetz R, Bartolucci A. Predictive value of magnetic resonance imaging in temporal lobe epilepsy surgery. *Arch Neurol* 1993; 50(1): 65–9.

10 Cascino GD. Advances in neuroimaging: Surgical localization. *Epilepsia* 2001; 42(1): 3–12.

11 Shorvon SD. Magnetic resonance imaging in epilepsy: The central clinical research questions. In: Shorvon SD, Fish DR, Andermann F, Bydder GM, Stefan H, eds. *Magnetic Resonance Scanning and Epilepsy*, 1st edn. New York/London: Plenum Press, 1994.

12 Thomas DG, Kitchen ND. Minimally invasive surgery neurosurgery. *BMJ* 1994; 8(308): 126–8.

13 Kitchen ND, Thomas DG. In: Stereotactic craniotomy. Pell MF, Thomas DG, eds. *Handbook of Stereotaxy Using the CRW Apparatus*. Baltimore: Williams and Warwick, 1994: 81–92.

14 Lemole GM, Henn JS, Riina HA, Spetzler RF. Cranial applications of frameless stereotaxy. *BNI Q* 2001; 17(1): 16–24.

15 McDonald JD, Chong BW, Lewine JD *et al.* Integration of preoperative and intraoperative functional brain mapping in a frameless stereotactic environment for lesions near eloquent cortex. Technical note. *J Neurosurg* 1999; 90(3): 591–8.

16 De La Porte C. Technical possibilities and limitations of stereotaxy. *Acta Neurochir (Wien)* 1993; 124: 3–6.

17 McEvoy AW, Porter DG, Bradford R, Wright A. Intra-operative localisation of skull base tumours. A case report using the ISG viewing wand in the management of trigeminal neuroma. *Postgrad Med J* 1999; 75(879): 35–8.

18 Tanaka T, Olivier A, Hashizume K, Hodozuka A, Nakai H. Image-guided epilepsy surgery. *Neurol Med Chir (Tokyo)* 1999; 39: 895–900.

19 Olivier A, Germano IM, Cukiert A, Peters T. Frameless stereotaxy for surgery of the epilepsies: preliminary experience. Technical note. *J Neurosurg* 1994; 81(4): 629–33.

20 Brommeland T, Hennig R. A new procedure for frameless computer navigated stereotaxy. *Acta Neurochir (Wien)* 2000; 142(4): 443–7.

21 Lawton MT, Spetzler RF. Clinical experience with a frameless stereotactic arm in intracranial neurosurgery. In: Alexander EI, Maciunas RJ, eds. *Advanced Neurosurgical Navigation*. New York: Thieme, 1999: 321–2.

22 Otsubo H, Hwang PA, Hunjan A *et al.* Use of frameless stereotaxy with location of electroencephalographic electrodes on three-dimensional computed tomographic images in epilepsy surgery. *J Clin Neurophysiol* 1995; 12(4): 363–71.

23 Sandeman DR, Patel N, Chandler C, Nelson RJ, Coakham HB, Griffith HB. Advances in image-directed neurosurgery: preliminary experience with the ISG Viewing Wand compared with the Leksell G frame. *Br J Neurosurg* 1994; 8(5): 529–44.

24 Stapleton SR, Kiriakopoulos E, Mikulis D *et al.* Combined utility of functional MRI, cortical mapping, and frameless stereotaxy in the resection of lesions in eloquent areas of brain in children. *Pediatr Neurosurg* 1997; 26(2): 68–82.

25 Barnett GH, Kormos DW, Steiner CP, Weisenberger J. Use of a frameless, armless stereotactic wand for brain tumor localization with two-dimensional and three-dimensional neuroimaging. *Neurosurgery* 1993; 33(4): 674–8.

26 Barnett GH, Kormos DW, Steiner CP, Weisenberger J. Intraoperative localization using an armless, frameless stereotactic wand. Technical note. *J Neurosurg* 1993; 78(3): 510–14.

27 Dorward NL, Alberti O, Palmer JD, Kitchen ND, Thomas DG. Accuracy of true frameless stereotaxy: in vivo measurement and laboratory phantom studies. Technical note. *J Neurosurg* 1999; 90(1): 160–8.

28 Germano IM, Villalobos H, Silvers A, Post KD. Clinical use of the optical digitizer for intracranial neuronavigation. *Neurosurgery* 1999; 45(2): 261–9.

29 Drake JM, Prudencio J, Holowaka S, Rutka JT, Hoffman HJ, Humphreys RP. Frameless stereotaxy in children. *Pediatr Neurosurg* 1994; 20(2): 152–9.

30 Ryan MJ, Erickson RK, Levin DN, Pelizzari CA, Macdonald RL, Dohrmann GJ. Frameless stereotaxy with real-time tracking of patient head movement and retrospective patient-image registration. *J Neurosurg* 1996; 85(2): 287–92.

31 Elias WJ, Chadduck JB, Alden TD, Laws ER, Jr. Frameless stereotaxy for transsphenoidal surgery. *Neurosurgery* 1999; 45(2): 271–5.

32 Kato A, Yoshimine T, Hayakawa T *et al.* A frameless, armless navigational system for computer-assisted neurosurgery. Technical note. *J Neurosurg* 1991; 74(5): 845–9.

33 Hall WA, Liu H, Martin AJ, Pozza CH, Maxwell RE, Truwit CL. Safety, efficacy, and functionality of high-field strength interventional magnetic resonance imaging for neurosurgery. *Neurosurgery* 2000; 46(3): 632–41.

34 Rubino GJ, Farahani K, McGill D, Van De Wiele B, Villablanca JP, Wang-Mathieson A. Magnetic resonance imaging-guided neurosurgery in the magnetic fringe fields: the next step in neuronavigation. *Neurosurgery* 2000; 46(3): 643–53.

35 Gering DT, Nabavi A, Kikinis R *et al.* An integrated visualization system for surgical planning and guidance using image fusion and an open MR. *J Magn Reson Imaging* 2001; 13(6): 967–75.

36 Staubert A, Vester M, Tronnier VM *et al.* Interventional MRI-guided brain biopsies using inductively coupled surface coils. *Magn Reson Med* 2000; 43(2): 278–83.

37 Tyler D, Mandybur G. Interventional MRI-guided stereotactic aspiration of acute/subacute intracerebral hematomas. *Stereotact Funct Neurosurg* 1999; 72 (2–4): 129–35.

38 Seifert V, Zimmermann M, Trantakis C *et al.* Open MRI-guided neurosurgery. *Acta Neurochir (Wien)* 1999; 141(5): 455–64.

39 Zimmermann M, Seifert V, Trantakis C *et al.* Open MRI-guided microsurgery of intracranial tumours. Preliminary experience using a vertical open MRI-scanner. *Acta Neurochir (Wien)* 2000; 142(2): 177–86.

40 Steinmeier R, Fahlbusch R, Ganslandt O *et al.* Intraoperative magnetic resonance imaging with the magnetom open scanner: concepts, neurosurgical indications, and procedures: a preliminary report. *Neurosurgery* 1998; 43(4): 739–47.

41 Lunsford LD, Kondziolka D, Bissonette DJ. Intraoperative imaging of the brain. *Stereotact Funct Neurosurg* 1996; 66(1–3): 58–64.

42 Koivukangas J, Louhisalmi Y, Alakuijala J, Oikarinen J. Ultrasound-controlled neuronavigator-guided brain surgery. *J Neurosurg* 1993; 79(1): 36–42.

43 Nakajima S, Atsumi H, Kikinis R *et al.* Use of cortical surface vessel registration for image-guided neurosurgery. *Neurosurgery* 1997; 40(6): 1201–8.

44 Roux FE, Boulanouar K, Ibarrola D, Berry I. Role pratique de l'IRM fonctionnelle en neurochirurgie. [Practical role of functional MRI in neurosurgery]. *Neurochirurgie* 2000; 46(1): 11–22.

45 Binder JR, Swanson SJ, Hammeke TA *et al.* Determination of language dominance using functional MRI: a comparison with the Wada test. *Neurology* 1996; 46(4): 978–84.

46 Worthington C, Vincent DJ, Bryant AE *et al.* Comparison of functional magnetic resonance imaging for language localization and intracarotid speech amytal testing in presurgical evaluation for intractable epilepsy. Preliminary results. *Stereotact Funct Neurosurg* 1997; 69(1–4 Pt 2): 197–201.

47 Benson RR, FitzGerald DB, LeSueur LL *et al.* Language dominance determined by whole brain functional MRI in patients with brain lesions. *Neurology* 1999; 52(4): 798–809.

48 Detre JA, Maccotta L, King D *et al.* Functional MRI lateralization of memory in temporal lobe epilepsy. *Neurology* 1998; 50(4): 926–32.

49 Righini A, de Divitiis O, Prinster A *et al.* Functional MRI: primary motor cortex localization in patients with brain tumors. *J Comput Assist Tomogr* 1996; 20(5): 702–8.

50 Lundquist P, Backlund EO, Sjoqvist L. Letter. *J Neuroimaging* 1997; 2(2): 131–3.

51 Duncan JD, Moss SD, Bandy DJ *et al.* Use of positron emission tomography for presurgical localization of eloquent brain areas in children with seizures. *Pediatr Neurosurg* 1997; 26(3): 144–56.

52 Achten E, Santens P, Boon P *et al.* Single-voxel proton MR spectroscopy and positron emission tomography for lateralization of refractory temporal lobe epilepsy. *Am J Neuroradiol* 1998; 19(1): 1–8.

53 Jackson GD, Connelly A, Cross JH, Gordon I, Gadian DG. Functional magnetic resonance imaging of focal seizures. *Neurology* 1994; 44(5): 850–6.

54 Warach S, Ives JR, Schlaug G *et al.* EEG-triggered echo-planar functional MRI in epilepsy. *Neurology* 1996; 47(1): 89–93.

55 Swartz BE, Halgren E, Delgado-Escueta AV *et al.* Neuroimaging in pa-

tients with seizures of probable frontal lobe origin. *Epilepsia* 1989; 30(5): 547–58.

56 O'Brien TJ, So EL, Mullan BP *et al.* Subtraction ictal SPECT co-registered to MRI improves clinical usefulness of SPECT in localizing the surgical seizure focus. *Neurology* 1998; 50(2): 445–54.

57 Mendes-Ribeiro JA, Soares R, Simoes-Ribeiro F, Guimaraes ML. Reduction in temporal *N*-acetylaspartate and creatine (or choline) ratio in temporal lobe epilepsy: does this ¹H-magnetic resonance spectroscopy finding mean poor seizure control? *J Neurol Neurosurg Psychiatr* 1998; 65(4): 518–22.

58 Garcia PA, Laxer KD, van der Grond J, Hugg JW, Matson GB, Weiner MW. Proton magnetic resonance spectroscopic imaging in patients with frontal lobe epilepsy. *Ann Neurol* 1995; 37(2): 279–81.

59 Stanley JA, Cendes F, Dubeau F, Andermann F, Arnold DL. Proton magnetic resonance spectroscopic imaging in patients with extratemporal epilepsy. *Epilepsia* 1998; 39(3): 267–73.

60 Cendes F, Caramanos Z, Andermann F, Dubeau F, Arnold DL. Proton magnetic resonance spectroscopic imaging and magnetic resonance imaging volumetry in the lateralization of temporal lobe epilepsy: a series of 100 patients. *Ann Neurol* 1997; 42(5): 737–46.

61 Rezai AR, Hund M, Kronberg E *et al.* The interactive use of magnetoencephalography in stereotactic image-guided neurosurgery. *Neurosurgery* 1996; 39(1): 92–102.

62 Bergstrom M, Kumlien E, Lilja A, Tyrefors N, Westerberg G, Langstrom B. Temporal lobe epilepsy visualized with PET with 11C-L-Deuterium-deprenyl – analysis of kinetic data. *Acta Neurol Scand* 1998; 98(4): 224–31.

63 Zubal IG, Spencer SS, Imam K, Seibyl J, Smith EO, Wisniewski G, Hoffer PB. Difference images calculated from ictal and interictal technetium-99m-HMPAO SPECT scans of epilepsy. *J Nucl Med* 1995; 36(4): 684–9.

64 Kuzniecky R, Hugg JW, Hetherington H *et al.* Relative utility of ¹H spectroscopic imaging and hippocampal volumetry in the lateralization of mesial temporal lobe epilepsy. *Neurology* 1998; 51(1): 66–71.

65 Holopainen IE, Valtonen ME, Komu ME *et al.* Proton spectroscopy in children with epilepsy and febrile convulsions. *Pediatr Neurol* 1998; 19(2): 93–9.

66 Talairach J, Bancaud J, Szikla G, Bonis A, Geier S, Vedrenne C. [New approach to the neurosurgery of epilepsy. Stereotaxic methodology and therapeutic results. 1. Introduction and history]. *Neurochirurgie* 1974; 20(1): 1–240.

67 Olivier A, Marchand E, Peters T *et al.* Depth electrode implantation at the Montreal Neurological Institute and Hospital. In: Engel J Jr, ed. *Surgical Treatment of the Epilepsies*, 1st edn. New York: Raven Press, 1987: 595–601.

68 Agbi C, Polkey CE. Calculation of coordinates for depth electrodes placed in temporal lobe structures visualized by oblique CT scan cuts. *Br J Neurosurg* 1990; 4(6): 517–21.

69 Lunsford LD, Latchaw RE, Vries JK. Stereotactic implantation of deep brain electrodes using computed tomography. *Neurosurgery* 1983; 13(3): 280–6.

70 Peters TM, Olivier A. CT aided stereotaxy for depth electrode implantation and biopsy. *Can J Neurol Sci* 1983; 10(3): 166–9.

71 Levesque MF, Zhang JX, Wilson CL *et al.* Stereotactic investigation of limbic epilepsy using a multimodal image analysis system. Technical note. *J Neurosurg* 1990; 73(5): 792–7.

72 Ross DA, Brunberg JA, Drury I, Henry TR. Intracerebral depth electrode monitoring in partial epilepsy: The morbidity and efficacy of placement using magnetic resonance image-guided stereotactic surgery. *Neurosurgery* 1996; 39(2): 327–34.

73 Kratimenos GP, Thomas DGT, Shorvon SD, Fish DR. Stereotactic insertion of intracerebral electrodes in the investigation of epilepsy. *Br J Neurosurg* 1993; 7: 45–52.

74 Lemieux L, Leduc A. Equivalent source estimation based on the calculation of the electric field from depth EEG data. *IEEE Trans Biomed Eng* 1992; 39(8): 805–17.

75 Lemieux L, Lester S, Fish D. Multimodality imaging and intracranial EEG display for stereotactic surgery planning in epilepsy. *Electroencephalogr Clin Neurophysiol* 1992; 82(6): 399–407.

76 Engel J Jr, Henry TR, Risinger MW *et al.* Presurgical evaluation for partial epilepsy: relative contributions of chronic depth-electrode recordings versus FDG-PET and scalp-sphenoidal ictal EEG. *Neurology* 1990; 40(11): 1670–7.

77 Van Buren JM. Complications of surgical procedures in the diagnosis and treatment of epilepsy. In: Engel J Jr, ed. *Surgical Treatment of Epilepsies*, 1st edn. New York: Raven Press, 1987: 465–75.

78 Pillay PK, Barnett G, Awad I. MRI-guided stereotactic placement of depth electrodes in temporal lobe epilepsy. *Br J Neurosurg* 1992; 6: 47–54.

79 Spencer DD, Spencer SS, Mattson RH, Williamson PD, Novelly RA. Access to the posterior medial temporal lobe structures in the surgical treatment of temporal lobe epilepsy. *Neurosurgery* 1984; 15(5): 667–71.

80 Gerber M, Henn JS, Manwaring K, Smith KA. Application of frameless stereotaxy to minimally invasive neurosurgery. *BNI Q* 2001; 17(1): 28–32.

81 Gill SS, Thomas DGT. A relocatable frame. *J Neurol Neurosurg Psychiatr* 1989; 52: 1460–1.

82 Kitchen ND, Thomas DGT. The GTC repeat stereotactic localiser. In: Pell MF, Thomas DGT, eds. *Handbook of Stereotaxy Using the CRW Apparatus*, 1st edn. Baltimore: Williams and Warwick, 1994: 171–8.

83 Neimeyer P. The transventricular amygdalohippocampectomy in temporal lobe epilepsy. In: Baldwin N, Bailey P, eds. *Temporal Lobe Epilepsy*. Springfield, Illinois: CC Thomas, 1958: 461–82.

84 Olivier A. Transcortical selective amygdalohippocampectomy in temporal lobe epilepsy. *Can J Neurol Sci* 2000; 27(S1): S68–S76.

85 Yasargil MG, Teddy PJ, Roth P. Selective amygdalohippocampectomy: operative anatomy and surgical technique. In: Symon L, ed. *Advances and Technical Standards in Neurosurgery*, 12th edn. New York: Springer, 1985: 93–123.

86 Hori T, Tabuchi S, Kurosaki M, Kondo S, Takenobu A, Watanabe T. Subtemporal amygdalohippocampectomy for treating medically intractable temporal lobe epilepsy. *Neurosurgery* 1993; 33(1): 50–6.

87 Kim HI, Olivier A, Jones-Gotman M, Primrose D, Andermann F. Corticoamygdalectomy in memory-impaired patients. *Stereotact Funct Neurosurg* 1992; 58(1–4): 162–7.

88 Dinner DS, Luders H, Lesser RP. Relationship of memory changes after temporal lobectomy and extent of resection. *Neurology* 1986; 36: 294–5.

89 Kelly PJ, Sharbrough FW, Kall BA, Goerss SJ. Magnetic resonance imaging-based computer-assisted stereotactic resection of the hippocampus and amygdala in patients with temporal lobe epilepsy. *Mayo Clin Proc* 1987; 62(2): 103–8.

90 Nayel MH, Awad IA, Luders H. Extent of mesiobasal resection determines outcome after temporal lobectomy for intractable complex partial seizures. *Neurosurgery* 1991; 29(1): 55–60.

91 Kitchen ND, Thomas DGT, Thompson PJ, Shorvon SD, Fish D. Open stereotactic selective amygdalohippocampectomy: indications, methods and results. *Epilepsia* 1993; 34(6): 105.

92 Goldstein LH, Polkey CE. Short-term cognitive changes after unilateral temporal lobectomy or unilateral amygdalo-hippocampectomy for the relief of temporal lobe epilepsy. *J Neurol Neurosurg Psychiatr* 1993; 56(2): 135–40.

93 Parrent AG, Lozano AM. Stereotactic surgery for temporal lobe epilepsy. *Can J Neurol Sci* 2000; 27(S1): S79–S84.

94 Wieser HG, Yasargil MG. Selective amygdalohippocampectomy as a surgical treatment of mesiobasal limbic epilepsy. *Surg Neurol* 1982; 17(6): 445–57.

95 Siegel AM, Wieser HG, Yasargil GM. Relationships between MR-imaged total amount of tissue removed, resection scores of specific mediobasal limbic subcompartments and clinical outcome following selective amygdalohippocampectomy. *Epilepsy Res* 1990; 6(1): 56–65.

96 Gerber M, Smith KA. Frameless stereotaxy and minimally invasive neurosurgery. *BNI Q* 2001; 17(1): 33–4.

97 Cascino GD, Kelly PJ, Hirschorn KA, Marsh WR, Sharbrough FW. Stereotactic resection of intra-axial cerebral lesions in partial epilepsy. *Mayo Clin Proc* 1990; 65(8): 1053–60.

98 Cascino GD, Kelly PJ, Sharbrough FW, Hulihan JF, Hirschorn KA, Trenerry MR. Long-term follow-up of stereotactic lesionectomy in partial epilepsy: predictive factors and electroencephalographic results. *Epilepsia* 1992; 33(4): 639–44.

99 Davis DH, Kelly PJ. Stereotactic resection of occult vascular malformations. *J Neurosurg* 1990; 72(5): 698–702.

100 Kitchen ND, Thompson PJ, Fish D, Shorvon SD, Harkness W, Thomas DGT. Neuropsychological sequelae after temporal neocortical lesionectomy: comparison with temporal lobectomy. *Epilepsia* 1993; 34(6): 71.

101 Yeh HS, Kashiwagi S, Tew JM Jr, Berger TS. Surgical management of epilepsy associated with cerebral arteriovenous malformations. *J Neurosurg* 1990; 72(2): 216–23.

102 Piepgras DG, Sundt TM, Ragoowansi AT, Stevens L. Seizure outcome in patients with surgically treated cerebral arteriovenous malformations. *J Neurosurg* 1993; 78(1): 5–11.

103 Jelsma RK, Bertrand CM, Martinez SN, Molina-Negro P. Stereotaxic treatment of frontal-lobe and centrencephalic epilepsy. *J Neurosurg* 1973; 39(1): 42–51.

104 Ojemann GA, Ward AA Jr. Stereotactic and other procedures for epilepsy. *Adv Neurol* 1975; 8: 241–63.

105 Gillingham FJ, Watson WS, Donaldson AA, Cairns VM. Stereotactic lesions for the control of intractable epilepsy. *Acta Neurochir (Wien)* 1976; 23 (Suppl.): 263–9.

106 Jinnai D, Mukawa J, Kobayashi K. Forel-H-tomy for the treatment of intractable epilepsy. *Acta Neurochir (Wien)* 1976; 23 (Suppl.): 159–65.

107 Mundinger F, Becker P, Groebner E, Bachschmid G. Late results of stereotactic surgery of epilepsy predominantly temporal lobetype. *Acta Neurochir (Wien)* 1976; 23 (Suppl.): 177–82.

108 Yoshii N. Follow-up study of epileptic patients following Forel-H-tomy. *Appl Neurophysiol* 1977; 40(1): 1–12.

109 Yap JC, Ramani SV. Stereotaxic treatment of seizure disorder. *J Clin Psychiatr* 1978; 39(3): 199–203.

110 Ganglberger JA. Additional new approach in treatment of temporal lobe epilepsy. *Acta Neurochir (Wien)* 1984; S33: 149–54.

111 Umbach W. Long-term results of fornicotomy for temporal epilepsy. *Confin Neurol* 1966; 27: 121–3.

112 Shi YC. Long-term follow-up stereotactic destruction of Forel's field-H in the treatment of intractable epilepsy. *Acta Neurochir (Wien)* 1992; 117: 112.

113 Narabayashi H, Mizutani T. Epileptic seizures and the stereotaxic amygdalotomy. *Confin Neurol* 1970; 32(2): 289–97.

114 Meyer CHA, Hitchcock ER. Radiofrequency amygdalotomy for aggressive behaviour and epilepsy. *Acta Neurochir (Wien)* 1992; 117: 111.

115 Patil AA, Andrews R, Torkelson R. Stereotactic volumetric radiofrequency lesioning of intracranial structures for control of intractable seizures. *Stereotact Funct Neurosurg* 1995; 64(3): 123–33.

116 Schwab RS, Sweet WH, Mark VH, Kjellberg RN, Ervin FR. Treatment of intractable temporal lobe epilepsy by stereotactic amygdala lesions. *Trans Am Neurol Assoc* 1965; 90: 12–19.

117 Heimburger RF, Small IF, Milstein V, Moore D. Stereotactic amygdalotomy for convulsive and behavioural disorders. *Appl Neurophysiol* 1978; 41: 43–51.

118 Vaernet K. Stereotaxic amygdalotomy in temporal lobe epilepsy. *Confin Neurol* 1972; 34(1): 176–83.

119 Flanigin HF, Nashold BS. Stereotactic lesions of the amygdala and hippocampus in epilepsy. *Acta Neurochir (Wien)* 1976; 23 (Suppl.): 235–9.

120 Mempel E, Witkiewicz B, Stadnicki R et al. The effect of medial amygdalotomy and anterior hippocampotomy on behavior and seizures in epileptic patients. *Acta Neurochir Suppl (Wien)* 1980; 30: 161–7.

121 Nadvornik P, Sramka M, Gajdosova D, Kokavec M. Longitudinal hippocampectomy. A new stereotaxic approach to the gyrus hippocampi. *Confin Neurol* 1975; 37(1–3): 245–8.

122 Talairach J, Szikla G. Destruction partielle amygdalohippocampique par l'yttrium 90 dans le traitement de certaines epilepsies rhinencephalique. *Neurochirurgie* 1965; 11: 233–40.

123 Patil AA, Torkelson AR. Minimally invasive surgical approach for intractable seizures. *Stereotact Funct Neurosurg* 1995; 65: 86–9.

124 Parrent AG, Blume WT. Stereotactic amygdalohippocampotomy for the treatment of medial temporal lobe epilepsy. *Epilepsia* 1999; 40: 1408–16.

125 Morillo LE, Ebner TJ, Bloedel JR. The early involvement of subcortical structures during the development of a cortical seizure focus. *Epilepsia* 1972; 13: 579–608.

126 Fisher RS, Uthman BM, Ramsey RE, Engel J Jr. Alternative surgical techniques for epilepsy. In: Engel J Jr, ed. *Surgical Treatment of the Epilepsies.* New York: Raven Press, 1993: 549–64.

127 Kondziolka D. Functional radiosurgery. *Neurosurgery* 1999; 44(1): 12–22.

128 Regis J, Bartolomei F, Rey M et al. Gamma knife surgery for mesial temporal lobe epilepsy. *Epilepsia* 1999; 40(11): 1551–6.

129 Leksell L. Cerebral radiosurgery. I. Gammathalanotomy in two cases of intractable pain. *Acta Chir Scand* 1968; 134(8): 585–95.

130 Leksell L. Sterotaxic radiosurgery in trigeminal neuralgia. *Acta Chir Scand* 1971; 137(4): 311–14.

131 Leksell L. Stereotactic radiosurgery. *J Neurol Neurosurg Psychiatr* 1983; 46(9): 797–803.

132 Dunoyer C, Ragheb J, Resnick T et al. The use of stereotactic radiosurgery to treat intractable childhood partial epilepsy. *Epilepsia* 2002; 43(3): 292–300.

133 Cmelak AJ, Abou-Khalil B, Konrad PE, Duggan D, Maciunas RJ. Low-dose stereotactic radiosurgery is inadequate for medically intractable mesial temporal lobe epilepsy: a case report. *Seizure* 2001; 10(6): 442–6.

134 Kurita H, Suzuki I, Shin M et al. Successful radiosurgical treatment of lesional epilepsy of mesial temporal origin. *Minim Invasive Neurosurg* 2001; 44(1): 43–6.

135 Kawai K, Suzuki I, Kurita H, Shin M, Arai N, Kirino T. Failure of low-dose radiosurgery to control temporal lobe epilepsy. *J Neurosurg* 2001; 95(5): 883–7.

136 Unger F, Schrottner O, Haselsberger K, Korner E, Ploier R, Pendl G. Gamma knife radiosurgery for hypothalamic hamartomas in patients with medically intractable epilepsy and precocious puberty. Report of two cases. *J Neurosurg* 2000; 92(4): 726–31.

137 Lindquist C, Kihlstrom L, Hellstrand E. Functional neurosurgery – a future for the gamma knife? *Stereotact Funct Neurosurg* 1991; 57(1–2): 72–81.

138 Heikkinen ER, Konnov B, Melnikov L et al. Relief of epilepsy by radiosurgery of cerebral arteriovenous malformations. *Stereotact Funct Neurosurg* 1989; 53(3): 157–66.

139 Steiner L, Lindquist C, Adler JR, Torner JC, Alves W, Steiner M. Clinical outcome of radiosurgery for cerebral arteriovenous malformations. *J Neurosurg* 1992; 77(1): 1–8.

140 Sutcliffe JC, Forster DMC, Walton L, Dias PS, Kemeny AA. Untoward clinical effects after stereotactic radiosurgery for intracranial arteriovenous malformations. *Br J Neurosurg* 1992; 6: 177–86.

141 Betti OO, Munari C, Rosler R. Stereotactic radiosurgery with the linear accelerator: treatment of arteriovenous malformations. *Neurosurgery* 1989; 24(3): 311–21.

142 Colombo F, Benedetti A, Pozza F, Marchetti C, Chierego G. Linear accelerator radiosurgery of cerebral arteriovenous malformations. *Neurosurgery* 1989; 24(6): 833–40.

143 Steinberg SK, Fabrikant JI, Marks MP. Stereotactic heavy-charged-particle Bragg-peak radiation for intracranial arteriovenous malformations. *N Engl J Med* 1990; 323: 96–101.

144 Lunsford LD, Kondziolka D, Flickinger JC et al. Stereotactic radiosurgery for arteriovenous malformations of the brain. *J Neurosurg* 1991; 75(4): 512–24.

145 Marraire JN, Awad IA. Intracranial cavernous malformations: lesion behaviour and management strategies. *Neurosurgery* 1995; 37: 605.

146 Kondziolka D, Lunsford LD, Flickinger JC, Kestle JR. Reduction of hemorrhage risk after stereotactic radiosurgery for cavernous malformations. *J Neurosurg* 1995; 83(5): 825–31.

147 Weil S, Tew J, Steiner L. Comparison of radiosurgery and microsurgery for the treatment of cavernous malformations of the brainstem. *J Neurosurg* 1995; 75: 32–9.

148 Karlsson B, Kihlstrom L, Lindquist C, Ericson K, Steiner L. Radiosurgery for cavernous malformations. *J Neurosurg* 1998; 88(2): 293–7.

149 Bartolomei F, Regis J, Kida Y et al. Gamma knife radiosurgery for epilepsy associated with cavernous hemangiomas: a retrospective study of 49 cases. *Stereotact Funct Neurosurg* 1999; 72 (Suppl. 1): 22–8.

150 Barcia Salorio JL, Roldan P, Hernandez G, Lopez GL. Radiosurgical treatment of epilepsy. *Appl Neurophysiol* 1985; 48(1–6): 400–3.

151 Rogers L, Morris H, Lupica K. Effect of cranial irradiation on seizure frequency in adults with low-grade astrocytoma and medically intractable epilepsy. *Neurology* 1993; 43: 1599–601.

152 Whang CJ, Kwon Y. Long-term follow-up of stereotactic gamma knife

radiosurgery in epilepsy. *Stereotact Funct Neurosurg* 1996; 66(S1): 349–56.

153 Regis J, Peragui JC, Rey M *et al.* First selective amygdalohippocampal radiosurgery for 'mesial temporal lobe epilepsy'. *Stereotact Funct Neurosurg* 1995; 64 (Suppl. 1): 193–201.

154 Regis J, Roberts DW. Gamma knife radiosurgery relative to microsurgery: Epilepsy. *Stereotact Funct Neurosurg* 1999; 72(S1): 11–21.

155 Regis J, Bartolomei F, Hayashi M, Roberts D, Chauvel P, Peragut JC. The role of gamma knife surgery in the treatment of severe epilepsies. *Epileptic Disord* 2000; 2(2): 113–22.

156 Barcia-Salorio JL, Barcia JA, Hernandez G, Lopez-Gomez L. Radiosurgery of epilepsy. Long-term results. *Acta Neurochir Suppl (Wien)* 1994; 62: 111–13.

157 Heikkinen ER, Heikkinen MI, Sotaniemi K. Stereotactic radiotherapy instead of conventional epilepsy surgery. A case report. *Acta Neurochir (Wien)* 1992; 119(1–4): 159–60.

158 Pendl G, Eder H, Schroettner O, Leber K. Corpus callosotomy with radiosurgery. *Neurosurgery* 1999; 45: 303–8.

159 Kitchen ND. Experimental and clinical studies on the putative therapeutic efficacy of cerebral irradiation (radiotherapy) in epilepsy. *Epilepsy Res* 1995; 20: 1–10.

160 Kondziolka D, Lunsford LD, Witt TC, Flickinger JC. The future of radiosurgery: Radiobiology, technology, and applications. *Surg Neurol* 2000; 54: 406–14.

161 Hadjipanayis CG, Levy EI, Niranjan A *et al.* Stereotactic radiosurgery for motor cortex region arteriovenous malformations. *Neurosurgery* 2001; 48(1): 70–6.

71 Complications of Epilepsy Surgery

C.E. Polkey

Epilepsy surgery involves invasive procedures during presurgical assessment as well as definitive surgical procedures; therefore the complications arising from all these procedures, which may involve disciplines other than neurosurgery, have to be considered. The precise definition of a complication is difficult; with certain procedures it is known that physical side-effects are inevitable and these will be described, as complication in addition to those that are unexpected. In addition, procedures such as craniotomy carry general complications, for example haemorrhage and infection, and these will be dealt with briefly. Except where relevant, I will not deal with more distant possible effects, such as DVT and pulmonary embolus. It should also be realized that certain groups may be at greater risk. In particular, major procedures in young children carry additional hazards. The relevant literature suggests that there are no additional risks in the older age group, generally more than 50 years old, although it is unusual to operate over the age of 60 years.

Complications of invasive procedures for presurgical assessment

The procedures with significant complications are the intracarotid sodium amytal (ISA) test and the insertion of intracranial electrodes. The electrode insertions themselves can be divided into minor and major electrode insertions.

ISA test

In the most usual and simplest form of the ISA test, the internal carotid arteries are cannulated via the femoral artery, the usual technique for cerebral angiography. This test is relatively safe, with complication rates of 1–3% for transient neurological complications and permanent neurological change in 0.1–0.3% [1]. The incidence is likely to be lower in patients undergoing presurgical assessment because in general they are young and free of arterial disease. Recent papers describing the standard ISA do not mention complications. For theoretical reasons, the standard test was thought to be unsatisfactory for assessing speech and memory, but not for looking for bilateral secondary synchrony. Therefore selective amytal tests, where smaller arteries are catheterized, have been described. Borchgrevinck *et al.* in Oslo suggested that catheterization of the middle cerebral trunk was more satisfactory [2]. Jack *et al.* first described selective catheterization of posterior cerebral branches, but this has given rise to some complications [3,4]. There are no problems described with an alternative procedure used by Wieser in Zurich [5]. In our unit over the last 25 years, we have performed at least 250 standard amytal tests with very little morbidity

and no mortality. One patient, aged 42, developed a mild paraparesis, which recovered over some months and was thought to be due to the dislodging of an atheromatous plaque from the lumbar aorta. In the same group there were five patients (<2%), in whom there was evidence of a mild hemiparesis that recovered within 2–36 h. They were all treated with steroids but not with anticoagulants.

Testing for bilateral secondary synchrony may require large amounts of intravenous barbiturate anaesthetic, even to the point of producing a silent EEG. There should be careful consultation with the anaesthetist about the care and monitoring of these patients, and especially their airway, during the test and recovery.

Invasive procedures for placing electrodes

Recording and documenting seizures by videotelemetry, irrespective of the electrodes used, can be troublesome. Constraints of time and finance usually make it necessary to reduce the patient's antiepileptic medication, or even remove it completely. This can result in secondary generalization of seizures, serial seizures and occasionally status epilepticus. Confusion, for which the patient can be amnesic, or occasionally a postictal psychosis, which may require treatment in addition to the restoration of antiepileptic medication, can accompany these.

To avoid repetition, it is convenient to discuss two other points of general interest. There is still a great deal of uncertainty about imaging intracranial electrodes with MRI. Most departments will refuse to examine patients with MRI who have steel or nichrome electrodes in place. Zhang *et al.* have shown that there is no undue heating of these electrodes in a 1.5-T MRI [6] and the Yale group have reported a substantial series in which no complications have been observed [7]. We have successfully used MRI to image platinum-based electrodes without any apparent difficulty. Our neuroradiologists examine plain X-rays to assess the proximity of electrodes and the possibility of their crossing before the MRI is performed. The second problem is the possibility of introducing diseases such as Creutzfeldt–Jakob disease, as was reported with the re-use of electrodes in 1977 [8]. The only way to avoid this is never to re-use the electrodes.

Minor invasive techniques

There are three minor invasive techniques used: sphenoid electrodes, epidural peg electrodes and foramen ovale electrodes. Although subtemporal strip electrodes are relatively minor, since they involve direct access to the subdural space they have been included in the 'major invasive techniques' section.

Sphenoidal electrodes

These are effectively extracranial electrodes and serious complications are rare.

Epidural peg electrodes

These are not commonly used. Pilcher *et al.* quote a personal report by Wylie in which bacterial colonization was seen in 22%, a haematoma on CT in one patient and two patients were rendered sufficiently anaemic to need a blood transfusion [9].

Foramen ovale electrodes

These are placed through the foramen ovale, and therefore through the fibres of the trigeminal nerve, to lie in the subarachnoid space in the ambient cistern. The method was introduced by Wieser [10] and taken up by a number of other groups. We have used this method in over 200 patients. The technique used is important; most centres regularly use smooth multicontact electrodes for this method inserted through an appropriate needle. The possible complications include nerve damage during insertion, haemorrhage within the subdural or subarachnoid space, usually of no significance, and misplacement of the electrode within the cerebral substance and infection. In our patients the commonest problems were facial swelling and transient pain or numbness in the trigeminal territory. This is related to the number of placements and the experience of the operator. In our patients, there were a small number, less than 2%, who were left with permanent numbness in trigeminal territory and only one with persistent facial pain. Misplacement of the electrodes is difficult to diagnose; the alignment of the electrode along a curved course, following the floor of the middle fossa, suggests correct placement, whereas a straight course suggests the electrode may have entered the cerebral substance. We have only noted penetration of the brain with clinical consequences on four occasions, two with serious consequences. In one case there was a disorder of eye movement, which recovered completely, and in the other there was a capsular haemorrhage which resulted in a permanent hemiparesis. Wieser *et al.* reported transient perioral dysaesthesia in 9% of patients, one case of pontine haemorrhage and one subarachnoid haemorrhage [11]. Schuler *et al.* have reported serious consequences in patients who have undergone previous temporal surgery [12]. There have been unpublished anecdotal reports of death and avulsion of the trigeminal nerve from use of this technique. We have had five cases of frank meningitis including one of unsuccessful insertion, all of which responded to appropriate treatment. Wyllie reports two cases of infection in 32 patients, in a survey by Pilcher *et al.* [9].

Major invasive techniques

Electrodes are placed within the subdural space, or within the cerebral substance (depth electrodes), or using combinations of both methods. These electrodes are used chiefly for recording but may also be used for stimulation. Provided the parameters of current and voltage are controlled, there are no known permanent consequences of such stimulation. Goldring and Gregorie have described the use of epidural mats [13].

Subdural electrodes

Most centres now use commercial electrodes for these investigations. They are well made, flexible and manufactured from platinum. Vast numbers of configurations are available, from strips containing only four contacts in-line to large arrays of 8×8 with a total of 64 contacts. The complications increase with increasing size and number of contacts, and duration of implantation. In all patients with indwelling electrodes, we have used antibiotic cover, usually with cefuroxime 750 mg twice daily, from the time of insertion until at least 24 h after removal.

In recent years we have preferred subdural strip electrodes to foramen ovale electrodes because the minor complication rate is less and the coverage of the temporal structures is more flexible. We have used these electrodes in over 100 bilateral implantations and have only encountered one problem. This was an acute subdural haematoma probably arising from rupture of a bridging vein associated with coughing and vomiting during recovery from anaesthetic. Regrettably the patient was left with a significant neurological deficit. Wyler *et al.* report no such complications in 300 cases [14]. Stephan *et al.* report one silent subdural haematoma in 49 patients implanted with strip electrodes [15].

More complications arise when larger subdural mats are used. Ninety-three patients have been implanted in our centre with 20, 32 or 64 contact mats and significant complications were seen in 22 patients (23.6%). The commonest complication was infection which was seen in 12 patients (12.9%); there was transient neurological deterioration in seven patients (7.5%) and significant subdural haematomas in only two patients (2.1%). The origin of the changes induced in the underlying brain by subdural grids is complex. Stephan *et al.* report a picture of aseptic meningitis which is severe in 27% [16]. Local cerebral swelling can be a problem, especially in patients who have been previously operated at that site, and in whom tedious dissection of adhesions has been necessary. Most of the infection is local within the wound, invariably in the extradural space, and clear meningitis or encephalitis has not been seen. The likelihood of infection increases with prolonged implantation, which should therefore be kept to a minimum. Swartz *et al.* in 1996 reported expected adverse events, including fever, CSF leakage, nausea and headache, in 41% of patients and unexpected in 5% [17].

Intracranial depth electrodes

Centres using these electrodes report an infection rate of about 2%. In 1993 Pilcher *et al.* reported 1.4% in 1582 patients pooled from eight centres [9].

The risk of haemorrhage depends upon the technique, which determines the direction of track and the structures at risk, and also the number of electrodes used. Insertion techniques use three routes, the orthogonal, axial and the posterior approach. In the orthogonal approach, especially around the insula in the temporal lobe, the major vessels are at risk and some groups insist that angiography is necessary. The axial approach tends to pass through areas which have fewer major vessels. The posterior approach, devised by Spencer, has produced visual field defects [18]. Data from Pilcher *et al.* in 1993, suggested that the orthogonal approach (1–2%) was safer than the axial approach (2–3%) possibly because of the use of angiography [9]. Clinically significant haematoma arose in three of our 57 patients (5.2%). However with changes of technique and materials, our risk has diminished to those described by other groups.

It would be logical to suppose that the complications of depth electrode insertion would relate to the number of electrodes implanted and therefore some groups, notably Van Veelen *et al.*, have used a combination of subdural and depth electrodes and report no complications in 28 patients [19].

Summary

Presurgical evaluation has both physical and intellectual complications generally proportional to the invasiveness of the techniques. They are also dependent upon the experience of the centre and our complication rate has improved with time. In general there are no deaths reported from presurgical evaluation procedures. Significant physical complications occur with more complex interventions in less than 5% of cases and the general level is 1–3%.

Therapeutic procedures

Most candidates for epilepsy surgery are free of chronic or severe medical problems. A high proportion of these procedures is intracranial and is therefore subject to the usual complications of craniotomy. In brief, and except where detailed under the individual procedures, they comprise haematomas (extradural, subdural and intracerebral), infection, possibly hydrocephalus and rarely air embolism and pulmonary embolism. These complications usually respond to appropriate treatment and do not usually influence the outcome of the surgery.

In modern epilepsy surgery operative mortality is commendably low. Typical figures from pooled data presented in 1993 and from an International League Against Epilepsy survey suggest a mortality between 0.5% and 1% with some centres having no deaths at all [9,20]. In a long series of patients from Vellore there were no deaths since 1960 [21], and in a series of 654 procedures from Sweden between 1990 and 1995 there was only one death from haematoma [22]. In the King's/Maudsley series from 1976 to 2001 there have been 818 procedures resulting in seven perioperative deaths (0.86%) and 20 late deaths (2.4%). These are detailed in Table 71.1. The late deaths were associated with seizures in 15 patients (75%); although most of these had poor postsurgical seizure control (Engel group 4A in 60%), there were six patients in group 1A who died during their first postoperative seizure, in some cases in the course of antiepileptic drug reduction.

The incidence of infection is relatively low, estimated at around 0.5% by Pilcher and Rusyniak [23]. In our series it is commoner when intracranial monitoring has been used. Occasionally the patient appears to have meningitis or a meningitic reaction, but more commonly the infection occurs in the extradural space, often involving the bone flap. Although there may be evidence of it in the immediate postoperative period, it can take months or even years to declare itself. Once established it will not be controlled until all the dead tissue and foreign material has been removed. It has been much less common in our patients since the use of absorbable deep sutures (Vicryl) and prophylactic antibiotics. If the mastoid air cells are uncovered in the course of a craniotomy for temporal lobectomy it is important to cover them immediately with a patch of pericra-

nium. No patient in our series has died or come to permanent harm from intracranial infection; it does not appear to affect the seizure outcome of the operation, but the misery it can cause to all parties should not be underestimated.

Intracranial resective surgery

In addition to the general neurosurgical complications described, it is necessary to examine the particular problems associated with specific resections; these generally produce physical neurological deficit, changes in intellectual ability or psychiatric morbidity. For this purpose we will divide specific resections into frontal, temporal, parietal and central, occipital resections and major resections and hemispherectomy. Where appropriate, reference will be made to additional complications from operating in the dominant hemisphere. The avoidance of complications by careful subpial dissection of the cortex (possibly using the Cavitron ultrasonic aspirator, or CUSA), and proper respect for the blood supply, arterial and venous, with skeletalization, are essential.

It is appropriate at this point to mention a rare complication of craniotomy involving the use of vacuum drains. In two patients, one undergoing anatomical hemispherectomy and the other a selective amygdalohippocampectomy by the trans-sylvian route, excessive pressure was inadvertently applied to the subgaleal drain. This caused traction on the brainstem across the tentorial hiatus, resulting in sudden and profound hypotension. In the first patient this resulted in a watershed infarct in the remaining hemisphere.

Frontal lobe resection

These are mostly unilateral frontal lobe resections; as far as I am aware bifrontal resections for epilepsy are rarely done. Proper technique should ensure no damage to the medial surface of the remaining hemisphere or its blood supply. Even with formal resection it is theoretically possible to avoid damage to the olfactory tract. Unless the resection encroaches upon the gyrus anterior to the precentral gyrus in a non-dominant hemisphere it is unlikely to produce any hemiparesis. In the dominant hemisphere the region of Broca's area must be respected and Comair *et al.* recommended that such resections should be carried out under local anaesthesia [24]. Cognitive effects, even with large resections, can be difficult to detect but have been described. However, the complications such as specific memory loss seen after bifrontal insults for other reasons are not seen in these patients. Likewise, provided the remaining frontal lobe is healthy, the gross personality changes seen with frontal lobe disease do not occur. The lack of gross intellectual and psychiatric complications from frontal lobe resections probably depends upon normal function in the remaining frontal lobe, but may also be illusory in that the number of patients undergoing frontal lobe surgery is small and the patients are seldom submitted either preoperatively or postoperatively to intellectual or psychiatric tests of sufficient complexity to reveal subtle deficits. Studies on our patients have revealed that they are impaired on an adaptation task [25], are poor on the use of strategy [26] and on changing from one dimension to another [27].

Table 71.1 Immediate and late deaths in 818 therapeutic operations for epilepsy at Maudsley/King's College Hospital 1976–2001

Age	Operation	Elapsed time	Seizure status	Cause of death
		Immediate deaths		
8 months	FL	Immediate	Not applicable	Air embolus
50	VNS	2 weeks	Not applicable	Pneumonia
51	TL	Immediate	Not applicable	Cerebral oedema
43	TL	2 weeks	Not applicable	Cerebral haemorrhage after anti-coagulation for DVT
30	ACS	1 week	Not applicable	Pneumonia
40	THSP	2 months	Not applicable	Chronic sepsis
17	THSP	Immediate	Not applicable	Cerebral oedema
		Late deaths		
22	TL	4 years	1A	Unclear—died in police custody
54	TL	5 years	4A	Seizure
41	TL	2 years	1A	Seizure
25	FR	10 years	4A	Seizure
23+	TL	6+years	3A	Seizure
25	SHSP	4 years	3A	Seizure—late Rasmussen's disease
29	TL	6 years	4A	Seizure
26	AHE	5 years	1A	Seizure
31	TL	11 years	1A	Seizure
32	TL	2 years	3A	Seizure
25	TL	0.5 years	1A	Seizure
19	TL	2 years	1A	Road accident
25	TL	3 years	4A	Status
21	TL	1 years	2A	Suicide
54	TL	17 years	3A	Natural causes
26	TL	8 years	4A	Unclear
36	TL	7 years	4A	Seizure
31	TL + VNS	9 years	4A	Seizure
28	Occipital resection	0.42 years	4A	Seizure
30	TL	8 years	3A	Seizure

ACS, anterior callosal section; AHE, anterior hippocampal excision; FL, frontal lobectomy; FR, frontal resection; SHSP, selective hemispherectomy; THSP, total hemispherectomy; TL, temporal lobectomy; VNS, vagal nerve stimulation.

Temporal lobe resections

Mortality and non-neurological morbidity

Peroperative mortality is low; in the latest review it is put at less than 1% with some centres such as MNI reporting no deaths in 526 cases [23]. In our own series there have been only two postoperative deaths in 451 operations since 1976 (0.44%), one patient developed a deep vein thrombosis and then haemorrhaged as a result of anticoagulant therapy and another patient had unexplained cerebral oedema at the end of uneventful surgery with no apparent cause at autopsy. Other non-neurological complications are acceptably low and perhaps the commonest is postoperative infection which was estimated at 0.5% in the Second Palm Desert Symposium [23]. Rare complications include distant haemorrhage in the cerebellum [28] and a middle fossa cyst causing raised pressure [29]. Seizures have also been described in the immediate postoperative period in about 20% of patients. If such seizures were similar to the preoperative ones, then they were of poor prognostic significance, otherwise not [30].

Late mortality following temporal lobe surgery is a different matter. Jensen notes that there is an excess mortality among those with chronic epilepsy, around 59.4 deaths per 1000 patients, and that suicide was a common cause of death in this group [31]. However, although the early postoperative deaths in the operated patients were low, there were 50 late deaths in 2282 patients, 21.9 per 1000 or around 2%; 31 of these were either suicide or epilepsy related, and these patients tended to be those who had not benefited from surgery. Taylor and Marsh reporting on the deaths in Falconer's series noted that there had been 37 deaths in 193 patients (19%) and 23 of these deaths were either in circumstances which related to epilepsy, or by suicide, half the suicides occurring in patients who were seizure free [32]. We investigated the survival status of 299 patients, from 305 consecutive temporal lobectomies, at the Maudsley Hospital. There were 20 late deaths (6.7%), six were sudden and unexpected (SUDEP). Both the overall death rate, one per 136 person-years (SMR 4.5) and the SUDEP rate, one per 455 person-years, were lower than those expected for a population with chronic epilepsy. There was excess mortality of patients who underwent right-sided resections for mesial temporal sclerosis [33].

Neurological sequelae

The neurological sequelae of temporal lobe resections are now acceptably low. Lesionectomy and neocortical removal is least likely to produce such problems so long as the superior temporal gyrus is respected. The sequelae of combined neocortical and deep removal and of selective mesial resections are similar and, on the whole, since the inception of temporal lobe surgery the complication rate has fallen. There is no point in a detailed history of this except to note that resection of the insular cortex was found at an early stage, by the MNI, to run a high risk of hemiparesis; this was called manipulation hemiplegia, because it probably resulted from manipulation of branches of the middle cerebral artery, without any increased improvement in seizure control [34]. The commonest neurological lobe resection complications are: a contralateral hemiparesis or hemiplegia, a contralateral visual field defect or a homolateral third nerve palsy or paresis. Pooled results, summarized in Table 71.2, are available from the two Palm Desert Symposia [23,35]. The hemiplegia or hemiparesis must be related mainly to vascular causes, especially in selective mesial resections, although the vascular injury is seldom apparent intraoperatively. In our series of temporal lobe resections the incidence was 2% in 400 operations, virtually all right-sided. In combined resections the risk varies between zero and 1–2%, being lower in larger series, and in selective amygdalohippocampectomy, the risk varies between less than 0.5% in the Zurich series to 4% in our series, and two transient hemiparesis (3.2%) in Renella's series [36].

Falconer and Wilson showed that the relationship between the length of a temporal lobe resection and the subsequent visual field cut was due to the course of the visual fibres around the temporal horn [37]. Such visual field defects relate to the disruption of the fibres in the roof of the temporal horn. Katz et al. in their analysis of postoperative MRI scans showed that the more lateral the resection the more likely it was to produce a deficit although there was no close correlation between the size of the resection and the severity of the visual field defect [38]. The size of the defect cannot be predicted with resections of less than 7.5 cm [23]. Spencer et al.'s extended

Table 71.2 Complications of temporal lobe resection — pooled data

Complication	1987[a]	1993[b]
Transient hemiparesis	0.7%	4%
Permanent hemiparesis	0.7%	<2%
IIIrd nerve palsy		<1%
Complete hemianopia	0.6%	3%
Speech disturbance	0.37%	2%
Non-neurological	1.4%	
Mortality	0.47%	<1%

[a] From [35].
[b] From [23].

lobectomy does not produce more visual field defects than the standard operation [39]. In our series, a complete field defect occurred in 12 operations among 440 (2.3%). A recent paper from Manji and Plant reports any field defect in about 50% of 24 patients with at least 24% failing the driving test criteria. This occurred in three patients who were seizure free [40].

Intellectual sequelae

This is a very complex matter which relates to the nature of the underlying pathology in the temporal lobe and the type of resection performed. The second Palm Desert Symposium reported that global amnesia was less than 1% [23]; the matter is reviewed in more detail in the same volume by Dodrill et al. [41].

A number of studies have shown that patients with predominantly unilateral sclerotic lesions of the temporal lobe tend to suffer less change in their intellectual performance as a result of anterior temporal lobectomy than those with other pathology or non-specific changes in the temporal lobe [42]. Ojemann and Dodrill have described the mapping of verbal memory under local anaesthesia at surgery in order to limit verbal memory loss (see Chapter 69) [43]. It was hoped that when selective amygdalohippocampectomy was introduced this would minimize the intellectual sequelae of temporal lobe resection. Renella noted slight deterioration in all aspects of intellectual performance in his small group of patients when they had left-sided operations, and the converse following right-sided operations [36]. Wieser notes that two main factors influenced improvement: the first was when the non-operated side subserved the function and the second was freedom from seizures [44]. The same findings as Renella are reported later by Wieser and suggest that right-sided operations result in an improvement in learning and memory whereas left-sided operations have the opposite effect [45]. Awad et al., using a method of quantitative analysis of postresection MRI scans, attempted to correlate resection with intellectual changes [39]. In contrast to Ojemann's experience they were unable to correlate the extent of lateral cortical resection with memory loss in the dominant temporal lobe, but the decrease in verbal memory correlated with the extent of resection in the mesial and basal quadrants, and a similar correlation was found with non-verbal memory and right-sided resections [38]. This is consistent with the earlier descriptions of material-specific deficits by Milner in 1958 [46]. We studied 42 patients undergoing either amygdalohippocampectomy or temporal lobectomy; all were left hemisphere dominant [47]. The side and type of operation were approximately equal. If seizures persisted, then there was a poor performance in the material-specific tasks performed by the target temporal lobe, a finding in line with those reported by others. It was also found that selective amygdalohippocampectomy had less effect on the functions of the target temporal lobe than anterior temporal lobectomy but the converse was true of the non-target temporal lobe. The patients in our series with non-specific changes in the resected specimen and persisting seizures is too small for formal analysis, but it is our impression that they all suffer considerable deterioration in cognitive function after operation, as suggested by Wieser [44]. A paper from Oxford suggests that there may be a cognitive advantage to selective amygdalohippocampectomy in the dominant hemisphere [48]. A comparison between the effects of neocortical excision alone, anterior temporal resection and selective amygdalohippocampectomy by the Zurich method concluded that disconnection of the mesial and lateral temporal structures resulted in a similar functional deficit [49].

Psychiatric consequences and social outcome

Behavioural changes in patients undergoing temporal lobe surgery are well documented, but the patient usually benefits from the surgery. The exception is psychotic illness, which may occur after temporal lobectomy.

Psychosis supervening on chronic epilepsy is usually a late event. Temporal lobe surgery, at any rate resective surgery, can produce a schizophreniform psychosis often associated with left-sided resections or a depressive illness more often associated with right-sided operations. In early series of temporal lobe resections the incidence of schizophreniform illness was relatively high, 12–15% [50]. In more recent studies, the incidence has been much lower, in our series around 2–3%. The connection with left-handed females with alien tissue lesions described by Taylor and Bruton [51] has not been generally confirmed although Andermann *et al.* recently reported similar findings in a population of patients with ganglioglioma [52]. Mace and Trimble note that both left-sided and right-sided operations may be followed by psychosis [53]. *De novo* postictal psychosis is described in 5.3% of 57 Finnish patients [54]. In a wider survey of patients with intractable epilepsy the most prevalent disorder was anxiety disorder (10.7%); a schizophreniform psychosis occurred in only 4.3% [55]. However in temporal lobe patients, it was only 1.3% [56].

A depressive illness following temporal lobe surgery is commoner, does not necessarily occur immediately after surgery and may require careful questioning to elicit the symptoms. Patients subjected to temporal lobe surgery already have a predisposition to suicide. In our own material suicide is relatively rare, one known case in 400 operations, but depression is much commoner; an informal survey suggests around 35% of patients, almost exclusively in non-dominant, usually right-sided resections. We have found it is rare after amygdalohippocampectomy and in children, although one 12-year-old child with a large resection developed clinical depression requiring treatment. Paradiso *et al.* put the incidence of depression in their 70 patients as 34% and found it was underrecognized and undertreated [57].

Central and parietal resections

Any resection from the central area, that is the primary motor or sensory area, must carry some risk of loss of their function, and this risk is related to the underlying pathology, which may have already produced a disability or displaced the cortex away. It is now possible to identify the motor and sensory cortex in the context of both normal and abnormal cortices. The sophisticated use of structural MRI has also enabled surgeons to distinguish lesions that are distinct from cortex, or displace it, from those which involve cortex or may contain functioning tissue. The central cortex can now be identified reliably on MRI both visually and using the callosal reference system and AC–PC coordinates [58]. Finally, functional MRI has now become more widespread and accurate. It has been verified in comparisons with transcranial magnetic stimulation [59] and anatomical criteria [60]. The gold standard of mapping by stimulation during chronic intracranial recording [14], or during surgery, has also been used for comparison.

In spite of these precautions unexpected deficits can occur. Although these could be due to wrong identification of the primary areas, it may also occur if secondary vascular damage takes place because an artery or vein passing through a resected area is damaged, a mechanism postulated by Olivier and Awad [58]. In the same review Olivier and Awad note that when there is no voluntary hand movement, position sense is absent and there is paresis of the lower limb, then the whole central area can be resected. It should be noted that it is equally important to identify the postcentral gyrus in order to avoid profound proprioceptive loss in the hand or arm which can be more disabling than pure motor loss. However in the resection of discrete lesions there may be no deficit or the deficit may be transient. The Paris group has described the outcome from frontocentral area resections. In a detailed review of 120 patients they note that 40% of patients were unchanged immediately after surgery and there was a minor defect in 15.8%, but in the remainder (44.2%) there was either a monoparesis or a major hemiplegia. At 1 year or more there was significant improvement or no change in 67.5%, a mild disability in 10% and an additional severe disability in 22.5% [61]. In another report describing 57 patients, there were eight patients in whom there was a discrete lesion; three of these underwent lesionectomy and the remaining five a corticectomy. There were mild deficits in only two of these patients [62]. Sandok and Cascino reported similar findings describing one monoparesis among 14 patients who underwent stereotactic lesionectomy in the peri-rolandic region [63]. In the dominant hemisphere resections from the posterior temporal/parietal region run the risk of receptive aphasia, dyslexia, dysgraphia and dyscalculia. For this reason resections from these areas are usually avoided.

Occipital resections

Occipital resections are rare and there are three series in the literature, the largest number of patients being 42. Recently Curatolo *et al.* have reported the use of intraoperative photic driving to identify central visual cortex; they describe two patients in whom they were able to preserve the central visual field [64]. In two series, it is noted that there were already preoperative visual field defects, 56% in one series [65] and 59% in the other [66]. In the second series the visual field defect was complete in all these patients and five others acquired a defect, also complete, making the overall incidence after operation of 76%. Bidzinksi *et al.* also noted that a complete occipital resection always produced some visual field defect [67]. However two patients undergoing occipital lesionectomy described by Cascino *et al.* had no defect [68]. Williamson *et al.* noted that most patients adapted to their visual field defect within 1 year of surgery [65]. However, persisting field defects with loss of central vision may be a disabling consequence.

Major resections

These are defined as resections which involve more than one anatomical lobe. The creation of such a space within the cranial cavity does not itself create any special problems, although the patients tend to be more constitutionally ill and cerebrally irritable postoperatively than those undergoing lesser resections. As far as the creation or persistence of neurological deficits, especially limb dysfunction such as hemiparesis or hemi-sensory loss, visual field defects or deterioration of speech function, is concerned, this is often related to the original pathology which may have produced such defects in any event. By and large they can only be judged for each individual patient, but with one exception they are unlikely to be substantially increased by the resection. The exception is any form of cortical dysplasia or hemimegalencephaly-type syndrome where function may be preserved in the presence of a severe epileptic disorder.

Hemispherectomy

Although hemispherectomy is a serious operation it is likely that the mortality rate of 6–8% quoted at the Second Palm Desert Symposium [9] probably includes series of patients operated upon over a long period of time; more recent series do not have such mortality. In a review of 333 patients by Holthausen et al., perioperative mortality was 1.5% [69]. In our own series of 53 operations there has been one immediate postoperative death (1.9%), Villemure et al. quote 4.8% for functional hemispherectomy and Delalande 1.9% for hemispherotomy [70].

It is impossible to discuss this topic without some reference to the various techniques available, which are aimed at reducing serious side-effects, and the underlying pathology, which determines the extent of the additional damage inflicted by the surgery. In practice patients coming to hemispherectomy or equivalent operation fall into three groups. First those with a major hemispheric insult at a very early age which is not progressive. Examples of this are *in utero* vascular occlusion and the consequences of a major venous thrombosis. These patients usually have a complete infantile hemiplegia and average to low cognitive function. Their neurological status is usually unchanged by surgery and their cognitive function can be unchanged or improved [71]. The second group are those with Rasmussen's disease [72] where the hemiplegia may not be complete and there may be no visual field defect. Furthermore because of the late onset, especially when the dominant hemisphere is involved, there may be irreversible cognitive changes, which are worsened by the surgery [73]. Lastly there is the group of patients with hemimegalencephaly where further deterioration may occur but is less likely than with Rasmussen's disease.

Complications with regard to technique relate to the difficulties of such a major operation in infants and young children and to the fate of the large space created. In infants and young children problems may arise with regard to blood loss which, even if the operation is conducted carefully, can be sufficient to require transfusion. The worst problem is venous bleeding which can be torrential and difficult to control in the short term. The position of the head is a compromise between too much elevation which risks air embolism and too little which increases venous pressure making haemostasis more difficult to secure. Two simple manoeuvres can help. The first is to ensure that all veins draining into major venous sinuses are divided close to the cortex leaving a suitable stump to coagulate, if the initial coagulation is not secure, and minimizing the risk of tearing the sinus. The second is to take particular care in the posterior dissection around the tentorium where tributaries may lead into the great vein of Galen or straight sinus. There is also a theoretical possibility that manoeuvres to control severe bleeding from the superior sagittal sinus could lead to thrombosis of this sinus although I have not seen it personally.

There are a number of variants of hemispherectomy which were devised to overcome the well-documented consequences of anatomical hemispherectomy as described by Krynauw [74]. However, the complications of haemosiderosis and associated conditions occur even with modern techniques [75]. One possible solution is a modified anatomical hemispherectomy, excluding the CSF pathways, as proposed by Adams [76]. Another possible solution is the functional hemispherectomy, which in its most recent form is the peri-insular operation proposed by Villemure and Mascott (see Chapter 66) [71]. Finally a more minimal operation, hemispherotomy, described in two separate forms by Delalande *et al.* and by Schramm *et al.*, also resolves this problem [78,79]. These modified operations still have their complications. The exact frequency is difficult to discern because some series extend over a considerable period of time. Typical of these is the report from Boston, describing 10 patients in whom blood loss was the main problem, of a magnitude necessitating ITU care. In addition they describe haemorrhage into the operation cavity and seizures [80]. A more recent report from Rome describes less severe complications, including anaemia in 12 of 15 patients. In eight patients a second surgical procedure was needed, including five shunts, all in children operated at less than 9 months of age [81]. In our own mixed series of 50 adults and children only four required shunts and there were four cases of severe postoperative infection requiring removal of the bone flap. In two of these there had been exploration with large subdural grids. In terms of operating time and blood loss, some form of hemispherotomy or the peri-insular hemispherectomy should be preferred. In Villemure's 63 patients undergoing functional hemispherotomy, three required shunts and one was complicated by infection [70]. In Delalande *et al.*'s 53 patients undergoing hemispherotomy, there were 10 shunts [70]. Finally Kestle *et al.* made an interesting comparison between hemidecortication in five patients and peri-insular hemispherotomy in 11 patients. On all measures such as blood loss, postoperative fever, ventriculoperitoneal shunt insertion and length of stay those patients subjected to peri-insular hemispherotomy did better [82].

Reoperation

All surgeons are familiar from their general neurosurgical practice with the technical difficulties of second or third operations at the same anatomical site. Awad *et al.* [83] were the first to outline specific difficulties of reoperation, and the matter has also been dealt with in detail by Germano *et al.* [84]. Awad *et al.* noted that anatomical structures will frequently become distorted and MRI and neuronavigation are obvious aids to countering this problem [83]. Vascular adhesions can form between the dura and cortex; these vessels may make a significant contribution to the blood supply of that cortex and therefore should be preserved as far as possible. Only one paper on reoperation, that by Salanova *et al.*, quotes morbidity where they had transient weakness in 28% and permanent neurological defects in 8% [85].

Functional surgery

These procedures can be divided into three groups: interruption of fibre tracts such as callosotomy and multiple subpial transection, stereotactic creation of lesions within the brain and stimulation of deep brain and other nervous system structures.

Callosal section

Complications from callosal section depend upon the extent of the section and the nature of the underlying disease process. When carried out as an alternative to hemispherectomy in unilateral hemisphere disease, it is clearly sensible to approach the midline from the damaged side. Also in those patients there is more likely to be mixed cerebral speech dominance which may have important consequences, as discussed below. Finally, planning the approach may be important and this will depend upon whether a total or partial section is intended. In any event the approach should be made so as to avoid interruption of major tributaries to the superior sagittal sinus.

The complications can be divided into acute and chronic. The complications are related to the extent of the resection being minimal with a truncal section, and greatest with an anterior two-thirds or total section. Venous ischaemia or even thrombosis, when unilateral, may manifest as a hemiparesis with the possible addition of focal seizures. There may be transient paresis, usually affecting one leg, due to retraction on the medial surface of the hemisphere. More serious however is the risk of akinetic mutism, probably the result of bilateral anterior cerebral artery spasm. In very early series, the complication rate was high but after the Dartmouth group modified their procedure by staging it, performing a less extensive callosotomy and using the operating microscope, the complication rate was much lower [86]. However, even in series published since the late 1980s there is still a significant incidence of both general complications and neurological complications, although the latter tend to be transient. Thus Kimball *et al.* reported three deaths in 52 operations including one air embolism and one extradural haematoma [87]. The MNI reporting 43 operations had no deaths but some complications in 16 patients including three patients with transient weakness of the right leg and four with decreased speech output, also transient [88]. In a French series of 26 children transient complications were recorded in 30%, all of which resolved within 3 months [89]. Phillips and Sakas reported four instances (20%) of transient hemiparesis, Quattrini *et al.* transient mutism in 27.8%, which always recovered completely [90,91]. In our own series of 28 patients undergoing anterior callosotomy there has been one peroperative death from pneumonia and two instances of acute anterior cerebral ischaemia, both of which recovered completely. We have had transient limb weakness in a few patients and an extradural haematoma in one. Therefore in summary the risk of death at callosotomy seems to be between zero and 6% and of permanent neurological deficit less than 5%, but of transient deficit up to 5%.

There are two important cognitive complications of callosal section. The first is a change in speech function in patients of mixed cerebral dominance for speech, where interhemispheric communication is essential for the proper comprehension and production of speech and related functions. This was first reported by Sass *et al.* [92]. It has been suggested, but is by no means the universal opinion, that a carotid amytal test to establish speech dominance should precede the surgery in every case, and the operation, especially total section, refused to those of mixed dominance.

The second potentially serious complication is that of posterior disconnection syndrome. This comprises a situation in which complex motor or organizational tasks, which require the combination of information from both hemispheres, become impossible. Sperry *et al.* first described this [93]. Sauerwein and Lassonde noted that the cognitive effects of callosal section were related to the location and extent of the section and the age of the patient at the time of operation. Posterior section resulted in sensory disconnection; total callosotomy introduced problems with bimanual coordination and apraxia of the non-dominant hand to verbal commands. Many of these symptoms subside and those that remain are not disabling [94]. In another paper describing 25 children, they note that the effects of callosal section were less in younger children [95]. Finally callosal section may produce an alteration in the patient's seizure pattern so that certain kinds of seizures such as myoclonic jerks or absent seizures may become more frequent.

Multiple subpial transection

Morrell *et al.* devised this procedure for use in eloquent areas of cortex, attempting to produce good seizure control with minimal functional disturbance [96]. Their experience is summarized in a review published in 1999. They report transient morbidity in the form of paresis and dysaesthesia lasting 2–3 weeks, although occasionally lasting some months. Permanent deficits were less common, occurring in only 14% of patients. In addition there were unrelated complications in four other patients bringing the overall complication rate to 19% [97]. Our own experience in 40 patients has been similar. There have been severe complications associated with patients who underwent resection as well as MST, there were six hemipareses (30%), four transient and with MST alone three hemipareses (27%), two transient. The Bonn group reports a lower complication rate with subtle changes recorded in five of 14 patients (35%) transected in eloquent areas [98].

Stereotactic lesions

The creation of lesions in apparently normal brain to control epilepsy by modification of brain activity has been proposed and performed for many years by a number of methods. Generally speaking they were directed to temporal and extratemporal targets. However these procedures are now not much used.

There are reports on the use of stereotactic radiosurgery in treating drug-resistant epilepsy due to mesial temporal sclerosis and hypothalamic hamartoma. The number of patients reported is small but there do not appear to be any of the particular complications of radiotherapy, such as radiation necrosis. Regis *et al.* reports three asymptomatic field defects in 25 patients with mesial temporal sclerosis treated with the gamma knife [99].

Stimulation

Clearly the use of chronic indwelling stimulating electrodes will run the risk of complications commonly associated with such apparatus. These must include implant failure and infection. These are relatively rare and occur with the same frequency as any other implanted device. When the stimulating electrodes are intracranial there is also the possibility of CSF leakage.

At present the only stimulation procedure in common use in epilepsy is stimulation of the left vagus nerve. The complications associated with this procedure fall into three groups. The stimulus is applied to the nerve intermittently and when 'on' produces minor side-effects that include voice change, usually hoarseness, coughing and occasionally shortness of breath. Many of these effects are related to the amplitude of stimulation and tend to become less obtrusive with time at a constant level of stimulation. Typical figures are those given by Morris and Mueller with hoarseness at 28% and paraesthesiae at 12% at 1 year and hoarseness at 19% and headache at 4.5% at 2 years and shortness of breath at 3.2% at 3 years [100]. In the same group low levels of infection were reported with an overall rate of 2.86% requiring explantation of the device in 1.76% [101].

There have been particular anxieties about cranial nerve function. It is suggested that patients with swallowing difficulties might aspirate. Both Murphy and Lundgren *et al.* reported this in a group of children [102,103]. Clearly the vocal cords are affected [104], and there are also isolated reports of a Horner's syndrome [105], and of glossopharyngeal neuralgia [106]. More important, however, are the potential effects on respiratory and cardiac function. In our series of over 120 implantations there has been one death and one serious morbidity from pneumonia in the postoperative period, unrelated to aspiration. Lotvall *et al.* have described deterioration in lung function in patients with chronic obstructive airways disease [107]. Malow *et al.* have shown adverse changes in respiration during stimulation when the patient is asleep and note that it is more significant in patients with obstructive airways disease [108]. Several groups now report bradycardia or asystole during intraoperative testing [109–111]. In our series of over 120 implantations this has occurred once. According to the manufacturers the incidence of this intraoperative event is 0.1% [109]. Current practice is to abort the procedure and remove the device.

Sudden death in epilepsy (SUDEP) has occurred in patients during vagus nerve stimulation, but it is the view of Fisher and Handforth that this is not more frequent than in a similar population of patients with severe epilepsy [112].

Deep brain stimulation for epilepsy has been directed at two targets, the cerebellum and the thalamic nuclei. Cerebellar stimulation was introduced by Cooper *et al.* [113] but subsequently shown to be ineffective [114]. Complications were rare; there were anecdotal reports of sudden death but these occur in epilepsy anyway.

Deep brain stimulation has also been applied to the thalamic nuclei and to the subthalamic nucleus. Studies are sparse and inconclusive. The same potential complications must exist as with stereotactic lesioning, mainly malposition of the electrodes and haemorrhage.

Risk management

In the surgical management of chronic drug-resistant epilepsy, the use of interventional procedures in presurgical evaluation, and the therapeutic procedures themselves, can never be without risk of significant physical, intellectual and psychiatric complications. I have dealt with ways of minimizing the occurrence of these risks. The impact of these complications spreads beyond the patient and surgeon to the family, referring physician, referring organization and society itself.

Because most epilepsy surgery or invasive diagnostic procedures are elective rather than involving decisions made under pressure of clinical circumstances, the concept and application of informed consent is especially important. A person taking such consent must be sufficiently senior and experienced, and the person giving consent must have understood the explanation and implications. It may be impossible to achieve this in one session, and extensive preoperative counselling is often necessary. It is especially important that any such discussion should include the particular experience or facilities of the group undertaking the procedure, since these will influence the possible frequency and severity of complications. The legal validity of the present operation consent form used in the UK is uncertain. It is commonsense to make sure that it is countersigned by the operating surgeon or equivalent. A written record that a discussion regarding the purpose of the procedure and possible complications has taken place should exist and if appropriate the actual complications should be listed. In the Sidaway legal case in the UK it was hoped that an objective frequency of any complication would be suggested above which the patient must be warned. However, after appeal to the House of Lords, it was stated that the surgeon must only warn of those complications about which a reasonable body of professional practitioners would warn the patient [115]. This is in keeping with the Bolam test, which uses the proposition that a practitioner cannot be accused of negligence if they act in accordance with practice accepted at the time by a responsible body of medical opinion [116].

Summary

1 The complications of epilepsy surgery must include the complications from invasive procedures used in presurgical assessment as well as those arising in relation to therapeutic interventions.
2 The ISA test has a low complication rate, less than 0.5%, in the classical form.
3 Intracranial electrodes have a complication rate which increases with the invasiveness and complexity of the procedure. Mortality is zero, but there is a significant complication rate from haemorrhage and infection of 2–5%.
4 Therapeutic procedures are divided into resective and functional operations. Overall perioperative mortality in large series of mixed procedures is 1% and overall mortality, including late deaths, is around 2–3%.
5 In resective surgery morbidity depends upon the size and site of the resection. It can be very low in non-eloquent areas such as the non-dominant frontal lobe; around 1% compared with greater than 30% in central and occipital regions.
6 In unilateral hemisphere disease the age of the patient, the underlying pathology and the operative technique employed will all affect the nature and severity of the potential complications.
7 In temporal lobe resections there are additional intellectual and behavioural consequences of the procedure dependent upon the preoperative status of the patient and the nature of the resection.

8 Reoperation and functional procedures such as callosotomy and multiple subpial transection also-carry significant risk.

9 Risk management, preoperative counselling and informed consent are critical.

References

1 Waugh JR, Sacharias N. Arteriographic complications in the DSA era [see comments]. *Radiology* 1992; 1: 243–6.
2 Borchgrevink HM, Nakstad PH, Bjorneas H, Bakke SJ. Superselective amytal anaesthesia by the medial and posterior cerebral arteries improved localisation of function in epileptic patients prior to neurosurgical intervention. *Epilepsia* 1993; 34(Suppl. 2): 34.
3 Jack CR, Nichols DA, Sharbrough FW, Marsh WR, Petersen RC. Selective posterior cerebral amytal test for evaluating memory function before surgery for temporal lobe seizure. *Radiology* 1988; 168: 787–93.
4 Rausch R, Silfvenius H, Wieser HG, Dodrill CB, Meador KJ, Jones-Gotman M. Intraarterial amobarbital procedures. In: Engel J, ed. *Surgical Treatment of the Epilepsies*. New York: Raven Press, 1993: 341–58.
5 Hajek M, Valavanis A, Yonekawa Y, Schiess R, Buck A, Wieser HG. Selective amobarbital test for the determination of language function in patients with epilepsy with frontal and posterior temporal brain lesions. *Epilepsia* 1998; 39(4): 389–98.
6 Zhang J, Wilson CL, Levesque MF, Behnke EJ, Lufkin RB. Temperature changes in nickel-chromium intracranial depth electrodes during MR scanning. *Am J Neuroradiol* 1993; 14: 497–500.
7 Davis LM, Spencer DD, Spencer SS, Bronen RA. MR imaging of implanted depth and subdural electrodes: is it safe? *Epilepsy Res* 1999; 35(2): 95–8.
8 Bernoulli C, Siegfried J, Baumgartner G *et al.* Danger of accidental person-to-person transmission of Creutzfeldt-Jakob disease by surgery. *Lancet* 1977; 8009: 478–9.
9 Pilcher WH, Roberts DW, Flanigin HF *et al.* Complications of epilepsy surgery. In: Engel J, ed. *Surgical Treatment of the Epilepsies*. New York: Raven Press, 1993: 565–81.
10 Siegfried J, Wieser HG, Stodieck SRG. Foramen ovale electrodes: A new technique enabling presurgical evaluation of patients with mesiobasal temporal lobe seizures. *Appl Neurophysiol* 1985; 48: 408–17.
11 Wieser HG, Quesney LF, Morris HH. Foramen ovale and peg electrodes. In: Engel J, ed. *Surgical Treatment of the Epilepsies*. New York: Raven Press, 1993: 331–9.
12 Schuler P, Neubauer U, Schulemann H, Stefan H. Brain-stem lesions in the course of a presurgical re-evaluation by foramen-ovale electrodes in temporal lobe epilepsy. *Electroencephalogr Clin Neurophysiol* 1993; 86: 301–2.
13 Goldring S, Gregorie EM. Surgical management of epilepsy using epidural mats to localise the seizure focus. *J Neurosurg* 1984; 60: 457–66.
14 Wyler AR, Walker G, Somes G. The morbidity of long term seizure monitoring using subdural strip recording. *J Neurosurg* 1991; 74: 734–7.
15 Stephan CL, Kepes JJ, SantaCruz K, Wilkinson SB, Fegley B, Osorio I. Spectrum of clinical and histopathologic responses to intracranial electrodes: from multifocal aseptic meningitis to multifocal hypersensitivity-type meningovasculitis. *Epilepsia* 2001; 42(7): 895–901.
16 Stephan CL, Kepes JJ, SantaCruz K, Wilkinson SB, Fegley B, Osorio I. Spectrum of clinical and histopathologic responses to intracranial electrodes: from multifocal aseptic meningitis to multifocal hypersensitivity-type meningovasculitis. *Epilepsia* 2001; 42(7): 895–901.
17 Swartz BE, Rich JR, Dwan PS *et al.* The safety and efficacy of chronically implanted subdural electrodes: a prospective study. *Surg Neurol* 1996; 46(1): 87–93.
18 Spencer DD. Depth electrode implantation at Yale University. In: Engel J, ed. *Surgical Treatment of the Epilepsies*. New York: Raven Press, 1993: 603–7.
19 Van Veelen CMW, Debets C, Van Huffelen AC *et al.* Combined use of subdural and intracerebral electrodes in preoperative evaluation of epilepsy. *Neurosurgery* 1990; 26: 93–101.
20 Wieser HG, Silfvenius H. Unpublished data.
21 Daniel RT, Chandy MJ. Epilepsy surgery: overview of forty years' experience. *Neurol India* 1999; 47(2): 98–103.
22 Rydenhag B, Silander HC. Complications of epilepsy surgery after 654 procedures in Sweden, September 1990–1995: a multicenter study based on the Swedish National Epilepsy Surgery Register. *Neurosurgery* 2001; 49(1): 51–6.
23 Pilcher WH, Rusyniak G. Complications of epilepsy surgery. In: Silberg DI, Ojemann GA, eds. *Epilepsy Surgery*. Philadelphia: W.B. Saunders, 1993: 311–25.
24 Comair Y, Choi HY, Van Ness PC. Neocortical resections. In: Engel JJ, Pedley TA, eds. *Epilepsy: A Comprehensive Textbook*. Philadelphia: Lippincott-Raven, 1998: 1819–28.
25 Canavan AGM, Passingham RE, Marsden CD, Quinn N, Wyke M, Polkey CE. Prism adaptation and other tasks involving spatial abilities in patients with Parkinson's disease, patients with frontal lobe lesions and patients with unilateral temporal lobectomies. *Neuropsychologia* 1990; 28: 969–84.
26 Owen AM, Morris RG, Sahakian BJ, Polkey CE, Robbins TW. Double dissociations of memory and executive functions in working memory tasks following frontal lobe excisions, temporal lobe excisions or amygdalo-hippocampectomy in man. *Brain* 1996; 119(Pt 5): 1597–615.
27 Owen AM, Roberts AC, Polkey CE, Sahakian BJ, Robbins TW. Extra-dimensional versus intra-dimensional set shifting performance following frontal lobe excisions, temporal lobe excisions or amygdalo-hippocampectomy in man. *Neuropsychologia* 1991; 10: 993–1006.
28 Toczek MT, Morrell MJ, Silverberg GA, Lowe GM. Cerebellar hemorrhage complicating temporal lobectomy. Report of four cases. *J Neurosurg* 1996; 85(4): 718–22.
29 Weaver JP, Phillips C, Horowitz SL, Benjamin S. Middle fossa cyst presenting as a delayed complication of temporal lobectomy: case report. *Neurosurgery* 1996; 38(5): 1047–50.
30 Malla BR, O'Brien TJ, Cascino GD *et al.* Acute postoperative seizures following anterior temporal lobectomy for intractable partial epilepsy. *J Neurosurg* 1998; 89(2): 177–82.
31 Jensen I. Temporal lobe epilepsy. Late mortality in patients treated with unilateral temporal lobe resections. *Acta Neurol Scand* 1975; 52: 374–80.
32 Taylor DC, Marsh SM. Implications of long-term follow-up studies in epilepsy: With a note on the cause of death. In: Penry JK, ed. *Epilepsy. The Eighth International Symposium*. New York: Raven Press, 1977: 27–34.
33 Hennessy MJ, Langan Y, Elwes RD, Binnie CD, Polkey CE, Nashef L. A study of mortality after temporal lobe epilepsy surgery. *Neurology* 1999; 53(6): 1276–83.
34 Penfield W, Lende RA, Rasmussen T. Manipulation hemiplegia, an untoward complication in the surgery of focal epilepsy. *J Neurosurg* 1961; 18: 769–76.
35 Van Buren JM. Complications of surgical procedures in the treatment and diagnosis of epilepsy. In: Engel J, ed. *Surgical Treatment of the Epilepsies*. New York: Raven Press, 1993: 465–75.
36 Renella RR. *Outcome of Surgery. Microsurgery of the Temporal Region*. Wien: Springer-Verlag, 1989: 158–64.
37 Falconer MA, Wilson JL. Visual field changes following anterior temporal lobectomy: their significance in relation to 'Meyer's loop' of the optic radiation. *Brain* 1958; 81: 1–14.
38 Katz A, Awad IA, Kong AK *et al.* Extent of resection in temporal lobectomy for epilepsy. II. Memory changes and neurologic complications. *Epilepsia* 1989; 30: 763–71.
39 Spencer DD, Spencer SS, Mattson RH, Williamson PD, Novelly RA. Access to the posterior medial temporal structures in the surgical treatment of temporal lobe epilepsy. *Neurosurgery* 1984; 15: 667–71.
40 Manji H, Plant GT. Epilepsy surgery, visual fields, and driving: a study of the visual field criteria for driving in patients after temporal lobe epilepsy surgery with a comparison of Goldmann and Esterman perimetry. *J Neurol Neurosurg Psychiatr* 2000; 68(1): 80–2.
41 Dodrill CB, Hermann BP, Rausch R, Chelune G, Oxbury S. Neuropsychological testing for assessing prognosis following epilepsy surgery. In: Engel J, ed. *Surgical Treatment of the Epilepsies*. New York: Raven Press, 1993: 263–71.
42 McMillan T, Powell GE, Janota I, Polkey CE. Relationship between neuropathology and cognitive functioning in temporal lobe patients. *J Neurol Neurosurg Psychiatr* 1987; 50: 167–76.

43 Ojemann GA, Dodrill CB. Verbal memory deficits after left temporal lobectomy for epilepsy: mechanism and intraoperative prediction. *J Neurosurg* 1985; 62: 101–7.

44 Wieser HG. Selective amygdalo-hippocampectomy for temporal lobe epilepsy. *Epilepsia* 1988; 29: S100–S113.

45 Wieser HG. Selective amygdalo-hippocampectomy: indications and follow-up. *Can J Neurol Sci* 1991; 4: 617–27.

46 Milner B. Psychological defects produced by temporal lobe excision. *Res Publ Assoc Res Nerv Men Dis* 1958; 36: 244–57.

47 Goldstein LH, Polkey CE. Short-term cognitive changes after unilateral temporal lobectomy or unilateral amygdalo-hippocampectomy for the relief of temporal lobe epilepsy. *J Neurol Neurosurg Psychiatr* 1993; 56: 135–40.

48 Renowden SA, Matkovic Z, Adams CB et al. Selective amygdalohippocampectomy for hippocampal sclerosis: postoperative MR appearance. *Am J Neuroradiol* 1995; 16(9): 1855–61.

49 Jones-Gotman M, Zatorre RJ, Olivier A et al. Learning and retention of words and designs following excision from medial or lateral temporal-lobe structures. *Neuropsychologia* 1997; 35(7): 963–73.

50 Jensen I, Larsen JK. Mental aspects of temporal lobe epilepsy: follow-up of 74 patients after resection of a temporal lobe. *J Neurol Neurosurg Psychiatr* 1979; 42: 256–65.

51 Taylor DC. Factors influencing the occurrence of schizophrenia-like psychosis in patients with temporal lobe epilepsy. *Psychol Med* 1975; 5: 249–54.

52 Andermann LF, Savard G, Meencke HJ, McLachlan R, Moshe S, Andermann F. Psychosis after resection of ganglioglioma or DNET: evidence for an association. *Epilepsia* 1999; 40(1): 83–7.

53 Mace CJ, Trimble MR. Psychosis following temporal lobe surgery: a report of six cases. *J Neurol Neurosurg Psychiatr* 1991; 54: 639–44.

54 Leinonen E, Tuunainen A, Lepola U. Postoperative psychoses in epileptic patients after temporal lobectomy. *Acta Neurol Scand* 1994; 90(6): 394–9.

55 Manchanda R, Schaefer B, McLachlan RS et al. Psychiatric disorders in candidates for surgery for epilepsy. *J Neurol Neurosurg Psychiatr* 1996; 61(1): 82–9.

56 Manchanda R, Miller H, McLachlan RS. Post-ictal psychosis after right temporal lobectomy. *J Neurol Neurosurg Psychiatr* 1993; 56: 277–9.

57 Paradiso S, Hermann BP, Blumer D, Davies K, Robinson RG. Impact of depressed mood on neuropsychological status in temporal lobe epilepsy. *J Neurol Neurosurg Psychiatr* 2001; 70(2): 180–5.

58 Olivier A, Awad IA. Extratemporal resections. In: Engel J, ed. *Surgical Treatment of the Epilepsies*. New York: Raven Press, 1993: 489–500.

59 Macdonell RA, Jackson GD, Curatolo JM et al. Motor cortex localization using functional MRI and transcranial magnetic stimulation. *Neurology* 1999; 53(7): 1462–7.

60 Yetkin FZ, Papke RA, Mark LP, Daniels DL, Mueller WM, Haughton VM. Location of the sensorimotor cortex: functional and conventional MR compared. *Am J Neuroradiol* 1995; 16(10): 2109–13.

61 Chassoux F, Devaux B, Landre E, Chodkiewicz JP, Talairach J, Chauvel P. Postoperative motor deficits and recovery after cortical resections. *Adv Neurol* 1999; 81: 189–99.

62 Devaux B, Chassoux F, Landre E et al. Chronic intractable epilepsy associated with a tumor located in the central region: functional mapping data and postoperative outcome. *Stereotact Funct Neurosurg* 1997; 69 (1–4 Pt 2): 229–38.

63 Sandok EK, Cascino GD. Surgical treatment for perirolandic lesional epilepsy. *Epilepsia* 1998; 39 (Suppl. 4): S42–S48.

64 Curatolo JM, Macdonell RA, Berkovic SF, Fabinyi GC. Intraoperative monitoring to preserve central visual fields during occipital corticectomy for epilepsy. *J Clin Neurosci* 2000; 7(3): 234–7.

65 Williamson PD, Thadani VM, Darcey TM, Spencer DD, Spencer SS, Mattson RH. Occipital lobe epilepsy: clinical characteristics, seizure spread patterns, and results of surgery. *Ann Neurol* 1992; 31: 3–13.

66 Salanova V, Andermann F, Olivier A, Rasmussen T, Quesney LF. Occipital lobe epilepsy: electroclinical manifestations, electrocorticography, cortical stimulation and outcome in 42 patients treated between 1930 and 1991. Surgery of occipital lobe epilepsy. *Brain* 1992; 115: 1655–80.

67 Bidzinski J, Bacia T, Ruzikowski E. The results of the surgical treatment of occipital lobe epilepsy. *Acta Neurochir Wien* 1992; 114: 128–30.

68 Cascino GD, Kelly PJ, Hirschorn KA, Marsh WR, Sharbrough FW. Stereotactic resection of intra-axial cerebral lesions in partial epilepsy. *Mayo Clin Proc* 1990; 65: 1053–60.

69 Holthausen H, May TW, Adams CBT et al. Seizures post hemispherectomy. In: Tuxhorn I, Holthausen H, Boenigk H, eds. *Paediatric Epilepsy Syndromes and their Surgical Treatment*. London: John Libbey & Co. Ltd, 1997: 749–73.

70 Villemure JG, Vernet O, Delalande O. Hemispheric disconnection: callosotomy and hemispherotomy. *Adv Tech Stand Neurosurg* 2000; 26: 25–78.

71 Beardsworth ED, Adams CBT. Modified hemispherectomy for epilepsy. Early results in 10 cases. *Br J Neurosurg* 1988; 2: 73–84.

72 Rasmussen T, Obozewski J, Lloyd-Smith D. Focal seizures due to chronic localised encephalitis. *Neurology* 1958; 8: 435–45.

73 Vargha-Khadem F, Polkey CE. A review of cognitive outcome after hemidecortication in humans. In: Rose FD, Johnson DA, eds. *Recovery from Brain Damage. Reflections and Directions*. New York: Plenum Press, 1993: 137–52.

74 Krynauw RA. Infantile hemiplegia treated by removing one cerebral hemisphere. *J Neurol Neurosurg Psychiatr* 1950; 13: 243–67.

75 Rasmussen T. Post-operative superficial hemosiderosis of the brain, its diagnosis, treatment and prevention. *Am Neurol Assoc* 1973; 98: 133–7.

76 Adams CBT. Hemispherectomy – a modification. *J Neurol Neurosurg Psychiatr* 1983; 46: 617–19.

77 Villemure JG, Mascott CR. Peri-insular hemispherotomy: surgical principles and anatomy. *Neurosurgery* 1995; 37(5): 975–81.

78 Delalande O, Pinard JM, Basdevant C, Plouin P, Dulac O. Hemispherotomy: a new procedure for hemispheric disconnection. *Epilepsia* 1993; 34 (Suppl. 2): 140.

79 Schramm J, Kral T, Clusmann H. Transsylvian keyhole functional hemispherectomy. *Neurosurgery* 2001; 49(4): 891–900.

80 Brian JE Jr, Deshpande JK, McPherson RW. Management of cerebral hemispherectomy in children. *J Clin Anesth* 1990; 2: 91–5.

81 Di Rocco C, Iannelli A. Hemimegalencephaly and intractable epilepsy: complications of hemispherectomy and their correlations with the surgical technique. A report on 15 cases. *Pediatr Neurosurg* 2000; 33(4): 198–207.

82 Kestle J, Connolly M, Cochrane D. Pediatric peri-insular hemispherotomy. *Pediatr Neurosurg* 2000; 32(1): 44–7.

83 Awad IA, Nayel MH, Luders H. Second operation after the failure of previous resection for epilepsy. *Neurosurgery* 1991; 28: 510–18.

84 Germano IM, Poulin N, Olivier A. Reoperation for recurrent temporal lobe epilepsy. *J Neurosurg* 1994; 81(1): 31–6.

85 Salanova V, Quesney LF, Rasmussen T, Andermann F, Olivier A. Reevaluation of surgical failures and the role of reoperation in 39 patients with frontal lobe epilepsy. *Epilepsia* 1994; 35(1): 70–80.

86 Wilson DH, Reeves AG, Gazzaniga M. 'Central' commissurotomy for intractabler generalised: Series two. *Neurology* 1982; 32: 687–97.

87 Kimball S, Walker GG, Wyler AR. Corpus callosotomy: Anterior versus staged anterior and posterior callosal sectioning. *Epilepsia* 1989; 30: 729.

88 Oguni H, Olivier A, Andermann F, Comair J. Anterior callosotomy in the treatment of medically intractable epilepsies: a study of 43 patients with a mean follow-up of 39 months. *Ann Neurol* 1991; 30: 357–64.

89 Pinard JM, Delande, Jambaque I, Chiron C, Plouin P, Dulac O. Anterior and total callosotomy in epileptic children: Prospective one-year follow-up study. *Epilepsia* 1991; 32 (Suppl. 1): 54.

90 Phillips J, Sakas DE. Anterior callosotomy for intractable epilepsy: outcome in a series of twenty patients. *Br J Neurosurg* 1996; 10(4): 351–6.

91 Quattrini A, Del Pesce M, Provinciali L et al. Mutism in 36 patients who underwent callosotomy for drug-resistant epilepsy. *J Neurosurg Sci* 1997; 41(1): 93–6.

92 Sass KJ, Spencer SS, Spencer DD, Novelly RA, Williamson PD, Mattson RH. Corpus callosotomy for epilepsy. II. Neurologic and neuropsychological outcome. *Neurology* 1988; 38: 24–8.

93 Gordon HW, Bogen JE, Sperry RW. Absence of deconnexion syndrome in two patients with partial section of the neocommissure. *Brain* 1971; 94: 327–36.

94 Sauerwein HC, Lassonde M. Neuropsychological alterations after split-brain surgery. *J Neurosurg Sci* 1997; 41(1): 59–66.

95 Lassonde M, Sauerwein C. Neuropsychological outcome of corpus cal-

losotomy in children and adolescents. *J Neurosurg Sci* 1997; 41(1): 67–73.

96 Morrell F, Whisler WW, Bleck TP. Multiple subpial transection. A new approach to the surgical treatment of focal epilepsy. *J Neurosurg* 1989; 70: 231–9.

97 Morrell F, Kanner AM, Toledo-Morrell L, Hoeppner T, Whisler WW. Multiple subpial transection. *Adv Neurol* 1999; 81: 259–70.

98 Hufnagel A, Zentner J, Fernandez G, Wolf HK, Schramm J, Elger CE. Multiple subpial transection for control of epileptic seizures: effectiveness and safety. *Epilepsia* 1997; 38(6): 678–88.

99 Regis J, Bartolomei F, Rey M, Hayashi M, Chauvel P, Peragut JC. Gamma knife surgery for mesial temporal lobe epilepsy. *J Neurosurg* 2000; 93 (Suppl. 3): 141–6.

100 Morris GL, III, Mueller WM. Long-term treatment with vagus nerve stimulation in patients with refractory epilepsy. The Vagus Nerve Stimulation Study Group E01-E05. *Neurology* 1999; 53(8): 1731–5.

101 Bruce DA, Alksne JA, Bernard A, Blume H, Fraser RAR, Li M. Implantation of a vagus nerve stimulator for refractory partial seizures: Surgical outcomes of 454 study patients. *Epilepsia* 1998; 39 (S6): 92.

102 Murphy JV. Left vagal nerve stimulation in children with medically refractory epilepsy. The Pediatric VNS Study Group. *J Pediatr* 1999; 134(5): 563–6.

103 Lundgren J, Ekberg O, Olsson R. Aspiration: a potential complication to vagus nerve stimulation. *Epilepsia* 1998; 39(9): 998–1000.

104 Lundy DS, Casiano RR, Landy HJ, Gallo J, Gallo B, Ramsey RE. Effects of vagal nerve stimulation on laryngeal function. *J Voice* 1993; 7(4): 359–64.

105 Kim W, Clancy RR, Liu GT. Horner syndrome associated with implantation of a vagus nerve stimulator. *Am J Ophthalmol* 2001; 131(3): 383–4.

106 Duhaime AC, Melamed S, Clancy RR. Tonsillar pain mimicking glossopharyngeal neuralgia as a complication of vagus nerve stimulation: case report. *Epilepsia* 2000; 41(7): 903–5.

107 Lotvall J, Lunde H, Augustinson LE, Hedner T, Svedmyr N, Ben Menachem E. Airway effects of direct left-sided cervical vagal stimulation in patients with complex partial seizures. *Epilepsy Res* 1994; 18(2): 149–54.

108 Malow BA, Edwards J, Marzec M, Sagher O, Fromes G. Effects of vagus nerve stimulation on respiration during sleep: a pilot study. *Neurology* 2000; 55(10): 1450–4.

109 Asconape JJ, Moore DD, Zipes DP, Hartman LM, Duffell WH Jr. Bradycardia and asystole with the use of vagus nerve stimulation for the treatment of epilepsy: a rare complication of intraoperative device testing. *Epilepsia* 1999; 40(10): 1452–4.

110 Lanska DJ. Ventricular asystole during vagus nerve stimulation for epilepsy in humans. *Neurology* 2000; 54(3): 775.

111 Lesser RP. Ventricular asystole during vagus nerve stimulation for epilepsy in humans. *Neurology* 2000; 54(3): 776.

112 Fisher RS, Handforth A. Reassessment: vagus nerve stimulation for epilepsy: a report of the Therapeutics and Technology Assessment Subcommittee of the American Academy of Neurology. *Neurology* 1999; 53(4): 666–9.

113 Cooper IS, Amin I, Riklan M, Waltz JM, Poon TP. Chronic cerebellar stimulation in epilepsy. Clinical and anatomical studies. *Arch Neurol* 1976; 33(8): 559–70.

114 Wright GDS, McLellan DL, Brice JG. A double-blind trial of chronic cerebellar stimulation in twelve patients with severe epilepsy. *J Neurol Neurosurg Psychiatr* 1985; 47: 769–74.

115 Sidaway *vs.* Governors Bethlem Royal Hospital. 1985. 1 AC 871.

116 Bolam *vs.* Friern Hospital Management Committee. 1957. 1 WLR 582.

72 Anaesthesia for Epilepsy Surgery

M. Smith

The surgical treatment of epilepsy requires a coordinated approach from the epileptologist, neurosurgeon, neurophysiologist and neuroanaesthetist. The anaesthetic technique must provide optimal operating conditions for the surgeon and the maintenance of a safe and comfortable environment for the patient. Other considerations include avoiding the precipitation of seizures and the effect of anaesthetic agents on the EEG, especially if the neurophysiologist needs to obtain high-quality intraoperative recordings. The aims of this chapter are to characterize the electroencephalographic effects of anaesthetic agents and to discuss anaesthetic techniques for epilepsy surgery. The role of the neuroanaesthetist is a challenging one, as the factors affecting operating conditions may adversely affect the ability to obtain clear and useful intraoperative electrophysiological data.

Anaesthetic agents and EEG

In 1886 Victor Horsley commented that he had not used ether in operations on man because it caused 'cerebral excitement' whereas chloroform on the other hand produced 'well-marked depression' [1]. Horsley did not employ ECoG during his operations but he did guide intraoperative decision making with cortical stimulation mapping. His concerns regarding anaesthesia are reiterated over a century later by the ongoing controversy over the choice of anaesthetic during surgical procedures for epilepsy. Most anaesthetic agents have both activating and inhibitory effects on electrocortical activity. They produce this biphasic effect in a dose-dependent manner, with activation of the EEG at low doses and EEG suppression at higher doses [2,3]. This section reviews the evidence relating to the electrocortical effects of anaesthetic agents with particular reference to the interpretation of the ECoG.

Inhalation anaesthetics

The halogenated inhalational anaesthetic agents in common usage are isoflurane, sevoflurane and desflurane with the older agents, halothane and enflurane, still being used in many parts of the world. The best measure of potency of inhalational agents is the minimum alveolar concentration (MAC) at 1 atmosphere, which is the concentration of the agent that produces immobility in 50% of subjects exposed to a standard surgical incision. The MAC in oxygen of halothane is 0.8%, enflurane 1.7%, isoflurane 1.2%, sevoflurane 1.8% and desflurane 6%. Many things affect the MAC but, in particular, it is lowered by the use of adjuvant agents such as opioids and nitrous oxide. Despite the chemical similarity of inhalational anaesthetics, their effects upon cerebral electrical activity are diverse.

Halothane

Halothane at 1.2 MAC causes replacement of the background α-frequencies with fast β-activity [4]. As inspired concentrations rise to 2.5 MAC, high-amplitude δ-activity predominates. Halothane does not induce epileptiform activity or clinical seizures, even in those with epilepsy [5]. Suppression of spike activity occurs at clinically useful concentrations of halothane [4,5], which also attenuates spikes produced by activating agents. It should therefore not be used when intraoperative ECoG is planned.

Enflurane

Enflurane is a halogenated ether that has the most potent activating properties of any volatile anaesthetic agent, especially in the presence of hypocarbia [6–8]. At low inspired concentrations, enflurane causes β-activity that is replaced by high-amplitude δ and θ waves as the inspired concentration rises. At higher concentrations (> 2.5 MAC), spike and polyspike activity is produced and, even during deep anaesthesia, burst-suppression is interspaced with polyspike activity [6,9]. Hypercarbia suppresses these activating effects [6,7]. Enflurane has been noted to produce generalized seizures in patients with no previous history of seizure activity [10,11]. This is most likely to occur during severe hypocarbia or when the inspired concentration of enflurane is rapidly raised [12]. There has been obvious concern over the use of this agent in patients with epilepsy, but there appears to be no greater risk of seizure generation than in the general population [13]. During ECoG, enflurane has been shown to extend the field of epileptiform discharges outside the area of spontaneous ictal activity [14] and bilateral activation of epileptiform discharges has been noted in the amygdala and hippocampus in patients with unilateral temporal lobe epilepsy [7,9]. Although some workers have used enflurane as an activating agent during diagnostic ECoG [15,16] others do not recommend it when corticography is used as a guide to tailored surgical resection because of potential spike extension [17].

Isoflurane

Isoflurane is chemically similar to enflurane but shows little, if any, proconvulsant activity. It produces a predictable, dose-dependent suppression of EEG activity [2]. Fast EEG activity is seen at low concentrations with bursts of high-voltage β-activity at 1 MAC. This progresses to burst-suppression at 1.5 MAC with the development of an isoelectric EEG at levels >2 MAC [18,19]. Epileptiform activity may be reduced or suppressed by low-dose isoflurane which has been used in the treatment of status epilepticus refractory to other agents [20,21]. It possibly also has suppressive effects on the ECoG and reduces the area of interictal spiking [14]. However, one study demonstrated that isoflurane has no significant effect on spike activity provided that inspired concentrations are maintained <1.25% with nitrous oxide concentrations within the 50–70% range [22]. Many centres performing epilepsy surgery under general anaesthesia have employed a combination of isoflurane and fentanyl, with and without nitrous oxide, and reported the ease with which diagnostic ECoG recordings, with maintenance of spike activity, can be obtained [23,24]. There is no good evidence for proconvulsant effects of isoflurane. Reports of 'seizure-like' movements occurring during isoflurane anaesthesia have either not been confirmed by EEG or have been complicated by the coadministration of nitrous oxide [25].

Sevoflurane

Sevoflurane is a fluorinated ether that was initially believed to have isoflurane-like effects on the EEG [26,27]. There is progression from high-amplitude slow wave activity to burst-suppression with increasing concentrations in animals [28] and in man [29]. Burst-suppression has been reported to occur between 1 and 2.15 MAC sevoflurane with no evidence of spike or seizure activity [26,27,29]. However, the electrophysiological effects of sevoflurane have not been fully characterized and there are conflicting reports of its EEG effects. Despite early studies in healthy volunteers, in which sevoflurane anaesthesia was not associated with excitation of the EEG [30,31], later studies have suggested that sevoflurane is associated both with activation of the EEG and seizure activity. There has been a report of EEG-confirmed seizure activity during deep sevoflurane anaesthesia in a non-epileptic patient [32]. Furthermore, seizure-like movements and EEG-recorded seizures have also been noted during induction of anaesthesia with sevoflurane [33–35]. In one study, EEG suppression with spikes, rhythmic polyspikes and periodic epileptiform discharges was recorded during induction of anaesthesia with 8% sevoflurane in children [35]. Scheller *et al.* noted brief epileptiform discharges and a clinical seizure in one of five dogs subjected to sevoflurane anaesthesia, and concluded that the EEG effects of sevoflurane reside between those of isoflurane and enflurane, with more similarity to isoflurane [27]. Sevoflurane administration produces spontaneous, high-amplitude spikes in cats [28] and interictal spike activity is increased with sevoflurane compared to equipotent doses of isoflurane in patients with refractory epilepsy [36,37]. Watts *et al.* noted that sevoflurane activation occurred relatively selectively at the pre-existing seizure focus [36] whereas extension of spike activity beyond the epileptogenic zone has also been reported [38]. Sevoflurane appears to activate interictal spike activity more selectively than enflurane, and this is not affected by other EEG-activating agents [36]. Hypocapnia has variably been reported to have no effect [36], to suppress [37] and to increase sevoflurane-induced EEG abnormalities [34]. Sevoflurane is widely used during neurosurgical anaesthesia and is likely to be a safe agent for use during epilepsy surgery. However, its effects on the ECoG require further clarification before it can be recommended during intraoperative ECoG localization of the epileptogenic zone [38].

Desflurane

Desflurane differs chemically from isoflurane only in the substitution of fluorine for chlorine. It produces similar EEG changes to equipotent concentrations of isoflurane in animals [39] and in man [40,41]. Increasing concentrations of desflurane initially decrease the frequency and increase the amplitude of the EEG [41], with prominent burst-suppression occurring at 1.24 MAC and higher [40]. At concentrations >2 MAC, desflurane results in regular attenuation of the EEG with interruption by periodic polyspiking [41]. At both 1.5 and 2.0 MAC desflurane, the EEG pattern initially observed changes to one with a faster background activity with time [41]. No epileptiform activity has been noted even in the presence of hypocapnia [40].

Nitrous oxide

Nitrous oxide is a gaseous anaesthetic agent that is used widely to potentiate the effect of inhalational or intravenous anaesthetics. Dose-dependent EEG changes occur at nitrous oxide concentrations above 25% [42]. Normal α-rhythm is replaced by low-amplitude, fast activity and at higher concentrations EEG slowing occurs and low-voltage θ-activity may be seen [43]. Nitrous oxide itself does not have convulsant properties under normal circumstances [42,43] but when used in combination with other agents may potentiate the specific effects of that agent on the EEG [19,44]. However, it may affect the interpretation of ECoG, as it can also suppress or even eliminate spike activity [45]. Some workers have warned against the use of nitrous oxide during surgery for epilepsy because, although it lowers the MAC of inhalational anaesthetic agents, it potentiates the suppressive effects of these agents on the ECoG [46,47]. Others merely recommend discontinuation of nitrous oxide 30 min prior to recording of ECoG [17] whereas others continue its administration [24].

Intravenous anaesthetic agents

Barbiturates

Barbiturates are intravenous anaesthetic agents with different hypnotic and anticonvulsant activity depending on the addition to the parent molecule of carbon side chains or sulphydryl groups. All barbiturates have similar effects on the EEG in normal patients [3]. Thiopentone is frequently used as an intravenous anaesthetic induction agent and has dose-dependent effects on the EEG. The normal α-rhythm is initially replaced by fast activity, with EEG suppression at increasing doses and burst-suppression, progressing to an isoelectric EEG during deep barbiturate anaesthesia [3,48]. It has been known since the earliest days of its use that thiopentone has proconvulsant activity at low doses [49]. It produces paroxysmal spike activity in epileptic patients [49,50] and is a potent β-activator in normal cortex [17]. However, in normal cortex adjacent to pathological tissue, there is either a focal reduction in induced β-activity or burst-suppression [51,52]. Such differential findings have been used as a diagnostic tool during planning for epilepsy surgery in some units [23] but others have noted more spike activation in the less epileptogenic temporal lobe and suggest that thiopentone is less reliable than ictal EEG in identifying resection margins [53,54]. At higher doses, thiopentone has potent anticonvulsant properties, producing burst-suppression and ultimately electrical silence. It has been widely used to treat postoperative seizures in neurosurgical patients [55] and has a role in the treatment of status epilepticus [56,57].

Methohexitone activates the EEG in patients with temporal lobe or primary generalized epilepsies [58]. It induces spikes, polyspikes and spike-and-wave activity in epileptogenic areas of patients with temporal lobe epilepsy [59–61] and does so more reliably than thiopentone [59,62]. Methohexitone has been used widely to induce focal spike-wave activity during diagnostic ECoG in instances when spikes do not occur spontaneously [61,63]. In one study, a small dose of methohexitone caused selective activation in 87% of cases during local or general anaesthesia [63]. Other anaesthetic agents do not suppress this spike activity and methohexitone is therefore a useful drug for stimulation during ECoG in the anaesthetized patient [62,63]. Concern has been raised that methohexitone may induce spikes outside the epileptogenic zone [60], although others are confident that this is not the case [63].

Propofol

Propofol is an intravenous anaesthetic agent with a pharmacological profile that allows smooth and rapid induction of anaesthesia and reliable and swift recovery. It is widely used for induction and maintenance of general anaesthesia in neurosurgical patients and is useful as a short acting sedative during awake craniotomy. Propofol causes dose-dependent, characteristic EEG changes with initial increase in amplitude of the α-rhythm followed by slowing into theta and δ-range and ultimately burst-suppression and an isoelectric EEG [64]. In the UK, the Committee of Safety of Medicines received 170 reports of 'convulsions' and excitatory movements during or after propofol anaesthesia between 1986 and 1992 [65]. During this period an estimated 8 million patients received propofol anaesthesia. Contemporaneous EEG recording has confirmed the epileptic nature of these seizures in a few cases [66] but not in the majority [67–69]. It has been suggested that propofol-induced abnormal motor movements might have a subcortical origin [70]. Despite these observations, propofol has been demonstrated to possess strong anticonvulsant actions [71] and has been used successfully to treat status epilepticus resistant to other therapies [57,72,73].

There have been many studies of the effects of propofol on the EEG and ECoG in patients with epilepsy with markedly different results. An early report described activation in temporal lobe epilepsy with the development of spikes, polyspikes and spike-and-wave complexes and suggested that activation occurred in previously quiescent areas of cortex [74]. However, Samra et al. examined the effects of subanaesthetic doses of propofol on the ECoG and did not observe epileptiform discharges [75]. Another study also reported no proconvulsant effect of propofol in awake patients during the early stages of epilepsy surgery, but a burst-suppression pattern was observed with higher doses of propofol [76]. Lack of EEG activation has also been noted during high-dose propofol infusion [77,78]. It has been suggested that the EEG activating effects of propofol might be caused by the coadministration of other medica-

tion. This view is supported by the findings of Hufnagel et al. who studied the effects of a bolus dose of propofol 50 mg, with and without fentanyl, and noted that epileptiform activity was only induced in the presence of fentanyl [79]. Activation of the ECoG by propofol during isoflurane anaesthesia, with and without coadministration of fentanyl, has also been reported [80,81]. In one of these studies, propofol produced activation of spike discharges at the site of pre-propofol discharge in 17 out of 20 patients and a more extensive distribution of activation was also seen in 15 patients [80]. Conversely, another group has suggested that propofol might mask epileptiform activity during seizure surgery [82]. These disparate reports on the effect of propofol on the ECoG are difficult to explain but can be minimized if propofol is discontinued at least 30 min before diagnostic corticography during general anaesthesia [80]. A recent study has also confirmed that propofol sedation during awake craniotomy does not interfere with ECoG during epilepsy surgery, provided that administration is suspended at least 15 min before recording [83].

Etomidate

Etomidate is an ultra short-acting, non-barbiturate, hypnotic anaesthetic which has now been superseded by other agents and is not widely used in anaesthetic practice. It has similar EEG effects to barbiturates, except that fast activity is less prominent throughout the EEG [84,85] and burst-suppression occurs only in about 25% of patients even at high doses [84]. Etomidate may activate the EEG in non-epileptic patients [86] although it is not proconvulsant under normal circumstances [84,85]. It commonly causes myoclonic movements during induction of, and recovery from, anaesthesia although these are not associated with epileptiform activity on the EEG [87,88]. In epileptic patients, however, etomidate generates interictal spiking [89,90] and has been reported to cause clinical seizures [91]. During ECoG, etomidate causes an increase in spike activity within a focal area [74] but may also extend epileptiform activity into nearby cortex [92]. Despite this finding, etomidate has been used to induce epileptiform activity during diagnostic ECoG because it reliably causes spike activation [23,89]. At larger doses, etomidate has strong anticonvulsant properties in animals and in man [93]. Although it has been used in the treatment of refractory status epilepticus [94], it has no place in the modern treatment of this condition [57].

Benzodiazepines

All benzodiazepines have similar effects on the EEG. Small doses, such as those used in premedication, produce high frequency β-activity and should be avoided prior to surgery for epilepsy. High-voltage β and θ activity can also be induced but burst-suppression is not seen [95]. Benzodiazepines do not induce EEG or clinical seizure activity in people without epilepsy or in most patients with epilepsy, except during rapid withdrawal [96,97]. However, benzodiazepines have been reported to cause brief episodes of EEG and clinical seizure activity in patients with Lennox–Gastaut syndrome [98]. Benzodiazepines are potent anticonvulsants and are widely used to treat epilepsy and status epilepticus [57,96]. Following acute administration, they also result in reduction in epileptiform spike activity and should be avoided if diagnostic ECoG is planned during epilepsy surgery [99].

Ketamine

Ketamine is an intravenous anaesthetic agent that simultaneously produces central nervous system (CNS) excitation and depression, manifest as a catatonic-like state. It is a potent analgesic and can provide surgical anaesthesia as a sole agent. However, its clinical indications are strictly limited. It has distinct effects on the EEG compared to other intravenous anaesthetic agents. It produces low-amplitude fast EEG activity (30–40 Hz) throughout all stages of anaesthesia and may lead to burst-suppression at very high doses (>2 mg/kg). There are no reports of epileptiform activity in non-epileptic patients [95,100–102] and reports of myoclonus and 'seizure-like' activity in children have not been correlated with EEG changes [102]. However, in patients with epilepsy, ketamine induces limbic seizure activity which may be associated with clinical seizures in up to 50% of cases [100,103] but this is not reliably associated with epileptiform activity on the scalp EEG [104]. Exacerbation of pre-existing epilepsy that lasted for several months after ketamine anaesthesia has been reported [105] although this effect has not been confirmed by other studies [100,106]. However, it is generally accepted that ketamine is contraindicated in people with epilepsy and it has no place during ECoG recording.

Local anaesthetics

Local anaesthetic drugs, particularly lidocaine, possess both pro- and anticonvulsant properties [3] due to differing sensitivities of inhibitory and excitatory neurones to their membrane-stabilizing effects [107]. This occurs in both those with and those without epilepsy. At low plasma concentrations, lidocaine has sedative and anticonvulsant-like actions [108], but excitatory effects and clinical seizures occur at higher concentrations [109]. CNS depression and coma occur at very high plasma levels. Lidocaine can generate epileptiform activity specifically in the limbic system associated with typical auras [110]. Overdose of local anaesthetic should be avoided in any patient, but it seems prudent to avoid doses in the upper range of normal during epilepsy surgery when diagnostic ECoG is planned [17].

Adjuvant agents

Opioid analgesics

Opioids are an important adjunct during general and local anaesthetic techniques for epilepsy surgery. Fentanyl is the most widely used intraoperative opioid in the UK. Alfentanil has limited application in neurosurgical anaesthesia, whereas remifentanil, an ultra-short acting synthetic opioid, is gaining in popularity in this field. In the USA, sufentanil is also available. All opioids produce similar EEG changes, characterized by an initial slowing followed by progression to high voltage δ-activity and marked slowing of the EEG at high doses. There are minimal EEG effects at usual clinical doses and most studies report no epileptiform activity [111–114]. In a study of patients undergoing coronary artery surgery, Kearse et al. compared the effects of high doses of fentanyl and sufentanil on the

EEG and attempted to determine a 'dosing effect' by giving each opioid in four divided doses [115]. Out of 20 patients 19 developed epileptiform activity, characterized by generalized single and multiphasic, low-to-moderate voltage spike discharges after the initial dose. With increasing serum concentrations of opioid, the number of spike discharges initially increased during the first and second dose intervals and then declined during the third and fourth.

Pethidine causes neurological side-effects including tremors, myoclonus and seizures that are attributed to the N-demethylated metabolite norpethidine [116]. Pethidine exhibits the lowest safety margin for convulsions of all opioids and should therefore be avoided during epilepsy surgery [117]. Low-dose fentanyl (1–8 µg/kg) is widely used during seizure surgery and only causes mild slowing of the EEG [118]. At moderate doses (25 µg/kg), Tempel-hoff et al. reported activation of the EEG in eight out of nine patients undergoing presurgical evaluation with epidural electrodes and suggested limiting the dose when ECoG is used to guide tailored surgical resection [119]. Alfentanil has been shown to increase epileptiform activity in patients with epilepsy [120–123] and, because it is short acting, has been recommended for localization of epileptogenic foci during epilepsy surgery [120]. The ease with which alfentanil is able to cause activation of epileptiform discharges was demonstrated in one study where activation occurred in 83% of patients with epilepsy following alfentanil infusion but in only 50% following methohexitone [121]. However, another group has cautioned against the use of alfentanil in patients with epilepsy because bolus administration produced epileptiform activity in three of five patients, with two having electrographic seizures [122]. Epileptiform activity was detected by depth electrodes and not by scalp electrodes in this study and further increase or spread of epileptiform activity did not occur despite cumulative bolus doses. Infusion of remifentanil has recently been shown to have a variable effect on ECoG in patients with epilepsy. Spike numbers were increased during remifentanil infusion in the presence of limited spontaneous spike activity, but spike frequency was not affected, or slightly reduced, if baseline spike activity was high [124]. The authors of this study concluded that remifentanil infusion could be continued during diagnostic ECoG recording.

There are many reports in the literature of seizures following low-, moderate- and high-dose opioid anaesthesia but none is correlated with epileptiform EEG activity [111–113]. Athetoid and other abnormal movements during opioid administration may represent myoclonus [125,126] or an exaggerated form of opioid-induced rigidity [113,114]. It has been suggested that such movements have a neocortical origin [112,114]. However, animal data suggest that the motor activity may result from seizures arising in the hippocampal region [127] and a study of six epileptic patients receiving 20–52 µg/kg of fentanyl reported epileptiform activity in perihippocampal electrodes which did not propagate to scalp electrodes [128]. The effect of low-dose fentanyl on interictal EcoG appears to be minimal, although this has not been addressed in formal clinical studies. Opioids will continue to form an integral part of the anaesthetic technique during epilepsy surgery but large doses should be avoided, particularly during diagnostic ECoG.

Droperidol

Droperidol is frequently used in combination with fentanyl for neuroleptanalgesia during awake craniotomy or in small doses for its antiemetic effect. Droperidol has no effect on the EEG when given alone [95] but when combined with fentanyl has a synergistic suppressive effect [17]. Low-dose droperidol combined with fentanyl increases α-activity, whereas doses sufficient to produce unconsciousness cause high-amplitude δ- and β-activities [118]. Depth electrode studies in animals confirm that droperidol/fentanyl combinations do not suppress limbic activity [129] and droperidol does not affect the nature of the baseline interictal spike activity when used as part of a neuroleptanalgesia technique for awake craniotomy [130]. Despite the absence of definitive studies in man, it seems likely that the small doses of droperidol used in clinical practice have little effect on the ECoG during awake craniotomy.

Muscle relaxants

Despite being ionized, the muscle relaxants used in clinical practice do cross the blood–brain barrier to a limited extent and enter the cerebrospinal fluid when given for sufficient time. However, this is unlikely to be of any clinical significance during the relatively short time periods that neuromuscular blocking drugs are administered during anaesthesia [131]. They have not been reported to cause EEG changes or clinical seizures [132] and different agents have similar effects on lidocaine-induced seizure threshold in cats [133]. Laudanosine, the primary metabolite of atracurium, has been noted to induce clinical seizure activity in animals [134] but it does not increase the threshold or incidence of lidocaine-induced seizures in cats compared to pancuronium or vecuronium [133]. Furthermore, the plasma laudanosine concentrations in patients given atracurium by bolus or by short-term infusion during surgery are significantly less than those required to induce epileptic activity in animals [131]. Even prolonged use of atracurium in critically ill patients on the ICU results in only moderate accumulation of laudanosine and no effects on the EEG [135].

Anticholinergics

The central cholinergic system is an important component in generating seizure activity and the tertiary-amine anticholinergic agents that are capable of crossing the blood–brain barrier might be expected to possess anticonvulsant activity. Atropine reduces epileptiform activity in patients with epilepsy [136] but, when used as premedication, has no effect on the EEG in normal subjects except for that normally associated with somnolence [95]. Hyoscine has also been reported to reduce spike activity in animals [137]. In epilepsy surgery, it is therefore preferable to use glycopyrrolate which has no CNS effects.

Anaesthetic techniques

Surgery for epilepsy may be performed under general anaesthesia using techniques with minimal effects upon normal or epileptiform electrocerebral activity. Alternatively, functional cortical mapping and intraoperative ECoG recording can be achieved in the awake patient using local anaesthesia and sedation. General considerations during anaesthesia for craniotomy for refractory epilepsy include the provision of a safe and comfortable environment for the patient, suitable operating conditions for the neurosurgeon, lack of

interference with intraoperative ECoG recordings and facilitation of intraoperative cortical mapping. Providing the conditions that simultaneously meet these requirements, using general or local anaesthesia with sedation, provides a significant challenge for the neuroanaesthetist [138]. The major decision over the choice of anaesthetic technique relates to whether it is necessary to have the patient awake for ECoG or cortical stimulation mapping. The increasing sophistication of preoperative investigation allowing accurate localization of areas of epileptogenesis and normal brain function, the introduction of minimally invasive surgery, smaller focal resections and the questionable value of ECoG and cortical mapping in relation to seizure outcome are changing the indications for local anaesthesia and sedation [139]. Indications that were previously absolute are now perhaps relative. There has been a trend towards increased use of tailored general anaesthesia as techniques with minimal effects on the EEG have been introduced [17,23,24].

Preoperative assessment

The preoperative visit of patients scheduled for epilepsy surgery is an essential part of the anaesthetic management. The patient's history should be assessed in relation to his or her epilepsy and any other concurrent medical problems. The type and pattern of seizures should be established as well as their frequency and precipitating factors. Previous and current antiepileptic therapy should also be noted. Complications of antiepileptic therapy have been discussed in detail elsewhere in this volume and those with significance to anaesthetists and surgeons should be carefully evaluated during the preoperative assessment. In particular, haematological and hepatic abnormalities must be excluded. An examination of the airway should be carried out, since airway control may be difficult in patients receiving chronic phenytoin therapy because of gingival hyperplasia and poor dentition.

During the preoperative visit the patient must also be prepared psychologically for the forthcoming operation. If awake craniotomy is planned, the sequence of events should be discussed in detail with the patient and the parts of the procedure which may be uncomfortable described. The effects of intraoperative stimulation testing, the potential for nausea following traction on the temporal lobe and the possibility of intraoperative seizures should be highlighted. If craniotomy under general anaesthesia is planned, the need to lighten anaesthesia during neurophysiological testing must be discussed. However, with modern techniques, the possibility of awareness is theoretical rather than real [17,24].

Premedication is rarely given. In particular, benzodiazepines should be avoided to minimize effects on intraoperative ECoG. Anticholinergic 'drying' agents are rarely necessary with modern induction techniques and should be avoided whenever possible. However, if anticholinergic premedication is crucial, glycopyrrolate should be chosen because of its lack of central effects. It is the authors practice to avoid premedication in all cases. Antiepileptic medication should be continued up to and including the day of surgery. Antiepileptic drug levels must be checked preoperatively and supplementary doses administered as required.

General anaesthesia

Many surgeons prefer to carry out epilepsy surgery in an awake patient [140] but most patients, on the other hand, prefer to undergo surgical procedures under general anaesthesia. Some patients, especially the paediatric population, cannot tolerate awake procedures under any circumstances. The majority of epilepsy surgery can be safely performed under general anaesthesia with continued ability to make excellent intraoperative electrophysiological recordings [17,23,24]. General anaesthesia has many benefits for the surgeon, including the provision of optimal operating conditions by the ability to control the arterial partial pressure of carbon dioxide and blood pressure, and the assurance of immobility. The advantage for the patient is, of course, unawareness of the whole procedure. Disadvantages of general anaesthesia include the sacrifice of intraoperative memory and language assessment.

Anaesthesia is induced with thiopentone or propofol and an intravenous opioid, usually fentanyl. The EEG effects of these short-acting induction agents have ended before ECoG is recorded. Tracheal intubation is achieved with the use of a short-acting non-depolarizing neuromuscular blocking agent such as vecuronium or atracurium. It is essential that coughing and straining, with consequent adverse effects on intracranial pressure, are avoided during endotracheal intubation. Anaesthesia is maintained with inhalational or intravenous agents and, despite their different cerebrovascular effects, both are suitable for elective neurosurgical procedures and have similar effects on short-term outcome [141]. Isoflurane and sevoflurane are widely used in neuroanaesthesia. Both are suitable for epilepsy surgery and may be administered in nitrous oxide and oxygen or in oxygen-enriched air. Some neuroranaesthetists avoid nitrous oxide because of its cerebral vasodilating and EEG effects [17]. Continuous infusion of propofol is now popular for maintenance of anaesthesia during neurosurgery [142] but it cannot be used as the sole hypnotic when intraoperative ECoG is planned because its administration must be suspended 15–30 min before recording to minimize effects on the ECoG [24,83]. During the initial craniotomy and dural opening, blood pressure may be controlled with additional doses of fentanyl (to a total of 5 µg/kg) and incremental doses of labetolol, a combined α- and β-adrenoreceptor antagonist. Remifentanil is becoming an increasingly popular agent during epilepsy surgery [126,143–145] because levels of analgesia can be easily titrated to maintain haemodynamic stability during changes in surgical stimulus.

Prior to ECoG recording the inspired concentration of isoflurane or sevoflurane should be maintained at levels <1 MAC to minimize EEG effects. Some prefer to discontinue nitrous oxide 30–50 min prior to ECoG recording [17] but others find it possible to obtain high quality recordings in the presence of nitrous oxide [24]. Reduction of inspired concentrations of volatile agent and discontinuation of nitrous oxide may produce light levels of anaesthesia but the concurrent use of remifentanil minimizes the risk of awareness. If the anaesthetic technique is relying on the maintenance of muscle relaxation to prevent movement or coughing, monitoring of neuromuscular function is mandatory because antiepileptic drugs can alter the response to neuromuscular-blocking drugs [146,147]. It is usually possible to obtain high-quality diagnostic EcoG recordings using this technique [23,24], but activating agents may be administered if adequate recordings cannot be obtained despite a reduction or discontinuation of the inhalational anaesthetic agent. Intraoperative EEG activation has been obtained with methohexitone [63], etomidate [3,90], enflurane [15,16], fentanyl and alfentanil [124]. Anaesthesia may be deepened after corticography by increasing the inspired concentration of volatile agent. It should be remembered that further ECoG recording may be required from electrodes placed over the amygdala or hippocampus after removal of the temporal lobe and at this time inhalational agent concentration should again be reduced.

The disadvantage of general anaesthesia is that it prevents intraoperative motor and speech mapping, but one technique has been described that allows limited mapping of motor function during balanced anaesthesia. The arm contralateral to the surgery was selectively isolated from the effect of neuromuscular blockade using a tourniquet and its motor response to cortical stimulation preserved [148]. The authors claimed that this technique assured patient immobility, shortened the stimulation time and precluded the development of clinical seizures whilst allowing localization of the appropriate area of motor cortex. Clearly this technique has very limited applicability and has not gained widespread acceptance.

Monitoring requirements are similar to those for general neurosurgical procedures and include continuous ECG, pulse oximetry, direct arterial blood pressure, end-tidal carbon dioxide tension, end-tidal inhalational agent concentration, neuromuscular function and temperature. A urinary catheter and nasogastric tube should be inserted after induction of anaesthesia if the surgery will be protracted. Attention must be paid to maintenance of normothermia by the use of a warming mattress, warming blanket and the administration of warmed intravenous fluids.

Local anaesthesia and sedation

The major disadvantage of general anaesthesia for epilepsy surgery is the inability to perform intraoperative cortical stimulation testing. In patients with dominant hemisphere lesions or epileptic foci whose resection margins impinge upon nearby eloquent areas, an awake procedure permits intraoperative sensorimotor mapping and neuropsychological assessment to help define resection margins [149,150].

The technique of awake craniotomy has evolved over many years. Initially, the procedure involved either local anaesthesia followed by general anaesthesia or various methods of intraoperative wake-up techniques [151]. In the 1960s, neuroleptanalgesia using phenoperidine and haloperidol was introduced [152] and, with the advent of fentanyl and droperidol, closer titration of dosing regimens became possible [153,154]. The introduction of short-acting agents such as propofol and remifentanil has given the neuroanaesthetist the ability to titrate sedation and analgesia more reliably, thereby allowing controllable sedation and rapid wake-up when required [76,143,145].

During awake craniotomy all members of the operating team should be briefed on their duties in advance, and patient management carefully planned so that the operation proceeds in a smooth and uneventful manner. The operating theatre becomes a crowded place during epilepsy surgery, particularly during neurophysiological monitoring, and staff movement should be kept to a minimum. Delays and technical problems must be avoided in the presence of an awake patient.

Intravenous and arterial cannulae are inserted under local anaesthesia, and continuous direct arterial blood pressure monitoring, ECG and pulse oximetry initiated. Separate, dedicated intravenous cannulae should be inserted for fluid replacement and sedative/analgesic infusions. A urinary catheter should be inserted if surgery will be prolonged. As the procedure can last for several hours, it is essential that the patient feels comfortable and thus should be carefully positioned on a well-padded table [155]. In particular, patients must be happy with the position of their head and, if a Mayfield head fixator is used, adequate local anaesthesia should be applied prior to application of the pins. The surgical drapes must be positioned to allow the anaesthetist to see and communicate freely with the patient during surgery and maintain continued access to the airway whilst preserving a sterile field for the neurosurgeon. The neuropsychologist also needs unimpeded access to the patient during intraoperative testing.

The techniques available for awake craniotomy include local anaesthesia and sedation or true asleep–awake–asleep techniques using general anaesthesia and intraoperative wake-up. For both techniques, the provision of adequate local anaesthesia using regional, field and dural blocks is essential. The surgeon performs field block of the scalp, using combinations of lidocaine and bupivacaine with epinephrine, after preparation of the operative site [153,155,156]. The skin, scalp, pericranium and periosteum of the outer table of the skull are all innervated by cutaneous nerves arising from branches of the trigeminal nerve. Subcutaneous infiltration with local anaesthetic in the manner of a field block, or over specific sensory nerve branches, effectively blocks afferent input from all layers of the scalp. The skull can be drilled and opened without discomfort to the patient, as it has no sensation itself. The dura, however, is innervated by branches from all three divisions of the trigeminal nerve, the recurrent meningeal branch of the vagus and by branches of the upper cervical roots. It must therefore be adequately anaesthetized by a local anaesthetic nerve block around the nerve trunk running with the middle meningeal artery, and also by a field block around the edges of the craniotomy. The local anaesthetic solutions deposited around the middle meningeal artery should not contain epinephrine. Large doses of local anaesthetic may be required for adequate analgesia and the potential for toxicity must be borne in mind.

Many patients find the early part of the craniotomy until dural opening distressing because of incomplete local anaesthesia or noise from power tools. It is appropriate to use intravenous sedation or general anaesthesia during this phase of the surgery. Sedation techniques have previously relied upon incremental fentanyl, titrated against sedation level and respiratory rate to a maximum of 5 μg/kg. Use of the newer opioids, sufentanil and alfentanil, does not appear to offer any benefit over fentanyl during awake procedures [157]. Some workers have suggested the addition of droperidol (up to 0.1 mg/kg) to provide conscious sedation [153,154] whereas others avoid large doses of droperidol, but administer a small (0.25–0.5 mg) antiemetic dose. More recently, infusions of propofol in conjunction with fentanyl have been used with great success for sedation during the early part of the craniotomy [24,76] and target controlled infusion of propofol has been recommended [158]. The propofol infusion is discontinued as the dura is being opened; the patient then returns to full consciousness and is able to cooperate with stimulation testing and neuropsychological assessment. Furthermore, any EEG affects are avoided if propofol is discontinued at least 15 min prior to corticography [83]. The use of patient-controlled sedation with propofol is also an effective alternative to

neuroleptanalgesia during awake epilepsy surgery and is associated with a lower incidence of intraoperative seizures but a higher incidence of transient respiratory depression [159]. Recently, remifentanil has been used in conjunction with propofol to provide analgesia during awake craniotomy [143–145]. The balance between achieving adequate sedation and analgesia without compromising ventilation and oxygenation may be more difficult when using potent opioids [145] but it is claimed that the safety of the technique can be increased using bispectral index monitoring to guide target-controlled infusions [144]. Furthermore, pharmacokinetic simulations have revealed that changes in infusion rates of propofol and remifentanil are quickly followed by changes in effect site concentrations which correspond well with the desired clinical changes in patient sedation and analgesia [143]. The combination of propofol and remifentanil is likely to be a major advance in the provision of sedation and analgesia during awake craniotomy. There has also been recent interest in the use of α_2-adrenoreceptor agonists during awake craniotomy because these agents provide sedation that is easily reversed with verbal stimulation and they do not suppress ventilation. Dexmedetomidine, a highly specific α_2-adrenoreceptor agonist, has been successfully used as an adjunct during awake craniotomy to provide sedation and analgesia sufficient to complete cortical mapping and tumour resection [160]. Some neuroanaesthetists still prefer to employ general anaesthesia with intraoperative wake-up and recommend using propofol [161], isoflurane, sevoflurane and desflurane [162–164] with and without nitrous oxide.

Management of the airway is of crucial importance, particularly during the sedation phase or if general anaesthesia and intraoperative wake-up are employed. Several methods of airway control have been described. One simple method, suitable for use during sedation techniques, employs topical anaesthesia of the nostrils with cocaine and insertion of a soft nasopharyngeal airway. This allows control of the airway during the sedation phase of the procedure and enables expired carbon dioxide to be monitored [24]. Supplemental oxygen may be administered via the contralateral nostril using one-half of a pair of nasal prongs. Alternatively, a commercially available double nasal cannula allows expired carbon dioxide monitoring from one nostril and administration of oxygen via the other but does not offer any means of airway control. The provision of general anaesthesia prior to intraoperative wake-up necessitates more reliable control of the airway. Several techniques using the laryngeal mask airway (LMA) have been described [161,163,165]. Some recommend use of the LMA only during the sedation phase of the procedure and remove it to allow patient participation during cortical mapping [161]. These authors claim that the LMA can be repositioned with ease for resedation. More recently, a technique that uses the LMA for the entire procedure has been described [163]. In this pilot study a preoperative communication system was established to facilitate intraoperative functional mapping with the LMA in situ but coughing and restlessness necessitated endotracheal intubation in some patients. A modified endotracheal tube that allows topical airway anaesthesia has also been utilized during asleep–awake–asleep procedures [164]. Prior to cortical mapping, the anaesthesia was discontinued and lidocaine injected into the airway via a catheter that was spirally attached to the endotracheal tube. After speech mapping, the patients were reintubated using a fibreoptic laryngoscope or an endotracheal tube changer. A cuffed oropharyngeal airway (COPA) has also been used as a method of airway control during awake craniotomy [162]. Following dural opening, anaesthesia was discontinued and the COPA removed to allow patient cooperation during cortical mapping. After definitive surgery anaesthesia was reinduced and the COPA was reinserted. No coughing or straining was reported and it was possible to reinsert the COPA in the lateral or supine positions. The use of airway instrumentation of any type brings the risk of coughing or straining and subsequent vomiting during lightening of anaesthesia or sedation. For this reason the author prefers to use sedation techniques and non-invasive methods of airway management whenever possible. Airway management is generally uneventful under such circumstances, although the use of sedation inevitably runs the risk of apnoea and airway obstruction. Patient position is crucial, with the lateral position being less likely to result in airway obstruction. Equipment for emergency airway control must always be available during the sedation phase of awake craniotomy. The options for emergency airway control include endotracheal intubation under direct vision, blind nasal intubation, fibreoptic nasotracheal intubation and insertion of an LMA.

Following cortical mapping and ECoG recording, the patient may be resedated or reanaesthetized for the surgical resection. However, many patients prefer to remain awake during the surgical resection and closure of the craniotomy when they realise that the procedure is completely painless.

Although awake craniotomy enables the neurosurgeon to perform precise functional mapping of the cortex, it is not without risk to the patient [166]. The most frequent complication is the development of generalized seizures during stimulation testing [154]. The development of intraoperative seizures in awake patients is a major problem which should be treated aggressively. The choice of anticonvulsant depends upon the stage of the surgery and the severity of the seizure. Prior to corticography, it is preferable to avoid long-acting antiepileptic drugs or benzodiazepines and a small dose of thiopentone or propofol is an appropriate choice [24,154]. Following corticography, any suitable agent may be chosen and it may also be necessary to administer also a top-up dose of the patient's regular long-acting antiepileptic drugs. Dysphoric reactions may also occur during awake craniotomy and these can lead to loss of control of a patient with an open craniotomy. Respiratory depression, due to seizures or sedative and analgesic infusions, leads to brain swelling if untreated. Airway obstruction is also a risk in the sedated, unintubated patient and this has been discussed earlier. Air embolism during awake craniotomy, possibly related to the generation of high negative intrathoracic pressures secondary to airway obstruction, has also been described [167]. Nausea and vomiting occurred in 8% of patients in one study [166] and is more likely during traction on the temporal lobe. Pulmonary aspiration is a rare consequence of intraoperative vomiting in unintubated patients. Despite these potential difficulties, few major problems are encountered during awake craniotomy and no mortality or morbidity related to the anaesthetic technique was reported in a review of over 1000 patients [168]. It is also a procedure that is well tolerated by the average adult patient [169].

Postoperative care

Following surgery, the patient should be nursed in a neurosurgical intensive care or high dependency unit and invasive monitoring should be continued into the postoperative period [55]. The risk of seizures is increased in the immediate few hours after surgery and can progress to status epilepticus. Seizures should be treated aggressively to avoid cerebral damage [21,57]. Because of a prolonged duration of action when given after other sedative/anaesthetic drugs, benzodiazepine administration may limit the ability to carry out a careful postictal neurological assessment. Thiopentone and propofol are readily available in the neurosurgical critical care unit and small doses rapidly and effectively terminate postoperative seizures and ensure swift recovery [55]. Plasma levels of long-acting anticonvulsant drugs should be checked and top-up doses administered as required. It may be necessary to add other anticonvulsants in the short term. A surgical cause for recurrent seizures in the postoperative period should be excluded by CT scanning.

Summary

Surgery for medically intractable epilepsy may be carried out under general anaesthesia or local anaesthesia and sedation. Careful choice of general anaesthetic technique allows intraoperative recording of diagnostic ECoG, whereas awake procedures additionally allow memory, language and sensorimotor mapping. The requirements to provide optimal operative conditions whilst retaining the ability to obtain high-quality intraoperative ECoG and maintain patient safety and comfort may be conflicting. The neuroanaesthetist plays a key role in the perioperative management of this challenging group of patients.

References

1 Horsley V. Brain surgery. *Br Med J* 1886; 2: 670–5.

2 Modica PA, Tempelhoff R, White PF. Pro- and anticonvulsant effects of anaesthetics (part I). *Anesth Analg* 1990; 70: 303–15.

3 Modica PA, Tempelhoff R, White PF. Pro- and anticonvulsant effects of anaesthetics (part II). *Anesth Analg* 1990; 70: 433–43.

4 Avramov MN, Murayama T, Shingu K, Mori K. Electroencephalographic changes during vital capacity breath induction with halothane. *Br J Anaesth* 1991; 66: 211–15.

5 Mecarelli O, De Feo MR, Romanini L, Calvisi V, D'Andrea E. EEG and clinical features in epileptic children during halothane anaesthesia. *Electroencephalogr Clin Neurophysiol* 1981; 52: 468–9.

6 Neigh JL, Garman JK, Harp JR. The electroencephalographic pattern during anaesthesia with ethrane: effects of the depth of anaesthesia, $PaCO_2$ and nitrous oxide. *Anesthesiology* 1971; 35: 482–7.

7 Lebowitz MH, Blitt CE, Dillon JB. Enflurane induced central nervous system excitation and its relation to carbon dioxide tension. *Anesth Analg* 1972; 51: 355–63.

8 Michenfelder JD, Cucchiara RF. Canine cerebral oxygen consumption during enflurane anaesthesia and its modification during induced seizures. *Anesthesiology* 1974; 40: 575–80.

9 Kavan EM, Julien RM, Lucero JJ. Electrographic alterations induced in limbic and sensory systems during induction of anaesthesia with halothane, methoxyflurane, diethyl ether, and enflurane. *Br J Anaesth* 1972; 44: 1234–9.

10 Ohm WW, Cullen BF, Amory DW, Kennedy RD. Delayed seizure activity following enflurane anesthesia. *Anesthesiology* 1975; 42: 367–8.

11 Grant IS. Delayed convulsions following enflurane anaesthesia. *Anaesthesia* 1986; 41: 1024–5.

12 Burchiel KJ, Stockard JJ, Claverly RK and Smith NT. Relationship of pre and post anaesthetic EEG abnormalities to enflurane-induced seizure activity. *Anesth Analg* 1977; 56: 509–14.

13 Opitz A, Oberwetter WD. Enflurane or halothane anesthesia for patients

with convulsive disorders? *Acta Anaesthesiol Scand* 1979; 71 (Suppl.): 43–7.

14 Ito BM, Sato S, Kupta C, Tran D. The effect of isoflurane and enflurane on the electrocorticogram of epileptic patients. *Neurology* 1988; 38: 924–8.

15 Flemming DC, Fitzpatrick J, Fariello RG, Dugg T, Hellman D, Hoff BH. Diagnostic activation of epileptogenic foci by enflurane. *Anesthesiology* 1980; 52: 431–3.

16 Michenfelder JD, ed. *Anaesthesia and the Brain.* New York: Churchill Livingstone, 1988.

17 Kraemer DL, Spencer DD. Anaesthesia in epilepsy surgery. In: Engel J Jr, ed. *Surgical Treatment of the Epilepsies.* New York: Raven Press Ltd, 1993.

18 Newberg LA, Milde JH, Michenfelder JD. Systemic and cerebral effects of isoflurane at and above concentrations that suppress cortical activity. *Anesthesiology* 1983; 59: 23–8.

19 Eger EI. Are seizures caused by isoflurane or nitrous oxide? *Anesthesiology* 1985; 62: 698–9.

20 Kofke WA, Young RS, Davis P *et al.* Isoflurane for refractory status epilepticus: a clinical series. *Anesthesiology* 1989; 71: 653–9.

21 Sakaki T, Abe K, Hoshida T *et al.* Isoflurane in the management of status epilepticus after surgery for lesions around the motor area. *Acta Neurochir* 1992; 116: 38–43.

22 Fiol ME, Boening JA, Cruz-Rodriguez R, Maxwell R. Effect of isoflurane (Forane) on intraoperative electrocorticogram. *Epilepsia* 1993; 34: 897–900.

23 Lüders HO. Protocols for surgery of epilepsy in different centers. In: Lüders HO, ed. *Epilepsy.* New York: Raven Press, 1992.

24 Smith M. Anaesthesia for epilepsy and stereotactic surgery. In: Walters JM, Ingram GS, Jenkinson, eds. *Anaesthesia and Intensive Care for the Neurosurgical Patient.* Oxford: Blackwell Scientific Publications, 1994.

25 Poulton TJ, Ellingston RJ. Seizure associated with induction of anesthesia with isoflurane. *Anesthesiology* 1984; 61: 471–6.

26 Scheller MS, Tateishi A, Drummond JC, Zornow MH. The effect of sevoflurane on cerebral blood flow, cerebral metabolic rate for oxygen, intracranial pressure and electroencephalogram are similar to those of isoflurane in the rabbit. *Anesthesiology* 1988; 68: 548–51.

27 Scheller MS, Nakakimura K, Fleischer JE, Zornow MH. Cerebral effects of sevoflurane in the dog: comparison with isoflurane and enflurane. *Br J Anaesth* 1990; 65: 388–92.

28 Osawa M, Shingu K, Murakawa M *et al.* Effects of sevoflurane on central nervous system electrical activity in cats. *Anesth Analg* 1994; 79: 52–7.

29 Artru AA, Lam AM, Johnson JO, Sperry RJ. Intracranial pressure, middle cerebral artery flow velocity and plasma inorganic fluoride concentrations in neurosurgical patients receiving sevoflurane or isoflurane. *Anesth Analg* 1997; 85: 587–92.

30 Holaday DA, Smith FR. Clinical characteristics and biotransformation of sevoflurane in healthy human volunteers. *Anesthesiology* 1981; 54: 100–6.

31 Avramov MN, Shingu K, Omatsu Y, Osawa M, Mori K. Effects of difference speed of induction with sevoflurane on the EEG in man. *J Anesth* 1987; 1: 1–7.

32 Ian JW, Richard GH, Matthew RC *et al.* Electroencephalographic evidence of seizure activity under deep sevoflurane anaesthesia. *Anesthesiology* 1997; 87: 1579–82.

33 Adachi M, Ikemoto Y, Kubo T, Takuma C. Seizure-like movements during induction of anaesthesia with sevoflurane. *Br J Anaesth* 1992; 68: 214–15.

34 Vakkuri A, Jantti V, Sarkela M, Lindgren L, Korttila K, Yli-Hankala A. Epileptiform EEG during sevoflurane mask induction: effect of delaying the onset of hyperventilation. *Acta Anaesthesiol Scand* 2000; 44: 713–19.

35 Vakkuri A, Yli-Hankala A, Sarkela M *et al.* Sevoflurane mask induction of anaesthesia is associated with epileptiform EEG in children. *Acta Anaesthesiol Scand* 2001; 45: 805–11.

36 Watts ADJ, Herrick IA, McLachlan RS, Craen RA, Gelb AW. The effect of sevoflurane and isoflurane anesthesia on interictal spike activity among patients with refractory epilepsy. *Anesth Analg* 1999; 89: 1275–81.

37 Iijima T, Nakamura Z, Iwao Y, Sankawa H. The epileptogenic properties of the volatile anesthestics sevoflurane and isoflurane in patients with epilepsy. *Anesth Analg* 2000; 91: 989–95.

38 Hisada K, Morioka T, Fukui K. Effects of sevoflurane and isoflurane on electrocorticographic activities in patients with temporal lobe epilepsy. *J Neurosurg Anaesth* 2001; 13: 333–7.

39 Rampil IJ, Weiskop RB, Brown JG. I-653 and isoflurane produce similar dose-related changes in the electroencephalogram of pigs. *Anesthesiology* 1988; 69: 298–302.

40 Rampil IJ, Lockhart SH, Eger EI. EEG effects of desflurane in humans. *Anesthesiology* 1991; 74: 434–9.

41 Lutz LJ, Milde JH, Milde LN. The cerebral functional, metabolic, and hemodynamic effects of desflurane in dogs. *Anesthesiology* 1990; 73: 125–31.

42 Faulconer A, Pender JW, Bickford RG. The influence of partial pressure of nitrous oxide on the depth of anaesthesia and the electroencephalogram in man. *Anesthesiology* 1994; 10: 601–9.

43 Horbein TF, Eger EI, Winter PM, Smith G, Wetstone D, Smith KH. The minimum alveolar concentration of nitrous oxide in man. *Anesth Analg* 1982; 61: 533–6.

44 Modica PA, Tempelhoff R. Seizures during emergence from anaesthesia. *Anesthesiology* 1989; 71: 296–300.

45 Gloor P. *Contributions of Electroencephalography and Electrocorticography to the Neurosurgical Treatment of the Epilepsies.* New York: Raven Press, 1975.

46 Stevens JE, Oshima E, Mori K. Effects of nitrous oxide on the epileptogenic property of enflurane in cats. *Br J Anaesth* 1983; 55: 145–53.

47 Ojemann GA, Engle J Jr. Acute and chronic intracranial recording and stimulation. In: Engel J Jr, ed. *Surgical Treatment of the Epilepsies.* New York: Raven Press, 1987.

48 Kiersey DK, Bickford RG, Faulconer A. Electroencephalographic patterns produced by thiopental sodium during surgical operations: description and classification. *Br J Anaesth* 1951; 23: 141–52.

49 Fuster B, Gibbs FL, Gibbs FA. Pentothal sleep as an aid to the diagnosis and localisation of seizure discharges of the psychomotor types. *Dis Nerv Syst* 1948; 9: 199–202.

50 Stoica I. Rapid electroencephalographic activation by small doses of natruimevaipan. *Epilepsia* 1965; 6: 54–66.

51 Lombroso CT, Erba G. Primary and secondary bilateral synchrony in epilepsy. A clinical and electroencephalographic study. *Arch Neurol* 1970; 22: 321–34.

52 Engel J, Driver MV, Falconer MA. Electrophysiological correlates of pathology and surgical results in temporal lobe epilepsy. *Brain* 1975; 98: 129–56.

53 Engel J, Pausch R, Lieb JP, Kuhl DE, Crandall PI I. Correlation of criteria used for localizing epileptogenic foci in patients considered for surgical therapy of epilepsy. *Ann Neurol* 1981; 9: 215–24.

54 Lieb JP, Babb TL, Engel J. Quantitative comparison of cell loss and thiopental-induced EEG changes in human epileptic hippocampus. *Epilepsia* 1989; 30: 147–56.

55 Smith M. Post-operative neurosurgical care. *Curr Anaesth Crit Care* 1994; 5: 29–35.

56 Partinen M, Kovanen J, Nilsson E. Status epilepticus treated by barbiturate anaesthesia with continuous monitoring of cerebral function. *Br Med J* 1981; 282: 520–1.

57 Chapman MG, Smith M, Hirsch NP. Status epilepticus. *Anaesthesia* 2001; 56: 648–59.

58 Gumpert J, Paul R. Activation of the electroencephalogram with intravenous Brietal (methohexitone): the findings in 100 cases. *J Neurol Neurosurg Psychiatr* 1971; 34: 646–8.

59 Paul R, Harris R. A comparison of methohexitone and thiopentone in electrocorticography. *J Neurol Neurosurg Psychiatry* 1970; 33: 100–4.

60 Austin EJ, Chatrian GE, Ojemann GA, Lettich E. Methohexital activation of epileptiform discharges in the human electrocorticogram. *Epilepsia* 1986; 27: 624.

61 Hufnagel A, Burr W, Elger CE, Madstawek J, Hefner G. Localization of the epileptogenic focus during methohexital-induced anaesthesia. *Epilepsia* 1992; 33: 271–84.

62 Hardiman O, Coughlan A, O'Moore B, Phillips J, Staunton H. Interictal spike localisation with methohexitone: preoperative activation and surgical follow-up. *Epilepsia* 1987; 28: 335–9.

63 Wyler AR, Richey ET, Atkinson RA, Hermann BP. Methohexital activation of epileptogenic foci during acute electrocorticography. *Epilepsia* 1987; 28: 490–4.

64 Mahla ME, Pashayan AG, Grundy BL, Mixson S, Richards RK, Day AL. Prolonged anaesthesia with propofol or isoflurane: intraoperative electroencephalographic patterns and postoperative recovery. *Semin Anesth* 1992; 11 (Suppl. 1): 31–2.

65 Committee on Safety of Medicines. Propofol and delayed convulsions. *Current Problems* 1992; 35: 2.

66 Makela JP, Iivanainen M, Pieninkeroinen IP, Waltimo O, Ladensuu M. Seizures associated with propofol anesthesia. *Epilepsia* 1993; 34: 832–5.

67 Jones GW, Boykett MH, Klok M. Propofol, opisthotonus and epilepsy. *Anaesthesia* 1988; 43: 904.

68 Victory RAP, Magee D. A case of convulsion after propofol anaesthesia. *Anaesthesia* 1988; 43: 904.

69 DeFriez CB, Wong HC. Seizures and opisthotonus after propofol anaesthesia. *Anesth Analg* 1992; 75: 630–2.

70 Boorgeat A, Dessigbourg C, Popovic V, Meier D, Blanchard M, Schwander D. Propofol and spontaneous movement: an EEG study. *Anesthesiology* 1991; 74: 24–7.

71 Lowson S, Gent JP, Goodchild CS. Anticonvulsant properties of propofol and thiopentone: comparison using two tests in laboratory mice. *Br J Anaesth* 1990; 64: 59–64.

72 MacKenzie SJ, Kapadia F, Grant IS. Propofol infusion for control of status epilepticus. *Anaesthesia* 1990; 45: 1043–5.

73 McBurney JW, Teiken PJ, Moon MR. Propofol for treating status epilepticus. *J Epilepsy* 1994; 7: 21–2.

74 Hodkinson BP, Frith RW, Mee EW. Propofol and the electroencephalogram. *Lancet* 1987; ii: 1518.

75 Samra SK, Sneyd JR, Ross DA, Henry TR. Effects of propofol sedation on seizures and intracranially recorded epileptiform activity in patients with partial epilepsy. *Anesthesiology* 1995; 82: 843–51.

76 Silbergeld DL, Mueller WM, Coley PS, Ojemann GA, Lettich E. Use of propofol (Diprivan) for awake craniotomies; technical note. *Surg Neurol* 1992; 38: 271–2.

77 Ebrahim ZY, Schubert A, Van Ness P, Wolgamuth B, Awad I. The effect of propofol on the electroencephalogram of patients with epilepsy. *Anesth Analg* 1994; 78: 275–9.

78 Cheng MA, Tempelhoff R, Silbergeld DL, Theard MA, Haines SK, Miller JW. Large-dose propofol alone in adult epileptic patients: electrocorticographic results. *Anesth Analg* 1996; 83: 169–74.

79 Hufnagel A, Aleger CE, Nadstawek J, Stueckel H, Boker DK. Specific response of the epileptic focus to anaesthesia with propofol. *J Epilepsy* 1990; 3: 37–45.

80 Smith M, Smith SJ, Scott CA, Harkness WFJ. Activation of the electrocorticogram by propofol during epilepsy surgery. *Br J Anaesth* 1996; 76: 499–502.

81 Hewitt PB, Chu DLK, Polkey CE, Binnie CD. Effect of propofol on the electrocorticogram in epileptic patients undergoing cortical resection. *Br J Anaesth* 1999; 82: 199–202.

82 Drummond JC, Iragui-Madoz VJ, Alksne JF, Kalkman CJ. Masking epileptiform activity by propofol during seizure surgery. *Anesthesiology* 1992; 76: 652–4.

83 Herrick IA, Craen RA, Gelb AW *et al.* Propofol sedation during awake craniotomy for seizures: electrocorticographic and epileptogenic effects. *Anesth Analg* 1997; 84: 1280–4.

84 Ghoneim MM, Yamada T. Etomidate: a clinical and electroencephalographic comparison with thiopental. *Anesth Analg* 1977; 56: 479–85.

85 Doenicke A, Loffler B, Kugler J, Suttmann H, Grote B. Plasma concentration and EEG after various regimens of etomidate. *Br J Anaesth* 1982; 54: 393–400.

86 Krieger W, Copperman J, Laxer KD. Seizures with etomidate anaesthesia. *Anesth Analg* 1985; 64: 1226–7.

87 Grant JS, Hutchinson G. Epileptiform seizures during prolonged etomidate sedation. *Lancet* 1983; ii: 511–12.

88 Laughlin TP, Newberg LA. Prolonged myoclonus after etomidate anaesthesia. *Anesth Analg* 1985; 64: 80–2.

89 Ebrahim ZY, DeBoer GE, Lüders H, Hahn JF, Lesser RP. Effect of etomidate on the electroencephalogram of patients with epilepsy. *Anesth Analg* 1986; 65: 1004–6.

90 Koerner MK, Laxer KD, Krieger W. Etomidate for the activation of epileptiform abnormalities. *Epilepsy* 1986; 27: 624.

91 Krieger W, Koerner M. Generalised grand mal seizure after recovery from uncomplicated fentanyl-etomidate anaesthesia. *Anesth Analg* 1987; 66: 284–5.

92 Gancher S, Laxer KD, Kreger W. Activation of epileptogenic activity by etomidate. *Anesthesiology* 1984; 61: 616–18.

93 Wauquier A. Profile of etomidate, a hypnotic, anticonvulsant and brain protective compound. *Anaesthesia* 1983; 38 (Suppl.): 26–33.

94 Hoffman P, Schockenhoff B. Etomidate as an anticonvulsive agent. *Anaesthetist* 1984; 33: 142–4.

95 Pichlmayr I, Lips U, Kunkel H. Electroencephalographic patterns induced by various anesthetics and perioperative influences. In: Pichlmayr I, Lips U, Kunkel H, eds. *The Electroencephalogram in Anaesthesia*. Berlin: Springer-Verlag, 1984.

96 Browne TR, Penny JK. Benzodiazepines in the treatment of epilepsy. *Epilepsia* 1973; 14: 277–310.

97 Wroblewski BA, Joseph AB. Intramuscular midazolam for treatment of acute seizures or behavioural episodes in patients with brain injuries. *J Neurol Neurosurg Psychiatr* 1992; 55: 328–9.

98 Tassinari CA, Dravet C, Roger J, Cano JP, Gastaut H. Tonic status epilepticus precipitated by intravenous benzodiazepine in five patients with Lennox–Gastaut syndrome. *Epilepsia* 1972; 12: 421–35.

99 Gotman J, Gloor P, Quesney LF, Olivier A. Correlations between EEG changes induced by diazepam and the localisation of epileptic spikes and seizures. *Electroencephalogr Clin Neurophysiol* 1982; 54: 614–21.

100 Corssen G, Little S, Tavakoli M. Ketamine and epilepsy. *Anesth Analg* 1974; 53: 319–35.

101 Schwartz MS, Virden S, Scott DF. Effects of ketamine on the electroencephalograph. *Anaesthesia* 1974; 29: 135–40.

102 Rosen I, Hagerdal M. Electroencephalographic study of children during ketamine anaesthesia. *Acta Anaesth Scand* 1976; 20: 32–9.

103 Winters WD. Epilepsy or anesthesia with ketamine. *Anesthesiology* 1972; 36: 309–12.

104 Ferrer-Allado T, Brechner VL, Dymond A, Cozen H, Crandall P. Ketamine induced electroconvulsive phenomena in the human limbic and thalamic regions. *Anesthesiology* 1973; 38: 333–44.

105 Bennett DR, Madsen JA, Jordan WS, Wiser WC. Ketamine anesthesia in brain damaged epileptics. *Neurology* 1973; 23: 449–60.

106 Celesia GC, Chen RC, Bamforth BJ. Effects of ketamine in epilepsy. *Neurology* 1975; 25: 169–72.

107 Wagman IH, DeJong RH, Prince DA. Effects of lidocaine on the central nervous system. *Anesthesiology* 1967; 28: 155–72.

108 Pascual J, Ciudad J, Berciano J. Role of lidocaine (lignocaine) in managing status epilepticus. *J Neurol Neurosurg Psychiatr* 1992; 55: 49–51.

109 Wagman IH, DeJong RH, Prince DA. Effects of lidocaine upon spontaneous cortical and subcortical electric activity. Production of seizure discharges. *Arch Neurol* 1968; 18: 277–90.

110 DeJong RG, Walts LF. Lidocaine-induced psychomotor seizures in man. *Acta Anaesthesiol Scand* 1966; 23 (Suppl.): 598–604.

111 Sebel PS, Bovill JG, Wauquier A, Rog P. Effects of high-dose fentanyl anesthesia on the electroencephalogram. *Anesthesiology* 1981; 55: 203–11.

112 Murkin JM, Moldenhauer CC, Hug CC, Epstein CM. Absence of seizures during induction of anaesthesia with high-dose fentanyl. *Anesth Analg* 1984; 63: 489–94.

113 Scott JC, Sarnquist FH. Seizure-like movements during a fentanyl infusion with absence of seizure activity in a simultaneous EEG recording. *Anesthesiology* 1985; 62: 812–14.

114 Smith NT, Benthuysen JL, Bickford RG *et al.* Seizures during opioid anesthetic induction: are they opioid-induced rigidity? *Anesthesiology* 1989; 71: 852–62.

115 Kearse LA, Koski G, Husain MV, Philbin DM, McPeck LK. Epileptiform activity during opioid anesthesia. *Electroencephalogr Clin Neurophysiol* 1993; 87: 374–9.

116 Kaiko RF, Foley KM, Grabinski PY *et al.* Central nervous system excitatory effects of meperidine in cancer patients. *Ann Neurol* 1983; 13: 180–5.

117 Goetting MG, Thirmam MJ. Neurotoxicity of meperidine. *Ann Emerg Med* 1985; 14: 1007–9.

118 Nilsson E, Ingvar DH. EEG findings in neuroleptanalgesia. *Acta Anaesthesiol Scand* 1967; 11: 121–7.

119 Tempelhoff R, Modica PA, Bernardo KL, Edwards I. Fentanyl-induced electrocorticographic seizures in patients with complex partial seizures. *J Neurosurg* 1992; 77: 201–8.

120 Manninen PH, Burke SJ, Wennberg R, Lozano AM, El Beheiry H. Intraoperative localization of an epileptogenic focus with alfentanil and fentanyl. *Anesth Analg* 1999; 88: 1101–6.

121 Keene DL, Roberts D, Splinter WM *et al*. Alfentanil mediated activation of epileptiform activity in the electrocorticogram during resection of epileptogenic foci. *Can J Neurol Sci* 1997; 24: 37–9.

122 Ross J, Kearse LA, Barlow MK, Houghton KJ, Cosgrove GR. Alfentanil-induced epileptiform activity: a simultaneous surface and depth electroencephalographic study in complex partial epilepsy. *Epilepsia* 2001; 42: 220–5.

123 Cascino GD, So EL, Sharbrough FW *et al*. Alfentanil-induced epileptiform activity in patients with partial epilepsy. *J Clin Neurophysiol* 1993; 10: 520–5.

124 Herrick IA, Craen RA, Blume WT, Novick T, Gelb AW. Sedative doses of remifentanil have minimal effects on ECoG spike activity during awake epilepsy surgery. *J Neurosurg Anesthesiol* 2002; 14: 55–8.

125 Bowdle TA. Myoclonus following sufentanil without EEG seizure activity. *Anesthesiology* 1987; 67: 593–5.

126 Goroszeniuk T, Albin M, Jones RM. Generalised grand mal seizure after recovery from uncomplicated fentanyl-etomidate anaesthesia. *Anesth Analg* 1986; 65: 979–81.

127 Tommasino C, Maekawa T, Shapiro HM. Fentanyl induced seizures activate subcortical brain metabolism. *Anesthesiology* 1984; 60: 283–90.

128 Tempelhoff R, Bernardo KL, Modica PA, Edwards I. Fentanyl-induced temporal lobe seizure activity recorded with epidural (including perihippocampal) electrodes. *Anesthesiology* 1990; 73 (Suppl.): A168.

129 Kavan EM, Reite ML, Rhodes JM, Adey WR. Effect of innovan on subcortical structures in monkeys. *Acta Anaesthesiol Scand* 1967; 11: 109–13.

130 Opitz A, Marschall M, Degan R, Koch D. General anesthesia in patients with epilepsy and status epilepticus. In: Delgado Escueta AV *et al*., eds. *Status Epilepticus: Mechanisms of Brain Damage and Treatment*. New York: Raven Press, 1983.

131 Chapple DJ, Miller AA, Ward JB, Wheatley PL. Cardiovascular and neurological effects of laudanosine. Studies in mice and rats and conscious and anesthetized dogs. *Br J Anaesth* 1987; 59: 218–25.

132 Lanier WL, Milde JH, Michenfelder JD. The cerebral effects of pancuronium and atracurium in halothane-anesthetized dogs. *Anesthesiology* 1985; 63: 589–97.

133 Lanier WL, Sharbrough FW, Michenfelder JD. Effects of atracurium, vecuronium or pancuronium pretreatment on lignocaine seizure thresholds in cats. *Br J Anaesth* 1988; 60: 74–80.

134 Tateishi A, Zornow MH, Scheller MS, Canfell PC. Electroencephalographic effects of laudanosine in an animal model of epilepsy. *Br J Anaesth* 1989; 62: 548–52.

135 Grigore AM, Brusco L, Kuroda M, Koorn R. Laudanosine and atracurium concentrations in a patient receiving long-term atracurium infusion. *Crit Care Med* 1998; 26: 180–3.

136 Toman JEP, Davis JP. The effects of drugs upon the electrical activity of the brain. *Pharmacol Rev* 1949; 1: 425–92.

137 Moorthy SS, Reddy RV, Paradise RR, Losasso AM, Gibbs PS. Reduction of enflurane-induced spike activity in by scopolamine. *Anesth Analg* 1980; 59: 417–20.

138 Herrick IA, Gelb AW. Anesthesia for temporal lobe epilepsy surgery. *Can J Neurol Sci* 2000; 27: S64–7.

139 Sahjpaul RL. Awake craniotomy: controversies, indications and techniques in the surgical treatment of temporal lobe epilepsy. *Can J Neurol Sci* 2000; 27: S55–63.

140 Larkin M. Neurosurgeons wake up to awake-brain surgery. *Lancet* 1999; 353: 1772.

141 Todd MM, Warner DS, Sokoll MD. A prospective, comparative trial of three anesthetics for elective supratentorial craniotomy. Propofol/fentanyl, isoflurane/nitrous oxide, and fentanyl/nitrous oxide. *Anesthesiology* 1993; 78: 1005–20.

142 Ravussin P, de Tribolet N, Wilder-Smith OH. Total intravenous anesthesia is best for neurological surgery. *J Neurosurg Anesthesiol* 1994; 6: 285–9.

143 Johnson KB, Egan TD. Remifentanil and propofol combination for awake craniotomy: case report with pharmacokinetic simulations. *J Neurosurg Anesthesiol* 1998; 10: 25–9.

144 Hans P, Bonhomme V, Born JD *et al*. Target-controlled infusion of propofol and remifentanil combined with bispectral index monitoring for awake craniotomy. *Anaesthesia* 2000; 55: 255–9.

145 Berkenstadt H, Perel A, Hadani M, Unofrievich I, Ram Z. Monitored anesthesia care using remifentanil and propofol for awake craniotomy. *J Neurosurg Anesthesiol* 2001; 13: 246–9.

146 Ornstein E, Matteo RS, Silverberg PA, Schwartz AE, Young WL, Diaz J. Chronic phenytoin therapy and non-depolarizing muscular blockade. *Anesthesiology* 1986; 63: A331.

147 Tempelhoff R, Modica PA, Jellish WS, Spitznagel EL. Resistance to atracurium-induced neuromuscular blockade in patients with intractable seizure disorders treated with anticonvulsants. *Anesth Analg* 1990; 71: 665–9.

148 Abou-Madi M, Trop D, Lenis S, Olivier A, Leblanc R. Selective neuromuscular blockade for intraoperative electrocorticography. *Appl Neurophysiol* 1987; 50: 386–9.

149 Penfield W, Pasquet A. Combined regional and general anaesthesia for craniotomy and cortical exploration. *Anaesth Analg* 1954; 33: 145–64.

150 Dreifus FE. Goals of surgery for epilepsy. In: *Surgical Treatment of the Epilepsies*. Engel J, ed. New York: Raven Press, 1987.

151 Pasquet A. Combined regional and general anesthesia for craniotomy and cortical exploration. Part II. Anaesthetic considerations. *Int Anesthsiol Clin* 1986; 24: 12–20.

152 Lassner J, Brown AS, Foldes FF *et al*. Symposium on neuroleptanalgesia. *Acta Anaesthesiol Scand Suppl* 1966; 25: 251–79.

153 Trop D. Conscious-sedation analgesia during the neurosurgical treatment of epilepsies – practice at the Montreal Neurological Institute. *Int Anesthesiol Clin* 1986; 24: 175–84.

154 Manninen P, Contreras J. Anaesthetic considerations for craniotomy in awake patients. *Int Anesthesiol Clin* 1986; 24: 157–74.

155 Girvin J. Neurosurgical considerations and general methods for craniotomy under local anaesthesia. *Int Anesthesiol Clin* 1986; 24: 89–114.

156 Geevarghese KP, Reiss SJ, Garretson HD. Alert anaesthesia for intracranial surgery. *Anesth Analg* 1989; 68: S97.

157 Gignac E, Manninen PH, Gelb AW. Comparison of fentanyl, sufentanil and alfentanil during awake craniotomy for epilepsy. *Can J Anaesth* 1993; 40: 421–4.

158 Huggins N. 'Diprifusor' for neurosurgical procedures. *Anaesthesia* 1998; 53 (Suppl.): 13–21.

159 Herrick IA, Craen RA, Gelb AW *et al*. Propofol sedation during awake craniotomy for seizures: patient-controlled administration versus neurolept analgesia. *Anesth Analg* 1997; 84: 1285–91.

160 Bekker AY, Kaufman B, Smir H, Doyle W. The use of dexmedetomidine infusion or awake craniotomy. *Anesth Analg* 2001; 92: 1251–3.

161 Fukaya C, Katayama Y, Yoshino A, Kobayashi K, Kasai M, Yamamotot T. Intraoperative wake-up procedure with propofol and laryngeal mask for optimal excision of brain tumour in eloquent areas. *J Clin Neurosci* 2001; 8: 253–5.

162 Audu P, Atkinson-Polise P, Loomba N. Cuffed oropharyngeal airway (COPA) in awake intracranial surgery (AICS). *J Neurosurg Anesthesiol* 2001; 13: 367.

163 Ling E, Parrish MB, Reddy KKV. Awake craniotomy for tumour resection using the laryngeal mask airway. *J Neurosurg Anesthesiol* 2001; 13: 368.

164 Huncke K, Van de Wiele B, Fried I, Rubinstein EH. The asleep-awake-asleep anesthetic technique for intraoperative language mapping. *Neurosurgery* 1998; 42: 1312–16.

165 Tongier WK, Joshi GP, Landers DF, Mickey B. Use of the laryngeal mask during awake craniotomy for tumour resection. *J Clin Anesth* 2000; 12: 592–4.

166 Archer DP, McKenna JMA, Morin L. Conscious-sedation analgesia during craniotomy for intractable epilepsy: a review of 354 cases. *Can J Anaesth* 1988; 35: 338–44.

167 Scuplak SM, Smith M, Harkness WF. Air embolism during awake craniotomy. *Anesthesia* 1995; 50: 338–40.

168 Rasmussen TB. Surgical treatment of complex-partial seizures: results, lessons and problems. *Epilepsia* 1983; 24: S65–76.

169 Danks RA, Rogers M, Aglio LS, Gugino LD, Black PM. Patient tolerance of craniotomy performed with a patient under local anesthesia and monitored conscious sedation. *Neurosurgery* 1998; 42: 28–34.

73 Vagus Nerve Stimulation

S.C. Schachter

Despite the introduction of numerous antiepileptic drugs (AEDs) over the past decade, partial onset seizures in many patients with epilepsy remain refractory to medical therapy at maximum tolerated dosages [1,2]. Vagus nerve stimulation or VNS (VNS Therapy; Cyberonics, Inc.), a new non-pharmacological antiepileptic therapy, was approved in 1997 by the US Food and Drug Administration for use as adjunctive therapy for adults and adolescents over 12 years of age whose partial onset seizures are refractory to antiepileptic medications. VNS is also approved in numerous European Union countries for use in reducing the frequency of seizures in patients of any age whose epileptic disorder is dominated by partial seizures (with and without secondary generalization) or generalized seizures. This chapter will review VNS Therapy and potential mechanisms of action, results of VNS efficacy studies and the safety and tolerability profile of this therapy.

VNS Therapy: the implantation procedure

The components of VNS Therapy (Fig. 73.1) are the programmable pulse generator, a bipolar lead, a programming wand with accompanying software, a tunnelling tool and hand-held magnets [3,4].

The Model 102 VNS Therapy pulse generator, which is usually implanted in the patient's upper left chest, is powered by a lithium carbon monofluoride battery that produces charge-balanced waveforms at constant current. The latest version of the hermetically sealed titanium generator weighs 25 g, and is 52 mm in diameter and 6.9 mm deep.

The stimulating electrodes, which connect via the alloy bipolar lead to the generator, are attached to the left vagus nerve and thereby convey the electrical signal produced by the generator to the vagus nerve. The bipolar lead has two connector pins at one end, which are plugged into the generator, and two separate helical silicone coils at the other end. Each helix has three turns; on the inside of the middle turn is a platinum ribbon coil that is welded to the lead wire.

The implantation procedure usually lasts between 30 min and 2 h, and is performed as same day surgery at some centres [5]. At other facilities, patients remain in the hospital the night after the implantation. The procedure, described in detail elsewhere [6], is typically performed under general anaesthesia to minimize the possibility that a seizure will disrupt the operation [7–9], though regional cervical blocks with the patient awake have also been used [10].

The initial incision is made over the anterior border of the left sternocleidomastoid muscle between the mastoid process and the clavicle. The vagus nerve is then identified in the carotid sheath in a posterior groove between the carotid artery and the jugular vein. Several centimetres of the nerve are mobilized using vessel loops to facilitate attachment of the helical coils. The second incision is made either in the left upper chest or further laterally near the axilla. A subcutaneous pouch is then made above this incision, into which the generator will eventually be inserted.

The tunnelling tool advances the electrode pins subcutaneously from the base of the cervical incision to the thoracic incision. The stimulating electrodes at the rostral end of the bipolar lead are then carefully attached to the exposed vagus nerve. The helical shape of the stimulating electrodes allows the surgeon to place the coils around the vagus nerve non-traumatically while ensuring mechanical contact between the middle coil and the nerve. The generator is then brought into the surgical field and attached to the electrode connector pins at the caudal end of the bipolar lead.

Before the generator is placed into the subcutaneous pouch and both incisions are closed, diagnostic tests are performed to check the system for proper operation. At most centres, the generator's output current is then set to 0 mA for the first 2 postoperative weeks, after which ramping up of the output current is initiated. Other centres begin stimulation within the first postoperative day.

Clinicians set the parameters for automatic stimulation via computer software, which are then transmitted by the programming wand using radiofrequency signals to the generator (Fig. 73.2, Table 73.1). Parameter settings for magnet-activated on-demand stimulation are also programmable (see below). The wand is further used to perform diagnostic checks of wand–generator communications, lead impedance, programmed current and an estimation of the remaining generator battery life.

The ramp-up procedure and settings for chronic, intermittent stimulation are individualized according to patient tolerance (see clinical use of VNS for epilepsy below). Besides intermittent stimulation, on-demand stimulation is achieved by the patient or a companion placing the supplied magnet on the patient's chest over the generator for several seconds. The stimulator settings employed for on-demand stimulation usually utilize a higher current and pulse width than those used for intermittent stimulation. Some patients have reported that on-demand stimulation interrupts a seizure or reduces its severity and/or duration, particularly if applied during the early phase of the seizure [11]. Patients can also turn off stimulation at any time by keeping the supplied magnet over the generator.

The generator in the Model 102 system is estimated to provide between 6 and 11 years of operation, after which it can be replaced with a minor procedure performed under local anaesthesia.

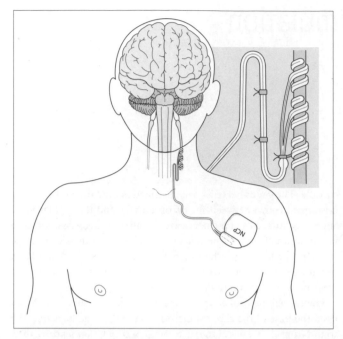

Fig. 73.1 Schematic drawing of the general placement of the NCP vagus nerve stimulation system and bipolar stimulating lead [121]. Cover design; reproduced with permission.

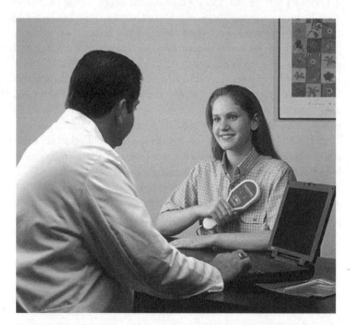

Fig. 73.2 Use of programming wand to adjust generator stimulator parameters. Courtesy of Cyberonics, Inc.

Vagus nerve anatomy and mechanism of action of VNS

The possible mechanism(s) of action of VNS are discussed in detail elsewhere [12,13] and are clearly different from those known to be associated with pharmacotherapy, such as effects on neuronal membrane ionic conductance or neurotransmitters and their receptors [14]. The vagus nerve is a mixed nerve with regard to fibre size

Table 73.1 Available stimulation parameter settings (Model 102 VNS Therapy)

Stimulation parameter	Available settings
Output current	0–3.5 mA ± 10%, in 0.25 mA steps
Signal frequency	1, 2, 5, 10, 15, 20, 25, 30 Hz
Pulse width	130, 250, 500, 750, 1000 µs ± 10%
Signal ON time	7, 14, 21, 30, 60 s
Signal OFF time	0.2, 0.3, 0.5, 0.8, 1.1, 1.8, 3 min, and 5–180 min (5–6 min in 5-min steps; 60–180 min in 30-min steps)

and direction of nerve transmission. Most vagal fibres are small-diameter unmyelinated C fibres; the rest are intermediate-diameter myelinated B fibres and large-diameter myelinated A fibres. Just as for other peripheral nerves, there are direct relationships between vagus fibre diameter and conduction velocity, and between fibre diameter and stimulation threshold. The threshold for C fibre activation is 10–100 times higher than for A fibre activation. As discussed below, the anticonvulsant effect of VNS in experimental animals generally requires C fibre stimulation.

Vagal efferents

Special visceral vagal efferents innervate the pharynx and the larynx, the latter via the recurrent laryngeal branches of the vagus nerve. The general visceral efferents supply parasympathetic innervation to the heart (resulting in slowing of the heart rate), lungs (bronchial constriction and pulmonary secretions) and gastrointestinal tract (increased peristalsis and secretions).

During development, the right and left vagal efferents establish asymmetrical connections with their visceral targets [15,16]. For example, the right vagus innervates the cardiac atria, whereas the left vagus primarily connects with the ventricles [16]. Furthermore, ventricular innervation is less dense than that of the atria, which may explain why left vagus stimulation is less likely than right vagus stimulation to affect adversely cardiac conduction [13].

Vagal afferents

Sensory vagal afferents comprise 80% of vagus fibres and transmit visceral sensation from the head, neck, thorax and abdomen [17,18]. The cell bodies of the vagus nerve in the nodose ganglion project to the nucleus of the solitary tract (NTS; Fig. 73.3). The NTS, in turn, projects to autonomic preganglionic and related somatic motor neurones in the medulla and spinal cord [19,20], and to the medullary reticular formation and the forebrain.

Most NTS output is relayed via the parabrachial nucleus (PBN), located in the dorsal pons lateral to the locus coeruleus (LC) [21], which sends efferents to the hypothalamus as well as the amygdala and orbitofrontal cortex. The PBN has direct input to several thalamic nuclei, including the ventroposterior parvocellular nucleus (which relays visceral sensation to the insular cortex [22]), and the intralaminar nuclei of the thalamus [23], which have widespread effects on cortical activity. Both the PBN and the NTS project to the hypothalamus, amygdala and basal forebrain. The lateral

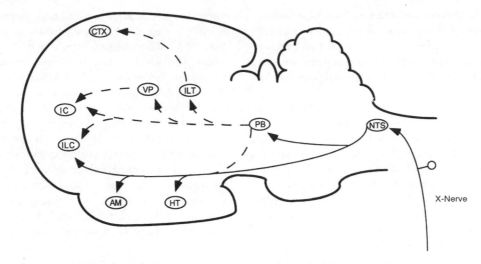

Fig. 73.3 A schematic drawing of the ascending pathways relaying information from the vagus nerve to the forebrain. All afferents in the vagus nerve (X Nerve) synapse in the nucleus of the solitary tract (NTS). The NTS provides an ascending pathway to the parabrachial nucleus (PB). The output from the PB is then supplemented by additional axons from the NTS in providing input to the hypothalamus (HT), bed nucleus of the stria terminalis and amygdala (AM), and the infralimbic cortex (ILC). These pathways allow vagus inputs to interact with autonomic, endocrine and emotional control. A second pathway from the PB goes directly to the thalamus and cortex. Some axons go to a visceral sensory relay nucleus in the ventroposterior thalamic complex (VP), which relays information about the internal body to the visceral sensory cortex in the insular area (IC). This is probably the pathway that relays sensation from vagus stimulation to conscious perception. Other axons from the PB go to the thalamic intralaminar and midline nuclei (ILT), which have extensive and diffuse projections throughout the cerebral cortex (CTX). This latter pathway may represent the point at which vagus stimulation interacts with pathways traditionally thought to control cortical synchronization and desynchronization. Reproduced with permission [13].

hypothalamus and basal forebrain, in turn, project diffusely to the cerebral cortex and influence overall cortical activity [24].

The impact of VNS on this anatomical circuitry has been studied with a variety of techniques, including fos immunoreactivity in animal models. The expression of fos, a nuclear protein that signals gene transcription, denotes neurones that become activated under controlled experimental conditions. In rats undergoing left VNS, increased fos is expressed in posterior cortical amygdaloid nucleus, cingulate and retrosplenial cortex, and ventromedial and arcuate hypothalamic nuclei; fos induction is also observed in the habenular nucleus of thalamus, vagus nerve nuclei and in the A5 and LC noradrenergic nuclei [25].

Physiological studies

Neurophysiological techniques, including EEG and evoked responses, provide supportive evidence that vagus stimulation influences NTS–PBN–thalamic circuitry [26–29]. In animals, VNS stimulation generates measurable evoked responses in the thalamus (ventroposterior complex and intralaminar regions), and in humans, VNS produces cortical evoked potentials. Carotid sinus pressure induces EEG slowing in experimental animals [29–31] and humans undergoing carotid surgery (independent of cardiovascular effects) [32]. Repetitive vagus stimulation in anaesthetized animals synchronizes or desynchronizes the EEG, depending on stimulus frequency, current strength and the vagal fibre types that are recruited, presumably via effects on the thalamus [33–35]. Similarly, high-frequency stimulation (> 30 Hz) of the NTS in animals desynchronizes the EEG, while slower stimulation (1–17 Hz) causes synchronization [29]. Inasmuch as seizures result from excessive cortical synchronization, these observations supported the hypoth-

esis that vagus stimulation disrupts the spread of seizures in animals by desynchronizing interconnected cortical regions. Furthermore, because EEG rhythms become synchronized when myelinated nerve fibres are stimulated and desynchronized when slower conducting, unmyelinated vagus nerve fibres are activated [36,37], each subpopulation of vagus afferents might have separate effects on thalamoforebrain regulation.

Whereas VNS has no obvious time-locked, acute effects on the EEG background rhythms of awake, asleep or anaesthetized humans [11,38,39], or in awake and freely moving rats [40], there is a suggestion it could influence paroxysmal activity. Olejniczak *et al.* reported the effect of VNS on interictal epileptiform activity in a patient with left temporal lobe onset seizures who underwent depth electrode monitoring [41]. Reduced epileptiform sharp waves from the left hippocampus were associated with 30-Hz stimulation, whereas 5-Hz stimulation was associated with an increase in epileptiform activity from the same site.

VNS-associated effects on human forebrain function have been studied with SPECT, PET and functional MRI (fMRI) [42–46]. Ring *et al.* obtained SPECT with particular attention to thalamic and insular regions in seven subjects treated for at least 6 months [42]. Rapid cycling stimulation (7 s on, 12 s off) was associated with decreased regional cerebral blood flow (rCBF) in the medial thalamic regions bilaterally. Vonck *et al.* also found evidence on SPECT scans of thalamic hypoperfusion with stimulation, though the degree of rCBF changes did not correlate with seizure reduction [46]. By contrast, Henry *et al.* found relationships using PET scans between bilateral thalamic changes and reductions in seizure frequency [47], as well as between stimulation parameters and both chronicity of stimulation and the volumes of activation and deactivation sites (Plate 73.4, shown in colour between pp. 670 and 671)

[48,49]. Bohning *et al.* demonstrated the feasibility of recording VNS-synchronized fMRI [45] in a cohort of nine patients enrolled in a depression protocol. They found blood oxygenation level dependent responses to VNS in bilateral orbitofrontal and parieto-occipital cortices, left temporal cortex, the hypothalamus and the left amygdala.

It is not clear which of these effects, if any, are related to the anticonvulsant mechanism of action of VNS. There are emerging clues, however. Krahl *et al.* showed that chemical lesions of the LC eliminated VNS-induced seizure suppression in rats, suggesting that the LC is critically involved in the mechanism of action of VNS, possibly through the release of norepinephrine [50]. Further, because increased γ-aminobutyric acid (GABA) transmission or decreased glutamate transmission in the rat mediocaudal NTS reduces susceptibility to limbic motor seizures [51], it is reasonable to hypothesize that VNS inhibits the rat NTS. The functional interrelationships between VNS, the LC and NTS inhibition remain to be elucidated.

Efficacy of VNS in animal models of epilepsy

VNS has been investigated in several animal models of epilepsy. In most of these studies, stimulation was applied just before or immediately after the onset of a seizure [37,52–54]. Other studies evaluated the relationship between cumulative duration of vagus stimulation and seizure prophylaxis [40,55].

In male rats, VNS prevented or reduced clonic seizures induced by intraperitoneal pentylenetetrazol (PTZ) and 3-mercaptopropionic acid (an inhibitor of GABA synthesis and release), as well as tonic-clonic seizures caused by maximal electroshock [37,53], especially with stimulus frequencies and pulse widths of 10–20 Hz and 0.5–1 ms, respectively. In this model, the effectiveness of VNS directly correlated with the fraction of C fibres stimulated, consistent with another study in male rats that showed penicillin-induced focal interictal spikes in male rats were reduced by 33% by direct C fibre stimulation [52]. Effectiveness also correlated inversely with the delay of stimulus from seizure onset—the greater the delay before vagus stimulation, the greater the seizure duration; therefore, stimulation worked best when applied as soon as possible after a seizure began.

In a dog model of strychnine-induced generalized seizures and PTZ-induced muscle tremors, VNS stopped seizures and tremors within 0.5–5 s when acutely applied [54]. Furthermore, VNS protected against seizures for a period that was four times longer than the duration of stimulation. Stimulation frequencies over 60 Hz were less effective than slower frequencies, consistent with other studies [37,53].

In a study of both the acute and prophylactic effects of on-demand and intermittent vagus stimulation, VNS was administered at the onset of each spontaneous seizure or at least every 3 h for 40 s in an alumina-gel monkey model of spontaneous partial and secondarily generalized seizures [55]. Seizures were completely controlled in two of four monkeys and decreased in frequency in the other two. Furthermore, the prophylactic anticonvulsant effect persisted into a stimulation-free period. No diminishment of interictal spike frequency was observed.

Takaya *et al.* demonstrated that VNS protected against experimentally induced seizures even when discontinued prior to seizure onset [40]. The anticonvulsant effect was nearly half-maximal

5 min after VNS was discontinued. In addition, they showed that 60 min of continuous VNS protected awake and freely moving rats from PTZ-induced seizures more effectively than 60 min of intermittent VNS with the same stimulation settings, and that intermittent stimulation was more effective than a single 1-min stimulus. It is impractical to apply continuous electrical stimulation to the vagus nerve due to safety considerations and limitations in battery life, but these results suggest that the stimulation parameters used to treat seizures in humans are reasonable (see below).

In cats, VNS applied during amygdaloid kindling significantly delayed the onset of seizures compared to controls and prevented the attainment of stage VI (generalized tonic-clonic convulsive seizures) [56]. The relevance of these results to patients with epilepsy is uncertain, particularly in light of evidence from clinical studies that is inconsistent with a kindling effect [57].

Efficacy studies in patients with epilepsy

Clinical studies of VNS began in 1988 with a pilot, single-blind trial of patients with refractory partial seizures who were not candidates for epilepsy surgery [10]. This was followed by the first pivotal trial of VNS (the E03 study), a multicentre, double-blind, randomized, parallel, active control trial of VNS in 114 patients with predominantly partial seizures [58–61]. The second pivotal clinical study was the E05 study, a multicentre, double-blind, randomized, parallel, active control trial of VNS in 199 patients with complex partial seizures [62]. In 1991, a compassionate use trial enrolled 124 patients with all types of intractable seizures (the E04 study) [63].

Add-on, double-blind, active-control, parallel-design trials (E03 and E05 studies)

Study designs

The E03 and E05 studies were multicentre, blinded, randomized, active control trials in patients with treatment-resistant partial onset seizures that compared two different VNS stimulation protocols: high stimulation (30 Hz, 30 s on, 5 min off, 500 ms pulse width) and low stimulation (1 Hz, 30 s on, 90–180 min off, 130 ms pulse width), which was expected to be less effective than high stimulation treatment.

Study candidates were monitored over a 12–16-week prospective baseline period during which seizures were counted and changes in AED dosages were allowed only to maintain appropriate concentrations or in response to drug toxicity. Patients who satisfied all inclusion and exclusion criteria were then implanted with the NCP system. Two weeks later, patients were randomized to receive either high or low stimulation. Over the next 2 weeks, patients randomized to the high stimulation group had their generator output current increased as high as tolerated, whereas those randomized to the low group had the current increased until stimulation could be perceived. Efficacy was then assessed during the remaining 12 weeks of the treatment phase. At the conclusion of the study, patients were eligible to enter long-term open studies.

Enrolment information

Participants in the E03 and E05 studies were at least 12 years old, had at least six seizures per month during the baseline period, and were taking one to three AEDs. In the E05 study, patients had to have partial seizures with alteration of consciousness.

In the E03 study, 125 patients participated; 114 completed the prospective baseline and were implanted. The average duration of epilepsy was 23 years for patients in the high group ($n = 54$) and 20 years for the low group ($n = 60$). Patients in both groups were taking a mean of 2.1 AEDs at study entry.

There were 254 participants in the E05 study; 55 discontinued from baseline for failing protocol eligibility and 199 were implanted. One patient was not randomized due to device infection, and two randomized patients (one in each treatment group) were excluded from the analysis for administrative reasons. The baseline characteristics for patients in both groups were similar and consistent with the E03 study.

Results

In both studies, the primary efficacy analysis was per cent change in total seizure frequency during treatment relative to baseline, comparing the high and low stimulation groups. In the E03 study, the high stimulation group had a mean reduction in seizure frequency of 24.5%, vs. 6.1% for the low stimulation group ($P = 0.01$). In the E05 study, the mean per cent decreases in seizure frequency during treatment compared to baseline were 28% and 15% for the high and low stimulation groups, respectively. The between-group comparison was statistically significant in favour of high stimulation ($P = 0.039$).

Secondary efficacy measures in both studies showed statistically significant effects in favour of high stimulation. In the E03 study, 31% of patients in the high stimulation group had at least 50% reduction in seizures compared to 13% of patients in the low stimulation group ($P = 0.02$). In the E05 study, 11% of patients in the high stimulation group had a reduction in seizure frequency greater than 75%, vs. 2% for patients in the low stimulation group ($P = 0.01$). In addition, both the high and the low stimulation groups showed a statistically and clinically significant difference in within-group mean per cent change in seizure frequency during treatment compared to baseline ($P < 0.0001$).

Long-term efficacy

DeGiorgio et al. prospectively evaluated seizure frequencies during a 12-month period in patients who had completed the E05 study, including patients who had been randomized to low stimulation during the E05 study but were then transitioned to high stimulation settings as tolerated [64]. The primary efficacy variable was the percentage change in total seizure frequency at 3 and 12 months compared to the 3-month preimplantation baseline. The median seizure reductions at 3 and 12 months were 34% and 45%, respectively ($P = 0.0001$, 12 months vs. 3 months). In addition, one in five patients had at least 75% or greater reduction in seizure frequency at 12 months. Retrospective analysis of changes in stimulation parameters showed that device changes were not the predominant predictor of increased efficacy after 12 months [65].

In a prospective study of 21 patients treated with VNS for a mean duration of 13.2 months, Tatum et al. showed that reductions in numbers or dosages of AEDs without loss of seizure control and

with improved patient satisfaction were possible in 15 (71%) [66]. In addition, seven patients were able to discontinue psychotropic drugs.

Other efficacy studies in epilepsy

Labar et al. reported on 24 patients with medication-resistant generalized seizures and only generalized epileptiform activity or generalized EEG slowing [63]. Epilepsy was idiopathic in seven patients and symptomatic in the remaining 17. Median seizure frequency was reduced by 46% after 3 months of stimulation compared to a 1-month baseline. Eleven patients had at least a 50% reduction in seizure frequency. The best responses to VNS occurred in patients with high baseline seizure rates and later ages of seizure onset.

Hosain et al. studied 13 patients with Lennox–Gastaut syndrome (age range 4–44 year, mean 16.7 year) and found a median seizure rate reduction of 52% during the first 6 months of treatment (range, 0–93%; $P = 0.04$) [67]. After 6 months of treatment, three patients had > 90% reduction in seizures, two had > 75% reduction, and one had > 50% reduction. No patient had a worsening of seizure frequency. Other anecdotal reports in patients with Lennox–Gastaut syndrome are encouraging [68–70].

Among 12 children aged 4–16 years with medically and surgically refractory seizures who were treated with VNS, five patients had a greater than 90% reduction in seizure frequency and four patients were able to reduce the number of AEDs used [71]. In another series of 16 children aged 4–19 years, six children experienced at least a 50% reduction in seizure frequency during the tenth to twelfth month of VNS [72].

Sixteen children with epileptic encephalopathy were treated with VNS and prospectively studied for changes in seizure frequency, EEG, adaptive behaviour, quality of life (QOL) and language performance [73]. One device was explanted due to infection. Of the remaining 15 children, four had at least 50% seizure reduction at 1 year following implant; conversely, two had at least a 50% increase in seizure frequency. Perceived treatment side-effects and general behaviour improved, and in six children, there was significant improvement in verbal performance that did not correlate with changes in seizure frequency.

VNS was studied in 60 children aged 3–18 with pharmacoresistant epilepsy; 27% of these children had generalized tonic-clonic seizures [74]. After 6 months of VNS treatment ($n = 55$), the median reduction in seizure frequency was 31%. The corresponding figures at 12 and 18 months were 34% ($n = 51$) and 42% ($n = 46$), respectively. None of the adverse events required discontinuation of stimulation. Patwardhan et al. reported reductions in atonic (80%), absence (65%), complex partial (48%) and generalized tonic-clonic (45%) seizures in an uncontrolled study of 38 children with a median follow-up period of 12 months (range, 10–18 months) [75].

Sirven et al. studied the efficacy, safety and tolerability of VNS for refractory epilepsy in 45 adults 50 years of age and older [76]. After 3 months of treatment, 12 patients had a > 50% decrease in seizure frequency; at 1 year, 21 of 31 patients had > 50% reduction. Side-effects were mild and transient, and QOL scores improved significantly during the first year of treatment.

Small open studies in selected populations have suggested efficacy of VNS in patients with bilateral independent temporal lobe epilepsy [77] and in developmentally disabled or mentally retarded patients with epilepsy [78].

Efficacy in other conditions

Clark *et al.* showed that VNS enhanced memory storage in rats when applied after the memory training [79]. Based on these findings, word recognition memory was studied in patients with epilepsy participating in VNS trials [80]. The patients were asked to read paragraphs that contained highlighted words. They then received either VNS or sham stimulation. Retention of verbal learning (word recognition) was significantly enhanced by VNS but not by sham stimulation; the authors suggested that vagus nerve activation modulates memory formation in a similar manner to arousal. The potential clinical relevance of this work to patients with epilepsy and memory dysfunction deserves further study. Pilot studies in patients with Alzheimer's disease are underway.

A 30-patient open study suggested that VNS has antidepressant effects in patients with treatment-resistant depression [81] without evidence of cognitive compromise [82]. This study was therefore extended to a total of 60 patients with chronic or recurrent depression (average duration 10 years) whose current episode had failed to respond to an average of 4.8 treatments [83]. After 3 months of VNS treatment, 40% of the patients had at least 50% improvement in the Hamilton Rating Scale for Depression total score ('responders') and 21% achieved complete remission of their depression. Over 90% of the patients with at least 50% improvement after 3 months of therapy maintained that response after 1 year. In addition, 18% of initial non-responders had at least 50% improvement after 1 year. A 21-site, double-blind, controlled study of VNS for 275 patients with chronic or recurrent depression did not show statistical superiority of VNS compared to sham over a 10-week double blind treatment phase and long-term follow-up is underway.

In 2001, VNS was approved in all European Union member countries and Canada for adults with treatment-resistant or treatment-intolerant chronic or recurrent depression, including major depressive disorders (unipolar depression) and manic depression (bipolar disorder).

In addition to the pilot studies in Alzheimer's disease, other pilot studies of obesity, rapid cycling bipolar disorder, obsessive–compulsive disorder, post-traumatic stress disorder, chronic migraine headaches and anxiety disorders are planned, underway or recently completed.

Safety and tolerability in patients with epilepsy

Mechanical and electrical safety

Though high frequency stimulation may be associated with tissue damage [4], there is no evidence that the stimulation parameters used clinically cause damage to the vagus nerve [7,84]. The NCP system has several built-in safety features that prevent excessive stimulation.

Environmental considerations

The antenna within the generator is controlled by radiofrequency signals transmitted by the programming wand. Nonetheless, neither the generator nor the electrode leads are affected by microwave transmission, cellular phones or airport security systems. Some restrictions do apply to MRI testing, however. Because the heat induced in the electrode leads by a body MRI could theoretically cause local tissue injury, body MRI scans are contraindicated. Brain MRI testing performed with a send-and-receive head coil appears to be safe under the conditions described in the physician's manual supplied by Cyberonics, Inc.

In a safety alert (27 August 2001), Cyberonics, Inc. cautioned against the use of short-wave diathermy, microwave diathermy or therapeutic ultrasound diathermy in patients implanted with the NCP system due to the possibility that the generator or lead could become hot and cause tissue damage or discomfort. At the time of the alert, there had been no reports of injuries related to these modalities in patients treated with VNS. Diagnostic ultrasound was not mentioned.

Safety and tolerability in the E03 and E05 studies

In the E03 study, safety and tolerability were evaluated with interviews, physical and neurological examinations, vital signs, electrocardiogram rhythm strips, Holter monitoring in a subset of 28 patients, gastric acid monitoring in 14 patients and AED concentrations. Similarly, safety and tolerability were evaluated in the E05 study with interviews, physical and neurological examinations, vital signs, Holter monitoring, pulmonary function tests, standard laboratory tests and urinalysis.

In the E03 study, the adverse events (side-effects) that occurred in at least 5% of patients in the high group during treatment were hoarseness (37%), throat pain (11%), coughing (7%), dyspnoea (6%), paraesthesia (6%) and muscle pain (6%). Hoarseness was the only adverse event that was reported significantly more often with high stimulation than with low stimulation.

In the E05 study, none of the serious adverse events that occurred during the treatment phase were judged to be probably or definitely due to VNS. Implantation-related adverse events all resolved and included left vocal cord paralysis (two patients), lower facial muscle paresis (two patients) and pain and fluid accumulation over the generator requiring aspiration (one patient). The perioperative adverse events that were reported by 10% or more patients included pain (29%), coughing (14%), voice alteration (13%), chest pain (12%) and nausea (10%). Following randomization, the adverse events that were reported by patients in the high group at some time during treatment which were significantly increased compared to baseline were voice alteration/hoarseness, cough, throat pain, non-specific pain, dyspnoea, paraesthesia, dyspepsia, vomiting and infection (Table 73.2). The only two adverse events that occurred significantly more often in the high group than the low group were dyspnoea and voice alteration. Adverse events in both treatment groups were rated as mild or moderate 99% of the time. There were no sedative, visual, affective or coordination side-effects, nor any cognitive changes as measured by the Wonderlic Personnel test, Digit Cancellation, the Stroop test and Symbol Digit Modalities [85]. No significant changes in Holter monitoring or pulmonary function tests were noted.

Two E05 patients had VNS discontinued during the treatment. One patient in the high group had two episodes of Cheyne–Stokes

Table 73.2 Treatment-phase adverse events among patients treated with low or high vagus nerve stimulation in the E05 study [62]

Adverse event	Low stimulation (n = 103) n (%)	High stimulation (n = 95) n (%)
Voice alteration	31 (30.1)	63 (66.3)
Cough	44 (42.7)	43 (45.3)
Pharyngitis	26 (25.2)	33 (34.7)
Pain	31 (30.1)	27 (28.4)
Dyspnoea	11 (10.7)	24 (25.3)
Headache	24 (23.3)	23 (24.2)
Dyspepsia	13 (12.6)	17 (17.9)
Vomiting	14 (13.6)	17 (17.9)
Paraesthesia	26 (25.2)	17 (17.9)
Nausea	21 (20.4)	14 (14.7)
Accidental injury	13 (12.6)	12 (12.6)
Fever	19 (18.4)	11 (11.6)
Infection	12 (11.7)	11 (11.6)

Only adverse events that occurred in more than 10% of high stimulation patients are listed.

respirations postictally; after the device was deactivated, two more episodes were reported and the patient's mother requested that the device be reactivated. One patient in the low group had the device deactivated due to a group of symptoms that the patient had experienced preimplantation as well as subsequent to device deactivation. No deaths occurred during either study.

Laboratory values

As would be predicted from a non-pharmacological therapy, there were no changes in haematology values or common chemistry values in either study. Similarly, there were no changes seen with AED concentrations.

Long-term safety and tolerability

Among a cohort of 444 patients who entered a long-term trial following participation in a short-term clinical study of VNS, 97% continued for at least 1 year, and 85% and 72% continued for at least 2 and 3 years, respectively [86]. The most commonly reported side-effects at the end of the first year of VNS were hoarseness (29%) and paraesthesia (12%); at the end of 2 years the most reported side-effects were hoarseness (19%) and cough (6%); and at 3 years, shortness of breath (3%) was the most frequent side-effect.

Hoppe *et al.* studied cognition in 36 adult patients before and at least 6 months after implantation using tests of attention, motor functioning, short-term memory, learning and memory and executive functions [87]. No evidence of cognitive worsening was found.

QOL was assessed in 136 adults before VNS initiation and 3 months afterwards in an open study [88]. Patients were categorized as responders (≥50% seizure reduction) and non-responders (<50% seizure reduction). Responders experienced statistically significant improvements in energy, memory, social aspects, mental

effects and fear of seizures; non-responders improved in down-heartedness and overall QOL. The results suggest a positive effect of VNS on QOL beyond changes in seizure frequency, though a placebo effect could not be completely excluded. In a related study by Malow *et al.*, 15 patients treated with VNS underwent polysomnography and multiple sleep latency tests [89]. Reduced daytime sleepiness and enhanced REM sleep were noted, even in subjects without reductions in seizure frequency.

The mortality rates and standardized mortality ratios of 1819 patients treated for 3176 person-years with VNS were contrasted with other epilepsy cohorts [90]. These rates and ratios were comparable with those of other young adults with refractory seizures who were not treated with VNS. Additionally, the incidence of definite and probable sudden unexpected death in epilepsy (SUDEP) was 4.1 per 1000 person-years, which were consistent with other non-VNS epilepsy cohorts. Interestingly, the rate of SUDEP was 5.5 per 1000 over the first 2 years of VNS treatment, and 1.7 per 1000 thereafter.

Cardiac arrhythmias attributable to VNS in patients undergoing chronic stimulation have not been described, though Frei and Osorio reported changes in heart rate and heart rate variability in a study of five subjects [91]. In another study, high strength stimulation produced no observable acute cardiorespiratory effects [92].

Six patients from VNS clinical studies and two patients who were implanted postapproval became pregnant while receiving VNS [93]. Five of the pregnancies resulted in full-term, healthy infants, including one set of twins. There was one spontaneous abortion, one unplanned pregnancy was terminated by an elective abortion and another pregnancy ended with an elective abortion because of abnormal fetal development that was attributed to AEDs.

The possible relationship of VNS to swallowing difficulties [72] was studied by barium swallow in a series of eight children [94]. Laryngeal penetration of barium was present in three patients without stimulation, and was caused by VNS in one other patient. Results from another small series of children treated with chronic VNS suggest that some children with severe mental and motor retardation who are dependent on assisted feeding may be at increased risk for aspiration if VNS occurs during feeding [95].

Several anecdotal reports of complications of VNS have appeared as the number of patients treated with VNS has rapidly grown. These reports include posture-dependent stimulation of the phrenic nerve [96], worsening of pre-existing obstructive sleep apnoea [97], exacerbation of preimplantation dysphoric disorders and psychotic episodes with VNS-associated seizure reduction [98] and transient asystole lasting up to 20 s in nine patients (0.1% of all implantations) during the intraoperative lead test [99–101]. The intraoperative lead test assesses stimulation function and system integrity by turning on the generator briefly at 1.0 mA, 500 μs and 20 Hz. Four patients had the device acutely explanted; the others were chronically stimulated without difficulty. There were no sequelae in any of the patients.

Effects on mood and behaviour in patients with epilepsy

Two recently published studies demonstrated mood improvements in patients with epilepsy treated with VNS for up to 6 months [102,103]. Though different mood scales were used, both studies included adults with long-standing, poorly controlled partial onset seizures, and in each study AEDs remained constant. In both studies, there was no significant association between seizure reduction and mood improvement, and in one study, there was no correlation between 'dose' of the VNS treatment and mood improvement ('dose' was calculated by multiplying per cent 'on' time by stimulus intensity) [103].

Hoppe *et al.* used self-report questionnaires and evaluated changes in mood and health-related QOL following 6 months of VNS treatment in 28 patients whose AED regimen was stable and who had low baseline depression scores [104]. Improvements in tenseness, negative arousal and dysphoria—but not of depression—were observed.

In an open 6-month study of 16 children with Lennox–Gastaut syndrome ($n = 12$), Doose's syndrome ($n = 3$) and myoclonic absence epilepsy ($n = 1$), Aldenkamp *et al.* observed increased independent behaviour, mood improvements and fewer symptoms of pervasive development disorders [105]. These behavioural effects were independent of changes in seizure frequency.

In four out of six patients with hypothalamic hamartomas, Murphy *et al.* reported 'striking' behavioural improvements, including one patient whose episodic rages could be terminated by magnet activation of the generator [106].

Clinical use of VNS for epilepsy

Most centres initiate programming within the first 2 postoperative weeks. Usual target stimulation parameters are shown in Table 73.3. Ramping up of the device typically occurs at outpatient follow-up visits every 1–2 weeks over the next several months. At these visits, the current is usually increased by 0.25 mA increments to the maximum tolerated settings or until reduction in seizure frequency exceeds 50% compared to the preimplantation baseline. If side-effects become intolerable or do not resolve following a change of stimulation parameters, the current is reduced by 0.25 mA increments as necessary. Reducing the pulse width may also improve tolerability [107].

Implanted patients should be counselled about the likely necessity of ongoing AED treatment, the possible delay in onset of efficacy and use of the supplied magnet to activate and turn off the generator. Stimulation can be stopped temporarily by securing the supplied magnet over the device with tape or by inserting the magnet in an athletic bra over the generator. This may be necessary, for example, if the patient wants to avoid hoarseness while speaking, during eating if pre-existing dysphagia is present, during intense exercise if the patient experiences dyspnoea while exercising, or at night if either stimulation-related discomfort or an exacerbation of sleep apnoea occurs.

If a patient's seizures have not satisfactorily improved with regard to frequency or severity after 6–9 months of stimulation, most clinicians would decrease the off time from 5 to 3 min. Subsequent staged reductions of the off time to 1.8 min and 0.2 min (with an associated decrease of on time to 7 s; 'rapid cycle') have been tried with success in some patients [108].

A minority of patients have the device explanted because of lack of sufficient efficacy. Based on the long-term efficacy studies it appears prudent to wait at least 12–18 months before deciding to remove the generator. Once the decision is made, the generator should first be turned off for several weeks or longer depending on the patient's preimplantation seizure frequency. If seizures worsen

Table 73.3 Usual initial target stimulation parameters for VNS stimulation in patients with epilepsy

Stimulation parameter	Setting
Output current	1.5 mA
Signal frequency	20–30 Hz
Pulse width	250–500 µs
Signal ON time	30 s
Signal OFF time	5 min

for no other apparent reason, then the device may have actually been efficacious for that particular patient and device removal should be reconsidered. Explantation can be performed as an outpatient procedure under local anaesthesia. Because dissecting the helical coils off the vagus nerve is laborious and there are no reported complications of leaving them in place, most surgeons do not explore and remove the stimulating electrodes during the explantation procedure.

By August 2003, over 22 000 patients had been implanted with VNS Therapy worldwide. Published data include 5-year results of treatment [109]. Experience has shown that the successful implementation of a VNS programme requires a coordinated team approach to facilitate patient education, surgical implantation and follow-up programming visits [110]. While the initial cost of VNS treatment compared to pharmacotherapy is high, these costs should be considered in light of reductions in direct medical expenses due to epilepsy within the first several years after implantation [111].

The application of VNS therapy will be enhanced once a measurable physiological response to VNS is identified that can be used to 'titrate' stimulation. In this regard, Koo *et al.* used EEG findings at 6 months postimplantation, including clustering and synchronization of epileptiform activity, to guide further VNS programming in 20 patients with impressive results [112].

The appropriate role of VNS in the treatment of epilepsy is under active discussion [113,114]. Many epileptologists now consider this therapy an option for patients (a) whose partial onset seizures adversely affect QOL despite trials with three or more AEDs that are appropriate for partial seizures and that have been titrated to maximally tolerated doses; and (b) who do not have surgically remediable partial seizures. The use of VNS in patients with generalized epilepsies at the present time is supported only by open, uncontrolled studies, though results are promising.

Summary

VNS is effective, safe and well tolerated in patients with long-standing, refractory partial onset seizures [115], and may be beneficial to patients with other forms of epilepsy, including Lennox–Gastaut syndrome [63,67,116] and for patients with depression. There has been no indication of tolerance to therapeutic effect in long-term, open studies. Efficacy results for other seizure types, and in children and the elderly are encouraging, but preliminary.

While relatively few patients with medically resistant epilepsy become seizure free with VNS, there are suggestions that efficacy and QOL further improve over time [60,64,66,117–120], though outcomes in long-term, open, unblinded studies should be interpreted cautiously. Given the possibility that efficacy may be delayed following implantation, it is prudent to wait at least 1 year, if not longer, before concluding that VNS has had no effect on seizure frequency or severity.

The most frequently encountered adverse effects occur during stimulation, are usually mild to moderate in severity and resolve with reduction in current intensity or spontaneously over time. Conspicuously absent with VNS stimulation therapy are the typical central nervous system side-effects of AEDs. Pending further studies, caution may be warranted when recommending VNS for patients with dysphagia, sleep apnoea and cardiac conduction disorders.

Further controlled studies should be performed to explore the use of VNS for generalized seizures and epilepsy syndromes. Additional controlled studies are also needed to determine (a) how VNS therapy can be individualized to maximize its effectiveness, either with intermittent stimulation or acutely with the magnet; (b) whether VNS complements AEDs or non-AEDs with particular mechanisms of action; (c) how to identify prospectively patients who are most likely to benefit from VNS; and (d) the efficacy and tolerability of adjunctive VNS compared with adjunctive AED therapy, particularly early in the course of epilepsy.

References

1 Lhatoo SD, Wong IC, Polizzi G, Sander JW. Long-term retention rates of lamotrigine, gabapentin, and topiramate in chronic epilepsy. *Epilepsia* 2000; 41(12): 1592–6.
2 Fisher RS, Vickrey BG, Gibson P *et al*. The impact of epilepsy from the patient's perspective II: views about therapy and health care. *Epilepsy Res* 2000; 41(1): 53–61.
3 Terry R, Tarver WB, Zabara J. An implantable neurocybernetic prosthesis system. *Epilepsia* 1990; 31 (Suppl. 2): S33–S37.
4 Terry RS, Tarver WB, Zabara J. The implantable neurocybernetic prosthesis system. *Pacing Clin Electrophysiol* 1991; 14(1): 86–93.
5 Schaefer PA, Rosenfeld WE, Lippmann SM. Same-day surgery for implanting vagal nerve stimulators: safe and decreased cost. *Epilepsia* 1998; 39 (Suppl. 6): 193.
6 DeGiorgio CM, Amar A, Apuzzo MLJ. Surgical anatomy, implantation technique, and operative complications. In: Schachter SC, Schmidt D, eds. *Vagus Nerve Stimulation*, 2nd edn. London: Martin Dunitz, 2001: 31–50.
7 Tarver WB, George RE, Maschino SE, Holder LK, Wernicke JF. Clinical experience with a helical bipolar stimulating lead. *Pacing Clin Electrophysiol* 1992; 15 (10 Pt 2): 1545–56.
8 Reid SA. Surgical technique for implantation of the neurocybernetic prosthesis. *Epilepsia* 1990; 31 (Suppl. 2): S38–S39.
9 Landy HJ, Ramsay RE, Slater J, Casiano RR, Morgan R. Vagus nerve stimulation for complex partial seizures: surgical technique, safety, and efficacy. *J Neurosurg* 1993; 78(1): 26–31.
10 Penry JK, Dean JC. Prevention of intractable partial seizures by intermittent vagal stimulation in humans: preliminary results. *Epilepsia* 1990; 31 (Suppl. 2): S40–S43.
11 Hammond EJ, Uthman BM, Reid SA, Wilder BJ. Electrophysiological studies of cervical vagus nerve stimulation in humans: I. EEG effects. *Epilepsia* 1992; 33(6): 1013–20.
12 Henry TR. Anatomical, experimental, and mechanistic investigations. In: Schachter SC, Schmidt D, ed. *Vagus Nerve Stimulation*, 2nd edn. London: Martin Dunitz, 2001: 1–30.
13 Schachter SC, Saper CB. Progress in epilepsy research: vagus nerve stimulation. *Epilepsia* 1998; 39: 677–86.
14 Schachter SC. Review of the mechanisms of action of antiepileptic drugs. *CNS Drugs* 1995; 4(6): 469–77.
15 Prechtl JC, Powley TL. Organization and distribution of the rat subdiaphragmatic vagus and associated paraganglia. *J Comp Neurol* 1985; 235: 182–95.
16 Saper CB, Kibbe MR, Hurley KM *et al*. Brain natriuretic peptide-like immunoreactive innervation of the cardiovascular and cerebrovascular systems in the rat. *Circ Res* 1990; 67: 1345–54.
17 Foley JO, DuBois F. Quantitative studies of the vagus nerve in the cat. I. The ratio of sensory and motor fibers. *J Comp Neurol* 1937; 67: 49–97.
18 Agostini E, Chinnock JE, Daly MD, Murray JG. Functional and histological studies of the vagus nerve and its branches to the heart, lungs, and abdominal viscera in the cat. *J Physiol (Lond)* 1957; 135: 182–205.
19 Loewy AD, Burton H. Nuclei of the solitary tract: efferent projections to the lower brain stem and spinal cord. *J Comp Neurol* 1978; 181: 421–50.
20 Ruggiero DA, Cravo SL, Arango V, Reis DJ. Central control of the circulation by the rostral ventrolateral reticular nucleus: anatomical substrates. *Prog Brain Res* 1989; 81: 49–79.
21 Saper CB. The central autonomic system. In: Paxinos G, ed. *The Rat Nervous System*, 2nd edn. San Diego: Academic Press, 1995: 107–31.
22 Cechetto DF, Saper CB. Evidence for a viscerotopic sensory representation in the cortex and thalamus in the rat. *J Comp Neurol* 1987; 262: 27–45.
23 Fulwiler CE, Saper CB. Subnuclear organization of the efferent connections of the parabrachial nucleus in the rat. *Brain Res Rev* 1984; 7: 229–59.
24 Saper CB. Diffuse cortical projection systems: anatomical organization and role in cortical function. In: Plum F, ed. *Handbook of Physiology. The Nervous System V*. Bethesda: American Physiological Society, 1987: 169–210.
25 Naritoku DK, Terry WJ, Helfert RH. Regional induction of *fos* immunoreactivity in the brain by anticonvulsant stimulation of the vagus nerve. *Epilepsy Res* 1995; 22(1): 53–62.
26 Bailey P, Bremer F. A sensory cortical representation of the vagus nerve. *J Neurophysiol* 1938; 1: 405–12.
27 Dell P, Olson R. Projections thalamiques, corticales, et cerebelleuses des afferences viscerales vagales. *CR Soc Seances Soc Biol Fil* 1951; 145: 1084–8.
28 Zanchetti A, Wang SC, Moruzzi G. The effect of vagal stimulation on the EEG pattern of the cat. *EEG Clin Neurophysiol* 1952; 4: 357–461.
29 Magnes J, Moruzzi G, Pompeiano O. Synchronization of the EEG produced by low frequency electrical stimulation of the region of the solitary tract. *Arch Ital Biol* 1961; 99: 33–67.
30 Bonvallet M, Dell P, Hiebel G. Tonus sympathetiques et activité electrique corticale. *EEG Clin Neurophysiol* 1954; 6: 119–44.
31 Garnier L. EEG modifications produced by gastric distention in cats. *CR Seances Soc Biol Fil* 1968; 162: 2164–8.
32 Bridgers SL, Spencer SS, Spencer DD, Sasaki CT. A cerebral effect of carotid sinus stimulation. Observation during intraoperative electroencephalographic monitoring. *Arch Neurol* 1985; 42: 574–7.
33 Chase MH, Sterman MB, Clemente CD. Cortical and subcortical patterns of response to afferent vagal stimulation. *Exp Neurol* 1966; 16: 36–49.
34 Chase MH, Nakamura Y, Clemente CD, Sterman MB. Afferent vagal stimulation: neurographic correlates of induced EEG synchronization and desynchronization. *Brain Res* 1967; 5: 236–49.
35 Chase MH, Nakamura Y, Clemente CD, Sterman MB. Cortical and subcortical EEG patterns of response to afferent abdominal vagal stimulation: neurographic correlates. *Physiol Behav* 1968; 3: 605–10.
36 Rutecki P. Anatomical, physiological, and theoretical basis for the antiepileptic effect of vagus nerve stimulation. *Epilepsia* 1990; 31 (Suppl. 2): S1–S6.
37 Woodbury DM, Woodbury JW. Effects of vagal stimulation on experimentally induced seizures in rats. *Epilepsia* 1990; 31 (Suppl. 2): S7–S19.
38 Hammond EJ, Uthman BM, Reid SA, Wilder BJ. Electrophysiologic studies of cervical vagus nerve stimulation in humans: II. Evoked potentials. *Epilepsia* 1992; 33(6): 1021–8.
39 Salinsky MC, Burchiel KJ. Vagus nerve stimulation has no effect on awake EEG rhythms in humans. *Epilepsia* 1993; 34(2): 299–304.
40 Takaya M, Terry WJ, Naritoku DK. Vagus nerve stimulation induces a sustained anticonvulsant effect. *Epilepsia* 1996; 37(11): 1111–16.
41 Olejniczak PW, Fisch BJ, Carey M, Butterbaugh G, Happel L, Tardo C.

The effect of vagus nerve stimulation on epileptiform activity recorded from hippocampal depth electrodes. *Epilepsia* 2001; 42(3): 423–9.

42 Ring HA, White S, Costa DC *et al*. A SPECT study of the effect of vagal nerve stimulation on thalamic activity in patients with epilepsy. *Seizure* 2000; 9(6): 380–4.

43 Garnett ES, Nahmias C, Scheffel A, Firnau G, Upton ARM. Regional cerebral blood flow in man manipulated by direct vagal stimulation. *Pacing Clin Electrophysiol* 1992; 15 (10 Pt 2): 1579–80.

44 Ko D, Heck C, Grafton S *et al*. Vagus nerve stimulation activates central nervous system structures in epileptic patients during PET H$_2$^{15}O blood flow imaging. *Neurosurgery* 1996; 39(2): 426–31.

45 Bohning DE, Lomarev MP, Denslow S, Nahas Z, Shastri A, George MS. Feasibility of vagus nerve stimulation-synchronized blood oxygenation level-dependent functional MRI. *Invest Radiol* 2001; 36(8): 470–9.

46 Vonck K, Boon P, Van Laere K *et al*. Acute single photon emission computed tomographic study of vagus nerve stimulation in refractory epilepsy. *Epilepsia* 2000; 41(5): 601–9.

47 Henry TR, Votaw JR, Pennell PB *et al*. Acute blood flow changes and efficacy of vagus nerve stimulation in partial epilepsy. *Neurology* 1999; 52(6): 1166–73.

48 Henry TR, Bakay RAE, Votaw JR *et al*. Brain blood flow alterations induced by therapeutic vagus nerve stimulation in partial epilepsy: I. Acute effects at high and low levels of stimulation. *Epilepsia* 1998; 39: 983–90.

49 Henry TR, Votaw JR, Bakay RAE *et al*. Vagus nerve stimulation-induced cerebral blood flow changes differ in acute and chronic therapy of complex partial seizures. *Epilepsia* 1998; 39 (Suppl. 6): 92.

50 Krahl SE, Clark KB, Smith DC, Browning RA. Locus coeruleus lesions suppress the seizure-attenuating effects of vagus nerve stimulation. *Epilepsia* 1998; 39: 709–14.

51 Walker BR, Easton A, Gale K. Regulation of limbic motor seizures by GABA and glutamate transmission in nucleus tractus solitarius. *Epilepsia* 1999; 40(8): 1051–7.

52 McLachlan RS. Suppression of interictal spikes and seizures by stimulation of the vagus nerve. *Epilepsia* 1993; 34(5): 918–23.

53 Woodbury JW, Woodbury DM. Vagal stimulation reduces the severity of maximal electroshock seizures in intact rats: use of a cuff electrode for stimulating and recording. *Pacing Clin Electrophysiol* 1991; 14(1): 94–107.

54 Zabara J. Inhibition of experimental seizures in canines by repetitive vagal stimulation. *Epilepsia* 1992; 33(6): 1005–12.

55 Lockard JS, Congdon WC, DuCharme LL. Feasibility and safety of vagal stimulation in monkey model. *Epilepsia* 1990; 31 (Suppl. 2): S20–S26.

56 Fernandez-Guardiola A, Martinez A, Valdes-Cruz A, Magdaleno-Madrigal VM, Martinez D, Fernandez-Mas R. Vagus nerve prolonged stimulation in cats: effects on epileptogenesis (amygdala electrical kindling): behavioral and electrographic changes. *Epilepsia* 1999; 40(7): 822–9.

57 Dasheiff RM, Sandberg T, Thompson J, Arrambide S. Vagal nerve stimulation does not unkindle seizures. *J Clin Neurophysiol* 2001; 18(1): 68–74.

58 Ben-Menachem E, Manon-Espaillat R, Ristanovic R *et al*. Vagus nerve stimulation for treatment of partial seizures: 1. A controlled study of effect on seizures. *Epilepsia* 1994; 35(3): 616–26.

59 Ramsay RE, Uthman BM, Augustinsson LE *et al*. Vagus nerve stimulation for treatment of partial seizures: 2. Safety, side effects, and tolerability. *Epilepsia* 1994; 35(3): 627–36.

60 George R, Salinsky M, Kuzniecky R *et al*. Vagus nerve stimulation for treatment of partial seizures: 3. Long-term follow-up on first 67 patients exiting a controlled study. *Epilepsia* 1994; 35(3): 637–43.

61 The Vagus Nerve Stimulation Study Group. A randomized controlled trial of chronic vagus nerve stimulation for treatment of medically intractable seizures. *Neurology* 1995; 45: 224–30.

62 Handforth A, DeGiorgio CM, Schachter SC *et al*. Vagus nerve stimulation therapy for partial-onset seizures: a randomized active-control trial. *Neurology* 1998; 51(1): 48–55.

63 Labar D, Murphy J, Tecoma E. Vagus nerve stimulation for medication-resistant generalized epilepsy. E04 VNS Study Group. *Neurology* 1999; 52(7): 1510–12.

64 DeGiorgio CM, Schachter SC, Handforth A *et al*. Prospective long-term

65 DeGiorgio CM, Thompson J, Lewis P *et al*. Vagus nerve stimulation: Analysis of device parameters in 154 patients during the long-term XE5 study. *Epilepsia* 2001; 42(8): 1017–20.

66 Tatum WO, Johnson KD, Goff S, Ferreira JA, Vale FL. Vagus nerve stimulation and drug reduction. *Neurology* 2001; 56(4): 561–3.

67 Hosain S, Nikalov B, Harden C, Li M, Fraser R, Labar D. Vagus nerve stimulation treatment for Lennox–Gastaut syndrome. *J Child Neurol* 2000; 15(8): 509–12.

68 Helmers SL, Al-Jayyousi M, Madsen J. Adjunctive treatment in Lennox–Gastaut syndrome using vagal nerve stimulation. *Epilepsia* 1998; 39 (Suppl. 6): 169.

69 Murphy JV, Hornig G. Chronic intermittent stimulation of the left vagal nerve in nine children with Lennox–Gastaut syndrome. *Epilepsia* 1998; 39 (Suppl. 6): 169.

70 Hornig G, Murphy JV. Vagal nerve stimulation: updated experience in 60 pediatric patients. *Epilepsia* 1998; 39 (Suppl. 6): 169.

71 Murphy JV, Hornig G, Schallert G. Left vagal nerve stimulation in children with refractory epilepsy. Preliminary observations. *Arch Neurol* 1995; 52(9): 886–9.

72 Lundgren J, Amark P, Blennow G, Stromblad LG, Wallstedt L. Vagus nerve stimulation in 16 children with refractory epilepsy. *Epilepsia* 1998; 39: 809–13.

73 Parker AP, Polkey CE, Binnie CD, Madigan C, Ferrie CD, Robinson RO. Vagal nerve stimulation in epileptic encephalopathies. *Pediatrics* 1999; 103 (4 Pt 1): 778–82.

74 Murphy JV. Left vagal nerve stimulation in children with medically refractory epilepsy. The Pediatric VNS Study Group. *J Pediatr* 1999; 134(5): 563–6.

75 Patwardhan RV, Stong B, Bebin EM, Mathisen J, Grabb PA. Efficacy of vagal nerve stimulation in children with medically refractory epilepsy. *Neurosurgery* 2000; 47(6): 1353–8.

76 Sirven JI, Sperling M, Naritoku D *et al*. Vagus nerve stimulation therapy for epilepsy in older adults. *Neurology* 2000; 54(5): 1179–82.

77 Alsaadi TM, Laxer KD, Barbaro NM, Marks WJ, Garcia PA. Vagus nerve stimulation for the treatment of bilateral independent temporal lobe epilepsy. *Epilepsia* 2001; 42(7): 954–6.

78 Andriola MR, Vitale SA. Vagus nerve stimulation in the developmentally disabled. *Epilepsy Behav* 2001; 2: 129–34.

79 Clark KB, Smith DC, Hassert DL, Browning RA, Naritoku DK, Jensen RA. Posttraining electrical stimulation of vagal afferents with concomitant vagal efferent inactivation enhances memory storage processes in the rat. *Neurobiol Learn Mem* 1998; 70(3): 364–73.

80 Clark KB, Naritoku DK, Smith DC, Browning RA, Jensen RA. Enhanced recognition memory following vagus nerve stimulation in human subjects. *Nat Neurosci* 1999; 2(1): 94–8.

81 Rush AJ, George MS, Sackeim HA *et al*. Vagus nerve stimulation (VNS) for treatment-resistant depression: A multicenter study. *Biol Psychiatr* 2000; 47: 276–86.

82 Sackeim HA, Keilp JG, Rush AJ *et al*. The effects of vagus nerve stimulation on cognitive performance in patients with treatment-resistant depression. *Neuropsychiatr Neuropsychol Behav Neurol* 2001; 14(1): 53–62.

83 Sackeim HA, Rush AJ, George MS *et al*. Vagus nerve stimulation (VNS^{TM}) for treatment-resistant depression: efficacy, side effects, and predictors for outcome. *Neuropsychopharmacology* 2001; 25: 713–28.

84 Agnew WF, McCreery DB. Considerations for safety with chronically implanted nerve electrodes. *Epilepsia* 1990; 31 (Suppl. 2): S27–S32.

85 Dodrill CB, Morris GL. Effects of vagal nerve stimulation on cognition and quality of life in epilepsy. *Epilepsy Behav* 2001; 2: 46–53.

86 Morris GL, Mueller WM. Long-term treatment with vagus nerve stimulation in patients with refractory epilepsy. *Neurology* 1999; 53(8): 1731–5.

87 Hoppe C, Helmstaedter C, Schermann J, Elger CE. No evidence for cognitive side effects after 6 months of vagus nerve stimulation in epilepsy patients. *Epilepsy Behav* 2001; 2: 351–6.

88 Cramer JA. Exploration of changes in health-related quality of life after 3 months of vagus nerve stimulation. *Epilepsy Behav* 2001; 2: 460–5.

89 Malow BA, Edwards J, Marzec M, Sagher O, Ross D, Fromes G. Vagus

nerve stimulation reduces daytime sleepiness in epilepsy patients. *Neurology* 2001; 57: 879–84.

90 Annegers JF, Coan SP, Hauser WA, Leestma J. Epilepsy, vagal nerve stimulation by the NCP system, all-cause mortality, and sudden, unexpected, unexplained death. *Epilepsia* 2000; 41(5): 549–53.

91 Frei MG, Osorio I. Left vagus nerve stimulation with the Neurocybernetic Prosthesis has complex effects on heart rate and on its variability in humans. *Epilepsia* 2001; 42(8): 1007–16.

92 Binks AP, Paydarfar D, Schachter SC, Guz A, Banzett RB. High strength stimulation of the vagus nerve in awake humans: a lack of cardiorespiratory effects. *Respir Physiol* 2001; 127: 125–33.

93 Ben-Menachem E, Ristanovic R, Murphy J. Gestational outcomes in patients with epilepsy receiving vagus nerve stimulation. *Epilepsia* 1998; 39 (Suppl. 6): 180.

94 Schallert G, Foster J, Lindquist N, Murphy JV. Chronic stimulation of the left vagal nerve in children: effect on swallowing. *Epilepsia* 1998; 39: 1113–14.

95 Lundgren J, Ekberg O, Olsson R. Aspiration: a potential complication to vagus nerve stimulation. *Epilepsia* 1998; 39: 998–1000.

96 Leijten FSS, Van Rijen PC. Stimulation of the phrenic nerve as a complication of vagus nerve pacing in a patient with epilepsy. *Neurology* 1998; 51: 1224–5.

97 Malow BA, Edwards J, Marzec M, Sagher O, Fromes G. Effects of vagus nerve stimulation on respiration during sleep: A pilot study. *Neurology* 2000; 55(10): 1450–4.

98 Blumer D, Davies K, Alexander A, Morgan S. Major psychiatric disorders subsequent to treating epilepsy by vagus nerve stimulation. *Epilepsy Behav* 2001; 2: 466–72.

99 Asconape JJ, Moore DD, Zipes DP, Hartman LM. Early experience with vagus nerve stimulation for the treatment of epilepsy: cardiac complications. *Epilepsia* 1998; 39 (Suppl. 6): 193.

100 Tatum WO, Moore DB, Stecker MM *et al*. Ventricular asystole during vagus nerve stimulation for epilepsy in humans. *Neurology* 1999; 52: 1267–9.

101 Andriola MR, Rosenzweig T, Vlay S. Vagus nerve stimulation (VNS): induction of asystole during implantation with subsequent successful stimulation. *Epilepsia* 2000; 41 (Suppl. 7): 223.

102 Elger G, Hoppe C, Falkai P, Rush AJ, Elger CE. Vagus nerve stimulation is associated with mood improvements in epilepsy patients. *Epilepsy Res* 2000; 42: 203–10.

103 Harden CL, Pulver MC, Ravdin LD, Nikolov B, Halper JP, Labar DR. A pilot study of mood in epilepsy patients treated with vagus nerve stimulation. *Epilepsy Behav* 2000; 1: 93–9.

104 Hoppe C, Helmstaedter C, Schermann J, Elger CE. Self-reported mood changes following 6 months of vagus nerve stimulation in epilepsy patients. *Epilepsy Behav* 2001; 2: 335–42.

105 Aldenkamp AP, Van de Veerdonk SHA, Majoie HJM *et al*. Effects of 6 months of treatment with vagus nerve stimulation on behavior in children with Lennox–Gastaut syndrome in an open clinical and nonrandomized study. *Epilepsy Behav* 2001; 2: 343–50.

106 Murphy JV, Wheless JW, Schmoll CM. Left vagal nerve stimulation in six patients with hypothalamic hamartomas. *Pediatr Neurol* 2000; 23: 167–8.

107 Liporace J, Hucko D, Morrow R *et al*. Vagal nerve stimulation: Adjustments to reduce painful side effects. *Neurology* 2001; 57: 885–6.

108 Naritoku DK, Handforth A, Labar DR, Gilmartin RC. Effects of reducing stimulation intervals on antiepileptic efficacy of vagus nerve stimulation (VNS). *Epilepsia* 1998; 39 (Suppl. 6): 194.

109 Ben-Menachem E, Hellstrom K, Waldton C, Augustinsson LE. Evaluation of refractory epilepsy treated with vagus nerve stimulation for up to 5 years. *Neurology* 1999; 52(6): 1265–7.

110 Doerksen K, Klassen L. Vagus nerve stimulation therapy: nurses role in a collaborative approach to a program. *Axone* 1998; 20(1): 6–9.

111 Boon P, Vonck K, D'Have M, O'Connor S, Vandekerckhove T, De Reuck J. Cost-benefit of vagus nerve stimulation for refractory epilepsy. *Acta Neurol Belg* 1999; 99: 275–80.

112 Koo BK, Ham SD, Canady A, Sood S. EEG changes with vagus nerve stimulation and clinical application of these changes to determine optimum stimulation parameters. *Epilepsia* 2000; 41 (Suppl. 7): 226.

113 McLachlan RS. Vagus nerve stimulation for treatment of seizures? Maybe. *Arch Neurol* 1998; 55: 232–3.

114 Chadwick D. Vagal-nerve stimulation for epilepsy. *Lancet* 2001; 357: 1726–7.

115 Ben-Menachem E. Vagus nerve stimulation for treatment of seizures? Yes. *Arch Neurol* 1998; 55: 231–2.

116 Rafael H, Moromizato P. Vagus nerve stimulation (VNS) may be useful in treating patients with symptomatic generalized epilepsy. *Epilepsia* 1998; 39(9): 1018.

117 Michael JE, Wegener K, Barnes DW. Vagus nerve stimulation for intractable seizures: one year follow-up. *J Neurosci Nurs* 1993; 25(6): 362–6.

118 Salinsky MC, Uthman BM, Ristanovic RK, Wernicke JF, Tarver WB. Vagus nerve stimulation for the treatment of medically intractable seizures. Results of a 1-year open-extension trial. *Arch Neurol* 1996; 53(11): 1176–80.

119 DeGiorgio CM, Handforth A, Schachter S. Multicenter double-blind crossover and 6-month follow-up study of vagus nerve stimulation for intractable partial seizures. *Epilepsia* 1998; 39 (Suppl. 6): 69.

120 Vonck K, Boon P, D'Have M, Vandekerckhove T, O'Connor S, De Reuck J. Long-term results of vagus nerve stimulation in refractory epilepsy. *Seizure* 1999; 8(6): 328–34.

Future Surgical Approaches to Epilepsy

K.E. Nilsen and H.R. Cock

In recent years, there have been considerable advances in epilepsy treatment. Yet up to a third of patients continue to experience seizures on maximal tolerated therapy [1], and therefore urgently require alternative treatment strategies [2]. Two such novel approaches are focal drug delivery and neuronal stem cell grafting. All the published studies to date are preclinical; these studies have been undertaken in a variety of experimental epilepsy models, all with certain limitations (see Chapter 8 and [3]). Nonetheless these provide a good basis from which future studies can be developed, with the hope of new treatment options for currently intractable patients. This chapter will consider the principles behind these focal treatment strategies, and will critically review current work.

Focal treatment principles

Systemic administration of antiepileptic drugs is frequently limited by dose-related side-effects due to actions both outside the central nervous system and also on non-epileptic brain regions. Clearly a system that permitted selective delivery of drugs to regions involved in seizure generation or propagation, rather than the whole brain, would be advantageous. Similarly, neuronal/stem cell grafts could also prove beneficial given their potential to effect long-term local changes in the neurochemical environment, and to alter the structure and function of local neuronal networks. For any focal approach, there are a variety of sites in the brain that could be targeted (Fig. 74.1). The most obvious, as for surgical resections, would be the epileptogenic zone, identified either by neuroimaging or electrophysiological means. Focal drug delivery or neuronal grafts could be applicable for those patients in whom resection or lesioning is not considered appropriate due to proximity to eloquent cortex. Secondly, when considering reflex epilepsies, such as photosensitive seizures, then targeting the trigger site (e.g. occipital cortex) might be effective. Finally, for patients with multiple foci, or without a clear focal onset, manipulation of key propagation pathways might prevent seizures or at least limit their clinical severity.

Focal drug delivery

The seizure focus

The majority of studies have investigated the effects of γ-aminobutyric (GABA)-ergic drugs at the seizure focus. Thus for example, in rats with seizures evoked by hippocampal bicuculline, a $GABA_A$ receptor antagonist [4], subsequent hippocampal infusions of diazepam significantly reduced the occurrence of clinical seizures and interictal EEG spiking. Focal diazepam has also proved equally effective in other focal epilepsy models such as the cobalt/systemic

pilocarpine model [5]. Several other compounds injected into the seizure focus in a variety of models have also demonstrated antiepileptic effects, at least in the short term (Table 74.1) [6–13]. Although in some studies partial beneficial effects were also observed with control injections of vehicle substances alone [4,7], suggesting a non-specific effect perhaps related to the effect of cannula placement *per se* (e.g. unintended ablation or lesioning of the focus), the majority demonstrate convincing antiepileptic effects from a wide range of pharmacological modulations directed to the seizure focus. However, in most of the experimental paradigms, local drug applications have a limited therapeutic time course, lasting at most hours. Thus these studies have largely been performed in acute seizure provocation models rather than more clinically appropriate models with spontaneous seizures. Furthermore, there is little opportunity to observe potential behavioural side-effects. Few studies have addressed the problem on a more long-term basis, although technological developments, including osmotic minipump systems or synthetic polymers can facilitate long-term drug delivery to discrete brain regions. A polymeric micro-disk containing thyrotrophin-releasing hormone (TRH) implanted into the seizure focus in amygdala-kindled rats retarded kindling development up to 50 days later, although no control values were shown for the latter half of the trial [11]. In this study the treatment was initiated prior to starting kindling, and therefore before an epileptogenic focus had developed. This would not thus be clinically applicable. However, a polymer-releasing adenosine, an endogenous inhibitory neuromodulator, implanted into the lateral ventricle of fully hippocampal-kindled rats has been shown to increase the seizure threshold for subsequent stimulations [12]. Adenosine was released for 17 days and the anticonvulsant effect on seizures progressively decreased over time, as the release of adenosine declined, and was absent by 14 days. Although undertaken in animals with an established increased seizure susceptibility, these studies still relied on acutely provoked rather than spontaneous seizures, but are nonetheless promising.

Very few longer-term studies have been undertaken in spontaneous seizure models. Remler and Marcussen [14] administered intravenous GABA to cats with a cobalt-induced focus and found little effect on the subsequent spontaneous seizures. However, if GABA was given after local radiation was used to permeabilize the blood–brain barrier directly over the seizure focus, there was a significant suppression of spike activity, maximal 7–9 days after irradiation. Radiation itself had no effect on the seizures and the procedure was well tolerated with no obvious loss of function. The authors interpret the clinical effects seen as representing local delivery of GABA to the seizure focus, although this was not directly confirmed. More recently, using the same model in rats, Tamargo *et al.*

[13] used a surgically implantable synthetic polymer designed to produce long-term, intracerebral delivery of phenytoin over the cortical seizure focus. *In vitro* studies demonstrated continuous release of phenytoin (0.2–0.7% loaded dose/week) for up to 1 year, with loading doses that would theoretically deliver for up to 3 years in total. The efficacy studies in the cobalt rats included behavioural and ECoG monitoring before and after implantation of phenytoin-loaded or sham polymers. In the treatment groups, both the incidence of clinical seizures (2/9 animals vs. 7/10) and the mean ECoG spike frequency (22/10 min vs. 70/10 min) were significantly reduced compared to the shams, with no observed behavioural side-effects. As the authors themselves point out, the *in vivo* studies were limited (over only 2 weeks), despite the potential for much longer-term phenytoin release, because the epilepsy in this model is self-limiting, and seizures remit spontaneously after 21 days or so. Nonetheless, the results are promising, and should be investigated in models with a more chronic seizure focus.

The trigger site

Another potential treatment site for some patients with reflex

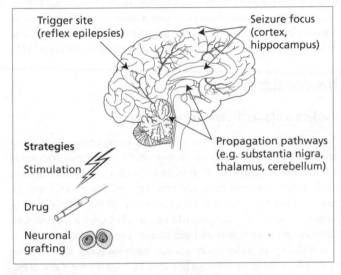

Fig. 74.1 Summary focal treatment strategies for refractory epilepsy.

epilepsies might be the brain area where seizures are triggered, and there are a number of established animal models of reflex epilepsies. In genetically epilepsy-prone rats (GEPRs) intense sound stimulation induces hyperlocomotion followed by clonic then tonic motor activity. These audiogenic seizures seem to be triggered from the inferior colliculus (IC) and can be suppressed for as long as 3 days with a group II glutamate metabotropic receptor agonist [15], and for shorter time periods with other agents (Table 74.2) [16,17]. Longer-term drug delivery to a trigger site was achieved with an implanted minipump in the photosensitive baboon, *Papio papio* [18]. In this model, intermittent light stimulation induces bilateral myoclonus preceded by paroxysmal discharges, the neural generation of which has been localized in the motor cortex and has human parallels in some primary generalized epilepsy syndromes. These photoconvulsive responses were blocked during chronic 7-day infusion of GABA into the motor cortex (seizure focus), but also to the occipital cortex (trigger site), believed to carry the motor cortex afferents necessary for the induction of paroxysmal discharges. Perhaps surprisingly, there were no observed behavioural effects in terms of either visual or motor function.

Propagation pathways

In patients without an identifiable seizure or trigger focus, focal therapies may still offer the chance of at least disrupting the spread of seizure activity around the brain by targeting known key propagation pathways. The substantia nigra (SN) has been shown to play a critical role in the spread of seizure activity [19–21]. In addition to electrical stimulation studies (see Chapter 73 and [22]), once again various focally directed pharmacological manipulations in this region have proved to have at least partial effects in experimental models (Table 74.3) [23–28]. However as lesioning of the SN had a similar effect in some studies [26], as does electrical stimulation, and not all the studies have adequate histological or pharmacodynamic data, it is not always clear that the results are due to specific pharmacological drug effects. In addition, in some studies the endpoints were purely EEG based, rather than clinical, although in others behavioural seizure severity was also significantly reduced. One significant potential limitation is that GABAergic manipulations of the SN in rats seem to result in consistent side-effects with unilateral applications producing turning and circling behaviour and bilat-

Table 74.1 Positive focal drug injection studies into the seizure focus in experimental epilepsy models

Antiepileptic agent	Seizure model	Reference
Taurine	Amygdala electrical kindling	[6]
Lidocaine hydrochloride	Pyriform cortex bicuculline	[7]
Serotonin agonists	Hippocampal electrical kindling (cats)	[8]
Diazepam	Hippocampal bicuculline; cortical cobalt; systemic pilocarpine	[4,5]
mGluR II agonists	Amygdala electrical kindling	[9]
Glutamate antagonists	Prepyriform cortex electrical kindling	[10]
TRH	Amygdala electrical kindling	[11]
Adenosine	Hippocampal electrical kindling	[12]
Phenytoin	Cortical cobalt	[13]

Positive focal drug injection studies into the seizure focus in experimental epilepsy models. All studies are in rat unless otherwise stated. mGluR II, metabotrophic glutamate receptor, group II; TRH, thyrotrophin-releasing hormone.

Table 74.2 Focal drug injection studies to trigger sites in experimental reflex epilepsy models

Antiepileptic agent	Injection site	Model	Reference
Glutamate antagonists	Inferior colliculus	GEPR	[17]
Muscimol	Inferior colliculus	GEPR	[16]
GABA	Motor or occipital cortex	Photosensitive baboon	[18]
mGluR II agonists	Inferior colliculus	GEPR	[15]

Focal drug injection studies to trigger sites in experimental reflex epilepsy models. mGluR II, metabotrophic glutamate receptor, group II.

Table 74.3 Focal drug injection studies to the substantia nigra in experimental epilepsy models

Antiepileptic agent	Model	Reference
Vigabatrin	Amygadala electrical kindling	[23]
Vigabatrin	Maximal electroshock; systemic pentylenetetrazole; focal bicuculline	[24]
Muscimol	Focal bicuculline	[25]
Muscimol	Amygdala electrical kindling	[26]
2-Chloroadenosine	GEPR; maximal electroshock	[27]
GABA	Amygdala electrical kindling	[28]
Glutamate antagonists	Focal bicuculline	[25]

Focal drug injection studies to the substantia nigra in experimental epilepsy models. All studies were in rats.

eral applications inducing increased gnawing and sniffing. How this might translate to man is not yet clear, but is obviously of concern. In addition, at best this approach aims to reduce seizure severity, rather than hoping for seizure freedom, and whether the benefits in all but a few individuals with severe frequent falls and convulsion would outweigh the risks involved is uncertain.

Seizure-stimulated drug release

In most patients all but very localized minor seizures are associated with a detectable EEG change at onset, and in some this may precede the clinical event by a matter of seconds. Therefore, a further step on from chronic focal drug delivery might be to link seizure onset with acute focal drug delivery, and this is an area under investigation. Using a computerized EEG detection system in rats, Stein et al. [29] set up a linked automated drug release system delivering diazepam into the seizure focus, which rapidly terminated seizure activity induced by hippocampal bicuculline. In terms of automated EEG detection this is a very preliminary study, and any such system in man would have to be very sophisticated to guarantee accuracy and protect against potential confounding factors, such as movement artefacts or triggering unnecessary release of drugs. However, for some patients with a reliable clinical aura of sufficient duration, patient-activated drug delivery systems might be devised.

As discussed, many of these studies have limitations, but nonetheless they demonstrate a proof in principle that focal neurochemical and pharmacological manipulations in the brain can be ef-

fective in suppressing seizure activity. This certainly opens a new therapeutic avenue for patients with identified but non-resectable seizure foci, and potentially also for others with poorly localized onset, by targeting known propagation or trigger pathways. However, even with the best of slow-release mechanisms or drug delivery systems, in the lifetime of an epilepsy patient repeated implantation or refill procedures would be needed, with the attendant increasing risks of complications. In this context grafting of neuronal stem cells, particularly given the potential to manipulate their later differentiation, and for genetic modification prior to implantation, might provide a more long-term solution. In addition, many epilepsies involve focal brain damage, which at least in principle might be repaired by neuronal grafts in the same way as has been applied to ischaemic brain damage [30] and neurodegenerative diseases [31].

Neuronal grafting

Repletion of specific neurotransmitters

A number of studies have been conducted in experimental epilepsy and seizure models to address the potential for neuronal grafting as a treatment for epilepsy. The majority with positive results have used similar experimental paradigms (Fig. 74.2) in which a specific neurotransmitter system is targeted using physical or chemical means. Lesions of the noradrenergic (NA), cholinergic and serotonergic system have all previously been shown to increase susceptibility to subsequent seizure provocations. This can be undertaken either in previously normal animals with subsequent electrical kindling, or in models with established seizure tendencies such as the GEPR in which audiogenic stimuli provoke seizures. Grafts, usually of same-species fetal origin, are then undertaken with the aim of replenishing the previously depleted neurotransmitter and restoring seizure susceptibility to control (predepletion) levels. This approach has been used targeting NA, cholinergic and serotonergic inputs to the hippocampus, in a variety of models, and the positive studies are summarized in Table 74.4 [32–41]. The results are not always easy to interpret, with differing models, variable graft–host integration and detail. For example Cassel et al. [36] tested the effect of grafting fetal basal forebrain cells, rich in acetylcholine (ACh), into the hippocampus of rats that had a depleted ACh system due to a lesion of the fimbria–fornix pathway. They found that ACh-grafted rats had a decreased susceptibility to audiogenic seizures but also that the same rats had an increased susceptibility to the convulsant pentylenetetrazol (PTZ). A followup study [37], which reported less graft-induced damage to the host and better graft integration, showed an increased susceptibility to

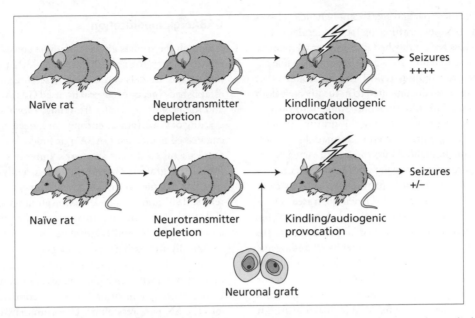

Fig. 74.2 Experimental paradigm for neurotransmitter depletion-repletion grafting studies. The same paradigm was also applied to GEPRs, with audiogenic seizure provocation rather than electrical kindling. (a) Naïve animals with no seizure susceptibility, following noradrenergic, cholinergic, or serotonergic depletion, have significantly increased seizure susceptibility with subsequent electrical kindling. (b) Neuronal grafts to restore the depleted neurotransmitter result in seizure susceptibility returning to that of control (unlesioned) animals.

Table 74.4 Neurotransmitter depletion-repletion grafting studies in experimental epilepsy models

Neurotransmitter modulation	Grafted cell type	Seizure model	Reference
6-OHDA, NA depletion	Fetal locus coeruleus	Hippocampal electrical kindling	[32–34]
6-OHDA, NA depletion	Fetal locus coeruleus	GEPR	[35]
Fimbra-fornix lesion (ACh depletion)	Fetal basal forebrain	Audiogenic provoked seizures Pentyelenetrazol provoked seizures	[36,37]
Surgical subcortical hippocampal deafferentation[a]	Fetal locus coeruleus	Picrotoxin seizures Perforant path stimulation	[38]
192-IgG Saporin, ACh depletion	Fetal basal forebrain	Hippocampal electrical kindling	[39]
5,7-DHT, serotonin depletion	Fetal raphe tissue	Hippocampal electrical kindling	[40]
5,7-DHT, serotonin depletion	Fetal raphe tissue	GEPRs	[41]

Neurotransmitter depletion—repletion grafting studies in experimental epilepsy models. All studies were in rats, and cells grafted either intracerebroventricularly, with migration to the hippocampus, or directly into the hippocampus. 5,7-DHT, 5,7-dihydroxytryptamine; 6-OHDA, 6-hydroxydopamine microinfusion; NA, noradrenaline.
[a] This procedure affects noradrenergic, cholinergic, GABAergic and serotonergic inputs to the hippocampus.

sound and a decreased susceptibility to PTZ after grafting. These conflicting results from the same group make it difficult to draw conclusions about the effects of grafting ACh cells on seizure activity in these models.

However, the remaining studies, particularly with respect to (NA) grafts, are largely consistent and show that after specific neurotransmitter lesioning, appropriate fetal grafting can restore the targeted neurotransmitter levels to near normal [42], and some host integration and synaptic connectivity occurs [32]. One group using NA grafts have further provided evidence that the functional effects of grafted cells are dependent on synaptic transmitter release

[33,34]. This may explain why merely increasing local NA levels using NA-releasing polymers [28] was not effective in earlier experiments. In addition, as long as grafts were undertaken before any seizures had been provoked, the seizure threshold, expected to have been reduced by the neurotransmitter depletion, is similarly returned to control (unlesioned) levels.

These studies illustrate the known potential of neuronal grafts in terms of neurochemical restoration. However, where the same grafts have been undertaken in animals not subjected to prior specific neurotransmitter lesioning, or where grafting has been undertaken only after the kindling process is complete and seizures have already occurred, for the most part no significant beneficial effects have been demonstrated. Thus, grafting of locus coeruleus (LC) cells after kindling seizures are established in 6-hydroxydopamine (OHDA) treated rats produced no significant effects [43], while LC grafts administered before kindling retard the development of seizures [32]. GEPRs have been documented to naturally have both widespread detriments in NA function and some serotonergic depletion before seizures occur [44]. Despite this grafting without additional specific neurotransmitter depletion has had disappointing results. Fetal LC tissue implanted into the lateral ventricles or IC (thought to be important in triggering audiogenic seizures) of naïve GEPRs results in at best minor improvements unlikely to be of clinical significance. Holmes et al. [45] demonstrated an increased latency to tonic phase, and a decreased duration of the clonic phase, of audiogenic seizures in grafted GEPRs compared to shams, but no other effects on kindling parameters or audiogenic seizure severity. Similarly in the same model others have reported no significant reduction in seizure severity with fetal LC [46], or raphe [41] grafts to the hippocampus, although the power of such studies is often limited by small numbers and considerable variation in graft survival and integration.

Thus overall the positive results from depletion-graft repletion studies may be interpreted as showing a protective effect of grafts in terms of abating early epileptogenic processes, which is of scientific value in terms of understanding pathophysiology. However, they cannot be considered of direct clinical relevance for human epilepsy, presenting only after seizures have occurred, and in which specific neurotransmitter deficiencies have not been identified. This highlights the importance of choosing appropriate experimental models to evaluate treatment effects.

NA grafting has also been assessed in models without specific known deficits and in whom spontaneous seizures occur, which might be considered more appropriate to human epilepsy. The pilocarpine rat model has initial status epilepticus, following which the animals develop chronic spontaneous temporal lobe seizures, with pathology similar to that of hippocampal sclerosis, and additional widespread limbic forebrain damage. Bilaterally grafting cell suspensions of fetal LC tissue into the hippocampus after status epilepticus in this model significantly reduced the number of spontaneous seizures in comparison to non-grafted animals and animals with grafts into the cerebellum or olfactory bulbs [47]. The decrease in seizure frequency, which occurred 6 weeks after grafting, when host integration would be expected to be maximal, was maintained for up to 15 weeks. However, it was not seen in all animals and crucially the study did not provide any histological evaluation of graft placement, survival, phenotype or integration. Thus, whether the apparent treatment effect was in any way related to neuronal grafts, as opposed to other non-specific focal effects, including hippocampal lesioning/destruction which is of known efficacy, is unclear and further studies have not been reported. In contrast, implanting LC cells bilaterally in to the hippocampus after pretreating with kainic acid (KA) which produces a similar clinical phenotype had no effect on subsequent kindling parameters [48]. However, the animals grafted with LC cells did have fewer spontaneous seizures after KA administration than controls, suggesting a mild treatment effect and illustrating that the outcome in provoked seizure models cannot necessarily be extrapolated to those with spontaneous seizures.

GABAergic modification

Although the studies above cannot be considered of direct clinical relevance, they do establish the principle that grafting neuronal cells into seizure models can modulate seizure susceptibility. With the established efficacy of several licensed GABAergic drugs in epilepsy, and the promising results from initial focal drug delivery studies, grafting of GABAergic neurones, or indeed any cell line specifically engineered to increase GABAergic function at the focus, might be a more useful treatment strategy. Numerous studies have demonstrated that grafts of GABAergic cells, usually derived from the fetal striatum, can survive, make axonal connections [49], restore GABA release [50] and restore levels of glutamatic acid decarboxylase (GAD) [51], an enzyme involved in the synthesis of GABA, in lesioned animals, and there have now been a number of studies specifically addressing this in epilepsy.

Fine et al. [52] increased seizure susceptibility by lesioning the caudate putamen with a glutamate receptor agonist, ibotenic acid, before grafting fetal striatal cells or a control graft of sciatic tissue into the SN pars reticulum. Unfortunately, both GABAergic and the sham/control sciatic nerve grafts reduced the severity of pilocarpine-induced seizures to almost that of the intact animal and the survival of grafted neurones was not evaluated. Thus this may represent a non-specific effect from lesioning the SN, although the treatment effects were slightly greater in the GABAergic grafted animals. Studies of fetal GABAergic grafts to the SN in fully kindled animals have been disappointing [53], producing only a transient initial increase in the threshold for eliciting focal epileptiform EEG activity, without any significant difference in clinical or electrographic seizure duration.

Thompson et al. [54] produced genetically engineered cell lines from conditionally immortalized neurones, specifically designed to increase production and release of GABA by driving GAD_{65} expression. GAD_{65} cells or control (sham) cells were grafted into either the anterior or posterior SN. GAD_{65} cells in the posterior SN appeared to have a proconvulsant effect, in that these animals more readily and reliably reached a fully kindled state than the controls. In contrast, although not significant when compared to sham grafts, GAD_{65} cells transplanted into the anterior SN appeared to retard kindling development. Thus, GABAergic modulation in the SN can give opposing results. Focal GABAergic drug studies suggest that this may reflect subtle variations not only in precise target site within the SN [55], but also in host age and in dose [56]. The influence of the SN on seizure propagation may also vary considerably in different models of epilepsy, and certainly much more work is needed to unravel these complex relationships before such approaches might become clinically applicable.

The same group [57] have also grafted these cells to the piriform cortex, believed to play a role in seizure propagation prior to limbic kindling in rats, with disappointing results in that only a very transient effect in seizure threshold prior to kindling was shown, with no significant difference on any parameters after kindling. The authors suggest that downregulation of GABA synthesis, GABA receptors, or decreased long-term neuronal survival might all contribute to this lack of effect—all of which could be problems in a clinical paradigm. This emphasizes the need to resolve such issues experimentally before clinical trials would be appropriate.

A more obvious approach, supported by the focal drug studies, might be to target GABA to the seizure focus, although the potential problems of downregulation would still apply. There have been few studies addressing this, perhaps because of technical problems relating to GABAergic graft survival in cortical brain regions [58]. Thompson *et al.* [59] published an abstract suggesting a beneficial effect of grafting genetically modified GABAergic cells to the seizure focus in hippocampally-kindled rats, with an additional capacity for *in vivo* regulation of the GAD_{65} expression (using doxycycline), but full details of this work have yet to be reported.

In the hippocampus, it seems direct grafts of GABAergic cell types are not the only way to increase local GABAergic interneurone numbers, and that this can occur as a secondary consequence of repairing other local circuitry. Shetty and Turner [60], using rats treated with unilateral intracerebroventricular KA, have reported eloquent and detailed histological studies which will be fully discussed in the next section. In the context of GABA, however, these demonstrate, along with specific CA3 pyramidal cell depletion, a loss of GAD-positive interneurones in the hippocampus, which appears to be reversed by grafts of mixed fetal hippocampal cells or grafts from the CA3 hippocampal subfield. The grafts themselves survive well and form connections with host tissue, but do not appear to be directly donating the restored GAD-positive cells. Of note, grafts from the CA1 subfield had no effect on GAD-positive interneurone numbers, suggesting it is a very specific effect. The authors interpret this as reflecting that the loss of CA3 afferents contributes to a secondary loss of the GAD protein expression, which is thus reversed by repleting CA3 cells. Unfortunately, these studies did not include any behavioural or functional experiments, so whether restoration of GAD-positive interneurones has any beneficial effect on seizure parameters remains unknown. Overall, these studies suggest that the transplantation of GABAergic cells or agents has potential as a treatment strategy and, although the availability of genetically engineered cells to promote local sustained GABA release is encouraging, these should be evaluated in appropriate experimental paradigms before studies in man are considered.

Hippocampal repair

Given the frequency of hippocampal sclerosis as a pathological substrate for epilepsy in man, and the well-established patterns of neuronal loss that these patients exhibit, many investigators have concentrated on the potential for neuronal grafts to repair this damage. Several animal models exist that mimic this pathology, usually with initial acutely provoked (electrical stimulation or chemical, e.g. KA, pilocarpine) status epilepticus followed by chronic spontaneous seizures.

Shetty, Turner and co-workers have published a series of eloquent studies in rats given unilateral intraventricular KA [60–68]. This typically results in significant loss of CA3 pyramidal cells, with relative preservation of CA1 and dentate granule cells. In this model, fetal hippocampal cells grafted into the lesioned hippocampus have shown good cell survival, with cells differentiating into mature neurones, and a restoration of total neuronal number with limited damage to the host hippocampus by the graft itself. In addition the grafts appear to reverse or prevent other secondary pathological consequences including aberrant sprouting of host mossy fibres into the dentate supragranular layer, thereby restoring the

damaged cytoarchitecture, possibly by providing appropriate target neurones [65]. As discussed above, GAD-positive interneurone numbers are also restored [60]. For good connectivity both the precise location of the graft within the hippocampus and the donor cell type appear to be important. Whilst in this series of detailed studies, all grafts (mixed hippocampus, CA1 or CA3 cells) showed good cell survival and sent projections to the ipsilateral septum, only grafted tissue located in the degenerated CA3 cell layer [63] and containing CA3 donor cells [66] contained neurones that established robust projections to the contralateral hippocampus. This projection pattern resembled that seen in intact animals. In addition, all donor cell types resembled those *in situ* [67] with CA1 cells being of a smaller pyramidal shape and well dispersed and CA3 cells being of larger pyramidal shape and clustered together. The specificity and success of neuronal grafting to the hippocampus clinically could, therefore, depend upon matching specific cells to specific lesion types, and as the authors point out, in contrast to the KA model, human hippocampal sclerosis involves damage to the CA1 region as well as the CA3 region and would therefore potentially require multiple grafts of appropriate cells [66].

A further problem is that in all these studies grafting was undertaken only 4 days after KA lesioning, as it had been previously found that grafts implanted after this time resulted in steadily decreasing cell survival [61]. When cells were grafted 45 days postlesion, and examined 1 month later, cell survival had fallen to 31% [68] in comparison with 69% at 4 days postlesion [67]. It is not known when hippocampal cell loss in epileptic patients occurs, but it is likely that any grafting would only be considered relatively late in the disease process, and inevitably after seizure onset. However, survival 1 month after grafting appeared to be a good predictor of long-term (1 year) cell survival [64] and even the lower survival levels appeared sufficient to result in structural repair of the local damage.

The biggest limitation of these studies, however, is that the model did not exhibit spontaneous behavioural seizures (Ashok Turner, personal communication, 2002), so no information on the potential therapeutic benefits of these grafts in terms of seizure outcome is available. It is also recognized that hippocampal cell death is neither necessary nor sufficient for epileptogenesis [69], so any repair that can be achieved may have little influence on the epilepsy, although it may affect other clinically important parameters such as memory function. Other groups have found that grafts to both the intact hippocampus [70] or to lesioned hippocampi [71] (subcortical deafferentation) may in themselves be epileptogenic, with both electrographic spiking and occasional behavioural seizures occurring in previously non-epileptic animals. These grafted animals were also more susceptible to picrotoxin-induced behavioural seizures than controls [38]. Thus, there are a number of concerns about the potential of attempted hippocampal repair as a strategy for neuronal grafting in epilepsy, particularly when balanced against the established efficacy of surgical resection of hippocampal foci in man.

Some studies have reported slightly more promising results. A study in a small number of amygdala-kindled rats showed that fetal hippocampal cells grafted near the CA2 region of the hippocampus reduced the severity of subsequent kindling-induced seizures to some extent in 80% of animals [72]. However, for most animals the seizure severity levels fluctuated with increasing number of stimulations, sometimes reaching pregraft levels. A very mild beneficial effect was also seen after transplanting hippocampal cells into the KA-degenerated hippocampus. Although grafting had no effect on subsequent kindling-induced seizures, there was a slight reduction in the number of spontaneous seizures following the KA administration [48]. Nonetheless, further studies to elucidate the role of neuronal cell loss in epileptogenesis, and of the potential for its repair as a treatment for epilepsy, are needed.

Conclusions

Epilepsy is a heterogeneous neurological condition and despite recent advances it seems likely there will remain a significant cohort of intractable patients for whom other treatment approaches need to be developed.

At present many of the focal treatment studies have been carried in experimental models with provoked seizures, and there are few in good models with spontaneous chronic seizures, in part reflecting the practical difficulties that long-term seizure monitoring in animals entails. However, current technology does enable video-EEG recording of small mammals on a long-term continuous basis [73] and software packages for semi-automated detection can be designed. Various models with frequent spontaneous seizures (e.g. [74]) might be considered more reflective of human refractory epilepsy and would perhaps be more appropriate for future studies.

Focal drug delivery systems certainly show promise, although more detailed long-term studies in a range of experimental models, and including behavioural outcomes, are needed. Neuronal grafting holds the promise of effecting potentially permanent local change and initial studies demonstrate the feasibility of both restoring neuronal loss, altering circuitry, or increasing local neurochemical concentrations, all of which might prove beneficial in epilepsy. However, in addition to the limitations posed by the models used, the most promising results have arisen when the time between the initial insult and transplantation was short; when specific known lesions and depletions were made prior to grafting, and the appropriate type of grafted cells was used to match the lesion; and when therapeutic intervention occurred prior to a chronic epileptic tendency being established. None of these scenarios can be applied to most clinical situations. In addition, many of the existing studies are inconclusive and difficult to interpret due to the relatively small number of animals used, the effects not always reaching significance, and due to the inevitable variations that occur in cell survival, axonal outgrowth, the disruption caused to host tissue and the size and placement of grafts between animals.

In both focal drug delivery and grafting studies, none have been of sufficient duration to establish whether even with a permanent therapeutic local manipulation the benefits might only be transient, given the known highly adaptable capacity of the brain in terms of receptor function and reorganization. The long-term ethical and safety aspects of using embryonic and/or genetically engineered cells lines also require further careful scrutiny, particularly for epilepsy patients, most of whom will may have a normal life expectancy. Nonetheless, focal treatment techniques in epilepsy offer a novel approach to an important clinical problem and the promise that, with ongoing work in this field in the years to come, more patients may lead seizure-free lives.

References

1 Cockerell OC, Johnson AL, Sander JW et al. Prognosis of epilepsy: a review and further analysis of the first nine years of the British National General Practice Study of Epilepsy, a prospective population-based study. Epilepsia 1997; 38 (1): 31–46.
2 Jacobs MP, Fischbach GD, Davis MR et al. Future directions for epilepsy research. Neurology 2001; 57 (9): 1536–42.
3 Kupferberg H. Animal models used in the screening of antiepileptic drugs. Epilepsia 2001; 42: 7–12.
4 Eder HG, Jones DB, Fisher RS. Local perfusion of diazepam attenuates interictal and ictal events in the bicuculline model of epilepsy in rats. Epilepsia 1997; 38 (5): 516–21.
5 Eder HG, Stein A, Fisher RS. Interictal and ictal activity in the rat cobalt/pilocarpine model of epilepsy decreased by local perfusion of diazepam. Epilepsy Res 1997; 29 (1): 17–24.
6 Uemura S, Ienaga K, Higashiura K et al. Effects of intraamygdaloid injection of taurine and valyltaurine on amygdaloid kindled seizure in rats. Jpn J Psychiatr Neurol 1991; 45 (2): 383–5.
7 Smith DC, Krahl SE, Browning RA et al. Rapid cessation of focally induced generalized seizures in rats through microinfusion of lidocaine hydrochloride into the focus. Epilepsia 1993; 34 (1): 43–53.
8 Wada Y, Nakamura M, Hasegawa H et al. Intra-hippocampal injection of 8-hydroxy-2-(di-n-propylamino)tetralin (8-OH-DPAT) inhibits partial and generalized seizures induced by kindling stimulation in cats. Neurosci Lett 1993; 159 (1–2): 179–82.
9 Attwell PJE, Koumentaki A, Croucher MJ et al. Specific group II metabotropic glutamate receptor activation inhibits the development of kindled epilepsy in rats. Brain Res 1998; 787 (2): 286–91.
10 Croucher MJ, Bradford HF, Sunter DC et al. Inhibition of the development of electrical kindling of the prepyriform cortex by daily focal injections of excitatory amino acid antagonists. Eur J Pharmac 1988; 152 (1–2): 29–38.
11 Kubek MJ, Liang D, Byrd KE et al. Prolonged seizure suppression by a single implantable polymeric-TRH microdisk preparation. Brain Res 1998; 809 (2): 189–97.
12 Boison D, Scheurer L, Tseng JL et al. Seizure suppression in kindled rats by intraventricular grafting of an adenosine releasing synthetic polymer. Exp Neurol 1999; 160 (1): 164–74.
13 Tamargo RJ, Rossell LA, Kossoff EH et al. The intracerebral administration of phenytoin using controlled-release polymers reduces experimental seizures in rats. Epilepsy Res 2002; 48 (3): 145–55.
14 Remler MP, Marcussen W. Radiation-controlled focal pharmacology in the therapy of experimental epilepsy. Epilepsia 1981; 22 (2): 153–9.
15 Tang E, Yip PK, Chapman AG et al. Prolonged anticonvulsant action of glutamate metabotropic receptor agonists in inferior colliculus of genetically epilepsy-prone rats. Eur J Pharmac 1997; 327 (2–3): 109–15.
16 Browning RA, Lanker ML, Faingold CL. Injections of noradrenergic and GABAergic agonists into the inferior colliculus: effects on audiogenic seizures in genetically epilepsy-prone rats. Epilepsy Res 1989; 4 (2): 119–25.
17 Meldrum B, Millan M, Patel S et al. Anti-epileptic effects of focal microinjection of excitatory amino acid antagonists. J Neural Transm 1988; 72 (3): 191–200.
18 Brailowsky S, Silva BC, Menini C et al. Effects of localized, chronic GABA infusions into different cortical areas of the photosensitive baboon, Papio papio. Electroencephalogr Clin Neurophysiol 1989; 72 (2): 147–56.
19 Bonhaus DW, Walters JR, McNamara JO. Activation of substantia nigra neurons: role in the propagation of seizures in kindled rats. J Neurosci 1986; 6 (10): 3024–30.
20 Gale K. Mechanisms of seizure control mediated by gamma-aminobutyric acid: role of the substantia nigra. Fed Proc 1985; 44 (8): 2414–24.
21 Morimoto K, Goddard GV. The substantia nigra is an important site for the containment of seizure generalization in the kindling model of epilepsy. Epilepsia 1987; 28 (1): 1–10.
22 Sabatino M, Gravante G, Ferraro G et al. Striatonigral suppression of focal hippocampal epilepsy. Neurosci Lett 1989; 98 (3): 285–90.
23 Löscher W, Czuczwar SJ, Jackler R et al. Effect of microinjections of

gamma-vinyl GABA or isoniazid into substantia-nigra on the development of amygdala kindling in rats. *Exp Neurol* 1987; 95 (3): 622–38.

24 Iadarola MJ, Gale K. Substantia nigra: site of anticonvulsant activity mediated by gamma-aminobutyric acid. *Science* 1982; 218 (4578): 1237–40.

25 Maggio R, Gale K. Seizures evoked from area tempestas are subject to control by GABA and glutamate receptors in substantia nigra. *Exp Neurol* 1989; 105 (2): 184–8.

26 McNamara JO, Galloway MT, Rigsbee LC *et al*. Evidence implicating substantia nigra in regulation of kindled seizure threshold. *J Neurosci* 1984; 4 (9): 2410–17.

27 De Sarro G, Meldrum BS, Reavill C. Anticonvulsant action of 2-amino-7-phosphonoheptanoic acid in the substantia nigra. *Eur J Pharmacol* 1984; 106 (1): 175–9.

28 Kokaia M, Aebischer P, Elmer E *et al*. Seizure suppression in kindling epilepsy by intracerebral implants of GABA- but not by noradrenaline-releasing polymer matrices. *Exp Brain Res* 1994; 100 (3): 385–94.

29 Stein AG, Eder HG, Blum DE *et al*. An automated drug delivery system for focal epilepsy. *Epilepsy Res* 2000; 39 (2): 103–14.

30 Sinden JD, Rashid-Doubell F, Kershaw TR *et al*. Recovery of spatial learning by grafts of a conditionally immortalized hippocampal neuroepithelial cell line into the ischaemia-lesioned hippocampus. *Neurosci* 1997; 81 (3): 599–608.

31 Kordower JH, Freeman TB, Chen EY *et al*. Fetal nigral grafts survive and mediate clinical benefit in a patient with Parkinson's disease. *Mov Disord* 1998; 13 (3): 383–93.

32 Barry DI, Kikvadze I, Brundin P *et al*. Grafted noradrenergic neurons suppress seizure development in kindling-induced epilepsy. *Proc Natl Acad Sci USA* 1987; 84 (23): 8712–15.

33 Bengzon J, Kokaia M, Brundin P *et al*. Seizure suppression in kindling epilepsy by intrahippocampal locus coeruleus grafts: evidence for an alpha-2-adrenoreceptor mediated mechanism. *Exp Brain Res* 1990; 81 (2): 433–7.

34 Kokaia M, Cenci MA, Elmer E *et al*. Seizure development and noradrenaline release in kindling epilepsy after noradrenergic reinnervation of the subcortically deafferented hippocampus by superior cervical ganglion or fetal locus coeruleus grafts. *Exp Neurol* 1994; 130 (2): 351–61.

35 Clough RW, Browning RA, Maring ML *et al*. Effects of intraventricular locus coeruleus transplants on seizure severity in genetically epilepsy-prone rats following depletion of brain norepinephrine. *J Neural Transplant Plast* 1994; 5 (1): 65–79.

36 Cassel JC, Kelche C, Will BE. Susceptibility to pentylenetetrazol-induced and audiogenic seizures in rats with selective fimbria-fornix lesions and intrahippocampal septal grafts. *Exp Neurol* 1987; 97 (3): 564–76.

37 Cassel JC, Kelche C, Will BE. Susceptibility to pentylenetetrazol-induced and audiogenic seizures in rats given aspirative lesions of the fimbria-fornix pathways followed by intrahippocampal grafts – a time course approach. *Restorative Neurol Neurosci* 1991; 3 (2): 55–64.

38 Buzsaki G, Ponomareff G, Bayardo F *et al*. Suppression and induction of epileptic activity by neuronal grafts. *Proc Natl Acad Sci USA* 1988; 85 (23): 9327–30.

39 Ferencz I, Kokaia M, Elmer E *et al*. Suppression of kindling epileptogenesis in rats by intrahippocampal cholinergic grafts. *Eur J Neurosci* 1998; 10 (1): 213–20.

40 Camu W, Marlier L, Lernernatoli M *et al*. Transplantation of serotonergic neurons into the 5,7-DHT-lesioned rat olfactory-bulb restores the parameters of kindling. *Brain Res* 1990; 518 (1–2): 23–30.

41 Clough R, Statnick M, Maring SM *et al*. Fetal raphe transplants reduce seizure severity in serotonin-depleted GEPRs. *Neuroreport* 1996; 8 (1): 341–6.

42 Bengzon J, Brundin P, Kalen P *et al*. Host regulation of noradrenaline release from grafts of seizure-suppressant locus coeruleus neurons. *Exp Neurol* 1991; 111 (1): 49–54.

43 Bengzon J, Kokaia Z, Lindvall O. Specific functions of grafted locus coeruleus neurons in the kindling model of epilepsy. *Exp Neurol* 1993; 122 (1): 143–54.

44 Dailey JW, Jobe PC. Indexes of noradrenergic function in the central nervous system of the seizure-naive genetically epilepsy-prone rats. *Epilepsia* 1986; 27 (6): 665–70.

45 Holmes GL, Thompson JL, Huh K *et al*. Effects of neural transplantation

on seizures in the immature genetically epilepsy-prone rat. *Exp Neurol* 1992; 116 (1): 52–63.

46 Clough RW, Browning RA, Maring ML *et al*. Intracerebral grafting of fetal dorsal pons in genetically epilepsy-prone rats: effects on audiogenic-induced seizures. *Exp Neurol* 1991; 112 (2): 195–9.

47 Bortolotto ZA, Calderazzo L, Cavalheiro EA. Some evidence that intrahippocampal grafting of noradrenergic neurons suppresses spontaneous seizures in epileptic rats. *Braz J Med Biol Res* 1990; 23 (12): 1267–9.

48 Holmes GL, Thompson JL, Huh K *et al*. Effect of neural transplants on seizure frequency and kindling in immature rats following kainic acid. *Brain Res Dev Brain Res* 1991; 64 (1–2): 47–56.

49 Wictorin K, Clarke DJ, Bolam JP *et al*. Fetal striatal neurons grafted into the ibotenate lesioned adult striatum: efferent projections and synaptic contacts in the host globus pallidus. *Neurosci* 1990; 37 (2): 301–15.

50 Sirinathsinghji DJ, Dunnett SB, Isacson O *et al*. Striatal grafts in rats with unilateral neostriatal lesions—II. In vivo monitoring of GABA release in globus pallidus and substantia nigra. *Neuroscience* 1988; 24 (3): 803–11.

51 Isacson O, Brundin P, Gage FH *et al*. Neural grafting in a rat model of Huntington's disease: progressive neurochemical changes after neostriatal ibotenate lesions and striatal tissue grafting. *Neurosci* 1985; 16 (4): 799–817.

52 Fine A, Meldrum BS, Patel S. Modulation of experimentally induced epilepsy by intracerebral grafts of fetal GABAergic neurons. *Neuropsychologia* 1990; 28 (6): 627–34.

53 Löscher W, Ebert U, Lehmann H *et al*. Seizure suppression in kindling epilepsy by grafts of fetal GABAergic neurons in rat substantia nigra. *J Neurosci Res* 1998; 51 (2): 196–209.

54 Thompson K, Anantharam V, Behrstock S *et al*. Conditionally immortalized cell lines, engineered to produce and release GABA, modulate the development of behavioral seizures. *Exp Neurol* 2000; 161 (2): 481–9.

55 Moshe SL, Brown LL, Kubova H *et al*. Maturation and segregation of brain networks that modify seizures. *Brain Res* 1994; 665 (1): 141–6.

56 Garant DS, Xu SG, Sperber EF *et al*. Age-related differences in the effects of GABA(A) agonists microinjected into rat substantia nigra—proconvulsant and anticonvulsant actions. *Epilepsia* 1995; 36 (10): 960–5.

57 Gernert M, Thompson KW, Loscher W *et al*. Genetically engineered GABA-producing cells demonstrate anticonvulsant effects and long-term transgene expression when transplanted into the central piriform cortex of rats. *Exp Neurol* 2002; 176 (1): 183–92.

58 Bragin A, Takacs J, Vinogradova O *et al*. Age-related loss of GABA-positive and GABA-negative neurons in neocortical transplants. *J Neural Transplant Plast* 1993; 4 (1): 53–9.

59 Thompson K, Guttman O, Tobin AJ. Doxycycline-dependent modulation of kindled seizures following hippocampal transplantation of cells engineered to produce GABA. *Soc Neurosci* 1999; 25: 846.

60 Shetty AK, Turner DA. Fetal hippocampal grafts containing CA3 cells restore host hippocampal glutamate decarboxylase-positive interneuron numbers in a rat model of temporal lobe epilepsy. *J Neurosci* 2000; 20 (23): 8788–801.

61 Shetty AK, Turner DA. Enhanced cell-survival in fetal hippocampal suspension transplants grafted to adult-rat hippocampus following kainate lesions – A 3-dimensional graft reconstruction study. *Neuroscience* 1995; 67 (3): 561–82.

62 Shetty AK, Turner DA. Development of fetal hippocampal grafts in intact and lesioned hippocampus. [Review] [355 refs]. *Prog Neurobiol* 1996; 50 (5–6): 597–653.

63 Shetty AK, Turner DA. Development of long-distance efferent projections from fetal hippocampal grafts depends upon pathway specificity and graft location in kainate-lesioned adult hippocampus. *Neuroscience* 1997; 76 (4): 1205–19.

64 Zaman V, Shetty AK. Fetal hippocampal CA3 cell grafts transplanted to lesioned CA3 region of the adult hippocampus exhibit long-term survival in a rat model of temporal lobe epilepsy. *Neurobiol Dis* 2001; 8 (6): 942–52.

65 Shetty AK, Turner DA. Fetal hippocampal cells grafted to kainate-lesioned CA3 region of adult hippocampus suppress aberrant supragranular sprouting of host mossy fibers. *Exp Neurol* 1997; 143 (2): 231–45.

66 Shetty AK, Zaman V, Turner DA. Pattern of long-distance projections

from fetal hippocampal field CA3 and CA1 cell grafts in lesioned CA3 of adult hippocampus follows intrinsic character of respective donor cells. *Neuroscience* 2000; 99 (2): 243–55.

67 Zaman V, Turner DA, Shetty AK. Survival of grafted fetal neural cells in kainic acid lesioned CA3 region of adult hippocampus depends upon cell specificity. *Exp Neurol* 2000; 161 (2): 535–61.

68 Zaman V, Turner DA, Shetty AK. Prolonged postlesion transplantation delay adversely influences survival of both homotopic and heterotopic fetal hippocampal cell grafts in kainate-lesioned CA3 region of adult hippocampus. *Cell Transplantation* 2001; 10 (1): 41–52.

69 Sutula TP, Pitkanen A, eds. *Do Seizures Damage the Brain? Progress in Brain Research*. Amsterdam: Elsevier Science, 2002: 135.

70 Buzsaki G, Masliah E, Chen LS *et al*. Hippocampal grafts into the intact brain induce epileptic patterns. *Brain Res* 1991; 554 (1–2): 30–7.

71 Buzsaki G, Bayardo F, Miles R *et al*. The grafted hippocampus: an epileptic focus. *Exp Neurol* 1989; 105 (1): 10–22.

72 Miyamoto O, Itano T, Yamamoto Y *et al*. Effect of embryonic hippocampal transplantation in amygdaloid kindled rat. *Brain Res* 1993; 603 (1): 143–7.

73 Bertram EH, Williamson JM, Cornett JF *et al*. Design and construction of a long-term continuous video-EEG monitoring unit for simultaneous recording of multiple small animals. *Brain Res Protocols* 1997; 2 (1): 85–97.

74 Nilsen KE, Walker MC, Cock HR. A rat model of cortical myoclonus and epilepsia partialis continua. *Epilepsia* 2002; 43 (Suppl. 7): 21.

Index

Page numbers in *italic* refer to figures and **bold** refer to tables

A

absence seizures
  in childhood absence epilepsy 13, 521
  choice of drugs in treatment of 142–4, **142**
  classification and symptomatology 5, 6–7
  in epilepsy with myoclonic absence 15
  prognosis 33
  treatment
    acetazolamide 337
    clonazepam 368
    ethosuximide 395–6
    lamotrigine 433
    levetiracetam 447
    topiramate 521
    trimethadione 565
    valproate 532
    see also individual antiepileptic drugs
absence status epilepticus, emergency treatment
    of
  atypical absence status epilepticus 236–7,
    235
  typical absence status epilepticus *228*, 235–6,
    235
accidental injury, risk in epilepsy 166
acetazolamide 334–44, **334**
  advantages **334**
  bioavailability **334**, 336
  clinical therapeutics and summary of
    use 342–3
  clinical trials and efficacy 337–40, **338–89**
    absence seizures 337
    catamenial seizures 340
    focal seizures 340
    generalized tonic-clonic seizures 337, 340
    myoclonic seizures 337
  cost of treatment xxxi
  disadvantages **334**
  dosage **334**, 340
  dosage interval **334**, 340
  drug interactions **334**, 336
  early use of xxviii, *xxix*, **xxx**
  elimination half-life 336, **334**
  excretion **334**, 336
  indications **334**, 336
  mechanism of action **334**, 335–6
  metabolism 336, **334**
  pharmacokinetics 336
  precautions and contraindications 342–3,
    342
  protein binding **334**
  side effects **334**, 341–2, **341**
    effect on bone 342
    effects of fetus and newborn 342
    idiosyncratic **341**
    increased incidence of kidney stones 341
    metabolic acidosis 341
    symptomatic 341
  time to peak blood levels 336, **334**

tolerance 340
volume of distribution 336, **334**
acetylcholine receptors in epileptogenesis 78
achondroplasia, risk of epilepsy 55
aciclovir, as cause of seizures 53
acquired causes of epilepsy 59, 60–2
  cerebral palsy and mental retardation 60
  cerebral tumours 62
  cerebrovascular disease 61
  CNS infections 60
  dementia 60
  demyelinating disorders 61
  drugs and toxic agents 53–4, **53**
  head trauma 61–2, **62**
  neurosurgery 62
  prenatal and perinatal risk factors **59**, 60
  vascular malformations 61
acquired epileptic aphasia *see* Landau-Kleffner
    syndrome
acrocallosal syndrome, risk of epilepsy 55
ACTH *see* adrenocorticotrophic hormone
acupuncture, in treatment of epilepsy 273–4
acute seizures, animal models of 108–9
  bicuculline 109
  6-Hz seizure model 109
  MES test 108–9
  PTZ test 109
acute symptomatic seizures 51–6, *52*, **53**
  causes of 52–3
  drugs and toxic agents 53–4, **53**
adrenocorticotrophic hormone (ACTH) 560–1
  biotransformation 560
  chemistry 560
  clinical efficacy 560–1
  clinical therapeutics 561
  drug interactions 560
  infantile epilepsy 183–4
  pharmacokinetics 560
  side effects 561
  West syndrome (infantile spasms) 183–4,
    191
adverse drug reactions 166–67
  avoidance of 139–40
  and choice of drug 144–5
  in learning-disabled patients 217, 220
  see also drug interactions; and individual
    antiepileptic drugs
AEDs *see* antiepileptic drugs
aetiology of epilepsy 50–63
  acquired causes of epilepsy 59, 60–2
    cerebral palsy and mental retardation 60
    cerebrovascular disease 61
    CNS infections 60
    dementia 60
    demyelinating disorders 61
    head trauma 61–2, **62**
    prenatal and perinatal risk factors 60
    vascular malformations 61

acute symptomatic seizures 51–6, *52*, **53**,
    55–6
  cerebral tumours 62
  definitions 50
  genetic causes and gene-environment
    relationship 55–6, 56–60, 57, 58
  idiopathic, cryptogenic and symptomatic
    epilepsy 50–1
  methodological issues 50
  neurosurgery 62
  as predictor of seizure remission 31
  well-defined populations 51
  see also specific aetiologies
age
  and epilepsy surgery 585
  and incidence of epilepsy 25
  and mortality due to epilepsy 35
  of onset of epilepsy
    as predictor of remission 31
    and risk of relapse 175–6
alcohol
  as cause of seizures 53
  cytochrome P450 induction **122**
allopurinol 561–2
  biotransformation 561
  chemistry 561
  clinical efficacy 561–2
  clinical therapeutics 562
  drug interactions 561
  mechanisms of action 561
  pharmacokinetics 561
  side effects 562
alopecia, in valproate therapy 534
alternative therapy *see* complementary and
    alternative therapy
Alzheimer's disease, risk of epilepsy **56**
amiodarone, cytochrome P450 inhibition **122**
amitriptyline, as cause of seizures 53
Ammon's horn sclerosis, MRI findings 642,
    643–44
  see also hippocampal sclerosis; temporal lobe
    epilepsy
AMPA receptors, as target for antiepileptic drug
    action 104
amphetamines, as cause of seizures 53, 54
anaesthesia
  in epilepsy surgery 861–72
    adjuvant agents 864–5
      anticholinergics 865
      droperidol 864–5
      muscle relaxants 865
      opioid analgesics 864
    general anaesthesia 865–6
    inhalation anaesthetics 861–2
      desflurane 862
      enflurane 861
      halothane 861
      isoflurane 861–2

anaesthesia (*cont'd*)
  nitrous oxide 862
  sevoflurane 862
  intravenous anaesthetics 862–4
    barbiturates 862–3
    benzodiazepines 863–4
    etomidate 863
    ketamine 864
    local anaesthetics 864
    propofol 863
  local anaesthesia and sedation 866–8
  postoperative care 868
  preoperative assessment 965
  in status epilepticus **234**
Angelman's syndrome, risk of epilepsy 55, 56, 224
animal models of epilepsy 107–13
  acute seizures 108–9
  chronic seizures 109–10
  drug resistance 86
  vagus nerve stimulation 876
  see also individual drugs
aniracetam **491**
anterior frontopolar seizures 10
anticholinergics, anaesthesia for epilepsy surgery 865
anticonvulsants *see* antiepileptic drugs
antiepileptic drug discovery 89–95
  current era 89–90
  differentiation of anticonvulsant activity 92–3
  future issues 94
  ideal model system 89
  identification of anticonvulsant activity 90–2, *90*, **91**, **92**
    6 Hz seizure test **92**
    MES and PTZ tests 90
  pharmacological profile and potential clinical utility 93
  recommendations for future developments 94
antiepileptic drugs
  aetiology of epilepsy 144
  age-dependent pharmacokinetics/pharmacodynamics 180–1, *181*
  animal models 107–12
  choice of 168–70, **170**, 317–33
    ease of use 146–7, **147**
    EEG features 144
    established epilepsy and continuing seizures 329–31, **329**
    learning disability 217–21, 218 **217**, **218**, **219**, **220**
    mechanisms of anticonvulsant action 146
    medical expertise available 145–6, *145*
    newly diagnosed partial onset seizures 328–9
    old versus new drugs 146
    partial epilepsy 317–33
    seizure type and epilepsy syndrome 142–4, **142**, *143*
    side-effect profile and patient characteristics 144–5
  clinical trials 568–75
  compliance 168
  cost of treatment **147**, 328, xxxi
  criteria for starting 167–8, **167**
  developmental toxicity 281–4
  drug discovery 89–95
  elderly patients 205–10
  focal drug delivery by surgical means 884–6
  formulation 147–9, *148*, **149**, 328
  historical aspects xvii, xix–xx, **xix**
  and infantile epilepsy 181

interactions *see* drug interactions
in vitro models 112–13
pharmacokinetics 328
polytherapy 47, 328
in pregnancy 286
randomized controlled trials 317–25
seizure-inducing effects 327
side effects 166–7, 326–7, **327**
targets for development **569**
targets of 96–107
teratogenicity 169, 327
  see also individual drugs; and treatment in specific situations
antipsychotic drugs, seizure-inducing properties 222–3, **223**
anxiety disorders, in epilepsy 258–9, **258**
Apert's syndrome, risk of epilepsy 55
aromatic anticonvulsant hypersensitivity syndrome 482
arteriovenous malformations 742–6
  classification **743**
  clinical features 742–3
  evaluation 743, *744*
  MRI abnormalities **641**, **646**
  surgical treatment 743–5
  stereotactic radiosurgery 842–3
associated disabilities of epilepsy *see* comorbidities
atonic seizures, classification and symptomatology 5, 8
  treatment *see individual antiepileptic drugs*
atypical absence seizures 5, 7
  treatment *see individual antiepileptic drugs*
atypical benign partial epilepsy 11
autosomal dominant nocturnal frontal lobe epilepsy (ADNFLE) **296**, 297–8
awake surgery 824–32
  functional mapping 826–7
  intraoperative electrocorticography 824–6
  technical aspects 827–30
    identification of eloquent cortex 828–30
    intraoperative electrocorticography 828
AWD131-138 568, **570**

B
Baltic myoclonic epilepsy *see* Unverricht-Lundborg disease
Bannayan-Riley-Ruvalcaba syndrome, risk of epilepsy 55
barbexaclone 472
barbiturates 461–74, **461**
  action at GABA receptors 101
  as cause of seizures 53
  cytochrome P450 induction **122**
  early use of **xxx**
  in intravenous anaesthesia in surgery 862–3
  structure *xxi*
  see also barbexaclone; metharbital; methylphenobarbitone; phenobarbitone; primidone; pentobarbital; thiopentone
Batten's disease 304
Beck Depression Inventory (BID), use in psychiatric assessment in epilepsy 717
Beckwith-Wiedemann syndrome, risk of epilepsy 55
behavioural disorder, influencing selection for epilepsy surgery 585
benign epilepsy of childhood with centrotemporal spikes (rolandic epilepsy; benign partial epilepsy of childhood with centrotemporal spikes)
  genetic risk and genetic counselling 300
  prognosis 33

symptomatology and EEG 11, 195, 300
treatment 195–6
  see also individual antiepileptic drugs
benign familial adult myoclonic epilepsy **296**, 298
benign familial infantile seizures **296**, 297
benign familial neonatal seizures 296–7, **296**
benign myoclonic epilepsy of infancy 13
benign neonatal convulsions 12
benign neonatal familial convulsions 12
benign partial epilepsy
  of childhood 11
  of infancy 11–12
  treatment *see individual antiepileptic drugs*
benign rolandic epilepsy *see* benign epilepsy of childhood with centrotemporal spikes
benzchlorpropamide
  early use of xxviii, *xxix*, xxx
  introduction of xvii
benzedrine xxv
benzodiazepine receptors, in PET scanning for presurgical evaluation 657–8
benzodiazepines 374–90
  action at GABA receptors 100–1
  action on sodium channels **97**
  as cause of seizures 53
  efficacy spectrum **142**
  in intravenous anaesthesia in epilepsy surgery 863–4
  mechanism of action 374–5
  molecular pharmacology of GABA receptors 375–8, **376**, *377*
  and oral contraception 279
  partial and inverse agonists 377–8
  seizure clusters 374
  short-acting 378–82
  status epilepticus 233, 374
    non-convulsive 235
  therapeutic range **156**
  tolerance and GABA receptor plasticity 378
  see also individual drugs
beta-blockers, as cause of seizures 53
bicuculline test, as experimental model of epilepsy 109, 501
  see also individual antiepileptic drugs
biofeedback, in treatment of epilepsy 270–1
birth control, effects of antiepileptic drugs 279
  see also individual antiepileptic drugs
bitemporal epilepsy, intracranial monitoring in 609–10
Blitz-Nick-Salaam Krampfe syndrome *see* West syndrome
blood level monitoring of antiepileptic drugs *see* therapeutic drug monitoring
Bloom's syndrome, risk of epilepsy 55
Borjeson-Forssman-Lehmann syndrome, risk of epilepsy 55
borotartrate xix
Bourneville's syndrome *see* tuberous sclerosis
Brachmann-de Lange syndrome, risk of epilepsy 55
brain slices as experimental model of epilepsy 112–13
brain malformations *see* cortical dysgenesis
brain plasticity, and hemispherectomy 795–6
brain tumour (cerebral tumours)
  as cause of epilepsy 62, 729–30
  mechanism of epileptogenesis 728–9, **729**
  paediatric surgery for 781
  pathology 729–31, **729**
    dysembryoplastic neuroepithelial tumours (DNETs) 730
    gangliogliomas 730
    hamartomas 730

meningiomas 730–1
tuberous sclerosis 730
presurgical evaluation 731–5
age at onset of seizures 731
clinical seizure characteristics 731
duration of seizure disorder 731
functional mapping 733
history and examination 731
intensive video scalp EEG monitoring 732
invasive cortical mapping 735
invasive monitoring 733
lesion detection 732
neuropsychological assessment 733
non-invasive mapping 733–5
MRI 732–3, **732**, 733–5
magnetoencephalography 735
positron emission tomography 734–5
SISCOM 734
SPECT 733–4
scalp EEG recording 731–2
surgery 728–41, 781
outcome 736–8
treatment 736
breastfeeding
and antiepileptic drugs 284–5, **285**
see also individual antiepileptic drugs
brilliant vital red **xix**
bromide 562–4
biotransformation 563
chemistry 562
clinical efficacy 563–4, *563*
clinical therapeutics 564
cost of treatment **xxxi**
drug interactions 563
early use of **xix, xxv, xxx**
mechanisms of action 562
pharmacokinetics 562–3
side effects 564
bruxism, in differential diagnosis of epilepsy 70
bupropion, as cause of seizures 53
busulphan, as cause of seizures 53

C
calcium ion channels
as antiepileptic drug target 98–100, **98**, **99**
and epileptogenesis 77–8, **77**
capillary malformations
as cause of epilepsy 747
treatment of 747
carabersat (SB-204269) 568–9, **570**
carbamazepine 168, **170**, 345–57, **345**
action on calcium channels **98**
action on monoaminergic
neurotransmission 107
action on sodium channels **97**
active metabolites **345**, 348
advantages **345**
benign epilepsy of childhood **191**
bioavailability **345**, 346–7
in breast milk **285**, 347
as cause of seizures 53
clinical efficacy **142**, 350–1, 484, 485
combination therapy 351
febrile seizures 351
idiopathic generalized epilepsies 350
localization-related epilepsies and partial
seizures 351
primary generalized tonic clonic
seizures 350
symptomatic generalized epilepsies and
secondarily generalized seizures 350–1
clinical therapeutics 356
cost of treatment **147**
cryptogenic/symptomatic partial epilepsy **191**

cytochrome P450 induction **122**
disadvantages **345**
dosage **345**, 356
dosage interval **345**, 356
drug interactions 129–30, 131–2, **345**, 348–9,
348, 349, 350, 454, 530
effect on drug-metabolizing enzymes **128**,
129–30
efficacy spectrum **142**, 350–1
elimination 131–2, **131**
half-life **152, 345**, 348
frequency of administration **148**, 356
generalized seizures **170**
indications **345**, 350–1, 356
infants and children 348
initial target dose **148, 345**, 356
late onset childhood idiopathic occipital
seizures **191**
learning-disabled patients 217
maintenance dose **148, 345**, 356
infants and children **153, 345**, 356
mechanism of action **345, 346**
metabolism **345**, *453*
and oral contraception **279**
overdose and intoxication 355
partial onset seizures **170**
pharmacoeconomic aspects 355
pharmacokinetics 346–50
absorption and distribution 346–7
determinants of plasma
concentrations 347–8
dosage forms 347
dosage regimens 347
food 347
in hepatic and renal disease 349–50
metabolism and elimination 348
moistured tablets 347
rectal administration 347
plasma clearance **345**, 348
in pregnancy 348
preparations **345**
protective index **404**
protein binding **131, 345**, 346
quality of life 355–6
in saliva and tears 347
side effects 217, 327, **345**, 351–5, *352*
dermatological and hypersensitivity
reactions 353
endocrinological effects 353–4
haematotoxicity 353
hepatotoxicity 353
miscellaneous side effects 354–5
neurotoxicity 352–3
teratogenicity 354
therapeutic range **156, 345**, 356
time to peak blood levels **345**, 346
titration rate **148**
volume of distribution **345**, 346
carbon monoxide, as cause of seizures 54
cardiac disease
as cause of seizures 250
treatment of seizures in 250
cardiofaciocutaneous syndrome, risk of
epilepsy 55
carnitine deficiency, contraindication to
ketogenic diet 264
causes of epilepsy 26–7, **26**, 50–63
cavernous haemangioma (cavernoma)
clinical features 734–6, *745*
MRI abnormalities 641, 646
stereotactic radiosurgery 843
surgical treatment of 745–6, *746*
central resection, complications resulting
from 854

cerebral abscess see pyogenic cerebral abscess
cerebral blood flow, in PET and SPECT
scanning 656
cerebral ischaemia, in differential diagnosis of
epilepsy 71
cerebral oedema, and invasive EEG 615
cerebral palsy, as a cause of epilepsy 60
cerebral tuberculoma
as cause of epilepsy 755–57
diagnosis 756–7
management 757
treatment of 755–7
cerebral tumours see brain tumour
cerebrovascular disease, as a cause of
epilepsy 31–2, 61
ceroid lipofuscinosis, risk of epilepsy 56
CGX-1007 (conantokin-G) 569–70, **570**
childhood epilepsy syndromes
acquired epileptic aphasia (Landau-Kleffner
syndrome) 16
benign neonatal convulsions 12–13
benign neonatal familial convulsions 12
benign partial epilepsy of childhood 11,
195–7
benign partial epilepsy in infancy 11–12
childhood absence epilepsy (pyknolepsy) 9,
13, 196–7, 521
childhood epilepsy with centrotemporal
spikes 9, 11
childhood epilepsy with occipital
paroxysms 12
chronic epilepsia partialis continua of
childhood 9, 12
early infantile epileptic encephalopathy with
suppression-burst 15
early myoclonic encephalopathy 15
epilepsy with continuous spike-waves during
slow-wave sleep 15, 16
epilepsy with myoclonic absences 15
epilepsy with myoclonic astatic seizures 14
febrile convulsions 16, 191–3
idiopathic epilepses 195–6
juvenile myoclonic epilepsy 13, 33, 197
Lennox-Gastaut syndrome see Lennox-
Gastaut syndrome
management of 190–200, **191**
MRI in 647–8
neonatal seizures 15–16
psychosocial effects 779
quality of life in 780
severe myoclonic epilepsy in infancy 15
surgery 779–89
brain tumours 781
developmental and intellectual
disabilities 786–7, **786, 787**
hypothalamic hamartoma and gelastic
epilepsy 782–3
infantile spasms 782
infants with partial epilepsy 786
Landau-Kleffner syndrome 782
malformations of cortical
development 780–1, **781**
preoperative evaluation 784, 78305
Rasmussen's encephalitis 783
rationale for 779–80, **780**
Sturge-Weber syndrome 781–2
tuberous sclerosis 781
symptomatic and cryptogenic partial 197–8
West syndrome see West syndrome
see also infantile epilepsy; juvenile epilepsies;
and individual antiepileptic drugs
children
epilepsy in see childhood epilepsy syndromes
general characteristics of epilepsy in 190–1

children (cont'd)
management of epilepsy in 190–200, **191**
benign partial epilepsy with centrotemporal spikes (BECTs) 195
childhood absence epilepsy 196–7
drugs of choice for paediatric syndromes 190–1, **191**
early onset benign childhood occipital epilepsy (EBOS) 196
febrile seizures 9, 16, 191–3, 301
juvenile myoclonic epilepsy 197
late onset benign idiopathic occipital epilepsy (LOE) 196
Lennox-Gastaut syndrome *see* Lennox-Gastaut syndrome
long term management and prophylaxis 192–3
idiopathic partial epilepsies of childhood 195–7
symptomatic and cryptogenic patial epilepsy 197–9
see also drug interactions; paediatric epilepsy surgery; individual drugs; individual surgical procedures; individual epilepsy syndromes; and treatment in specific situations
chiropractic therapy, in treatment of epilepsy 274–5
chlorambucil, as cause of seizures 53
chlormethiazole, status epilepticus 233
chlorpromazine, seizure-inducing properties **223**
choice of AED *see* antiepileptic drugs; medical treatment
Christian's syndrome, risk of epilepsy 55
chromosomal inheritance 291–2, **293**
chronic epilepsia partialis continua of childhood 9, 12
chronic seizures, animal models of 109–10
kindling 109–10
post-status epilepticus 110
cimetidine, as cause of seizures 54
cingulate seizures, symptomatology 10
ciprofloxacin, cytochrome P450 inhibition **122**
circuits in epileptogenesis 78–82
intrinsically bursting-operated 79
seizure-dependent rearrangements 79–81, *80*
thalamocortical circuitry *81*
classification of epileptic syndromes 8–11, **9**, **10**
frontal lobe epilepsies 10–11, **10**
occipital lobe epilepsies 11
parietal lobe epilepsies 11
temporal lobe epilepsies 10
classification of seizure types 3–8, **4–5**, **7**
absence seizures 6–7
atonic seizures 8
atypical absence seizures 7
clonic seizures 7
complex partial seizures 6
generalized seizures 6
myoclonic seizures 7
partial seizures 3
psychic symptoms 6
simple partial seizures 3, 5–6
tonic seizures 7
tonic-clonic seizures 7–8
unclassified seizures 8
clobazam 170, 358–64, **358**
active metabolites 358, 360
advantages **358**
bioavailability **358**, 359
biotransformation 360
in breast milk 285
clinical efficacy 485

cost of treatment **147**
disadvantages 358
dosage **358**, 362
dosage interval **358**, 362
dose and clinical therapeutics 362
drug interactions **358**, 360, 454
efficacy 361–2, **361**
elimination half-life **152**, **358**, 359
frequency of administration 148, 362
generalized seizures **170**
indications 358, 361–62
initial target dose **148**
Lennox-Gastaut syndrome **191**, 362
maintenance dose **148**
infants and children **153**
mechanism of action 358, 359
metabolism 358, 360
mode of action 359
partial onset seizures **170**
pharmacokinetics 359–60
preparations **358**
protein binding **358**, 362
side effects **358**, 360–1
status epilepticus, non-convulsive 235, 362
startle seizures 362
time to peak blood levels **358**
titration rate **148**
toxicity 360–1, **360**
clonazepam 170, 365–73, **365**
absence seizures 368
advantages 365
bioavailability 365, 366
in breast milk 285
chemistry and metabolism 366
disadvantages 365
dosage 365
dosage interval 365
drug interactions 365, 367–8
elimination half-life **152**, 365, 367
generalized seizures **170**
indications 365, 368–70
infantile spasms 369
Landau-Kleffner syndrome 369
Lennox-Gastaut syndrome 369
maintenance dose, infants and children **153**
mechanism of action 365, 367
metabolism 365, 366
myoclonic seizures 369
neonatal seizures 369–70
partial onset seizures **170**, 369
pharmacodynamics 367–8
pharmacokinetics 366–7
absorption, distribution and excretion 366–7
plasma concentration, half-life and seizure control 367
plasma clearance 365, 367
in pregnancy 370
preparations 365
protein binding 365, 366
reflex epilepsy 370
side effects 365, 370
status epilepticus 233, 370
therapeutic range 365, 367
time to peak blood levels 365, 366
tolerance 368
tonic-clonic seizures 368–9
volume of distribution 365, 366
withdrawal effects 368
clonic seizures
classification and symptomatology **5**, **7**
treatment *see individual antiepileptic drugs*
clorazepate 382–3
clinical applications 383

drug interactions 383
pharmacokinetics 383
side effects 383
structure *377*
clozapine, as cause of seizures 53, **223**
CNS infections
as a cause of epilepsy 32, 60
surgical treatment of 747–58
cocaine, as cause of seizures 53, 54
Cockayne's syndrome, risk of epilepsy 55
Coffin-Lowry syndrome, risk of epilepsy 55
Cohen's syndrome, risk of epilepsy 55
comorbidities
epidemiology of 27–8, *27*
learning disabilities 27
motor disabilities 27–8
other associated disabilities 28
as predictors of remission 31
complementary and alternative therapy 269–76
acupuncture 273–4
chiropractic treatment 274–5
dietary measures
food sensitivity 272
naturopathy 273
nutritional supplements 272–3
exercise 271–2
herbal medicine 272
homoeopathy 273
music 272
psychological treatments
EEG biofeedback 270–1
hypnosis 269–70
meditation and yoga 270
psychiatric interventions 270
relaxation 270
transcranial magnetic stimulation 274
complex epilepsies, genetic influences in 298–300, **299**
complex inheritance 295
complex partial seizures *see* partial seizures and epilepsies
complex partial status epilepticus 228, 236
see also status epilepticus, emergency treatment of
compliance
blood level monitoring 158
in the elderly patient 210
drug treatment in established epilepsy 329, 330
learning-disabled patients 216–17, **217**
initiation of treatment 168
impact in the investigation of epilepsy 581
pyogenic cerebral abscess *750*
computerized tomography
in presurgical assessment 581, **581**, 593
stereotactic surgery 834–6, 838–9
connective tissue diseases, treatment of seizures in 249–50
contraception, oral
effect of antiepileptic drugs 279, **279**
see also pharmacokinetic drug interactions; and individual antiepileptic drugs
convulsive status epilepticus 230–5
acidosis 231
aetiology 231
diagnosis 230
drug treatment 232–5, **233**, 237–40
emergency investigations 231
intensive care 232
medical complications 231
medical management 230–2
intravenous glucose and thiamine 231
intravenous lines 231

oxygen and cardiorespiratory
  resuscitation 231
pressor therapy 232
monitoring 231, 232
physiological changes 231–2
refractory 234–5, **234**
corpus callosum section 798–811
anatomy 798
anterior callosotomy 807
complete callosotomy 808
complications 856
EEG in presurgical evaluation 605–6, *804*
follow-up 806–8
neurophysiology 798–800, *799*
neuropsychiatric aspects 808
outcome **801, 802, 803**
posterior callosotomy 807–8
presurgical evaluation 800–5, **801–3**, *804*
surgery 805–6, *806*
vagus nerve stimulation 806, *807*
variations on technique 805
cortical dysgenesis
EEG in 605
MRI in 591, **593**, *593*, 643, 644–6, *644*
paediatric epilepsy surgery 780–1, *781*
surgery of 763–4, 780–1
  dysembryoplastic neuroepithelia tumours
    (DNETs) 767–68
  focal cortical dysplasia 765–6
  lissencephaly 767
  outcome of 763–5, **764, 765**
  periventricular heterotopia 766
  polymicrogyria and schizencephaly 767
  subcortical heterotopia 766–7
cortical dysplasia *see* cortical dysgenesis
cortical stimulation for presurgical
    assessment 619–20
advantages and disadvantages 619–20
technical aspects 619
use of 619
corticosteroids, use in infantile epilepsy 183–4
cost of antiepileptic drugs **xxxi**, **147**, 328
counselling **171**
childhood epilepsy 192
genetic *see* genetic counselling
preconception 285–6
presurgical 595
cri-du-chat syndrome, risk of epilepsy 55
Crouzon's syndrome, risk of epilepsy 55
cryptogenic epilepsies
generalized 14–15
  epilepsy with myoclonic absences 15
  epilepsy with myoclonic astatic seizures 14
  Lennox-Gastaut syndrome 14
  West syndrome 14
incidence and prevalence 50–1
localisational related 10
cumulative incidence of epilepsy 25
CT *see* computerized tomography
cyclosporin, as cause of seizures 53
cyprofloxacine, as cause of seizures 53
Cysticercus cellulosae see
    neurocysticercosis 753
cytochrome P450 121–3, **122**

D
dBA/2J mouse, as experimental model of
    epilepsy 112
dementia, as a cause of epilepsy 60
demyelinating disorders, as a cause of
    epilepsy 61
dentatorubropallidoluysian atrophy, risk of
    epilepsy 56
depression in epilepsy 258–9, **258**

depth electrodes in presurgical assessment of
    epilepsy 610–12
advantages
  access 611
  accuracy of placement 612
  seizure cure 612
complications of 612, 850–1
disadvantages
  damage to brain parenchyma 612
  epileptogenesis 612
  haemorrhage 612
  infection 612
  restricted sampling 612
extratemporal epilepsy 611
medial temporal lobe epilepsy *611*
neocortical temporal lobe epilepsy 611
technical aspects 610
desflurane, as anaesthesia for epilepsy
    surgery 862
Design Fluence test 701–2, *702, 703*
desipramine, as cause of seizures 53
developed countries
incidence of epilepsy 25
prevalence of epilepsy 21–2, **22**
developing countries
incidence of epilepsy 25, **26**
mortality of epilepsy 36–7
prevalence of epilepsy 22, **23**
developmental toxicity of antiepileptic
    drugs 281–4, 327
growth retardation 282–3
major congenital malformations 281–2, **281,
    282**
mechanisms of 283–4
minor anomalies and fetal AED
    syndromes 282
psychomotor development 283
sensitive periods **284**
dexedrine
cost of treatment **xxxi**
early use of **xxv**
diagnosis of epilepsy
implications for starting treatment 161–2
elderly onset seizures 202–4, **203**
newly diagnosed epilepsy, treatment
    of 161–73
see also differential diagnosis of epilepsy
dialysis encephalopathy, and epilepsy 247
Diamox *see* acetazolamide
diazepam 378–80
acute seizure treatment 222, *222*
clinical applications
  chronic epilepsies 380
  febrile convulsions 379–80
  serial seizures 380
  status epilepticus 237–38, 379–80
drug interactions 379
early onset benign occipital seizures **191**
febrile seizures **191**, 191–2, 380
pharmacokinetics 378–9, *379*
rectal 379–80
side effects **360**, 379
status epilepticus 237–8, 379–80
  convulsive **233**
structure 377
dietary measures in treatment of epilepsy
    272–3
see also ketogenic diet
differential diagnosis of epilepsy 64–73, **162**
cerebral ischaemia 71
endocrine/metabolic abnormalities 71
general approach to 64–6
migraine 69–70
movement disorders 71

non-epileptic seizures 68–9
panic disorders 69
sleep disorders 70
syncope 67–8
transient global amnesia 71–2
vertigo 70–1
Dilantin *see* phenytoin
diphenylhydantoin *see* phenytoin
dipole source modelling 665–79
clinical relevance 678
forward and inverse problems 666
ictal discharges 678, 679
instantaneous dipoles 667
interictal spikes 668–78
  dipole sources and intracranial
    recordings 672, 674–8, *674–7*
  dipole sources and MRI lesions 671–2,
    673
  dipole sources and PET metabolic
    abnormalities 672
  frontal lobe epilepsy 670–1
  temporal lobe epilepsy 668, 670, *670*
modelling of conductive volume 665–6
modelling of sources 665
multiple spatiotemporal dipoles 667
preprocessing of data
  average-spike topography 666–7, *666*
  spike averaging 666
principle 665
projection of sources onto 3D MRI 667
quality of solution and accuracy of
    localization 667–8, *668*
disulfiram, cytochrome P450 inhibition **122**
DNET *see* dysembryoplastic neuroepithelial
    tumour
Doose's syndrome 14
dopamine, as target for antiepileptic drug
    action 106
dorsolateral frontal seizures,
    symptomatology 11
doublecortin gene 766
Down syndrome, risk of epilepsy 55, **56**
doxepin, as cause of seizures 53
Dravet's syndrome 15
management 185–6
droperidol, in anaesthesia for epilepsy
    surgery 864–5
drug discovery *see* antiepileptic drug discovery
drug interactions 120–36, 328
pharmacodynamic 134
pharmacokinetic 120–33
  antiepileptic drugs 128–33
  mechanisms of 120–8
see also pharmacokinetic drug interactions;
    and individual drugs
drug resistance in epilepsy 84–8
animal models 86
causes of 84
drug resistance proteins
  overexpression of 8586–7
  physiological expression of 85–6
drug-induced seizures 53–4, **53**
dual pathology 610, 768–71
Dubowitz's syndrome, risk of epilepsy 55
dysembryoplastic neuroepithelial tumour
    (DNET, DNT)
MRI abnormalities **641**, 646
surgery 730, 767–8

E
EAA receptors, in epileptogenesis 78
early infantile epileptic encephalopathy with
    suppression-burst 15
early myoclonic encephalopathy 15

Echinococcus see hydatid disease
EEG *see* electroencephalography
EEG biofeedback 270–1
EEG correlated fMRI *see* functional magnetic
    resonance imaging
elderly onset seizures 201–14
  diagnosis of 202–4, **203**
  epidemiology 201
  future research **212**
  impact of seizures 201–2
  investigations **204**
  management 204–10
    choice of drug 205–8, **209**
    compliance 210, **211**
    dosage of drug 209–10
    prescribing strategies 208–10, **209**
    start of treatment 205
    therapeutic drug monitoring 210
  patient services 211–12
  prognosis 210–11
    mortality 211
    seizure control 210–11
    withdrawal of drugs 211
  special features of 202, **202**
  underlying cause 203–4
  see also individual antiepileptic drugs
electrical status epilepticus during slow wave
    sleep *228*
electroclinical syndrome 175
electrocorticography 620–1
  awake surgery 824–6
  brain tumours 735
  frontal lobe epilepsy 620–1
  intraoperative 828
  structural lesions 621
  technical aspects 620
  temporal lobe epilepsy 620
  use of 620
electroencephalography
  intracranial 594–5, 837–40
    see also intracranial monitoring
  prediction of relapse after drug
    withdrawal 176
  relationship to prognosis 32–3
  scalp *see* scalp EEG
emergency treatment 227–43
  epilepsia partialis continua 237
  myoclonic status epilepticus in coma 237
  serial seizures 230
  status epilepticus *see* status epilepticus
encephalocraniocutaneous lipomatosis, risk of
    epilepsy 55
encephalopathy, as side effect of
    valproate 533–4
endocrine abnormalities, in differential diagnosis
    of epilepsy 71
enflurane
  as anaesthesia for epilepsy surgery 861
  as cause of seizures 53
enzyme induction, as a cause of drug
    interaction **122**, 124–5
enzyme inhibition, as a cause of drug
    interaction **122**, 123–4
ephedrine **xix**
epidemiology of epilepsy 21–9
  incidence 24–6
    age specific 25
    cumulative incidence 25
    epileptic syndromes 25–6
    ethnicity and socioeconomic factors 25
    gender 25
    less developed countries 25, **26**
    more developed countries 25
    seizure type 25

  of sudden death 45–6
  prevalence 21–4
    ethnicity 23
    gender 22
    less developed countries 22, **23**
    more developed countries 21–2, **22**
    prevalence of epileptic syndormes 24
    seizure types 23–4
    socioeconomic factors 23
  time trends 28–9
epidural electrodes *617*
  advantages of 617
  complications 850
  disadvantages of 617
  technical aspects 617
Epilepsia
  early days xvii–xviii
  postwar decade xxiii–xxv
epilepsia partialis continua, emergency
    treatment of *228*, *237*
epilepsy with continuous spike-waves during
    slow-wave sleep 15–16, *228*
epilepsy (EL) mouse, as experimental model of
    epilepsy 112
epilepsy with myoclonic absences 15
epilepsy surgery
  anaesthesia 861–72
    adjuvant agents 864–5
    general anaesthesia 865–6
    inhalation anaesthetics 861–2
    intravenous anaesthetics 862–4
    local anaesthesia and sedation 866–8
    postoperative care 868
    preoperative assessment 965
  awake surgery 824–32
    functional mapping 826–7
    intraoperative electrocorticography 824–6
    technical aspects 827–30
  complications 849–60
    invasive procedures for presurgical
      assessment 849–51
      electrode placement 849
      epidural peg electrodes 849
      foramen ovale electrodes 850
      intracranial depth electrodes 850–1
      ISA test 849
      sphenoidal electrodes 850
      subdural electrodes 850
    therapeutic procedures 851–7
      corpus callosum section (callosal
        section) 856
      central and parietal resections 854
      frontal lobe resection 851
      functional surgery 855–6
      hemispherectomy 855
      intracranial resective surgery 851
      major resections 854–5
      multiple subpial transection 856
      occipital resections 854
      reoperation 855
      risk management 857
      sterotactic lesions 856
      stimulation 856–7
      temporal lobe resections 852–4, **853**
  corpus callosum section 798–811
    anatomy 798
    anterior callosotomy 807
    complete callosotomy 808
    complications 856
    follow-up 806–8
    neurophysiology 798–800, *799*
    neuropsychiatric aspects 808
    posterior callosotomy 807–8
    presurgical evaluation 800–5, **801–3**, *804*

    scalp EEG 605–6
    surgery 805–6, *806*
    vagus nerve stimulation 806
    variations on technique 805
  cortical dysgenesis 763–74
    dysembryoplastic neuroeipthelia
      tumours 767–8
    focal cortical dysplasia 765–6
    lissencephaly 767
    outcome of 763–5, **764**, **765**
    periventricular heterotopia 766
    polymicrogyria and schizencephaly 767
    scalp EEG 605
    subcortical heterotopia 766–7
  early procedures **582**
  epilepsy surgery centres 596, *597*
  future approaches 884–92
    focal drug delivery 884–6, *885*, *886*
    neuronal grafting 886–90, *887*
  hemispherectomy 790–7
    anatomical 793
    and brain plasticity 795–6
    complications 855
    functional 793
    hemicorticectomy 793
    hemidecortication 793
    hemispherotomy 793
    indications for 790–3, **791**, *792*
    modified 793
    outcome 795
    peri-insular hemispherectomy 793–4, *794*
    surgical morbidity 794–5
  hippocampal sclerosis 723–7
    methods 723–6, **724**, *725*
    outcome 726
  historical background 579–82, **582**
  infective lesions 747–58
    cerebral tuberculoma 755–7
    hydatid disease 757–8
    neurocysticercosis 753–5
    pyogenic cerebral abscess 747–53
  learning-disabled patients 221–2
    indications for 813–14, *815–18*
    multiple subpial transection 812–23
      complications 856
    physiology 812–13
    results 820–1, *821*
    surgical technique 814–20, *819*
  need for 582–3, **583**
  paediatric 779–89
    brain tumours 781
    developmental and intellectual
      disabilities 786–7, **786**, **787**
    early infantile epileptic encephalopathy 783
    hypothalamic hamartoma and gelastic
      epilepsy 782–3
    infantile spasms 782
    infants with partial epilepsy 786
    Landau-Kleffner syndrome 782
    malformations of cortical
      development 780–1, **781**
    preoperative evaluation 783–5, **784**
    Rasmussen's encephalitis 783
    rationale for 779–80, **780**
    Sturge-Weber syndrome 781–2
    tuberous sclerosis 781
  post-traumatic epilepsy 775–8
  postoperative care 596–8, **597**
  presurgical evaluation *see* presurgical
    evaluation
  remission after 178
  risk of 584
  stereotactic surgery 833–48
    ablation and stimulation for epilepsy 841–2

as aid to conventional surgery 837–41, *838,*
    839
  complications 849–51, 855–7
  frame-based *834*
  frameless 834–7, *835, 836*
  multimodality imaging 837
  radiosurgery 842–4
surgical planning meeting 595–6, *596*
temporal lobe epilepsy 586–8
timing of 585
types of 583, *584*
vascular lesions 742–7
epileptic syndromes
  classification of 8–11, **9, 10**
  incidence of 25–6
  prevalence of 24
  see also childhood epilepsy syndromes;
        individual drugs; and individual
        syndromes
epileptogenesis
  acetylcholine receptors in 78
  and brain tumours 728–9, **729**
  dual pathology 610, 768–71
  EAA receptors in 78
  electrode-induced 612
  GABA receptors in 78
  mechanism of 74–83
    circuit involvement 78–82
      intrinsically bursting-operated
          circuits 79
      seizure-dependent circuit
          rearrangements 79–81, *80*
      thalamocortical circuitry *81*
    ligand-gated channels 78
    membrane ion channels 74–8
      calcium channels 77–8, *77*
      potassium channels 76–7
      sodium channels 75–6, *75, 76*
      voltage gated channels 75–8, *75*
  prevention of 140–1
  thalamocortical circuitry *81*
epileptogenic zone, definition 585–6
epoxide hydrolases, in drug interactions 123
ergotamine xix
erythromycin, cytochrome P450 inhibition **122**
established epilepsy, approach to drug
        treatment 329–31
ethnicity
  incidence of epilepsy 25
  prevalence of epilepsy 23
ethosuximide 391–402, **391**
  6 Hz seizure test 92
  absorption
    in animals 393
    in humans 393–4
  action on calcium channels 98
  advantages 391
  adverse reactions 391, 396–8
  anticonvulsant activity 92
  bioavailability 391, 393
  biotransformations *392*
  in breast milk 285
  as cause of seizures 53
  childhood absence epilepsy 191
  clinical efficacy 395–6
  clinical therapeutics 398–9
  cost of treatment xxxi, **147**
  disadvantages 391
  distribution
    in animals 393
    in humans 394
  dosage 391, 398–9
  dosage interval 391, 398–9
  dose and titration rate 398–9

drug interactions 132, **391**, 394–5, 530
effect on drug-metabolizing enzymes **128**
efficacy
  absence seizures 395
  absence status epilepticus 395–6
  experimental epilepsy 393
  human epilepsy 395–6
efficacy spectrum **142**, 395–6
elimination 131, 132
  in animals 393
  half-life **152, 391**, 394
  in humans 394
experimental studies 393
frequency of administration 148
generalized seizures 170
indications 391, 395–6
initial target dose 148
juvenile absence epilepsy 191, 396
laboratory monitoring 399
maintenance dose 148
  infants and children 153
mechanism of action 391, 392
metabolism
  in animals 393
  in humans 391, 393
and oral contraception 279
overdose 398
pharmacokinetics 393–5
  in liver and renal disease 395
  racemic mixtures 393
plasma clearance 391, 394
preparations 391
protective index 404
protein binding 131, 391
side effects 396–8, **396**
  dermatological 397
  gastrointestinal 396
  haematological 397, 398
  neurological 396–7
  psychiatric 397
structure 392
therapeutic range 156, **391**, 399
time to peak blood levels **391**, 393–4
titration rate 148
volume of distribution 391
ethotoin 564
etomidate
  as cause of seizures 53
  in intravenous anaesthesia in epilepsy
      surgery 863
exercise, in treatment of epilepsy 271–2
extratemporal epilepsy
  ictal EEG 632
  intracranial monitoring
    depth electrodes 611
    subdural grid electrodes 616
    subdural strip electrodes 613
  see also frontal lobe epilepsy; occipital lobe
      epilepsy; parietal lobe epilepsy; and
      individual conditions

F

familial temporal lobe epilepsy 300
fasoracetam *491*
febrile seizures 9, 16
  genetic counselling 300–1
  infants 187
  management 191–3, 379–80, 382
  status epilepticus, *228*
  see also hippocampal sclerosis; temporal lobe
      epilepsy
felbamate 403–9, **403**
  absorption and distribution 404
  advantages **403**

adverse reactions 403, 405–6
bioavailability **403**
biotransformation and excretion 404
clinical efficacy 406–7
  partial seizures 406–7
cost of treatment **147**
cytochrome P450 induction 122
cytochrome P450 inhibition 122
disadvantages **403**
dosage **403**, 407–8
dosage interval 403
drug interactions 129, 130, 132, **403**, 405,
    407, 454, 530
effect on drug-metabolizing enzymes 128,
    129, 130
efficacy spectrum **142**
elimination 131, 132, 405
  half-life **152, 403,** 404
excretion 403, 404
frequency of administration 148, **403**
indications **403**, 408
initial target dose 148, **403**, 407–8
laboratory testing 407
learning-disabled patients 218–19, **218, 219**
maintenance dose 148, **403**, 407–8
  infants and children 153
measurement 404–5
mechanism of action 403, 404
metabolism 403, 404
and oral contraception 279
plasma clearance 403, 405
preparations 403
protective index 404
protein binding 131, **403**, 404
starting therapy 407–8
therapeutic range 156, **403**, 405
time to peak blood levels **403**, 404
titration rate 148
toxicity 405–6, **406**
volume of distribution 403
fertility, in epilepsy 277–9
  choice of AEDs 279
  polycystic ovary syndrome 278–9
  reproductive dysfunction 277–8
fetal AED syndromes 282
fetus, effects of maternal seizures on 279–80
fluconazole, cytochrome P450 inhibition **122**
flumazenil, structure *377*
fluoxetine
  as cause of seizures 53
  cytochrome P450 inhibition **122**
fluvoxamine, cytochrome P450 inhibition **122**
fMRI *see* Functional magnetic resonance imaging
focal cortical dysplasia
  MRI abnormalities 641, *643, 645–6*
  surgery 765–6
  see also cortical dysgenesis
focal drug delivery by surgical means 884–6
  propagation pathways 885–6, *886*
  seizure focus 884–5, *884*
  seizure-stimulated drug release 886
  trigger site 885, *886*
focal structural lesions
  scalp EEG 604–5
  see also individual conditions
folate deficiency induced by antiepileptic
      drugs 327
  see also individual antiepileptic drugs
folate supplements during pregnancy in
      epilepsy 285
food sensitivity 272
foramen ovale electrodes 618–19
  advantages 618
  complications 850

foramen ovale electrodes (*cont'd*)
 disadvantages 618–19
 technical aspects *618*
 use of 618
foscarnet, as cause of seizures 53
fosphenytoin 233–4, 238, 410–17, **410**
 action on calcium channels 98
 active metabolites **410**
 advantages **410**
 bioavailability *411*
 chemical stability 412
 in children 414
 clinical efficacy in acute seizures and status
   epilepticus 233–4, **233**, 238, 414–15
 clinical therapeutics 415–16
 clinical trials in acute seizures and status
   epilepticus
    intramuscular 412–14, *413*
    intravenous 412
 cost considerations 415
 disadvantages **410**
 distribution 411–12
 dosage **410**, 415
 elimination half-life **410**
 indications **410**, 414–15
 mechanism of action **410**
 medication errors 415
 metabolism **410**
 physical and chemical properties 410–11
 preparations **410**
 protein binding 411
 side effects **410**
 status epilepticus 233–4, **233**, 238, 412–15
 therapeutic range **410**
 see also phenytoin
fragile X syndrome, risk of epilepsy 55, 224
frontal lobe epilepsy
 autosomal dominant frontal lobe epilepsy
   (ADNFLE) **296**, 297–8
 classification 10–11, *10*
 complications of surgery in 851
 dipole source modelling 670–1
 intracranial monitoring 620–1
    cortical stimulation 619
    corticography 620–1
    depth electrodes 611
    interictal EEG 622–3
    ictal EEG 632
    subdural grid electrodes 613
    subdural strip electrodes 613
 PET scanning 658
 neuropsychological assessment 700–4
 scalp EEG 604–5
 SPECT scanning 660
 symptomatology 10–11, *10*
 see also autosomal dominant frontal lobe
   epilepsy; multiple subpial transection;
   corpus callosum section; awake
   surgery; stereotactic surgery; individual
   conditions, investigatory methods and
   surgical procedures
frontal lobe function 700–4
 Design Fluency test 701–2, *702*, *703*
 Modified Card Sorting test 701
 motor tasks 704
 Stroop test 702–3
 Tower of London test 703–4
 Wisconsin Card Sorting test 701
functional deficit zone, MRI 649
functional magnetic resonance imaging 595,
   690–2
 in children 784
 EEG-correlated 684–90
    ictal 686

interictal 686–7, **688**, *689*
 interleaved 685, *686*
 limitations of 687–90, *690*
 methodology 684–6, *684*, *685*, *686*
language lateralization 691
memory 691–2
motor function 690–1
simultaneous 685–6
see also magnetic resonance imaging

G
GABA 100–4, *100*, *102*, *103*, *104*
 uptake and breakdown 101–3, *102*, *103*
GABA receptors
 antagonists, partial agonists and inverse
   agonists *377*
 and epilepsy 376
 and epileptogenesis 78
 GABA$_A$ receptors 100–1
 GABA$_B$ receptors 101
 molecular biology 375–8
 α subunits 376–7
 plasticity 378
 subunit composition 375–6, *376*
 as target for antiepileptic drug action 78,
   100–4, *100*, *102*, *103*, *104*
gabapentin 170, 418–24, **418**
 absorption 420
 action on calcium channels 98
 administration and dosage 423
 advantages **418**
 animal toxicology 420
 bioavailability **418**, 420
 in breast milk **285**
 as cause of seizures 53
 chemistry 419
 clinical efficacy
    childhood partial seizures 421–2
    long-term efficacy and safety studies 421
    monotherapy 421
    open-label studies 421
    randomized controlled trials 421
 cost of treatment **147**
 disadvantages **418**
 distribution 420
 dosage **418**, 423
 dosage interval **418**, 423
 drug interactions 132–3, **418**, 420, 530
 effect on drug-metabolizing enzymes **128**
 efficacy spectrum **142**
 elderly onset seizures 208
 elimination 131, 132–3, 420
    half-life **152**, **418**
 excretion **418**, 420
 frequency of administration **148**, 423
 improvement/success rates 325
 indications **418**, 421–2
 initial target dose **148**, 421–2, 423
 learning-disabled patients 218, 219
 maintenance dose **148**, 422–2, 423
    infants and children 153
 mechanism of action **418**
 mechanisms of action 419–20, **419**
 metabolism 420
 number-needed-to-treat *323*
 odds ratio *322*, *323*
 and oral contraception 279
 partial onset seizures 170
 pharmacokinetics 420–1
 plasma clearance **418**, 420
 preparations **418**
 protein binding 131, **418**, 420
 side effects **418**, 422, *422*
 teratogenicity 420–1

therapeutic range **156**, **418**, 420
time to peak blood levels **418**, 420
titration rate **148**
volume of distribution **418**, 420
gamma knife, stereotactic radiosurgery 842–4
ganaxolone 570
ganciclovir, as cause of seizures 53
ganglioglioma, as cause of epilepsy 730
 MRI abnormalities **641**, *646*
Gaucher's disease, as cause of epilepsy 56
gelastic epilepsy
 MRI abnormalities in hypothalamic
   hamartoma **641**, *647*
 surgery of 782–3
Gemonil *see* metharbital
gender
 incidence of epilepsy 25
 and mortality 35
 as predictor of remission 30–1
 prevalence of epilepsy 22
generalized epilepsies
 classification and symptomatology 12–16
 cryptogenic/symptomatic 14–15
    epilepsy with myoclonic absences 15
    epilepsy with myoclonic astatic seizures 14
    Lennox-Gastaut syndrome 14
    West syndrome 14
 idiopathic with age-related onset 12–13
    benign myoclonic epilepsy in infancy 13
    benign neonatal convulsions 12
    benign neonatal familial convulsions 12
    childhood absence epilepsy 13
    epilepsy with grand mal seizures on
      awakening 13
    juvenile myoclonic epilepsy 13
 relapse after drug withdrawal 175–7, *177*
 symptomatic with age-related onset 15
 undetermined type 15–16
generalized epilepsy with febrile seizures plus
   (GEFS+) 298, **296**
generalized seizures, classification 6
 see also absence seizures; atypical absence
   seizures; clonic seizures; generalized
   tonic clonic seizures; myoclonic
   seizures; tonic seizures
generalized tonic clonic seizures
 choice of drugs in treatment of 142–4, **142**
 classification and definition 6, 12–13
 drug treatment with
    acetazolamide 337, 338–9, 340
    allopurinol 561–62
    bromide 563–64
    carbamazepine 350–1
    clobazam 361–2
    clonazepam 368–9
    ethotoin 564
    lamotrigine 432, 433
    levetiracetam 447
    oxcarbazepine 454–6, **455**. **456**
    phenobarbitone 465
    phenytoin 484–5
    primidone 471
    rufinamide 504–5
    topiramate 519, 520–1
    valproate 532–3
    zonisamide 552–5, **552**, **553**, **554**
 see also partial seizures and epilepsies;
   individual epilepsy surgical procedures
genetic absence epilepsy rats from Strasbourg
   (GAERS)
 as experimental model of epilepsy 111–12
 as test for antiepileptic drug discovery 93
genetic counselling 290–306
 communication 291

febrile seizures 300–1
genetic syndromes including epilepsy 301–4, **301, 302**
  progressive myoclonus epilepsies 301–4, **301, 302**
heterogeneous disorder, epilepsy as 295–6
idiopathic epilepsies 296–300
  complex 298–300, **299**
  mendelian 296–8, **296**
  severe myoclonic epilepsy of infancy 300
individual syndromes
  autosomal dominant nocturnal frontal lobe epilepsy (ADNFLE) 297–8, **296**
  benign familial adult myoclonic epilepsy 298, **296**
  benign familial infantile seizures 297, **296**
  benign familial neonatal seizures 296–7, **296**
benign childhood epilepsy with centrotemporal spikes (Rolandic epilepsy) 300, **299**
familial temporal lobe epilepsy 300, **299**
febrile seizure 300–1
generalised epilepsy and febrile seizures plus (GEFS+) 298, **296**
idiopathic generalized epilepsies 299–300, **299**
idiopathic partial epilepsies 200, **299**
progressive myoclonus epilepsy 301–4, **302**
  Lafora's disease **302**
  MERRF 303, **302**
  neuronal ceroid lipofuscinoses 303–4, **302**
  sialidosis 303, **302**
  Unverricht-Lundborg disease **302**
severe myoclonic epilepsy of infancy (SMEI) 300
mode of inheritance 291–5, **292**
  chromosomal inheritance 291–2
  complex inheritance 295
  mendelian inheritance 292–4, **293**, *294*, **296**
  mitochondrial inheritance 294–5, *295*
  X-linked inheritance 294
pedigree as diagnostic tool 290, *291*
risk assessment 290–1
see also individual epilepsy syndromes
genetic disorders, risk of epilepsy 55–6
genetic models 110–12
  convulsive seizures 112
    DBA/2J mice 112
    epilepsy mouse 112
    genetically epilepsy-prone rat 112
    spontaneous epileptic rat 112
  non-convulsive epilepsy 110–12
    genetic absence epilepsy rats from Strasbourg 111–12
    lethargic mouse 111
    stargazer mouse 111
    tottering mouse 111
genetically epilepsy-prone rat (GEPR), as experimental model of epilepsy 112
genetics 55–6, 56–60, 57, 58, 59
  generalized tonic-clonic seizures 59–60
  idiopathic epilepsies
    with complex inheritance 58–9, *58*
    with simple mendelian inheritance 57–8, *57*
  mechanisms of inheritance 55–6, *56*
  multiorgan hereditary disorders 56–7
glucose transporter protein deficiency, ketogenic diet in 264
glutamate 104–5, **104**
glutamate receptors
  AMPA and kainite receptors 104

metabotropic receptors 105
  NMDA receptors 104
  as target for antiepileptic drug action 104–5, **104**
glutamic acid decarboxylase 100
glycogen storage disease, risk of epilepsy 55
grand mal seizures, on awakening 13

H
Hallermann-Streiff syndrome, risk of epilepsy 55
Hallervorden-Spatz disease, risk of epilepsy 56
haloperidol, as cause of seizures 53, **223**
halothane, as anaesthesia for epilepsy surgery 861
hamartoma, as cause of epilepsy 730
  see also hypothalamic hamartoma; neoplastic lesions
harkoseride 570, 571
head trauma, as a cause of epilepsy 32, 61–2, **62**
hemidecortication 793
hemimegalencephaly, MRI abnormalities **641**, *643*, 646
hemispherectomy 790–7
  anatomical 793
  and brain plasticity 795–6
  complications 854
  functional 793
  hemicorticectomy 793
  hemispherotomy 793
  indications for and patient selection 790–3, **791**, *792*
  modified 793
  outcome 795
  peri-insular hemispherectomy 793–4, *794*
  surgical morbidity 794–5
hemispherotomy 793
  peri-insular 793–4, *794*
hepatic disease, treatment of seizures 248
hepatic porphyrias
  drug treatment of seizures 248–9
  ketogenic diet 264
herbal medicines in treatment of epilepsy 272
heroin, as cause of seizures 53, 54
Hibicon *see* benzchlorpropamide
hippocampal relaxometry 648
hippocampal sclerosis
  EEG scalp 601–4, *602*, *603*
    bilateral hippocampal sclerosis 604
    dual pathology 591, **593**, *593* 604,
    isolated hippocampal sclerosis 602–4, *603*
  EEG invasive 609–10, 611, 622, 623–9
  MRI 590–3, *594*, **641**, *642*, 643–4
  pathological findings 587
  resective surgery
    methods 723–6, **724**, *725*
    outcome 726
    selection of patients for 586–8
  stereotactic surgery 840–1
  surgery 723–7
  symptomatology of seizures in 587–8
  see also partial seizures and epilepsy; temporal lobe epilepsy; and individual investigatory techniques
hippocampal slices, as experimental models of epilepsy 112–13
hippocampal volimetry, MRI in presurgical evaluation 591, *584*, 648
historical aspects of medical treatment of epilepsy between 1938 and 1955 xvi–xxxiii
holoprosencephaly, risk of epilepsy 55
homocystinuria, risk of epilepsy 55
homoeopathy, in treatment of epilepsy 273

Horsley, Sir Victor *579*
Hospital Anxiety and Depression Scale (HADS), use in psychiatric assessment in epilepsy 717
hydantoins **xxx**
  see also mephenytoin; phenytoin
hydatid disease 757–8
  diagnosis 757–8
  management 758
5-hydroxytryptamine, as target for antiepileptic drug actio 107
hyperammonaemic encephalopathy 534
hypnosis in treatment of epilepsy 269–70
hypophosphatasia, risk of epilepsy 55
hypothalamic hamartoma
  MRI abnormalities **641**, 647
  surgery 782–3
6-Hz seizure model, as experimental model of epilepsy 109
hysterical seizures *see* non-epileptic seizures

I
ictal EEG
  invasive EEG
    extratemporal epilepsy 632
    medial temporal lobe epilepsy 623–9, *624–9*
    neocortical temporal lobe epilepsy 629–32, *630*, *631*
  scalp EEG 589–90, *591*, 601
  video-EEG telemetry 589–90
ictal onset zone
  definition 585–6
  fMRI 686
idiopathic epilepsies 10
  idiopathic partial epilepsies of childhood 195–96
    benign partial epilepsy with cetnrotemporal spikes (BECTs) 195
    early onset benign childhood occipital epilepsy (EBOS) 196
    late onset benign idiopathic occipital epilepsy (LOE) 196
  with complex inheritance 58–9, *58*
  idiopathic generalized epilepsies 12–13, 299–300
    benign myoclonic epilepsy in infancy 13
    benign neonatal convulsions 12
    benign neonatal familial convulsions 12
    childhood absence epilepsy 13, 196–97
    epilepsy with grand mal seizures on awakening 13
    juvenile absence epilepsy 196–7
    juvenile myoclonic epilepsy 13, 197
  genetic counselling
    complex epilepsies 298–300, **299**
    mendelian epilepsies 296–8, **296**
    severe myoclonic epilepsy of infancy 300
  incidence and prevalence 50–1
  of infancy 187
  localization-related 11–12
  partial 300
  with simple mendelian inheritance 57–8, *57*
  see also individual epilepsy syndromes
imipramine, as cause of seizures 53
in vitro experimental models of epilepsy 112–13
incidence of epilepsy 24–6, *25*
  age-specific incidence *25*
  cumulative incidence *25*
  epileptic syndromes 25–6
  ethnicity and socioeconomic factors *25*
  gender *25*
  less developed countries 25, **26**
  more developed countries 25

incidence of epilepsy (*cont'd*)
  seizure types 25
  of sudden death 45–6
indinavir, cytochrome P450 inhibition **122**
infantile epilepsy 180–9
  age-dependent pharmacokinetics and
      pharmacodynamics 180
  benign myoclonic 13
  benign partial 11–12
  characteristics of 181
  effects of antiepileptic drugs on 181
  epileptic encephalopathies 15
      management of 181–5, *182*
  febrile seizures 187
  idiopathic epilepsies 187
  infantile spasms *see* West syndrome
  initiation of treatment 187
  maintenance doses of antiepileptic drugs **153**
  management of infantile epilepsy
      syndromes 181–7
  myoclonic epilepsy in non-progressive
      encephalopathy encephalopathy 15
    management 186
  pharmacokinetics and
      pharmacodynamics 180–1, *181*
  tolerability and side effect profile 180–1
  severe myoclonic epilepsy of infancy (Dravet's
      syndrome; SMEI) 15, 185–6
    management 185–6
  surgery 782
  symptomatic partial epilepsies 186–7
  treatment *see individual drugs*
  West syndrome *see* West syndrome
  see also individual epilepsy syndromes
infantile spasm *see* West syndrome
infective lesions 747–58
  cerebral tuberculoma 755–7
  hydatid disease 757–8
  neurocysticercosis 753–5
  pyogenic cerebral abscess 747–53
interictal EEG
  invasive EEG
    extrahippocampal epilepsies 622–3
    medial temporal lobe epilepsy 622
  scalp EEG 588–9, 601–6
interictal psychosis 257
International Classification of Epilepsies and
    Epileptic Syndromes **9**, 161
International Classification of Epileptic
    Seizures 161
International League Against Epilepsy
  international congresses of **xviii**
  member chapters **xvii**
  officers and members **xvii**
intracarotid amobarbital procedure (sodium
    amytal test) 594, 710–12
  in children 785
  complications 849
intracranial depth electrodes *see* depth electrodes
intracranial monitoring (invasive EEG) 594–5,
    609–34
  aim of intracranial EEG in presurgical
      assessment 594–5
  background 621–2
  in children 783–4, **784**
  combined studies 616
  cortical stimulation 619–20
    advantages and disadvantages 619–20
    technical aspects 619
    use of 619
  depth electrodes 610–12, 837–40
    advantages of 611–12
    complications 851–2
    disadvantages of 612

extratemporal epilepsy 611
  medial temporal lobe epilepsy *611*
  neocortical temporal lobe epilepsy 611
  stereotactic implantation 837–40
  technical aspects 610–11
electrocorticography 620–1
  frontal lobe epilepsy 620–1
  structural lesions 621
  technical aspects 620
  temporal epilepsy 620
epidural electrodes *617*
  advantages of 617
  complications 850
  disadvantages of 617
  technical aspects 617
foramen ovale electrodes 618–19
  advantages 618
  complications 850
  disadvantages 618–19
  technical aspects *618*
  use of 618
ictal EEG 590–600, 623–32
  extratemporal epilepsy 632
  medial temporal lobe epilepsy 560, 601–4,
      602, 623–9, *624–9*
  neocortical temporal lobe epilepsy 560,
      629–32, *630*, *631*
  indications for 609–10
    dual pathology 610
    lesional epilepsy 610
    medial temporal lobe epilepsy 609–10
    non-lesional extratemporal epilepsies 610
    non-lesional, non-medial temporal lobe
        epilepsy 610
  interictal EEG 622–3
    extrahippocampal epilepsies 622–3
    medial temporal lobe epilepsy 622
  interpretation of invasive EEG 622–32
  non-epileptiform findings 622
  recording sessions 621
  subdural grid electrodes 614–16
    advantages 615
    disadvantages 615–16
    technical aspects 614–15, *614*
    use of 615
  subdural strip electrodes 612–14
    advantages 613
    disadvantages 613–14
    extratemporal epilepsy 613
    technical aspects 612–13
    temporal lobe epilepsy *613*
intracranial resective surgery, complications
    of 851–5
  see also individual operative techniques
intractable epilepsy, definition of 584
intrinsic optical imaging 680–4
  age dependence of seizures 681
  clinical studies 682
  energy associated with seizure activity 682
  epileptiform activity 681
  near-infrared spectroscopy 682–4, *683*
  optical physics 680–1
  origin and spread of seizures 681
  physiological processes 680–1
iphosphamide, as cause of seizures 53
irritative zone
  definition of 585–6
  MRI 648, 686
isoflurane, as anaesthesia for epilepsy
    surgery 861–2
isoniazid
  as cause of seizures 53
  cytochrome P450 induction **122**
itraconazole, cytochrome P450 inhibition **122**

J
juvenile absence epilepsy 196–7
juvenile myoclonic epilepsy 13, 197
  prognosis 33
  treatment 447, 471, 532

K
kainate receptors, as target for antiepileptic drug
    action 104
ketamine, anaesthesia for epilepsy surgery 864
ketoconazole, cytochrome P450 inhibition **122**
ketogenic diet 222, 262–8
  calculation of 264–5
  discontinuation of 266
  early use of **xix**, xx
  handling of increased seizures 266
  history 262
  indications and contraindications for 264,
      264
  initiation of 264–5, **265**, **266**
  mechanisms of action 262–3, *263*
  outcomes 263–4
  side-effects 266–7, **266**
kindling
  as experimental model of epilepsy 109–10
  as test in antiepileptic drug discovery **91**,
      92–3, **92**
  see also individual antiepileptic drugs
Kojewnikow's syndrome 9, 12
Krabbe's disease, risk of epilepsy 55, *56*
Krebs' cycle *100*
Kufs' disease, genetic counselling in 304

L
Lafora's disease as cause of epilepsy, genetic
    counselling in 57, 302–3, **302**
lamotrigine 170, 425–42, **425**
  6 Hz seizure test **92**
  absorption 427–8
  action on calcium channels **98**
  action on sodium channels **97**
  advantages **425**
  anticonvulsant activity **92**
  bioavailability **425**, 427–8
  in breast milk **285**, 429
  child development effects 436
  childhood absence epilepsy **191**
  clinical efficacy 485
    absence seizures 433
    active control study 431–2
    generalized epilepsy 433
    generalized tonic clonic seizures 433
    Lennox-Gastaut syndrome 433
    mood disorders 433
    myoclonus and myoclonic syndromes 433
    newly diagnosed patients 432, **432**
    partial seizures 431–2, **431**
    paediatric mixed seizures 433
    use with valproate 432–3
  clinical therapeutics 436–7
    adjunctive therapy with enzyme-inducing
        AEDs 437
    adjunctive therapy with valproate 436–7
    monotherapy 437
  concentration and effect 429–30
  cost of treatment **147**
  disadvantages **425**
  distribution 427–8
  dosage **425**, 436–8
  dosage interval **425**, 436–8
  drug interactions 133, 430, **425**, **530**
  drug-metabolizing enzymes, effects on **128**,
      430
  EEG, effects on 427

efficacy spectrum 142
elderly onset seizures 207
elimination 131, 133, 428–9
    half-life 152, 425, 428
experimental studies
    animal seizure models 426–7
    cognitive and psychomotor effects 427
    EEG in epileptic patients 427
frequency of administration 148
generalized seizures 170
improvement/success rates 325
indications 425, 431–3
initial target dose 148, 436–7
juvenile absence epilepsy 191
juvenile myoclonic epilepsy 191
laboratory monitoring 429–30, 437
learning-disabled patients 218, 219
Lennox-Gastaut syndrome 191, 433
long-term therapy 437
maintenance dose 148, 436–7
    infants and children 153, 436–7
mechanism of action 425, 426
metabolism 425, 428–9, 430
number-needed-to-treat 323
odds ratio 322, 323
and oral contraception 279, 431
overdose 436
partial onset seizures 170
pharmacokinetics 427–31, 428, 429
    effects of coadministered drugs on 430
    effects on pharmacokinetics of
        coadministered drugs 430
    interactions 430–1
    oral contraceptives 431
plasma clearance 425, 428–9, 428
preparations 425
protein binding 131, 425, 427–8
quality of life 433
renal impairment, effects on metabolism 429
side effects 425, 434–6, 434, 435
    idiosyncratic 434–5
    multiorgan failure 436
    rash 434–5, 435
    sudden unexplained death 436
teratogenicity 436
therapeutic range 156, 425, 429–30
time to peak blood levels 425, 428
titration rate 148
volume of distribution 425, 428
Landau-Kleffner syndrome 9, 11, 15, 16, 228
    multiple subpial transection 813–14, 815–18
    surgery 782
    treatment with clonazepam 369
Langer-Giedion syndrome, risk of epilepsy 55
learning disabilities 215–26
    acute seizure treatment with diazepam 222,
        222
    and adverse drug reactions 217, 220
    association with epilepsy 27
    choice of antiepileptic drugs 217–21, 217,
        218, 219, 220
    compliance 216–17, 217
    concomitant psychopharmacological
        treatment 222–3, 223
    medical aspects 215, 216
    multidisciplinary approach 215
    non-pharmacological treatment
        epilepsy surgery 221–2
        ketogenic diet 222
        vagus nerve stimulation 222
    prognosis 223–4
    prophylactic treatment 216–21
        and alteration of disease process 221
        CNS side-effects 220

new AEDs 218–20, 218, 219
older AEDs 217–18, 217
paradoxical effects 220–1, 220
psychological and cognitive aspects 216
social and educational aspects 216
see also ketogenic diet; individual antiepileptic
    drugs; and individual surgical
    procedures
Leigh's syndrome, risk of epilepsy 55
Lennox-Gastaut syndrome 8, 9, 14, 24, 193–5
    causes 193
    choice of drug 142–4, 142, 194–5
    prognosis 33
    treatment 194–5, 264, 362, 369, 384, 433,
        509, 519, 520, 532, 533, 544, 554, 560
    see also corpus callosal section; and specific
        causes
lesionectomy, stereotactic 841
    see also individual conditions
lethargic mouse
    as experimental model of epilepsy 111
    as test in antiepileptic drug discovery 93
levetiracetam 170, 443–50, 443
    6 Hz seizure test 92
    action on calcium channels 98
    advantages 443
    anticonvulsant activity 92
    bioavailability 443, 444
    chemical properties 443–4
    clinical therapeutics 449
    cost of treatment 147
    disadvantages 443
    dosage 443, 449
    dosage interval 443, 449
    drug interactions 133, 443, 445, 530
    effect on drug-metabolizing enzymes 128, 445
    efficacy 142
        absence seizures 447
        generalized tonic clonic seizures 447
        juvenile myoclonic epilepsy 447
        myoclonic seizures 447
        photosensitivity 447
        refractory partial seizures 445–7, 446
    elderly onset seizures 208
    elimination 131, 133, 445
        half-life 152, 443, 445
    frequency of administration 149
    improvement/success rates 325
    indications 443, 445–7
    initial target dose 149, 449
    learning-disabled patients 218, 219
    maintenance dose 149, 449
        infants and children 153
    metabolism 443, 445
    number-needed-to-treat 323, 324
    odds ratio 322, 323
    and oral contraception 279
    overdose 449
    partial onset seizures 170
    pharmacokinetics 444–5
    plasma clearance 443, 445
    preclinical data 444
    preparations 443
    protein binding 131
    renal impairment, effect on dosage 445, 445
    serum levels 445
    side effects 443, 447–9, 448, 449
        in children 448–9, 449
        idiosyncratic 448
    structure 491
    teratogenicity 448
    therapeutic range 156
    time to peak blood levels 443, 444
    titration rate 149

tolerance 449
    volume of distribution 443, 444–5
ligand-gated channels, and epileptogenesis 78
lignocaine
    as cause of seizures 53
    status epilepticus 238
        convulsive 233
limbic encephalitis, MRI appearances 644
lissencephaly
    EEG 605
    risk of epilepsy 55
    surgery 767
liver disease, treatment of seizures in 248
local anaesthesia in epilepsy surgery 864,
    866–7
localization-related syndromes 11
    symptomatology
        idiopathic 11–12
        symptomatic 12
lorazepam 380–1
    clinical applications
        alcohol withdrawal seizures 381
        chronic epilepsies 381
        serial seizures 381
        status epilepticus 381
    drug interactions 380
    pharmacokinetics 380
    side effects 380–1
    status epilepticus 238
        convulsive 233
    structure 377
Lyell's syndrome caused by antiepileptic
    drugs 326

M
magnetic resonance imaging (MRI) 581, 590–3,
    592, 593, 594, 640–51
    brain tumours 732–3, 732
    in children 647–8, 783, 784
    epileptogenic area 648–9
        functional deficit zone 649
        irritative zone 648
        pacemaker zone 649
    future perspectives 649
    hippocampal relaxometry 648
    hippocampal volimetry 648
    impact of 581
    localization of eloquent areas 649
    negative results 586, 605
    pyogenic cerebral abscess 750
    quantitative 648
    as screening test 586
    structural imaging 640–7, 641
        Ammon's horn sclerosis 642–3, 642,
            643
        dysembryoplastic neuroepithelial tumour
            (DNT)/ganglioglioma 646
        focal cortical dysplasia 644, 645–6, 645,
            646
        focal polymicrogyria/pachygyria 646
        hemimegalencephaly 646
        hypothalamic hamartomas 647
        limbic encephalitis 644
        malformations of cortical
            development 644–6, 644
        neurocutaneous syndromes 647
        nodular heterotopia 646, 647
        post-traumatic lesions 647
        protocols 641
        Rasmussen's encephalitis 647
        vascular abnormalities 646–7
magnetic resonance spectroscopy 648
    brain tumours 735
    pyogenic cerebral abscess 751

magnetoencephalography (MEG) 635–9
  applications of
    evoked activity 636
    spontaneous activity 636–8
    brain tumours 735
  method 635–6
malaria, cerebral, phenobarbitone therapy
      in 466
malformations of cortical development *see*
      cortical dysgenesis
maprotiline, as cause of seizures 53
Marshall-Smith syndrome, risk of epilepsy 55
maximal electroshock test (MES test)
  as experimental model of epilepsy 108–9
  as test in antiepileptic drug discovery 90,
      90–2, **91**, **92**, 93
  see also individual antiepileptic drugs
medial temporal lobe epilepsy *see* temporal lobe
      epilepsy
medial temporal lobe function,
      neuropsychological assessment 707
medical treatment, principles of
  aims of 139–41
    avoidance of adverse drug reactions 140
    avoidance of obstruction to patient's
        life 140
    avoidance of side-effects 139–40
    complete seizure control 139
    prevention of epileptogenesis 140–1
    reduction of mortality and morbidity 140
    reduction of seizure severity 139
    suppression of subclinical epileptic
        activity 140
  assessment of response 153
  choice of drug 142–55, 168–70, **170**, 317–33
    aetiology of epilepsy 144
    cost of treatment **147**
    ease of use 146–7, **147**
    EEG features 144
    mechanism of anticonvulsant action 146
    medical expertise available 145–6, *145*
    old versus new drugs 146
    partial epilepsy 317–33
    seizure type and epilepsy syndrome 142–4,
        142, *143*
    side-effect profiles and patient's
        characteristics 144–5
  drug formulation 147–9, *148*, **149**
  failure of 153–5
    alternative monotherapy 153–4
    combination therapy 154–5
  general principles 139–60
  individualization of dosage 150–3
    dosage adjustments 151–2
    dose optimization 152–3
    frequency of administration 148–9, 150–1
    initial target maintenance dose 148–9, 150
    rate of dose escalation 148–9, 150
  and natural history of epilepsy 38
  polytherapy 47
  route of administration 147–9, *148*, **149**
  therapeutic drug monitoring 155–8
    individualized drug concentrations 156–7,
        157
    monitoring of unbound drug
        concentrations 157–8
    therapeutic range 155–6, **156**
    timing of blood samples 155
    value of 157
    when to measure drug concentrations 158
  when to start 141–2
    seizures with specific triggers 141
    single seizure 141
    two or more unprovoked seizures 141

  see also newly diagnosed epilepsy
  see also antiepileptic drugs; and individual
        antiepileptic drugs
meditation, in treatment of epilepsy 270
mefloquine, as cause of seizures 53
MEG *see* magnetoencephalography
MELAS syndrome, as cause of epilepsy 12, 56,
      57
membrane ion channels in epileptogenesis 7408
  calcium channels 77–8, 77
  potassium channels 76–7
  sodium channels 75–6, 75, 76
memory assessment 707–10, *708*, 709
  matched learning tasks 708–10, *708*, *709*
  non-verbal learning and memory tests 710
  traditional tests 707–8, *708*
mendelian inheritance 292–4, **293**, *294*, **296**
meningioma 730–1
Menkes disease, risk of epilepsy 55
mental retardation, association with epilepsy 60
meperidine, as cause of seizures 53, 54
mephenytoin 564
  cost of treatment xxxi
  early use of xxv–xxvi, *xxv*, **xxv**, xxx
  introduction of **xvii**
  structure *xxi*
meprobamate, as cause of seizures 53
MERRF syndrome, as cause of epilepsy 56, 57,
      302, 303
MES test *see* maximal electroshock test
Mesantoin *see* mephenytoin
metabolic abnormalities, in differential diagnosis
      of epilepsy 71
metabotropic glutamate receptors, as target for
      antiepileptic drug action 104
metharbital 471
  cost of treatment xxxi
  early use of xxviii
  introduction of **xvii**
methylbarbitone, early use of **xxv**
methylene blue **xix**
methylphenobarbitone 471–2
methylphenyl barbituric acid **xxx**
methylphenylethyl barbituric acid **xxx**
mexyletine, as cause of seizures 53
miconazole, cytochrome P450 inhibition **122**
midazolam 381–2
  clinical applications
    febrile seizures 382
    serial seizures 382
    status epilepticus 239–40, 382
  drug interactions 382
  pharmacokinetics 381–2
  side effects 382
  status epilepticus 238–9
    convulsive **233**
    refractory **234**
  structure 377
migraine, in differential diagnosis of
      epilepsy 69–70, **162**
Miller-Dieker syndrome, risk of epilepsy 55, 56,
      182
Milontin *see* phensuximide
Minnesota Multiple Personality Inventory
      (MPPI), use in psychiatric assessment in
      epilepsy 717
mitochondrial disease
  contraindication to ketogenic diet **264**
  myoclonic epilepsy *see* MELAS syndrome;
      MERRF syndrome
mitochondrial inheritance 294–5, *295*, *293*
Modified Card Sorting test 701
monoamine oxidase inhibitors, as cause of
      ·seizures 53

monoamines, as target for antiepileptic drug
      action 106
monotherapy, advantages over combination
      therapy 330
Morrell hooks, multiple subpial transection *819*
mortality of epilepsy 33–8
  by aetiology 35
  by age and gender 35
  by duration of epilepsy 35–6
  by seizure type 36
  cause-specific 36–7, **37**
  elderly onset epilepsy 211
  epidemiological studies 34
  less developed countries 36–7
  measures of 34
  mortality ratios **34**
  population-based studies 34–5
  reduction of 140
  relative survivorship 36
  risk in early epilepsy 165–6
  selected epilepsy populations 35
  trends over time 37
  see also sudden death in epilepsy (SUDEP)
motor cortex seizures, symptomatology 11
motor disabilities associated with epilepsy 27–8
motor tasks 704
movement disorders, in differential diagnosis of
      epilepsy 71
Mozart effect, complementary therapy for
      epilepsy 272
MRI *see* magnetic resonance imaging
multiple subpial transection 812–23
  complications 856
  indications for 813–14
    Landau-Kleffner syndrome 813–14,
        815–18
    multilobar or bihemispheric foci 814
    resections involving eloquent cortex 813
  physiology 812–13
  results 820–1, *821*
  surgical technique 814–20, *819*
muscle relaxants, anaesthesia for epilepsy
      surgery 865
music therapy for epilepsy 272
myoclonic absences, epilepsy with 15
myoclonic astatic epilepsy 14, *228*
myoclonic seizures
  choice of drug in treatment of 142–4, **142**
  infantile 15, 180–1, 185–6
  progressive moyclonus epilepsies 301–4, **302**,
      492–3
  relapse after drug withdrawal 175–7, **177**
  symptomatology 5, 7
  treatment
    acetazolamide 337, **338–9**
    bromide 563
    clonazepam 368, 369
    lamotrigine 433
    levetiracetam 447
    piracetam 491–3, *492*
myoclonic status epilepticus
  emergency treatment of *228*, 237
    see also status epilepticus, emergency
        treatment
  in coma, treatment of *228*, 236
myoclonus epilepsy and red-ragged fibres *see*
      MERFF syndrome
Mysoline *see* primidone

N

nalidixic acid, as cause of seizures 53
naloxone, as cause of seizures 53
narcolepsy, in differential diagnosis of
      epilepsy 70

National Hospital, Queen Square, in history of
epilepsy surgery 579, *580*
naturopathy, as treatment for epilepsy 273
near-infrared spectroscopy 682–4, *683*
nebracetam *491*
nefazodone, cytochrome P450 inhibition **122**
nefiracetam *491*
neocortical temporal lobe epilepsy *see* temporal
lobe epilepsy
neonates, seizures in
benign convulsions 12
benign familial convulsions 12
seizure types 15
status epilepticus 228
treatment *see individual drugs*
neoplastic lesions *see* brain tumours
neuroacanthocytosis, risk of epilepsy 56
Neurobehavioral Inventory (NBI), use in
psychiatric assessment in epilepsy
717
neurocutaneous syndromes
MRI abnormalities 647
see also individual syndromes
neurocysticercosis 753–5
diagnosis 753–5, **754**
management *756*
neurofibromatosis, risk of epilepsy 55
neurological examination, related to prognosis in
epilepsy 32
neuronal ceroid lipofuscinoses, as cause of
epilepsy **302**, 303–4
neuronal grafting 886–90
GABAergic modification 888–9
hippocampal repair 889–90
repletion of specific neurotransmitters 886–8,
887
neuropsychological assessment *see* psychological
assessment, in presurgical evaluation
neurosurgery, as a cause of epilepsy 62, 245–8
aneurysm and aneurysm surgery 245
prophylaxis after neurosurgery 246
ventricular shunt 246
newly diagnosed epilepsy 161–73, 328–9
approach to drug treatment 328–9
choice of drug 142–7, 168–70, 328–9
in the elderly 205–10
women's issues 169–70
counselling **171**
criteria for starting therapy 142–7, 167–8,
167
likelihood of compliance 168
patient's wishes 167
type of seizures or syndrome 168
diagnosis 161–2, **162**
initiation of treatment in infantile
epilepsies 187
initiation of treatment in the elderly
patient 205–10
principles of treatment 328–9, **329**
provoking factors for seizures 170–1, **170**
rationale for treatment 162–7
effect of repeated seizures on recurrence
risk 164
effect of treatment on long-term
prognosis 165
effect of treatment on recurrence risk 164–5
psychosocial morbidity 166
risk of injury 166
risk of mortality 165–6
risk of recurrence after first seizure 162–4,
162, **163**
side effects of drugs 166–7
starting medication **170**
see also individual antiepileptic drugs

night terrors, in differential diagnosis of
epilepsy 70
nipecotic acid, and GABA transporter
inhibition 101
nitrazepam 383–4
clinical applications 384
drug interactions 383–4
pharmacokinetics 383
side effects 383–4
structure *377*
nitrous oxide, as anaesthesia for epilepsy
surgery 862
NMDA receptors, as target for antiepileptic drug
action 104–5
nodular heterotopia, MRI abnormalities **641**,
643, 646
non-convulsive epilepsy, genetic models 110–12
non-convulsive status epilepticus 235–7
diagnosis 235
treatment 235–7, **235**
non-convulsive status epilepticus in coma 236
non-epileptic attack disorder *see* non-epileptic
seizures
non-epileptic seizures 307–13
diagnosis and treatment 310–12
historical features 310–11
neuropsychological testing 311
video-EEG monitoring 311
in differential diagnosis of epilepsy 68–9,
301–10
epidemiology and cost 310
physiological non-epileptic events 307–9,
308, 309
psychogenic non-epileptic seizures 309–10
referral for surgery 585
terminology and classification 307
Noonan's syndrome, risk of epilepsy 55
noradrenaline, as target of antiepileptic drug
action 107
norfloxacine, as cause of seizures 53
nortriptyline, as cause of seizures 53
NPS 1776 570, *571*
number-needed-to-treat, in comparative
evaluation of antiepileptic
drugs 323–4, *323, 324*
nutritional supplements, as treatment of
epilepsy 272–3

O

occipital lobe epilepsies, symptomatology 11
occipital lobe function, neuropsychological
testing of 705–6
occipital lobe resections, stereotactic
surgery 854
*see also individual conditions and individual
investigatory methods*
Ohtahara syndrome 15, *783*
omeprazole
cytochrome P450 induction **122**
cytochrome P450 inhibition **122**
opercular frontal lobe seizures,
symptomatology 11
opiate receptors in PET scanning 657
opioid analgesics in epilepsy surgery 864
oral contraceptive pill, reduced efficacy with
AED therapy 169–70
orbitofrontal seizures, symptomatology 10
organic mental disorders in epilepsy 255–6, **256**
osteochondrodysplasias, risk of epilepsy 55
osteopetrosis, risk of epilepsy 55
oxcarbazepine 169, **170**, 451–60, **451**
absorption 452
action on calcium channels 98
action on sodium channels 97

active metabolites **451**, 452
advantages **451**
bioavailability **451**, 452
in breast milk 285
chemistry 452
children, treatment in 456, 458–9
clinical therapeutics 458–9
conversion from carbamazepine 458
dose initiation 458
dosing interval 459
maintenance treatment and serum
levels 458–9
monitoring of serum sodium 459
cost of treatment 147
cytochrome P450 induction **122**, 453
disadvantages **451**
distribution 452
dosage **451**, 458–9
dosage interval **451**, 459
drug interactions 130, 133, **451**, 453–4, **454**,
530
effect on drug-metabolizing enzymes **128**,
130, 453
efficacy in partial seizures 142, 454–6, **454**,
455, 456
adjunctive therapy **456**
compared to AEDs **455**
compared to carbamazepine 454–5
monotherapy in refractory patients 455–6
elderly onset seizures 207–8
elimination **131**, 133, 453
half-life **152**, **451**
frequency of administration 149, 459
improvement/success rates 325
indications **451**
initial target dose 149
learning-disabled patients 218, *219*
maintenance dose 149, 458–9
infants and children 153
mechanism of action **451**, 452
metabolism **451**, 452, *453*
number-needed-to-treat *323*
odds ratio *322, 323*
and oral contraception 279, 453
overdose 457
partial onset seizures 170
pharmacokinetics 452–3
plasma concentrations 453
preparations **451**
protein binding **131**, **451**
side effects **451**, 457–8, **457**
cognitive effects 458
gastrointestinal 457
hyponatraemia 457
rash 457
special populations 458
therapeutic range 156, **451**
time to peak blood levels **451**, 452
titration rate 149
tolerance 456
toxicology 452
volume of distribution **451**, 452
oxiracetam *491*

P

pacemaker zone, MRI 649
pachygyria, MRI appearances **641**, *646*
panic disorders, in differential diagnosis of
epilepsy 69, **162**
Paradione *see* paramethadione
paraldehyde 230, 564–5
clinical therapeutics 565
mechanisms of action 564
pharmacokinetics and clinical efficacy 564–5

paraldehyde (*cont'd*)
  side effects 565
  status epilepticus 233
paramethadione
  cost of treatment xxxi
  early use of xxv, xxvii, xxx
  introduction of xvii
parasomnias, in differential diagnosis of
      epilepsy 70
parietal lobe epilepsies, symptomatology 11
parietal lobe function, neuropsychological
      testing of 705
parietal lobe resections, stereotactic surgery
      854
see also individual conditions; individual
      investigatory methods
Parkinson's disease, risk of epilepsy 56, 535
paroxysmal nocturnal dystonia, in differential
      diagnosis of epilepsy 70
partial seizures and epilepsies
  approach to treatment 329–31
  choice of drugs in treatment of 142–4, **142**,
      317–33
  classification and symptomatology 3, 4
  infantile partial epilepsies of 180–1, 186–7
  idiopathic partial epilepsies of
      childhood 195–6
  mortality 36
  status epilepticus *228, 236*
  symptomatic and cryptogenic partial epilepsies
      of childhood 197–9
  treatment of partial seizures 317–33
    acetazolamide 340, **338–9**
    allopurinol 561–2
    bromide 563–4
    carbamazepine 351
    clobazam 361–2
    clonazepam 369
    felbamate 406–7
    gabapentin 421–2
    ganaxolone 570
    harkoseride 571
    lamotrigine 431–2, **431**
    levetiracetam 445–47, **446**
    oxcarbazepine 454–56, **455, 456**
    phenacemide 565
    phenobarbitone 465
    phenytoin 484–5
    primidone 471
    pregabalin 497–8
    retigabine 572
    rufinamide 504–5
    talamparel 573
    topiramate 517–19, 520–1
    valproate 531–2
    vigabatrin 542–3
    zonisamide 552–5, **552, 553, 554**
  see also medical treatment; and individual
      antiepileptic drugs, epilepsy
      syndromes, surgical procedures and
      investigatory methods
patient selection for surgery, principles of 584–6
  intractable epilepsy 584
  learning disability, behavioural disorder and
      psychosis 585
  medical fitness and age 585
  non-epileptic seizures 585
  quality of life gain 584–5
  seizure outcome and risk of surgery 584
  temporal lobe surgery 586–8
    causative aetiologies and pathologies 587
    symptomatology 587–8
  see also individual conditions, surgical
      techniques and investigatory methods

pavor nocturnes, in differential diagnosis of
      epilepsy 70
penicillins, as cause of seizures 53
pentobarbitone, in treatment of refractory status
      epilepticus **234**, 240
pentylenetetrazole test 501
  as experimental model of epilepsy 109
  as test in antiepileptic drug discovery 90–2,
      90, **91, 92,** 93
  see also individual antiepileptic drugs
perinatal risk factors for epilepsy 60
periventricular heterotopia 766
  MRI appearances **641, 646**
  surgery of 766
  see also cortical dysgenesis
perphenazine
  cytochrome P450 inhibition 122
  seizure-inducing properties 223
personality disorders associated with
      epilepsy 259–60
PET *see* positron emission tomography
Pfeiffer's syndrome, risk of epilepsy 55
pharmacodynamic drug interactions 134
pharmacodynamics, age-dependent 180–1,
      181
pharmacokinetic drug interactions 120–33
  antiepileptic drugs 128–33
  effects of antiepileptics on pharmacokinetics of
      other drugs 128–30, **128**
  effects of other drugs on pharmacokinetics of
      antiepileptics 130–3, **131**
  individual drugs
    acetazolamide **334**, 336
    bromide 563
    carbamazepine 129–30, 131–2, **345,**
      348–9, **348, 349, 350, 454,** 530
    clobazam 358, 360, 454
    clonazepam 337–8, **365,** 366–8
    diazepam 379
    ethosuximide 132, **391,** 394–5, 530
    felbamate 129, 130, 132, **403,** 405, 407,
      403, **405, 454,** 530
    gabapentin 132–3, **418,** 420, 530
    lamotrigine 133, **425,** 430, 530
    levetiracetam 133, **443,** 445, 530
    lorazepam 380
    midazolam 382
    oxcarbazepine 130, 133, **451,** 453–4, **454,**
      530
    phenobarbital 129–30, 131, **454, 461,**
      464–5, 530
    phenytoin 129–30, 131, 480–1, **454, 475,**
      480, 481, 530
    primidone 131, **470**–1
    rufinamide 503
    tiagabine 122, **507, 530,** 508–9
    topiramate 129, 131, 133, **517, 515**
    valproate 128–9, 131, **454,** 530–1, **530,**
      528
    vigabatrin 133, **541**–2, **530, 540,**
    zonisamade 133, **530, 548,** 552
  mechanisms of 120–8
    enzyme induction 124–5, 127
    enzyme inhibition 123–7
    enzyme systems 121–3, **122**
      cytochrome P450 121–3, **122, 128**
      epoxide hydrolases 123
      uridine diphosphate
          glucuronosyltransferases 123
    metabolically based 120–7
      active or toxic metabolite 126
      extent and clinical relevance of 126–7,
          126, 127
      predictability of 125–6

      therapeutic index of substrate 126
      protein binding displacement 127–8, *128,*
          130
pharmacokinetics
  age-dependent 180–1, *181*
  in pregnancy 280–1
  in status epilepticus 229–30, *229*
  see also individual drugs
phenacemide 565
  cost of treatment xxxi
  early use of xxviii
  introduction of xvii
phenacetylurea, early use of xxv
phencyclidine, as cause of seizures 53, 54
phenobarbitone 170, 462–9
  absorption *463,* 463
  action on calcium channels 98
  action on sodium channels 97
  advantages **461**
  bioavailability **461,** 463
  in breast milk 285
  chemistry 462
  clinical efficacy in partial and generalized
      seizures 465–6, 484
    adults and children 465
    cerebral malaria 466
    febrile seizures 466
    generalized seizures 170, 476
    neonatal seizures 465–6, **465**
    status epilepticus 233–4, **233,** 235, 239,
      466
  clinical therapeutics 469
  cost of treatment xxxi, 147
  dependence and withdrawal 467
  disadvantages **461**
  distribution 463
  dosage **461,** 469
  dosage interval **461,** 469
  drug interactions 129–30, 131, **454, 461,**
      464–5, 530
  early use of xix, xxv
  effect on drug-metabolizing enzymes 128,
      129–30
  efficacy spectrum **142,** 465–6
  elimination 131, 464
    half-life 152, **461**
  frequency of administration **149,** 469
    indications **461,** 465–6
  initial target dose **149,** 469
  learning-disabled patients 217
  maintenance dose **149,** 469
    infants and children 153
  mechanism of action **461,** 462
  metabolism **461,** 463–4
  and oral contraception 279
  overdose 467, *468*
  partial onset seizures 170, 465–6
  pharmacokinetics 463–4
  plasma clearance **461,** 463
  preparations **461**
  protein binding 131, **461,** 463
  side effects 217, 327, **461,** 466–9
    connective tissue disorders 467
    haematological 467
    hypersensitivity 467
    metabolic bone disorders 467
    neurotoxicity 466–7
  structure *xxi,* 462
  teratogenicity 467, 469
  therapeutic range 156, **461,** 469, *469*
  time to peak blood levels **461,** 463
  titration rate 149
  volume of distribution **461,** 463
phenothiazines, as cause of seizures 53

phensuximide
  cost of treatment **xxxi**
  early use of xxvii
  introduction of **xvii**
phenthenylate, introduction of **xvii**
Phenurone *see* phenacemide
phenylacetylurea **xxx**
phenylbutazone, cytochrome P450
      inhibition **122**
phenylethyl barbituric acid **xxx**
phenylpropanolamine, as cause of seizures 53
phenytoin 170, 475–88, **475**
  6 Hz seizure test **92**
  absorption 477
  action on calcium channels 98
  action on monoaminergic
      neurotransmission 107
  action on sodium channels 97
  advantages **475**
  anticonvulsant activity **92**
  bioavailability 475, 477
  in breast milk 285, 477
  as cause of seizures 53
  chemistry 476
  clinical effectiveness, partial seizures and
      generalized tonic clonic seizures 484–5
  clinical effectiveness compared with
    carbamazepine 484, 485
    clobazam 485
    lamotrigine 485
    phenobarbitone 484
    primidone 484
    valproate 485
  clinical therapeutics 485–6
  cost of treatment **xxxi**, 147
  cytochrome P450 induction **122**
  disadvantages **475**
  distribution 477
  dosage 475, 485–6
  dosage interval 475, 485–6
  drug interactions 129–30, 131, 454, **475**,
    480–1, **480, 481**, 530
  early use of xix, xx–xxiii, **xxv, xxx**
  effect on drug-metabolizing enzymes **128**,
    129–30, 477–81
  efficacy spectrum 142, 484–6
  electrophysiological effects 477
  elimination 131, 477–8, 478
    half-life 152, 475, 479, 477–80
  generalized seizures 170, 484–5
  hydroxylator status, effects on
    metabolism 478
  indications 475, 484–5
  introduction of **xvii**
  learning-disabled patients 217
  maintenance dose 149, 485–6
    infants and children 153, 486
  mechanism of action **475**
  metabolism **475**
  molecular mechanisms 476–7
  and oral contraception 279, 480
  partial onset seizures 170, 484–5
  pharmacodynamics 476–7
  pharmacokinetics 477–80
    clinical 478–80, *479*
  plasma clearance 475, 479, 478–80
  pregnancy, effects on phenytoin
    metabolism 479–80
  preparations **475**
  protective index 404
  protein binding 131, 475, 477
  side effects 217, 327, 475, 481–4
    aromatic anticonvulsant hypersensitivity
      syndrome 482

    bone 482–3
    cardiovascular system 483
    folates 483
    gums 482
    lymphoid tissue 483
    nervous system 482
    skin 482
  status epilepticus 233–4, 239–40, 478, 486,
    233, 235
  structure *xxi*, 476
  teratogenicity 483–4
  therapeutic range 156, 475, 478–80, 485
  time to peak blood levels 475
  titration rate 149, 485–6
  volume of distribution 475, 477, **479**
phethenylate xxviii
picrotoxin test, as an experimental test in
    antiepileptic drug discovery 92
  see also individual antiepileptic drugs
piracetam 489–95, **489**
  absorption 491–2
  administration and dosage 494
  advantages **489**
  bioavailability 489, 490–1
  clinical efficacy 491–3, *492*
  disadvantages **489**
  dosage 489, 494
  dosage interval 489, 494
  drug interactions 489, 491
  elimination half-life 489, 491
  excretion 489, 491
  indications 489, 491–3
  licensed indications 490
  mechanism of action 490
  pharmacology and pharmacokinetics 490–1,
    491, 492
  preparations **489**
  side effects 489, 493–4
  structure *491*
  time to peak blood levels 489, 490–1
  volume of distribution 489, 491
polycystic ovary syndrome, and antiepileptic
    drugs 278–9, 535
polymicrogyria
  MRI abnormalities **641**, *643*, 646
  surgery 767
  see also cortical dysgenesis
polytherapy 328
  as risk factor for sudden death 47
  in therapy of epilepsy 154–5, 328, 330
  see also pharmacokinetic drug interactions;
    and individual drugs
population-based studies
  aetiology of epilepsy 51
  incidence of epilepsy 25
  mortality 34–5, 36
  prevalence of epilepsy 21–2, **23**
  prognosis of epilepsy **30**
porphyria, treatment of seizures in 248–9
positron emission tomography 595, 652–8
  brain tumours 734–5
  cerebral blood flow 656
  in children 785
  glucose metabolism 653–6, *654*
  method 652–3
  radiolabelled molecules for **653**
  receptor studies 656–8
    benzodiazepine receptors 657–8
    opiate receptors 657
post-neurosurgical seizures 62, 245–6
post-traumatic epilepsy 32, 61–2, **62**, 244–5,
    775–9
  mechanisms of 775
  MRI abnormalities **641**, 647

  surgery 775–8
postictal psychosis 257, 258
postnatal risk factors for epilepsy 60
postoperative care after epilepsy surgery 596–7,
  597
potassium ion channels
  and epileptogenesis 76–7
  as target for antiepileptic drug action 105–6
Prader-Willi syndrome, risk of epilepsy 55, 56
pramiracetam *491*
pregabalin 496–9, **496**
  advantages **496**
  animal models of epilepsy 497
  bioavailability 496, 497
  clinical efficacy 497–8
  clinical therapeutics 499
  cytochrome P450 enzymes, lack of effect
    on 497
  disadvantages **496**
  dosage 496, 499
  dosage interval 496, 499
  elimination half-life 496, 497
  excretion 496, 497
  indications 496, 497–8
  pharmacokinetics 497
  pharmacology 496–7
  pregnancy 497
  preparations **496**
  side effects 496, 498
  time to peak blood levels 496, 497
  volume of distribution **496**
pregnancy 279–87
  breastfeeding 284–5, **285**
  complications 281
  developmental toxicity of AEDs 281–4, 327
    growth retardation 284–5
    major congenital malformations 281–2,
      281, 282
    mechanism of teratogenic effects 283–4
    minor anomalies and fetal AED
      syndrome 282
    psychomotor development 283
    sensitive periods *283*
  effects of maternal seizures on fetus 279–80
  folate supplementation 285
  management during
    AED treatment 286
    delivery and labour 287
    prenatal diagnosis 286–7
    puerperium 287
    vitamin supplementation 285, 287
  pharmacokinetics of AEDs during 280–1
  preconception counselling 285–6
  seizure control during pregnancy and
    delivery **280**
  treatment of women of childbearing age 287
  vitamin K supplementation 285
  see also individual antiepileptic drugs
prenatal diagnosis, risk of congenital anomalies
    due to antiepileptic drugs 286–7
prenatal risk factors for epilepsy 60
presurgical evaluation for epilepsy surgery
  aims, process and procedures 583–95
  brain tumours 731–5
    age at onset of seizures 731
    clinical seizure characteristics 731
    duration of seizure disorder 731
    functional mapping 733
    history and examination 731
    intensive video scalp EEG monitoring 732
    invasive cortical mapping 735
    invasive monitoring 733
    lesion detection 732
    MRI 732–3, **732**

presurgical evaluation for epilepsy surgery
(*cont'd*)
  neuropsychological assessment 733
  non-invasive mapping 733–5
  scalp EEG recording 731–2
 dipole source modelling 665–79
  clinical relevance 678
  forward and inverse problems 666
  ictal discharges 678, 679
  instantaneous dipoles 667
  interictal spikes 668–78
  modelling of conductive volume 665–6
  modelling of sources 665
  multiple spatiotemporal dipoles 667
  preprocessing of data 666–7, 666
  principle, 665
  projection of sources onto 3D MRI 667
  quality of solution and accuracy of
   localization 667–8, 668
 functional magnetic resonance imaging 690–2
  EEG-correlated 684–90
  language lateralization 691
  memory 691–2
  motor function 690–1
  simultaneous 685–6
 intracranial monitoring (invasive
  EEG) 609–34
  background 621–2
  combined studies 616
  cortical stimulation 619–20
  depth electrodes 610–12
  electrocorticography 620–1
  epidural electrodes 617
  foramen ovale electrodes 618–19
  ictal EEG 623–32
  indications for 609–10
  interictal EEG 622–3
  non-epileptiform findings 622
  recording sessions 621
  subdural grid electrodes 614–16
  subdural strip electrodes 612–14
 intrinsic optical imaging 680–4
  age dependence of seizures 681
  clinical studies 682
  energy associated with seizure activity 682
  epileptiform activity 681
  near-infrared spectroscopy 682–4, 683
  optical physics 680–1
  origin and spread of seizures 681
  physiological processes 680–1
 investigation, approach to 585–6
  aetiology and syndrome 586
  concordance in 586
  epileptogenic, irritative and ictal onset
   zones 585–6
 magnetoencephalography 635–9
  evoked activity 636
  method 635–6
  spontaneous activity 636–8
 MRI 590–3, 592, 593, 594, 640–51
  in children 647–8
  future perspectives 649
  imaging of epileptogenic area 648–9
  localization of eloquent areas 649
  quantitative 648
  screening investigation 586
  structural imaging 640–7
 organizational aspects 595–8
  epilepsy surgery centers 596, 597
  postoperative care and follow up 596–8,
   597
  surgery planning meeting 595–6, 596
 paediatric surgery 783–5
  functional MRI 785

  functional neuroimaging 784
  intracarotid amobarbital procedure 785
  invasive EEG monitoring 783–4, 794
  MRI 783, 784
  positron emission tomography 785
  SPECT 785
 patient selection, principles of 584–6
  estimation of seizure outcome and risk of
   surgery 584
  intractable epilepsy 584
  learning disability, behavioural disorder and
   psychosis 585
  medical fitness and age 585
  non-epileptic seizures 585
  quality of life gain 584–5
  temporal lobe surgery 586–8
 positron emission tomography 652–8
  in brain tumours 734–5
  cerebral blood flow 656
  in children 785
  glucose metabolism 653–6, 654
  method 652–3
  radiolabelled molecules for 653
  receptor studies 656–8
 protocol for 588–95, 589
  counselling 595
  functional imaging 595
  intracranial EEG 594–5
  medical history and examination 588
  MRI and other imaging modalities 590–3
  neuropsychological assessment 593–4
  psychiatric assessment 588
  scalp EEG 588–9
  sodium amytal (Wada) test 594
 psychiatric assessment 716–22
  how to assess 717
  neuropsychiatric contraindications for
   surgery 718
  neuropsychiatric indications for
   surgery 718
  postsurgery period 718–19
  reasons for 717–18, 718
  risk of poor psychiatric outcome 719–20,
   720
  special groups 719
  what to assess 716
  when to assess 717
  whom to assess 716–17
 psychological testing 699–715
  evaluation of frontal lobe function 700–4,
   702, 703
  evaluation of occipital lobes 705–6
  evaluation of parietal lobes 705
  evaluation of temporal neocortex 706–7
  intracarotid amobarbital
   procedure 710–12
  memory assessment 707–10, 708, 709
  potential pitfalls 700
  site of dysfunction 699
 scalp EEG 588–90, 590, 591, 599–608
  evaluation for corpus callosal
   section 605–6
  focal structural lesions 604–5
  hemispherectomy 605
  hippocampal sclerosis 602–4, 603
  ictal recordings 589–90, 591, 601
  malformations of cortical development 605
  medial temporal lobe epilepsy 601–2, 602
  MRI-negative cases 605
  scalp electrodes 599–600
  seizure activation and drug withdrawal 601
  types of 600–1
single photon emission computed
  tomography 659–60

  SISCOM 692–3
prevalence of epilepsy 21–4
 more developed countries 21–2, 22
  epileptic syndromes 24
  ethnicity 23
  gender 22
  less developed countries 22, 23
  seizure types 23–4
  socioeconomic factors 23
primidone 170, 469–72
 absorption 470
 advantages 461
 bioavailability 461
 chemistry 469
 clinical efficacy in generalized or partial
  seizures 471, 484
  juvenile myoclonic epilepsy 471
 clinical therapeutics 471
 cost of treatment xxxi, 147
 disadvantages 461
 distribution 470
 dosage 461
 dosage interval 461
 drug interactions 461, 470–1, 470, 530
 early use of *xxvii*
 effect on drug-metabolizing enzymes 128
 efficacy spectrum 142
 elimination 131, 470
  half-life 152, 461
 frequency of administration 149
 generalized seizures 170
 indications 461
 initial target dose 149
 introduction of xvii
 maintenance dose 149
  infants and children 153
 mechanism of action 461, 469
 metabolism 461, 470
 overdose 471
 partial onset seizures 170
 pharmacokinetics 470
 plasma clearance 461
 preparations 461
 protein binding 461
 side effects 461
 therapeutic range 156, 461
 time to peak blood levels 461
 titration rate 149
 toxicity 471
 volume of distribution 461
 see also Phenobarbitone
prognosis of epilepsy 29–33
 cumulative remission of seizures 30
 early 29
 effect of treatment on 165
 in elderly patients 210–11, **211**
 initial seizure frequency 30
 in largely untreated populations 37
 late with overall remission 29
 learning-disabled patients 223–4
 population-based studies 30
 predictors of remission 30–3
 time to enter remission 29–30, 30
prominal, early use of xix
propafenone, cytochrome P450 inhibition 122
propofol
 as cause of seizures 53, 54
 in intravenous anaesthesia for epilepsy
  surgery 863
 status epilepticus 239–40
  refractory 234
prostigmine xix
protein binding and drug interactions 127–8,
  128

antiepileptic drugs as displacers 130
monitoring of unbound drug
    concentrations 157–8
protriptyline, as cause of seizures 53
provocation of seizures, influence on
    treatment 170–1
psychiatric assessment, in presurgical
    evaluation 588, 716–22
  how to assess 717
  neuropsychiatric contraindications for
      surgery 718
  neuropsychiatric indications for surgery 718
  postsurgery period 718–19
  reasons for 717–18, 718
  risk of poor psychiatric outcome 719–20, 720
  special groups 719
  what to assess 716
  when to assess 717
  whom to assess 716–17
psychiatric disorders, in epilepsy 255–61
  depression and anxiety disorders 257–8, 257
  epilepsy-associated neuropsychology 260
  organic mental disorders 255–6, 256
  personality disorders 259–60
  psychological therapies 260
  psychosis 256–7
  see also psychoses
psychiatric interventions, as treatment in
    epilepsy 260, 271
  see also psychiatric disorders in epilepsy
psychological testing in presurgical
    evaluation 593–4, 699–715
  aim of neuropsychological assessment 593–4
  evaluation of frontal lobe function 700–4
    Design Fluency test 701–2, 702, 703
    Modified Card Sorting test 701
    motor tasks 704
    Stroop test 702–3
    Tower of London test 703–4
    Wisconsin Card Sorting test 701
  evaluation of occipital lobes 705–6
  evaluation of parietal lobes 705
  evaluation of temporal neocortex 706–7
  intracarotid amobarbital procedure (WADA
      test) 710–12
    language dominance 711
    memory 711
    non-invasive procedures 712
    present status and utility 711–12
  memory assessment 707–10, 708, 709
    matched learning tasks 708–10, 708, 709
    non-verbal learning and memory tests 710
    traditional tests 707–8, 708
  potential pitfalls 700
  site of dysfunction 699
psychological therapies as treatment for
    epilepsy 260
psychoses 256–8, 257
  alternative 257
  interictal 257
  postictal 257, 258
  presentation 256
  influence on the section of patients for epilepsy
      surgery 585
  treatment 257–8
psychosocial morbidity of epilepsy 166
PTZ test see pentylenetetrazole test
pyknolepsy see Children, absence epilepsy
pyogenic cerebral abscess 747–53
  diagnosis 749
  laboratory diagnosis 749–50
  microbiology 749
  outcome 752–3
  predisposing factors 748–9

contiguous spread 748
haematogenous spread 748
postoperative abscess 748
trauma 748–9
radiological diagnosis 750–1, 751
surgical management 751–2
pyridoxine dependency 8
pyruvate carboxylase deficiency 264
pyruvate decarboxylase deficiency 264, 264

Q
quality of life, outcome, paediatric epilepsy
    surgery 780
Quality of Life in Epilepsy (QOLIE), use in
    psychiatric assessment in epilepsy 717
quality of life gain
  carbamazepine 355–6
  epilepsy surgery 584–5
  lamotrigine 433
Questionnaire for Expectations and Beliefs about
    Epilepsy Surgery, use in psychiatric
    assessment in epilepsy 717
quinidine, cytochrome P450 inhibition 122

R
radiosurgery, stereotactic 842–4
randomized controlled trials (RCTs) 317–25
  advantages of 317–18
  comparison of AEDs using
    meta-analysis 321–2
    number-needed-to-treat 323–4, 323, 324
    odds ratio 322–3, 322, 323
    retention rates and sustained efficacy
        measures 324–5, 325, 326
    success rates, improvement rates, problems
        rates, complaint rates and summary
        complaint scores 324, 325
  limitations of 318–19
    artificiality of clinical setting 319
    fixed dosage 319
    inclusion of only partial seizures 319
    inclusion of selected populations 318–19
    lack of comparative data 318
    primary efficacy measures of limited clinical
        value 318
    recording of side-effects 319
    short duration of trials 318
  primary efficacy endpoints 319–21
    responder rates 320–1, 320, 321
    seizure frequency reduction 319–20, 320
    survival analyses and time to event 321
  see also individual antiepileptic drugs
Rasmussen's encephalitis 561
  MRI appearances 641, 647
  surgery 783
reading epilepsy 12
recurrence of seizures
  effect of repeated seizures on risk of 164
  effect of treatment after first seizures on risk
      of 164–5
  risk after first seizure 162–4, 163
rehabilitation after epilepsy surgery 719
relapse of seizures
  prediction of 176–7, 177
  prognosis after 177–8
  risk of 174–6, 175
    age at onset 175–6
    EEG 176
    electroclinical syndrome 175
    influence of individual drugs 176
    response to treatment 176
    seizure type 175
    severity of epilepsy 176
    status epilepticus 176

underlying aetiology 176
  see also recurrence of seizures
relaxation therapy as treatment for epilepsy
    271
REM behaviour disorders, in differential
    diagnosis of epilepsy 70
remission of seizures in epilepsy
  after epilepsy surgery 178
  length of, before drug withdrawal 174
  management of patients in seizure
      remission 174–9
  prediction of relapse, following drug
      withdrawal 176–7, 177
  predictors of 30–3
    aetiology 31
    age at onset 31
    CNS infections 32
    comorbidities 31
    EEG 32–3
    gender 30–1
    neurological examination 32
    seizure type 32
    status epilepticus 32
    after stroke 31–2
    after trauma 32
  prognosis after relapse following drug
      withdrawal 177–8
  relapse after 33
  risk of relapse of seizures 174–6, 175
    age at onset 175–6
    drug withdrawal 176
    EEG 176
    electroclinical syndrome 175
    response to individual drugs and
        treatment 176
    seizure type 175
    severity of epilepsy 176
    status epilepticus 176
    underlying aetiology 176
  seizure-free period to consider drug
      withdrawal 174
  time to enter 29–30, 30
renal failure, treatment of seizures in 246–8
reoperation, after seizure recurrence following
    initial surgery 854
reproduction, aspects related to epilepsy
    treatment 277–89
  birth control 279
  see also individual antiepileptic drugs
  fertility 277–9
    choice of AEDs 279
    polycystic ovary syndrome 278–9
    reproductive dysfunction 277–8
  pregnancy in epilepsy see pregnancy
retigabine 570, 571–2
  action on potassium channels 106
Rett's syndrome, risk of epilepsy 56, 57
Reye's syndrome, use of antiepileptic drugs
    in 248
rifampicin, cytochrome P450 induction 122
risk assessment in genetic counselling 290–1
risk factors for epilepsy
  genetic disorders 55–6
  injury 166
  mortality in early epilepsy 165–6
  prenatal and perinatal 60
  see also individual conditions
risperidone, seizure-inducing properties 223
ritonavir, cytochrome P450 inhibition 122
Robinow's syndrome, risk of epilepsy 55
rolandic epilepsy see benign epilepsy of
    childhood with centrotemporal spikes
Rubinstein-Taybi syndrome, risk of epilepsy
    55

rufinamide 500–6, **500**
  absorption and bioavailability 501–3, *502, 503*
  advantages **500**
  bioavailability **500**, 501–2
  chemical characteristics 500–1
  children, pharmacokinetics 502–3
  clinical efficacy 504
  disadvantages **500**
  dosage **500**
  dosage interval **500**
  drug interactions **500**, 503
  efficacy and safety data 504–5, **504**
  elimination half-life **500**, 502, 504
  excretion **500**, 501–2
  indications **500**, 504
  level determination 503
  mechanism of action **500**, 501
  metabolism **500**, 501–3
  multiple dose studies 503–4
  non-epileptic use 505
  pharmacokinetics 501–4
  preparations **500**
  protein binding **500**, 501
  side effects **500**, 504–5, **504**
  time to peak blood levels **500**, **501–3**
  toxicology 503

S
Saethre-Chotzen syndrome, risk of epilepsy **55**
safinamide **570**, 572
Saiko-Keishi-To, as treatment for epilepsy 272
saquinavir, cytochrome P450 inhibition **122**
scalp EEG in presurgical evaluation 588–90, *590, 591*, 599–608
  brain tumours 731–2
  evaluation for corpus callosal section 605–6
  focal structural lesions 604–5
  hemispherectomy 605
  hippocampal sclerosis
    bilateral 604
    dual pathology 604
    isolated 602–4, *603*
  ictal recordings 589–90, *591*, 601
  malformations of cortical development 605
  medial temporal lobe epilepsy 601–2, *602*
  MRI-negative cases 605
  scalp electrodes, technical considerations 599–600
  seizure activation and drug withdrawal 601
  types of 600–1
  see also childhood epilepsy syndromes; epilepsy syndromes; individual conditions, syndromes and surgical procedures
scalp EEG electrodes, technical considerations 599–600
schizencephaly, surgical treatment of 767
secondarily generalized seizures, *see* generalised tonic clonic seizures, partal seizures and epilepsies
sedation in anaesthesia for epilepsy surgery 866–8
seizure frequency, epidemiology of 28
seizure type 23–4
  and choice of drug 142–4, **142**, *143*
  classification *see* classification of seizure types
  incidence 25
  and mortality 36
  and prediction of remission 32
  and prevalence 23–4
  and risk of relapse 175
  see also individual seizure types
serial seizures, emergency treatment of 230

serum level monitoring of antiepileptic drugs *see* therapeutic drug monitoring
severe myoclonic epilepsy of infancy, genetic counselling 300
sevoflurane, as anaesthesia for surgery 862
sialidoses, as cause of myoclonic epilepsy 302, 303
side effects of antiepileptic drugs
  comparison of in antiepileptic drug trials 324–5
  in infantile epilepsy 180–81
  severe irreversible and longer-term side-effects 326–7
  seizure inducing effects 327
  teratogenicity *see* developmental toxicity of antiepileptic drugs
  see also adverse drug reactions; and individual antiepileptic drugs
simple partial seizures, classification and symptomatology 3, **4**, 5–6
  see also partial seizures and epilepsies
single photon emission computed tomography (SPECT) 595, 659–60
  brain tumours 733–4
  in children 785
SISCOM *see* Subtraction Ictal SPECT Coregistered on MRI
SLE, treatment of seizures in 248–9
sleep disorders, in differential diagnosis of epilepsy 70, **162**
Smith-Golabi-Behmel syndrome, risk of epilepsy **55**
Smith-Lemli-Opitz syndrome, risk of epilepsy **55**
socioeconomic factors
  incidence of epilepsy 25
  prevalence of epilepsy 23
sodium amytal test *see* intracarotid amobarbital procedure
sodium ion channels
  as antiepileptic drug target 96–8, **97**, *98*
  and epileptogenesis 75–6, *75, 76*
sodium valproate *see* valproate
Sotos' syndrome, risk of epilepsy **55**
SPD421 **570**, 572–3
SPECT *see* single photon emission computed tomography
sphenoidal electrodes, complications of 850
spontaneous epileptic rat (SER), as experimental model of epilepsy 112
standardized mortality ratio 43, 166
stargazer mouse model, as experimental model of epilepsy 111
State-Trait Anxiety Inventory, use in psychiatric assessment in epilepsy 717
status epilepticus
  as animal model of experimental epilepsy 110
  emergency treatment of 227–43
    absence status epilepticus 235–7
    atypical absence status epilepticus 236–7
    typical absence status epilepticus 235–6
  classification of **228**
  complex partial status epilepticus 236
  convulsive status epilepticus 230–5
    drug treatment 232–5, **233**, **234**
    medical management and complications 230–2
  drug pharmacokinetics and pharmacodynamics 229–30, *229*
  drug responsiveness 230
  drugs used in 237–9
    ACTH and corticosteroids 237
    chlormethiazole 234, **233**
    clobazam 236, 362

clonazepam 390, **233**
diazepam 237–8, 378–80, 232–3, 236 **233**
fosphenytoin 233–4, 236, 238, 412, 414–15, **233**
lignocaine 233, 238, **233**
lorazepam 233–4, 238, 380–1, 236 **233**
midazolam 238–9, 234, 382, **233**, **234**
paraldehyde 564–5, **233**
pentobarbital 240, **234**
phenobarbital 233–4, 239, 466, **233**
phenytoin 233–4, 239–40, 478, 486, **233**, **235**
propofol 234, 239–40, **233**, **234**
thiopentone 233–40, **233**, **234**
valproate **233**, **235**, 236, 533
mid-1930s **xix**
epilepsia partialis continua 237
myclonic status epilepticus in coma 237
neuronal damage 227–8
non-convulsive status epilepticus 235–7, **235**
  diagnosis 235
  treatment 235–7
non-convulsive status epilepticus in coma 236
in pregnancy 280
as predictor of prognosis in epilepsy 30
and risk of relapse 176
serial seizures (premonitory phase) 230
tonic status epilepticus 228, 230–5, 237
treatment *see individual drugs*
see also individual antiepileptic drugs
stereotactic surgery 833–48
  ablation and stimulation for epilepsy 841–2
  as aid to conventional surgery 837–41, *838, 839*
    depth electrodes and stereotactic EEG 837–40, *838, 839*
    stereotactic amygdalohippocampectomy 840–1
    stereotactic craniotomy and lesionectomy 841
  complications 856
  Cosman-Roberts-Wells base ring *836*
  frame-based *834*
  frameless 834–7, *835, 836*
  multimodality imaging 837
  radiosurgery 842–4
Stevens-Johnson syndrome due to antiepileptic drugs 326
stiripentol 185
stroke *see* cerebrovascular disease
Stroop test 702–3
Sturge-Weber syndrome
  as cause of epilepsy 57
  MRI abnormalities **641**, *646, 647*
  risk of epilepsy **55**
  surgery of 781–2
subcortical heterotopia
  MRI appearances **641**
  surgery in 766–7
subdural grid electrodes 614–16
  advantages 615
  disadvantages
    cerebral oedema 615
    haemorrhage 615
    impact on recorded signals 616
    infection 615
    neurological deficits 615–16
    restricted sampling 615
    surgical complications 615
  technical aspects 614–15, *614*
  use of 615
subdural strip electrodes 612–14
  advantages 613
  complications 850

disadvantages
  inaccurate placement 613–14
  restricted sampling 613
  surgical complications 614
extratemporal epilepsy 613
technical aspects 612–13
temporal lobe epilepsy *613*
Subjective Handicap of Epilepsy (SHE), use in
      psychiatric assessment in epilepsy 717
subtraction ictal SPECT coregistered on
      MRI 692–3
  use in surgery of brain tumours 734
sudden death in epilepsy (SUDEP) 37, 43–9
  and antiepileptic drug treatment 47
  causes of **44**
  clinical implications 47
  definitions 43–4, **44**
  future research 47–8, **48**
  general and neuropathological changes 45
  historical perspective 43
  incidence studies 45–6, *46*
  pathophysiological mechanisms 44–5
  prevention of **48**
  risk factors and case-control studies 46–7
  see also mortality of epilepsy
SUDEP *see* Sudden death
sulfaphenazole, cytochrome P450
      inhibition **122**
supplementary motor seizures,
      symptomatology 10
surgery *see* epilepsy surgery
symptomatic epilepsies 10
  generalized 14–15
    epilepsy with myoclonic absences 15
    epilepsy with myoclonic astatic seizures 14
    Lennox-Gastaut syndrome 14
    non-specific aetiology 15
    West syndrome 14
  incidence and prevalence 50–1
  localization-related 12
symptoms and signs in epileptic seizures 3–8
syncope 67–8
  confusion with seizures **162**
systemic lupus erythematosus 249–50

T
talampanel **570**, 573
temporal lobe epilepsy
  aetiology and pathology 587
  dipole source modelling 668, 670, *670*
  familial 611
  intracranial monitoring 594–5, 609–10, 611,
      613, 616, 618, 620, 622–32, *624–9,
      630–1,* 783–4
  lateral, aetiology and symptomatology 587,
      588
    intracranial EEG
      combined studies 616
      depth electrodes 611
      ictal 629–32, *630–1*
      indications for 595, 620
      interictal 622–3
      subdural electrodes 613
    MRI 590–3
    psychological testing 706–7
    scalp EEG 588–90, 604
  medial, aetiology and symptomatology 587–8
    intracranial EEG monitoring 609–10
      depth electrodes 611, *611*
      ictal EEG 623–9, *624–9*
      interictal EEG 622
      indications for 609–10
    MRI 590–93, *594*, **641**, *642,* 643–4, 648
    psychological testing in 707–10

scalp EEG 588–90, 601–2, *602*
surgical treatment
  hippocampal sclerosis, surgery of 723–7
  stereotactic amygdalohippocampectomy
      840–1
  stereotactic radiosurgery 643–4
  symptomatology 587–8
neocortical *see* lateral
PET scanning in 653–5, *654, 658*
protocol for presurgical assessment 588–95
selection of patients for temporal lobe
      surgery 586–8
SPECT scanning in 659–60
surgical treatment of
  awake surgery 825–6, *826–7,* 828–30
  complications 852–4
    intellectual sequelae 853–4
    mortality and non-neurological
        morbidity 852–3
    neurological sequelae **853**
    psychiatric consequences and social
        outcome 854
  hippocampal sclerosis, surgery of 723–7
    methods 723–6, **724,** *725*
  stereotactic surgery 840–1
  stereotactic radiosurgery 843–4
  symptomatology 10, 586–8, *587–8*
  see also hippocampal sclerosis; individual
      presurgical investigatory techniques;
      and surgery of specific conditions
temporal neocortical function,
      neuropsychological assessment
      of 706–7
teratogenicity *see* developmental toxicity of
      antiepileptic drugs; and individual
      antiepileptic drugs
theophylline, as cause of seizures 53
therapeutic drug monitoring 155–8
  in the elderly 210
  individualized drug concentrations 156–7,
      157
  monitoring of unbound drug
      concentrations 157–8
  therapeutic range 155–6, **156**
  timing of blood samples 155
  value of 157
  when to measure drug concentrations 158
  see also individual antiepileptic drugs
therapeutic index 126
Thiantoin *see* phenthenylate; phethenylate
thiopentone, use in status epilepticus 234, 240
thioridazine
  cytochrome P450 inhibition **122**
  seizure-inducing properties 223
tiagabine 102, 103, **170,** 507–14, **507**
  advantages 507
  bioavailability 507, 508
  clinical efficacy in partial seizures 509–11,
      509
    as monotherapy 510–11
    in paediatric patients 511
    randomized controlled trials 509–10, **509**
  clinical therapeutics 512–13
  cost of treatment **147**
  disadvantages 507
  dosage 507, 512–13
  dosage interval 507, 512–13
  drug interactions 122, 507, 530, 508–9
  effect on drug-metabolizing
      enzymes **128,** 508
  efficacy spectrum 142, 509–11
  elderly onset seizures 208
  elimination 131, 133, 508–9
    half-life 152, 507, 508–9

experimental studies 508
frequency of administration **149,** 512–13
improvement/success rates 325
indications 507, 509–11
initial target dose **149,** 513
learning-disabled patients **218,** 219
maintenance dose **149,** 513
  infants and children 153, 511
mechanism of action 507, 508
metabolism 507, 508
number-needed-to-treat *323*
odds ratio *322, 323*
and oral contraception 279, 508
partial onset seizures 170, 509–11
pharmacokinetics 508–9
plasma clearance 507
preparations 507
protein binding 131, 507, 508
side effects 507, 511–12, *511*
therapeutic range **156,** 507
time to peak blood levels 507
titration rate **149**
volume of distribution 507
ticlopidine, cytochrome P450 inhibition **122**
Todd's paralysis 3, 7, 11
tonic seizures, classification and
      symptomatology 5, 7
  treatment *see individual antiepileptic drugs*
  see also Lennox Gastaut Syndrome; and
      individual drugs
tonic-clonic seizures
  classification and symptomatology 7–8, *7,*
      59–60
  mortality 36
  treatment *see individual antiepileptic drugs*
  see also generalised tonic clonic seizures
topiramate 170, 515–27, *515*
  action on calcium channels 98
  action on sodium channels 97
  advantages 515
  adverse events 521–4, **522**
    cognitive effects 522–3
    weight loss 523
  bioavailability 515, 516
  in children 523–4
  clinical efficacy 517–21
    childhood absence epilepsy 521
    Lennox-Gastaut syndrome 519
    open-label experience 520–1
    partial seizures 517–19, 520–1
    primary generalized tonic-clonic
        seizures 519, 520–1
    randomized controlled trials 517–20, *518*
    recently diagnosed epilepsy 519–20
    refractory epilepsy 517–18, 521
    refractory partial onset seizures 518, 519,
        520–1
    West's syndrome 521
  clinical therapeutics 524–5
  cost of treatment **147**
  cytochrome P450 induction **122**
  cytochrome P450 inhibition **122**
  disadvantages 515
  dosage 515, 524–5
  dosage interval 515
  drug interactions 129, 131, 133, **515,** 530–1,
      530
  effect on drug-metabolizing enzymes **128,**
      129, 130
  efficacy spectrum 142, 517–21
  elderly onset seizures 208
  elimination 131, 133, 516–17
    half-life 152, 515, 516–17
  excretion 515, 516–17

topiramate (*cont'd*)
experimental studies 516
frequency of administration **149**
generalized seizures **170**, 519
improvement/success rates **325**
indications **515**, 517–21
infantile epilepsy 185–6
initial target dose **149**, 524–5
learning-disabled patients 218, 219
Lennox-Gastaut syndrome **191**, 519
maintenance dose **149**, 524–5
  infants and children **153**
mechanism of action **515**, 516
neuroprotection 524
number-needed-to-treat *323*, *324*
odds ratio *322*, *323*
and oral contraception 279, 517
partial onset seizures **170**, 517–21
pharmacokinetics 516–17
  in children 517
  in elderly 517
  impaired hepatic function 517
  impaired renal function 517
plasma clearance **515**, 516–17
in pregnancy 523
preparations 515
protein binding **131**, 515, 516
side effects **515**, 521–4, 552
therapeutic range **156**, 515
time to peak blood levels **515**, 516
titration rate **149**, 524–5
volume of distribution 515
tottering mouse, as experimental model of
    epilepsy 111
transcranial magnetic stimulation, in treatment
    of epilepsy 274
transient global ischaemia, in differential
    diagnosis of epilepsy 71–2
transplant patients, seizures in 250–1, *251*
Treacher-Collins syndrome, risk of epilepsy 55
treatment of epilepsy *see* medical treatment;
    epilepsy surgery; and antiepileptic
    drugs
Tridione *see* trimethadione
trimethadione 565
  cost of treatment **xxxi**
  early use of **xxv**, *xxvi*
  introduction of **xvii**
trisomy 13 syndrome, risk of epilepsy 55
trisomy 18 syndrome, risk of epilepsy 55
troleandomycin, cytochrome P450
    inhibition **122**
tuberous sclerosis 730
  MRI abnormalities **641**, 647
  risk of epilepsy 55
  surgery of 781

U

unclassified seizures 5, 8
Unverricht-Lundborg disease, as cause of
    epilepsy 57, 302, **302**
uridine diphosphate glucuronosyltransferases, in
    drug interactions 123

V

vagus nerve anatomy 874–6
  physiological studies 875–6
  vagal afferents 874–5, *875*
  vagal efferents 874
vagus nerve stimulation 222, 260, 806, *807*,
    873–83
  clinical use **880**
  efficacy 878
    in animal models 876

in patients with epilepsy 876–8
  implantation procedure 873–4, *874*
  safety and tolerability 878–80
    adverse events 879
    effects on mood and behaviour 879–80
    environmental considerations 878
    long-term 879
    mechanical and electrical safety 878
valproate 168, 170, **528–39**, *528*
  6 Hz seizure test 92
  absorption and distribution 529
  action on monoaminergic
      neurotransmission 107
  action on sodium channels 97
  advantages **528**
  age effects 519
  anticonvulsant activity **92**
  benign epilepsy of childhood **191**
  bioavailability **528**, 529, *529*
  in breast milk 285, 529
  childhood absence epilepsy **191**, 532
  clinical efficacy 485, 531–3
    generalised epilepsies 532–3
    localization-related epilepsies 531–2
    seizure-epilepsy prophylaxis 533
    status epilepticus 533
  clinical therapeutics 535–7, *536*
    contraindications and precautions 536
    dosages 535, 536
    therapeutic range 535–6
  cost of treatment **147**
  cryptogenic/symptomatic partial
      epilepsy **191**, 531–2
  cytochrome P450 inhibition **122**
  disadvantages **528**
  dosage 528, 535
  dosage interval 528, 535
  drug interactions 128–9, **131**, 454, 530–1,
      530, *528*
  effect on drug-metabolizing enzymes 128–9,
      128
  efficacy spectrum **142**, 531–3
  elimination **131**, 132, 529
    half-life **152**, 528, 529, *529*
  experimental studies 529
  frequency of administration **149**
  generalized seizures **170**, 532–3
  indications **528**, 531–3, 536–7
  initial target dose **149**, 535
  juvenile absence epilepsy **191**, 532
  juvenile myoclonic epilepsy **191**, 532
  learning-disabled patients 217
  Lennox-Gastaut syndrome **191**, 532
  maintenance dose **149**, 535
    infants and children **153**
  mechanism of action 528, 529
  metabolism 528, 529, *529*
  and oral contraception 279, 531
  partial onset seizures **170**, 531–3
  pharmacodynamics 520
  pharmacokinetics 529–31, *529*
    age effects 519
    diabetes mellitus 520
    hepatic disease 519–20
    renal disease 520
  plasma clearance 528, 529
  in pregnancy 520, 536
  preparations **528**
  protective index 404
  protein binding **131**, 528, 529
  as protein binding displacer 130
  side effects 217, 327, **528**, 533–5
    alopecia 534
    blood disorders 534

bone resorption 535
  central nervous system 533–4
  hepatotoxicity 534–5
  hyperammonaemic encephalopathy 534
  pancreatitis 534
  parkinsonism 535
  polycystic ovarian syndrome 535
  stimulation of HIV virus 535
  weight gain 534
  status epilepticus 233, 235, 236, 533
  therapeutic range **156**, 528, 535–6
  time to peak blood levels 528, 529
  titration rate **149**, 535
  volume of distribution 528, 529
valproic acid *see* Valproate
valrocemide 570, 573–4
vascular lesions
  aetiology of epilepsy 61
  arteriovenous malformations *see*
      arteriovenous malformations
  capillary malformations 747
  cavernous haemangioma (cavernoma) *see*
      cavernous haemangioma
  MRI abnormalities *645*, 646–7
  surgery of 742–7
  venous malformations 746–7
  see also cerebrovascular disease
vasculitis, treatment of seizures in 249
venous malformations, clinical features and
    surgery of 746–7
vertigo, in differential diagnosis of epilepsy 70–1
vigabatrin *102*, *103*, 169, **540–7**, *540*
  advantages **540**
  adverse events 545–6
  animal studies 542
  bioavailability **540**, 541
  as cause of seizures 53
  clinical studies 542–5
    adults 544–5
    infants and children 542–3
    Lennox-Gastaut syndrome 544
    partial seizures 542–43
    long-term efficacy 545
    West syndrome 543–4
  cost of treatment **147**
  disadvantages **540**
  dosage 540, 545
  dosage interval 540, 545
  drug interactions 133, 530, 540, 541–2
  drug monitoring 542
  effect on drug-metabolizing enzymes **128**
  efficacy spectrum **142**, 542–5
  elderly onset seizures 208
  elimination **131**, 133, 541
    half-life **152**, 540, 541
  excretion 540, 541
  frequency of administration **149**, 545
  improvement/success rates **325**
  indications **540**
  infantile epilepsy 184
  initial target dose **149**, 545
  learning-disabled patients 218, 219
  maintenance dose **149**, 545
    infants and children **153**, 543
  mechanism of action 540, 541
  number-needed-to-treat *323*
  odds ratio *322*, *323*
  and oral contraception 279,
  pharmacokinetics 541
  pharmacology 541
  plasma clearance 540
  preparations **540**
  protein binding **131**, 541
  side effects 327, 540, 545–6

depression and psychosis 545
   visual field constriction 545–6
therapeutic range 156
time to peak blood levels 540, 541
titration rate 149
volume of distribution 540, 541
West syndrome 191
vitamin supplements 287
   vitamin K 285
voltage gated channels, and
      epileptogenesis 75–8, 75

W

Wada test (intracarotid amobarbital
      procedure) 594, 710–12
   in children 785
   complications 849
Weaver's syndrome, risk of epilepsy 55
West syndrome (infantile spasm)
   drug treatment 181–5, 362, 363, 384, 521,
      532, 543–4, 554, 560, 570
   idiopathic 183
   management 181–5, 182
      ACTH and corticosteroids 183–4
      antiepileptic drugs 183
      vigabatrin 184
   prevalence 24
   prognosis 33
   surgery 782
   status epilepticus 228
   symptomatology 8, 9, 14
   see also individual antiepileptic drugs
Wilson's disease 248
   risk of epilepsy 56
   treatment of epilepsy in 248

Wisconsin Card Sorting test 701
withdrawal of antiepileptic drugs 158–9
   in the elderly 211
   in patients with learning disability 224
   in patients whose epilepsy is in
      remission 158–9, 174–8
   when changing therapy 330–31
   see also individual antiepileptic drugs
Wolf-Hirschhorn syndrome, risk of epilepsy 55,
   56

X

X-linked inheritance, genetic counselling 294
xeroderma pigmentosum, risk of epilepsy 55

Y

yoga, in treatment of epilepsy 270

Z

Zellweger's syndrome, as a cause of epilepsy 56
zidovudine, as cause of seizures 53
zonisamide 170, 548–59, 548
   action on calcium channels 98
   action on monoaminergic
      neurotransmission 107
   action on sodium channels 97
   advantages 548
   bioavailability 548, 551–2
   chemistry 549
   clinical therapeutics 557
   disadvantages 548
   dosage 548, 552–6
   dosage interval 548
   drug interactions 530, 548, 552
   effect on drug-metabolizing enzymes 128

efficacy in partial and generalized
      seizures 552–4, 552, 553, 554
   long-term 555–6
efficacy spectrum 142, 552–6
elderly onset seizures 208
elimination 131, 133, 552
   half-life 152, 548, 552
frequency of administration 149
improvement/success rates 325
indications 548, 552–6, 557
initial target dose 149
learning-disabled patients 218, 219
maintenance dose 149
   infants and children 153
metabolism 548, 552
number-needed-to-treat 323
odds ratio 322, 323
partial onset seizures 170, 552–4, 555, 557
pharmacokinetics 551–2
pharmacology 549–51
   anticonvulsant properties 549
   free radical scavenging and
      neuroprotection 550–1
   mechanism of anticonvulsant
      action 549–50
preclinical toxicity 551
preparations 548
protein binding 131, 548, 551–2
safety 556–7, 556
side effects 548, 556–7
therapeutic range 156, 548
time to peak blood levels 548, 551
titration rate 149